Pediatric Clinical Practice Guidelines & Policies

A Compendium of Evidence-based Research for Pediatric Practice

20th Edition

American Academy of Pediatrics
345 Park Blvd
Itasca, IL 60143
www.aap.org

AMERICAN ACADEMY OF PEDIATRICS
PUBLISHING STAFF

Mary Lou White
Chief Product and Services Officer/SVP, Membership, Marketing, and Publishing

Mark Grimes
Vice President, Publishing

Jennifer McDonald
Senior Editor, Digital Publishing

Sean Rogers
Digital Content Specialist

Leesa Levin-Doroba
Production Manager, Practice Management

Peg Mulcahy
Manager, Art Direction and Production

Linda Smessaert, MSIMC
Senior Marketing Manager, Professional Resources

Mary Louise Carr
Marketing Manager, Clinical Publications

The American Academy of Pediatrics is an organization of 67,000 primary care pediatricians, pediatric medical subspecialists, and pediatric surgical specialists dedicated to the health, safety, and well-being of infants, children, adolescents, and young adults.

The recommendations in this publication do not indicate an exclusive course of treatment or serve as a standard of medical care. Variations, taking into account individual circumstances, may be appropriate.

Products are mentioned for informational purposes only. Inclusion in this publication does not imply endorsement by the American Academy of Pediatrics.

Every effort has been made to ensure that the drug selection and dosage set forth in this publication are in accordance with the current recommendations and practice at the time of publication. It is the responsibility of the health care professional to check the package insert of each drug for any change in indications and dosage and for added warnings and precautions.

This publication has been developed by the American Academy of Pediatrics. The authors, editors, and contributors are expert authorities in the field of pediatrics. No commercial involvement of any kind has been solicited or accepted in the development of the content of this publication.

© 2020 American Academy of Pediatrics

All rights reserved. No part of this publication may be reproduced, stored in a retrieval system, or transmitted in any form or by any means—electronic, mechanical, photocopying, recording, or otherwise—without prior written permission from the publisher (locate title at http://ebooks.aappublications.org and click on © Get permissions; you may also fax the permissions editor at 847/434-8780 or email permissions@aap.org).
First edition published 2001; 20th, 2020.

Printed in the United States of America

9-5/1119
MA0961
ISBN: 978-1-61002-392-4
eBook: 978-1-61002-393-1
ISSN: 1942-2024

INTRODUCTION TO *PEDIATRIC CLINICAL PRACTICE GUIDELINES & POLICIES: A COMPENDIUM OF EVIDENCE-BASED RESEARCH FOR PEDIATRIC PRACTICE*

Clinical practice guidelines have long provided physicians with evidence-based decision-making tools for managing common pediatric conditions. Policy statements issued and endorsed by the American Academy of Pediatrics (AAP) are developed to provide physicians with a quick reference guide to the AAP position on child health care issues. We have combined these 2 authoritative resources into 1 comprehensive manual/eBook resource to provide easy access to important clinical and policy information.

This manual contains

- Clinical practice guidelines from the AAP, plus related recommendation summaries, *ICD-10-CM* coding information, and AAP patient education handouts
- Clinical practice guidelines endorsed by the AAP, including abstracts where applicable
- Full text of all 2019 AAP policy statements, clinical reports, and technical reports
- Policy statements, clinical reports, and technical reports issued or endorsed through December 2019, including abstracts where applicable

The eBook, which is available via the code on the inside cover of this manual, builds on content of the manual and points to the full text of all AAP

- Clinical practice guidelines
- Policy statements
- Clinical reports
- Technical reports
- Endorsed clinical practice guidelines and policies

For easy reference within this publication, dates when AAP clinical practice guidelines, policy statements, clinical reports, and technical reports first appeared in the AAP journal *Pediatrics* are provided. In 2009, the online version of *Pediatrics* at http://pediatrics.aappublications.org became the official journal of record; therefore, date of online publication is given for policies from 2010 to present.

Additional information about AAP policy can be found in a variety of professional publications such as

Red Book®, 31st Edition, and *Red Book*® *Online* (http://redbook.solutions.aap.org)

Pediatric Nutrition, 8th Edition

Medications in Pediatrics: A Compendium of AAP Clinical Practice Guidelines and Policies

Injury and Violence Prevention: A Compendium of AAP Clinical Practice Guidelines and Policies

Adolescent Health: A Compendium of AAP Clinical Practice Guidelines and Policies

Pediatric Mental Health: A Compendium of AAP Clinical Practice Guidelines and Policies

Neonatal Care: A Compendium of AAP Clinical Practice Guidelines and Policies

Guidelines for Air and Ground Transport of Neonatal and Pediatric Patients, 4th Edition

Guidelines for Perinatal Care, 8th Edition

Pediatric Environmental Health, 4th Edition

To order these and other pediatric resources, please call 866/843-2271 or visit http://shop.aap.org/books.

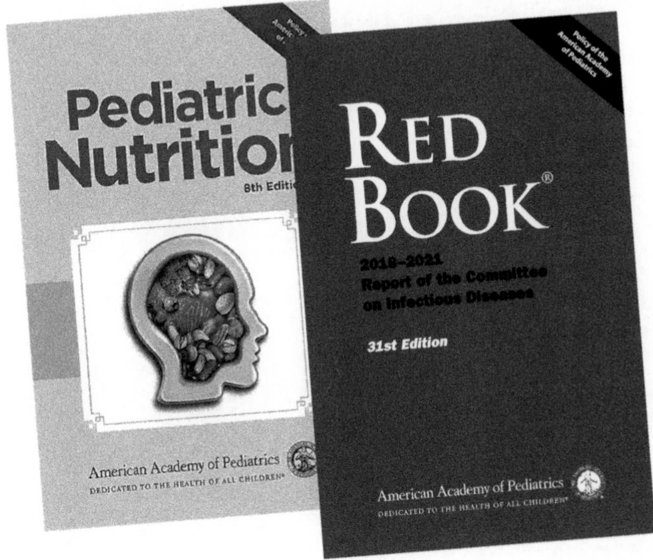

All policy statements, clinical reports, and technical reports from the American Academy of Pediatrics automatically expire 5 years after publication unless reaffirmed, revised, or retired at or before that time. Please check the American Academy of Pediatrics website at www.aap.org for up-to-date reaffirmations, revisions, and retirements.

AMERICAN ACADEMY OF PEDIATRICS

The American Academy of Pediatrics (AAP) and its member pediatricians dedicate their efforts and resources to the health, safety, and well-being of infants, children, adolescents, and young adults. The AAP has approximately 67,000 members in the United States, Canada, and Latin America. Members include pediatricians, pediatric medical subspecialists, and pediatric surgical specialists.

Core Values. ***We believe***

- In the inherent worth of all children; they are our most enduring and vulnerable legacy.
- Children deserve optimal health and the highest quality health care.
- Pediatricians, pediatric medical subspecialists, and pediatric surgical specialists are the best qualified to provide child health care.
- Multidisciplinary teams including patients and families are integral to delivering the highest quality health care.

The AAP is the organization to advance child health and well-being and the profession of pediatrics.

Vision. Children have optimal health and well-being and are valued by society. American Academy of Pediatrics members practice the highest quality health care and experience professional satisfaction and personal well-being.

Mission. The mission of the AAP is to attain optimal physical, mental, and social health and well-being for all infants, children, adolescents, and young adults. To accomplish this mission, the AAP shall support the professional needs of its members.

Table of Contents

Sleep Apnea

Urinary Tract Infection

PPI AAP Partnership for Policy Implementation See Appendix 1.

SECTION 2
ENDORSED CLINICAL PRACTICE GUIDELINES

Autism Spectrum Disorder

Cardiovascular Health

Cerebral Palsy

Cerumen Impaction

Congenital Muscular Dystrophy

Depression

Duchenne Muscular Dystrophy

Dysplasia of the Hip

Food Allergy

Hemorrhage

HIV

Hypotension

Infantile Spasms

Intravascular Catheter-Related Infections

Medullary Thyroid Carcinoma

Migraine Headache

Palliative Care

Positional Plagiocephaly

Rhinoplasty

PPI AAP Partnership for Policy Implementation See Appendix 1.

SECTION 4

CURRENT POLICIES FROM THE AMERICAN ACADEMY OF PEDIATRICS

SECTION 5

ENDORSED POLICIES

SECTION 1

Clinical Practice Guidelines

From the American Academy of Pediatrics

- *Clinical Practice Guidelines*
  EVIDENCE-BASED DECISION-MAKING TOOLS FOR MANAGING COMMON PEDIATRIC CONDITIONS

- *Quick Reference Tools*
  TOOLS FOR IMPLEMENTING AMERICAN ACADEMY OF PEDIATRICS GUIDELINES IN YOUR PRACTICE AND AT THE POINT OF CARE

FOREWORD

To promote the practice of evidence-based medicine and to improve the health outcomes of children, the American Academy of Pediatrics (AAP) provides physicians with evidence-based guidelines for managing common pediatric conditions. The AAP has established an organizational process and methodology for the development, implementation, and improvement of these clinical practice guidelines.

The evidence-based approach to developing clinical practice guidelines begins by systematically reviewing and synthesizing the literature to provide the scientific basis for guideline recommendations. Clinical practice guideline teams with stakeholder representation systematically develop recommendations by carefully considering the evidence, risk, benefits, and patient and caregiver preferences. Each clinical practice guideline undergoes a thorough peer-review process before publication. The AAP supports efforts to implement the recommendations into practice and to evaluate whether they are leading to improved outcomes. Every 5 years, each clinical practice guideline and the scientific literature are reevaluated by the subcommittee to ensure that the recommendations are based on the most up-to-date science.

American Academy of Pediatrics clinical practice guidelines are designed to provide physicians with an analytic framework for evaluating and treating common pediatric conditions and are not intended as an exclusive course of treatment or standard of care. The AAP recognizes circumstances in which there is a lack of definitive data and relies on expert consensus in cases in which data do not exist. American Academy of Pediatrics clinical practice guidelines allow for flexibility and adaptability at the local and patient levels to address unique circumstances and should not replace sound clinical judgment.

If you have any questions about current or future clinical practice guidelines, please contact Kymika Okechukwu, senior manager of evidence-based medicine initiatives at the AAP, at 630/626-6317 or via email at kokechukwu@aap.org.

To order copies of patient education resources that accompany each guideline, please call the AAP at 866/843-2271 or visit http://shop.aap.org/books.

Joel Tieder, MD, MPH, FAAP
Chairperson, Council on Quality Improvement and Patient Safety

Clinical Practice Guideline for the Diagnosis, Evaluation, and Treatment of Attention-Deficit/ Hyperactivity Disorder in Children and Adolescents

- *Clinical Practice Guideline*
  - *PPI: AAP Partnership for Policy Implementation*
    See Appendix 1 for more information.

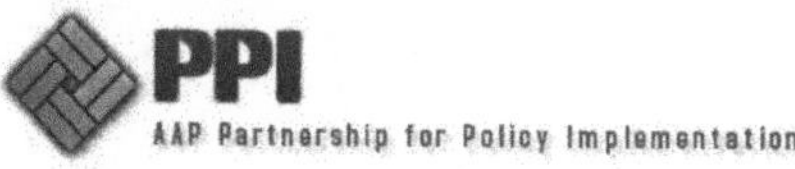

CLINICAL PRACTICE GUIDELINE

American Academy of Pediatrics

DEDICATED TO THE HEALTH OF ALL CHILDREN™

Clinical Practice Guideline for the Diagnosis, Evaluation, and Treatment of Attention-Deficit/Hyperactivity Disorder in Children and Adolescents

Mark L. Wolraich, MD, FAAP,[a] Joseph F. Hagan, Jr, MD, FAAP,[b,c] Carla Allan, PhD,[d,e] Eugenia Chan, MD, MPH, FAAP,[f,g] Dale Davison, MSpEd, PCC,[h,i] Marian Earls, MD, MTS, FAAP,[j,k] Steven W. Evans, PhD,[l,m] Susan K. Flinn, MA,[n] Tanya Froehlich, MD, MS, FAAP,[o,p] Jennifer Frost, MD, FAAFP,[q,r] Joseph R. Holbrook, PhD, MPH,[s] Christoph Ulrich Lehmann, MD, FAAP,[t] Herschel Robert Lessin, MD, FAAP,[u] Kymika Okechukwu, MPA,[v] Karen L. Pierce, MD, DFAACAP,[w,x] Jonathan D. Winner, MD, FAAP,[y] William Zurhellen, MD, FAAP,[z] SUBCOMMITTEE ON CHILDREN AND ADOLESCENTS WITH ATTENTION-DEFICIT/HYPERACTIVE DISORDER

abstract

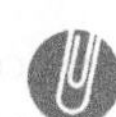

Attention-deficit/hyperactivity disorder (ADHD) is 1 of the most common neurobehavioral disorders of childhood and can profoundly affect children's academic achievement, well-being, and social interactions. The American Academy of Pediatrics first published clinical recommendations for evaluation and diagnosis of pediatric ADHD in 2000; recommendations for treatment followed in 2001. The guidelines were revised in 2011 and published with an accompanying process of care algorithm (PoCA) providing discrete and manageable steps by which clinicians could fulfill the clinical guideline's recommendations. Since the release of the 2011 guideline, the *Diagnostic and Statistical Manual of Mental Disorders* has been revised to the fifth edition, and new ADHD-related research has been published. These publications do not support dramatic changes to the previous recommendations. Therefore, only incremental updates have been made in this guideline revision, including the addition of a key action statement related to diagnosis and treatment of comorbid conditions in children and adolescents with ADHD. The accompanying process of care algorithm has also been updated to assist in implementing the guideline recommendations. Throughout the process of revising the guideline and algorithm, numerous systemic barriers were identified that restrict and/or hamper pediatric clinicians' ability to adopt their recommendations. Therefore, the subcommittee created a companion article (available in the Supplemental Information) on systemic barriers to the care of children and adolescents with ADHD, which identifies the major systemic-level barriers and presents recommendations to address those barriers; in this article, we support the recommendations of the clinical practice guideline and accompanying process of care algorithm.

[a]Section of Developmental and Behavioral Pediatrics, University of Oklahoma, Oklahoma City, Oklahoma; [b]Department of Pediatrics, The Robert Larner, MD, College of Medicine, The University of Vermont, Burlington, Vermont; [c]Hagan, Rinehart, and Connolly Pediatricians, PLLC, Burlington, Vermont; [d]Division of Developmental and Behavioral Health, Department of Pediatrics, Children's Mercy Kansas City, Kansas City, Missouri; [e]School of Medicine, University of Missouri-Kansas City, Kansas City, Missouri; [f]Division of Developmental Medicine, Boston Children's Hospital, Boston, Massachusetts; [g]Harvard Medical School, Harvard University, Boston, Massachusetts; [h]Children and Adults with Attention-Deficit/Hyperactivity Disorder, Lanham, Maryland; [i]Dale Davison, LLC, Skokie, Illinois; [j]Community Care of North Carolina, Raleigh, North Carolina; [k]School of Medicine, University of North Carolina, Chapel Hill, North Carolina; [l]Department of Psychology, Ohio University, Athens, Ohio; [m]Center for Intervention Research in Schools, Ohio University, Athens, Ohio; [n]American Academy of Pediatrics, Alexandria, Virginia; [o]Department of Pediatrics, University of Cincinnati, Cincinnati, Ohio; [p]Cincinnati Children's Hospital Medical Center, Cincinnati, Ohio; [q]Swope Health Services, Kansas City, Kansas; [r]American Academy of Family Physicians, Leawood, Kansas; [s]National Center on Birth Defects and Developmental Disabilities, Centers for Disease Control and Prevention, Atlanta, Georgia; [t]Departments of Biomedical Informatics and Pediatrics, Vanderbilt University, Nashville, Tennessee; [u]The Children's Medical Group, Poughkeepsie, New York;

To cite: Wolraich ML, Hagan JF, Allan C, et al. AAP SUBCOMMITTEE ON CHILDREN AND ADOLESCENTS WITH ATTENTION-DEFICIT/HYPERACTIVE DISORDER. Clinical Practice Guideline for the Diagnosis, Evaluation, and Treatment of Attention-Deficit/Hyperactivity Disorder in Children and Adolescents. *Pediatrics.* 2019;144(4):e20192528

INTRODUCTION

This article updates and replaces the 2011 clinical practice guideline revision published by the American Academy of Pediatrics (AAP), "Clinical Practice Guideline: Diagnosis and Evaluation of the Child with Attention-Deficit/Hyperactivity Disorder."[1] This guideline, like the previous document, addresses the evaluation, diagnosis, and treatment of attention-deficit/hyperactivity disorder (ADHD) in children from age 4 years to their 18th birthday, with special guidance provided for ADHD care for preschool-aged children and adolescents. (Note that for the purposes of this document, "preschool-aged" refers to children from age 4 years to the sixth birthday.) Pediatricians and other primary care clinicians (PCCs) may continue to provide care after 18 years of age, but care beyond this age was not studied for this guideline.

Since 2011, much research has occurred, and the *Diagnostic and Statistical Manual of Mental Disorders, Fifth Edition (DSM-5)*, has been released. The new research and *DSM-5* do not, however, support dramatic changes to the previous recommendations. Hence, this new guideline includes only incremental updates to the previous guideline. One such update is the addition of a key action statement (KAS) about the diagnosis and treatment of coexisting or comorbid conditions in children and adolescents with ADHD. The subcommittee uses the term "comorbid," to be consistent with the *DSM-5*.

Since 2011, the release of new research reflects an increased understanding and recognition of ADHD's prevalence and epidemiology; the challenges it raises for children and families; the need for a comprehensive clinical resource for the evaluation, diagnosis, and treatment of pediatric ADHD; and the barriers that impede the implementation of such a resource. In response, this guideline is supported by 2 accompanying documents, available in the Supplemental Information: (1) a process of care algorithm (PoCA) for the diagnosis and treatment of children and adolescents with ADHD and (2) an article on systemic barriers to the care of children and adolescents with ADHD. These supplemental documents are designed to aid PCCs in implementing the formal recommendations for the evaluation, diagnosis, and treatment of children and adolescents with ADHD. Although this document is specific to children and adolescents in the United States in some of its recommendations, international stakeholders can modify specific content (ie, educational laws about accommodations, etc) as needed. (Prevention is addressed in the Mental Health Task Force recommendations.[2])

PoCA for the Diagnosis and Treatment of Children and Adolescents With ADHD

In this revised guideline and accompanying PoCA, we recognize that evaluation, diagnosis, and treatment are a continuous process. The PoCA provides recommendations for implementing the guideline steps, although there is less evidence for the PoCA than for the guidelines. The section on evaluating and treating comorbidities has also been expanded in the PoCA document.

Systems Barriers to the Care of Children and Adolescents With ADHD

There are many system-level barriers that hamper the adoption of the best-practice recommendations contained in the clinical practice guideline and the PoCA. The procedures recommended in this guideline necessitate spending more time with patients and their families, developing a care management system of contacts with school and other community stakeholders, and providing continuous, coordinated care to the patient and his or her family. There is some evidence that African American and Latino children are less likely to have ADHD diagnosed and are less likely to be treated for ADHD. Special attention should be given to these populations when assessing comorbidities as they relate to ADHD and when treating for ADHD symptoms.[3] Given the nationwide problem of limited access to mental health clinicians,[4] pediatricians and other PCCs are increasingly called on to provide services to patients with ADHD and to their families. In addition, the AAP holds that primary care pediatricians should be prepared to diagnose and manage mild-to-moderate ADHD, anxiety, depression, and problematic substance use, as well as co-manage patients who have more severe conditions with mental health professionals. Unfortunately, third-party payers seldom pay appropriately for these time-consuming services.[5,6]

To assist pediatricians and other PCCs in overcoming such obstacles, the companion article on systemic barriers to the care of children and adolescents with ADHD reviews the barriers and makes recommendations to address them to enhance care for children and adolescents with ADHD.

ADHD EPIDEMIOLOGY AND SCOPE

Prevalence estimates of ADHD vary on the basis of differences in research methodologies, the various age groups being described, and changes in diagnostic criteria over time.[7] Authors of a recent meta-analysis calculated a pooled worldwide ADHD prevalence of 7.2% among children[8]; estimates from some community-based samples are somewhat higher, at 8.7% to 15.5%.[9,10] National survey data from 2016 indicate that 9.4% of children in the United States 2 to 17 years of age have ever had an ADHD diagnosis, including 2.4% of children 2 to 5 years of age.[11] In that national survey, 8.4% of children 2 to 17 years of age currently had ADHD, representing 5.4 million children.[11] Among children and adolescents with current ADHD, almost two-thirds were taking medication, and approximately half had received behavioral treatment of ADHD in the past year. Nearly one quarter had received neither type of treatment of ADHD.[11]

Symptoms of ADHD occur in childhood, and most children with ADHD will continue to have symptoms and impairment through adolescence and into adulthood. According to a 2014 national survey, the median age of diagnosis was 7 years; approximately one-third of children were diagnosed before 6 years of age.[12] More than half of these children were first diagnosed by a PCC, often a pediatrician.[12] As individuals with ADHD enter adolescence, their overt hyperactive and impulsive symptoms tend to decline, whereas their inattentive symptoms tend to persist.[13,14] Learning and language problems are common comorbid conditions with ADHD.[15]

Boys are more than twice as likely as girls to receive a diagnosis of ADHD,[9,11,16] possibly because hyperactive behaviors, which are easily observable and potentially disruptive, are seen more frequently in boys. The majority of both boys and girls with ADHD also meet diagnostic criteria for another mental disorder.[17,18] Boys are more likely to exhibit externalizing conditions like oppositional defiant disorder or conduct disorder.[17,19,20] Recent research has established that girls with ADHD are more likely than boys to have a comorbid internalizing condition like anxiety or depression.[21]

Although there is a greater risk of receiving a diagnosis of ADHD for children who are the youngest in their class (who are therefore less developmentally capable of compensating for their weaknesses), for most children, retention is not beneficial.[22]

METHODOLOGY

As with the original 2000 clinical practice guideline and the 2011 revision, the AAP collaborated with several organizations to form a subcommittee on ADHD (the subcommittee) under the oversight of the AAP Council on Quality Improvement and Patient Safety.

The subcommittee's membership included representation of a wide range of primary care and subspecialty groups, including primary care pediatricians, developmental-behavioral pediatricians, an epidemiologist from the Centers for Disease Control and Prevention; and representatives from the American Academy of Child and Adolescent Psychiatry, the Society for Pediatric Psychology, the National Association of School Psychologists, the Society for Developmental and Behavioral Pediatrics (SDBP), the American Academy of Family Physicians, and Children and Adults with Attention-Deficit/Hyperactivity Disorder (CHADD) to provide feedback on the patient/parent perspective.

This subcommittee met over a 3.5-year period from 2015 to 2018 to review practice changes and newly identified issues that have arisen since the publication of the 2011 guidelines. The subcommittee members' potential conflicts were identified and taken into consideration in the group's deliberations. No conflicts prevented subcommittee member participation on the guidelines.

Research Questions

The subcommittee developed a series of research questions to direct an evidence-based review sponsored by 1 of the Evidence-based Practice Centers of the US Agency for Healthcare Research and Quality (AHRQ).[23] These questions assessed 4 diagnostic areas and 3 treatment areas on the basis of research published in 2011 through 2016.

The AHRQ's framework was guided by key clinical questions addressing diagnosis as well as treatment interventions for children and adolescents 4 to 18 years of age.

The first clinical questions pertaining to ADHD diagnosis were as follows:

1. What is the comparative diagnostic accuracy of approaches that can be used in the primary care practice setting or by specialists to diagnose ADHD among children younger than 7 years of age?
2. What is the comparative diagnostic accuracy of EEG, imaging, or executive function approaches that can be used in the primary care practice setting or by specialists to diagnose ADHD among individuals aged 7 to their 18th birthday?
3. What are the adverse effects associated with being labeled correctly or incorrectly as having ADHD?
4. Are there more formal neuropsychological, imaging, or genetic tests that improve the diagnostic process?

The treatment questions were as follows:

1. What are the comparative safety and effectiveness of pharmacologic and/or nonpharmacologic treatments of ADHD in improving outcomes associated with ADHD?
2. What is the risk of diversion of pharmacologic treatment?
3. What are the comparative safety and effectiveness of different monitoring strategies to evaluate the effectiveness of treatment or changes in ADHD status (eg, worsening or resolving symptoms)?

In addition to this review of the research questions, the subcommittee considered information from a review of evidence-based psychosocial treatments for children and adolescents with ADHD[24] (which, in some cases, affected the evidence grade) as well as updated information on prevalence from the Centers for Disease Control and Prevention.

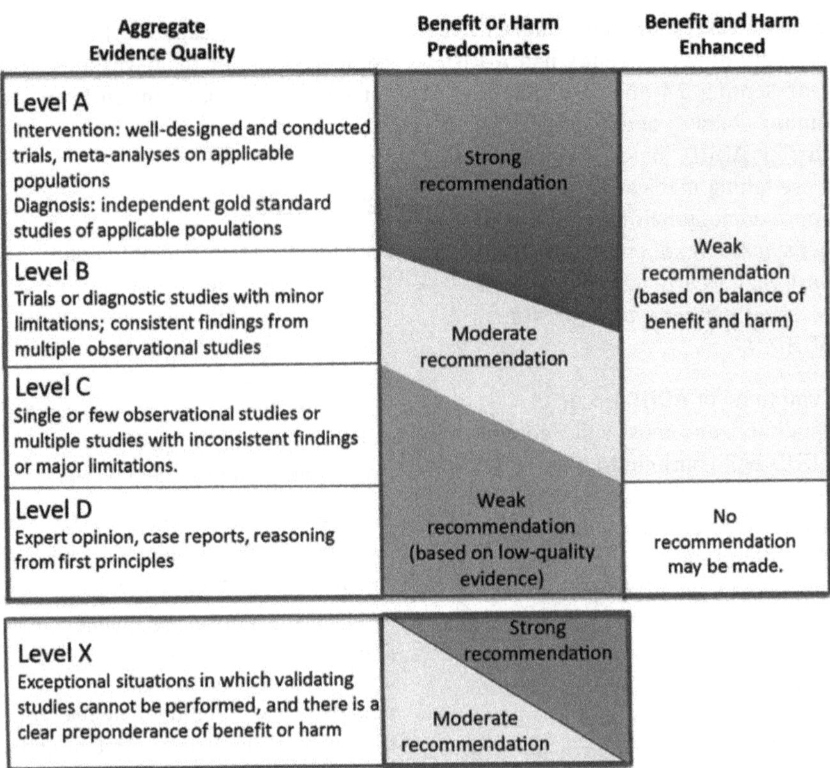

FIGURE 1
AAP rating of evidence and recommendations.

Evidence Review

This article followed the latest version of the evidence base update format used to develop the previous 3 clinical practice guidelines.[24–26] Under this format, studies were only included in the review when they met a variety of criteria designed to ensure the research was based on a strong methodology that yielded confidence in its conclusions.

The level of efficacy for each treatment was defined on the basis of child-focused outcomes related to both symptoms and impairment. Hence, improvements in behaviors on the part of parents or teachers, such as the use of communication or praise, were not considered in the review. Although these outcomes are important, they address how treatment reaches the child or adolescent with ADHD and are, therefore, secondary to changes in the child's behavior. Focusing on improvements in the child or adolescent's symptoms and impairment emphasizes the disorder's characteristics and manifestations that affect children and their families.

The treatment-related evidence relied on a recent review of literature from 2011 through 2016 by the AHRQ of citations from Medline, Embase, PsycINFO, and the Cochrane Database of Systematic Reviews.

The original methodology and report, including the evidence search and review, are available in their entirety and as an executive summary at https://effectivehealthcare.ahrq.gov/sites/default/files/pdf/cer-203-adhd-final_0.pdf.

The evidence is discussed in more detail in published reports and articles.[25]

Guideline Recommendations and Key Action Statements

The AAP policy statement, "Classifying Recommendations for Clinical Practice Guidelines," was followed in designating aggregate evidence quality levels for the available evidence (see Fig 1).[27] The AAP policy statement is consistent with the grading recommendations advanced by the University of Oxford Centre for Evidence Based Medicine.

The subcommittee reached consensus on the evidence, which was then used to develop the clinical practice guideline's KASs.

When the scientific evidence was at least "good" in quality and demonstrated a preponderance of benefits over harms, the KAS provides a "strong recommendation" or "recommendation."[27] Clinicians should follow a "strong recommendation" unless a clear and compelling rationale for an alternative approach is present; clinicians are prudent to follow a "recommendation" but are advised to remain alert to new information and be sensitive to patient preferences[27] (see Fig 1).

When the scientific evidence comprised lower-quality or limited data and expert consensus or high-quality evidence with a balance between benefits and harms, the KAS provides an "option" level of recommendation. Options are clinical interventions that a reasonable health care provider might or might not wish to implement in the practice.[27] Where the evidence was lacking, a combination of evidence and expert consensus would be used, although this did not occur in these guidelines, and all KASs achieved a "strong recommendation" level except for KAS 7, on comorbidities, which received a recommendation level (see Fig 1).

As shown in Fig 1, integrating evidence quality appraisal with an assessment of the anticipated balance between benefits and harms leads to a designation of a strong recommendation, recommendation, option, or no recommendation.

Once the evidence level was determined, an evidence grade was assigned. AAP policy stipulates that the evidence supporting each KAS be prospectively identified, appraised, and summarized, and an explicit link between quality levels and the grade of recommendation must be defined. Possible grades of recommendations range from "A" to "D," with "A" being the highest:

- grade A: consistent level A studies;
- grade B: consistent level B or extrapolations from level A studies;
- grade C: level C studies or extrapolations from level B or level C studies;
- grade D: level D evidence or troublingly inconsistent or inconclusive studies of any level; and
- level X: not an explicit level of evidence as outlined by the Centre for Evidence-Based Medicine. This level is reserved for interventions that are unethical or impossible to test in a controlled or scientific fashion and for which the preponderance of benefit or harm is overwhelming, precluding rigorous investigation.

Guided by the evidence quality and grade, the subcommittee developed 7 KASs for the evaluation, diagnosis, and treatment of ADHD in children and adolescents (see Table 1).

These KASs provide for consistent and high-quality care for children and adolescents who may have symptoms suggesting attention disorders or problems as well as for their families. In developing the 7 KASs, the subcommittee considered the requirements for establishing the diagnosis; the prevalence of ADHD; the effect of untreated ADHD; the efficacy and adverse effects of treatment; various long-term outcomes; the importance of coordination between pediatric and mental health service providers; the value of the medical home; and the common occurrence of comorbid conditions, the importance of addressing them, and the effects of not treating them.

The subcommittee members with the most epidemiological experience assessed the strength of each recommendation and the quality of evidence supporting each draft KAS.

Peer Review

The guidelines and PoCA underwent extensive peer review by more than 30 internal stakeholders (eg, AAP committees, sections, councils, and task forces) and external stakeholder groups identified by the subcommittee. The resulting comments were compiled and reviewed by the chair and vice chair; relevant changes were incorporated into the draft, which was then reviewed by the full subcommittee.

KASS FOR THE EVALUATION, DIAGNOSIS, TREATMENT, AND MONITORING OF CHILDREN AND ADOLESCENTS WITH ADHD

KAS 1

The pediatrician or other PCC should initiate an evaluation for ADHD for any child or adolescent age 4 years to the 18th birthday who presents with academic or behavioral problems and symptoms of inattention, hyperactivity, or impulsivity (Table 2). (Grade B: strong recommendation.)

The basis for this recommendation is essentially unchanged from the previous guideline. As noted, ADHD is the most common neurobehavioral disorder of childhood, occurring in approximately 7% to 8% of children and youth.[8,18,28,29] Hence, the number of children with this condition is far greater than can be managed by the mental health system.[4] There is evidence that appropriate diagnosis can be accomplished in the primary care setting for children and adolescents.[30,31] Note that there is insufficient evidence to recommend diagnosis or treatment for children younger than 4 years (other than parent training in behavior management [PTBM], which does not require a diagnosis to be applied); in instances in which ADHD-like symptoms in children younger than 4 years bring substantial impairment, PCCs can consider making a referral for PTBM.

KAS 2

To make a diagnosis of ADHD, the PCC should determine that *DSM-5* criteria have been met, including documentation of symptoms and impairment in more than 1 major setting (ie, social, academic, or occupational), with information obtained primarily from reports from parents or guardians, teachers, other school personnel, and mental health clinicians who are involved in the child or adolescent's care. The PCC should also rule out any alternative cause (Table 3). (Grade B: strong recommendation.)

The American Psychiatric Association developed the *DSM-5* using expert consensus and an expanding research foundation.[32] The *DSM-5* system is used by professionals in psychiatry, psychology, health care systems, and primary care; it is also well established with third-party payers.

TABLE 1 Summary of KASs for Diagnosing, Evaluating, and Treating ADHD in Children and Adolescents

KASs	Evidence Quality, Strength of Recommendation
KAS 1: The pediatrician or other PCC should initiate an evaluation for ADHD for any child or adolescent age 4 years to the 18th birthday who presents with academic or behavioral problems and symptoms of inattention, hyperactivity, or impulsivity.	Grade B, strong recommendation
KAS 2: To make a diagnosis of ADHD, the PCC should determine that *DSM-5* criteria have been met, including documentation of symptoms and impairment in more than 1 major setting (ie, social, academic, or occupational), with information obtained primarily from reports from parents or guardians, teachers, other school personnel, and mental health clinicians who are involved in the child or adolescent's care. The PCC should also rule out any alternative cause.	Grade B, strong recommendation
KAS 3: In the evaluation of a child or adolescent for ADHD, the PCC should include a process to at least screen for comorbid conditions, including emotional or behavioral conditions (eg, anxiety, depression, oppositional defiant disorder, conduct disorders, substance use), developmental conditions (eg, learning and language disorders, autism spectrum disorders), and physical conditions (eg, tics, sleep apnea).	Grade B, strong recommendation
KAS 4: ADHD is a chronic condition; therefore, the PCC should manage children and adolescents with ADHD in the same manner that they would children and youth with special health care needs, following the principles of the chronic care model and the medical home.	Grade B, strong recommendation
KAS 5a: For preschool-aged children (age 4 years to the sixth birthday) with ADHD, the PCC should prescribe evidence-based PTBM and/or behavioral classroom interventions as the first line of treatment, if available.	Grade A, strong recommendation for PTBM
Methylphenidate may be considered if these behavioral interventions do not provide significant improvement and there is moderate-to-severe continued disturbance in the 4- through 5-year-old child's functioning. In areas in which evidence-based behavioral treatments are not available, the clinician needs to weigh the risks of starting medication before the age of 6 years against the harm of delaying treatment.	Grade B, strong recommendation for methylphenidate
KAS 5b. For elementary and middle school-aged children (age 6 years to the 12th birthday) with ADHD, the PCC should prescribe FDA-approved medications for ADHD, along with PTBM and/or behavioral classroom intervention (preferably both PTBM and behavioral classroom interventions). Educational interventions and individualized instructional supports, including school environment, class placement, instructional placement, and behavioral supports, are a necessary part of any treatment plan and often include an IEP or a rehabilitation plan (504 plan).	Grade A, strong recommendation for medications Grade A, strong recommendation for training and behavioral treatments for ADHD with family and school
KAS 5c. For adolescents (age 12 years to the 18th birthday) with ADHD, the PCC should prescribe FDA-approved medications for ADHD with the adolescent's assent. The PCC is encouraged to prescribe evidence-based training interventions and/or behavioral interventions as treatment of ADHD, if available. Educational interventions and individualized instructional supports, including school environment, class placement, instructional placement, and behavioral supports, are a necessary part of any treatment plan and often include an IEP or a rehabilitation plan (504 plan).	Grade A, strong recommendation for medications Grade A, strong recommendation for training and behavioral treatments for ADHD with the family and school
KAS 6. The PCC should titrate doses of medication for ADHD to achieve maximum benefit with tolerable side effects.	Grade B, strong recommendation
KAS 7. The PCC, if trained or experienced in diagnosing comorbid conditions, may initiate treatment of such conditions or make a referral to an appropriate subspecialist for treatment. After detecting possible comorbid conditions, if the PCC is not trained or experienced in making the diagnosis or initiating treatment, the patient should be referred to an appropriate subspecialist to make the diagnosis and initiate treatment.	Grade C, recommendation

The *DSM-5* criteria define 4 dimensions of ADHD:

1. attention-deficit/hyperactivity disorder primarily of the inattentive presentation (ADHD/I) (314.00 [F90.0]);
2. attention-deficit/hyperactivity disorder primarily of the hyperactive-impulsive presentation (ADHD/HI) (314.01 [F90.1]);
3. attention-deficit/hyperactivity disorder combined presentation (ADHD/C) (314.01 [F90.2]); and
4. ADHD other specified and unspecified ADHD (314.01 [F90.8]).

As with the previous guideline recommendations, the *DSM-5* classification criteria are based on the best available evidence for ADHD diagnosis and are the standard most frequently used by clinicians and researchers to render the diagnosis and document its appropriateness for a given child. The use of neuropsychological testing has not been found to improve diagnostic accuracy in most cases, although it may have benefit in clarifying the child or adolescent's learning strengths and weaknesses. (See the

TABLE 2 KAS 1: The pediatrician or other PCC should initiate an evaluation for ADHD for any child or adolescent age 4 years to the 18th birthday who presents with academic or behavioral problems and symptoms of inattention, hyperactivity, or impulsivity. (Grade B: strong recommendation.)

Aggregate evidence quality	Grade B
Benefits	ADHD goes undiagnosed in a considerable number of children and adolescents. Primary care clinicians' more-rigorous identification of children with these problems is likely to decrease the rate of undiagnosed and untreated ADHD in children and adolescents.
Risks, harm, cost	Children and adolescents in whom ADHD is inappropriately diagnosed may be labeled inappropriately, or another condition may be missed, and they may receive treatments that will not benefit them.
Benefit-harm assessment	The high prevalence of ADHD and limited mental health resources require primary care pediatricians and other PCCs to play a significant role in the care of patients with ADHD and assist them to receive appropriate diagnosis and treatment. Treatments available have good evidence of efficacy, and a lack of treatment has the risk of impaired outcomes.
Intentional vagueness	There are limits between what a PCC can address and what should be referred to a subspecialist because of varying degrees of skills and comfort levels present among the former.
Role of patient preferences	Success with treatment is dependent on patient and family preference, which need to be taken into account.
Exclusions	None.
Strength	Strong recommendation.
Key references	Wolraich et al[31]; Visser et al[28]; Thomas et al[8]; Egger et al[30]

PoCA for more information on implementing this KAS.)

Special Circumstances: Preschool-Aged Children (Age 4 Years to the Sixth Birthday)

There is evidence that the diagnostic criteria for ADHD can be applied to preschool-aged children.[33–39] A review of the literature, including the multisite study of the efficacy of methylphenidate in preschool-aged children, found that the *DSM-5* criteria could appropriately identify children with ADHD.[25]

To make a diagnosis of ADHD in preschool-aged children, clinicians should conduct a clinical interview with parents, examine and observe the child, and obtain information from parents and teachers through *DSM*-based ADHD rating scales.[40] Normative data are available for the *DSM-5*–based rating scales for ages 5 years to the 18th birthday.[41] There are, however, minimal changes in the specific behaviors from the *DSM-IV*, on which all the other *DSM*-based ADHD rating scales obtained normative data. Both the ADHD Rating Scale-IV and the Conners Rating Scale have preschool-age normative data based on the *DSM-IV*. The specific behaviors in the *DSM-5* criteria for ADHD are the same for all children younger than 18 years (ie, preschool-aged children, elementary and middle school–aged children, and adolescents) and are only minimally different from the *DSM-IV*. Hence, if clinicians do not have the ADHD Rating Scale-5 or the ADHD Rating Scale-IV Preschool Version,[42] any other *DSM*-based scale can be used to provide a systematic method for collecting information from parents and teachers, even in the absence of normative data.

Pediatricians and other PCCs should be aware that determining the presence of key symptoms in this age group has its challenges, such as

TABLE 3 KAS 2: To make a diagnosis of ADHD, the PCC should determine that *DSM-5* criteria have been met, including documentation of symptoms and impairment in more than 1 major setting (ie, social, academic, or occupational), with information obtained primarily from reports from parents or guardians, teachers, other school personnel, and mental health clinicians who are involved in the child or adolescent's care. The PCC should also rule out any alternative cause. (Grade B: strong recommendation.)

Aggregate evidence quality	Grade B
Benefits	Use of the *DSM-5* criteria has led to more uniform categorization of the condition across professional disciplines. The criteria are essentially unchanged from the *Diagnostic and Statistical Manual of Mental Disorders, Fourth Edition (DSM-IV)*, for children up to their 18th birthday, except that *DSM-IV* required onset prior to age 7 for a diagnosis, while *DSM-5* requires onset prior to age 12.
Risks, harm, cost	The *DSM-5* does not specifically state that symptoms must be beyond expected levels for developmental (rather than chronologic) age to qualify for an ADHD diagnosis, which may lead to some misdiagnoses in children with developmental disorders.
Benefit-harm assessment	The benefits far outweigh the harm.
Intentional vagueness	None.
Role of patient preferences	Although there is some stigma associated with mental disorder diagnoses, resulting in some families preferring other diagnoses, the need for better clarity in diagnoses outweighs this preference.
Exclusions	None.
Strength	Strong recommendation.
Key references	Evans et al[25]; McGoey et al[42]; Young[43]; Sibley et al[46]

observing symptoms across multiple settings as required by the *DSM-5*, particularly among children who do not attend a preschool or child care program. Here, too, focused checklists can be used to aid in the diagnostic evaluation.

PTBM is the recommended primary intervention for preschool-aged children with ADHD as well as children with ADHD-like behaviors whose diagnosis is not yet verified. This type of training helps parents learn age-appropriate developmental expectations, behaviors that strengthen the parent-child relationship, and specific management skills for problem behaviors. Clinicians do not need to have made an ADHD diagnosis before recommending PTBM because PTBM has documented effectiveness with a wide variety of problem behaviors, regardless of etiology. In addition, the intervention's results may inform the subsequent diagnostic evaluation. Clinicians are encouraged to recommend that parents complete PTBM, if available, before assigning an ADHD diagnosis.

After behavioral parent training is implemented, the clinician can obtain information from parents and teachers through *DSM-5*–based ADHD rating scales. The clinician may obtain reports about the parents' ability to manage their children and about the child's core symptoms and impairments. Referral to an early intervention program or enrolling in a PTBM program can help provide information about the child's behavior in other settings or with other observers. The evaluators for these programs and/or early childhood special education teachers may be useful observers, as well.

Special Circumstances: Adolescents (Age 12 Years to the 18th Birthday)

Obtaining teacher reports for adolescents is often more challenging than for younger children because many adolescents have multiple teachers. Likewise, an adolescent's parents may have less opportunity to observe their child's behaviors than they did when the child was younger. Furthermore, some problems experienced by children with ADHD are less obvious in adolescents than in younger children because adolescents are less likely to exhibit overt hyperactive behavior. Of note, adolescents' reports of their own behaviors often differ from other observers because they tend to minimize their own problematic behaviors.[43–45]

Despite these difficulties, clinicians need to try to obtain information from at least 2 teachers or other sources, such as coaches, school guidance counselors, or leaders of community activities in which the adolescent participates.[46] For the evaluation to be successful, it is essential that adolescents agree with and participate in the evaluation. Variability in ratings is to be expected because adolescents' behavior often varies between different classrooms and with different teachers. Identifying reasons for any variability can provide valuable clinical insight into the adolescent's problems.

Note that, unless they previously received a diagnosis, to meet *DSM-5* criteria for ADHD, adolescents must have some reported or documented manifestations of inattention or hyperactivity/impulsivity before age 12. Therefore, clinicians must establish that an adolescent had manifestations of ADHD before age 12 and strongly consider whether a mimicking or comorbid condition, such as substance use, depression, and/or anxiety, is present.[46]

In addition, the risks of mood and anxiety disorders and risky sexual behaviors increase during adolescence, as do the risks of intentional self-harm and suicidal behaviors.[31] Clinicians should also be aware that adolescents are at greater risk for substance use than are younger children.[44,45,47] Certain substances, such as marijuana, can have effects that mimic ADHD; adolescent patients may also attempt to obtain stimulant medication to enhance performance (ie, academic, athletic, etc) by feigning symptoms.[48]

Trauma experiences, posttraumatic stress disorder, and toxic stress are additional comorbidities and risk factors of concern.

Special Circumstances: Inattention or Hyperactivity/Impulsivity (Problem Level)

Teachers, parents, and child health professionals typically encounter children who demonstrate behaviors relating to activity level, impulsivity, and inattention but who do not fully meet *DSM-5* criteria. When assessing these children, diagnostic criteria should be closely reviewed, which may require obtaining more information from other settings and sources. Also consider that these symptoms may suggest other problems that mimic ADHD.

Behavioral interventions, such as PTBM, are often beneficial for children with hyperactive/impulsive behaviors who do not meet full diagnostic criteria for ADHD. As noted previously, these programs do not require a specific diagnosis to be beneficial to the family. The previous guideline discussed the diagnosis of problem-level concerns on the basis of the *Diagnostic and Statistical Manual for Primary Care (DSM-PC), Child and Adolescent Version*,[49] and made suggestions for treatment and care. The *DSM-PC* was published in 1995, however, and it has not been revised to be compatible with the *DSM-5*. Therefore, the *DSM-PC* cannot be used as a definitive source for diagnostic codes related to ADHD and comorbid conditions, although it can be used conceptually as a resource for enriching the understanding of problem-level manifestations.

KAS 3

In the evaluation of a child or adolescent for ADHD, the PCC should include a process to at least screen for comorbid conditions, including emotional or behavioral conditions (eg, anxiety, depression, oppositional defiant disorder, conduct disorders, substance use), developmental conditions (eg, learning and language disorders, autism spectrum disorders), and physical conditions (eg, tics, sleep apnea) (Table 4). (Grade B: strong recommendation.)

The majority of both boys and girls with ADHD also meet diagnostic criteria for another mental disorder.[17,18] A variety of other behavioral, developmental, and physical conditions can be comorbid in children and adolescents who are evaluated for ADHD, including emotional or behavioral conditions or a history of these problems. These include but are not limited to learning disabilities, language disorder, disruptive behavior, anxiety, mood disorders, tic disorders, seizures, autism spectrum disorder, developmental coordination disorder, and sleep disorders.[50–66] In some cases, the presence of a comorbid condition will alter the treatment of ADHD.

The SDBP is developing a clinical practice guideline to support clinicians in the diagnosis of treatment of "complex ADHD," which includes ADHD with comorbid developmental and/or mental health conditions.[67]

Special Circumstances: Adolescents (Age 12 Years to the 18th Birthday)

At a minimum, clinicians should assess adolescent patients with newly diagnosed ADHD for symptoms and signs of substance use, anxiety, depression, and learning disabilities. As noted, all 4 are common comorbid conditions that affect the treatment approach. These comorbidities make it important for the clinician to consider sequencing psychosocial and medication treatments to maximize the impact on areas of greatest risk and impairment while monitoring for possible risks such as stimulant abuse or suicidal ideation.

KAS 4

ADHD is a chronic condition; therefore, the PCC should manage children and adolescents with ADHD in the same manner that they would children and youth with special health care needs, following the principles of the chronic care model and the medical home (Table 5). (Grade B: strong recommendation.)

As in the 2 previous guidelines, this recommendation is based on the evidence that for many individuals, ADHD causes symptoms and dysfunction over long periods of time, even into adulthood. Available treatments address symptoms and function but are usually not curative. Although the chronic illness model has not been specifically studied in children and adolescents with ADHD, it has been effective for other chronic conditions, such as asthma.[68] In addition, the medical home model has been accepted as the preferred standard of care for children with chronic conditions.[69]

The medical home and chronic illness approach may be particularly beneficial for parents who also have ADHD themselves. These parents can benefit from extra support to help them follow a consistent schedule for medication and behavioral programs.

Authors of longitudinal studies have found that ADHD treatments are frequently not maintained over time[13] and impairments persist into adulthood.[70] It is indicated in prospective studies that patients with ADHD, whether treated or not, are at increased risk for early death, suicide, and increased psychiatric

TABLE 4 KAS 3: In the evaluation of a child or adolescent for ADHD, the PCC should include a process to at least screen for comorbid conditions, including emotional or behavioral conditions (eg, anxiety, depression, oppositional defiant disorder, conduct disorders, substance use), developmental conditions (eg, learning and language disorders, autism spectrum disorders), and physical conditions (eg, tics, sleep apnea). (Grade B: strong recommendation.)

Aggregate evidence quality	Grade B
Benefits	Identifying comorbid conditions is important in developing the most appropriate treatment plan for the child or adolescent with ADHD.
Risks, harm, cost	The major risk is misdiagnosing the comorbid condition(s) and providing inappropriate care.
Benefit-harm assessment	There is a preponderance of benefits over harm.
Intentional vagueness	None.
Role of patient preferences	None.
Exclusions	None.
Strength	Strong recommendation.
Key references	Cuffe et al[51]; Pastor and Reuben[52]; Bieiderman et al[53]; Bieiderman et al[54]; Bieiderman et al[72]; Crabtree et al[57]; LeBourgeois et al[58]; Chan[115]; Newcorn et al[60]; Sung et al[61]; Larson et al[66]; Mahajan et al[65]; Antshel et al[64]; Rothenberger and Roessner[63]; Froehlich et al[62]

TABLE 5 KAS 4: ADHD is a chronic condition; therefore, the PCC should manage children and adolescents with ADHD in the same manner that they would children and youth with special health care needs, following the principles of the chronic care model and the medical home. (Grade B: strong recommendation.)

Aggregate evidence quality	Grade B
Benefits	The recommendation describes the coordinated services that are most appropriate to manage the condition.
Risks, harm, cost	Providing these services may be more costly.
Benefit-harm assessment	There is a preponderance of benefits over harm.
Intentional vagueness	None.
Role of patient preferences	Family preference in how these services are provided is an important consideration, because it can increase adherence.
Exclusions	None
Strength	Strong recommendation.
Key references	Brito et al[69]; Biederman et al[72]; Scheffler et al[74]; Barbaresi et al[75]; Chang et al[71]; Chang et al[78]; Lichtenstein et al[77]; Harstad and Levy[80]

comorbidity, particularly substance use disorders.[71,72] They also have lower educational achievement than those without ADHD[73,74] and increased rates of incarceration.[75–77] Treatment discontinuation also places individuals with ADHD at higher risk for catastrophic outcomes, such as motor vehicle crashes[78,79]; criminality, including drug-related crimes[77] and violent reoffending[76]; depression[71]; interpersonal issues[80]; and other injuries.[81,82]

To continue providing the best care, it is important for a treating pediatrician or other PCC to engage in bidirectional communication with teachers and other school personnel as well as mental health clinicians involved in the child or adolescent's care. This communication can be difficult to achieve and is discussed in both the PoCA and the section on systemic barriers to the care of children and adolescents with ADHD in the Supplemental Information, as is the medical home model.[69]

Special Circumstances: Inattention or Hyperactivity/Impulsivity (Problem Level)

Children with inattention or hyperactivity/impulsivity at the problem level, as well as their families, may also benefit from the chronic illness and medical home principles.

Recommendations for the Treatment of Children and Adolescents With ADHD: KAS 5a, 5b, and 5c

Recommendations vary depending on the patient's age and are presented for the following age ranges:

a. preschool-aged children: age 4 years to the sixth birthday;

b. elementary and middle school–aged children: age 6 years to the 12th birthday; and

c. adolescents: age 12 years to the 18th birthday.

The KASs are presented, followed by information on medication, psychosocial treatments, and special circumstances.

KAS 5a

For preschool-aged children (age 4 years to the sixth birthday) with ADHD, the PCC should prescribe evidence-based behavioral PTBM and/or behavioral classroom interventions as the first line of treatment, if available (grade A: strong recommendation). Methylphenidate may be considered if these behavioral interventions do not provide significant improvement and there is moderate-to-severe continued disturbance in the 4- through 5-year-old child's functioning. In areas in which evidence-based behavioral treatments are not available, the clinician needs to weigh the risks of starting medication before the age of 6 years against the harm of delaying treatment (Table 6). (Grade B: strong recommendation.)

A number of special circumstances support the recommendation to initiate PTBM as the first treatment of preschool-aged children (age 4 years to the sixth birthday) with ADHD.[25,83] Although it was limited to children who had moderate-to-severe dysfunction, the largest multisite study of methylphenidate use in preschool-aged children revealed symptom improvements after PTBM alone.[83] The overall evidence for PTBM among preschoolers is strong.

PTBM programs for preschool-aged children are typically group programs and, although they are not always paid for by health insurance, they may be relatively low cost. One evidence-based PTBM, parent-child interaction therapy, is a dyadic therapy for parent and child. The PoCA contains criteria for the clinician's use to assess the quality of PTBM programs. If the child attends preschool, behavioral classroom interventions are also recommended. In addition, preschool programs (such as Head Start) and ADHD-focused organizations (such as CHADD[84]) can also provide behavioral supports. The issues related to referral, payment, and communication are discussed in the section on systemic barriers in the Supplemental Information.

TABLE 6 KAS 5a: For preschool-aged children (age 4 years to the sixth birthday) with ADHD, the PCC should prescribe evidence-based behavioral PTBM and/or behavioral classroom interventions as the first line of treatment, if available (grade A: strong recommendation). Methylphenidate may be considered if these behavioral interventions do not provide significant improvement and there is moderate-to-severe continued disturbance in the 4- through 5-year-old child's functioning. In areas in which evidence-based behavioral treatments are not available, the clinician needs to weigh the risks of starting medication before the age of 6 years against the harm of delaying treatment (grade B: strong recommendation).

Aggregate evidence quality	Grade A for PTBM; Grade B for methylphenidate
Benefits	Given the risks of untreated ADHD, the benefits outweigh the risks.
Risks, harm, cost	Both therapies increase the cost of care; PTBM requires a high level of family involvement, whereas methylphenidate has some potential adverse effects.
Benefit-harm assessment	Both PTBM and methylphenidate have relatively low risks; initiating treatment at an early age, before children experience repeated failure, has additional benefits. Thus, the benefits outweigh the risks.
Intentional vagueness	None.
Role of patient preferences	Family preference is essential in determining the treatment plan.
Exclusions	None.
Strength	Strong recommendation.
Key references	Greenhill et al[83]; Evans et al[25]

In areas in which evidence-based behavioral treatments are not available, the clinician needs to weigh the risks of starting methylphenidate before the age of 6 years against the harm of delaying diagnosis and treatment. Other stimulant or nonstimulant medications have not been adequately studied in children in this age group with ADHD.

KAS 5b

For elementary and middle school–aged children (age 6 years to the 12th birthday) with ADHD, the PCC should prescribe US Food and Drug Administration (FDA)–approved medications for ADHD, along with PTBM and/or behavioral classroom intervention (preferably both PTBM and behavioral classroom interventions). Educational interventions and individualized instructional supports, including school environment, class placement, instructional placement, and behavioral supports, are a necessary part of any treatment plan and often include an Individualized Education Program (IEP) or a rehabilitation plan (504 plan) (Table 7). (Grade A: strong recommendation for medications; grade A: strong recommendation for PTBM training and behavioral treatments for ADHD implemented with the family and school.)

The evidence is particularly strong for stimulant medications; it is sufficient, but not as strong, for atomoxetine, extended-release guanfacine, and extended-release clonidine, in that order (see the Treatment section, and see the PoCA for more information on implementation).

KAS 5c

For adolescents (age 12 years to the 18th birthday) with ADHD, the PCC should prescribe FDA-approved medications for ADHD with the adolescent's assent (grade A: strong recommendation). The PCC is encouraged to prescribe evidence-based training interventions and/or behavioral interventions as treatment of ADHD, if available. Educational interventions and individualized instructional supports, including school environment, class placement, instructional placement, and behavioral supports, are a necessary part of any treatment plan and often include an IEP or a rehabilitation plan (504 plan) (Table 8). (Grade A: strong recommendation.)

Transition to adult care is an important component of the chronic care model for ADHD. Planning for the transition to adult care is an ongoing process that may culminate after high school or, perhaps, after college. To foster a smooth transition, it is best to introduce components at the start of high school, at about 14 years of age, and specifically focus during the 2 years preceding high school completion.

Psychosocial Treatments

Some psychosocial treatments for children and adolescents with ADHD have been demonstrated to be effective for the treatment of ADHD, including behavioral therapy and training interventions.[24–26,85] The diversity of interventions and outcome measures makes it challenging to assess a meta-analysis of psychosocial treatment's effects alone or in association with medication treatment. As with medication treatment, the long-term positive effects of psychosocial treatments have yet to be determined. Nonetheless, ongoing adherence to psychosocial treatment is a key contributor to its beneficial effects, making implementation of a chronic care model for child health important to ensure sustained adherence.[86]

Behavioral therapy involves training adults to influence the contingencies in an environment to improve the behavior of a child or adolescent in that setting. It can help parents and school personnel learn how to effectively prevent and respond to adolescent behaviors such as

TABLE 7 KAS 5b: For elementary and middle school–aged children (age 6 years to the 12th birthday) with ADHD, the PCC should prescribe US Food and Drug Administration (FDA)–approved medications for ADHD, along with PTBM and/or behavioral classroom intervention (preferably both PTBM and behavioral classroom interventions). Educational interventions and individualized instructional supports, including school environment, class placement, instructional placement, and behavioral supports, are a necessary part of any treatment plan and often include an Individualized Education Program (IEP) or a rehabilitation plan (504 plan). (Grade A: strong recommendation for medications; grade A: strong recommendation for PTBM training and behavioral treatments for ADHD implemented with the family and school.)

Aggregate evidence quality	Grade A for Treatment with FDA-Approved Medications; Grade A for Training and Behavioral Treatments for ADHD With the Family and School.
Benefits	Both behavioral therapy and FDA-approved medications have been shown to reduce behaviors associated with ADHD and to improve function.
Risks, harm, cost	Both therapies increase the cost of care. Psychosocial therapy requires a high level of family and/or school involvement and may lead to increased family conflict, especially if treatment is not successfully completed. FDA-approved medications may have some adverse effects and discontinuation of medication is common among adolescents.
Benefit-harm assessment	Given the risks of untreated ADHD, the benefits outweigh the risks.
Intentional vagueness	None.
Role of patient preferences	Family preference, including patient preference, is essential in determining the treatment plan and enhancing adherence.
Exclusions	None.
Strength	Strong recommendation.
Key references	Evans et al[25]; Barbaresi et al[73]; Jain et al[103]; Brown and Bishop[104]; Kambeitz et al[105]; Bruxel et al[106]; Kieling et al[107]; Froehlich et al[108]; Joensen et al[109]

interrupting, aggression, not completing tasks, and not complying with requests. Behavioral parent and classroom training are well-established treatments with preadolescent children.[25,87,88] Most studies comparing behavior therapy to stimulants indicate that stimulants have a stronger immediate effect on the 18 core symptoms of ADHD. Parents, however, were more satisfied with the effect of behavioral therapy, which addresses symptoms and functions in addition to ADHD's core symptoms. The positive effects of behavioral therapies tend to persist, but the positive effects of medication cease when medication stops. Optimal care is likely to occur when both therapies are used, but the decision about therapies is heavily dependent on acceptability by, and feasibility for, the family.

Training interventions target skill development and involve repeated practice with performance feedback over time, rather than modifying behavioral contingencies in a specific setting. Less research has been conducted on training interventions compared to behavioral treatments; nonetheless, training interventions are well-established treatments to target disorganization of materials and time that are exhibited by most youth with ADHD; it is likely that they will benefit younger children, as well.[25,89] Some training interventions, including social skills training, have not been shown to be effective for children with ADHD.[25]

TABLE 8 KAS 5c: For adolescents (age 12 years to the 18th birthday) with ADHD, the PCC should prescribe FDA-approved medications for ADHD with the adolescent's assent (grade A: strong recommendation). The PCC is encouraged to prescribe evidence-based training interventions and/or behavioral interventions as treatment of ADHD, if available. Educational interventions and individualized instructional supports, including school environment, class placement, instructional placement, and behavioral supports, are a necessary part of any treatment plan and often include an IEP or a rehabilitation plan (504 plan). (Grade A: strong recommendation.)

Aggregate evidence quality	Grade A for Medications; Grade A for Training and Behavioral Therapy
Benefits	Training interventions, behavioral therapy, and FDA-approved medications have been demonstrated to reduce behaviors associated with ADHD and to improve function.
Risks, harm, cost	Both therapies increase the cost of care. Psychosocial therapy requires a high level of family and/or school involvement and may lead to unintended increased family conflict, especially if treatment is not successfully completed. FDA-approved medications may have some adverse effects, and discontinuation of medication is common among adolescents.
Benefit-harm assessment	Given the risks of untreated ADHD, the benefits outweigh the risks.
Intentional vagueness	None.
Role of patient preferences	Family preference, including patient preference, is likely to predict engagement and persistence with a treatment.
Exclusions	None.
Strength	Strong recommendation.
Key references	Evans et al[25]; Webster-Stratton et al[87]; Evans et al[95]; Fabiano et al[93]; Sibley and Graziano et al[94]; Langberg et al[96]; Schultz et al[97]; Brown and Bishop[104]; Kambeitz et al[105]; Bruxel et al[106]; Froehlich et al[108]; Joensen et al[109]

Some nonmedication treatments for ADHD-related problems have either too little evidence to recommend them or have been found to have little or no benefit. These include mindfulness, cognitive training, diet modification, EEG biofeedback, and supportive counseling. The suggestion that cannabidiol oil has any effect on ADHD is anecdotal and has not been subjected to rigorous study. Although it is FDA approved, the efficacy for external trigeminal nerve stimulation (eTNS) is documented by one 5-week randomized controlled trial with just 30 participants receiving eTNS.[90] To date, there is no long-term safety and efficacy evidence for eTNS. Overall, the current evidence supporting treatment of ADHD with eTNS is sparse and in no way approaches the robust strength of evidence documented for established medication and behavioral treatments for ADHD; therefore, it cannot be recommended as a treatment of ADHD without considerably more extensive study on its efficacy and safety.

Special Circumstances: Adolescents

Much less research has been published on psychosocial treatments with adolescents than with younger children. PTBM has been modified to include the parents and adolescents in sessions together to develop a behavioral contract and improve parent-adolescent communication and problem-solving (see above).[91] Some training programs also include motivational interviewing approaches. The evidence for this behavioral family approach is mixed and less strong than PTBM with pre-adolescent children.[92–94] Adolescents' responses to behavioral contingencies are more varied than those of younger children because they can often effectively obstruct behavioral contracts, increasing parent-adolescent conflict.

Training approaches that are focused on school functioning skills have consistently revealed benefits for adolescents.[95–97] The greatest benefits from training interventions occur when treatment is continued over an extended period of time, performance feedback is constructive and frequent, and the target behaviors are directly applicable to the adolescent's daily functioning.

Overall, behavioral family approaches may be helpful to some adolescents and their families, and school-based training interventions are well established.[25,94] Meaningful improvements in functioning have not been reported from cognitive behavioral approaches.

Medication for ADHD

Preschool-aged children may experience increased mood lability and dysphoria with stimulant medications.[83] None of the nonstimulants have FDA approval for use in preschool-aged children. For elementary school–aged students, the evidence is particularly strong for stimulant medications and is sufficient, but less strong, for atomoxetine, extended-release guanfacine, and extended-release clonidine (in that order). The effect size for stimulants is 1.0 and for nonstimulants is 0.7. An individual's response to methylphenidate verses amphetamine is idiosyncratic, with approximately 40% responding to both and about 40% responding to only 1. The subtype of ADHD does not appear to be a predictor of response to a specific agent. For most adolescents, stimulant medications are highly effective in reducing ADHD's core symptoms.[73]

Stimulant medications have an effect size of around 1.0 (effect size = [treatment M − control M)/control SD]) for the treatment of ADHD.[98] Among nonstimulant medications, 1 selective norepinephrine reuptake inhibitor, atomoxetine,[99,100] and 2 selective α-2 adrenergic agonists, extended-release guanfacine[101,102] and extended-release clonidine,[103] have also demonstrated efficacy in reducing core symptoms among school-aged children and adolescents, although their effect sizes, —around 0.7 for all 3, are less robust than that of stimulant medications. Norepinephrine reuptake inhibitors and α-2 adrenergic agonists are newer medications, so, in general, the evidence base supporting them is considerably less than that for stimulants, although it was adequate for FDA approval.

A free list of the currently available, FDA-approved medications for ADHD is available online at www.ADHDMedicationGuide.com. Each medication's characteristics are provided to help guide the clinician's prescription choice. With the expanded list of medications, it is less likely that PCCs need to consider the off-label use of other medications. The section on systemic barriers in the Supplemental Information provides suggestions for fostering more realistic and effective payment and communication systems.

Because of the large variability in patients' response to ADHD medication, there is great interest in pharmacogenetic tools that can help clinicians predict the best medication and dose for each child or adolescent. At this time, however, the available scientific literature does not provide sufficient evidence to support their clinical utility given that the genetic variants assayed by these tools have generally not been fully studied with respect to medication effects on ADHD-related symptoms and/or impairment, study findings are inconsistent, or effect sizes are not of sufficient size to ensure clinical utility.[104–109] For that reason, these pharmacogenetics tools are not recommended. In addition, these tests may cost thousands of dollars and are typically not covered by insurance. For a pharmacogenetics tool to be recommended for clinical use, studies would need to reveal (1) the genetic variants assayed have consistent, replicated associations with medication response; (2) knowledge about a patient's genetic profile would change clinical decision-making, improve outcomes and/or reduce costs or burden; and (3) the acceptability of the test's operating characteristics has been demonstrated (eg, sensitivity, specificity, and reliability).

Side Effects

Stimulants' most common short-term adverse effects are appetite loss, abdominal pain, headaches, and sleep disturbance. The Multimodal Treatment of Attention Deficit Hyperactivity Disorder (MTA) study results identified stimulants as having a more persistent effect on decreasing growth velocity compared to most previous studies.[110] Diminished growth was in the range of 1 to 2 cm from predicted adult height. The results of the MTA study were particularly noted among children who were on higher and more consistently administered doses of stimulants.[110] The effects diminished by the third year of treatment, but no compensatory rebound growth was observed.[110] An uncommon significant adverse effect of stimulants is the occurrence of hallucinations and other psychotic symptoms.[111]

Stimulant medications, on average, increase patient heart rate (HR) and blood pressure (BP) to a mild and clinically insignificant degree (average increases: 1–2 beats per minute for HR and 1–4 mm Hg for systolic and diastolic BP).[112] However, because stimulants have been linked to more substantial increases in HR and BP in a subset of individuals (5%–15%), clinicians are encouraged to monitor these vital signs in patients receiving stimulant treatment.[112] Although concerns have been raised about sudden cardiac death among children and adolescents using stimulant and medications,[113] it is an extremely rare occurrence. In fact, stimulant medications have not been shown to increase the risk of sudden death beyond that observed in children who are not receiving stimulants.[114–118] Nevertheless, before initiating therapy with stimulant medications, it is important to obtain the child or adolescent's history of specific cardiac symptoms in addition to the family history of sudden death, cardiovascular symptoms, Wolff-Parkinson-White syndrome, hypertrophic cardiomyopathy, and long QT syndrome. If any of these risk factors are present, clinicians should obtain additional evaluation to ascertain and address potential safety concerns of stimulant medication use by the child or adolescent.[112,114]

Among nonstimulants, the risk of serious cardiovascular events is extremely low, as it is for stimulants. The 3 nonstimulant medications that are FDA approved to treat ADHD (ie, atomoxetine, guanfacine, and clonidine) may be associated with changes in cardiovascular parameters or other serious cardiovascular events. These events could include increased HR and BP for atomoxetine and decreased HR and BP for guanfacine and clonidine. Clinicians are recommended to not only obtain the personal and family cardiac history, as detailed above, but also to perform additional evaluation if risk factors are present before starting nonstimulant medications (ie, perform an electrocardiogram [ECG] and possibly refer to a pediatric cardiologist if the ECG is not normal).[112]

Additional adverse effects of atomoxetine include initial somnolence and gastrointestinal tract symptoms, particularly if the dosage is increased too rapidly, and decreased appetite.[119–122] Less commonly, an increase in suicidal thoughts has been found; this is noted by an FDA black box warning. Extremely rarely, hepatitis has been associated with atomoxetine. Atomoxetine has also been linked to growth delays compared to expected trajectories in the first 1 to 2 years of treatment, with a return to expected measurements after 2 to 3 years of treatment, on average. Decreases were observed among those who were taller or heavier than average before treatment.[123]

For extended-release guanfacine and extended-release clonidine, adverse effects include somnolence, dry mouth, dizziness, irritability, headache, bradycardia, hypotension, and abdominal pain.[30,124,125] Because rebound hypertension after abrupt guanfacine and clonidine discontinuation has been observed,[126] these medications should be tapered off rather than suddenly discontinued.

Adjunctive Therapy

Adjunctive therapies may be considered if stimulant therapy is not fully effective or limited by side effects. Only extended-release guanfacine and extended-release clonidine have evidence supporting their use as adjunctive therapy with stimulant medications sufficient to have achieved FDA approval.[127] Other medications have been used in combination on an off-label basis, with some limited evidence available to support the efficacy and safety of using atomoxetine in combination with stimulant medications to augment treatment of ADHD.[128]

Special Circumstances: Preschool-Aged Children (Age 4 Years to the Sixth Birthday)

If children do not experience adequate symptom improvement with PTBM, medication can be prescribed for those with moderate-to-severe ADHD. Many young children with ADHD may require medication to achieve maximum improvement; methylphenidate is the recommended first-line pharmacologic treatment of preschool children because of the lack of sufficient rigorous study in the preschool-aged population for nonstimulant ADHD medications and dextroamphetamine. Although amphetamine is the only medication with FDA approval for use in children younger than 6 years, this authorization was issued at a time when approval criteria were less stringent than current requirements. Hence, the available evidence regarding dextroamphetamine's use in preschool-aged children with ADHD is not adequate to recommend it as an initial ADHD medication treatment at this time.[80]

No nonstimulant medication has received sufficient rigorous study in the preschool-aged population to be recommended for treatment of ADHD of children 4 through 5 years of age.

Although methylphenidate is the ADHD medication with the strongest evidence for safety and efficacy in preschool-aged children, it should be noted that the evidence has not yet met the level needed for FDA approval. Evidence for the use of methylphenidate consists of 1 multisite study of 165 children[83] and 10 other smaller, single-site studies ranging from 11 to 59 children, for a total of 269 children.[129] Seven of the 10 single-site studies revealed efficacy for methylphenidate in preschoolers. Therefore, although there is moderate evidence that methylphenidate is safe and effective in preschool-aged children, its use in this age group remains on an "off-label" basis.

With these caveats in mind, before initiating treatment with medication, the clinician should assess the severity of the child's ADHD. Given current data, only preschool-aged children with ADHD and moderate-to-severe dysfunction should be considered for medication. Severity criteria are symptoms that have persisted for at least 9 months; dysfunction that is manifested in both home and other settings, such as preschool or child care; and dysfunction that has not responded adequately to PTBM.[83]

The decision to consider initiating medication at this age depends, in part, on the clinician's assessment of the estimated developmental impairment, safety risks, and potential consequences if medications are not initiated. Other considerations affecting the treatment of preschool-aged children with stimulant medications include the lack of information and experience about their longer-term effects on growth and brain development, as well as the potential for other adverse effects in this population. It may be helpful to obtain consultation from a mental health specialist with specific experience with preschool-aged children, if possible.

Evidence suggests that the rate of metabolizing methylphenidate is slower in children 4 through 5 years of age, so they should be given a low dose to start; the dose can be increased in smaller increments. Maximum doses have not been adequately studied in preschool-aged children.[83]

Special Circumstances: Adolescents (Age 12 Years to the 18th Birthday)

As noted, before beginning medication treatment of adolescents with newly diagnosed ADHD, clinicians should assess the patient for symptoms of substance use. If active substance use is identified, the clinician should refer the patient to a subspecialist for consultative support and guidance.[2,130–134]

In addition, diversion of ADHD medication (ie, its use for something other than its intended medical purposes) is a special concern among adolescents.[135] Clinicians should monitor the adolescent's symptoms and prescription refill requests for signs of misuse or diversion of ADHD medication, including by parents, classmates, or other acquaintances of the adolescent. The majority of states now require prescriber participation in prescription drug monitoring programs, which can be helpful in identifying and preventing diversion activities. They may consider prescribing nonstimulant medications that minimize abuse potential, such as atomoxetine and extended-release guanfacine or extended-release clonidine.

Given the risks of driving for adolescents with ADHD, including crashes and motor vehicle violations, special concern should be taken to provide medication coverage for symptom control while driving.[79,136,137] Longer-acting or late-afternoon, short-acting medications may be helpful in this regard.[138]

Special Circumstances: Inattention or Hyperactivity/Impulsivity (Problem Level)

Medication is not appropriate for children whose symptoms do not meet *DSM-5* criteria for ADHD. Psychosocial treatments may be appropriate for these children and adolescents. As noted, psychosocial treatments do not require a specific diagnosis of ADHD, and many of the studies on the efficacy of PTBM included children who did not have a specific psychiatric or ADHD diagnosis.

Combination Treatments

Studies indicate that behavioral therapy has positive effects when it is combined with medication for pre-adolescent children.[139] (The combined effects of training interventions and medication have not been studied.)

In the MTA study, researchers found that although the combination of behavioral therapy and stimulant medication was not significantly more effective than treatment with medication alone for ADHD's core symptoms, after correcting for multiple tests in the primary analysis,[139] a secondary analysis of a combined measure of parent and teacher ratings of ADHD symptoms did find a significant advantage for the combination, with a small effect of $d = 0.28$.[140] The combined treatment also offered greater improvements on academic and conduct measures, compared to medication alone, when the ADHD was comorbid with anxiety and the child or adolescent lived in a lower socioeconomic environment.

In addition, parents and teachers of children who received combined therapy reported that they were significantly more satisfied with the treatment plan. Finally, the combination of medication management and behavioral therapy allowed for the use of lower stimulant dosages, possibly reducing the risk of adverse effects.[141]

School Programming and Supports

Encouraging strong family-school partnerships helps the ADHD management process.[142] Psychosocial treatments that include coordinating efforts at school and home may enhance the effects.

Children and adolescents with ADHD may be eligible for services as part of a 504 Rehabilitation Act Plan (504 plan) or special education IEP under the "other health impairment" designation in the Individuals with Disability Education Act (IDEA).[143] (ADHD qualifies as a disability under a 504 plan. It does not qualify under an IEP unless its severity impairs the child's ability to learn. See the PoCA for more details.) It is helpful for clinicians to be aware of the eligibility criteria in their states and school districts to advise families of their options. Eligibility decisions can vary considerably between school districts, and school professionals' independent determinations might not agree with the recommendations of outside clinicians.

There are essentially 2 categories of school-based services for students with ADHD. The first category includes interventions that are intended to help the student independently meet age-appropriate academic and behavioral expectations. Examples of these interventions include daily report cards, training interventions, point systems, and academic remediation of skills. If successful, the student's impairment will resolve, and the student will no longer need services.

The second category is intended to provide changes in the student's program so his or her ADHD-related problems no longer result in failure and cause distress to parents, teachers, and the student.[144] These services are referred to as "accommodations" and include extended time to complete tests and assignments, reduced homework demands, the ability to keep study materials in class, and provision of the teacher's notes to the student. These services are intended to allow the student to accomplish his work successfully and communicate that the student's impairment is acceptable. Accommodations make the student's impairment acceptable and are separate from interventions aimed at improving the students' skills or behaviors. In the absence of such interventions, long-term accommodations may lead to reduced expectations and can lead to the need for accommodations to be maintained throughout the student's education.

Encouraging strong family-school partnerships helps the ADHD management process, and addressing social determinants of health is essential to these partnerships.[145,146] Psychosocial treatments that include coordinating efforts at school and home may enhance the effects.

KAS 6

The PCC should titrate doses of medication for ADHD to achieve maximum benefit with tolerable side effects (Table 9). (Grade B: strong recommendation.)

The MTA study is the landmark study comparing effects of methylphenidate and behavioral treatments in children with ADHD. Investigators compared treatment effects in 4 groups of children who received optimal medication management, optimal behavioral management, combined medication and behavioral management, or community treatment. Children in the optimal medication management and combined medication and behavioral management groups underwent a systematic trial with 4 different doses of methylphenidate, with results suggesting that when this full range of doses is administered, more than 70% of children and adolescents with ADHD are methylphenidate responders.[140]

Authors of other reports suggest that more than 90% of patients will have a beneficial response to 1 of the psychostimulants if a range of medications from both the methylphenidate and amphetamine and/or dextroamphetamine classes

TABLE 9 KAS 6: The PCC should titrate doses of medication for ADHD to achieve maximum benefit with tolerable side effects. (Grade B: strong recommendation.)

Aggregate evidence quality	Grade B
Benefits	The optimal dose of medication is required to reduce core symptoms to, or close to, the levels of children without ADHD.
Risks, harm, cost	Higher levels of medication increase the chances of side effects.
Benefit-harm assessment	The importance of adequately treating ADHD outweighs the risk of adverse effects.
Intentional vagueness	None.
Role of patient preferences	The families' preferences and comfort need to be taken into consideration in developing a titration plan, as they are likely to predict engagement and persistence with a treatment.
Exclusions	None
Strength	Strong recommendation
Key references	Jensen et al[140]; Solanto[147]; Brinkman et al[149]

are tried.[147] Of note, children in the MTA study who received care in the community as usual, either from a clinician they chose or to whom their family had access, showed less beneficial results compared with children who received optimal medication management. The explanation offered by the study investigators was that the community treatment group received lower medication doses and less frequent monitoring than the optimal medication management group.

A child's response to stimulants is variable and unpredictable. For this reason, it is recommended to titrate from a low dose to one that achieves a maximum, optimal effect in controlling symptoms without adverse effects. Calculating the dose on the basis of milligrams per kilogram has not usually been helpful because variations in dose have not been found to be related to height or weight. In addition, because stimulant medication effects are seen rapidly, titration can be accomplished in a relatively short time period. Stimulant medications can be effectively titrated on a 7-day basis, but in urgent situations, they may be effectively titrated in as few as 3 days.[140]

Parent and child and adolescent education is an important component in the chronic illness model to ensure cooperation in efforts to achieve appropriate titration, remembering that the parents themselves may be significantly challenged by ADHD.[148,149] The PCC should alert parents and children that changing medication dose and occasionally changing a medication may be necessary for optimal medication management, may require a few months to achieve optimal success, and that medication efficacy should be monitored at regular intervals.

By the 3-year (ie, 36-month) follow-up to the MTA interventions, there were no differences among the 4 groups (ie, optimal medications management, optimal behavioral management, a combination of medication and behavioral management, and community treatment). This equivalence in poststudy outcomes may, however, have been attributable to convergence in ongoing treatments received for the 4 groups. After the initial 14-month intervention, the children no longer received the careful monthly monitoring provided by the study and went back to receiving care from their community providers; therefore, they all effectively received a level of ongoing care consistent with the "community treatment" study arm of the study. After leaving the MTA trial, medications and doses varied for the children who had been in the optimal medication management or combined medication and behavioral management groups, and a number stopped taking ADHD medication. On the other hand, some children who had been in the optimal behavioral management group started taking medication after leaving the trial. The results further emphasize the need to treat ADHD as a chronic illness and provide continuity of care and, where possible, provide a medical home.[140]

See the PoCA for more on implementation of this KAS.

KAS 7

The PCC, if trained or experienced in diagnosing comorbid conditions, may initiate treatment of such conditions or make a referral to an appropriate subspecialist for treatment. After detecting possible comorbid conditions, if the PCC is not trained or experienced in making the diagnosis or initiating treatment, the patient should be referred to an appropriate subspecialist to make the diagnosis and initiate treatment (Table 10). (Grade C: recommendation.)

The effect of comorbid conditions on ADHD treatment is variable. In some cases, treatment of the ADHD may resolve the comorbid condition. For example, treatment of ADHD may lead to improvement in coexisting aggression and/or oppositional defiant, depressive, or anxiety symptoms.[150,151]

Sometimes, however, the comorbid condition may require treatment in addition to the ADHD treatment. If the PCC is confident of his or her ability to diagnose and treat certain comorbid conditions, the PCC may do so. The PCC may benefit from additional consultative support and guidance from a mental health subspecialist or may need to refer a child with ADHD and comorbid conditions, such as severe mood or anxiety disorders, to subspecialists for assessment and management. The subspecialists could include child and adolescent psychiatrists, clinical child psychologists, developmental-behavioral pediatricians, neurodevelopmental disability physicians, child neurologists, or child- or school-based evaluation teams.

IMPLEMENTATION: PREPARING THE PRACTICE

It is generally the role of the primary care pediatrician to manage mild-to-moderate ADHD, anxiety, depression, and substance use. The AAP statement "The Future of Pediatrics: Mental Health Competencies for Pediatric Primary Care" describes the competencies needed in both pediatric primary and specialty care to address the social-emotional and mental health needs of children and families.[152] Broadly, these include incorporating mental health content and tools into health promotion, prevention, and primary care intervention, becoming knowledgeable about use of evidence-based treatments, and participating as a team member and comanaging with pediatric and mental health specialists.

The recommendations made in this guideline are intended to be integrated with the broader mental health algorithm developed as part of the AAP Mental Health Initiatives.[2,133,153] Pediatricians have unique opportunities

TABLE 10 KAS 7: The PCC, if trained or experienced in diagnosing comorbid conditions, may initiate treatment of such conditions or make a referral to an appropriate subspecialist for treatment. After detecting possible comorbid conditions, if the PCC is not trained or experienced in making the diagnosis or initiating treatment, the patient should be referred to an appropriate subspecialist to make the diagnosis and initiate treatment. (Grade C: recommendation.)

Aggregate evidence quality	Grade C
Benefits	Clinicians are most effective when they know the limits of their practice to diagnose comorbid conditions and are aware of resources in their community.
Risks, harm, cost	Under-identification or inappropriate identification of comorbidities can lead to inadequate or inappropriate treatments.
Benefit-harm assessment	The importance of adequately identifying and addressing comorbidities outweighs the risk of inappropriate referrals or treatments.
Intentional vagueness	None.
Role of patient preferences	The families' preferences and comfort need to be taken into consideration in identifying and treating or referring their patients with comorbidities, as they are likely to predict engagement and persistence with a treatment.
Exclusions	None.
Strength	Recommendation.
Key references	Pliszka et al[150]; Pringsheim et al[151]

to identify conditions, including ADHD, intervene early, and partner with both families and specialists for the benefit of children's health. A wealth of useful information is available at the AAP Mental Health Initiatives Web site (https://www.aap.org/en-us/advocacy-and-policy/aap-health-initiatives/Mental-Health/Pages/Tips-For-Pediatricians.aspx).

It is also important for PCCs to be aware of health disparities and social determinants that may impact patient outcomes and strive to provide culturally appropriate care to all children and adolescents in their practice.[145,146,154,155]

The accompanying PoCA provides supplemental information to support PCCs as they implement this guideline's recommendations. In particular, the PoCA describes steps for preparing the practice that provide useful recommendations to clinicians. For example, the PoCA includes information about using standardized rating scales to diagnose ADHD, assessing for comorbid conditions, documenting all aspects of the diagnostic and treatment procedures in the patient's records, monitoring the patient's treatment and outcomes, and providing families with written management plans.

The AAP acknowledges that some PCCs may not have the training, experience, or resources to diagnose and treat children and adolescents with ADHD, especially if severity or comorbid conditions make these patients complex to manage. In these situations, comanagement with specialty clinicians is recommended. The SDBP is developing a guideline to address such complex cases and aid pediatricians and other PCCs to manage these cases; the SDBP currently expects to publish this document in 2019.[67]

AREAS FOR FUTURE RESEARCH

There is a need to conduct research on topics pertinent to the diagnosis and treatment of ADHD, developmental variations, and problems in children and adolescents in primary care. These research opportunities include the following:

- assessment of ADHD and its common comorbidities: anxiety, depression, learning disabilities, and autism spectrum disorder;
- identification and/or development of reliable instruments suitable for use in primary care to assess the nature or degree of functional impairment in children and adolescents with ADHD and to monitor improvement over time;
- refinement of developmentally informed assessment procedures for evaluating ADHD in preschoolers;
- study of medications and other therapies used clinically but not FDA approved for ADHD;
- determination of the optimal schedule for monitoring children and adolescents with ADHD, including factors for adjusting that schedule according to age, symptom severity, and progress reports;
- evaluation of the effectiveness and adverse effects of medications used in combination, such as a stimulant with an α-adrenergic agent, selective serotonin reuptake inhibitor, or atomoxetine;
- evaluation of processes of care to assist PCCs to identify and treat comorbid conditions;
- evaluation of the effectiveness of various school-based interventions;
- comparisons of medication use and effectiveness in different ages, including both harms and benefits;
- development of methods to involve parents, children, and adolescents in their own care and improve adherence to both psychosocial and medication treatments;
- conducting research into psychosocial treatments, such as cognitive behavioral therapy and cognitive training, among others;

- development of standardized and documented tools to help primary care providers identify comorbid conditions;
- development of effective electronic and Web-based systems to help gather information to diagnose and monitor children and adolescents with ADHD;
- improvements to systems for communicating with schools, mental health professionals, and other community agencies to provide effective collaborative care;
- development of more objective measures of performance to more objectively monitor aspects of severity, disability, or impairment;
- assessment of long-term outcomes for children in whom ADHD was first diagnosed at preschool ages; and
- identification and implementation of ideas to address the barriers that hamper the implementation of these guidelines and the PoCA.

CONCLUSIONS

Evidence is clear with regard to the legitimacy of the diagnosis of ADHD and the appropriate diagnostic criteria and procedures required to establish a diagnosis, identify comorbid conditions, and effectively treat with both psychosocial and pharmacologic interventions. The steps required to sustain appropriate treatments and achieve successful long-term outcomes remain challenging, however.

As noted, this clinical practice guideline is supported by 2 accompanying documents available in the Supplemental Information: the PoCA and the article on systemic barriers to the car of children and adolescents with ADHD. Full implementation of the guideline's KASs, the PoCA, and the recommendations to address barriers to care may require changes in office procedures and the identification of community resources. Fully addressing systemic barriers requires identifying local, state, and national entities with which to partner to advance solutions and manifest change.[156]

SUBCOMMITTEE ON CHILDREN AND ADOLESCENTS WITH ADHD (OVERSIGHT BY THE COUNCIL ON QUALITY IMPROVEMENT AND PATIENT SAFETY)

Mark L. Wolraich, MD, FAAP, Chairperson, Section on Developmental Behavioral Pediatrics
Joseph F. Hagan Jr, MD, FAAP, Vice Chairperson, Section on Developmental Behavioral Pediatrics
Carla Allan, PhD, Society of Pediatric Psychology
Eugenia Chan, MD, MPH, FAAP, Implementation Scientist
Dale Davison, MSpEd, PCC, Parent Advocate, Children and Adolescents with Attention-Deficit/Hyperactivity Disorder
Marian Earls, MD, MTS, FAAP, Mental Health Leadership Work Group
Steven W. Evans, PhD, Clinical Psychologist
Tanya Froehlich, MD, FAAP, Section on Developmental Behavioral Pediatrics/Society for Developmental and Behavioral Pediatrics
Jennifer Frost, MD, FAAFP, American Academy of Family Physicians
Joseph R. Holbrook, PhD, MPH, Epidemiologist, Centers for Disease Control and Prevention
Herschel Robert Lessin, MD, FAAP, Section on Administration and Practice Management
Karen L. Pierce, MD, DFAACAP, American Academy of Child and Adolescent Psychiatry
Christoph Ulrich Lehmann, MD, FAAP, Partnership for Policy Implementation
Jonathan D. Winner, MD, FAAP, Committee on Practice and Ambulatory Medicine
William Zurhellen, MD, FAAP, Section on Administration and Practice Management

STAFF

Kymika Okechukwu, MPA, Senior Manager, Evidence-Based Medicine Initiatives
Jeremiah Salmon, MPH, Program Manager, Policy Dissemination and Implementation

CONSULTANT

Susan K. Flinn, MA, Medical Editor

ABBREVIATIONS

AAP: American Academy of Pediatrics
ADHD: attention-deficit/hyperactivity disorder
ADHD/C: attention-deficit/hyperactivity disorder combined presentation
ADHD/HI: attention-deficit/hyperactivity disorder primarily of the hyperactive-impulsive presentation
ADHD/I: attention-deficit/hyperactivity disorder primarily of the inattentive presentation
AHRQ: Agency for Healthcare Research and Quality
BP: blood pressure
CHADD: Children and Adults with Attention-Deficit/Hyperactivity Disorder
DSM-5: *Diagnostic and Statistical Manual of Mental Disorders, Fifth Edition*
DSM-IV: *Diagnostic and Statistical Manual of Mental Disorders Fourth Edition*
DSM-PC: *Diagnostic and Statistical Manual for Primary Care*
ECG: electrocardiogram
eTNS: external trigeminal nerve stimulation
FDA: US Food and Drug Administration
HR: heart rate
IDEA: Individuals with Disability Education Act
IEP: Individualized Education Program
KAS: key action statement
MTA: The Multimodal Treatment of Attention Deficit Hyperactivity Disorder
PCC: primary care clinician
PoCA: process of care algorithm
PTBM: parent training in behavior management
SDBP: Society for Developmental and Behavioral Pediatrics

[v]American Academy of Pediatrics, Itasca, Illinois; [w]American Academy of Child and Adolescent Psychiatry, Washington, District of Columbia; [x]Feinberg School of Medicine, Northwestern University, Chicago, Illinois; [y]Atlanta, Georgia; and [z]Holderness, New Hampshire

The guidance in this report does not indicate an exclusive course of treatment or serve as a standard of medical care. Variations, taking into account individual circumstances, may be appropriate.

All clinical practice guidelines from the American Academy of Pediatrics automatically expire 5 years after publication unless reaffirmed, revised, or retired at or before that time.

The findings and conclusions in this report are those of the authors and do not necessarily represent the official position of the Centers for Disease Control and Prevention. Dr Holbrook was not an author of the accompanying supplemental section on barriers to care.

This document is copyrighted and is property of the American Academy of Pediatrics and its Board of Directors. All authors have filed conflict of interest statements with the American Academy of Pediatrics. Any conflicts have been resolved through a process approved by the Board of Directors. The American Academy of Pediatrics has neither solicited nor accepted any commercial involvement in the development of the content of this publication.

DOI: https://doi.org/10.1542/peds.2019-2528

Address correspondence to Mark L. Wolraich, MD, FAAP. Email: mark-wolraich@ouhsc.edu

PEDIATRICS (ISSN Numbers: Print, 0031-4005; Online, 1098-4275).

Copyright © 2019 by the American Academy of Pediatrics

FINANCIAL DISCLOSURE: The authors have indicated they have no financial relationships relevant to this article to disclose.

FUNDING: No external funding.

POTENTIAL CONFLICT OF INTEREST: All authors have filed conflict of interest statements with the American Academy of Pediatrics. Any conflicts have been resolved through a process approved by the American Academy of Pediatrics board of directors. Dr Allan reports a relationship with ADDitude Magazine; Dr Chan reports relationships with TriVox Health and Wolters Kluwer; Dr Lehmann reports relationships with International Medical Informatics Association, Springer Publishing, and Thieme Publishing Group; Dr Wolraich reports a Continuing Medical Education trainings relationship with the Resource for Advancing Children's Health Institute; the other authors have indicated they have no potential conflicts of interest to disclose.

REFERENCES

1. American Academy of Pediatrics. Subcommittee on Attention-Deficit/Hyperactivity Disorder, Steering Committee on Quality Improvement and Management. ADHD: Clinical guideline for the diagnosis, evaluation, and treatment of attention-deficit/hyperactivity disorder in children and adolescents. *Pediatrics*. 2011;128(5):1007–1022
2. American Academy of Pediatrics Task Force on Mental Health. *Addressing Mental Health Concerns in Primary Care: A Clinician's Toolkit [CD-ROM]*. Elk Grove Village, IL: American Academy of Pediatrics; 2010
3. Pastor PN, Reuben CA. Racial and ethnic differences in ADHD and LD in young school-age children: parental reports in the National Health Interview Survey. *Public Health Rep*. 2005;120(4):383–392
4. US Department of Health and Human Services; Health Resources and Services Administration. Designated health professional shortage areas statistics: designated HPSA quarterly summary. Rockville, MD: Health Resources and Services Administration; 2018
5. Pelech D, Hayford T. Medicare advantage and commercial prices for mental health services. *Health Aff (Millwood)*. 2019;38(2):262–267
6. Melek SP, Perlman D, Davenport S. *Differential Reimbursement of Psychiatric Services by Psychiatrists and Other Medical Providers*. Seattle, WA: Milliman;2017
7. Holbrook JR, Bitsko RH, Danielson ML, Visser SN. Interpreting the prevalence of mental disorders in children: tribulation and triangulation. *Health Promot Pract*. 2017;18(1):5–7
8. Thomas R, Sanders S, Doust J, Beller E, Glasziou P. Prevalence of attention-deficit/hyperactivity disorder: a systematic review and meta-analysis. *Pediatrics*. 2015;135(4). Available at: www.pediatrics.org/cgi/content/full/135/4/e994
9. Wolraich ML, McKeown RE, Visser SN, et al. The prevalence of ADHD: its diagnosis and treatment in four school districts across two states. *J Atten Disord*. 2014;18(7):563–575
10. Rowland AS, Skipper BJ, Umbach DM, et al. The prevalence of ADHD in a population-based sample. *J Atten Disord*. 2015;19(9):741–754
11. Danielson ML, Bitsko RH, Ghandour RM, Holbrook JR, Kogan MD, Blumberg SJ. Prevalence of parent-reported ADHD diagnosis and associated treatment among U.S. children and adolescents, 2016. *J Clin Child Adolesc Psychol*. 2018;47(2):199–212
12. Visser SN, Zablotsky B, Holbrook JR, et al. *National Health Statistics Reports, No 81: Diagnostic Experiences of Children with Attention-Deficit/Hyperactivity Disorder*. Hyattsville, MD: National Center for Health Statistics; 2015
13. Molina BS, Hinshaw SP, Swanson JM, et al; MTA Cooperative Group. The MTA at 8 years: prospective follow-up of children treated for combined-type ADHD in a multisite study. *J Am Acad Child Adolesc Psychiatry*. 2009;48(5):484–500
14. Holbrook JR, Cuffe SP, Cai B, et al. Persistence of parent-reported ADHD symptoms from childhood through adolescence in a community sample. *J Atten Disord*. 2016;20(1):11–20

15. Mueller KL, Tomblin JB. Examining the comorbidity of language disorders and ADHD. *Top Lang Disord.* 2012;32(3): 228–246

16. Pastor PN, Reuben CA, Duran CR, Hawkins LD. *Association Between Diagnosed ADHD and Selected Characteristics Among Children Aged 4–17 Years: United States, 2011–2013. NCHS Data Brief, No. 201.* Hyattsville, MD: National Center for Health Statistics; 2015

17. Elia J, Ambrosini P, Berrettini W. ADHD characteristics: I. Concurrent co-morbidity patterns in children & adolescents. *Child Adolesc Psychiatry Ment Health.* 2008;2(1):15

18. Centers for Disease Control and Prevention (CDC). Mental health in the United States. Prevalence of diagnosis and medication treatment for attention-deficit/hyperactivity disorder--United States, 2003. *MMWR Morb Mortal Wkly Rep.* 2005;54(34):842–847

19. Cuffe SP, Visser SN, Holbrook JR, et al. ADHD and psychiatric comorbidity: functional outcomes in a school-based sample of children [published online ahead of print November 25, 2015]. *J Atten Disord.* doi:10.1177/1087054715613437

20. Gaub M, Carlson CL. Gender differences in ADHD: a meta-analysis and critical review. *J Am Acad Child Adolesc Psychiatry.* 1997;36(8):1036–1045

21. Tung I, Li JJ, Meza JI, et al. Patterns of comorbidity among girls with ADHD: a meta-analysis. *Pediatrics.* 2016;138(4): e20160430

22. Layton TJ, Barnett ML, Hicks TR, Jena AB. Attention deficit-hyperactivity disorder and month of school enrollment. *N Engl J Med.* 2018;379(22): 2122–2130

23. Kemper AR, Maslow GR, Hill S, et al. *Attention Deficit Hyperactivity Disorder: Diagnosis and Treatment in Children and Adolescents. Comparative Effectiveness Reviews, No. 203.* Rockville, MD: Agency for Healthcare Research and Quality; 2018

24. Pelham WE Jr, Wheeler T, Chronis A. Empirically supported psychosocial treatments for attention deficit hyperactivity disorder. *J Clin Child Psychol.* 1998;27(2):190–205

25. Evans SW, Owens JS, Wymbs BT, Ray AR. Evidence-based psychosocial treatments for children and adolescents with attention deficit/hyperactivity disorder. *J Clin Child Adolesc Psychol.* 2018;47(2):157–198

26. Pelham WE Jr, Fabiano GA. Evidence-based psychosocial treatments for attention-deficit/hyperactivity disorder. *J Clin Child Adolesc Psychol.* 2008;37(1): 184–214

27. American Academy of Pediatrics Steering Committee on Quality Improvement and Management. Classifying recommendations for clinical practice guidelines. *Pediatrics.* 2004;114(3):874–877

28. Visser SN, Lesesne CA, Perou R. National estimates and factors associated with medication treatment for childhood attention-deficit/hyperactivity disorder. *Pediatrics.* 2007;119(suppl 1):S99–S106

29. Centers for Disease Control and Prevention (CDC). Increasing prevalence of parent-reported attention-deficit/hyperactivity disorder among children–United States, 2003 and 2007. *MMWR Morb Mortal Wkly Rep.* 2010;59(44):1439–1443

30. Egger HL, Kondo D, Angold A. The epidemiology and diagnostic issues in preschool attention-deficit/hyperactivity disorder: a review. *Infants Young Child.* 2006;19(2):109–122

31. Wolraich ML, Wibbelsman CJ, Brown TE, et al. Attention-deficit/hyperactivity disorder among adolescents: a review of the diagnosis, treatment, and clinical implications. *Pediatrics.* 2005;115(6): 1734–1746

32. American Psychiatric Association. *Diagnostic and Statistical Manual of Mental Disorders (DSM-5).* 5th ed. Arlington, VA: American Psychiatric Association; 2013

33. Lahey BB, Pelham WE, Stein MA, et al. Validity of DSM-IV attention-deficit/hyperactivity disorder for younger children. *J Am Acad Child Adolesc Psychiatry.* 1998;37(7):695–702

34. Pavuluri MN, Luk SL, McGee R. Parent reported preschool attention deficit hyperactivity: measurement and validity. *Eur Child Adolesc Psychiatry.* 1999;8(2):126–133

35. Harvey EA, Youngwirth SD, Thakar DA, Errazuriz PA. Predicting attention-deficit/hyperactivity disorder and oppositional defiant disorder from preschool diagnostic assessments. *J Consult Clin Psychol.* 2009;77(2): 349–354

36. Keenan K, Wakschlag LS. More than the terrible twos: the nature and severity of behavior problems in clinic-referred preschool children. *J Abnorm Child Psychol.* 2000;28(1):33–46

37. Gadow KD, Nolan EE, Litcher L, et al. Comparison of attention-deficit/hyperactivity disorder symptom subtypes in Ukrainian schoolchildren. *J Am Acad Child Adolesc Psychiatry.* 2000;39(12):1520–1527

38. Sprafkin J, Volpe RJ, Gadow KD, Nolan EE, Kelly K. A DSM-IV-referenced screening instrument for preschool children: the Early Childhood Inventory-4. *J Am Acad Child Adolesc Psychiatry.* 2002;41(5):604–612

39. Poblano A, Romero E. ECI-4 screening of attention deficit-hyperactivity disorder and co-morbidity in Mexican preschool children: preliminary results. *Arq Neuropsiquiatr.* 2006;64(4):932–936

40. American Academy of Pediatrics. *Mental Health Screening and Assessment Tools for Primary Care.* Elk Grove Village, IL: American Academy of Pediatrics; 2012. Available at: https://www.aap.org/en-us/advocacy-and-policy/aap-health-initiatives/Mental-Health/Documents/MH_ScreeningChart.pdf. Accessed September 8, 2019

41. DuPaul GJ, Power TJ, Anastopoulos AD, Reid R. *ADHD Rating Scale – 5 for Children and Adolescents: Checklists, Norms, and Clinical Interpretation.* 2nd ed. New York, NY: Guilford Press; 2016

42. McGoey KE, DuPaul GJ, Haley E, Shelton TL. Parent and teacher ratings of attention-deficit/hyperactivity disorder in preschool: the ADHD rating scale-IV preschool version. *J Psychopathol Behav Assess.* 2007;29(4):269–276

43. Young J. Common comorbidities seen in adolescents with attention-deficit/hyperactivity disorder. *Adolesc Med State Art Rev.* 2008;19(2):216–228, vii

44. Freeman RD; Tourette Syndrome International Database Consortium. Tic disorders and ADHD: answers from

a world-wide clinical dataset on Tourette syndrome. *Eur Child Adolesc Psychiatry.* 2007;16(suppl 1):15–23

45. Riggs PD. Clinical approach to treatment of ADHD in adolescents with substance use disorders and conduct disorder. *J Am Acad Child Adolesc Psychiatry.* 1998;37(3):331–332
46. Sibley MH, Pelham WE, Molina BSG, et al. Diagnosing ADHD in adolescence. *J Consult Clin Psychol.* 2012;80(1): 139–150
47. Kratochvil CJ, Vaughan BS, Stoner JA, et al. A double-blind, placebo-controlled study of atomoxetine in young children with ADHD. *Pediatrics.* 2011;127(4). Available at: www.pediatrics.org/cgi/content/full/127/4/e862
48. Harrison AG, Edwards MJ, Parker KC. Identifying students faking ADHD: preliminary findings and strategies for detection. *Arch Clin Neuropsychol.* 2007; 22(5):577–588
49. Wolraich ML, Felice ME, Drotar DD. *The Classification of Child and Adolescent Mental Conditions in Primary Care: Diagnostic and Statistical Manual for Primary Care (DSM-PC), Child and Adolescent Version.* Elk Grove Village, IL: American Academy of Pediatrics; 1996
50. Rowland AS, Lesesne CA, Abramowitz AJ. The epidemiology of attention-deficit/hyperactivity disorder (ADHD): a public health view. *Ment Retard Dev Disabil Res Rev.* 2002;8(3):162–170
51. Cuffe SP, Moore CG, McKeown RE. Prevalence and correlates of ADHD symptoms in the national health interview survey. *J Atten Disord.* 2005; 9(2):392–401
52. Pastor PN, Reuben CA. Diagnosed attention deficit hyperactivity disorder and learning disability: United States, 2004-2006. *Vital Health Stat 10.* 2008; 10(237):1–14
53. Biederman J, Faraone SV, Wozniak J, Mick E, Kwon A, Aleardi M. Further evidence of unique developmental phenotypic correlates of pediatric bipolar disorder: findings from a large sample of clinically referred preadolescent children assessed over the last 7 years. *J Affect Disord.* 2004; 82(suppl 1):S45–S58
54. Biederman J, Kwon A, Aleardi M, et al. Absence of gender effects on attention deficit hyperactivity disorder: findings in nonreferred subjects. *Am J Psychiatry.* 2005;162(6):1083–1089
55. Biederman J, Ball SW, Monuteaux MC, et al. New insights into the comorbidity between ADHD and major depression in adolescent and young adult females. *J Am Acad Child Adolesc Psychiatry.* 2008;47(4):426–434
56. Biederman J, Melmed RD, Patel A, McBurnett K, Donahue J, Lyne A. Long-term, open-label extension study of guanfacine extended release in children and adolescents with ADHD. *CNS Spectr.* 2008;13(12):1047–1055
57. Crabtree VM, Ivanenko A, Gozal D. Clinical and parental assessment of sleep in children with attention-deficit/hyperactivity disorder referred to a pediatric sleep medicine center. *Clin Pediatr (Phila).* 2003;42(9):807–813
58. LeBourgeois MK, Avis K, Mixon M, Olmi J, Harsh J. Snoring, sleep quality, and sleepiness across attention-deficit/hyperactivity disorder subtypes. *Sleep.* 2004;27(3):520–525
59. Chan E, Zhan C, Homer CJ. Health care use and costs for children with attention-deficit/hyperactivity disorder: national estimates from the Medical Expenditure Panel Survey. *Arch Pediatr Adolesc Med.* 2002;156(5):504–511
60. Newcorn JH, Miller SR, Ivanova I, et al. Adolescent outcome of ADHD: impact of childhood conduct and anxiety disorders. *CNS Spectr.* 2004;9(9): 668–678
61. Sung V, Hiscock H, Sciberras E, Efron D. Sleep problems in children with attention-deficit/hyperactivity disorder: prevalence and the effect on the child and family. *Arch Pediatr Adolesc Med.* 2008;162(4):336–342
62. Froehlich TE, Fogler J, Barbaresi WJ, Elsayed NA, Evans SW, Chan E. Using ADHD medications to treat coexisting ADHD and reading disorders: a systematic review. *Clin Pharmacol Ther.* 2018;104(4):619–637
63. Rothenberger A, Roessner V. The phenomenology of attention-deficit/hyperactivity disorder in tourette syndrome. In: Martino D, Leckman JF, eds. *Tourette Syndrome.* New York, NY: Oxford University Press; 2013:26–49
64. Antshel KM, Zhang-James Y, Faraone SV. The comorbidity of ADHD and autism spectrum disorder. *Expert Rev Neurother.* 2013;13(10):1117–1128
65. Mahajan R, Bernal MP, Panzer R, et al; Autism Speaks Autism Treatment Network Psychopharmacology Committee. Clinical practice pathways for evaluation and medication choice for attention-deficit/hyperactivity disorder symptoms in autism spectrum disorders. *Pediatrics.* 2012;130(suppl 2):S125–S138
66. Larson K, Russ SA, Kahn RS, Halfon N. Patterns of comorbidity, functioning, and service use for US children with ADHD, 2007. *Pediatrics.* 2011;127(3): 462–470
67. Society for Developmental and Behavioral Pediatrics. ADHD special interest group. Available at: www.sdbp.org/committees/sig-adhd.cfm. Accessed September 8, 2019
68. Medical Home Initiatives for Children With Special Needs Project Advisory Committee. American Academy of Pediatrics. The medical home. *Pediatrics.* 2002;110(1 pt 1):184–186
69. Brito A, Grant R, Overholt S, et al. The enhanced medical home: the pediatric standard of care for medically underserved children. *Adv Pediatr.* 2008;55:9–28
70. Sibley MH, Swanson JM, Arnold LE, et al; MTA Cooperative Group. Defining ADHD symptom persistence in adulthood: optimizing sensitivity and specificity. *J Child Psychol Psychiatry.* 2017;58(6): 655–662
71. Chang Z, D'Onofrio BM, Quinn PD, Lichtenstein P, Larsson H. Medication for attention-deficit/hyperactivity disorder and risk for depression: a nationwide longitudinal cohort study. *Biol Psychiatry.* 2016;80(12):916–922
72. Biederman J, Monuteaux MC, Spencer T, Wilens TE, Faraone SV. Do stimulants protect against psychiatric disorders in youth with ADHD? A 10-year follow-up study. *Pediatrics.* 2009;124(1):71–78
73. Barbaresi WJ, Katusic SK, Colligan RC, Weaver AL, Jacobsen SJ. Modifiers of long-term school outcomes for children with attention-deficit/hyperactivity disorder: does treatment with

stimulant medication make a difference? Results from a population-based study. *J Dev Behav Pediatr.* 2007; 28(4):274–287

74. Scheffler RM, Brown TT, Fulton BD, Hinshaw SP, Levine P, Stone S. Positive association between attention-deficit/hyperactivity disorder medication use and academic achievement during elementary school. *Pediatrics.* 2009; 123(5):1273–1279

75. Barbaresi WJ, Colligan RC, Weaver AL, Voigt RG, Killian JM, Katusic SK. Mortality, ADHD, and psychosocial adversity in adults with childhood ADHD: a prospective study. *Pediatrics.* 2013;131(4):637–644

76. Chang Z, Lichtenstein P, Långström N, Larsson H, Fazel S. Association between prescription of major psychotropic medications and violent reoffending after prison release. *JAMA.* 2016; 316(17):1798–1807

77. Lichtenstein P, Halldner L, Zetterqvist J, et al. Medication for attention deficit-hyperactivity disorder and criminality. *N Engl J Med.* 2012;367(21):2006–2014

78. Chang Z, Quinn PD, Hur K, et al. Association between medication use for attention-deficit/hyperactivity disorder and risk of motor vehicle crashes. *JAMA Psychiatry.* 2017;74(6):597–603

79. Chang Z, Lichtenstein P, D'Onofrio BM, Sjölander A, Larsson H. Serious transport accidents in adults with attention-deficit/hyperactivity disorder and the effect of medication: a population-based study. *JAMA Psychiatry.* 2014;71(3):319–325

80. Harstad E, Levy S; Committee on Substance Abuse. Attention-deficit/hyperactivity disorder and substance abuse. *Pediatrics.* 2014;134(1). Available at: www.pediatrics.org/cgi/content/full/134/1/e293

81. Dalsgaard S, Leckman JF, Mortensen PB, Nielsen HS, Simonsen M. Effect of drugs on the risk of injuries in children with attention deficit hyperactivity disorder: a prospective cohort study. *Lancet Psychiatry.* 2015;2(8):702–709

82. Raman SR, Marshall SW, Haynes K, Gaynes BN, Naftel AJ, Stürmer T. Stimulant treatment and injury among children with attention deficit hyperactivity disorder: an application of the self-controlled case series study design. *Inj Prev.* 2013;19(3):164–170

83. Greenhill L, Kollins S, Abikoff H, et al. Efficacy and safety of immediate-release methylphenidate treatment for preschoolers with ADHD. *J Am Acad Child Adolesc Psychiatry.* 2006;45(11): 1284–1293

84. Children and Adults with Attention-Deficit/Hyperactivity Disorder. CHADD. Available at: www.chadd.org. Accessed September 8, 2019

85. Sonuga-Barke EJ, Daley D, Thompson M, Laver-Bradbury C, Weeks A. Parent-based therapies for preschool attention-deficit/hyperactivity disorder: a randomized, controlled trial with a community sample. *J Am Acad Child Adolesc Psychiatry.* 2001;40(4):402–408

86. Van Cleave J, Leslie LK. Approaching ADHD as a chronic condition: implications for long-term adherence. *J Psychosoc Nurs Ment Health Serv.* 2008;46(8):28–37

87. Webster-Stratton CH, Reid MJ, Beauchaine T. Combining parent and child training for young children with ADHD. *J Clin Child Adolesc Psychol.* 2011;40(2):191–203

88. Shepard SA, Dickstein S. Preventive intervention for early childhood behavioral problems: an ecological perspective. *Child Adolesc Psychiatr Clin N Am.* 2009;18(3):687–706

89. Evans SW, Langberg JM, Egan T, Molitor SJ. Middle school-based and high school-based interventions for adolescents with ADHD. *Child Adolesc Psychiatr Clin N Am.* 2014;23(4):699–715

90. McGough JJ, Sturm A, Cowen J, et al. Double-blind, sham-controlled, pilot study of trigeminal nerve stimulation for attention-deficit/hyperactivity disorder. *J Am Acad Child Adolesc Psychiatry.* 2019;58(4):403–411.e3

91. Robin AL, Foster SL. *The Guilford Family Therapy Series. Negotiating Parent–Adolescent Conflict: A Behavioral–Family Systems Approach.* New York, NY: Guilford Press; 1989

92. Barkley RA, Guevremont DC, Anastopoulos AD, Fletcher KE. A comparison of three family therapy programs for treating family conflicts in adolescents with attention-deficit hyperactivity disorder. *J Consult Clin Psychol.* 1992;60(3):450–462

93. Fabiano GA, Schatz NK, Morris KL, et al. Efficacy of a family-focused intervention for young drivers with attention-deficit hyperactivity disorder. *J Consult Clin Psychol.* 2016;84(12):1078–1093

94. Sibley MH, Graziano PA, Kuriyan AB, et al. Parent-teen behavior therapy + motivational interviewing for adolescents with ADHD. *J Consult Clin Psychol.* 2016;84(8):699–712

95. Evans SW, Langberg JM, Schultz BK, et al. Evaluation of a school-based treatment program for young adolescents with ADHD. *J Consult Clin Psychol.* 2016;84(1):15–30

96. Langberg JM, Dvorsky MR, Molitor SJ, et al. Overcoming the research-to-practice gap: a randomized trial with two brief homework and organization interventions for students with ADHD as implemented by school mental health providers. *J Consult Clin Psychol.* 2018; 86(1):39–55

97. Schultz BK, Evans SW, Langberg JM, Schoemann AM. Outcomes for adolescents who comply with long-term psychosocial treatment for ADHD. *J Consult Clin Psychol.* 2017;85(3): 250–261

98. Newcorn JH, Kratochvil CJ, Allen AJ, et al; Atomoxetine/Methylphenidate Comparative Study Group. Atomoxetine and osmotically released methylphenidate for the treatment of attention deficit hyperactivity disorder: acute comparison and differential response. *Am J Psychiatry.* 2008;165(6): 721–730

99. Cheng JY, Chen RY, Ko JS, Ng EM. Efficacy and safety of atomoxetine for attention-deficit/hyperactivity disorder in children and adolescents-meta-analysis and meta-regression analysis. *Psychopharmacology (Berl).* 2007; 194(2):197–209

100. Michelson D, Allen AJ, Busner J, et al. Once-daily atomoxetine treatment for children and adolescents with attention deficit hyperactivity disorder: a randomized, placebo-controlled study. *Am J Psychiatry.* 2002;159(11): 1896–1901

101. Biederman J, Melmed RD, Patel A, et al; SPD503 Study Group. A randomized,

double-blind, placebo-controlled study of guanfacine extended release in children and adolescents with attention-deficit/hyperactivity disorder. *Pediatrics*. 2008;121(1). Available at: www.pediatrics.org/cgi/content/full/121/1/e73

102. Sallee FR, Lyne A, Wigal T, McGough JJ. Long-term safety and efficacy of guanfacine extended release in children and adolescents with attention-deficit/hyperactivity disorder. *J Child Adolesc Psychopharmacol*. 2009;19(3):215–226

103. Jain R, Segal S, Kollins SH, Khayrallah M. Clonidine extended-release tablets for pediatric patients with attention-deficit/hyperactivity disorder. *J Am Acad Child Adolesc Psychiatry*. 2011;50(2):171–179

104. Brown JT, Bishop JR. Atomoxetine pharmacogenetics: associations with pharmacokinetics, treatment response and tolerability. *Pharmacogenomics*. 2015;16(13):1513–1520

105. Kambeitz J, Romanos M, Ettinger U. Meta-analysis of the association between dopamine transporter genotype and response to methylphenidate treatment in ADHD. *Pharmacogenomics J*. 2014;14(1):77–84

106. Bruxel EM, Akutagava-Martins GC, Salatino-Oliveira A, et al. ADHD pharmacogenetics across the life cycle: new findings and perspectives. *Am J Med Genet B Neuropsychiatr Genet*. 2014;165B(4):263–282

107. Kieling C, Genro JP, Hutz MH, Rohde LA. A current update on ADHD pharmacogenomics. *Pharmacogenomics*. 2010;11(3):407–419

108. Froehlich TE, McGough JJ, Stein MA. Progress and promise of attention-deficit hyperactivity disorder pharmacogenetics. *CNS Drugs*. 2010;24(2):99–117

109. Joensen B, Meyer M, Aagaard L. Specific genes associated with adverse events of methylphenidate use in the pediatric population: a systematic literature review. *J Res Pharm Pract*. 2017;6(2):65–72

110. Swanson JM, Elliott GR, Greenhill LL, et al. Effects of stimulant medication on growth rates across 3 years in the MTA follow-up. *J Am Acad Child Adolesc Psychiatry*. 2007;46(8):1015–1027

111. Mosholder AD, Gelperin K, Hammad TA, Phelan K, Johann-Liang R. Hallucinations and other psychotic symptoms associated with the use of attention-deficit/hyperactivity disorder drugs in children. *Pediatrics*. 2009;123(2):611–616

112. Cortese S, Holtmann M, Banaschewski T, et al; European ADHD Guidelines Group. Practitioner review: current best practice in the management of adverse events during treatment with ADHD medications in children and adolescents. *J Child Psychol Psychiatry*. 2013;54(3):227–246

113. Avigan M. *Review of AERS Data From Marketed Safety Experience During Stimulant Therapy: Death, Sudden Death, Cardiovascular SAEs (Including Stroke). Report No. D030403*. Silver Spring, MD: Food and Drug Administration, Center for Drug Evaluation and Research; 2004

114. Perrin JM, Friedman RA, Knilans TK; Black Box Working Group; Section on Cardiology and Cardiac Surgery. Cardiovascular monitoring and stimulant drugs for attention-deficit/hyperactivity disorder. *Pediatrics*. 2008;122(2):451–453

115. McCarthy S, Cranswick N, Potts L, Taylor E, Wong IC. Mortality associated with attention-deficit hyperactivity disorder (ADHD) drug treatment: a retrospective cohort study of children, adolescents and young adults using the general practice research database. *Drug Saf*. 2009;32(11):1089–1096

116. Gould MS, Walsh BT, Munfakh JL, et al. Sudden death and use of stimulant medications in youths. *Am J Psychiatry*. 2009;166(9):992–1001

117. Cooper WO, Habel LA, Sox CM, et al. ADHD drugs and serious cardiovascular events in children and young adults. *N Engl J Med*. 2011;365(20):1896–1904

118. Schelleman H, Bilker WB, Strom BL, et al. Cardiovascular events and death in children exposed and unexposed to ADHD agents. *Pediatrics*. 2011;127(6):1102–1110

119. Garnock-Jones KP, Keating GM. Atomoxetine: a review of its use in attention-deficit hyperactivity disorder in children and adolescents. *Paediatr Drugs*. 2009;11(3):203–226

120. Reed VA, Buitelaar JK, Anand E, et al. The safety of atomoxetine for the treatment of children and adolescents with attention-deficit/hyperactivity disorder: a comprehensive review of over a decade of research. *CNS Drugs*. 2016;30(7):603–628

121. Bangs ME, Tauscher-Wisniewski S, Polzer J, et al. Meta-analysis of suicide-related behavior events in patients treated with atomoxetine. *J Am Acad Child Adolesc Psychiatry*. 2008;47(2):209–218

122. Bangs ME, Jin L, Zhang S, et al. Hepatic events associated with atomoxetine treatment for attention-deficit hyperactivity disorder. *Drug Saf*. 2008;31(4):345–354

123. Spencer TJ, Kratochvil CJ, Sangal RB, et al. Effects of atomoxetine on growth in children with attention-deficit/hyperactivity disorder following up to five years of treatment. *J Child Adolesc Psychopharmacol*. 2007;17(5):689–700

124. Elbe D, Reddy D. Focus on guanfacine extended-release: a review of its use in child and adolescent psychiatry. *J Can Acad Child Adolesc Psychiatry*. 2014;23(1):48–60

125. Croxtall JD. Clonidine extended-release: in attention-deficit hyperactivity disorder. *Paediatr Drugs*. 2011;13(5):329–336

126. Vaughan B, Kratochvil CJ. Pharmacotherapy of pediatric attention-deficit/hyperactivity disorder. *Child Adolesc Psychiatr Clin N Am*. 2012;21(4):941–955

127. Hirota T, Schwartz S, Correll CU. Alpha-2 agonists for attention-deficit/hyperactivity disorder in youth: a systematic review and meta-analysis of monotherapy and add-on trials to stimulant therapy. *J Am Acad Child Adolesc Psychiatry*. 2014;53(2):153–173

128. Treuer T, Gau SS, Méndez L, et al. A systematic review of combination therapy with stimulants and atomoxetine for attention-deficit/hyperactivity disorder, including patient characteristics, treatment strategies, effectiveness, and tolerability. *J Child Adolesc Psychopharmacol*. 2013;23(3):179–193

129. Greenhill LL, Posner K, Vaughan BS, Kratochvil CJ. Attention deficit hyperactivity disorder in preschool children. *Child Adolesc Psychiatr Clin N Am.* 2008;17(2):347–366, ix

130. Wilens TE, Spencer TJ. Understanding attention-deficit/hyperactivity disorder from childhood to adulthood. *Postgrad Med.* 2010;122(5):97–109

131. Foy JM, ed. Psychotropic medications in primary care. In: *Mental Health Care of Children and Adolescents: A Guide for Primary Care Clinicians.* Itasca, IL: American Academy of Pediatrics; 2018: 315–374

132. Wilens TE, Adler LA, Adams J, et al. Misuse and diversion of stimulants prescribed for ADHD: a systematic review of the literature. *J Am Acad Child Adolesc Psychiatry.* 2008;47(1): 21–31

133. American Academy of Pediatrics. Mental health initiatives. Available at: https://www.aap.org/en-us/advocacy-and-policy/aap-health-initiatives/Mental-Health/Pages/default.aspx. Accessed September 8, 2019

134. Levy S, Campbell MD, Shea CL, DuPont R. Trends in abstaining from substance use in adolescents: 1975-2014. *Pediatrics.* 2018;142(2):e20173498

135. Graff Low K, Gendaszek AE. Illicit use of psychostimulants among college students: a preliminary study. *Psychol Health Med.* 2002;7(3):283–287

136. Barkley RA, Cox D. A review of driving risks and impairments associated with attention-deficit/hyperactivity disorder and the effects of stimulant medication on driving performance. *J Safety Res.* 2007;38(1):113–128

137. Jerome L, Habinski L, Segal A. Attention-deficit/hyperactivity disorder (ADHD) and driving risk: a review of the literature and a methodological critique. *Curr Psychiatry Rep.* 2006;8(5): 416–426

138. Cox DJ, Merkel RL, Moore M, Thorndike F, Muller C, Kovatchev B. Relative benefits of stimulant therapy with OROS methylphenidate versus mixed amphetamine salts extended release in improving the driving performance of adolescent drivers with attention-deficit/hyperactivity disorder. *Pediatrics.* 2006;118(3). Available at: www.pediatrics.org/cgi/content/full/118/3/e704

139. The MTA Cooperative Group; Multimodal Treatment Study of Children with ADHD. A 14-month randomized clinical trial of treatment strategies for attention-deficit/hyperactivity disorder. *Arch Gen Psychiatry.* 1999;56(12):1073–1086

140. Jensen PS, Hinshaw SP, Swanson JM, et al. Findings from the NIMH Multimodal Treatment Study of ADHD (MTA): implications and applications for primary care providers. *J Dev Behav Pediatr.* 2001;22(1):60–73

141. Pelham WE Jr, Gnagy EM. Psychosocial and combined treatments for ADHD. *Ment Retard Dev Disabil Res Rev.* 1999; 5(3):225–236

142. Homer CJ, Klatka K, Romm D, et al. A review of the evidence for the medical home for children with special health care needs. *Pediatrics.* 2008;122(4). Available at: www.pediatrics.org/cgi/content/full/122/4/e922

143. Davila RR, Williams ML, MacDonald JT. Memorandum on clarification of policy to address the needs of children with attention deficit disorders within general and/or special education. In: Parker HC, ed. *The ADD Hyperactivity Handbook for Schools.* Plantation, FL: Impact Publications Inc; 1991:261–268

144. Harrison JR, Bunford N, Evans SW, Owens JS. Educational accommodations for students with behavioral challenges: a systematic review of the literature. *Rev Educ Res.* 2013;83(4): 551–597

145. Committee on Pediatric Workforce. Enhancing pediatric workforce diversity and providing culturally effective pediatric care: implications for practice, education, and policy making. *Pediatrics.* 2013;132(4). Available at: www.pediatrics.org/cgi/content/full/132/4/e1105

146. Berman RS, Patel MR, Belamarich PF, Gross RS. Screening for poverty and poverty-related social determinants of health. *Pediatr Rev.* 2018;39(5):235–246

147. Solanto MV. Neuropsychopharmacological mechanisms of stimulant drug action in attention-deficit hyperactivity disorder: a review and integration. *Behav Brain Res.* 1998;94(1):127–152

148. Wagner E. Chronic disease management: what will it take to improve care for chronic illness? *Effect Clin Pract.* 1998;1(1):2–4

149. Brinkman WB, Sucharew H, Majcher JH, Epstein JN. Predictors of medication continuity in children with ADHD. *Pediatrics.* 2018;141(6):e20172580

150. Pliszka SR, Crismon ML, Hughes CW, et al; Texas Consensus Conference Panel on Pharmacotherapy of Childhood Attention Deficit Hyperactivity Disorder. The Texas Children's Medication Algorithm Project: revision of the algorithm for pharmacotherapy of attention-deficit/hyperactivity disorder. *J Am Acad Child Adolesc Psychiatry.* 2006;45(6):642–657

151. Pringsheim T, Hirsch L, Gardner D, Gorman DA. The pharmacological management of oppositional behaviour, conduct problems, and aggression in children and adolescents with attention-deficit hyperactivity disorder, oppositional defiant disorder, and conduct disorder: a systematic review and meta-analysis. Part 1: psychostimulants, alpha-2 agonists, and atomoxetine. *Can J Psychiatry.* 2015; 60(2):42–51

152. Committee on Psychosocial Aspects of Child and Family Health and Task Force on Mental Health. Policy statement--The future of pediatrics: mental health competencies for pediatric primary care. *Pediatrics.* 2009;124(1):410–421

153. Foy JM, ed. Algorithm: a process for integrating mental health care into pediatric practice. In: *Mental Health Care of Children and Adolescents: A Guide for Primary Care Clinicians.* Itasca, IL: American Academy of Pediatrics; 2018:815

154. Cheng TL, Emmanuel MA, Levy DJ, Jenkins RR. Child health disparities: what can a clinician do? *Pediatrics.* 2015;136(5):961–968

155. Stein F, Remley K, Laraque-Arena D, Pursley DM. New resources and strategies to advance the AAP's values of diversity, inclusion, and health equity. *Pediatrics.* 2018;141(4):e20180177

156. American Academy of Pediatrics, Committee on Child Health Financing. Scope of health care benefits for children from birth through age 26. *Pediatrics.* 2012;129(1):185–189

Supplemental Information

ALGORITHM

IMPLEMENTING THE KEY ACTION STATEMENTS OF THE AAP ADHD CLINICAL PRACTICE GUIDELINES: AN ALGORITHM AND EXPLANATION FOR PROCESS OF CARE FOR THE EVALUATION, DIAGNOSIS, TREATMENT, AND MONITORING OF ADHD IN CHILDREN AND ADOLESCENTS

I. INTRODUCTION

Practice guidelines provide a broad outline of the requirements for high-quality, evidence-based care. The AAP "Clinical Practice Guideline: Diagnosis and Evaluation of the Child With Attention-Deficit/Hyperactivity Disorder" provides the evidence-based processes for caring for children and adolescents with ADHD symptoms or diagnosis. This document supplements that guideline. It provides a PoCA that details processes to implement the guidelines; describes procedures for the evaluation, treatment, and monitoring of children and adolescents with ADHD; and addresses practical issues related to the provision of ADHD-related care within a typical, busy pediatric practice. The algorithm is entirely congruent with the guidelines and is based on the practical experience and expert advice of clinicians who are experienced in the diagnosis and management of children and adolescents with ADHD. Unlike the guidelines, this algorithm is based primarily on expert opinion and has a less robust evidence base because of the lack of clinical studies specifically addressing this approach. Understanding that providing appropriate care to children with ADHD in a primary care setting faces a number of challenges and barriers, the subcommittee has also provided an additional article describing needed changes to address barriers to care (found in the Supplemental Information).

In this algorithm, we describe a continuous process; as such, its constituent steps are not intended to be completed in a single office visit or in a specific number of visits. Evaluation, treatment, and monitoring are ongoing processes to be addressed throughout the child's and adolescent's care within the practice and in transition planning as the adolescent moves into the adult care system. Many factors will influence the pace of the process, including the experience of the PCC, the practice's volume, the longevity of the relationship between the PCC and family, the severity of concerns, the availability of academic records and school input, the family's schedule, and the payment structure.

An awareness of the AAP "Primary Care Approach to Mental Health Care Algorithm," which is available on the AAP Mental Health Initiatives Web site, will enhance the integration of the procedures described in this document (http://www.aap.org/mentalhealth). That algorithm describes the process to integrate an initial psychosocial assessment at well visits and a brief mental health update at acute and chronic care visits. Mental health concerns, including symptoms of inattention and impulsivity, may present when (1) elicited during the initial psychosocial assessment at a routine well visit, (2) elicited during a brief mental health update at an acute or chronic visit, or (3) presented during a visit triggered by a family or school concern.

When concerns are identified, the algorithm describes the process of conducting a brief primary care intervention, secondary screening, diagnostic assessment, treatment, and follow-up. Like this document, the mental health algorithm is intended to present a process that may involve more than 1 visit and may be completed over time.

This algorithm assumes that the primary care practice has adopted the initial psychosocial assessment and mental health update, as described by the AAP Mental Health Initiatives.[153] It begins with steps paralleling the secondary assessment of the general mental health algorithm. Both algorithms focus on the care team and include the family as a part of that team.

In light of the prevalence of ADHD, the severe consequences of untreated ADHD, and the availability of effective ADHD treatments, the AAP recommends that every child and adolescent identified with signs or symptoms suggestive of ADHD be evaluated for ADHD or other conditions that may share its symptomatology. Documenting all aspects of the diagnostic and treatment procedures in the patient's records will improve the ability of the

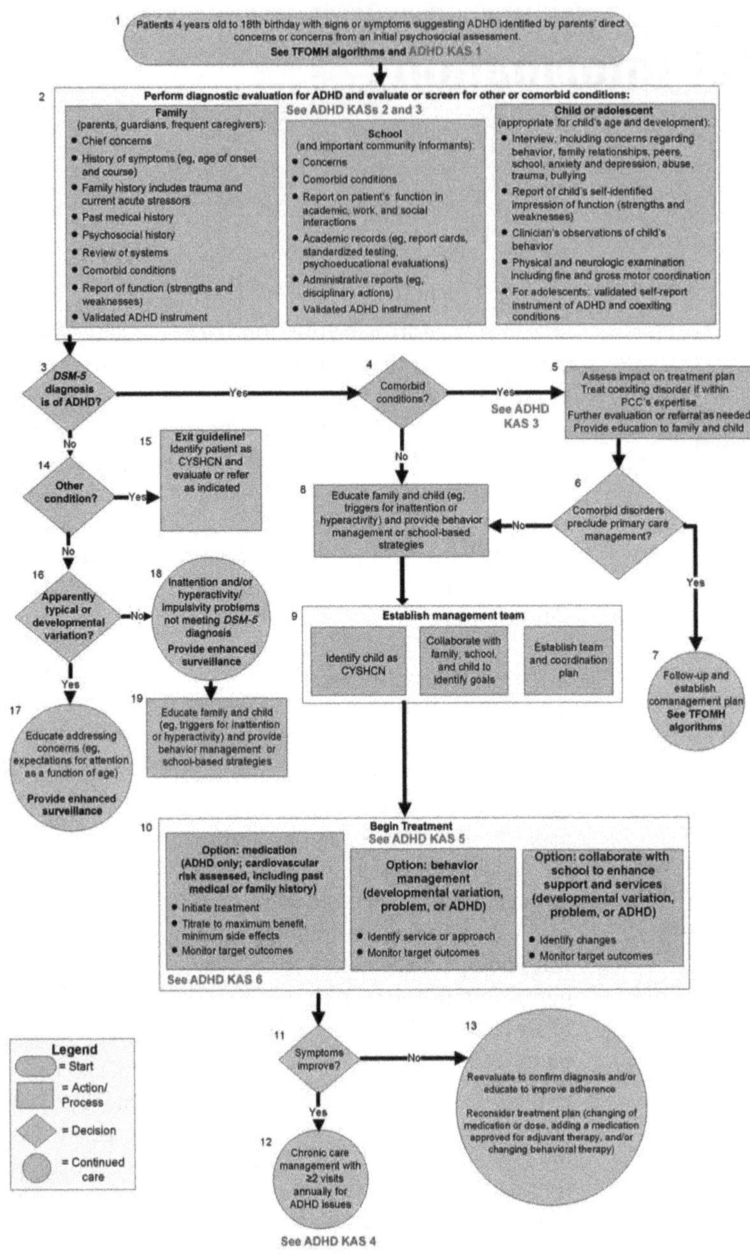

SUPPLEMENTAL FIGURE 2

ADHD care algorithm. CYSHCN, children and youth with special health care needs; TFOMH, Task Force on Mental Health.

pediatrician to best treat children with ADHD.

II. EVALUATION FOR ADHD

II a. A Child or Adolescent Presents With Signs and Symptoms Suggesting ADHD

The algorithm's steps can be implemented when a child or adolescent presents to a PCC for an assessment for ADHD. This may occur in a variety of ways.

Pediatricians and other PCCs traditionally have long-standing relationships with the child and family, which foster the opportunity to identify concerns early on. The young child may have a history of known ADHD risks, such as having parents who have been diagnosed with ADHD or having extremely low birth weight. In those instances, the PCC would monitor for emerging issues.

Many parents bring their child or adolescent to the PCC with specific concerns about the child's or adolescent's ability to sustain attention, curb activity levels, and/or inhibit impulsivity at home, school, or in the community. In many instances, the parents may express concerns about behaviors and characteristics

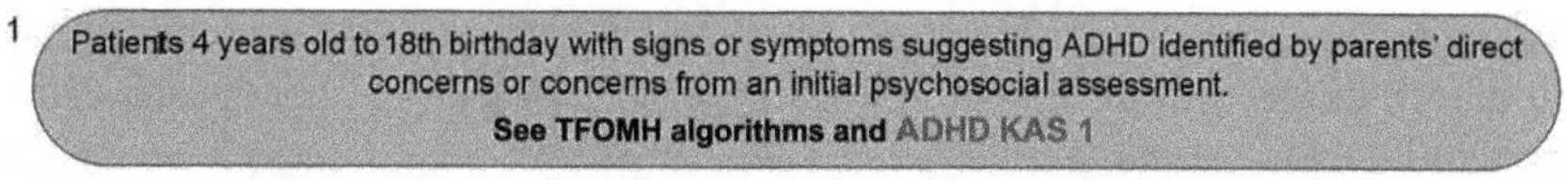

1 Patients 4 years old to 18th birthday with signs or symptoms suggesting ADHD identified by parents' direct concerns or concerns from an initial psychosocial assessment.
See TFOMH algorithms and ADHD KAS 1

SUPPLEMENTAL FIGURE 3
Evaluate for ADHD. TFOMH, Task Force on Mental Health.

that are associated with ADHD but may not mention the core ADHD symptoms. For example, parents may report that their child is getting poor grades, does not perform well in team sports (despite being athletic), has few friends, or is moody and quick to anger. These children and adolescents may have difficulty remaining organized; planning activities; or inhibiting their initial thoughts, actions, or emotions, which are behaviors that fall under the umbrella of executive functioning (ie, planning, prioritizing, and producing) or cognitive control. Problems with executive functions may be correlated with ADHD and are common among children and adolescents with ADHD. As recommended by Bright Futures (a national health promotion and prevention initiative led by the AAP[157]), routine psychosocial screening at preventive visits may identify concerns on the part of parent or another clinician (see below for more information on co-occurring conditions.)

Finally, parents may bring a child to a PCC for ADHD evaluation on the basis of the recommendation of a teacher, tutor, coach, etc.

(See the ADHD guideline's KAS 1.)

II b. Perform a Diagnostic Evaluation for ADHD and Evaluate or Screen for Comorbid Disorders

When a child or adolescent presents with concerns about ADHD, as described above, the clinician should initiate an evaluation for ADHD. (See the ADHD guideline's KASs 2 and 3.)

II c. Gather Information From the Family

As noted previously, the recommendations in the accompanying guideline are intended to be integrated with the broader mental health algorithm developed as part of the AAP Mental Health Initiatives.[2,133,153] It is also important for pediatricians and other PCCs to be aware of health disparities and social determinants that may affect patient outcomes and to provide culturally appropriate care to all children and adolescents in their practice, including during the initial evaluation and assessment of the patient's condition.[145,146,154,155,158]

Ideally, the PCC's office staff obtains information from the family about the visit's purpose at scheduling so that an extended visit or multiple visits can be made available for the initial ADHD evaluation. This also increases the efficiency of an initial evaluation. Data on the child's or adolescent's symptoms and functioning can be gathered from parents, school personnel, and other sources before the visit. Parents can be given rating scales that are to be completed before the visit by teachers, coaches, and others who interact with the child. This strategy allows the PCC to focus on the most pertinent issues for that child or adolescent and family at the time of the visit. (See later discussion for more information on rating scales.) Note that schools will not release data to pediatric providers without written parental consent.

During the office evaluation session, the PCC reviews the patient's medical, family, and psychosocial history. Developmental history is presumed to be part of the patient's medical

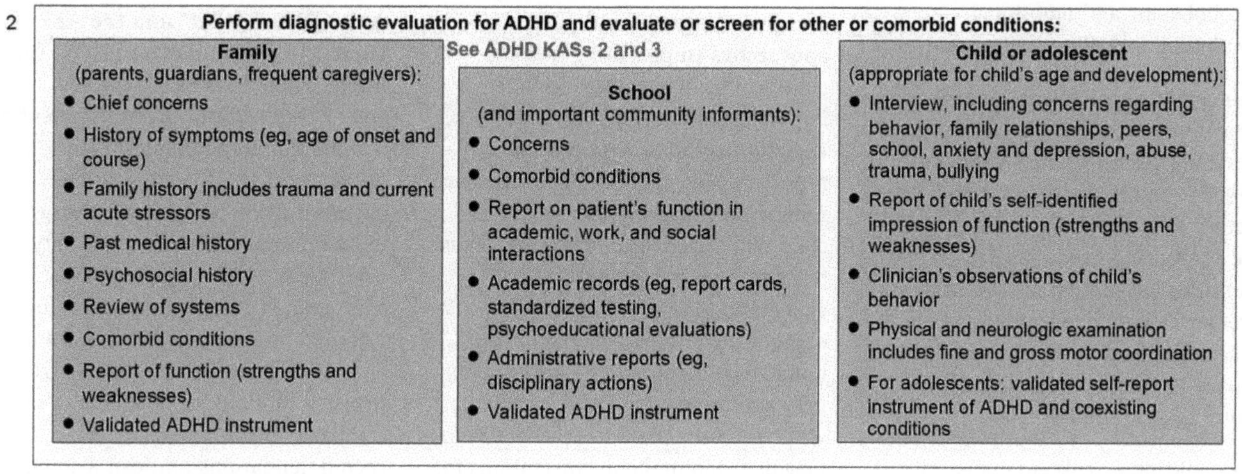

2 **Perform diagnostic evaluation for ADHD and evaluate or screen for other or comorbid conditions:**
See ADHD KASs 2 and 3

Family
(parents, guardians, frequent caregivers):
- Chief concerns
- History of symptoms (eg, age of onset and course)
- Family history includes trauma and current acute stressors
- Past medical history
- Psychosocial history
- Review of systems
- Comorbid conditions
- Report of function (strengths and weaknesses)
- Validated ADHD instrument

School
(and important community informants):
- Concerns
- Comorbid conditions
- Report on patient's function in academic, work, and social interactions
- Academic records (eg, report cards, standardized testing, psychoeducational evaluations)
- Administrative reports (eg, disciplinary actions)
- Validated ADHD instrument

Child or adolescent
(appropriate for child's age and development):
- Interview, including concerns regarding behavior, family relationships, peers, school, anxiety and depression, abuse, trauma, bullying
- Report of child's self-identified impression of function (strengths and weaknesses)
- Clinician's observations of child's behavior
- Physical and neurologic examination includes fine and gross motor coordination
- For adolescents: validated self-report instrument of ADHD and coexisting conditions

SUPPLEMENTAL FIGURE 4
Perform a diagnostic evaluation for ADHD and evaluate or screen for comorbid disorders

history. Family members (including parents, guardians, and other frequent caregivers) are asked to identify their chief concerns and provide a history of the onset, frequency, and duration of problem behaviors, situations that increase or decrease the problems, previous treatments and their results, and the caregivers' understanding of the issues. It is important to assess behaviors and conditions that are frequent side effects of stimulant medication (ie, sleep difficulties, tics, nail-biting, skin-picking, headaches, stomachaches, or afternoon irritability) and preexisting conditions, so they are not confused with the frequent side effects of stimulants. This enables the PCC to compare changes if medication is initiated later.

A sound assessment of symptoms and functioning in major areas can be used to construct an educational and behavioral profile that includes the child's strengths and talents. Many children with ADHD exhibit enthusiasm, exuberance, creativity, flexibility, the ability to detect and quickly respond to subtle changes in the environment, a sense of humor, a desire to please, etc. The most common areas of functioning affected by ADHD include academic achievement; relationships with peers, parents, siblings, and adult authority figures; participation in recreational activities, such as sports; and behavior and emotional regulation, including risky behavior.

The child's and family's histories can provide information about the status of symptoms and functioning and help determine age of onset and other factors that may be associated with the presenting problems. It also identifies any potential traumatic events that the child may have experienced, such as a family death, separation from the family, or physical or mental abuse.

The child or adolescent's medical history can help identify factors associated with ADHD, such as prenatal and perinatal complications and exposures (eg, preterm delivery, maternal hypertension, prenatal alcohol exposure), childhood exposures, and head trauma.

The family history includes any medical syndromes, developmental delays, cognitive limitations, learning disabilities, trauma or toxic stress, or mental illness in the patient and family members, including ADHD, mood, anxiety, and bipolar disorders. Ask what the family has already tried, what works, and what does not work to avoid wasting time on interventions that have already been attempted unsuccessfully. Parental tobacco and substance use, including their use prenatally, are relevant risk factors for, and correlate with, ADHD.[159] ADHD is highly heritable and is often seen in other family members who may or may not have been formally diagnosed with ADHD. For this reason, asking about family members' school experience, including time and task management, grades, and highest grade level achieved, can aid in treatment decisions.

The psychosocial history is important in any ADHD evaluation and usually includes queries about environmental factors, such as family stress and problematic relationships, which sometime contribute to the child or adolescent's overall functioning. The caregivers' current and past approaches to parenting and the child's misbehavior can provide important information that may explain discrepancies between reporters. For example, parents may reduce their expectations for their child with ADHD as a means to relieve parenting stress. When these expectations are reduced (eg, eliminating chores, not monitoring homework completion, etc), parents may experience far fewer problems with the child than do teachers who may have maintained expectations for the child to complete tasks and follow rules. Knowing the parents' approach to parenting may help the PCC understand differences in ratings completed by parents versus teachers.

Further evidence for an ADHD diagnosis includes an inability to independently complete daily routines in an age-appropriate manner as well as multiple and short-lasting friendships, trouble keeping and/or making friends, staying up late to complete assignments, and late, incomplete, and/or lost assignments. Somatic symptoms and school avoidance are more common among girls and may mask an ADHD diagnosis. With information obtained from the parents and school personnel, the PCC can make a clinical judgment about the effect of the core and associated ADHD symptoms on academic achievement, classroom performance, family and social relationships, independent functioning, and safety and/or unintentional injuries.

If other issues exist, such as self-injuries, comorbid mental health issues also need to be evaluated. Possible areas of functional impairment that require evaluation include domains such as self-perception, leisure activities, and self-care (ie, bathing, toileting, dressing, and eating). Additional guidance regarding functional assessment is available through the AAP ADHD Toolkit[2] and the AAP Mental Health Initiatives.[133,160] The ADHD Toolkit[2] is being revised concurrently with the development of these updated guidelines. After publication, the toolkit may be accessed at https://www.aap.org/en-us/professional-resources/quality-improvement/Pages/Quality-Improvement-Implementation-Guide.aspx. Additionally, a new Education in Quality Improvement for Pediatric Practice Module was developed on the basis of the new clinical recommendations and can also be accessed by using the same link above.

The patient needs to be screened for hearing and/or visual problems because these can mimic inattention. A full review of systems may reveal other symptoms or disorders, such as sleep disturbances, absence seizures, or tic disorders, which may assist in formulating a differential diagnosis and/or developing management plans. Internal feelings such as anxiety and depression can occur but may not be noticeable to parents and teachers, so it is important to elicit feedback about them from the patient as well.

The information gathered from this diagnostic interview, combined with the data from the rating scales (see below), provides an excellent foundation for determining the presence of symptoms and impairment criteria needed to diagnose ADHD.

II d. Use Parent Rating Scales and Other Tools

Rating scales that use the *DSM-5* criteria for ADHD can help obtain the information that will contribute to making a diagnosis. Rating scales for parents that use *DSM-5* criteria for ADHD are helpful in obtaining the core symptoms required to make a diagnosis on the basis of the *DSM-5*.[161] Because changes in the 18 core symptoms are essentially unchanged from *DSM-IV* criteria, *DSM-IV*–based rating scales can be used if *DSM-5* rating scales are not readily available. Some of these symptom rating scales include symptoms of commonly comorbid conditions and measures of impairment in a variety of domains that are also required for a diagnosis.[41,162] Some available measures are limited because they provide only a global rating.[163,164]

Caregiver and teacher endorsement of the requisite number of ADHD symptoms on the rating scales is not sufficient for diagnosis. A rating scale documents the presence of inattention, hyperactivity, and impulsivity symptoms but not whether these symptoms are actually attributable to ADHD versus a mimicking condition. Caregivers may misread or misunderstand some of the behaviors. Furthermore, rating scales do not inform the PCC about contextual influences that may account for the symptoms and impairment. Likewise, broadband rating scales that assess general mental health functioning do not provide reliable and valid indications of ADHD diagnoses, although they can help to screen for concurrent behavioral conditions.[165]

Nevertheless, parent ratings provide valuable information on their perspective of the child's symptoms and impairment and add information about normative levels of the parents' perspectives, which help the PCC determine the degree with which the problems are or are not in the typical range for the child's age and sex. Finally, broad rating scales that assess general mental health functioning do not provide sufficient information about all the ADHD core symptoms but may help screen for the concurrent behavioral conditions.[165]

To address the rating scales' limitations, pediatricians and other PCCs need to interview parents and may need to review documents such as report cards and standardized test results and historical records of detentions, suspensions, and/or expulsions from school, which can serve as evidence of functional impairment. Further evidence may include difficulty developing and maintaining lasting friendships. This information is discussed below.

II e. Gather Information From School and Community Informants

Information from parents is not the only source that informs diagnostic decisions for children and adolescents because a key criterion for an ADHD diagnosis is the display of symptoms and impairments in multiple settings. Gathering data from other adults who regularly interact with the child or adolescent being evaluated provides rich additional information for the evaluation.

The information from various sources may be inconsistent because parents and teachers observe the children at different times and under different circumstances, as described previously.[166] Disagreement may result from differences in students' behavior and performance in different classrooms, their relationship with the teachers, or variations in teachers' expectations, as well as training in or experience with behavior management. Classes with high homework demands or classes with less structure are often the most problematic for students with ADHD. Investigating these inconsistencies can lead to hypotheses about the child that help inform the eventual clinical diagnoses and treatment decisions.[167]

Teachers and Other School Personnel

Teachers and other school personnel can provide critically important information because they develop a rich sense of the typical range of behaviors within a specific age group over time. School and classrooms settings provide the greatest social and performance expectations that potentially tax children and adolescents with ADHD. Parents and older children may be the best sources for identifying the school personnel who can best complete rating scales for an ADHD evaluation.

The value of school ratings increases as children age because parents often have less detailed information about their child's behavior and performance at school as the student moves into the higher grades. With elementary and middle school children, the classroom teacher is usually the best source; he or she may be the only source necessary. Other school staff, such as a special education teacher or school counselor, may be valuable sources of information. Direct communication with a school psychologist and/or school counselor may provide additional information on the child's functioning within the context of the classroom and school.

In secondary schools, students interact with many teachers who often instruct >100 students daily. As a result, high school teachers may not know the students as well as elementary and middle school teachers do. Parents and students may be encouraged to choose the 2 or 3 teachers who they believe know the student best and solicit their input (eg, math and English teachers or, for children or adolescents with learning disabilities, a teacher in an area of strong function and a teacher in an area of weak function). Regardless of the presence of a learning disability, it is helpful to obtain feedback from the teacher of the class in which the child or adolescent is having the most difficulty. The ADHD Toolkit provides materials relevant to school data collection.

Teachers may communicate their major concerns using questionnaires or verbally in person, via secure e-mail (if available), or over the telephone. It is important to ask an appropriate school representative to complete a validated ADHD instrument or behavior scale based on the *DSM-5* criteria for ADHD. A school representative's report might include information about any comorbid or alternative conditions, including disruptive behavior disorders, depression and anxiety disorders, tics, or learning disabilities. As noted, some parent rating scales have a version for teachers and assess symptoms and impairment in multiple domains.[41] Teacher rating scales exist that specifically target behavior and performance at school,[168] which provide a comprehensive and detailed description of a student's school functioning relative to normative data.

In addition to the academic information, it is important to request information characterizing the child or adolescent's level of functioning with regard to peer, teacher, and other authority figure relationships, ability to follow directions, organizational skills, history of classroom disruption, and assignment completion.

Academic Records

In addition to ratings from teachers and other school staff, academic records are sometimes available to inform a PCC's evaluation. These records include report cards; results from reading, math, and written expression standardized tests; and other assessments of academic competencies. If a child were referred for an evaluation for special education services, his or her file is likely to contain a report on the evaluation, which can be useful during an ADHD evaluation. School records pertaining to office discipline referrals, suspensions, absences, and detentions can provide valuable information about social function and behavioral regulation. Parents often keep report cards from early grades, which can provide valuable information about age of onset for children older than 12 years. Teachers in primary grades often provide information pertaining to important information about the history of the presenting problems.

Other Community Sources

It can be helpful to obtain information not only from school professionals but also from additional sources, such as grandparents, faith-based organization group leaders, scouting leaders, sports coaches, and others. Depending on the areas in which the child or adolescent exhibits impairment, these adults may be able to provide a valuable perspective on the nature of the presenting problems, although the accuracy of their reporting has not been studied.

II f. Gather Information From the Child or Adolescent

Another source of information is from the child or adolescent. This information is often collected but carries less weight than information from other sources because of children's and adolescents' limited ability to accurately report their strengths and weaknesses, including those associated with ADHD.[169] As a result, information gathered from the child about specific ADHD behaviors may do little to inform the presence or absence of symptoms and impairments because evidence suggests that children tend to minimize their problems and blame others for concerns.[170]

Nevertheless, self-report may provide other values. First, self-report is the primary means by which one can screen for internalizing conditions such as depression and anxiety. The AAP Mental Health Initiatives[133] and the *Guidelines for Adolescent Depression in Primary Care*[171–173] recommend the use of validated diagnostic rating scales for adolescent mood and anxiety disorders for clinicians who wish to use this format.[174–178] As measures of internal mental disorders, these data are likely to be more valid than the reports of adults about their children's behaviors.

Second, youth with ADHD are prone to talk impulsively and excessively when adults show an interest in them. They may share useful information about the home or classroom that parents and teachers do not know or impart. In addition, many share their experience with risky and dangerous behaviors that may be unknown to the adults in their lives. This information can be critical in both determining a diagnosis and designing treatment.

Third, even if little information of value is obtained, the fact that the PCC takes the time to meet alone and ask questions of the child or adolescents demonstrates respect and lays the foundation for collaboration in the decision-making and treatment process to follow. This relationship building is particularly important for adolescents.

Fourth, by gaining an understanding of the child's perspective, the PCC can anticipate the likely acceptance or resistance to treatment.

Interviewing the child or adolescent provides many important benefits beyond the possibility of informing the diagnosis and warrants its inclusion in the evaluation. For example, part of this interview includes asking the child or adolescent to identify personal goals (eg, What do you want to be when you grow up? What do you think that requires? How can we help you get there?). It is helpful when children perceive the pediatrician and other PCCs as seeking to help them achieve their goals rather than arbitrarily labeling them as deficient, defective, or needing to be fixed in some way.

II g. Clinical Observations and Physical Examination of the Child or Adolescent

The physical and neurologic examination needs to be comprehensive to determine if further medical or developmental assessments are indicated. Baseline height, weight, BP, and pulse measurements are required to be recorded in the medical record. It is important to look for behaviors that are consistent with ADHD's symptoms, including the child's level of attention, activity, and impulsivity during the encounter. Yet, ADHD is context dependent, and for this reason, behaviors and core symptoms that are seen in other settings are often not observed during an office visit.[179] Although the presence of hyperactivity and inattention during an office visit may provide supporting evidence of ADHD symptoms, their absence is not considered evidence that the child does not have ADHD.

Observations of a broad range of behaviors can be important for considering their contribution to the presenting problems and the potential diagnosis of other conditions. Careful attention to these various behaviors can provide useful information when beginning the next step involving making diagnostic decisions. For example, hearing and visual acuity problems can often lead to inattention and overactivity at school. Attending to concerns about anxiety is also important given that young children may become overactive when they are in anxiety-provoking situations like a clinic visit.

In addition, observing the child's language skills is important because difficulties with language can be a symptom of a language disorder and predictor of subsequent reading problems. This observation is particularly important with young children given that language disorders may present as problems with sustaining attention and impulsivity. A language disorder may also involve pragmatic usage or the social use of language, which can contribute to social impairment. If the PCC, family, and/or school have concerns about receptive, expressive, or pragmatic language, it is important to make a referral for a formal speech and language evaluation. Dysmorphic features also need to be noted because symptoms of ADHD are similar to characteristics of children with some prenatal exposures and genetic syndromes (eg, fetal alcohol exposure,[180,181] fragile X syndrome).

Many children with ADHD have poor coordination, which may be severe enough to warrant a diagnosis of developmental coordination disorder and referral to occupational and/or physical therapy. Findings of poor coordination can affect how well the child performs in competitive sports, a frequent source of social interactions for children, and can adversely affect the child's writing skills. Detecting any motor or verbal tics is important as well, particularly because the use of stimulant medications may cause or exacerbate tics.

Finally, it is important to evaluate the child's cardiovascular status because cardiovascular health must be considered if ADHD medication becomes an option. Cardiac illness is rare, and more evidence is required to determine if children or adolescents with ADHD are at increased risk when taking ADHD medications. Nevertheless, before initiating therapy with stimulant medications, it is important to obtain the child or adolescent's history of specific cardiac symptoms, as well as the family history of sudden death, cardiovascular symptoms, Wolff-Parkinson-White syndrome, hypertrophic cardiomyopathy, and long QT syndrome. If any of these risk factors are present, clinicians should obtain additional evaluation with an ECG and possibly consult with a pediatric cardiologist.

II h. Gather Information About Conditions That Mimic or Are Comorbid With ADHD

It is important for the PCC to obtain information about the status and history of conditions that may mimic or are comorbid with ADHD, such as depression, anxiety disorders, and posttraumatic stress disorder. Several validated rating scales are within the public domain and can help identify comorbid conditions. Examples include the Pediatric Symptom Checklist-17 as a screen for depression and anxiety[182]; the Screen for Child Anxiety Related Emotional Disorders, more specifically for anxiety disorders[176]; the Patient Health Questionnaire modified for adolescents; the Screening to Brief Intervention tool[183,184]; and the Child and Adolescent Trauma Screen for exposure to trauma.[185] All include questionnaire forms for both parents and patients.[2] The results help the PCC assess the extent to which reported impairment and/or distress are associated with ADHD versus comorbid conditions. These conditions are described in greater detail later.

Safety and Serious Mental Illness Concerns

PCCs may be asked to complete mental health or safety assessments, particularly for adolescents. Assessment requests may come from schools or other settings after a behavioral crisis, aggressive behavior, or destructive behaviors have occurred. With patient or guardian consent, information may be shared regarding diagnosis and current treatment strategies. Pediatricians and other PCCs are encouraged to exercise caution when asked to predict the likelihood of future behaviors in the absence of detailed understanding of the environment in which the behaviors occurred. Self-injurious behaviors or threats of self-harm are serious concerns that, when possible, should immediately be referred to community mental health crisis services or experienced child mental health professionals. PCCs are encouraged to provide further monitoring of the child or adolescent with these comorbidities.

III. MAKING DIAGNOSTIC DECISIONS

After gathering all of the relevant available information, the PCC will consider an ADHD diagnosis as well as a diagnosis of other related and/or comorbid disorders. The primary decision-making process involves comparing the information obtained to the *DSM-5* criteria for ADHD. Although this assessment is straightforward, there are some issues the PCC needs to consider, including development, sex, and other disorders that may fit the presenting problems better than ADHD (see below for more on these issues).

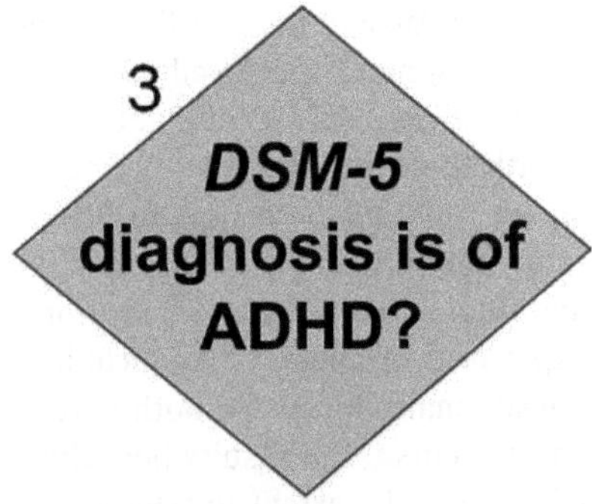

SUPPLEMENTAL FIGURE 5
Making diagnostic decisions.

III a. DSM-5 Criteria for ADHD

The *DSM-5* criteria define 4 dimensions of ADHD:

1. ADHD/I (314.00 [F90.0]);
2. ADHD/HI (314.01 [F90.1]);
3. ADHD/C (314.01 [F90.2]); and
4. ADHD other specified and unspecified ADHD (314.01 [F90.8]).

To make a diagnosis of ADHD, the PCC needs to establish that 6 or more (5 or more if the adolescent is 17 years or older) core symptoms are present in either or both of the inattention dimension and/or the hyperactivity-impulsivity dimension and occur inappropriately often. The core symptoms and dimensions are presented in Supplemental Table 2.

- ADHD/I: having at least 6 of 9 inattention behaviors and less than 6 hyperactive-impulsive behaviors;
- ADHD/HI: having at least 6 of 9 hyperactive-impulsive behaviors and less than 6 inattention behaviors;
- ADHD/C: having at least 6 of 9 behaviors in both the inattention and hyperactive-impulsive dimensions; and
- ADHD other specified and unspecified ADHD: These categories are meant for children who meet many of the criteria for ADHD, but not the full criteria, and who have significant impairment. "ADHD other specified" is used if the PCC specifies those criteria that have not been met; "unspecified ADHD" is used if the PCC does not specify these criteria.

In school-aged children and adolescents, diagnostic criteria for ADHD include documentation of the following criteria:

- At least 6 of the 9 behaviors described in the inattentive domain occur often, and to a degree, that is inconsistent with the child's developmental age. (For adolescents 17 years and older, documentation of at least 5 of the 9 behaviors is required.)
- At least 6 of the 9 behaviors described in the hyperactive-impulsive domain occur often, and to a degree, that is inconsistent with the child's developmental age. (For adolescents 17 years and older, documentation of at least 5 of the 9 behaviors is required.)
- Several inattentive or hyperactive-impulsive symptoms were present before age 12 years.
- There is clear evidence that the child's symptoms interfere with or reduce the quality of his or her social, academic, and/or occupational functioning.
- The symptoms have persisted for at least 6 months.
- The symptoms are not attributable to another physical, situational, or mental health condition.

Clear evidence exists that these criteria are appropriate for preschool-aged children (ie, age 4 years to the sixth birthday), elementary and middle school-aged children (ie, age 6 years to the 12th birthday), and adolescents (ie, age 12 years to the 18th birthday).[30,31] *DSM-5* criteria have also been updated to better describe how inattentive and hyperactive-impulsive symptoms present in older adolescents and adults.

DSM-5 criteria require evidence of symptoms before age 12 years. In some cases, however, parents and teachers may not recognize ADHD symptoms until the child is older than 12 years, when school tasks and responsibilities become more challenging and exceed the child's ability to perform effectively in school. For these children, history can often identify an earlier age of onset of some ADHD symptoms. Delayed recognition may also be seen more often in ADHD/I, which is more commonly diagnosed in girls.

If symptoms arise suddenly without previous history, the PCC needs to consider other conditions, including mood or anxiety disorders, substance use, head trauma, physical or sexual abuse, neurodegenerative disorders, sleep disorders (including sleep apnea), or a major psychological stress in the family or school (such as bullying). In adolescents and young adults, PCCs are encouraged to consider the potential for false reporting and misrepresentation of symptoms to obtain medications for other than appropriate medicinal use (ie, diversion, secondary gain). The majority of states now require prescriber participation in prescription drug monitoring programs, which can be helpful in identifying and preventing diversion activities. Pediatricians and other PCCs may consider prescribing nonstimulant medications that minimize abuse potential, such as atomoxetine and extended-release guanfacine or extended-release clonidine.

In the absence of other concerns and findings on prenatal or medical history, further diagnostic testing will not help to reach an ADHD diagnosis. Compared to clinical interviews, standardized psychological tests, such as computerized attention tests, have not been found to reliably differentiate between youth with and without ADHD.[187,188] Appropriate further assessment is indicated if an underlying etiology is suspected. Imaging studies or screening for high lead levels and abnormal thyroid hormone levels can be pursued if they are suggested by other historic or physical information, such as history or symptoms of a tumor or significant brain injury. When children experience trauma, their evaluation needs to include the consideration of both the trauma and ADHD because they can co-occur and can exacerbate ADHD symptoms. Toxic stress has shown to be associated with the incidence of pediatric ADHD, but the conclusion that ADHD is a manifestation of this stress has not been demonstrated.[188]

Patients with ADHD commonly have comorbid conditions, such as oppositional defiant disorder, anxiety, depression, and language and learning disabilities. These conditions may present with ADHD symptoms and need evaluation because their treatment may relieve symptoms. Additionally, some conditions may present with ADHD symptoms and respond to treatment of the primary condition, such as sleep disorders, absence seizures, and hyperthyroidism. (Comorbid conditions are discussed later in this document.)

In addition, the behavioral characteristics specified in the *DSM-5* remain subjective and may be interpreted differently by various observers. Rates of ADHD and its treatment have been found to be different for different racial and/or ethnic groups.[50,189] Cultural norms and the expectations of parents or teachers may influence reporting of symptoms. Hence, the clinician benefits from being sensitive to cultural differences about the appropriateness of behaviors and perceptions of mental health conditions.[145,155]

After the diagnostic evaluation, a PCC will be able to answer the following questions:

- How many inattentive and hyperactive/impulsive behavior criteria for ADHD does the child or adolescent manifest across major settings of his or her life?
- Have these criteria been present for 6 months or longer?
- Was the onset of these or similar behaviors present before the child's 12th birthday?
- What functional impairments are caused by these behaviors?
- Could any other condition be a better explanation for the behaviors?
- Is there evidence of comorbid problems or disorders?

On the basis of this information, the clinician is usually able to arrive at a preliminary diagnosis of whether the child or adolescents has ADHD or not. (For children and adolescents who do not receive an ADHD diagnosis, see below.)

III b. Developmental Considerations

Considerations About the Child or Adolescent's Age

Although the diagnostic criteria for ADHD are the same for children up to age 17 years, developmental considerations affect the interpretation of whether a symptom is present. Before school age, the primary set of distinguishing symptoms involve hyperactivity, although this can be difficult to identify as outside of the normal range given the large variability in this young age group. Similarly, difficulties sustaining attention are difficult to determine with young children because of considerable variability in presentation and the limited demands for children in this age group to sustain attention over time. (See below for more information on developmental delays.)

Some children demonstrate hyperactivity and inattention that are clearly beyond the normal range. They may experience substantial impairment to an extent that baby-sitters or child care agencies refuse to care for them, parents are unable to take them shopping or to restaurants, or they routinely engage in dangerous or risky behaviors. In these extreme cases, the PCC may be able to make the decision for an ADHD diagnosis more quickly than other scenarios that require a thorough assessment. For other young children, the diagnosis will be less obvious, and developmental and environmental issues may lead the PCC to be cautious in making an ADHD diagnosis. In these situations, monitoring for the emergence or clarification of ADHD symptoms and/or providing a diagnosis of other specified *ADHD* or unspecified *ADHD* are appropriate options.

Adolescence is another developmental period when developmental considerations are warranted. Beginning at age 17 years, there are only 5 symptoms of inattention and/or 5 symptoms of hyperactivity/impulsivity required for an ADHD diagnosis. Hyperactivity typically diminishes for most children during adolescence, but problems associated with impulsivity can be dangerous and can include impaired driving, substance use, risky sexual behavior, and suicide. Disorganization of time and resources can be associated with substantial academic problems at school. Parent-child conflict and disengagement from school can provide a context that contributes toward poor long-term outcomes. Comorbid depression and conduct disorder are common but do not negate the importance of diagnosing ADHD when the developmental path warrants it and the ADHD symptoms exacerbate problems associated with the comorbid conditions.

Adolescence is the first developmental period for which age of onset of symptoms must be documented before 12 years. School records and parent reports are often the richest source for making this determination. It is important to try to identify adolescents (or their parents) who are pursuing a diagnosis of ADHD for secondary gains such as school accommodations, standardized testing accommodations, and/or stimulant prescriptions. In addition, impairment sometimes emerges when expectations for the adolescent markedly increase or when accommodations are removed. The teenager's level of functioning may stay the same, but when faced with the expectations of advanced placement courses or a part-time job, failure to keep pace with increasing expectations may lead to concerns that warrant an evaluation for ADHD. These examples emphasize the importance of determining an early age of onset.

Considerations About the Child or Adolescent's Sex

ADHD is diagnosed in boys about twice as often as it is diagnosed in girls. There are many hypotheses about reasons for this difference; the primary reason appears to simply be that the disorder is more common in boys than girls. Some have raised concerns that the difference may be attributable to variances in society's expectations for boys versus girls or underdiagnosis in girls, but these reasons are unlikely to account for the large difference in diagnoses. Hence, no adjustment is needed in terms of the standards for girls to meet the criteria for an ADHD diagnosis compared with boys.

Girls are less likely to exhibit hyperactivity symptoms, which are the most easily observable of all ADHD symptoms, particularly in younger patients. This fact may account for a portion of the difference in diagnosis between girls and boys. As a result, it is important to fully consider a diagnosis of ADHD, predominantly inattentive presentation, when evaluating girls.

Symptoms of inattention alone can complicate the diagnosis because inattention is 1 of the most common symptoms across all disorders in the *DSM-5*. After puberty, it is more common for depression and anxiety to be diagnosed in girls than in boys, and symptoms of inattention may be a result of these disorders as well as ADHD. Examining the age of onset and considering other distinguishing features, such as avoidance and anhedonia, can help the PCC clarify this challenging differential when evaluating girls for ADHD. For example, does the inattention occur primarily in anxiety-provoking situations or when the child or adolescent is experiencing periods of low mood and then remit when the anxiety or mood improves?

III c. Consideration of Comorbid Conditions

If other disorders are suspected or detected during the diagnostic evaluation, an assessment of the urgency of these conditions and their impact on the ADHD treatment plan should be made. Comorbid conditions provide unique challenges for treatment planning. Urgent conditions need to be addressed immediately with services capable of handling crisis situations. These conditions include suicidal thoughts or acts and other behaviors with the potential to severely injure the child, adolescent, and/or other people, including severe temper outbursts or child abuse. Note that adolescents are potentially more likely to provide honest answers if the PCC asks sensitive questions in the absence of the parents and may respond more readily to rating scales that assess mood or anxiety. In addition, substance use disorders require immediate attention and may precede or coincide with beginning treatment of ADHD. Additional information is available in the complex ADHD guideline published by the SDBP.[67]

Evidence shows that comorbid conditions may improve with treatment of ADHD, including oppositional behaviors and anxiety.[140] For example, children with ADHD and comorbid anxiety disorders may find that addressing the ADHD symptoms with

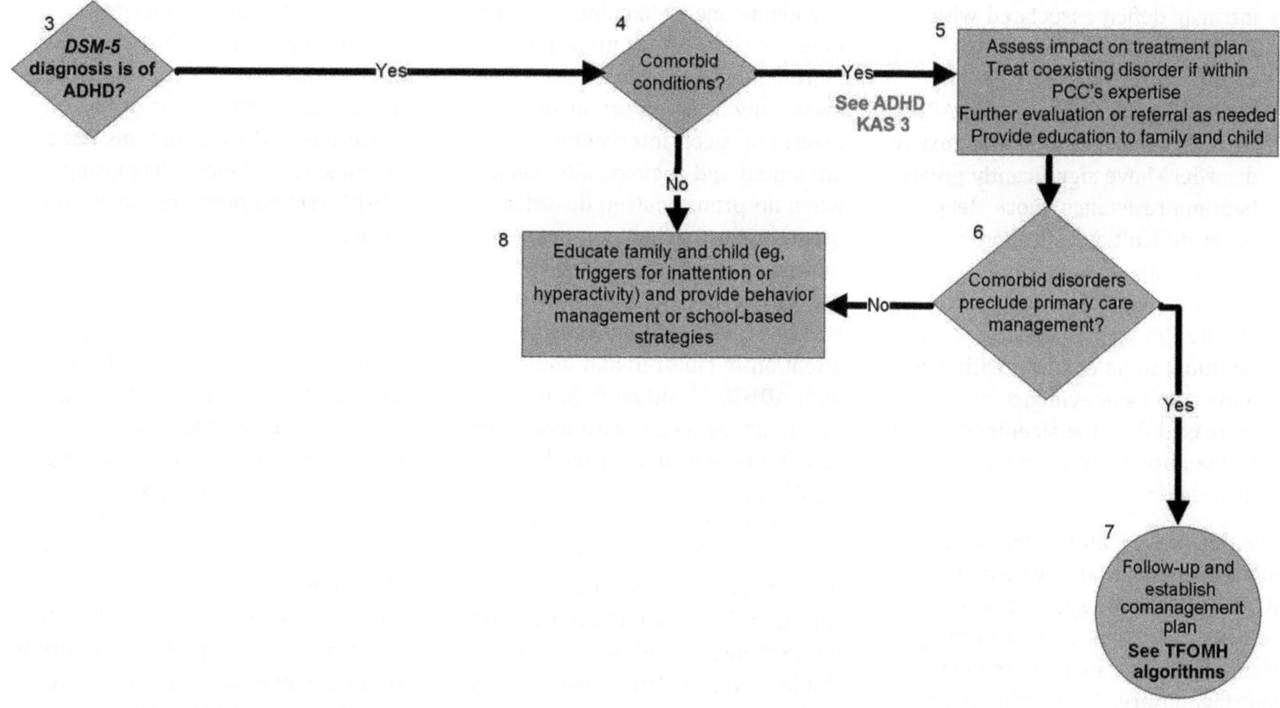

SUPPLEMENTAL FIGURE 6
Consideration of comorbid conditions. TFOMH, Task Force on Mental Health.

medications also decreases anxiety or mood symptoms. Other children may require additional therapeutic treatments to treat the ADHD adequately and treat comorbid conditions, including cognitive behavioral therapy (CBT), academic interventions, or different and/or additional medications.

The PCC may evaluate and treat the comorbid disorder if it is within his or her training and expertise. In addition, the PCC can provide education to the family and child or adolescent about triggers for inattention and/or hyperactivity. If the PCC requires the advice of a subspecialist, the clinician is encouraged to consider carefully when to initiate treatment of ADHD. In some cases, it may be advisable to delay the start of medication until the role of each member of the treatment team is established (see below). Integrated care models can be helpful (see www.integratedcareforkids.org).

The following are brief discussions of sleep disorders, psychiatric disorders, emotion dysregulation, exposure to trauma, and learning disabilities, all of which can manifest in manners similar to ADHD and can complicate making a diagnosis.

(See the ADHD guideline's KAS 3.)

Sleep Disorders

Sleepiness impairs most people's ability to sustain attention and often leads to caffeine consumption to counter these effects. In the same way, sleep disturbance can lead to symptoms and impairment that mimic or exacerbate ADHD symptoms. A child with ADHD may have difficulty falling asleep because of the busy thoughts caused by ADHD. Some sleep disorders are frequently associated with ADHD or present as symptoms of inattention, hyperactivity, and impulsivity, such as obstructive sleep apnea syndrome and restless legs syndrome and/or periodic limb movement disorder (RLS/PLMD).[190–193]

The differential diagnosis of insomnia in children and adolescents with ADHD includes the following:

- inadequate sleep hygiene (eg, inconsistent bedtimes and wake times, absence of a bedtime routine, electronics in the bedroom, caffeine use)[194];
- ADHD medication (stimulant and nonstimulant) effects:
  - o direct effects on sleep architecture: prolonged sleep onset, latency, and decreased sleep duration, increased night wakings[195–197]; and
  - o indirect effects: inadequate control of ADHD symptoms in the evening and medication withdrawal or rebound symptoms[198,199];
- sleep problems associated with comorbid psychiatric conditions (eg, anxiety and mood disorders, disruptive behavior disorders)[200];
- circadian-based phase delay in sleep-wake patterns, which have been shown to occur in some children with ADHD, resulting in both prolonged sleep onset and difficulty waking in the morning[201]; and

- intrinsic deficit associated with ADHD. Authors of numerous studies have reported that nonmedicated children with ADHD without comorbid mood or anxiety disorders have significantly greater bedtime resistance, more sleep onset difficulties, and more frequent night awakenings when compared with typically developing children in control groups.[202] In addition, some children with ADHD appear to have evidence of increased daytime sleepiness, even in the absence of a primary sleep disorder.[202–204]

For this reason, all children and adolescents who are evaluated for ADHD need to be systematically screened for symptoms of primary sleep disorders, such as frequent snoring, observed breathing pauses, restless sleep, urge to move one's legs at night, and excessive daytime sleepiness. (Issues of access to these services are discussed in the accompanying section, Systemic Barriers to the Care of Children and Adolescents with ADHD.) In addition, screenings generally include primary sleep disorders' risk factors, such as adenotonsillar hypertrophy, asthma and allergies, obesity, a family history of RLS/PLMD, and iron deficiency.[199] Sleep assessment measures that have been shown to be useful in the pediatric primary care practice setting include brief screening tools[205] and parent-report surveys.[206,207] Overnight polysomnography is generally required for children who have symptoms suggestive of and/or risk factors for obstructive sleep apnea syndrome and RLS/PLMD.[208,209]

If the results suggest the presence of a sleep disorder, the PCC needs to obtain a comprehensive sleep history, including assessment of the environment in which the child sleeps; the cohabitants in the room; the bedtime routine, including its initiation, how long it takes for the child fall asleep, sleep duration, and any night-time awakenings; and what time the child wakes up in the morning and his or her state when awakening. It is important to determine sleep interventions attempted and their results. Even when no primary sleep disorders occur, modest reductions in sleep duration or increases in sleep disruption may be associated with increased, detectable problems with attention in children and adolescents with ADHD.[210] Although fully disentangling sleep disruption from ADHD may not be possible because significant sleep problems and their associated impairment are often comorbid with ADHD, sleep disruptions often warrant consideration as an additional target for treatment. In addition, some children with ADHD appear to show evidence of increased daytime sleepiness, even in the absence of a primary sleep disorder.[203,204] Significant sleep problems and their associated impairment are often comorbid with ADHD and, for many children, are considered as an additional target for treatment.

A variety of issues need to be considered when determining if sleep problems constitute an additional diagnosis of insomnia disorder or are linked to ADHD-related treatment issues. First, a child's sleep can be affected if he or she is already taking stimulant medication or regularly consuming caffeine. The dosage and timing of this consumption needs to be tracked and manipulated to examine its effects; simple modifications of timing and dosage of stimulant consumption can improve sleep onset, duration, and quality. Second, sleep problems can occur from inadequate sleep health and/or hygiene[194] or from other disorders, such as anxiety and mood disorders, when the rumination and worry associated with them impairs or disrupts the child's sleep. Restructuring behavior preceding and at bedtime can dramatically improve sleep and diminish associated impairments. These potential causes of sleep disturbance and the related impairments that mimic or exacerbate ADHD symptoms need to be considered before diagnosing ADHD, related problems, or insomnia disorder.

Trauma

Children with ADHD are at higher-than-normal risk of experiencing some forms of trauma, including corporal punishment and accidents (often because of their risk-taking behaviors). In addition, posttraumatic stress disorder may manifest some similar symptoms. Depending on the child, the trauma may have been a one-time event or one to which they are consistently exposed. Exposure to trauma may exacerbate or lead to symptoms shared by trauma disorders and ADHD (eg, inattention). As a result, when evaluating a child for ADHD, obtaining a brief trauma history and screening for indicators of impairing responses to trauma can be helpful. Although a trauma history does not inform the diagnosis of ADHD, it may identify an alternative diagnosis and inform treatment and other interventions, including referral for trauma-focused therapy and reporting suspected abuse.

Mental Health Conditions

In children or adolescents who have coexisting mild depression, anxiety, or obsessive-compulsive disorder, the PCC may undertake the treatment of all disorders if doing so is within his or her abilities. Another option is to collaborate with a mental health clinician to treat the coexisting condition while the PCC oversees the ADHD treatment. As a third option, the consulting specialists may advise about the treatment of the coexisting condition to the extent that the PCC is comfortable treating both ADHD and the coexisting problems. With some coexisting psychiatric disorders, such as severe anxiety, depression, autism, schizophrenia, obsessive-compulsive disorder, oppositional defiant disorder, conduct disorder, and bipolar disorder, a comanaging developmental-behavioral pediatrician or child and adolescent psychiatrist might take responsibility for treatment of both ADHD and the coexisting illness.

Many children with ADHD exhibit emotion dysregulation, which is considered to be a common feature of the disorder and one that is potentially related to other executive functioning deficits.[211] A child exhibiting emotion dysregulation with either or both positive (eg, exuberance) or negative (eg, anger) emotions along with symptoms of ADHD can be considered as a good candidate for an ADHD diagnosis. Sometimes behavior related to emotion dysregulation can lead the PCC to consider other diagnoses such as disruptive mood dysregulation disorder, intermittent explosive disorder, and bipolar disorder. All 3 may be diagnosed with ADHD. Intermittent explosive disorder and bipolar disorder are rare in children, and data are currently inadequate to know the prevalence of disruptive mood dysregulation disorder. Given the base rates, these other diagnoses are unlikely, although they do occur in childhood. If the PCC has any uncertainty about making these distinctions, referring the child to a clinical child psychologist or child mental health professionals may be warranted.

Learning Disabilities

Learning disabilities frequently co-occur with ADHD and can lead to symptoms and impairment that are similar to those in children with ADHD. As a result, screening for learning disabilities' presence, such as via the Vanderbilt ADHD Rating Scale,[212] is important given that treatment of ADHD and learning disabilities differ markedly.

Learning disabilities involve impairment related to learning specific academic content, usually reading or math, although there is increased awareness about disorders of written expression. The impairment is not attributable to difficulties with sustaining attention; however, some children with learning disabilities have trouble sustaining attention in class because they cannot keep up and then disengage. A careful evaluation for learning disabilities includes achievement testing, cognitive ability testing, and measures of the child's learning in response to evidence-based instruction. Such thorough evaluations are typically not available in a PCC practice. If screening suggests the possibility of learning disabilities, the PCC can help advise parents on how to obtain school psychoeducational evaluations or refer the child to a psychologist or other specialist trained in conducting these evaluations.

The PCC's attention is directed to language skills in preschool-aged and young school-aged children because difficulties in language skills can be a symptom of a language disorder and predictor of subsequent reading problems. Language disorders may present as problems with attention and impulsivity. Likewise, social interactions need to be noted during the examination because they may be impaired when the child or adolescent's language skills are delayed or disordered.

Children who have intellectual or other developmental disabilities may have ADHD, but assessment of these patients is more difficult because a diagnosis of ADHD would only be appropriate if the child or adolescent's level of inattention or hyperactivity/impulsivity is disproportionate to his or her developmental rather than chronological age. Therefore, assessment of ADHD in individuals with intellectual disabilities requires input from the child or adolescent's education specialists, school psychologists, and/or independent psychologists. Although it is important to attempt to differentiate whether the presenting problems are associated with learning disabilities, ADHD, or something else, it is important to consider the possibility that a child has multiple disorders. Pediatricians and other PCCs who are involved in assessing ADHD in children with intellectual disabilities will need to collaborate closely with school or independent psychologists.

Summary

Overall, there are many factors that influence a diagnostic decision. Frequently, these decisions must be made without the benefit of all of the relevant information described. Family and cultural issues that affect parents' expectations for their child and perceptions about mental health can further complicate this process. Poverty, family history, access to care, and many other factors that a PCC will probably not know when making the diagnosis can also be formative in the child's presenting problems.[145,146,154,155,158] The PCC will wisely remain sensitive to individual variations in parents' beliefs, values, and perception of their culture and community when completing the assessment and determining a diagnosis. These factors add complexities to the assessment and diagnostic process and make a good evaluation and diagnosis a function of clinical experience, judgment, and a foundation in science.

IV. TREATMENT

If the child meets the *DSM-5* criteria for ADHD, including commensurate functional disabilities, progress through the PoCA.

(See the AHDH guideline's KASs 5 and 6.)

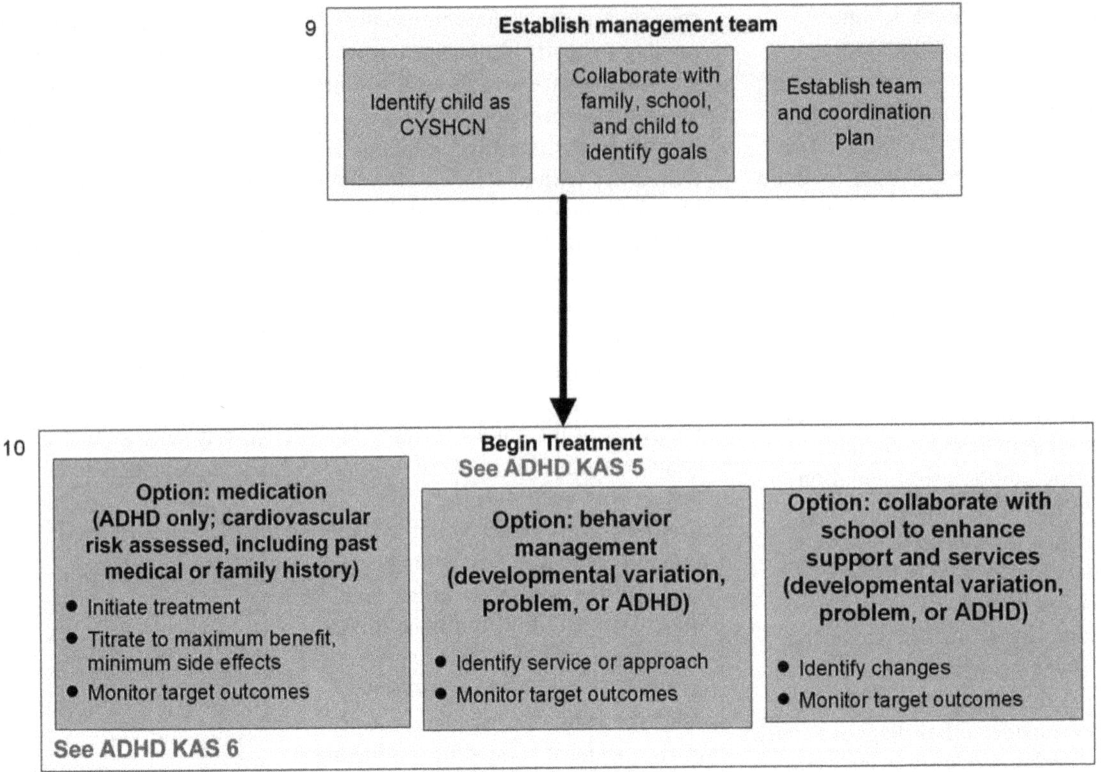

SUPPLEMENTAL FIGURE 7
Treatment. CYSHCN, children and youth with special health care needs.

IV a. Establish Management Team: Identify the Patient as a Child With Special Health Care Needs

Any child who meets the criteria for ADHD is considered a "child or youth with special health care needs"; these children are best managed in a medical home.[213–217] In addition, the AAP encourages clinicians to develop systems to allow the medical home to meet all needs of children with chronic illnesses. These needs and strategies for meeting them are discussed in further detail in AAP resources such as the Building Your Medical Home toolkit and Addressing Concerns in Primary Care: A Clinician's Toolkit. Care in the medical home is reviewed in the AAP publication *Bright Futures: Guidelines for Health Supervision of Infants, Children, and Adolescents, Fourth Edition*. Pediatricians and other PCCs who provide effective medical homes identify family strengths and recognize the importance of parents in the care team.[218–221] The PCC may provide education about the disorder and treatment options, medication, and/or psychosocial treatment and monitor response to treatments over time as well as the child's development.

IV b. Establish Management Team: Collaborate With Family, School, and Child to Identify Target Goals

ADHD is a chronic illness; hence, education for both the child or adolescent and other family members is a critical element in the care plan. Family education involves all members of the family, including the provision of developmentally age-appropriate information for the affected child or adolescent and any siblings. Topics may include the disorder's potential causes and typical symptoms, the assessment process; common coexisting disorders; ADHD's effect on school performance and social participation; long-term sequelae; and treatment options and their potential benefits, adverse effects, and long-term outcomes. It is important to address the patient's self-concept and clarify that having ADHD does not mean that the child is less smart than others. At every stage, education must continue in a manner consistent with the child or adolescent's level of understanding.

The emphasis for parental education is on helping parents understand the disorder, how to obtain additional accurate information about ADHD and treatments, and how to effectively advocate for their child. This may include addressing parental concerns about labeling the child or adolescent with a disorder by providing information on the benefits of diagnosis and treatment.

Some guidance about effective parenting strategies may be helpful, but PTBM is likely to be most beneficial for most parents (see the section on Psychosocial Treatments). Pediatricians and other PCCs are encouraged to be cognizant of the challenges families may face to attend such training, including taking time off from work and covering the costs associated with the intervention.

Parents may benefit from learning about optimal ways to partner with schools, particularly their child's teachers, and become part of the educational and intervention teams. Educating parents about special education and other services can be helpful, but school interventions and advocacy may be best aided by partnering closely with an advocate or clinician experienced in working with schools (see the Psychosocial Treatment section). With the parent's permission, the clinician may provide educators at the school with information from the evaluation that will help the school determine eligibility for special education services or accommodations and/or develop appropriate services.

In addition, it is helpful to provide assistance to the parent or other caregiver in understanding and using any relevant electronic health record (EHR) system. Sometimes, the health literacy gap around EHRs can lead to confusion and frustration on the family's side. Also, providing information on community resources, such as other health care providers or specialists, can be beneficial in addressing fragmentation and communication barriers.

Family education continues throughout the course of treatment and includes anticipatory guidance in areas such as transitions (eg, from elementary to middle school, middle to high school, and high school to college or employment); working with schools; and developmental challenges that may be affected by ADHD, including driving, sexual activity, and substance use and abuse. For parents who are interested in understanding the developmental aspects of children's understanding about ADHD (ie, causes, manifestations, treatments), several AAP publications may be useful.[222–224]

Although having a child diagnosed with ADHD can sometimes provide relief for families, it is important to check on the parents' well-being. Having a disruptive child who has trouble interacting with others can be stressful for parents, and learning that their child has a disorder sometimes gives them something to blame other than themselves. Helping families cope with parenting challenges or making referrals for services to address their stress or depression can be an important part of care. These concerns are particularly relevant when a parent has ADHD or associated conditions. Parents may require support balancing the needs of their child with ADHD and their other children's needs. Advocacy and support groups such as the National Resource on ADHD (a program of CHADD: https://chadd.org/about/about-nrc/) and the Attention Deficit Disorder Association (www.add.org) can provide information and support for families. There also may be local support organizations. The ADHD Toolkit provides lists of educational resources including Internet-based resources, organizations, and books that may be useful to parents and children.

IV c. Establish Management Team: Establish Team and Coordination Plan

Treatment Team

The optimal treatment team includes everyone involved in the care of the child: the child, parents, teachers, PCC, therapists, subspecialists, and other adults (such as coaches or faith leaders) who will be actively engaged in supporting and monitoring the treatment of ADHD.[218–221] It is helpful for the PCC or another assigned care coordinator to make each team member aware of his or her role, the process and timing of routine and as-needed communication strategies, and expectations for reports (ie, frequency, scope). Collaboration with school personnel goes beyond the initial report of diagnosis and is best facilitated by agreement on a standardized, reliable communication system. Although there are obstacles to achieving this level of coordination, if successful, it enhances care and improves outcomes for the child. (See Systemic Barriers to the Care of Children and Adolescents With ADHD section in the Supplemental Information for a discussion of systemic challenges.)

Treatment Goals

Management plans include the establishment of treatment goals for the areas of concern, such as those most commonly affected by ADHD: academic performance; relationships with peers, parents, and siblings; and safety. It is not necessary to develop goals in every area at once. Families might be encouraged to identify up to 3 of the most impairing areas to address initially. Parents and the child or adolescent can add other targets as indicated by their relative importance. Other goals may be identified using the International Classification of Function, Disability, and Health analysis conducted in the diagnostic phase of the clinical pathway. This process increases the understanding of ADHD's effects on each family member and may lead to improved collaboration in developing a few specific and measurable outcomes. It is helpful to incorporate a child's strengths and resilience when considering target goals and generating the treatment plan. Academic or school goals require the input of teachers and other personnel for both identification and measurement.

Establishing measurable goals in interpersonal domains and improving behavior in unstructured settings may be particularly important. Wherever possible, progress should be quantifiable to monitor the frequency of behaviors. The number of achieved and missed goals per day can be recorded by the parent, child, and/or teacher. Charts may be suggested as strategies to record events so that parents, teachers, children, and PCCs can agree on how much progress has been made building success in a systematic and measurable way. Keeping the focus on progress toward the identified goals can keep all family members engaged, provide a rubric for measuring response to various treatments, and offer a vehicle for rewarding success. Such strategies can help a family accurately assess and see progress of behavior changes. A single-page daily report card can be used to identify and monitor 4 or 5 behaviors that affect function at school and the card can be shared with parents. Other strategies and tools are available to clinicians in the AAP *ADHD Provider Toolkit, Third Edition*,[225] and for parents, *ADHD: What Every Parent Needs to Know*.[226]

As treatment proceeds, in addition to using a *DSM-5*–based ADHD rating scale to monitor core symptom changes, formal and informal queries can be made in the areas affected by ADHD. At every visit, it is helpful for the PCC to gradually further empower children and adolescents so they are able to be full partners in the treatment plan by adolescence. Data from school are helpful at these visits, including rating scales completed by the child or adolescent's teacher, grades, daily behavior ratings (when available), and formal test results.

Management Plan

In addition to educating the family, the PCC can consider developing a management plan that, over time, addresses the following questions:

- Does the family need further assistance in understanding the core symptoms of ADHD and the child or adolescent's target symptoms and coexisting conditions?
- Does the family need support in learning how to establish, measure, and monitor target goals?
- Have the family's goals been identified and addressed in the care plan?
- Does the family have an understanding of effective behavior management techniques for responding to tantrums, oppositional behavior, and/or poor compliance with requests or commands?
- Does the family need help on normalizing peer and family relationships?
- Does the child need help in academic areas? If so, has a formal evaluation been performed and reviewed to distinguish work production problems secondary to ADHD or attributable to coexisting learning or language disabilities?
- Does the child or adolescent need assistance in achieving independence in self-help or schoolwork?
- Does the child or adolescent or family require help with optimizing, organizing, planning, or managing schoolwork?
- Does the family need help in recognizing, understanding, or managing coexisting conditions?
- Does the family have a plan to educate the child or adolescent systematically about ADHD and its treatment, as well as the child's own strengths and weaknesses?
- Does the family have a plan to empower the child or adolescent with the knowledge and understanding that will increase their adherence to treatments? Has that plan been initiated, and is it pitched at the child or adolescent's developmental level?
- Does the family have a copy of a care plan that summarizes the evaluation findings and treatment recommendations?
- Does the follow-up plan provide comprehensive, coordinated, family-centered, and culturally competent ongoing care?
- Does the family have any needed referrals to specialists to provide additional evaluations, treatments, and support?
- Does the family have a plan for the transition from pediatric to adult care that provides the transitioning youth with the necessary ADHD self-management skills, understanding of health care and educational privacy laws, identified adult clinician to continue his or her ADHD care, and health insurance coverage?

IV d. Treatment: Medication, Psychosocial Treatment, and Collaboration With the School to Enhance Support Services

The decision about the most acceptable treatment of the child rests with the family and its decisions about treatment. The PCC needs to encourage that this decision is based on accurate and adequate information, which often involves correcting misinformation or unwarranted concerns about medication. If the family still declines medication treatment, the PCC can encourage all other types of effective treatment and provide appropriate monitoring (families who decline medication are discussed in more detail below).

Pediatricians and other PCCs need to educate families about the benefits and characteristics of evidence-based ADHD psychosocial treatment and explicitly communicate that play therapy and sensory-related therapies have not been demonstrated to be effective. Likewise, for children younger than 7 years, individual CBT lacks demonstrated effectiveness; CBT has some, but not strong, evidence for children 7 to 17 years of age. Families should be made aware that for psychosocial treatments to be effective, the therapist needs to work with the family (not just the child or adolescent) on setting and maintaining routines, discipline and reward-related procedures, training programs, and creating a home environment that will bring out the best in the child and minimize ADHD-related dysfunction.

(See the ADHD guideline KASs 5 and 6.)

Treatment: Medication

This treatment option is restricted to children and adolescents who meet diagnostic criteria for ADHD.

The FDA has approved stimulant medications (ie, methylphenidate and amphetamines) and several nonstimulant medications for the treatment of ADHD in children and adolescents. New brands of methylphenidate and amphetamines continue to be introduced, including longer-acting products, various isomeric products, and delayed-release products. Hence, it is increasingly unlikely that pediatricians and other PCCs need to consider the off-label use of other medications. A free and continually updated list of medications is available at www.adhdmedicationguide.com. (See the ADHD guideline for information on off-label use.)

With the expanded choices and considerations of the clinical effects comes the reality that clinical choices are often heavily restricted by insurance coverage. Some, but not all, of the problems include changes in insurance and formulary that preclude the use of certain medications or force a stable patient to change medications, step therapy requirements that may delay effective treatment, and financial barriers that preclude a patient's use of newer drugs or those not preferred by the payer. (See Systemic Barriers to the Care of Children and Adolescents with ADHD section in the Supplemental Information for a discussion of this issue.)

The choice of stimulant medication formulation depends on such factors as the efficacy of each agent for a given child, the preferred length of coverage, whether a child can swallow pills or capsules, and out-of-pocket costs. The extended-release formulations are generally more expensive than the immediate-release formulations. Families and children may prefer them, however, because of the benefits of consistent and sustained coverage with fewer daily administrations. Long-acting formulations usually avoid the need for school-based administration of ADHD medication. Better coverage with fewer daily administrations leads to greater convenience to the family and is linked with increased adherence to the medication management plan.[227]

Some patients, particularly adolescents, may require more than 12 hours of coverage daily to ensure adequate focus and concentration during the evening, when they are more likely to be studying and/or driving. In these cases, a nonstimulant medication or short-acting preparation of stimulant medication may be used in the evening in addition to a long-acting preparation in the morning. Of note, stimulant medication treatment of individuals with ADHD has been linked to better driving performance and a significant reduced risk of motor vehicle crashes.[78]

The ease with which preparations can be administered and the minimization of adverse effects are key quality-of-life factors and are important concerns for children, adolescents, and their parents. When making medication recommendations, PCCs have to consider the time of day when the targeted symptoms occur, when homework is usually done, whether medication remains active when teenagers are driving, whether medication alters sleep initiation, and risk status for substance use or stimulant misuse or diversion.

All FDA-approved stimulant medications are methylphenidate or amphetamine compounds and have similar desired and adverse effects. Given the extensive evidence of efficacy and safety, these drugs remain the first choice in medication treatment. The decision about what compound a PCC prescribes first should be made on the basis of individual clinician and family preferences and the child's age. Some children will respond better to, or experience more adverse effects with, 1 of the 2 stimulants groups (ie, methylphenidate or amphetamine) over another. Because this cannot be determined in advance, medication trials are appropriate. If a trial with 1 group is unsuccessful because of poor efficacy or significant adverse effects, a medication trial with medication from the other group should be undertaken. At least half of children who fail to respond to 1 stimulant medication have a positive response to the alternative medication.[228]

Of note, recent meta-analyses have documented some subtle group-level differences in amphetamine and/or dextroamphetamine and methylphenidate response. Authors of 1 such analysis found that, on average, youth with ADHD who were treated with either amphetamine- or methylphenidate-based medications showed improvement in ADHD symptoms.[229] There was a marginally larger improvement in clinicians' ADHD symptom ratings for amphetamine-based versus methylphenidate-based preparations.[229] This meta-analysis indicated that overall adverse effects (including sleep problems and emotional side effects) were more prominent among those using amphetamine-based preparations. The findings were corroborated by a 2018 meta-analysis in which authors found that amphetamine and/or dextroamphetamine worsened emotional lability compared to the premedication baseline. Authors of the meta-analysis found there was a tendency for methylphenidate to reduce irritability and anxiety compared to the patients' premedication ratings.[230] Among individual patients, medication's efficacy and adverse effects can vary from these averages.

Families who are concerned about the use of stimulants or the potential for their abuse and/or diversion may choose to start with atomoxetine, extended-release guanfacine, or extended-release clonidine. In addition, those not responding to either stimulant group may still respond to atomoxetine, extended-release guanfacine, or extended-release clonidine.

There is a black box warning on atomoxetine about the possibility of suicidal ideation when initiating medication management. Early symptoms of suicidal ideation may include thinking about self-harm and increasing agitation. If there are any concerns about suicidal ideation in children prescribed atomoxetine, further evaluation (ie, using the Patient Health Questionnaire-9 rating scale, asking about suicidal ideation, reviewing presence of firearms in the home, determining if there is good communication between the patient and parents or trusted adults, etc), reconsideration about the use of atomoxetine, and more frequent monitoring should be considered; referral to a mental health clinician may be necessary.

Atomoxetine is a selective norepinephrine reuptake inhibitor that may demonstrate maximum response after approximately 4 to 6 weeks of use, although some patients experience modest benefits after 1 week of atomoxetine treatment. Extended-release guanfacine and extended-release clonidine are α-2A adrenergic agonists that may demonstrate maximum response in about 2 to 4 weeks. It is worth making families aware that symptom change is more gradual with atomoxetine and α-2A adrenergic agonists than the rapid effect seen with stimulant medications. Atomoxetine may cause gastrointestinal tract symptoms and sedation early on, so it is recommended to prescribe half the treatment dose (0.5 mg/kg) for the first week. Appetite suppression can also occur. Both α-2A agonists can cause the adverse effect of somnolence. It is recommended that α-2A agonists be tapered when discontinued to prevent possible rebound hypertension.

In patients who only respond partially to stimulant medications, it is possible to combine stimulant and nonstimulant α-2 agonist medications to obtain better efficacy (see Medication for ADHD section in the clinical practice guideline). It is helpful to ask the family if they have any previous experience with any of the medications because a previous good or bad experience in other family members may indicate a willingness or reluctance to use 1 type or a specific stimulant medication. When there is concern about possible use or diversion of the medication or a strong family preference against stimulant medication, an FDA-approved nonstimulant medication may be considered as the first choice of medication.

Medications that use a microbead technology can be opened and sprinkled on food and are, therefore, suitable for children who have difficulty swallowing tablets or capsules. For patients who are unable to swallow pills, alternative options include immediate- and extended-release methylphenidate and amphetamine in a liquid and chewable form, a methylphenidate transdermal patch, and an orally disintegrating tablet.

It is often helpful to inform families that the initial medication titration process may take several weeks to complete, medication changes can be made on a weekly basis, and subsequent changes in medication may be necessary. Completion of ADHD rating scales before dose adjustment helps promote measurement-based treatment. The usual procedure is to begin with a low dose of medication and titrate to the dose that provides maximum benefit and minimal adverse effects. Core symptom reduction can be seen immediately with stimulant medication initiation, but improvements in function require more time to manifest. Stimulant medications can be effectively titrated with changes occurring in a 3- to 7-day period. During the first month of treatment, the medication dose may be titrated with a weekly or biweekly follow-up. The increasing doses can be provided either by prescriptions that allow dose adjustments upward or, for some of medications, by 1 prescription of tablets or capsules of the same strength with instructions to administer progressively higher amounts by doubling or tripling the initial dose.

Another approach, similar to the one used in the MTA study,[228] is for parents to be directed to administer different doses of the same preparation, each for 1 week at a time (eg, Saturday through Friday). At the end of each week, feedback from parents and teachers and/or *DSM-5*–based ADHD rating scales can be obtained through a phone interview, fax, or a secure electronic system. In addition to the ADHD rating scale, parents and teachers can be asked to review adverse effects and progress on target goals.

Follow-up Visits

A face-to face follow-up visit is recommended at about the fourth week after starting the medication. At this visit, the PCC reviews the child or adolescent's responses to the varying doses and monitors adverse effects, pulse, BP, and weight. To promote progress in controlling symptoms is maintained, PCCs will continue to monitor levels of core symptoms and improvement in specified target goals. ADHD rating scales should be completed at each visit, particularly before any changes in medication and/or dose.

In the first year of treatment, face-to-face visits to the PCC are recommended to occur on a monthly basis until consistent and optimal response has been achieved, then they should occur every 3 months. Subsequent face-to-face visits will be dependent on the response; they typically occur quarterly but need to occur at least twice annually until it is clear that target goals are progressing and that symptoms have stabilized. Thereafter, visits occur periodically as determined by the family and the PCC. After several years, if the child or adolescent is doing well and wants to attempt a trial off of the medication, this can be initiated.

Results from the MTA study suggest that there are some children who, after 3 years of medication treatment, continue to improve even if the medication is discontinued.[13] These findings suggest that children who are stable in their improvement of ADHD symptoms may be given a trial off medication after extended periods of use to determine if medication is still needed. This process is best undertaken with close monitoring of the child's core symptoms and function at home, in school, and in the community. If pharmacologic interventions do not improve the child or adolescent's symptoms, the diagnosis needs to be reassessed (see Treatment Failure section).

Whenever possible, improvements in core symptoms and target goals should be monitored in an objective way (eg, an increase from 40% goal attainment to 80% per week; see the ADHD Toolkit for more information). Core symptoms can be monitored with 1 of the *DSM-5*–based ADHD rating scales.

Pediatricians and other PCCs are encouraged to educate parents that although medications can be effective in facilitating schoolwork, they have not been shown to be effective in addressing learning disabilities or a child's level of motivation. A child or adolescent who continues to experience academic underachievement after attaining some control of his or her ADHD behavioral symptoms needs to be assessed for a coexisting condition. Such coexisting conditions include learning and language disabilities, other mental health disorders, and other psychosocial stressors. This assessment is part of the initial assessment in children who present with difficulties in keeping up with their schoolwork and grades and who are rated as having problems in the 3 academic areas (ie, reading, writing, and math).

Treatment: Psychosocial Treatment

Two types of psychosocial treatments are well established for children and adolescents with ADHD, including some behavioral treatments and training.[25]

Behavioral Treatments

There is a great deal of evidence supporting the use of behavioral treatments for preschool-aged and elementary and middle school–aged children, including several types of PTBM and classroom interventions (see the clinical practice guideline for more information). There are multiple PTBM programs available, which are reviewed in the ADHD Toolkit.[225]

Evidence-based PTBM training typically begins with 7 to 12 weekly group or individual sessions with a trained or certified therapist. Although PTBM treatments differ, the primary focus is on helping parents improve the methods they use to reward and motivate their child to reduce the behavioral difficulties posed by ADHD and improve their child's behavior. Therapists help parents establish consistent relationships or contingencies between the child's specific behaviors and the parents' use of rewards or logical consequences for misbehavior. These treatments typically use specific directed praise, point systems, time-outs, and privileges to shape behavior. Parents learn how to effectively communicate expectations and responses to desirable and undesirable behaviors.

PTBM programs offer specific techniques for reinforcing adaptive and positive behaviors and decreasing or eliminating inappropriate behaviors, which alter the motivation of the child or adolescent to control attention, activity, and impulsivity. These programs emphasize establishing positive interactions between parents and children, shaping children's behaviors through praising and strengths spotting, giving successful commands, and reinforcing positive behaviors. They help parents to extinguish inappropriate behaviors through ignoring, to identify behaviors that are most appropriately handled through natural consequences, and to use natural consequences in in a responsible way.

These programs all emphasize teaching self-control and building positive family relationships. If parents strongly disagree about behavior management or have contentious relationships, parenting programs will likely be unsuccessful.

Depending on the severity of the child or adolescent's behaviors and the capabilities of the parents, group or individual training programs will be required. Programs may also include support for maintenance and relapse prevention.

Although all effective parenting uses behavioral techniques, applying these strategies to children or adolescents with ADHD requires additional rigor, adherence, and persistence, compared with children without the disorder. Some PTBM programs include additional components such as education about ADHD, development and other related issues, motivational interviewing, and support for parents coping with a child with ADHD.

PTBM training has been modified for use with adolescents to incorporate a family therapy approach that includes communication, problem-solving, and negotiation. Initially developed for adolescents with a wide range of problems,[94,231] this approach has been modified for adolescents with ADHD.[94,233] The approach's effects are not as large as with PTBM training with children, but clear benefits have been reported; this is a feasible clinic-based approach that warrants a referral, if available.

Although PTBM training is typically effective, such programs may not be available in many areas (see Systemic Barriers to the Care of Children and Adolescents with ADHD section in the Supplemental Information for further discussion of this issue[153]). Factors that may diminish PTBM's effects and/or render them ineffective include the time commitment required to attend sessions and practice the recommendations at home, particularly given other competing demands for the family's time. Parental disagreements about implementing the PTBM program, conflicts between parents, and separated parents who share caretaking responsibilities can adversely affect the results. Careful monitoring of progress and follow-up by the therapist or PCC can reduce the likelihood of these risks. PTBM training may not be covered by health insurance (insurance issues are discussed in the Systemic Barriers to the Care of Children and Adolescents With ADHD section).

Training Interventions

Training interventions are likely to be effective with children and adolescents with ADHD. These interventions involve targeting specific deficiencies in skills such as study, organization, and interpersonal skills. Effective training approaches involve targeting a set of behaviors that are useful to the child in daily life and providing extensive training, practice, and coaching over an extended period of time. For some children, the combination of behavioral treatments and training may be most effective. Psychosocial treatments are applicable for children who have problems with inattentive or hyperactive/impulsive behaviors but do not meet the *DSM-5* criteria for a diagnosis of ADHD.

Many of the behavioral and training treatments described above can be provided at school. Coaching, which has emerged as a treatment modality over the last decade, can be a useful alternative to clinic- or school-based treatments. There has yet to be rigorous studies to support its benefits, although it has good face validity. Currently, there is no standardized training or certification for coaches.

Other Considerations

PCCs can make recommendations about treatments that are most likely to help a child or adolescent with ADHD and discourage the use of nonmedication treatments that are unlikely to be effective. Pediatricians and other PCCs are encouraged to discuss what parents have tried in the past and what has been beneficial for the child and his or her family.

Treatments for which there is insufficient evidence include large doses of vitamins and other dietary alterations, vision and/or visual training, chelation, EEG biofeedback, and working memory (ie, cognitive training) programs.[25] To date, there is insufficient evidence to determine that these therapies lead to changes in ADHD's core symptoms or functioning. There is a lack of information about the safety of many of these alternative therapies. Although there is some minimal information that significant doses of essential fatty acids may help with ADHD symptoms, further study on effectiveness, negative impacts, and adverse effects is needed before it can be considered a recommended treatment.[233]

As noted, some therapies that are effective for other disorders are not supported for use with children or adolescents with ADHD. These include CBT (which has documented effectiveness for the treatment of anxiety and depressive disorders), play therapy, social skills training, and interpersonal talk therapy. Although it is possible that these treatments may improve ADHD symptoms in a specific child or adolescent, they are less likely to do so compared to evidence-based treatments. As a result, the PCC should discourage use of these approaches. If these ineffective treatments are attempted before evidence-based modalities, parents may erroneously conclude that all mental health treatments are ineffective. For example, if CBT or play therapy does not help their child's ADHD, parents may dismiss other treatments, like PTBM, which could be helpful. Parents also may discount CBT if it subsequently is recommended for an emerging anxiety disorder.

Pediatricians and other PCCs are unlikely to be effective in providing psychosocial treatment unless they are specifically trained, have trained staff, are colocated with a therapist, or dedicate multiple visits to providing this treatment. Clinicians may have difficulty determining if the therapists listed in the patient's health insurance plan have the requisite skills to provide evidence-based, psychosocial ADHD-related treatment. This determination is important because many therapists focus on a play therapy or interpersonal talk therapy, which have not been shown to be effective in treating the impairments associated with ADHD.

Pediatricians and other PCCs may want to develop a resource list of local therapists, agencies, and other mental health clinicians who can treat these impairments. Clinicians might request references from other parents of children with ADHD, professional organizations (eg, the Association for Behavioral and Cognitive Therapies), and ADHD advocacy organizations (eg, CHADD). Parents who have read authoritatively written books about psychosocial treatment may be in a better position to know what they are looking for in a therapist. Some of these resources are available in the ADHD Toolkit[225] and in *ADHD: What Every Parent Needs to Know*[226] as well as other online sources.[226,234–236] Unfortunately, lack of insurance coverage, availability, and accessibility of effective services may limit the implementation of this process (see Systemic Barriers to the Care of Children and Adolescents with ADHD section in the Supplemental Information for further discussion).

Treatment: Collaborate With School to Enhance Support and Services

School-based approaches have demonstrated both short- and long-term benefits for at least 1 year beyond treatment.[95,97] Schools can implement behavioral or training interventions that directly target ADHD symptoms and interventions to enhance academic and social functioning. Schools may use strategies to enhance communication with families, such as daily behavior report cards. All schools should have specialists (eg, school psychologists, counselors, special educators) who can observe the child or adolescent, identify triggers and reinforcers, and support teachers in improving the classroom environment. School specialists can recommend accommodations to address ADHD symptoms, such as untimed testing, testing in less distracting environments, and routine reminders. As children and adolescents get older, their executive functioning skills continue developing. Thus, their delays may decrease, and they may no longer need the accommodations. Alternatively, further intervention may be indicated to facilitate the development of these independent skills.

It is helpful for PCCs to be aware of the eligibility criteria for 504 Rehabilitation Act and the IDEA support in their state and local school districts.[143] It is helpful to understand the process for referral and the specific individuals to contact about these issues. Providing this information to parents will support their efforts to secure classroom adaptations for their child or adolescent, including the use of empirically supported academic interventions to address the achievement difficulties that are often associated with ADHD symptoms.

Educate Parents About School Services

School is often the place where many problems of a child or adolescent with ADHD occur. Although services are available through special education, IDEA, and Section 504 plans, classroom teachers can help students with ADHD. Students with ADHD are most likely to succeed in effectively managed classrooms in which teachers provide engaging instruction, support their students, and implement rules consistently. School staff can sometimes consult with classroom teachers to help them improve their skills in these areas. In many schools, parents can ask the principal for a specific teacher for their child the following academic year.

In some schools, teachers may implement activities to help a student before he or she is considered for special services, including a daily report card, organization interventions, behavioral point systems, and coordinating with the parents, such as using Web sites or portal systems for communication. Individualized behavioral interventions, if implemented well and consistently, are some of the most effective interventions for children with ADHD. In addition to individualized interventions, encouraging parents to increase communication with the teacher can help parents reinforce desirable behavior at school.

If these approaches are not adequate or teachers are unwilling to provide them, parents can be encouraged to write to the principal or the director of special education requesting an evaluation for special education services. An evaluation from a PCC can help this evaluation process but is unlikely to replace it. A child who has an ADHD diagnosis may be eligible for special education services in the category of "other health impaired." Depending on the specific nature of a child's impairment at school, he or she may be eligible for the categories of "emotional and behavioral disorders" or "specific learning disability." The category of eligibility does not affect the services available to the child but usually reflect the nature of the problems that resulted in his or her eligibility for special education services.

Although a PCC may recommend that a child is eligible for special education and specific services, these are only recommendations, as specific evaluation procedures and criteria for eligibility are determined by each school district within federal guidelines. If the ADHD is severe and interfering with school performance, services are usually provided under the other health impaired category. It is important for PCCs to avoid using language in the report that could alienate people in the school or create conflict between the parents and school staff. After school staff complete the evaluation, a meeting will be held to review the results of all evaluation information (including the PCC report) and determine the student's eligibility for an IEP or a 504 plan. If they wish, the parents may invite others to attend the meeting. Some communities have individuals who are trained to help parents effectively advocate for services; being aware of existing resources, if they exist, can help the PCC refer parents to them. Additional details about eligibility are usually available on the Web sites of the school district and the state department of education.

A PCC can help educate the parents about the types of services they can request at the meeting. There are generally 2 categories of services. Some of the most common services are often referred to as accommodations, including extending time on tests, reducing homework, or providing a child with class notes from the teacher or a peer. These services reduce the expectations for a child and can quickly eliminate school problems. For example, if a child is failing classes because he or she is not completing homework and the teacher stops assigning the child homework, then the child's grade in the class is likely to improve quickly. Similarly, parent-child conflict regarding homework will quickly cease. Although these outcomes are desirable, if discontinuing the expectation for completing homework results does not help improve the student's ability to independently complete tasks outside school, which is an important life skill, it may not be beneficial. Although appealing, these services may not improve and in some cases may decrease the child's long-term competencies. They need to be considered with this in mind.

The second set of services consists of interventions that enhance the student's competencies. These take much more work to implement than the services described above and do not solve the problem nearly as quickly. Although appealing, these services may decrease the child's long-term competencies if they are not combined with interventions that are aimed at improving the student's skills and behaviors. Accommodations need to be considered with this broader context in mind. The advantage of interventions is that many students improve their competencies and become able to independently meet age-appropriate expectations over time (for more information on this approach, see information on the Life Course Model[237]).[238] Interventions include organization interventions, daily report cards, and training study skills. The following school-based interventions have been found to be effective in improving academic and interpersonal skills for students with ADHD: Challenging Horizons Program,[95] Child Life and Attention Skills Program,[239] and Homework and Organization Planning Skills.[96] If these are available in area schools, it is important to encourage their use.

V. AGE-RELATED ISSUES

V a. Preschool-Aged Children (Age 4 Years to the Sixth Birthday)

Clinicians can initiate treatment of preschool-aged children with ADHD (ie, children age 4 years to the sixth birthday) with PTBM training and assess for other developmental problems, especially with language. If children continue to have moderate-to-severe dysfunction, the PCC needs to reevaluate the extent to which the parents can implement the therapy; the PCC can also consider prescribing methylphenidate, as described previously. Titration should start with a small dose of immediate-release methylphenidate because preschool-aged children metabolize medication at a slower rate. They have shown lower optimal milligrams-per-kilogram daily doses than older children and may be more sensitive to emotional side effects such as irritability and crying.[83,98]

Currently, dextroamphetamine is the only FDA-approved ADHD medication to treat preschool-aged children. However, when dextroamphetamine received FDA approval, the criteria were less stringent than they are now, so there is only sparse evidence to support its safety and efficacy in this age group. There is more abundant evidence that methylphenidate is safe and efficacious for preschool-aged children with ADHD. For this reason, methylphenidate is the first-line recommended ADHD medication treatment of this age group despite not having FDA approval.[28]

The Preschool ADHD Treatment Study,[83] the landmark trial documenting methylphenidate's safety and efficacy in this age group, included children with moderate-to-severe dysfunction. Therefore, the recommendation for methylphenidate treatment is reserved for children with significant, rather than mild, ADHD-related impairment. In the Preschool ADHD Treatment Study trial, moderate-to-severe impairment was defined as having symptoms present for at least 9 months and clear impairment in both the home and child care and/or preschool settings that did not respond to an appropriate intervention.

There is limited published evidence of the safety and efficacy for the preschool-aged group of atomoxetine, extended-release guanfacine, or extended-release clonidine. None of these nonstimulant medications have FDA approval for this age group.[47]

V b. Adolescents (Age 12 Years to the 18th Birthday)

Pediatricians and other PCCs may increase medication adherence and engagement in the treatment process by closely involving adolescents (age 12 years to the 18th birthday) in medication treatment decisions. Collaborating with the adolescent to determine if the medication is beneficial can help align outcome measures with the adolescent's own goals. Special attention ought to be paid to provide medication coverage at times when the adolescent may exhibit risky behaviors, such as when he or she is driving or spending unsupervised time with friends. Longer-acting or late-afternoon administration of nonstimulant medications or short-acting medications may be helpful.

If pediatricians and other PCCs begin transitioning children to be increasingly responsible for treatment decisions during early adolescence, then transitioning to a primary care physician who specializes in care for adults will be a natural continuation of that process when the adolescent reaches the highest grades in high school. Preparation for the transition to adulthood is an important step that includes planning for transferring care, adapting treatment to new activities and schedules, and educating the patient about effective ways to obtain insurance and engage in services.

Counseling for adolescents around medication issues needs to include dealing with resistance to treatment and empowering the patient to take charge of and own his or her medication management as much as possible. Techniques of motivational interviewing may be useful in improving adherence.[240]

In addition to the numerous developmental changes encountered when working with adolescents, PCCs should assess adolescent patients with ADHD for symptoms of substance use or abuse before beginning medication treatment. If substance use is revealed, the patient should stop the use. Referral for treatment of substance use must be provided before beginning treatment of ADHD (see the clinical practice guideline). Pediatricians and other PCCs should pay careful attention to potential substance use and misuse and diversion of medications. Screening for signs of substance use is important in the care of all adolescents and, depending on the amount of use, may lead a PCC to recommend treatment of substance use. Extensive use or abuse may result in concerns about continuing medication treatment of ADHD until the abuse is resolved. Similar concerns and consideration of discontinuing medication treatment of ADHD could emerge if there is evidence that the adolescent is misusing or diverting medications for other than its intended medical purposes. Pediatricians and other PCCs are encouraged to monitor symptoms and prescription refills for signs of misuse or diversion of ADHD medication. Diversion of ADHD medication is a special concern among adolescents.[132]

When misuse or diversion is a concern, the PCC might consider prescribing nonstimulant medications with much less abuse potential, such as atomoxetine, extended-release guanfacine, or extended-release clonidine. It is more difficult but not impossible to extract the methylphenidate or amphetamine for abuse from the stimulant medications lisdexamfetamine, dermal methylphenidate, and osmotic-release oral system methylphenidate, although these preparations still have some potential for abuse or misuse.

PCCs should be aware that short-acting, mixed amphetamine salts are the most commonly misused or diverted ADHD medication. It is important to note that diversion and misuse of ADHD medications may be committed by individuals who have close contact with or live in the same house as the adolescent, not necessarily by the adolescent him- or herself; this is especially true for college-aged adolescents. Pediatricians and other PCCs are encouraged to discuss safe storage practices, such as lockboxes for controlled substances, when used by college-aged adolescents.

VI. MONITORING

Pediatricians and other PCCs should regularly monitor all aspects of ADHD treatment, including the following:

- systematic reassessment of core symptoms and function;
- regular reassessment of target goals;
- family satisfaction with the care it is receiving from other clinicians and therapists, if applicable;
- provision of anticipatory guidance, further child or adolescent and family education, and transition planning as needed and appropriate;
- occurrence and quality of care coordination to meet the needs of the child or adolescent and family;
- confirmation of adherence to any prescribed medication regimen, with adjustments made as needed;
- HR, BP, height, and weight monitoring; and
- furthering the therapeutic relationship with the child or adolescent and empowering families and children or adolescents to be strong, informed advocates.

Some treatment monitoring can occur during general health care visits if the PCC inquires about the child or adolescent's progress toward target goals, adherence to medication and behavior therapy, concerns, and

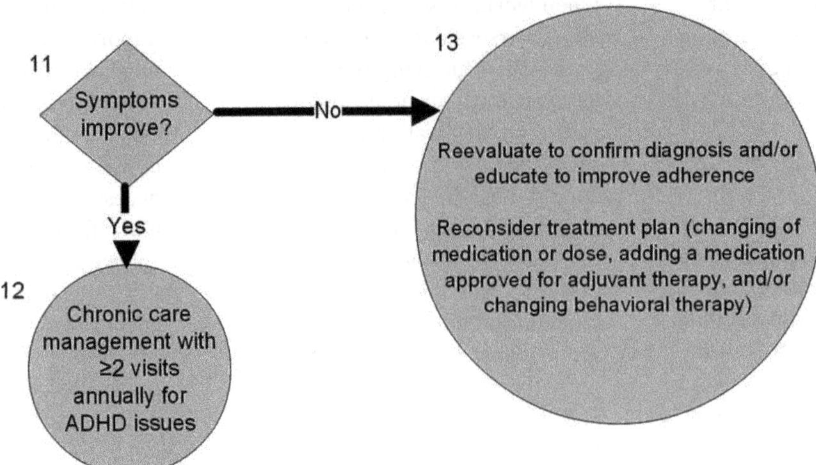

SUPPLEMENTAL FIGURE 8
Monitoring.

changes. This extra time and evaluation effort may generate an evaluate and management (E/M) code along with the well-child care code and may result in an additional cost to the family (see the section on barriers, specifically the compensation section[153]). Monitoring of a child or adolescent with inattention or hyperactivity/impulsivity problems can help to ensure prompt treatment should symptoms worsen to the extent that a diagnosis of ADHD is warranted.

As treatment proceeds, in addition to using a *DSM-5*–based ADHD rating scale to monitor core symptom changes, the PCC can make formal and informal queries in the areas of function most commonly affected by ADHD: academic achievement; peer, parent, or sibling relationships; and risk-taking behavior. Progress can be measured by monitoring the target goals established in collaboration with the child and family. Checklists completed by the school can facilitate medication monitoring. Data from the school, including ADHD symptom ratings completed by the teacher as well as grades and any other formal testing, are helpful at these visits. Screening for substance use and sleep problems is best continued throughout treatment because these problems can emerge at any time. At every visit, it is helpful to gradually further empower children to become full partners in their treatment plan by adolescence.

In the early stages of treatment, after a successful titration period, the frequency of follow-up visits will depend on adherence, coexisting conditions, family willingness, and persistence of symptoms. As noted, a general guide for visits to the PCC is for these visits to occur initially on a monthly basis, then at least quarterly for the first year of treatment. More frequent visits may be necessary if comorbid conditions are present. Visits then need be held preferably quarterly but at least twice each year, with additional phone contact monitoring at the time of medication refill requests. Ongoing communication with the school regarding medication and services is needed.

There is little evidence establishing the optimal, practical follow-up regimen. It is likely that the regimen will need to be tailored to the individual child or adolescent and family needs on the basis of clinical judgment. Follow-up may incorporate electronic collection of rating scales, telehealth, or use of remote monitoring of symptoms and impairment. The time-intensive nature of this process, insurance restrictions, and lack of payment may be significant barriers to adoption (see Systemic Barriers to the Care of Children and Adolescents with ADHD section in the Supplemental Information for more information on this issue).

(See the ADHD guideline's KAS 4.)

VI A. TREATMENT FAILURE

ADHD treatment failure may be a sign of inadequate dosing, lack of patient or family information or compliance, and/or incorrect or incomplete diagnosis. Family conflict and parental psychopathology can also contribute to treatment failure.

In the event of treatment failure, the PCC is advised to repeat the full diagnostic evaluation with increased attention to the possibility of another condition or comorbid conditions that mimic or are associated with ADHD, such as sleep disorders, autism spectrum disorders, or epilepsy (eg, absence epilepsy or partial seizures). Treatment failure may also arise from a new acute stressor or from an unrecognized or underappreciated traumatic event. A coexisting learning disability may cause an apparent treatment failure. In the case of a child or adolescent previously diagnosed with problem-level inattention or hyperactivity, repeating the diagnostic evaluation may result in a diagnosis of ADHD, which would allow for increased school support and the inclusion of medication in the treatment plan. A forthcoming complex ADHD guideline from the SDBP will provide additional information on diagnostic evaluation and treatment of children and adolescents with ADHD treatment failure and/or ADHD that is complicated by coexisting developmental or mental health conditions.

Treatment failure could result from poor adherence to the treatment plan. Increased monitoring and education, especially by including the patient, may increase adherence. It is helpful to try to identify the issues restricting adherence, including lack of information about or understanding of the treatment plan. It is also important to recognize that cultural factors may impact the patient's treatment and outcomes.

If the child continues to struggle despite the school's interventions and treatment of ADHD, further psychoeducational, neuropsychological, and/or language assessments are necessary to evaluate for a learning, language, or processing disorder. The clinician may recommend evaluation by an independent psychologist or neuropsychologist.

VII. CHILDREN AND ADOLESCENTS FOR WHOM AN ADHD DIAGNOSIS IS NOT MADE

If the evaluation identifies or suggests another disorder is the cause of the concerning signs and symptoms, it is appropriate to exit this algorithm.

VII a. Other Condition

The subsequent approach is dictated by the evaluation's results. If the PCC has the expertise and ability to evaluate and treat the other or comorbid condition, he or she may do so. Many collaborative care models exist to help facilitate a pediatrician's comfort with comorbidity, as well as programs that teach pediatricians to manage comorbidities. It is important for the PCC to frame the referral questions clearly if a referral is made. A comanagement plan must be established that addresses the family's and child or adolescent's ongoing needs for education and general and specialty health care. Resources from the AAP Mental Health Initiatives and the forthcoming complex ADHD clinical practice guideline from the SDBP may be helpful.[67,133,241]

VII b. Apparently Typical or Developmental Variation

Evaluation may reveal that the child or adolescent's inattention, activity level, and impulsivity are within the typical range of development, mildly or inconsistently elevated in comparison with his or her peers, or is not associated with any functional impairment in behavior, academics, social skills, or other domains. The clinician can probe further to determine if the parents' concerns are attributable to other issues in the family, such as parental tension or drug use by a family member; whether they are caused by other issues in school, such as social pressures or bullying; or whether they are within the spectrum of typical development.

In talking with parents, it may help to explain that ADHD differs from a condition like pregnancy, which is a "yes" or "no" condition. With ADHD, behaviors follow a spectrum from variations on typical behavior, to atypical behaviors that cause problems but are not severe enough to be considered a disorder, to consistent behaviors that are severe enough to be considered a disorder. With problematic behaviors, it is helpful for the PCC to provide education about both the range of typical development and strategies to improve the child or adolescent's behaviors. A schedule of enhanced surveillance absolves the family of the need to reinitiate contact if the situation deteriorates. If a recommendation for continued routine systematic surveillance is made by the PCC, it is important to provide reassurance that ongoing concerns can be revisited at future primary care visits.

VII c. Children and Adolescents With Inattention or Hyperactivity/Impulsivity (Problem Level)

Children and adolescents whose symptoms do not meet the criteria for diagnosis of ADHD may still encounter some difficulties or mild impairment in some settings, as described in the *DSM-PC, Child and Adolescent Version*.[49] For these patients, enhanced surveillance is recommended. PCCs are encouraged to provide education for both the patient and his or her family, specifically about triggers for inattention and/or hyperactivity as well as behavior management strategies.

Medication is not appropriate for children and adolescents whose symptoms do not meet *DSM-5* criteria for diagnosis of ADHD, but PTBM does not require a diagnosis of ADHD to be recommended.

VIII. COMPLEMENTARY AND ALTERNATIVE THERAPIES AND/OR INTEGRATIVE MEDICINE

Families of children and adolescents with ADHD increasingly ask their pediatrician and other PCCs about complementary and alternative therapies. These include megavitamins and other dietary alterations, vision and/or visual training, chelation, EEG biofeedback, and working memory (eg, cognitive training) programs.[242] As noted, there is insufficient evidence to suggest that these therapies lead to changes in ADHD's core symptoms or function.

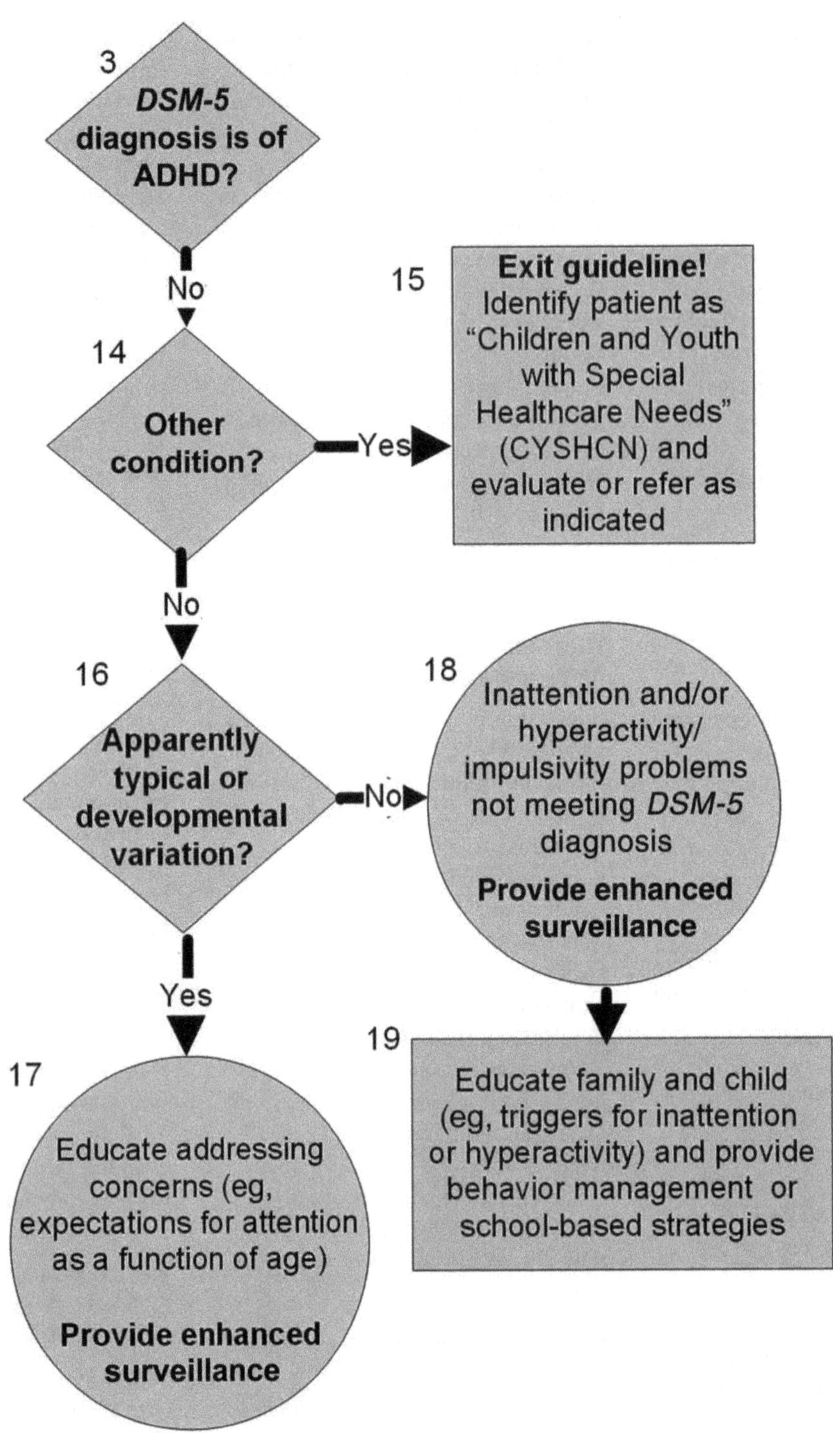

SUPPLEMENTAL FIGURE 9

Children and adolescents for whom an ADHD diagnosis is not made. CYSHCN, children and youth with special health care needs.

For many complementary and alternative therapies, limited information is available about their safety. Both chelation and megavitamins have been proven to cause adverse effects and are contraindicated.[243,244] For these reasons, complementary and alternative therapies are not recommended.

Pediatricians and other PCCs can play a constructive role in helping families make thoughtful treatment choices by reviewing the goals and/or effects claimed for a given treatment, the state of evidence to support or discourage use of the treatment, and known or potential adverse effects. If families are interested in trying complementary and alternative treatments, it is helpful to have them define specific measurable goals to monitor the treatment's impact. Families also need to be strongly encouraged to use evidence-based interventions while they explore complementary and alternative treatments. PCCs have to respect families' interests and preferences while they address and answer questions about complementary and alternative therapies.

Pediatricians and other PCCs should ask about additional therapies that families may be administering to adequately monitor for drug interactions. Parents and children or adolescents who do not feel that their choices in health care are respected by their PCCs may be less likely to communicate about complementary or alternative therapies and/or integrative medicine.

IX. IMPLEMENTATION ISSUES: PREPARING THE PRACTICE

Implementation of the process described in this algorithm can be enhanced with preparation of the practice to meet the needs of children and adolescents with ADHD. This preparation includes both internal practice characteristics and relationships within the community. (More detail can be found in the AAP Mental Health Initiatives' resources.[133,245])

The following office procedures and resources will help practices facilitate the steps in this algorithm:

- developing a packet of ADHD questionnaires and rating scales for parents and teachers to complete before a scheduled visit;
- allotting adequate time for ADHD-related visits;
- determining billing and documentation procedures and monitoring insurance payments to appropriately capture the services rendered to the extent possible;
- implementing methods to track and follow patients (see Systemic Barriers to the Care of Children and Adolescents with ADHD section in the Supplemental Information for more information on this issue);
- asking questions during all clinical encounters and promoting patient education materials (ie, brochures and posters) that alert parents and patients that appropriate issues to discuss with the PCC include problem behaviors, school problems, and concerns about attention and hyperactivity;
- developing an office system for monitoring and titrating medication, including communication with parents and teachers. For stimulant medications, which are controlled substances requiring new, monthly prescriptions, it is necessary to develop a monitoring and refill process including periodic review of the state's database of controlled substance prescriptions (any such system is based on the PCC's assessment of family organization, phone access, and parent-teacher communication effectiveness); and
- using the ADHD Toolkit resources.

Establishing relations with schools and other agencies can facilitate communication and establish clear expectations when collaborating on care for a child. A community-level system that reflects consensus among district school staff and local PCCs for key elements of diagnosis, interventions, and ongoing communication can help to provide consistent, well-coordinated, and cost-effective care. A community-based system with schools relieves the individual PCC from negotiating with each school about care and communication regarding each patient. Offices that have incorporated medical home principles are ideal for establishing this kind of community-level system. Although achieving the level of coordination described below is ideal and takes consistent effort over the years, especially in areas with multiple separate school systems, some aspects may be achieved relatively quickly and will enhance services for children.

The key elements for a community-based collaborative system include consensus on the following:

- a clear and organized process by which an evaluation can be initiated when concerns are identified either by parents or school personnel;
- a packet of information completed by parents and teachers about each child and/or adolescent referred to the PCC;
- a contact person at the practice to receive information from parents and teachers at the time of evaluation and during follow-up;
- an assessment process to investigate coexisting conditions;
- a directory of evidence-based interventions available in the community;
- an ongoing process for follow-up visits, phone calls, teacher reports, and medication refills;
- availability of forms for collecting and exchanging information;
- a plan for keeping school staff and PCCs up to date on the process; and
- awareness of the network of mental health providers in your area and establishments of collaborative relationships with them.

The PCC may face challenges to developing such a collaborative process. For example, a PCC is typically caring for children from more than 1 school system, a school system may be large and not easily accessed, schools may have limited staff and resources to complete assessments, or scheduling may make it difficult for the PCC to communicate with school personnel. Further complicating these efforts is the fact that many providers encounter a lack of recognition and payment for the time involved in coordinating care. These barriers may hamper efforts to provide the internal resources within a practice and coordination across schools and other providers that are described above; nevertheless, some pediatricians and other PCCs have found ways to lessen some of these obstacles (see Systemic Barriers to the Care of Children and Adolescents with ADHD section in the Supplemental Information for more information on overcoming challenges).

In the case of multiple or large school systems in a community, the PCC may want to begin with 1 school psychologist or principal, or several practices can initiate contact collectively with a community school system. Agreement among the clinicians on the components of a good evaluation process facilitates cooperation and communication with the school toward common goals. Agreement on behavior rating scales used can facilitate completion by school personnel. Standard communication forms that monitor progress and specific interventions can be exchanged among the school and the pediatric office to share information. Collaborative systems can extend to other providers who may comanage care with a PCC. Such providers may include a mental health professional who sees the child or adolescent for psychosocial interventions or a specialist to address difficult cases, such as a developmental-behavioral pediatrician, child and adolescent psychiatrist, child neurologist, neurodevelopmental disability physician, or psychologist. The AAP Mental Health Initiatives provide a full discussion of collaborative relationships with mental health professionals, including colocation and integrated models, in its Chapter Action Kit and PediaLink Module.[133,241]

Achieving this infrastructure in the practice and the coordination across schools and other providers will enhance the PCC's ability to implement the treatment guidelines and this algorithm. Achieving these ideals is not necessary for providing care consistent with these practices, however.

X. CONCLUSIONS

ADHD is the most common neurobiological disorder of children and adolescents. Untreated or undertreated ADHD can have far-reaching and serious consequences for the child or adolescent's health and well-being. Fortunately, effective treatments are available, as are methods for assessing and diagnosing ADHD in children and adolescents. The AAP is committed to supporting primary care physicians in providing quality care to children and adolescents with ADHD and their families. This algorithm represents a portion of that commitment and an effort to assist pediatricians and other PCCs to deliver care that meets the quality goals of the practice guideline. This PoCA, in combination with the guideline and Systemic Barriers to the Care of Children and Adolescents With ADHD section below, is intended to provide support and guidance in what is currently the best evidence-based care for their patients with ADHD. Additional support and guidance can be obtained through the work and publications of the AAP Mental Health Initiatives.[133,241]

BARRIERS

SYSTEMIC BARRIERS TO THE CARE OF CHILDREN AND ADOLESCENTS WITH ADHD

INTRODUCTION

The AAP strives to improve the quality of care provided by PCCs through quality improvement initiatives including developing, promulgating, and regularly revising evidence-based clinical practice guidelines. The AAP has published a revision to its 2011 guideline on evaluating, diagnosing, and treating ADHD on the basis of the latest scientific evidence (see main article). This latest revision of the clinical practice guideline is accompanied by a PoCA (also found in the Supplemental Information), which outlines the applicable diagnostic and treatment processes needed to implement the guidelines. This section, which is a companion to the clinical guideline and PoCA, outlines common barriers that impede ADHD care and provides suggested strategies for clinicians seeking to improve care for children and adolescents with ADHD and work with other concerned public and private organizations, health care payers, government entities, state insurance regulators, and other stakeholders.

ADHD is the most common childhood neurobehavioral disorder in the United States and the second most commonly diagnosed childhood condition after asthma.[246] The *DSM-5* criteria define 4 dimensions of ADHD:

1. ADHD/I (314.00 [F90.0]);
2. ADHD/HI (314.01 [F90.1]);
3. ADHD/C (314.01 [F90.2]); and
4. ADHD other specified and unspecified ADHD (314.01 [F90.8]).

National survey data from 2016 reveal that 9.4% of 2- to 17-year-old US children received an ADHD diagnosis during childhood, and 8.4% currently have ADHD.[247] Prevalence estimates from community-based samples are somewhat higher, ranging from 8.7% to 15.5%.[9,10] Most children with ADHD (67%) had at least 1 other comorbidity, and 18% had 3 or more comorbidities, such as mental health disorders and/or learning disorders. These comorbidities increase the complexity of the diagnostic and treatment processes.[66]

The majority of care for children and adolescents with ADHD is provided by the child's PCC, particularly when the ADHD is uncomplicated in nature. In addition, families typically have a high degree of confidence and trust in pediatricians' ability to provide this professional care. Because of the high prevalence of ADHD in children and adolescents, it is essential that PCCs, particularly pediatricians, be able to diagnose, treat, and coordinate this care or identify an appropriate clinician who can provide this needed care. Despite having a higher prevalence than other conditions that PCCs see and manage, such as urinary tract infections and sports injuries, ADHD is often viewed as different from other pediatric conditions and beyond the purview of primary care. In addition, several barriers to care hamper effective and timely diagnosis and treatment of these children and adolescents and must be addressed and corrected to achieve optimum outcomes for these children.[153] These barriers include the following:

1. limited access to care because of inadequate developmental-behavioral and mental health care training during residencies and other clinical training and shortages of consultant specialists and referral resources;
2. inadequate payment for needed services and payer coverage limitations for needed medications;
3. challenges in practice organization and staffing; and
4. fragmentation of care and resulting communication barriers.

Addressing these barriers from a clinical and policy standpoint will enhance clinicians' ability to provide high-quality care for children and adolescents who are being evaluated and/or treated for ADHD. Strategies for improvement in the delivery of care to patients with ADHD and their families are offered for consideration for practice and for advocacy.

BARRIERS TO HIGH-QUALITY CARE FOR CHILDREN AND ADOLESCENTS WITH ADHD

Multiple barriers exist in the primary medical care of children and adolescents that are impediments to excellent ADHD care.

Limited Access to Care Because of Inadequate Developmental-Behavioral and Mental Health Care Training During Pediatric Residency and Other Clinical Training Programs and Shortages of Consultant Specialists and Referral Resources

There is an overall lack of adequate pediatric residency and other training programs for pediatric clinicians on developmental-behavioral and mental health conditions, including ADHD. The current curriculum and the nature of pediatric training still focus on the diagnosis and treatment of inpatient and intensive care conditions despite the fact that many primary care pediatricians spend less and less time providing these services, which are increasingly managed by pediatric hospitalists and intensive care specialists. Pediatric and family medicine residents do not receive sufficient training in the diagnosis and treatment of developmental-behavioral and mental health conditions, including ADHD, despite the high frequency in which they will encounter these conditions in their practices.[152,248]

SUPPLEMENTAL TABLE 2 Core Symptoms of ADHD From the *DSM-5*

Inattention Dimension	Hyperactivity-Impulsivity Dimension	
	Hyperactivity	Impulsivity
Careless mistakes	Fidgeting	Blurting answers before questions completed
Difficulty sustaining attention	Unable to stay seated	Difficulty awaiting turn
Seems not to listen	Moving excessively (restless)	Interrupting and/or intruding on others
Fails to finish tasks	Difficulty engaging in leisure activities quietly	—
Difficulty organizing	"On the go"	—
Avoids tasks requiring sustained attention	Talking excessively	—
Loses things	—	—
Easily distracted	—	—
Forgetful	—	—

Adapted from American Psychiatric Association. *Diagnostic and Statistical Manual of Mental Disorders. 5th ed.* Washington, DC: American Psychiatric Association; 2000:59–60. —, *not applicable.*

In addition, many experienced pediatric clinicians believe that general pediatric and family medicine residencies do not fully ensure that clinicians who enter primary care practice have the organizational tools to develop, join, or function in medical home settings and address chronic developmental and behavioral conditions like ADHD.[152] The current funding of residency and other training programs for pediatric clinicians and the needs of hospitals tend to limit those aspects of training. The training challenges are subsequently not sufficiently addressed by practicing pediatric and family medicine practitioners, in part because of the limited number and varying quality of continuing medical education (CME) opportunities and quality improvement projects focused on medical home models and/or the chronic care of developmental and behavioral pediatric and mental health conditions.

The lack of training is compounded by the national shortage of child and adolescent psychiatrists and developmental-behavioral pediatricians: the United States has only 8300 child psychiatrists[249] and 662 developmental-behavioral pediatricians.[250] The additional training required for child psychiatry and developmental-behavioral pediatrics certification increases education time and costs yet results in little or no return on this investment in terms of increased compensation for these specialists.[249] Given the high cost of medical school and the increasing educational debt incurred by graduating medical students, physicians lack a financial incentive to add the extra years of training required for these specialties.[251] As a result, there are insufficient numbers of mental health professionals, including child psychiatrists and developmental-behavioral pediatricians, to serve as subspecialty referral options and/or provide PCCs with consultative support to comanage their patients effectively.

The specialist shortage is exacerbated by the geographically skewed distribution of extant child psychiatrists and developmental-behavioral pediatricians who are concentrated in academic medical centers and urban environments. Almost three quarters (74%) of US counties have no child and adolescent psychiatrists; almost half (44%) do not even have any pediatricians.[252] As a result, many PCCs lack an adequate pool of pediatric behavioral and mental health specialists who can accept referrals to treat complicated pediatric ADHD patients and an adequate pool of behavioral therapists to provide evidence-based behavioral interventions. The result is that patients must often travel untenable distances and endure long waits to obtain these specialty services.

Suggested Strategies for Change to Address Limited Access to Care: Policy-Oriented Strategies for Change

- Promote changes in pediatric and family medicine residency curricula to devote more time to developmental, behavioral, learning, and mental health issues with a focus on prevention, early detection, assessment, diagnosis, and treatment. Changes in the national and individual training program requirements and in funding of training should foster practitioners' understanding of the family perspective; promote communication skills, including motivational interviewing; and bolster understanding and readiness in the use of behavioral interventions and medication as treatment options for ADHD.
- Emphasize teaching and practice activities within general pediatric residencies and other clinical training, so pediatricians and other PCCs gain the skills and ability they need to function within a medical home setting.
- Support pediatric primary care mental health specialist certification for advanced practice registered nurses through the

Pediatric Nursing Certification Board to provide advanced practice care to help meet evidence-based needs of children or adolescents with ADHD.

- Encourage the development and maintenance of affordable programs to provide CME and other alternative posttraining learning opportunities on behavioral and developmental health, including ADHD. These opportunities will help stakeholders, including PCCs, mental health clinicians, and educators, become more comfortable in providing such services within the medical home and/or educational settings.
- Develop, implement, and support collaborative care models that facilitate PCCs' rapid access to behavioral and mental health expertise and consultation. Examples include integration (such as collaborative care or colocation), on-call consultation, and support teams such as the Massachusetts Child Psychiatry Access Program,[253] the "Project Teach Initiative" of the New York State Department of Mental Health,[254] and Project Extension for Community Healthcare Outcomes, a collaborative model of medical education and care management that can be targeted to pediatric mental health.[255] In addition, federal funding had provided grants to18 states to develop Child Psychiatry Access Programs through Health Resources and Services Administration's Pediatric Mental Health Care Access Program.[256,257] Promote incentives such as loan forgiveness to encourage medical students to enter the fields of child and adolescent psychiatry and developmental and behavioral pediatrics, particularly for those who are willing to practice in underserved communities.
- Expand posttraining opportunities to include postpediatric portal programs, which provide alternative ways to increase number of child and adolescent psychiatrists.

Inadequate Payment for Needed Services and Payer Coverage Limitations for Needed Medications

Although proper diagnostic and procedure codes currently exist for ADHD care in pediatrics, effective and adequate third-party payment is not guaranteed for any covered services.[258] In addition, many payment mechanisms impede the delivery of comprehensive ADHD care. These impediments include restrictions to medication treatment choices such as step therapy, previous approval, narrow formularies, and frequent formulary changes. Some payers define ADHD as a "mental health problem" and implement a "carve-out" health insurance benefit that bars PCCs from participation.[259] This designation results in denial of coverage for primary care ADHD services. Some payers have restrictive service and/or medication approval practices that prevent patients from receiving or continuing needed care and treatment. Examples include approval of only a limited number of specialist visits, limited ADHD medication options, mandatory step therapy, frequent formulary changes resulting in clinical destabilization, and disproportionally high out-of-pocket copays for mental health care or psychotropic medications.

Payments for mental health and cognitive services are frequently lower than equivalents (by relative value unit measurement) paid for physical health care services, particularly those entailing specific procedures.[258] Longer and more frequent visits are often necessary to successfully address ADHD, yet time-based billing yields lower payment compared to multiple shorter visits. These difficulties financially limit a practice's ability to provide these needed services. Payments for E/M codes for chronic care are often insufficient to cover the staff and clinician time needed to provide adequate care. Furthermore, many payers deny payment for the use of rating scales, which are the currently recommended method for monitoring ADHD patients. The use of rating scales takes both the PCC's time and the practice's organizational resources. Arbitrary denial of payment is a disincentive to the provisions of this essential and appropriate service.

Finally, payers commonly decline to pay or provide inadequate payment for care coordination services. Yet, office staff and clinicians are asked to spend large amounts of uncompensated time on these activities, including communicating with parents, teachers, and other stakeholders. Proposed new practice structures such as accountable care organizations (ACOs) are predicated on value-based services and may provide new financial mechanisms to support expanded care coordination services. Originally implemented for Medicare, all-payer ACO models are under development in many states. To date, however, the specifics of these ACO models have not been delineated, and their effectiveness has not yet been documented.[260]

The seemingly arbitrary and ever-changing standards for approval of services; the time-consuming nature of previous approval procedures; and restrictive, opaque pharmacy rules combine to create substantial barriers that result in many PCCs declining to care for children and adolescents with ADHD.[252] According to a recent AAP Periodic Survey of Fellows, 41% of pediatricians reported that "inadequate reimbursement is a major barrier to providing mental health counseling."[258] Of note, 46% reported that they would be interested in hiring mental health clinicians in their practice "if payment and financial resources were not an issue."[258]

Payers' practices regarding medication approval also create challenges for treating pediatric ADHD. In conflict with best-practice or evidence-based guidelines, payers commonly favor 1 ADHD medication and refuse to approve others, even when the latter may be more appropriate for a specific patient. Decisions seem to be made on cost, which at times can be variable. Certain drugs may be allowed only after review processes; others are refused for poorly delineated reasons. Reviewers of insurance denial appeals often lack pediatric experience and are unfamiliar with the effect of the patient's coexisting condition(s) or developmental stage on the medication choice. Step therapy protocols that require specific medications at treatment initiation may require patients to undergo time-consuming treatment failures before an effective therapy can be started. Changes to formularies may force medication changes on patients whose ADHD had been well-controlled, leading to morbidity or delays in finding alternative covered medications that might be equally effective in restoring clinical control.

Similarly, payers may inappropriately insist that a newer replacement drug be used in a patient whose ADHD has been well-controlled by another drug of the same or similar class. The assumption that generic psychoactive preparations are equal to brand-name compounds in efficacy and duration of action is not always accurate.[261] Although generic substitution is generally appropriate, a change in a patient's response may necessitate return to the nongeneric formulation. In addition, because of the variation in covered medications across insurance companies, when a family changes health plans, clinicians have to spend more time to clarify treatments and reduce family stress and their economic burden.

Suggested Strategies for Change to Address Inadequate Payment and Payer Coverage Limitations: Policy-Oriented Strategies

- Revise payment systems to reflect the time and cognitive effort required by primary care, developmental-behavioral, and mental health clinicians to diagnose, treat, and manage pediatric ADHD and compensate these services at levels that incentivize and support their use.
- Support innovative partnerships between payers and clinicians to facilitate high-quality ADHD care. As new payment models are proposed, include input from practicing clinicians to inform insurance plans' understanding of the resources needed to provide comprehensive ADHD care.
- Require that payers' medical directors who review pediatric ADHD protocols and medication formularies either have pediatric expertise or seek such expertise before making decisions that affect the management of pediatric patients with ADHD.
- Advocate that health care payers' rules for approval of developmental-behavioral and mental health care services and medications are consistent with best-practice recommendations based on scientific evidence such as the AAP ADHD guideline. Payers should not use arbitrary step-based medication approval practices or force changes to a patient's stable and effective medication plans because of cost-based formulary changes.
- Advocate for better monitoring by the FDA of ADHD medication generic formulations to verify their equivalency to brand-name preparations in terms of potency and delivery.
- Partner with CHADD and other parent support groups to help advocate for positive changes in payers' rules; these organizations provide a strong voice from families who face the challenges on a day-to-day basis.

Challenges in Practice Organization

ADHD is a chronic condition. Comprehensive ADHD care requires additional clinician time for complex visits, consultation and communication with care team members, and extended staff time to coordinate delivery of chronic care. Children and adolescents with ADHD have a special health care condition and should be cared for in a manner similar to that of other children and youth with special health care needs.[262] Such care is ideally delivered by practices that are established as patient- and family-centered medical homes. Yet, the number of patient- and family-centered medical homes is insufficient to meet the needs of many children with ADHD and their families. Pediatricians and other PCCs who have not adopted a patient- and family-centered medical home model may benefit from the use of similar systems to facilitate ADHD management. For more information, see the recommendations and descriptions from the AAP and the American Academy of Family Medicine regarding medical homes.[262]

Caring for children and adolescents with ADHD requires practices to modify office systems to address their patients' mental health care needs. Specifically, practices need to be familiar with local area mental health referral options, where available, and communicate these options to families. Once a referral has been made, the office flow needs to support communication with other ADHD care team members.[263] Other team members, especially those in mental health, need to formally communicate with the referring clinician in a bidirectional process.

Making a referral does not always mean that the patient is able to access care, however. Practices need to consider that many families face difficulties in following through with referrals for ADHD diagnosis and treatment. These difficulties may arise for a variety of reasons, including lack of insurance coverage, lengthy wait lists for mental health providers, transportation difficulties, reluctance to engage with an unfamiliar care system, cultural factors, and/or the perceived stigma of receiving mental health–specific services.[145,146,155,158]

Many of these barriers can be addressed by the integration of mental health services within primary care practices and other innovative collaborative care models. These models can help increase the opportunities for families to receive care in a familiar and accessible location and provide a "warm hand off" of the patient into the mental health arena. The implementation of these models can be hindered by cost; collaboration with mental health agencies may be fruitful.

Another challenge is the difficulty in determining which mental health subspecialists use evidence-based treatments for ADHD. Pediatricians and other PCCs can increase the likelihood that families receive evidence-based services by establishing a referral network of clinicians who are known to use evidence-based practices and educating parents about effective psychosocial treatments for children and adolescents to help them be wise consumers. It is also important to be cognizant of the fact that for some families, accessing these services may present challenges, such as the need to take time off from work or cover any program costs.

Finding professionals who use evidence-based treatments is of the utmost importance, because exposure to non–evidence-based treatments has the potential to harm patients in several ways. First, the treatment is less likely to be effective and may be harmful (eg, adverse events can and do occur in psychosocial treatments).[264] Second, the effort and money spent on ineffective treatment interferes with the ability to meaningfully engage in evidence-based treatments. Finally, when a treatment does not yield benefits, families are likely to become disillusioned with psychosocial treatments generally, even those that are evidence-based, decreasing the likelihood of future engagement. Each of these harms may place the child at greater risk of problematic outcomes over time.

Suggested Strategies to Address Challenges in Practice Organization

Clinician-Focused Implementation Strategies

- Develop ADHD-specific office workflows, as detailed in the Preparing the Practice section of the PoCA (see Supplemental Information).
- Ensure that the practice is welcoming and inclusive to patients and families of all backgrounds and cultures.
- Enable office systems to support communication with parents, education professionals, and mental health specialists, possibly through electronic communication systems (discussed below).
- Consider office certification as a patient- and family-centered medical home.
- If certification as a patient- and family-centered medical home is not feasible, implement medical home policies and procedures, including care conferences and management. Explore care management opportunities, including adequate resourcing and payment, with third-party payers.
- Identify and establish relationships with mental health consultation and referral sources in the community and within region, if available, and investigate integration of services as well as the resources to support them.
- Promote communication between ADHD care team members by integrating health and mental health services and using collaborative care model treatments when possible.
- Be aware of the community mental health crisis providers' referral processes and be prepared to educate families about evidence-based psychosocial treatments for ADHD across the life span.

Policy-Oriented Suggested Strategies

- Encourage efforts to support the development and maintenance of patient- and family-centered medical homes or related systems to enable patients with chronic complex disorders to receive comprehensive care.
- Support streamlined, coordinated ADHD care across systems by providing incentives for the integration of health and mental health services and collaborative care models.

Fragmentation of Care and Resulting Communication Barriers

Multiple team members provide care for children and adolescents with ADHD, including those in the fields of physical health, mental health, and education. Each of these systems has its own professional standards and terminologies, environments, and hierarchical systems. Moreover, they protect communication via different privacy rules: the Health Insurance Portability and Accountability Act (HIPAA)[265] for the physical and mental health systems and the Family Educational Rights and Privacy Act (FERPA)[266] for the education system. These factors complicate communication not only within but also across these fields. The lack of communication interferes with clinicians' abilities to make accurate diagnoses of ADHD and co-occurring conditions, monitor progress in symptom reduction when providing treatment, identify patient resources, and coordinate the most effective services for children and adolescents with ADHD.

Electronic systems can help address these communication barriers by facilitating asynchronous communication among stakeholders. This is particularly useful for disparate stakeholders, such as parents, teachers, and clinicians, who often cannot all be available simultaneously for a telephone or in-person conference. Electronic systems can also facilitate the timely completion and submission of standardized ADHD rating scales, which are the best tools to assess and treat the condition.[267] Because implementation of electronic systems lies partially within the PCC's control, additional information is provided below on the strengths and weaknesses of a variety of such systems, including telemedicine.

Stand-alone Software Platforms and EHRs

Stand-alone software platforms and EHRs have the potential to improve communication and care coordination among ADHD care team members. Commercially available stand-alone software platforms typically use electronic survey interfaces (either Web or mobile) to collect rating data from parents and teachers, use algorithms to score the data, and display the results cross-sectionally or longitudinally for the clinician's review. Advantages of stand-alone platforms include the fact that they are designed specifically for ADHD care and can be accessed via the Internet through computers and mobile devices. Once implemented, these user-friendly systems allow parents, teachers, and practitioners from multiple disciplines or practices to conveniently complete rating scales remotely. Stand-alone platforms also offer the ability to customize rating scales and their frequency of use for individual patients. Submitted data are stored automatically in a database, mitigating the transcription errors that are often associated with manual data entry. Data are available for clinical care, quality improvement, or research, including quality metrics.

A substantial downside to stand-alone ADHD care systems is the lack of data integration into EHRs. Practitioners must log in to disparate systems for different facets of patient care: the stand-alone system to track ADHD symptoms and the EHR to track medications records, visit notes, and patient or family phone calls. To achieve data accuracy in the 2 different systems, the practitioner must copy medication information from the EHR into the stand-alone system and ADHD symptom and adverse effect ratings from the stand-alone system into the EHR. In addition, stand-alone systems require clinicians to log in before each visit to review the relevant ADHD care data. Patients may use a variety of ADHD stand-alone tracking systems, requiring the PCC to remember several accounts and passwords in addition to his or her own office and hospital EHR systems, creating an added burden that may reduce enthusiasm for such platforms. Finally, stand-alone systems typically charge fees to support the maintenance of servers, cybersecurity, and technical and customer support functionalities.

An issue over which the PCC has little control is the fact that other stakeholders may use stand-alone systems inconsistently. Parents (who may themselves have ADHD) must log in to the platform and complete the requisite ADHD rating scales. Teachers may be required to log in and complete the evaluation process, often for several students, on top of their other obligations. The fact that different pediatricians may use different systems, each with their own log-in and interface, adds to the activity's complexity, particularly for teachers who need to report on multiple students to a variety of PCCs.

EHRs for ADHD Management

EHRs can be adapted to improve the timely collection of parent and teacher ratings of ADHD symptoms, impairment, and medication adverse effects. Some EHRs use an electronic survey functionality or patient portal, similar to that provided by ADHD care stand-alone systems, to allow parents' access to online rating scales. A clear advantage of these EHR systems is that they increase the ability to access documentation about an individual patient's past treatment modalities and medications in the same place as information about his or her ADHD symptoms. The functionality of these EHRs may facilitate other care-related activities, including evidence-based decision support, quality improvement efforts, and outcomes reporting.[268]

Despite these benefits, there are numerous limitations to managing ADHD care with EHRs. First, health care systems' confidentiality barriers often prevent teachers from entering ratings directly into the child's medical record. The large number and heterogeneity of EHR systems and their lack of interoperability are additional barriers to their use for ADHD care.[269] Even when institutions use the same vendor's EHR, exchanging respective ADHD documentation among a variety of clinicians and therapists is frequently impossible.[270] The inability to share information and the lack of interoperability often results in incomplete information in the EHR about a given patient's interventions, symptoms, impairments, and adverse effects over time. Systems for tracking and comparing these aspects of a patient's care are not standard for most EHR packages. The ability to construct templates that are congruent with a clinician's workflow may be limited by the EHR itself. ADHD functionality must often be custom-built for each organization, a cumbersome, expensive, and lengthy process, resulting in lost productivity, clinical effectiveness, and revenue.

General Issues With ADHD Electronic Tracking Systems

EHRs have been linked to increased clinician stress. For this reason, it is important to consider the potential for added burden when either stand-alone or EHR-embedded systems are used to facilitate ADHD care.[271] Although the use of electronic ADHD systems to monitor patients remotely may be advantageous, clinicians and practices may not be equipped or staffed to manage the burden of additional clinical information arriving between visits (ie, intervisit data).

Clinicians must also consider the liability associated with potentially actionable information that families may report electronically without realizing the information might not be reviewed in real time. Examples of such liabilities include a severe medication adverse effect, free-text report of suicidal ideation, and sudden deterioration in ADHD symptoms and/or functioning. In addition, parents and teachers may receive numerous requests to complete rating scales, leading them to experience "survey fatigue" and ignore the requests to complete these scales. Conversely, they may forget how to use the system if they engage with it on an infrequent basis. Some parents or teachers may be uncomfortable using electronic systems and within the medical home might prefer paper rating scales, and others may not have ready access to electronic systems or the Internet.

Telemedicine for ADHD Management

Telemedicine is a new and rapidly growing technology that has the potential, when properly implemented within the medical home, to expand access to care and to improve clinicians' ability to communicate with schools, consultants, care management team members, and especially patients and parents.[213,272,273] Well-run telemedicine programs offer some promise as a way to deliver evidence-based psychosocial treatments, although few evidence-based programs have been tested via telemental health trials.[274,275] Telemedicine is one of the foundations of the new advanced medical home and offers advantages as follows:

- offering communication opportunities (either face-to-face and synchronous as a conversation or asynchronous as messaging), which can be prescheduled to minimize interruption of office flow;
- enabling communication on a one-on-one basis or one-to-many basis (for conference situations);
- replacing repeated office visits for patient follow-up and monitoring, which reduces time and the need for patients to travel to the PCC's office;
- facilitating digital storage of the telemedicine episode and its incorporation into multiple EHR systems as part of the patient record; and
- enhancing cooperation among all parties in the evaluation and treatment processes.

Telemedicine has great potential but needs to be properly implemented and integrated into the practice workflow to achieve maximum effectiveness and flexibility. Although some new state insurance regulations mandate payment for telemedicine services, such mandates have not yet been implemented in all states, limiting telemedicine's utility. Finally, payment for services needs to include the added cost of equipment and staff to provide them.

Suggested Strategies to Address Fragmentation of Care and Resulting Communication Barriers

Clinician-Focused Implementation Strategies

- Ensure the practice is aware of, and in compliance with, HIPAA and FERPA policies, as well as confidentiality laws and cybersecurity safeguards that impact EHRs' communication with school personnel and parents.[276]
- Maintain open lines of communication with all team members involved in the patient's ADHD care within the practical limits of existing systems, time, and economic constraints. As noted,

team members include teachers, other school personnel, clinicians, and mental health practitioners. This activity involves a team-based approach and agreeing on a communication method and process to track ADHD interventions, symptoms, impairments, and adverse effects over time. Communication can be accomplished through a variety of means, including electronic systems, face-to-face meetings, conference calls, emails, and/or faxes.

- Consider using electronic communication via stand-alone ADHD management systems and electronic portals, after evaluating EHR interoperability and other administrative considerations.
- Integrate electronic ADHD systems into the practice's clinical workflow: decide who will review the data and when, how actionable information will be flagged and triaged, how information and related decision-making will be documented in the medical record, etc.
- Set and clarify caregivers' expectations about the practice's review of information provided electronically versus actionable information that should be communicated directly by phone.
- Promote the implementation of telemedicine for ADHD management in states where payment for such services is established; ensure the telemedicine system chosen is patient centered, HIPAA and FERPA compliant, and practice enhancing.

Policy-Oriented Suggested Strategies

- Promote the development of mechanisms for online communication to enhance ADHD care collaboration, including electronic portals and stand-alone ADHD software systems, to serve as communication platforms for families, health professionals, mental health professionals, and educators. Ideally, these portals would be integrated with the most commonly used EHR systems.
- Advocate for regulations that mandate a common standard of interoperability for certified EHR systems. Interoperability facilitates the use of EHRs as a common repository of ADHD care information and communication platform for ADHD care team members.[276]
- Advocate for exceptions to HIPAA and FERPA regulations to allow more communication between education and health and mental health practitioners while maintaining privacy protections.
- Ensure that billing, coding, and payment systems provide adequate resources and time for clinicians to communicate with teachers and mental health clinicians, as discussed previously.
- Provide incentives for integration of health and mental health services, collaborative care models, and telemedicine to facilitate communication among ADHD care team members, including telemedicine services that cross state lines.
- Fund research in telehealth to learn more about who responds well to these approaches and whether telehealth is feasible for underserved populations.

CONCLUSIONS

Appropriate and comprehensive ADHD care requires a well-trained and adequately resourced multidisciplinary workforce, with office workflows that are organized to provide collaborative services that are consistent with a chronic care model and to promote communication among treatment team members.[277-280] Many barriers in the current health care system must be addressed to support this care.

First and foremost, the shortage of clinicians, such as child and adolescent psychiatrists and developmental-behavioral pediatricians who provide consultation and referral ADHD care, must also be addressed. The shortages are driven by the lack of residency and other training programs for pediatric clinicians in the management of ADHD and other behavioral health issues, the lack of return on investment in the additional training and debt required to specialize in this area, and inadequate resourcing at all levels of ADHD care. The shortage is exacerbated by geographic maldistribution of practitioners and lack of adequate mental health training as a whole during residency and in CME projects. These challenges must be addressed on a system-wide level.

A significant review and change in the ADHD care payment for cognitive services is required to ensure that practitioners are backed by appropriate resources that support the provision of high-quality ADHD care. The lack of adequate compensation for ADHD care is a major challenge to reaching children and adolescents with the care they need. Improved payment is a major need to encourage primary care clinicians to train in ADHD subspecialty care and incentivize child and adolescent psychiatry and developmental-behavioral pediatrics practitioners to provide ADHD care in the primary care setting, so the provision of such care does not result in financial hardship for the families or the practice. Improvement should also include changes to payer policies to improve compensation for care coordination services and mental health care.

Because the pediatrician is often the first contact for a parent seeking help for a child with symptoms that may be caused by ADHD, barriers to payment need to be addressed before providing these time-consuming services. Some insurance plans direct all claims with a diagnosis reported by *International Classification of Diseases, 10th Revision, Clinical Modification* codes F01–F99 to their mental and behavioral health benefits system. Because pediatricians are generally not included in networks for mental and behavioral health plans, this can create delays or denials of payment. This is not always the case, though, and with a little preventive footwork, practices can identify policy guidelines for plans that are commonly seen in the practice patient population.

The first step in identifying coverage for services to diagnose or treat ADHD is to determine what payment guidelines have been published by plans that contract with your practice. Many health plans post their payment guidelines on their Web sites, but even when publicly available, the documents do not always clearly address whether payment for primary care diagnosis and management of ADHD are covered. It may be necessary to send a written inquiry to provider relations and the medical director of a plan seeking clarification of what diagnoses and procedure codes should pass through the health benefit plan's adjudication system without denial or crossover to a mental health benefit plan. It is important to recognize that even with documentation that the plan covers primary care services related to ADHD, claims adjudication is an automated process that may erroneously cause denials. Billing and payment reconciliation staff should always refer such denials for appeal.

Once plans that do and do not provide medical benefits for the diagnosis and treatment of ADHD have been identified, advocacy to the medical directors of those plans that do not recognize the role of the medical home in mental health care can be initiated. The AAP template letter, Increasing Access to Mental Health Care, is a resource for this purpose. Practices should also be prepared to offer advance notice to parents when their plan is likely to deny or pay out of network for services. A list of referral sources for mental and behavioral health is also helpful for parents whose financial limitations may require alternative choices and for patients who may require referral for additional evaluation.

For services rendered, identify the codes that represent covered diagnoses and services and be sure that these codes are appropriately linked and reported on claims.

When ADHD is suspected but not yet diagnosed, symptoms such as attention and concentration deficit (R41.840) should be reported. Screening for ADHD in the absence of signs or symptoms may be reported with code Z13.4, encounter for screening for certain developmental disorders in childhood. *Current Procedural Terminology* codes 96110 and 96112 to 96113 should be reported for developmental screening and testing services.

Services related to diagnosis and management of ADHD are more likely to be paid under the patient's medical benefits when codes reported are not those for psychiatric or behavioral health services. Reporting of E/M service codes based on face-to-face time of the visit when more than 50% of that time was spent in counseling or coordination of care will likely be more effective than use of codes such as 90791, psychiatric diagnostic evaluation. *Current Procedural Terminology* E/M service guidelines define counseling as a discussion with a patient or family concerning 1 or more of the following areas:

- diagnostic results, impressions, or recommended diagnostic studies;
- prognosis;
- risks and benefits of management (treatment) options;
- instructions for management (treatment) or follow-up;
- importance of compliance with chosen management (treatment) options;
- risk factor reduction; and
- patient and family education.

Finally, staff should track claim payment trends for services related to ADHD, including the number of claims requiring appeal and status of appeal determinations to inform future advocacy efforts and practice policy.

Many AAP chapters have developed pediatric councils that meet with payers on pediatric coding issues. Sharing your experiences with your chapter pediatric council will assist in its advocacy efforts. AAP members can also report carrier issues on the AAP Hassle Factor Form.

These system-wide barriers are challenging, if not impossible, for individual practitioners to address on their own. Practice organization and communication changes can be made, however, that have the potential to improve access to ADHD care. Clinicians and other practitioners can implement the office work-flow recommendations made in the Preparing the Practice section of the updated PoCA (see Supplemental Information). Implementing a patient- and family-centered medical home model, colocating health and mental health services, and adopting collaborative care models can also help overcome communication barriers and minimize fragmentation of care. It is noted that these models must be adequately resourced to be effective.

Finally, practitioners can implement innovative communication and record-keeping solutions to overcome barriers to ADHD care. Potential solutions could include the use of EHRs, other electronic systems, and high-quality telemedicine to support enhanced communication and record-keeping on the part of myriad ADHD care team members. These solutions can also aid with monitoring treatment responses on the part of the child or adolescent with ADHD. Telemedicine also has the distinct benefit of compensating for the maldistribution of specialists and other clinicians who can treat pediatric ADHD.

Many stakeholders have a role in addressing the barriers that prevent children and adolescents from receiving needed evidenced-based treatment of ADHD. Pediatric councils, the national AAP, and state and local AAP chapters must be advocates for broad changes in training, CME, and payment policies to overcome the systemic challenges that hamper access to care. On an individual level, practitioners can effect change in their own practice systems and professional approaches and implement systems that address fragmentation of care and communication. Practitioners are important agents for change in ADHD care. The day-to-day interactions that practitioners have with patients, families, educators, payers, state insurance regulators, and others can foster comprehensive, contemporary, and effective care that becomes a pillar of advocacy and change.

SUBCOMMITTEE ON CHILDREN AND ADOLESCENTS WITH ATTENTION-DEFICIT/HYPERACTIVITY DISORDER

The Council on Quality Improvement and Patient Safety oversees the Subcommittee

Mark L. Wolraich, MD, FAAP (Chairperson: Section on Developmental Behavioral Pediatrics).

Joseph F. Hagan, Jr, MD, FAAP (Vice Chairperson: Section on Developmental Behavioral Pediatrics).

Carla Allan, PhD (Society of Pediatric Psychology).

Eugenia Chan, MD, MPH, FAAP (Implementation Scientist).

Dale Davison, MSpEd, PCC (Parent Advocate, Children and Adults with ADHD).

Marian Earls, MD, MTS, FAAP (Mental Health Leadership Work Group).

Steven W. Evans, PhD (Clinical Psychologist).

Tanya Froehlich, MD, FAAP (Section on Developmental Behavioral Pediatrics/Society for Developmental and Behavioral Pediatrics).

Jennifer L. Frost, MD, FAAFP (American Academy of Family Physicians).

Herschel R. Lessin, MD, FAAP, Section on Administration and Practice Management).

Karen L. Pierce, MD, DFAACAP (American Academy of Child and Adolescent Psychiatry).

Christoph Ulrich Lehmann, MD, FAAP (Partnership for Policy Implementation).

Jonathan D. Winner, MD, FAAP (Committee on Practice and Ambulatory Medicine).

William Zurhellen, MD, FAAP (Section on Administration and Practice Management).

STAFF

Kymika Okechukwu, MPA, Senior Manager, Evidence-Based Medicine Initiatives

Jeremiah Salmon, MPH, Program Manager, Policy Dissemination and Implementation

CONSULTANT

Susan K. Flinn, MA, Medical Editor

SUPPLEMENTAL REFERENCES

157. Bright Futures Available at: https://brightfutures.aap.org. Accessed September 8, 2019

158. American Academy of Pediatrics. AAP Diversity and Inclusion Statement. *Pediatrics.* 2018;141(4): e20180193

159. Chronis AM, Lahey BB, Pelham WE Jr, Kipp HL, Baumann BL, Lee SS. Psychopathology and substance abuse in parents of young children with attention-deficit/hyperactivity disorder. *J Am Acad Child Adolesc Psychiatry.* 2003;42(12):1424–1432

160. Foy JM, ed. Iterative Mental Health Assessement, Appendix 2: Mental Health Tools for Pediatrics. In: *Mental Health Care of Children and Adolescents: A Guide for Primary Care Clinicians.* Itasca, IL: American Academy of Pediatrics; 2018:817–868

161. Wolraich ML, Bard DE, Neas B, Doffing M, Beck L. The psychometric properties of the Vanderbilt attention-deficit hyperactivity disorder diagnostic teacher rating scale in a community population. *J Dev Behav Pediatr.* 2013;34(2):83–93

162. Bard DE, Wolraich ML, Neas B, Doffing M, Beck L. The psychometric properties of the Vanderbilt attention-deficit hyperactivity disorder diagnostic parent rating scale in a community population. *J Dev Behav Pediatr.* 2013;34(2):72–82

163. Goodman R. The extended version of the Strengths and Difficulties Questionnaire as a guide to child psychiatric caseness and consequent burden. *J Child Psychol Psychiatry.* 1999;40(5):791–799

164. Shaffer D, Gould MS, Brasic J, et al. A children's global assessment scale (CGAS). *Arch Gen Psychiatry.* 1983; 40(11):1228–1231

165. Brown RT, Freeman WS, Perrin JM, et al. Prevalence and assessment of attention-deficit/hyperactivity disorder in primary care settings. *Pediatrics.* 2001;107(3). Available at:

www.pediatrics.org/cgi/content/full/107/3/E43

166. Evans SW, Allen J, Moore S, Strauss V. Measuring symptoms and functioning of youth with ADHD in middle schools. *J Abnorm Child Psychol.* 2005;33(6): 695–706

167. Wolraich ML, Lambert EW, Bickman L, Simmons T, Doffing MA, Worley KA. Assessing the impact of parent and teacher agreement on diagnosing attention-deficit hyperactivity disorder. *J Dev Behav Pediatr.* 2004;25(1):41–47

168. DiPerna JC, Elliott SN. *Academic Competence Evaluation Scales (ACES).* San Antonio, TX: The Psychological Corporation; 2000

169. Smith BH, Pelham WE, Gnagy E, Molina B, Evans S. The reliability, validity, and unique contributions of self-report by adolescents receiving treatment for attention-deficit/hyperactivity disorder. *J Consult Clin Psychol.* 2000; 68(3):489–499

170. Hoza B, Pelham WE Jr, Dobbs J, Owens JS, Pillow DR. Do boys with attention-deficit/hyperactivity disorder have positive illusory self-concepts? *J Abnorm Psychol.* 2002;111(2): 268–278

171. Zuckerbrot RA, Cheung AH, Jensen PS, Stein RE, Laraque D; GLAD-PC Steering Group. Guidelines for adolescent depression in primary care (GLAD-PC): I. Identification, assessment, and initial management. *Pediatrics.* 2007;120(5). Available at: www.pediatrics.org/cgi/content/full/120/5/e1299

172. Cheung AH, Zuckerbrot RA, Jensen PS, Ghalib K, Laraque D, Stein RE; GLAD-PC Steering Group. Guidelines for adolescent depression in primary care (GLAD-PC): II. Treatment and ongoing management. *Pediatrics.* 2007;120(5). Available at: www.pediatrics.org/cgi/content/full/120/5/e1313

173. Foy JM, ed. Low Mood, Appendix 2: Mental Health Tools for Pediatrics. In: *Mental Health Care of Children and Adolescents: A Guide for Primary Care Clinicians.* Itasca, IL: American Academy of Pediatrics; 2018:817–868

174. The Center for Adolescent Substance Use Research, Children's Hospital Boston. *CRAFFT: Screening Adolescents for Alcohol and Drugs.* Boston, MA: Children's Hospital Boston; 2001. Available at: http://www.childrenshospital.org/~/media/microsites/ceasar/2016-2sided-crafft-card_clinician-interview.ashx?la=en. Accessed September 8, 2019

175. Levy S, Weiss R, Sherritt L, et al. An electronic screen for triaging adolescent substance use by risk levels. *JAMA Pediatr.* 2014;168(9): 822–828

176. University of Pittsburgh Child and Adolescent Bipolar Spectrum Services. Instruments: Screen for Child Anxiety Related Emotional Disorders (SCARED). Available at: https://www.pediatricbipolar.pitt.edu/resources/instruments. Accessed September 8, 2019

177. Kovacs M. *CDI 2: Children's Depression Inventory.* 2nd ed. North Tonawanda, NY: Multi-Health Systems Assessments; 2018. Available at: https://www.mhs.com/MHS-Assessment?prodname=cdi2. Accessed September 8, 2019

178. Richardson LP, McCauley E, Grossman DC, et al. Evaluation of the Patient Health Questionnaire-9 Item for detecting major depression among adolescents. *Pediatrics.* 2010;126(6): 1117–1123

179. Sleator EK, Ullmann RK. Can the physician diagnose hyperactivity in the office? *Pediatrics.* 1981;67(1):13–17

180. American Academy of Pediatrics. Fetal alcohol spectrum disorders program: toolkit. Available at: https://www.aap.org/en-us/advocacy-and-policy/aap-health-initiatives/fetal-alcohol-spectrum-disorders-toolkit/Pages/default.aspx. Accessed September 8, 2019

181. Hagan JF Jr, Balachova T, Bertrand J, et al; Neurobehavioral Disorder Associated With Prenatal Alcohol Exposure Workgroup; American Academy of Pediatrics. Neurobehavioral disorder associated with prenatal alcohol exposure. *Pediatrics.* 2016;138(4):e20151553

182. Gardner W, Murphy M, Childs G, et al. The PSC-17: a brief pediatric symptom checklist including psychosocial problem subscales: a report from PROS and ASPN. *Ambul Child Health.* 1999;5:225–236

183. National Institutes of Health. *Screening to Brief Intervention (S2BI).* Bethesda, MD: National Institute on Drug Abuse. Available at: https://www.drugabuse.gov/ast/s2bi/#/. Accessed September 8, 2019

184. Levy SJ, Williams JF; Committee on Substance Use and Prevention. Substance use screening, brief intervention, and referral to treatment. *Pediatrics.* 2016;138(1): e20161211

185. University of Washington Harborview Center for Sexual Assault and Traumatic Stress. Standardized measures. Available at: https://depts.washington.edu/hcsats/PDF/TF-%20CBT/pages/assessment.html. Accessed September 8, 2019

186. Gordon M, Barkley RA, Lovett B. Tests and observational measures. In: Barkley RA, ed. *Attention-Deficit Hyperactivity Disorder Third Edition: A Handbook for Diagnosis and Treatment.* 3rd ed. New York, NY: Guilford Press; 2005:369–388

187. Edwards MC, Gardner ES, Chelonis JJ, Schulz EG, Flake RA, Diaz PF. Estimates of the validity and utility of the Conners' Continuous Performance Test in the assessment of inattentive and/or hyperactive-impulsive behaviors in children. *J Abnorm Child Psychol.* 2007;35(3):393–404

188. Li J, Olsen J, Vestergaard M, Obel C. Attention-deficit/hyperactivity disorder in the offspring following prenatal maternal bereavement: a nationwide follow-up study in Denmark. *Eur Child Adolesc Psychiatry.* 2010;19(10): 747–753

189. Angold A, Erkanli A, Egger HL, Costello EJ. Stimulant treatment for children: a community perspective. *J Am Acad Child Adolesc Psychiatry.* 2000;39(8): 975–984; discussion 984–994

190. Konofal E, Lecendreux M, Cortese S. Sleep and ADHD. *Sleep Med.* 2010; 11(7):652–658

191. Gozal D, Kheirandish-Gozal L. Neurocognitive and behavioral morbidity in children with sleep disorders. *Curr Opin Pulm Med.* 2007; 13(6):505–509

192. Capdevila OS, Kheirandish-Gozal L, Dayyat E, Gozal D. Pediatric obstructive sleep apnea: complications, management, and long-term

outcomes. *Proc Am Thorac Soc.* 2008; 5(2):274–282

193. Cortese S, Konofal E, Lecendreux M, et al. Restless legs syndrome and attention-deficit/hyperactivity disorder: a review of the literature. *Sleep.* 2005;28(8):1007–1013

194. Weiss MD, Wasdell MB, Bomben MM, Rea KJ, Freeman RD. Sleep hygiene and melatonin treatment for children and adolescents with ADHD and initial insomnia. *J Am Acad Child Adolesc Psychiatry.* 2006;45(5):512–519

195. Stein MA, Sarampote CS, Waldman ID, et al. A dose-response study of OROS methylphenidate in children and adolescents with attention-deficit/hyperactivity disorder. *Pediatrics.* 2003;112(5). Available at: www.pediatrics.org/cgi/content/full/112/5/e404

196. Corkum P, Panton R, Ironside S, Macpherson M, Williams T. Acute impact of immediate release methylphenidate administered three times a day on sleep in children with attention-deficit/hyperactivity disorder. *J Pediatr Psychol.* 2008;33(4): 368–379

197. O'Brien LM, Ivanenko A, Crabtree VM, et al. The effect of stimulants on sleep characteristics in children with attention deficit/hyperactivity disorder. *Sleep Med.* 2003;4(4): 309–316

198. Owens J, Sangal RB, Sutton VK, Bakken R, Allen AJ, Kelsey D. Subjective and objective measures of sleep in children with attention-deficit/hyperactivity disorder. *Sleep Med.* 2009;10(4):446–456

199. Owens JA. A clinical overview of sleep and attention-deficit/hyperactivity disorder in children and adolescents. *J Can Acad Child Adolesc Psychiatry.* 2009;18(2):92–102

200. Mick E, Biederman J, Jetton J, Faraone SV. Sleep disturbances associated with attention deficit hyperactivity disorder: the impact of psychiatric comorbidity and pharmacotherapy. *J Child Adolesc Psychopharmacol.* 2000;10(3):223–231

201. van der Heijden KB, Smits MG, van Someren EJ, Boudewijn Gunning W. Prediction of melatonin efficacy by pretreatment dim light melatonin onset in children with idiopathic chronic sleep onset insomnia. *J Sleep Res.* 2005;14(2):187–194

202. Cortese S, Faraone SV, Konofal E, Lecendreux M. Sleep in children with attention-deficit/hyperactivity disorder: meta-analysis of subjective and objective studies. *J Am Acad Child Adolesc Psychiatry.* 2009;48(9):894–908

203. Golan N, Shahar E, Ravid S, Pillar G. Sleep disorders and daytime sleepiness in children with attention-deficit/hyperactive disorder. *Sleep.* 2004;27(2):261–266

204. Lecendreux M, Konofal E, Bouvard M, Falissard B, Mouren-Siméoni MC. Sleep and alertness in children with ADHD. *J Child Psychol Psychiatry.* 2000;41(6): 803–812

205. Owens JA, Dalzell V. Use of the 'BEARS' sleep screening tool in a pediatric residents' continuity clinic: a pilot study. *Sleep Med.* 2005;6(1):63–69

206. Chervin RD, Hedger K, Dillon JE, Pituch KJ. Pediatric sleep questionnaire (PSQ): validity and reliability of scales for sleep-disordered breathing, snoring, sleepiness, and behavioral problems. *Sleep Med.* 2000;1(1):21–32

207. Owens JA, Spirito A, McGuinn M. The Children's Sleep Habits Questionnaire (CSHQ): psychometric properties of a survey instrument for school-aged children. *Sleep.* 2000;23(8):1043–1051

208. Aurora RN, Zak RS, Karippot A, et al; American Academy of Sleep Medicine. Practice parameters for the respiratory indications for polysomnography in children. *Sleep (Basel).* 2011;34(3):379–388

209. Aurora RN, Lamm CI, Zak RS, et al. Practice parameters for the non-respiratory indications for polysomnography and multiple sleep latency testing for children. *Sleep (Basel).* 2012;35(11):1467–1473

210. Gruber R, Wiebe S, Montecalvo L, Brunetti B, Amsel R, Carrier J. Impact of sleep restriction on neurobehavioral functioning of children with attention deficit hyperactivity disorder. *Sleep (Basel).* 2011;34(3):315–323

211. Bunford N, Evans SW, Wymbs F. ADHD and emotion dysregulation among children and adolescents. *Clin Child Fam Psychol Rev.* 2015;18(3):185–217

212. Langberg JM, Vaughn AJ, Brinkman WB, Froehlich T, Epstein JN. Clinical utility of the Vanderbilt ADHD Rating Scale for ruling out comorbid learning disorders. *Pediatrics.* 2010;126(5). Available at: www.pediatrics.org/cgi/content/full/126/5/e1033

213. Kressly SJ. Extending the medical home to meet your patients' mental health needs: is telehealth the answer? *Pediatrics.* 2019;143(3): e20183765

214. Dudek E, Henschen E, Finkle E, Vyas S, Fiszbein D, Shukla A. Improving continuity in a patient centered medical home. *Pediatrics.* 2018;142(1): 366

215. Dessie AS, Hirway P, Gjelsvik A. Children with developmental, behavioral, or emotional problems are less likely to have a medical home. *Pediatrics.* 2018;141(1):23

216. Foy JM. The medical home and integrated behavioral health. *Pediatrics.* 2015;135(5):930–931

217. Ader J, Stille CJ, Keller D, Miller BF, Barr MS, Perrin JM. The medical home and integrated behavioral health: advancing the policy agenda. *Pediatrics.* 2015;135(5):909–917

218. American Academy of Pediatrics. Collaboration in practice: implementing team-based care. *Pediatrics.* 2016;138(2):e20161486

219. Kressley SJ. Team-based care for children: who should be included and who should lead? *AAP News.* July 24, 2017. Available at: https://www.aappublications.org/news/2017/07/24/TeamBased072417. Accessed September 8, 2019

220. Katkin JP, Kressly SJ, Edwards AR, et al; Task Force on Pediatric Practice Change. Guiding principles for team-based pediatric care. *Pediatrics.* 2017; 140(2):e20171489

221. Godoy L, Hodgkinson S, Robertson HA, et al. Increasing mental health engagement from primary care: the potential role of family navigation. *Pediatrics.* 2019;143(4):e20182418

222. Wolraich ML, Hagan JF Jr. *ADHD: What Every Parent Needs to Know.* 3rd ed.

Itasca, IL: American Academy of Pediatrics; 2019. Available at: https://shop.aap.org/adhd-paperback/. Accessed September 8, 2019

223. American Academy of Pediatrics. *Understanding ADHD.* Itasca, IL: American Academy of Pediatrics; 2017. Available at: https://shop.aap.org/understanding-adhd-brochure-50pk-brochure/. Accessed September 8, 2019

224. HealthyChildren.org. ADHD. 2018. Available at: https://www.healthychildren.org/English/health-issues/conditions/adhd/Pages/default.aspx. Accessed September 8, 2019

225. American Academy of Pediatrics. *ADHD Provider Toolkit.* 3rd ed. In production

226. Reiff MI. *ADHD: What Every Parent Needs to Know.* 2nd ed. Elk Grove Village, IL: American Academy of Pediatrics; 2011

227. Charach A, Fernandez R. Enhancing ADHD medication adherence: challenges and opportunities. *Curr Psychiatry Rep.* 2013;15(7):371

228. Greenhill LL, Abikoff HB, Arnold LE, et al. Medication treatment strategies in the MTA Study: relevance to clinicians and researchers. *J Am Acad Child Adolesc Psychiatry.* 1996;35(10):1304–1313

229. Cortese S, Adamo N, Del Giovane C, et al. Comparative efficacy and tolerability of medications for attention-deficit hyperactivity disorder in children, adolescents, and adults: a systematic review and network meta-analysis. *Lancet Psychiatry.* 2018;5(9):727–738

230. Pozzi M, Carnovale C, Peeters GGAM, et al. Adverse drug events related to mood and emotion in paediatric patients treated for ADHD: a meta-analysis. *J Affect Disord.* 2018;238:161–178

231. Robin AL, Foster SL. *Negotiating Parent Adolescent Conflict: A Behavioral-Family Systems Approach.* New York, NY: Guilford Press; 1989

232. Barkley RA, Edwards G, Laneri M, Fletcher K, Metevia L. The efficacy of problem-solving communication training alone, behavior management training alone, and their combination for parent-adolescent conflict in teenagers with ADHD and ODD. *J Consult Clin Psychol.* 2001;69(6):926–941

233. Bloch MH, Qawasmi A. Omega-3 fatty acid supplementation for the treatment of children with attention-deficit/hyperactivity disorder symptomatology: systematic review and meta-analysis. *J Am Acad Child Adolesc Psychiatry.* 2011;50(10):991–1000

234. Understood.org. Get personalized recommendations for you and your child. Available at: https://www.understood.org/en/learning-attention-issues/treatments-approaches/working-with-clinicians. Accessed September 8, 2019

235. ImpactADHD. Free resources for parents. Available at: https://impactadhd.com/resources/free-impactadhd-resources-for-parents/. Accessed September 8, 2019

236. ImpactADHD. ImpactADHD. Available at: https://www.youtube.com/user/ImpactADHD. Accessed September 8, 2019

237. Halfon N, Forrest CB, Lerner RM, Faustman EM. *Handbook of Life Course Health Development.* Cham, Switzerland: Springer; 2018

238. Evans SW, Owens JS, Mautone JA, DuPaul GJ, Power TJ. Toward a comprehensive, Life Course Model of care for youth with ADHD. In: Weist M, Lever N, Bradshaw C, Owens J, eds. *Handbook of School Mental Health.* 2nd ed. New York, NY: Springer; 2014:413–426

239. Pfiffner LJ, Hinshaw SP, Owens E, et al. A two-site randomized clinical trial of integrated psychosocial treatment for ADHD-inattentive type. *J Consult Clin Psychol.* 2014;82(6):1115–1127

240. Charach A, Volpe T, Boydell KM, Gearing RE. A theoretical approach to medication adherence for children and youth with psychiatric disorders. *Harv Rev Psychiatry.* 2008;16(2):126–135

241. Foy JM, ed. *Mental Health Care of Children and Adolescents: A Guide for Primary Care Clinicians.* Itasca, IL: American Academy of Pediatrics; 2018

242. Chan E. Complementary and alternative medicine in developmental-behavioral pediatrics. In: Wolraich ML, Drotar DD, Dworkin PH, Perrin EC, eds. *Developmental-Behavioral Pediatrics: Evidence and Practice.* Philadelphia, PA: Mosby Elsevier; 2008:259–280

243. Chan E. The role of complementary and alternative medicine in attention-deficit hyperactivity disorder. *J Dev Behav Pediatr.* 2002;23(suppl 1):S37–S45

244. James S, Stevenson SW, Silove N, Williams K. Chelation for autism spectrum disorder (ASD). *Cochrane Database Syst Rev.* 2015;(5):CD010766

245. Foy JM, ed. Office and network systems to support mental health care. In: *Mental Health Care of Children and Adolescents: A Guide for Primary Care Clinicians.* Itasca, IL: American Academy of Pediatrics; 2018:73–126

246. kidsdata.org. *Children With Special Health Care Needs, by Condition (California & U.S. Only).* Palo Alto, CA: Lucille Packard Foundation for Children's Health; 2010. Available at: https://www.kidsdata.org/topic/486/special-needs-condition/table#fmt=640&loc=1,2&tf=74&ch=152,1039,854,154,845,1040,1041,858,157,158,1042,1043,160,161,861,1044,1045,1046,165,166. Accessed September 8, 2019

247. Danielson ML, Visser SN, Gleason MM, Peacock G, Claussen AH, Blumberg SJ. A national profile of attention-deficit hyperactivity disorder diagnosis and treatment among US children aged 2 to 5 years. *J Dev Behav Pediatr.* 2017;38(7):455–464

248. American Academy of Pediatrics. Mental health initiatives: residency curriculum. Available at: https://www.aap.org/en-us/advocacy-and-policy/aap-health-initiatives/Mental-Health/Pages/Residency-Curriculum.aspx. Accessed September 8, 2019

249. American Academy of Child & Adolescent Psychiatry. *Workforce Issues.* Washington, DC: American Academy of Child & Adolescent Psychiatry; 2016. Available at: https://www.aacap.org/aacap/Resources_for_Primary_Care/Workforce_Issues.aspx. Accessed September 8, 2019

250. Thomas CR, Holzer CE III. The continuing shortage of child and adolescent psychiatrists. *J Am Acad Child Adolesc Psychiatry.* 2006;45(9): 1023–1031

251. Rohlfing J, Navarro R, Maniya OZ, Hughes BD, Rogalsky DK. Medical student debt and major life choices other than specialty. *Med Educ Online.* 2014;19:25603

252. Centers for Disease Control and Prevention. *ADHD: Behavioral Health Services – Where They Are and Who Provides Them.* Atlanta, GA: Centers for Disease Control and Prevention; 2018. Available at: https://www.cdc.gov/ncbddd/adhd/stateprofiles-providers/index.html. Accessed September 8, 2019

253. Massachusetts Child Psychiatry Access Program. MCPAP: connecting primary care with child psychiatry. Available at: https://www.mcpap.com. Accessed September 8, 2019

254. Project Training and Education for the Advancement of Children's Health. Project TEACH (Training and Education for the Advancement of Children's Health). 2018. Available at: https://projectteachny.org/. Accessed September 8, 2019

255. Project Extension for Community Healthcare Outcomes. About ECHO. Available at: https://echo.unm.edu/about-echo/. Accessed September 8, 2019

256. Health Resources and Services Administration, Maternal and Child Health Bureau. Pediatric mental health care access program. Available at: https://mchb.hrsa.gov/training/projects.asp?program=34. Accessed July 2, 2019

257. National Network of Child Psychiatry Access Programs. Integrating mental and behavioral health care for every child. Available at: https://nncpap.org/. Accessed July 2, 2019

258. Horwitz SM, Storfer-Isser A, Kerker BD, et al. Barriers to the identification and management of psychosocial problems: changes from 2004 to 2013. *Acad Pediatr.* 2015;15(6):613–620

259. American Academy of Child and Adolescent Psychiatry Committee on Health Care Access and Economics Task Force on Mental Health. Improving mental health services in primary care: reducing administrative and financial barriers to access and collaboration [published correction appears in *Pediatrics. 2009;123(6):1611]. Pediatrics.* 2009;123(4):1248–1251

260. Centers for Medicare and Medicaid Services. *Accountable Care Organizations (ACOs).* Baltimore, MD: Centers for Medicare and Medicaid Services; 2018. Available at: https://www.cms.gov/Medicare/Medicare-Fee-for-Service-Payment/ACO/. Accessed September 8, 2019

261. Fallu A, Dabouz F, Furtado M, Anand L, Katzman MA. A randomized, double-blind, cross-over, phase IV trial of oros-methylphenidate (CONCERTA(®)) and generic novo-methylphenidate ER-C (NOVO-generic). *Ther Adv Psychopharmacol.* 2016;6(4):237–251

262. Hagan JF, Shaw JS, Duncan PM, eds. *Bright Futures Guidelines for Health Supervision of Infants, Children, and Adolescents.* 4th ed. Elk Grove Village, IL: American Academy of Pediatrics; 2017

263. Foy JM, Kelleher KJ, Laraque D; American Academy of Pediatrics Task Force on Mental Health. Enhancing pediatric mental health care: strategies for preparing a primary care practice.*Pediatrics.* 2010;125(suppl 3): S87–S108

264. Allan C, Chacko A. Adverse events in behavioral parent training for children with ADHD: an under-appreciated phenomenon. *ADHD Rep.* 2018;26(1):4–9

265. US Department of Health and Human Services. Health information privacy. Available at: https://www.hhs.gov/hipaa/index.html. Accessed September 8, 2019

266. US Department of Education. *Family Educational Rights and Privacy Act (FERPA).* Washington, DC: Department of Education; 2018. Available at: https://www2.ed.gov/policy/gen/guid/fpco/ferpa/index.html. Accessed September 8, 2019

267. Epstein JN, Langberg JM, Lichtenstein PK, Kolb R, Altaye M, Simon JO. Use of an Internet portal to improve community-based pediatric ADHD care: a cluster randomized trial. *Pediatrics.* 2011;128(5). Available at: www.pediatrics.org/cgi/content/full/128/5/e1201

268. Centers for Medicare and Medicaid Services. *Electronic Health Records.* Baltimore, MD: Centers for Medicare and Medicaid Services; 2012. Available at: https://www.cms.gov/Medicare/E-Health/EHealthRecords/index.html. Accessed September 8, 2019

269. Ohno-Machado L. Electronic health record systems: risks and benefits. *J Am Med Inform Assoc.* 2014;21(e1):e1

270. Koppel R, Lehmann CU. Implications of an emerging EHR monoculture for hospitals and healthcare systems. *J Am Med Inform Assoc.* 2015;22(2):465–471

271. Babbott S, Manwell LB, Brown R, et al. Electronic medical records and physician stress in primary care: results from the MEMO Study. *J Am Med Inform Assoc.* 2014;21(e1):e100–e106

272. Burke BL Jr, Hall RW; Section on Telehealth Care. Telemedicine: pediatric applications. *Pediatrics.* 2015;136(1). Available at: www.pediatrics.org/cgi/content/full/136/1/e293

273. Marcin JP, Rimsza ME, Moskowitz WB; Committee on Pediatric Workforce. The use of telemedicine to address access and physician workforce shortages. *Pediatrics.* 2015;136(1): 202–209

274. Sibley MH, Comer JS, Gonzalez J. Delivering parent-teen therapy for ADHD through videoconferencing: a preliminary investigation. *J Psychopathol Behav Assess.* 2017; 39(3):467–485

275. Comer JS, Furr JM, Miguel EM, et al. Remotely delivering real-time parent training to the home: an initial randomized trial of Internet-delivered parent-child interaction therapy (I-PCIT). *J Consult Clin Psychol.* 2017;85(9): 909–917

276. American Academy of Child and Adolescent Psychiatry; American Academy of Pediatrics. HIPAA privacy rule and provider to provider communication. Available at: https://www.aap.org/en-us/advocacy-and-policy/aap-health-initiatives/Mental-Health/Pages/HIPAA-Privacy-Rule-and-Provider-to-Provider-Communication.aspx. Accessed September 8, 2019

277. Kolko DJ, Campo J, Kilbourne AM, Hart J, Sakolsky D, Wisniewski S. Collaborative care outcomes for

pediatric behavioral health problems: a cluster randomized trial. *Pediatrics*. 2014;133(4). Available at: www.pediatrics.org/cgi/content/full/133/4/e981

278. Pordes E, Gordon J, Sanders LM, Cohen E. Models of care delivery for children with medical complexity. *Pediatrics*. 2018;141(suppl 3): S212–S223

279. Silverstein M, Hironaka LK, Walter HJ, et al. Collaborative care for children with ADHD symptoms: a randomized comparative effectiveness trial. *Pediatrics*. 2015;135(4). Available at: www.pediatrics.org/cgi/content/full/135/4/e858

280. Liddle M, Birkett K, Bonjour A, Risma K. A collaborative approach to improving health care for children with developmental disabilities. *Pediatrics*. 2018;142(6):e20181136

Attention-Deficit/Hyperactivity Disorder Clinical Practice Guideline Quick Reference Tools

- Action Statement Summary
  — Clinical Practice Guideline for the Diagnosis, Evaluation, and Treatment of Attention-Deficit/Hyperactivity Disorder in Children and Adolescents
- *ICD-10-CM* Coding Quick Reference for ADHD
- Bonus Features
  — ADHD Coding Fact Sheet for Primary Care Physicians
  — Continuum Model for ADHD
- AAP Patient Education Handouts
  — *ADHD—What Is Attention-Deficit/Hyperactivity Disorder?*
  — *What Are the Symptoms of Attention-Deficit/Hyperactivity Disorder?*
  — *How Is Attention-Deficit/Hyperactivity Disorder Diagnosed?*
  — *What Causes Attention-Deficit/Hyperactivity Disorder and How Is It Treated?*

Action Statement Summary

Clinical Practice Guideline for the Diagnosis, Evaluation, and Treatment of Attention-Deficit/Hyperactivity Disorder in Children and Adolescents

Key Action Statement 1

The pediatrician or other PCC should initiate an evaluation for ADHD for any child or adolescent age 4 years to the 18th birthday who presents with academic or behavioral problems and symptoms of inattention, hyperactivity, or impulsivity. (Grade B: strong recommendation.)

Key Action Statement 2

To make a diagnosis of ADHD, the PCC should determine that *DSM-5* criteria have been met, including documentation of symptoms and impairment in more than 1 major setting (ie, social, academic, or occupational), with information obtained primarily from reports from parents or guardians, teachers, other school personnel, and mental health clinicians who are involved in the child or adolescent's care. The PCC should also rule out any alternative cause. (Grade B: strong recommendation.)

Key Action Statement 3

In the evaluation of a child or adolescent for ADHD, the PCC should include a process to at least screen for comorbid conditions, including emotional or behavioral conditions (eg, anxiety, depression, oppositional defiant disorder, conduct disorders, substance use), developmental conditions (eg, learning and language disorders, autism spectrum disorders), and physical conditions (eg, tics, sleep apnea). (Grade B: strong recommendation.)

Key Action Statement 4

ADHD is a chronic condition; therefore, the PCC should manage children and adolescents with ADHD in the same manner that they would children and youth with special health care needs, following the principles of the chronic care model and the medical home. (Grade B: strong recommendation.)

Key Action Statement 5a

For preschool-aged children (age 4 years to the sixth birthday) with ADHD, the PCC should prescribe evidence-based behavioral PTBM and/or behavioral classroom interventions as the first line of treatment, if available (grade A: strong recommendation). Methylphenidate may be considered if these behavioral interventions do not provide significant improvement and there is moderate-to-severe continued disturbance in the 4- through 5-year-old child's functioning. In areas in which evidence-based behavioral treatments are not available, the clinician needs to weigh the risks of starting medication before the age of 6 years against the harm of delaying treatment. (Grade B: strong recommendation.)

Key Action Statement 5b

For elementary and middle school–aged children (age 6 years to the 12th birthday) with ADHD, the PCC should prescribe US Food and Drug Administration (FDA)–approved medications for ADHD, along with PTBM and/or behavioral classroom intervention (preferably both PTBM and behavioral classroom interventions). Educational interventions and individualized instructional supports, including school environment, class placement, instructional placement, and behavioral supports, are a necessary part of any treatment plan and often include an Individualized Education Program (IEP) or a rehabilitation plan (504 plan). (Grade A: strong recommendation for medications; grade A: strong recommendation for PTBM training and behavioral treatments for ADHD implemented with the family and school.)

Key Action Statement 5c

For adolescents (age 12 years to the 18th birthday) with ADHD, the PCC should prescribe FDA-approved medications for ADHD with the adolescent's assent (grade A: strong recommendation). The PCC is encouraged to prescribe evidence-based training interventions and/or behavioral interventions as treatment of ADHD, if available. Educational interventions and individualized instructional supports, including school environment, class placement, instructional placement, and behavioral supports, are a necessary part of any treatment plan and often include an IEP or a rehabilitation plan (504 plan). (Grade A: strong recommendation.)

Key Action Statement 6

The PCC should titrate doses of medication for ADHD to achieve maximum benefit with tolerable side effects. (Grade B: strong recommendation.)

Key Action Statement 7

The PCC, if trained or experienced in diagnosing comorbid conditions, may initiate treatment of such conditions or make a referral to an appropriate subspecialist for treatment. After detecting possible comorbid conditions, if the PCC is not trained or experienced in making the diagnosis or initiating treatment, the patient should be referred to an appropriate subspecialist to make the diagnosis and initiate treatment. (Grade C: recommendation.)

Coding Quick Reference for ADHD	
ICD-10-CM	
F90.0	Attention-deficit hyperactivity disorder, predominantly inattentive type
F90.1	Attention-deficit hyperactivity disorder, predominantly hyperactive type

ADHD Coding Fact Sheet for Primary Care Physicians

Current Procedural Terminology (CPT®) (Procedure) Codes

Initial assessment usually involves a lot of time in determining the differential diagnosis, a diagnostic plan, and potential treatment options. Therefore, most pediatricians will report either an office or an outpatient evaluation and management (E/M) code using time as the key factor or a consultation code for the initial assessment.

Physician E/M Services

***99201** Office or other outpatient visit, *new*[a] patient; self limited or minor problem, 10 min.
***99202** low to moderate severity problem, 20 min.
***99203** moderate severity problem, 30 min.
***99204** moderate to high severity problem, 45 min.
***99205** high severity problem, 60 min.
***99211** Office or other outpatient visit, *established* patient; minimal problem, 5 min.
***99212** self limited or minor problem, 10 min.
***99213** low to moderate severity problem, 15 min.
***99214** moderate severity problem, 25 min.
***99215** moderate to high severity problem, 40 min.
***99241** Office or other outpatient *consultation*,[b–d] new or established patient; self-limited or minor problem, 15 min.
***99242** low severity problem, 30 min.
***99243** moderate severity problem, 45 min.
***99244** moderate to high severity problem, 60 min.
***99245** moderate to high severity problem, 80 min.
***+99354** Prolonged physician services in office or other outpatient setting, with direct patient contact; first hour (*use in conjunction with time-based codes* **99201–99215**, **99241–99245**, **99301–99350**, **90837**)
***+99355** each additional 30 min. (*use in conjunction with* **99354**)

- Used when a physician provides prolonged services beyond the usual service (ie, beyond the typical time).
- Time spent does not have to be continuous.
- Prolonged service of less than 15 minutes beyond the first hour or less than 15 minutes beyond the final 30 minutes is not reported separately.
- If reporting E/M service according to time and not key factors (history, examination, and medical decision-making), the physician must reach the typical time in the highest code in the code set being reported (eg, **99205**, **99215**, **99245**) before face-to-face prolonged services can be reported.
- Refer to *CPT* for clinical staff prolonged services.

[a] A new patient is one who has not received any professional services (face-to-face services) rendered by physicians and other qualified health care professionals who may report E/M services using 1 or more specific *CPT* codes from the physician/qualified health care professional, or another physician/qualified health care professional of the exact same specialty and subspecialty who belongs to the same group practice, within the past 3 years.

[b] Use of these codes (**99241–99245**) requires the following actions:
1. Written or verbal request for consultation is documented in the medical record.
2. Consultant's opinion and any services ordered or performed are documented in the medical record.
3. Consultant's opinion and any services that are performed are prepared in a written report, which is sent to the requesting physician or other appropriate source.

[c] Patients/parents may not initiate a consultation.

[d] For more information on consultation code changes for 2010, see www.aap.org/en-us/professional-resources/practice-transformation/getting-paid/Coding-at-the-AAP/Pages/ADHD-Coding-Fact-Sheet.aspx.

• New *CPT* code
▲ Revised *CPT* code
+ Codes are *add-on codes*, meaning they are reported separately in addition to the appropriate code for the service provided.
* Indicates a *CPT*-approved telemedicine service.

CPT® copyright 2019 American Medical Association. All rights reserved.

Reporting E/M Services Using "Time"

- When counseling or coordination of care dominates (>50%) the physician/patient or family encounter (face-to-face time in the office or other outpatient setting or floor/unit time in the hospital or nursing facility), **time shall** be considered the key or controlling factor to qualify for a particular level of E/M services.
- This includes time spent with parties who have assumed responsibility for the care of the patient or decision-making, whether or not they are family members (eg, foster parents, person acting in loco parentis, legal guardian). The extent of counseling or coordination of care must be documented in the medical record.
- For coding purposes, face-to-face time for these services is defined as only that time that the physician spends face-to-face with the patient or family. This includes the time in which the physician performs such tasks as obtaining a history, performing an examination, and counseling the patient.
- When codes are ranked in sequential typical times (eg, office-based E/M services, consultation codes) and the actual time is between 2 typical times, the code with the typical time closest to the actual time is used.
  - **Example:** A physician sees an established patient in the office to discuss the current attention-deficit/hyperactivity disorder (ADHD) medication the patient was placed on. The total face-to-face time was 22 minutes, of which 15 minutes was spent in counseling the mom and patient. Because more than 50% of the total time was spent in counseling, the physician would report the E/M service according to time. The physician would report **99214** instead of **99213** because the total face-to-face time was closer to **99214** (25 minutes) than **99213** (15 minutes).

ADHD Follow-up During a Routine Preventive Medicine Service

- A good time to follow up with a patient regarding his or her ADHD could be during a preventive medicine service.
- If the follow-up requires little additional work on behalf of the physician, it should be reported under the preventive medicine service, rather than as a separate service.
- If the follow-up work requires an additional E/M service in addition to the preventive medicine service, it should be reported as a separate service.
- Chronic conditions should be reported only if they are separately addressed.
- When reporting a preventive medicine service in addition to an office-based E/M service and the services are significant and separately identifiable, modifier **25** will be required on the office-based E/M service.
  - **Example:** A 12-year-old established patient presents for his routine preventive medicine service and, while he and Mom are there, Mom asks about changing his ADHD medication because of some side effects he is experiencing. The physician completes the routine preventive medicine check and then addresses the mom's concerns in a separate service. The additional E/M service takes 15 minutes, of which the physician spends about 10 minutes in counseling and coordinating care; therefore, the E/M service is reported according to time.
    - Code **99394** and **99213-25** account for both E/M services and link each to the appropriate *International Classification of Diseases, 10th Revision, Clinical Modification (ICD-10-CM)* code.
    - Modifier **25** is required on the problem-oriented office visit code (eg, **99213**) when it is significant and separately identifiable from another service.

Physician Non–face-to-face Services

99339 Care Plan Oversight—Individual physician supervision of a patient (patient not present) in home, domiciliary or rest home (e.g., assisted living facility) requiring complex and multidisciplinary care modalities involving regular physician development and/or revision of care plans, review of subsequent reports of patient status, review of related laboratory and other studies, communication (including telephone calls) for purposes of assessment or care decisions with health care professional(s), family member(s), surrogate decision maker(s) (e.g., legal guardian) and/or key caregiver(s) involved in patient's care, integration of new information into the medical treatment plan and/or adjustment of medical therapy, within a calendar month; 15–29 minutes

99340 30 minutes or more

99358 Prolonged physician services without direct patient contact; first hour

+99359 each additional 30 min. (+ *use in conjunction with* **99358**)

99367 Medical team conference by physician with interdisciplinary team of health care professionals, patient and/or family not present, 30 minutes or more

Telephone Care

99441 Telephone evaluation and management to patient, parent or guardian not originating from a related E/M service within the previous 7 days nor leading to an E/M service or procedure within the next 24 hours or soonest available appointment; 5–10 minutes of medical discussion

99442 11–20 minutes of medical discussion

99443 21–30 minutes of medical discussion

99444 Online E/M service provided by a physician or other qualified health care professional to an established patient, guardian or health care provider not originating from a related E/M service provided within the previous 7 days, using the internet or similar electronic communications network

Digital Online E/M Services

Are patient-initiated services with physicians or other advanced practitioners (NP/PA).

Require evaluation, assessment, and management of the patient.

The patient must be established, but the condition can be new.

The digital communication must take place over a secure platform which allows digital communication.

Online digital E/M services are reported once for the *cumulative time* devoted to the service, which includes

- review of the initial inquiry,
- review of patient records or data pertinent to assessment of the patient's problem,
- interaction with clinical staff focused on the patient's problem, development of management plans, including generation of prescriptions or ordering of tests, and subsequent communication with the patient through online, telephone, email, or other digitally supported communication during a seven-day period.

The seven-day period begins with the personal review of the patient-generated inquiry.

Online digital E/M services require permanent documentation storage

•99421 Online digital evaluation and management service, for an established patient, for up to 7 days, cumulative time during the 7 days; 5-10 minutes

•99422 11–20 minutes

•99423 21 or more minutes

Care Management Services

Codes are selected according to the amount of time spent by clinical staff (**99490**)/physician (**99491**) providing care coordination activities. *CPT* clearly defines which activities are care coordination activities. To report chronic care management codes, you must

1. Provide 24/7 access to physicians or other qualified health care professionals or clinical staff.
2. Use a standardized methodology to identify patients who require chronic complex care coordination services.
3. Have an internal care coordination process/function whereby a patient identified as meeting the requirements for these services starts receiving them in a timely manner.
4. Use a form and format in the medical record that is standardized within the practice.
5. Be able to engage and educate patients and caregivers, as well as coordinate care among all service professionals, as appropriate for each patient (also applies to code **99490** under NPP services).

99491 Chronic care management services, provided personally by a physician or other qualified health care professional, at least 30 minutes of physician or other qualified health care professional time, per calendar month, with the following required elements:

- multiple (two or more) chronic conditions expected to last at least 12 months, or until the death of the patient;
- chronic conditions place the patient at significant risk of death, acute exacerbation/decompensation, or functional decline;
- comprehensive care plan established, implemented, revised, or monitored.

Psychiatry

+90785 Interactive complexity (Use in conjunction with codes for diagnostic psychiatric evaluation [**90791**, **90792**], psychotherapy [**90832**, **90834**, **90837**], psychotherapy when performed with an evaluation and management service [**90833**, **90836**, **90838**, **99201–99255**, **99304–99337**, **99341–99350**], and group psychotherapy [**90853**])

Psychiatric Diagnostic or Evaluative Interview Procedures

90791 Psychiatric diagnostic interview examination evaluation

90792 Psychiatric diagnostic evaluation with medical services

Psychotherapy

***90832** Psychotherapy, 30 min with patient;

***+90833** with medical E/M (Use in conjunction with **99201–99255**, **99304–99337**, **99341–99350**)

***90834** Psychotherapy, 45 min with patient;

***+90836** with medical E/M services (Use in conjunction with **99201–99255**, **99304–99337**, **99341–99350**)

***90837** Psychotherapy, 60 min with patient;

***+90838** with medical E/M services (Use in conjunction with **99201–99255**, **99304–99337**, **99341–99350**)

+90785 Interactive complexity (Use in conjunction with codes for diagnostic psychiatric evaluation [**90791**, **90792**], psychotherapy [**90832**, **90834**, **90837**], psychotherapy when performed with an evaluation and manage-

---

• New *CPT* code
▲ Revised *CPT* code
+ Codes are *add-on codes*, meaning they are reported separately in addition to the appropriate code for the service provided.
* Indicates a *CPT*-approved telemedicine service.

CPT® copyright 2019 American Medical Association. All rights reserved.

ment service [**90833**, **90836**, **90838**, **99201–99255**, **99304–99337**, **99341–99350**], and group psychotherapy [**90853**])

- Refers to specific communication factors that complicate the delivery of a psychiatric procedure. Common factors include more difficult communication with discordant or emotional family members and engagement of young and verbally undeveloped or impaired patients. Typical encounters include
  - — Patients who have other individuals legally responsible for their care
  - — Patients who request others to be present or involved in their care such as translators, interpreters, or additional family members
  - — Patients who require the involvement of other third parties such as child welfare agencies, schools, or probation officers

***90846** Family psychotherapy (without patient present), 50 min

***90847** Family psychotherapy (conjoint psychotherapy) (with patient present), 50 min

Other Psychiatric Services/Procedures

90863 Pharmacologic management, including prescription and review of medication, when performed with psychotherapy services (Use in conjunction with **90832**, **90834**, **90837**)

- For pharmacologic management with psychotherapy services performed by a physician or other qualified health care professional who may report E/M codes, use the appropriate E/M codes (**99201–99255**, **99281–99285**, **99304–99337**, **99341–99350**) and the appropriate psychotherapy with E/M service (**90833**, **90836**, **90838**).

90887 Interpretation or explanation of results of psychiatric, other medical exams, or other accumulated data to family or other responsible persons, or advising them how to assist patient

90889 Preparation of reports on patient's psychiatric status, history, treatment, or progress (other than for legal or consultative purposes) for other physicians, agencies, or insurance carriers

97127 Therapeutic interventions that focus on cognitive function (eg, attention, memory, reasoning, executive function, problem solving, and/or pragmatic functioning) and compensatory strategies to manage the performance of an activity (eg, managing time or schedules, initiating, organizing and sequencing tasks), direct (one-on-one) patient contact

Developmental/Psychological Testing

96110 Developmental screening, with scoring and documentation, per standardized instrument (Do not use for ADHD screens or assessments)

96112 Developmental test administration (including assessment of fine and/or gross motor, language, cognitive level, social, memory and/or executive functions by standardized developmental instruments when performed), by physician or other qualified health care professional, with interpretation and report; first hour

+96113 each additional 30 minutes (Report with **96112**)

***96116** Neurobehavioral status examination (clinical assessment of thinking, reasoning and judgment [eg, acquired knowledge, attention, language, memory, planning and problem solving, and visual spatial abilities]), by physician or other qualified health care professional, both face-to-face time with the patient and time interpreting test results and preparing the report; first hour

***96121** each additional hour (Report with **96116**)

96127 Brief emotional/behavioral assessment (eg, depression inventory, attention-deficit/hyperactivity disorder [ADHD] scale), with scoring and documentation, per standardized instrument

96130 Psychological testing evaluation services by physician or other qualified health care professional, including integration of patient data, interpretation of standardized test results and clinical data, clinical decision making, treatment planning and report, and interactive feedback to the patient, family member(s) or caregiver(s), when performed; first hour

+96131 each additional hour (code with **96130**)

96136 Psychological or neuropsychological test administration and scoring by physician or other qualified health care professional, two or more tests, any method; first 30 minutes

+96137 each additional 30 minutes

Nonphysician Provider (NPP) Services

99366 Medical team conference with interdisciplinary team of health care professionals, face-to-face with patient and/or family, 30 minutes or more, participation by a nonphysician qualified health care professional

99368 Medical team conference with interdisciplinary team of health care professionals, patient and/or family not present, 30 minutes or more, participation by a nonphysician qualified health care professional

96146 Psychological or neuropsychological test administration, with single automated, standardized instrument via electronic platform, with automated result only

Health and Behavior (Re-) Assessment and Intervention

The following codes are reported to describe services offered to patients who present with primary *physical illnesses, diagnoses,* or *symptoms* and may benefit from assessments and interventions that focus on the psychological and/or psychosocial factors related to the patient's health status.

•96156 Health behavior assessment, or re-assessment (ie, health-focused clinical interview, behavioral observations, clinical decision making)

•96158 Health behavior intervention, individual, face-to-face; initial 30 minutes

•+96159 each additional 15 minutes (code with **96158**)

•96164 Health behavior intervention, group (2 or more patients), face-to-face; initial 30 minutes

•+96165 each additional 15 minutes (code with **96164**)

•96167 Health behavior intervention, family (with the patient present), face-to-face; initial 30 minutes

•+96168 each additional 15 minutes (code with **96167**)

•96170 Health behavior intervention, family (without the patient present), face-to-face; initial 30 minutes

•+96171 each additional 15 minutes (code with **96170**)

Non–face-to-face Services: NPP

98966 Telephone assessment and management service provided by a qualified nonphysician health care professional to an established patient, parent or guardian not originating from a related assessment and management service provided within the previous seven days nor leading to an assessment and management service or procedure within the

• New *CPT* code
▲ Revised *CPT* code
+ Codes are *add-on codes,* meaning they are reported separately in addition to the appropriate code for the service provided.
* Indicates a *CPT*-approved telemedicine service.

CPT® copyright 2019 American Medical Association. All rights reserved.

next 24 hours or soonest available appointment; 5–10 minutes of medical discussion

98967 11–20 minutes of medical discussion

98968 21–30 minutes of medical discussion

98969 Online assessment and management service provided by a qualified nonphysician health care professional to an established patient or guardian not originating from a related assessment and management service provided within the previous seven days nor using the internet or similar electronic communications network

NPP Online Digital E/M Service

Reported only once per 7 days.

Report these codes for qualified health care professionals such as speech pathologists, registered dieticians, or physical therapists.

Do not report for physician's or advanced practitioners (NP/PA).

For additional information see codes **99421–99423** in this resource or refer to the *CPT* manual.

•98970 Qualified nonphysician health care professional online digital evaluation and management service, for an established patient, for up to 7 days, cumulative time during the 7 days; 5–10 minutes

•98971 11–20 minutes

•98972 21 or more minutes

Clinical Staff Services

99490 *Chronic care management services,* at least 20 minutes of clinical staff time directed by a physician or other qualified health care professional, per calendar month, with the following required elements:

- multiple (two or more) chronic conditions expected to last at least 12 months, or until the death of the patient;
- chronic conditions place the patient at significant risk of death, acute exacerbation/decompensation, or functional decline;
- comprehensive care plan established, implemented, revised, or monitored.

Chronic care management services are provided when medical needs or psychosocial needs (or both types of needs) of the patient require establishing, implementing, revising, or monitoring the care plan. If 20 minutes is not met within a calendar month, you do not report chronic care management. Refer to code **99491** in this resource and *CPT* for more information.

Clinical Staff

99484 Care management services for *behavioral health conditions,* at least 20 minutes of clinical staff time, directed by a physician or other qualified health care professional, per calendar month, with the following required elements:

- initial assessment or follow-up monitoring, including the use of applicable validated rating scales;
- behavioral health care planning in relation to behavioral/ psychiatric health problems, including revision for patients who are not progressing or whose status changes;
- facilitating and coordinating treatment such as psychotherapy, pharmacotherapy, counseling and/ or psychiatric consultation; and
- continuity of care with a designated member of the care team.
- Do not report in conjunction with psychiatric collaborative care management codes (**99492, 99493, 99494**) for the same calendar month.

99492 Initial psychiatric collaborative care management, first 70 minutes in the first calendar month of behavioral health care manager activities, in consultation with a psychiatric consultant, and directed by the treating physician or other qualified health care professional, with the following required elements:

- outreach to and engagement in treatment of a patient directed by the treating physician or other qualified health care professional;
- initial assessment of the patient, including administration of validated rating scales, with the development of an individualized treatment plan;
- review by the psychiatric consultant with modifications of the plan if recommended;
- entering patient in a registry and tracking patient follow-up and progress using the registry, with appropriate documentation, and participation in weekly caseload consultation with the psychiatric consultant; and
- provision of brief interventions using evidence-based techniques such as behavioral activation, motivational interviewing, and other focused treatment strategies.

99493 Subsequent psychiatric collaborative care management, first 60 minutes in a subsequent month of behavioral health care manager activities, in consultation with a psychiatric consultant, and directed by the treating physician or other qualified health care professional, with the following required elements:

- tracking patient follow-up and progress using the registry, with appropriate documentation;
- participation in weekly caseload consultation with the psychiatric consultant;
- ongoing collaboration with and coordination of the patient's mental health care with the treating physician or other qualified health care professional and any other treating mental health providers;
- additional review of progress and recommendations for changes in treatment, as indicated, including medications, based on recommendations provided by the psychiatric consultant;
- provision of brief interventions using evidence-based techniques such as behavioral activation, motivational interviewing, and other focused treatment strategies;
- monitoring of patient outcomes using validated rating scales; and
- relapse prevention planning with patients as they achieve remission of symptoms and/or other treatment goals and are prepared for discharge from active treatment.

+99494 Initial or subsequent psychiatric collaborative care management, each additional 30 minutes in a calendar month of behavioral health care manager activities, in consultation with a psychiatric consultant, and directed by the treating physician or other qualified health care professional (Use **99494** in conjunction with **99492, 99493**)

Miscellaneous Services

99071 Educational supplies, such as books, tapes, or pamphlets, provided by the physician for the patient's education at cost to the physician

• New *CPT* code
▲ Revised *CPT* code
+ Codes are *add-on codes,* meaning they are reported separately in addition to the appropriate code for the service provided.
* Indicates a *CPT*-approved telemedicine service.

CPT® copyright 2019 American Medical Association. All rights reserved.

ICD-10-CM Codes

- Use as many diagnosis codes that apply to document the patient's complexity and report the patient's symptoms or adverse environmental circumstances (or both).
- Once a definitive diagnosis is established, report any appropriate definitive diagnosis codes as the primary codes, plus any other symptoms that the patient is exhibiting as secondary diagnoses that are not part of the usual disease course or are considered incidental.

Depressive Disorders

F34.1 Dysthymic disorder (depressive personality disorder, dysthymia neurotic depression)
F39 Mood (affective) disorder, unspecified
F30.8 Other manic episode

Anxiety Disorders

F06.4 Anxiety disorder due to known physiological conditions
F40.10 Social phobia, unspecified
F40.11 Social phobia, generalized
F40.8 Phobic anxiety disorders, other (phobic anxiety disorder of childhood)
F40.9 Phobic anxiety disorder, unspecified
F41.1 Generalized anxiety disorder
F41.9 Anxiety disorder, unspecified

Feeding and Eating Disorders/Elimination Disorders

F50.89 Eating disorders, other
F50.9 Eating disorder, unspecified
F98.0 Enuresis not due to a substance or known physiological condition
F98.1 Encopresis not due to a substance or known physiological condition
F98.3 Pica (infancy or childhood)

Impulse Disorders

F63.9 Impulse disorder, unspecified

Trauma- and Stressor-Related Disorders

F43.20 Adjustment disorder, unspecified
F43.21 Adjustment disorder with depressed mood
F43.22 Adjustment disorder with anxiety
F43.23 Adjustment disorder with mixed anxiety and depressed mood
F43.24 Adjustment disorder with disturbance of conduct

Neurodevelopmental/Other Developmental Disorders

F70 Mild intellectual disabilities
F71 Moderate intellectual disabilities
F72 Severe intellectual disabilities
F73 Profound intellectual disabilities
F79 Unspecified intellectual disabilities
F80.0 Phonological (speech) disorder (speech-sound disorder)
F80.1 Expressive language disorder
F80.2 Mixed receptive-expressive language disorder
F80.4 Speech and language developmental delay due to hearing loss (code also hearing loss)
F80.81 Stuttering
F80.82 Social pragmatic communication disorder
F80.89 Other developmental disorders of speech and language
F80.9 Developmental disorder of speech and language, unspecified
F81.0 Specific reading disorder
F81.2 Mathematics disorder
F81.89 Other developmental disorders of scholastic skills
F82 Developmental coordination disorder
F84.0 Autistic disorder (Autism spectrum disorder)
F88 Specified delays in development; other
F89 Unspecified delay in development
F81.9 Developmental disorder of scholastic skills, unspecified

Behavioral/Emotional Disorders

F90.0 Attention-deficit hyperactivity disorder, predominantly inattentive type
F90.1 Attention-deficit hyperactivity disorder, predominantly hyperactive type
F90.8 Attention-deficit hyperactivity disorder, other type
F90.9 Attention-deficit hyperactivity disorder, unspecified type
F91.1 Conduct disorder, childhood-onset type
F91.2 Conduct disorder, adolescent-onset type
F91.3 Oppositional defiant disorder
F91.9 Conduct disorder, unspecified
F93.0 Separation anxiety disorder
F93.8 Other childhood emotional disorders (relationship problems)
F93.9 Childhood emotional disorder, unspecified
F94.9 Childhood disorder of social functioning, unspecified
F95.0 Transient tic disorder
F95.1 Chronic motor or vocal tic disorder
F95.2 Tourette's disorder
F95.9 Tic disorder, unspecified
F98.8 Other specified behavioral and emotional disorders with onset usually occurring in childhood and adolescence (nail-biting, nose-picking, thumb-sucking)

Other

F07.81 Postconcussional syndrome
F07.89 Personality and behavioral disorders due to known physiological condition, other
F07.9 Personality and behavioral disorder due to known physiological condition, unspecified
F45.41 Pain disorder exclusively related to psychological factors
F48.8 Nonpsychotic mental disorders, other (neurasthenia)
F48.9 Nonpsychotic mental disorders, unspecified
F51.01 Primary insomnia
F51.02 Adjustment insomnia
F51.03 Paradoxical insomnia
F51.04 Psychophysiologic insomnia
F51.05 Insomnia due to other mental disorder (Code also associated mental disorder)
F51.09 Insomnia, other (not due to a substance or known physiological condition)
F51.3 Sleepwalking [somnambulism]
F51.4 Sleep terrors [night terrors]
F51.8 Other sleep disorders
F93.8 Childhood emotional disorders, other
R46.89 Other symptoms and signs involving appearance and behavior

Substance-Related and Addictive Disorders

If a provider documents multiple patterns of use, only 1 should be reported. Use the following hierarchy: use–abuse–dependence

• New *CPT* code
▲ Revised *CPT* code
+ Codes are *add-on codes,* meaning they are reported separately in addition to the appropriate code for the service provided.
* Indicates a *CPT*-approved telemedicine service.

CPT® copyright 2019 American Medical Association. All rights reserved.

(eg, if use and dependence are documented, only code for dependence).

When a minus symbol (-) is included in codes **F10–F17**, a last character is required. Be sure to include the last character from the following list:

0 anxiety disorder

2 sleep disorder

8 other disorder

9 unspecified disorder

Alcohol

F10.10 Alcohol abuse, uncomplicated (alcohol use disorder, mild)
F10.14 Alcohol abuse with alcohol-induced mood disorder
F10.159 Alcohol abuse with alcohol-induced psychotic disorder, unspecified
F10.18- Alcohol abuse with alcohol-induced
F10.19 Alcohol abuse with unspecified alcohol-induced disorder
F10.20 Alcohol dependence, uncomplicated
F10.21 Alcohol dependence, in remission
F10.24 Alcohol dependence with alcohol-induced mood disorder
F10.259 Alcohol dependence with alcohol-induced psychotic disorder, unspecified
F10.28- Alcohol dependence with alcohol-induced
F10.29 Alcohol dependence with unspecified alcohol-induced disorder
F10.94 Alcohol use, unspecified with alcohol-induced mood disorder
F10.959 Alcohol use, unspecified with alcohol-induced psychotic disorder, unspecified
F10.98- Alcohol use, unspecified with alcohol-induced
F10.99 Alcohol use, unspecified with unspecified alcohol-induced disorder

Cannabis

F12.10 Cannabis abuse, uncomplicated (cannabis use disorder, mild)
F12.18- Cannabis abuse with cannabis-induced
F12.19 Cannabis abuse with unspecified cannabis-induced disorder
F12.20 Cannabis dependence, uncomplicated
F12.21 Cannabis dependence, in remission
F12.28- Cannabis dependence with cannabis-induced
F12.29 Cannabis dependence with unspecified cannabis-induced disorder
F12.90 Cannabis use, unspecified, uncomplicated
F12.98- Cannabis use, unspecified with
F12.99 Cannabis use, unspecified with unspecified cannabis-induced disorder

Sedatives

F13.10 Sedative, hypnotic or anxiolytic abuse, uncomplicated (sedative, hypnotic, or anxiolytic use disorder, mild)
F13.129 Sedative, hypnotic or anxiolytic abuse with intoxication, unspecified
F13.14 Sedative, hypnotic or anxiolytic abuse with sedative, hypnotic or anxiolytic-induced mood disorder
F13.18- Sedative, hypnotic or anxiolytic abuse with sedative, hypnotic or anxiolytic-induced
F13.21 Sedative, hypnotic or anxiolytic dependence, in remission
F13.90 Sedative, hypnotic or anxiolytic use, unspecified, uncomplicated
F13.94 Sedative, hypnotic or anxiolytic use, unspecified with sedative, hypnotic or anxiolytic-induced mood disorder
F13.98- Sedative, hypnotic or anxiolytic use, unspecified with sedative, hypnotic or anxiolytic-induced
F13.99 Sedative, hypnotic or anxiolytic use, unspecified with unspecified sedative, hypnotic or anxiolytic-induced disorder

Stimulants (eg, caffeine, amphetamines)

F15.10 Other stimulant (amphetamine-related disorders or caffeine) abuse, uncomplicated (amphetamine, other or unspecified type substance use disorder, mild)
F15.14 Other stimulant (amphetamine-related disorders or caffeine) abuse with stimulant-induced mood disorder
F15.18- Other stimulant (amphetamine-related disorders or caffeine) abuse with stimulant-induced
F15.19 Other stimulant (amphetamine-related disorders or caffeine) abuse with unspecified stimulant-induced disorder
F15.20 Other stimulant (amphetamine-related disorders or caffeine) dependence, uncomplicated
F15.21 Other stimulant (amphetamine-related disorders or caffeine) dependence, in remission
F15.24 Other stimulant (amphetamine-related disorders or caffeine) dependence with stimulant-induced mood disorder
F15.28- Other stimulant (amphetamine-related disorders or caffeine) dependence with stimulant-induced
F15.29 Other stimulant (amphetamine-related disorders or caffeine) dependence with unspecified stimulant-induced disorder
F15.90 Other stimulant (amphetamine-related disorders or caffeine) use, unspecified, uncomplicated
F15.94 Other stimulant (amphetamine-related disorders or caffeine) use, unspecified with stimulant-induced mood disorder
F15.98- Other stimulant (amphetamine-related disorders or caffeine) use, unspecified with stimulant-induced
F15.99 Other stimulant (amphetamine-related disorders or caffeine) use, unspecified with unspecified stimulant-induced disorder

Nicotine (eg, cigarettes)

F17.200 Nicotine dependence, unspecified, uncomplicated (tobacco use disorder, mild, moderate or severe)
F17.201 Nicotine dependence, unspecified, in remission
F17.203 Nicotine dependence, unspecified, with withdrawal
F17.20- Nicotine dependence, unspecified, with
F17.210 Nicotine dependence, cigarettes, uncomplicated
F17.211 Nicotine dependence, cigarettes, in remission
F17.213 Nicotine dependence, cigarettes, with withdrawal
F17.218- Nicotine dependence, cigarettes, with

Symptoms, Signs, and Ill-defined Conditions

Use these codes in absence of a definitive mental diagnosis or when the sign or symptom is not part of the disease course or is considered incidental.

G47.9 Sleep disorder, unspecified
H90.0 Conductive hearing loss, bilateral
H90.11 Conductive hearing loss, unilateral, right ear, with unrestricted hearing on the contralateral side
H90.12 Conductive hearing loss, unilateral, left ear, with unrestricted hearing on the contralateral side

• New *CPT* code
▲ Revised *CPT* code
+ Codes are *add-on codes*, meaning they are reported separately in addition to the appropriate code for the service provided.
* Indicates a *CPT*-approved telemedicine service.

CPT® copyright 2019 American Medical Association. All rights reserved.

H90.A1- Conductive hearing loss, unilateral, with restricted hearing on the contralateral side
H90.A2- Sensorineural hearing loss, unilateral, with restricted hearing on the contralateral side
H90.A3- Mixed conductive and sensorineural hearing loss, unilateral, with restricted hearing on the contralateral side
(Codes under category **H90** require a 6th digit: 1–right ear, 2–left ear)
K11.7 Disturbance of salivary secretions
K59.00 Constipation, unspecified
N39.44 Nocturnal enuresis
R10.0 Acute abdomen pain
R11.11 Vomiting without nausea
R11.2 Nausea with vomiting, unspecified
R19.7 Diarrhea, unspecified
R21 Rash, NOS
R25.0 Abnormal head movements
R25.1 Tremor, unspecified
R25.3 Twitching, NOS
R25.8 Other abnormal involuntary movements
R25.9 Unspecified abnormal involuntary movements
R27.8 Other lack of coordination (excludes ataxia)
R27.9 Unspecified lack of coordination
R41.83 Borderline intellectual functioning
R42 Dizziness
R48.0 Alexia/dyslexia, NOS
R51 Headache
R62.0 Delayed milestone in childhood
R62.52 Short stature (child)
R63.3 Feeding difficulties
R63.4 Abnormal weight loss
R63.5 Abnormal weight gain
R68.2 Dry mouth, unspecified
T56.0X1A Toxic effect of lead and its compounds, accidental (unintentional), initial encounter

Z Codes

Z codes represent reasons for encounters. Categories **Z00–Z99** are provided for occasions when circumstances other than a disease, an injury, or an external cause classifiable to categories **A00–Y89** are recorded as *diagnoses* or *problems*. This can arise in 2 main ways.

1. When a person who may or may not be sick encounters the health services for some specific purpose, such as to receive limited care or service for a current condition, to donate an organ or tissue, to receive prophylactic vaccination (immunization), or to discuss a problem that is, in itself, not a disease or an injury
2. When some circumstance or problem is present that influences the person's health status but is not, in itself, a current illness or injury

Z55.0 Illiteracy and low-level literacy
Z55.2 Failed school examinations
Z55.3 Underachievement in school
Z55.4 Educational maladjustment and discord with teachers and classmates
Z55.8 Other problems related to education and literacy
Z55.9 Problems related to education and literacy, unspecified
(**Z55** codes exclude those conditions reported with **F80–F89**)
Z60.4 Social exclusion and rejection
Z60.8 Other problems related to social environment
Z60.9 Problem related to social environment, unspecified
Z62.0 Inadequate parental supervision and control
Z62.21 Foster care status (child welfare)
Z62.6 Inappropriate (excessive) parental pressure
Z62.810 Personal history of physical and sexual abuse in childhood
Z62.811 Personal history of psychological abuse in childhood
Z62.820 Parent-biological child conflict
Z62.821 Parent-adopted child conflict
Z62.822 Parent-foster child conflict
Z63.72 Alcoholism and drug addiction in family
Z63.8 Other specified problems related to primary support group
Z65.3 Problems related to legal circumstances
Z71.89 Counseling, other specified
Z71.9 Counseling, unspecified
Z72.0 Tobacco use
Z77.011 Contact with and (suspected) exposure to lead
Z79.899 Other long term (current) drug therapy
Z81.0 Family history of intellectual disabilities (conditions classifiable to **F70–F79**)
Z81.8 Family history of other mental and behavioral disorders
Z83.2 Family history of diseases of the blood and blood-forming organs (anemia) (conditions classifiable to **D50–D89**)
Z86.2 Personal history of diseases of the blood and blood-forming organs
Z86.39 Personal history of other endocrine, nutritional, and metabolic disease
Z86.59 Personal history of other mental and behavioral disorders
Z86.69 Personal history of other diseases of the nervous system and sense organs
Z87.09 Personal history of other diseases of the respiratory system
Z87.19 Personal history of other diseases of the digestive system
Z87.798 Personal history of other (corrected) congenital malformations
Z87.820 Personal history of traumatic brain injury
Z91.128 Patient's intentional underdosing of medication regimen for other reason (report drug code)
Z91.138 Patient's unintentional underdosing of medication regimen for other reason (report drug code)
Z91.14 Patient's other noncompliance with medication regimen
Z91.19 Patient's noncompliance with other medical treatment and regimen
Z91.411 Personal history of adult psychological abuse

• New *CPT* code
▲ Revised *CPT* code
+ Codes are *add-on codes*, meaning they are reported separately in addition to the appropriate code for the service provided.
* Indicates a *CPT*-approved telemedicine service.

CPT® copyright 2019 American Medical Association. All rights reserved.

Continuum Model for ADHD

The following continuum model from *Coding for Pediatrics 2020* has been devised to express the various levels of service for ADHD. This model demonstrates the cumulative effect of the key criteria for each level of service using a single diagnosis as the common denominator. It also shows the importance of other variables, such as patient age, duration and severity of illness, social contexts, and comorbid conditions, that often have key roles in pediatric cases.

Quick Reference for Codes Used in Continuum for ADHD—Established Patients[a]

E/M Code Level	History	Examination	MDM	Time
99211[b]	NA	NA	NA	5 min
99212	Problem-focused	Problem-focused	Straightforward	10 min
99213	Expanded problem-focused	Expanded problem-focused	Low	15 min
99214	Detailed	Detailed	Moderate	25 min
99215	Comprehensive	Comprehensive	High	40 min

Abbreviations: ADHD, attention-deficit/hyperactivity disorder; E/M, evaluation and management; MDM, medical decision-making; NA, not applicable.
[a] Use of a code level requires that you meet or exceed 2 of the 3 key components on the basis of medical necessity.
[b] Low level E/M service that may not require the presence of a physician.

Adapted from American Academy of Pediatrics. *Coding for Pediatrics 2020: A Manual for Pediatric Documentation and Payment*. 25th ed. Itasca, IL: American Academy of Pediatrics; 2020.

CPT® copyright 2019 American Medical Association. All rights reserved.

Continuum Model for Attention-Deficit/Hyperactivity Disorder

Code selection at any level above **99211** may be based on time when documentation states that more than 50% of the total face-to-face time of the encounter is spent in counseling and/or coordination of care. Select the code with the typical time closest to the total face-to-face time.

CPT® Code Vignette	History	Physical Examination (systems)	Medical Decision-making (2 of 3 diagnoses, data, risk)
99211 Nurse visit to check growth or blood pressure prior to renewing prescription for psychoactive drugs	No specific key components required. Must indicate continuation of physician's plan of care, medical necessity, assessment, and/or education provided. CC: Check growth or blood pressure. HPI: Existing medications and desired/undesired effects. Documentation of height, weight, and blood pressure. Assessment: Doing well. Obtained physician approval for prescription refill. Keep appointment with physician in 1 month.		
99212 (Typical time: 10 min) Visit to recheck recent weight loss in patient with established ADHD otherwise stable on stimulant medication	**Problem focused** CC: Weight loss, ADHD HPI: Appetite, signs and symptoms, duration since last weight check	**Problem focused** 1. Constitutional (weight, blood pressure, overall appearance)	**Straightforward** 1. Stable established problem 2. No tests ordered/data reviewed 3. Risk: 1 chronic illness with side effects of treatment and prescription drug management
99213 (Typical time: 15 min) 3- to 6-month visit for child with ADHD who is presently doing well using medication and without other problems	**Expanded problem focused** CC: ADHD HPI: Effect of medication on appetite, mood, sleep, quality of schoolwork (eg, review report cards) ROS: Neurologic (no tics) PFSH: Review of medications	**Expanded problem focused** 1. Constitutional (temperature, weight, blood pressure) 2. Neurologic 3. Psychiatric (alert and oriented, mood and affect)	**Low complexity** 1. Stable established problem 2. Data reviewed: Rating scale results and feedback materials from teacher 3. Risk: Prescription drug management *or* Time: Documented faced-to-face time and >50% spent in counseling and/or coordination and context of discussion of 6-month treatment plan with adjustment of medication
99214 (Typical time: 25 min) Follow-up evaluation of an established patient with ADHD with failure to improve on medication and/or weight loss and new symptoms of depression	**Detailed** CC: ADHD with failure to improve HPI: Signs and symptoms since start of medication; modifying factors; quality of schoolwork (eg, review report cards) ROS: Gastrointestinal and psychiatric PFSH: Current medications; allergies; school attendance; substance use	**Detailed** 1. General multisystem examination with details of affected systems (2–7 systems in all) or detailed single organ system examination of neurologic system	**Moderate complexity** 1. Established problem, not improving with current therapy, and new problem without additional workup planned 2. Data reviewed: Rating scale results and feedback materials from teacher; depression screening score 3. Risk: Prescription drug management *or* Time: Documented face-to-face time with >50% spent in discussion of possible interventions, including, but not limited to 1. Educational intervention 2. Alteration in medications 3. Obtaining drug levels 4. Psychiatric intervention 5. Behavioral modification program

Continuum Model for Attention-Deficit/Hyperactivity Disorder (*continued*)

Code selection at any level above **99211** may be based on time when documentation states that more than 50% of the total face-to-face time of the encounter is spent in counseling and/or coordination of care. Select the code with the typical time closest to the total face-to-face time.

CPT® Code Vignette	History	Physical Examination (systems)	Medical Decision-making (2 of 3 diagnoses, data, risk)
99215 (Typical time: 40 min) Initial evaluation of an established patient experiencing difficulty in classroom, home, or social situation and suspected of having ADHD	**Comprehensive** CC: Difficulty in school, home, and social situations HPI: Signs and symptoms, duration, modifying factors, severity ROS: Constitutional, eyes, ENMT, cardiovascular, respiratory, musculoskeletal, integumentary, neurological, psychiatric, endocrine	Comprehensive examination of ≥8 systems or comprehensive neurologic/psychiatric examination (1997 guidelines)	**High complexity** 1. New problem with additional workup 2. Tests ordered and data reviewed: ADHD assessment instruments; history obtained from parents; and case discussion with another provider (eg, school counselor) 3. Risk: Undiagnosed new problem

Abbreviations: ADHD, attention-deficit/hyperactivity disorder; CC, chief complaint; CPT, Current Procedural Terminology; *ENMT, ears, nose, mouth, throat; HPI, history of present illness; PFSH, past, family, and social history; ROS, review of systems.*

ADHD—What is Attention Deficit/ Hyperactivity Disorder?

Almost all children can experience times of decreased attention and/or increased activity. However, for some children, decreased attention and/or increased activity is more than an occasional problem. Read on for information from the American Academy of Pediatrics about attention deficit/hyperactivity disorder (ADHD).

What is ADHD?

ADHD is a condition of the brain that makes it difficult for children to manage their attention, activity, and impulses. It is one of the most common chronic conditions of childhood. It affects 6% to 12% of school-aged children. ADHD is diagnosed about 3 times more often in boys than in girls (who more frequently have the inattentive type that goes unnoticed). The condition affects children in specific ways.

Children with attention-deficit/hyperactivity disorder (ADHD) have neurobehavioral problems that can interfere with their daily lives. An impulsive nature may put them into physical danger. Children with ADHD may speed about in constant motion, make noise nonstop, refuse to wait their turn, or crash into things. At other times, they may drift as if in a daydream, be unable to pay attention, or be unable to or finish what they start because they are paying attention to another thought or something they see. Those who have trouble paying attention may have trouble learning. Keep in mind that not all children with ADHD have all the symptoms. Each child is unique. For example, some may only have problems paying attention, while others may have problems with both attention and activity.

Recognition is important as early as possible to help minimize or prevent serious, lifelong problems, such as difficulty in school, at home, or at work and/or difficulty in making and keeping friends. Children with ADHD may have trouble getting along with siblings and other children. They may be labeled "bad kids."

If your child has ADHD, effective treatment is available. Your child's doctor can offer a long-term treatment plan to help your child lead a happy and healthy life. As a parent, you have a very important role in this treatment.

Visit HealthyChildren.org for more information.

Resources

American Academy of Pediatrics

www.AAP.org and www.HealthyChildren.org

Here is a list of ADHD support groups and resources. Also, your child's doctor may know about specific resources in your community.

ADDA (Attention Deficit Disorder Association)

www.add.org

CHADD (Children and Adults with Attention-Deficit/ Hyperactivity Disorder)—The National Resource Center on ADHD

800/233-4050

www.chadd.org

Center for Parent Information and Resources

www.parentcenterhub.org

National Institute of Mental Health

866/615-6464 www.nimh.nih.gov

Tourette Association of America

888/4-TOURET (486-8738)

www.tourette.org

From Your Doctor 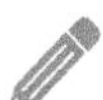

American Academy of Pediatrics
DEDICATED TO THE HEALTH OF ALL CHILDREN®

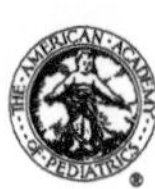

healthychildren.org
Powered by pediatricians. Trusted by parents. from the American Academy of Pediatrics

The American Academy of Pediatrics (AAP) is an organization of 67,000 primary care pediatricians, pediatric medical subspecialists, and pediatric surgical specialists dedicated to the health, safety, and well-being of infants, children, adolescents, and young adults.

Adapted from the American Academy of Pediatrics patient education booklet, *Understanding ADHD: Information for Parents About Attention-Deficit/Hyperactivity Disorder.* Any websites, brand names, products, or manufacturers are mentioned for informational and identification purposes only and do not imply an endorsement by the American Academy of Pediatrics (AAP). The AAP is not responsible for the content of external resources. Information was current at the time of publication. The information contained in this publication should not be used as a substitute for the medical care and advice of your pediatrician. There may be variations in treatment that your pediatrician may recommend based on individual facts and circumstances.

© 2020 American Academy of Pediatrics. All rights reserved.

ADHD—What are the Symptoms of Attention Deficit/Hyperactivity Disorder?

Are you concerned your child may have attention deficit/hyperactivity disorder (ADHD)? Read on for information from the American Academy of Pediatrics about the symptoms and types of ADHD.

What are the symptoms of ADHD?

Children with ADHD have symptoms that fall into 3 groups: inattention, hyperactivity, and impulsivity. See Table 1.

Table 1. Symptoms of ADHD

Symptom	How a Child With This Symptom May Behave
Inattention	Often has a hard time paying attention; daydreams
	Often does not seem to listen
	Is easily distracted from work or play
	Often does not seem to notice details; makes careless mistakes
	Frequently does not follow through on instructions or finish tasks
	Is disorganized
	Frequently loses a lot of important things
	Often forgets things
	Frequently avoids doing things that require ongoing mental efforts
Hyperactivity	Is in constant motion, as if "driven by a motor"
	Has trouble staying seated
	Frequently squirms and fidgets
	Talks a lot
	Often runs, jumps, and climbs when this is not permitted
	Has trouble playing quietly
Impulsivity	Frequently acts and speaks without thinking
	May run into the street without looking for traffic first
	Frequently has trouble taking turns
	Cannot wait for things
	Often calls out an answer before the question is complete
	Frequently interrupts others

Are there different types of ADHD?

Children with ADHD may have one or more of the symptoms listed in Table 1. The symptoms are usually classified as the following types of ADHD:

- Inattentive only (formerly known as attention-deficit disorder [ADD])—Children with this form of ADHD are not overly active. Because they do not disrupt the classroom or other activities, their symptoms may not be noticed. Among girls with ADHD, this form is more common.
- Hyperactive-impulsive—Children with this type of ADHD have increased activity and impulsivity with typical attention spans. This is the least common type and often occurs in younger children.
- Combined inattentive-hyperactive-impulsive—Children with this type of ADHD have all 3 symptoms. It is the type most people think of when they think of ADHD.

How can I tell if my child has ADHD?

Remember, it is common for all children to show some of these symptoms from time to time. Your child may be reacting to stress at school or at home. He may be bored or going through a difficult stage of life. It does not mean he has ADHD.

Sometimes a teacher is the first to notice inattention, hyperactivity, and/or impulsivity and will inform the parents.

Visit HealthyChildren.org for more information.

From Your Doctor 

American Academy of Pediatrics 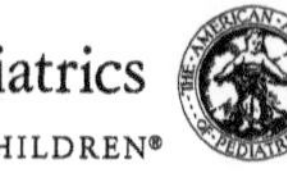

DEDICATED TO THE HEALTH OF ALL CHILDREN®

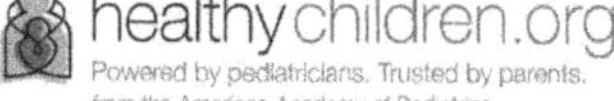

The American Academy of Pediatrics (AAP) is an organization of 67,000 primary care pediatricians, pediatric medical subspecialists, and pediatric surgical specialists dedicated to the health, safety, and well-being of infants, children, adolescents, and young adults.

Adapted from the American Academy of Pediatrics patient education booklet, *Understanding ADHD: Information for Parents About Attention-Deficit/Hyperactivity Disorder.* The information contained in this publication should not be used as a substitute for the medical care and advice of your pediatrician. There may be variations in treatment that your pediatrician may recommend based on individual facts and circumstances.

© 2020 American Academy of Pediatrics. All rights reserved.

ADHD — What are the Symptoms of Attention-Deficit/Hyperactivity Disorder?

ADHD—How is Attention Deficit/ Hyperactivity Disorder Diagnosed?

There is no single test for attention deficit/hyperactivity disorder (ADHD). Diagnosis requires several steps and involves gathering information from multiple sources. You, your child, your child's school, and other caregivers should be involved in observing your child. Read on for information from the American Academy of Pediatrics about diagnosing ADHD.

How is ADHD diagnosed?

Your child's or teen's doctor will determine whether your child or teen has ADHD by using standard guidelines developed by the American Academy of Pediatrics specifically for children, teens, and young adults 4 to 18 years of age.

It is difficult to diagnose ADHD in children younger than 4 years. This is because younger children change very rapidly. It is also more difficult to diagnose ADHD once a child becomes a teen.

Children with ADHD show signs of inattention, hyperactivity, and/or impulsivity in specific ways. Your child's doctor will consider how your child's actions compare with that of other children his age, using the information reported about your child by you, his teacher, and any other caregivers who spend time with your child, such as coaches, grandparents, or child care workers.

Here are guidelines used to confirm a diagnosis of ADHD.

- Some symptoms occur in 2 or more settings such as home, school, and social situations and cause some impairment.
- In a child or teen 4 to 17 years of age, 6 or more symptoms must be identified.
- In a teen or young adult 17 years and older, 5 or more symptoms must be identified.
- Symptoms significantly impair your child's ability to function in some daily activities, such as doing schoolwork, maintaining relationships with parents and siblings, building relationships with friends, or having the ability to function in groups such as sports teams.

Your child's doctor will conduct a physical and neurological examination. A full medical history will be needed to put your child's action into context and screen for other conditions that may affect behavior. Your child's doctor will also talk with your child about how he acts and feels.

Your child's doctor may refer your child to a pediatric subspecialist or mental health professionals if there are concerns of

- Intellectual disability (previously called mental retardation)
- Developmental disorders, such as in speech, coordination, or learning
- Chronic illness being treated with a medication that may interfere with learning
- Trouble seeing and/or hearing
- History of abuse
- Major anxiety or major depression
- Severe aggression
- Possible seizure disorder
- Possible sleep disorder

How can parents help with the diagnosis?

As a parent, you will provide crucial information about your child's actions and how they affect life at home, in school, and in other social settings. Your child's doctor will want to know what symptoms your child is showing, how long the symptoms have occurred, and how these affect him and your family. You will likely be asked to fill in checklists or rating scales about your child's actions.

In addition, sharing your family history can offer important clues about your child's behavior.

How will my child's school be involved?

For an accurate diagnosis, your child's doctor will need to get information about your child directly from his classroom teacher or another school professional. Children at least 4 years and older spend many of their waking hours at preschool or school. Teachers provide valuable insights. Your child's teacher may write a report or discuss the following topics with your child's doctor:

- Your child's actions in the classroom
- Your child's learning patterns
- How long the symptoms have been a problem
- How the symptoms are affecting your child's progress at school
- Ways the classroom program is being adapted to help your child
- Whether other conditions may be affecting the symptoms
- If there are evaluations and help the school can provide

In addition, your child's doctor may want to see report cards, standardized tests, and samples of your child's schoolwork.

How will others who care for my child be involved?

Other caregivers may also provide important information about your child's actions. Former teachers, religious and scout leaders, grandparents, or coaches may have valuable input. If your child is homeschooled, it is especially important to assess his actions in settings outside the home.

Your child may not behave the same way at home as he does in other settings. Direct information about the way your child acts in more than one setting is a requirement to make a diagnosis. It is important to consider other possible causes of your child's symptoms in these settings.

In some cases, other mental health care professionals, such as child psychologists or psychiatrists, may also need to be involved in gathering information for the diagnosis.

Are there other tests for ADHD?

You may have heard theories about other tests for ADHD. There are no other proven diagnostic tests at this time.

Many theories have been presented, but studies have shown that the following evaluations add little value in diagnosing the disorder:

- Screening for thyroid problems
- Computerized continuous performance tests
- Brain imaging studies, such as computed tomography (CT) and magnetic resonance imaging (MRI)
- Electroencephalography (EEG) or brain-wave testing

While these evaluations are not helpful in diagnosing ADHD, your child's doctor may see other signs or symptoms in your child that warrant additional tests.

What are coexisting conditions?

As part of the diagnosis, your child's doctor will look for other conditions that cause the same types of symptoms as ADHD. Your child may simply have a different condition or ADHD combined with another condition (a coexisting condition). Most children with a diagnosis of ADHD have at least one additional condition.

Common coexisting conditions include

- **Learning disabilities**—Learning disabilities are conditions that make it difficult for a child to master specific skills, such as reading or math. ADHD is not a learning disability per se. However, ADHD can make it hard for a child to learn and do well in school. Diagnosing learning disabilities requires conducting evaluations, such as intelligence quotient (IQ) and academic achievement tests, and it requires educational interventions. The school will usually be able to assess whether your child has a learning disability and what his educational needs are.
- **Oppositional defiant disorder or conduct disorder**—Up to 35% of children with ADHD may have inappropriate actions because of an oppositional defiant or conduct disorder.
  - Children with oppositional defiant disorder tend to lose their temper easily and to annoy people on purpose, and they can be defiant and hostile toward authority figures.
  - Children with conduct disorder may break rules, destroy property, be suspended or expelled from school, violate the rights of other people, or show cruelty to other children or animals.
  - Children with coexisting conduct disorder are at higher risk of having trouble with the law or having substance use problems than children who have only ADHD. Studies show that this type of coexisting condition is more common among children with the combined type of ADHD.
- **Anxiety disorders**—About 25% of children with ADHD also have anxiety disorders. Children with anxiety disorders have extreme feelings of fear, worry, or panic that make it difficult to function. These disorders can produce physical symptoms such as racing pulse, sweating, diarrhea, and nausea. Counseling and/or different medication may be needed to treat these coexisting conditions.
- **Mood disorders, including depression**—About 18% of children with ADHD also have mood disorders, usually depression and less commonly bipolar disorder (formerly called manic depressive disorder). There may be a family history of these conditions. Coexisting mood disorders may put children and teens at higher risk for self-harm or suicide, especially during the teen years. These disorders are more common among children with inattentive or combined type of ADHD. Children with mood disorders or depression often require additional interventions or a different type of medication than those typically used to treat ADHD.
- **Language disorders**—Children with ADHD may have difficulty with how they use language. This is referred to as a pragmatic language disorder. It may not show up with standard tests of language. A speech-language clinician can detect it by observing how a child uses language in his day-to-day activities.

Visit HealthyChildren.org for more information.

From Your Doctor

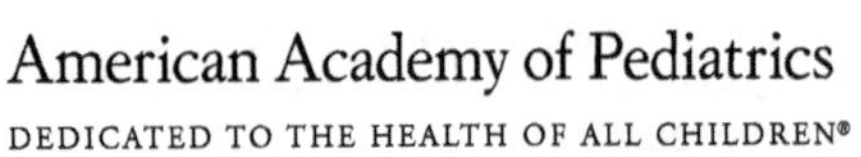

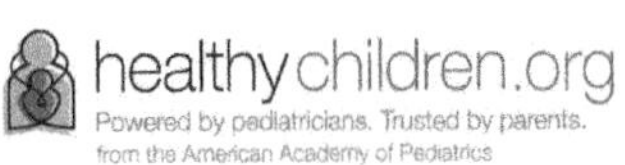

The American Academy of Pediatrics (AAP) is an organization of 67,000 primary care pediatricians, pediatric medical subspecialists, and pediatric surgical specialists dedicated to the health, safety, and well-being of infants, children, adolescents, and young adults.

Adapted from the American Academy of Pediatrics patient education booklet, *Understanding ADHD: Information for Parents About Attention-Deficit/Hyperactivity Disorder.* Information applies to all sexes and genders; however, for easier reading, pronouns such as he are used in this publication. The information contained in this publication should not be used as a substitute for the medical care and advice of your pediatrician. There may be variations in treatment that your pediatrician may recommend based on individual facts and circumstances.

© 2020 American Academy of Pediatrics. All rights reserved.

ADHD—What Causes Attention Deficit/ Hyperactivity Disorder and How Is It Treated?

Understanding attention deficit/hyperactivity disorder (ADHD) helps you understand how it affects your child. Read on for information from the American Academy of Pediatrics about the causes and treatments for ADHD.

What causes ADHD?

ADHD is one of the most studied conditions of childhood, and it may be caused by a number of things.

Research to date has shown

- ADHD is a neurobiological condition whose symptoms can also depend on the child's environment.
- A lower level of activity in the parts of the brain that control attention and activity level may be associated with ADHD.
- ADHD often runs in families.
- In very rare cases, toxins in the environment may lead to ADHD-like symptoms. For instance, lead in the body can affect child development.
- Significant head injuries may cause ADHD-like symptoms in some children.
- Preterm birth increases the risk of developing ADHD.
- Prenatal substance exposures, such as to alcohol or nicotine from smoking, increase the risk of developing ADHD-like symptoms.

There is no scientific evidence that ADHD is caused by

- Eating too much sugar
- Food additives or food colorings
- Allergies
- Immunizations

How is ADHD treated?

Once the diagnosis is confirmed, the outlook for most children who receive treatment of ADHD is encouraging. There is no specific cure for ADHD, but many treatment options are available to manage the condition. Some children and adults learn to compensate for the symptoms as they mature so that they no longer require treatment.

Each child's treatment must be tailored to meet his individual needs. In most cases, treatment of ADHD should include A long-term management plan with

- Target outcomes for behavior
  - Follow-up activities
  - Monitoring
  - Education about ADHD
- Teamwork among doctors, parents, teachers, caregivers, other health care professionals, and the child
- Behavioral parent training
- Behavioral school programs
- Medication

Treatment of ADHD is based on the same principles that are used to treat other chronic conditions, such as asthma or diabetes. Long-term planning for many children is needed. Families must manage chronic conditions continually. In the case of ADHD, schools and other caregivers must also be involved in managing the condition.

Educating the people involved with your child is a key part of treatment of ADHD. As a parent, you will need to learn about the condition. Read about it and talk with people who understand it. This will help you manage the ways ADHD affects your child and your family day to day. It will also help your child learn to help himself.

What are target outcomes?

At the beginning of treatment, your child's doctor should help your family set up to 3 target outcomes (goals) for your child. These target outcomes will guide the treatment plan. Your child's target outcomes should be chosen to help him function as well as possible at home, at school, and in your community. You and your child should identify what is preventing him from succeeding.

Here are examples of target outcomes.

- Improved relationships with parents, siblings, teachers, and friends—for example, fewer arguments with siblings or being invited more often to friends' houses or parties
- Better schoolwork practices—for example, completing all classwork or homework assignments
- More independence in self-care or homework—for example, getting ready for school in the morning without supervision
- Improved self-esteem, such as feeling that he can get his work done
- Fewer disruptive actions—for example, decreasing the number of times he refuses to obey rules
- Safer behavior in the community—for example, being careful when crossing streets

The target outcomes should be

- Realistic
- Something your child will be able to do
- Behaviors that you can observe and count (with rating scales when possible)

Your child's treatment plan will be set up to help achieve these goals.

Visit HealthyChildren.org for more information.

American Academy of Pediatrics
DEDICATED TO THE HEALTH OF ALL CHILDREN®

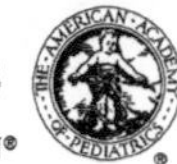

healthychildren.org
Powered by pediatricians. Trusted by parents.
from the American Academy of Pediatrics

The American Academy of Pediatrics (AAP) is an organization of 67,000 primary care pediatricians, pediatric medical subspecialists, and pediatric surgical specialists dedicated to the health, safety, and well-being of infants, children, adolescents, and young adults.

Adapted from the American Academy of Pediatrics patient education booklet, *Understanding ADHD: Information for Parents About Attention-Deficit/Hyperactivity Disorder.* The information contained in this publication should not be used as a substitute for the medical care and advice of your pediatrician. There may be variations in treatment that your pediatrician may recommend based on individual facts and circumstances.

© 2020 American Academy of Pediatrics. All rights reserved.

Brief Resolved Unexplained Events (Formerly Apparent Life-Threatening Events) and Evaluation of Lower-Risk Infants

- *Clinical Practice Guideline*
  - *PPI: AAP Partnership for Policy Implementation See Appendix 1 for more information.*

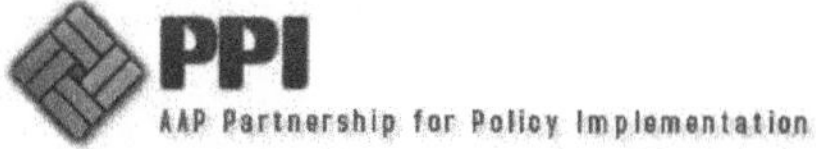

- *Executive Summary*
  - *PPI: AAP Partnership for Policy Implementation See Appendix 1 for more information.*

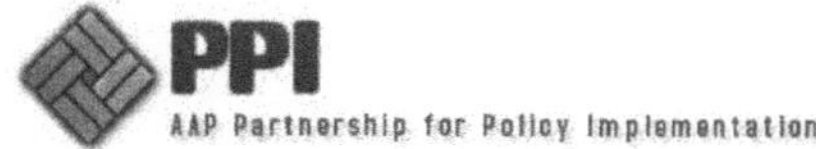

CLINICAL PRACTICE GUIDELINE Guidance for the Clinician in Rendering Pediatric Care

American Academy of Pediatrics

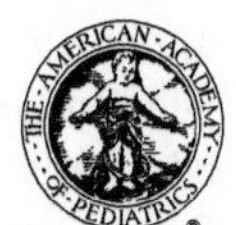

DEDICATED TO THE HEALTH OF ALL CHILDREN™

Brief Resolved Unexplained Events (Formerly Apparent Life-Threatening Events) and Evaluation of Lower-Risk Infants

Joel S. Tieder, MD, MPH, FAAP, Joshua L. Bonkowsky, MD, PhD, FAAP, Ruth A. Etzel, MD, PhD, FAAP, Wayne H. Franklin, MD, MPH, MMM, FAAP, David A. Gremse, MD, FAAP, Bruce Herman, MD, FAAP, Eliot S. Katz, MD, FAAP, Leonard R. Krilov, MD, FAAP, J. Lawrence Merritt II, MD, FAAP, Chuck Norlin, MD, FAAP, Jack Percelay, MD, MPH, FAAP, Robert E. Sapién, MD, MMM, FAAP, Richard N. Shiffman, MD, MCIS, FAAP, Michael B.H. Smith, MB, FRCPCH, FAAP, for the SUBCOMMITTEE ON APPARENT LIFE THREATENING EVENTS

abstract

This is the first clinical practice guideline from the American Academy of Pediatrics that specifically applies to patients who have experienced an apparent life-threatening event (ALTE). This clinical practice guideline has 3 objectives. First, it recommends the replacement of the term ALTE with a new term, brief resolved unexplained event (BRUE). Second, it provides an approach to patient evaluation that is based on the risk that the infant will have a repeat event or has a serious underlying disorder. Finally, it provides management recommendations, or key action statements, for lower-risk infants. The term BRUE is defined as an event occurring in an infant younger than 1 year when the observer reports a sudden, brief, and now resolved episode of ≥1 of the following: (1) cyanosis or pallor; (2) absent, decreased, or irregular breathing; (3) marked change in tone (hyper- or hypotonia); and (4) altered level of responsiveness. A BRUE is diagnosed only when there is no explanation for a qualifying event after conducting an appropriate history and physical examination. By using this definition and framework, infants younger than 1 year who present with a BRUE are categorized either as (1) a lower-risk patient on the basis of history and physical examination for whom evidence-based recommendations for evaluation and management are offered or (2) a higher-risk patient whose history and physical examination suggest the need for further investigation and treatment but for whom recommendations are not offered. This clinical practice guideline is intended to foster a patient- and family-centered approach to care, reduce unnecessary and costly medical interventions, improve patient outcomes, support implementation, and provide direction for future research. Each key action statement indicates a level of evidence, the benefit-harm relationship, and the strength of recommendation.

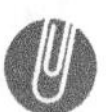

This document is copyrighted and is property of the American Academy of Pediatrics and its Board of Directors. All authors have filed conflict of interest statements with the American Academy of Pediatrics. Any conflicts have been resolved through a process approved by the Board of Directors. The American Academy of Pediatrics has neither solicited nor accepted any commercial involvement in the development of the content of this publication.

The guidance in this report does not indicate an exclusive course of treatment or serve as a standard of medical care. Variations, taking into account individual circumstances, may be appropriate.

All clinical practice guidelines from the American Academy of Pediatrics automatically expire 5 years after publication unless reaffirmed, revised, or retired at or before that time.

DOI: 10.1542/peds.2016-0590

PEDIATRICS (ISSN Numbers: Print, 0031-4005; Online, 1098-4275).

Copyright © 2016 by the American Academy of Pediatrics

To cite: Tieder JS, Bonkowsky JL, Etzel RA, et al. Brief Resolved Unexplained Events (Formerly Apparent Life-Threatening Events) and Evaluation of Lower-Risk Infants. *Pediatrics.* 2016;137(5):e20160590

INTRODUCTION

This clinical practice guideline applies to infants younger than 1 year and is intended for pediatric clinicians. This guideline has 3 primary objectives. First, it recommends the replacement of the term apparent life-threatening event (ALTE) with a new term, brief resolved unexplained event (BRUE). Second, it provides an approach to patient evaluation that is based on the risk that the infant will have a recurring event or has a serious underlying disorder. Third, it provides evidence-based management recommendations, or key action statements, for lower-risk patients whose history and physical examination are normal. It does not offer recommendations for higher-risk patients whose history and physical examination suggest the need for further investigation and treatment (because of insufficient evidence or the availability of clinical practice guidelines specific to their presentation). This clinical practice guideline also provides implementation support and suggests directions for future research.

The term ALTE originated from a 1986 National Institutes of Health Consensus Conference on Infantile Apnea and was intended to replace the term "near-miss sudden infant death syndrome" (SIDS).[1] An ALTE was defined as "an episode that is frightening to the observer and that is characterized by some combination of apnea (central or occasionally obstructive), color change (usually cyanotic or pallid but occasionally erythematous or plethoric), marked change in muscle tone (usually marked limpness), choking, or gagging. In some cases, the observer fears that the infant has died."[2] Although the definition of ALTE eventually enabled researchers to establish that these events are separate entities from SIDS, the clinical application of this classification, which describes a constellation of observed, subjective, and nonspecific symptoms, has raised significant challenges for clinicians and parents in the evaluation and care of these infants.[3] Although a broad range of disorders can present as an ALTE (eg, child abuse, congenital abnormalities, epilepsy, inborn errors of metabolism, and infections), for a majority of infants who appear well after the event, the risk of a serious underlying disorder or a recurrent event is extremely low.[2]

CHANGE IN TERMINOLOGY AND DIAGNOSIS

The imprecise nature of the original ALTE definition is difficult to apply to clinical care and research.[3] As a result, the clinician is often faced with several dilemmas. First, under the ALTE definition, the infant is often, but not necessarily, asymptomatic on presentation. The evaluation and management of symptomatic infants (eg, those with fever or respiratory distress) need to be distinguished from that of asymptomatic infants. Second, the reported symptoms under the ALTE definition, although often concerning to the caregiver, are not intrinsically life-threatening and frequently are a benign manifestation of normal infant physiology or a self-limited condition. A definition needs enough precision to allow the clinician to base clinical decisions on events that are characterized as abnormal after conducting a thorough history and physical examination. For example, a constellation of symptoms suggesting hemodynamic instability or central apnea needs to be distinguished from more common and less concerning events readily characterized as periodic breathing of the newborn, breath-holding spells, dysphagia, or gastroesophageal reflux (GER). Furthermore, events defined as ALTEs are rarely a manifestation of a more serious illness that, if left undiagnosed, could lead to morbidity or death. Yet, the perceived potential for recurring events or a serious underlying disorder often provokes concern in caregivers and clinicians.[2,4,5] This concern can compel testing or admission to the hospital for observation, which can increase parental anxiety and subject the patient to further risk and does not necessarily lead to a treatable diagnosis or prevention of future events. A more precise definition could prevent the overuse of medical interventions by helping clinicians distinguish infants with lower risk. Finally, the use of ALTE as a diagnosis may reinforce the caregivers' perceptions that the event was indeed "life-threatening," even when it most often was not. For these reasons, a replacement of the term ALTE with a more specific term could improve clinical care and management.

In this clinical practice guideline, a more precise definition is introduced for this group of clinical events: brief resolved unexplained event (BRUE). The term BRUE is intended to better reflect the transient nature and lack of clear cause and removes the "life-threatening" label. The authors of this guideline recommend that the term ALTE no longer be used by clinicians to describe an event or as a diagnosis. Rather, the term BRUE should be used to describe events occurring in infants younger than 1 year of age that are characterized by the observer as "brief" (lasting <1 minute but typically <20–30 seconds) and "resolved" (meaning the patient returned to baseline state of health after the event) and with a reassuring history, physical examination, and vital signs at the time of clinical evaluation by trained medical providers (Table 1). For example, the presence of respiratory symptoms or fever would preclude classification of an event as a BRUE. BRUEs are also "unexplained," meaning that a clinician is unable to explain the cause of the event after an appropriate history and physical examination. Similarly, an event characterized as choking or gagging associated with spitting up is not included in the BRUE definition, because clinicians will want to pursue the cause of vomiting, which may be related to GER, infection, or central nervous system (CNS) disease. However, until BRUE-specific codes are available, for billing and coding purposes, it is reasonable to apply the ALTE International Classification of Diseases, 9th Revision, and International Classification of Diseases, 10th revision, codes to patients determined to have experienced a BRUE (see section entitled "Dissemination and Implementation").

BRUE DEFINITION

Clinicians should use the term BRUE to describe an event occurring in an infant <1 year of age when the observer reports a sudden, brief, and now resolved episode of ≥1 of the following:

- **cyanosis or pallor**
- **absent, decreased, or irregular breathing**
- **marked change in tone (hyper- or hypotonia)**
- **altered level of responsiveness**

Moreover, clinicians should diagnose a BRUE only when there is no explanation for a qualifying event after conducting an appropriate history and physical examination (Tables 2 and 3).

TABLE 1 BRUE Definition and Factors for Inclusion and Exclusion

	Includes	Excludes
Brief	Duration <1 min; typically 20–30 s	Duration ≥1 min
Resolved	Patient returned to his or her baseline state of health after the event	At the time of medical evaluation:
	Normal vital signs	Fever or recent fever
	Normal appearance	Tachypnea, bradypnea, apnea
		Tachycardia or bradycardia
		Hypotension, hypertension, or hemodynamic instability
		Mental status changes, somnolence, lethargy
		Hypotonia or hypertonia
		Vomiting
		Bruising, petechiae, or other signs of injury/trauma
		Abnormal weight, growth, or head circumference
		Noisy breathing (stridor, sturgor, wheezing)
		Repeat event(s)
Unexplained	Not explained by an identifiable medical condition	Event consistent with GER, swallow dysfunction, nasal congestion, etc
		History or physical examination concerning for child abuse, congenital airway abnormality, etc
Event Characterization		
Cyanosis or pallor	Central cyanosis: blue or purple coloration of face, gums, trunk	Acrocyanosis or perioral cyanosis
	Central pallor: pale coloration of face or trunk	Rubor
Absent, decreased, or irregular breathing	Central apnea	Periodic breathing of the newborn
	Obstructive apnea	Breath-holding spell
	Mixed obstructive apnea	
Marked change in tone (hyper- or hypotonia)	Hypertonia	Hypertonia associated with crying, choking, or gagging due to GER or feeding problems
	Hypotonia	Tone changes associated with breath-holding spell
		Tonic eye deviation or nystagmus
		Tonic-clonic seizure activity
		Infantile spasms
Altered responsiveness	Loss of consciousness	Loss of consciousness associated with breath-holding spell
	Mental status change	
	Lethargy	
	Somnolence	
	Postictal phase	

Differences between the terms ALTE and BRUE should be noted. First, the BRUE definition has a strict age limit. Second, an event is only a BRUE if there is no other likely explanation. Clinical symptoms such as fever, nasal congestion, and increased work of breathing may indicate temporary airway obstruction from viral infection. Events characterized as choking after vomiting may indicate a gastrointestinal cause, such as GER. Third, a BRUE diagnosis is based on the clinician's characterization of features of the event and not on a caregiver's perception that the event was life-threatening. Although such perceptions are understandable and important to address, such risk can only be assessed after the event has been objectively characterized by a clinician. Fourth, the clinician should determine whether the infant had episodic cyanosis or pallor, rather than just determining whether "color change" occurred. Episodes of rubor or redness are not consistent with BRUE, because they are common in healthy infants. Fifth, BRUE expands the respiratory criteria beyond "apnea" to include absent breathing, diminished breathing, and other breathing irregularities. Sixth, instead of the less specific criterion of "change in muscle tone," the clinician should determine whether there was marked change in tone, including hypertonia or hypotonia. Seventh, because choking and gagging usually indicate common diagnoses such as GER or respiratory infection, their presence suggests an event was not a BRUE. Finally, the use of "altered level of responsiveness" is a new criterion, because it can be an important component of an episodic but serious cardiac, respiratory, metabolic, or neurologic event.

For infants who have experienced a BRUE, a careful history and physical examination are necessary to characterize the event, assess the risk of recurrence, and determine the presence of an underlying disorder (Tables 2 and 3). The recommendations provided in this guideline focus on infants with a lower risk of a subsequent event or serious underlying disorder (see section entitled "Risk Assessment: Lower- Versus Higher-Risk BRUE"). In the absence of identifiable risk factors, infants are at lower risk and laboratory studies, imaging studies, and other diagnostic procedures are unlikely to be useful or necessary. However, if the clinical history or physical examination reveals abnormalities, the patient may be at higher risk and further evaluation should focus on the specific areas of concern. For example,

- possible child abuse may be considered when the event history is reported inconsistently or is incompatible with the child's developmental age, or when, on physical examination, there is unexplained bruising or a torn labial or lingual frenulum;
- a cardiac arrhythmia may be considered if there is a family history of sudden, unexplained death in first-degree relatives; and
- infection may be considered if there is fever or persistent respiratory symptoms.

TABLE 2 Historical Features To Be Considered in the Evaluation of a Potential BRUE

Features To Be Considered
Considerations for possible child abuse:
Multiple or changing versions of the history/circumstances
History/circumstances inconsistent with child's developmental stage
History of unexplained bruising
Incongruence between caregiver expectations and child's developmental stage, including assigning negative attributes to the child
History of the event
General description
Who reported the event?
Witness of the event? Parent(s), other children, other adults? Reliability of historian(s)?
State immediately before the event
Where did it occur (home/elsewhere, room, crib/floor, etc)?
Awake or asleep?
Position: supine, prone, upright, sitting, moving?
Feeding? Anything in the mouth? Availability of item to choke on? Vomiting or spitting up?
Objects nearby that could smother or choke?
State during the event
Choking or gagging noise?
Active/moving or quiet/flaccid?
Conscious? Able to see you or respond to voice?
Muscle tone increased or decreased?
Repetitive movements?
Appeared distressed or alarmed?
Breathing: yes/no, struggling to breathe?
Skin color: normal, pale, red, or blue?
Bleeding from nose or mouth?
Color of lips: normal, pale, or blue?
End of event
Approximate duration of the event?
How did it stop: with no intervention, picking up, positioning, rubbing or clapping back, mouth-to-mouth, chest compressions, etc?
End abruptly or gradually?
Treatment provided by parent/caregiver (eg, glucose-containing drink or food)?
911 called by caregiver?
State after event
Back to normal immediately/gradually/still not there?
Before back to normal, was quiet, dazed, fussy, irritable, crying?
Recent history
Illness in preceding day(s)?
If yes, detail signs/symptoms (fussiness, decreased activity, fever, congestion, rhinorrhea, cough, vomiting, diarrhea, decreased intake, poor sleep)
Injuries, falls, previous unexplained bruising?
Past medical history
Pre-/perinatal history
Gestational age
Newborn screen normal (for IEMs, congenital heart disease)?
Previous episodes/BRUE?
Reflux? If yes, obtain details, including management
Breathing problems? Noisy ever? Snoring?
Growth patterns normal?
Development normal? Assess a few major milestones across categories, any concerns about development or behavior?
Illnesses, injuries, emergencies?
Previous hospitalization, surgery?
Recent immunization?
Use of over-the-counter medications?
Family history
Sudden unexplained death (including unexplained car accident or drowning) in first- or second-degree family members before age 35, and particularly as an infant?
Apparent life-threatening event in sibling?
Long QT syndrome?
Arrhythmia?

TABLE 2 Continued

Features To Be Considered
Inborn error of metabolism or genetic disease?
Developmental delay?
Environmental history
Housing: general, water damage, or mold problems?
Exposure to tobacco smoke, toxic substances, drugs?
Social history
Family structure, individuals living in home?
Housing: general, mold?
Recent changes, stressors, or strife?
Exposure to smoke, toxic substances, drugs?
Recent exposure to infectious illness, particularly upper respiratory illness, paroxysmal cough, pertussis?
Support system(s)/access to needed resources?
Current level of concern/anxiety; how family manages adverse situations?
Potential impact of event/admission on work/family?
Previous child protective services or law enforcement involvement (eg, domestic violence, animal abuse), alerts/reports for this child or others in the family (when available)?
Exposure of child to adults with history of mental illness or substance abuse?

The key action statements in this clinical practice guideline do not apply to higher-risk patients but rather apply only to infants who meet the lower-risk criteria by having an otherwise normal history and physical examination.

RISK ASSESSMENT: LOWER- VERSUS HIGHER-RISK BRUE

Patients who have experienced a BRUE may have a recurrent event or an undiagnosed serious condition (eg, child abuse, pertussis, etc) that confers a risk of adverse outcomes. Although this risk has been difficult to quantify historically and no studies have fully evaluated patient-centered outcomes (eg, family experience survey), the systematic review of the ALTE literature identified a subset of BRUE patients who are unlikely to have a recurrent event or undiagnosed serious conditions, are at lower risk of adverse outcomes, and can likely be managed safely without extensive diagnostic evaluation or hospitalization.[3] In the systematic review of ALTE studies in which it was possible to identify BRUE patients, the following characteristics most consistently conferred higher risk: infants <2 months of age, those with a history of prematurity, and those with more than 1 event. There was generally an increased risk from prematurity in infants born at <32 weeks' gestation, and the risk attenuated once infants born at <32 weeks' gestation reached 45 weeks' postconceptional age. Two ALTE studies evaluated the duration of the event.[6,7] Although duration did not appear to be predictive of hospital admission, it was difficult to discern a BRUE population from the heterogeneous ALTE populations. Nonetheless, most events were less than one minute. By consensus, the subcommittee established <1 minute as the upper limit of a "brief event," understanding that objective, verifiable measurements were rarely, if ever, available. Cariopulmonary resuscitation (CPR) was identified as a risk factor in the older ALTE studies and confirmed in a recent study,[6] but it was unclear how the need for CPR was determined. Therefore, the committee agreed by consensus that the need for CPR should be determined by trained medical providers.

PATIENT FACTORS THAT DETERMINE A LOWER RISK

To be designated lower risk, the following criteria should be met (see Fig 1):

- Age >60 days
- Prematurity: gestational age ≥32 weeks and postconceptional age ≥45 weeks
- First BRUE (no previous BRUE ever and not occurring in clusters)
- Duration of event <1 minute
- No CPR required by trained medical provider
- No concerning historical features (see Table 2)
- No concerning physical examination findings (see Table 3)

Infants who have experienced a BRUE who do not qualify as lower-risk patients are, by definition, at higher risk. Unfortunately, the outcomes data from ALTE studies in the heterogeneous higher-risk population are unclear and preclude the derivation of evidence-based recommendations regarding management. Thus, pending further research, this guideline does not provide recommendations for the management of the higher-risk infant. Nonetheless, it is important for clinicians and researchers to recognize that some studies suggest that higher-risk BRUE patients may be more likely to have a serious underlying cause, recurrent event, or an adverse outcome. For example, infants younger than 2 months who experience a BRUE may be more likely to have a congenital or infectious cause and be at higher risk of an adverse outcome. Infants who have experienced multiple events or a concerning social assessment for child abuse may warrant increased observation to better document the events or contextual factors. A list of differential diagnoses for BRUE patients is provided in Supplemental Table 6.

METHODS

In July 2013, the American Academy of Pediatrics (AAP) convened a multidisciplinary subcommittee composed of primary care clinicians

TABLE 3 Physical Examination Features To Be Considered in the Evaluation of a Potential BRUE

Physical Examination
General appearance
Craniofacial abnormalities (mandible, maxilla, nasal)
Age-appropriate responsiveness to environment
Growth variables
Length, weight, occipitofrontal circumference
Vital signs
Temperature, pulse, respiratory rate, blood pressure, oxygen saturation
Skin
Color, perfusion, evidence of injury (eg, bruising or erythema)
Head
Shape, fontanelles, bruising or other injury
Eyes
General, extraocular movement, pupillary response
Conjunctival hemorrhage
Retinal examination, if indicated by other findings
Ears
Tympanic membranes
Nose and mouth
Congestion/coryza
Blood in nares or oropharynx
Evidence of trauma or obstruction
Torn frenulum
Neck
Mobility
Chest
Auscultation, palpation for rib tenderness, crepitus, irregularities
Heart
Rhythm, rate, auscultation
Abdomen
Organomegaly, masses, distention
Tenderness
Genitalia
Any abnormalities
Extremities
Muscle tone, injuries, limb deformities consistent with fracture
Neurologic
Alertness, responsiveness
Response to sound and visual stimuli
General tone
Pupillary constriction in response to light
Presence of symmetrical reflexes
Symmetry of movement/tone/strength

and experts in the fields of general pediatrics, hospital medicine, emergency medicine, infectious diseases, child abuse, sleep medicine, pulmonary medicine, cardiology, neurology, biochemical genetics, gastroenterology, environmental health, and quality improvement. The subcommittee also included a parent representative, a guideline methodologist/informatician, and an epidemiologist skilled in systematic reviews. All panel members declared potential conflicts on the basis of the AAP policy on Conflict of Interest and Voluntary Disclosure. Subcommittee members repeated this process annually and upon publication of the guideline. All potential conflicts of interest are listed at the end of this document. The project was funded by the AAP.

The subcommittee performed a comprehensive review of the literature related to ALTEs from 1970 through 2014. Articles from 1970 through 2011 were identified and evaluated by using "Management of Apparent Life Threatening Events in Infants: A Systematic Review," authored by the Society of Hospital Medicine's ALTE Expert Panel (which included 4 members of the subcommittee).[3] The subcommittee partnered with the Society of Hospital Medicine Expert Panel and a librarian to update the original systematic review with articles published through December 31, 2014, with the use of the same methodology as the original systematic review. PubMed, Cumulative Index to Nursing and Allied Health Literature, and Cochrane Library databases were searched for studies involving children younger than 24 months by using the stepwise approach specified in the Preferred Reporting Items for Systematic Reviews and Meta-Analyses (PRISMA) statement.[8] Search terms included "ALTE(s)," "apparent life threatening event(s)," "life threatening event(s)," "near miss SIDS" or "near miss sudden infant death syndrome," "aborted crib death" or "aborted sudden infant death syndrome," and "aborted SIDS" or "aborted cot death" or "infant death, sudden." The Medical Subject Heading "infantile apparent life-threatening event," introduced in 2011, was also searched but did not identify additional articles.

In updating the systematic review published in 2012, pairs of 2 subcommittee members used validated methodology to independently score the newly identified abstracts from English-language articles (n = 120) for relevance to the clinical questions (Supplemental Fig 3).[9,10] Two independent reviewers then critically appraised the full text of the identified articles (n = 23) using a structured data collection form based on published guidelines for evaluating medical literature.[11,12] They recorded each study's relevance to the clinical question, research design, setting, time period covered, sample size, patient eligibility criteria, data source, variables collected, key results, study

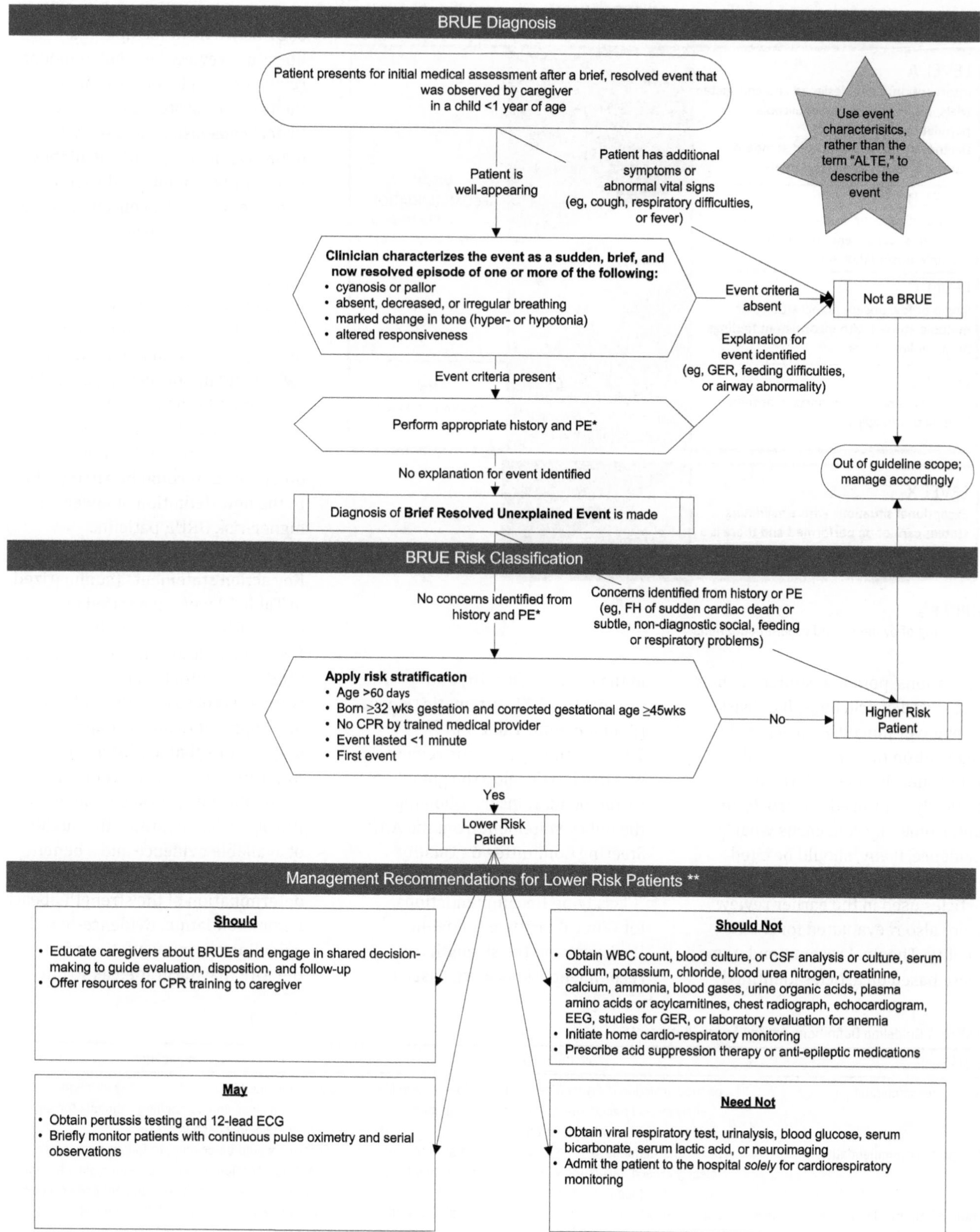

FIGURE 1

Diagnosis, risk classification, and recommended management of a BRUE. *See Tables 3 and 4 for the determination of an appropriate and negative FH and PE. **See Fig 2 for the AAP method for rating of evidence and recommendations. CSF, cerebrospinal fluid; FH, family history; PE, physical examination; WBC, white blood cell.

Figure 1, shown here, has been updated per the erratum at http://pediatrics.aappublications.org/content/138/2/e20161487.

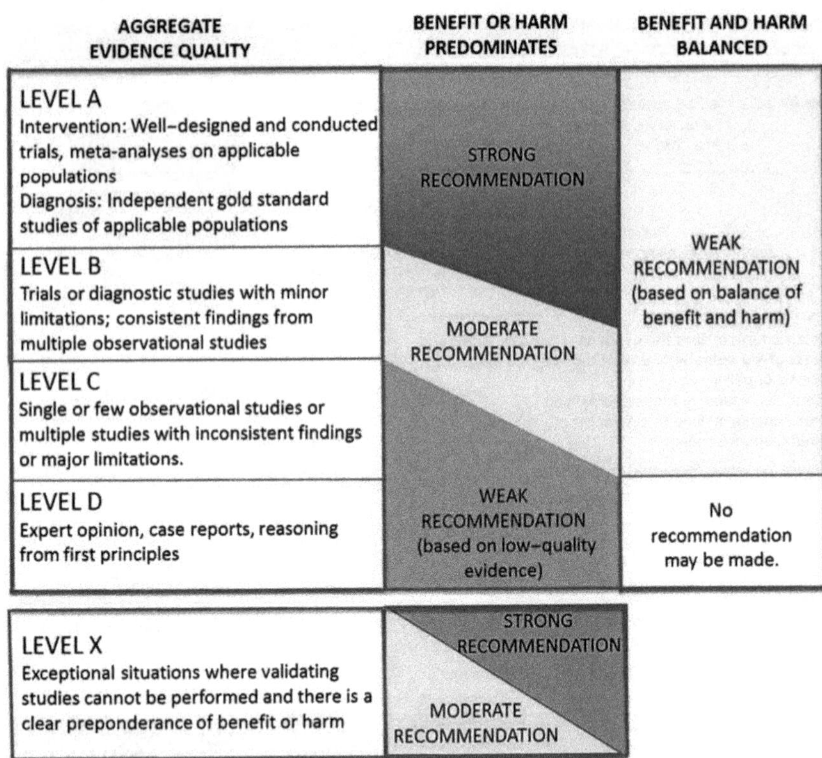

FIGURE 2
AAP rating of evidence and recommendations.

limitations, potential sources of bias, and stated conclusions. If at least 1 reviewer judged an article to be relevant on the basis of the full text, subsequently at least 2 reviewers critically appraised the article and determined by consensus what evidence, if any, should be cited in the systematic review. Selected articles used in the earlier review were also reevaluated for their quality. The final recommendations were based on articles identified in the updated (n = 18) and original (n = 37) systematic review (Supplemental Table 7).[6,7,13–28] The resulting systematic review was used to develop the guideline recommendations by following the policy statement from the AAP Steering Committee on Quality Improvement and Management, "Classifying Recommendations for Clinical Practice Guidelines."[29] Decisions and the strength of recommendations were based on a systematic grading of the quality of evidence from the updated literature review by 2 independent reviewers and incorporation of the previous systematic review. Expert consensus was used when definitive data were not available. If committee members disagreed with the rest of the consensus, they were encouraged to voice their concern until full agreement was reached. If full agreement could not be reached, each committee member reserved the right to state concern or disagreement in the publication (which did not occur). Because the recommendations of this guideline were based on the ALTE literature, we relied on the studies and outcomes that could be attributable to the new definition of lower- or higher-risk BRUE patients.

Key action statements (summarized in Table 5) were generated by using BRIDGE-Wiz (Building Recommendations in a Developers Guideline Editor), an interactive software tool that leads guideline development teams through a series of questions that are intended to create clear, transparent, and actionable key action statements.[30] BRIDGE-Wiz integrates the quality of available evidence and a benefit-harm assessment into the final determination of the strength of each recommendation. Evidence-based guideline recommendations from the AAP may be graded as strong,

TABLE 4 Guideline Definitions for Key Action Statements

Statement	Definition	Implication
Strong recommendation	A particular action is favored because anticipated benefits clearly exceed harms (or vice versa) and quality of evidence is excellent or unobtainable.	Clinicians should follow a strong recommendation unless a clear and compelling rationale for an alternative approach is present.
Moderate recommendation	A particular action is favored because anticipated benefits clearly exceed harms (or vice versa) and the quality of evidence is good but not excellent (or is unobtainable).	Clinicians would be prudent to follow a moderate recommendation but should remain alert to new information and sensitive to patient preferences.
Weak recommendation (based on low-quality evidence)	A particular action is favored because anticipated benefits clearly exceed harms (or vice versa), but the quality of evidence is weak.	Clinicians would be prudent follow a weak recommendation but should remain alert to new information and very sensitive to patient preferences.
Weak recommendation (based on balance of benefits and harms)	Weak recommendation is provided when the aggregate database shows evidence of both benefit and harm that appear to be similar in magnitude for any available courses of action.	Clinicians should consider the options in their decision-making, but patient preference may have a substantial role.

TABLE 5 Summary of Key Action Statements for Lower-Risk BRUEs

When managing an infant aged >60 d and <1 y and who, on the basis of a thorough history and physical examination, meets criteria for having experienced a lower-risk BRUE, clinicians:	Evidence Quality; Strength of Recommendation
1. Cardiopulmonary evaluation	
1A. Need not admit infants to the hospital solely for cardiorespiratory monitoring.	B; Weak
1B. May briefly monitor patients with continuous pulse oximetry and serial observations.	D; Weak
1C. Should not obtain a chest radiograph.	B; Moderate
1D. Should not obtain a measurement of venous or arterial blood gas.	B; Moderate
1E. Should not obtain an overnight polysomnograph.	B; Moderate
1F. May obtain a 12-lead electrocardiogram.	C; Weak
1G. Should not obtain an echocardiogram.	C; Moderate
1H. Should not initiate home cardiorespiratory monitoring.	B; Moderate
2. Child abuse evaluation	
2A. Need not obtain neuroimaging (CT, MRI, or ultrasonography) to detect child abuse.	C; Weak
2B. Should obtain an assessment of social risk factors to detect child abuse.	C; Moderate
3. Neurologic evaluation	
3A. Should not obtain neuroimaging (CT, MRI, or ultrasonography) to detect neurologic disorders.	C; Moderate
3B. Should not obtain an EEG to detect neurologic disorders.	C; Moderate
3C. Should not prescribe antiepileptic medications for potential neurologic disorders.	C; Moderate
4. Infectious disease evaluation	
4A. Should not obtain a WBC count, blood culture, or cerebrospinal fluid analysis or culture to detect an occult bacterial infection.	B; Strong
4B. Need not obtain a urinalysis (bag or catheter).	C; Weak
4C. Should not obtain chest radiograph to assess for pulmonary infection.	B; Moderate
4D. Need not obtain respiratory viral testing if rapid testing is available.	C; Weak
4E. May obtain testing for pertussis.	B; Weak
5. Gastrointestinal evaluation	
5A. Should not obtain investigations for GER (eg, upper gastrointestinal tract series, pH probe, endoscopy, barium contrast study, nuclear scintigraphy, and ultrasonography).	C; Moderate
5B. Should not prescribe acid suppression therapy.	C; Moderate
6. IEM evaluation	
6A. Need not obtain measurement of serum lactic acid or serum bicarbonate.	C; Weak
6B. Should not obtain a measurement of serum sodium, potassium, chloride, blood urea nitrogen, creatinine, calcium, or ammonia.	C; Moderate
6C. Should not obtain a measurement of venous or arterial blood gases.	C; Moderate
6D. Need not obtain a measurement of blood glucose.	C; Weak
6E. Should not obtain a measurement of urine organic acids, plasma amino acids, or plasma acylcarnitines.	C; Moderate
7. Anemia evaluation	
7A. Should not obtain laboratory evaluation for anemia.	C; Moderate
8. Patient- and family-centered care	
8A. Should offer resources for CPR training to caregiver.	C; Moderate
8B. Should educate caregivers about BRUEs.	C; Moderate
8C. Should use shared decision-making.	C; Moderate

CPR, cardiopulmonary resuscitation; CT, computed tomography; GER, gastroesophageal reflux; WBC, white blood cell.

moderate, weak based on low-quality evidence, or weak based on balance between benefits and harms. Strong and moderate recommendations are associated with "should" and "should not" recommendation statements, whereas weak recommendation may be recognized by use of "may" or "need not" (Fig 2, Table 4).

A strong recommendation means that the committee's review of the evidence indicates that the benefits of the recommended approach clearly exceed the harms of that approach (or, in the case of a strong negative recommendation, that the harms clearly exceed the benefits) and that the quality of the evidence supporting this approach is excellent. Clinicians are advised to follow such guidance unless a clear and compelling rationale for acting in a contrary manner is present. A moderate recommendation means that the committee believes that the benefits exceed the harms (or, in the case of a negative recommendation, that the harms exceed the benefits), but the quality of the evidence on which this recommendation is based is not as strong. Clinicians are also encouraged to follow such guidance but also should be alert to new information and sensitive to patient preferences.

A weak recommendation means either that the evidence quality that exists is suspect or that well-designed, well-conducted studies have shown little clear advantage to one approach versus another. Weak recommendations offer clinicians flexibility in their decision-making regarding appropriate practice, although they may set boundaries on alternatives. Family and patient preference should have a substantial role in influencing clinical

1A. Clinicians Need Not Admit Infants Presenting With a Lower-Risk BRUE to the Hospital Solely for Cardiorespiratory Monitoring (Grade B, Weak Recommendation)

Aggregate Evidence Quality	Grade B
Benefits	Reduce unnecessary testing and caregiver/infant anxiety Avoid consequences of false-positive result, health care–associated infections, and other patient safety risks
Risks, harm, cost	May rarely miss a recurrent event or diagnostic opportunity for rare underlying condition
Benefit-harm assessment	The benefits of reducing unnecessary testing, nosocomial infections, and false-positive results, as well as alleviating caregiver and infant anxiety, outweigh the rare missed diagnostic opportunity for an underlying condition
Intentional vagueness	None
Role of patient preferences	Caregiver anxiety and access to quality follow-up care may be important considerations in determining whether a hospitalization for cardiovascular monitoring is indicated
Exclusions	None
Strength	Weak recommendation (because of equilibrium between benefits and harms)
Key references	31, 32

1B. Clinicians May Briefly Monitor Infants Presenting With a Lower-Risk BRUE With Continuous Pulse Oximetry and Serial Observations (Grade D, Weak Recommendation)

Aggregate Evidence Quality	Grade D
Benefits	Identification of hypoxemia
Risks, harm, cost	Increased costs due to monitoring over time and the use of hospital resources False-positive results may lead to subsequent testing and hospitalization False reassurance from negative test results
Benefit-harm assessment	The potential benefit of detecting hypoxemia outweighs the harm of cost and false results
Intentional vagueness	Duration of time to monitor patients with continuous pulse oximetry and the number and frequency of serial observations may vary
Role of patient preferences	Level of caregiver concern may influence the duration of oximetry monitoring
Exclusions	None
Strength	Weak recommendation (based on low quality of evidence)
Key references	33, 36

decision-making, particularly when recommendations are expressed as weak. Key action statements based on that evidence and expert consensus are provided. A summary is provided in Table 5.

The practice guideline underwent a comprehensive review by stakeholders before formal approval by the AAP, including AAP councils, committees, and sections; selected outside organizations; and individuals identified by the subcommittee as experts in the field. All comments were reviewed by the subcommittee and incorporated into the final guideline when appropriate.

This guideline is intended for use primarily by clinicians providing care for infants who have experienced a BRUE and their families. This guideline may be of interest to parents and payers, but it is not intended to be used for reimbursement or to determine insurance coverage. This guideline is not intended as the sole source of guidance in the evaluation and management of BRUEs but rather is intended to assist clinicians by providing a framework for clinical decision-making.

KEY ACTION STATEMENTS FOR LOWER-RISK BRUE

1. Cardiopulmonary

1A. Clinicians Need Not Admit Infants Presenting With a Lower-Risk BRUE to the Hospital Solely for Cardiorespiratory Monitoring (Grade B, Weak Recommendation)

Infants presenting with an ALTE often have been admitted for observation and testing. Observational data indicate that 12% to 14% of infants presenting with a diagnosis of ALTE had a subsequent event or condition that required hospitalization.[7,31] Thus, research has sought to identify risk factors that could be used to identify infants likely to benefit from hospitalization. A long-term follow-up study in infants hospitalized with an ALTE showed that no infants subsequently had SIDS but 11% were victims of child abuse and 4.9% had adverse neurologic outcomes (see 3. Neurology).[32] The ALTE literature supports that infants presenting with a lower-risk BRUE do not have an increased rate of cardiovascular or other events during admission and hospitalization may not be required, but close follow-up is recommended. Careful outpatient follow-up is advised (repeat clinical history and physical examination within 24 hours after the initial evaluation) to identify infants with ongoing medical concerns that would indicate further evaluation and treatment.

Al-Kindy et al[33] used documented monitoring in 54% of infants admitted for an ALTE (338 of 625) and identified 46 of 338 (13.6%) with "extreme" cardiovascular events (central apnea >30 seconds, oxygen saturation <80% for 10 seconds, decrease in heart rate <50–60/minutes for 10 seconds on the basis of postconceptional age). However, no adverse outcomes were noted for any of their cohort (although whether there is a protective effect of observation alone is not known). Some of the infants with extreme events developed symptoms of upper respiratory infection 1 to 2 days after the ALTE presentation. The risk factors for "extreme" events were prematurity, postconceptional age <43 weeks, and (presence of) upper respiratory infection symptoms. Importantly, infants with a postconceptional age >48 weeks were not documented as having an extreme event in this cohort. A previous longitudinal study also identified "extreme" events that occurred with comparable frequency in otherwise normal term infants and that were not statistically increased in term infants with a history of ALTE.[34]

Preterm infants have been shown to have more serious events, although an ALTE does not further increase that risk compared with asymptomatic preterm infants without ALTE.[34] Claudius and Keens[31] performed an observational prospective study in 59 infants presenting with ALTE who had been born at >30 weeks' gestation and had no significant medical illness. They evaluated factors in the clinical history and physical examination that, according to the authors, would warrant hospital admission on the basis of adverse outcomes (including recurrent cardiorespiratory events, infection, child abuse, or any life-threatening condition). Among these otherwise well infants, those with multiple ALTEs or age <1 month experienced adverse outcomes necessitating hospitalization. Prematurity was also a risk factor predictive of subsequent adverse events after an ALTE. Paroxysmal decreases in oxygen saturation in infants immediately before and during viral illnesses have been well documented.[33,35] However, the significance of these brief hypoxemic events has not been established.

1B. Clinicians May Briefly Monitor Infants Presenting With a Lower-Risk BRUE With Continuous Pulse Oximetry and Serial Observations (Grade D, Weak Recommendation)

A normal physical examination, including vital signs and oximetry, is needed for a patient who has experienced a BRUE to be considered lower-risk. An evaluation at a single point in time may not be as accurate as a longer interval of observation. Unfortunately, there are few data to suggest the optimal duration of this period, the value of repeat examinations, and the effect of false-positive evaluations on family-centered care. Several studies have documented intermittent episodes of hypoxemia after admission for ALTE.[7,31,33] Pulse oximetry identified more infants with concerning paroxysmal events than cardiorespiratory monitoring alone.[33] However, occasional oxygen desaturations are commonly observed in normal infants, especially during sleep.[36] Furthermore, normative oximetry data are dependent on the specific machine, averaging interval, altitude, behavioral state, and postconceptional age. Similarly, there may be considerable variability in the vital signs and the clinical appearance of an infant. Pending further research into this important issue, clinicians may choose to monitor and provide serial examinations of infants in the lower-risk group for a brief period of time, ranging from 1 to 4 hours, to establish that the vital signs, physical examination, and symptomatology remain stable.

1C. Clinicians Should Not Obtain a Chest Radiograph in Infants Presenting With a Lower-Risk BRUE (Grade B, Moderate Recommendation)

Infectious processes can precipitate apnea. In 1 ALTE study, more than 80% of these infections involved the respiratory tract.[37] Most, but not all, infants with significant lower respiratory tract infections will be symptomatic at the time of ALTE presentation. However, 2 studies have documented pneumonia in infants presenting with ALTE and an otherwise noncontributory history and physical examination.[4,37] These rare exceptions have generally been in infants younger than 2 months and would have placed them in the higher-risk category for a BRUE in this guideline. Similarly, Davies and Gupta[38] reported that 9 of 65 patients (ages unknown) who had ALTEs had abnormalities on chest radiography (not fully specified) despite no suspected respiratory disorder on clinical history or physical examination. Some of the radiographs were performed up to 24 hours after presentation. Davies and Gupta further reported that 33% of infants with ALTEs that were ultimately associated with a respiratory disease had a normal initial respiratory examination.[38] Kant et al[18] reported that 2 of 176 infants discharged after admission for ALTE died within 2 weeks, both of pneumonia. One infant had a normal chest radiograph initially; the other, with a history of prematurity, had a "possible" infiltrate. Thus, most experience has shown that a chest radiograph in otherwise well-appearing infants rarely alters clinical management.[7] Careful follow-up within 24 hours is important in infants with a nonfocal clinical history and physical examination to identify those who will ultimately have a lower respiratory tract infection diagnosed.

1D. Clinicians Should Not Obtain Measurement of Venous or Arterial Blood Gases in Infants Presenting With a Lower-Risk BRUE (Grade B, Moderate Recommendation)

Blood gas measurements have not been shown to add significant clinical information in otherwise well-appearing infants presenting with an ALTE.[4] Although not part of

1C. Clinicians Should Not Obtain Chest Radiograph in Infants Presenting With a Lower-Risk BRUE (Grade B, Moderate Recommendation)

Aggregate Evidence Quality	Grade B
Benefits	Reduce costs, unnecessary testing, radiation exposure, and caregiver/infant anxiety Avoid consequences of false-positive results
Risks, harm, cost	May rarely miss diagnostic opportunity for early lower respiratory tract or cardiac disease
Benefit-harm assessment	The benefits of reducing unnecessary testing, radiation exposure, and false-positive results, as well as alleviating caregiver and infant anxiety, outweigh the rare missed diagnostic opportunity for lower respiratory tract or cardiac disease
Intentional vagueness	None
Role of patient preferences	Caregiver may express concern regarding a longstanding breathing pattern in his/her infant or a recent change in breathing that might influence the decision to obtain chest radiography
Exclusions	None
Strength	Moderate recommendation
Key references	4, 37

1D. Clinicians Should Not Obtain Measurement of Venous or Arterial Blood Gases in Infants Presenting With a Lower-Risk BRUE (Grade B, Moderate Recommendation)

Aggregate Evidence Quality	Grade B
Benefits	Reduce costs, unnecessary testing, pain, risk of thrombosis, and caregiver/infant anxiety Avoid consequences of false-positive results
Risks, harm, cost	May miss rare instances of hypercapnia and acid-base imbalances
Benefit-harm assessment	The benefits of reducing unnecessary testing and false-positive results, as well as alleviating caregiver and infant anxiety, outweigh the rare missed diagnostic opportunity for hypercapnia and acid-base imbalances
Intentional vagueness	None
Role of patient preferences	None
Exclusions	None
Strength	Moderate recommendation
Key reference	4

this guideline, future research may demonstrate that blood gases are helpful in select infants with a higher risk BRUE to support the diagnosis of pulmonary disease, control-of-breathing disorders, or inborn errors of metabolism (IEMs).

1E. Clinicians Should Not Obtain an Overnight Polysomnograph in Infants Presenting With a Lower-Risk BRUE (Grade B, Moderate Recommendation)

Polysomnography consists of 8 to 12 hours of documented monitoring, including EEG, electro-oculography, electromyography, nasal/oral airflow, electrocardiography, end-tidal carbon dioxide, chest/abdominal excursion, and oximetry. Polysomnography is considered by many to be the gold standard for identifying obstructive sleep apnea (OSA), central sleep apnea, and periodic breathing and may identify seizures. Some data have suggested using polysomnography in infants presenting with ALTEs as a means to predict the likelihood of recurrent significant cardiorespiratory events. A study in which polysomnography was performed in a cohort of infants with ALTEs (including recurrent episodes) reported that polysomnography may reveal respiratory pauses of >20 seconds or brief episodes of bradycardia that are predictive of ensuing events over the next several months.[40] However, without a control population, the clinical significance of these events is uncertain, because respiratory pauses are frequently observed in otherwise normal infants.[35] Similarly, Kahn and Blum[41] reported that 10 of 71 infants with a clinical history of "benign" ALTEs had an abnormal polysomnograph, including periodic breathing (7 of 10) or obstructive apnea (4 of 100), but specific data were not presented. These events were not found in a control group of 181 infants. The severity of the periodic breathing (frequency of arousals and extent of oxygen desaturation) could not be evaluated from these data. Daniëls et al[42] performed polysomnography in 422 infants with ALTEs and identified 11 infants with significant bradycardia, OSA, and/or oxygen desaturation. Home monitoring revealed episodes of bradycardia (<50 per minute) in 7 of 11 infants and concluded that polysomnography is a useful modality. However, the clinical history, physical examination, and laboratory findings were not presented. GER has also been associated with specific episodes of severe bradycardia in monitored infants.[43] Overall, most polysomnography studies have shown minimal or nonspecific findings in infants presenting with ALTEs.[44,45] Polysomnography studies generally have not been predictive of ALTE recurrence and do not identify those infants at risk of SIDS.[46] Thus, the routine use of polysomnography in infants presenting with a lower-risk BRUE is likely to have a low diagnostic yield and is unlikely to lead to changes in therapy.

OSA has been occasionally associated with ALTEs in many series, but not all.[39,47–49] The use of overnight polysomnography to evaluate for OSA should be guided by an assessment of risk on the basis of a

1E. Clinicians Should Not Obtain an Overnight Polysomnograph in Infants Presenting With a Lower-Risk BRUE (Grade B, Moderate Recommendation)

Aggregate Evidence Quality	Grade B
Benefits	Reduce costs, unnecessary testing, and caregiver/infant anxiety Avoid consequences of false-positive results
Risks, harm, cost	May miss rare instances of hypoxemia, hypercapnia, and/or bradycardia that would be detected by polysomnography
Benefit-harm assessment	The benefits of reducing unnecessary testing and false-positive results, as well as alleviating caregiver and infant anxiety, outweigh the rare missed diagnostic opportunity for hypoxemia, hypercapnia, and/or bradycardia
Intentional vagueness	None
Role of patient preferences	Caregivers may report concern regarding some aspects of their infant's sleep pattern that may influence the decision to perform polysomnography
Exclusions	None
Strength	Moderate recommendation
Key reference	39

1F. Clinicians May Obtain a 12-Lead Electrocardiogram for Infants Presenting With Lower-Risk BRUE (Grade C, Weak Recommendation)

Aggregate Evidence Quality	Grade C
Benefits	May identify BRUE patients with channelopathies (long QT syndrome, short QT syndrome, and Brugada syndrome), ventricular pre-excitation (Wolff-Parkinson-White syndrome), cardiomyopathy, or other heart disease
Risks, harm, cost	False-positive results may lead to further workup, expert consultation, anxiety, and cost False reassurance from negative results Cost and availability of electrocardiography testing and interpretation
Benefit-harm assessment	The benefit of identifying patients at risk of sudden cardiac death outweighs the risk of cost and false results
Intentional vagueness	None
Role of patient preferences	Caregiver may decide not to have testing performed
Exclusions	None
Strength	Weak recommendation (because of equilibrium between benefits and harms)
Key references	4, 16

comprehensive clinical history and physical examination.[50] Symptoms of OSA, which may be subtle or absent in infants, include snoring, noisy respirations, labored breathing, mouth breathing, and profuse sweating.[51] Occasionally, infants with OSA will present with failure to thrive, witnessed apnea, and/or developmental delay.[52] Snoring may be absent in younger infants with OSA, including those with micrognathia. In addition, snoring in otherwise normal infants is present at least 2 days per week in 11.8% and at least 3 days per week in 5.3% of infants.[53] Some infants with OSA may be asymptomatic and have a normal physical examination.[54] However, some studies have reported a high incidence of snoring in infants with (26%–44%) and without (22%–26%) OSA, making the distinction difficult.[55] Additional risk factors for infant OSA include prematurity, maternal smoking, bronchopulmonary dysplasia, obesity, and specific medical conditions including laryngomalacia, craniofacial abnormalities, neuromuscular weakness, Down syndrome, achondroplasia, Chiari malformations, and Prader-Willi syndrome.[34,56–58]

1F. Clinicians May Obtain a 12-Lead Electrocardiogram for Infants Presenting With Lower-Risk BRUE (Grade C, Weak Recommendation)

ALTE studies have examined screening electrocardiograms (ECGs). A study by Brand et al[4] found no positive findings on 24 ECGs performed on 72 patients (33%) without a contributory history or physical examination. Hoki et al[16] reported a 4% incidence of cardiac disease found in 485 ALTE patients; ECGs were performed in 208 of 480 patients (43%) with 3 of 5 abnormal heart rhythms identified by the ECG and the remaining 2 showing structural heart disease. Both studies had low positive-predictive values of ECGs (0% and 1%, respectively). Hoki et al had a negative predictive value of 100% (96%–100%), and given the low prevalence of disease, there is little need for further testing in patients with a negative ECG.

Some cardiac conditions that may present as a BRUE include channelopathies (long QT syndrome, short QT syndrome, Brugada syndrome, and catecholaminergic polymorphic ventricular tachycardia), ventricular pre-excitation (Wolff-Parkinson-White syndrome), and cardiomyopathy/myocarditis (hypertrophic cardiomyopathy, dilated cardiomyopathy). Resting ECGs are ineffective in identifying patients with catecholaminergic polymorphic ventricular tachycardia. Family history is important in identifying individuals with channelopathies.

Severe potential outcomes of any of these conditions, if left undiagnosed or untreated, include sudden death or neurologic injury.[59] However, many patients do not ever experience symptoms in their lifetime and adverse outcomes are uncommon. A genetic autopsy study in infants who died of SIDS in Norway showed an association between 9.5% and 13.0% of infants with abnormal

1G. Clinicians Should Not Obtain an Echocardiogram in Infants Presenting With Lower-Risk BRUE (Grade C, Moderate Recommendation)

Aggregate Evidence Quality	Grade C
Benefits	Reduce costs, unnecessary testing, caregiver/infant anxiety, and sedation risk Avoid consequences of false-positive results
Risks, harm, cost	May miss rare diagnosis of cardiac disease
Benefit-harm assessment	The benefits of reducing unnecessary testing and sedation risk, as well as alleviating caregiver and infant anxiety, outweigh the rare missed diagnostic opportunity for cardiac causes
Intentional vagueness	Abnormal cardiac physical examination reflects the clinical judgment of the clinician
Role of patient preferences	Some caregivers may prefer to have echocardiography performed
Exclusions	Patients with an abnormal cardiac physical examination
Strength	Moderate recommendation
Key references	4, 16

1H. Clinicians Should Not Initiate Home Cardiorespiratory Monitoring in Infants Presenting With a Lower-Risk BRUE (Grade B, Moderate Recommendation)

Aggregate Evidence Quality	Grade B
Benefits	Reduce costs, unnecessary testing, and caregiver/infant anxiety Avoid consequences of false-positive results
Risks, harm, cost	May rarely miss an infant with recurrent central apnea or cardiac arrhythmias
Benefit-harm assessment	The benefits of reducing unnecessary testing and false-positive results, as well as alleviating caregiver and infant anxiety, outweigh the rare missed diagnostic opportunity for recurrent apnea or cardiac arrhythmias
Intentional vagueness	None
Role of patient preferences	Caregivers will frequently request monitoring be instituted after an ALTE in their infant; a careful explanation of the limitations and disadvantages of this technology should be given
Exclusions	None
Strength	Moderate recommendation
Key reference	34

or novel gene findings at the long QT loci.[60] A syncopal episode, which could present as a BRUE, is strongly associated with subsequent sudden cardiac arrest in patients with long QT syndrome.[61] The incidence and risk in those with other channelopathies have not been adequately studied. The incidence of sudden cardiac arrest in patients with ventricular pre-excitation (Wolff-Parkinson-White syndrome) is 3% to 4% over the lifetime of the individual.[62]

1G. Clinicians Should Not Obtain an Echocardiogram in Infants Presenting With Lower-Risk BRUE (Grade C, Moderate Recommendation)

Cardiomyopathy (hypertrophic and dilated cardiomyopathy) and myocarditis could rarely present as a lower-risk BRUE and can be identified with echocardiography. The cost of an echocardiogram is high and accompanied by sedation risks.

In a study in ALTE patients, Hoki et al[16] did not recommend echocardiography as an initial cardiac test unless there are findings on examination or from an echocardiogram consistent with heart disease. The majority of abnormal echocardiogram findings in their study were not perceived to be life-threatening or related to a cause for the ALTE (eg, septal defects or mild valve abnormalities), and they would have been detected on echocardiogram or physical examination. Brand et al[4] reported 32 echocardiograms in 243 ALTE patients and found only 1 abnormal echocardiogram, which was suspected because of an abnormal history and physical examination (double aortic arch).

1H. Clinicians Should Not Initiate Home Cardiorespiratory Monitoring in Infants Presenting With a Lower-Risk BRUE (Grade B, Moderate Recommendation)

The use of ambulatory cardiorespiratory monitors in infants presenting with ALTEs has been proposed as a modality to identify subsequent events, reduce the risk of SIDS, and alert caregivers of the need for intervention. Monitors can identify respiratory pauses and bradycardia in many infants presenting with ALTE; however, these events are also occasionally observed in otherwise normal infants.[34,40] In addition, infant monitors are prone to artifact and have not been shown to improve outcomes or prevent SIDS or improve neurodevelopmental outcomes.[63] Indeed, caregiver anxiety may be exacerbated with the use of infant monitors and potential false alarms. The overwhelming majority of monitor-identified alarms, including many with reported clinical symptomatology, do not reveal abnormalities on cardiorespiratory recordings.[64–66] Finally, there are several studies showing a lack of correlation between ALTEs and SIDS.[24,32]

Kahn and Blum[41] monitored 50 infants considered at "high risk" of SIDS and reported that 80% had alarms at home. All infants with alarms had at least 1 episode of parental intervention motivated by the alarms, although the authors acknowledged that some cases of parental intervention may have been attributable to parental anxiety. Nevertheless, the stimulated infants did not die of SIDS or require rehospitalization and therefore it was concluded that monitoring resulted in successful resuscitation, but this was not firmly established. Côté et al[40] reported "significant events" involving central apnea and bradycardia with long-term monitoring. However, these events were later shown to be frequently present in otherwise well infants.[34] There are insufficient data to support the use of commercial infant monitoring devices marketed directly to parents for the purposes of SIDS prevention.[63] These monitors may be prone to false alarms, produce anxiety, and disrupt sleep. Furthermore, these machines are frequently used without a medical support system and in the absence of specific training to respond to alarms. Although it is beyond the scope of this clinical practice guideline, future research may show that home monitoring (cardiorespiratory and/or oximetry) is appropriate for some infants with higher-risk BRUE.

2. Child Abuse

2A. Clinicians Need Not Obtain Neuroimaging (Computed Tomography, MRI, or Ultrasonography) To Detect Child Abuse in Infants Presenting With a Lower-Risk BRUE (Grade C, Weak Recommendation)

2B. Clinicians Should Obtain an Assessment of Social Risk Factors To Detect Child Abuse in Infants Presenting With a Lower-Risk BRUE (Grade C, Moderate Recommendation)

Child abuse is a common and serious cause of an ALTE. Previous research has suggested that this occurs in up to 10% of ALTE cohorts.[3,67] Abusive head trauma is the most common form of child maltreatment associated with an ALTE. Other forms of child abuse that can present as an ALTE, but would not be identified by radiologic evaluations, include caregiver-fabricated illness (formally known as Münchausen by proxy), smothering, and poisoning.

Children who have experienced child abuse, most notably abusive head trauma, may present with a BRUE. Four studies reported a low incidence (0.54%–2.5%) of abusive head trauma in infants presenting to the emergency department with an ALTE.[22,37,67,69] If only those patients meeting lower-risk BRUE criteria were included, the incidence of abusive head trauma would have been <0.3%. Although missing abusive head trauma can result in significant morbidity and mortality, the yield of performing neuroimaging to screen for abusive head trauma is extremely low and has associated risks of sedation and radiation exposure.[32,70]

Unfortunately, the subtle presentation of child abuse may lead to a delayed diagnosis of abuse and result in significant morbidity and mortality.[70] A thorough history and physical examination is the best way to identify infants at risk of these

2A. Clinicians Need Not Obtain Neuroimaging (Computed Tomography, MRI, or Ultrasonography) To Detect Child Abuse in Infants Presenting With a Lower-Risk BRUE (Grade C, Weak Recommendation)

Aggregate Evidence Quality	Grade C
Benefits	Decrease cost Avoid sedation, radiation exposure, consequences of false-positive results
Risks, harm, cost	May miss cases of child abuse and potential subsequent harm
Benefit-harm assessment	The benefits of reducing unnecessary testing, sedation, radiation exposure, and false-positive results, as well as alleviating caregiver and infant anxiety, outweigh the rare missed diagnostic opportunity for child abuse
Intentional vagueness	None
Role of patient preferences	Caregiver concerns may lead to requests for CNS imaging
Exclusions	None
Strength	Weak recommendation (based on low quality of evidence)
Key references	3, 67

2B. Clinicians Should Obtain an Assessment of Social Risk Factors To Detect Child Abuse in Infants Presenting With a Lower-Risk BRUE (Grade C, Moderate Recommendation)

Aggregate Evidence Quality	Grade C
Benefits	Identification of child abuse May benefit the safety of other children in the home May identify other social risk factors and needs and help connect caregivers with appropriate resources (eg, financial distress)
Risks, harm, cost	Resource intensive and not always available, particularly for smaller centers Some social workers may have inadequate experience in child abuse assessment May decrease caregiver's trust in the medical team
Benefit-harm assessment	The benefits of identifying child abuse and identifying and addressing social needs outweigh the cost of attempting to locate the appropriate resources or decreasing the trust in the medical team
Intentional vagueness	None
Role of patient preferences	Caregivers may perceive social services involvement as unnecessary and intrusive
Exclusions	None
Strength	Moderate recommendation
Key reference	68

conditions.[67,71] Significant concerning features for child abuse (especially abusive head trauma) can include a developmentally inconsistent or discrepant history provided by the caregiver(s), a previous ALTE, a recent emergency service telephone call, vomiting, irritability, or bleeding from the nose or mouth.[67,71]

Clinicians and medical team members (eg, nurses and social workers) should obtain an assessment of social risk factors in infants with a BRUE, including negative attributions to and unrealistic expectations of the child, mental health problems, domestic violence/intimate partner violence, social service involvement, law enforcement involvement, and substance abuse.[68] In addition, clinicians and medical team members can help families identify and use resources that may expand and strengthen their network of social support.

In previously described ALTE cohorts, abnormal physical findings were associated with an increased risk of abusive head trauma. These findings include bruising, subconjunctival hemorrhage, bleeding from the nose or mouth, and a history of rapid head enlargement or head circumference >95th percentile.[67,70–74] It is important to perform a careful physical examination to identify subtle findings of child abuse, including a large or full/bulging anterior fontanel, scalp bruising or bogginess, oropharynx or frenula damage, or skin findings such as bruising or petechiae, especially on the trunk, face, or ears. A normal physical examination does not rule out the possibility of abusive head trauma. Although beyond the scope of this guideline, it is important for the clinician to note that according to the available evidence, brain neuroimaging is probably indicated in patients who qualify as higher-risk because of concerns about abuse resulting from abnormal history or physical findings.[67]

A social and environmental assessment should evaluate the risk of intentional poisoning, unintentional poisoning, and environmental exposure (eg, home environment), because these can be associated with the symptoms of ALTEs in infants.[75–78] In 1 study, 8.4% of children presenting to the emergency department after an ALTE were found to have a clinically significant, positive comprehensive toxicology screen.[76] Ethanol or other drugs have also been associated with ALTEs.[79] Pulmonary hemorrhage can be caused by environmental exposure to moldy, water-damaged homes; it would usually present with hemoptysis and thus probably would not qualify as a BRUE.[80]

3. Neurology

3A. Clinicians Should Not Obtain Neuroimaging (Computed Tomography, MRI, or Ultrasonography) To Detect Neurologic Disorders in Infants Presenting With a Lower-Risk BRUE (Grade C, Moderate Recommendation)

Epilepsy or an abnormality of brain structure can present as a lower-risk BRUE. CNS imaging is 1 method for evaluating whether underlying abnormalities of brain development or structure might have led to the BRUE. The long-term risk of a diagnosis of neurologic disorders ranges from 3% to 11% in historical cohorts of ALTE patients.[2,32] One retrospective study in 243 ALTE patients reported that CNS imaging contributed to a neurologic diagnosis in 3% to 7% of patients.[4] However, the study population included all ALTEs, including those with a significant past medical history, non–well-appearing infants, and those with tests ordered as part of the emergency department evaluation.

In a large study of ALTE patients, the utility of CNS imaging studies in potentially classifiable lower-risk BRUE patients was found to be low.[32] The cohort of 471 patients was followed both acutely and long-term for the development of epilepsy and other neurologic disorders, and the sensitivity and positive-predictive value of abnormal CNS imaging for subsequent development of epilepsy was 6.7% (95% confidence interval [CI]: 0.2%–32%) and 25% (95% CI: 0.6%–81%), respectively.

The available evidence suggests minimal utility of CNS imaging to evaluate for neurologic disorders, including epilepsy, in lower-risk patients. This situation is particularly true for pediatric epilepsy, in which even if a patient is determined ultimately to have seizures/epilepsy, there is no evidence of benefit from starting therapy after the first seizure compared with starting therapy after a second seizure in terms of achieving seizure remission.[81–83] However, our recommendations for BRUEs are not based on any prospective studies and only on a single retrospective study. Future work should track both short- and long-term neurologic outcomes when considering this issue.

3B. Clinicians Should Not Obtain an EEG To Detect Neurologic Disorders in Infants Presenting With a Lower-Risk BRUE (Grade C, Moderate Recommendation)

Epilepsy may first present as a lower-risk BRUE. The long-term risk of epilepsy ranges from 3% to 11% in historical cohorts of ALTE patients.[2,32] EEG is part of the typical evaluation for diagnosis of seizure disorders. However, the utility of obtaining an EEG routinely was found to be low in 1 study.[32] In a cohort of 471 ALTE patients followed both acutely and long-term for the development of epilepsy, the sensitivity and positive-predictive value of an abnormal EEG for subsequent development of epilepsy was 15% (95% CI: 2%–45%) and 33% (95% CI: 4.3%–48%), respectively. In contrast, another retrospective study in 243 ALTE patients reported that EEG contributed to a neurologic diagnosis in 6% of patients.[4] This study

3A. Clinicians Should Not Obtain Neuroimaging (Computed Tomography, MRI, or Ultrasonography) To Detect Neurologic Disorders in Infants Presenting With a Lower-Risk BRUE (Grade C, Moderate Recommendation)

Aggregate Evidence Quality	Grade C
Benefits	Reduce unnecessary testing, radiation exposure, sedation, caregiver/infant anxiety, and costs Avoid consequences of false-positive results
Risks, harm, cost	May rarely miss diagnostic opportunity for CNS causes of BRUEs May miss unexpected cases of abusive head trauma
Benefit-harm assessment	The benefits of reducing unnecessary testing, radiation exposure, sedation, and false-positive results, as well as alleviating caregiver and infant anxiety, outweigh the rare missed diagnostic opportunity for CNS cause
Intentional vagueness	None
Role of patient preferences	Caregivers may seek reassurance from neuroimaging and may not understand the risks from radiation and sedation
Exclusions	None
Strength	Moderate recommendation
Key references	2, 32, 81

3B. Clinicians Should Not Obtain an EEG To Detect Neurologic Disorders in Infants Presenting With a Lower-Risk BRUE (Grade C, Moderate Recommendation)

Aggregate Evidence Quality	Grade C
Benefits	Reduce unnecessary testing, sedation, caregiver/infant anxiety, and costs Avoid consequences of false-positive or nonspecific results
Risks, harm, cost	Could miss early diagnosis of seizure disorder
Benefit-harm assessment	The benefits of reducing unnecessary testing, sedation, and false-positive results, as well as alleviating caregiver and infant anxiety, outweigh the rare missed diagnostic opportunity for epilepsy
Intentional vagueness	None
Role of patient preferences	Caregivers may seek reassurance from an EEG, but they may not appreciate study limitations and the potential of false-positive results
Exclusions	None
Strength	Moderate recommendation
Key references	32, 84, 85

population differed significantly from that of Bonkowsky et al[32] in that all ALTE patients with a significant past medical history and non–well-appearing infants were included in the analysis and that tests ordered in the emergency department evaluation were also included in the measure of EEG yield.

A diagnosis of seizure is difficult to make from presenting symptoms of an ALTE.[30] Although EEG is recommended by the American Academy of Neurology after a first-time nonfebrile seizure, the yield and sensitivity of an EEG after a first-time ALTE in a lower-risk child are low.[86] Thus, the evidence available suggests no utility for routine EEG to evaluate for epilepsy in a lower-risk BRUE. However, our recommendations for BRUEs are based on no prospective studies and on only a single retrospective study. Future work should track both short- and long-term epilepsy when considering this issue.

Finally, even if a patient is determined ultimately to have seizures/epilepsy, the importance of an EEG for a first-time ALTE is low, because there is little evidence that shows a benefit from starting therapy after the first seizure compared with after a second seizure in terms of achieving seizure remission.[81–83,85]

3C. Clinicians Should Not Prescribe Antiepileptic Medications for Potential Neurologic Disorders in Infants Presenting With a Lower-Risk BRUE (Grade C, Moderate Recommendation)

Once epilepsy is diagnosed, treatment can consist of therapy with an antiepileptic medication. In a cohort of 471 ALTE patients followed both acutely and long-term for the development of epilepsy, most patients who developed epilepsy had a second event within 1 month of their initial presentation.[32,87] Even if a patient is determined ultimately to have seizures/epilepsy, there is no evidence of benefit from starting therapy after the first seizure compared with starting therapy after a second seizure in terms of achieving seizure remission.[81–83,85] Sudden unexpected death in epilepsy (SUDEP) has a frequency close to 1 in 1000 patient-years, but the risks of SUDEP are distinct from ALTEs/BRUEs and include adolescent age and presence of epilepsy for more than 5 years. These data do not support prescribing an antiepileptic medicine for a first-time possible seizure because of a concern for SUDEP. Thus, the evidence available for ALTEs suggests lack of benefit for starting an antiepileptic medication for a lower-risk BRUE. However, our recommendations for BRUEs are based on no prospective studies and on only a single retrospective study. Future work should track both short- and long-term epilepsy when considering this issue.

4. Infectious Diseases

4A. Clinicians Should Not Obtain a White Blood Cell Count, Blood Culture, or Cerebrospinal Fluid Analysis or Culture To Detect an Occult Bacterial Infection in Infants Presenting With a Lower-Risk BRUE (Grade B, Strong Recommendation)

Some studies reported that ALTEs are the presenting complaint of an invasive infection, including bacteremia and/or meningitis

3C. Clinicians Should Not Prescribe Antiepileptic Medications for Potential Neurologic Disorders in Infants Presenting With a Lower-Risk BRUE (Grade C, Moderate Recommendation)

Aggregate Evidence Quality	Grade C
Benefits	Reduce medication adverse effects and risks, avoid treatment with unproven efficacy, and reduce cost
Risks, harm, cost	Delay in treatment of epilepsy could lead to subsequent BRUE or seizure
Benefit-harm assessment	The benefits of reducing medication adverse effects, avoiding unnecessary treatment, and reducing cost outweigh the risk of delaying treatment of epilepsy
Intentional vagueness	None
Role of patient preferences	Caregivers may feel reassured by starting a medicine but may not understand the medication risks
Exclusions	None
Strength	Moderate recommendation
Key references	32, 85, 87

4A. Clinicians Should Not Obtain a White Blood Cell Count, Blood Culture, or Cerebrospinal Fluid Analysis or Culture To Detect an Occult Bacterial Infection in Infants Presenting With a Lower-Risk BRUE (Grade B, Strong Recommendation)

Aggregate Evidence Quality	Grade B
Benefits	Reduce unnecessary testing, pain, exposure, caregiver/infant anxiety, and costs Avoid unnecessary antibiotic use and hospitalization pending culture results Avoid consequences of false-positive results/contaminants
Risks, harm, cost	Could miss serious bacterial infection at presentation
Benefit-harm assessment	The benefits of reducing unnecessary testing, pain, exposure, costs, unnecessary antibiotic use, and false-positive results, as well as alleviating caregiver and infant anxiety, outweigh the rare missed diagnostic opportunity for a bacterial infection
Intentional vagueness	None
Role of patient preferences	Caregiver concerns over possible infectious etiology may lead to requests for antibiotic therapy
Exclusions	None
Strength	Strong recommendation
Key references	4, 37, 88

detected during the initial workup. However, on further review of such cases with serious bacterial infections, these infants did not qualify as lower-risk BRUEs, because they had risk factors (eg, age <2 months) and/or appeared ill and had abnormal findings on physical examination (eg, meningeal signs, nuchal rigidity, hypothermia, shock, respiratory failure) suggesting a possible severe bacterial infection. After eliminating those cases, it appears extremely unlikely that meningitis or sepsis will be the etiology of a lower-risk BRUE.[2–4,37,88,89] Furthermore, performing these tests for bacterial infection may then lead the clinician to empirically treat with antibiotics with the consequent risks of medication adverse effects, intravenous catheters, and development of resistant organisms. Furthermore, false-positive blood cultures (eg, coagulase negative staphylococci, *Bacillus* species, *Streptococcus viridans)* are likely to occur at times, leading to additional testing, longer hospitalization and antibiotic use, and increased parental anxiety until they are confirmed as contaminants.

Thus, the available evidence suggests that a complete blood cell count, blood culture, and lumbar puncture are not of benefit in infants with the absence of risk factors or findings from the patient's history, vital signs, and physical examination (ie, a lower-risk BRUE).

4B. Clinicians Need Not Obtain a Urinalysis (Bag or Catheter) in Infants Presenting With a Lower-Risk BRUE (Grade C, Weak Recommendation)

Case series of infants with ALTEs have suggested that a urinary tract infection (UTI) may be detected at the time of first ALTE presentation in up to 8% of cases.[3,4,37,88] Claudius et al[88] provided insight into 17 cases of certain (n = 13) or possible (n = 4) UTI. However, 14 of these cases would not meet the criteria for a lower-risk BRUE on the basis of age younger than 2 months or being ill-appearing and/or having fever at presentation.

Furthermore, these studies do not always specify the method of urine collection, urinalysis findings, and/or the specific organisms and colony-forming units per milliliter of the isolates associated with the reported UTIs that would confirm the diagnosis. AAP guidelines for the diagnosis and management of UTIs in children 2 to 24 months of age assert that the diagnosis of UTI requires "*both* urinalysis results that suggest infection (pyuria and/ or bacteruria) *and* the presence of at least 50 000 colony-forming units/mL of a uropathogen cultured from a urine specimen obtained through catheterization or suprapubic aspirate."[90] Thus, it seems unlikely for a UTI to present as a lower-risk BRUE.

Pending more detailed studies that apply a rigorous definition of UTI to infants presenting with a lower-risk BRUE, a screening urinalysis need not be obtained routinely. If it is decided to evaluate the infant for a possible UTI, then a urinalysis can be obtained but should only be followed up with a culture if the urinalysis has

4B. Clinicians Need Not Obtain a Urinalysis (Bag or Catheter) in Infants Presenting With a Lower-Risk BRUE (Grade C, Weak Recommendation)

Aggregate Evidence Quality	Grade C
Benefits	Reduce unnecessary testing, pain, iatrogenic infection, caregiver/infant anxiety, and costs Avoid consequences of false-positive results Avoid delay from time it takes to obtain a bag urine
Risks, harm, cost	May delay diagnosis of infection
Benefit-harm assessment	The benefits of reducing unnecessary testing, iatrogenic infection, pain, costs, and false-positive results, as well as alleviating caregiver and infant anxiety, outweigh the rare missed diagnostic opportunity for a urinary tract infection
Intentional vagueness	None
Role of patient preferences	Caregiver concerns may lead to preference for testing
Exclusions	None
Strength	Weak recommendation (based on low quality of evidence)
Key references	4, 88

4C. Clinicians Should Not Obtain a Chest Radiograph To Assess for Pulmonary Infection in Infants Presenting With a Lower-Risk BRUE (Grade B, Moderate Recommendation)

Aggregate Evidence Quality	Grade B
Benefits	Reduce costs, unnecessary testing, radiation exposure, and caregiver/infant anxiety Avoid consequences of false-positive results
Risks, harm, cost	May miss early lower respiratory tract infection
Benefit-harm assessment	The benefits of reducing unnecessary testing, radiation exposure, and false-positive results, as well as alleviating caregiver and infant anxiety, outweigh the rare missed diagnostic opportunity for pulmonary infection
Intentional vagueness	None
Role of patient preferences	Caregiver concerns may lead to requests for a chest radiograph
Exclusions	None
Strength	Moderate recommendation
Key references	4, 18, 37

abnormalities suggestive of possible infection (eg, increased white blood cell count, positive nitrates, and/or leukocyte esterase).

4C. Clinicians Should Not Obtain a Chest Radiograph To Assess for Pulmonary Infection in Infants Presenting With a Lower-Risk BRUE (Grade B, Moderate Recommendation)

Chest radiography is unlikely to yield clinical benefit in a well-appearing infant presenting with a lower-risk BRUE. In the absence of abnormal respiratory findings (eg, cough, tachypnea, decreased oxygen saturation, auscultatory changes), lower respiratory tract infection is unlikely to be present.

Studies in children presenting with an ALTE have described occasional cases with abnormal findings on chest radiography in the absence of respiratory findings on history or physical examination.[4,37] However, the nature of the abnormalities and their role in the ALTE presentation in the absence of further details about the radiography results make it difficult to interpret the significance of these observations. For instance, descriptions of increased interstitial markings or small areas of atelectasis would not have the same implication as a focal consolidation or pleural effusion.

Kant et al,[18] in a follow-up of 176 children admitted for an ALTE, reported that 2 infants died within 2 weeks of discharge and both were found to have pneumonia on postmortem examination. This observation does not support the potential indication for an initial radiograph. In fact, one of the children had a normal radiograph during the initial evaluation. The finding of pneumonia on postmortem examination may reflect an agonal aspiration event. Brand et al[4] reported 14 cases of pneumonia identified at presentation in their analysis of 95 cases of ALTEs. However, in 13 of the patients, findings suggestive of lower respiratory infection, such as tachypnea, stridor, retractions, use of accessory muscles, or adventitious sounds on auscultation, were detected at presentation, leading to the request for chest radiography.

4D. Clinicians Need Not Obtain Respiratory Viral Testing If Rapid Testing Is Available in Infants Presenting With a Lower-Risk BRUE (Grade C, Weak Recommendation)

Respiratory viral infections (especially with respiratory syncytial virus [RSV]) have been reported as presenting with apnea or an ALTE, with anywhere from 9% to 82% of patients tested being positive for RSV.[2,4,37,88] However, this finding was observed predominantly in children younger than 2 months and/or those who were born prematurely. Recent data suggest that apnea or an ALTE presentation is not unique to RSV and may be seen with a spectrum of respiratory viral infections.[90] The data in ALTE cases do not address the potential role of other respiratory viruses in ALTEs or BRUEs.

In older children, respiratory viral infection would be expected to present with symptoms ranging from upper respiratory to lower respiratory tract infection rather than as an isolated BRUE. A history of respiratory symptoms and illness exposure; findings of congestion and/or cough, tachypnea, or lower respiratory tract abnormalities; and local epidemiology regarding currently circulating viruses are

4D. Clinicians Need Not Obtain Respiratory Viral Testing If Rapid Testing Is Available in Infants Presenting With a Lower-Risk BRUE (Grade C, Weak Recommendation)

Aggregate Evidence Quality	Grade C
Benefits	Reduce costs, unnecessary testing, and caregiver/infant discomfort Avoid false-negative result leading to missed diagnosis and false reassurance
Risks, harm, cost	Failure to diagnose a viral etiology Not providing expectant management for progression and appropriate infection control interventions for viral etiology
Benefit-harm assessment	The benefits of reducing unnecessary testing, pain, costs, false reassurance, and false-positive results, as well as alleviating caregiver and infant anxiety and challenges associated with providing test results in a timely fashion, outweigh the rare missed diagnostic opportunity for a viral infection
Intentional vagueness	"Rapid testing"; time to results may vary
Role of patient preferences	Caregiver may feel reassured by a specific viral diagnosis
Exclusions	None
Strength	Weak recommendation (based on low-quality evidence)
Key references	4, 37, 91

4E. Clinicians May Obtain Testing for Pertussis in Infants Presenting With a Lower-Risk BRUE (Grade B, Weak Recommendation)

Aggregate Evidence Quality	Grade B
Benefits	Identify a potentially treatable infection Monitor for progression of symptoms, additional apneic episodes Potentially prevent secondary spread and/or identify and treat additional cases
Risks, harm, cost	Cost of test Discomfort of nasopharyngeal swab False-negative results leading to missed diagnosis and false reassurance Rapid testing not always available False reassurance from negative results
Benefit-harm assessment	The benefits of identifying and treating pertussis and preventing apnea and secondary spread outweigh the cost, discomfort, and consequences of false test results and false reassurance; the benefits are greatest in at-risk populations (exposed, underimmunized, endemic, and during outbreaks)
Intentional vagueness	None
Role of patient preferences	Caregiver may feel reassured if a diagnosis is obtained and treatment can be implemented
Exclusions	None
Strength	Weak recommendation (based on balance of benefit and harm)
Key reference	93

considerations in deciding whether to order rapid testing for respiratory viruses. Because lower-risk BRUE patients do not have these symptoms, clinicians need not perform such testing.

In addition, until recently and in reports of ALTE patients to date, RSV testing was performed by using antigen detection tests. More recently, automated nucleic acid amplification-based tests have entered clinical practice. These assays are more sensitive than antigen detection tests and can detect multiple viruses from a single nasopharyngeal swab. The use of these tests in future research may allow better elucidation of the role of respiratory viruses in patients presenting with an ALTE in general and whether they play a role in BRUEs.

As a cautionary note, detection of a virus in a viral multiplex assay may not prove causality, because some agents, such as rhinovirus and adenovirus, may persist for periods beyond the acute infection (up to 30 days) and may or may not be related to the present episode.[92] In a lower-risk BRUE without respiratory symptoms testing for viral infection may not be indicated, but in the presence of congestion and/or cough, or recent exposure to a viral respiratory infection, such testing may provide useful information regarding the cause of the child's symptoms and for infection control management. Anticipatory guidance and arranging close follow-up at the initial presentation could be helpful if patients subsequently develop symptoms of a viral infection.

4E. Clinicians May Obtain Testing for Pertussis in Infants Presenting With a Lower-Risk BRUE (Grade B, Weak Recommendation)

Pertussis infection has been reported to cause ALTEs in infants, because it can cause gagging, gasping, and color change followed by respiratory pause. Such infants can be afebrile and may not develop cough or lower respiratory symptoms for several days afterward.

The decision to test a lower-risk BRUE patient for pertussis should consider potential exposures, vaccine history (including intrapartum immunization of the mother as well as the infant's vaccination history), awareness of pertussis activity in the community, and turnaround time for results. Polymerase chain reaction testing for pertussis on a nasopharyngeal specimen, if available, offers the advantage of rapid turnaround time to results.[94] Culture for the organism requires selective media and will take days to yield results but may still be useful in the face of identified risk of exposure. In patients in whom there is a high index of suspicion on the basis of the aforementioned risk factors, clinicians may consider prolonging the observation period and starting empirical antibiotics while awaiting test results (more information is available from the Centers for Disease Control and Prevention).[95]

5. Gastroenterology

5A. Clinicians Should Not Obtain Investigations for GER (eg, Upper Gastrointestinal Series, pH Probe, Endoscopy, Barium Contrast Study, Nuclear Scintigraphy, and Ultrasonography) in Infants Presenting With a Lower-Risk BRUE (Grade C, Moderate Recommendation)

GER occurs in more than two-thirds of infants and is the topic of discussion with pediatricians at one-quarter of all routine 6-month infant visits.[96] GER can lead to airway obstruction, laryngospasm, or aspiration. Although ALTEs that can be attributed to GER symptoms (eg, choking after spitting up) qualify as an ALTE according to the National Institutes of Health definition, importantly, they do not qualify as a BRUE.

5A. Clinicians Should Not Obtain Investigations for GER (eg, Upper Gastrointestinal Series, pH Probe, Endoscopy, Barium Contrast Study, Nuclear Scintigraphy, and Ultrasonography) in Infants Presenting With a Lower-Risk BRUE (Grade C, Moderate Recommendation)

Aggregate Evidence Quality	Grade C
Benefits	Reduce unnecessary testing, procedural complications (sedation, intestinal perforation, bleeding), pain, radiation exposure, caregiver/infant anxiety, and costs Avoid consequences of false-positive results
Risks, harm, cost	Delay diagnosis of rare but serious gastrointestinal abnormalities (eg, tracheoesophageal fistula) Long-term morbidity of repeated events (eg, chronic lung disease)
Benefit-harm assessment	The benefits of reducing unnecessary testing, complications, radiation, pain, costs, and false-positive results, as well as alleviating caregiver and infant anxiety, outweigh the rare missed diagnostic opportunity for a gastrointestinal abnormality or morbidity from repeat events
Intentional vagueness	None
Role of patient preferences	Caregiver may be reassured by diagnostic evaluation of GER
Exclusions	None
Strength	Moderate recommendation
Key references	96, 97

GER may still be a contributing factor to a lower-risk BRUE if the patient's GER symptoms were not witnessed or well described by caregivers. However, the available evidence suggests no utility of routine diagnostic testing to evaluate for GER in these patients. The brief period of observation that occurs during an upper gastrointestinal series is inadequate to rule out the occurrence of pathologic reflux at other times, and the high prevalence of nonpathologic reflux that often occurs during the study can encourage false-positive diagnoses. In addition, the observation of the reflux of a barium column into the esophagus during gastrointestinal contrast studies may not correlate with the severity of GER or the degree of esophageal mucosal inflammation in patients with reflux esophagitis. Routine performance of an upper gastrointestinal series to diagnose GER is not justified and should be reserved to screen for anatomic abnormalities associated with vomiting (which is a symptom that precludes the diagnosis of a lower-risk BRUE).[98] Gastroesophageal scintigraphy scans for reflux of ^{99m}Tc-labeled solids or liquids into the esophagus or lungs after the administration of the test material into the stomach. The lack of standardized techniques and age-specific normal values limits the usefulness of this test. Therefore, gastroesophageal scintigraphy is not recommended in the routine evaluation of pediatric patients with GER symptoms or a lower-risk BRUE.[97] Multiple intraluminal impedance (MII) is useful for detecting both acidic and nonacidic reflux, thereby providing a more detailed picture of esophageal events than pH monitoring. Combined pH/MII testing is evolving into the test of choice to detect temporal relationships between specific symptoms and the reflux of both acid and nonacid gastric contents. In particular, MII has been used in recent years to investigate how GER correlates with respiratory symptoms, such as apnea or cough. Performing esophageal pH +/- impedance monitoring is not indicated in the routine evaluation of infants presenting with a lower-risk BRUE, although it may be considered in patients with recurrent BRUEs and GER symptoms even if these occur independently.

Problems with the coordination of feedings can lead to ALTEs and BRUEs. In a study in Austrian newborns, infants who experienced an ALTE had a more than twofold increase in feeding difficulties (multivariate relative risk: 2.5; 95% CI: 1.3–4.6).[99] In such patients, it is likely that poor suck-swallow-breathe coordination triggered choking or laryngospasm. A clinical speech therapy evaluation may help to evaluate any concerns for poor coordination swallowing with feeding.

5B. Clinicians Should Not Prescribe Acid Suppression Therapy for Infants Presenting With a Lower-Risk BRUE (Grade C, Moderate Recommendation)

The available evidence suggests no proven efficacy of acid suppression therapy for esophageal reflux in patients presenting with a lower-risk BRUE. Acid suppression therapy with H2-receptor antagonists or proton

5B. Clinicians Should Not Prescribe Acid Suppression Therapy for Infants Presenting With a Lower-Risk BRUE (Grade C, Moderate Recommendation)

Aggregate Evidence Quality	Grade C
Benefits	Reduce unnecessary medication use, adverse effects, and cost from treatment with unproven efficacy
Risks, harm, cost	Delay treatment of rare but undiagnosed gastrointestinal disease, which could lead to complications (eg, esophagitis)
Benefit-harm assessment	The benefits of reducing medication adverse effects, avoiding unnecessary treatment, and reducing cost outweigh the risk of delaying treatment of gastrointestinal disease
Intentional vagueness	None
Role of patient preferences	Caregiver concerns may lead to requests for treatment
Exclusions	None
Strength	Moderate recommendation
Key reference	98

pump inhibitors may be indicated in selected pediatric patients with GER disease (GERD), which is diagnosed in patients when reflux of gastric contents causes troublesome symptoms or complications.[98] Infants with spitting up or throat-clearing coughs that are not troublesome do not meet diagnostic criteria for GERD. Indeed, the inappropriate administration of acid suppression therapy may have harmful adverse effects because it exposes infants to an increased risk of pneumonia or gastroenteritis.[100]

GER leading to apnea is not always clinically apparent and can be the cause of a BRUE. Acid reflux into the esophagus has been shown to be temporally associated with oxygen desaturation and obstructive apnea, suggesting that esophageal reflux may be one of the underlying conditions in selected infants presenting with BRUEs.[101] Respiratory symptoms are more likely to be associated with GER when gross emesis occurs at the time of a BRUE, when episodes occur while the infant is awake and supine (sometimes referred to as "awake apnea"), and when a pattern of obstructive apnea is observed while the infant is making respiratory efforts without effective air movement.[102]

Wenzl et al[103] reported a temporal association between 30% of the nonpathologic, short episodes of central apnea and GER by analyzing combined data from simultaneous esophageal and cardiorespiratory monitoring. These findings cannot be extrapolated to pathologic infant apnea and may represent a normal protective cessation of breathing during regurgitation. Similarly, Mousa et al[104] analyzed data from 527 apneic events in 25 infants and observed that only 15.2% were temporally associated with GER. Furthermore, there was no difference in the linkage between apneic events and acid reflux (7.0%) and nonacid reflux (8.2%). They concluded that there is little evidence for an association between acid reflux or nonacid reflux and the frequency of apnea. Regression analysis revealed a significant association between apnea and reflux in 4 of 25 infants. Thus, in selected infants, a clear temporal relationship between apnea and ALTE can be shown. However, larger studies have not proven a causal relationship between pathologic apnea and GER.[105]

As outlined in the definition of a BRUE, when an apparent explanation for the event, such as GER, is evident at the time of initial evaluation, the patient should be managed as appropriate for the clinical situation. However, BRUEs can be caused by episodes of reflux-related laryngospasm (sometimes referred to as "silent reflux"), which may not be clinically apparent at the time of initial evaluation. Laryngospasm may also occur during feeding in the absence of GER. Measures that have been shown to be helpful in the nonpharmacologic management of GER in infants include avoiding overfeeding, frequent burping during feeding, upright positioning in the caregiver's arms after feeding, and avoidance of secondhand smoke.[106] Thickening feedings with commercially thickened formula for infants without milk-protein intolerance does not alter esophageal acid exposure detected by esophageal pH study but has been shown to decrease the frequency of regurgitation. Given the temporal association observed between GER and respiratory symptoms in selected infants, approaches that decrease the height of the reflux column, the volume of refluxate, and the frequency of reflux episodes may theoretically be beneficial.[98] Combined pH/MII testing has shown that, although the frequency of reflux events is unchanged with thickened formula, the height of the column of refluxate is decreased. Studies have shown that holding the infant on the caregiver's shoulders for 10 to 20 minutes to allow for adequate burping after a feeding before placing the infant in the "back to sleep position" can decrease the frequency of GER in infants. In contrast, placing an infant in a car seat or in other semisupine positions, such as in an infant carrier, exacerbates esophageal reflux and should be avoided.[98] The frequency of GER has been reported to be decreased in breastfed compared with formula-fed infants. Thus, the benefits of breastfeeding are preferred over the theoretical effect of thickened formula feeding, so exclusive breastfeeding should be encouraged whenever possible.

6. Inborn Errors of Metabolism

6A. Clinicians Need Not Obtain Measurement of Serum Lactic Acid or Serum Bicarbonate To Detect an IEM in Infants Presenting With a Lower-Risk BRUE (Grade C, Weak Recommendation)

6B. Clinicians Should Not Obtain a Measurement of Serum Sodium, Potassium, Chloride, Blood Urea Nitrogen, Creatinine, Calcium, or Ammonia To Detect an IEM on Infants Presenting With a Lower-Risk BRUE (Grade C, Moderate Recommendation)

6C. Clinicians Should Not Obtain a Measurement of Venous or Arterial Blood Gases To Detect an IEM in Infants Presenting With Lower-Risk BRUE (Grade C, Moderate Recommendation)

6D. Clinicians Need Not Obtain a Measurement of Blood Glucose To Detect an IEM in Infants Presenting With a Lower-Risk BRUE (Grade C, Weak Recommendation)

6E. Clinicians Should Not Obtain Measurements of Urine Organic Acids, Plasma Amino Acids, or Plasma Acylcarnitines To Detect an IEM in Infants Presenting With a Lower-Risk BRUE (Grade C, Moderate Recommendation)

IEMs are reported to cause an ALTE in 0% to 5% of cases.[2,27,38,99,107,108] On the basis of the information provided by the authors for these patients, it seems unlikely that events could have been classified as a lower-risk BRUE, either because the patient had a positive history or physical examination or a recurrent event. The most commonly reported disorders include fatty acid oxidation disorders or urea cycle disorders.[107,109] In cases of vague or resolved symptoms, a careful history can help determine whether the infant had not received previous treatment (eg, feeding after listlessness for suspected hypoglycemia). These rare circumstances could include milder or later-onset presentations of IEMs.

Infants may be classified as being at a higher risk of BRUE because of a family history of an IEM, developmental disabilities, SIDS, or a medical history of abnormal newborn screening results, unexplained infant death, age younger than 2 months, a prolonged event (>1 minute), or multiple events without an explanation. Confirmation that a newborn screen is complete and is negative is an important aspect of the medical history, but the clinician must consider that not all potential disorders are included in current newborn screening panels in the United States.

6A. Clinicians Need Not Obtain Measurement of Serum Lactic Acid or Serum Bicarbonate To Detect an IEM in Infants Presenting With a Lower-Risk BRUE (Grade C, Weak Recommendation)

Aggregate Evidence Quality	Grade C
Benefits	Reduce unnecessary testing, caregiver/infant anxiety, and costs Avoid consequences of false-positive or nonspecific results
Risks, harm, cost	May miss detection of an IEM
Benefit-harm assessment	The benefits of reducing unnecessary testing, cost, and false-positive results, as well as alleviating caregiver and infant anxiety, outweigh the rare missed diagnostic opportunity for an IEM
Intentional vagueness	Detection of higher lactic acid or lower bicarbonate levels should be considered to have a lower likelihood of being a false-positive result and may warrant additional investigation
Role of patient preferences	Caregiver concerns may lead to requests for diagnostic testing
Exclusions	None
Strength	Weak recommendation (based on low-quality evidence)
Key reference	38

6B. Clinicians Should Not Obtain a Measurement of Serum Sodium, Potassium, Chloride, Blood Urea Nitrogen, Creatinine, Calcium, or Ammonia To Detect an IEM on Infants Presenting With a Lower-Risk BRUE (Grade C, Moderate Recommendation)

Aggregate Evidence Quality	Grade C
Benefits	Reduce costs, unnecessary testing, pain, and caregiver/infant anxiety Avoid consequences of false-positive results
Risks, harm, cost	May miss detection of an IEM
Benefit-harm assessment	The benefits of reducing unnecessary testing, cost, and false-positive results, as well as alleviating caregiver and infant anxiety, outweigh the rare missed diagnostic opportunity for an IEM
Intentional vagueness	None
Role of patient preferences	Caregiver concerns may lead to requests for diagnostic testing
Exclusions	None
Strength	Moderate recommendation
Key reference	4

Lactic Acid

Measurement of lactic acid can result in high false-positive rates if the sample is not collected properly, making the decision to check a lactic acid problematic. In addition, lactic acid may be elevated because of metabolic abnormalities attributable to other conditions, such as sepsis, and are not specific for IEMs.

Only 2 studies evaluated the specific measurement of lactic acid.[27,38] Davies and Gupta[38] reported 65 infants with consistent laboratory evaluations and found that 54% of infants had a lactic acid >2 mmol/L but only 15% had levels >3 mmol/L. The latter percentage of infants are more likely to be clinically significant and less likely to reflect a false-positive result. Five of 7 infants with a lactic acid >3 mmol/L had a "specific, serious diagnosis," although the specifics of these diagnoses were not included and no IEM was

6C. Clinicians Should Not Obtain a Measurement of Venous or Arterial Blood Gases To Detect an IEM in Infants Presenting With Lower-Risk BRUE (Grade C, Moderate Recommendation)

Aggregate Evidence Quality	Grade C
Benefits	Reduce costs, unnecessary testing, pain, risk of thrombosis, and caregiver/infant anxiety Avoid consequences of false-positive results
Risks, harm, cost	May miss detection of an IEM
Benefit-harm assessment	The benefits of reducing unnecessary testing, cost, and false-positive results, as well as alleviating caregiver and infant anxiety, outweigh the rare missed diagnostic opportunity for an IEM
Intentional vagueness	None
Role of patient preferences	Caregiver concerns may lead to requests for diagnostic testing
Exclusions	None
Strength	Moderate recommendation
Key reference	4

6D. Clinicians Need Not Obtain a Measurement of Blood Glucose To Detect an IEM in Infants Presenting With a Lower-Risk BRUE (Grade C, Weak Recommendation)

Aggregate Evidence Quality	Grade C
Benefits	Reduce costs, unnecessary testing, pain, risk of thrombosis, and caregiver/infant anxiety Avoid consequences of false-positive results
Risks, harm, cost	May miss rare instances of hypoglycemia attributable to undiagnosed IEM
Benefit-harm assessment	The benefits of reducing unnecessary testing, cost, and false-positive results, as well as alleviating caregiver and infant anxiety, outweigh the rare missed diagnostic opportunity for an IEM
Intentional vagueness	Measurement of glucose is often performed immediately through a simple bedside test; no abnormalities have been reported in asymptomatic infants, although studies often do not distinguish between capillary or venous measurement
Role of patient preferences	Caregiver concerns may lead to requests for diagnostic testing
Exclusions	None
Strength	Weak recommendation (based on low-quality evidence)
Key reference	4

confirmed in this study. This study also reported a 20% positive yield of testing for a bicarbonate <20 mmol/L and commented that there was a trend for lower bicarbonate and higher lactic acid levels in those with a recurrent event or a definitive diagnosis. The second publication[27] found no elevations of lactate in 4 of 49 children who had an initial abnormal venous blood gas, of which all repeat blood gas measurements were normal.

Serum Bicarbonate

Abnormal serum bicarbonate levels have been studied in 11 infants, of whom 7 had a diagnosis of sepsis or seizures.[38] Brand et al[4] studied 215 infants who had bicarbonate measured and found only 9 abnormal results, and only 3 of these contributed to the final diagnosis. Although unknown, it is most likely that the event in those infants would not have been classified as a BRUE under the new classification, because those infants were most likely symptomatic on presentation.

Serum Glucose

Abnormal blood glucose levels were evaluated but not reported in 3 studies.[4,38,110] Although abnormalities of blood glucose can occur from various IEMs, such as medium-chain acyl–coenzyme A dehydrogenase deficiency or other fatty acid oxidation disorders, their prevalence has not been increased in SIDS and near-miss SIDS but could be considered as a cause of higher-risk BRUEs.[111] It is important to clarify through a careful medical history evaluation that the infant was not potentially hypoglycemic at discovery of the event and improved because of enteral treatment, because these disorders will not typically self-resolve without intervention (ie, feeding).

Serum Electrolytes and Calcium

ALTE studies evaluating the diagnostic value of electrolytes, including sodium, potassium, blood urea nitrogen, and creatinine, reported the rare occurrence of abnormalities, ranging from 0% to 4.3%.[4,38,110] Abnormal calcium levels have been reported in 0% to 1.5% of infants with ALTE, although these reports did not provide specific causes of hypocalcemia. Another study reported profound vitamin D deficiency with hypocalcemia in 5 of 25 infants with a diagnosis of an ALTE over a 2-year period in Saudi Arabia.[4,21,38,110] In lower-risk BRUE infants, clinicians should not obtain a calcium measurement unless the clinical history raises suspicion of hypocalcemia (eg, vitamin D deficiency or hypoparathyroidism).

Ammonia

Elevations of ammonia are typically associated with persistent symptoms and recurring events, and therefore testing would not be indicated in lower-risk BRUEs. Elevations of ammonia were reported in 11 infants (7 whom had an IEM) in a report of infants with recurrent ALTE and SIDS, limiting extrapolation to lower-risk BRUEs.[109] Elevations of ammonia >100 mmol/L were found in 4% of 65 infants, but this publication did not document a confirmed IEM.[38] Weiss et al[27] reported no abnormal elevations of ammonia in 4 infants with abnormal venous blood gas.

Venous or Arterial Blood Gas

Blood gas abnormalities leading to a diagnosis have not been reported in previous ALTE studies. Brand et al[4] reported 53 of 60 with positive findings, with none contributing to the final diagnosis. Weiss et al[27] reported 4 abnormal findings of 49 completed, all of which were normal on repeat measurements (along with normal lactate and ammonia levels). Blood gas detection is a routine test performed in acutely symptomatic patients who are being evaluated for suspected IEMs and may be considered in higher-risk BRUEs.

Urine Organic Acids, Plasma Amino Acids, Plasma Acylcarnitines

The role of advanced screening for IEMs has been reported in only 1 publication. Davies and Gupta[38] reported abnormalities of urine organic acids in 2% of cases and abnormalities of plasma amino acids in 4% of cases. Other reports have described an "unspecified metabolic screen" that was abnormal in 4.5% of cases but did not provide further description of specifics within that "screen."[4] Other reports have frequently included the descriptions of ALTEs with urea cycle disorders, organic acidemias, lactic acidemias, and fatty acid oxidation disorders such as medium chain acyl–coenzyme A dehydrogenase deficiency but did not distinguish between SIDS and near-miss SIDS.[107,109,111] Specific testing of urine organic acids, plasma amino acids, or plasma acylcarnitines may have a role in patients with a higher-risk BRUE.

6E. Clinicians Should Not Obtain Measurements of Urine Organic Acids, Plasma Amino Acids, or Plasma Acylcarnitines To Detect an IEM in Infants Presenting With a Lower-Risk BRUE (Grade C, Moderate Recommendation)

Aggregate Evidence Quality	Grade C
Benefits	Reduce costs, unnecessary testing, pain, risk of thrombosis, and caregiver/infant anxiety Avoid consequences of false-positive results
Risks, harm, cost	May miss detection of an IEM
Benefit-harm assessment	The benefits of reducing unnecessary testing, cost, and false-positive results, as well as alleviating caregiver and infant anxiety, outweigh the rare missed diagnostic opportunity for an IEM
Intentional vagueness	Lower-risk BRUEs will have a very low likelihood of disease, but these tests may be indicated in rare cases in which there is no documentation of a newborn screen being performed
Role of patient preferences	Caregiver concerns may lead to requests for diagnostic testing
Exclusions	None
Strength	Moderate recommendation
Key references	4, 38

7A. Clinicians Should Not Obtain Laboratory Evaluation for Anemia in Infants Presenting With a Lower-Risk BRUE (Grade C, Moderate Recommendation)

Aggregate Evidence Quality	Grade C
Benefits	Reduce costs, unnecessary testing, pain, risk of thrombosis, and caregiver/infant anxiety Avoid consequences of false-positive results
Risks, harm, cost	May miss diagnosis of anemia
Benefit-harm assessment	The benefits of reducing unnecessary testing, cost, and false-positive results, as well as alleviating caregiver and infant anxiety, outweigh the missed diagnostic opportunity for anemia
Intentional vagueness	None
Role of patient preferences	Caregivers may be reassured by testing
Exclusions	None
Strength	Moderate recommendation
Key reference	22

7. Anemia

7A. Clinicians Should Not Obtain Laboratory Evaluation for Anemia in Infants Presenting With a Lower-Risk BRUE (Grade C, Moderate Recommendation)

Anemia has been associated with ALTEs in infants, but the significance and causal association with the event itself are unclear.[38,112,113] Normal hemoglobin concentrations have also been reported in many other ALTE populations.[69,112,114] Brand et al[4] reported an abnormal hemoglobin in 54 of 223 cases, but in only 2 of 159 was the hemoglobin concentration associated with the final diagnosis (which was abusive head injury in both). Parker and Pitetti[22] also reported that infants who presented with ALTEs and ultimately were determined to be victims of child abuse were more likely to have a lower mean hemoglobin (10.6 vs 12.7 g/dL; $P = .02$).

8. Patient- and Family-Centered Care

8A. Clinicians Should Offer Resources for CPR Training to Caregivers (Grade C, Moderate Recommendation)

The majority of cardiac arrests in children result from a respiratory deterioration. Bystander CPR has been reported to have been conducted in 37% to 48% of pediatric out-of-hospital cardiac arrests and in 34% of respiratory arrests.[116] Bystander CPR results in significant improvement in 1-month survival rates in both cardiac and respiratory arrest.[117–119]

Although lower-risk BRUEs are neither a cardiac nor a respiratory arrest, the AAP policy statement on CPR recommends that pediatricians advocate for life-support training for caregivers and the general public.[115] A technical report that accompanies the AAP policy statement on CPR proposes that this can improve overall community health.[115] CPR training has not been shown to increase caregiver anxiety, and in fact, caregivers have reported a sense of empowerment.[120–122] There are many accessible and effective methods for CPR training (eg, e-learning).

8A. Clinicians Should Offer Resources for CPR Training to Caregivers (Grade C, Moderate Recommendation)

Aggregate Evidence Quality	Grade C
Benefits	Decrease caregiver anxiety and increase confidence Benefit to society
Risks, harm, cost	May increase caregiver anxiety Cost and availability of training
Benefit-harm assessment	The benefits of decreased caregiver anxiety and increased confidence, as well as societal benefits, outweigh the increase in caregiver anxiety, cost, and resources
Intentional vagueness	None
Role of patient preferences	Caregiver may decide not to seek out the training
Exclusions	None
Strength	Moderate recommendation
Key reference	115

8B. Clinicians Should Educate Caregivers About BRUEs (Grade C, Moderate Recommendation)

Pediatric providers are an important source of this health information and can help guide important conversations around BRUEs. A study by Feudtner et al[123] identified 4 groups of attributes of a "good parent": (1) making sure the child feels loved, (2) focusing on the child's health, (3) advocating for the child and being informed, and (4) ensuring the child's spiritual well-being. Clinicians should be the source of information for caregivers. Informed caregivers can advocate for their child in all of the attribute areas/domains, and regardless of health literacy levels, prefer being offered choices and being asked for information.[124] A patient- and family-centered care approach results in better health outcomes.[125,126]

8B. Clinicians Should Educate Caregivers About BRUEs (Grade C, Moderate Recommendation)

Aggregate Evidence Quality	Grade C
Benefits	Improve caregiver empowerment and health literacy and decrease anxiety May reduce unnecessary return visits Promotion of the medical home
Risks, harm, cost	Increase caregiver anxiety and potential for caregiver intimidation in voicing concerns Increase health care costs and length of stay
Benefit-harm assessment	The benefits of decreased caregiver anxiety and increased empowerment and health literacy outweigh the increase in cost, length of stay, and caregiver anxiety and intimidation
Intentional vagueness	None
Role of patient preferences	Caregiver may decide not to listen to clinician
Exclusions	None
Strength	Moderate recommendation
Key references	None

8C. Clinicians Should Use Shared Decision-Making for Infants Presenting With a Lower-Risk BRUE (Grade C, Moderate Recommendation)

Shared decision-making is a partnership between the clinician and the patient and family.[125,126] The general principles of shared decision-making are as follows: (1) information sharing, (2) respect and honoring differences, (3) partnership and collaboration, (4) negotiation, and (5) care in the context of family and community.[125] The benefits include improved care and outcomes; improved patient, family, and clinician satisfaction; and better use of health resources.[126] It is advocated for by organizations such as the AAP and the Institute of Medicine.[126,127] The 5 principles can be applied to all aspects of the infant who has experienced a BRUE, through each step (assessment, stabilization, management, disposition, and follow-up). Shared decision-making will empower families and foster a stronger clinician-patient/family alliance as they make decisions together in the face of a seemingly uncertain situation.

DISSEMINATION AND IMPLEMENTATION

Dissemination and implementation efforts are needed to facilitate guideline use across pediatric medicine, family medicine, emergency medicine, research, and patient/family communities.[128] The following general approaches and a Web-based toolkit are proposed for the dissemination and implementation of this guideline.

8C. Clinicians Should Use Shared Decision-Making for Infants Presenting With a Lower-Risk BRUE (Grade C, Moderate Recommendation)

Aggregate Evidence Quality	Grade C
Benefits	Improve caregiver empowerment and health literacy and decrease anxiety May reduce unnecessary return visits Promotion of the medical home
Risks, harm, cost	Increase cost, length of stay, and caregiver anxiety and intimidation in voicing concerns
Benefit-harm assessment	The benefits of decreased caregiver anxiety and unplanned return visits and increased empowerment, health, literacy, and medical home promotion outweigh the increase in cost, length of stay, and caregiver anxiety and information
Intentional vagueness	None
Role of patient preferences	Caregiver may decide not to listen to clinician
Exclusions	None
Strength	Moderate recommendation
Key references	None

1. Education

Education will be partially achieved through the AAP communication outlets and educational services (*AAP News, Pediatrics,* and PREP). Further support will be sought from stakeholder organizations (American Academy of Family Physicians, American College of Emergency Physicians, American Board of Pediatrics, Society of Hospital Medicine). A Web-based toolkit (to be published online) will include caregiver handouts and a shared decision-making tool to facilitate patient- and family-centered care. Efforts will address appropriate disease classification and diagnosis coding.

2. Integration of Clinical Workflow

An algorithm is provided (Fig 1) for diagnosis and management. Structured history and physical examination templates also are provided to assist in addressing all of the relevant risk factors for BRUEs (Tables 2 and 3). Order sets and modified documents will be hosted on a Web-based learning platform that promotes crowd-sourcing.

3. Administrative and Research

International Classification of Diseases, 9th Revision, and International Classification of Diseases, 10th Revision, diagnostic codes are used for billing, quality improvement, and research; and new codes for lower- and higher-risk BRUEs will need to be developed. In the interim, the current code for an ALTE (799.82) will need to be used for billing purposes. Efforts will be made to better reflect present knowledge and to educate clinicians and payers in appropriate use of codes for this condition.

4. Quality Improvement

Quality improvement initiatives that provide Maintenance of Certification credit, such as the AAP's PREP and EQIPP courses, or collaborative opportunities through the AAP's Quality Improvement Innovation Networks, will engage clinicians in the use and improvement of the guideline. By using proposed quality measures, adherence and outcomes can be assessed and benchmarked with others to inform continual improvement efforts. Proposed measures include process evaluation (use of definition and evaluation), outcome assessment (family experience and diagnostic outcomes), and balancing issues (cost and length of visit). Future research will need to be conducted to validate any measures.

FUTURE RESEARCH

The transition in nomenclature from the term ALTE to BRUE after 30 years reflects the expanded understanding of the etiology and consequences of this entity. Previous research has been largely retrospective or observational in nature, with little long-term follow-up data available. The more-precise definition, the classification of lower- and higher-risk groups, the recommendations for the lower-risk group, and the implementation toolkit will serve as the basis for future research. Important areas for future prospective research include the following.

1. Epidemiology

- Incidence of BRUEs in all infants (in addition to those seeking medical evaluation)
- Influence of race, gender, ethnicity, seasonality, environmental exposures, and socioeconomic status on incidence and outcomes

2. Diagnosis

- Use and effectiveness of the BRUE definition
- Screening tests and risk of UTI
- Quantify and better understand risk in higher- and lower-risk groups
- Risk and benefit of screening tests
- Risk and benefit and optimal duration of observation and monitoring periods
- Effect of prematurity on risk
- Appropriate indications for subspecialty referral
- Early recognition of child maltreatment
- Importance of environmental history taking
- Role of human psychology on accuracy of event characterization

- Type and length of monitoring in the acute setting

3. Pathophysiology

- Role of abnormalities of swallowing, laryngospasm, GER, and autonomic function

4. Outcomes

- Patient- and family-centered outcomes, including caregiver satisfaction, anxiety, and family dynamics (eg, risk of vulnerable child syndrome)
- Long-term health and cognitive consequences

5. Treatment

- Empirical GER treatment on recurrent BRUEs
- Caregiver education strategies, including basic life support, family-centered education, and postpresentation clinical visits

6. Follow-up

- Strategies for timely follow-up and surveillance

SUBCOMMITTEE ON BRIEF RESOLVED UNEXPLAINED EVENTS (FORMERLY REFERRED TO AS APPARENT LIFE THREATENING EVENTS) (OVERSIGHT BY THE COUNCIL ON QUALITY IMPROVEMENT AND PATIENT SAFETY)

Joel S. Tieder, MD, MPH, FAAP, Chair (no financial conflicts, published research related to BRUEs/ALTEs)
Joshua L. Bonkowsky, MD, PhD, FAAP, Pediatric Neurologist
Ruth A. Etzel, MD, PhD, FAAP, Pediatric Epidemiologist
Wayne H. Franklin, MD, MPH, MMM, FAAP, Pediatric Cardiologist
David A. Gremse, MD, FAAP, Pediatric Gastroenterologist
Bruce Herman, MD, FAAP, Child Abuse and Neglect
Eliot Katz, MD, FAAP, Pediatric Pulmonologist
Leonard R. Krilov, MD, FAAP, Pediatric Infectious Diseases
J. Lawrence Merritt II, MD, FAAP, Clinical Genetics and Biochemical Genetics
Chuck Norlin, MD, FAAP, Pediatrician
Robert E. Sapién, MD, MMM, FAAP, Pediatric Emergency Medicine
Richard Shiffman, MD, FAAP, Partnership for Policy Implementation Representative
Michael B.H. Smith, MB, FRCPCH, FAAP, Hospital Medicine
Jack Percelay, MD, MPH, FAAP, Liaison, Society for Hospital Medicine

STAFF

Kymika Okechukwu, MPA

ABBREVIATIONS

AAP: American Academy of Pediatrics
ALTE: apparent life-threatening event
BRUE: brief resolved unexplained event
CI: confidence interval
CNS: central nervous system
CPR: cardiopulmonary resuscitation
ECG: electrocardiogram
GER: gastroesophageal reflux
IEM: inborn error of metabolism
MII: multiple intraluminal impedance
OSA: obstructive sleep apnea
RSV: respiratory syncytial virus
SIDS: sudden infant death syndrome
SUDEP: sudden unexpected death in epilepsy
UTI: urinary tract infection

REFERENCES

1. National Institutes of Health Consensus Development Conference on Infantile Apnea and Home Monitoring, Sept 29 to Oct 1, 1986. *Pediatrics*. 1987;79(2):292–299
2. McGovern MC, Smith MB. Causes of apparent life threatening events in infants: a systematic review. *Arch Dis Child*. 2004;89(11):1043–1048
3. Tieder JS, Altman RL, Bonkowsky JL, et al Management of apparent life-threatening events in infants: a systematic review. *J Pediatr*. 2013;163(1):94–99, e91–e96
4. Brand DA, Altman RL, Purtill K, Edwards KS. Yield of diagnostic testing in infants who have had an apparent life-threatening event. *Pediatrics*. 2005;115(4):885–893
5. Green M. Vulnerable child syndrome and its variants. *Pediatr Rev*. 1986;8(3):75–80
6. Kaji AH, Claudius I, Santillanes G, et al. Apparent life-threatening event: multicenter prospective cohort study to develop a clinical decision rule for admission to the hospital. *Ann Emerg Med*. 2013;61(4):379–387.e4
7. Mittal MK, Sun G, Baren JM. A clinical decision rule to identify infants with apparent life-threatening event who can be safely discharged from the emergency department. *Pediatr Emerg Care*. 2012;28(7):599–605
8. Moher D, Liberati A, Tetzlaff J, Altman DG; PRISMA Group. Preferred reporting items for systematic reviews and meta-analyses: the PRISMA statement. *Ann Intern Med*. 2009;151(4):264–269, W64
9. Haynes RB, Cotoi C, Holland J, et al; McMaster Premium Literature Service (PLUS) Project. Second-order peer review of the medical literature for clinical practitioners. *JAMA*. 2006;295(15):1801–1808
10. Lokker C, McKibbon KA, McKinlay RJ, Wilczynski NL, Haynes RB. Prediction of citation counts for clinical articles at two years using data available within three weeks of publication: retrospective cohort study. *BMJ*. 2008;336(7645):655–657
11. Laupacis A, Wells G, Richardson WS, Tugwell P; Evidence-Based Medicine Working Group. Users' guides to the medical literature. V. How to use an article about prognosis. *JAMA*. 1994;272(3):234–237
12. Jaeschke R, Guyatt G, Sackett DL. Users' guides to the medical literature. III. How to use an article about a diagnostic test. A. Are the results of the study valid? Evidence-Based Medicine Working Group. *JAMA*. 1994;271(5):389–391
13. Anjos AM, Nunes ML. Prevalence of epilepsy and seizure disorders as causes of apparent life-threatening event (ALTE) in children admitted to a tertiary hospital. *Arq Neuropsiquiatr*. 2009;67(3a 3A):616–620

14. Doshi A, Bernard-Stover L, Kuelbs C, Castillo E, Stucky E. Apparent lifethreatening event admissions and gastroesophageal reflux disease: the value of hospitalization. *Pediatr Emerg Care*. 2012;28(1):17–21

15. Franco P, Montemitro E, Scaillet S, et al. Fewer spontaneous arousals in infants with apparent life-threatening event. *Sleep*. 2011;34(6):733–743

16. Hoki R, Bonkowsky JL, Minich LL, Srivastava R, Pinto NM. Cardiac testing and outcomes in infants after an apparent life-threatening event. *Arch Dis Child*. 2012;97(12):1034–1038

17. Kaji AH, Santillanes G, Claudius I, et al. Do infants less than 12 months of age with an apparent life-threatening event need transport to a pediatric critical care center? *Prehosp Emerg Care*. 2013;17(3):304–311

18. Kant S, Fisher JD, Nelson DG, Khan S. Mortality after discharge in clinically stable infants admitted with a fi rsttime apparent life-threatening event. *Am J Emerg Med*. 2013;31(4):730–733

19. Miano S, Castaldo R, Ferri R, et al. Sleep cyclic alternating pattern analysis in infants with apparent life-threatening events: a daytime polysomnographic study. *Clin Neurophysiol*. 2012;123(7):1346–1352

20. Mittal MK, Donda K, Baren JM. Role of pneumography and esophageal pH monitoring in the evaluation of infants with apparent life-threatening event: a prospective observational study. *Clin Pediatr (Phila)*. 2013;52(4):338–343

21. Mosalli RM, Elsayed YY, Paes BA. Acute life threatening events associated with hypocalcemia and vitamin D defi ciency in early infancy: a single center experience from the Kingdom of Saudi Arabia. *Saudi Med J*. 2011;32(5):528–530

22. Parker K, Pitetti R. Mortality and child abuse in children presenting with apparent life-threatening events. *Pediatr Emerg Care*. 2011;27(7):591–595

23. Poets A, Urschitz MS, Steinfeldt R, Poets CF. Risk factors for early sudden deaths and severe apparent lifethreatening events. *Arch Dis Child Fetal Neonatal Ed*. 2012;97(6):F395–F397

24. Semmekrot BA, van Sleuwen BE, Engelberts AC, et al. Surveillance study of apparent life-threatening events (ALTE) in the Netherlands. *Eur J Pediatr*. 2010;169(2):229–236

25. Tieder JS, Altman RL, Bonkowsky JL, et al. Management of apparent life-threatening events in infants: a systematic review. *J Pediatr*. 2013;163(1):94–9.e1, 6

26. Wasilewska J, Sienkiewicz-Szłapka E, Kuźbida E, Jarmołowska B, Kaczmarski M, Kostyra E. The exogenous opioid peptides and DPPIV serum activity in infants with apnoea expressed as apparent life threatening events (ALTE). *Neuropeptides*. 2011;45(3):189–195

27. Weiss K, Fattal-Valevski A, Reif S. How to evaluate the child presenting with an apparent life-threatening event? *Isr Med Assoc J*. 2010;12(3):154–157

28. Zimbric G, Bonkowsky JL, Jackson WD, Maloney CG, Srivastava R. Adverse outcomes associated with gastroesophageal reflux disease are rare following an apparent life-threatening event. *J Hosp Med*. 2012;7(6):476–481

29. American Academy of Pediatrics Steering Committee on Quality Improvement and Management. Classifying recommendations for clinical practice guidelines. *Pediatrics*. 2004;114(3):874–877

30. Shiffman RN, Michel G, Rosenfeld RM, Davidson C. Building better guidelines with BRIDGE-Wiz: development and evaluation of a software assistant to promote clarity, transparency, and implementability. *J Am Med Inform Assoc*. 2012;19(1):94–101

31. Claudius I, Keens T. Do all infants with apparent life-threatening events need to be admitted? *Pediatrics*. 2007;119(4):679–683

32. Bonkowsky JL, Guenther E, Filloux FM, Srivastava R. Death, child abuse, and adverse neurological outcome of infants after an apparent lifethreatening event. *Pediatrics*. 2008;122(1):125–131

33. Al-Kindy HA, Gelinas JF, Hatzakis G, Cote A. Risk factors for extreme events in infants hospitalized for apparent life-threatening events. *J Pediatr*. 2009;154(3):332–337, 337.e1–337.e2

34. Ramanathan R, Corwin MJ, Hunt CE, et al; Collaborative Home Infant Monitoring Evaluation (CHIME) Study Group. Cardiorespiratory events recorded on home monitors: comparison of healthy infants with those at increased risk for SIDS. *JAMA*. 2001;285(17):2199–2207

35. Poets CF, Stebbens VA, Alexander JR, Arrowsmith WA, Salfield SA, Southall DP. Hypoxaemia in infants with respiratory tract infections. *Acta Paediatr*. 1992;81(6–7):536–541

36. Hunt CE, Corwin MJ, Lister G, et al; Collaborative Home Infant Monitoring Evaluation (CHIME) Study Group. Longitudinal assessment of hemoglobin oxygen saturation in healthy infants during the first 6 months of age. *J Pediatr*. 1999;135(5):580–586

37. Altman RL, Li KI, Brand DA. Infections and apparent life-threatening events. *Clin Pediatr (Phila)*. 2008;47(4):372–378

38. Davies F, Gupta R. Apparent life threatening events in infants presenting to an emergency department. *Emerg Med J*. 2002;19(1):11–16

39. Guilleminault C, Ariagno R, Korobkin R, et al. Mixed and obstructive sleep apnea and near miss for sudden infant death syndrome: 2. Comparison of near miss and normal control infants by age. *Pediatrics*. 1979;64(6):882–891

40. Côté A, Hum C, Brouillette RT, Themens M. Frequency and timing of recurrent events in infants using home cardiorespiratory monitors. *J Pediatr*. 1998;132(5):783–789

41. Kahn A, Blum D. Home monitoring of infants considered at risk for the sudden infant death syndrome: four years' experience (1977-1981). *Eur J Pediatr*. 1982;139(2):94–100

42. Daniëls H, Naulaers G, Deroost F, Devlieger H. Polysomnography and home documented monitoring of cardiorespiratory pattern. *Arch Dis Child*. 1999;81(5):434–436

43. Marcus CL, Hamer A. Significance of isolated bradycardia detected

by home monitoring. *J Pediatr.* 1999;135(3):321–326

44. Rebuffat E, Groswasser J, Kelmanson I, Sottiaux M, Kahn A. Polygraphic evaluation of night-to-night variability in sleep characteristics and apneas in infants. *Sleep.* 1994;17(4):329–332
45. Horemuzova E, Katz-Salamon M, Milerad J. Increased inspiratory effort in infants with a history of apparent life-threatening event. *Acta Paediatr.* 2002;91(3):280–286; discussion: 260–261
46. Schechtman VL, Harper RM, Wilson AJ, Southall DP. Sleep state organization in normal infants and victims of the sudden infant death syndrome. *Pediatrics.* 1992;89(5 Pt 1):865–870
47. Arad-Cohen N, Cohen A, Tirosh E. The relationship between gastroesophageal reflux and apnea in infants. *J Pediatr.* 2000;137(3):321–326
48. Harrington C, Kirjavainen T, Teng A, Sullivan CE. Altered autonomic function and reduced arousability in apparent life-threatening event infants with obstructive sleep apnea. *Am J Respir Crit Care Med.* 2002;165(8):1048–1054
49. Guilleminault C, Pelayo R, Leger D, Philip P. Apparent life-threatening events, facial dysmorphia and sleep-disordered breathing. *Eur J Pediatr.* 2000;159(6):444–449
50. Aurora RN, Zak RS, Karippot A, et al; American Academy of Sleep Medicine. Practice parameters for the respiratory indications for polysomnography in children. *Sleep.* 2011;34(3):379–388
51. Kahn A, Groswasser J, Sottiaux M, Rebuffat E, Franco P. Mechanisms of obstructive sleep apneas in infants. *Biol Neonate.* 1994;65(3–4):235–239
52. Leiberman A, Tal A, Brama I, Sofer S. Obstructive sleep apnea in young infants. *Int J Pediatr Otorhinolaryngol.* 1988;16(1):39–44
53. Montgomery-Downs HE, Gozal D. Sleep habits and risk factors for sleep-disordered breathing in infants and young toddlers in Louisville, Kentucky. *Sleep Med.* 2006;7(3):211–219
54. Brouillette RT, Fernbach SK, Hunt CE. Obstructive sleep apnea in infants and children. *J Pediatr.* 1982;100(1):31–40
55. Kahn A, Groswasser J, Sottiaux M, et al. Clinical symptoms associated with brief obstructive sleep apnea in normal infants. *Sleep.* 1993;16(5):409–413
56. Kahn A, Groswasser J, Sottiaux M, et al. Prenatal exposure to cigarettes in infants with obstructive sleep apneas. *Pediatrics.* 1994;93(5):778–783
57. Kahn A, Mozin MJ, Rebuffat E, et al. Sleep pattern alterations and brief airway obstructions in overweight infants. *Sleep.* 1989;12(5):430–438
58. Fajardo C, Alvarez J, Wong A, Kwiatkowski K, Rigatto H. The incidence of obstructive apneas in preterm infants with and without bronchopulmonary dysplasia. *Early Hum Dev.* 1993;32(2–3):197–206
59. Horigome H, Nagashima M, Sumitomo N, et al. Clinical characteristics and genetic background of congenital long-QT syndrome diagnosed in fetal, neonatal, and infantile life: a nationwide questionnaire survey in Japan. *Circ Arrhythm Electrophysiol.* 2010;3(1):10–17
60. Arnestad M, Crotti L, Rognum TO, et al. Prevalence of long-QT syndrome gene variants in sudden infant death syndrome. *Circulation.* 2007;115(3):361–367
61. Goldenberg I, Moss AJ, Peterson DR, et al. Risk factors for aborted cardiac arrest and sudden cardiac death in children with the congenital long-QT syndrome. *Circulation.* 2008;117(17):2184–2191
62. Munger TM, Packer DL, Hammill SC, et al. A population study of the natural history of Wolff-Parkinson-White syndrome in Olmsted County, Minnesota, 1953-1989. *Circulation.* 1993;87(3):866–873
63. American Academy of Pediatrics, Committee on Fetus and Newborn. Apnea, sudden infant death syndrome, and home monitoring. *Pediatrics.* 2003;111(4 pt 1):914–917
64. Krongrad E, O'Neill L. Near miss sudden infant death syndrome episodes? A clinical and electrocardiographic correlation. *Pediatrics.* 1986;77(6):811–815
65. Nathanson I, O'Donnell J, Commins MF. Cardiorespiratory patterns during alarms in infants using apnea/bradycardia monitors. *Am J Dis Child.* 1989;143(4):476–480
66. Weese-Mayer DE, Brouillette RT, Morrow AS, Conway LP, Klemka-Walden LM, Hunt CE. Assessing validity of infant monitor alarms with event recording. *J Pediatr.* 1989;115(5 pt 1):702–708
67. Guenther E, Powers A, Srivastava R, Bonkowsky JL. Abusive head trauma in children presenting with an apparent life-threatening event. *J Pediatr.* 2010;157(5):821–825
68. Pierce MC, Kaczor K, Thompson R. Bringing back the social history. *Pediatr Clin North Am.* 2014;61(5):889–905
69. Pitetti RD, Maffei F, Chang K, Hickey R, Berger R, Pierce MC. Prevalence of retinal hemorrhages and child abuse in children who present with an apparent life-threatening event. *Pediatrics.* 2002;110(3):557–562
70. Jenny C, Hymel KP, Ritzen A, Reinert SE, Hay TC. Analysis of missed cases of abusive head trauma. *JAMA.* 1999;281(7):621–626
71. Southall DP, Plunkett MC, Banks MW, Falkov AF, Samuels MP. Covert video recordings of life-threatening child abuse: lessons for child protection. *Pediatrics.* 1997;100(5):735–760
72. Sugar NF, Taylor JA, Feldman KW; Puget Sound Pediatric Research Network. Bruises in infants and toddlers: those who don't cruise rarely bruise. *Arch Pediatr Adolesc Med.* 1999;153(4):399–403
73. Harper NS, Feldman KW, Sugar NF, Anderst JD, Lindberg DM; Examining Siblings To Recognize Abuse Investigators. Additional injuries in young infants with concern for abuse and apparently isolated bruises. *J Pediatr.* 2014;165(2):383–388, e1
74. DeRidder CA, Berkowitz CD, Hicks RA, Laskey AL. Subconjunctival hemorrhages in infants and children: a sign of nonaccidental trauma. *Pediatr Emerg Care.* 2013;29(2):222–226
75. Buck ML, Blumer JL. Phenothiazine-associated apnea in two siblings. *DICP.* 1991;25(3):244–247
76. Hardoin RA, Henslee JA, Christenson CP, Christenson PJ, White M. Colic

medication and apparent life-threatening events. *Clin Pediatr (Phila)*. 1991;30(5):281–285

77. Hickson GB, Altemeier WA, Martin ED, Campbell PW. Parental administration of chemical agents: a cause of apparent life-threatening events. *Pediatrics*. 1989;83(5):772–776

78. Pitetti RD, Whitman E, Zaylor A. Accidental and nonaccidental poisonings as a cause of apparent life-threatening events in infants. *Pediatrics*. 2008;122(2). Available at: www.pediatrics.org/cgi/content/full/122/2/e359

79. McCormick T, Levine M, Knox O, Claudius I. Ethanol ingestion in two infants under 2 months old: a previously unreported cause of ALTE. *Pediatrics*. 2013;131(2). Available at: www.pediatrics.org/cgi/content/full/131/2/e604

80. Dearborn DG, Smith PG, Dahms BB, et al. Clinical profile of 30 infants with acute pulmonary hemorrhage in Cleveland. *Pediatrics*. 2002;110(3):627–637

81. Leone MA, Solari A, Beghi E; First Seizure Trial (FIRST) Group. Treatment of the first tonic-clonic seizure does not affect long-term remission of epilepsy. *Neurology*. 2006;67(12):2227–2229

82. Musicco M, Beghi E, Solari A, Viani F; First Seizure Trial (FIRST) Group. Treatment of first tonic-clonic seizure does not improve the prognosis of epilepsy. *Neurology*. 1997;49(4):991–998

83. Camfield P, Camfield C, Smith S, Dooley J, Smith E. Long-term outcome is unchanged by antiepileptic drug treatment after a first seizure: a 15-year follow-up from a randomized trial in childhood. *Epilepsia*. 2002;43(6):662–663

84. Gilbert DL, Buncher CR. An EEG should not be obtained routinely after first unprovoked seizure in childhood. *Neurology*. 2000;54(3):635–641

85. Arts WF, Geerts AT. When to start drug treatment for childhood epilepsy: the clinical-epidemiological evidence. *Eur J Paediatr Neurol*. 2009;13(2):93–101

86. Hirtz D, Ashwal S, Berg A, et al. Practice parameter: evaluating a first nonfebrile seizure in children: report of the Quality Standards Subcommittee of the American Academy of Neurology, The Child Neurology Society, and The American Epilepsy Society. *Neurology*. 2000;55(5):616–623

87. Bonkowsky JL, Guenther E, Srivastava R, Filloux FM. Seizures in children following an apparent life-threatening event. *J Child Neurol*. 2009;24(6):709–713

88. Claudius I, Mittal MK, Murray R, Condie T, Santillanes G. Should infants presenting with an apparent life-threatening event undergo evaluation for serious bacterial infections and respiratory pathogens? *J Pediatr*. 2014;164(5):1231–1233, e1

89. Mittal MK, Shofer FS, Baren JM. Serious bacterial infections in infants who have experienced an apparent life-threatening event. *Ann Emerg Med*. 2009;54(4):523–527

90. Roberts KB; Subcommittee on Urinary Tract Infection, Steering Committee on Quality Improvement and Management. Urinary tract infection: clinical practice guideline for the diagnosis and management of the initial UTI in febrile infants and children 2 to 24 months. *Pediatrics*. 2011;128(3):595–610

91. Schroeder AR, Mansbach JM, Stevenson M, et al. Apnea in children hospitalized with bronchiolitis. *Pediatrics*. 2013;132(5). Available at: www.pediatrics.org/cgi/content/full/132/5/e1194

92. Loeffelholz MJ, Trujillo R, Pyles RB, et al. Duration of rhinovirus shedding in the upper respiratory tract in the first year of life. *Pediatrics*. 2014;134(6):1144–1150

93. Crowcroft NS, Booy R, Harrison T, et al. Severe and unrecognised: pertussis in UK infants. *Arch Dis Child*. 2003;88(9):802–806

94. Centers for Disease Control and Prevention. Pertussis (whooping cough): diagnostic testing. Available at: www.cdc.gov/pertussis/clinical/diagnostic-testing/index.html. Accessed June 26, 2015

95. Centers for Disease Control and Prevention. Pertussis (whooping cough): treatment. Available at: www.cdc.gov/pertussis/clinical/treatment.html. Accessed June 26, 2015

96. Campanozzi A, Boccia G, Pensabene L, et al. Prevalence and natural history of gastroesophageal reflux: pediatric prospective survey. *Pediatrics*. 2009;123(3):779–783

97. Lightdale JR, Gremse DA; American Academy of Pediatrics, Section on Gastroenterology, Hepatology, and Nutrition. Gastroesophageal reflux: management guidance for the pediatrician. *Pediatrics*. 2013;131(5). Available at: www.pediatrics.org/cgi/content/full/131/5/e1684

98. Vandenplas Y, Rudolph CD, Di Lorenzo C, et al; North American Society for Pediatric Gastroenterology Hepatology and Nutrition; European Society for Pediatric Gastroenterology Hepatology and Nutrition. Pediatric gastroesophageal reflux clinical practice guidelines: joint recommendations of the North American Society for Pediatric Gastroenterology, Hepatology, and Nutrition (NASPGHAN) and the European Society for Pediatric Gastroenterology, Hepatology, and Nutrition (ESPGHAN). *J Pediatr Gastroenterol Nutr*. 2009;49(4):498–547

99. Kiechl-Kohlendorfer U, Hof D, Peglow UP, Traweger-Ravanelli B, Kiechl S. Epidemiology of apparent life threatening events. *Arch Dis Child*. 2005;90(3):297–300

100. Chung EY, Yardley J. Are there risks associated with empiric acid suppression treatment of infants and children suspected of having gastroesophageal reflux disease? *Hosp Pediatr*. 2013;3(1):16–23

101. Herbst JJ, Minton SD, Book LS. Gastroesophageal reflux causing respiratory distress and apnea in newborn infants. *J Pediatr*. 1979;95(5 pt 1):763–768

102. Orenstein SR. An overview of reflux-associated disorders in infants: apnea, laryngospasm, and aspiration. *Am J Med*. 2001;111(suppl 8A):60S–63S

103. Wenzl TG, Schenke S, Peschgens T, Silny J, Heimann G, Skopnik H. Association of

apnea and nonacid gastroesophageal reflux in infants: investigations with the intraluminal impedance technique. *Pediatr Pulmonol.* 2001;31(2):144–149

104. Mousa H, Woodley FW, Metheney M, Hayes J. Testing the association between gastroesophageal reflux and apnea in infants. *J Pediatr Gastroenterol Nutr.* 2005;41(2):169–177

105. Kahn A, Rebuffat E, Sottiaux M, Dufour D, Cadranel S, Reiterer F. Lack of temporal relation between acid reflux in the proximal oesophagus and cardiorespiratory events in sleeping infants. *Eur J Pediatr.* 1992;151(3):208–212

106. Orenstein SR, McGowan JD. Efficacy of conservative therapy as taught in the primary care setting for symptoms suggesting infant gastroesophageal reflux. *J Pediatr.* 2008;152(3): 310–314

107. Kahn A; European Society for the Study and Prevention of Infant Death. Recommended clinical evaluation of infants with an apparent life-threatening event: consensus document of the European Society for the Study and Prevention of Infant Death, 2003. *Eur J Pediatr.* 2004;163(2):108–115

108. Veereman-Wauters G, Bochner A, Van Caillie-Bertrand M. Gastroesophageal reflux in infants with a history of near-miss sudden infant death. *J Pediatr Gastroenterol Nutr.* 1991;12(3): 319–323

109. Arens R, Gozal D, Williams JC, Ward SL, Keens TG. Recurrent apparent life-threatening events during infancy: a manifestation of inborn errors of metabolism. *J Pediatr.* 1993;123(3):415–418

110. See CC, Newman LJ, Berezin S, et al. Gastroesophageal reflux-induced hypoxemia in infants with apparent life-threatening event(s). *Am J Dis Child.* 1989;143(8):951–954

111. Penzien JM, Molz G, Wiesmann UN, Colombo JP, Bühlmann R, Wermuth B. Medium-chain acyl-CoA dehydrogenase deficiency does not correlate with apparent life-threatening events and the sudden infant death syndrome: results from phenylpropionate loading tests and DNA analysis. *Eur J Pediatr.* 1994;153(5):352–357

112. Pitetti RD, Lovallo A, Hickey R. Prevalence of anemia in children presenting with apparent life-threatening events. *Acad Emerg Med.* 2005;12(10):926–931

113. Gray C, Davies F, Molyneux E. Apparent life-threatening events presenting to a pediatric emergency department. *Pediatr Emerg Care.* 1999;15(3):195–199

114. Poets CF, Samuels MP, Wardrop CA, Picton-Jones E, Southall DP. Reduced haemoglobin levels in infants presenting with apparent life-threatening events—a retrospective investigation. *Acta Paediatr.* 1992;81(4):319–321

115. Pyles LA, Knapp J; American Academy of Pediatrics Committee on Pediatric Emergency Medicine. Role of pediatricians in advocating life support training courses for parents and the public. *Pediatrics.* 2004;114(6). Available at: www.pediatrics.org/cgi/content/full/114/6/e761

116. Tunik MG, Richmond N, Treiber M, et al. Pediatric prehospital evaluation of NYC respiratory arrest survival (PHENYCS). *Pediatr Emerg Care.* 2012;28(9):859–863

117. Foltin GL, Richmond N, Treiber M, et al. Pediatric prehospital evaluation of NYC cardiac arrest survival (PHENYCS). *Pediatr Emerg Care.* 2012;28(9):864–868

118. Akahane M, Tanabe S, Ogawa T, et al. Characteristics and outcomes of pediatric out-of-hospital cardiac arrest by scholastic age category. *Pediatr Crit Care Med.* 2013;14(2): 130–136

119. Atkins DL, Everson-Stewart S, Sears GK, et al; Resuscitation Outcomes Consortium Investigators. Epidemiology and outcomes from out-of-hospital cardiac arrest in children: the Resuscitation Outcomes Consortium Epistry-Cardiac Arrest. *Circulation.* 2009;119(11): 1484–1491

120. McLauchlan CA, Ward A, Murphy NM, Griffith MJ, Skinner DV, Camm AJ. Resuscitation training for cardiac patients and their relatives—its effect on anxiety. *Resuscitation.* 1992;24(1):7–11

121. Higgins SS, Hardy CE, Higashino SM. Should parents of children with congenital heart disease and life-threatening dysrhythmias be taught cardiopulmonary resuscitation? *Pediatrics.* 1989;84(6):1102–1104

122. Dracup K, Moser DK, Taylor SE, Guzy PM. The psychological consequences of cardiopulmonary resuscitation training for family members of patients at risk for sudden death. *Am J Public Health.* 1997;87(9):1434–1439

123. Feudtner C, Walter JK, Faerber JA, et al. Good-parent beliefs of parents of seriously ill children. *JAMA Pediatr.* 2015;169(1):39–47

124. Yin HS, Dreyer BP, Vivar KL, MacFarland S, van Schaick L, Mendelsohn AL. Perceived barriers to care and attitudes towards shared decision-making among low socioeconomic status parents: role of health literacy. *Acad Pediatr.* 2012;12(2):117–124

125. Kuo DZ, Houtrow AJ, Arango P, Kuhlthau KA, Simmons JM, Neff JM. Family-centered care: current applications and future directions in pediatric health care. *Matern Child Health J.* 2012;16(2):297–305

126. American Academy of Pediatrics, Committee on Hospital Care; Institute for Patient- and Family-Centered Care. Patient- and family-centered care and the pediatrician's role. *Pediatrics.* 2012;129(2):394–404

127. Institute of Medicine. *Crossing the Quality Chasm: A New Health System for the 21st Century.* Washington, DC: Institute of Medicine, Committee on Quality Healthcare in America National Academies Press; 2001

128. Pronovost PJ. Enhancing physicians' use of clinical guidelines. *JAMA.* 2013;310(23):2501–2502

CLINICAL PRACTICE GUIDELINE Guidance for the Clinician in Rendering Pediatric Care

American Academy of Pediatrics 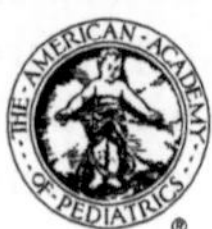

DEDICATED TO THE HEALTH OF ALL CHILDREN™

Brief Resolved Unexplained Events (Formerly Apparent Life-Threatening Events) and Evaluation of Lower-Risk Infants: Executive Summary

Joel S. Tieder, MD, MPH, FAAP, Joshua L. Bonkowsky, MD, PhD, FAAP, Ruth A. Etzel, MD, PhD, FAAP, Wayne H. Franklin, MD, MPH, MMM, FAAP, David A. Gremse, MD, FAAP, Bruce Herman, MD, FAAP, Eliot S. Katz, MD, FAAP, Leonard R. Krilov, MD, FAAP, J. Lawrence Merritt II, MD, FAAP, Chuck Norlin, MD, FAAP, Jack Percelay, MD, MPH, FAAP, Robert E. Sapién, MD, MMM, FAAP, Richard N. Shiffman, MD, MCIS, FAAP, Michael B.H. Smith, MB, FRCPCH, FAAP, SUBCOMMITTEE ON APPARENT LIFE THREATENING EVENTS

EXECUTIVE SUMMARY

This clinical practice guideline has 2 primary objectives. First, it recommends the replacement of the term "apparent life-threatening event" (ALTE) with a new term, "brief resolved unexplained event" (BRUE). Second, it provides an approach to evaluation and management that is based on the risk that the infant will have a repeat event or has a serious underlying disorder.

Clinicians should use the term BRUE to describe an event occurring in an infant younger than 1 year when the observer reports a sudden, brief, and now resolved episode of ≥1 of the following: (1) cyanosis or pallor; (2) absent, decreased, or irregular breathing; (3) marked change in tone (hyper- or hypotonia); and (4) altered level of responsiveness. Moreover, clinicians should diagnose a BRUE only when there is no explanation for a qualifying event after conducting an appropriate history and physical examination (see Tables 2 and 3 in www.pediatrics.org/cgi/doi/10.1542/peds.2016-0590). Among infants who present for medical attention after a BRUE, the guideline identifies (1) lower-risk patients on the basis of history and physical examination, for whom evidence-based guidelines for evaluation and management are offered, and (2) higher-risk patients, whose history and physical examination suggest the need for further investigation, monitoring, and/or treatment, but for whom recommendations are not offered (because of insufficient evidence or the availability of guidance from other clinical practice guidelines specific to their presentation or diagnosis). Recommendations in this guideline apply only to lower-risk patients,

This document is copyrighted and is property of the American Academy of Pediatrics and its Board of Directors. All authors have filed conflict of interest statements with the American Academy of Pediatrics. Any conflicts have been resolved through a process approved by the Board of Directors. The American Academy of Pediatrics has neither solicited nor accepted any commercial involvement in the development of the content of this publication.

The guidance in this report does not indicate an exclusive course of treatment or serve as a standard of medical care. Variations, taking into account individual circumstances, may be appropriate.

All clinical practice guidelines from the American Academy of Pediatrics automatically expire 5 years after publication unless reaffirmed, revised, or retired at or before that time.

DOI: 10.1542/peds.2016-0591

PEDIATRICS (ISSN Numbers: Print, 0031-4005; Online, 1098-4275).

Copyright © 2016 by the American Academy of Pediatrics

To cite: Tieder JS, Bonkowsky JL, Etzel RA, et al. Brief Resolved Unexplained Events (Formerly Apparent Life-Threatening Events) and Evaluation of Lower-Risk Infants: Executive Summary. *Pediatrics.* 2016;137(5):e20160591

who are defined by (1) age >60 days; (2) gestational age ≥32 weeks and postconceptional age ≥45 weeks; (3) occurrence of only 1 BRUE (no prior BRUE ever and not occurring in clusters); (4) duration of BRUE <1 minute; (5) no cardiopulmonary resuscitation by trained medical provider required; (6) no concerning historical features; and (7) no concerning physical examination findings (Fig 1). This clinical practice guideline also provides implementation support and suggests directions for future research.

The term ALTE originated from a 1986 National Institutes of Health Consensus Conference on Infantile Apnea and was intended to replace the term "near-miss sudden infant death syndrome (SIDS)."[1] An ALTE was defined as "[a]n episode that is frightening to the observer and that is characterized by some combination of apnea (central or occasionally obstructive), color change (usually cyanotic or pallid but occasionally erythematous or plethoric), marked change in muscle tone (usually marked limpness), choking, or gagging. In some cases, the observer fears that the infant has died."[2] Although the definition of ALTE enabled researchers to establish over time that these events were a separate entity from SIDS, the clinical application of this classification, which describes a constellation of observed, subjective, and nonspecific symptoms, has raised significant challenges for clinicians and parents in the evaluation and care of these infants.[3] Although a broad range of disorders can present as an ALTE (eg, child abuse, congenital abnormalities, epilepsy, inborn errors of metabolism, and infections), for a majority of well-appearing infants, the risk of a recurrent event or a serious underlying disorder is extremely low.

ALTEs can create a feeling of uncertainty in both the caregiver and the clinician. Clinicians may feel compelled to perform tests and hospitalize the patient even though this may subject the patient to unnecessary risk and is unlikely to lead to a treatable diagnosis or prevent future events.[2,4,5] Understanding the risk of an adverse outcome for an infant who has experienced an ALTE has been difficult because of the nonspecific nature and variable application of the ALTE definition in research. A recent systematic review of nearly 1400 ALTE publications spanning 4 decades concluded that risk of a subsequent or underlying disorder could not be quantified because of the variability in case definitions across studies.[3] Although there are history and physical examination factors that can determine lower or higher risk, it is clear that the term ALTE must be replaced to advance the quality of care and improve research.

This guideline is intended for use primarily by clinicians providing care for infants who have experienced a BRUE, as well as their families. The guideline may be of interest to payers, but it is not intended to be used for reimbursement or to determine insurance coverage. This guideline is not intended as the sole source of guidance in the evaluation and management of BRUEs and specifically does not address higher-risk BRUE patients. Rather, it is intended to assist clinicians by providing a framework for clinical decision making. It is not intended to replace clinical judgment, and these recommendations may not provide the only appropriate approach to the management of this problem.

This guideline is intended to provide a patient- and family-centered approach to care, reduce unnecessary and costly medical interventions, and improve patient outcomes. It includes recommendations for diagnosis, risk-based stratification, monitoring, disposition planning, effective communication with the patient and family, guideline implementation and evaluation, and future research. In addition, it aims to help clinicians determine the presence of a serious underlying cause and a safe disposition by alerting them to the most significant features of the clinical history and physical examination on which to base an approach for diagnostic testing and hospitalization. Key action statements are summarized in Table 1.

SUBCOMMITTEE ON BRIEF RESOLVED UNEXPLAINED EVENTS (FORMERLY REFERRED TO AS APPARENT LIFE THREATENING EVENTS); OVERSIGHT BY THE COUNCIL ON QUALITY IMPROVEMENT AND PATIENT SAFETY

Joel S. Tieder, MD, MPH, FAAP, Chair
Joshua L. Bonkowsky, MD, PhD, FAAP, Pediatric Neurologist
Ruth A. Etzel, MD, PhD, FAAP, Pediatric Epidemiologist
Wayne H. Franklin, MD, MPH, MMM, FAAP, Pediatric Cardiologist
David A. Gremse, MD, FAAP, Pediatric Gastroenterologist
Bruce Herman, MD, FAAP, Child Abuse and Neglect
Eliot Katz, MD, FAAP, Pediatric Pulmonologist
Leonard R. Krilov, MD, FAAP, Pediatric Infectious Diseases
J. Lawrence Merritt, II, MD, FAAP, Clinical Genetics and Biochemical Genetics
Chuck Norlin, MD, FAAP, Pediatrician
Robert E. Sapién, MD, MMM, FAAP, Pediatric Emergency Medicine
Richard Shiffman, MD, FAAP, Partnership for Policy Implementation Representative
Michael B.H. Smith, MB, FRCPCH, FAAP, Hospital Medicine

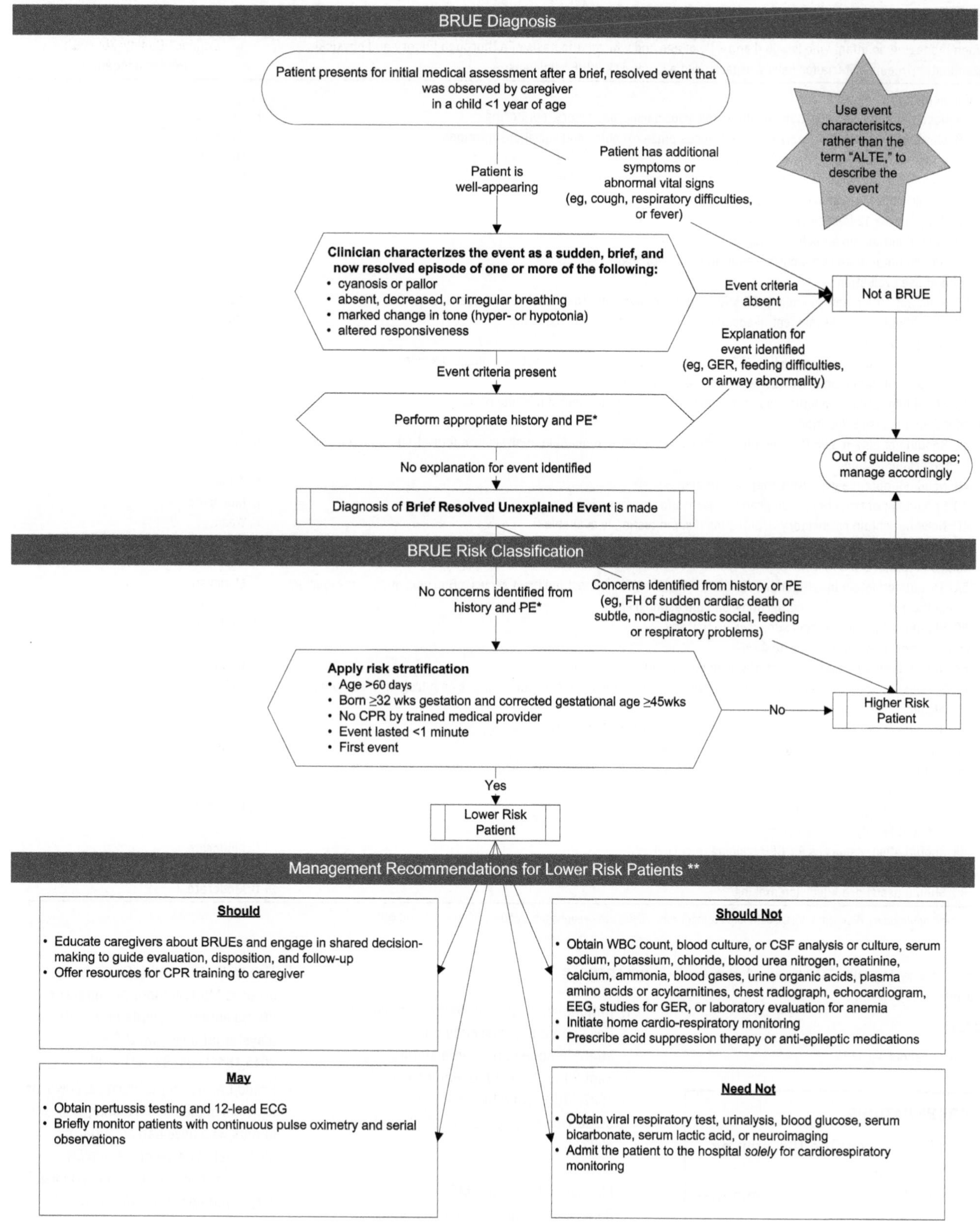

FIGURE 1

Diagnosis, risk classification, and recommended management of a BRUE. *Refer to Tables 3 and 4 in www.pediatrics.org/cgi/doi/10.1542/peds.2016-0591 for the determination of an appropriate and negative history and PE. **Refer to Figure 2 in www.pediatrics.org/cgi/doi/10.1542/peds.2016-0591 for the American Academy of Pediatrics method for rating of evidence and recommendations. CPR, cardiopulmonary resuscitation; CSF, cerebrospinal fluid; ECG, electrocardiogram; FH, family history; GER, gastroesophageal reflux; PE, physical examination; WBC, white blood cell.

Figure 1, shown here, has been updated per the erratum at http://pediatrics.aappublications.org/content/138/2/e20161488.

TABLE 1 Summary of Key Action Statements for Lower-Risk BRUEs

When managing an infant who is >60 d and <1 y of age and who, on the basis of a thorough history and physical examination, meets criteria for having experienced a lower-risk BRUE, clinicians:	Evidence Quality; Strength of Recommendation
1. Cardiopulmonary Evaluation	
1A. Need not admit infants to the hospital solely for cardiorespiratory monitoring.	B; Weak
1B. May briefly monitor patients with continuous pulse oximetry and serial observations.	D; Weak
1C. Should not obtain chest radiograph.	B; Moderate
1D. Should not obtain a measurement of venous or arterial blood gas.	B; Moderate
1E. Should not obtain an overnight polysomnograph.	B; Moderate
1F. May obtain a 12-lead electrocardiogram.	C; Weak
1G. Should not obtain an echocardiogram.	C; Moderate
1H. Should not initiate home cardiorespiratory monitoring.	B; Moderate
2. Child Abuse Evaluation	
2A. Need not obtain neuroimaging (CT, MRI, or ultrasonography) to detect child abuse.	C; Weak
2B. Should obtain an assessment of social risk factors to detect child abuse.	C; Moderate
3. Neurologic Evaluation	
3A. Should not obtain neuroimaging (CT, MRI, or ultrasonography) to detect neurologic disorders.	C; Moderate
3B. Should not obtain an EEG to detect neurologic disorders.	C; Moderate
3C. Should not prescribe antiepileptic medications for potential neurologic disorders.	C; Moderate
4. Infectious Disease Evaluation	
4A. Should not obtain a WBC count, blood culture, or cerebrospinal fluid analysis or culture to detect an occult bacterial infection.	B; Strong
4B. Need not obtain a urinalysis (bag or catheter).	C; Weak
4C. Should not obtain chest radiograph to assess for pulmonary infection.	B; Moderate
4D. Need not obtain respiratory viral testing if rapid testing is available.	C; Weak
4E. May obtain testing for pertussis.	B; Weak
5. Gastrointestinal Evaluation	
5A. Should not obtain investigations for GER (eg, upper gastrointestinal tract series, pH probe, endoscopy, barium contrast study, nuclear scintigraphy, and ultrasonography).	C; Moderate
5B. Should not prescribe acid suppression therapy.	C; Moderate
6. Inborn Error of Metabolism Evaluation	
6A. Need not obtain measurement of serum lactic acid or serum bicarbonate.	C; Weak
6B. Should not obtain a measurement of serum sodium, potassium, chloride, blood urea nitrogen, creatinine, calcium, or ammonia.	C; Moderate
6C. Should not obtain a measurement of venous or arterial blood gases.	C; Moderate
6D. Need not obtain a measurement of blood glucose.	C; Weak
6E. Should not obtain measurements of urine organic acids, plasma amino acids, or plasma acylcarnitines.	C; Moderate
7. Anemia Evaluation	
7A. Should not obtain laboratory evaluation for anemia.	C; Moderate
8. Patient- and Family-Centered Care	
8A. Should offer resources for CPR training to caregiver.	C; Moderate
8B. Should educate caregivers about BRUEs.	C; Moderate
8C. Should use shared decision making.	C; Moderate

CPR, cardiopulmonary resuscitation; CT, computed tomography; GER, gastroesophageal reflux; WBC, white blood cell.

Jack Percelay, MD, MPH, FAAP, Liaison, Society for Hospital Medicine

STAFF

Kymika Okechukwu, MPA

ABBREVIATIONS

ALTE: apparent life-threatening event
BRUE: brief resolved unexplained event
SIDS: sudden infant death syndrome

REFERENCES

1. National Institutes of Health Consensus Development Conference on Infantile Apnea and Home Monitoring, Sept 29 to Oct 1, 1986. *Pediatrics*. 1987;79(2). Available at: www.pediatrics.org/cgi/content/full/79/2/e292
2. McGovern MC, Smith MB. Causes of apparent life threatening events in infants: a systematic review. *Arch Dis Child*. 2004;89(11):1043–1048
3. Tieder JS, Altman RL, Bonkowsky JL, et al Management of apparent life-threatening events in infants: a systematic review. *J Pediatr*. 2013;163(1):94–99, e91–e96
4. Brand DA, Altman RL, Purtill K, Edwards KS. Yield of diagnostic testing in infants who have had an apparent life-threatening event. *Pediatrics*. 2005;115(4). Available at: www.pediatrics.org/cgi/content/full/115/4/e885
5. Green M. Vulnerable child syndrome and its variants. *Pediatr Rev*. 1986; 8(3):75–80

Brief Resolved Unexplained Events Clinical Practice Guideline Quick Reference Tools

- Action Statement Summary
  — Brief Resolved Unexplained Events (Formerly Apparent Life-Threatening Events) and Evaluation of Lower-Risk Infants
- *ICD-10-CM* Coding Quick Reference for Brief Resolved Unexplained Events
- AAP Patient Education Handout
  — *Brief Resolved Unexplained Event: What Parents and Caregivers Need to Know*

Action Statement Summary

Brief Resolved Unexplained Events (Formerly Apparent Life-Threatening Events) and Evaluation of Lower-Risk Infants

Key Action Statement 1

Cardiopulmonary

Key Action Statement 1A

Clinicians need not admit infants presenting with a lower-risk BRUE to the hospital solely for cardiorespiratory monitoring (grade B, weak recommendation)

Key Action Statement 1B

Clinicians may briefly monitor infants presenting with a lower-risk BRUE with continuous pulse oximetry and serial observations (grade D, weak recommendation)

Key Action Statement 1C

Clinicians should not obtain a chest radiograph in infants presenting with a lower-risk BRUE (grade B, moderate recommendation)

Key Action Statement 1D

Clinicians should not obtain measurement of venous or arterial blood gases in infants presenting with a lower-risk BRUE (grade B, moderate recommendation)

Key Action Statement 1E

Clinicians should not obtain an overnight polysomnograph in infants presenting with a lower-risk BRUE (grade B, moderate recommendation)

Key Action Statement 1F

Clinicians may obtain a 12-lead electrocardiogram for infants presenting with lower-risk BRUE (grade C, weak recommendation)

Key Action Statement 1G

Clinicians should not obtain an echocardiogram in infants presenting with lower-risk BRUE (grade C, moderate recommendation)

Key Action Statement 1H

Clinicians should not initiate home cardiorespiratory monitoring in infants presenting with a lower-risk BRUE (grade B, moderate recommendation)

Key Action Statement 2

Child abuse

Key Action Statement 2A

Clinicians need not obtain neuroimaging (computed tomography, MRI, or ultrasonography) to detect child abuse in infants presenting with a lower-risk BRUE (grade C, weak recommendation)

Key Action Statement 2B

Clinicians should obtain an assessment of social risk factors to detect child abuse in infants presenting with a lower-risk BRUE (grade C, moderate recommendation)

Key Action Statement 3

Neurology

Key Action Statement 3A

Clinicians should not obtain neuroimaging (computed tomography, MRI, or ultrasonography) to detect neurologic disorders in infants presenting with a lower-risk BRUE (grade C, moderate recommendation)

Key Action Statement 3B

Clinicians should not obtain an EEG to detect neurologic disorders in infants presenting with a lower-risk BRUE (grade C, moderate recommendation)

Key Action Statement 3C

Clinicians should not prescribe antiepileptic medications for potential neurologic disorders in infants presenting with a lower-risk BRUE (grade C, moderate recommendation)

Key Action Statement 4

Infectious diseases

Key Action Statement 4A

Clinicians should not obtain a white blood cell count, blood culture, or cerebrospinal fluid analysis or culture to detect an occult bacterial infection in infants presenting with a lower-risk BRUE (grade B, strong recommendation)

Key Action Statement 4B

Clinicians need not obtain a urinalysis (bag or catheter) in infants presenting with a lower-risk BRUE (grade C, weak recommendation)

Key Action Statement 4C

Clinicians should not obtain a chest radiograph to assess for pulmonary infection in infants presenting with a lower-risk BRUE (grade B, moderate recommendation)

Key Action Statement 4D

Clinicians need not obtain respiratory viral testing if rapid testing is available in infants presenting with a lower-risk BRUE (grade C, weak recommendation)

Key Action Statement 4E

Clinicians may obtain testing for pertussis in infants presenting with a lower-risk BRUE (grade B, weak recommendation)

Key Action Statement 5

Gastroenterology

Key Action Statement 5A

Clinicians should not obtain investigations for GER (eg, upper gastrointestinal series, pH probe, endoscopy, barium contrast study, nuclear scintigraphy, and ultrasonography) in infants presenting with a lower-risk BRUE (grade C, moderate recommendation)

Key Action Statement 5B

Clinicians should not prescribe acid suppression therapy for infants presenting with a lower-risk BRUE (grade C, moderate recommendation)

Key Action Statement 6

Inborn errors of metabolism

Key Action Statement 6A

Clinicians need not obtain measurement of serum lactic acid or serum bicarbonate to detect an IEM in infants presenting with a lower-risk BRUE (grade C, weak recommendation)

Key Action Statement 6B

Clinicians should not obtain a measurement of serum sodium, potassium, chloride, blood urea nitrogen, creatinine, calcium, or ammonia to detect an IEM in infants presenting with a lower-risk BRUE (grade C, moderate recommendation)

Key Action Statement 6C

Clinicians should not obtain a measurement of venous or arterial blood gases to detect an IEM in infants presenting with lower-risk BRUE (grade C, moderate recommendation)

Key Action Statement 6D

Clinicians need not obtain a measurement of blood glucose to detect an IEM in infants presenting with a lower-risk BRUE (grade C, weak recommendation)

Key Action Statement 6E

Clinicians should not obtain measurements of urine organic acids, plasma amino acids, or plasma acylcarnitines to detect an IEM in infants presenting with a lower-risk BRUE (grade C, moderate recommendation)

Key Action Statement 7

Anemia

Key Action Statement 7A

Clinicians should not obtain laboratory evaluation for anemia in infants presenting with a lower-risk BRUE (grade C, moderate recommendation)

Key Action Statement 8

Patient- and family-centered care

Key Action Statement 8A

Clinicians should offer resources for CPR training to caregivers (grade C, moderate recommendation)

Key Action Statement 8B

Clinicians should educate caregivers about BRUEs (grade C, moderate recommendation)

Key Action Statement 8C

Clinicians should use shared decision-making for infants presenting with a lower-risk BRUE (grade C, moderate recommendation)

Coding Quick Reference for Brief Resolved Unexplained Events
ICD-10-CM
R68.13 Apparent life threatening event (ALTE) in infant (includes brief resolved unexplained events [BRUE])

Brief Resolved Unexplained Event:
What Parents and Caregivers Need to Know

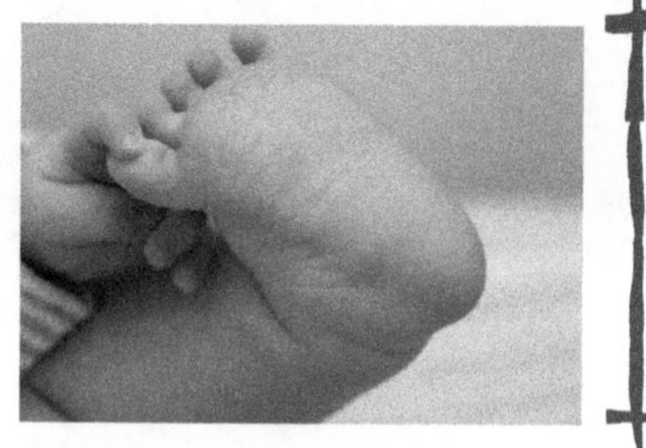

What is a brief resolved unexplained event?

A **b**rief **r**esolved **u**nexplained **e**vent (or BRUE for short) occurs suddenly and can be scary for parents and caregivers. A brief resolved unexplained event is a diagnosis made after your baby's doctor or health care professional has examined your baby and determined that there was no known concerning cause for the event.

When a brief resolved unexplained event occurs, babies may seem to stop breathing, their skin color may change to pale or blue, their muscles may relax or tighten, or they may seem to pass out. After a brief period of time, they recover (with or without any medical help) and are soon back to normal.

Though we can never say that a baby who has had a brief resolved unexplained event is at *no* risk for future problems, we can say that babies are at lower risk if

- They are older than 60 days.
- They were born on time (not premature).
- They did not need CPR (cardiopulmonary resuscitation) by a health care professional.
- The brief resolved unexplained event lasted less than 1 minute.
- This was their only such event.

Frequently asked questions after a brief resolved unexplained event

Q: Why did my baby have this event?

A: Your baby's doctor was unable to find a cause based on the results of your baby's examination and cannot tell you why this event happened. If it happens again or your baby develops additional problems, contact your baby's doctor or health care professional. The doctor may decide to have your baby return for another visit.

Q: Should my baby stay in the hospital?

A: Babies who are felt to be at lower risk by their doctors or health care professionals do not need to stay in the hospital. They are safe to go home without doing blood tests or imaging that uses x-rays, and they do not need home monitoring of their heart or lungs.

Q: Does having a brief resolved unexplained event increase my baby's risk for sudden infant death syndrome (SIDS)?

A: No—though the causes of SIDS are not known, events like these do not increase the risk of SIDS. For all babies, it is important to create a safe home and sleeping environment. Your baby should not be exposed to smoky environments. Visit **www.HealthyChildren.org/safesleep** to learn more about how to create a safe sleeping environment for your baby.

Q: What should I do if it happens again?

A: If you are worried that this new event is life threatening, call 911 or your local emergency numbers. If not, call your baby's doctor if you have any questions or worries and to let the doctor know about the event.

Q: Does my baby need extra care after having a brief resolved unexplained event? Is my baby more delicate or weak?

A: No special care is needed. Continue to love and care for your baby as you normally do.

A few important reminders for parents and caregivers of healthy infants

- Remember to take your baby to regular well-child visits to help keep your child healthy and safe.
- Though your baby is not more likely to need it, it is a good idea for everyone who cares for an infant to learn CPR. If you know CPR, you may also use it one day to help someone else in need. For classes near you, contact your child's doctor, the American Red Cross, the American Heart Association, or a national or local organization that offers training.

Listing of resources does not imply an endorsement by the American Academy of Pediatrics (AAP). The AAP is not responsible for the content of external resources. Information was current at the time of publication.

The information contained in this publication should not be used as a substitute for the medical care and advice of your pediatrician. There may be variations in treatment that your pediatrician may recommend based on individual facts and circumstances.

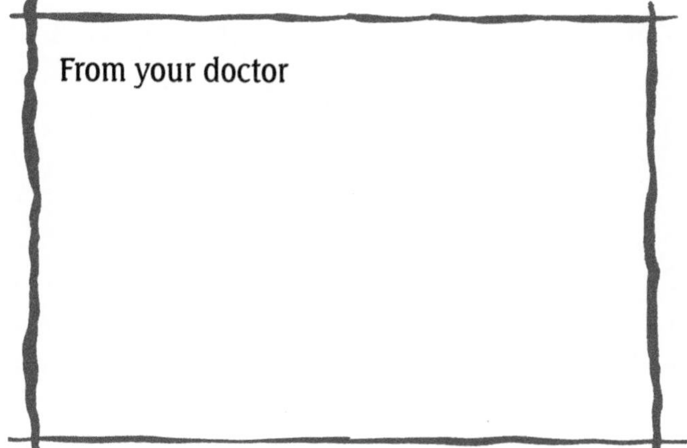

American Academy of Pediatrics

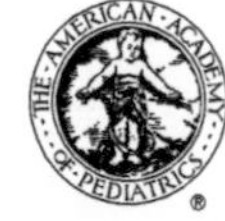

DEDICATED TO THE HEALTH OF ALL CHILDREN™

The American Academy of Pediatrics (AAP) is an organization of 64,000 primary care pediatricians, pediatric medical subspecialists, and pediatric surgical specialists dedicated to the health, safety, and well-being of all infants, children, adolescents, and young adults.

American Academy of Pediatrics
Web site—www.HealthyChildren.org

© 2016 American Academy of Pediatrics.
All rights reserved.

The Diagnosis, Management, and Prevention of Bronchiolitis

- *Clinical Practice Guideline*
  - *PPI: AAP Partnership for Policy Implementation See Appendix 1 for more information.*

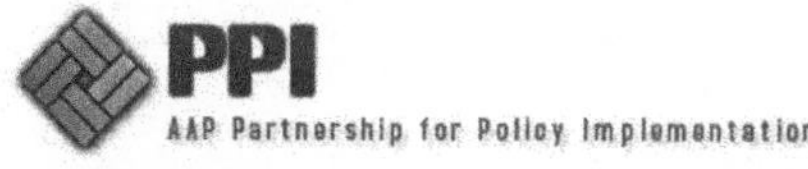

CLINICAL PRACTICE GUIDELINE

Clinical Practice Guideline: The Diagnosis, Management, and Prevention of Bronchiolitis

abstract

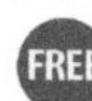

This guideline is a revision of the clinical practice guideline, "Diagnosis and Management of Bronchiolitis," published by the American Academy of Pediatrics in 2006. The guideline applies to children from 1 through 23 months of age. Other exclusions are noted. Each key action statement indicates level of evidence, benefit-harm relationship, and level of recommendation. Key action statements are as follows: *Pediatrics* 2014;134:e1474–e1502

DIAGNOSIS

1a. Clinicians should diagnose bronchiolitis and assess disease severity on the basis of history and physical examination (Evidence Quality: B; Recommendation Strength: Strong Recommendation).

1b. Clinicians should assess risk factors for severe disease, such as age less than 12 weeks, a history of prematurity, underlying cardiopulmonary disease, or immunodeficiency, when making decisions about evaluation and management of children with bronchiolitis (Evidence Quality: B; Recommendation Strength: Moderate Recommendation).

1c. When clinicians diagnose bronchiolitis on the basis of history and physical examination, radiographic or laboratory studies should not be obtained routinely (Evidence Quality: B; Recommendation Strength: Moderate Recommendation).

TREATMENT

2. Clinicians should not administer albuterol (or salbutamol) to infants and children with a diagnosis of bronchiolitis (Evidence Quality: B; Recommendation Strength: Strong Recommendation).

3. Clinicians should not administer epinephrine to infants and children with a diagnosis of bronchiolitis (Evidence Quality: B; Recommendation Strength: Strong Recommendation).

4a. Nebulized hypertonic saline should not be administered to infants with a diagnosis of bronchiolitis in the emergency department (Evidence Quality: B; Recommendation Strength: Moderate Recommendation).

4b. Clinicians may administer nebulized hypertonic saline to infants and children hospitalized for bronchiolitis (Evidence Quality: B; Recommendation Strength: Weak Recommendation [based on randomized controlled trials with inconsistent findings]).

Shawn L. Ralston, MD, FAAP, Allan S. Lieberthal, MD, FAAP, H. Cody Meissner, MD, FAAP, Brian K. Alverson, MD, FAAP, Jill E. Baley, MD, FAAP, Anne M. Gadomski, MD, MPH, FAAP, David W. Johnson, MD, FAAP, Michael J. Light, MD, FAAP, Nizar F. Maraqa, MD, FAAP, Eneida A. Mendonca, MD, PhD, FAAP, FACMI, Kieran J. Phelan, MD, MSc, Joseph J. Zorc, MD, MSCE, FAAP, Danette Stanko-Lopp, MA, MPH, Mark A. Brown, MD, Ian Nathanson, MD, FAAP, Elizabeth Rosenblum, MD, Stephen Sayles III, MD, FACEP, and Sinsi Hernandez-Cancio, JD

KEY WORDS

bronchiolitis, infants, children, respiratory syncytial virus, evidence-based, guideline

ABBREVIATIONS

AAP—American Academy of Pediatrics
AOM—acute otitis media
CI—confidence interval
ED—emergency department
KAS—Key Action Statement
LOS—length of stay
MD—mean difference
PCR—polymerase chain reaction
RSV—respiratory syncytial virus
SBI—serious bacterial infection

This document is copyrighted and is property of the American Academy of Pediatrics and its Board of Directors. All authors have filed conflict of interest statements with the American Academy of Pediatrics. Any conflicts have been resolved through a process approved by the Board of Directors. The American Academy of Pediatrics has neither solicited nor accepted any commercial involvement in the development of the content of this publication.

The recommendations in this report do not indicate an exclusive course of treatment or serve as a standard of medical care. Variations, taking into account individual circumstances, may be appropriate.

All clinical practice guidelines from the American Academy of Pediatrics automatically expire 5 years after publication unless reaffirmed, revised, or retired at or before that time.

Dedicated to the memory of Dr Caroline Breese Hall.

www.pediatrics.org/cgi/doi/10.1542/peds.2014-2742

doi:10.1542/peds.2014-2742

PEDIATRICS (ISSN Numbers: Print, 0031-4005; Online, 1098-4275).

Copyright © 2014 by the American Academy of Pediatrics

5. Clinicians should not administer systemic corticosteroids to infants with a diagnosis of bronchiolitis in any setting (Evidence Quality: A; Recommendation Strength: Strong Recommendation).

6a. Clinicians may choose not to administer supplemental oxygen if the oxyhemoglobin saturation exceeds 90% in infants and children with a diagnosis of bronchiolitis (Evidence Quality: D; Recommendation Strength: Weak Recommendation [based on low level evidence and reasoning from first principles]).

6b. Clinicians may choose not to use continuous pulse oximetry for infants and children with a diagnosis of bronchiolitis (Evidence Quality: D; Recommendation Strength: Weak Recommendation [based on low-level evidence and reasoning from first principles]).

7. Clinicians should not use chest physiotherapy for infants and children with a diagnosis of bronchiolitis (Evidence Quality: B; Recommendation Strength: Moderate Recommendation).

8. Clinicians should not administer antibacterial medications to infants and children with a diagnosis of bronchiolitis unless there is a concomitant bacterial infection, or a strong suspicion of one (Evidence Quality: B; Recommendation Strength: Strong Recommendation).

9. Clinicians should administer nasogastric or intravenous fluids for infants with a diagnosis of bronchiolitis who cannot maintain hydration orally (Evidence Quality: X; Recommendation Strength: Strong Recommendation).

PREVENTION

10a. Clinicians should not administer palivizumab to otherwise healthy infants with a gestational age of 29 weeks, 0 days or greater (Evidence Quality: B; Recommendation Strength: Strong Recommendation).

10b. Clinicians should administer palivizumab during the first year of life to infants with hemodynamically significant heart disease or chronic lung disease of prematurity defined as preterm infants <32 weeks 0 days' gestation who require >21% oxygen for at least the first 28 days of life (Evidence Quality: B; Recommendation Strength: Moderate Recommendation).

10c. Clinicians should administer a maximum 5 monthly doses (15 mg/kg/dose) of palivizumab during the respiratory syncytial virus season to infants who qualify for palivizumab in the first year of life (Evidence Quality: B; Recommendation Strength: Moderate Recommendation).

11a. All people should disinfect hands before and after direct contact with patients, after contact with inanimate objects in the direct vicinity of the patient, and after removing gloves (Evidence Quality: B; Recommendation Strength: Strong Recommendation).

11b. All people should use alcohol-based rubs for hand decontamination when caring for children with bronchiolitis. When alcohol-based rubs are not available, individuals should wash their hands with soap and water (Evidence Quality: B; Recommendation Strength: Strong Recommendation).

12a. Clinicians should inquire about the exposure of the infant or child to tobacco smoke when assessing infants and children for bronchiolitis (Evidence Quality: C; Recommendation Strength: Moderate Recommendation).

12b. Clinicians should counsel caregivers about exposing the infant or child to environmental tobacco smoke and smoking cessation when assessing a child for bronchiolitis (Evidence Quality: B; Recommendation Strength: Strong).

13. Clinicians should encourage exclusive breastfeeding for at least 6 months to decrease the morbidity of respiratory infections. (Evidence Quality: B; Recommendation Strength: Moderate Recommendation).

14. Clinicians and nurses should educate personnel and family members on evidence-based diagnosis, treatment, and prevention in bronchiolitis. (Evidence Quality: C; observational studies; Recommendation Strength: Moderate Recommendation).

INTRODUCTION

In October 2006, the American Academy of Pediatrics (AAP) published the clinical practice guideline "Diagnosis and Management of Bronchiolitis."[1] The guideline offered recommendations ranked according to level of evidence and the benefit-harm relationship. Since completion of the original evidence review in July 2004, a significant body of literature on bronchiolitis has been published. This update of the 2006 AAP bronchiolitis guideline evaluates published evidence, including that used in the 2006 guideline as well as evidence published since 2004. Key action statements (KASs) based on that evidence are provided.

The goal of this guideline is to provide an evidence-based approach to the diagnosis, management, and prevention of bronchiolitis in children from 1 month through 23 months of age. The guideline is intended for pediatricians, family physicians, emergency medicine specialists, hospitalists, nurse practitioners, and physician assistants who care for these children. The guideline does not apply to children with immunodeficiencies, including those with HIV infection or recipients of solid organ or hematopoietic stem cell transplants. Children with underlying respiratory illnesses, such as recurrent wheezing, chronic neonatal lung disease (also known as bronchopulmonary dysplasia), neuromuscular disease, or cystic fibrosis and those with hemodynamically significant congenital heart disease are excluded from the sections on management unless otherwise noted but are included in the discussion of prevention. This guideline will not address long-term sequelae of bronchiolitis, such as recurrent wheezing or risk of asthma, which is a field with a large and distinct literature.

Bronchiolitis is a disorder commonly caused by viral lower respiratory tract infection in infants. Bronchiolitis is characterized by acute inflammation, edema, and necrosis of epithelial cells lining small airways, and increased mucus production. Signs and symptoms typically begin with rhinitis and cough, which may progress to tachypnea, wheezing, rales, use of accessory muscles, and/or nasal flaring.[2]

Many viruses that infect the respiratory system cause a similar constellation of signs and symptoms. The most common etiology of bronchiolitis is respiratory syncytial virus (RSV), with the highest incidence of infection occurring between December and March in North America; however, regional variations occur[3] (Fig 1).[4] Ninety percent of children are infected with RSV in the first 2 years of life,[5] and up to 40% will experience lower respiratory tract infection during the initial infection.[6,7] Infection with RSV does not grant permanent or long-term immunity, with reinfections common throughout life.[8] Other viruses that cause bronchiolitis include human rhinovirus, human metapneumovirus, influenza, adenovirus, coronavirus, human, and parainfluenza viruses. In a study of inpatients and outpatients with bronchiolitis,[9] 76% of patients had RSV, 39% had human rhinovirus, 10% had influenza, 2% had coronavirus, 3% had human metapneumovirus, and 1% had parainfluenza viruses (some patients had coinfections, so the total is greater than 100%).

Bronchiolitis is the most common cause of hospitalization among infants during the first 12 months of life. Approximately 100 000 bronchiolitis admissions occur annually in the United States at an estimated cost of $1.73 billion.[10] One prospective, population-based study sponsored by the Centers for Disease Control and Prevention reported the average RSV hospitalization rate was 5.2 per 1000 children younger than 24 months of age during the 5-year period between 2000 and 2005.[11] The highest age-specific rate of RSV hospitalization occurred among infants between 30 days and 60 days of age (25.9 per 1000 children). For preterm infants (<37 weeks' gestation), the RSV hospitalization rate was 4.6 per 1000 children, a number similar to the RSV hospitalization rate for term infants of 5.2 per 1000. Infants born at <30 weeks' gestation had the highest hospitalization rate at 18.7 children per 1000, although the small number of infants born before 30 weeks' gestation make this number unreliable. Other studies indicate the RSV hospitalization rate in extremely

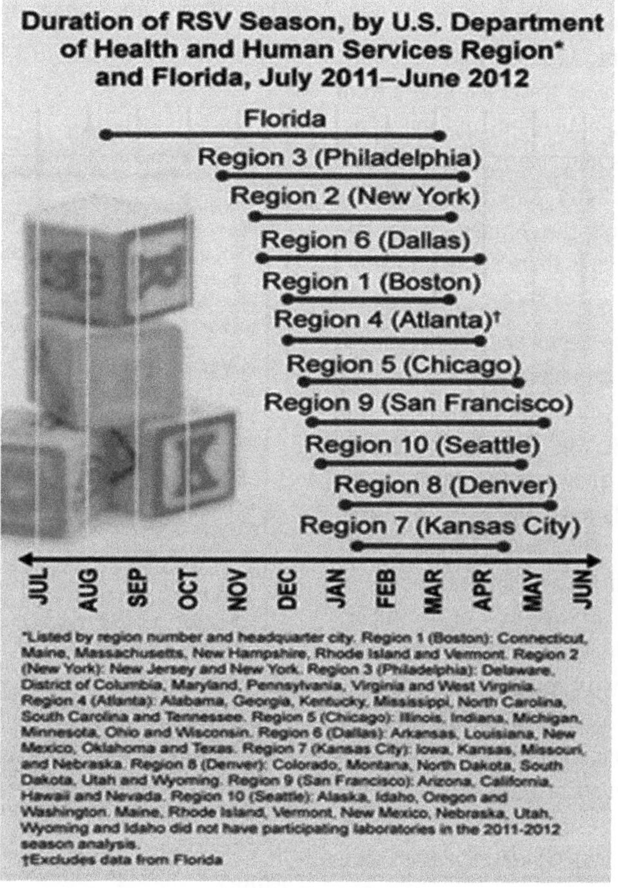

FIGURE 1

RSV season by US regions. Centers for Disease Control and Prevention. RSV activity—United States, July 2011–Jan 2013. *MMWR Morb Mortal Wkly Rep.* 2013;62(8):141–144.

preterm infants is similar to that of term infants.[12,13]

METHODS

In June 2013, the AAP convened a new subcommittee to review and revise the 2006 bronchiolitis guideline. The subcommittee included primary care physicians, including general pediatricians, a family physician, and pediatric subspecialists, including hospitalists, pulmonologists, emergency physicians, a neonatologist, and pediatric infectious disease physicians. The subcommittee also included an epidemiologist trained in systematic reviews, a guideline methodologist/informatician, and a parent representative. All panel members reviewed the AAP Policy on Conflict of Interest and Voluntary Disclosure and were given an opportunity to declare any potential conflicts. Any conflicts can be found in the author listing at the end of this guideline. All funding was provided by the AAP, with travel assistance from the American Academy of Family Physicians, the American College of Chest Physicians, the American Thoracic Society, and the American College of Emergency Physicians for their liaisons.

The evidence search and review included electronic database searches in *The Cochrane Library*, Medline via Ovid, and CINAHL via EBSCO. The search strategy is shown in the Appendix. Related article searches were conducted in PubMed. The bibliographies of articles identified by database searches were also reviewed by 1 of 4 members of the committee, and references identified in this manner were added to the review. Articles included in the 2003 evidence report on bronchiolitis in preparation of the AAP 2006 guideline2 also were reviewed. In addition, the committee reviewed articles published after completion of the systematic review for these updated guidelines. The current literature review encompasses the period from 2004 through May 2014.

The evidence-based approach to guideline development requires that the evidence in support of a policy be identified, appraised, and summarized and that an explicit link between evidence and recommendations be defined. Evidence-based recommendations reflect the quality of evidence and the balance of benefit and harm that is anticipated when the recommendation is followed. The AAP policy statement "Classifying Recommendations for Clinical Practice"[14] was followed in designating levels of recommendation (Fig 2; Table 1).

A draft version of this clinical practice guideline underwent extensive peer review by committees, councils, and sections within AAP; the American Thoracic Society, American College of Chest Physicians, American Academy of Family Physicians, and American College of Emergency Physicians; other outside organizations; and other individuals identified by the subcommittee as experts in the field. The resulting comments were reviewed by the subcommittee and, when appropriate, incorporated into the guideline.

This clinical practice guideline is not intended as a sole source of guidance in the management of children with bronchiolitis. Rather, it is intended to assist clinicians in decision-making. It is not intended to replace clinical judgment or establish a protocol for the care of all children with bronchiolitis. These recommendations may not provide the only appropriate approach to the management of children with bronchiolitis.

All AAP guidelines are reviewed every 5 years.

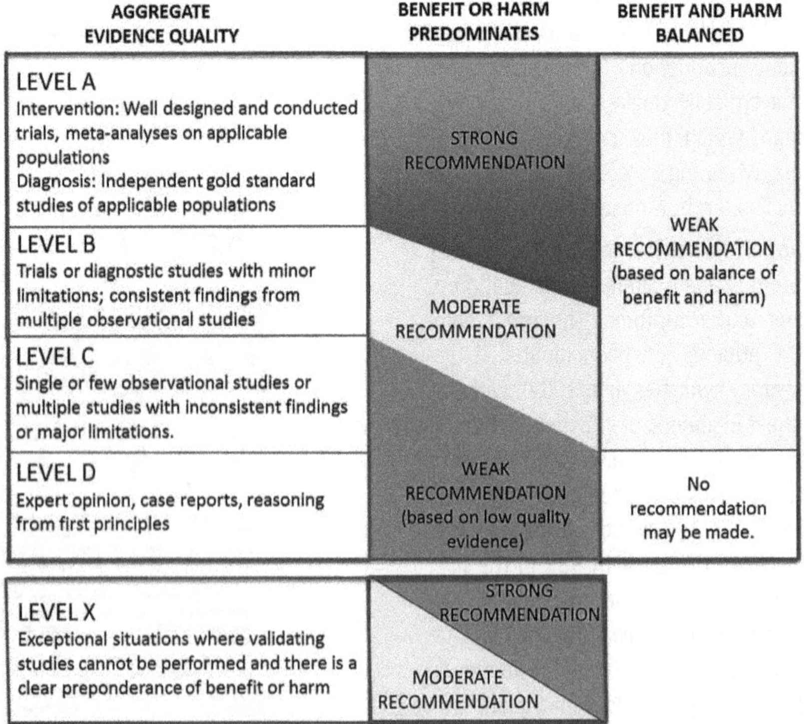

FIGURE 2

Integrating evidence quality appraisal with an assessment of the anticipated balance between benefits and harms leads to designation of a policy as a strong recommendation, moderate recommendation, or weak recommendation.

TABLE 1 Guideline Definitions for Evidence-Based Statements

Statement	Definition	Implication
Strong recommendation	A particular action is favored because anticipated benefits clearly exceed harms (or vice versa), and quality of evidence is excellent or unobtainable.	Clinicians should follow a strong recommendation unless a clear and compelling rationale for an alternative approach is present.
Moderate recommendation	A particular action is favored because anticipated benefits clearly exceed harms (or vice versa), and the quality of evidence is good but not excellent (or is unobtainable).	Clinicians would be prudent to follow a moderate recommendation but should remain alert to new information and sensitive to patient preferences.
Weak recommendation (based on low-quality evidence	A particular action is favored because anticipated benefits clearly exceed harms (or vice versa), but the quality of evidence is weak.	Clinicians would be prudent to follow a weak recommendation but should remain alert to new information and very sensitive to patient preferences.
Weak recommendation (based on balance of benefits and harms)	Weak recommendation is provided when the aggregate database shows evidence of both benefit and harm that appear similar in magnitude for any available courses of action	Clinicians should consider the options in their decision making, but patient preference may have a substantial role.

DIAGNOSIS

Key Action Statement 1a

Clinicians should diagnose bronchiolitis and assess disease severity on the basis of history and physical examination (Evidence Quality: B; Recommendation Strength: Strong Recommendation).

Action Statement Profile KAS 1a

Aggregate evidence quality	B
Benefits	Inexpensive, noninvasive, accurate
Risk, harm, cost	Missing other diagnoses
Benefit-harm assessment	Benefits outweigh harms
Value judgments	None
Intentional vagueness	None
Role of patient preferences	None
Exclusions	None
Strength	Strong recommendation
Differences of opinion	None

Key Action Statement 1b

Clinicians should assess risk factors for severe disease, such as age <12 weeks, a history of prematurity, underlying cardiopulmonary disease, or immunodeficiency, when making decisions about evaluation and management of children with bronchiolitis (Evidence Quality: B; Recommendation Strength: Moderate Recommendation).

Action Statement Profile KAS 1b

Aggregate evidence quality	B
Benefits	Improved ability to predict course of illness, appropriate disposition
Risk, harm, cost	Possible unnecessary hospitalization parental anxiety
Benefit-harm assessment	Benefits outweigh harms
Value judgments	None
Intentional vagueness	"Assess" is not defined
Role of patient preferences	None
Exclusions	None
Strength	Moderate recommendation
Differences of opinion	None

Key Action Statement 1c

When clinicians diagnose bronchiolitis on the basis of history and physical examination, radiographic or laboratory studies should not be obtained routinely (Evidence Quality: B; Recommendation Strength: Moderate Recommendation).

Action Statement Profile KAS 1b

Aggregate evidence quality	B
Benefits	Decreased radiation exposure, noninvasive (less procedure-associated discomfort), decreased antibiotic use, cost savings, time saving
Risk, harm, cost	Misdiagnosis, missed diagnosis of comorbid condition
Benefit-harm assessment	Benefits outweigh harms
Value judgments	None
Intentional vagueness	None
Role of patient preferences	None
Exclusions	Infants and children with unexpected worsening disease
Strength	Moderate recommendation
Differences of opinion	None

The main goals in the history and physical examination of infants presenting with wheeze or other lower respiratory tract symptoms, particularly in the winter season, is to differentiate infants with probable viral bronchiolitis from those with other disorders. In addition, an estimate of disease severity (increased respiratory rate, retractions, decreased oxygen saturation) should be made. Most clinicians recognize bronchiolitis as a constellation of clinical signs and symptoms occurring in children younger than 2 years, including a viral upper respiratory tract prodrome followed by increased respiratory effort and wheezing. Clinical signs and symptoms of bronchiolitis consist of rhinorrhea, cough, tachypnea, wheezing, rales, and increased respiratory effort manifested as grunting, nasal flaring, and intercostal and/or subcostal retractions.

The course of bronchiolitis is variable and dynamic, ranging from transient events, such as apnea, to progressive respiratory distress from lower airway obstruction. Important issues to assess in the history include the effects of respiratory symptoms on mental status, feeding, and hydration. The clinician should assess the ability of the family to care for the child and to return for further evaluation if needed. History of underlying conditions, such as prematurity, cardiac disease, chronic pulmonary disease, immunodeficiency, or episodes of previous wheezing, should be identified. Underlying conditions that may be associated with an increased risk of progression to severe disease or mortality include hemodynamically significant congenital heart disease, chronic lung disease (bronchopulmonary dysplasia), congenital anomalies,[15–17] in utero smoke exposure,[18] and the presence of an immunocompromising state.[19,20] In addition, genetic abnormalities have been associated with more severe presentation with bronchiolitis.[21]

Assessment of a child with bronchiolitis, including the physical examination, can be complicated by variability in the disease state and may require serial observations over time to fully assess the child's status. Upper airway obstruction contributes to work of breathing. Suctioning and positioning may decrease the work of breathing and improve the quality of the examination. Respiratory rate in otherwise healthy children changes considerably over the first year of life.[22–25] In hospitalized children, the 50th percentile for respiratory rate decreased from 41 at 0 to 3 months of age to 31 at 12 to 18 months of age.[26] Counting respiratory rate over the course of 1 minute is more accurate than shorter observations.[27] The presence of a normal respiratory rate suggests that risk of significant viral or bacterial lower respiratory tract infection or pneumonia in an infant is low (negative likelihood ratio approximately 0.5),[27–29] but the presence of tachypnea does not distinguish between viral and bacterial disease.[30,31]

The evidence relating the presence of specific findings in the assessment of bronchiolitis to clinical outcomes is limited. Most studies addressing this issue have enrolled children when presenting to hospital settings, including a large, prospective, multicenter study that assessed a variety of outcomes from the emergency department (ED) and varied inpatient settings.[18,32,33] Severe adverse events, such as ICU admission and need for mechanical ventilation, are uncommon among children with bronchiolitis and limit the power of these studies to detect clinically important risk factors associated with disease progression.[16,34,35] Tachypnea, defined as a respiratory rate ≥70 per minute, has been associated with increased risk of severe disease in some studies[35–37] but not others.[38] Many scoring systems have been developed in an attempt to objectively quantify respiratory distress, although none has achieved widespread acceptance and few have demonstrated any predictive validity, likely because of the substantial temporal variability in physical findings in infants with bronchiolitis.[39]

Pulse oximetry has been rapidly adopted into clinical assessment of children with bronchiolitis on the basis of data suggesting that it reliably detects hypoxemia not suspected on physical examination[36,40]; however, few studies have assessed the effectiveness of pulse oximetry to predict clinical outcomes. Among inpatients, perceived need for supplemental oxygen on the basis of pulse oximetry has been associated with prolonged hospitalization, ICU admission, and mechanical ventilation.[16,34,41] Among outpatients, available evidence differs on whether mild reductions in pulse oximetry (<95% on room air) predict progression of disease or need for a return observational visit.[38]

Apnea has been reported to occur with a wide range of prevalence estimates and viral etiologies.[42,43] Retrospective, hospital-based studies have included a high proportion of infants with risk factors, such as prematurity or neuromuscular disease, that may have biased the prevalence estimates. One large study found no apnea events for infants assessed as low risk by using several risk factors: age >1 month for full-term infants or 48 weeks' postconceptional age for preterm infants, and absence of any previous apneic event at presentation to the hospital.[44] Another large multicenter study found no association between the specific viral agent and risk of apnea in bronchiolitis.[42]

The literature on viral testing for bronchiolitis has expanded in recent years with the availability of sensitive polymerase chain reaction (PCR) assays. Large studies of infants hospitalized for bronchiolitis have consistently found that 60% to 75% have positive test results for RSV, and have noted coinfections in up to one-third of infants.[32,33,45] In the event an infant receiving monthly prophylaxis is hospitalized with bronchiolitis, testing should be performed to determine if RSV is the etiologic agent. If a breakthrough RSV infection is determined to be present based on antigen detection or other assay, monthly palivizumab prophylaxis should be discontinued because of the very low likelihood of a second RSV infection in the same year. Apart from this setting, routine virologic testing is not recommended.

Infants with non-RSV bronchiolitis, in particular human rhinovirus, appear to have a shorter courses and may represent a different phenotype associated with repeated wheezing.[32] PCR assay results should be interpreted cautiously, given that the assay may detect prolonged viral shedding from an unrelated previous illness, particularly with rhinovirus. In contrast, RSV detected by PCR assay almost always is associated with disease. At the individual patient level, the value of identifying a specific viral etiology causing bronchiolitis has not been demonstrated.[33]

Current evidence does not support routine chest radiography in children with bronchiolitis. Although many infants with bronchiolitis have abnormalities on chest radiography, data are insufficient to demonstrate that chest radiography correlates well with disease severity. Atelectasis on chest radiography was associated with increased risk of severe disease in 1 outpatient study.[16] Further studies, including 1 randomized trial, suggest children with suspected lower respiratory tract infection who had radiography performed were more likely to receive antibiotics without any difference in outcomes.[46,47] Initial radiography should be reserved for cases in which respiratory effort is severe enough to warrant ICU admission or where signs of an airway complication (such as pneumothorax) are present.

TREATMENT

ALBUTEROL

Key Action Statement 2

Clinicians should not administer albuterol (or salbutamol) to infants and children with a diagnosis of bronchiolitis (Evidence Quality: B; Recommendation Strength: Strong Recommendation).

Action Statement Profile KAS 2

Aggregate evidence quality	B
Benefits	Avoid adverse effects, avoid ongoing use of ineffective medication, lower costs
Risk, harm, cost	Missing transient benefit of drug
Benefit-harm assessment	Benefits outweigh harms
Value judgments	Overall ineffectiveness outweighs possible transient benefit
Intentional vagueness	None
Role of patient preferences	None
Exclusions	None
Strength	Strong recommendation
Differences of opinion	None
Notes	This guideline no longer recommends a trial of albuterol, as was considered in the 2006 AAP bronchiolitis guideline

Although several studies and reviews have evaluated the use of bronchodilator medications for viral bronchiolitis, most randomized controlled trials have failed to demonstrate a consistent benefit from α- or β-adrenergic agents. Several meta-analyses and systematic reviews[48–53] have shown that bronchodilators may improve clinical symptom scores, but they do not affect disease resolution, need for hospitalization, or length of stay (LOS). Because clinical scores may vary from one observer to the next[39,54] and do not correlate with more objective measures, such as pulmonary function tests,[55] clinical scores are not validated measures of the efficacy of bronchodilators. Although transient improvements in clinical score have been observed, most infants treated with bronchodilators will not benefit from their use.

A recently updated Cochrane systematic review assessing the impact of bronchodilators on oxygen saturation, the primary outcome measure, reported 30 randomized controlled trials involving 1992 infants in 12 countries.[56] Some studies included in this review evaluated agents other than albuterol/salbutamol (eg, ipratropium and metaproterenol) but did not include epinephrine. Small sample sizes, lack of standardized methods for outcome evaluation (eg, timing of assessments), and lack of standardized intervention (various bronchodilators, drug dosages, routes of administration, and nebulization delivery systems) limit the interpretation of these studies. Because of variable study designs as well as the inclusion of infants who had a history of previous wheezing in some studies, there was considerable heterogeneity in the studies. Sensitivity analysis (ie, including only studies at low risk of bias) significantly reduced heterogeneity measures for oximetry while having little effect on the overall effect size of oximetry (mean difference [MD] −0.38, 95% confidence interval [CI] −0.75 to 0.00). Those studies showing benefit[57–59] are methodologically weaker than other studies and include older children with recurrent wheezing. Results of the Cochrane review indicated no benefit in the clinical course of infants with bronchiolitis who received bronchodilators. The potential adverse effects (tachycardia and tremors) and cost of these agents outweigh any potential benefits.

In the previous iteration of this guideline, a trial of β-agonists was included as an option. However, given the greater strength of the evidence demonstrating no benefit, and that there is no well-established way to determine an "objective method of response" to bronchodilators in bronchiolitis, this option has been removed. Although it is true that a small subset of children with bronchiolitis may have reversible airway obstruction resulting from smooth muscle constriction, attempts to define a subgroup of responders have not been successful to date. If a clinical trial of bronchodilators is undertaken, clinicians should note that the variability of the disease process, the host's airway, and the clinical assessments, particularly scoring, would limit the clinician's ability to observe a clinically relevant response to bronchodilators.

Chavasse et al[60] reviewed the available literature on use of β-agonists for children younger than 2 years with recurrent wheezing. At the time of that review, there were 3 studies in the outpatient setting, 2 in the ED, and 3 in the pulmonary function laboratory setting. This review concluded there were no clear benefits from the use of β-agonists in this population. The authors noted some conflicting evidence, but further study was recommended only if the population could be clearly defined and meaningful outcome measures could be identified.

The population of children with bronchiolitis studied in most trials of bronchodilators limits the ability to make recommendations for all clinical scenarios. Children with severe disease or with respiratory failure were generally excluded from these trials, and this evidence cannot be generalized to these situations. Studies using pulmonary function tests show no effect of albuterol among infants hospitalized with bronchiolitis.[56,61] One study in a critical care setting showed a small decrease in inspiratory resistance after albuterol in one group and levalbuterol in another group, but therapy was accompanied by clinically significant tachycardia.[62] This small clinical change occurring with significant adverse effects does not justify recommending albuterol for routine care.

EPINEPHRINE

Key Action Statement 3

Clinicians should not administer epinephrine to infants and children with a diagnosis of bronchiolitis (Evidence Quality: B; Recommendation Strength: Strong Recommendation).

Action Statement Profile KAS 3

Aggregate evidence quality	B
Benefits	Avoiding adverse effects, lower costs, avoiding ongoing use of ineffective medication
Risk, harm, cost	Missing transient benefit of drug
Benefit-harm assessment	Benefits outweigh harms
Value judgments	The overall ineffectiveness outweighs possible transient benefit
Intentional vagueness	None
Role of patient preferences	None
Exclusions	Rescue treatment of rapidly deteriorating patients
Strength	Strong recommendation
Differences of opinion	None

Epinephrine is an adrenergic agent with both β- and α-receptor agonist activity that has been used to treat upper and lower respiratory tract illnesses both as a systemic agent and directly into the respiratory tract, where it is typically administered as a nebulized solution. Nebulized epinephrine has been administered in the racemic form and as the purified L-enantiomer, which is commercially available in the United States for intravenous use. Studies in other diseases, such as croup, have found no difference in efficacy on the basis of preparation,[63] although the comparison has not been specifically studied for bronchiolitis. Most studies have compared L-epinephrine to placebo or albuterol. A recent Cochrane meta-analysis by Hartling et al[64] systematically evaluated the evidence on this topic and found no evidence for utility in the inpatient setting. Two large, multicenter randomized trials comparing nebulized epinephrine to placebo[65] or albuterol[66] in the hospital setting found no improvement in LOS or other inpatient outcomes. A recent, large multicenter trial found a similar lack of efficacy compared with placebo and further demonstrated longer LOS when epinephrine was used on a fixed schedule compared with an as-needed schedule.[67] This evidence suggests epinephrine should not be used in children hospitalized for bronchiolitis, except potentially as a rescue agent in severe disease, although formal study is needed before a recommendation for the use of epinephrine in this setting.

The role of epinephrine in the outpatient setting remains controversial. A major addition to the evidence base came from the Canadian Bronchiolitis Epinephrine Steroid Trial.[68] This multicenter randomized trial enrolled 800 patients with bronchiolitis from 8 EDs and compared hospitalization rates over a 7-day period. This study had 4 arms: nebulized epinephrine plus oral dexamethasone, nebulized epinephrine plus oral placebo, nebulized placebo plus oral dexamethasone, and nebulized placebo plus oral placebo. The group of patients who received epinephrine concomitantly with corticosteroids had a lower likelihood of hospitalization by day 7 than the double placebo group, although this effect was no longer statistically significant after adjusting for multiple comparisons.

The systematic review by Hartling et al[64] concluded that epinephrine reduced hospitalizations compared with placebo on the day of the ED visit but not overall. Given that epinephrine has a transient effect and home administration is not routine practice, discharging an infant after observing a response in a monitored setting raises concerns for subsequent progression of illness. Studies have not found a difference in revisit rates, although the numbers of revisits are small and may not be adequately powered for this outcome. In summary, the current state of evidence does not support a routine role for epinephrine for bronchiolitis in outpatients, although further data may help to better define this question.

HYPERTONIC SALINE

Key Action Statement 4a

Nebulized hypertonic saline should not be administered to infants with a diagnosis of bronchiolitis in the emergency department (Evidence Quality: B; Recommendation Strength: Moderate Recommendation).

Action Statement Profile KAS 4a

Aggregate evidence quality	B
Benefits	Avoiding adverse effects, such as wheezing and excess secretions, cost
Risk, harm, cost	None
Benefit-harm assessment	Benefits outweigh harms
Value judgments	None
Intentional vagueness	None
Role of patient preferences	None
Exclusions	None
Strength	Moderate recommendation
Differences of opinion	None

Key Action Statement 4b

Clinicians may administer nebulized hypertonic saline to infants and children hospitalized for bronchiolitis (Evidence Quality: B; Recommendation Strength: Weak Recommendation [based on randomized controlled trials with inconsistent findings]).

Action Statement Profile KAS 4b

Aggregate evidence quality	B
Benefits	May shorten hospital stay if LOS is >72 h
Risk, harm, cost	Adverse effects such as wheezing and excess secretions; cost
Benefit-harm assessment	Benefits outweigh harms for longer hospital stays
Value judgments	Anticipating an individual child's LOS is difficult. Most US hospitals report an average LOS of <72 h for patients with bronchiolitis. This weak recommendation applies only if the average length of stay is >72 h
Intentional vagueness	This weak recommendation is based on an average LOS and does not address the individual patient.
Role of patient preferences	None
Exclusions	None
Strength	Weak
Differences of opinion	None

Nebulized hypertonic saline is an increasingly studied therapy for acute viral bronchiolitis. Physiologic evidence suggests that hypertonic saline increases mucociliary clearance in both normal and diseased lungs.[69–71] Because the pathology in bronchiolitis involves airway inflammation and resultant mucus plugging, improved mucociliary clearance should be beneficial, although there is only indirect evidence to support such an assertion. A more specific theoretical mechanism of action has been proposed on the basis of the concept of rehydration of the airway surface liquid, although again, evidence remains indirect.[72]

A 2013 Cochrane review[73] included 11 trials involving 1090 infants with mild to moderate disease in both inpatient and emergency settings. There were 6 studies involving 500 inpatients providing data for the analysis of LOS with an aggregate 1-day decrease reported, a result largely driven by the inclusion of 3 studies with relatively long mean length of stay of 5 to 6 days. The analysis of effect on clinical scores included 7 studies involving 640 patients in both inpatient and outpatient settings and demonstrated incremental positive effect with each day posttreatment from day 1 to day 3 (−0.88 MD on day 1, −1.32 MD on day 2, and −1.51 MD on day 3). Finally, Zhang et al[73] found no effect on hospitalization rates in the pooled analysis of 1 outpatient and 3 ED studies including 380 total patients.

Several randomized trials published after the Cochrane review period further informed the current guideline recommendation. Four trials evaluated admission rates from the ED, 3 using 3% saline and 1 using 7% saline.[74–76] A single trial[76] demonstrated a difference in admission rates from the ED favoring hypertonic saline, although the other 4 studies were concordant with the studies included in the Cochrane review. However, contrary to the studies included in the Cochrane review, none of the more recent trials reported improvement in LOS and, when added to the older studies for an updated meta-analysis, they significantly attenuate the summary estimate of the effect on LOS.[76,77] Most of the trials included in the Cochrane review occurred in settings with typical LOS of more than 3 days in their usual care arms. Hence, the significant decrease in LOS noted by Zhang et al[73] may not be generalizable to the United States where the average LOS is 2.4 days.[10] One other ongoing clinical trial performed in the United States, unpublished except in abstract form, further supports the observation that hypertonic saline does not decrease LOS in settings where expected stays are less than 3 days.[78]

The preponderance of the evidence suggests that 3% saline is safe and effective at improving symptoms of mild to moderate bronchiolitis after 24 hours of use and reducing hospital LOS in settings in which the duration of stay typically exceeds 3 days. It has not been shown to be effective at reducing hospitalization in emergency settings or in areas where the length of usage is brief. It has not been studied in intensive care settings, and most trials have included only patients with mild to moderate disease. Most studies have used a 3% saline concentration, and most have combined it with bronchodilators with each dose; however, there is retrospective evidence that the rate of adverse events is similar without bronchodilators,[79] as well as prospective evidence extrapolated from 2 trials without bronchodilators.[79,80] A single study was performed in the ambulatory outpatient setting[81]; however, future studies in the United States should focus on sustained usage on the basis of pattern of effects discerned in the available literature.

CORTICOSTEROIDS

Key Action Statement 5

Clinicians should not administer systemic corticosteroids to infants with a diagnosis of bronchiolitis in any setting (Evidence Quality: A; Recommendation Strength: Strong Recommendation).

Action Statement Profile KAS 5

Aggregate evidence quality	A
Benefits	No clinical benefit, avoiding adverse effects
Risk, harm, cost	None
Benefit-harm assessment	Benefits outweigh harms
Value judgments	None
Intentional vagueness	None
Role of patient preferences	None
Exclusions	None
Strength	Strong recommendation
Differences of opinion	None

Although there is good evidence of benefit from corticosteroids in other respiratory diseases, such as asthma and croup,[82–84] the evidence on corticosteroid use in bronchiolitis is negative. The most recent Cochrane systematic review shows that corticosteroids do not significantly reduce outpatient admissions when compared with placebo (pooled risk ratio, 0.92; 95% CI, 0.78 to 1.08; and risk ratio, 0.86; 95% CI, 0.7 to 1.06, respectively) and do not reduce LOS for inpatients (MD −0.18 days; 95% CI −0.39 to 0.04).[85] No other comparisons showed relevant differences for either primary or secondary outcomes. This review contained 17 trials with 2596 participants and included 2 large ED-based randomized trials, neither of which showed reductions in hospital admissions with treatment with corticosteroids as compared with placebo.[69,86]

One of these large trials, the Canadian Bronchiolitis Epinephrine Steroid Trial, however, did show a reduction in hospitalizations 7 days after treatment with combined nebulized epinephrine and oral dexamethasone as compared with placebo.[69] Although an unadjusted analysis showed a relative risk for hospitalization of 0.65 (95% CI 0.45 to 0.95; P = .02) for combination therapy as compared with placebo, adjustment for multiple comparison rendered the result insignificant (P = .07). These results have generated considerable controversy.[87] Although there is no standard recognized rationale for why combination epinephrine and dexamethasone would be synergistic in infants with bronchiolitis, evidence in adults and children older than 6 years with asthma shows that adding inhaled long-acting β agonists to moderate/high doses of inhaled corticosteroids allows reduction of the corticosteroid dose by, on average, 60%.[88] Basic science studies focused on understanding the interaction between β agonists and corticosteroids have shown potential mechanisms for why simultaneous administration of these drugs could be synergistic.[89–92] However, other bronchiolitis trials of corticosteroids administered by using fixed simultaneous bronchodilator regimens have not consistently shown benefit[93–97]; hence, a recommendation regarding the benefit of combined dexamethasone and epinephrine therapy is premature.

The systematic review of corticosteroids in children with bronchiolitis cited previously did not find any differences in short-term adverse events as compared with placebo.[86] However, corticosteroid therapy may prolong viral shedding in patients with bronchiolitis.[17]

In summary, a comprehensive systematic review and large multicenter randomized trials provide clear evidence that corticosteroids alone do not provide significant benefit to children with bronchiolitis. Evidence for potential benefit of combined corticosteroid and agents with both α- and β-agonist activity is at best tentative, and additional large trials are needed to clarify whether this therapy is effective.

Further, although there is no evidence of short-term adverse effects from corticosteroid therapy, other than prolonged viral shedding, in infants and children with bronchiolitis, there is inadequate evidence to be certain of safety.

OXYGEN

Key Action Statement 6a

Clinicians may choose not to administer supplemental oxygen if the oxyhemoglobin saturation exceeds 90% in infants and children with a diagnosis of bronchiolitis (Evidence Quality: D; Recommendation Strength: Weak Recommendation [based on low-level evidence and reasoning from first principles]).

Action Statement Profile KAS 6a

Benefits	Decreased hospitalizations, decreased LOS
Risk, harm, cost	Hypoxemia, physiologic stress, prolonged LOS, increased hospitalizations, increased LOS, cost
Benefit-harm assessment	Benefits outweigh harms
Value judgments	Oxyhemoglobin saturation >89% is adequate to oxygenate tissues; the risk of hypoxemia with oxyhemoglobin saturation >89% is minimal
Intentional vagueness	None
Role of patient preferences	Limited
Exclusions	Children with acidosis or fever
Strength	Weak recommendation (based on low-level evidence/ reasoning from first principles)
Differences of opinion	None

Key Action Statement 6b

Clinicians may choose not to use continuous pulse oximetry for infants and children with a diagnosis of bronchiolitis (Evidence Quality: C; Recommendation Strength: Weak Recommendation [based on lower-level evidence]).

Action Statement Profile KAS 6b

Aggregate evidence quality	C
Benefits	Shorter LOS, decreased alarm fatigue, decreased cost
Risk, harm, cost	Delayed detection of hypoxemia, delay in appropriate weaning of oxygen
Benefit-harm assessment	Benefits outweigh harms
Value judgments	None
Intentional vagueness	None
Role of patient preferences	Limited
Exclusions	None
Strength	Weak recommendation (based on lower level of evidence)
Differences of opinion	None

Although oxygen saturation is a poor predictor of respiratory distress, it is associated closely with a perceived need for hospitalization in infants with bronchiolitis.[98,99] Additionally, oxygen saturation has been implicated as a primary determinant of LOS in bronchiolitis.[40,100,101]

Physiologic data based on the oxyhemoglobin dissociation curve (Fig 3) demonstrate that small increases in arterial partial pressure of oxygen are associated with marked improvement in pulse oxygen saturation when the latter is less than 90%; with pulse oxygen saturation readings greater than 90% it takes very large elevations in arterial partial pressure of oxygen to affect further increases. In infants and children with bronchiolitis, no data exist to suggest such increases result in any clinically significant difference in physiologic function, patient symptoms, or clinical outcomes. Although it is well understood that acidosis, temperature, and 2,3-diphosphoglutarate influence the oxyhemoglobin dissociation curve, there has never been research to demonstrate how those influences practically affect infants with hypoxemia. The risk of hypoxemia must be weighed against the risk of hospitalization when making any decisions about site of care. One study of hospitalized children with bronchiolitis, for example, noted a 10% adverse error or near-miss rate for harm-causing interventions.[103] There are no studies on the effect of short-term, brief periods of hypoxemia such as may be seen in bronchiolitis. Transient hypoxemia is common in healthy infants.[104] Travel of healthy children even to moderate altitudes of 1300 m results in transient sleep desaturation to an average of 84% with no known adverse consequences.[105] Although children with chronic hypoxemia do incur developmental and behavioral problems, children who suffer intermittent hypoxemia from diseases such as asthma do not have impaired intellectual abilities or behavioral disturbance.[106–108]

Supplemental oxygen provided for infants not requiring additional respiratory support is best initiated with nasal prongs, although exact measurement of fraction of inspired oxygen is unreliable with this method.[109]

Pulse oximetry is a convenient method to assess the percentage of hemoglobin bound by oxygen in children. Pulse oximetry has been erroneously used in bronchiolitis as a proxy for respiratory distress. Accuracy of pulse oximetry is poor, especially in the 76% to 90% range.[110] Further, it has been well demonstrated that oxygen saturation has much less impact on respiratory drive than carbon dioxide concentrations in the blood.[111] There is very poor correlation between respiratory distress and oxygen saturations among infants with lower respiratory tract infections.[112] Other than cyanosis, no published clinical sign, model, or score accurately identifies hypoxemic children.[113]

Among children admitted for bronchiolitis, continuous pulse oximetry measurement is not well studied and potentially problematic for children who do not require oxygen. Transient desaturation is a normal phenomenon in healthy infants. In 1 study of 64 healthy infants between 2 weeks and 6 months of age, 60% of these infants exhibited a transient oxygen desaturation below 90%, to values as low as 83%.[105] A retrospective study of the role of continuous measurement of oxygenation in infants hospitalized with bronchiolitis found that 1 in 4 patients incur unnecessarily prolonged hospitalization as a result of a perceived need for oxygen outside of other symptoms[40] and no evidence of benefit was found.

Pulse oximetry is prone to errors of measurement. Families of infants hospitalized with continuous pulse oximeters are exposed to frequent alarms that

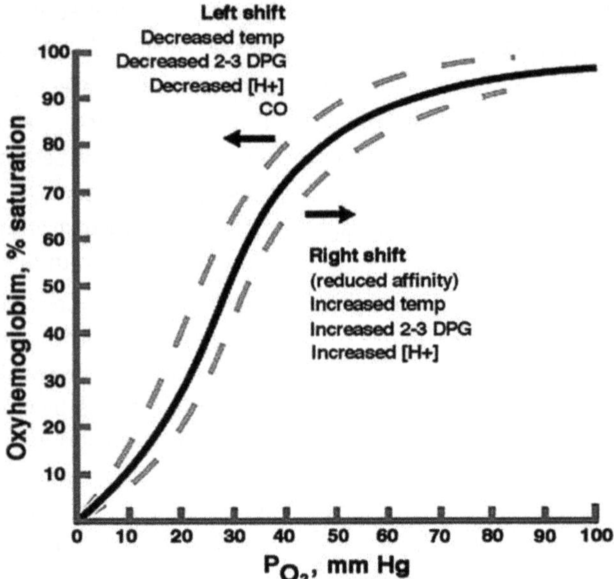

FIGURE 3

Oxyhemoglobin dissociation curve showing percent saturation of hemoglobin at various partial pressures of oxygen (reproduced with permission from the educational Web site www.anaesthesiauk.com).[102]

may negatively affect sleep. Alarm fatigue is recognized by The Joint Commission as a contributor toward in-hospital morbidity and mortality.[114] One adult study demonstrated very poor documentation of hypoxemia alerts by pulse oximetry, an indicator of alarm fatigue.[115] Pulse oximetry probes can fall off easily, leading to inaccurate measurements and alarms.[116] False reliance on pulse oximetry may lead to less careful monitoring of respiratory status. In one study, continuous pulse oximetry was associated with increased risk of minor adverse events in infants admitted to a general ward.[117] The pulse oximetry–monitored patients were found to have less-effective surveillance of their severity of illness when controlling for other variables.

There are a number of new approaches to oxygen delivery in bronchiolitis, 2 of which are home oxygen and high-frequency nasal cannula. There is emerging evidence for the role of home oxygen in reducing LOS or admission rate for infants with bronchiolitis, including 2 randomized trials.[118,119] Most of the studies have been performed in areas of higher altitude, where prolonged hypoxemia is a prime determinant of LOS in the hospital.[120,121] Readmission rates may be moderately higher in patients discharged with home oxygen; however, overall hospital use may be reduced,[122] although not in all settings.[123] Concerns have been raised that home pulse oximetry may complicate care or confuse families.[124] Communication with follow-up physicians is important, because primary care physicians may have difficulty determining safe pulse oximetry levels for discontinuation of oxygen.[125] Additionally, there may be an increased demand for follow-up outpatient visits associated with home oxygen use.[124]

Use of humidified, heated, high-flow nasal cannula to deliver air-oxygen mixtures provides assistance to infants with bronchiolitis through multiple proposed mechanisms.[126] There is evidence that high-flow nasal cannula improves physiologic measures of respiratory effort and can generate continuous positive airway pressure in bronchiolitis.[127–130] Clinical evidence suggests it reduces work of breathing[131,132] and may decrease need for intubation,[133–136] although studies are generally retrospective and small. The therapy has been studied in the ED[136,137] and the general inpatient setting,[134,138] as well as the ICU. The largest and most rigorous retrospective study to date was from Australia,[138] which showed a decline in intubation rate in the subgroup of infants with bronchiolitis (n = 330) from 37% to 7% after the introduction of high-flow nasal cannula, while the national registry intubation rate remained at 28%. A single pilot for a randomized trial has been published to date.[139] Although promising, the absence of any completed randomized trial of the efficacy of high-flow nasal cannula in bronchiolitis precludes specific recommendations on it use at present. Pneumothorax is a reported complication.

CHEST PHYSIOTHERAPY

Key Action Statement 7

Clinicians should not use chest physiotherapy for infants and children with a diagnosis of bronchiolitis (Evidence Quality: B; Recommendation Strength: Moderate Recommendation).

Action Statement Profile KAS 7

Aggregate evidence quality	B
Benefits	Decreased stress from therapy, reduced cost
Risk, harm, cost	None
Benefit-harm assessment	Benefits outweigh harms
Value judgments	None
Intentional vagueness	None
Role of patient preferences	None
Exclusions	None
Strength	Moderate recommendation
Differences of opinion	None

Airway edema, sloughing of respiratory epithelium into airways, and generalized hyperinflation of the lungs, coupled with poorly developed collateral ventilation, put infants with bronchiolitis at risk for atelectasis. Although lobar atelectasis is not characteristic of this disease, chest radiographs may show evidence of subsegmental atelectasis, prompting clinicians to consider ordering chest physiotherapy to promote airway clearance. A Cochrane Review[140] found 9 randomized controlled trials that evaluated chest physiotherapy in hospitalized patients with bronchiolitis. No clinical benefit was found by using vibration or percussion (5 trials)[141–144] or passive expiratory techniques (4 trials).[145–148] Since that review, a study[149] of the passive expiratory technique found a small, but significant reduction in duration of oxygen therapy, but no other benefits.

Suctioning of the nasopharynx to remove secretions is a frequent practice in infants with bronchiolitis. Although suctioning the nares may provide temporary relief of nasal congestion or upper airway obstruction, a retrospective study reported that deep suctioning[150] was associated with longer LOS in hospitalized infants 2 to 12 months of age. The same study also noted that lapses of greater than 4 hours in noninvasive, external nasal suctioning were also associated with longer LOS. Currently, there are insufficient data to make a recommendation about suctioning, but it appears that routine use of "deep" suctioning[151,153] may not be beneficial.

ANTIBACTERIALS

Key Action Statement 8

Clinicians should not administer antibacterial medications to infants and children with a diagnosis of bronchiolitis unless there is a concomitant bacterial infection, or a strong suspicion of one. (Evidence Quality: B; Recommendation Strength: Strong Recommendation).

Action Statement Profile KAS 8

Aggregate evidence quality	B
Benefits	Fewer adverse effects, less resistance to antibacterial agents, lower cost
Risk, harm, cost	None
Benefit-harm assessment	Benefits outweigh harms
Value judgments	None
Intentional vagueness	Strong suspicion is not specifically defined and requires clinician judgment. An evaluation for the source of possible serious bacterial infection should be completed before antibiotic use
Role of patient preferences	None
Exclusions	None
Strength	Strong recommendation
Differences of opinion	None

Infants with bronchiolitis frequently receive antibacterial therapy because of fever,[152] young age,[153] and concern for secondary bacterial infection.[154] Early randomized controlled trials[155,156] showed no benefit from routine antibacterial therapy for children with bronchiolitis. Nonetheless, antibiotic therapy continues to be overused in young infants with bronchiolitis because of concern for an undetected bacterial infection. Studies have shown that febrile infants without an identifiable source of fever have a risk of bacteremia that may be as high as 7%. However, a child with a distinct viral syndrome, such as bronchiolitis, has a lower risk (much less than 1%) of bacterial infection of the cerebrospinal fluid or blood.[157]

Ralston et al[158] conducted a systematic review of serious bacterial infections (SBIs) occurring in hospitalized febrile infants between 30 and 90 days of age with bronchiolitis. Instances of bacteremia or meningitis were extremely rare. Enteritis was not evaluated. Urinary tract infection occurred at a rate of approximately 1%, but asymptomatic bacteriuria may have explained this finding. The authors concluded routine screening for SBI among hospitalized febrile infants with bronchiolitis between 30 and 90 days of age is not justified. Limited data suggest the risk of bacterial infection in hospitalized infants with bronchiolitis younger than 30 days of age is similar to the risk in older infants. An abnormal white blood cell count is not useful for predicting a concurrent SBI in infants and young children hospitalized with RSV lower respiratory tract infection.[159] Several retrospective studies support this conclusion.[160–166] Four prospective studies of SBI in patients with bronchiolitis and/or RSV infections also demonstrated low rates of SBI.[167–171]

Approximately 25% of hospitalized infants with bronchiolitis have radiographic evidence of atelectasis, and it may be difficult to distinguish between atelectasis and bacterial infiltrate or consolidation.[169] Bacterial pneumonia in infants with bronchiolitis without consolidation is unusual.[170] Antibiotic therapy may be justified in some children with bronchiolitis who require intubation and mechanical ventilation for respiratory failure.[172,173]

Although acute otitis media (AOM) in infants with bronchiolitis may be attributable to viruses, clinical features generally do not permit differentiation of viral AOM from those with a bacterial component.[174] Two studies address the frequency of AOM in patients with bronchiolitis. Andrade et al[175] prospectively identified AOM in 62% of 42 patients who presented with bronchiolitis. AOM was present in 50% on entry to the study and developed in an additional 12% within 10 days. A subsequent report[176] followed 150 children hospitalized for bronchiolitis for the development of AOM. Seventy-nine (53%) developed AOM, two-thirds within the first 2 days of hospitalization. AOM did not influence the clinical course or laboratory findings of bronchiolitis. The current AAP guideline on AOM[177] recommends that a diagnosis of AOM should include bulging of the tympanic membrane. This is based on bulging being the best indicator for the presence of bacteria in multiple tympanocentesis studies and on 2 articles comparing antibiotic to placebo therapy that used a bulging tympanic membrane as a necessary part of the diagnosis.[178,179] New studies are needed to determine the incidence of AOM in bronchiolitis by using the new criterion of bulging of the tympanic membrane. Refer to the AOM guideline[180] for recommendations regarding the management of AOM.

NUTRITION AND HYDRATION

Key Action Statement 9

Clinicians should administer nasogastric or intravenous fluids for infants with a diagnosis of bronchiolitis who cannot maintain hydration orally (Evidence Quality: X; Recommendation Strength: Strong Recommendation).

Action Statement Profile KAS 9

Aggregate evidence quality	X
Benefits	Maintaining hydration
Risk, harm, cost	Risk of infection, risk of aspiration with nasogastric tube, discomfort, hyponatremia, intravenous infiltration, overhydration
Benefit-harm assessment	Benefits outweigh harms
Value judgments	None
Intentional vagueness	None
Role of patient preferences	Shared decision as to which mode is used
Exclusions	None
Strength	Strong recommendation
Differences of opinion	None

The level of respiratory distress attributable to bronchiolitis guides the indications for fluid replacement. Conversely, food intake in the previous 24 hours may be a predictor of oxygen saturation among infants with bronchiolitis. One study found that food intake at less than 50% of normal for the previous 24 hours is associated with a pulse oximetry value of <95%.[180] Infants with mild respiratory distress may require only observation, particularly if feeding remains unaffected. When the respiratory rate exceeds 60 to 70 breaths per minute, feeding may be compromised, particularly if nasal secretions are copious. There is limited evidence to suggest coordination of breathing with swallowing may be impaired among infants with bronchiolitis.[181] These infants may develop increased nasal flaring, retractions, and prolonged expiratory wheezing when fed and may be at increased risk of aspiration.[182]

One study estimated that one-third of infants hospitalized for bronchiolitis require fluid replacement.[183] One case series[184] and 2 randomized trials,[185,186] examined the comparative efficacy and safety of the intravenous and nasogastric routes for fluid replacement. A pilot trial in Israel that included 51 infants younger than 6 months demonstrated no significant differences in the duration of oxygen needed or time to full oral feeds between infants receiving intravenous 5% dextrose in normal saline solution or nasogastric breast milk or formula.[187] Infants in the intravenous group had a shorter LOS (100 vs 120 hours) but it was not statistically significant. In a larger open randomized trial including infants between 2 and 12 months of age and conducted in Australia and New Zealand, there were no significant differences in rates of admission to ICUs, need for ventilatory support, and adverse events between 381 infants assigned to nasogastric hydration and 378 infants assigned to intravenous hydration.[188] There was a difference of 4 hours in mean LOS between the intravenous group (82.2 hours) and the nasogastric group (86.2 hours) that was not statistically significant. The nasogastric route had a higher success rate of insertion than the intravenous route. Parental satisfaction scores did not differ between the intravenous and nasogastric groups. These studies suggest that infants who have difficulty feeding safely because of respiratory distress can receive either intravenous or nasogastric fluid replacement; however, more evidence is needed to increase the strength of this recommendation.

The possibility of fluid retention related to production of antidiuretic hormone has been raised in patients with bronchiolitis.[187–189] Therefore, receipt of hypotonic fluid replacement and maintenance fluids may increase the risk of iatrogenic hyponatremia in these infants. A recent meta-analysis demonstrated that among hospitalized children requiring maintenance fluids, the use of hypotonic fluids was associated with significant hyponatremia compared with isotonic fluids in older children.[190] Use of isotonic fluids, in general, appears to be safer.

PREVENTION

Key Action Statement 10a

Clinicians should not administer palivizumab to otherwise healthy

infants with a gestational age of 29 weeks, 0 days or greater (Evidence Quality: B; Recommendation Strength: Strong Recommendation).

Action Statement Profile KAS 10a

Aggregate evidence quality	B
Benefits	Reduced pain of injections, reduced use of a medication that has shown minimal benefit, reduced adverse effects, reduced visits to health care provider with less exposure to illness
Risk, harm, cost	Minimal increase in risk of RSV hospitalization
Benefit-harm assessment	Benefits outweigh harms
Value judgments	None
Intentional vagueness	None
Role of patient preferences	Parents may choose to not accept palivizumab
Exclusions	Infants with chronic lung disease of prematurity and hemodynamically significant cardiac disease (as described in KAS 10b)
Strength	Recommendation
Differences of opinion	None
Notes	This KAS is harmonized with the AAP policy statement on palivizumab

Key Action Statement 10b

Clinicians should administer palivizumab during the first year of life to infants with hemodynamically significant heart disease or chronic lung disease of prematurity defined as preterm infants <32 weeks, 0 days' gestation who require >21% oxygen for at least the first 28 days of life (Evidence Quality: B; Recommendation Strength: Moderate Recommendation).

Action Statement Profile KAS 10b

Aggregate evidence quality	B
Benefits	Reduced risk of RSV hospitalization
Risk, harm, cost	Injection pain; increased risk of illness from increased visits to clinician office or clinic; cost; side effects from palivizumab
Benefit-harm assessment	Benefits outweigh harms
Value judgments	None
Intentional vagueness	None
Role of patient preferences	Parents may choose to not accept palivizumab
Exclusions	None
Strength	Moderate recommendation
Differences of opinion	None
Notes	This KAS is harmonized with the AAP policy statement on palivizumab[191,192]

Key Action Statement 10c

Clinicians should administer a maximum 5 monthly doses (15 mg/kg/dose) of palivizumab during the RSV season to infants who qualify for palivizumab in the first year of life (Evidence Quality: B, Recommendation Strength: Moderate Recommendation).

Action Statement Profile KAS 10c

Aggregate evidence quality	B
Benefits	Reduced risk of hospitalization; reduced admission to ICU
Risk, harm, cost	Injection pain; increased risk of illness from increased visits to clinician office or clinic; cost; adverse effects of palivizumab
Benefit-harm assessment	Benefits outweigh harms
Value judgments	None
Intentional vagueness	None
Role of patient preferences	None
Exclusions	Fewer doses should be used if the bronchiolitis season ends before the completion of 5 doses; if the child is hospitalized with a breakthrough RSV, monthly prophylaxis should be discontinued
Strength	Moderate recommendation
Differences of opinion	None
Notes	This KAS is harmonized with the AAP policy statement on palivizumab[191,192]

Detailed evidence to support the policy statement on palivizumab and this palivizumab section can be found in the technical report on palivizumab.[192]

Palivizumab was licensed by the US Food and Drug Administration in June 1998 largely on the basis of results of 1 clinical trial.[193] The results of a second clinical trial among children with congenital heart disease were reported in December 2003.[194] No other prospective, randomized, placebo-controlled trials have been conducted in any subgroup. Since licensure of palivizumab, new peer-reviewed publications provide greater insight into the epidemiology of disease caused by RSV.[195–197] As a result of new data, the Bronchiolitis Guideline Committee and the Committee on Infectious Diseases have updated recommendations for use of prophylaxis.

PREMATURITY

Monthly palivizumab prophylaxis should be restricted to infants born before 29 weeks, 0 days' gestation, except for infants who qualify on the basis of congenital heart disease or chronic lung disease of prematurity. Data show that infants born at or after 29 weeks, 0 days' gestation have an RSV hospitalization rate similar to the rate of full-term infants.[11,198] Infants with a gestational age of 28 weeks, 6 days or less who will be younger than 12 months at the start of the RSV season should receive a maximum of 5 monthly doses of palivizumab or until the end of the RSV season, whichever comes first. Depending on the month of birth, fewer than 5 monthly doses will provide protection for most infants for the duration of the season.

CONGENITAL HEART DISEASE

Despite the large number of subjects enrolled, little benefit from palivizumab prophylaxis was found in the industry-sponsored cardiac study among infants in the cyanotic group (7.9% in control group versus 5.6% in palivizumab group, or 23 fewer hospitalizations per1000 children; *P* = .285).[197] In the acyanotic group (11.8% vs 5.0%), there were 68 fewer RSV hospitalizations per 1000 prophylaxis recipients (*P* = .003).[197,199,200]

CHRONIC LUNG DISEASE OF PREMATURITY

Palivizumab prophylaxis should be administered to infants and children younger than 12 months who develop chronic lung disease of prematurity, defined as a requirement for 28 days of more than 21% oxygen beginning at birth. If a child meets these criteria and is in the first 24 months of life and continues to require supplemental oxygen, diuretic therapy, or chronic corticosteroid therapy within 6 months of the start of the RSV season, monthly prophylaxis should be administered for the remainder of the season.

NUMBER OF DOSES

Community outbreaks of RSV disease usually begin in November or December, peak in January or February, and end by late March or, at times, in April.[4] Figure 1 shows the 2011–2012 bronchiolitis season, which is typical of most years. Because 5 monthly doses will provide more than 24 weeks of protective serum palivizumab concentration, administration of more than 5 monthly doses is not recommended within the continental United States. For infants who qualify for 5 monthly doses, initiation of prophylaxis in November and continuation for a total of 5 doses will provide protection into April.[201] If prophylaxis is initiated in October, the fifth and final dose should be administered in February, and protection will last into March for most children.

SECOND YEAR OF LIFE

Because of the low risk of RSV hospitalization in the second year of life, palivizumab prophylaxis is not recommended for children in the second year of life with the following exception. Children who satisfy the definition of chronic lung disease of infancy and continue to require supplemental oxygen, chronic corticosteroid therapy, or diuretic therapy within 6 months of the onset of the second RSV season may be considered for a second season of prophylaxis.

OTHER CONDITIONS

Insufficient data are available to recommend routine use of prophylaxis in children with Down syndrome, cystic fibrosis, pulmonary abnormality, neuromuscular disease, or immune compromise.

Down Syndrome

Routine use of prophylaxis for children in the first year of life with Down syndrome is not recommended unless the child qualifies because of cardiac disease or prematurity.[202]

Cystic Fibrosis

Routine use of palivizumab prophylaxis in patients with cystic fibrosis is not recommended.[203,204] Available studies indicate the incidence of RSV hospitalization in children with cystic fibrosis is low and unlikely to be different from children without cystic fibrosis. No evidence suggests a benefit from palivizumab prophylaxis in patients with cystic fibrosis. A randomized clinical trial involving 186 children with cystic fibrosis from 40 centers reported 1 subject in each group was hospitalized because of RSV infection. Although this study was not powered for efficacy, no clinically meaningful differences in outcome were reported.[205] A survey of cystic fibrosis center directors published in 2009 noted that palivizumab prophylaxis is not the standard of care for patients with cystic fibrosis.[206] If a neonate is diagnosed with cystic fibrosis by newborn screening, RSV prophylaxis should not be administered if no other indications are present. A patient with cystic fibrosis with clinical evidence of chronic lung disease in the first year of life may be considered for prophylaxis.

Neuromuscular Disease and Pulmonary Abnormality

The risk of RSV hospitalization is not well defined in children with pulmonary abnormalities or neuromuscular disease that impairs ability to clear secretions from the lower airway because of ineffective cough, recurrent gastroesophageal tract reflux, pulmonary malformations, tracheoesophageal fistula, upper airway conditions, or conditions requiring tracheostomy. No data on the relative risk of RSV hospitalization are available for this cohort. Selected infants with disease or congenital anomaly that impairs their ability to clear secretions from the lower airway because of ineffective cough may be considered for prophylaxis during the first year of life.

Immunocompromised Children

Population-based data are not available on the incidence or severity of RSV hospitalization in children who undergo solid organ or hematopoietic stem cell transplantation, receive chemotherapy, or are immunocompromised because of other conditions. Prophylaxis may be considered for hematopoietic stem cell transplant patients who undergo transplantation and are profoundly immunosuppressed during the RSV season.[207]

MISCELLANEOUS ISSUES

Prophylaxis is not recommended for prevention of nosocomial RSV disease in the NICU or hospital setting.[208,209]

No evidence suggests palivizumab is a cost-effective measure to prevent recurrent wheezing in children. Prophylaxis should not be administered to reduce recurrent wheezing in later years.[210,211]

Monthly prophylaxis in Alaska Native children who qualify should be determined by locally generated data regarding season onset and end.

Continuation of monthly prophylaxis for an infant or young child who experiences breakthrough RSV hospitalization is not recommended.

HAND HYGIENE

Key Action Statement 11a

All people should disinfect hands before and after direct contact with patients, after contact with inanimate objects in the direct vicinity of the patient, and after removing gloves (Evidence Quality: B; Recommendation Strength: Strong Recommendation).

Action Statement Profile KAS 11a

Aggregate evidence quality	B
Benefits	Decreased transmission of disease
Risk, harm, cost	Possible hand irritation
Benefit-harm assessment	Benefits outweigh harms
Value judgments	None
Intentional vagueness	None
Role of patient preferences	None
Exclusions	None
Strength	Strong recommendation
Differences of opinion	None

Key Action Statement 11b

All people should use alcohol-based rubs for hand decontamination when caring for children with bronchiolitis. When alcohol-based rubs are not available, individuals should wash their hands with soap and water (Evidence Quality: B; Recommendation Strength: Strong Recommendation).

Action Statement Profile KAS 11b

Aggregate evidence quality	B
Benefits	Less hand irritation
Risk, harm, cost	If there is visible dirt on the hands, hand washing is necessary; alcohol-based rubs are not effective for *Clostridium difficile*, present a fire hazard, and have a slight increased cost
Benefit-harm assessment	Benefits outweigh harms
Value judgments	None
Intentional vagueness	None
Role of patient preferences	None
Exclusions	None
Strength	Strong recommendation
Differences of opinion	None

Efforts should be made to decrease the spread of RSV and other causative agents of bronchiolitis in medical settings, especially in the hospital. Secretions from infected patients can be found on beds, crib railings, tabletops, and toys.[12] RSV, as well as many other viruses, can survive better on hard surfaces than on porous surfaces or hands. It can remain infectious on counter tops for ≥6 hours, on gowns or paper tissues for 20 to 30 minutes, and on skin for up to 20 minutes.[212]

It has been shown that RSV can be carried and spread to others on the hands of caregivers.[213] Studies have shown that health care workers have acquired infection by performing activities such as feeding, diaper change, and playing with the RSV-infected infant. Caregivers who had contact only with surfaces contaminated with the infants' secretions or touched inanimate objects in patients' rooms also acquired RSV. In these studies, health care workers contaminated their hands (or gloves) with RSV and inoculated their oral or conjunctival mucosa.[214] Frequent hand washing by health care workers has been shown to reduce the spread of RSV in the health care setting.[215]

The Centers for Disease Control and Prevention published an extensive review of the hand-hygiene literature and made recommendations as to indications for hand washing and hand antisepsis.[216] Among the recommendations are that hands should be disinfected before and after direct contact with every patient, after contact with inanimate objects in the direct vicinity of the patient, and before putting on and after removing gloves. If hands are not visibly soiled, an alcohol-based rub is preferred. In guidelines published in 2009, the World Health Organization also recommended alcohol-based hand-rubs as the standard for hand hygiene in health care.[217] Specifically, systematic reviews show them to remove organisms more effectively, require less time, and irritate skin less often than hand washing with soap or other antiseptic agents and water. The availability of bedside alcohol-based solutions increased compliance with hand hygiene among health care workers.[214]

When caring for hospitalized children with clinically diagnosed bronchiolitis, strict adherence to hand decontamination and use of personal protective equipment (ie, gloves and gowns) can reduce the risk of cross-infection in the health care setting.[215]

Other methods of infection control in viral bronchiolitis include education of personnel and family members, surveillance for the onset of RSV season, and wearing masks when anticipating exposure to aerosolized secretions while performing patient care activities. Programs that implement the aforementioned principles, in conjunction with effective hand decontamination and cohorting of patients, have been shown to reduce the spread of RSV in the health care setting by 39% to 50%.[218,219]

TOBACCO SMOKE

Key Action Statement 12a

Clinicians should inquire about the exposure of the infant or child to tobacco smoke when assessing infants and children for bronchiolitis (Evidence Quality: C; Recommendation Strength: Moderate Recommendation).

Action Statement Profile KAS 12a

Aggregate evidence quality	C
Benefits	Can identify infants and children at risk whose family may benefit from counseling, predicting risk of severe disease
Risk, harm, cost	Time to inquire
Benefit-harm assessment	Benefits outweigh harms
Value judgments	None
Intentional vagueness	None
Role of patient preferences	Parent may choose to deny tobacco use even though they are, in fact, users
Exclusions	None
Strength	Moderate recommendation
Differences of opinion	None

Key Action Statement 12b

Clinicians should counsel caregivers about exposing the infant or child to environmental tobacco smoke and smoking cessation when assessing a child for bronchiolitis (Evidence Quality: B; Recommendation Strength: Strong Recommendation).

Action Statement Profile KAS 12b

Aggregate evidence quality	B
Benefits	Reinforces the detrimental effects of smoking, potential to decrease smoking
Risk, harm, cost	Time to counsel
Benefit-harm assessment	Benefits outweigh harms
Value judgments	None
Intentional vagueness	None
Role of patient preferences	Parents may choose to ignore counseling
Exclusions	None
Strength	Moderate recommendation
Differences of opinion	None
Notes	Counseling for tobacco smoke prevention should begin in the prenatal period and continue in family-centered care and at all well-infant visits

Tobacco smoke exposure increases the risk and severity of bronchiolitis. Strachan and Cook[220] first delineated the effects of environmental tobacco smoke on rates of lower respiratory tract disease in infants in a meta-analysis including 40 studies. In a more recent systematic review, Jones et al[221] found a pooled odds ratio of 2.51 (95% CI 1.96 to 3.21) for tobacco smoke exposure and bronchiolitis hospitalization among the 7 studies specific to the condition. Other investigators have consistently reported tobacco smoke exposure increases both severity of illness and risk of hospitalization for bronchiolitis.[222–225] The AAP issued a technical report on the risks of secondhand smoke in 2009. The report makes recommendations regarding effective ways to eliminate or reduce secondhand smoke exposure, including education of parents.[226]

Despite our knowledge of this important risk factor, there is evidence to suggest health care providers identify fewer than half of children exposed to tobacco smoke in the outpatient, inpatient, or ED settings.[227–229] Furthermore, there is evidence that counseling parents in these settings is well received and has a measurable impact. Rosen et al[230] performed a meta-analysis of the effects of interventions in pediatric settings on parental cessation and found a pooled risk ratio of 1.3 for cessation among the 18 studies reviewed.

In contrast to many of the other recommendations, protecting children from tobacco exposure is a recommendation that is primarily implemented outside of the clinical setting. As such, it is critical that parents are fully educated about the importance of not allowing smoking in the home and that smoke lingers on clothes and in the environment for prolonged periods.[231] It should be provided in plain language and in a respectful, culturally effective manner that is family centered, engages parents as partners in their child's health, and factors in their literacy, health literacy, and primary language needs.

BREASTFEEDING

Key Action Statement 13

Clinicians should encourage exclusive breastfeeding for at least 6 months to decrease the morbidity of respiratory infections (Evidence Quality: Grade B; Recommendation Strength: Moderate Recommendation).

Action Statement Profile KAS 13

Aggregate evidence quality	B
Benefits	May reduce the risk of bronchiolitis and other illnesses; multiple benefits of breastfeeding unrelated to bronchiolitis
Risk, harm, cost	None
Benefit-harm assessment	Benefits outweigh risks
Value judgments	None
Intentional vagueness	None
Role of patient preferences	Parents may choose to feed formula rather than breastfeed
Exclusions	None
Strength	Moderate recommendation
Notes	Education on breastfeeding should begin in the prenatal period

In 2012, the AAP presented a general policy on breastfeeding.[232] The policy statement was based on the proven benefits of breastfeeding for at least 6 months. Respiratory infections were shown to be significantly less common in breastfed children. A primary resource was a meta-analysis from the Agency for Healthcare Research and Quality that showed an overall 72% reduction in the risk of hospitalization secondary to respiratory diseases in infants who were exclusively breastfed for 4 or more months compared with those who were formula fed.[233]

The clinical evidence also supports decreased incidence and severity of illness in breastfed infants with bronchiolitis. Dornelles et al[234] concluded that the duration of exclusive breastfeeding was inversely related to the length of oxygen use and the length of hospital stay in previously healthy infants with acute bronchiolitis. In a large prospective study in Australia, Oddy et al[235] showed that breastfeeding for less than 6 months was associated with an increased risk for 2 or more medical visits and hospital admission for wheezing lower respiratory illness. In Japan, Nishimura et al[236] looked at 3 groups of RSV-positive infants defined as full, partial, or token breastfeeding. There were no significant differences in the hospitalization rate among the 3 groups; however, there were significant differences in the duration of hospitalization and the rate of requiring oxygen therapy, both favoring breastfeeding.

FAMILY EDUCATION

Key Action Statement 14

Clinicians and nurses should educate personnel and family members on evidence-based diagnosis, treatment, and prevention in bronchiolitis (Evidence Quality: C; observational studies; Recommendation Strength; Moderate Recommendation).

Action Statement Profile KAS 14

Aggregate evidence quality	C
Benefits	Decreased transmission of disease, benefits of breastfeeding, promotion of judicious use of antibiotics, risks of infant lung damage attributable to tobacco smoke
Risk, harm, cost	Time to educate properly
Benefit-harm assessment	Benefits outweigh harms
Value judgments	None
Intentional vagueness	Personnel is not specifically defined but should include all people who enter a patient's room
Role of patient preferences	None
Exclusions	None
Strength	Moderate recommendation
Differences of opinion	None

Shared decision-making with parents about diagnosis and treatment of bronchiolitis is a key tenet of patient-centered care. Despite the absence of effective therapies for viral bronchiolitis, caregiver education by clinicians may have a significant impact on care patterns in the disease. Children with bronchiolitis typically suffer from symptoms for 2 to 3 weeks, and parents often seek care in multiple settings during that time period.[237] Given that children with RSV generally shed virus for 1 to 2 weeks and from 30% to 70% of family members may become ill,[238,239] education about prevention of transmission of disease is key. Restriction of visitors to newborns during the respiratory virus season should be considered. Consistent evidence suggests that parental education is helpful in the promotion of judicious use of antibiotics and that clinicians may misinterpret parental expectations about therapy unless the subject is openly discussed.[240–242]

FUTURE RESEARCH NEEDS

- Better algorithms for predicting the course of illness
- Impact of clinical score on patient outcomes
- Evaluating different ethnic groups and varying response to treatments
- Does epinephrine alone reduce admission in outpatient settings?
- Additional studies on epinephrine in combination with dexamethasone or other corticosteroids
- Hypertonic saline studies in the outpatient setting and in in hospitals with shorter LOS
- More studies on nasogastric hydration
- More studies on tonicity of intravenous fluids

- Incidence of true AOM in bronchiolitis by using 2013 guideline definition
- More studies on deep suctioning and nasopharyngeal suctioning
- Strategies for monitoring oxygen saturation
- Use of home oxygen
- Appropriate cutoff for use of oxygen in high altitude
- Oxygen delivered by high-flow nasal cannula
- RSV vaccine and antiviral agents
- Use of palivizumab in special populations, such as cystic fibrosis, neuromuscular diseases, Down syndrome, immune deficiency
- Emphasis on parent satisfaction/patient-centered outcomes in all research (ie, not LOS as the only measure)

SUBCOMMITTEE ON BRONCHIOLITIS (OVERSIGHT BY THE COUNCIL ON QUALITY IMPROVEMENT AND PATIENT SAFETY, 2013–2014)

Shawn L. Ralston, MD, FAAP: Chair, Pediatric Hospitalist (no financial conflicts; published research related to bronchiolitis)

Allan S. Lieberthal, MD, FAAP: Chair, General Pediatrician with Expertise in Pulmonology (no conflicts)

Brian K. Alverson, MD, FAAP: Pediatric Hospitalist, AAP Section on Hospital Medicine Representative (no conflicts)

Jill E. Baley, MD, FAAP: Neonatal-Perinatal Medicine, AAP Committee on Fetus and Newborn Representative (no conflicts)

Anne M. Gadomski, MD, MPH, FAAP: General Pediatrician and Research Scientist (no financial conflicts; published research related to bronchiolitis including Cochrane review of bronchodilators)

David W. Johnson, MD, FAAP: Pediatric Emergency Medicine Physician (no financial conflicts; published research related to bronchiolitis)

Michael J. Light, MD, FAAP: Pediatric Pulmonologist, AAP Section on Pediatric Pulmonology Representative (no conflicts)

Nizar F. Maraqa, MD, FAAP: Pediatric Infectious Disease Physician, AAP Section on Infectious Diseases Representative (no conflicts)

H. Cody Meissner, MD, FAAP: Pediatric Infectious Disease Physician, AAP Committee on Infectious Diseases Representative (no conflicts)

Eneida A. Mendonca, MD, PhD, FAAP, FACMI: Informatician/Academic Pediatric Intensive Care Physician, Partnership for Policy Implementation Representative (no conflicts)

Kieran J. Phelan, MD, MSc: General Pediatrician (no conflicts)

Joseph J. Zorc, MD, MSCE, FAAP: Pediatric Emergency Physician, AAP Section on Emergency Medicine Representative (no financial conflicts; published research related to bronchiolitis)

Danette Stanko-Lopp, MA, MPH: Methodologist, Epidemiologist (no conflicts)

Mark A. Brown, MD: Pediatric Pulmonologist, American Thoracic Society Liaison (no conflicts)

Ian Nathanson, MD, FAAP: Pediatric Pulmonologist, American College of Chest Physicians Liaison (no conflicts)

Elizabeth Rosenblum, MD: Academic Family Physician, American Academy of Family Physicians liaison (no conflicts).

Stephen Sayles, III, MD, FACEP: Emergency Medicine Physician, American College of Emergency Physicians Liaison (no conflicts)

Sinsi Hernández-Cancio, JD: Parent/Consumer Representative (no conflicts)

STAFF

Caryn Davidson, MA
Linda Walsh, MAB

REFERENCES

1. American Academy of Pediatrics Subcommittee on Diagnosis and Management of Bronchiolitis. Diagnosis and management of bronchiolitis. *Pediatrics*. 2006;118(4):1774–1793
2. Agency for Healthcare Research and Quality. Management of Bronchiolitis in Infants and Children. Evidence Report/Technology Assessment No. 69. Rockville, MD: Agency for Healthcare Research and Quality; 2003. AHRQ Publication No. 03-E014
3. Mullins JA, Lamonte AC, Bresee JS, Anderson LJ. Substantial variability in community respiratory syncytial virus season timing. *Pediatr Infect Dis J*. 2003;22(10):857–862
4. Centers for Disease Control and Prevention. Respiratory syncytial virus activity—United States, July 2011-January 2013. *MMWR Morb Mortal Wkly Rep*. 2013;62(8):141–144
5. Greenough A, Cox S, Alexander J, et al. Health care utilisation of infants with chronic lung disease, related to hospitalisation for RSV infection. *Arch Dis Child*. 2001;85(6):463–468
6. Parrott RH, Kim HW, Arrobio JO, et al. Epidemiology of respiratory syncytial virus infection in Washington, D.C. II. Infection and disease with respect to age, immunologic status, race and sex. *Am J Epidemiol*. 1973;98(4):289–300
7. Meissner HC. Selected populations at increased risk from respiratory syncytial virus infection. *Pediatr Infect Dis J*. 2003;22(suppl 2):S40–S44, discussion S44–S45
8. Shay DK, Holman RC, Roosevelt GE, Clarke MJ, Anderson LJ. Bronchiolitis-associated mortality and estimates of respiratory syncytial virus-associated deaths among US children, 1979-1997. *J Infect Dis*. 2001;183(1):16–22
9. Miller EK, Gebretsadik T, Carroll KN, et al. Viral etiologies of infant bronchiolitis, croup and upper respiratory illness during 4 consecutive years. *Pediatr Infect Dis J*. 2013;32(9):950–955
10. Hasegawa K, Tsugawa Y, Brown DF, Mansbach JM, Camargo CA Jr. Trends in bronchiolitis hospitalizations in the United States, 2000-2009. *Pediatrics*. 2013;132(1):28–36
11. Hall CB, Weinberg GA, Blumkin AK, et al. Respiratory syncytial virus-associated hospitalizations among children less than 24 months of age. *Pediatrics*. 2013;132(2). Available at: www.pediatrics.org/cgi/content/full/132/2/e341
12. Hall CB. Nosocomial respiratory syncytial virus infections: the "Cold War" has not ended. *Clin Infect Dis*. 2000;31(2):590–596
13. Stevens TP, Sinkin RA, Hall CB, Maniscalco WM, McConnochie KM. Respiratory syncytial virus and premature infants born at 32 weeks' gestation or earlier: hospitalization and economic implications of prophylaxis. *Arch Pediatr Adolesc Med*. 2000;154(1):55–61
14. American Academy of Pediatrics Steering Committee on Quality Improvement and Management. Classifying recommendations for clinical practice guidelines. *Pediatrics*. 2004;114(3):874–877

15. Ricart S, Marcos MA, Sarda M, et al. Clinical risk factors are more relevant than respiratory viruses in predicting bronchiolitis severity. *Pediatr Pulmonol.* 2013;48(5):456–463
16. Shaw KN, Bell LM, Sherman NH. Outpatient assessment of infants with bronchiolitis. *Am J Dis Child.* 1991;145(2):151–155
17. Hall CB, Powell KR, MacDonald NE, et al. Respiratory syncytial viral infection in children with compromised immune function. *N Engl J Med.* 1986;315(2):77–81
18. Mansbach JM, Piedra PA, Stevenson MD, et al; MARC-30 Investigators. Prospective multicenter study of children with bronchiolitis requiring mechanical ventilation. *Pediatrics.* 2012;130(3). Available at: www.pediatrics.org/cgi/content/full/130/3/e492
19. Prescott WA Jr, Hutchinson DJ. Respiratory syncytial virus prophylaxis in special populations: is it something worth considering in cystic fibrosis and immunosuppression? *J Pediatr Pharmacol Ther.* 2011;16(2):77–86
20. Armstrong D, Grimwood K, Carlin JB, et al. Severe viral respiratory infections in infants with cystic fibrosis. *Pediatr Pulmonol.* 1998;26(6):371–379
21. Alvarez AE, Marson FA, Bertuzzo CS, Arns CW, Ribeiro JD. Epidemiological and genetic characteristics associated with the severity of acute viral bronchiolitis by respiratory syncytial virus. *J Pediatr (Rio J).* 2013;89(6):531–543
22. Iliff A, Lee VA. Pulse rate, respiratory rate, and body temperature of children between two months and eighteen years of age. *Child Dev.* 1952;23(4):237–245
23. Rogers MC. Respiratory monitoring. In: Rogers MC, Nichols DG, eds. *Textbook of Pediatric Intensive Care.* Baltimore, MD: Williams & Wilkins; 1996:332–333
24. Berman S, Simoes EA, Lanata C. Respiratory rate and pneumonia in infancy. *Arch Dis Child.* 1991;66(1):81–84
25. Fleming S, Thompson M, Stevens R, et al. Normal ranges of heart rate and respiratory rate in children from birth to 18 years of age: a systematic review of observational studies. *Lancet.* 2011;377(9770):1011–1018
26. Bonafide CP, Brady PW, Keren R, Conway PH, Marsolo K, Daymont C. Development of heart and respiratory rate percentile curves for hospitalized children. *Pediatrics.* 2013;131(4). Available at: www.pediatrics.org/cgi/content/full/131/4/e1150
27. Margolis P, Gadomski A. The rational clinical examination. Does this infant have pneumonia? *JAMA.* 1998;279(4):308–313
28. Mahabee-Gittens EM, Grupp-Phelan J, Brody AS, et al. Identifying children with pneumonia in the emergency department. *Clin Pediatr (Phila).* 2005;44(5):427–435
29. Brooks AM, McBride JT, McConnochie KM, Aviram M, Long C, Hall CB. Predicting deterioration in previously healthy infants hospitalized with respiratory syncytial virus infection. *Pediatrics.* 1999;104(3 pt 1): 463–467
30. Neuman MI, Monuteaux MC, Scully KJ, Bachur RG. Prediction of pneumonia in a pediatric emergency department. *Pediatrics.* 2011;128(2):246–253
31. Shah S, Bachur R, Kim D, Neuman MI. Lack of predictive value of tachypnea in the diagnosis of pneumonia in children. *Pediatr Infect Dis J.* 2010;29(5):406–409
32. Mansbach JM, McAdam AJ, Clark S, et al. Prospective multicenter study of the viral etiology of bronchiolitis in the emergency department. *Acad Emerg Med.* 2008;15(2): 111–118
33. Mansbach JM, Piedra PA, Teach SJ, et al; MARC-30 Investigators. Prospective multicenter study of viral etiology and hospital length of stay in children with severe bronchiolitis. *Arch Pediatr Adolesc Med.* 2012;166(8):700–706
34. Navas L, Wang E, de Carvalho V, Robinson J; Pediatric Investigators Collaborative Network on Infections in Canada. Improved outcome of respiratory syncytial virus infection in a high-risk hospitalized population of Canadian children. *J Pediatr.* 1992;121(3):348–354
35. Wang EE, Law BJ, Stephens D. Pediatric Investigators Collaborative Network on Infections in Canada (PICNIC) prospective study of risk factors and outcomes in patients hospitalized with respiratory syncytial viral lower respiratory tract infection. *J Pediatr.* 1995;126(2):212–219
36. Chan PW, Lok FY, Khatijah SB. Risk factors for hypoxemia and respiratory failure in respiratory syncytial virus bronchiolitis. *Southeast Asian J Trop Med Public Health.* 2002;33(4):806–810
37. Roback MG, Baskin MN. Failure of oxygen saturation and clinical assessment to predict which patients with bronchiolitis discharged from the emergency department will return requiring admission. *Pediatr Emerg Care.* 1997;13(1):9–11
38. Lowell DI, Lister G, Von Koss H, McCarthy P. Wheezing in infants: the response to epinephrine. *Pediatrics.* 1987;79(6):939–945
39. Destino L, Weisgerber MC, Soung P, et al. Validity of respiratory scores in bronchiolitis. *Hosp Pediatr.* 2012;2(4):202–209
40. Schroeder AR, Marmor AK, Pantell RH, Newman TB. Impact of pulse oximetry and oxygen therapy on length of stay in bronchiolitis hospitalizations. *Arch Pediatr Adolesc Med.* 2004;158(6):527–530
41. Dawson KP, Long A, Kennedy J, Mogridge N. The chest radiograph in acute bronchiolitis. *J Paediatr Child Health.* 1990;26 (4):209–211
42. Schroeder AR, Mansbach JM, Stevenson M, et al. Apnea in children hospitalized with bronchiolitis. *Pediatrics.* 2013;132(5). Available at: www.pediatrics.org/cgi/content/full/132/5/e1194
43. Ralston S, Hill V. Incidence of apnea in infants hospitalized with respiratory syncytial virus bronchiolitis: a systematic review. *J Pediatr.* 2009;155(5):728–733
44. Willwerth BM, Harper MB, Greenes DS. Identifying hospitalized infants who have bronchiolitis and are at high risk for apnea. *Ann Emerg Med.* 2006;48(4):441–447
45. García CG, Bhore R, Soriano-Fallas A, et al. Risk factors in children hospitalized with RSV bronchiolitis versus non-RSV bronchiolitis. *Pediatrics.* 2010;126(6). Available at: www.pediatrics.org/cgi/content/full/126/6/e1453
46. Swingler GH, Hussey GD, Zwarenstein M. Randomised controlled trial of clinical outcome after chest radiograph in ambulatory acute lower-respiratory infection in children. *Lancet.* 1998;351(9100):404–408
47. Schuh S, Lalani A, Allen U, et al. Evaluation of the utility of radiography in acute bronchiolitis. *J Pediatr.* 2007;150(4):429–433
48. Kellner JD, Ohlsson A, Gadomski AM, Wang EE. Efficacy of bronchodilator therapy in bronchiolitis. A meta-analysis. *Arch Pediatr Adolesc Med.* 1996;150(11):1166–1172
49. Flores G, Horwitz RI. Efficacy of beta2-agonists in bronchiolitis: a reappraisal and meta-analysis. *Pediatrics.* 1997;100(2 pt 1):233–239
50. Hartling L, Wiebe N, Russell K, Patel H, Klassen TP. A meta-analysis of randomized controlled trials evaluating the efficacy of epinephrine for the treatment of acute viral bronchiolitis. *Arch Pediatr Adolesc Med.* 2003;157(10):957–964
51. King VJ, Viswanathan M, Bordley WC, et al. Pharmacologic treatment of bronchiolitis in infants and children: a systematic review. *Arch Pediatr Adolesc Med.* 2004;158 (2):127–137
52. Zorc JJ, Hall CB. Bronchiolitis: recent evidence on diagnosis and management. *Pediatrics.* 2010;125(2):342–349
53. Wainwright C. Acute viral bronchiolitis in children—a very common condition with few therapeutic options. *Paediatr Respir Rev.* 2010;11(1):39–45, quiz 45

54. Walsh P, Caldwell J, McQuillan KK, Friese S, Robbins D, Rothenberg SJ. Comparison of nebulized epinephrine to albuterol in bronchiolitis. *Acad Emerg Med.* 2008;15(4):305–313
55. Scarlett EE, Walker S, Rovitelli A, Ren CL. Tidal breathing responses to albuterol and normal saline in infants with viral bronchiolitis. *Pediatr Allergy Immunol Pulmonol.* 2012;25(4):220–225
56. Gadomski AM, Scribani MB. Bronchodilators for bronchiolitis. *Cochrane Database Syst Rev.* 2014;(6):CD001266
57. Mallol J, Barrueto L, Girardi G, et al. Use of nebulized bronchodilators in infants under 1 year of age: analysis of four forms of therapy. *Pediatr Pulmonol.* 1987;3(5):298–303
58. Lines DR, Kattampallil JS, Liston P. Efficacy of nebulized salbutamol in bronchiolitis. *Pediatr Rev Commun.* 1990;5(2):121–129
59. Alario AJ, Lewander WJ, Dennehy P, Seifer R, Mansell AL. The efficacy of nebulized metaproterenol in wheezing infants and young children. *Am J Dis Child.* 1992;146(4):412–418
60. Chavasse RJPG, Seddon P, Bara A, McKean MC. Short acting beta2-agonists for recurrent wheeze in children under two years of age. *Cochrane Database Syst Rev.* 2009;(2):CD002873
61. Totapally BR, Demerci C, Zureikat G, Nolan B. Tidal breathing flow-volume loops in bronchiolitis in infancy: the effect of albuterol [ISRCTN47364493]. *Crit Care.* 2002;6(2):160–165
62. Levin DL, Garg A, Hall LJ, Slogic S, Jarvis JD, Leiter JC. A prospective randomized controlled blinded study of three bronchodilators in infants with respiratory syncytial virus bronchiolitis on mechanical ventilation. *Pediatr Crit Care Med.* 2008;9(6):598–604
63. Bjornson C, Russell K, Vandermeer B, Klassen TP, Johnson DW. Nebulized epinephrine for croup in children. *Cochrane Database Syst Rev.* 2013;(10):CD006619
64. Hartling L, Fernandes RM, Bialy L, et al. Steroids and bronchodilators for acute bronchiolitis in the first two years of life: systematic review and meta-analysis. *BMJ.* 2011;342:d1714
65. Wainwright C, Altamirano L, Cheney M, et al. A multicenter, randomized, double-blind, controlled trial of nebulized epinephrine in infants with acute bronchiolitis. *N Engl J Med.* 2003;349(1):27–35
66. Patel H, Gouin S, Platt RW. Randomized, double-blind, placebo-controlled trial of oral albuterol in infants with mild-to-moderate acute viral bronchiolitis. *J Pediatr.* 2003;142(5):509–514
67. Skjerven HO, Hunderi JO, Brügmann-Pieper SK, et al. Racemic adrenaline and inhalation strategies in acute bronchiolitis. *N Engl J Med.* 2013;368(24):2286–2293
68. Plint AC, Johnson DW, Patel H, et al; Pediatric Emergency Research Canada (PERC). Epinephrine and dexamethasone in children with bronchiolitis. *N Engl J Med.* 2009;360(20):2079–2089
69. Wark PA, McDonald V, Jones AP. Nebulised hypertonic saline for cystic fibrosis. *Cochrane Database Syst Rev.* 2005;(3):CD001506
70. Daviskas E, Anderson SD, Gonda I, et al. Inhalation of hypertonic saline aerosol enhances mucociliary clearance in asthmatic and healthy subjects. *Eur Respir J.* 1996;9(4):725–732
71. Sood N, Bennett WD, Zeman K, et al. Increasing concentration of inhaled saline with or without amiloride: effect on mucociliary clearance in normal subjects. *Am J Respir Crit Care Med.* 2003;167(2):158–163
72. Mandelberg A, Amirav I. Hypertonic saline or high volume normal saline for viral bronchiolitis: mechanisms and rationale. *Pediatr Pulmonol.* 2010;45(1):36–40
73. Zhang L, Mendoza-Sassi RA, Wainwright C, Klassen TP. Nebulized hypertonic saline solution for acute bronchiolitis in infants. *Cochrane Database Syst Rev.* 2008;(4):CD006458
74. Jacobs JD, Foster M, Wan J, Pershad J. 7% Hypertonic saline in acute bronchiolitis: a randomized controlled trial. *Pediatrics.* 2014;133(1). Available at: www.pediatrics.org/cgi/content/full/133/1/e8
75. Wu S, Baker C, Lang ME, et al. Nebulized hypertonic saline for bronchiolitis: a randomized clinical trial. *JAMA Pediatr.* 2014;168(7):657–663
76. Florin TA, Shaw KN, Kittick M, Yakscoe S, Zorc JJ. Nebulized hypertonic saline for bronchiolitis in the emergency department: a randomized clinical trial. *JAMA Pediatr.* 2014;168(7):664–670
77. Sharma BS, Gupta MK, Rafik SP. Hypertonic (3%) saline vs 0.93% saline nebulization for acute viral bronchiolitis: a randomized controlled trial. *Indian Pediatr.* 2013;50(8):743–747
78. Silver AH. Randomized controlled trial of the efficacy of nebulized 3% saline without bronchodilators for infants admitted with bronchiolitis: preliminary data [abstr E-PAS2014:2952.685]. Paper presented at: Pediatric Academic Societies Annual Meeting; May 3–6, 2014; Vancouver, British Columbia, Canada
79. Ralston S, Hill V, Martinez M. Nebulized hypertonic saline without adjunctive bronchodilators for children with bronchiolitis. *Pediatrics.* 2010;126(3). Available at: www.pediatrics.org/cgi/content/full/126/3/e520
80. Luo Z, Liu E, Luo J, et al. Nebulized hypertonic saline/salbutamol solution treatment in hospitalized children with mild to moderate bronchiolitis. *Pediatr Int.* 2010;52(2):199–202
81. Sarrell EM, Tal G, Witzling M, et al. Nebulized 3% hypertonic saline solution treatment in ambulatory children with viral bronchiolitis decreases symptoms. *Chest.* 2002;122(6):2015–2020
82. Rowe BH, Spooner C, Ducharme FM, Bretzlaff JA, Bota GW. Early emergency department treatment of acute asthma with systemic corticosteroids. *Cochrane Database Syst Rev.* 2001;(1):CD002178
83. Smith M, Iqbal S, Elliott TM, Everard M, Rowe BH. Corticosteroids for hospitalised children with acute asthma. *Cochrane Database Syst Rev.* 2003;(2):CD002886
84. Russell KF, Liang Y, O'Gorman K, Johnson DW, Klassen TP. Glucocorticoids for croup. *Cochrane Database Syst Rev.* 2011;(1):CD001955
85. Fernandes RM, Bialy LM, Vandermeer B, et al. Glucocorticoids for acute viral bronchiolitis in infants and young children. *Cochrane Database Syst Rev.* 2013;(6):CD004878
86. Corneli HM, Zorc JJ, Mahajan P, et al; Bronchiolitis Study Group of the Pediatric Emergency Care Applied Research Network (PECARN). A multicenter, randomized, controlled trial of dexamethasone for bronchiolitis [published correction appears in *N Engl J Med* 2008;359(18):1972]. *N Engl J Med.* 2007;357(4):331–339
87. Frey U, von Mutius E. The challenge of managing wheezing in infants. *N Engl J Med.* 2009;360(20):2130–2133
88. Gibson PG, Powell H, Ducharme F. Long-acting beta2-agonists as an inhaled corticosteroid-sparing agent for chronic asthma in adults and children. *Cochrane Database Syst Rev.* 2005;(4):CD005076
89. Barnes PJ. Scientific rationale for using a single inhaler for asthma control. *Eur Respir J.* 2007;29(3):587–595
90. Giembycz MA, Kaur M, Leigh R, Newton R. A Holy Grail of asthma management: toward understanding how long-acting beta (2)-adrenoceptor agonists enhance the clinical efficacy of inhaled corticosteroids. *Br J Pharmacol.* 2008;153(6):1090–1104
91. Kaur M, Chivers JE, Giembycz MA, Newton R. Long-acting beta2-adrenoceptor agonists synergistically enhance glucocorticoid-dependent transcription in human airway

epithelial and smooth muscle cells. *Mol Pharmacol.* 2008;73(1):203–214

92. Holden NS, Bell MJ, Rider CF, et al. β2-Adrenoceptor agonist-induced RGS2 expression is a genomic mechanism of bronchoprotection that is enhanced by glucocorticoids. *Proc Natl Acad Sci U S A.* 2011;108(49):19713–19718
93. Schuh S, Coates AL, Binnie R, et al. Efficacy of oral dexamethasone in outpatients with acute bronchiolitis. *J Pediatr.* 2002;140(1):27–32
94. Bentur L, Shoseyov D, Feigenbaum D, Gorichovsky Y, Bibi H. Dexamethasone inhalations in RSV bronchiolitis: a double-blind, placebo-controlled study. *Acta Paediatr.* 2005;94(7):866–871
95. Kuyucu S, Unal S, Kuyucu N, Yilgor E. Additive effects of dexamethasone in nebulized salbutamol or L-epinephrine treated infants with acute bronchiolitis. *Pediatr Int.* 2004;46(5):539–544
96. Mesquita M, Castro-Rodríguez JA, Heinichen L, Fariña E, Iramain R. Single oral dose of dexamethasone in outpatients with bronchiolitis: a placebo controlled trial. *Allergol Immunopathol (Madr).* 2009; 37(2):63–67
97. Alansari K, Sakran M, Davidson BL, Ibrahim K, Alrefai M, Zakaria I. Oral dexamethasone for bronchiolitis: a randomized trial. *Pediatrics.* 2013;132(4). Available at: www.pediatrics.org/cgi/content/full/132/4/e810
98. Mallory MD, Shay DK, Garrett J, Bordley WC. Bronchiolitis management preferences and the influence of pulse oximetry and respiratory rate on the decision to admit. *Pediatrics.* 2003;111(1). Available at: www.pediatrics.org/cgi/content/full/111/1/e45
99. Corneli HM, Zorc JJ, Holubkov R, et al; Bronchiolitis Study Group for the Pediatric Emergency Care Applied Research Network. Bronchiolitis: clinical characteristics associated with hospitalization and length of stay. *Pediatr Emerg Care.* 2012; 28(2):99–103
100. Unger S, Cunningham S. Effect of oxygen supplementation on length of stay for infants hospitalized with acute viral bronchiolitis. *Pediatrics.* 2008;121(3):470–475
101. Cunningham S, McMurray A. Observational study of two oxygen saturation targets for discharge in bronchiolitis. *Arch Dis Child.* 2012;97(4):361–363
102. Anaesthesia UK. Oxygen dissociation curve. Available at: http://www.anaesthesiauk.com/SearchRender.aspx?DocId=1419&Index=D%3a\dtSearch\UserData\AUK&HitCount=19&hits=4+5+d+e+23+24+37+58+59+a7+a8+14a+14b+17e+180+181+1a9+1aa+1d4 Accessed July 15, 2014
103. McBride SC, Chiang VW, Goldmann DA, Landrigan CP. Preventable adverse events in infants hospitalized with bronchiolitis. *Pediatrics.* 2005;116(3):603–608
104. Hunt CE, Corwin MJ, Lister G, et al; Collaborative Home Infant Monitoring Evaluation (CHIME) Study Group. Longitudinal assessment of hemoglobin oxygen saturation in healthy infants during the first 6 months of age. *J Pediatr.* 1999;135(5):580–586
105. Gavlak JC, Stocks J, Laverty A, et al. The Young Everest Study: preliminary report of changes in sleep and cerebral blood flow velocity during slow ascent to altitude in unacclimatised children. *Arch Dis Child.* 2013;98(5):356–362
106. O'Neil SL, Barysh N, Setear SJ. Determining school programming needs of special population groups: a study of asthmatic children. *J Sch Health.* 1985;55 (6):237–239
107. Bender BG, Belleau L, Fukuhara JT, Mrazek DA, Strunk RC. Psychomotor adaptation in children with severe chronic asthma. *Pediatrics.* 1987;79(5):723–727
108. Rietveld S, Colland VT. The impact of severe asthma on schoolchildren. *J Asthma.* 1999;36(5):409–417
109. Sung V, Massie J, Hochmann MA, Carlin JB, Jamsen K, Robertson CF. Estimating inspired oxygen concentration delivered by nasal prongs in children with bronchiolitis. *J Paediatr Child Health.* 2008;44 (1-2):14–18
110. Ross PA, Newth CJL, Khemani RG. Accuracy of pulse oximetry in children. *Pediatrics.* 2014;133(1):22–29
111. Hasselbalch KA. Neutralitatsregulation und reizbarkeit des atemzentrums in ihren Wirkungen auf die koklensaurespannung des Blutes. *Biochem Ztschr.* 1912;46:403–439
112. Wang EE, Milner RA, Navas L, Maj H. Observer agreement for respiratory signs and oximetry in infants hospitalized with lower respiratory infections. *Am Rev Respir Dis.* 1992;145(1):106–109
113. Rojas MX, Granados Rugeles C, Charry-Anzola LP. Oxygen therapy for lower respiratory tract infections in children between 3 months and 15 years of age. *Cochrane Database Syst Rev.* 2009;(1):CD005975
114. Mitka M. Joint commission warns of alarm fatigue: multitude of alarms from monitoring devices problematic. *JAMA.* 2013;309(22):2315–2316
115. Bowton DL, Scuderi PE, Harris L, Haponik EF. Pulse oximetry monitoring outside the intensive care unit: progress or problem? *Ann Intern Med.* 1991;115(6):450–454
116. Groothuis JR, Gutierrez KM, Lauer BA. Respiratory syncytial virus infection in children with bronchopulmonary dysplasia. *Pediatrics.* 1988;82(2):199–203
117. Voepel-Lewis T, Pechlavanidis E, Burke C, Talsma AN. Nursing surveillance moderates the relationship between staffing levels and pediatric postoperative serious adverse events: a nested case-control study. *Int J Nurs Stud.* 2013;50(7):905–913
118. Bajaj L, Turner CG, Bothner J. A randomized trial of home oxygen therapy from the emergency department for acute bronchiolitis. *Pediatrics.* 2006;117(3):633–640
119. Tie SW, Hall GL, Peter S, et al. Home oxygen for children with acute bronchiolitis. *Arch Dis Child.* 2009;94(8):641–643
120. Halstead S, Roosevelt G, Deakyne S, Bajaj L. Discharged on supplemental oxygen from an emergency department in patients with bronchiolitis. *Pediatrics.* 2012;129(3). Available at: www.pediatrics.org/cgi/content/full/129/3/e605
121. Sandweiss DR, Mundorff MB, Hill T, et al. Decreasing hospital length of stay for bronchiolitis by using an observation unit and home oxygen therapy. *JAMA Pediatr.* 2013;167(5):422–428
122. Flett KB, Breslin K, Braun PA, Hambidge SJ. Outpatient course and complications associated with home oxygen therapy for mild bronchiolitis. *Pediatrics.* 2014;133(5):769–775
123. Gauthier M, Vincent M, Morneau S, Chevalier I. Impact of home oxygen therapy on hospital stay for infants with acute bronchiolitis. *Eur J Pediatr.* 2012;171(12):1839–1844
124. Bergman AB. Pulse oximetry: good technology misapplied. *Arch Pediatr Adolesc Med.* 2004;158(6):594–595
125. Sandweiss DR, Kadish HA, Campbell KA. Outpatient management of patients with bronchiolitis discharged home on oxygen: a survey of general pediatricians. *Clin Pediatr (Phila).* 2012;51(5):442–446
126. Dysart K, Miller TL, Wolfson MR, Shaffer TH. Research in high flow therapy: mechanisms of action. *Respir Med.* 2009;103 (10):1400–1405
127. Milési C, Baleine J, Matecki S, et al. Is treatment with a high flow nasal cannula effective in acute viral bronchiolitis? A physiologic study [published correction appears in *Intensive Care Med.* 2013;39(6): 1170]. *Intensive Care Med.* 2013;39(6): 1088–1094

128. Arora B, Mahajan P, Zidan MA, Sethuraman U. Nasopharyngeal airway pressures in bronchiolitis patients treated with high-flow nasal cannula oxygen therapy. *Pediatr Emerg Care*. 2012;28(11):1179–1184
129. Spentzas T, Minarik M, Patters AB, Vinson B, Stidham G. Children with respiratory distress treated with high-flow nasal cannula. *J Intensive Care Med*. 2009;24(5):323–328
130. Hegde S, Prodhan P. Serious air leak syndrome complicating high-flow nasal cannula therapy: a report of 3 cases. *Pediatrics*. 2013;131(3). Available at: www.pediatrics.org/cgi/content/full/131/3/e939
131. Pham TM, O'Malley L, Mayfield S, Martin S, Schibler A. The effect of high flow nasal cannula therapy on the work of breathing in infants with bronchiolitis [published online ahead of print May 21, 2014]. *Pediatr Pulmonol*. doi:doi:10.1002/ppul.23060
132. Bressan S, Balzani M, Krauss B, Pettenazzo A, Zanconato S, Baraldi E. High-flow nasal cannula oxygen for bronchiolitis in a pediatric ward: a pilot study. *Eur J Pediatr*. 2013;172(12):1649–1656
133. Ganu SS, Gautam A, Wilkins B, Egan J. Increase in use of non-invasive ventilation for infants with severe bronchiolitis is associated with decline in intubation rates over a decade. *Intensive Care Med*. 2012;38(7):1177–1183
134. Wing R, James C, Maranda LS, Armsby CC. Use of high-flow nasal cannula support in the emergency department reduces the need for intubation in pediatric acute respiratory insufficiency. *Pediatr Emerg Care*. 2012;28(11):1117–1123
135. McKiernan C, Chua LC, Visintainer PF, Allen H. High flow nasal cannulae therapy in infants with bronchiolitis. *J Pediatr*. 2010; 156(4):634–638
136. Schibler A, Pham TM, Dunster KR, et al. Reduced intubation rates for infants after introduction of high-flow nasal prong oxygen delivery. *Intensive Care Med*. 2011;37 (5):847–852
137. Kelly GS, Simon HK, Sturm JJ. High-flow nasal cannula use in children with respiratory distress in the emergency department: predicting the need for subsequent intubation. *Pediatr Emerg Care*. 2013;29(8): 888–892
138. Kallappa C, Hufton M, Millen G, Ninan TK. Use of high flow nasal cannula oxygen (HFNCO) in infants with bronchiolitis on a paediatric ward: a 3-year experience. *Arch Dis Child*. 2014;99(8):790–791
139. Hilliard TN, Archer N, Laura H, et al. Pilot study of vapotherm oxygen delivery in moderately severe bronchiolitis. *Arch Dis Child*. 2012;97(2):182–183
140. Roqué i Figuls M, Giné-Garriga M, Granados Rugeles C, Perrotta C. Chest physiotherapy for acute bronchiolitis in paediatric patients between 0 and 24 months old. *Cochrane Database Syst Rev*. 2012;(2): CD004873
141. Aviram M, Damri A, Yekutielli C, Bearman J, Tal A. Chest physiotherapy in acute bronchiolitis [abstract]. *Eur Respir J*. 1992; 5(suppl 15):229–230
142. Webb MS, Martin JA, Cartlidge PH, Ng YK, Wright NA. Chest physiotherapy in acute bronchiolitis. *Arch Dis Child*. 1985;60(11): 1078–1079
143. Nicholas KJ, Dhouieb MO, Marshal TG, Edmunds AT, Grant MB. An evaluation of chest physiotherapy in the management of acute bronchiolitis: changing clinical practice. *Physiotherapy*. 1999;85(12):669–674
144. Bohé L, Ferrero ME, Cuestas E, Polliotto L, Genoff M. Indications of conventional chest physiotherapy in acute bronchiolitis [in Spanish]. *Medicina (B Aires)*. 2004;64 (3):198–200
145. De Córdoba F, Rodrigues M, Luque A, Cadrobbi C, Faria R, Solé D. Fisioterapia respiratória em lactentes com bronquiolite: realizar ou não? *Mundo Saúde*. 2008; 32(2):183–188
146. Gajdos V, Katsahian S, Beydon N, et al. Effectiveness of chest physiotherapy in infants hospitalized with acute bronchiolitis: a multicenter, randomized, controlled trial. *PLoS Med*. 2010;7(9):e1000345
147. Rochat I, Leis P, Bouchardy M, et al. Chest physiotherapy using passive expiratory techniques does not reduce bronchiolitis severity: a randomised controlled trial. *Eur J Pediatr*. 2012;171(3):457–462
148. Postiaux G, Louis J, Labasse HC, et al. Evaluation of an alternative chest physiotherapy method in infants with respiratory syncytial virus bronchiolitis. *Respir Care*. 2011;56(7):989–994
149. Sánchez Bayle M, Martín Martín R, Cano Fernández J, et al. Chest physiotherapy and bronchiolitis in the hospitalised infant. Double-blind clinical trial [in Spanish]. *An Pediatr (Barc)*. 2012;77(1):5–11
150. Mussman GM, Parker MW, Statile A, Sucharew H, Brady PW. Suctioning and length of stay in infants hospitalized with bronchiolitis. *JAMA Pediatr*. 2013;167(5): 414–421
151. Weisgerber MC, Lye PS, Li SH, et al. Factors predicting prolonged hospital stay for infants with bronchiolitis. *J Hosp Med*. 2011;6(5):264–270
152. Nichol KP, Cherry JD. Bacterial-viral interrelations in respiratory infections of children. *N Engl J Med*. 1967;277(13):667–672
153. Field CM, Connolly JH, Murtagh G, Slattery CM, Turkington EE. Antibiotic treatment of epidemic bronchiolitis—a double-blind trial. *BMJ*. 1966;1(5479):83–85
154. Antonow JA, Hansen K, McKinstry CA, Byington CL. Sepsis evaluations in hospitalized infants with bronchiolitis. *Pediatr Infect Dis J*. 1998;17(3):231–236
155. Friis B, Andersen P, Brenøe E, et al. Antibiotic treatment of pneumonia and bronchiolitis. A prospective randomised study. *Arch Dis Child*. 1984;59(11):1038–1045
156. Greenes DS, Harper MB. Low risk of bacteremia in febrile children with recognizable viral syndromes. *Pediatr Infect Dis J*. 1999;18(3):258–261
157. Spurling GK, Doust J, Del Mar CB, Eriksson L. Antibiotics for bronchiolitis in children. *Cochrane Database Syst Rev*. 2011;(6): CD005189
158. Ralston S, Hill V, Waters A. Occult serious bacterial infection in infants younger than 60 to 90 days with bronchiolitis: a systematic review. *Arch Pediatr Adolesc Med*. 2011;165(10):951–956
159. Purcell K, Fergie J. Lack of usefulness of an abnormal white blood cell count for predicting a concurrent serious bacterial infection in infants and young children hospitalized with respiratory syncytial virus lower respiratory tract infection. *Pediatr Infect Dis J*. 2007;26(4):311–315
160. Purcell K, Fergie J. Concurrent serious bacterial infections in 2396 infants and children hospitalized with respiratory syncytial virus lower respiratory tract infections. *Arch Pediatr Adolesc Med*. 2002;156(4):322–324
161. Purcell K, Fergie J. Concurrent serious bacterial infections in 912 infants and children hospitalized for treatment of respiratory syncytial virus lower respiratory tract infection. *Pediatr Infect Dis J*. 2004; 23(3):267–269
162. Kuppermann N, Bank DE, Walton EA, Senac MO Jr, McCaslin I. Risks for bacteremia and urinary tract infections in young febrile children with bronchiolitis. *Arch Pediatr Adolesc Med*. 1997;151(12):1207–1214
163. Titus MO, Wright SW. Prevalence of serious bacterial infections in febrile infants with respiratory syncytial virus infection. *Pediatrics*. 2003;112(2):282–284
164. Melendez E, Harper MB. Utility of sepsis evaluation in infants 90 days of age or younger with fever and clinical bronchiolitis. *Pediatr Infect Dis J*. 2003;22(12): 1053–1056
165. Hall CB, Powell KR, Schnabel KC, Gala CL, Pincus PH. Risk of secondary bacterial

infection in infants hospitalized with respiratory syncytial viral infection. *J Pediatr.* 1988;113(2):266–271

166. Hall CB. Respiratory syncytial virus: a continuing culprit and conundrum. *J Pediatr.* 1999;135(2 pt 2):2–7
167. Davies HD, Matlow A, Petric M, Glazier R, Wang EE. Prospective comparative study of viral, bacterial and atypical organisms identified in pneumonia and bronchiolitis in hospitalized Canadian infants. *Pediatr Infect Dis J.* 1996;15(4):371–375
168. Levine DA, Platt SL, Dayan PS, et al; Multicenter RSV-SBI Study Group of the Pediatric Emergency Medicine Collaborative Research Committee of the American Academy of Pediatrics. Risk of serious bacterial infection in young febrile infants with respiratory syncytial virus infections. *Pediatrics.* 2004;113(6):1728–1734
169. Kellner JD, Ohlsson A, Gadomski AM, Wang EE. Bronchodilators for bronchiolitis. *Cochrane Database Syst Rev.* 2000;(2):CD001266
170. Pinto LA, Pitrez PM, Luisi F, et al. Azithromycin therapy in hospitalized infants with acute bronchiolitis is not associated with better clinical outcomes: a randomized, double-blinded, and placebo-controlled clinical trial. *J Pediatr.* 2012;161(6):1104–1108
171. McCallum GB, Morris PS, Chang AB. Antibiotics for persistent cough or wheeze following acute bronchiolitis in children. *Cochrane Database Syst Rev.* 2012;(12):CD009834
172. Levin D, Tribuzio M, Green-Wrzesinki T, et al. Empiric antibiotics are justified for infants with RSV presenting with respiratory failure. *Pediatr Crit Care.* 2010;11(3):390–395
173. Thorburn K, Reddy V, Taylor N, van Saene HK. High incidence of pulmonary bacterial co-infection in children with severe respiratory syncytial virus (RSV) bronchiolitis. *Thorax.* 2006;61(7):611–615
174. Gomaa MA, Galal O, Mahmoud MS. Risk of acute otitis media in relation to acute bronchiolitis in children. *Int J Pediatr Otorhinolaryngol.* 2012;76(1):49–51
175. Andrade MA, Hoberman A, Glustein J, Paradise JL, Wald ER. Acute otitis media in children with bronchiolitis. *Pediatrics.* 1998;101(4 pt 1):617–619
176. Shazberg G, Revel-Vilk S, Shoseyov D, Ben-Ami A, Klar A, Hurvitz H. The clinical course of bronchiolitis associated with acute otitis media. *Arch Dis Child.* 2000;83(4):317–319
177. Lieberthal AS, Carroll AE, Chonmaitree T, et al. The diagnosis and management of acute otitis media [published correction appears in *Pediatrics.* 2014;133(2):346]. *Pediatrics.* 2013;131(3). Available at: www.pediatrics.org/cgi/content/full/131/3/e964
178. Hoberman A, Paradise JL, Rockette HE, et al. Treatment of acute otitis media in children under 2 years of age. *N Engl J Med.* 2011;364(2):105–115
179. Tähtinen PA, Laine MK, Huovinen P, Jalava J, Ruuskanen O, Ruohola A. A placebo-controlled trial of antimicrobial treatment for acute otitis media. *N Engl J Med.* 2011;364(2):116–126
180. Corrard F, de La Rocque F, Martin E, et al. Food intake during the previous 24 h as a percentage of usual intake: a marker of hypoxia in infants with bronchiolitis: an observational, prospective, multicenter study. *BMC Pediatr.* 2013;13:6
181. Pinnington LL, Smith CM, Ellis RE, Morton RE. Feeding efficiency and respiratory integration in infants with acute viral bronchiolitis. *J Pediatr.* 2000;137(4):523–526
182. Khoshoo V, Edell D. Previously healthy infants may have increased risk of aspiration during respiratory syncytial viral bronchiolitis. *Pediatrics.* 1999;104(6):1389–1390
183. Kennedy N, Flanagan N. Is nasogastric fluid therapy a safe alternative to the intravenous route in infants with bronchiolitis? *Arch Dis Child.* 2005;90(3):320–321
184. Sammartino L, James D, Goutzamanis J, Lines D. Nasogastric rehydration does have a role in acute paediatric bronchiolitis. *J Paediatr Child Health.* 2002;38(3):321–322
185. Kugelman A, Raibin K, Dabbah H, et al. Intravenous fluids versus gastric-tube feeding in hospitalized infants with viral bronchiolitis: a randomized, prospective pilot study. *J Pediatr.* 2013;162(3):640–642.e1
186. Oakley E, Borland M, Neutze J, et al; Paediatric Research in Emergency Departments International Collaborative (PREDICT). Nasogastric hydration versus intravenous hydration for infants with bronchiolitis: a randomised trial. *Lancet Respir Med.* 2013;1(2):113–120
187. Gozal D, Colin AA, Jaffe M, Hochberg Z. Water, electrolyte, and endocrine homeostasis in infants with bronchiolitis. *Pediatr Res.* 1990;27(2):204–209
188. van Steensel-Moll HA, Hazelzet JA, van der Voort E, Neijens HJ, Hackeng WH. Excessive secretion of antidiuretic hormone in infections with respiratory syncytial virus. *Arch Dis Child.* 1990;65(11):1237–1239
189. Rivers RP, Forsling ML, Olver RP. Inappropriate secretion of antidiuretic hormone in infants with respiratory infections. *Arch Dis Child.* 1981;56(5):358–363
190. Wang J, Xu E, Xiao Y. Isotonic versus hypotonic maintenance IV fluids in hospitalized children: a meta-analysis. *Pediatrics.* 2014;133(1):105–113
191. American Academy of Pediatrics, Committee on Infectious Diseases and Bronchiolitis Guidelines Committee. Policy statement: updated guidance for palivizumab prophylaxis among infants and young children at increased risk of hospitalization for respiratory syncytial virus infection. *Pediatrics.* 2014;134(2):415–420
192. American Academy of Pediatrics; Committee on Infectious Diseases and Bronchiolitis Guidelines Committee. Technical report: updated guidance for palivizumab prophylaxis among infants and young children at increased risk of hospitalization for respiratory syncytial virus infection. *Pediatrics.* 2014;134(2):e620–e638.
193. IMpact-RSV Study Group. Palivizumab, a humanized respiratory syncytial virus monoclonal antibody, reduces hospitalization from respiratory syncytial virus infection in high-risk infants. The IMpact-RSV Study Group. *Pediatrics.* 1998;102(3):531–537
194. Feltes TF, Cabalk AK, Meissner HC, et al. Palivizumab prophylaxis reduces hospitalization due to respiratory syncytial virus in young children with hemodynamically significant congenital heart disease. *J Pediatr.* 2003;143(4):532–540
195. Andabaka T, Nickerson JW, Rojas-Reyes MX, Rueda JD, Bacic VV, Barsic B. Monoclonal antibody for reducing the risk of respiratory syncytial virus infection in children. *Cochrane Database Syst Rev.* 2013;(4):CD006602
196. Wang D, Bayliss S, Meads C. Palivizumab for immunoprophylaxis of respiratory syncytial virus (RSV) bronchiolitis in high-risk infants and young children: a systematic review and additional economic modelling of subgroup analyses. *Health Technol Assess.* 2011;1(5):iii–iv, 1–124
197. Hampp C, Kauf TL, Saidi AS, Winterstein AG. Cost-effectiveness of respiratory syncytial virus prophylaxis in various indications. *Arch Pediatr Adolesc Med.* 2011;165(6):498–505
198. Hall CB, Weinberg GA, Iwane MK, et al. The burden of respiratory syncytial virus infection in young children. *N Engl J Med.* 2009;360(6):588–598
199. Dupenthaler A, Ammann RA, Gorgievski-Hrisoho M, et al. Low incidence of respiratory syncytial virus hospitalisations in haemodynamically significant congenital

heart disease. *Arch Dis Child.* 2004;89:961–965

200. Geskey JM, Thomas NJ, Brummel GL. Palivizumab in congenital heart disease: should international guidelines be revised? *Expert Opin Biol Ther.* 2007;7(11):1615–1620
201. Robbie GJ, Zhao L, Mondick J, Losonsky G, Roskos LK. Population pharmacokinetics of palivizumab, a humanized anti-respiratory syncytial virus monoclonal antibody, in adults and children. *Antimicrob Agents Chemother.* 2012;56(9):4927–4936
202. Megged O, Schlesinger Y. Down syndrome and respiratory syncytial virus infection. *Pediatr Infect Dis J.* 2010;29(7):672–673
203. Robinson KA, Odelola OA, Saldanha IJ, Mckoy NA. Palivizumab for prophylaxis against respiratory syncytial virus infection in children with cystic fibrosis. *Cochrane Database Syst Rev.* 2012;(2):CD007743
204. Winterstein AG, Eworuke E, Xu D, Schuler P. Palivizumab immunoprophylaxis effectiveness in children with cystic fibrosis. *Pediatr Pulmonol.* 2013;48(9):874–884
205. Cohen AH, Boron ML, Dingivan C. A phase IV study of the safety of palivizumab for prophylaxis of RSV disease in children with cystic fibrosis [abstract]. *American Thoracic Society Abstracts,* 2005 International Conference; 2005. p. A178
206. Giusti R. North American synagis prophylaxis survey. *Pediatr Pulmonol.* 2009;44(1):96–98
207. El Saleeby CM, Somes GW, DeVincenzo HP, Gaur AH. Risk factors for severe respiratory syncytial virus disease in children with cancer: the importance of lymphopenia and young age. *Pediatrics.* 2008;121(2):235–243
208. Berger A, Obwegeser E, Aberle SW, Langgartner M, Popow-Kraupp T. Nosocomial transmission of respiratory syncytial virus in neonatal intensive care and intermediate care units. *Pediatr Infect Dis J.* 2010;29(7):669–670
209. Ohler KH, Pham JT. Comparison of the timing of initial prophylactic palivizumab dosing on hospitalization of neonates for respiratory syncytial virus. *Am J Health Syst Pharm.* 2013;70(15):1342–1346
210. Blanken MO, Robers MM, Molenaar JM, et al. Respiratory syncytial virus and recurrent wheeze in healthy preterm infants. *N Engl J Med.* 2013;368(19):1794–1799
211. Yoshihara S, Kusuda S, Mochizuki H, Okada K, Nishima S, Simões EAF; C-CREW Investigators. Effect of palivizumab prophylaxis on subsequent recurrent wheezing in preterm infants. *Pediatrics.* 2013;132(5):811–818
212. Hall CB, Douglas RG Jr, Geiman JM. Possible transmission by fomites of respiratory syncytial virus. *J Infect Dis.* 1980;141(1):98–102
213. Sattar SA, Springthorpe VS, Tetro J, Vashon R, Keswick B. Hygienic hand antiseptics: should they not have activity and label claims against viruses? *Am J Infect Control.* 2002;30(6):355–372
214. Picheansathian W. A systematic review on the effectiveness of alcohol-based solutions for hand hygiene. *Int J Nurs Pract.* 2004;10(1):3–9
215. Hall CB. The spread of influenza and other respiratory viruses: complexities and conjectures. *Clin Infect Dis.* 2007;45(3):353–359
216. Boyce JM, Pittet D; Healthcare Infection Control Practices Advisory Committee; HICPAC/SHEA/APIC/IDSA Hand Hygiene Task Force; Society for Healthcare Epidemiology of America/Association for Professionals in Infection Control/Infectious Diseases Society of America. Guideline for Hand Hygiene in Health-Care Settings. Recommendations of the Healthcare Infection Control Practices Advisory Committee and the HICPAC/SHEA/APIC/IDSA Hand Hygiene Task Force. *MMWR Recomm Rep.* 2002;51(RR-16):1–45, quiz CE1–CE4
217. World Health Organization. Guidelines on hand hygiene in health care. Geneva, Switzerland: World Health Organization; 2009. Available at: http://whqlibdoc.who.int/publications/2009/9789241597906_eng.pdf. Accessed July 15, 2014
218. Karanfil LV, Conlon M, Lykens K, et al. Reducing the rate of nosocomially transmitted respiratory syncytial virus. [published correction appears in Am J Infect Control. 1999;27(3):303] *Am J Infect Control.* 1999;27(2):91–96
219. Macartney KK, Gorelick MH, Manning ML, Hodinka RL, Bell LM. Nosocomial respiratory syncytial virus infections: the cost-effectiveness and cost-benefit of infection control. *Pediatrics.* 2000;106(3):520–526
220. Strachan DP, Cook DG. Health effects of passive smoking. 1. Parental smoking and lower respiratory illness in infancy and early childhood. *Thorax.* 1997;52(10):905–914
221. Jones LL, Hashim A, McKeever T, Cook DG, Britton J, Leonardi-Bee J. Parental and household smoking and the increased risk of bronchitis, bronchiolitis and other lower respiratory infections in infancy: systematic review and meta-analysis. *Respir Res.* 2011;12:5
222. Bradley JP, Bacharier LB, Bonfiglio J, et al. Severity of respiratory syncytial virus bronchiolitis is affected by cigarette smoke exposure and atopy. *Pediatrics.* 2005;115(1). Available at: www.pediatrics.org/cgi/content/full/115/1/e7
223. Al-Shawwa B, Al-Huniti N, Weinberger M, Abu-Hasan M. Clinical and therapeutic variables influencing hospitalisation for bronchiolitis in a community-based paediatric group practice. *Prim Care Respir J.* 2007;16(2):93–97
224. Carroll KN, Gebretsadik T, Griffin MR, et al. Maternal asthma and maternal smoking are associated with increased risk of bronchiolitis during infancy. *Pediatrics.* 2007;119(6):1104–1112
225. Semple MG, Taylor-Robinson DC, Lane S, Smyth RL. Household tobacco smoke and admission weight predict severe bronchiolitis in infants independent of deprivation: prospective cohort study. *PLoS ONE.* 2011;6(7):e22425
226. Best D; Committee on Environmental Health; Committee on Native American Child Health; Committee on Adolescence. From the American Academy of Pediatrics: Technical report—Secondhand and prenatal tobacco smoke exposure. *Pediatrics.* 2009;124(5). Available at: www.pediatrics.org/cgi/content/full/124/5/e1017
227. Wilson KM, Wesgate SC, Best D, Blumkin AK, Klein JD. Admission screening for secondhand tobacco smoke exposure. *Hosp Pediatr.* 2012;2(1):26–33
228. Mahabee-Gittens M. Smoking in parents of children with asthma and bronchiolitis in a pediatric emergency department. *Pediatr Emerg Care.* 2002;18(1):4–7
229. Dempsey DA, Meyers MJ, Oh SS, et al. Determination of tobacco smoke exposure by plasma cotinine levels in infants and children attending urban public hospital clinics. *Arch Pediatr Adolesc Med.* 2012;166(9):851–856
230. Rosen LJ, Noach MB, Winickoff JP, Hovell MF. Parental smoking cessation to protect young children: a systematic review and meta-analysis. *Pediatrics.* 2012;129(1):141–152
231. Matt GE, Quintana PJ, Destaillats H, et al. Thirdhand tobacco smoke: emerging evidence and arguments for a multidisciplinary research agenda. *Environ Health Perspect.* 2011;119(9):1218–1226
232. Section on Breastfeeding. Breastfeeding and the use of human milk. *Pediatrics.* 2012;129(3). Available at: www.pediatrics.org/cgi/content/full/129/3/e827
233. Ip S, Chung M, Raman G, et al. *Breastfeeding and Maternal and Infant Health Outcomes in Developed Countries.* Rockville,

MD: Agency for Healthcare Research and Quality; 2007

234. Dornelles CT, Piva JP, Marostica PJ. Nutritional status, breastfeeding, and evolution of infants with acute viral bronchiolitis. *J Health Popul Nutr.* 2007;25(3):336–343

235. Oddy WH, Sly PD, de Klerk NH, et al. Breast feeding and respiratory morbidity in infancy: a birth cohort study. *Arch Dis Child.* 2003;88(3):224–228

236. Nishimura T, Suzue J, Kaji H. Breastfeeding reduces the severity of respiratory syncytial virus infection among young infants: a multi-center prospective study. *Pediatr Int.* 2009;51(6):812–816

237. Petruzella FD, Gorelick MH. Duration of illness in infants with bronchiolitis evaluated in the emergency department. *Pediatrics.* 2010;126(2):285–290

238. von Linstow ML, Eugen-Olsen J, Koch A, Winther TN, Westh H, Hogh B. Excretion patterns of human metapneumovirus and respiratory syncytial virus among young children. *Eur J Med Res.* 2006;11(8):329–335

239. Sacri AS, De Serres G, Quach C, Boulianne N, Valiquette L, Skowronski DM. Transmission of acute gastroenteritis and respiratory illness from children to parents. *Pediatr Infect Dis J.* 2014;33(6):583–588

240. Taylor JA, Kwan-Gett TS, McMahon EM Jr. Effectiveness of an educational intervention in modifying parental attitudes about antibiotic usage in children. *Pediatrics.* 2003;111 (5 pt 1). Available at: www.pediatrics.org/cgi/content/full/111/5pt1/e548

241. Kuzujanakis M, Kleinman K, Rifas-Shiman S, Finkelstein JA. Correlates of parental antibiotic knowledge, demand, and reported use. *Ambul Pediatr.* 2003;3(4):203–210

242. Mangione-Smith R, McGlynn EA, Elliott MN, Krogstad P, Brook RH. The relationship between perceived parental expectations and pediatrician antimicrobial prescribing behavior. *Pediatrics.* 1999;103(4 pt 1):711–718

APPENDIX 1 SEARCH TERMS BY TOPIC

Introduction

MedLine

(("bronchiolitis"[MeSH]) OR ("respiratory syncytial viruses"[MeSH]) NOT "bronchiolitis obliterans"[All Fields])

1. and exp Natural History/
2. and exp Epidemiology/
3. and (exp economics/ or exp "costs and cost analysis"/ or exp "cost allocation"/ or exp cost-benefit analysis/ or exp "cost control"/ or exp "cost of illness"/ or exp "cost sharing"/ or exp health care costs/ or exp health expenditures/)
4. and exp Risk Factors/

Limit to English Language AND Humans AND ("all infant (birth to 23 months)" or "newborn infant (birth to 1 month)" or "infant (1 to 23 months)")

CINAHL

(MM "Bronchiolitis+") AND ("natural history" OR (MM "Epidemiology") OR (MM "Costs and Cost Analysis") OR (MM "Risk Factors"))

The Cochrane Library

Bronchiolitis AND (epidemiology OR risk factor OR cost)

Diagnosis/Severity

MedLine

exp BRONCHIOLITIS/di [Diagnosis] OR exp Bronchiolitis, Viral/di [Diagnosis]

limit to English Language AND ("all infant (birth to 23 months)" or "newborn infant (birth to 1 month)" or "infant (1 to 23 months)")

CINAHL

(MH "Bronchiolitis/DI")

The Cochrane Library

Bronchiolitis AND Diagnosis

*Upper Respiratory Infection Symptoms

MedLine

(exp Bronchiolitis/ OR exp Bronchiolitis, Viral/) AND exp *Respiratory Tract Infections/

Limit to English Language

Limit to "all infant (birth to 23 months)" OR "newborn infant (birth to 1 month)" OR "infant (1 to 23 months)")

CINAHL

(MM "Bronchiolitis+") AND (MM "Respiratory Tract Infections+")

The Cochrane Library

Bronchiolitis AND Respiratory Infection

Inhalation Therapies

*Bronchodilators & Corticosteroids

MedLine

(("bronchiolitis"[MeSH]) OR ("respiratory syncytial viruses"[MeSH]) NOT "bronchiolitis obliterans"[All Fields])

AND (exp Receptors, Adrenergic, β-2/ OR exp Receptors, Adrenergic, β/ OR exp Receptors, Adrenergic, β-1/ OR β adrenergic*.mp. OR exp ALBUTEROL/ OR levalbuterol.mp. OR exp EPINEPHRINE/ OR exp Cholinergic Antagonists/ OR exp IPRATROPIUM/ OR exp Anti-Inflammatory Agents/ OR ics.mp. OR inhaled corticosteroid*.mp. OR exp Adrenal Cortex Hormones/ OR exp Leukotriene Antagonists/ OR montelukast.mp. OR exp Bronchodilator Agents/)

Limit to English Language AND ("all infant (birth to 23 months)" or "newborn infant (birth to 1 month)" or "infant (1 to 23 months)")

CINAHL

(MM "Bronchiolitis+") AND (MM "Bronchodilator Agents")

The Cochrane Library

Bronchiolitis AND (bronchodilator OR epinephrine OR albuterol OR salbutamol OR corticosteroid OR steroid)

*Hypertonic Saline

MedLine

(("bronchiolitis"[MeSH]) OR ("respiratory syncytial viruses"[MeSH]) NOT "bronchiolitis obliterans"[All Fields])

AND (exp Saline Solution, Hypertonic/ OR (aerosolized saline.mp. OR (exp AEROSOLS/ AND exp Sodium Chloride/)) OR (exp Sodium Chloride/ AND exp "Nebulizers and Vaporizers"/) OR nebulized saline.mp.)

Limit to English Language

Limit to "all infant (birth to 23 months)" OR "newborn infant (birth to 1 month)" OR "infant (1 to 23 months)")

CINAHL

(MM "Bronchiolitis+") AND (MM "Saline Solution, Hypertonic")

The Cochrane Library

Bronchiolitis AND Hypertonic Saline

Oxygen

MedLine

(("bronchiolitis"[MeSH]) OR ("respiratory syncytial viruses"[MeSH]) NOT "bronchiolitis obliterans"[All Fields])

1. AND (exp Oxygen Inhalation Therapy/ OR supplemental oxygen.mp. OR oxygen saturation.mp. OR *Oxygen/ad, st [Administration & Dosage, Standards] OR oxygen treatment.mp.)
2. AND (exp OXIMETRY/ OR oximeters.mp.) AND (exp "Reproducibility of Results"/ OR reliability.mp. OR function.mp. OR technical specifications.mp.) OR (percutaneous measurement*.mp. OR exp Blood Gas Analysis/)

Limit to English Language

Limit to "all infant (birth to 23 months)" OR "newborn infant (birth to 1 month)" OR "infant (1 to 23 months)")

CINAHL

(MM "Bronchiolitis+") AND

((MM "Oxygen Therapy") OR (MM "Oxygen+") OR (MM "Oxygen Saturation") OR (MM "Oximetry+") OR (MM "Pulse Oximetry") OR (MM "Blood Gas Monitoring, Transcutaneous"))

The Cochrane Library

Bronchiolitis AND (oxygen OR oximetry)

Chest Physiotherapy and Suctioning

MedLine

(("bronchiolitis"[MeSH]) OR ("respiratory syncytial viruses"[MeSH]) NOT "bronchiolitis obliterans"[All Fields])

1. AND (Chest physiotherapy.mp. OR (exp Physical Therapy Techniques/ AND exp Thorax/))
2. AND (Nasal Suction.mp. OR (exp Suction/))

Limit to English Language

Limit to "all infant (birth to 23 months)" OR "newborn infant (birth to 1 month)" OR "infant (1 to 23 months)")

CINAHL

(MM "Bronchiolitis+")

1. AND ((MH "Chest Physiotherapy (Saba CCC)") OR (MH "Chest Physical Therapy+") OR (MH "Chest Physiotherapy (Iowa NIC)"))
2. AND (MH "Suctioning, Nasopharyngeal")

The Cochrane Library

Bronchiolitis AND (chest physiotherapy OR suction*)

Hydration

MedLine

(("bronchiolitis"[MeSH]) OR ("respiratory syncytial viruses"[MeSH]) NOT "bronchiolitis obliterans"[All Fields])

AND (exp Fluid Therapy/ AND (exp infusions, intravenous OR exp administration, oral))

Limit to English Language

Limit to ("all infant (birth to 23 months)" or "newborn infant (birth to 1 month)" or "infant (1 to 23 months)")

CINAHL

(MM "Bronchiolitis+") AND

((MM "Fluid Therapy+") OR (MM "Hydration Control (Saba CCC)") OR (MM "Hydration (Iowa NOC)"))

The Cochrane Library

Bronchiolitis AND (hydrat* OR fluid*)

SBI and Antibacterials

MedLine

(("bronchiolitis"[MeSH]) OR ("respiratory syncytial viruses"[MeSH]) NOT "bronchiolitis obliterans"[All Fields])

AND

(exp Bacterial Infections/ OR exp Bacterial Pneumonia/ OR exp Otitis Media/ OR exp Meningitis/ OR exp *Anti-bacterial Agents/ OR exp Sepsis/ OR exp Urinary Tract Infections/ OR exp Bacteremia/ OR exp Tracheitis OR serious bacterial infection.mp.)

Limit to English Language

Limit to ("all infant (birth to 23 months)" or "newborn infant (birth to 1 month)" or "infant (1 to 23 months)")

CINAHL

(MM "Bronchiolitis+") AND

((MM "Pneumonia, Bacterial+") OR (MM "Bacterial Infections+") OR (MM "Otitis Media+") OR (MM "Meningitis, Bacterial+") OR (MM "Antiinfective Agents+") OR (MM "Sepsis+") OR (MM "Urinary Tract Infections+") OR (MM "Bacteremia"))

The Cochrane Library

Bronchiolitis AND (serious bacterial infection OR sepsis OR otitis media OR meningitis OR urinary tract infection or bacteremia OR pneumonia OR antibacterial OR antimicrobial OR antibiotic)

Hand Hygiene, Tobacco, Breastfeeding, Parent Education

MedLine

(("bronchiolitis"[MeSH]) OR ("respiratory syncytial viruses"[MeSH]) NOT "bronchiolitis obliterans"[All Fields])

1. AND (exp Hand Disinfection/ OR hand decontamination.mp. OR handwashing.mp.)
2. AND exp Tobacco/
3. AND (exp Breast Feeding/ OR exp Milk, Human/ OR exp Bottle Feeding/)

Limit to English Language

Limit to ("all infant (birth to 23 months)" or "newborn infant (birth to 1 month)" or "infant (1 to 23 months)")

CINAHL

(MM "Bronchiolitis+")

1. AND (MH "Handwashing+")
2. AND (MH "Tobacco+")
3. AND (MH "Breast Feeding+" OR MH "Milk, Human+" OR MH "Bottle Feeding+")

The Cochrane Library

Bronchiolitis

1. AND (Breast Feeding OR breastfeeding)
2. AND tobacco
3. AND (hand hygiene OR handwashing OR hand decontamination)

Bronchiolitis Clinical Practice Guideline Quick Reference Tools

- Action Statement Summary
  — The Diagnosis, Management, and Prevention of Bronchiolitis
- *ICD-10-CM* Coding Quick Reference for Bronchiolitis
- AAP Patient Education Handout
  — *Bronchiolitis and Your Young Child*

Action Statement Summary

The Diagnosis, Management, and Prevention of Bronchiolitis

Key Action Statement 1a

Clinicians should diagnose bronchiolitis and assess disease severity on the basis of history and physical examination (Evidence Quality: B; Recommendation Strength: Strong Recommendation).

Key Action Statement 1b

Clinicians should assess risk factors for severe disease, such as age <12 weeks, a history of prematurity, underlying cardiopulmonary disease, or immunodeficiency, when making decisions about evaluation and management of children with bronchiolitis (Evidence Quality: B; Recommendation Strength: Moderate Recommendation).

Key Action Statement 1c

When clinicians diagnose bronchiolitis on the basis of history and physical examination, radiographic or laboratory studies should not be obtained routinely (Evidence Quality: B; Recommendation Strength: Moderate Recommendation).

Key Action Statement 2

Clinicians should not administer albuterol (or salbutamol) to infants and children with a diagnosis of bronchiolitis (Evidence Quality: B; Recommendation Strength: Strong Recommendation).

Key Action Statement 3

Clinicians should not administer epinephrine to infants and children with a diagnosis of bronchiolitis (Evidence Quality: B; Recommendation Strength: Strong Recommendation).

Key Action Statement 4a

Nebulized hypertonic saline should not be administered to infants with a diagnosis of bronchiolitis in the emergency department (Evidence Quality: B; Recommendation Strength: Moderate Recommendation).

Key Action Statement 4b

Clinicians may administer nebulized hypertonic saline to infants and children hospitalized for bronchiolitis (Evidence Quality: B; Recommendation Strength: Weak Recommendation [based on randomized controlled trials with inconsistent findings]).

Key Action Statement 5

Clinicians should not administer systemic corticosteroids to infants with a diagnosis of bronchiolitis in any setting (Evidence Quality: A; Recommendation Strength: Strong Recommendation).

Key Action Statement 6a

Clinicians may choose not to administer supplemental oxygen if the oxyhemoglobin saturation exceeds 90% in infants and children with a diagnosis of bronchiolitis (Evidence Quality: D; Recommendation Strength: Weak Recommendation [based on low-level evidence and reasoning from first principles]).

Key Action Statement 6b

Clinicians may choose not to use continuous pulse oximetry for infants and children with a diagnosis of bronchiolitis (Evidence Quality: C; Recommendation Strength: Weak Recommendation [based on lower-level evidence]).

Key Action Statement 7

Clinicians should not use chest physiotherapy for infants and children with a diagnosis of bronchiolitis (Evidence Quality: B; Recommendation Strength: Moderate Recommendation).

Key Action Statement 8

Clinicians should not administer antibacterial medications to infants and children with a diagnosis of bronchiolitis unless there is a concomitant bacterial infection, or a strong suspicion of one. (Evidence Quality: B; Recommendation Strength: Strong Recommendation).

Key Action Statement 9

Clinicians should administer nasogastric or intravenous fluids for infants with a diagnosis of bronchiolitis who cannot maintain hydration orally (Evidence Quality: X; Recommendation Strength: Strong Recommendation).

Key Action Statement 10a

Clinicians should not administer palivizumab to otherwise healthy infants with a gestational age of 29 weeks, 0 days or greater (Evidence Quality: B; Recommendation Strength: Strong Recommendation).

Key Action Statement 10b

Clinicians should administer palivizumab during the first year of life to infants with hemodynamically significant heart disease or chronic lung disease of prematurity defined as preterm infants <32 weeks, 0 days' gestation who require >21% oxygen for at least the first 28 days of life (Evidence Quality: B; Recommendation Strength: Moderate Recommendation).

Key Action Statement 10c

Clinicians should administer a maximum 5 monthly doses (15 mg/kg/dose) of palivizumab during the RSV season to infants who qualify for palivizumab in the first year of life (Evidence Quality: B, Recommendation Strength: Moderate Recommendation).

Key Action Statement 11a

All people should disinfect hands before and after direct contact with patients, after contact with inanimate objects in the direct vicinity of the patient, and after removing gloves (Evidence Quality: B; Recommendation Strength: Strong Recommendation).

Key Action Statement 11b

All people should use alcohol-based rubs for hand decontamination when caring for children with bronchiolitis. When alcohol-based rubs are not available, individuals should wash their hands with soap and water (Evidence Quality: B; Recommendation Strength: Strong Recommendation).

Key Action Statement 12a

Clinicians should inquire about the exposure of the infant or child to tobacco smoke when assessing infants and children for bronchiolitis (Evidence Quality: C; Recommendation Strength: Moderate Recommendation).

Key Action Statement 12b

Clinicians should counsel caregivers about exposing the infant or child to environmental tobacco smoke and smoking cessation when assessing a child for bronchiolitis (Evidence Quality: B; Recommendation Strength: Strong Recommendation).

Key Action Statement 13

Clinicians should encourage exclusive breastfeeding for at least 6 months to decrease the morbidity of respiratory infections (Evidence Quality: Grade B; Recommendation Strength: Moderate Recommendation).

Key Action Statement 14

Clinicians and nurses should educate personnel and family members on evidence-based diagnosis, treatment, and prevention in bronchiolitis (Evidence Quality: C; observational studies; Recommendation Strength; Moderate Recommendation).

Coding Quick Reference for Bronchiolitis
ICD-10-CM
J21.0 Acute bronchiolitis due to syncytial virus
J21.1 Acute bronchiolitis due to human metapneumovirus
J21.8 Acute bronchiolitis due to other specified organisms
J21.9 Acute bronchiolitis, unspecified

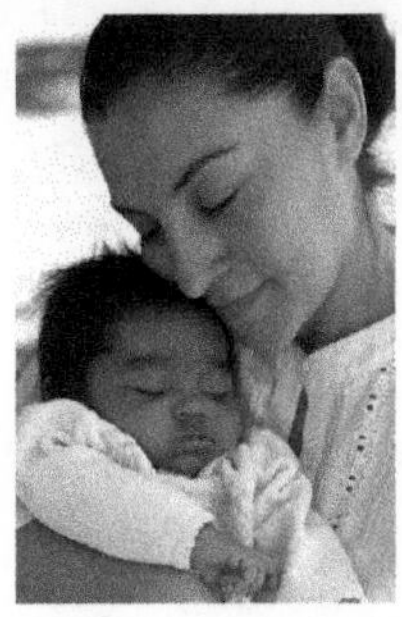

Bronchiolitis and Your Young Child

Bronchiolitis is a common respiratory illness among infants. One of its symptoms is trouble breathing, which can be scary for parents and young children. Read on for more information from the American Academy of Pediatrics about bronchiolitis, its causes, signs and symptoms, how to treat it, and how to prevent it.

What is bronchiolitis?

Bronchiolitis is an infection that causes the small breathing tubes of the lungs (bronchioles) to swell. This blocks airflow through the lungs, making it hard to breathe. It occurs most often in infants because their airways are smaller and more easily blocked than in older children. Bronchiolitis is not the same as bronchitis, which is an infection of the larger, more central airways that typically causes problems in adults.

What causes bronchiolitis?

Bronchiolitis is caused by one of several respiratory viruses such as influenza, respiratory syncytial virus (RSV), parainfluenza, and human metapneumovirus. Other viruses can also cause bronchiolitis.

Infants with RSV infection are more likely to get bronchiolitis with wheezing and difficulty breathing. Most adults and many older children with RSV infection only get a cold. RSV is spread by contact with an infected person's mucus or saliva (respiratory droplets produced during coughing or wheezing). It often spreads through families and child care centers. (See "How can you prevent your baby from getting bronchiolitis?")

What are the signs and symptoms of bronchiolitis?

Bronchiolitis often starts with signs of a cold, such as a runny nose, mild cough, and fever. After 1 or 2 days, the cough may get worse and an infant will begin to breathe faster. Your child may become dehydrated if he cannot comfortably drink fluids.

If your child shows any signs of troubled breathing or dehydration, call your child's doctor.

Signs of troubled breathing

- He may widen his nostrils and squeeze the muscles under his rib cage to try to get more air into and out of his lungs.
- When he breathes, he may grunt and tighten his stomach muscles.
- He will make a high-pitched whistling sound, called a wheeze, when he breathes out.
- He may have trouble drinking because he may have trouble sucking and swallowing.
- If it gets very hard for him to breathe, you may notice a bluish tint around his lips and fingertips. This tells you his airways are so blocked that there is not enough oxygen getting into his blood.

Signs of dehydration

- Drinking less than normal
- Dry mouth
- Crying without tears
- Urinating less often than normal

Can bronchiolitis be treated at home?

There is no specific treatment for RSV or other viruses that cause bronchiolitis. Antibiotics are not helpful because they treat illnesses caused by bacteria, not viruses. However, you can try to ease your child's symptoms.

To relieve a stuffy nose

- Thin the mucus using saline nose drops recommended by your child's doctor. Never use nonprescription nose drops that contain medicine.
- Clear your baby's nose with a suction bulb.Squeeze the bulb first. Gently put the rubber tip into one nostril, and slowly release the bulb. This suction will draw the clogged mucus out of the nose. This works best when your baby is younger than 6 months.

To relieve fever

Give your baby acetaminophen. (Follow the recommended dosage for your baby's age.) Do not give your baby aspirin because it has been associated with Reye syndrome, a disease that affects the liver and brain. Check with your child's doctor first before giving any other cold medicines.

To prevent dehydration

Make sure your baby drinks lots of fluid. She may want clear liquids rather than milk or formula. She may feed more slowly or not feel like eating because she is having trouble breathing.

Bronchiolitis and children with severe chronic illness

Bronchiolitis may cause more severe illness in children who have a chronic illness. If you think your child has bronchiolitis and she has any of the following conditions, call her doctor:

- Cystic fibrosis
- Congenital heart disease
- Chronic lung disease (seen in some infants who were on breathing machines or respirators as newborns)
- Immune deficiency disease (eg, acquired immunodeficiency syndrome [AIDS])
- Organ or bone marrow transplant
- A cancer for which she is receiving chemotherapy

How will your child's doctor treat bronchiolitis?

Your child's doctor will evaluate your child and advise you on nasal suctioning, fever control, and observation, as well as when to call back.

Some children with bronchiolitis need to be treated in a hospital for breathing problems or dehydration. Breathing problems may need to be treated with oxygen and medicine. Dehydration is treated with a special liquid diet or intravenous (IV) fluids.

In very rare cases when these treatments aren't working, an infant might have to be put on a respirator. This is usually only temporary until the infection is gone.

How can you prevent your baby from getting bronchiolitis?

The best steps you can follow to reduce the risk that your baby becomes infected with RSV or other viruses that cause bronchiolitis include

- Make sure everyone washes their hands before touching your baby.
- Keep your baby away from anyone who has a cold, fever, or runny nose.
- Avoid sharing eating utensils and drinking cups with anyone who has a cold, fever, or runny nose.

If you have questions about the treatment of bronchiolitis, call your child's doctor.

From Your Doctor

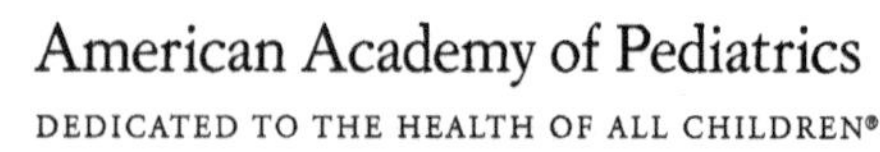

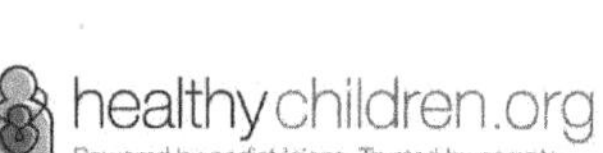

The American Academy of Pediatrics (AAP) is an organization of 67,000 primary care pediatricians, pediatric medical subspecialists, and pediatric surgical specialists dedicated to the health, safety, and well-being of all infants, children, adolescents, and young adults.

The persons whose photographs are depicted in this publication are professional models. They have no relation to the issues discussed. Any characters they are portraying are fictional. The information contained in this publication should not be used as a substitute for the medical care and advice of your pediatrician. There may be variations in treatment that your pediatrician may recommend based on individual facts and circumstances.

© 2019 American Academy of Pediatrics. All rights reserved.

Management of Newly Diagnosed Type 2 Diabetes Mellitus (T2DM) in Children and Adolescents

- *Clinical Practice Guideline*

CLINICAL PRACTICE GUIDELINE

Management of Newly Diagnosed Type 2 Diabetes Mellitus (T2DM) in Children and Adolescents

abstract

Over the past 3 decades, the prevalence of childhood obesity has increased dramatically in North America, ushering in a variety of health problems, including type 2 diabetes mellitus (T2DM), which previously was not typically seen until much later in life. The rapid emergence of childhood T2DM poses challenges to many physicians who find themselves generally ill-equipped to treat adult diseases encountered in children. This clinical practice guideline was developed to provide evidence-based recommendations on managing 10- to 18-year-old patients in whom T2DM has been diagnosed. The American Academy of Pediatrics (AAP) convened a Subcommittee on Management of T2DM in Children and Adolescents with the support of the American Diabetes Association, the Pediatric Endocrine Society, the American Academy of Family Physicians, and the Academy of Nutrition and Dietetics (formerly the American Dietetic Association). These groups collaborated to develop an evidence report that served as a major source of information for these practice guideline recommendations. The guideline emphasizes the use of management modalities that have been shown to affect clinical outcomes in this pediatric population. Recommendations are made for situations in which either insulin or metformin is the preferred first-line treatment of children and adolescents with T2DM. The recommendations suggest integrating lifestyle modifications (ie, diet and exercise) in concert with medication rather than as an isolated initial treatment approach. Guidelines for frequency of monitoring hemoglobin A1c (HbA1c) and finger-stick blood glucose (BG) concentrations are presented. Decisions were made on the basis of a systematic grading of the quality of evidence and strength of recommendation. The clinical practice guideline underwent peer review before it was approved by the AAP. This clinical practice guideline is not intended to replace clinical judgment or establish a protocol for the care of all children with T2DM, and its recommendations may not provide the only appropriate approach to the management of children with T2DM. Providers should consult experts trained in the care of children and adolescents with T2DM when treatment goals are not met or when therapy with insulin is initiated. The AAP acknowledges that some primary care clinicians may not be confident of their ability to successfully treat T2DM in a child because of the child's age, coexisting conditions, and/or other concerns. At any point at which a clinician feels he or she is not adequately trained or is uncertain about treatment, a referral to a pediatric medical subspecialist should be made. If a diagnosis of T2DM is made by a pediatric medical subspecialist, the primary care clinician should develop a comanagement strategy with the subspecialist to ensure that the child continues to receive appropriate care consistent with a medical home model in which the pediatrician partners with parents to ensure that all health needs are met. *Pediatrics* 2013;131:364–382

Kenneth C. Copeland, MD, Janet Silverstein, MD, Kelly R. Moore, MD, Greg E. Prazar, MD, Terry Raymer, MD, CDE, Richard N. Shiffman, MD, Shelley C. Springer, MD, MBA, Vidhu V. Thaker, MD, Meaghan Anderson, MS, RD, LD, CDE, Stephen J. Spann, MD, MBA, and Susan K. Flinn, MA

KEY WORDS

diabetes, type 2 diabetes mellitus, childhood, youth, clinical practice guidelines, comanagement, management, treatment

ABBREVIATIONS

AAP—American Academy of Pediatrics
AAFP—American Academy of Family Physicians
BG—blood glucose
FDA—US Food and Drug Administration
HbA1c—hemoglobin A1c
PES—Pediatric Endocrine Society
T1DM—type 1 diabetes mellitus
T2DM—type 2 diabetes mellitus
TODAY—Treatment Options for type 2 Diabetes in Adolescents and Youth

This document is copyrighted and is property of the American Academy of Pediatrics and its Board of Directors. All authors have filed conflict of interest statements with the American Academy of Pediatrics. Any conflicts have been resolved through a process approved by the Board of Directors. The American Academy of Pediatrics has neither solicited nor accepted any commercial involvement in the development of the content of this publication.

The recommendations in this report do not indicate an exclusive course of treatment or serve as a standard of medical care. Variations, taking into account individual circumstances, may be appropriate.

All clinical practice guidelines from the American Academy of Pediatrics automatically expire 5 years after publication unless reaffirmed, revised, or retired at or before that time.

www.pediatrics.org/cgi/doi/10.1542/peds.2012-3494

doi:10.1542/peds.2012-3494

PEDIATRICS (ISSN Numbers: Print, 0031-4005; Online, 1098-4275).

Copyright © 2013 by the American Academy of Pediatrics

Key action statements are as follows:

1. Clinicians must ensure that insulin therapy is initiated for children and adolescents with T2DM who are ketotic or in diabetic ketoacidosis and in whom the distinction between types 1 and 2 diabetes mellitus is unclear and, in usual cases, should initiate insulin therapy for patients
   a. who have random venous or plasma BG concentrations ≥250 mg/dL; or
   b. whose HbA1c is >9%.

2. In all other instances, clinicians should initiate a lifestyle modification program, including nutrition and physical activity, and start metformin as first-line therapy for children and adolescents at the time of diagnosis of T2DM.

3. The committee suggests that clinicians monitor HbA1c concentrations every 3 months and intensify treatment if treatment goals for finger-stick BG and HbA1c concentrations are not being met (intensification is defined in the Definitions box).

4. The committee suggests that clinicians advise patients to monitor finger-stick BG (see Key Action Statement 4 in the guideline for further details) concentrations in patients who
   a. are taking insulin or other medications with a risk of hypoglycemia; or
   b. are initiating or changing their diabetes treatment regimen; or
   c. have not met treatment goals; or
   d. have intercurrent illnesses.

5. The committee suggests that clinicians incorporate the Academy of Nutrition and Dietetics' *Pediatric Weight Management Evidence-Based Nutrition Practice Guidelines* in their dietary or nutrition counseling of patients with T2DM at the time of diagnosis and as part of ongoing management.

6. The committee suggests that clinicians encourage children and adolescents with T2DM to engage in moderate-to-vigorous exercise for at least 60 minutes daily and to limit nonacademic "screen time" to less than 2 hours a day.

Definitions

Adolescent: an individual in various stages of maturity, generally considered to be between 12 and 18 years of age.

Childhood T2DM: disease in the child who typically

- is overweight or obese (BMI ≥85th–94th and >95th percentile for age and gender, respectively);
- has a strong family history of T2DM;
- has substantial residual insulin secretory capacity at diagnosis (reflected by normal or elevated insulin and C-peptide concentrations);
- has insidious onset of disease;
- demonstrates insulin resistance (including clinical evidence of polycystic ovarian syndrome or acanthosis nigricans);
- lacks evidence for diabetic autoimmunity (negative for autoantibodies typically associated with T1DM). These patients are more likely to have hypertension and dyslipidemia than are those with T1DM.

Clinician: any provider within his or her scope of practice; includes medical practitioners (including physicians and physician extenders), dietitians, psychologists, and nurses.
Diabetes: according to the American Diabetes Association criteria, defined as

1. HbA1c ≥6.5% (test performed in an appropriately certified laboratory); or
2. fasting (defined as no caloric intake for at least 8 hours) plasma glucose ≥126 mg/dL (7.0 mmol/L); or
3. 2-hour plasma glucose ≥200 mg/dL (11.1 mmol/L) during an oral glucose tolerance test performed as described by the World Health Organization by using a glucose load containing the equivalent of 75 g anhydrous glucose dissolved in water; or
4. a random plasma glucose ≥200 mg/dL (11.1 mmol/L) with symptoms of hyperglycemia.

(In the absence of unequivocal hyperglycemia, criteria 1–3 should be confirmed by repeat testing.)

Diabetic ketoacidosis: acidosis resulting from an absolute or relative insulin deficiency, causing fat breakdown and formation of β hydroxybutyrate. Symptoms include nausea, vomiting, dehydration, Kussmaul respirations, and altered mental status.

Fasting blood glucose: blood glucose obtained before the first meal of the day and after a fast of at least 8 hours.

Glucose toxicity: The effect of high blood glucose causing both insulin resistance and impaired β-cell production of insulin.

Intensification: Increase frequency of blood glucose monitoring and adjustment of the dose and type of medication in an attempt to normalize blood glucose concentrations.

Intercurrent illnesses: Febrile illnesses or associated symptoms severe enough to cause the patient to stay home from school and/or seek medical care.

Microalbuminuria: Albumin:creatinine ratio ≥30 mg/g creatinine but <300 mg/g creatinine.

Moderate hyperglycemia: blood glucose = 180–250 mg/dL.

Moderate-to-vigorous exercise: exercise that makes the individual breathe hard and perspire and that raises his or her heart rate. An easy way to define exercise intensity for patients is the "talk test": during moderate physical activity a person can talk, but not sing. During vigorous activity, a person cannot talk without pausing to catch a breath.

Obese: BMI ≥95th percentile for age and gender.

Overweight: BMI between the 85th and 94th percentile for age and gender.

Prediabetes: Fasting plasma glucose ≥100–125 mg/dL or 2-hour glucose concentration during an oral glucose tolerance test ≥126 but <200 mg/dL or an HbA1c of 5.7% to 6.4%.

Severe hyperglycemia: blood glucose >250 mg/dL.

Thiazolidinediones (TZDs): Oral hypoglycemic agents that exert their effect at least in part by activation of the peroxisome proliferator-activated receptor γ.

Type 1 diabetes mellitus (T1DM): Diabetes secondary to autoimmune destruction of β cells resulting in absolute (complete or near complete) insulin deficiency and requiring insulin injections for management.

Type 2 diabetes mellitus (T2DM): The investigators' designation of the diagnosis was used for the purposes of the literature review. The committee acknowledges the distinction between T1DM and T2DM in this population is not always clear cut, and clinical judgment plays an important role. Typically, this diagnosis is made when hyperglycemia is secondary to insulin resistance accompanied by impaired β-cell function resulting in inadequate insulin production to compensate for the degree of insulin resistance.

Youth: used interchangeably with "adolescent" in this document.

INTRODUCTION

Over the past 3 decades, the prevalence of childhood obesity has increased dramatically in North America,[1–5] ushering in a variety of health problems, including type 2 diabetes mellitus (T2DM), which previously was not typically seen until much later in life. Currently, in the United States, up to 1 in 3 new cases of diabetes mellitus diagnosed in youth younger than 18 years is T2DM (depending on the ethnic composition of the patient population),[6,7] with a disproportionate representation in ethnic minorities[8,9] and occurring most commonly among youth between 10 and 19 years of age.[5,10] This trend is not limited to the United States but is occurring internationally[11]; it is projected that by the year 2030, an estimated 366 million people worldwide will have diabetes mellitus.[12]

The rapid emergence of childhood T2DM poses challenges to many physicians who find themselves generally ill-equipped to treat adult diseases encountered in children. Most diabetes education materials designed for pediatric patients are directed primarily to families of children with type 1 diabetes mellitus (T1DM) and emphasize insulin treatment and glucose monitoring, which may or may not be appropriate for children with

T2DM.[13,14] The National Diabetes Education Program TIP sheets (which can be ordered or downloaded from www.yourdiabetesinfo.org or ndep.nih.gov) provide guidance on healthy eating, physical activity, and dealing with T2DM in children and adolescents, but few other resources are available that are directly targeted at youth with this disease.[15] Most medications used for T2DM have been tested for safety and efficacy only in people older than 18 years, and there is scant scientific evidence for optimal management of children with T2DM.[16,17] Recognizing the scarcity of evidence-based data, this report provides a set of guidelines for the management and treatment of children with T2DM that is based on a review of current medical literature covering a period from January 1, 1990, to July 1, 2008.

Despite these limitations, the practicing physician is likely to be faced with the need to provide care for children with T2DM. Thus, the American Academy of Pediatrics (AAP), the Pediatric Endocrine Society (PES), the American Academy of Family Physicians (AAFP), American Diabetes Association, and the Academy of Nutrition and Dietetics (formerly the American Dietetic Association) partnered to develop a set of guidelines that might benefit endocrinologists and generalists, including pediatricians and family physicians alike. This clinical practice guideline may not provide the only appropriate approach to the management of children with T2DM. It is not expected to serve as a sole source of guidance in the management of children and adolescents with T2DM, nor is it intended to replace clinical judgment or establish a protocol for the care of all children with this condition. Rather, it is intended to assist clinicians in decision-making.

Primary care providers should endeavor to obtain the requisite skills to care for children and adolescents with T2DM, and should communicate and work closely with a diabetes team of subspecialists when such consultation is available, practical, and appropriate. The frequency of such consultations will vary, but should usually be obtained at diagnosis and then at least annually if possible. When treatment goals are not met, the committee encourages clinicians to consult with an expert trained in the care of children and adolescents with T2DM.[18,19] When first-line therapy (eg, metformin) fails, recommendations for intensifying therapy should be generally the same for pediatric and adult populations. The picture is constantly changing, however, as new drugs are introduced, and some drugs that initially appeared to be safe demonstrate adverse effects with wider use. Clinicians should, therefore, remain alert to new developments with regard to treatment of T2DM. Seeking the advice of an expert can help ensure that the treatment goals are appropriately set and that clinicians benefit from cutting-edge treatment information in this rapidly changing area.

The Importance of Family-Centered Diabetes Care

Family structure, support, and education help inform clinical decision-making and negotiations with the patient and family about medical preferences that affect medical decisions, independent of existing clinical recommendations. Because adherence is a major issue in any lifestyle intervention, engaging the family is critical not only to maintain needed changes in lifestyle but also to foster medication adherence.[20–22] The family's ideal role in lifestyle interventions varies, however, depending on the child's age. Behavioral interventions in younger children have shown a favorable effect. With adolescents, however, interventions based on target-age behaviors (eg, including phone or Internet-based interventions as well as face-to-face or peer-enhanced activities) appear to foster better results, at least for weight management.[23]

Success in making lifestyle changes to attain therapeutic goals requires the initial and ongoing education of the patient and the entire family about healthy nutrition and exercise. Any behavior change recommendations must establish realistic goals and take into account the families' health beliefs and behaviors. Understanding the patient and family's perception of the disease (and overweight status) before establishing a management plan is important to dispel misconceptions and promote adherence.[24] Because T2DM disproportionately affects minority populations, there is a need to ensure culturally appropriate, family-centered care along with ongoing education.[25–28] Several observational studies cite the importance of addressing cultural issues within the family.[20–22]

Restrictions in Creating This Document

In developing these guidelines, the following restrictions governed the committee's work:

- Although the importance of diabetes detection and screening of at-risk populations is acknowledged and referenced, the guidelines are restricted to patients meeting the diagnostic criteria for diabetes (eg, this document focuses on treatment postdiagnosis). Specifically, this document and its recommendations do not pertain to patients with impaired fasting plasma glucose (100–125 mg/dL) or impaired glucose tolerance (2-hour oral glucose tolerance test plasma glucose: 140–200 mg/dL) or isolated insulin resistance.
- Although it is noted that the distinction between types 1 and 2 diabetes mellitus in children may be

difficult,[29,30] these recommendations pertain specifically to patients 10 to less than 18 years of age with T2DM (as defined above).

- Although the importance of high-risk care and glycemic control in pregnancy, including pregravid glycemia, is affirmed, the evidence considered and recommendations contained in this document do not pertain to diabetes in pregnancy, including diabetes in pregnant adolescents.
- Recommended screening schedules and management tools for select comorbid conditions (hypertension, dyslipidemia, nephropathy, microalbuminuria, and depression) are provided as resources in the accompanying technical report.[31] These therapeutic recommendations were adapted from other recommended guideline documents with references, without an independent assessment of their supporting evidence.

METHODS

A systematic review was performed and is described in detail in the accompanying technical report.[31] To develop the clinical practice guideline on the management of T2DM in children and adolescents, the AAP convened the Subcommittee on Management of T2DM in Children and Adolescents with the support of the American Diabetes Association, the PES, the AAFP, and the Academy of Nutrition and Dietetics. The subcommittee was co-chaired by 2 pediatric endocrinologists preeminent in their field and included experts in general pediatrics, family medicine, nutrition, Native American health, epidemiology, and medical informatics/guideline methodology. All panel members reviewed the AAP policy on Conflict of Interest and Voluntary Disclosure and declared all potential conflicts (see conflicts statements in the Task Force member list).

These groups partnered to develop an evidence report that served as a major source of information for these practice guideline recommendations.[31] Specific clinical questions addressed in the evidence review were as follows: (1) the effectiveness of treatment modalities for T2DM in children and adolescents, (2) the efficacy of pharmaceutical therapies for treatment of children and adolescents with T2DM, (3) appropriate recommendations for screening for comorbidities typically associated with T2DM in children and adolescents, and (4) treatment recommendations for comorbidities of T2DM in children and adolescents. The accompanying technical report contains more information on comorbidities.[31]

Epidemiologic project staff searched Medline, the Cochrane Collaboration, and Embase. MESH terms used in various combinations in the search included diabetes, mellitus, type 2, type 1, treatment, prevention, diet, pediatric, T2DM, T1DM, NIDDM, metformin, lifestyle, RCT, meta-analysis, child, adolescent, therapeutics, control, adult, obese, gestational, polycystic ovary syndrome, metabolic syndrome, cardiovascular, dyslipidemia, men, and women. In addition, the Boolean operators NOT, AND, OR were included in various combinations. Articles addressing treatment of diabetes mellitus were prospectively limited to those that were published in English between January 1990 and June 2008, included abstracts, and addressed children between the ages of 120 and 215 months with an established diagnosis of T2DM. Studies in adults were considered for inclusion if >10% of the study population was 45 years of age or younger. The Medline search limits included the following: clinical trial; meta-analysis; randomized controlled trial; review; child: 6–12 years; and adolescent: 13–18 years. Additional articles were identified by review of reference lists of relevant articles and ongoing studies recommended by a technical expert advisory group. All articles were reviewed for compliance with the search limitations and appropriateness for inclusion in this document.

Initially, 199 abstracts were identified for possible inclusion, of which 52 were retained for systematic review. Results of the literature review were presented in evidence tables and published in the final evidence report. An additional literature search of Medline and the Cochrane Database of

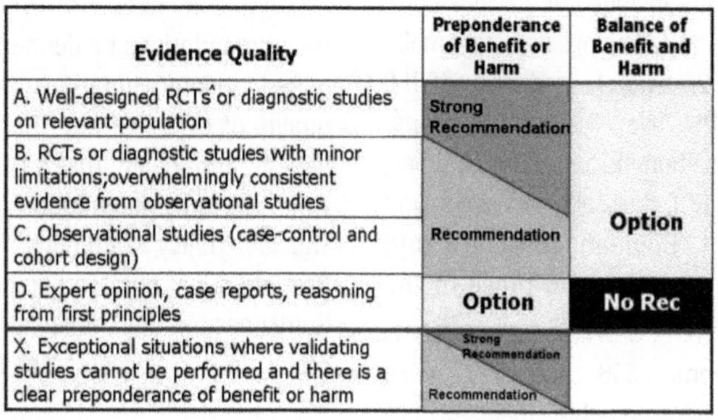

Evidence Quality	Preponderance of Benefit or Harm	Balance of Benefit and Harm
A. Well-designed RCTs* or diagnostic studies on relevant population	Strong Recommendation	Option
B. RCTs or diagnostic studies with minor limitations;overwhelmingly consistent evidence from observational studies		
C. Observational studies (case-control and cohort design)	Recommendation	
D. Expert opinion, case reports, reasoning from first principles	Option	No Rec
X. Exceptional situations where validating studies cannot be performed and there is a clear preponderance of benefit or harm	Strong Recommendation / Recommendation	

FIGURE 1

Evidence quality. Integrating evidence quality appraisal with an assessment of the anticipated balance between benefits and harms if a policy is carried out leads to designation of a policy as a strong recommendation, recommendation, option, or no recommendation.[32] RCT, randomized controlled trial; Rec, recommendation.

TABLE 1 Definitions and Recommendation Implications

Statement	Definition	Implication
Strong recommendation	A *strong recommendation* in favor of a particular action is made when the anticipated benefits of the recommended intervention clearly exceed the harms (as a strong recommendation against an action is made when the anticipated harms clearly exceed the benefits) and the quality of the supporting evidence is excellent. In some clearly identified circumstances, strong recommendations may be made when high-quality evidence is impossible to obtain and the anticipated benefits strongly outweigh the harms.	Clinicians should follow a strong recommendation unless a clear and compelling rationale for an alternative approach is present.
Recommendation	A *recommendation* in favor of a particular action is made when the anticipated benefits exceed the harms but the quality of evidence is not as strong. Again, in some clearly identified circumstances, recommendations may be made when high-quality evidence is impossible to obtain but the anticipated benefits outweigh the harms.	Clinicians would be prudent to follow a recommendation but should remain alert to new information and sensitive to patient preferences.
Option	*Options* define courses that may be taken when either the quality of evidence is suspect or carefully performed studies have shown little clear advantage to 1 approach over another.	Clinicians should consider the option in their decision-making, and patient preference may have a substantial role.
No recommendation	*No recommendation* indicates that there is a lack of pertinent published evidence and that the anticipated balance of benefits and harms is presently unclear.	Clinicians should be alert to new published evidence that clarifies the balance of benefit versus harm.

It should be noted that, because childhood T2DM is a relatively recent medical phenomenon, there is a paucity of evidence for many or most of the recommendations provided. In some cases, supporting references for a specific recommendation are provided that do not deal specifically with childhood T2DM, such as T1DM, childhood obesity, or childhood "prediabetes," or that were not included in the original comprehensive search. Committee members have made every effort to identify those references that did not affect or alter the level of evidence for specific recommendations.

Systematic Reviews was performed in July 2009 for articles discussing recommendations for screening and treatment of 5 recognized comorbidities of T2DM: cardiovascular disease, dyslipidemia, retinopathy, nephropathy, and peripheral vascular disease. Search criteria were the same as for the search on treatment of T2DM, with the inclusion of the term "type 1 diabetes mellitus." Search terms included, in various combinations, the following: diabetes, mellitus, type 2, type 1, pediatric, T2DM, T1DM, NIDDM, hyperlipidemia, retinopathy, microalbuminuria, comorbidities, screening, RCT, meta-analysis, child, and adolescent. Boolean operators and search limits mirrored those of the primary search.

An additional 336 abstracts were identified for possible inclusion, of which 26 were retained for systematic review. Results of this subsequent literature review were also presented in evidence tables and published in the final evidence report. An epidemiologist appraised the methodologic quality of the research before it was considered by the committee members.

The evidence-based approach to guideline development requires that the evidence in support of each key action statement be identified, appraised, and summarized and that an explicit link between evidence and recommendations be defined. Evidence-based recommendations reflect the quality of evidence and the balance of benefit and harm that is anticipated when the recommendation is followed. The AAP policy statement, "Classifying Recommendations for Clinical Practice Guidelines,"[32] was followed in designating levels of recommendation (see Fig 1 and Table 1).

To ensure that these recommendations can be effectively implemented, the Guidelines Review Group at Yale Center for Medical Informatics provided feedback on a late draft of these recommendations, using the GuideLine Implementability Appraisal.[33] Several potential obstacles to successful implementation were identified and resolved in the final guideline. Evidence was incorporated systematically into 6 key action statements about appropriate management facilitated by BRIDGE-Wiz software (Building Recommendations in a Developer's Guideline Editor; Yale Center for Medical Informatics).

A draft version of this clinical practice guideline underwent extensive peer review by 8 groups within the AAP, the American Diabetes Association, PES, AAFP, and the Academy of Nutrition and Dietetics. Members of the subcommittee were invited to distribute the draft to other representatives and committees within their specialty organizations. The resulting comments were reviewed by the subcommittee and incorporated into the guideline, as appropriate. All AAP guidelines are reviewed every 5 years.

KEY ACTION STATEMENTS

Key Action Statement 1

Clinicians must ensure that insulin therapy is initiated for children and adolescents with T2DM who are ketotic or in diabetic ketoacidosis and in whom the distinction between T1DM and T2DM is unclear; and, in usual cases, should initiate insulin therapy for patients:

a. who have random venous or plasma BG concentrations ≥250 mg/dL; or

b. whose HbA1c is >9%.

(Strong Recommendation: evidence quality X, validating studies cannot be performed, and C, observational studies and expert opinion; preponderance of benefit over harm.)

Action Statement Profile KAS 1

Aggregate evidence quality	X (validating studies cannot be performed)
Benefits	Avoidance of progression of diabetic ketoacidosis (DKA) and worsening metabolic acidosis; resolution of acidosis and hyperglycemia; avoidance of coma and/or death. Quicker restoration of glycemic control, potentially allowing islet β cells to "rest and recover," increasing long-term adherence to treatment; avoiding progression to DKA if T1DM. Avoiding hospitalization. Avoidance of potential risks associated with the use of other agents (eg, abdominal discomfort, bloating, loose stools with metformin; possible cardiovascular risks with sulfonylureas).
Harms/risks/cost	Potential for hypoglycemia, insulin-induced weight gain, cost, patient discomfort from injection, necessity for BG testing, more time required by the health care team for patient training.
Benefits-harms assessment	Preponderance of benefit over harm.
Value judgments	Extensive clinical experience of the expert panel was relied on in making this recommendation.
Role of patient preferences	Minimal.
Exclusions	None.
Intentional vagueness	None.
Strength	Strong recommendation.

The presentation of T2DM in children and adolescents varies according to the disease stage. Early in the disease, before diabetes diagnostic criteria are met, insulin resistance predominates with compensatory high insulin secretion, resulting in normoglycemia. Over time, β cells lose their ability to secrete adequate amounts of insulin to overcome insulin resistance, and hyperglycemia results. Early in this process, blood glucose (BG) concentrations may be normal much of the time and the patient likely will be asymptomatic. At this stage, the disease may only be detected by abnormal BG concentrations identified during screening. As insulin secretion declines further, the patient is likely to develop symptoms of hyperglycemia, occasionally with ketosis or frank ketoacidosis. High glucose concentrations can cause a reversible toxicity to islet β cells that contributes further to insulin deficiency. Of adolescents in whom T2DM is subsequently diagnosed, 5% to 25% present with ketoacidosis.[34]

Diabetic ketoacidosis must be treated with insulin and fluid and electrolyte replacement to prevent worsening metabolic acidosis, coma, and death. Children and adolescents with symptoms of hyperglycemia (polyuria, polydipsia, and polyphagia) who are diagnosed with diabetes mellitus should be evaluated for ketosis (serum or urine ketones) and, if positive, for ketoacidosis (venous pH), even if their phenotype and risk factor status (obesity, acanthosis nigricans, positive family history of T2DM) suggests T2DM. Patients in whom ketoacidosis is diagnosed require immediate treatment with insulin and fluid replacement in an inpatient setting under the supervision of a physician who is experienced in treating this complication.

Youth and adolescents who present with T2DM with poor glycemic control (BG concentrations ≥250 mg/dL or HbA1c >9%) but who lack evidence of ketosis or ketoacidosis may also benefit from initial treatment with insulin, at least on a short-term basis.[34] This allows for quicker restoration of glycemic control and, theoretically, may allow islet β cells to "rest and recover."[35,36] Furthermore, it has been noted that initiation of insulin may increase long-term adherence to treatment in children and adolescents with T2DM by enhancing the patient's perception of the seriousness of the disease.[7,37–40] Many patients with T2DM can be weaned gradually from insulin therapy and subsequently managed with metformin and lifestyle modification.[34]

As noted previously, in some children and adolescents with newly diagnosed diabetes mellitus, it may be difficult to distinguish between type 1 and type 2 disease (eg, an obese child presenting with ketosis).[39,41] These patients are best managed initially with insulin therapy while appropriate tests are performed to differentiate between T1DM and T2DM. The care of children and adolescents who have either newly diagnosed T2DM or undifferentiated-type diabetes and who require initial insulin treatment should be supervised by a physician experienced in treating diabetic patients with insulin.

Key Action Statement 2

In all other instances, clinicians should initiate a lifestyle modification program, including nutrition

and physical activity, and start metformin as first-line therapy for children and adolescents at the time of diagnosis of T2DM. (Strong recommendation: evidence quality B; 1 RCT showing improved outcomes with metformin versus lifestyle; preponderance of benefits over harms.)

Action Statement Profile KAS 2

Aggregate evidence quality	B (1 randomized controlled trial showing improved outcomes with metformin versus lifestyle combined with expert opinion).
Benefit	Lower HbA1c, target HbA1c sustained longer, less early deterioration of BG, less chance of weight gain, improved insulin sensitivity, improved lipid profile.
Harm (of using metformin)	Gastrointestinal adverse effects or potential for lactic acidosis and vitamin B_{12} deficiency, cost of medications, cost to administer, need for additional instruction about medication, self-monitoring blood glucose (SMBG), perceived difficulty of insulin use, possible metabolic deterioration if T1DM is misdiagnosed and treated as T2DM, potential risk of lactic acidosis in the setting of ketosis or significant dehydration. It should be noted that there have been no cases reported of vitamin B_{12} deficiency or lactic acidosis with the use of metformin in children.
Benefits-harms assessment	Preponderance of benefit over harm.
Value judgments	Committee members valued faster achievement of BG control over not medicating children.
Role of patient preferences	Moderate; precise implementation recommendations likely will be dictated by patient preferences regarding healthy nutrition, potential medication adverse reaction, exercise, and physical activity.
Exclusions	Although the recommendation to start metformin applies to all, certain children and adolescents with T2DM will not be able to tolerate metformin. In addition, certain older or more debilitated patients with T2DM may be restricted in the amount of moderate-to-vigorous exercise they can perform safely. Nevertheless, this recommendation applies to the vast majority of children and adolescents with T2DM.
Intentional vagueness	None.
Policy level	Strong recommendation.

Metformin as First-Line Therapy

Because of the low success rate with diet and exercise alone in pediatric patients diagnosed with T2DM, metformin should be initiated along with the promotion of lifestyle changes, unless insulin is needed to reverse glucose toxicity in the case of significant hyperglycemia or ketoacidosis (see Key Action Statement 1). Because gastrointestinal adverse effects are common with metformin therapy, the committee recommends starting the drug at a low dose of 500 mg daily, increasing by 500 mg every 1 to 2 weeks, up to an ideal and maximum dose of 2000 mg daily in divided doses.[41] It should be noted that the main gastrointestinal adverse effects (abdominal pain, bloating, loose stools) present at initiation of metformin often are transient and often disappear completely if medication is continued. Generally, doses higher than 2000 mg daily do not provide additional therapeutic benefit.[34,42,43] In addition, the use of extended-release metformin, especially with evening dosing, may be considered, although data regarding the frequency of adverse effects with this preparation are scarce. Metformin is generally better tolerated when taken with food. It is important to recognize the paucity of credible RCTs in adolescents with T2DM. The evidence to recommend initiating metformin at diagnosis along with lifestyle changes comes from 1 RCT, several observational studies, and consensus recommendations.

Lifestyle modifications (including nutrition interventions and increased physical activity) have long been the cornerstone of therapy for T2DM. Yet, medical practitioners recognize that effecting these changes is both challenging and often accompanied by regression over time to behaviors not conducive to maintaining the target range of BG concentrations. In pediatric patients, lifestyle change is most likely to be successful when a multidisciplinary approach is used and the entire family is involved. (Encouragement of healthy eating and physical exercise are discussed in Key Action Statements 5 and 6.) Unfortunately, efforts at lifestyle change often fail for a variety of reasons, including high rates of loss to follow-up; a high rate of depression in teenagers, which affects adherence; and peer pressure to participate in activities that often center on unhealthy eating.

Expert consensus is that fewer than 10% of pediatric T2DM patients will attain their BG goals through lifestyle interventions alone.[6,35,44] It is possible that the poor long-term success rates observed from lifestyle interventions stem from patients' perception that the intervention is not important because medications are not being prescribed. One might speculate that prescribing medications, particularly insulin therapy, may convey a greater degree of concern for the patient's health and the seriousness of the diagnosis, relative to that conveyed when medications are not needed, and that improved treatment adherence and follow-up may result from the use of medication. Indeed, 2 prospective observational studies revealed that treatment with lifestyle modification alone is associated with a higher rate of loss to follow-up than that found in patients who receive medication.[45]

Before initiating treatment with metformin, a number of important considerations must be taken into account. First, it is important to determine whether the child with a new diagnosis has T1DM or T2DM, and it is critical to err on the side of caution if there is any uncertainty. The 2009 *Clinical Practice Consensus Guidelines on Type 2 Diabetes in Children and Adolescents* from the International Society for Pediatric and Adolescent Diabetes provides more information on the classification of diabetes in children and adolescents with new diagnoses.[46] If the diagnosis is unclear (as may be the case when an obese child with diabetes presents also with ketosis), the adolescent must be treated with insulin until the T2DM diagnosis is confirmed.[47] Although it is recognized that some children with newly diagnosed T2DM may respond to metformin alone, the committee believes that the presence of either ketosis or ketoacidosis dictates an absolute initial requirement for insulin replacement. (This is addressed in Key Action Statement 1.)

Although there is little debate that a child presenting with significant hyperglycemia and/or ketosis requires insulin, children presenting with more modest levels of hyperglycemia (eg, random BG of 200–249 mg/dL) or asymptomatic T2DM present additional therapeutic challenges to the clinician. In such cases, metformin alone, insulin alone, or metformin with insulin all represent reasonable options. Additional agents are likely to become reasonable options for initial pharmacologic management in the near future. Although metformin and insulin are the only antidiabetic agents currently approved by the US Food and Drug Administration (FDA) for use in children, both thiazolidinediones and incretins are occasionally used in adolescents younger than 18 years.[48]

Metformin is recommended as the initial pharmacologic agent in adolescents presenting with mild hyperglycemia and without ketonuria or severe hyperglycemia. In addition to improving hepatic insulin sensitivity, metformin has a number of practical advantages over insulin:

- Potential weight loss or weight neutrality.[37,48]
- Because of a lower risk of hypoglycemia, less frequent finger-stick BG measurements are required with metformin, compared with insulin therapy or sulfonylureas.[37,42,49–51]
- Improves insulin sensitivity and may normalize menstrual cycles in females with polycystic ovary syndrome. (Because metformin may also improve fertility in patients with polycystic ovary syndrome, contraception is indicated for sexually active patients who wish to avoid pregnancy.)
- Taking pills does not have the discomfort associated with injections.
- Less instruction time is required to start oral medication, making it is easier for busy practitioners to prescribe.
- Adolescents do not always accept injections, so oral medication might enhance adherence.[52]

Potential advantages of insulin over metformin for treatment at diabetes onset include the following:

- Metabolic control may be achieved more rapidly with insulin compared with metformin therapy.[37]
- With appropriate education and targeting the regimen to the individual, adolescents are able to accept and use insulin therapy with improved metabolic outcomes.[53]
- Insulin offers theoretical benefits of improved metabolic control while preserving β-cell function or even reversing β-cell damage.[34,35]
- Initial use of insulin therapy may convey to the patient a sense of seriousness of the disease.[7,53]

Throughout the writing of these guidelines, the authors have been following the progress of the National Institute of Diabetes and Digestive and Kidney Diseases–supported Treatment Options for type 2 Diabetes in Adolescents and Youth (TODAY) trial,[54] designed to compare standard (metformin alone) therapy versus more aggressive therapy as the initial treatment of youth with recent-onset T2DM. Since the completion of these guidelines, results of the TODAY trial have become available and reveal that metformin alone is inadequate in effecting sustained glycemic control in the majority of youth with diabetes. The study also revealed that the addition of rosiglitazone to metformin is superior to metformin alone in preserving glycemic control. Direct application of these findings to clinical practice is problematic, however, because rosiglitazone is not FDA-approved for use in children, and its use, even in adults, is now severely restricted by the FDA because of serious adverse effects reported in adults. Thus, the results suggest that therapy that is more aggressive than metformin monotherapy may be required in these adolescents to prevent loss of glycemic control, but they do not provide specific guidance because it is not known whether the effect of the additional agent was specific to rosiglitazone or would be seen with the addition of other agents. Unfortunately, there are limited data for the use of other currently available oral or injected hypoglycemic agents in this age range, except for insulin. Therefore, the writing group for these guidelines continues to recommend metformin as first-line therapy in this age group but with close monitoring for glycemic deterioration and the early addition of insulin or another pharmacologic agent if needed.

Lifestyle Modification, Including Nutrition and Physical Activity

Although lifestyle changes are considered indispensable to reaching treatment goals in diabetes, no significant data from RCTs provide information on success rates with such an approach alone.

A potential downside for initiating lifestyle changes alone at T2DM onset is potential loss of patients to follow-up and worse health outcomes. The value of lifestyle modification in the management of adolescents with T2DM is likely forthcoming after a more detailed analysis of the lifestyle intervention arm of the multicenter TODAY trial becomes available.[54] As noted previously, although it was published after this guideline was developed, the TODAY trial indicated that results from the metformin-plus-lifestyle intervention were not significantly different from either metformin alone or the metformin-plus-rosiglitazone intervention in maintaining glycemic control over time.[54]

Summary

As noted previously, metformin is a safe and effective agent for use at the time of diagnosis in conjunction with lifestyle changes. Although observational studies and expert opinion strongly support lifestyle changes as a key component of the regimen in addition to metformin, randomized trials are needed to delineate whether using lifestyle options alone is a reasonable first step in treating any select subgroups of children with T2DM.

Key Action Statement 3

The committee suggests that clinicians monitor HbA1c concentrations every 3 months and intensify treatment if treatment goals for BG and HbA1c concentrations are not being met. (Option: evidence quality D; expert opinion and studies in children with T1DM and in adults with T2DM; preponderance of benefits over harms.)

Action Statement Profile KAS 3

Aggregate evidence quality	D (expert opinion and studies in children with T1DM and in adults with T2DM; no studies have been performed in children and adolescents with T2DM).
Benefit	Diminishing the risk of progression of disease and deterioration resulting in hospitalization; prevention of microvascular complications of T2DM.
Harm	Potential for hypoglycemia from overintensifying treatment to reach HbA1c target goals; cost of frequent testing and medical consultation; possible patient discomfort.
Benefits-harms assessment	Preponderance of benefits over harms.
Value judgments	Recommendation dictated by widely accepted standards of diabetic care.
Role of patient preferences	Minimal; recommendation dictated by widely accepted standards of diabetic care.
Exclusions	None.
Intentional vagueness	Intentional vagueness in the recommendation as far as setting goals and intensifying treatment attributable to limited evidence.
Policy level	Option.

HbA1c provides a measure of glycemic control in patients with diabetes mellitus and allows an estimation of the individual's average BG over the previous 8 to 12 weeks. No RCTs have evaluated the relationship between glycemic control and the risk of developing microvascular and/or macrovascular complications in children and adolescents with T2DM. A number of studies of children with T1DM[55–57] and adults with T2DM have, however, shown a significant relationship between glycemic control (as measured by HbA1c concentration) and the risk of microvascular complications (eg, retinopathy, nephropathy, and neuropathy).[58,59] The relationship between HbA1c concentration and risk of microvascular complications appears to be curvilinear; the lower the HbA1c concentration, the lower the downstream risk of microvascular complications, with the greatest risk reduction seen at the highest HbA1c concentrations.[57]

It is generally recommended that HbA1c concentrations be measured every 3 months.[60] For adults with T1DM, the American Diabetes Association recommends target HbA1c concentrations of less than 7%; the American Association of Clinical Endocrinologists recommends target concentrations of less than 6.5%. Although HbA1c target concentrations for children and adolescents with T1DM are higher,[13] several review articles suggest target HbA1c concentrations of less than 7% for children and adolescents with T2DM.[40,61–63] The committee concurs that, ideally, target HbA1c concentration should be less than 7% but notes that specific goals must be achievable for the individual patient and that this concentration may not be applicable for all patients. For patients in whom a target concentration of less than 7% seems unattainable, individualized goals should be set, with the ultimate goal of reaching guideline target concentrations. In addition, in the absence of hypoglycemia, even lower HbA1c target concentrations can be considered on the basis of an absence of hypoglycemic events and other individual considerations.

When concentrations are found to be above the target, therapy should be intensified whenever possible, with the goal of bringing the concentration to target. Intensification activities may include, but are not limited to, increasing the frequency of clinic visits, engaging in more frequent BG monitoring, adding 1 or more antidiabetic agents, meeting with a registered dietitian and/or diabetes educator, and increasing attention to diet and exercise regimens. Patients whose HbA1c concentrations remain relatively stable may only need to be tested every 6 months. Ideally, real-time HbA1c concentrations should be available at the time of the patient's visit with the clinician to allow the physician and patient and/or parent to discuss intensification of therapy during the visit, if needed.

Key Action Statement 4

The committee suggests that clinicians advise patients to monitor finger-stick BG concentrations in those who

a. are taking insulin or other medications with a risk of hypoglycemia; or
b. are initiating or changing their diabetes treatment regimen; or
c. have not met treatment goals; or
d. have intercurrent illnesses.

(Option: evidence quality D; expert consensus. Preponderance of benefits over harms.)

Action Statement Profile KAS 4

Aggregate evidence quality	D (expert consensus).
Benefit	Potential for improved metabolic control, improved potential for prevention of hypoglycemia, decreased long-term complications.
Harm	Patient discomfort, cost of materials.
Benefits-harms assessment	Benefit over harm.
Value judgments	Despite lack of evidence, there were general committee perceptions that patient safety concerns related to insulin use or clinical status outweighed any risks from monitoring.
Role of patient preferences	Moderate to low; recommendation driven primarily by safety concerns.
Exclusions	None.
Intentional vagueness	Intentional vagueness in the recommendation about specific approaches attributable to lack of evidence and the need to individualize treatment.
Policy level	Option.

Glycemic control correlates closely with the frequency of BG monitoring in adolescents with T1DM.[64,65] Although studies evaluating the efficacy of frequent BG monitoring have not been conducted in children and adolescents with T2DM, benefits have been described in insulin-treated adults with T2DM who tested their BG 4 times per day, compared with adults following a less frequent monitoring regimen.[66] These data support the value of BG monitoring in adults treated with insulin, and likely are relevant to youth with T2DM as well, especially those treated with insulin, at the onset of the disease, when treatment goals are not met, and when the treatment regimen is changed. The committee believes that current (2011) ADA recommendations for finger-stick BG monitoring apply to most youth with T2DM[67]:

- Finger-stick BG monitoring should be performed 3 or more times daily for patients using multiple insulin injections or insulin pump therapy.
- For patients using less-frequent insulin injections, noninsulin therapies, or medical nutrition therapy alone, finger-stick BG monitoring may be useful as a guide to the success of therapy.
- To achieve postprandial glucose targets, postprandial finger-stick BG monitoring may be appropriate.

Recognizing that current practices may not always reflect optimal care, a 2004 survey of practices among members of the PES revealed that 36% of pediatric endocrinologists asked their pediatric patients with T2DM to monitor BG concentrations twice daily; 12% asked patients to do so once daily; 13% asked patients to do so 3 times per day; and 12% asked patients to do so 4 times daily.[61] The questionnaire provided to the pediatric endocrinologists did not ask about the frequency of BG monitoring in relationship to the diabetes regimen, however.

Although normoglycemia may be difficult to achieve in adolescents with T2DM, a fasting BG concentration of 70 to 130 mg/dL is a reasonable target for most. In addition, because postprandial hyperglycemia has been associated with increased risk of cardiovascular events in adults, postprandial BG testing may be valuable in select patients. BG concentrations obtained 2 hours after meals (and paired with pre-meal concentrations) provide an index of glycemic excursion, and may be useful in improving glycemic control, particularly for the patient whose fasting plasma glucose is normal but whose HbA1c is not at target.[68] Recognizing the limited evidence for benefit of FSBG testing in this population, the committee provides suggested guidance for testing frequency, tailored to the medication regimen, as follows:

BG Testing Frequency for Patients With Newly Diagnosed T2DM: Fasting, Premeal, and Bedtime Testing

The committee suggests that all patients with newly diagnosed T2DM, regardless of prescribed treatment plan, should perform finger-stick BG monitoring before meals (including a morning fasting concentration) and at bedtime until reasonable metabolic control is achieved.[69] Once BG concentrations are at target levels, the frequency of monitoring can be modified depending on the medication used, the regimen's intensity, and the patient's metabolic control. Patients who are prone to marked hyperglycemia or hypoglycemia or who are on a therapeutic regimen associated with increased risk of hypoglycemia will require continued frequent BG testing. Expectations for frequency and timing of BG monitoring should be clearly defined through shared goal-setting between the patient and clinician. The adolescent and family members should be given a written action plan stating the medication regimen, frequency and timing of expected BG monitoring, as well as follow-up instructions.

BG Testing Frequency for Patients on Single Insulin Daily Injections and Oral Agents

Single bedtime long-acting insulin: The simplest insulin regimen consists of a single injection of long-acting insulin at bedtime (basal insulin only). The appropriateness of the insulin dose for patients using this regimen is best defined by the fasting/prebreakfast BG test. For patients on this insulin regimen, the committee suggests daily fasting BG measurements. This regimen is associated with some risk of hypoglycemia (especially overnight or fasting hypoglycemia) and may not provide adequate insulin coverage for mealtime ingestions throughout the day, as reflected by fasting BG concentrations in target, but daytime readings above target. In such cases, treatment with meglitinide (Prandin [Novo Nordisk Pharmaceuticals] or Starlix [Novartis Pharmaceuticals]) or a short-acting insulin before meals (see below) may be beneficial.

Oral agents: Once treatment goals are met, the frequency of monitoring can be decreased; however, the committee recommends some continued BG testing for all youth with T2DM, at a frequency determined within the clinical context (e.g. medication regimen, HbA1c, willingness of the patient, etc.). For example, an infrequent or intermittent monitoring schedule may be adequate when the patient is using exclusively an oral agent associated with a low risk of hypoglycemia and if HbA1c concentrations are in the ideal or non-diabetic range. A more frequent monitoring schedule should be advised during times of illness or if symptoms of hyperglycemia or hypoglycemia develop.

Oral agent plus a single injection of a long-acting insulin: Some youth with T2DM can be managed successfully with a single injection of long-acting insulin in conjunction with an oral agent. Twice a day BG monitoring (fasting plus a second BG concentration – ideally 2-hour post prandial) often is recommended, as long as HbA1c and BG concentrations remain at goal and the patient remains asymptomatic.

BG Testing Frequency for Patients Receiving Multiple Daily Insulin Injections (eg, Basal Bolus Regimens): Premeal and Bedtime Testing

Basal bolus regimens are commonly used in children and youth with T1DM and may be appropriate for some youth with T2DM as well. They are the most labor intensive, providing both basal insulin plus bolus doses of short-acting insulin at meals. Basal insulin is provided through either the use of long-acting, relatively peak-free insulin (by needle) or via an insulin pump. Bolus insulin doses are given at meal-time, using one of the rapid-acting insulin analogs. The bolus dose is calculated by using a correction algorithm for the premeal BG concentration as well as a "carb ratio," in which 1 unit of a rapid-acting insulin analog is given for "X" grams of carbohydrates ingested (see box below). When using this method, the patient must be willing and able to count the number of grams of carbohydrates in the meal and divide by the assigned "carb ratio (X)" to know how many units of insulin should be taken. In addition, the patient must always check BG concentrations before the meal to determine how much additional insulin should be given as a correction dose using an algorithm assigned by the care team if the fasting BG is not in target. Insulin pumps are based on this concept of "basal-bolus" insulin administration and have the capability of calculating a suggested bolus dosage, based on inputted grams of carbohydrates and BG concentrations. Because the BG value determines the amount of insulin to be given at each meal, the recommended testing frequency for patients on this regimen is before every meal.

Box 1 Example of Basal Bolus Insulin Regimen

If an adolescent has a BG of 250 mg/dL, is to consume a meal containing 60 g of carbohydrates, with a carbohydrate ratio of 1:10 and an assigned correction dose of 1:25>125 (with 25 being the insulin sensitivity and 125 mg/dL the target blood glucose level), the mealtime bolus dose of insulin would be as follows:

60 g/10 "carb ratio" =

6 units rapid-acting insulin for meal

plus

(250–125)/25 = 125/25 =

5 units rapid-acting insulin for correction

Thus, total bolus insulin coverage at mealtime is: **11 U** (6 + 5) of rapid-acting insulin.

Key Action Statement 5

The committee suggests that clinicians incorporate the Academy of Nutrition and Dietetics' *Pediatric Weight Management Evidence-Based Nutrition Practice Guidelines* in the nutrition counseling of patients with T2DM both at the time of diagnosis and as part of ongoing management. (Option; evidence quality D; expert opinion; preponderance of benefits over harms. Role of patient preference is dominant.)

Action Statement Profile KAS 5

Aggregate evidence quality	D (expert opinion).
Benefit	Promotes weight loss; improves insulin sensitivity; contributes to glycemic control; prevents worsening of disease; facilitates a sense of well-being; and improves cardiovascular health.
Harm	Costs of nutrition counseling; inadequate reimbursement of clinicians' time; lost opportunity costs vis-a-vis time and resources spent in other counseling activities.
Benefits-harms assessment	Benefit over harm.
Value judgments	There is a broad societal agreement on the benefits of dietary recommendations.
Role of patient preference	Dominant. Patients may have different preferences for how they wish to receive assistance in managing their weight-loss goals. Some patients may prefer a referral to a nutritionist while others might prefer accessing online sources of help. Patient preference should play a significant role in determining an appropriate weight-loss strategy.
Exclusions	None.
Intentional vagueness	Intentional vagueness in the recommendation about specific approaches attributable to lack of evidence and the need to individualize treatment.
Policy level	Option.

Consuming more calories than one uses results in weight gain and is a major contributor to the increasing incidence of T2DM in children and adolescents. Current literature is inconclusive about a single best meal plan for patients with diabetes mellitus, however, and studies specifically addressing the diet of children and adolescents with T2DM are limited. Challenges to making recommendations stem from the small sample size of these studies, limited specificity for children and adolescents, and difficulties in generalizing the data from dietary research studies to the general population.

Although evidence is lacking in children with T2DM, numerous studies have been conducted in overweight children and adolescents, because the great majority of children with T2DM are obese or overweight at diagnosis.[26] The committee suggests that clinicians encourage children and adolescents with T2DM to follow the Academy of Nutrition and Dietetics' recommendations for maintaining healthy weight to promote health and reduce obesity in this population. The committee recommends that clinicians refer patients to a registered dietitian who has expertise in the nutritional needs of youth with T2DM. Clinicians should incorporate the Academy of Nutrition and Dietetics' *Pediatric Weight Management Evidence-Based Nutrition Practice Guidelines*, which describe effective, evidence-based treatment options for weight management, summarized below (A complete list of these recommendations is accessible to health care professionals at: http://www.andevidencelibrary.com/topic.cfm?cat=4102&auth=1.)

According to the Academy of Nutrition and Dietetics' guidelines, when incorporated with lifestyle changes, balanced macronutrient diets at 900 to 1200 kcal per day are associated with both short- and long-term (eg, ≥ 1 year) improvements in weight status and body composition in children 6 to 12 years of age.[70] These calorie recommendations are to be incorporated with lifestyle changes, including increased activity and possibly medication. Restrictions of no less than 1200 kcal per day in adolescents 13 to 18 years old result in improved weight status and body composition as well.[71] The Diabetes Prevention Program demonstrated that participants assigned to the intensive lifestyle-intervention arm had a reduction in daily energy intake of 450 kcal and a 58% reduction in progression to diabetes at the 2.8-year follow-up.[71] At the study's end, 50% of the lifestyle-arm participants had achieved the goal weight loss of at least 7% after the 24-week curriculum and 38% showed weight loss of at least 7% at the time of their most recent visit.[72] The Academy of Nutrition and Dietetics recommends that protein-sparing, modified-fast (ketogenic) diets be restricted to children who are >120% of their ideal body weight and who have a serious medical complication that would benefit from rapid weight loss.[71] Specific recommendations are for the intervention to be short-term (typically 10 weeks) and to be conducted under the supervision of a multidisciplinary team specializing in pediatric obesity.

Regardless of the meal plan prescribed, some degree of nutrition education must be provided to maximize adherence and positive results. This education should encourage patients to follow healthy eating patterns, such as consuming 3 meals with planned snacks per day, not eating while watching television or using computers, using smaller plates to make portions appear larger, and leaving small amounts of food on the plate.[73] Common dietary recommendations to reduce calorie intake and to promote weight loss in children include the following: (1) eating regular meals and snacks; (2) reducing portion sizes; (3) choosing calorie-free beverages, except for milk; (4) limiting juice to 1 cup per day; (5) increasing consumption of fruits and vegetables; (6) consuming 3 or 4 servings of low-fat dairy products per day; (7) limiting intake of high-fat foods; (8) limiting frequency and size of snacks; and (9) reducing calories consumed in fast-food meals.[74]

Key Action Statement 6

The committee suggests that clinicians encourage children and adolescents with T2DM to engage in moderate-to-vigorous exercise for at least 60 minutes daily and to limit nonacademic screen time to less than 2 hours per day. (Option: evidence quality D, expert opinion and evidence from studies of metabolic syndrome and obesity; preponderance of benefits over harms. Role of patient preference is dominant.)

Action Statement Profile KAS 6

Aggregate evidence quality	D (expert opinion and evidence from studies of metabolic syndrome and obesity).
Benefit	Promotes weight loss; contributes to glycemic control; prevents worsening of disease; facilitates the ability to perform exercise; improves the person's sense of well-being; and fosters cardiovascular health.
Harm	Cost for patient of counseling, food, and time; costs for clinician in taking away time that could be spent on other activities; inadequate reimbursement for clinician's time.
Benefits-harms assessment	Preponderance of benefit over harm.
Value judgments	Broad consensus.
Role of patient preference	Dominant. Patients may seek various forms of exercise. Patient preference should play a significant role in creating an exercise plan.
Exclusions	Although certain older or more debilitated patients with T2DM may be restricted in the amount of moderate-to-vigorous exercise they can perform safely, this recommendation applies to the vast majority of children and adolescents with T2DM.
Intentional vagueness	Intentional vagueness on the sequence of follow-up contact attributable to the lack of evidence and the need to individualize care.
Policy level	Option.

Recommendations From the Academy of Nutrition and Dietetics

Pediatric Weight Management Evidence-Based Nutrition Practice Guidelines

Recommendation	Strength
Interventions to reduce pediatric obesity should be multicomponent and include diet, physical activity, nutritional counseling, and parent or caregiver participation.	Strong
A nutrition prescription should be formulated as part of the dietary intervention in a multicomponent pediatric weight management program.	Strong
Dietary factors that may be associated with an increased risk of overweight are increased total dietary fat intake and increased intake of calorically sweetened beverages.	Strong
Dietary factors that may be associated with a decreased risk of overweight are increased fruit and vegetable intake.	Strong
A balanced macronutrient diet that contains no fewer than 900 kcal per day is recommended to improve weight status in children aged 6–12 y who are medically monitored.	Strong
A balanced macronutrient diet that contains no fewer than 1200 kcal per day is recommended to improve weight status in adolescents aged 13–18 y who are medically monitored.	Strong
Family diet behaviors that are associated with an increased risk of pediatric obesity are parental restriction of highly palatable foods, consumption of food away from home, increased meal portion size, and skipping breakfast.	Fair

Engaging in Physical Activity

Physical activity is an integral part of weight management for prevention and treatment of T2DM. Although there is a paucity of available data from children and adolescents with T2DM, several well-controlled studies performed in obese children and adolescents at risk of metabolic syndrome and T2DM provide guidelines for physical activity. (See the Resources section for tools on this subject.) A summary of the references supporting the evidence for this guideline can be found in the technical report.[31]

At present, moderate-to-vigorous exercise of at least 60 minutes daily is recommended for reduction of BMI and improved glycemic control in patients with T2DM.[75] "Moderate to vigorous exercise" is defined as exercise that makes the individual breathe hard and perspire and that raises his or her heart rate. An easy way to define exercise intensity for patients is the "talk test"; during moderate physical activity a person can talk but not sing. During vigorous activity, a person cannot talk without pausing to catch a breath.[76]

Adherence may be improved if clinicians provide the patient with a written prescription to engage in physical activity, including a "dose" describing ideal duration, intensity, and frequency.[75] When prescribing physical exercise, clinicians are encouraged to be sensitive to the needs of children, adolescents, and their families. Routine, organized exercise may be beyond the family's logistical and/or financial means, and some families may not be able to provide structured exercise programs for their children. It is most helpful to recommend an individualized approach that can be incorporated into the daily routine, is tailored to the patients' physical abilities and preferences, and recognizes the families' circumstances.[77] For example, clinicians might recommend only daily walking, which has been shown to improve weight loss and insulin sensitivity in adults with T2DM[78] and may constitute "moderate to vigorous activity" for some children with T2DM. It is also important to recognize that the recommended 60 minutes of exercise do not have to be accomplished in 1 session but can be completed through several, shorter increments (eg, 10–15 minutes). Patients should be encouraged to identify a variety of forms of activity that can be performed both easily and frequently.[77] In addition, providers should be cognizant of the potential need to adjust the medication dosage, especially if the patient is receiving insulin, when initiating an aggressive physical activity program.

Reducing Screen Time

Screen time contributes to a sedentary lifestyle, especially when the child or adolescent eats while watching television or playing computer games. The US Department of Health and Human Services recommends that individuals limit "screen time" spent watching television and/or using computers and handheld devices to less than 2 hours per day unless the use is related to work or homework.[79] Physical activity may be gained either through structured games and sports or through everyday activities, such as walking, ideally with involvement of the parents as good role models.

Increased screen time and food intake and reduced physical activity are associated with obesity. There is good evidence that modifying these factors can help prevent T2DM by reducing the individual's rate of weight gain. The evidence profile in pediatric patients with T2DM is inadequate at this time, however. Pending new data, the committee suggests that clinicians follow the AAP Committee on Nutrition's guideline, *Prevention of Pediatric Overweight and Obesity.* The guideline recommends restricting nonacademic screen time to a maximum of 2 hours per day and discouraging the presence of video screens and television sets in children's bedrooms.[80–82] The American Medical Association's Expert Panel on Childhood Obesity has endorsed this guideline.

Valuable recommendations for enhancing patient health include the following:

- With patients and their families, jointly determining an individualized plan that includes specific goals to reduce sedentary behaviors and increase physical activity.
- Providing a written prescription for engaging in 60-plus minutes of moderate-to-vigorous physical activities per day that includes dose, timing, and duration. It is important for clinicians to be sensitive to the needs of children, adolescents, and their families in encouraging daily physical exercise. Graded duration of exercise is recommended for those youth who cannot initially be active for 60 minutes daily, and the exercise may be accomplished through several, shorter increments (eg, 10–15 minutes).
- Incorporating physical activities into children's and adolescents' daily routines. Physical activity may be gained either through structured games and sports or through everyday activities, such as walking.
- Restricting nonacademic screen time to a maximum of 2 hours per day.
- Discouraging the presence of video screens and television sets in children's bedrooms.

Conversations pertaining to the Key Action Statements should be clearly documented in the patient's medical record.

AREAS FOR FUTURE RESEARCH

As noted previously, evidence for medical interventions in children in general is scant and is especially lacking for interventions directed toward children who have developed diseases not previously seen commonly in youth, such as childhood T2DM. Recent studies such as the Search for Diabetes in Youth Study (SEARCH)—an observational multicenter study in 2096 youth with T2DM funded by the Centers for Disease Control and Prevention and the National Institute of Diabetes and Digestive and Kidney Diseases—now provide a detailed description of childhood diabetes. Subsequent trials will describe the short-term and enduring effects of specific interventions on the progression of the disease with time.

Although it is likely that children and adolescents with T2DM have an aggressive form of diabetes, as reflected by the age of onset, future research should determine whether the associated comorbidities and complications of diabetes also are more aggressive in pediatric populations than in adults and if they are more or less responsive to therapeutic interventions. Additional research should explore whether early introduction of insulin or the use of particular oral agents will preserve β-cell function in these children, and whether recent technologic advances (such as continuous glucose monitoring and insulin pumps) will benefit this population. Additional issues that require further study include the following:

- To delineate whether using lifestyle options without medication is a reliable first step in treating selected children with T2DM.
- To determine whether BG monitoring should be recommended to all children and youth with T2DM, regardless of therapy used; what the optimal frequency of BG monitoring is for pediatric patients on the basis of treatment regimen; and which subgroups will be able to successfully maintain glycemic goals with less frequent monitoring.
- To explore the efficacy of school- and clinic-based diet and physical activity interventions to prevent and manage pediatric T2DM.
- To explore the association between increased "screen time" and reduced physical activity with respect to T2DM's risk factors.

RESOURCES

Several tools are available online to assist providers in improving patient adherence to lifestyle modifications, including examples of activities to be recommended for patients:

- The American Academy of Pediatrics:
  - www.healthychildren.org
  - www.letsmove.gov
  - Technical Report: Management of Type 2 Diabetes Mellitus in Children and Adolescents.[31]
    - Includes an overview and screening tools for a variety of comorbidities.
  - Gahagan S, Silverstein J; Committee on Native American Child Health and Section on Endocrinology. Clinical report: prevention and treatment of type 2 diabetes mellitus in children, with special emphasis on American Indian and Alaska Native Children. *Pediatrics.* 2003;112 (4):e328–e347. Available at: http://www.pediatrics.org/cgi/content/full/112/4/e328[63]
    - Fig 3 presents a screening tool for microalbumin.
  - Bright Futures: http://brightfutures.aap.org/
  - Daniels SR, Greer FR; Committee on Nutrition. Lipid screening and cardiovascular health in childhood. *Pediatrics.* 2008;122 (1):198–208. Available at:
- The American Diabetes Association: www.diabetes.org
  - Management of dyslipidemia in children and adolescents with diabetes. *Diabetes Care.* 2003;26(7):2194–2197. Available at: http://care.diabetesjournals.org/content/26/7/2194.full
- Academy of Nutrition and Dietetics:
  - http://www.eatright.org/childhoodobesity/
  - http://www.eatright.org/kids/
  - http://www.eatright.org/cps/rde/xchg/ada/hs.xsl/index.html
  - Pediatric Weight Management Evidence-Based Nutrition Practice Guidelines: http://www.adaevidencelibrary.com/topic.cfm?cat=2721
- American Heart Association:
  - American Heart Association *Circulation.* 2006 Dec 12;114(24):2710-2738. Epub 2006 Nov 27. Review.
- Centers for Disease Control and Prevention:
  - http://www.cdc.gov/obesity/childhood/solutions.html
  - BMI and other growth charts can be downloaded and printed from the CDC Web site: http://www.cdc.gov/growthcharts.
  - Center for Epidemiologic Studies Depression Scale (CES-D): http://www.chcr.brown.edu/pcoc/cesdscale.pdf; see attachments
- *Diagnostic and Statistical Manual of Mental Disorders.* 4th ed. Washington, DC: American Psychiatric Association; 1994
- Let's Move Campaign: www.letsmove.gov
- The Reach Institute. *Guidelines for Adolescent Depression in Primary Care (GLAD-PC) Toolkit,* 2007. Contains a listing of the criteria for major depressive disorder as defined by the DSM-IV-TR. Available at: http://www.gladpc.org
- The National Heart, Lung, and Blood Institute (NHLBI) hypertension guidelines: http://www.nhlbi.nih.gov/guidelines/hypertension/child_tbl.htm
- The National Diabetes Education Program and TIP sheets (including tip sheets on youth transitioning to adulthood and adult providers, Staying Active, Eating Healthy, Ups and Downs of Diabetes, etc): www.ndep.nih.gov or www.yourdiabetesinfo.org

- National High Blood Pressure Education Program Working Group on High Blood Pressure in Children and Adolescents, The Fourth Report on the Diagnosis, Evaluation, and Treatment of High Blood Pressure in Children and Adolescents: *Pediatrics*. 2004;114:555–576. Available at: http://pediatrics.aappublications.org/content/114/Supplement_2/555.long
- National Initiative for Children's Healthcare Quality (NICHQ): childhood obesity section: http://www.nichq.org/childhood_obesity/index.html
- The National Institute of Child Health and Human Development (NICHD): www.NICHD.org
- President's Council on Physical Fitness and Sports: http://www.presidentschallenge.org/home_kids.aspx
- US Department of Agriculture's "My Pyramid" Web site:
- http://www.choosemyplate.gov/
- http://fnic.nal.usda.gov/lifecycle-nutrition/child-nutrition-and-health

SUBCOMMITTEE ON TYPE 2 DIABETES (OVERSIGHT BY THE STEERING COMMITTEE ON QUALITY IMPROVEMENT AND MANAGEMENT, 2008–2012)

Kenneth Claud Copeland, MD, FAAP: Co-chair —Endocrinology and Pediatric Endocrine Society Liaison (2009: Novo Nordisk, Genentech, Endo [National Advisory Groups]; 2010: Novo Nordisk [National Advisory Group]); published research related to type 2 diabetes

Janet Silverstein, MD, FAAP: Co-chair—Endocrinology and American Diabetes Association Liaison (small grants with Pfizer, Novo Nordisk, and Lilly; grant review committee for Genentech; was on an advisory committee for Sanofi Aventis, and Abbott Laboratories for a 1-time meeting); published research related to type 2 diabetes

Kelly Roberta Moore, MD, FAAP: General Pediatrics, Indian Health, AAP Committee on Native American Child Health Liaison (board member of the Merck Company Foundation Alliance to Reduce Disparities in Diabetes. Their national program office is the University of Michigan's Center for Managing Chronic Disease.)

Greg Edward Prazar, MD, FAAP: General Pediatrics (no conflicts)

Terry Raymer, MD, CDE: Family Medicine, Indian Health Service (no conflicts)

Richard N. Shiffman, MD, FAAP: Partnership for Policy Implementation Informatician, General Pediatrics (no conflicts)

Shelley C. Springer, MD, MBA, FAAP: Epidemiologist (no conflicts)

Meaghan Anderson, MS, RD, LD, CDE: Academy of Nutrition and Dietetics Liaison (formerly a Certified Pump Trainer for Animas)

Stephen J. Spann, MD, MBA, FAAFP: American Academy of Family Physicians Liaison (no conflicts)

Vidhu V. Thaker, MD, FAAP: QuIIN Liaison, General Pediatrics (no conflicts)

CONSULTANT

Susan K. Flinn, MA: Medical Writer (no conflicts)

STAFF

Caryn Davidson, MA

REFERENCES

1. Centers for Disease Control and Prevention. Data and Statistics. Obesity rates among children in the United States. Available at: www.cdc.gov/obesity/childhood/prevalence.html. Accessed August 13, 2012
2. Copeland KC, Chalmers LJ, Brown RD. Type 2 diabetes in children: oxymoron or medical metamorphosis? *Pediatr Ann*. 2005;34(9):686–697
3. Narayan KM, Boyle JP, Thompson TJ, Sorensen SW, Williamson DF. Lifetime risk for diabetes mellitus in the United States. *JAMA*. 2003;290(14):1884–1890
4. Chopra M, Galbraith S, Darnton-Hill I. A global response to a global problem: the epidemic of overnutrition. *Bull World Health Organ*. 2002;80(12):952–958
5. Liese AD, D'Agostino RB, Jr, Hamman RF, et al; SEARCH for Diabetes in Youth Study Group. The burden of diabetes mellitus among US youth: prevalence estimates from the SEARCH for Diabetes in Youth Study. *Pediatrics*. 2006;118(4):1510–1518
6. Silverstein JH, Rosenbloom AL. Type 2 diabetes in children. *Curr Diab Rep*. 2001;1(1):19–27
7. Pinhas-Hamiel O, Zeitler P. Clinical presentation and treatment of type 2 diabetes in children. *Pediatr Diabetes*. 2007;8(suppl 9):16–27
8. Dabelea D, Bell RA, D'Agostino RB Jr, et al; Writing Group for the SEARCH for Diabetes in Youth Study Group. Incidence of diabetes in youth in the United States. *JAMA*. 2007;297(24):2716–2724
9. Mayer-Davis EJ, Bell RA, Dabelea D, et al; SEARCH for Diabetes in Youth Study Group. The many faces of diabetes in American youth: type 1 and type 2 diabetes in five race and ethnic populations: the SEARCH for Diabetes in Youth Study. *Diabetes Care*. 2009;32(suppl 2):S99–S101
10. Copeland KC, Zeitler P, Geffner M, et al; TODAY Study Group. Characteristics of adolescents and youth with recent-onset type 2 diabetes: the TODAY cohort at baseline. *J Clin Endocrinol Metab*. 2011;96(1):159–167
11. Narayan KM, Williams R. Diabetes—a global problem needing global solutions. *Prim Care Diabetes*. 2009;3(1):3–4
12. Wild S, Roglic G, Green A, Sicree R, King H. Global prevalence of diabetes: estimates for the year 2000 and projections for 2030. *Diabetes Care*. 2004;27(5):1047–1053
13. Silverstein J, Klingensmith G, Copeland K, et al; American Diabetes Association. Care of children and adolescents with type 1 diabetes: a statement of the American Diabetes Association. *Diabetes Care*. 2005;28(1):186–212
14. Pinhas-Hamiel O, Zeitler P. Barriers to the treatment of adolescent type 2 diabetes—a survey of provider perceptions. *Pediatr Diabetes*. 2003;4(1):24–28
15. Moore KR, McGowan MK, Donato KA, Kollipara S, Roubideaux Y. Community resources for promoting youth nutrition and physical activity. *Am J Health Educ*. 2009;40(5):298–303
16. Zeitler P, Epstein L, Grey M, et al; The TODAY Study Group. Treatment Options for type 2 diabetes mellitus in Adolescents and Youth: a study of the comparative efficacy of metformin alone or in combination with rosiglitazone or lifestyle intervention in adolescents with type 2 diabetes mellitus. *Pediatr Diabetes*. 2007;8(2):74–87
17. Kane MP, Abu-Baker A, Busch RS. The utility of oral diabetes medications in type 2

diabetes of the young. *Curr Diabetes Rev.* 2005;1(1):83–92

18. De Berardis G, Pellegrini F, Franciosi M, et al. Quality of care and outcomes in type 2 diabetes patientes. *Diabetes Care.* 2004;27 (2):398–406
19. Ziemer DC, Miller CD, Rhee MK, et al. Clinical inertia contributes to poor diabetes control in a primary care setting. *Diabetes Educ.* 2005;31(4):564–571
20. Bradshaw B. The role of the family in managing therapy in minority children with type 2 diabetes mellitus. *J Pediatr Endocrinol Metab.* 2002;15(suppl 1):547–551
21. Pinhas-Hamiel O, Standiford D, Hamiel D, Dolan LM, Cohen R, Zeitler PS. The type 2 family: a setting for development and treatment of adolescent type 2 diabetes mellitus. *Arch Pediatr Adolesc Med.* 1999; 153(10):1063–1067
22. Mulvaney SA, Schlundt DG, Mudasiru E, et al. Parent perceptions of caring for adolescents with type 2 diabetes. *Diabetes Care.* 2006;29(5):993–997
23. Summerbell CD, Ashton V, Campbell KJ, Edmunds L, Kelly S, Waters E. Interventions for treating obesity in children. *Cochrane Database Syst Rev.* 2003;(3):CD001872
24. Skinner AC, Weinberger M, Mulvaney S, Schlundt D, Rothman RL. Accuracy of perceptions of overweight and relation to self-care behaviors among adolescents with type 2 diabetes and their parents. *Diabetes Care.* 2008;31(2):227–229
25. American Diabetes Association. Type 2 diabetes in children and adolescents. *Diabetes Care.* 2000;23(3):381–389
26. Pinhas-Hamiel O, Zeitler P. Type 2 diabetes in adolescents, no longer rare. *Pediatr Rev.* 1998;19(12):434–435
27. Fagot-Campagna A, Pettitt DJ, Engelgau MM, et al. Type 2 diabetes among North American children and adolescents: an epidemiologic review and a public health perspective. *J Pediatr.* 2000;136(5):664–672
28. Rothman RL, Mulvaney S, Elasy TA, et al. Self-management behaviors, racial disparities, and glycemic control among adolescents with type 2 diabetes. *Pediatrics.* 2008;121(4). Available at: www.pediatrics.org/cgi/content/full/121/4/e912
29. Scott CR, Smith JM, Cradock MM, Pihoker C. Characteristics of youth-onset noninsulin-dependent diabetes mellitus and insulin-dependent diabetes mellitus at diagnosis. *Pediatrics.* 1997;100(1):84–91
30. Libman IM, Pietropaolo M, Arslanian SA, LaPorte RE, Becker DJ. Changing prevalence of overweight children and adolescents at onset of insulin-treated diabetes. *Diabetes Care.* 2003;26(10):2871–2875
31. Springer SC, Copeland KC, Silverstein J, et al. Technical report: management of type 2 diabetes mellitus in children and adolescents. *Pediatrics.* 2012, In press
32. American Academy of Pediatrics Steering Committee on Quality Improvement and Management. Classifying recommendations for clinical practice guidelines. *Pediatrics.* 2004;114(3):874–877
33. Shiffman RN, Dixon J, Brandt C, et al. The GuideLine Implementability Appraisal (GLIA): development of an instrument to identify obstacles to guideline implementation. *BMC Med Inform Decis Mak.* 2005;5:23
34. Gungor N, Hannon T, Libman I, Bacha F, Arslanian S. Type 2 diabetes mellitus in youth: the complete picture to date. *Pediatr Clin North Am.* 2005;52(6):1579–1609
35. Daaboul JJ, Siverstein JH. The management of type 2 diabetes in children and adolescents. *Minerva Pediatr.* 2004;56(3):255–264
36. Kadmon PM, Grupposo PA. Glycemic control with metformin or insulin therapy in adolescents with type 2 diabetes mellitus. *J Pediatr Endocrinol.* 2004;17(9):1185–1193
37. Owada M, Nitadori Y, Kitagawa T. Treatment of NIDDM in youth. *Clin Pediatr (Phila).* 1998;37(2):117–121
38. Pinhas-Hamiel O, Zeitler P. Advances in epidemiology and treatment of type 2 diabetes in children. *Adv Pediatr.* 2005;52: 223–259
39. Jones KL, Haghi M. Type 2 diabetes mellitus in children and adolescence: a primer. *Endocrinologist.* 2000;10:389–396
40. Kawahara R, Amemiya T, Yoshino M, et al. Dropout of young non-insulin-dependent diabetics from diabetic care. *Diabetes Res Clin Pract.* 1994;24(3):181–185
41. Kaufman FR. Type 2 diabetes mellitus in children and youth: a new epidemic. *J Pediatr Endocrinol Metab.* 2002;15(suppl 2): 737–744
42. Garber AJ, Duncan TG, Goodman AM, Mills DJ, Rohlf JL. Efficacy of metformin in type II diabetes: results of a double-blind, placebo-controlled, dose-response trial. *Am J Med.* 1997;103(6):491–497
43. Dabelea D, Pettitt DJ, Jones KL, Arslanian SA. Type 2 diabetes mellitus in minority children and adolescents: an emerging problem. *Endocrinol Metabo Clin North Am.* 1999;28(4):709–729
44. Miller JL, Silverstein JH. The management of type 2 diabetes mellitus in children and adolescents. *J Pediatr Endocrinol Metab.* 2005;18(2):111–123
45. Reinehr T, Schober E, Roth CL, Wiegand S, Holl R; DPV-Wiss Study Group. Type 2 diabetes in children and adolescents in a 2-year follow-up: insufficient adherence to diabetes centers. *Horm Res.* 2008;69(2):107–113
46. Rosenbloom AL, Silverstein JH, Amemiya S, Zeitler P, Klingensmith GJ. Type 2 diabetes in children and adolescents. *Pediatr Diabetes.* 2009;10(suppl 12):17–32
47. Zuhri-Yafi MI, Brosnan PG, Hardin DS. Treatment of type 2 diabetes mellitus in children and adolescents. *J Pediatr Endocrinol Metab.* 2002;15(suppl 1):541–546
48. Rapaport R, Silverstein JH, Garzarella L, Rosenbloom AL. Type 1 and type 2 diabetes mellitus in childhood in the United States: practice patterns by pediatric endocrinologists. *J Pediatr Endocrinol Metab.* 2004;17 (6):871–877
49. Glaser N, Jones KL. Non-insulin-dependent diabetes mellitus in children and adolescents. *Adv Pediatr.* 1996;43:359–396
50. Miller JL, Silverstein JH. The treatment of type 2 diabetes mellitus in youth: which therapies? *Treat Endocrinol.* 2006;5(4):201–210
51. Silverstein JH, Rosenbloom AL. Treatment of type 2 diabetes mellitus in children and adolescents. *J Pediatr Endocrinol Metab.* 2000;13(suppl 6):1403–1409
52. Dean H. Treatment of type 2 diabetes in youth: an argument for randomized controlled studies. *Paediatr Child Health (Oxford).* 1999;4(4):265–270
53. Sellers EAC, Dean HJ. Short-term insulin therapy in adolescents with type 2 diabetes mellitus. *J Pediatr Endocrinol Metab.* 2004; 17(11):1561–1564
54. Zeitler P, Hirst K, Pyle L, et al; TODAY Study Group. A clinical trial to maintain glycemic control in youth with type 2 diabetes. *N Engl J Med.* 2012;366(24):2247–2256
55. White NH, Cleary PA, Dahms W, Goldstein D, Malone J, Tamborlane WV; Diabetes Control and Complications Trial (DCCT)/Epidemiology of Diabetes Interventions and Complications (EDIC) Research Group. Beneficial effects of intensive therapy of diabetes during adolescence: outcomes after the conclusion of the Diabetes Control and Complications Trial (DCCT). *J Pediatr.* 2001;139(6):804–812
56. The Diabetes Control and Complications Trial Research Group. The effect of intensive treatment of diabetes on the development and progression of long-term complications in insulin-dependent diabetes mellitus. *N Engl J Med.* 1993;329(14):977–986
57. Orchard TJ, Olson JC, Erbey JR, et al. Insulin resistance-related factors, but not glycemia, predict coronary artery disease in type 1 diabetes: 10-year follow-up data from the Pittsburgh Epidemiology of Diabetes Complications Study. *Diabetes Care.* 2003;26(5):1374–1379

58. UK Prospective Diabetes Study Group. U.K. prospective diabetes study 16. Overview of 6 years' therapy of type II diabetes: a progressive disease. *Diabetes*. 1995;44(11): 1249–1258

59. Shichiri M, Kishikawa H, Ohkubo Y, Wake N. Long-term results of the Kumamoto Study on optimal diabetes control in type 2 diabetic patients. *Diabetes Care*. 2000;23 (suppl 2):B21–B29

60. Baynes JW, Bunn HF, Goldstein D, et al; National Diabetes Data Group. National Diabetes Data Group: report of the expert committee on glucosylated hemoglobin. *Diabetes Care*. 1984;7(6):602–606

61. Dabiri G, Jones K, Krebs J, et al. Benefits of rosiglitazone in children with type 2 diabetes mellitus [abstract]. *Diabetes*. 2005; A457

62. Ponder SW, Sullivan S, McBath G. Type 2 diabetes mellitus in teens. *Diabetes Spectrum*. 2000;13(2):95–119

63. Gahagan S, Silverstein J, and the American Academy of Pediatrics Committee on Native American Child Health. Prevention and treatment of type 2 diabetes mellitus in children, with special emphasis on American Indian and Alaska Native children. *Pediatrics*. 2003;112(4). Available at: www.pediatrics.org/cgi/content/full/112/4/e328

64. Levine BS, Anderson BJ, Butler DA, Antisdel JE, Brackett J, Laffel LM. Predictors of glycemic control and short-term adverse outcomes in youth with type 1 diabetes. *J Pediatr*. 2001;139(2):197–203

65. Haller MJ, Stalvey MS, Silverstein JH. Predictors of control of diabetes: monitoring may be the key. *J Pediatr*. 2004;144(5):660–661

66. Murata GH, Shah JH, Hoffman RM, et al; Diabetes Outcomes in Veterans Study (DOVES). Intensified blood glucose monitoring improves glycemic control in stable, insulin-treated veterans with type 2 diabetes: the Diabetes Outcomes in Veterans Study (DOVES). *Diabetes Care*. 2003;26(6): 1759–1763

67. American Diabetes Association. Standards of medical care in diabetes—2011. *Diabetes Care*. 2011;34(suppl 1):S11–S61

68. Hanefeld M, Fischer S, Julius U, et al. Risk factors for myocardial infarction and death in newly detected NIDDM: the Diabetes Intervention Study, 11-year follow-up. *Diabetologia*. 1996;39(12):1577–1583

69. Franciosi M, Pellegrini F, De Berardis G, et al; QuED Study Group. The impact of blood glucose self-monitoring on metabolic control and quality of life in type 2 diabetic patients: an urgent need for better educational strategies. *Diabetes Care*. 2001;24 (11):1870–1877

70. American Dietetic Association. Recommendations summary: pediatric weight management (PWM) using protein sparing modified fast diets for pediatric weight loss. Available at: www.adaevidencelibrary.com/template.cfm?template=guide_-summary&key=416. Accessed August 13, 2012

71. Knowler WC, Barrett-Connor E, Fowler SE, et al; Diabetes Prevention Program Research Group. Reduction in the incidence of type 2 diabetes with lifestyle intervention or metformin. *N Engl J Med*. 2002;346(6): 393–403

72. Willi SM, Martin K, Datko FM, Brant BP. Treatment of type 2 diabetes in childhood using a very-low-calorie diet. *Diabetes Care*. 2004;27(2):348–353

73. Berry D, Urban A, Grey M. Management of type 2 diabetes in youth (part 2). *J Pediatr Health Care*. 2006;20(2):88–97

74. Loghmani ES. Nutrition therapy for overweight children and adolescents with type 2 diabetes. *Curr Diab Rep*. 2005;5(5):385–390

75. McGavock J, Sellers E, Dean H. Physical activity for the prevention and management of youth-onset type 2 diabetes mellitus: focus on cardiovascular complications. *Diab Vasc Dis Res*. 2007;4(4):305–310

76. Centers for Disease Control and Prevention. Physical activity for everyone: how much physical activity do you need? Atlanta, GA: Centers for Disease Control and Prevention; 2008. Available at: www.cdc.gov/physicalactivity/everyone/guidelines/children.html. Accessed August 13, 2012

77. Pinhas-Hamiel O, Zeitler P. A weighty problem: diagnosis and treatment of type 2 diabetes in adolescents. *Diabetes Spectrum*. 1997;10(4):292–298

78. Yamanouchi K, Shinozaki T, Chikada K, et al. Daily walking combined with diet therapy is a useful means for obese NIDDM patients not only to reduce body weight but also to improve insulin sensitivity. *Diabetes Care*. 1995;18(6):775–778

79. National Heart, Lung, and Blood Institute, US Department of Health and Human Services, National Institutes of Health. Reduce screen time. Available at: www.nhlbi.nih.gov/health/public/heart/obesity/wecan/reduce-screen-time/index.htm. Accessed August 13, 2012

80. Krebs NF, Jacobson MS; American Academy of Pediatrics Committee on Nutrition. Prevention of pediatric overweight and obesity. *Pediatrics*. 2003;112(2):424–430

81. American Academy of Pediatrics Committee on Public Education. American Academy of Pediatrics: children, adolescents, and television. *Pediatrics*. 2001;107(2):423–426

82. American Medical Association. Appendix. Expert Committee recommendations on the assessment, prevention, and treatment of child and adolescent overweight and obesity. Chicago, IL: American Medical Association; January 25, 2007. Available at: www.ama-assn.org/ama1/pub/upload/mm/433/ped_obesity_recs.pdf. Accessed August 13, 2012

ERRATA

Several inaccuracies occurred in the American Academy of Pediatrics "Clinical Practice Guideline: Management of Newly Diagnosed Type 2 Diabetes Mellitus (T2DM) in Children and Adolescents" published in the February 2013 issue of *Pediatrics* (2013;131[2]:364–382).

On page 366 in the table of definitions, "Prediabetes" should be defined as "Fasting plasma glucose ≥100–125 mg/dL or 2-hour glucose concentration during an oral glucose tolerance test of ≥140 but <200 mg/dL or an HbA1c of 5.7% to 6.4%."

On page 378, middle column, under "Reducing Screen Time," the second sentence should read as follows: "The US Department of Health and Human Services reflects the American Academy of Pediatrics policies by recommending that individuals limit "screen time" spent watching television and/or using computers and handheld devices to <2 hours per day unless the use is related to work or homework."[79–81,83]

Also on page 378, middle column, in the second paragraph under "Reducing Screen Time," the fourth sentence should read: "Pending new data, the committee suggests that clinicians follow the policy statement 'Children, Adolescents, and Television' from the AAP Council on Communications and Media (formerly the Committee on Public Education)." The references cited in the next sentence should be 80–83.

Reference 82 should be replaced with the following reference: Barlow SE; Expert Committee. Expert committee recommendations regarding the prevention, assessment, and treatment of child and adolescent overweight and obesity: summary report. *Pediatrics.* 2007;120(suppl 4):S164–S192

Finally, a new reference 83 should be added: American Academy of Pediatrics, Council on Communications and Media. Policy statement: children, adolescents, obesity, and the media. *Pediatrics.* 2011;128(1):201–208

doi:10.1542/peds.2013-0666

Diabetes Clinical Practice Guideline Quick Reference Tools

- Action Statement Summary
  — Management of Newly Diagnosed Type 2 Diabetes Mellitus (T2DM) in Children and Adolescents
- *ICD-10-CM* Coding Quick Reference for Type 2 Diabetes Mellitus
- AAP Patient Education Handout
  — *Type 2 Diabetes: Tips for Healthy Living*

Action Statement Summary

Management of Newly Diagnosed Type 2 Diabetes Mellitus (T2DM) in Children and Adolescents

Key Action Statement 1

Clinicians must ensure that insulin therapy is initiated for children and adolescents with T2DM who are ketotic or in diabetic ketoacidosis and in whom the distinction between T1DM and T2DM is unclear; and, in usual cases, should initiate insulin therapy for patients:

- who have random venous or plasma BG concentrations ≥250 mg/dL; or
- whose HbA1c is >9%.

(Strong Recommendation: evidence quality X, validating studies cannot be performed, and C, observational studies and expert opinion; preponderance of benefit over harm.)

Key Action Statement 2

In all other instances, clinicians should initiate a lifestyle modification program, including nutrition and physical activity, and start metformin as first-line therapy for children and adolescents at the time of diagnosis of T2DM. (Strong recommendation: evidence quality B; 1 RCT showing improved outcomes with metformin versus lifestyle; preponderance of benefits over harms.)

Key Action Statement 3

The committee suggests that clinicians monitor HbA1c concentrations every 3 months and intensify treatment if treatment goals for BG and HbA1c concentrations are not being met. (Option: evidence quality D; expert opinion and studies in children with T1DM and in adults with T2DM; preponderance of benefits over harms.)

Key Action Statement 4

The committee suggests that clinicians advise patients to monitor finger-stick BG concentrations in those who

- are taking insulin or other medications with a risk of hypoglycemia; or
- are initiating or changing their diabetes treatment regimen; or
- have not met treatment goals; or
- have intercurrent illnesses.

(Option: evidence quality D; expert consensus. Preponderance of benefits over harms.)

Key Action Statement 5

The committee suggests that clinicians incorporate the Academy of Nutrition and Dietetics' *Pediatric Weight Management Evidence-Based Nutrition Practice Guidelines* in the nutrition counseling of patients with T2DM both at the time of diagnosis and as part of ongoing management. (Option; evidence quality D; expert opinion; preponderance of benefits over harms. Role of patient preference is dominant.)

Key Action Statement 6

The committee suggests that clinicians encourage children and adolescents with T2DM to engage in moderate-to-vigorous exercise for at least 60 minutes daily and to limit nonacademic screen time to less than 2 hours per day. (Option: evidence quality D, expert opinion and evidence from studies of metabolic syndrome and obesity; preponderance of benefits over harms. Role of patient preference is dominant.)

Coding Quick Reference for Type 2 Diabetes Mellitus	
ICD-10-CM	
E11.649	Type 2 diabetes mellitus with hypoglycemia without coma
E11.65	Type 2 diabetes mellitus with hyperglycemia
E11.8	Type 2 diabetes mellitus with unspecified complications
E11.9	Type 2 diabetes mellitus without complications
E13.9	Other specified diabetes mellitus without complications
Use codes above (**E11.8–E13.9**). *ICD-10-CM* does not discern between controlled and uncontrolled.	

Type 2 Diabetes: Tips for Healthy Living

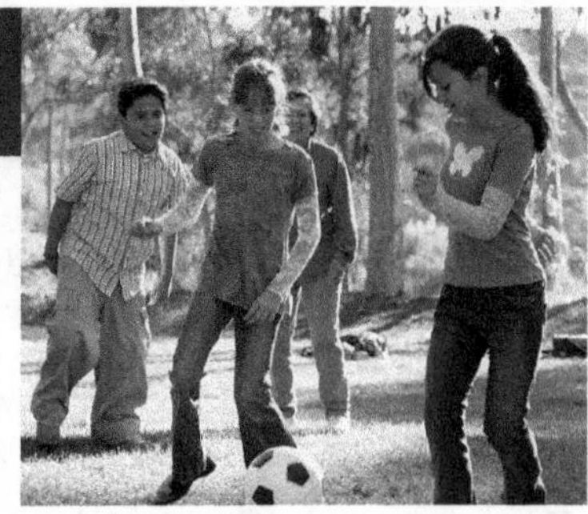

Children with type 2 diabetes can live a healthy life. If your child has been diagnosed with type 2 diabetes, your child's doctor will talk with you about the importance of lifestyle and medication in keeping your child's blood glucose (blood sugar) levels under control.

Read on for information from the American Academy of Pediatrics (AAP) about managing blood glucose and creating plans for healthy living.

What is blood glucose?

Glucose is found in the blood and is the body's main source of energy. The food your child eats is broken down by the body into glucose. Glucose is a type of sugar that gives energy to the cells in the body.

The cells need the help of insulin to take the glucose from the blood to the cells. Insulin is made by an organ called the pancreas.

In children with type 2 diabetes, the pancreas does not make enough insulin and the cells don't use the insulin very well.

Why is it important to manage blood glucose levels?

Glucose will build up in the blood if it cannot be used by the cells. High blood glucose levels can damage many parts of the body, such as the eyes, kidneys, nerves, and heart.

Your child's blood glucose levels may need to be checked on a regular schedule to make sure the levels do not get too high. Your child's doctor will tell you what your child's blood glucose level should be. You and your child will need to learn how to use a glucose meter. Blood glucose levels can be quickly and easily measured using a glucose meter. First, a lancet is used to prick the skin; then a drop of blood from your child's finger is placed on a test strip that is inserted into the meter.

Are there medicines for type 2 diabetes?

Insulin in a shot or another medicine by mouth may be prescribed by your child's doctor if needed to help control your child's blood glucose levels. If your child's doctor has prescribed a medicine, it's important that your child take it as directed. Side effects from certain medicines may include bloating or gassiness. Check with your child's doctor if you have questions.

Along with medicines, your child's doctor will suggest changes to your child's diet and encourage your child to be physically active.

Tips for healthy living

A healthy diet and staying active are especially important for children with type 2 diabetes. Your child's blood glucose levels are easier to manage when you child is at a healthy weight.

Create a plan for eating healthy

Talk with your child's doctor and registered dietitian about a meal plan that meets the needs of your child. The following tips can help you select foods that are healthy and contain a high content of nutrients (protein, vitamins, and minerals):

- Eat at least 5 servings of fruits and vegetables each day.
- Include high-fiber, whole-grain foods such as brown rice, whole-grain pasta, corns, peas, and breads and cereals at meals. Sweet potatoes are also a good choice.
- Choose lower-fat or fat-free toppings like grated low-fat parmesan cheese, salsa, herbed cottage cheese, nonfat/low-fat gravy, low-fat sour cream, low-fat salad dressing, or yogurt.
- Select lean meats such as skinless chicken and turkey, fish, lean beef cuts (round, sirloin, chuck, loin, lean ground beef—no more than 15% fat content), and lean pork cuts (tenderloin, chops, ham). Trim off all visible fat. Remove skin from cooked poultry before eating.
- Include healthy oils such as canola or olive oil in your diet. Choose margarine and vegetable oils without trans fats made from canola, corn, sunflower, soybean, or olive oils.
- Use nonstick vegetable sprays when cooking.
- Use fat-free cooking methods such as baking, broiling, grilling, poaching, or steaming when cooking meat, poultry, or fish.
- Serve vegetable- and broth-based soups, or use nonfat (skim) or low-fat (1%) milk or evaporated skim milk when making cream soups.
- Use the Nutrition Facts label on food packages to find foods with less saturated fat per serving. Pay attention to the serving size as you make choices. Remember that the percent daily values on food labels are based on portion sizes and calorie levels for adults.

Create a plan for physical activity

Physical activity, along with proper nutrition, promotes lifelong health. Following are some ideas on how to get fit:

- **Encourage your child to be active at least 1 hour a day.** Active play is the best exercise for younger children! Parents can join their children and have fun while being active too. School-aged child should participate every day in 1 hour or more of moderate to vigorous physical activity that is right for their age, is enjoyable, and involves a variety of activities.
- **Limit television watching and computer use.** The AAP discourages TV and other media use by children younger than 2 years and encourages interactive play. For older children, total entertainment screen time should be limited to less than 1 to 2 hours per day.
- **Keep an activity log.** The use of activity logs can help children and teens keep track of their exercise programs and physical activity. Online tools can be helpful.

- **Get the whole family involved.** It is a great way to spend time together. Also, children who regularly see their parents enjoying sports and physical activity are more likely to do so themselves.
- **Provide a safe environment.** Make sure your child's equipment and chosen site for the sport or activity are safe. Make sure your child's clothing is comfortable and appropriate.

For more information

National Diabetes Education Program

http://ndep.nih.gov

Listing of resources does not imply an endorsement by the American Academy of Pediatrics (AAP). The AAP is not responsible for the content of the resources mentioned in this publication. Web site addresses are as current as possible, but may change at any time.

The persons whose photographs are depicted in this publication are professional models. They have no relation to the issues discussed. Any characters they are portraying are fictional.

The information contained in this publication should not be used as a substitute for the medical care and advice of your pediatrician. There may be variations in treatment that your pediatrician may recommend based on individual facts and circumstances.

From your doctor

American Academy of Pediatrics

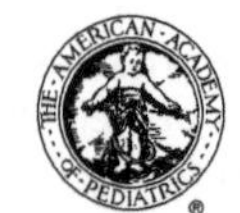

DEDICATED TO THE HEALTH OF ALL CHILDREN™

The American Academy of Pediatrics is an organization of 60,000 primary care pediatricians, pediatric medical subspecialists, and pediatric surgical specialists dedicated to the health, safety, and well-being of infants, children, adolescents, and young adults.

American Academy of Pediatrics
Web site—www.HealthyChildren.org

Copyright © 2013
American Academy of Pediatrics
All rights reserved.

Early Detection of Developmental Dysplasia of the Hip

- *Clinical Practice Guideline*

AMERICAN ACADEMY OF PEDIATRICS

Committee on Quality Improvement, Subcommittee on Developmental Dysplasia of the Hip

Clinical Practice Guideline: Early Detection of Developmental Dysplasia of the Hip

ABSTRACT. ***Developmental dysplasia of the hip*** **is the preferred term to describe the condition in which the femoral head has an abnormal relationship to the acetabulum. Developmental dysplasia of the hip includes frank dislocation (luxation), partial dislocation (subluxation), instability wherein the femoral head comes in and out of the socket, and an array of radiographic abnormalities that reflect inadequate formation of the acetabulum. Because many of these findings may not be present at birth, the term** ***developmental*** **more accurately reflects the biologic features than does the term** ***congenital.*** **The disorder is uncommon. The earlier a dislocated hip is detected, the simpler and more effective is the treatment. Despite newborn screening programs, dislocated hips continue to be diagnosed later in infancy and childhood,[1-11] in some instances delaying appropriate therapy and leading to a substantial number of malpractice claims. The objective of this guideline is to reduce the number of dislocated hips detected later in infancy and childhood. The target audience is the primary care provider. The target patient is the healthy newborn up to 18 months of age, excluding those with neuromuscular disorders, myelodysplasia, or arthrogryposis.**

ABBREVIATIONS. DDH, developmental dysplasia of the hip; AVN, avascular necrosis of the hip.

BIOLOGIC FEATURES AND NATURAL HISTORY

Understanding the developmental nature of developmental dysplasia of the hip (DDH) and the subsequent spectrum of hip abnormalities requires a knowledge of the growth and development of the hip joint.[12] Embryologically, the femoral head and acetabulum develop from the same block of primitive mesenchymal cells. A cleft develops to separate them at 7 to 8 weeks' gestation. By 11 weeks' gestation, development of the hip joint is complete. At birth, the femoral head and the acetabulum are primarily cartilaginous. The acetabulum continues to develop postnatally. The growth of the fibrocartilaginous rim (the labrum) that surrounds the bony acetabulum deepens the socket. Development of the femoral head and acetabulum are intimately related, and normal adult hip joints depend on further growth of these structures. Hip dysplasia may occur in utero, perinatally, or during infancy and childhood.

The acronym DDH includes hips that are unstable, subluxated, dislocated (luxated), and/or have malformed acetabula. A hip is *unstable* when the tight fit between the femoral head and the acetabulum is lost and the femoral head is able to move within (subluxated) or outside (dislocated) the confines of the acetabulum. A *dislocation* is a complete loss of contact of the femoral head with the acetabulum. Dislocations are divided into 2 types: teratologic and typical.[12] *Teratologic dislocations* occur early in utero and often are associated with neuromuscular disorders, such as arthrogryposis and myelodysplasia, or with various dysmorphic syndromes. The *typical dislocation* occurs in an otherwise healthy infant and may occur prenatally or postnatally.

During the immediate newborn period, laxity of the hip capsule predominates, and, if clinically significant enough, the femoral head may spontaneously dislocate and relocate. If the hip spontaneously relocates and stabilizes within a few days, subsequent hip development usually is normal. If subluxation or dislocation persists, then structural anatomic changes may develop. A deep concentric position of the femoral head in the acetabulum is necessary for normal development of the hip. When not deeply reduced (subluxated), the labrum may become everted and flattened. Because the femoral head is not reduced into the depth of the socket, the acetabulum does not grow and remodel and, therefore, becomes shallow. If the femoral head moves further out of the socket (dislocation), typically superiorly and laterally, the inferior capsule is pulled upward over the now empty socket. Muscles surrounding the hip, especially the adductors, become contracted, limiting abduction of the hip. The hip capsule constricts; once this capsular constriction narrows to less than the diameter of the femoral head, the hip can no longer be reduced by manual manipulative maneuvers, and operative reduction usually is necessary.

The hip is at risk for dislocation during 4 periods: 1) the 12th gestational week, 2) the 18th gestational week, 3) the final 4 weeks of gestation, and 4) the postnatal period. During the 12th gestational week, the hip is at risk as the fetal lower limb rotates medially. A dislocation at this time is termed teratologic. All elements of the hip joint develop abnor-

The recommendations in this statement do not indicate an exclusive course of treatment or serve as a standard of medical care. Variations, taking into account individual circumstances, may be appropriate.

The Practice Guideline, "Early Detection of Developmental Dysplasia of the Hip," was reviewed by appropriate committees and sections of the American Academy of Pediatrics (AAP) including the Chapter Review Group, a focus group of office-based pediatricians representing each AAP District: Gene R. Adams, MD; Robert M. Corwin, MD; Diane Fuquay, MD; Barbara M. Harley, MD; Thomas J. Herr, MD, Chair; Kenneth E. Matthews, MD; Robert D. Mines, MD; Lawrence C. Pakula, MD; Howard B. Weinblatt, MD; and Delosa A. Young, MD. The Practice Guideline was also reviewed by relevant outside medical organizations as part of the peer review process.
PEDIATRICS (ISSN 0031 4005). Copyright © 2000 by the American Academy of Pediatrics.

mally. The hip muscles develop around the 18th gestational week. Neuromuscular problems at this time, such as myelodysplasia and arthrogryposis, also lead to teratologic dislocations. During the final 4 weeks of pregnancy, mechanical forces have a role. Conditions such as oligohydramnios or breech position predispose to DDH.[13] Breech position occurs in ~3% of births, and DDH occurs more frequently in breech presentations, reportedly in as many as 23%. The frank breech position of hip flexion and knee extension places a newborn or infant at the highest risk. Postnatally, infant positioning such as swaddling, combined with ligamentous laxity, also has a role.

The true incidence of dislocation of the hip can only be presumed. There is no "gold standard" for diagnosis during the newborn period. Physical examination, plane radiography, and ultrasonography all are fraught with false-positive and false-negative results. Arthrography (insertion of contrast medium into the hip joint) and magnetic resonance imaging, although accurate for determining the precise hip anatomy, are inappropriate methods for screening the newborn and infant.

The reported incidence of DDH is influenced by genetic and racial factors, diagnostic criteria, the experience and training of the examiner, and the age of the child at the time of the examination. Wynne-Davies[14] reported an increased risk to subsequent children in the presence of a diagnosed dislocation (6% risk with healthy parents and an affected child, 12% risk with an affected parent, and 36% risk with an affected parent and 1 affected child). DDH is not always detectable at birth, but some newborn screening surveys suggest an incidence as high as 1 in 100 newborns with evidence of instability, and 1 to 1.5 cases of dislocation per 1000 newborns. The incidence of DDH is higher in girls. Girls are especially susceptible to the maternal hormone relaxin, which may contribute to ligamentous laxity with the resultant instability of the hip. The left hip is involved 3 times as commonly as the right hip, perhaps related to the left occiput anterior positioning of most nonbreech newborns. In this position, the left hip resides posteriorly against the mother's spine, potentially limiting abduction.

PHYSICAL EXAMINATION

DDH is an evolving process, and its physical findings on clinical examination change.[12,15,16] The newborn must be relaxed and preferably examined on a firm surface. Considerable patience and skill are required. The physical examination changes as the child grows older. No signs are pathognomonic for a dislocated hip. The examiner must look for asymmetry. Indeed, bilateral dislocations are more difficult to diagnose than unilateral dislocations because symmetry is retained. Asymmetrical thigh or gluteal folds, better observed when the child is prone, apparent limb length discrepancy, and restricted motion, especially abduction, are significant, albeit not pathognomonic signs. With the infant supine and the pelvis stabilized, abduction to 75° and adduction to 30° should occur readily under normal circumstances.

The 2 maneuvers for assessing hip stability in the newborn are the Ortolani and Barlow tests. The Ortolani elicits the sensation of the dislocated hip reducing, and the Barlow detects the unstable hip dislocating from the acetabulum. The Ortolani is performed with the newborn supine and the examiner's index and middle fingers placed along the greater trochanter with the thumb placed along the inner thigh. The hip is flexed to 90° but not more, and the leg is held in neutral rotation. The hip is gently abducted while lifting the leg anteriorly. With this maneuver, a "clunk" is felt as the dislocated femoral head reduces into the acetabulum. This is a positive Ortolani sign. The Barlow provocative test is performed with the newborn positioned supine and the hips flexed to 90°. The leg is then gently adducted while posteriorly directed pressure is placed on the knee. A palpable clunk or sensation of movement is felt as the femoral head exits the acetabulum posteriorly. This is a positive Barlow sign. The Ortolani and Barlow maneuvers are performed 1 hip at a time. Little force is required for the performance of either of these tests. The goal is not to prove that the hip can be dislocated. Forceful and repeated examinations can break the seal between the labrum and the femoral head. These strongly positive signs of Ortolani and Barlow are distinguished from a large array of soft or equivocal physical findings present during the newborn period. High-pitched clicks are commonly elicited with flexion and extension and are inconsequential. A dislocatable hip has a rather distinctive clunk, whereas a subluxable hip is characterized by a feeling of looseness, a sliding movement, but without the true Ortolani and Barlow clunks. Separating true dislocations (clunks) from a feeling of instability and from benign adventitial sounds (clicks) takes practice and expertise. This guideline recognizes the broad range of physical findings present in newborns and infants and the confusion of terminology generated in the literature. By 8 to 12 weeks of age, the capsule laxity decreases, muscle tightness increases, and the Barlow and Ortolani maneuvers are no longer positive regardless of the status of the femoral head. In the 3-month-old infant, limitation of abduction is the most reliable sign associated with DDH. Other features that arouse suspicion include asymmetry of thigh folds, a positive Allis or Galeazzi sign (relative shortness of the femur with the hips and knees flexed), and discrepancy of leg lengths. These physical findings alert the examiner that abnormal relationships of the femoral head to the acetabulum (dislocation and subluxation) *may* be present.

Maldevelopments of the acetabulum alone (acetabular dysplasia) can be determined only by imaging techniques. Abnormal physical findings may be absent in an infant with acetabular dysplasia but no subluxation or dislocation. Indeed, because of the confusion, inconsistencies, and misuse of language in the literature (eg, an Ortolani sign called a click by some and a clunk by others), this guideline uses the following definitions.

- A *positive examination* result for DDH is the Barlow or Ortolani sign. This is the clunk of dislocation or reduction.
- An *equivocal examination* or *warning signs* include an array of physical findings that may be found in children with DDH, in children with another orthopaedic disorder, or in children who are completely healthy. These physical findings include asymmetric thigh or buttock creases, an apparent or true short leg, and limited abduction. These signs, used singly or in combination, serve to raise the pediatrician's index of suspicion and act as a threshold for referral. Newborn soft tissue hip clicks are not predictive of DDH[17] but may be confused with the Ortolani and Barlow clunks by some screening physicians and thereby be a reason for referral.

IMAGING

Radiographs of the pelvis and hips have historically been used to assess an infant with suspected DDH. During the first few months of life when the femoral heads are composed entirely of cartilage, radiographs have limited value. Displacement and instability may be undetectable, and evaluation of acetabular development is influenced by the infant's position at the time the radiograph is performed. By 4 to 6 months of age, radiographs become more reliable, particularly when the ossification center develops in the femoral head. Radiographs are readily available and relatively low in cost.

Real-time ultrasonography has been established as an accurate method for imaging the hip during the first few months of life.[15,18–25] With ultrasonography, the cartilage can be visualized and the hip can be viewed while assessing the stability of the hip and the morphologic features of the acetabulum. In some clinical settings, ultrasonography can provide information comparable to arthrography (direct injection of contrast into the hip joint), without the need for sedation, invasion, contrast medium, or ionizing radiation. Although the availability of equipment for ultrasonography is widespread, accurate results in hip sonography require training and experience. Although expertise in pediatric hip ultrasonography is increasing, this examination may not always be available or obtained conveniently. Ultrasonographic techniques include *static evaluation* of the morphologic features of the hip, as popularized in Europe by Graf,[26] and a *dynamic evaluation*, as developed by Harcke[20] that assesses the hip for stability of the femoral head in the socket, as well as static anatomy. Dynamic ultrasonography yields more useful information. With both techniques, there is considerable interobserver variability, especially during the first 3 weeks of life.[7,27]

Experience with ultrasonography has documented its ability to detect abnormal position, instability, and dysplasia not evident on clinical examination. Ultrasonography during the first 4 weeks of life often reveals the presence of minor degrees of instability and acetabular immaturity. Studies[7,28,29] indicate that nearly all these mild early findings, which will not be apparent on physical examination, resolve spontaneously without treatment. Newborn screening with ultrasonography has required a high frequency of reexamination and results in a large number of hips being unnecessarily treated. One study[23] demonstrates that a screening process with higher false-positive results also yields increased prevention of late cases. Ultrasonographic screening of all infants at 4 to 6 weeks of age would be expensive, requiring considerable resources. This practice is yet to be validated by clinical trial. *Consequently, the use of ultrasonography is recommended as an adjunct to the clinical evaluation.* It is the technique of choice for clarifying a physical finding, assessing a high-risk infant, and monitoring DDH as it is observed or treated. Used in this selective capacity, it can guide treatment and may prevent overtreatment.

PRETERM INFANTS

DDH may be unrecognized in prematurely born infants. When the infant has cardiorespiratory problems, the diagnosis and management are focused on providing appropriate ventilatory and cardiovascular support, and careful examination of the hips may be deferred until a later date. The most complete examination the infant receives may occur at the time of discharge from the hospital, and this single examination may not detect subluxation or dislocation. Despite the medical urgencies surrounding the preterm infant, it is critical to examine the entire child.

METHODS FOR GUIDELINE DEVELOPMENT

Our goal was to develop a practice parameter by using a process that would be based whenever possible on available evidence. The methods used a combination of expert panel, decision modeling, and evidence synthesis[30] (see the Technical Report available on *Pediatrics electronic pages* at www.pediatrics.org). The predominant methods recommended for such evidence synthesis are generally of 2 types: a *data-driven* method and a *model-driven*[31,32] method. In data-driven methods, the analyst finds the best data available and induces a conclusion from these data. A model-driven method, in contrast, begins with an effort to define the context for evidence and then searches for the data as defined by that context. Data-driven methods are useful when the quality of evidence is high. A careful review of the medical literature revealed that the published evidence about DDH did not meet the criteria for high quality. There was a paucity of randomized clinical trials.[8] We decided, therefore, to use the model-driven method.

A decision model was constructed based on the perspective of practicing clinicians and determining the best strategy for screening and diagnosis. The target child was a full-term newborn with no obvious orthopaedic abnormalities. We focused on the various options available to the pediatrician* for the detection of DDH, including screening by physical examination, screening by ultrasonography, and episodic screening during health supervision. Because

*In this guideline, the term *pediatrician* includes the range of pediatric primary care providers, eg, family practitioners and pediatric nurse practitioners.

the detection of a dislocated hip usually results in referral by the pediatrician, and because management of DDH is not in the purview of the pediatrician's care, treatment options are not included. We also included in our model a wide range of options for detecting DDH during the first year of life if the results of the newborn screen are negative.

The outcomes on which we focused were a dislocated hip at 1 year of age as the major morbidity of the disease and avascular necrosis of the hip (AVN) as the primary complication of DDH treatment. AVN is a loss of blood supply to the femoral head resulting in abnormal hip development, distortion of shape, and, in some instances, substantial morbidity. Ideally, a gold standard would be available to define DDH at any point in time. However, as noted, no gold standard exists except, perhaps, arthrography of the hip, which is an inappropriate standard for use in a detection model. Therefore, we defined outcomes in terms of the *process of care*. We reviewed the literature extensively. The purpose of the literature review was to provide the probabilities required by the decision model since there were no randomized clinical trials. The article or chapter title and the abstracts were reviewed by 2 members of the methodology team and members of the subcommittee. Articles not rejected were reviewed, and data were abstracted that would provide evidence for the probabilities required by the decision model. As part of the literature abstraction process, the evidence quality in each article was assessed. A computer-based literature search, hand review of recent publications, or examination of the reference section for other articles ("ancestor articles") identified 623 articles; 241 underwent detailed review, 118 of which provided some data. Of the 100 ancestor articles, only 17 yielded useful articles, suggesting that our accession process was complete. By traditional epidemiologic standards,[33] the quality of the evidence in this set of articles was uniformly low. There were few controlled trials and few studies of the follow-up of infants for whom the results of newborn examinations were negative. When the evidence was poor or lacking entirely, extensive discussions among members of the committee and the expert opinion of outside consultants were used to arrive at a consensus. No votes were taken. Disagreements were discussed, and consensus was achieved.

The available evidence was distilled in 3 ways. First, estimates were made of DDH at birth in infants without risk factors. These estimates constituted the baseline risk. Second, estimates were made of the rates of DDH in the children with risk factors. These numbers guide clinical actions: rates that are too high might indicate referral or different follow-up despite negative physical findings. Third, each screening strategy (pediatrician-based, orthopaedist-based, and ultrasonography-based) was scored for the estimated number of children given a diagnosis of DDH at birth, at mid-term (4–12 months of age), and at late-term (12 months of age and older) and for the estimated number of cases of AVN incurred, assuming that all children given a diagnosis of DDH would be treated. These numbers suggest the best strategy, balancing DDH detection with incurring adverse effects.

The baseline estimate of DDH based on orthopaedic screening was 11.5/1000 infants. Estimates from pediatric screening were 8.6/1000 and from ultrasonography were 25/1000. The 11.5/1000 rate translates into a rate for not-at-risk boys of 4.1/1000 boys and a rate for not-at-risk girls of 19/1000 girls. These numbers derive from the facts that the relative risk—the rate in girls divided by the rate in boys across several studies—is 4.6 and because infants are split evenly between boys and girls, so $.5 \times 4.1/1000 + .5 \times 19/1000 = 11.5/1000$.[34,35] We used these baseline rates for calculating the rates in other risk groups. Because the relative risk of DDH for children with a positive family history (first-degree relatives) is 1.7, the rate for boys with a positive family history is $1.7 \times 4.1 = 6.4/1000$ boys, and for girls with a positive family history, $1.7 \times 19 = 32/1000$ girls. Finally, the relative risk of DDH for breech presentation (of all kinds) is 6.3, so the risk for breech boys is $7.0 \times 4.1 = 29/1000$ boys and for breech girls, $7.0 \times 19 = 133/1000$ girls. These numbers are summarized in Table 1.

These numbers suggest that boys without risk or those with a family history have the lowest risk; girls without risk and boys born in a breech presentation have an intermediate risk; and girls with a positive family history, and especially girls born in a breech presentation, have the highest risks. Guidelines, considering the risk factors, should follow these risk profiles. Reports of newborn screening for DDH have included various screening techniques. In some, the screening clinician was an orthopaedist, in

TABLE 1. Relative and Absolute Risks for Finding a Positive Examination Result at Newborn Screening by Using the Ortolani and Barlow Signs

Newborn Characteristics	Relative Risk of a Positive Examination Result	Absolute Risk of a Positive Examination Result per 1000 Newborns With Risk Factors
All newborns	. . .	11.5
Boys	1.0	4.1
Girls	4.6	19
Positive family history	1.7	
Boys	. . .	6.4
Girls	. . .	32
Breech presentation	7.0	
Boys	. . .	29
Girls	. . .	133

TABLE 2. Newborn Strategy*

Outcome	Orthopaedist PE	Pediatrician PE	Ultrasonography
DDH in newborn	12	8.6	25
DDH at ~6 mo of age	.1	.45	.28
DDH at 12 mo of age or more	.16	.33	.1
AVN at 12 mo of age	.06	.1	.1

* PE indicates physical examination. Outcome per 1000 infants initially screened.

others, a pediatrician, and in still others, a physiotherapist. In addition, screening has been performed by ultrasonography. In assessing the expected effect of each strategy, we estimated the newborn DDH rates, the mid-term DDH rates, and the late-term DDH rates for each of the 3 strategies, as shown in Table 2. We also estimated the rate of AVN for DDH treated before 2 months of age (2.5/1000 treated) and after 2 months of age (109/1000 treated). We could not distinguish the AVN rates for children treated between 2 and 12 months of age from those treated later. Table 2 gives these data. The total cases of AVN per strategy are calculated, assuming that all infants with positive examination results are treated.

Table 2 shows that a strategy using pediatricians to screen newborns would give the lowest newborn rate but the highest mid- and late-term DDH rates. To assess how much better an ultrasonography-only screening strategy would be, we could calculate a cost-effectiveness ratio. In this case, the "cost" of ultrasonographic screening is the number of "extra" newborn cases that probably include children who do not need to be treated. (The cost from AVN is the same in the 2 strategies.) By using these cases as the cost and the number of later cases averted as the effect, a ratio is obtained of 71 children treated neonatally because of a positive ultrasonographic screen for each later case averted. Because this number is high, and because the presumption of better late-term efficacy is based on a single study, we do not recommend ultrasonographic screening at this time.

RECOMMENDATIONS AND NOTES TO ALGORITHM (Fig 1)

1. **All newborns are to be screened by physical examination**. The evidence† for this recommendation is good. The expert consensus‡ is strong. Although initial screening by orthopaedists§ would be optimal (Table 2), it is doubtful that if widely practiced, such a strategy would give the same good results as those published from pediatric orthopaedic research centers. **It is recommended that screening be done by a properly trained health care provider** (eg, physician, pediatric nurse practitioner, physician assistant, or physical therapist). (Evidence for this recommendation is strong.) A number of studies performed by properly trained nonphysicians report results indistinguishable from those performed by physicians.[36] The examination after discharge from the neonatal intensive care unit should be performed as a newborn examination with appropriate screening. **Ultrasonography of all newborns is not recommended.** (Evidence is fair; consensus is strong.) Although there is indirect evidence to support the use of ultrasonographic screening of all newborns, it is not advocated because it is operator-dependent, availability is questionable, it increases the rate of treatment, and interobserver variability is high. There are probably some increased costs. We considered a strategy of "no newborn screening." This arm is politically indefensible because screening newborns is inherent in pediatrician's care. The technical report details this limb through decision analysis. Regardless of the screening method used for the newborn, DDH is detected in 1 in 5000 infants at 18 months of age.[3] The evidence and consensus for newborn screening remain strong.

†In this guideline, evidence is listed as good, fair, or poor based on the methodologist's evaluation of the literature quality. (See the Technical Report.)

‡Opinion or consensus is listed as *strong* if opinion of the expert panel was unanimous or *mixed* if there were dissenting points of view.

§In this guideline, the term *orthopaedist* refers to an orthopaedic surgeon with expertise in pediatric orthopaedic conditions.

Newborn Physical Examination and Treatment

2. **If a positive Ortolani or Barlow sign is found in the newborn examination, the infant should be referred to an orthopaedist**. Orthopaedic referral is recommended when the Ortolani sign is unequivocally positive (a clunk). Orthopaedic referral is not recommended for any softly positive finding in the examination (eg, hip click without dislocation). The precise time frame for the newborn to be evaluated by the orthopaedist cannot be determined from the literature. However, the literature suggests that the majority of "abnormal" physical findings of hip examinations at birth (clicks and clunks) will resolve by 2 weeks; therefore, consultation and possible initiation of treatment are recommended by that time. The data recommending that all those with a positive Ortolani sign be referred to an orthopaedist are limited, but expert panel consensus, nevertheless, was strong, because pediatricians do not have the training to take full responsibility and because true Ortolani clunks are rare and their management is more appropriately performed by the orthopaedist.

If the results of the physical examination at birth are "equivocally" positive (ie, soft click, mild asymmetry, but neither an Ortolani nor a Barlow sign is present), then a follow-up hip examination by the pediatrician in 2 weeks is recommended. (Evidence is good; consensus is strong.) The available data suggest that most clicks resolve by 2 weeks and that these "benign hip clicks" in the newborn period do

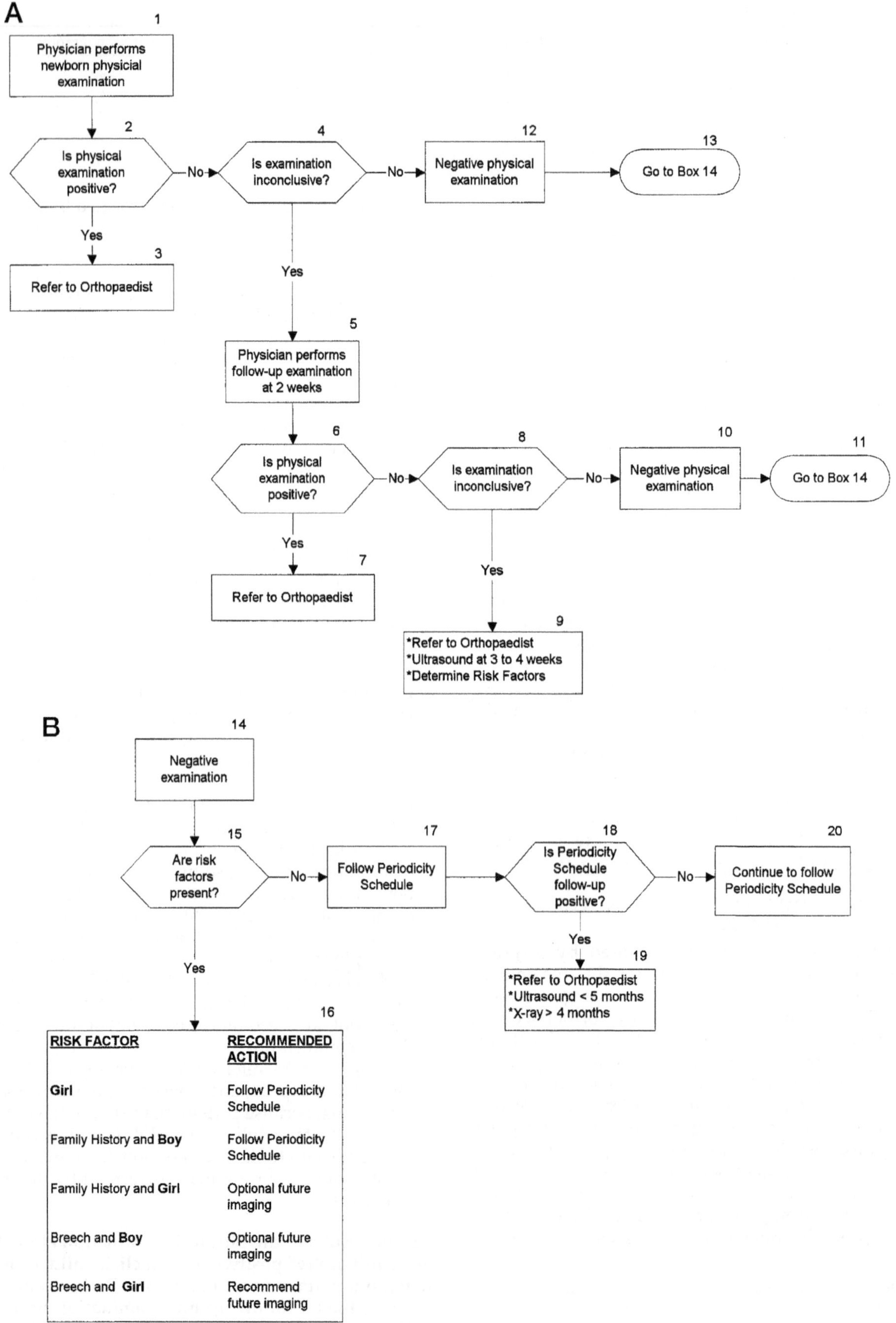

Fig 1. Screening for developmental hip dysplasia—clinical algorithm.

not lead to later hip dysplasia.[9,17,28,37] Thus, for an infant with softly positive signs, the pediatrician should reexamine the hips at 2 weeks before making referrals for orthopaedic care or ultrasonography. We recognize the concern of pediatricians about adherence to follow-up care regimens, but this concern regards all aspects of health maintenance and is not a reason to request ultrasonography or other diagnostic study of the newborn hips.

3. **If the results of the newborn physical examination are positive (ie, presence of an Ortolani or a Barlow sign), ordering an ultrasonographic examination of the newborn is not recommended**. (Evidence is poor; opinion is strong.) Treatment decisions are not influenced by the results of ultrasonography but are based on the results of the physical examination. The treating physician may use a variety of imaging studies during clinical management. **If the results of the newborn physical examination are positive, obtaining a radiograph of the newborn's pelvis and hips is not recommended** (evidence is poor; opinion is strong), because they are of limited value and do not influence treatment decisions.

The use of triple diapers when abnormal physical signs are detected during the newborn period is not recommended. (Evidence is poor; opinion is strong.) Triple diaper use is common practice despite the lack of data on the effectiveness of triple diaper use; and, in instances of frank dislocation, the use of triple diapers may delay the initiation of more appropriate treatment (such as with the Pavlik harness). Often, the primary care pediatrician may not have performed the newborn examination in the hospital. The importance of communication cannot be overemphasized, and triple diapers may aid in follow-up as a reminder that a possible abnormal physical examination finding was present in the newborn.

2-Week Examination

4. **If the results of the physical examination are positive (eg, positive Ortolani or Barlow sign) at 2 weeks, refer to an orthopaedist**. (Evidence is strong; consensus is strong.) Referral is urgent but is not an emergency. Consensus is strong that, as in the newborn, the presence of an Ortolani or Barlow sign at 2 weeks warrants referral to an orthopaedist. An Ortolani sign at 2 weeks may be a new finding or a finding that was not apparent at the time of the newborn examination.

5. **If at the 2-week examination the Ortolani and Barlow signs are absent but physical findings raise suspicions, consider referral to an orthopaedist or request ultrasonography at age 3 to 4 weeks**. Consensus is mixed about the follow-up for softly positive or equivocal findings at 2 weeks of age (eg, adventitial click, thigh asymmetry, and apparent leg length difference). Because it is necessary to confirm the status of the hip joint, the pediatrician can consider referral to an orthopaedist or for ultrasonography if the constellation of physical findings raises a high level of suspicion. However, if the physical findings are minimal, continuing follow-up by the periodicity schedule with focused hip examinations is also an option, provided risk factors are considered. (See "Recommendations" 7 and 8.)

6. **If the results of the physical examination are negative at 2 weeks, follow-up is recommended at the scheduled well-baby periodic examinations**. (Evidence is good; consensus is strong.)

7. **Risk factors. If the results of the newborn examination are negative (or equivocally positive), risk factors may be considered.**[13,21,38–41] Risk factors are a study of thresholds to act.[42] Table 1 gives the risk of finding a positive Ortolani or Barlow sign at the time of the initial newborn screening. If this examination is negative, the absolute risk of there being a true dislocated hip is greatly reduced. Nevertheless, the data in Table 1 may influence the pediatrician to perform confirmatory evaluations. Action will vary based on the individual clinician. The following recommendations are made (evidence is strong; opinion is strong):
   - **Girl** (newborn risk of 19/1000). When the results of the newborn examination are negative or equivocally positive, hips should be reevaluated at 2 weeks of age. If negative, continue according to the periodicity schedule; if positive, refer to an orthopaedist or for ultrasonography at 3 weeks of age.
   - **Infants with a positive family history of DDH** (newborn risk for boys of 9.4/1000 and for girls, 44/1000). When the results of the newborn examination in boys are negative or equivocally positive, hips should be reevaluated at 2 weeks of age. If negative, continue according to the periodicity schedule; if positive, refer to an orthopaedist or for ultrasonography at 3 weeks of age. In girls, the absolute risk of 44/1000 may exceed the pediatrician's threshold to act, and imaging with an ultrasonographic examination at 6 weeks of age or a radiograph of the pelvis at 4 months of age is recommended.
   - **Breech presentation** (newborn risk for boys of 26/1000 and for girls, 120/1000). **For negative or equivocally positive newborn examinations, the infant should be reevaluated at regular intervals (according to the periodicity schedule) if the examination results remain negative**. Because an absolute risk of 120/1000 (12%) probably exceeds most pediatricians' threshold to act, imaging with an ultrasonographic examination at 6 weeks of age or with a radiograph of the pelvis and hips at 4 months of age is recommended. In addition, because some reports show a high incidence of hip abnormalities detected at an older age in children born breech, this imaging strategy remains an option for all children born breech, not just girls. These hip abnormalities are, for the most part, inadequate development of the acetabulum. Acetabular dysplasia is best found by a radiographic examination at 6 months of age or older. A

suggestion of poorly formed acetabula may be observed at 6 weeks of age by ultrasonography, but the best study remains a radiograph performed closer to 6 months of age. Ultrasonographic newborn screening of all breech infants will not eliminate the possibility of later acetabular dysplasia.

8. **Periodicity. The hips must be examined at every well-baby visit according to the recommended periodicity schedule for well-baby examinations (2–4 days for newborns discharged in less than 48 hours after delivery, by 1 month, 2 months, 4 months, 6 months, 9 months, and 12 months of age).** If at any time during the follow-up period DDH is suspected because of an abnormal physical examination or by a parental complaint of difficulty diapering or abnormal appearing legs, the pediatrician must confirm that the hips are stable, in the sockets, and developing normally. Confirmation can be made by a focused physical examination when the infant is calm and relaxed, by consultation with another primary care pediatrician, by consultation with an orthopaedist, by ultrasonography if the infant is younger than 5 months of age, or by radiography if the infant is older than 4 months of age. (Between 4 and 6 months of age, ultrasonography and radiography seem to be equally effective diagnostic imaging studies.)

DISCUSSION

DDH is an important term because it accurately reflects the biologic features of the disorder and the susceptibility of the hip to become dislocated at various times. Dislocated hips always will be diagnosed later in infancy and childhood because not every dislocated hip is detectable at birth, and hips continue to dislocate throughout the first year of life. Thus, this guideline requires that the pediatrician follow *a process of care for the detection of DDH*. The process recommended for early detection of DDH includes the following:

- Screen all newborns' hips by physical examination.
- Examine all infants' hips according to a periodicity schedule and follow-up until the child is an established walker.
- Record and document physical findings.
- Be aware of the changing physical examination for DDH.
- If physical findings raise suspicion of DDH, or if parental concerns suggest hip disease, confirmation is required by expert physical examination, referral to an orthopaedist, or by an age-appropriate imaging study.

When this process of care is followed, the number of dislocated hips diagnosed at 1 year of age should be minimized. However, the problem of late detection of dislocated hips will not be eliminated. The results of screening programs have indicated that 1 in 5000 children have a dislocated hip detected at 18 months of age or older.[3]

TECHNICAL REPORT

The Technical Report is available from the American Academy of Pediatrics from several sources. The Technical Report is published in full-text on *Pediatrics electronic pages*. It is also available in a compendium of practice guidelines that contains guidelines and evidence reports together. The objective was to create a recommendation to pediatricians and other primary care providers about their role as screeners for detecting DDH. The patients are a theoretical cohort of newborns. A model-based method using decision analysis was the foundation. Components of the approach include:

- Perspective: primary care provider
- Outcomes: DDH and AVN
- Preferences: expected rates of outcomes
- Model: influence diagram assessed from the subcommittee and from the methodology team with critical feedback from the subcommittee
- Evidence sources: Medline and EMBase (detailed in "Methods" section)
- Evidence quality: assessed on a custom, subjective scale, based primarily on the fit of the evidence in the decision model

The results are detailed in the "Methods" section. Based on the raw evidence and Bayesian hierarchical meta-analysis,[34,35] estimates for the incidence of DDH based on the type of screener (orthopaedist vs pediatrician); the odds ratio for DDH given risk factors of sex, family history, and breech presentation; and estimates for late detection and AVN were determined and are detailed in the "Methods" section and in Tables 1 and 2.

The decision model (reduced based on available evidence) suggests that orthopaedic screening is optimal, but because orthopaedists in the published studies and in practice would differ in pediatric expertise, the supply of pediatric orthopaedists is relatively limited, and the difference between orthopaedists and pediatricians is statistically insignificant, we conclude that pediatric screening is to be recommended. The place for ultrasonography in the screening process remains to be defined because of the limited data available regarding late diagnosis in ultrasonography screening to permit definitive recommendations.

These data could be used by others to refine the conclusion based on costs, parental preferences, or physician style. Areas for research are well defined by our model-based method. All references are in the Technical Report.

RESEARCH QUESTIONS

The quality of the literature suggests many areas for research, because there is a paucity of randomized clinical trials and case-controlled studies. The following is a list of possibilities:

1. Minimum diagnostic abilities of a screener. Although there are data for pediatricians in general, few, if any, studies evaluated the abilities of an individual examiner. What should the minimum

sensitivity and specificity be, and how should they be assessed?

2. Intercurrent screening. There were few studies on systemic processes for screening after the newborn period.[2,43,44] Although several studies assessed postneonatal DDH, the data did not specify how many examinations were performed on each child before the abnormal result was found.
3. Trade-offs. Screening always results in false-positive results, and these patients suffer the adverse effects of therapy. How many unnecessary AVNs are we—families, physicians, and society—willing to tolerate from a screening program for every appropriately treated infant in whom late DDH was averted? This assessment depends on people's values and preferences and is not strictly an epidemiologic issue.
4. Postneonatal DDH after ultrasonographic screening. Although we concluded that ultrasonographic screening did not result in fewer diagnoses of postneonatal DDH, that conclusion was based on only 1 study.[36] Further study is needed.
5. Cost-effectiveness. If ultrasonographic screening reduces the number of postneonatal DDH diagnoses, then there will be a cost trade-off between the resources spent up front to screen everyone with an expensive technology, as in the case of ultrasonography, and the resources spent later to treat an expensive adverse event, as in the case of physical examination-based screening. The level at which the cost per case of postneonatal DDH averted is no longer acceptable is a matter of social preference, not of epidemiology.

ACKNOWLEDGMENTS

We acknowledge and appreciate the help of our methodology team, Richard Hinton, MD, Paola Morello, MD, and Jeanne Santoli, MD, who diligently participated in the literature review and abstracting the articles into evidence tables, and the subcommittee on evidence analysis.

We would also like to thank Robert Sebring, PhD, for assisting in the management of this process; Bonnie Cosner for managing the workflow; and Chris Kwiat, MLS, from the American Academy of Pediatrics Bakwin Library, who performed the literature searches.

Committee on Quality Improvement, 1999–2000
Charles J. Homer, MD, MPH, Chairperson
Richard D. Baltz, MD
Gerald B. Hickson, MD
Paul V. Miles, MD
Thomas B. Newman, MD, MPH
Joan E. Shook, MD
William M. Zurhellen, MD

Betty A. Lowe, MD, Liaison, National Association of Children's Hospitals and Related Institutions (NACHRI)
Ellen Schwalenstocker, MBA, Liaison, NACHRI
Michael J. Goldberg, MD, Liaison, Council on Sections
Richard Shiffman, MD, Liaison, Section on Computers and Other Technology
Jan Ellen Berger, MD, Liaison, Committee on Medical Liability
F. Lane France, MD, Committee on Practice and Ambulatory Medicine

Subcommittee on Developmental Dysplasia of the Hip, 1999–2000
Michael J. Goldberg, MD, Chairperson
Section on Orthopaedics
Theodore H. Harcke, MD
Section on Radiology
Anthony Hirsch, MD
Practitioner
Harold Lehmann, MD, PhD
Section on Epidemiology
Dennis R. Roy, MD
Section on Orthopaedics
Philip Sunshine, MD
Section on Perinatology

Consultant
Carol Dezateux, MB, MPH

REFERENCES

1. Bjerkreim I, Hagen O, Ikonomou N, Kase T, Kristiansen T, Arseth P. Late diagnosis of developmental dislocation of the hip in Norway during the years 1980–1989. *J Pediatr Orthop B.* 1993;2:112–114
2. Clarke N, Clegg J, Al-Chalabi A. Ultrasound screening of hips at risk for CDH: failure to reduce the incidence of late cases. *J Bone Joint Surg Br.* 1989;71:9–12
3. Dezateux C, Godward C. Evaluating the national screening programme for congenital dislocation of the hip. *J Med Screen.* 1995;2:200–206
4. Hadlow V. Neonatal screening for congenital dislocation of the hip: a prospective 21-year survey. *J Bone Joint Surg Br.* 1988;70:740–743
5. Krikler S, Dwyer N. Comparison of results of two approaches to hip screening in infants. *J Bone Joint Surg Br.* 1992;74:701–703
6. Macnicol M. Results of a 25-year screening programme for neonatal hip instability. *J Bone Joint Surg Br.* 1990;72:1057–1060
7. Marks DS, Clegg J, Al-Chalabi AN. Routine ultrasound screening for neonatal hip instability: can it abolish late-presenting congenital dislocation of the hip? *J Bone Joint Surg Br.* 1994;76:534–538
8. Rosendahl K, Markestad T, Lie R. Congenital dislocation of the hip: a prospective study comparing ultrasound and clinical examination. *Acta Paediatr.* 1992;81:177–181
9. Sanfridson J, Redlund-Johnell I, Uden A. Why is congenital dislocation of the hip still missed? Analysis of 96,891 infants screened in Malmo 1956–1987. *Acta Orthop Scand.* 1991;62:87–91
10. Tredwell S, Bell H. Efficacy of neonatal hip examination. *J Pediatr Orthop.* 1981;1:61–65
11. Yngve D, Gross R. Late diagnosis of hip dislocation in infants. *J Pediatr Orthop.* 1990;10:777–779
12. Aronsson DD, Goldberg MJ, Kling TF, Roy DR. Developmental dysplasia of the hip. *Pediatrics.* 1994;94:201–212
13. Hinderaker T, Daltveit AK, Irgens LM, Uden A, Reikeras O. The impact of intra-uterine factors on neonatal hip instability: an analysis of 1,059,479 children in Norway. *Acta Orthop Scand.* 1994;65:239–242
14. Wynne-Davies R. Acetabular dysplasia and familial joint laxity: two etiological factors in congenital dislocation of the hip: a review of 589 patients and their families. *J Bone Joint Surg Br.* 1970;52:704–716
15. De Pellegrin M. Ultrasound screening for congenital dislocation of the hip: results and correlations between clinical and ultrasound findings. *Ital J Orthop Traumatol.* 1991;17:547–553
16. Stoffelen D, Urlus M, Molenaers G, Fabry G. Ultrasound, radiographs, and clinical symptoms in developmental dislocation of the hip: a study of 170 patients. *J Pediatr Orthop B.* 1995;4:194–199
17. Bond CD, Hennrikus WL, Della Maggiore E. Prospective evaluation of newborn soft tissue hip clicks with ultrasound. *J Pediatr Orthop.* 1997;17:199–201
18. Bialik V, Wiener F, Benderly A. Ultrasonography and screening in developmental displacement of the hip. *J Pediatr Orthop B.* 1992;1:51–54
19. Castelein R, Sauter A. Ultrasound screening for congenital dysplasia of the hip in newborns: its value. *J Pediatr Orthop.* 1988;8:666–670
20. Clarke NMP, Harcke HT, McHugh P, Lee MS, Borns PF, MacEwen GP. Real-time ultrasound in the diagnosis of congenital dislocation and dysplasia of the hip. *J Bone Joint Surg Br.* 1985;67:406–412
21. Garvey M, Donoghue V, Gorman W, O'Brien N, Murphy J. Radiographic screening at four months of infants at risk for congenital hip dislocation. *J Bone Joint Surg Br.* 1992;74:704–707
22. Langer R. Ultrasonic investigation of the hip in newborns in the diagnosis of congenital hip dislocation: classification and results of a screening program. *Skeletal Radiol.* 1987;16:275–279

23. Rosendahl K, Markestad T, Lie RT. Ultrasound screening for developmental dysplasia of the hip in the neonate: the effect on treatment rate and prevalence of late cases. *Pediatrics*. 1994;94:47–52
24. Terjesen T. Ultrasound as the primary imaging method in the diagnosis of hip dysplasia in children aged <2 years. *J Pediatr Orthop B*. 1996;5: 123–128
25. Vedantam R, Bell M. Dynamic ultrasound assessment for monitoring of treatment of congenital dislocation of the hip. *J Pediatr Orthop*. 1995;15: 725–728
26. Graf R. Classification of hip joint dysplasia by means of sonography. *Arch Orthop Trauma Surg*. 1984;102:248–255
27. Berman L, Klenerman L. Ultrasound screening for hip abnormalities: preliminary findings in 1001 neonates. *Br Med J (Clin Res Ed)*. 1986;293: 719–722
28. Castelein R, Sauter A, de Vlieger M, van Linge B. Natural history of ultrasound hip abnormalities in clinically normal newborns. *J Pediatr Orthop*. 1992;12:423–427
29. Clarke N. Sonographic clarification of the problems of neonatal hip stability. *J Pediatr Orthop*. 1986;6:527–532
30. Eddy DM. The confidence profile method: a Bayesian method for assessing health technologies. *Operations Res*. 1989;37:210–228
31. Howard RA, Matheson JE. Influence diagrams. In: Matheson JE, ed. *Readings on the Principles and Applications of Decision Analysis*. Menlo Park, CA: Strategic Decisions Group; 1981:720–762
32. Nease RF, Owen DK. Use of influence diagrams to structure medical decisions. *Med Decis Making*. 1997;17:265–275
33. Guyatt GH, Sackett DL, Sinclair JC, Hayward R, Cook DJ, Cook RJ. Users' guide to the medical literature, IX: a method for grading health care recommendations. *JAMA*. 1995;274:1800–1804
34. Gelman A, Carlin JB, Stern HS, Rubin DB. *Bayesian Data Analysis*. London, UK: Chapman and Hall; 1997
35. Spiegelhalter D, Thomas A, Best N, Gilks W. *BUGS 0.5: Bayesian Inference Using Gibbs Sampling Manual, II*. Cambridge, MA: MRC Biostatistics Unit, Institute of Public Health; 1996. Available at: http://www.mrc-bsu.cam.ac.uk/bugs/software/software.html
36. Fiddian NJ, Gardiner JC. Screening for congenital dislocation of the hip by physiotherapists: results of a ten-year study. *J Bone Joint Surg Br*. 1994;76:458–459
37. Dunn P, Evans R, Thearle M, Griffiths H, Witherow P. Congenital dislocation of the hip: early and late diagnosis and management compared. *Arch Dis Child*. 1992;60:407–414
38. Holen KJ, Tegnander A, Terjesen T, Johansen OJ, Eik-Nes SH. Ultrasonographic evaluation of breech presentation as a risk factor for hip dysplasia. *Acta Paediatr*. 1996;85:225–229
39. Jones D, Powell N. Ultrasound and neonatal hip screening: a prospective study of "high risk" babies. *J Bone Joint Surg Br*. 1990;72:457–459
40. Teanby DN, Paton RW. Ultrasound screening for congenital dislocation of the hip: a limited targeted programme. *J Pediatr Orthop*. 1997;17: 202–204
41. Tonnis D, Storch K, Ulbrich H. Results of newborn screening for CDH with and without sonography and correlation of risk factors. *J Pediatr Orthop*. 1990;10:145–152
42. Pauker SG, Kassirer JP. The threshold approach to clinical decision making. *N Engl J Med*. 1980;302:1109–1117
43. Bower C, Stanley F, Morgan B, Slattery H, Stanton C. Screening for congenital dislocation of the hip by child-health nurses in western Australia. *Med J Aust*. 1989;150:61–65
44. Franchin F, Lacalendola G, Molfetta L, Mascolo V, Quagliarella L. Ultrasound for early diagnosis of hip dysplasia. *Ital J Orthop Traumatol*. 1992;18:261–269

ADDENDUM TO REFERENCES FOR THE DDH GUIDELINE

New information is generated constantly. Specific details of this report must be changed over time.

New articles (additional articles 1–7) have been published since the completion of our literature search and construction of this Guideline. These articles taken alone might seem to contradict some of the Guideline's estimates as detailed in the article and in the Technical Report. However, taken in context with the literature synthesis carried out for the construction of this Guideline, our estimates remain intact and no conclusions are obviated.

ADDITIONAL ARTICLES

1. Bialik V, Bialik GM, Blazer S, Sujov P, Wiener F, Berant M. Developmental dysplasia of the hip: a new approach to incidence. *Pediatrics*. 1999;103:93–99
2. Clegg J, Bache CE, Raut VV. Financial justification for routine ultrasound screening of the neonatal hip. *J Bone Joint Surg*. 1999;81-B:852–857
3. Holen KJ, Tegnander A, Eik-Nes SH, Terjesen T. The use of ultrasound in determining the initiation in treatment in instability of the hips in neonates. *J Bone Joint Surg*. 1999;81-B:846–851
4. Lewis K, Jones DA, Powell N. Ultrasound and neonatal hip screening: the five-year results of a prospective study in high risk babies. *J Pediatr Orthop*. 1999;19:760–762
5. Paton RW, Srinivasan MS, Shah B, Hollis S. Ultrasound screening for hips at risk in developmental dysplasia: is it worth it? *J Bone Joint Surg*. 1999;81-B:255–258
6. Sucato DJ, Johnston CE, Birch JG, Herring JA, Mack P. Outcomes of ultrasonographic hip abnormalities in clinically stable hips. *J Pediatr Orthop*. 1999;19:754–759
7. Williams PR, Jones DA, Bishay M. Avascular necrosis and the aberdeen splint in developmental dysplasia of the hip. *J Bone Joint Surg*. 1999;81-B:1023–1028

Dysplasia of the Hip Clinical Practice Guideline Quick Reference Tools

- Recommendation Summary
  — Early Detection of Developmental Dysplasia of the Hip
- *ICD-10-CM* Coding Quick Reference for Dysplasia of the Hip
- AAP Patient Education Handout
  — *Hip Dysplasia (Developmental Dysplasia of the Hip)*

Recommendation Summary

Early Detection of Developmental Dysplasia of the Hip

Recommendation 1

A. All newborns are to be screened by physical examination. (The evidence for this recommendation is good. The expert consensus is strong.)

B. It is recommended that screening be done by a properly trained health care provider (eg, physician, pediatric nurse practitioner, physician assistant, or physical therapist). (Evidence for this recommendation is strong.)

C. Ultrasonography of all newborns is not recommended. (Evidence is fair; consensus is strong.)

Recommendation 2

A. If a positive Ortolani or Barlow sign is found in the newborn examination, the infant should be referred to an orthopaedist. (The data recommending that all those with a positive Ortolani sign be referred to an orthopaedist are limited, but expert panel consensus, nevertheless, was strong….)

B. If the results of the physical examination at birth are "equivocally" positive (ie, soft click, mild asymmetry, but neither an Ortolani nor a Barlow sign is present), then a follow-up hip examination by the pediatrician in 2 weeks is recommended. (Evidence is good; consensus is strong.)

Recommendation 3

A. If the results of the newborn physical examination are positive (ie, presence of an Ortolani or a Barlow sign), ordering an ultrasonographic examination of the newborn is not recommended. (Evidence is poor; opinion is strong.)

B. If the results of the newborn physical examination are positive, obtaining a radiograph of the newborn's pelvis and hips is not recommended. (Evidence is poor; opinion is strong.)

C. The use of triple diapers when abnormal physical signs are detected during the newborn period is not recommended. (Evidence is poor; opinion is strong.)

Recommendation 4

If the results of the physical examination are positive (eg, positive Ortolani or Barlow sign) at 2 weeks, refer to an orthopaedist. (Evidence is strong; consensus is strong.)

Recommendation 5

If at the 2-week examination the Ortolani and Barlow signs are absent but physical findings raise suspicions, consider referral to an orthopaedist or request ultrasonography at age 3 to 4 weeks.

Recommendation 6

If the results of the physical examination are negative at 2 weeks, follow-up is recommended at the scheduled well-baby periodic examinations. (Evidence is good; consensus is strong.)

Recommendation 7

Risk factors. If the results of the newborn examination are negative (or equivocally positive), risk factors may be considered. The following recommendations are made (evidence is strong; opinion is strong):

A. Girl (newborn risk of 19/1000). When the results of the newborn examination are negative or equivocally positive, hips should be reevaluated at 2 weeks of age. If negative, continue according to the periodicity schedule; if positive, refer to an orthopaedist or for ultrasonography at 3 weeks of age.

B. Infants with a positive family history of DDH (newborn risk for boys of 9.4/1000 and for girls, 44/1000). When the results of the newborn examination in boys are negative or equivocally positive, hips should be reevaluated at 2 weeks of age. If negative, continue according to the periodicity schedule; if positive, refer to an orthopaedist or for ultrasonography at 3 weeks of age. In girls, the absolute risk of 44/1000 may exceed the pediatrician's threshold to act, and imaging with an ultrasonographic examination at 6 weeks of age or a radiograph of the pelvis at 4 months of age is recommended.

C. Breech presentation (newborn risk for boys of 26/1000 and for girls, 120/1000). For negative or equivocally positive newborn examinations, the infant should be reevaluated at regular intervals (according to the periodicity schedule) if the examination results remain negative.

Recommendation 8

Periodicity. The hips must be examined at every well-baby visit according to the recommended periodicity schedule for well-baby examinations (2–4 days for newborns discharged in less than 48 hours after delivery, by 1 month, 2 months, 4 months, 6 months, 9 months, and 12 months of age).

Coding Quick Reference for Dysplasia of the Hip	
ICD-10-CM	
Q65.0-	Congenital dislocation of hip, unilateral
Q65.1	Congenital dislocation of hip, bilateral
Q65.3-	Congenital partial dislocation of hip, unilateral
Q65.4	Congenital partial dislocation of hip, bilateral
Q65.6	Congenital unstable hip (Congenital dislocatable hip)
Q65.89	Other specified congenital deformities of hip

Symbol "-" requires a fifth character; **1** = right; **2** = left.

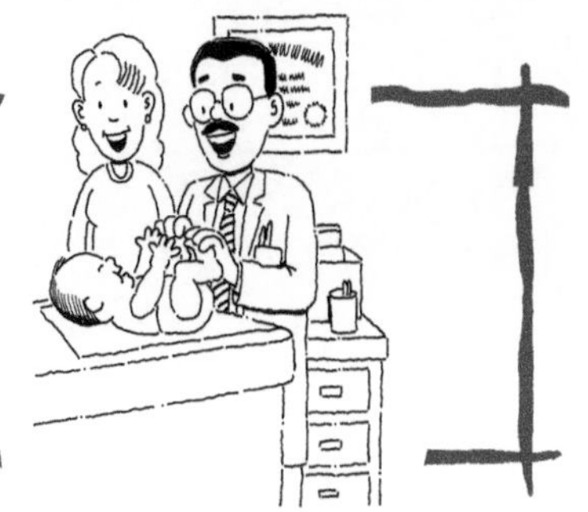

Hip Dysplasia

(Developmental Dysplasia of the Hip)

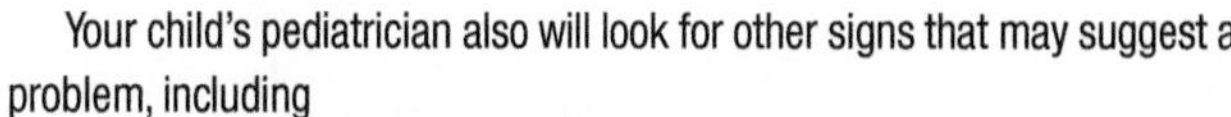

Hip dysplasia (developmental dysplasia of the hip) is a condition in which a child's upper thighbone is dislocated from the hip socket. It can be present at birth or develop during a child's first year of life.

Hip dysplasia is not always detectable at birth or even during early infancy. In spite of careful screening of children for hip dysplasia during regular well-child exams, a number of children with hip dysplasia are not diagnosed until after they are 1 year old.

Hip dysplasia is rare. However, if your baby is diagnosed with the condition, quick treatment is important.

What causes hip dysplasia?

No one is sure why hip dysplasia occurs (or why the left hip dislocates more often than the right hip). One reason may have to do with the hormones a baby is exposed to before birth. While these hormones serve to relax muscles in the pregnant mother's body, in some cases they also may cause a baby's joints to become too relaxed and prone to dislocation. This condition often corrects itself in several days, and the hip develops normally. In some cases, these dislocations cause changes in the hip anatomy that need treatment.

Who is at risk?

Factors that may increase the risk of hip dysplasia include

- Sex—more frequent in girls
- Family history—more likely when other family members have had hip dysplasia
- Birth position—more common in infants born in the breech position
- Birth order—firstborn children most at risk for hip dysplasia

Detecting hip dysplasia

Your pediatrician will check your newborn for hip dysplasia right after birth and at every well-child exam until your child is walking normally.

During the exam, your child's pediatrician will carefully flex and rotate your child's legs to see if the thighbones are properly positioned in the hip sockets. This does not require a great deal of force and will not hurt your baby.

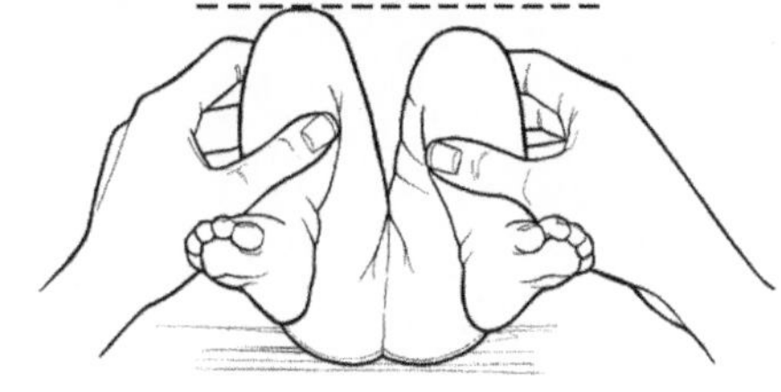

© Molly Borman

Your child's pediatrician also will look for other signs that may suggest a problem, including

- Limited range of motion in either leg
- One leg is shorter than the other
- Thigh or buttock creases appear uneven or lopsided

If your child's pediatrician suspects a problem with your child's hip, you may be referred to an orthopedic specialist who has experience treating hip dysplasia.

Treating hip dysplasia

Early treatment is important. The sooner treatment begins, the simpler it will be. In the past parents were told to double or triple diaper their babies to keep the legs in a position where dislocation was unlikely. *This practice is not recommended.* The diapering will not prevent hip dysplasia and will only delay effective treatment. Failure to treat this condition can result in permanent disability.

If your child is diagnosed with hip dysplasia before she is 6 months old, she will most likely be treated with a soft brace (such as the Pavlik harness) that holds the legs flexed and apart to allow the thighbones to be secure in the hip sockets.

The orthopedic consultant will tell you how long and when your baby will need to wear the brace. Your child also will be examined frequently during this time to make sure that the hips remain normal and stable.

In resistant cases or in older children, hip dysplasia may need to be treated with a combination of braces, casts, traction, or surgery. Your child will be admitted to the hospital if surgery is necessary. After surgery, your child will be placed in a hip spica cast for about 3 months. A hip spica cast is a hard cast that immobilizes the hips and keeps them in the correct position. When the cast is removed, your child will need to wear a removable hip brace for several more months.

Pavlik Harness

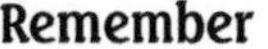

Remember

If you have any concerns about your child's walking, talk with his pediatrician. If the cause is hip dysplasia, prompt treatment is important.

The information contained in this publication should not be used as a substitute for the medical care and advice of your pediatrician. There may be variations in treatment that your pediatrician may recommend based on individual facts and circumstances.

American Academy of Pediatrics

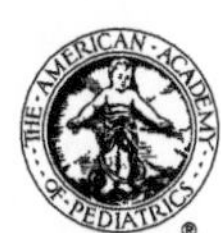

DEDICATED TO THE HEALTH OF ALL CHILDREN™

The American Academy of Pediatrics is an organization of 60,000 primary care pediatricians, pediatric medical subspecialists, and pediatric surgical specialists dedicated to the health, safety, and well-being of infants, children, adolescents, and young adults.

American Academy of Pediatrics
Web site—www.aap.org

Copyright © 2003
American Academy of Pediatrics

Febrile Seizures: Clinical Practice Guideline for the Long-term Management of the Child With Simple Febrile Seizures

- *Clinical Practice Guideline*

CLINICAL PRACTICE GUIDELINE

Febrile Seizures: Clinical Practice Guideline for the Long-term Management of the Child With Simple Febrile Seizures

Steering Committee on Quality Improvement and Management, Subcommittee on Febrile Seizures

ABSTRACT

Febrile seizures are the most common seizure disorder in childhood, affecting 2% to 5% of children between the ages of 6 and 60 months. Simple febrile seizures are defined as brief (<15-minute) generalized seizures that occur once during a 24-hour period in a febrile child who does not have an intracranial infection, metabolic disturbance, or history of afebrile seizures. This guideline (a revision of the 1999 American Academy of Pediatrics practice parameter [now termed clinical practice guideline] "The Long-term Treatment of the Child With Simple Febrile Seizures") addresses the risks and benefits of both continuous and intermittent anticonvulsant therapy as well as the use of antipyretics in children with simple febrile seizures. It is designed to assist pediatricians by providing an analytic framework for decisions regarding possible therapeutic interventions in this patient population. It is not intended to replace clinical judgment or to establish a protocol for all patients with this disorder. Rarely will these guidelines be the only approach to this problem. *Pediatrics* 2008;121:1281–1286

www.pediatrics.org/cgi/doi/10.1542/peds.2008-0939

doi:10.1542/peds.2008-0939

All clinical reports from the American Academy of Pediatrics automatically expire 5 years after publication unless reaffirmed, revised, or retired at or before that time.

The guidance in this report does not indicate an exclusive course of treatment or serve as a standard of medical care. Variations, taking into account individual circumstances, may be appropriate.

Key Word
fever

Abbreviation
AAP—American Academy of Pediatrics

PEDIATRICS (ISSN Numbers: Print, 0031-4005; Online, 1098-4275). Copyright © 2008 by the American Academy of Pediatrics

The expected outcomes of this practice guideline include:

1. optimizing practitioner understanding of the scientific basis for using or avoiding various proposed treatments for children with simple febrile seizures;
2. improving the health of children with simple febrile seizures by avoiding therapies with high potential for adverse effects and no demonstrated ability to improve children's long-term outcomes;
3. reducing costs by avoiding therapies that will not demonstrably improve children's long-term outcomes; and
4. helping the practitioner educate caregivers about the low risks associated with simple febrile seizures.

The committee determined that with the exception of a high rate of recurrence, no long-term effects of simple febrile seizures have been identified. The risk of developing epilepsy in these patients is extremely low, although slightly higher than that in the general population. No data, however, suggest that prophylactic treatment of children with simple febrile seizures would reduce the risk, because epilepsy likely is the result of genetic predisposition rather than structural damage to the brain caused by recurrent simple febrile seizures. Although antipyretics have been shown to be ineffective in preventing recurrent febrile seizures, there is evidence that continuous anticonvulsant therapy with phenobarbital, primidone, or valproic acid and intermittent therapy with diazepam are effective in reducing febrile-seizure recurrence. The potential toxicities associated with these agents, however, outweigh the relatively minor risks associated with simple febrile seizures. As such, the committee concluded that, on the basis of the risks and benefits of the effective therapies, neither continuous nor intermittent anticonvulsant therapy is recommended for children with 1 or more simple febrile seizures.

INTRODUCTION

Febrile seizures are seizures that occur in febrile children between the ages of 6 and 60 months who do not have an intracranial infection, metabolic disturbance, or history of afebrile seizures. Febrile seizures are subdivided into 2 categories: simple and complex. Simple febrile seizures last for less than 15 minutes, are generalized (without a focal component), and occur once in a 24-hour period, whereas complex febrile seizures are prolonged (>15 minutes), are focal, or occur more than once in 24 hours.[1] Despite the frequency of febrile seizures (2%–5%), there is no unanimity of opinion about management options. This clinical practice guideline addresses potential therapeutic interventions in neurologically normal children with simple febrile seizures. It is not intended for patients with complex febrile seizures and does not pertain to children with previous neurologic insults, known central nervous system abnormalities, or a history of afebrile seizures. This clinical practice guideline is a revision of a 1999 American Academy of Pediatrics (AAP) clinical practice parameter, "The Long-term Treatment of the Child With Simple Febrile Seizures."[2]

For a child who has experienced a simple febrile seizure, there are potentially 4 adverse outcomes that theoretically may be altered by an effective therapeutic agent: (1) decline in IQ; (2) increased risk of epilepsy; (3) risk of recurrent febrile seizures; and (4) death. Neither a decline in IQ, academic performance or neurocognitive inattention nor behavioral abnormalities have been shown to be a consequence of recurrent simple febrile seizures.[3] Ellenberg and Nelson[4] studied 431 children who experienced febrile seizures and observed no significant difference in their learning compared with sibling controls. In a similar study by Verity et al,[5] 303 children with febrile seizures were compared with control children. No difference in learning was identified, except in those children who had neurologic abnormalities before their first seizure.

The second concern, increased risk of epilepsy, is more complex. Children with simple febrile seizures have approximately the same risk of developing epilepsy by the age of 7 years as does the general population (ie, 1%).[6] However, children who have had multiple simple febrile seizures, are younger than 12 months at the time of their first febrile seizure, and have a family history of epilepsy are at higher risk, with generalized afebrile seizures developing by 25 years of age in 2.4%.[7] Despite this fact, no study has demonstrated that successful treatment of simple febrile seizures can prevent this later development of epilepsy, and there currently is no evidence that simple febrile seizures cause structural damage to the brain. Indeed, it is most likely that the increased risk of epilepsy in this population is the result of genetic predisposition.

In contrast to the slightly increased risk of developing epilepsy, children with simple febrile seizures have a high rate of recurrence. The risk varies with age. Children younger than 12 months at the time of their first simple febrile seizure have an approximately 50% probability of having recurrent febrile seizures. Children older than 12 months at the time of their first event have an approximately 30% probability of a second febrile seizure; of those who do have a second febrile seizure, 50% have a chance of having at least 1 additional recurrence.[8]

Finally, there is a theoretical risk of a child dying during a simple febrile seizure as a result of documented injury, aspiration, or cardiac arrhythmia, but to the committee's knowledge, it has never been reported.

In summary, with the exception of a high rate of recurrence, no long-term adverse effects of simple febrile seizures have been identified. Because the risks associated with simple febrile seizures, other than recurrence, are so low and because the number of children who have febrile seizures in the first few years of life is so high, to be commensurate, a proposed therapy would need to be exceedingly low in risks and adverse effects, inexpensive, and highly effective.

METHODS

To update the clinical practice guideline on the treatment of children with simple febrile seizures, the AAP reconvened the Subcommittee on Febrile Seizures. The committee was chaired by a child neurologist and consisted of a neuroepidemiologist, 2 additional child neurologists, and a practicing pediatrician. All panel members reviewed and signed the AAP voluntary disclosure and conflict-of-interest form. The guideline was reviewed by members of the AAP Steering Committee on Quality Improvement and Management; members of the AAP Sections on Neurology, Pediatric Emergency Medicine, Developmental and Behavioral Pediatrics, and Epidemiology; members of the AAP Committees on Pediatric Emergency Medicine and Medical Liability and Risk Management; members of the AAP Councils on Children With Disabilities and Community Pediatrics; and members of outside organizations including the Child Neurology Society and the American Academy of Neurology.

A comprehensive review of the evidence-based literature published since 1998 was conducted with the aim of addressing possible therapeutic interventions in the management of children with simple febrile seizures. The review focused on both the efficacy and potential adverse effects of the proposed treatments. Decisions were made on the basis of a systematic grading of the quality of evidence and strength of recommendations.

The AAP established a partnership with the University of Kentucky (Lexington, KY) to develop an evidence report, which served as a major source of information for these practice-guideline recommendations. The specific issues addressed were (1) effectiveness of continuous anticonvulsant therapy in preventing recurrent febrile seizures, (2) effectiveness of intermittent anticonvulsant therapy in preventing recurrent febrile seizures, (3) effectiveness of antipyretics in preventing recurrent febrile seizures, and (4) adverse effects of either continuous or intermittent anticonvulsant therapy.

In the original practice parameter, more than 300 medical journal articles reporting studies of the natural history of simple febrile seizures or the therapy of these seizures were reviewed and abstracted.[2] An additional 65 articles were reviewed and abstracted for the update. Emphasis was placed on articles that differentiated simple febrile seizures from other types of seizures, that carefully matched treatment and control groups, and that described adherence to the drug regimen. Tables were constructed from the 65 articles that best fit these criteria. A more comprehensive review of the literature on which this report is based can be found in a forthcoming technical report (the initial technical report can be accessed at http://aappolicy.aappublications.org/cgi/content/full/pediatrics;103/6/e86). The technical report also will contain dosing information.

The evidence-based approach to guideline development requires that the evidence in support of a recommendation be identified, appraised, and summarized and that an explicit link between evidence and recommendations be defined. Evidence-based recommendations reflect the quality of evidence and the balance of benefit and harm that is

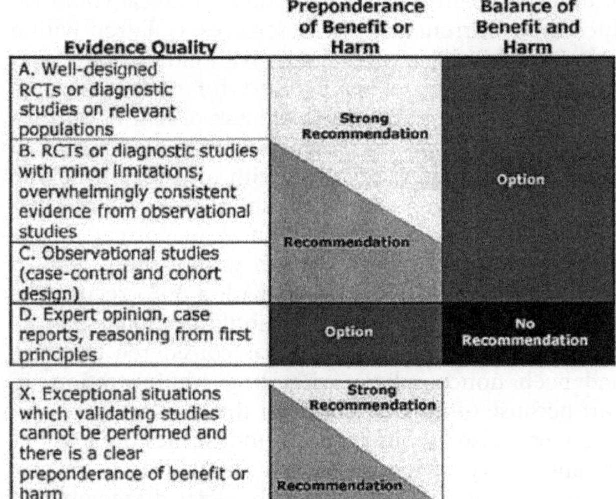

FIGURE 1
Integrating evidence-quality appraisal with an assessment of the anticipated balance between benefits and harms if a policy is conducted leads to designation of a policy as a strong recommendation, recommendation, option, or no recommendation. RCT indicates randomized, controlled trial.

anticipated when the recommendation is followed. The AAP policy statement "Classifying Recommendations for Clinical Practice Guidelines"[9] was followed in designating levels of recommendations (see Fig 1 and Table 1).

RECOMMENDATION

On the basis of the risks and benefits of the effective therapies, neither continuous nor intermittent anticonvulsant therapy is recommended for children with 1 or more simple febrile seizures.

- Aggregate evidence quality: B (randomized, controlled trials and diagnostic studies with minor limitations).
- Benefit: prevention of recurrent febrile seizures, which are not harmful and do not significantly increase the risk for development of future epilepsy.
- Harm: adverse effects including rare fatal hepatotoxicity (especially in children younger than 2 years who are also at greatest risk of febrile seizures), thrombocytopenia, weight loss and gain, gastrointestinal disturbances, and pancreatitis with valproic acid and hyperactivity, irritability, lethargy, sleep disturbances, and hypersensitivity reactions with phenobarbital; lethargy, drowsiness, and ataxia for intermittent diazepam as well as the risk of masking an evolving central nervous system infection.
- Benefits/harms assessment: preponderance of harm over benefit.
- Policy level: recommendation.

BENEFITS AND RISKS OF CONTINUOUS ANTICONVULSANT THERAPY

Phenobarbital

Phenobarbital is effective in preventing the recurrence of simple febrile seizures.[10] In a controlled double-blind study, daily therapy with phenobarbital reduced the rate of subsequent febrile seizures from 25 per 100 subjects per year to 5 per 100 subjects per year.[11] For the agent to be effective, however, it must be given daily and maintained in the therapeutic range. In a study by Farwell et al,[12] for example, children whose phenobarbital levels were in the therapeutic range had a reduction in recurrent seizures, but because noncompliance was so high, an overall benefit with phenobarbital therapy was not identified.

The adverse effects of phenobarbital include hyperactivity, irritability, lethargy, sleep disturbances, and hypersensitivity reactions. The behavioral adverse effects

TABLE 1 Guideline Definitions for Evidence-Based Statements

Statement	Definition	Implication
Strong recommendation	A strong recommendation in favor of a particular action is made when the anticipated benefits of the recommended intervention clearly exceed the harms (as a strong recommendation against an action is made when the anticipated harms clearly exceed the benefits) and the quality of the supporting evidence is excellent. In some clearly identified circumstances, strong recommendations may be made when high-quality evidence is impossible to obtain and the anticipated benefits strongly outweigh the harms.	Clinicians should follow a strong recommendation unless a clear and compelling rationale for an alternative approach is present.
Recommendation	A recommendation in favor of a particular action is made when the anticipated benefits exceed the harms but the quality of evidence is not as strong. Again, in some clearly identified circumstances, recommendations may be made when high-quality evidence is impossible to obtain but the anticipated benefits outweigh the harms.	Clinicians would be prudent to follow a recommendation but should remain alert to new information and sensitive to patient preferences.
Option	Options define courses that may be taken when either the quality of evidence is suspect or carefully performed studies have shown little clear advantage to 1 approach over another.	Clinicians should consider the option in their decision-making, and patient preference may have a substantial role.
No recommendation	No recommendation indicates that there is a lack of pertinent published evidence and that the anticipated balance of benefits and harms is presently unclear.	Clinicians should be alert to new published evidence that clarifies the balance of benefit versus harm.

may occur in up to 20% to 40% of patients and may be severe enough to necessitate discontinuation of the drug.[13–16]

Primidone

Primidone, in doses of 15 to 20 mg/kg per day, has also been shown to reduce the recurrence rate of febrile seizures.[17,18] It is of interest that the derived phenobarbital level in a Minigawa and Miura study[17] was below therapeutic (16 μg/mL) in 29 of the 32 children, suggesting that primidone itself may be active in preventing seizure recurrence. As with phenobarbital, adverse effects include behavioral disturbances, irritability, and sleep disturbances.[18]

Valproic Acid

In randomized, controlled studies, only 4% of children taking valproic acid, as opposed to 35% of control subjects, had a subsequent febrile seizure. Therefore, valproic acid seems to be at least as effective in preventing recurrent simple febrile seizures as phenobarbital and significantly more effective than placebo.[19–21]

Drawbacks to therapy with valproic acid include its rare association with fatal hepatotoxicity (especially in children younger than 2 years, who are also at greatest risk of febrile seizures), thrombocytopenia, weight loss and gain, gastrointestinal disturbances, and pancreatitis. In studies in which children received valproic acid to prevent recurrence of febrile seizures, no cases of fatal hepatotoxicity were reported.[15]

Carbamazepine

Carbamazepine has not been shown to be effective in preventing the recurrence of simple febrile seizures. Antony and Hawke[13] compared children who had been treated with therapeutic levels of either phenobarbital or carbamazepine, and 47% of the children in the carbamazepine-treated group had recurrent seizures compared with only 10% of those in the phenobarbital group. In another study, Camfield et al[22] treated children (whose conditions failed to improve with phenobarbital therapy) with carbamazepine. Despite good compliance, 13 of the 16 children treated with carbamazepine had a recurrent febrile seizure within 18 months. It is theoretically possible that these excessively high rates of recurrences might have been attributable to adverse effects of carbamazepine.

Phenytoin

Phenytoin has not been shown to be effective in preventing the recurrence of simple febrile seizures, even when the agent is in the therapeutic range.[23,24] Other anticonvulsants have not been studied for the continuous treatment of simple febrile seizures.

BENEFITS AND RISKS OF INTERMITTENT ANTICONVULSANT THERAPY

Diazepam

A double-blind controlled study of patients with a history of febrile seizures demonstrated that administration of oral diazepam (given at the time of fever) could reduce the recurrence of febrile seizures. Children with a history of febrile seizures were given either oral diazepam (0.33 mg/kg, every 8 hours for 48 hours) or a placebo at the time of fever. The risk of febrile seizures per person-year was decreased 44% with diazepam.[25] In a more recent study, children with a history of febrile seizures were given oral diazepam at the time of fever and then compared with children in an untreated control group. In the oral diazepam group, there was an 11% recurrence rate compared with a 30% recurrence rate in the control group.[26] It should be noted that all children for whom diazepam was considered a failure had been noncompliant with drug administration, in part because of adverse effects of the medication.

There is also literature that demonstrates the feasibility and safety of interrupting a simple febrile seizure lasting less than 5 minutes with rectal diazepam and with both intranasal and buccal midazolam.[27,28] Although these agents are effective in terminating the seizure, it is questionable whether they have any long-term influence on outcome. In a study by Knudsen et al,[29] children were given either rectal diazepam at the time of fever or only at the onset of seizure. Twelve-year follow-up found that the long-term prognosis of the children in the 2 groups did not differ regardless of whether treatment was aimed at preventing seizures or treating them.

A potential drawback to intermittent medication is that a seizure could occur before a fever is noticed. Indeed, in several of these studies, recurrent seizures were likely attributable to failure of method rather than failure of the agent.

Adverse effects of oral and rectal diazepam[26] and both intranasal and buccal midazolam include lethargy, drowsiness, and ataxia. Respiratory depression is extremely rare, even when given by the rectal route.[28,30] Sedation caused by any of the benzodiazepines, whether administered by the oral, rectal, nasal, or buccal route, have the potential of masking an evolving central nervous system infection. If used, the child's health care professional should be contacted.

BENEFITS AND RISKS OF INTERMITTENT ANTIPYRETICS

No studies have demonstrated that antipyretics, in the absence of anticonvulsants, reduce the recurrence risk of simple febrile seizures. Camfield et al[11] treated 79 children who had had a first febrile seizure with either a placebo plus antipyretic instruction (either aspirin or acetaminophen) versus daily phenobarbital plus antipyretic instruction (either aspirin or acetaminophen). Recurrence risk was significantly lower in the phenobarbital-treated group, suggesting that antipyretic instruction, including the use of antipyretics, is ineffective in preventing febrile-seizure recurrence.

Whether antipyretics are given regularly (every 4 hours) or sporadically (contingent on a specific body-temperature elevation) does not influence outcome. Acetaminophen was either given every 4 hours or only for temperature elevations of more than 37.9°C in 104 children. The incidence of febrile episodes did not differ significantly between the 2 groups, nor did the early recurrence of febrile seizures. The authors determined that administering prophylactic acetaminophen during febrile episodes was ineffective in preventing or reducing fever and in preventing febrile-seizure recurrence.[31]

In a randomized double-blind placebo-controlled trial, acetaminophen was administered along with low-dose oral diazepam.[32] Febrile-seizure recurrence was not reduced, compared with control groups. As with acetaminophen, ibuprofen also has been shown to be ineffective in preventing recurrence of febrile seizures.[33–35]

In general, acetaminophen and ibuprofen are considered to be safe and effective antipyretics for children. However, hepatotoxicity (with acetaminophen) and respiratory failure, metabolic acidosis, renal failure, and coma (with ibuprofen) have been reported in children after overdose or in the presence of risk factors.[36,37]

CONCLUSIONS

The subcommittee has determined that a simple febrile seizure is a benign and common event in children between the ages of 6 and 60 months. Nearly all children have an excellent prognosis. The committee concluded that although there is evidence that both continuous antiepileptic therapy with phenobarbital, primidone, or valproic acid and intermittent therapy with oral diazepam are effective in reducing the risk of recurrence, the potential toxicities associated with antiepileptic drugs outweigh the relatively minor risks associated with simple febrile seizures. As such, long-term therapy is not recommended. In situations in which parental anxiety associated with febrile seizures is severe, intermittent oral diazepam at the onset of febrile illness may be effective in preventing recurrence. Although antipyretics may improve the comfort of the child, they will not prevent febrile seizures.

SUBCOMMITTEE ON FEBRILE SEIZURES, 2002–2008

Patricia K. Duffner, MD, Chairperson
Robert J. Baumann, MD, Methodologist
Peter Berman, MD
John L. Green, MD
Sanford Schneider, MD

STEERING COMMITTEE ON QUALITY IMPROVEMENT AND MANAGEMENT, 2007–2008

Elizabeth S. Hodgson, MD, Chairperson
Gordon B. Glade, MD
Norman "Chip" Harbaugh, Jr, MD
Thomas K. McInerny, MD
Marlene R. Miller, MD, MSc
Virginia A. Moyer, MD, MPH
Xavier D. Sevilla, MD
Lisa Simpson, MB, BCh, MPH
Glenn S. Takata, MD

LIAISONS

Denise Dougherty, PhD
Agency for Healthcare Research and Quality
Daniel R. Neuspiel, MD
Section on Epidemiology
Ellen Schwalenstocker, MBA
National Association of Children's Hospitals and Related Institutions

STAFF

Caryn Davidson, MA

REFERENCES

1. Nelson KB, Ellenberg JH. Prognosis in children with febrile seizures. *Pediatrics.* 1978;61(5):720–727
2. American Academy of Pediatrics, Committee on Quality Improvement, Subcommittee on Febrile Seizures. The long-term treatment of the child with simple febrile seizures. *Pediatrics.* 1999;103(6 pt 1):1307–1309
3. Chang YC, Guo NW, Huang CC, Wang ST, Tsai JJ. Neurocognitive attention and behavior outcome of school age children with a history of febrile convulsions: a population study. *Epilepsia.* 2000;41(4):412–420
4. Ellenberg JH, Nelson KB. Febrile seizures and later intellectual performance. *Arch Neurol.* 1978;35(1):17–21
5. Verity CM, Butler NR, Golding J. Febrile convulsions in a national cohort followed up from birth. II: medical history and intellectual ability at 5 years of age. *BMJ.* 1985;290(6478):1311–1315
6. Nelson KB, Ellenberg JH. Predictors of epilepsy in children who have experienced febrile seizures. *N Engl J Med.* 1976;295(19):1029–1033
7. Annegers JF, Hauser WA, Shirts SB, Kurland LT. Factors prognostic of unprovoked seizures after febrile convulsions. *N Engl J Med.* 1987;316(9):493–498
8. Berg AT, Shinnar S, Darefsky AS, et al. Predictors of recurrent febrile seizures: a prospective cohort study. *Arch Pediatr Adolesc Med.* 1997;151(4):371–378
9. American Academy of Pediatrics, Steering Committee on Quality Improvement and Management. Classifying recommendations for clinical practice guidelines. *Pediatrics.* 2004;114(3):874–877
10. Wolf SM, Carr A, Davis DC, Davidson S, et al. The value of phenobarbital in the child who has had a single febrile seizure: a controlled prospective study. *Pediatrics.* 1977;59(3):378–385
11. Camfield PR, Camfield CS, Shapiro SH, Cummings C. The first febrile seizure: antipyretic instruction plus either phenobarbital or placebo to prevent recurrence. *J Pediatr.* 1980;97(1):16–21
12. Farwell JR, Lee JY, Hirtz DG, Sulzbacher SI, Ellenberg JH, Nelson KB. Phenobarbital for febrile seizures: effects on intelligence and on seizure recurrence [published correction appears in *N Engl J Med.* 1992;326(2):144]. *N Engl J Med.* 1990;322(6):364–369
13. Antony JH, Hawke SHB. Phenobarbital compared with carbamazepine in prevention of recurrent febrile convulsions. *Am J Dis Child.* 1983;137(9):892–895
14. Knudsen Fu, Vestermark S. Prophylactic diazepam or phenobarbitone in febrile convulsions: a prospective, controlled study. *Arch Dis Child.* 1978;53(8):660–663
15. Lee K, Melchior JC. Sodium valproate versus phenobarbital in the prophylactic treatment of febrile convulsions in childhood. *Eur J Pediatr.* 1981;137(2):151–153
16. Camfield CS, Chaplin S, Doyle AB, Shapiro SH, Cummings C, Camfield PR. Side effects of phenobarbital in toddlers: behavioral and cognitive aspects. *J Pediatr.* 1979;95(3):361–365
17. Minagawa K, Miura H. Phenobarbital, primidone and sodium valproate in the prophylaxis of febrile convulsions. *Brain Dev.* 1981;3(4):385–393
18. Herranz JL, Armijo JA, Arteaga R. Effectiveness and toxicity of phenobarbital, primidone, and sodium valproate in the pre-

vention of febrile convulsions, controlled by plasma levels. *Epilepsia.* 1984;25(1):89–95
19. Wallace SJ, Smith JA. Successful prophylaxis against febrile convulsions with valproic acid or phenobarbitone. *BMJ.* 1980; 280(6211):353–354
20. Mamelle N, Mamelle JC, Plasse JC, Revol M, Gilly R. Prevention of recurrent febrile convulsions: a randomized therapeutic assay—sodium valproate, phenobarbitone and placebo. *Neuropediatrics.* 1984;15(1):37–42
21. Ngwane E, Bower B. Continuous sodium valproate or phenobarbitone in the prevention of "simple" febrile convulsions. *Arch Dis Child.* 1980;55(3):171–174
22. Camfield PR, Camfield CS, Tibbles JA. Carbamazepine does not prevent febrile seizures in phenobarbital failures. *Neurology.* 1982;32(3):288–289
23. Bacon CJ, Hierons AM, Mucklow JC, Webb JK, Rawlins MD, Weightman D. Placebo-controlled study of phenobarbitone and phenytoin in the prophylaxis of febrile convulsions. *Lancet.* 1981;2(8247):600–604
24. Melchior JC, Buchthal F, Lennox Buchthal M. The ineffectiveness of diphenylhydantoin in preventing febrile convulsions in the age of greatest risk, under 3 years. *Epilepsia.* 1971;12(1): 55–62
25. Rosman NP, Colton T, Labazzo J, et al. A controlled trial of diazepam administered during febrile illnesses to prevent recurrence of febrile seizures. *N Engl J Med.* 1993;329(2):79–84
26. Verrotti A, Latini G, di Corcia G, et al. Intermittent oral diazepam prophylaxis in febrile convulsions: its effectiveness for febrile seizure recurrence. *Eur J Pediatr Neurol.* 2004;8(3): 131–134
27. Lahat E, Goldman M, Barr J, Bistritzer T, Berkovitch M. Comparison of intranasal midazolam with intravenous diazepam for treating febrile seizures in children: prospective randomized study. *BMJ.* 2000;321(7253):83–86
28. McIntyre J, Robertson S, Norris E, et al. Safety and efficacy of buccal midazolam versus rectal diazepam for emergency treatment of seizures in children: a randomized controlled trial. *Lancet.* 2005;366(9481):205–210
29. Knudsen FU, Paerregaard A, Andersen R, Andresen J. Long term outcome of prophylaxis for febrile convulsions. *Arch Dis Child.* 1996;74(1):13–18
30. Pellock JM, Shinnar S. Respiratory adverse events associated with diazepam rectal gel. *Neurology.* 2005;64(10):1768–1770
31. Schnaiderman D, Lahat E, Sheefer T, Aladjem M. Antipyretic effectiveness of acetaminophen in febrile seizures: ongoing prophylaxis versus sporadic usage. *Eur J Pediatr.* 1993;152(9): 747–749
32. Uhari M, Rantala H, Vainionpaa L, Kurttila R. Effect of acetaminophen and of low dose intermittent doses of diazepam on prevention of recurrences of febrile seizures. *J Pediatr.* 1995; 126(6):991–995
33. van Stuijvenberg M, Derksen-Lubsen G, Steyerberg EW, Habbema JDF, Moll HA. Randomized, controlled trial of ibuprofen syrup administered during febrile illnesses to prevent febrile seizure recurrences. *Pediatrics.* 1998;102(5). Available at: www.pediatrics.org/cgi/content/full/102/5/e51
34. van Esch A, Van Steensel-Moll HA, Steyerberg EW, Offringa M, Habbema JDF, Derksen-Lubsen G. Antipyretic efficacy of ibuprofen and acetaminophen in children with febrile seizures. *Arch Pediatr Adolesc Med.* 1995;149(6):632–637
35. van Esch A, Steyerberg EW, Moll HA, et al. A study of the efficacy of antipyretic drugs in the prevention of febrile seizure recurrence. *Ambul Child Health.* 2000;6(1):19–26
36. Easley RB, Altemeier WA. Central nervous system manifestations of an ibuprofen overdose reversed by naloxone. *Pediatr Emerg Care.* 2000;16(1):39–41
37. American Academy of Pediatrics, Committee on Drugs. Acetaminophen toxicity in children. *Pediatrics.* 2001;108(4): 1020–1024

Febrile Seizures: Guideline for the Neurodiagnostic Evaluation of the Child With a Simple Febrile Seizure

- *Clinical Practice Guideline*

Clinical Practice Guideline—Febrile Seizures: Guideline for the Neurodiagnostic Evaluation of the Child With a Simple Febrile Seizure

SUBCOMMITTEE ON FEBRILE SEIZURES

KEY WORD
seizure

ABBREVIATIONS
AAP—American Academy of Pediatrics
Hib—*Haemophilus influenzae* type b
EEG—electroencephalogram
CT—computed tomography

The recommendations in this report do not indicate an exclusive course of treatment or serve as a standard of medical care. Variations, taking into account individual circumstances, may be appropriate.

This document is copyrighted and is property of the American Academy of Pediatrics and its Board of Directors. All authors have filed conflict of interest statements with the American Academy of Pediatrics. Any conflicts have been resolved through a process approved by the Board of Directors. The American Academy of Pediatrics has neither solicited nor accepted any commercial involvement in the development of the content of this publication.

www.pediatrics.org/cgi/doi/10.1542/peds.2010-3318
doi:10.1542/peds.2010-3318

All clinical practice guidelines from the American Academy of Pediatrics automatically expire 5 years after publication unless reaffirmed, revised, or retired at or before that time.

PEDIATRICS (ISSN Numbers: Print, 0031-4005; Online, 1098-4275).

Copyright © 2011 by the American Academy of Pediatrics

abstract

OBJECTIVE: To formulate evidence-based recommendations for health care professionals about the diagnosis and evaluation of a simple febrile seizure in infants and young children 6 through 60 months of age and to revise the practice guideline published by the American Academy of Pediatrics (AAP) in 1996.

METHODS: This review included search and analysis of the medical literature published since the last version of the guideline. Physicians with expertise and experience in the fields of neurology and epilepsy, pediatrics, epidemiology, and research methodologies constituted a subcommittee of the AAP Steering Committee on Quality Improvement and Management. The steering committee and other groups within the AAP and organizations outside the AAP reviewed the guideline. The subcommittee member who reviewed the literature for the 1996 AAP practice guidelines searched for articles published since the last guideline through 2009, supplemented by articles submitted by other committee members. Results from the literature search were provided to the subcommittee members for review. Interventions of direct interest included lumbar puncture, electroencephalography, blood studies, and neuroimaging. Multiple issues were raised and discussed iteratively until consensus was reached about recommendations. The strength of evidence supporting each recommendation and the strength of the recommendation were assessed by the committee member most experienced in informatics and epidemiology and graded according to AAP policy.

CONCLUSIONS: Clinicians evaluating infants or young children after a simple febrile seizure should direct their attention toward identifying the cause of the child's fever. Meningitis should be considered in the differential diagnosis for any febrile child, and lumbar puncture should be performed if there are clinical signs or symptoms of concern. For any infant between 6 and 12 months of age who presents with a seizure and fever, a lumbar puncture is an option when the child is considered deficient in *Haemophilus influenzae* type b (Hib) or *Streptococcus pneumoniae* immunizations (ie, has not received scheduled immunizations as recommended), or when immunization status cannot be determined, because of an increased risk of bacterial meningitis. A lumbar puncture is an option for children who are pretreated with antibiotics. In general, a simple febrile seizure does not usually require further evaluation, specifically electroencephalography, blood studies, or neuroimaging. *Pediatrics* 2011;127:389–394

DEFINITION OF THE PROBLEM

This practice guideline provides recommendations for the neurodiagnostic evaluation of neurologically healthy infants and children 6 through 60 months of age who have had a simple febrile seizure and present for evaluation within 12 hours of the event. It replaces the 1996 practice parameter.[1] This practice guideline is not intended for patients who have had complex febrile seizures (prolonged, focal, and/or recurrent), and it does not pertain to children with previous neurologic insults, known central nervous system abnormalities, or history of afebrile seizures.

TARGET AUDIENCE AND PRACTICE SETTING

This practice guideline is intended for use by pediatricians, family physicians, child neurologists, neurologists, emergency physicians, nurse practitioners, and other health care providers who evaluate children for febrile seizures.

BACKGROUND

A febrile seizure is a seizure accompanied by fever (temperature ≥ 100.4°F or 38°C[2] by any method), without central nervous system infection, that occurs in infants and children 6 through 60 months of age. Febrile seizures occur in 2% to 5% of all children and, as such, make up the most common convulsive event in children younger than 60 months. In 1976, Nelson and Ellenberg,[3] using data from the National Collaborative Perinatal Project, further defined febrile seizures as being either simple or complex. Simple febrile seizures were defined as primary generalized seizures that lasted for less than 15 minutes and did not recur within 24 hours. Complex febrile seizures were defined as focal, prolonged (≥15 minutes), and/or recurrent within 24 hours. Children who had simple febrile seizures had no evidence of increased mortality, hemiplegia, or mental retardation. During follow-up evaluation, the risk of epilepsy after a simple febrile seizure was shown to be only slightly higher than that of the general population, whereas the chief risk associated with simple febrile seizures was recurrence in one-third of the children. The authors concluded that simple febrile seizures are benign events with excellent prognoses, a conclusion reaffirmed in the 1980 consensus statement from the National Institutes of Health.[3,4]

The expected outcomes of this practice guideline include the following:

1. Optimize clinician understanding of the scientific basis for the neurodiagnostic evaluation of children with simple febrile seizures.
2. Aid the clinician in decision-making by using a structured framework.
3. Optimize evaluation of the child who has had a simple febrile seizure by detecting underlying diseases, minimizing morbidity, and reassuring anxious parents and children.
4. Reduce the costs of physician and emergency department visits, hospitalizations, and unnecessary testing.
5. Educate the clinician to understand that a simple febrile seizure usually does not require further evaluation, specifically electroencephalography, blood studies, or neuroimaging.

METHODOLOGY

To update the clinical practice guideline on the neurodiagnostic evaluation of children with simple febrile seizures,[1] the American Academy of Pediatrics (AAP) reconvened the Subcommittee on Febrile Seizures. The committee was chaired by a child neurologist and consisted of a neuroepidemiologist, 3 additional child neurologists, and a practicing pediatrician. All panel members reviewed and signed the AAP voluntary disclosure and conflict-of-interest form. No conflicts were reported. Participation in the guideline process was voluntary and not paid. The guideline was reviewed by members of the AAP Steering Committee on Quality Improvement and Management; members of the AAP Section on Administration and Practice Management, Section on Developmental and Behavioral Pediatrics, Section on Epidemiology, Section on Infectious Diseases, Section on Neurology, Section on Neurologic Surgery, Section on Pediatric Emergency Medicine, Committee on Pediatric Emergency Medicine, Committee on Practice and Ambulatory Medicine, Committee on Child Health Financing, Committee on Infectious Diseases, Committee on Medical Liability and Risk Management, Council on Children With Disabilities, and Council on Community Pediatrics; and members of outside organizations including the Child Neurology Society, the American Academy of Neurology, the American College of Emergency Physicians, and members of the Pediatric Committee of the Emergency Nurses Association.

A comprehensive review of the evidence-based literature published from 1996 to February 2009 was conducted to discover articles that addressed the diagnosis and evaluation of children with simple febrile seizures. Preference was given to population-based studies, but given the scarcity of such studies, data from hospital-based studies, groups of young children with febrile illness, and comparable groups were reviewed. Decisions were made on the basis of a systematic grading of the quality of evidence and strength of recommendations.

In the original practice parameter,[1] 203 medical journal articles were reviewed and abstracted. An additional 372 articles were reviewed and abstracted for this update. Emphasis was placed on articles that differentiated simple febrile seizures from other types of seizures. Tables were constructed from the 70 articles that best fit these criteria.

The evidence-based approach to guideline development requires that the evidence in support of a recommendation be identified, appraised, and summarized and that an explicit link between

Evidence Quality	Preponderance of Benefit or Harm	Balance of Benefit and Harm
A. Well-designed RCTs or diagnostic studies on relevant population	Strong	Option
B. RCTs or diagnostic studies with minor limitations; overwhelmingly consistent evidence from observational studies	Strong / Rec	Option
C. Observational studies (case-control and cohort design)	Rec	Option
D. Expert opinion, case reports, reasoning from first principles	Option	No Rec
X. Exceptional situations for which validating studies cannot be performed and there is a clear preponderance of benefit or harm	Strong / Rec	

FIGURE 1

Integrating evidence quality appraisal with an assessment of the anticipated balance between benefits and harms if a policy is carried out leads to designation of a policy as a strong recommendation, recommendation, option, or no recommendation. RCT indicates randomized controlled trial; Rec, recommendation.

evidence and recommendations be defined. Evidence-based recommendations reflect the quality of evidence and the balance of benefit and harm that is anticipated when the recommendation is followed. The AAP policy statement "Classifying Recommendations for Clinical Practice Guidelines"[5] was followed in designating levels of recommendations (see Fig 1).

KEY ACTION STATEMENTS

Action Statement 1

Action Statement 1a

A lumbar puncture should be performed in any child who presents with a seizure and a fever and has meningeal signs and symptoms (eg, neck stiffness, Kernig and/or Brudzinski signs) or in any child whose history or examination suggests the presence of meningitis or intracranial infection.

- Aggregate evidence level: B (overwhelming evidence from observational studies).
- Benefits: Meningeal signs and symptoms strongly suggest meningitis, which, if bacterial in etiology, will likely be fatal if left untreated.
- Harms/risks/costs: Lumbar puncture is an invasive and often painful procedure and can be costly.
- Benefits/harms assessment: Preponderance of benefit over harm.
- Value judgments: Observational data and clinical principles were used in making this judgment.
- Role of patient preferences: Although parents may not wish to have their child undergo a lumbar puncture, health care providers should explain that if meningitis is not diagnosed and treated, it could be fatal.
- Exclusions: None.
- Intentional vagueness: None.
- Policy level: Strong recommendation.

Action Statement 1b

In any infant between 6 and 12 months of age who presents with a seizure and fever, a lumbar puncture is an option when the child is considered deficient in *Haemophilus influenzae* type b (Hib) or *Streptococcus pneumoniae* immunizations (ie, has not received scheduled immunizations as recommended) or when immunization status cannot be determined because of an increased risk of bacterial meningitis.

- Aggregate evidence level: D (expert opinion, case reports).
- Benefits: Meningeal signs and symptoms strongly suggest meningitis, which, if bacterial in etiology, will likely be fatal or cause significant long-term disability if left untreated.
- Harms/risks/costs: Lumbar puncture is an invasive and often painful procedure and can be costly.
- Benefits/harms assessment: Preponderance of benefit over harm.
- Value judgments: Data on the incidence of bacterial meningitis from before and after the existence of immunizations against Hib and *S pneumoniae* were used in making this recommendation.
- Role of patient preferences: Although parents may not wish their child to undergo a lumbar puncture, health care providers should explain that in the absence of complete immunizations, their child may be at risk of having fatal bacterial meningitis.
- Exclusions: This recommendation applies only to children 6 to 12 months of age. The subcommittee felt that clinicians would recognize symptoms of meningitis in children older than 12 months.
- Intentional vagueness: None.
- Policy level: Option.

Action Statement 1c

A lumbar puncture is an option in the child who presents with a seizure and fever and is pretreated with antibiotics, because antibiotic treatment can mask the signs and symptoms of meningitis.

- Aggregate evidence level: D (reasoning from clinical experience, case series).
- Benefits: Antibiotics may mask meningeal signs and symptoms but may be insufficient to eradicate meningitis; a diagnosis of meningitis, if bacterial in etiology, will likely be fatal if left untreated.
- Harms/risks/costs: Lumbar puncture is an invasive and often painful procedure and can be costly.

- Benefits/harms assessment: Preponderance of benefit over harm.
- Value judgments: Clinical experience and case series were used in making this judgment while recognizing that extensive data from studies are lacking.
- Role of patient preferences: Although parents may not wish to have their child undergo a lumbar puncture, medical providers should explain that in the presence of pretreatment with antibiotics, the signs and symptoms of meningitis may be masked. Meningitis, if untreated, can be fatal.
- Exclusions: None.
- Intentional vagueness: Data are insufficient to define the specific treatment duration necessary to mask signs and symptoms. The committee determined that the decision to perform a lumbar puncture will depend on the type and duration of antibiotics administered before the seizure and should be left to the individual clinician.
- Policy level: Option.

The committee recognizes the diversity of past and present opinions regarding the need for lumbar punctures in children younger than 12 months with a simple febrile seizure. Since the publication of the previous practice parameter,[1] however, there has been widespread immunization in the United States for 2 of the most common causes of bacterial meningitis in this age range: Hib and *S pneumoniae*. Although compliance with all scheduled immunizations as recommended does not completely eliminate the possibility of bacterial meningitis from the differential diagnosis, current data no longer support routine lumbar puncture in well-appearing, fully immunized children who present with a simple febrile seizure.[6–8] Moreover, although approximately 25% of young children with meningitis have seizures as the presenting sign of the disease, some are either obtunded or comatose when evaluated by a physician for the seizure, and the remainder most often have obvious clinical signs of meningitis (focal seizures, recurrent seizures, petechial rash, or nuchal rigidity).[9–11] Once a decision has been made to perform a lumbar puncture, then blood culture and serum glucose testing should be performed concurrently to increase the sensitivity for detecting bacteria and to determine if there is hypoglycorrhachia characteristic of bacterial meningitis, respectively.

Recent studies that evaluated the outcome of children with simple febrile seizures have included populations with a high prevalence of immunization.[7,8] Data for unimmunized or partially immunized children are lacking. Therefore, lumbar puncture is an option for young children who are considered deficient in immunizations or those in whom immunization status cannot be determined. There are also no definitive data on the outcome of children who present with a simple febrile seizure while already on antibiotics. The authors were unable to find a definition of "pretreated" in the literature, so they consulted with the AAP Committee on Infectious Diseases. Although there is no formal definition, pretreatment can be considered to include systemic antibiotic therapy by any route given within the days before the seizure. Whether pretreatment will affect the presentation and course of bacterial meningitis cannot be predicted but will depend, in part, on the antibiotic administered, the dose, the route of administration, the drug's cerebrospinal fluid penetration, and the organism causing the meningitis. Lumbar puncture is an option in any child pretreated with antibiotics before a simple febrile seizure.

Action Statement 2

An electroencephalogram (EEG) should not be performed in the evaluation of a neurologically healthy child with a simple febrile seizure.

- Aggregate evidence level: B (overwhelming evidence from observational studies).
- Benefits: One study showed a possible association with paroxysmal EEGs and a higher rate of afebrile seizures.[12]
- Harms/risks/costs: EEGs are costly and may increase parental anxiety.
- Benefits/harmsassessment: Preponderance of harm over benefit.
- Value judgments: Observational data were used for this judgment.
- Role of patient preferences: Although an EEG might have limited prognostic utility in this situation, parents should be educated that the study will not alter outcome.
- Exclusions: None.
- Intentional vagueness: None.
- Policy level: Strong recommendation.

There is no evidence that EEG readings performed either at the time of presentation after a simple febrile seizure or within the following month are predictive of either recurrence of febrile seizures or the development of afebrile seizures/epilepsy within the next 2 years.[13,14] There is a single study that found that a paroxysmal EEG was associated with a higher rate of afebrile seizures.[12] There is no evidence that interventions based on this test would alter outcome.

Action Statement 3

The following tests should not be performed routinely for the sole purpose of identifying the cause of a simple febrile seizure: measurement of serum electrolytes, calcium, phosphorus, magnesium, or blood glucose or complete blood cell count.

- Aggregate evidence level: B (overwhelming evidence from observational studies).
- Benefits: A complete blood cell count may identify children at risk for bacte-

remia; however, the incidence of bacteremia in febrile children younger than 24 months is the same with or without febrile seizures.

- Harms/risks/costs: Laboratory tests may be invasive and costly and provide no real benefit.
- Benefits/harms assessment: Preponderance of harm over benefit.
- Value judgments: Observational data were used for this judgment.
- Role of patient preferences: Although parents may want blood tests performed to explain the seizure, they should be reassured that blood tests should be directed toward identifying the source of their child's fever.
- Exclusions: None.
- Intentional vagueness: None.
- Policy level: Strong recommendation.

There is no evidence to suggest that routine blood studies are of benefit in the evaluation of the child with a simple febrile seizure.[15–18] Although some children with febrile seizures have abnormal serum electrolyte values, their condition should be identifiable by obtaining appropriate histories and performing careful physical examinations. It should be noted that as a group, children with febrile seizures have relatively low serum sodium concentrations. As such, physicians and caregivers should avoid overhydration with hypotonic fluids.[18] Complete blood cell counts may be useful as a means of identifying young children at risk of bacteremia. It should be noted, however, that the incidence of bacteremia in children younger than 24 months with or without febrile seizures is the same. When fever is present, the decision regarding the need for laboratory testing should be directed toward identifying the source of the fever rather than as part of the routine evaluation of the seizure itself.

Action Statement 4

Neuroimaging should not be performed in the routine evaluation of the child with a simple febrile seizure.

- Aggregate evidence level: B (overwhelming evidence from observational studies).
- Benefits: Neuroimaging might provide earlier detection of fixed structural lesions, such as dysplasia, or very rarely, abscess or tumor.
- Harms/risks/costs: Neuroimaging tests are costly, computed tomography (CT) exposes children to radiation, and MRI may require sedation.
- Benefits/harms assessment: Preponderance of harm over benefit.
- Value judgments: Observational data were used for this judgment.
- Role of patient preferences: Although parents may want neuroimaging performed to explain the seizure, they should be reassured that the tests carry risks and will not alter outcome for their child.
- Exclusions: None.
- Intentional vagueness: None.
- Policy level: Strong recommendation.

The literature does not support the use of skull films in evaluation of the child with a febrile seizure.[15,19] No data have been published that either support or negate the need for CT or MRI in the evaluation of children with simple febrile seizures. Data, however, show that CT scanning is associated with radiation exposure that may escalate future cancer risk. MRI is associated with risks from required sedation and high cost.[20,21] Extrapolation of data from the literature on the use of CT in neurologically healthy children who have generalized epilepsy has shown that clinically important intracranial structural abnormalities in this patient population are uncommon.[22,23]

CONCLUSIONS

Clinicians evaluating infants or young children after a simple febrile seizure should direct their attention toward identifying the cause of the child's fever. Meningitis should be considered in the differential diagnosis for any febrile child, and lumbar puncture should be performed if the child is ill-appearing or if there are clinical signs or symptoms of concern. A lumbar puncture is an option in a child 6 to 12 months of age who is deficient in Hib and *S pneumoniae* immunizations or for whom immunization status is unknown. A lumbar puncture is an option in children who have been pretreated with antibiotics. In general, a simple febrile seizure does not usually require further evaluation, specifically EEGs, blood studies, or neuroimaging.

SUBCOMMITTEE ON FEBRILE SEIZURES, 2002–2010

Patricia K. Duffner, MD (neurology, no conflicts)
Peter H. Berman, MD (neurology, no conflicts)
Robert J. Baumann, MD (neuroepidemiology, no conflicts)
Paul Graham Fisher, MD (neurology, no conflicts)
John L. Green, MD (general pediatrics, no conflicts)
Sanford Schneider, MD (neurology, no conflicts)

STAFF

Caryn Davidson, MA

OVERSIGHT BY THE STEERING COMMITTEE ON QUALITY IMPROVEMENT AND MANAGEMENT, 2009–2011

REFERENCES

1. American Academy of Pediatrics, Provisional Committee on Quality Improvement and Subcommittee on Febrile Seizures. Practice parameter: the neurodiagnostic evaluation of a child with a first simple febrile seizure. *Pediatrics*. 1996;97(5): 769–772; discussion 773–775
2. Michael Marcy S, Kohl KS, Dagan R, et al; Brighton Collaboration Fever Working Group. Fever as an adverse event following immunization: case definition and guidelines of data collection, analysis, and presentation. *Vaccine*. 2004;22(5–6):551–556
3. Nelson KB, Ellenberg JH. Predictors of epilepsy in children who have experienced febrile seizures. *N Engl J Med*. 1976;295(19): 1029–1033
4. Consensus statement: febrile seizures—long-term management of children with fever-associated seizures. *Pediatrics*. 1980; 66(6):1009–1012
5. American Academy of Pediatrics, Steering Committee on Quality Improvement and Management. Classifying recommendations for clinical practice guidelines. *Pediatrics*. 2004;114(3):874–877
6. Trainor JL, Hampers LC, Krug SE, Listernick R. Children with first-time simple febrile seizures are at low risk of serious bacterial illness. *Acad Emerg Med*. 2001;8(8):781–787
7. Shaked O, Peña BM, Linares MY, Baker RL. Simple febrile seizures: are the AAP guidelines regarding lumbar puncture being followed? *Pediatr Emerg Care*. 2009;25(1): 8–11
8. Kimia AA, Capraro AJ, Hummel D, Johnston P, Harper MB. Utility of lumbar puncture for first simple febrile seizure among children 6 to 18 months of age. *Pediatrics*. 2009; 123(1):6–12
9. Warden CR, Zibulewsky J, Mace S, Gold C, Gausche-Hill M. Evaluation and management of febrile seizures in the out-of-hospital and emergency department settings. *Ann Emerg Med*. 2003;41(2):215–222
10. Rutter N, Smales OR. Role of routine investigations in children presenting with their first febrile convulsion. *Arch Dis Child*. 1977; 52(3):188–191
11. Green SM, Rothrock SG, Clem KJ, Zurcher RF, Mellick L. Can seizures be the sole manifestation of meningitis in febrile children? *Pediatrics*. 1993;92(4):527–534
12. Kuturec M, Emoto SE, Sofijanov N, et al. Febrile seizures: is the EEG a useful predictor of recurrences? *Clin Pediatr (Phila)*. 1997; 36(1):31–36
13. Frantzen E, Lennox-Buchthal M, Nygaard A. Longitudinal EEG and clinical study of children with febrile convulsions. *Electroencephalogr Clin Neurophysiol*. 1968;24(3): 197–212
14. Thorn I. The significance of electroencephalography in febrile convulsions. In: Akimoto H, Kazamatsuri H, Seino M, Ward A, eds. *Advances in Epileptology: XIIIth International Epilepsy Symposium*. New York, NY: Raven Press; 1982:93–95
15. Jaffe M, Bar-Joseph G, Tirosh E. Fever and convulsions: indications for laboratory investigations. *Pediatrics*. 1981;67(5): 729–731
16. Gerber MA, Berliner BC. The child with a "simple" febrile seizure: appropriate diagnostic evaluation. *Am J Dis Child*. 1981; 135(5):431–443
17. Heijbel J, Blom S, Bergfors PG. Simple febrile convulsions: a prospective incidence study and an evaluation of investigations initially needed. *Neuropadiatrie*. 1980;11(1): 45–56
18. Thoman JE, Duffner PK, Shucard JL. Do serum sodium levels predict febrile seizure recurrence within 24 hours? *Pediatr Neurol*. 2004;31(5):342–344
19. Nealis GT, McFadden SW, Ames RA, Ouellette EM. Routine skull roentgenograms in the management of simple febrile seizures. *J Pediatr*. 1977;90(4):595–596
20. Stein SC, Hurst RW, Sonnad SS. Meta-analysis of cranial CT scans in children: a mathematical model to predict radiation-induced tumors associated with radiation exposure that may escalate future cancer risk. *Pediatr Neurosurg*. 2008;44(6): 448–457
21. Brenner DJ, Hall EJ. Computed tomography: an increasing source of radiation exposure. *N Engl J Med*. 2007;357(22):2277–2284
22. Yang PJ, Berger PE, Cohen ME, Duffner PK. Computed tomography and childhood seizure disorders. *Neurology*. 1979;29(8): 1084–1088
23. Bachman DS, Hodges FJ, Freeman JM. Computerized axial tomography in chronic seizure disorders of childhood. *Pediatrics*. 1976;58(6):828–832

Febrile Seizures Clinical Practice Guidelines Quick Reference Tools

- Recommendation Summaries
  - Febrile Seizures: Clinical Practice Guideline for the Long-term Management of the Child With Simple Febrile Seizures
  - Febrile Seizures: Guideline for the Neurodiagnostic Evaluation of the Child With a Simple Febrile Seizure
- *ICD-10-CM* Coding Quick Reference for Febrile Seizures
- AAP Patient Education Handout
  - *Febrile Seizures*

Recommendation Summaries

Febrile Seizures: Clinical Practice Guideline for the Long-term Management of the Child With Simple Febrile Seizures

On the basis of the risks and benefits of the effective therapies, neither continuous nor intermittent anticonvulsant therapy is recommended for children with 1 or more simple febrile seizures.

- Aggregate evidence quality: B (randomized, controlled trials and diagnostic studies with minor limitations).
- Benefit: prevention of recurrent febrile seizures, which are not harmful and do not significantly increase the risk for development of future epilepsy.
- Harm: adverse effects including rare fatal hepatotoxicity (especially in children younger than 2 years who are also at greatest risk of febrile seizures), thrombocytopenia, weight loss and gain, gastrointestinal disturbances, and pancreatitis with valproic acid and hyperactivity, irritability, lethargy, sleep disturbances, and hypersensitivity reactions with phenobarbital; lethargy, drowsiness, and ataxia for intermittent diazepam as well as the risk of masking an evolving central nervous system infection.
- Benefits/harms assessment: preponderance of harm over benefit.
- Policy level: recommendation.

Febrile Seizures: Guideline for the Neurodiagnostic Evaluation of the Child With a Simple Febrile Seizure

Action Statement 1a

A lumbar puncture should be performed in any child who presents with a seizure and a fever and has meningeal signs and symptoms (eg, neck stiffness, Kernig and/or Brudzinski signs) or in any child whose history or examination suggests the presence of meningitis or intracranial infection.

Action Statement 1b

In any infant between 6 and 12 months of age who presents with a seizure and fever, a lumbar puncture is an option when the child is considered deficient in *Haemophilus influenzae* type b (Hib) or *Streptococcus pneumoniae* immunizations (ie, has not received scheduled immunizations as recommended) or when immunization status cannot be determined because of an increased risk of bacterial meningitis.

Action Statement 1c

A lumbar puncture is an option in the child who presents with a seizure and fever and is pretreated with antibiotics, because antibiotic treatment can mask the signs and symptoms of meningitis.

Action Statement 2

An electroencephalogram (EEG) should not be performed in the evaluation of a neurologically healthy child with a simple febrile seizure.

Action Statement 3

The following tests should not be performed routinely for the sole purpose of identifying the cause of a simple febrile seizure: measurement of serum electrolytes, calcium, phosphorus, magnesium, or blood glucose or complete blood cell count.

Action Statement 4

Neuroimaging should not be performed in the routine evaluation of the child with a simple febrile seizure.

Coding Quick Reference for Febrile Seizures
ICD-10-CM
R56.00 Simple febrile convulsions
R56.01 Complex febrile convulsions

Febrile Seizures

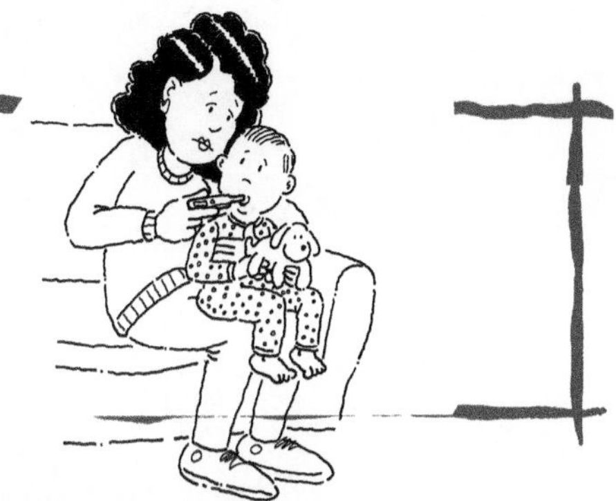

In some children, fevers can trigger seizures. Febrile seizures occur in 2% to 5% of all children between the ages of 6 months and 5 years. Seizures, sometimes called "fits" or "spells," are frightening, but they usually are harmless. Read on for information from the American Academy of Pediatrics that will help you understand febrile seizures and what happens if your child has one.

What is a febrile seizure?

A febrile seizure usually happens during the first few hours of a fever. The child may look strange for a few moments, then stiffen, twitch, and roll his eyes. He will be unresponsive for a short time, his breathing will be disturbed, and his skin may appear a little darker than usual. After the seizure, the child quickly returns to normal. Seizures usually last less than 1 minute but, although uncommon, can last for up to 15 minutes.

Febrile seizures rarely happen more than once within a 24-hour period. Other kinds of seizures (ones that are not caused by fever) last longer, can affect only one part of the body, and may occur repeatedly.

What do I do if my child has a febrile seizure?

If your child has a febrile seizure, act immediately to prevent injury.

- Place her on the floor or bed away from any hard or sharp objects.
- Turn her head to the side so that any saliva or vomit can drain from her mouth.
- Do not put anything into her mouth; she will not swallow her tongue.
- Call your child's doctor.
- If the seizure does not stop after 5 minutes, call 911 or your local emergency number.

Will my child have more seizures?

Febrile seizures tend to run in families. The risk of having seizures with other episodes of fever depends on the age of your child. Children younger than 1 year of age at the time of their first seizure have about a 50% chance of having another febrile seizure. Children older than 1 year of age at the time of their first seizure have only a 30% chance of having a second febrile seizure.

Will my child get epilepsy?

Epilepsy is a term used for multiple and recurrent seizures. Epileptic seizures are not caused by fever. Children with a history of febrile seizures are at only a slightly higher risk of developing epilepsy by age 7 than children who have not had febrile seizures.

Are febrile seizures dangerous?

While febrile seizures may be very scary, they are harmless to the child. Febrile seizures do not cause brain damage, nervous system problems, paralysis, intellectual disability (formerly called mental retardation), or death.

How are febrile seizures treated?

If your child has a febrile seizure, call your child's doctor right away. He or she will want to examine your child in order to determine the cause of your child's fever. It is more important to determine and treat the cause of the fever rather than the seizure. A spinal tap may be done to be sure your child does not have a serious infection like meningitis, especially if your child is younger than 1 year of age.

In general, doctors do not recommend treatment of a simple febrile seizure with preventive medicines. However, this should be discussed with your child's doctor. In cases of prolonged or repeated seizures, the recommendation may be different.

Medicines like acetaminophen and ibuprofen can help lower a fever, but they do not prevent febrile seizures. Your child's doctor will talk with you about the best ways to take care of your child's fever.

If your child has had a febrile seizure, do not fear the worst. These types of seizures are not dangerous to your child and do not cause long-term health problems. If you have concerns about this issue or anything related to your child's health, talk with your child's doctor.

The information contained in this publication should not be used as a substitute for the medical care and advice of your pediatrician. There may be variations in treatment that your pediatrician may recommend based on individual facts and circumstances.

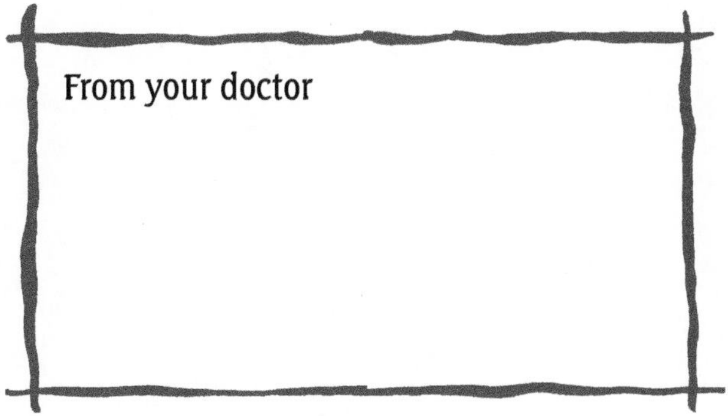

American Academy of Pediatrics

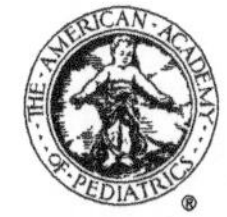

DEDICATED TO THE HEALTH OF ALL CHILDREN™

The American Academy of Pediatrics is an organization of 60,000 primary care pediatricians, pediatric medical subspecialists, and pediatric surgical specialists dedicated to the health, safety, and well-being of infants, children, adolescents, and young adults.

American Academy of Pediatrics
Web site—www.HealthyChildren.org

Copyright © 1999
American Academy of Pediatrics, Updated 1/12
All rights reserved.

Clinical Practice Guideline for Screening and Management of High Blood Pressure in Children and Adolescents

- *Clinical Practice Guideline*
  - *PPI: AAP Partnership for Policy Implementation*
    See Appendix 1 for more information.

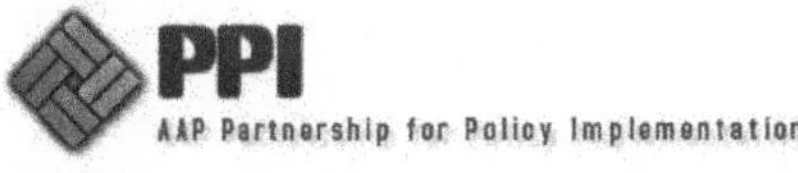

CLINICAL PRACTICE GUIDELINE Guidance for the Clinician in Rendering Pediatric Care

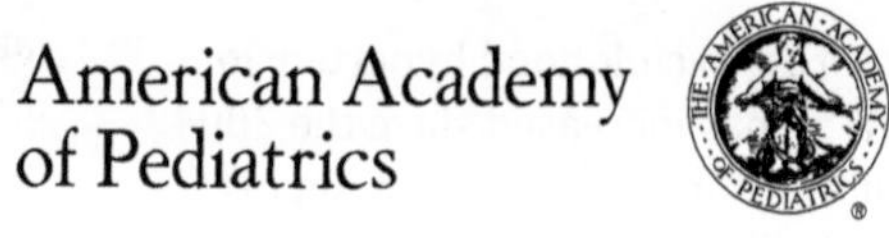

Clinical Practice Guideline for Screening and Management of High Blood Pressure in Children and Adolescents

Joseph T. Flynn, MD, MS, FAAP,[a] David C. Kaelber, MD, PhD, MPH, FAAP, FACP, FACMI,[b] Carissa M. Baker-Smith, MD, MS, MPH, FAAP, FAHA,[c] Douglas Blowey, MD,[d] Aaron E. Carroll, MD, MS, FAAP,[e] Stephen R. Daniels, MD, PhD, FAAP,[f] Sarah D. de Ferranti, MD, MPH, FAAP,[g] Janis M. Dionne, MD, FRCPC,[h] Bonita Falkner, MD,[i] Susan K. Flinn, MA,[j] Samuel S. Gidding, MD,[k] Celeste Goodwin,[l] Michael G. Leu, MD, MS, MHS, FAAP,[m] Makia E. Powers, MD, MPH, FAAP,[n] Corinna Rea, MD, MPH, FAAP,[o] Joshua Samuels, MD, MPH, FAAP,[p] Madeline Simasek, MD, MSCP, FAAP,[q] Vidhu V. Thaker, MD, FAAP,[r] Elaine M. Urbina, MD, MS, FAAP,[s] SUBCOMMITTEE ON SCREENING AND MANAGEMENT OF HIGH BLOOD PRESSURE IN CHILDREN

abstract

These pediatric hypertension guidelines are an update to the 2004 "Fourth Report on the Diagnosis, Evaluation, and Treatment of High Blood Pressure in Children and Adolescents." Significant changes in these guidelines include (1) the replacement of the term "prehypertension" with the term "elevated blood pressure," (2) new normative pediatric blood pressure (BP) tables based on normal-weight children, (3) a simplified screening table for identifying BPs needing further evaluation, (4) a simplified BP classification in adolescents ≥13 years of age that aligns with the forthcoming American Heart Association and American College of Cardiology adult BP guidelines, (5) a more limited recommendation to perform screening BP measurements only at preventive care visits, (6) streamlined recommendations on the initial evaluation and management of abnormal BPs, (7) an expanded role for ambulatory BP monitoring in the diagnosis and management of pediatric hypertension, and (8) revised recommendations on when to perform echocardiography in the evaluation of newly diagnosed hypertensive pediatric patients (generally only before medication initiation), along with a revised definition of left ventricular hypertrophy. These guidelines include 30 Key Action Statements and 27 additional recommendations derived from a comprehensive review of almost 15 000 published articles between January 2004 and July 2016. Each Key Action Statement includes level of evidence, benefit-harm relationship, and strength of recommendation. This clinical practice guideline, endorsed by the American Heart Association, is intended to foster a patient- and family-centered approach to care, reduce unnecessary and costly medical interventions, improve patient diagnoses and outcomes, support implementation, and provide direction for future research.

[a]Dr. Robert O. Hickman Endowed Chair in Pediatric Nephrology, Division of Nephrology, Department of Pediatrics, University of Washington and Seattle Children's Hospital, Seattle, Washington; [b]Departments of Pediatrics, Internal Medicine, Population and Quantitative Health Sciences, Center for Clinical Informatics Research and Education, Case Western Reserve University and MetroHealth System, Cleveland, Ohio; [c]Division of Pediatric Cardiology, School of Medicine, University of Maryland, Baltimore, Maryland; [d]Children's Mercy Hospital, University of Missouri-Kansas City and Children's Mercy Integrated Care Solutions, Kansas City, Missouri; [e]Department of Pediatrics, School of Medicine, Indiana University, Bloomington, Indiana; [f]Department of Pediatrics, School of Medicine, University of Colorado-Denver and Pediatrician in Chief, Children's Hospital Colorado, Aurora, Colorado; [g]Director, Preventive Cardiology Clinic, Boston Children's Hospital, Department of Pediatrics, Harvard Medical School, Boston, Massachusetts; [h]Division of Nephrology, Department of Pediatrics, University of British Columbia and British Columbia Children's Hospital, Vancouver, British Columbia, Canada; Departments of [i]Medicine and Pediatrics, Sidney Kimmel Medical College, Thomas Jefferson University, Philadelphia, Pennsylvania; [j]Consultant, American Academy of Pediatrics, Washington, District of Columbia; [k]Cardiology Division Head, Nemours Cardiac Center, Alfred I. duPont Hospital for Children, Wilmington, Delaware; [l]National Pediatric Blood Pressure Awareness Foundation, Prairieville, Louisiana; Departments of [m]Pediatrics and Biomedical Informatics and Medical Education, University of Washington, University of Washington Medicine and Information Technology Services, and Seattle Children's Hospital,

To cite: Flynn JT, Kaelber DC, Baker-Smith CM, et al. Clinical Practice Guideline for Screening and Management of High Blood Pressure in Children and Adolescents. *Pediatrics.* 2017;140(3):e20171904

1. INTRODUCTION

1. Scope of the Clinical Practice Guideline

Interest in childhood hypertension (HTN) has increased since the 2004 publication of the "Fourth Report on the Diagnosis, Evaluation, and Treatment of High Blood Pressure in Children and Adolescents" (Fourth Report).[1] Recognizing ongoing evidence gaps and the need for an updated, thorough review of the relevant literature, the American Academy of Pediatrics (AAP) and its Council on Quality Improvement and Patient Safety developed this practice guideline to provide an update on topics relevant to the diagnosis, evaluation, and management of pediatric HTN. It is primarily directed at clinicians caring for children and adolescents in the outpatient setting. This guideline is endorsed by the American Heart Association.

When it was not possible to identify sufficient evidence, recommendations are based on the consensus opinion of the expert members of the Screening and Management of High Blood Pressure in Children Clinical Practice Guideline Subcommittee (henceforth, "the subcommittee"). The subcommittee intends to regularly update this guideline as new evidence becomes available. Implementation tools for this guideline are available on the AAP Web site (https://www.aap.org/en-us/about-the-aap/Committees-Councils-Sections/coqips/Pages/Implementation-Guide.aspx).

1.1 Methodology

The subcommittee was co-chaired by a pediatric nephrologist and a general pediatrician and consisted of 17 members, including a parent representative. All subcommittee members were asked to disclose relevant financial or proprietary conflicts of interest for members or their family members at the start of and throughout the guideline preparation process. Potential conflicts of interest were addressed and resolved by the AAP. A detailed list of subcommittee members and affiliations can be found in the Consortium section at the end of this article. A listing of subcommittee members with conflicts of interest will be included in the forthcoming technical report.

The subcommittee epidemiologist created a detailed content outline, which was reviewed and approved by the subcommittee. The outline contained a list of primary and secondary topics generated to guide a thorough literature search and meet the goal of providing an up-to-date systemic review of the literature pertaining to the diagnosis, management, and treatment of pediatric HTN as well as the prevalence of pediatric HTN and its associated comorbidities.

Of the topics covered in the outline, ~80% were researched by using a Patient, Intervention/Indicator, Comparison, Outcome, and Time (PICOT) format to address the following key questions:

1. How should systemic HTN (eg, primary HTN, renovascular HTN, white coat hypertension [WCH], and masked hypertension [MH]) in children be diagnosed, and what is the optimal approach to diagnosing HTN in children and adolescents?
2. What is the recommended workup for pediatric HTN? How do we best identify the underlying etiologies of secondary HTN in children?
3. What is the optimal goal systolic blood pressure (SBP) and/or diastolic blood pressure (DBP) for children and adolescents?
4. In children 0 to 18 years of age, how does treatment with lifestyle versus antihypertensive agents influence indirect measures of cardiovascular disease (CVD) risk, such as carotid intimamedia thickness (cIMT), flow-mediated dilation (FMD), left ventricular hypertrophy (LVH), and other markers of vascular dysfunction?

To address these key questions, a systematic search and review of literature was performed. The initial search included articles published between the publication of the Fourth Report (January 2004) and August 2015. The process used to conduct the systematic review was consistent with the recommendations of the Institute of Medicine for systematic reviews.[2]

For the topics not researched by using the PICOT format, separate searches were conducted. Not all topics (eg, economic aspects of pediatric HTN) were appropriate for the PICOT format. A third and final search was conducted at the time the Key Action Statements (KASs) were generated to identify any additional relevant articles published between August 2015 and July 2016. (See Table 1 for a complete list of KASs.)

A detailed description of the methodology used to conduct the literature search and systematic review for this clinical practice guideline will be included in the forthcoming technical report. In brief, reference selection involved a multistep process. First, 2 subcommittee members reviewed the titles and abstracts of references identified for each key question. The epidemiologist provided a deciding vote when required. Next, 2 subcommittee members and the epidemiologist conducted full-text reviews of the selected articles. Although many subcommittee members have extensively published articles on topics covered in this guideline, articles were not preferentially selected on the basis of authorship.

Articles selected at this stage were mapped back to the relevant main topic in the outline. Subcommittee members were then assigned to

TABLE 1 Summary of KASs for Screening and Management of High BP in Children and Adolescents

KAS	Evidence Quality, Strength of Recommendation
1. BP should be measured annually in children and adolescents ≥3 y of age.	C, moderate
2. BP should be checked in all children and adolescents ≥3 y of age at every health care encounter if they have obesity, are taking medications known to increase BP, have renal disease, a history of aortic arch obstruction or coarctation, or diabetes.	C, moderate
3. Trained health care professionals in the office setting should make a diagnosis of HTN if a child or adolescent has auscultatory-confirmed BP readings ≥95th percentile at 3 different visits.	C, moderate
4. Organizations with EHRs used in an office setting should consider including flags for abnormal BP values, both when the values are being entered and when they are being viewed.	C, weak
5. Oscillometric devices may be used for BP screening in children and adolescents. When doing so, providers should use a device that has been validated in the pediatric age group. If elevated BP is suspected on the basis of oscillometric readings, confirmatory measurements should be obtained by auscultation.	B, strong
6. ABPM should be performed for confirmation of HTN in children and adolescents with office BP measurements in the elevated BP category for 1 year or more or with stage 1 HTN over 3 clinic visits.	C, moderate
7. Routine performance of ABPM should be strongly considered in children and adolescents with high-risk conditions (see Table 12) to assess HTN severity and determine if abnormal circadian BP patterns are present, which may indicate increased risk for target organ damage.	B, moderate
8. ABPM should be performed by using a standardized approach (see Table 13) with monitors that have been validated in a pediatric population, and studies should be interpreted by using pediatric normative data.	C, moderate
9. Children and adolescents with suspected WCH should undergo ABPM. Diagnosis is based on the presence of mean SBP and DBP <95th percentile and SBP and DBP load <25%.	B, strong
10. Home BP monitoring should not be used to diagnose HTN, MH, or WCH but may be a useful adjunct to office and ambulatory BP measurement after HTN has been diagnosed.	C, moderate
11. Children and adolescents ≥6 y of age do not require an extensive evaluation for secondary causes of HTN if they have a positive family history of HTN, are overweight or obese, and/or do not have history or physical examination findings (Table 14) suggestive of a secondary cause of HTN.	C, moderate
12. Children and adolescents who have undergone coarctation repair should undergo ABPM for the detection of HTN (including MH).	B, strong
13. In children and adolescents being evaluated for high BP, the provider should obtain a perinatal history, appropriate nutritional history, physical activity history, psychosocial history, and family history and perform a physical examination to identify findings suggestive of secondary causes of HTN.	B, strong
14. Clinicians should not perform electrocardiography in hypertensive children and adolescents being evaluated for LVH.	B, strong
15-1. It is recommended that echocardiography be performed to assess for cardiac target organ damage (LV mass, geometry, and function) at the time of consideration of pharmacologic treatment of HTN.	C, moderate
15-2. LVH should be defined as LV mass >51 g/m$^{2.7}$ (boys and girls) for children and adolescents older than age 8 y and defined by LV mass >115 g/BSA for boys and LV mass >95 g/BSA for girls.	
15-3. Repeat echocardiography may be performed to monitor improvement or progression of target organ damage at 6- to 12-mo intervals. Indications to repeat echocardiography include persistent HTN despite treatment, concentric LV hypertrophy, or reduced LV ejection fraction.	
15-4. In patients without LV target organ injury at initial echocardiographic assessment, repeat echocardiography at yearly intervals may be considered in those with stage 2 HTN, secondary HTN, or chronic stage 1 HTN incompletely treated (noncompliance or drug resistance) to assess for the development of worsening LV target organ injury.	
16. Doppler renal ultrasonography may be used as a noninvasive screening study for the evaluation of possible RAS in normal-wt children and adolescents ≥8 y of age who are suspected of having renovascular HTN and who will cooperate with the procedure.	C, moderate
17. In children and adolescents suspected of having RAS, either CTA or MRA may be performed as noninvasive imaging studies. Nuclear renography is less useful in pediatrics and should generally be avoided.	D, weak
18. Routine testing for MA is not recommended for children and adolescents with primary HTN.	C, moderate
19. In children and adolescents diagnosed with HTN, the treatment goal with nonpharmacologic and pharmacologic therapy should be a reduction in SBP and DBP to <90th percentile and <130/80 mm Hg in adolescents ≥ 13 years old.	C, moderate
20. At the time of diagnosis of elevated BP or HTN in a child or adolescent, clinicians should provide advice on the DASH diet and recommend moderate to vigorous physical activity at least 3 to 5 d per week (30–60 min per session) to help reduce BP.	C, weak
21. In hypertensive children and adolescents who have failed lifestyle modifications (particularly those who have LV hypertrophy on echocardiography, symptomatic HTN, or stage 2 HTN without a clearly modifiable factor [eg, obesity]), clinicians should initiate pharmacologic treatment with an ACE inhibitor, ARB, long-acting calcium channel blocker, or thiazide diuretic.	B, moderate
22. ABPM may be used to assess treatment effectiveness in children and adolescents with HTN, especially when clinic and/or home BP measurements indicate insufficient BP response to treatment.	B, moderate
23-1. Children and adolescents with CKD should be evaluated for HTN at each medical encounter.	B, strong
23-2. Children or adolescents with both CKD and HTN should be treated to lower 24-hr MAP <50th percentile by ABPM.	
23-3. Regardless of apparent control of BP with office measures, children and adolescents with CKD and a history of HTN should have BP assessed by ABPM at least yearly to screen for MH.	
24. Children and adolescents with CKD and HTN should be evaluated for proteinuria.	B, strong
25. Children and adolescents with CKD, HTN, and proteinuria should be treated with an ACE inhibitor or ARB.	B, strong

TABLE 1 Continued

KAS	Evidence Quality, Strength of Recommendation
26. Children and adolescents with T1DM or T2DM should be evaluated for HTN at each medical encounter and treated if BP ≥95th percentile or >130/80 mm Hg in adolescents ≥13 y of age.	C, moderate
27. In children and adolescents with acute severe HTN and life-threatening symptoms, immediate treatment with short-acting antihypertensive medication should be initiated, and BP should be reduced by no more than 25% of the planned reduction over the first 8 h.	Expert opinion, D, weak
28. Children and adolescents with HTN may participate in competitive sports once hypertensive target organ effects and cardiovascular risk have been assessed.	C, moderate
29. Children and adolescents with HTN should receive treatment to lower BP below stage 2 thresholds before participation in competitive sports.	C, moderate
30. Adolescents with elevated BP or HTN (whether they are receiving antihypertensive treatment) should typically have their care transitioned to an appropriate adult care provider by 22 y of age (recognizing that there may be individual cases in which this upper age limit is exceeded, particularly in the case of youth with special health care needs). There should be a transfer of information regarding HTN etiology and past manifestations and complications of the patient's HTN.	X, strong

writing teams that evaluated the evidence quality for selected topics and generated appropriate KASs in accordance with an AAP grading matrix (see Fig 1 and the detailed discussion in the forthcoming technical report).[3] Special working groups were created to address 2 specific topics for which evidence was lacking and expert opinion was required to generate KASs, "Definition of HTN" and "Definition of LVH." References for any topics not covered by the key questions were selected on the basis of additional literature searches and reviewed by the epidemiologist and subcommittee members assigned to the topic. When applicable, searches were conducted by using the PICOT format.

In addition to the 30 KASs listed above, this guideline also contains 27 additional recommendations that are based on the consensus expert opinion of the subcommittee members. These recommendations, along with their locations in the document, are listed in Table 2.

2. EPIDEMIOLOGY AND CLINICAL SIGNIFICANCE

2.1 Prevalence of HTN in Children

Information on the prevalence of high blood pressure (BP) in children is largely derived from data from the NHANES and typically is based on a single BP measurement session. These surveys, conducted since 1988, indicate that there has been an increase in the prevalence of childhood high BP, including both HTN and elevated BP.[4,5] High BP is consistently greater in boys (15%–19%) than in girls (7%–12%). The prevalence of high BP is higher among Hispanic and non-Hispanic African American children compared with non-Hispanic white children, with higher rates among adolescents than among younger children.[6]

However, in a clinical setting and with repeated BP measurements, the prevalence of confirmed HTN is lower in part because of inherent BP variability as well as an adjustment to the experience of having BP measured (also known as the accommodation effect). Therefore, the actual prevalence of clinical HTN in children and adolescents is ~3.5%.[7,8] The prevalence of persistently elevated BP (formerly termed "prehypertension," including BP values from the 90th to 94th percentiles or between 120/80 and 130/80 mm Hg in adolescents) is also ~2.2% to 3.5%, with higher rates among children and adolescents who have overweight and obesity.[7,9]

Data on BP tracking from childhood to adulthood demonstrate that higher BP in childhood correlates with higher BP in adulthood and the onset of HTN in young adulthood. The strength of the tracking relationship is stronger in older children and adolescents.[10] Trajectory data on BP (including repeat measurements from early childhood into midadulthood) confirm the association of elevated BP in adolescence with HTN in early adulthood[11] and that normal BP in childhood is associated with a lack of HTN in midadulthood.[11]

2.2 Awareness, Treatment, and Control of HTN in Children

Of the 32.6% of US adults who have HTN, almost half (17.2%) are not aware they have HTN; even among those who are aware of their condition, only approximately half (54.1%) have controlled BP.[12] Unfortunately, there are no large studies in which researchers have systematically studied BP awareness or control in youth, although an analysis of prescribing patterns from a nationwide prescription drug provider found an increase in the number of prescriptions written for high BP in youth from 2004 to 2007.[13]

The SEARCH for Diabetes in Youth study found that only 7.4% of youth with type 1 diabetes mellitus (T1DM) and 31.9% of youth with type 2 diabetes mellitus (T2DM) demonstrated knowledge of their BP status.[14] Even after becoming aware of the diagnosis, only 57.1% of patients with T1DM and 40.6% of patients with T2DM achieved good BP control.[14] The HEALTHY Primary Prevention Trial of Risk Factors for

TABLE 2 Additional Consensus Opinion Recommendations and Text Locations

Recommendation	CPG Section(s)
1. Follow the revised classification scheme in Table 3 for childhood BP levels, including the use of the term "elevated BP," the new definition of stage 2 HTN, and the use of similar BP levels as adults for adolescents ≥13 y of age.	3.1
2. Use simplified BP tables (Table 4) to screen for BP values that may require further evaluation by a clinician.	3.2a
3. Use reference data on neonatal BP from ref 80 to identify elevated BP values in neonates up to 44 wk postmenstrual age and BP curves from the 1987 Second Task Force report to identify elevated BP values in infants 1–12 mo of age.	3.3
4. Use the standardized technique for measuring BP by auscultation described in Table 7 and Fig 2 (including appropriate cuff size, extremity, and patient positioning) to obtain accurate BP values.	4.1
5. If the initial BP at an office visit is elevated, as described in Fig 3, obtain 2 additional BP measurements at the same visit and average them; use the averaged auscultatory BP measurement to determine the patient's BP category.	4.1
6. Oscillometric devices are used to measure BP in infants and toddlers until they are able to cooperate with auscultatory BP. Follow the same rules for BP measurement technique and cuff size as for older children.	4.1a
7. Measure BP at every health care encounter in children <3 y of age if they have an underlying condition listed in Table 9 that increases their risk for HTN.	4.2
8. After a patient's BP has been categorized, follow Table 11 for when to obtain repeat BP readings, institute lifestyle changes, or proceed to a workup for HTN.	4.3
9. When an oscillometric BP reading is elevated, obtain repeat readings, discard the first reading, and average subsequent readings to approximate auscultatory BP.	4.5
10. Wrist and forearm BP measurements should not be used in children and adolescents for the diagnosis or management of HTN.	4.6
11. Use ABPM to evaluate high-risk patients (those with obesity, CKD, or repaired aortic coarctation) for potential MH.	4.7a, 4.8
12. Routine use of BP readings obtained in the school setting is not recommended for diagnosis of HTN in children and adolescents.	4.10
13. Use the history and physical examination to identify possible underlying causes of HTN, such as heart disease, kidney disease, renovascular disease, endocrine HTN (Table 15), drug-induced HTN (Table 8), and OSAS-associated HTN (Table 18).	5.2–5.4, 5.7, 9.2
14. Suspect monogenic HTN in patients with a family history of early-onset HTN, hypokalemia, suppressed plasma renin, or an elevated ARR.	5.8
15. Obtain laboratory studies listed in Table 10 to evaluate for underlying secondary causes of HTN when indicated.	6.4
16. Routine use of vascular imaging, such as carotid intimal-media measurements or PWV measurements, is not recommended in the evaluation of HTN in children and adolescents.	6.7
17. Suspect renovascular HTN in selected children and adolescents with stage 2 HTN, significant diastolic HTN, discrepant kidney sizes on ultrasound, hypokalemia on screening laboratories, or an epigastric and/or upper abdominal bruit on physical examination.	6.8a
18. Routine measurement of serum UA is not recommended for children and adolescents with elevated BP.	6.9
19. Offer intensive weight-loss programs to hypertensive children and adolescents with obesity; consider using MI as an adjunct to the treatment of obesity.	7.2c
20. Follow-up children and adolescents treated with antihypertensive medications every 4–6 wk until BP is controlled, then extend the interval. Follow-up every 3–6 mo is appropriate for patients treated with lifestyle modification only.	7.3c
21. Evaluate and treat children and adolescents with apparent treatment-resistant HTN in a similar manner to that recommended for adults with resistant HTN.	7.4
22. Treat hypertensive children and adolescents with dyslipidemia according to current, existing pediatric lipid guidelines.	9.1
23. Use ABPM to evaluate for potential HTN in children and adolescents with known or suspected OSAS.	9.2
24. Racial, ethnic, and sex differences need not be considered in the evaluation and management of children and adolescents with HTN.	10
25. Use ABPM to evaluate BP in pediatric heart- and kidney-transplant recipients.	11.3

Type 2 Diabetes in Middle-School Youth, which examined a school-based intervention designed to reduce cardiovascular (CV) risk among middle school students, found the prevalence of stage 1 or 2 HTN to be ~9.5%.[15] There was no significant reduction in HTN in the control group after the intervention; the intervention group saw a reduction in the prevalence of HTN of ~1%, leaving 8.5% with BP still above the ideal range.

Researchers in a number of small, single-center studies have evaluated BP control in children and adolescents with HTN. One study found that lifestyle change and medications produced adequate BP control in 46 of 65 youth (70%) with HTN.[16] Another study in which researchers used ambulatory blood pressure monitoring (ABPM) to assess BP control among a group of 38 children (of whom 84% had chronic kidney disease [CKD]) found that only 13 children (34%) achieved adequate BP control even among those who received more than 1 drug.[17] A similar study found that additional drugs did increase rates of BP control in children with CKD, however.[18]

2.3 Prevalence of HTN Among Children With Various Chronic Conditions

It is well recognized that HTN rates are higher in children with certain chronic conditions, including children with obesity, sleep-disordered breathing (SDB), CKD, and those born preterm. These are described below.

2.3a Children With Obesity

HTN prevalence ranges from 3.8% to 24.8% in youth with overweight and obesity. Rates of HTN increase in a graded fashion with increasing adiposity.[19–24] Similar relationships are seen between HTN and increasing waist circumference.[4,25,26] Systematic reviews of 63 studies on BMI[27] and 61 studies on various measures

TABLE 2 Continued

Recommendation	CPG Section(s)
26. Reasonable strategies for HTN prevention include the maintenance of a normal BMI, consuming a DASH-type diet, avoidance of excessive sodium consumption, and regular vigorous physical activity.	13.2
27. Provide education about HTN to patients and their parents to improve patient involvement in their care and better achieve therapeutic goals.	15.2, 15.3

Based on the expert opinion of the subcommittee members (level of evidence = D; strength of recommendations = weak).
CPG, clinical practice guideline.

of abdominal adiposity[28] have shown associations between these conditions and HTN. Obesity is also associated with a lack of circadian variability of BP,[29,30] with up to 50% of children who have obesity not experiencing the expected nocturnal BP dip.[31–33]

Studies have shown that childhood obesity is also related to the development of future HTN.[22] Elevated BMI as early as infancy is associated with higher future BP.[34] This risk appears to increase with obesity severity; there is a fourfold increase in BP among those with severe obesity (BMI >99th percentile) versus a twofold increase in those with obesity (BMI 95th–98th percentiles) compared with normal-weight children and adolescents.[35]

Collectively, the results of these cross-sectional and longitudinal studies firmly establish an increasing prevalence of HTN with increasing BMI percentile. The study results also underscore the importance of monitoring BP in all children with overweight and/or obesity at every clinical encounter.

Obesity in children with HTN may be accompanied by additional cardiometabolic risk factors (eg, dyslipidemia and disordered glucose metabolism)[36,37] that may have their own effects on BP or may represent comorbid conditions arising from the same adverse lifestyle behaviors.[25,38] Some argue that the presence of multiple risk factors, including obesity and HTN, leads to far greater increases in CV risk than is explained by the individual risk factors alone. Although this phenomenon has been hard to demonstrate definitively, the Strong Heart Study did show that American Indian adolescents with multiple cardiometabolic risk factors had a higher prevalence of LVH (43.2% vs 11.7%), left atrial dilation (63.1% vs 21.9%; $P < .001$), and reduced LV systolic and diastolic function compared with those without multiple cardiometabolic risk factors.[39] Notably, both obesity and HTN were drivers of these CV abnormalities, with obesity being a stronger determinant of cardiac abnormalities than HTN (odds ratio, 4.17 vs 1.03).

2.3b Children With SDB

SDB occurs on a spectrum that includes (1) primary snoring, (2) sleep fragmentation, and (3) obstructive sleep apnea syndrome (OSAS). Researchers in numerous studies have identified an association between SDB and HTN in the pediatric population.[40–42] Studies suggest that children who sleep 7 hours or less per night are at increased risk for HTN.[43] Small studies of youth with sleep disorders have found the prevalence of high BP to range between 3.6% and 14%.[40,41] The more severe the OSAS, the more likely a child is to have HTN.[44,45] Even inadequate duration of sleep and poor-quality sleep have been associated with elevated BP.[43]

2.3c Children With CKD

There are well-established pathophysiologic links between childhood HTN and CKD. Certain forms of CKD can lead to HTN, and untreated HTN can lead to CKD in adults, although evidence for the latter in pediatric patients is lacking. Among children and adolescents with CKD, ~50% are known to be hypertensive.[46–48] In children and adolescents with end-stage renal disease (either those on dialysis or after transplant), ~48% to 79% are hypertensive, with 20% to 70% having uncontrolled HTN.[49–53] Almost 20% of pediatric HTN may be attributable to CKD.[54]

2.3d Children With History of Prematurity

Abnormal birth history—including preterm birth and low birth weight—has been identified as a risk factor for HTN and other CVD in adults[55]; only low birth weight has been associated with elevated BP in the pediatric age range.[56] One retrospective cohort study showed a prevalence of HTN of 7.3% among 3 year olds who were born preterm.[57] Researchers in another retrospective case series noted a high prevalence of HTN in older children with a history of preterm birth.[58] It also appears that preterm birth may result in abnormal circadian BP patterns in childhood.[59] These data are intriguing but limited. Further study is needed to determine how often preterm birth results in childhood HTN.

2.4 Importance of Diagnosing HTN in Children and Adolescents

Numerous studies have shown that elevated BP in childhood increases the risk for adult HTN and metabolic syndrome.[10,60–62] Youth with higher BP levels in childhood are also more likely to have persistent HTN as adults.[60,63] One recent study found that adolescents with elevated BP progressed to HTN at a rate of 7% per year, and elevated BMI predicted sustained BP elevations.[64] In addition, young patients with HTN are likely to experience accelerated vascular aging. Both autopsy[65] and imaging studies[66] have demonstrated BP-related CV damage in youth. These intermediate markers of CVD (eg, increased LV mass,[67] cIMT,[68] and pulse wave velocity [PWV][69]) are known to predict CV events in adults, making it crucial to diagnose and treat HTN early.

Eighty million US adults (1 in 3) have HTN, which is a major contributor to CVD.[12] Key contributors to CV health have been identified by the American Heart Association (AHA) as "Life's Simple 7," including 4 ideal health behaviors (not smoking, normal BMI, physical activity at goal levels, and a healthy diet) and 3 ideal health factors (untreated, normal total cholesterol; normal fasting blood glucose; and normal untreated BP, defined in childhood as ≤90th percentile or <120/80 mm Hg). Notably, elevated BP is the least common abnormal health factor in children and adolescents[70]; 89% of youth (ages 12–19 years) are in the ideal BP category.[6]

Given the prevalence of known key contributors in youth (ie, tobacco exposure, obesity, inactivity, and nonideal diet[12,71]), adult CVD likely has its origins in childhood. One-third of US adolescents report having tried a cigarette in the past 30 days.[72] Almost half (40%–48%) of teenagers have elevated BMI, and the rates of severe obesity (BMI >99th percentile) continue to climb, particularly in girls and adolescents.[73–75] Physical activity measured by accelerometry shows less than half of school-aged boys and only one-third of school-aged girls meet the goal for ideal physical activity levels.[72] More than 80% of youth 12 to 19 years of age have a poor diet (as defined by AHA metrics for ideal CV health); only ~10% eat adequate fruits and vegetables, and only ~15% consume <1500 mg per day of sodium, both of which are key dietary determinants of HTN.[76]

Finally, measuring BP at routine well-child visits enables the early detection of primary HTN as well as the detection of asymptomatic HTN secondary to another underlying disorder. Early detection of HTN is vital given the greater relative prevalence of secondary causes of HTN in children compared with adults.

TABLE 3 Updated Definitions of BP Categories and Stages

For Children Aged 1–13 y	For Children Aged ≥13 y
Normal BP: <90th percentile	Normal BP: <120/<80 mm Hg
Elevated BP: ≥90th percentile to <95th percentile or 120/80 mm Hg to <95th percentile (whichever is lower)	Elevated BP: 120/<80 to 129/<80 mm Hg
Stage 1 HTN: ≥95th percentile to <95th percentile + 12 mmHg, or 130/80 to 139/89 mm Hg (whichever is lower)	Stage 1 HTN: 130/80 to 139/89 mm Hg
Stage 2 HTN: ≥95th percentile + 12 mm Hg, or ≥140/90 mm Hg (whichever is lower)	Stage 2 HTN: ≥140/90 mm Hg

3. DEFINITION OF HTN

3.1 Definition of HTN (1–18 Years of Age)

Given the lack of outcome data, the current definition of HTN in children and adolescents is based on the normative distribution of BP in healthy children.[1] Because it is a major determinant of BP in growing children, height has been incorporated into the normative data since the publication of the 1996 Working Group Report.[1] BP levels should be interpreted on the basis of sex, age, and height to avoid misclassification of children who are either extremely tall or extremely short. It should be noted that the normative data were collected by using an auscultatory technique,[1] which may provide different values than measurement obtained by using oscillometric devices or from ABPM.

In the Fourth Report, "normal blood pressure" was defined as SBP and DBP values <90th percentile (on the basis of age, sex, and height percentiles). For the preadolescent, "prehypertension" was defined as SBP and/or DBP ≥90th percentile and <95th percentile (on the basis of age, sex, and height tables). For adolescents, "prehypertension" was defined as BP ≥120/80 mm Hg to <95th percentile, or ≥90th and <95th percentile, whichever was lower. HTN was defined as average clinic measured SBP and/or DBP ≥95th percentile (on the basis of age, sex, and height percentiles) and was further classified as stage 1 or stage 2 HTN.

There are still no data to identify a specific level of BP in childhood that leads to adverse CV outcomes in adulthood. Therefore, the subcommittee decided to maintain a statistical definition for childhood HTN. The staging criteria have been revised for stage 1 and stage 2 HTN for ease of implementation compared with the Fourth Report. For children ≥13 years of age, this staging scheme will seamlessly interface with the 2017 AHA and American College of Cardiology (ACC) adult HTN guideline.* Additionally, the term "prehypertension" has been replaced by the term "elevated blood pressure," to be consistent with the AHA and ACC guideline and convey the importance of lifestyle measures to prevent the development of HTN (see Table 3).

3.2 New BP Tables

New normative BP tables based on normal-weight children are included with these guidelines (see Tables 4 and 5). Similar to the tables in the

*Whelton PK, Carey RM, Aranow WS, et al. ACC/AHA/APPA/ABC/ACPM/AGS/APhA/ASH/ASPC/NMA/PCNA Guideline for the prevention, detection, evaluation and managament of high blood pressure in adults: A report of the American College of Cardiology/American Heart Association Task Force on Clinical Practice Guidelines. *Hypertension*. 2017, In press.

Fourth Report,[1] they include SBP and DBP values arranged by age, sex, and height (and height percentile). These values are based on auscultatory measurements obtained from ~50 000 children and adolescents. A new feature in these tables is that the BP values are categorized according to the scheme presented in Table 3 as normal (50th percentile), elevated BP (>90th percentile), stage 1 HTN (≥95th percentile), and stage 2 HTN (≥95th percentile + 12 mm Hg). Additionally, actual heights in centimeters and inches are provided.

Unlike the tables in the Fourth Report,[1] the BP values in these tables do not include children and adolescents with overweight and obesity (ie, those with a BMI ≥85th percentile); therefore, they represent normative BP values for normal-weight youth. The decision to create these new tables was based on evidence of the strong association of both overweight and obesity with elevated BP and HTN. Including patients with overweight and obesity in normative BP tables was thought to create bias. The practical effect of this change is that the BP values in Tables 4 and 5 are several millimeters of mercury lower than in the similar tables in the Fourth Report.[1] These tables are based on the same population data excluding participants with overweight and obesity, and the same methods used in the Fourth Report.[1] The methods and results have been published elsewhere.[77] For researchers and others interested in the equations used to calculate the tables' BP values, detailed methodology and the Statistical Analysis System (SAS) code can be found at: http://sites.google.com/a/channing.harvard.edu/bernardrosner/pediatric-blood-press/childhood-blood-pressure.

There are slight differences between the actual percentile-based values in these tables and the cut-points in Table 3, particularly for teenagers ≥13 years of age. Clinicians should understand that the scheme in Table 3 was chosen to align with the new adult guideline and facilitate the management of older adolescents with high BP. The percentile-based values in Tables 4 and 5 are provided to aid researchers and others interested in a more precise classification of BP.

3.2a. Simplified BP Table

This guideline includes a new, simplified table for initial BP screening (see Table 6) based on the 90th percentile BP for age and sex for children at the 5th percentile of height, which gives the values in the table a negative predictive value of >99%.[78] This simplified table is designed as a screening tool only for the identification of children and adolescents who need further evaluation of their BP starting with repeat BP measurements. It should not be used to diagnose elevated BP or HTN by itself. To diagnose elevated BP or HTN, it is important to locate the actual cutoffs in the complete BP tables because the SBP and DBP cutoffs may be as much as 9 mm Hg higher depending on a child's age and length or height. A typical-use case for this simplified table is for nursing staff to quickly identify BP that may need further evaluation by a clinician. For adolescents ≥13 years of age, a threshold of 120/80 mm Hg is used in the simplified table regardless of sex to align with adult guidelines for the detection of elevated BP.

3.3 Definition of HTN in the Neonate and Infant (0–1 Year of Age)

Although a reasonably strict definition of HTN has been developed for older children, it is more difficult to define HTN in neonates given the well-known changes in BP that occur during the first few weeks of life.[79] These BP changes can be significant in preterm infants, in whom BP depends on a variety of factors, including postmenstrual age, birth weight, and maternal conditions.[80] In an attempt to develop a more standardized approach to the HTN definition in preterm and term neonates, Dionne et al[79] compiled available data on neonatal BP and generated a summary table of BP values, including values for the 95th and 99th percentiles for infants from 26 to 44 weeks' postmenstrual age. The authors proposed that by using these values, a similar approach to that used to identify older children with elevated BP can be followed in neonates, even in those who are born preterm.

At present, no alternative data have been developed, and no outcome data are available on the consequences of high BP in this population; thus, it is reasonable to use these compiled BP values in the assessment of elevated BP in newborn infants. Of note, the 1987 "Report of the Second Task Force on Blood Pressure Control in Children" published curves of normative BP values in older infants up to 1 year of age.[81] These normative values should continue to be used given the lack of more contemporary data for this age group.

4. MEASUREMENT OF BP

4.1 BP Measurement Technique

BP in childhood may vary considerably between visits and even during the same visit. There are many potential etiologies for isolated elevated BP in children and adolescents, including such factors as anxiety and recent caffeine intake.[82] BP generally decreases with repeated measurements during a single visit,[83] although the variability may not be large enough to affect BP classification.[84] BP measurements can also vary across visits[64,85]; one study in adolescents found that only 56% of the sample had the same HTN stage on 3 different occasions.[8] Therefore, it is important to obtain multiple measurements over time before diagnosing HTN.

TABLE 4 BP Levels for Boys by Age and Height Percentile

Age (y)	BP Percentile	SBP (mm Hg)							DBP (mm Hg)						
		Height Percentile or Measured Height							Height Percentile or Measured Height						
		5%	10%	25%	50%	75%	90%	95%	5%	10%	25%	50%	75%	90%	95%
1	Height (in)	30.4	30.8	31.6	32.4	33.3	34.1	34.6	30.4	30.8	31.6	32.4	33.3	34.1	34.6
	Height (cm)	77.2	78.3	80.2	82.4	84.6	86.7	87.9	77.2	78.3	80.2	82.4	84.6	86.7	87.9
	50th	85	85	86	86	87	88	88	40	40	40	41	41	42	42
	90th	98	99	99	100	100	101	101	52	52	53	53	54	54	54
	95th	102	102	103	103	104	105	105	54	54	55	55	56	57	57
	95th + 12 mm Hg	114	114	115	115	116	117	117	66	66	67	67	68	69	69
2	Height (in)	33.9	34.4	35.3	36.3	37.3	38.2	38.8	33.9	34.4	35.3	36.3	37.3	38.2	38.8
	Height (cm)	86.1	87.4	89.6	92.1	94.7	97.1	98.5	86.1	87.4	89.6	92.1	94.7	97.1	98.5
	50th	87	87	88	89	89	90	91	43	43	44	44	45	46	46
	90th	100	100	101	102	103	103	104	55	55	56	56	57	58	58
	95th	104	105	105	106	107	107	108	57	58	58	59	60	61	61
	95th + 12 mm Hg	116	117	117	118	119	119	120	69	70	70	71	72	73	73
3	Height (in)	36.4	37	37.9	39	40.1	41.1	41.7	36.4	37	37.9	39	40.1	41.1	41.7
	Height (cm)	92.5	93.9	96.3	99	101.8	104.3	105.8	92.5	93.9	96.3	99	101.8	104.3	105.8
	50th	88	89	89	90	91	92	92	45	46	46	47	48	49	49
	90th	101	102	102	103	104	105	105	58	58	59	59	60	61	61
	95th	106	106	107	107	108	109	109	60	61	61	62	63	64	64
	95th + 12 mm Hg	118	118	119	119	120	121	121	72	73	73	74	75	76	76
4	Height (in)	38.8	39.4	40.5	41.7	42.9	43.9	44.5	38.8	39.4	40.5	41.7	42.9	43.9	44.5
	Height (cm)	98.5	100.2	102.9	105.9	108.9	111.5	113.2	98.5	100.2	102.9	105.9	108.9	111.5	113.2
	50th	90	90	91	92	93	94	94	48	49	49	50	51	52	52
	90th	102	103	104	105	105	106	107	60	61	62	62	63	64	64
	95th	107	107	108	108	109	110	110	63	64	65	66	67	67	68
	95th + 12 mm Hg	119	119	120	120	121	122	122	75	76	77	78	79	79	80
5	Height (in)	41.1	41.8	43.0	44.3	45.5	46.7	47.4	41.1	41.8	43.0	44.3	45.5	46.7	47.4
	Height (cm)	104.4	106.2	109.1	112.4	115.7	118.6	120.3	104.4	106.2	109.1	112.4	115.7	118.6	120.3
	50th	91	92	93	94	95	96	96	51	51	52	53	54	55	55
	90th	103	104	105	106	107	108	108	63	64	65	65	66	67	67
	95th	107	108	109	109	110	111	112	66	67	68	69	70	70	71
	95th + 12 mm Hg	119	120	121	121	122	123	124	78	79	80	81	82	82	83
6	Height (in)	43.4	44.2	45.4	46.8	48.2	49.4	50.2	43.4	44.2	45.4	46.8	48.2	49.4	50.2
	Height (cm)	110.3	112.2	115.3	118.9	122.4	125.6	127.5	110.3	112.2	115.3	118.9	122.4	125.6	127.5
	50th	93	93	94	95	96	97	98	54	54	55	56	57	57	58
	90th	105	105	106	107	109	110	110	66	66	67	68	68	69	69
	95th	108	109	110	111	112	113	114	69	70	70	71	72	72	73
	95th + 12 mm Hg	120	121	122	123	124	125	126	81	82	82	83	84	84	85
7	Height (in)	45.7	46.5	47.8	49.3	50.8	52.1	52.9	45.7	46.5	47.8	49.3	50.8	52.1	52.9
	Height (cm)	116.1	118	121.4	125.1	128.9	132.4	134.5	116.1	118	121.4	125.1	128.9	132.4	134.5
	50th	94	94	95	97	98	98	99	56	56	57	58	58	59	59
	90th	106	107	108	109	110	111	111	68	68	69	70	70	71	71
	95th	110	110	111	112	114	115	116	71	71	72	73	73	74	74
	95th + 12 mm Hg	122	122	123	124	126	127	128	83	83	84	85	85	86	86

TABLE 4 Continued

Age (y)	BP Percentile	SBP (mm Hg)							DBP (mm Hg)						
		Height Percentile or Measured Height							Height Percentile or Measured Height						
		5%	10%	25%	50%	75%	90%	95%	5%	10%	25%	50%	75%	90%	95%
8	Height (in)	47.8	48.6	50	51.6	53.2	54.6	55.5	47.8	48.6	50	51.6	53.2	54.6	55.5
	Height (cm)	121.4	123.5	127	131	135.1	138.8	141	121.4	123.5	127	131	135.1	138.8	141
	50th	95	96	97	98	99	99	100	57	57	58	59	59	60	60
	90th	107	108	109	110	111	112	112	69	70	70	71	72	72	73
	95th	111	112	112	114	115	116	117	72	73	73	74	75	75	75
	95th + 12 mm Hg	123	124	124	126	127	128	129	84	85	85	86	87	87	87
9	Height (in)	49.6	50.5	52	53.7	55.4	56.9	57.9	49.6	50.5	52	53.7	55.4	56.9	57.9
	Height (cm)	126	128.3	132.1	136.3	140.7	144.7	147.1	126	128.3	132.1	136.3	140.7	144.7	147.1
	50th	96	97	98	99	100	101	101	57	58	59	60	61	62	62
	90th	107	108	109	110	112	113	114	70	71	72	73	74	74	74
	95th	112	112	113	115	116	118	119	74	74	75	76	76	77	77
	95th + 12 mm Hg	124	124	125	127	128	130	131	86	86	87	88	88	89	89
10	Height (in)	51.3	52.2	53.8	55.6	57.4	59.1	60.1	51.3	52.2	53.8	55.6	57.4	59.1	60.1
	Height (cm)	130.2	132.7	136.7	141.3	145.9	150.1	152.7	130.2	132.7	136.7	141.3	145.9	150.1	152.7
	50th	97	98	99	100	101	102	103	59	60	61	62	63	63	64
	90th	108	109	111	112	113	115	116	72	73	74	74	75	75	76
	95th	112	113	114	116	118	120	121	76	76	77	77	78	78	78
	95th + 12 mm Hg	124	125	126	128	130	132	133	88	88	89	89	90	90	90
11	Height (in)	53	54	55.7	57.6	59.6	61.3	62.4	53	54	55.7	57.6	59.6	61.3	62.4
	Height (cm)	134.7	137.3	141.5	146.4	151.3	155.8	158.6	134.7	137.3	141.5	146.4	151.3	155.8	158.6
	50th	99	99	101	102	103	104	106	61	61	62	63	63	63	63
	90th	110	111	112	114	116	117	118	74	74	75	75	75	76	76
	95th	114	114	116	118	120	123	124	77	78	78	78	78	78	78
	95th + 12 mm Hg	126	126	128	130	132	135	136	89	90	90	90	90	90	90
12	Height (in)	55.2	56.3	58.1	60.1	62.2	64	65.2	55.2	56.3	58.1	60.1	62.2	64	65.2
	Height (cm)	140.3	143	147.5	152.7	157.9	162.6	165.5	140.3	143	147.5	152.7	157.9	162.6	165.5
	50th	101	101	102	104	106	108	109	61	62	62	62	62	63	63
	90th	113	114	115	117	119	121	122	75	75	75	75	75	76	76
	95th	116	117	118	121	124	126	128	78	78	78	78	78	79	79
	95th + 12 mm Hg	128	129	130	133	136	138	140	90	90	90	90	90	91	91
13	Height (in)	57.9	59.1	61	63.1	65.2	67.1	68.3	57.9	59.1	61	63.1	65.2	67.1	68.3
	Height (cm)	147	150	154.9	160.3	165.7	170.5	173.4	147	150	154.9	160.3	165.7	170.5	173.4
	50th	103	104	105	108	110	111	112	61	60	61	62	63	64	65
	90th	115	116	118	121	124	126	126	74	74	74	75	76	77	77
	95th	119	120	122	125	128	130	131	78	78	78	78	80	81	81
	95th + 12 mm Hg	131	132	134	137	140	142	143	90	90	90	90	92	93	93
14	Height (in)	60.6	61.8	63.8	65.9	68.0	69.8	70.9	60.6	61.8	63.8	65.9	68.0	69.8	70.9
	Height (cm)	153.8	156.9	162	167.5	172.7	177.4	180.1	153.8	156.9	162	167.5	172.7	177.4	180.1
	50th	105	106	109	111	112	113	113	60	60	62	64	65	66	67
	90th	119	120	123	126	127	128	129	74	74	75	77	78	79	80
	95th	123	125	127	130	132	133	134	77	78	79	81	82	83	84
	95th + 12 mm Hg	135	137	139	142	144	145	146	89	90	91	93	94	95	96

TABLE 4 Continued

Age (y)	BP Percentile	SBP (mm Hg)							DBP (mm Hg)						
		Height Percentile or Measured Height							Height Percentile or Measured Height						
		5%	10%	25%	50%	75%	90%	95%	5%	10%	25%	50%	75%	90%	95%
15	Height (in)	62.6	63.8	65.7	67.8	69.8	71.5	72.5	62.6	63.8	65.7	67.8	69.8	71.5	72.5
	Height (cm)	159	162	166.9	172.2	177.2	181.6	184.2	159	162	166.9	172.2	177.2	181.6	184.2
	50th	108	110	112	113	114	114	114	61	62	64	65	66	67	68
	90th	123	124	126	128	129	130	130	75	76	78	79	80	81	81
	95th	127	129	131	132	134	135	135	78	79	81	83	84	85	85
	95th + 12 mm Hg	139	141	143	144	146	147	147	90	91	93	95	96	97	97
16	Height (in)	63.8	64.9	66.8	68.8	70.7	72.4	73.4	63.8	64.9	66.8	68.8	70.7	72.4	73.4
	Height (cm)	162.1	165	169.6	174.6	179.5	183.8	186.4	162.1	165	169.6	174.6	179.5	183.8	186.4
	50th	111	112	114	115	115	116	116	63	64	66	67	68	69	69
	90th	126	127	128	129	131	131	132	77	78	79	80	81	82	82
	95th	130	131	133	134	135	136	137	80	81	83	84	85	86	86
	95th + 12 mm Hg	142	143	145	146	147	148	149	92	93	95	96	97	98	98
17	Height (in)	64.5	65.5	67.3	69.2	71.1	72.8	73.8	64.5	65.5	67.3	69.2	71.1	72.8	73.8
	Height (cm)	163.8	166.5	170.9	175.8	180.7	184.9	187.5	163.8	166.5	170.9	175.8	180.7	184.9	187.5
	50th	114	115	116	117	117	118	118	65	66	67	68	69	70	70
	90th	128	129	130	131	132	133	134	78	79	80	81	82	82	83
	95th	132	133	134	135	137	138	138	81	82	84	85	86	86	87
	95th + 12 mm Hg	144	145	146	147	149	150	150	93	94	96	97	98	98	99

Use percentile values to stage BP readings according to the scheme in Table 3 (elevated BP: ≥90th percentile; stage 1 HTN: ≥95th percentile; and stage 2 HTN: ≥95th percentile + 12 mm Hg). The 50th, 90th, and 95th percentiles were derived by using quantile regression on the basis of normal-weight children (BMI <85th percentile).[77]

TABLE 5 BP Levels for Girls by Age and Height Percentile

Age (y)	BP Percentile	SBP (mm Hg)							DBP (mm Hg)						
		Height Percentile or Measured Height							Height Percentile or Measured Height						
		5%	10%	25%	50%	75%	90%	95%	5%	10%	25%	50%	75%	90%	95%
1	Height (in)	29.7	30.2	30.9	31.8	32.7	33.4	33.9	29.7	30.2	30.9	31.8	32.7	33.4	33.9
	Height (cm)	75.4	76.6	78.6	80.8	83	84.9	86.1	75.4	76.6	78.6	80.8	83	84.9	86.1
	50th	84	85	86	86	87	88	88	41	42	42	43	44	45	46
	90th	98	99	99	100	101	102	102	54	55	56	56	57	58	58
	95th	101	102	102	103	104	105	105	59	59	60	60	61	62	62
	95th + 12 mm Hg	113	114	114	115	116	117	117	71	71	72	72	73	74	74
2	Height (in)	33.4	34	34.9	35.9	36.9	37.8	38.4	33.4	34	34.9	35.9	36.9	37.8	38.4
	Height (cm)	84.9	86.3	88.6	91.1	93.7	96	97.4	84.9	86.3	88.6	91.1	93.7	96	97.4
	50th	87	87	88	89	90	91	91	45	46	47	48	49	50	51
	90th	101	101	102	103	104	105	106	58	58	59	60	61	62	62
	95th	104	105	106	106	107	108	109	62	63	63	64	65	66	66
	95th + 12 mm Hg	116	117	118	118	119	120	121	74	75	75	76	77	78	78
3	Height (in)	35.8	36.4	37.3	38.4	39.6	40.6	41.2	35.8	36.4	37.3	38.4	39.6	40.6	41.2
	Height (cm)	91	92.4	94.9	97.6	100.5	103.1	104.6	91	92.4	94.9	97.6	100.5	103.1	104.6
	50th	88	89	89	90	91	92	93	48	48	49	50	51	53	53
	90th	102	103	104	104	105	106	107	60	61	61	62	63	64	65
	95th	106	106	107	108	109	110	110	64	65	65	66	67	68	69
	95th + 12 mm Hg	118	118	119	120	121	122	122	76	77	77	78	79	80	81
4	Height (in)	38.3	38.9	39.9	41.1	42.4	43.5	44.2	38.3	38.9	39.9	41.1	42.4	43.5	44.2
	Height (cm)	97.2	98.8	101.4	104.5	107.6	110.5	112.2	97.2	98.8	101.4	104.5	107.6	110.5	112.2
	50th	89	90	91	92	93	94	94	50	51	51	53	54	55	55
	90th	103	104	105	106	107	108	108	62	63	64	65	66	67	67
	95th	107	108	109	109	110	111	112	66	67	68	69	70	70	71
	95th + 12 mm Hg	119	120	121	121	122	123	124	78	79	80	81	82	82	83
5	Height (in)	40.8	41.5	42.6	43.9	45.2	46.5	47.3	40.8	41.5	42.6	43.9	45.2	46.5	47.3
	Height (cm)	103.6	105.3	108.2	111.5	114.9	118.1	120	103.6	105.3	108.2	111.5	114.9	118.1	120
	50th	90	91	92	93	94	95	96	52	52	53	55	56	57	57
	90th	104	105	106	107	108	109	110	64	65	66	67	68	69	70
	95th	108	109	109	110	111	112	113	68	69	70	71	72	73	73
	95th + 12 mm Hg	120	121	121	122	123	124	125	80	81	82	83	84	85	85
6	Height (in)	43.3	44	45.2	46.6	48.1	49.4	50.3	43.3	44	45.2	46.6	48.1	49.4	50.3
	Height (cm)	110	111.8	114.9	118.4	122.1	125.6	127.7	110	111.8	114.9	118.4	122.1	125.6	127.7
	50th	92	92	93	94	96	97	97	54	54	55	56	57	58	59
	90th	105	106	107	108	109	110	111	67	67	68	69	70	71	71
	95th	109	109	110	111	112	113	114	70	71	72	72	73	74	74
	95th + 12 mm Hg	121	121	122	123	124	125	126	82	83	84	84	85	86	86
7	Height (in)	45.6	46.4	47.7	49.2	50.7	52.1	53	45.6	46.4	47.7	49.2	50.7	52.1	53
	Height (cm)	115.9	117.8	121.1	124.9	128.8	132.5	134.7	115.9	117.8	121.1	124.9	128.8	132.5	134.7
	50th	92	93	94	95	97	98	99	55	55	56	57	58	59	60
	90th	106	106	107	109	110	111	112	68	68	69	70	71	72	72
	95th	109	110	111	112	113	114	115	72	72	73	73	74	74	75
	95th + 12 mm Hg	121	122	123	124	125	126	127	84	84	85	85	86	86	87

TABLE 5 Continued

Age (y)	BP Percentile	SBP (mm Hg)							DBP (mm Hg)						
		Height Percentile or Measured Height							Height Percentile or Measured Height						
		5%	10%	25%	50%	75%	90%	95%	5%	10%	25%	50%	75%	90%	95%
8	Height (in)	47.6	48.4	49.8	51.4	53	54.5	55.5	47.6	48.4	49.8	51.4	53	54.5	55.5
	Height (cm)	121	123	126.5	130.6	134.7	138.5	140.9	121	123	126.5	130.6	134.7	138.5	140.9
	50th	93	94	95	97	98	99	100	56	56	57	59	60	61	61
	90th	107	107	108	110	111	112	113	69	70	71	72	72	73	73
	95th	110	111	112	113	115	116	117	72	73	74	74	75	75	75
	95th + 12 mm Hg	122	123	124	125	127	128	129	84	85	86	86	87	87	87
9	Height (in)	49.3	50.2	51.7	53.4	55.1	56.7	57.7	49.3	50.2	51.7	53.4	55.1	56.7	57.7
	Height (cm)	125.3	127.6	131.3	135.6	140.1	144.1	146.6	125.3	127.6	131.3	135.6	140.1	144.1	146.6
	50th	95	95	97	98	99	100	101	57	58	59	60	60	61	61
	90th	108	108	109	111	112	113	114	71	71	72	73	73	73	73
	95th	112	112	113	114	116	117	118	74	74	75	75	75	75	75
	95th + 12 mm Hg	124	124	125	126	128	129	130	86	86	87	87	87	87	87
10	Height (in)	51.1	52	53.7	55.5	57.4	59.1	60.2	51.1	52	53.7	55.5	57.4	59.1	60.2
	Height (cm)	129.7	132.2	136.3	141	145.8	150.2	152.8	129.7	132.2	136.3	141	145.8	150.2	152.8
	50th	96	97	98	99	101	102	103	58	59	59	60	61	61	62
	90th	109	110	111	112	113	115	116	72	73	73	73	73	73	73
	95th	113	114	114	116	117	119	120	75	75	76	76	76	76	76
	95th + 12 mm Hg	125	126	126	128	129	131	132	87	87	88	88	88	88	88
11	Height (in)	53.4	54.5	56.2	58.2	60.2	61.9	63	53.4	54.5	56.2	58.2	60.2	61.9	63
	Height (cm)	135.6	138.3	142.8	147.8	152.8	157.3	160	135.6	138.3	142.8	147.8	152.8	157.3	160
	50th	98	99	101	102	104	105	106	60	60	60	61	62	63	64
	90th	111	112	113	114	116	118	120	74	74	74	74	74	75	75
	95th	115	116	117	118	120	123	124	76	77	77	77	77	77	77
	95th + 12 mm Hg	127	128	129	130	132	135	136	88	89	89	89	89	89	89
12	Height (in)	56.2	57.3	59	60.9	62.8	64.5	65.5	56.2	57.3	59	60.9	62.8	64.5	65.5
	Height (cm)	142.8	145.5	149.9	154.8	159.6	163.8	166.4	142.8	145.5	149.9	154.8	159.6	163.8	166.4
	50th	102	102	104	105	107	108	108	61	61	61	62	64	65	65
	90th	114	115	116	118	120	122	122	75	75	75	75	76	76	76
	95th	118	119	120	122	124	125	126	78	78	78	78	79	79	79
	95th + 12 mm Hg	130	131	132	134	136	137	138	90	90	90	90	91	91	91
13	Height (in)	58.3	59.3	60.9	62.7	64.5	66.1	67	58.3	59.3	60.9	62.7	64.5	66.1	67
	Height (cm)	148.1	150.6	154.7	159.2	163.7	167.8	170.2	148.1	150.6	154.7	159.2	163.7	167.8	170.2
	50th	104	105	106	107	108	108	109	62	62	63	64	65	65	66
	90th	116	117	119	121	122	123	123	75	75	75	76	76	76	76
	95th	121	122	123	124	126	126	127	79	79	79	79	80	80	81
	95th + 12 mm Hg	133	134	135	136	138	138	139	91	91	91	91	92	92	93
14	Height (in)	59.3	60.2	61.8	63.5	65.2	66.8	67.7	59.3	60.2	61.8	63.5	65.2	66.8	67.7
	Height (cm)	150.6	153	156.9	161.3	165.7	169.7	172.1	150.6	153	156.9	161.3	165.7	169.7	172.1
	50th	105	106	107	108	109	109	109	63	63	64	65	66	66	66
	90th	118	118	120	122	123	123	123	76	76	76	76	77	77	77
	95th	123	123	124	125	126	127	127	80	80	80	80	81	81	82
	95th + 12 mm Hg	135	135	136	137	138	139	139	92	92	92	92	93	93	94

TABLE 5 Continued

Age (y)	BP Percentile	SBP (mm Hg)							DBP (mm Hg)						
		Height Percentile or Measured Height							Height Percentile or Measured Height						
		5%	10%	25%	50%	75%	90%	95%	5%	10%	25%	50%	75%	90%	95%
15	Height (in)	59.7	60.6	62.2	63.9	65.6	67.2	68.1	59.7	60.6	62.2	63.9	65.6	67.2	68.1
	Height (cm)	151.7	154	157.9	162.3	166.7	170.6	173	151.7	154	157.9	162.3	166.7	170.6	173
	50th	105	106	107	108	109	109	109	64	64	64	65	66	67	67
	90th	118	119	121	122	123	123	124	76	76	76	77	77	78	78
	95th	124	124	125	126	127	127	128	80	80	80	81	82	82	82
	95th + 12 mm Hg	136	136	137	138	139	139	140	92	92	92	93	94	94	94
16	Height (in)	59.9	60.8	62.4	64.1	65.8	67.3	68.3	59.9	60.8	62.4	64.1	65.8	67.3	68.3
	Height (cm)	152.1	154.5	158.4	162.8	167.1	171.1	173.4	152.1	154.5	158.4	162.8	167.1	171.1	173.4
	50th	106	107	108	109	109	110	110	64	64	65	66	66	67	67
	90th	119	120	122	123	124	124	124	76	76	76	77	78	78	78
	95th	124	125	125	127	127	128	128	80	80	80	81	82	82	82
	95th + 12 mm Hg	136	137	137	139	139	140	140	92	92	92	93	94	94	94
17	Height (in)	60.0	60.9	62.5	64.2	65.9	67.4	68.4	60.0	60.9	62.5	64.2	65.9	67.4	68.4
	Height (cm)	152.4	154.7	158.7	163.0	167.4	171.3	173.7	152.4	154.7	158.7	163.0	167.4	171.3	173.7
	50th	107	108	109	110	110	110	111	64	64	65	66	66	66	67
	90th	120	121	123	124	124	125	125	76	76	77	77	78	78	78
	95th	125	125	126	127	128	128	128	80	80	80	81	82	82	82
	95th + 12 mm Hg	137	137	138	139	140	140	140	92	92	92	93	94	94	94

Use percentile values to stage BP readings according to the scheme in Table 3 (elevated BP: ≥90th percentile; stage 1 HTN: ≥95th percentile; and stage 2 HTN: ≥95th percentile + 12 mm Hg). The 50th, 90th, and 95th percentiles were derived by using quantile regression on the basis of normal-weight children (BMI <85th percentile).[77]

The initial BP measurement may be oscillometric (on a calibrated machine that has been validated for use in the pediatric population) or auscultatory (by using a mercury or aneroid sphygmomanometer[86,87]). (Validation status for oscillometric BP devices, including whether they are validated in the pediatric age group, can be checked at www.dableducational.org.) BP should be measured in the right arm by using standard measurement practices unless the child has atypical aortic arch anatomy, such as right aortic arch and aortic coarctation or left aortic arch with aberrant right subclavian artery (see Table 7). Other important aspects of proper BP measurement are illustrated in an AAP video available at http://youtu.be/JLzkNBpqwi0. Care should be taken that providers follow an accurate and consistent measurement technique.[88,89]

An appropriately sized cuff should be used for accurate BP measurement.[83] Researchers in 3 studies in the United Kingdom and 1 in Brazil documented the lack of availability of an appropriately sized cuff in both the inpatient and outpatient settings.[91–94] Pediatric offices should have access to a wide range of cuff sizes, including a thigh cuff for use in children and adolescents with severe obesity. For children in whom the appropriate cuff size is difficult to determine, the midarm circumference (measured as the midpoint between the acromion of the scapula and olecranon of the elbow, with the shoulder in a neutral position and the elbow flexed to 90°[86,95,96]) should be obtained for an accurate determination of the correct cuff size (see Fig 2 and Table 7).[95]

If the initial BP is elevated (≥90th percentile), providers should perform 2 additional oscillometric or auscultatory BP measurements at the same visit and average them. If using auscultation, this averaged measurement is used to determine the child's BP category (ie, normal,

TABLE 6 Screening BP Values Requiring Further Evaluation

Age, y	BP, mm Hg			
	Boys		Girls	
	Systolic	DBP	Systolic	DBP
1	98	52	98	54
2	100	55	101	58
3	101	58	102	60
4	102	60	103	62
5	103	63	104	64
6	105	66	105	67
7	106	68	106	68
8	107	69	107	69
9	107	70	108	71
10	108	72	109	72
11	110	74	111	74
12	113	75	114	75
≥13	120	80	120	80

elevated BP, stage 1 HTN, or stage 2 HTN). If the averaged oscillometric reading is ≥90th percentile, 2 auscultatory measurements should be taken and averaged to define the BP category (see Fig 3).

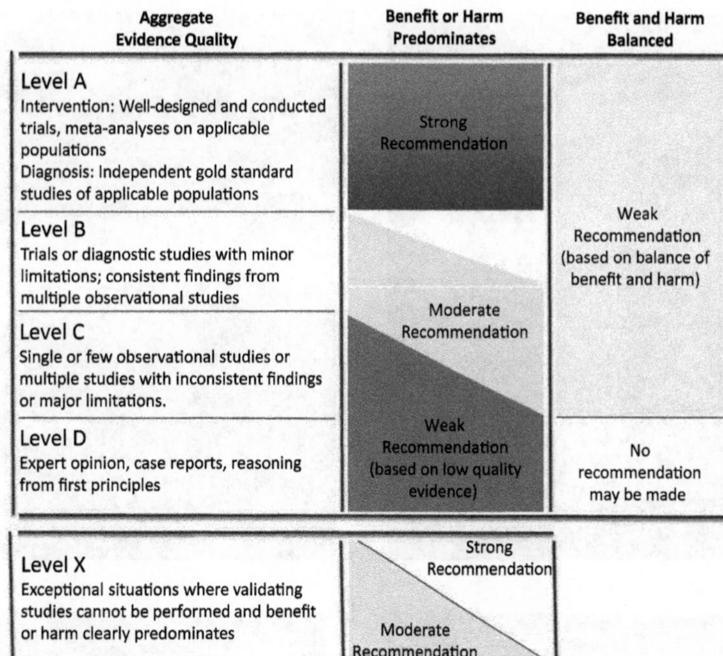

FIGURE 1
AAP grading matrix.

4.1a Measurement of BP in the Neonate

Multiple methods are available for the measurement of BP in hospitalized neonates, including direct intra-arterial measurements using indwelling catheters as well as indirect measurements using the oscillometric technique. In the office, however, the oscillometric technique typically is used at least until the infant is able to cooperate with manual BP determination (which also depends on the ability of the individual measuring the BP to obtain auscultatory BP in infants and toddlers). Normative values for neonatal and infant BP have generally been determined in the right upper arm with the infant supine, and a similar approach should be followed in the outpatient setting.

As with older children, proper cuff size is important in obtaining accurate BP readings in neonates. The cuff bladder length should encircle 80% to 100% of the arm circumference; a cuff bladder with a width-to-arm circumference ratio of 0.45 to 0.55 is recommended.[79,97,98] Offices that will be obtaining BP measurements in neonates need to have a variety of cuff sizes available. In addition, the oscillometric device used should be validated in neonates and programmed to have an initial inflation value appropriate for infants (generally ≤120 mm Hg). Auscultation becomes technically feasible once the infant's upper arm is large enough for the smallest cuff available for auscultatory devices. Measurements are best taken when the infant is in a calm state; multiple readings may be needed if the first

TABLE 7 Best BP Measurement Practices

1. The child should be seated in a quiet room for 3–5 min before measurement, with the back supported and feet uncrossed on the floor.
2. BP should be measured in the right arm for consistency, for comparison with standard tables, and to avoid a falsely low reading from the left arm in the case of coarctation of the aorta. The arm should be at heart level,[90] supported, and uncovered above the cuff. The patient and observer should not speak while the measurement is being taken.
3. The correct cuff size should be used. The bladder length should be 80%–100% of the circumference of the arm, and the width should be at least 40%.
4. For an auscultatory BP, the bell of the stethoscope should be placed over the brachial artery in the antecubital fossa, and the lower end of the cuff should be 2–3 cm above the antecubital fossa. The cuff should be inflated to 20–30 mm Hg above the point at which the radial pulse disappears. Overinflation should be avoided. The cuff should be deflated at a rate of 2–3 mm Hg per second. The first (phase I Korotkoff) and last (phase V Korotkoff) audible sounds should be taken as SBP and DBP. If the Korotkoff sounds are heard to 0 mm Hg, the point at which the sound is muffled (phase IV Korotkoff) should be taken as the DBP, or the measurement repeated with less pressure applied over the brachial artery. The measurement should be read to the nearest 2 mm Hg.
5. To measure BP in the legs, the patient should be in the prone position, if possible. An appropriately sized cuff should be placed midthigh and the stethoscope placed over the popliteal artery. The SBP in the legs is usually 10%–20% higher than the brachial artery pressure.

Adapted from Pickering TG, Hall JE, Appel LJ, et al. Recommendations for blood pressure measurement in humans and experimental animals: part 1: blood pressure measurement in humans: a statement for professionals from the Subcommittee of Professional and Public Education of the American Heart Association Council on High Blood Pressure Research. *Circulation*. 2005;111(5):697–716.

A

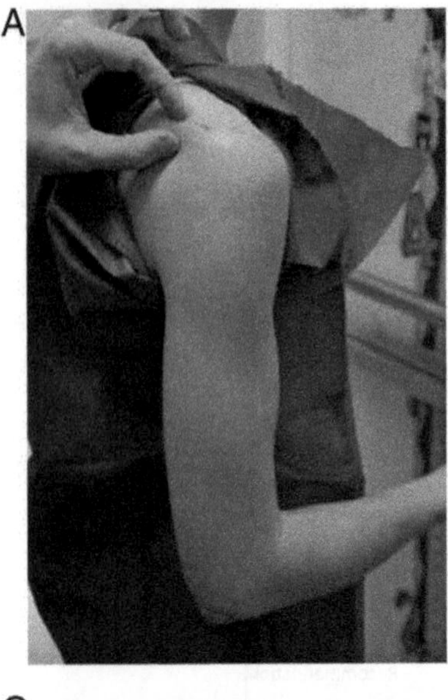

B

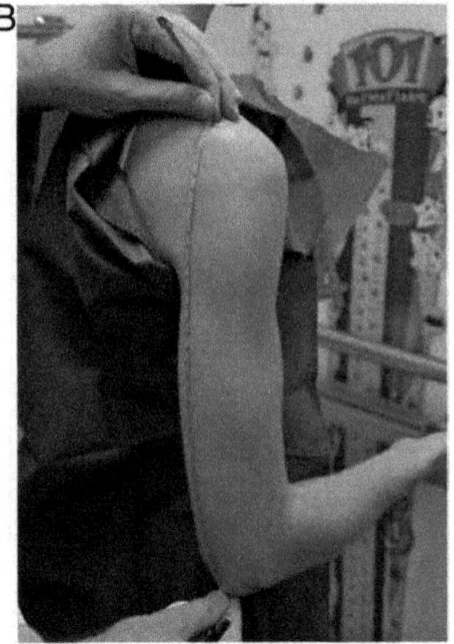

C

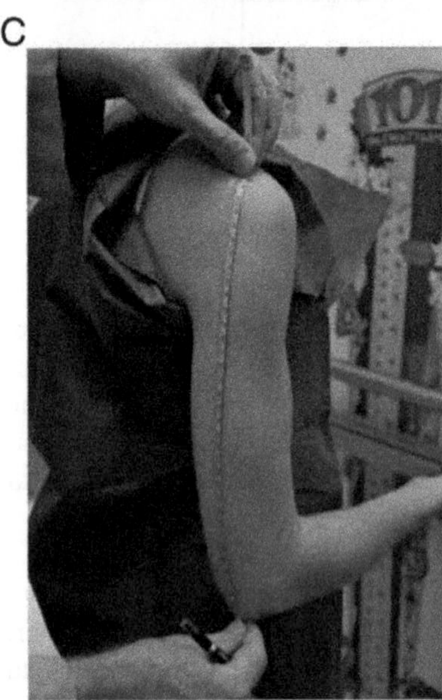

D

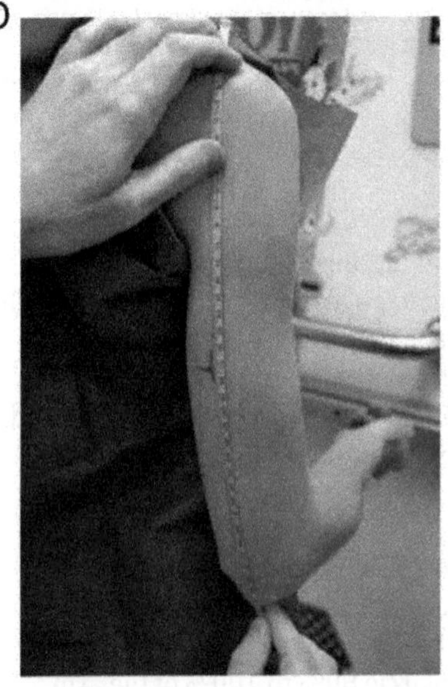

FIGURE 2
Determination of proper BP cuff size.[95] A, Marking spine extending from acromion process. B, Correct tape placement for upper arm length. C, Incorrect tape placement for upper arm length. D, Marking upper arm length midpoint.

reading is elevated, similar to the technique recommended for older children.[99,100]

4.2 BP Measurement Frequency

It remains unclear what age is optimal to begin routine BP measurement in children, although available data suggest that prevention and intervention efforts should begin at a young age.[10,60,101–106] The subcommittee believes that the recommendation to measure BP in the ambulatory setting beginning at 3 years of age should remain unchanged.[1] For otherwise healthy children, however, BP need only be measured annually rather than during every health care encounter.

Some children should have BP measured at every health encounter, specifically those with obesity (BMI ≥95 percentile),[5,27,107–109] renal disease,[46] diabetes,[110,111] aortic arch obstruction or coarctation, or those who are taking medications known to increase BP (see Table 8 and the "Secondary Causes: Medication-related" section of this guideline).[112,113]

Children younger than 3 years should have BP measurements taken at well-child care visits if they are at increased risk for developing HTN (see Table 9).[1]

Key Action Statement 1

BP should be measured annually in children and adolescents ≥3 years of age (grade C, moderate recommendation).

Key Action Statement 2

BP should be checked in all children and adolescents ≥3 years of age at every health care encounter if they have obesity, are taking medications known to increase BP, have renal disease, a history of aortic arch obstruction or coarctation, or diabetes (see Table 9) (grade C, moderate recommendation).

4.3 Patient Management on the Basis of Office BP

4.3a Normal BP

If BP is normal or normalizes after repeat readings (ie, BP <90th percentile), then no additional action is needed. Practitioners should measure the BP at the next routine well-child care visit.

4.3b Elevated BP

1. If the BP reading is at the elevated BP level (Table 3), lifestyle interventions should be recommended (ie, healthy diet, sleep, and physical activity); the measurement should be repeated in 6 months by auscultation. Nutrition and/or weight management referral should be considered as appropriate;
2. If BP remains at the elevated BP level after 6 months, upper and lower extremity BP should be checked (right arm, left arm, and 1 leg), lifestyle counseling should be repeated, and BP should be

Key Action Statement 1. BP should be measured annually in children and adolescents ≥3 years of age (grade C, moderate recommendation).

Aggregate Evidence Quality	Grade C
Benefits	Early detection of asymptomatic HTN; prevention of short- and long-term HTN-related morbidity
Risks, harm, cost	Overtesting, misclassification, unnecessary treatment, discomfort from BP measurement procedure, time involved in measuring BP
Benefit–harm assessment	Benefit of annual BP measurement exceeds potential harm
Intentional vagueness	None
Role of patient preferences	Increased visit time, discomfort of cuff
Exclusions	None
Strength	Moderate recommendation
Key references	10,60,102,103

Key Action Statement 2. BP should be checked in all children and adolescents ≥3 years of age at every health care encounter if they have obesity, are taking medications known to increase BP, have renal disease, a history of aortic arch obstruction or coarctation, or diabetes (see Table 9) (grade C, moderate recommendation).

Aggregate Evidence Quality	Grade C
Benefits	Early detection of HTN and prevention of CV morbidity in predisposed children and adolescents
Risks, harm, cost	Time for and difficulty of conducting measurements
Benefit–harm assessment	Benefits exceed harm
Intentional vagueness	Frequency of evaluation
Role of patient preferences	Increased visit time, discomfort of cuff
Exclusions	Children and adolescents who are not at increased risk for HTN
Strength	Moderate recommendation
Key references	27,46,107,110–112

rechecked in 6 months (ie, at the next well-child care visit) by auscultation;

3. If BP continues at the elevated BP level after 12 months (eg, after 3 auscultatory measurements), ABPM should be ordered (if available), and diagnostic evaluation should be conducted (see Table 10 for a list of screening tests and the populations in which they should be performed). Consider subspecialty referral (ie, cardiology or nephrology) (see Table 11); and
4. If BP normalizes at any point, return to annual BP screening at well-child care visits.

4.3c Stage 1 HTN

1. If the BP reading is at the stage 1 HTN level (Table 3) and the patient is asymptomatic, provide lifestyle counseling and recheck the BP in 1 to 2 weeks by auscultation;
2. If the BP reading is still at the stage 1 level, upper and lower extremity BP should be checked (right arm, left arm, and 1 leg), and BP should be rechecked in 3 months by auscultation. Nutrition and/or weight management referral should be considered as appropriate; and
3. If BP continues to be at the stage 1 HTN level after 3 visits, ABPM should be ordered (if available), diagnostic evaluation should be conducted, and treatment should be initiated. Subspecialty referral should be considered (see Table 11).

4.3d Stage 2 HTN

1. If the BP reading is at the stage 2 HTN level (Table 3), upper and lower extremity BP should be checked (right arm, left arm, and 1 leg), lifestyle recommendations given, and the BP measurement should be repeated within 1 week. Alternatively, the patient could be referred to subspecialty care within 1 week;
2. If the BP reading is still at the stage 2 HTN level when repeated, then diagnostic evaluation, including ABPM, should be conducted and treatment should be initiated, or the patient should

TABLE 8 Common Pharmacologic Agents Associated With Elevated BP in Children

Over-the-counter drugs	Decongestants
	Caffeine
	Nonsteroidal anti-inflammatory drugs
	Alternative therapies, herbal and nutritional supplements
Prescription drugs	Stimulants for attention-deficit/hyperactivity disorder
	Hormonal contraception
	Steroids
	Tricyclic antidepressants
Illicit drugs	Amphetamines
	Cocaine

Adapted from the Fourth Report.[1]

TABLE 9 Conditions Under Which Children Younger Than 3 Years Should Have BP Measured

History of prematurity <32 week's gestation or small for gestational age, very low birth weight, other neonatal complications requiring intensive care, umbilical artery line
Congenital heart disease (repaired or unrepaired)
Recurrent urinary tract infections, hematuria, or proteinuria
Known renal disease or urologic malformations
Family history of congenital renal disease
Solid-organ transplant
Malignancy or bone marrow transplant
Treatment with drugs known to raise BP
Other systemic illnesses associated with HTN (neurofibromatosis, tuberous sclerosis, sickle cell disease,[114] etc)
Evidence of elevated intracranial pressure

Adapted from Table 3 in the Fourth Report.[1]

Key Action Statement 3. Trained health care professionals in the office setting should make a diagnosis of HTN if a child or adolescent has auscultatory-confirmed BP readings ≥95th percentile on 3 different visits (grade C, moderate recommendation).

Aggregate Evidence Quality	Grade C
Benefits	Early detection of HTN; prevention of CV morbidity in predisposed children and adolescents; identification of secondary causes of HTN
Risks, harm, cost	Overtesting, misclassification, unnecessary treatment, discomfort from BP measurement, time involved in taking BP
Benefit–harm assessment	Benefits of repeated BP measurement exceeds potential harm
Intentional vagueness	None
Role of patient preferences	Families may have varying levels of concern about elevated BP readings and may request evaluation on a different time line
Exclusions	None
Strength	Moderate recommendation
Key references	8,84,85

be referred to subspecialty care within 1 week (see Table 11); and

3. If the BP reading is at the stage 2 HTN level and the patient is symptomatic, or the BP is >30 mm Hg above the 95th percentile (or >180/120 mm Hg in an adolescent), refer to an immediate source of care, such as an emergency department (ED).

Key Action Statement 3

Trained health care professionals in the office setting should make a diagnosis of HTN if a child or adolescent has auscultatory-confirmed BP readings ≥95th percentile on 3 different visits (grade C, moderate recommendation).

4.4 Use of Electronic Health Records

Studies have demonstrated that primary care providers frequently fail to measure BP and often underdiagnose HTN.[85,115,116] One analysis using nationally representative survey data found that providers measured BP at only 67% of preventive visits for children 3 to 18 years of age. Older children and children with overweight or obesity were more likely to be screened.[117] In a large cohort study of 14 187 children, 507 patients met the criteria for HTN, but only 131 (26%) had the diagnosis documented in their electronic health records (EHRs). Elevated BP was only recognized in 11% of cases.[7]

It is likely that the low rates of screening and diagnosis of pediatric HTN are related, at least in part, to the need to use detailed reference tables incorporating age, sex, and height to classify BP levels.[118] Studies have shown that using health information technology can increase adherence to clinical guidelines and improve practitioner performance.[119–121] In fact, applying decision support in conjunction with an EHR in adult populations has also been associated with improved BP screening, recognition, medication prescribing, and control; pediatric data are limited, however.[122–125] Some studies failed to show improvement in BP screening or control,[122,126] but given the inherent complexity in the interpretation of pediatric BP measurements, EHRs should be designed to flag abnormal values both at the time of measurement and on entry into the EHR.

Key Action Statement 4

Organizations with EHRs used in an office setting should consider including flags for abnormal BP values both when the values are being entered and when they are being viewed (grade C, weak recommendation).

Key Action Statement 4. Organizations with EHRs used in an office setting should consider including flags for abnormal BP values both when the values are being entered and when they are being viewed (grade C, weak recommendation).

Aggregate Evidence Quality	Grade C
Benefits	Improved rate of screening and recognition of elevated BP
Risks, harm, cost	Cost of EHR development, alert fatigue
Benefit–harm assessment	Benefit of EHR flagging of elevated BP outweighs harm from development cost and potential for alert fatigue
Intentional vagueness	None
Role of patient preferences	None
Exclusions	None
Strength	Weak recommendation (because of a lack of pediatric data)
Key references	7,117,120,125

4.5 Oscillometric Versus Auscultatory (Manual) BP Measurement

Although pediatric normative BP data are based on auscultatory measurements, oscillometric BP devices have become commonplace in health care settings.[127] Ease of use, a lack of digit preference, and automation are all perceived benefits of using oscillometric devices. Unlike auscultatory measurement, however, oscillometric devices measure the oscillations transmitted from disrupted arterial flow by using the cuff as a transducer to determine mean arterial pressure (MAP). Rather than directly measuring any pressure that correlates to SBP or DBP, the device uses a proprietary algorithm to calculate these values from the directly measured MAP.[127] Because the algorithms vary for different brands of oscillometric devices, there is no standard oscillometric BP.[128]

Researchers in several studies have evaluated the accuracy of oscillometric devices[127,129–134] and compared auscultatory and

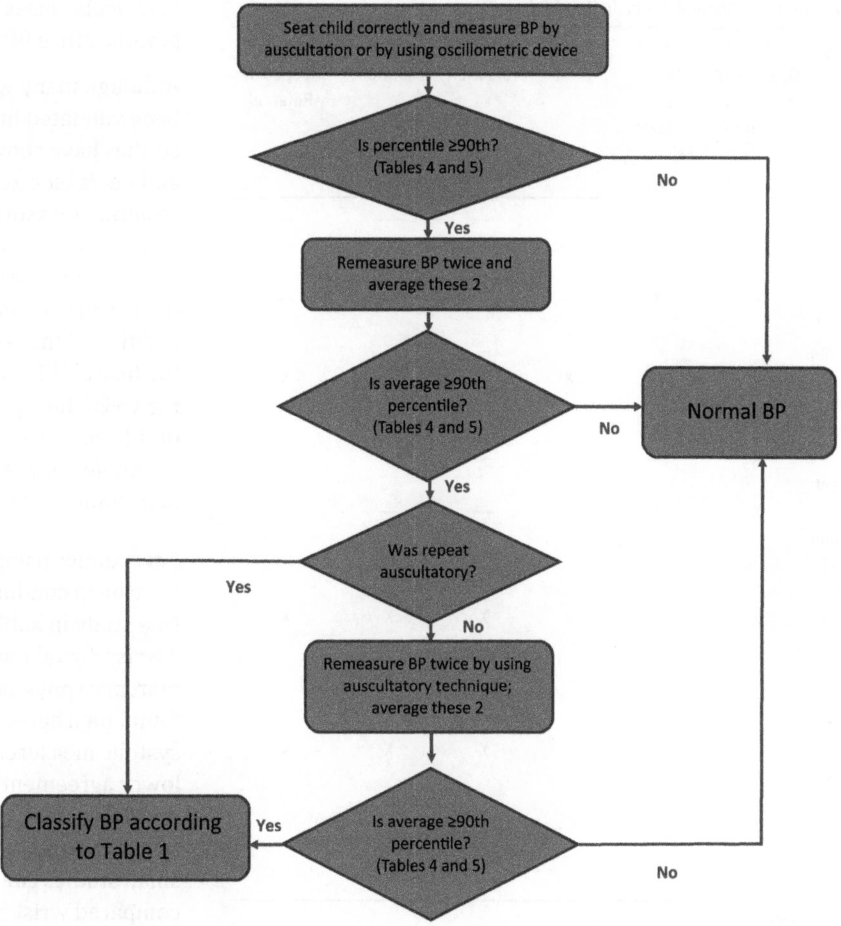

FIGURE 3
Modified BP measurement algorithm.

oscillometric readings' ability to predict target organ damage.[135] These studies demonstrated that oscillometric devices systematically overestimate SBP and DBP compared with values obtained by auscultation.[129,133] BP status potentially can be misclassified because of the different values obtained by these 2 methods, which may be magnified in the office setting.[86,88,129] Target organ damage (such as increased LV mass and elevated PWV) was best predicted by BPs obtained by auscultation.[135]

A major issue with oscillometric devices is that there appears to be great within-visit variation with inaccurately high readings obtained on initial measurement.[136] An elevated initial oscillometric reading should be ignored and repeat measures averaged to approximate values obtained by auscultation.

TABLE 10 Screening Tests and Relevant Populations

Patient Population	Screening Tests
All patients	Urinalysis
	Chemistry panel, including electrolytes, blood urea nitrogen, and creatinine
	Lipid profile (fasting or nonfasting to include high-density lipoproteina and total cholesterol)
	Renal ultrasonography in those <6 y of age or those with abnormal urinalysis or renal function
In the obese (BMI >95th percentile) child or adolescent, in addition to the above	Hemoglobin A1c (accepted screen for diabetes)
	Aspartate transaminase and alanine transaminase (screen for fatty liver)
	Fasting lipid panel (screen for dyslipidemia)
Optional tests to be obtained on the basis of history, physical examination, and initial studies	Fasting serum glucose for those at high risk for diabetes mellitus
	Thyroid-stimulating hormone
	Drug screen
	Sleep study (if loud snoring, daytime sleepiness, or reported history of apnea)
	Complete blood count, especially in those with growth delay or abnormal renal function

Adapted from Wiesen J, Adkins M, Fortune S, et al. Evaluation of pediatric patients with mild-to-moderate hypertension: yield of diagnostic testing. *Pediatrics*. 2008;122(5). Available at: www.pediatrics.org/cgi/content/full/122/5/e988.

Key Action Statement 5

Oscillometric devices may be used for BP screening in children

TABLE 11 Patient Evaluation and Management According to BP Level

BP Category (See Table 3)	BP Screening Schedule	Lifestyle Counseling (Weight and Nutrition)	Check Upper and Lower Extremity BP	ABPM[a]	Diagnostic Evaluation[b]	Initiate Treatment[c]	Consider Subspecialty Referral
Normal	Annual	X	—	—	—	—	—
Elevated BP	Initial measurement	X	—	—	—	—	—
	Second measurement: repeat in 6 mo	X	X	—	—	—	—
	Third measurement: repeat in 6 mo	X	—	X	X	—	X
Stage 1 HTN	Initial measurement	X	—	—	—	—	—
	Second measurement: repeat in 1–2 wk	X	X	—	—	—	—
	Third measurement: repeat in 3 mo	X	—	X	X	X	X
Stage 2 HTN[d]	Initial measurement	X	X	—	—	—	—
	Second measurement: repeat, refer to specialty care within 1 wk	X	—	X	X	X	X

X, recommended intervention; —, not applicable.
[a] ABPM is done to confirm HTN before initiating a diagnostic evaluation.
[b] See Table 15 for recommended studies.
[c] Treatment may be initiated by a primary care provider or subspecialist.
[d] If the patient is symptomatic or BP is >30 mm Hg above the 95th percentile (or >180/120 mm Hg in an adolescent), send to an ED.

and adolescents. When doing so, providers should use a device that has been validated in the pediatric age group. If elevated BP is suspected on the basis of oscillometric readings, confirmatory measurements should be obtained by auscultation (grade B, strong recommendation).

Key Action Statement 5. Oscillometric devices may be used for BP screening in children and adolescents. When doing so, providers should use a device that has been validated in the pediatric age group. If elevated BP is suspected on the basis of oscillometric readings, confirmatory measurements should be obtained by auscultation (grade B, strong recommendation).

Aggregate Evidence Quality	Grade B
Benefits	Use of auscultatory readings prevents potential misclassification of patients as hypertensive because of inaccuracy of oscillometric devices
Risks, harm, cost	Auscultation requires more training and experience and has flaws such as digit preference
Benefit–harm assessment	Benefit exceeds harm
Intentional vagueness	None
Role of patient preferences	Patients may prefer the convenience of oscillometric monitors
Exclusions	None
Strength	Strong recommendation
Key references	86,88,128–136

4.6 Forearm and/or Wrist BP Measurement

Wrist monitors have several potential advantages when compared with arm devices. They are smaller; they can be placed more easily; and, because wrist diameter is less affected by BMI, they do not need to be modified for patients with obesity.[83,137] Several studies in adults have found excellent reproducibility of wrist BP measurements, equivalence to readings obtained by mercury sphygmomanometers or ABPM, and better correlation with left ventricular mass index (LVMI) than systolic office BP.[138,139]

Although many wrist devices have been validated in adults,[140–142] some studies have shown greater variation and decreased accuracy in the resulting measurements.[143–146] These negative outcomes may possibly result from differences in the number of measurements taken,[139] the position of the wrist in relation to the heart,[147] flexion or extension of the wrist during measurement,[148] or differences in pulse pressure.[149] Technologies are being developed to help standardize wrist position.[150,151]

Few studies using wrist monitors have been conducted in children. One study in adolescents compared a wrist digital monitor with a mercury sphygmomanometer and found high agreement between systolic measurements but lower agreement for diastolic measurements, which was clinically relevant.[152] Researchers in 2 small studies conducted in PICUs compared wrist monitors with indwelling arterial lines and found good agreement between the 2 measurement modalities.[153,154] No large comparative studies or formal validation studies of wrist monitors have been conducted in children, however. Because of limited data, the use of wrist and forearm monitors is not recommended in the diagnosis or

TABLE 12 High-Risk Conditions for Which ABPM May Be Useful

Condition	Rationale
Secondary HTN	Severe ambulatory HTN or nocturnal HTN indicates higher likelihood of secondary HTN[161,167]
CKD or structural renal abnormalities	Evaluate for MH or nocturnal HTN,[168–172] better control delays progression of renal disease[173]
T1DM and T2DM	Evaluate for abnormal ABPM patterns,[174,175] better BP control delays the development of MA[176–178]
Solid-organ transplant	Evaluate for MH or nocturnal HTN, better control BP[179–188]
Obesity	Evaluate for WCH and MH[23,189–192]
OSAS	Evaluate for nondipping and accentuated morning BP surge[43,46,193,194]
Aortic coarctation (repaired)	Evaluate for sustained HTN and MH[58,112,113]
Genetic syndromes associated with HTN (neurofibromatosis, Turner syndrome, Williams syndrome, coarctation of the aorta)	HTN associated with increased arterial stiffness may only be manifest with activity during ABPM[58,195]
Treated hypertensive patients	Confirm 24-h BP control[155]
Patient born prematurely	Evaluate for nondipping[196]
Research, clinical trials	To reduce sample size[197]

TABLE 13 Recommended Procedures for the Application of ABPM

Procedure	Recommendation
Device	Should be validated by the Association for the Advancement of Medical Instrumentation or the British Hypertension Society for use in children
	May be oscillometric or auscultatory
Application	Trained personnel should apply the monitor
	Correct cuff size should be selected
	Right and left arm and a lower extremity BP should be obtained to rule out coarctation of the aorta
	Use nondominant arm unless there is large difference in size between the left arm and right arm, then apply to the arm with the higher BP
	Take readings every 15–20 min during the day and every 20–30 min at night
	Compare (calibrate) the device to resting BP measured by the same technique (oscillometric or auscultatory)
	Record time of medications, activity, and sleep
Assessment	A physician who is familiar with pediatric ABPM should interpret the results
	Interpret only recordings of adequate quality. Minimum of 1 reading per hour, 40–50 for a full day, 65%–75% of all possible recordings
	Edit outliers by inspecting for biologic plausibility, edit out calibration measures
	Calculate mean BP, BP load (% of readings above threshold), and dipping (% decline in BP from wake to sleep)
	Interpret with pediatric ABPM normal data by sex and height
	Use AHA staging schema[155]
	Consider interpretation of 24-h, daytime, and nighttime MAP, especially in patients with CKD[173,198]

Adapted from Flynn JT, Daniels SR, Hayman LL, et al; American Heart Association Atherosclerosis, Hypertension and Obesity in Youth Committee of the Council on Cardiovascular Disease in the Young. Update: ambulatory blood pressure monitoring in children and adolescents: a scientific statement from the American Heart Association. *Hypertension*. 2014;63(5):1116–1135.

management of HTN in children and adolescents at this time.

4.7 ABPM

An ambulatory BP monitor consists of a BP cuff attached to a box slightly larger than a cell phone, which records BP periodically (usually every 20–30 minutes) throughout the day and night; these data are later downloaded to a computer for analysis.[155]

ABPM has been recommended by the US Preventive Services Task Force for the confirmation of HTN in adults before starting treatment.[156] Although a growing number of pediatric providers have access to ABPM, there are still gaps in access and knowledge regarding the optimal application of ABPM to the evaluation of children's BP.[155,157] For example, there are currently no reference data for children whose height is <120 cm. Because no outcome data exist linking ABPM data from childhood to hard CV events in adulthood, recommendations either rely largely on surrogate outcome markers or are extrapolated from adult studies.

However, sufficient data exist to demonstrate that ABPM is more accurate for the diagnosis of HTN than clinic-measured BP,[158,159] is more predictive of future BP,[160] and can assist in the detection of secondary HTN.[161] Furthermore, increased LVMI and LVH correlate more strongly with ABPM parameters than casual BP.[162–166] In addition, ABPM is more reproducible than casual or home BP measurements.[159] For these reasons, the routine application of ABPM is recommended, when available, as indicated below (see also Tables 12 and 13). Obtaining ABPM may require referral to a specialist.

Key Action Statement 6

ABPM should be performed for the confirmation of HTN in children and adolescents with office BP measurements in the elevated BP category for 1 year or more or with stage 1 HTN over 3 clinic visits (grade C, moderate recommendation).

For technical reasons, ABPM may need to be limited to children ≥5 years of age who can tolerate the procedure and those for whom reference data are available.

Key Action Statement 7

The routine performance of ABPM should be strongly considered in children and adolescents with high-risk conditions (see Table 12) to assess HTN severity and determine if abnormal circadian BP patterns are present, which may indicate increased risk for target organ damage (grade B, moderate recommendation).

Key Action Statement 8

ABPM should be performed by using a standardized approach (see Table 13) with monitors that have been validated in a pediatric population, and studies should be interpreted by using pediatric normative data (grade C, moderate recommendation).

4.7a Masked Hypertension

MH occurs when patients have normal office BP but elevated BP on ABPM, and it has been found in 5.8% of unselected children studied by ABPM.[199] There is growing evidence that compared with those with normal 24-hour BP, these patients have significant risk for end organ hypertensive damage.[200,203] Patients who are at risk of MH include patients with obesity and secondary forms of HTN, such as CKD or repaired aortic coarctation. MH is particularly prevalent in patients with CKD[48] and is associated with target organ damage.[203] Children with CKD should be periodically evaluated using ABPM for MH as part of routine CKD management.[201,204–206]

4.7b White Coat Hypertension

WCH is defined as BP ≥95th percentile in the office or clinical setting but <95th percentile outside of the office or clinical setting. WCH is diagnosed by ABPM when the mean SBP and DBP are <95th percentile and SBP and DBP load are <25%; load is defined as the percentage of valid ambulatory BP measurements above a set threshold value (eg, 95th percentile) for age, sex, and height.[155,156,206] It is estimated that up to half of children who are evaluated for elevated office BP have WCH.[207,208]

In adults, compared with normotension, WCH is associated with only a slightly increased risk of adverse outcomes but at a much lower risk compared with those with established HTN.[209] Most (but not all) studies suggest that WCH is not associated with increased LV mass.[200,207,210] Although the distinction between WCH and true HTN is important, abnormal BP response to exercise and increased LVM has been found to occur in children with WCH.[207] Furthermore, the identification of WCH may reduce costs by reducing the number of additional tests performed and decreasing the number of children who are exposed to antihypertensive medications.[208] Children and adolescents with WCH should have screening BP measured at regular well-child care visits with consideration of a repeat ABPM in 1 to 2 years.

Key Action Statement 9

Children and adolescents with suspected WCH should undergo ABPM. Diagnosis is based on the presence of mean SBP and DBP <95th percentile and SBP and DBP load <25% (grade B, strong recommendation).

4.8 Measurement in Children With Obesity

Accurate BP measurement can be challenging in individuals with obesity. [23,211,212] Elevated BMI in children and adolescents is associated with an increase in the midarm circumference,[96] requiring the use of a larger cuff to obtain accurate BP measurements.[83] During NHANES 2007–2010, among children 9 to 11 years of age with obesity, one-third of boys and one-quarter of girls required an adult BP cuff, and a fraction required a large adult cuff or an adult thigh cuff for an accurate measurement of BP.[213] Researchers in studies of adults have also noted the influence of the conical upper arm shape on BP measurements in people with obesity.[214,215] ABPM is a valuable tool in the diagnosis of HTN in children with obesity because of the discrepancies between casual and

Key Action Statement 6. ABPM should be performed for the confirmation of HTN in children and adolescents with office BP measurements in the elevated BP category for 1 year or more or with stage 1 HTN over 3 clinic visits (grade C, moderate recommendation).

Aggregate Evidence Quality	Grade C
Benefits	Avoids unnecessarily exposing youth with WCH to extensive diagnostic testing or medication
Risks, harm, cost	Risk of discomfort to patient. Some insurance plans may not reimburse for the test
Benefit–harm assessment	The risk of ABPM is lower than the risk of unnecessary treatment. The use of ABPM has also been shown to be more cost-effective than other approaches to diagnosing HTN
Intentional vagueness	None
Role of patient preferences	Some patients may prefer repeat office or home measurements to ABPM
Exclusions	None
Strength	Moderate recommendation
Key references	23,155,158,159

Key Action Statement 7. The routine performance of ABPM should be strongly considered in children and adolescents with high-risk conditions (see Table 12) to assess HTN severity and determine if abnormal circadian BP patterns are present, which may indicate increased risk for target organ damage (grade B, moderate recommendation).

Aggregate Evidence Quality	Grade B
Benefits	Improved 24-h control of BP improves outcomes. Recognition of MH or nocturnal HTN might lead to therapeutic changes that will limit end organ damage
Risks, harm, cost	Risk of discomfort to patient. Some insurance plans may not reimburse for the test. The risk of diagnosing and labeling a patient as having MH or nocturnal HTN might lead to increased anxiety and cost of evaluation
Benefit–harm assessment	The risk of ABPM is much lower than the risk of inadequate treatment
Intentional vagueness	Frequency at which normal or abnormal ABPM should be repeated is not known
Role of patient preferences	Some patients may prefer repeat office or home measurements to ABPM
Exclusions	None
Strength	Moderate recommendation
Key references	47,155,199–202

Key Action Statement 8. ABPM should be performed by using a standardized approach (see Table 13) with monitors that have been validated in a pediatric population, and studies should be interpreted by using pediatric normative data (grade C, moderate recommendation).

Aggregate Evidence Quality	Grade C
Benefits	Validated monitors applied and interpreted correctly will provide the most accurate results
Risks, harm, cost	Risk of discomfort to patient. Some insurance plans may not reimburse for the test. Monitors validated in the pediatric population and expertise in reading pediatric ABPM may not be universally available
Benefit–harm assessment	There is substantial evidence showing incorrect application or interpretation reduces the accuracy of results
Intentional vagueness	None
Role of patient preferences	Some patients may prefer repeat office or home measurements to ABPM
Exclusions	None
Strength	Moderate recommendation
Key references	155

ambulatory BP[23,33] and the higher prevalence of MH.[26,29,155,216,217]

4.9. At-Home Measurement

Home measurement (or self-monitoring) of BP has advantages over both office and ambulatory monitoring, including convenience and the ability to obtain repeated measurements over time.[83,218] Furthermore, automated devices with memory capacity are straightforward to use and avoid potential problems, such as observer bias, inaccurate reporting, and terminal digit preference (ie, overreporting of certain digits, like 0, as the terminal digit in recording BP).[219,220]

Numerous studies have shown that it is feasible for families to conduct repeated measurements at home.[221–223] Home BP measurements appear to be more reproducible than those conducted in the office, likely because of the familiarity of the home environment and greater comfort with repeated measurements.[159,223,224] Inaccuracies occur when measurements obtained at home are either excluded or inappropriately recorded.[219] Inconsistencies in home, office, and ambulatory BP measurements seem to be influenced by both age and HTN status, with ABPM tending to be higher than home BP measurements in children.[222,225–227] Home BP measurements show no consistent pattern when compared with office measurements.[228–230]

There are several practical concerns with the use of home BP measurement, however. The only normative data available are from the relatively small Arsakeion School study.[231] In addition, only a few automated devices have been validated for use in the pediatric population, and available cuff sizes for them are limited. Furthermore, there is no consensus regarding how many home measurements across what period of time are needed to evaluate BP.

Key Action Statement 10

Home BP monitoring should not be used to diagnose HTN, MH, or WCH but may be a useful adjunct to office and ambulatory BP measurement after HTN has been diagnosed (grade C, moderate recommendation).

4.10 School Measurement and the Role of School-Based Health Professionals

There is limited evidence to support school-based measurement of children's BP.[8,232] Observational studies demonstrate that school measurements can be reliable[233] and that longitudinal follow-up is feasible.[8,232,234] Available data do not distinguish between the efficacy of school-based screening programs in which measurements are obtained by trained clinical personnel (not a school nurse) versus measurements obtained by the school nurse. Because of insufficient evidence and a lack of established protocols, the routine use of school-based measurements to diagnose HTN cannot be recommended. However, school-based BP measurement can be a useful tool to identify children who require formal evaluation as well as a helpful adjunct in the monitoring of diagnosed HTN. Note: School-based health clinics are considered part of

Key Action Statement 9. Children and adolescents with suspected WCH should undergo ABPM. Diagnosis is based on the presence of mean SBP and DBP <95th percentile and SBP and DBP load <25% (grade B, strong recommendation).

Aggregate Evidence Quality	Grade B (Evidence Level A in Adults)
Benefits	Improved diagnosis of WCH and the benefit of fewer additional laboratory tests and/or treatment of primary HTN. Costs might be reduced if the treatment of those misdiagnosed as hypertensive is prevented
Risks, harm, cost	Additional costs; costs may not be covered by insurance companies. The ambulatory BP monitor is uncomfortable for some patients
Benefit–harm assessment	Benefit exceeds risk
Intentional vagueness	None
Role of patient preferences	Important; some patients may not want to undergo ABPM. Benefits of the procedure should be reviewed with families to assist in decision-making
Exclusions	None
Strength	Strong recommendation
Key references	206

Key Action Statement 10. Home BP monitoring should not be used to diagnose HTN, MH, or WCH but may be a useful adjunct to office and ambulatory BP measurement after HTN has been diagnosed (grade C, moderate recommendation).

Aggregate Evidence Quality	Grade C
Benefits	Convenient, cost-effective, widely available, can be used over time
Risks, harm, cost	Risk of inaccurate diagnosis. Unclear what norms or schedule should be used. Few validated devices in children, and cuff sizes are limited
Benefit–harm assessment	Benefits outweigh harm when used as an adjunctive measurement technique
Intentional vagueness	None
Role of patient preferences	Patients may find home BP more convenient and accessible than office or ambulatory BP
Exclusions	None
Strength	Moderate recommendation
Key references	159,221–225,227,230

systems of pediatric primary care, and these comments would not apply to them.

5. PRIMARY AND SECONDARY CAUSES OF HTN

5.1 Primary HTN

Primary HTN is now the predominant diagnosis for hypertensive children and adolescents seen in referral centers in the United States,[235,236] although single-center studies from outside the United States still find primary HTN to be uncommon.[237] Although prospective, multicenter studies are generally lacking, at least one large study in which researchers used insurance claims data confirmed that primary HTN is significantly more common than secondary HTN among American youth.[238]

General characteristics of children with primary HTN include older age (≥6 years),[239,240] positive family history (in a parent and/or grandparent) of HTN,[236,237,240] and overweight and/or obesity.[16,236,237,239] Severity of BP elevation has not differed significantly between children with primary and secondary HTN in some studies,[235,237] but DBP elevation appears to be more predictive of secondary HTN,[239,240] whereas systolic HTN appears to be more predictive of primary HTN.[236,239]

Key Action Statement 11

Children and adolescents ≥6 years of age do not require an extensive evaluation for secondary causes of HTN if they have a positive family history of HTN, are overweight or obese, and/or do not have history or physical examination findings (Table 14) suggestive of a secondary cause of HTN (grade C, moderate recommendation).

5.2 Secondary Causes: Renal and/or Renovascular

Renal disease and renovascular disease are among the most common secondary causes of HTN in children. Renal parenchymal disease and renal structural abnormalities accounted for 34% to 79% of patients with secondary HTN in 3 retrospective, single-center case series, and renovascular disease was present in 12% to 13%.[101,240,241] The literature suggests that renal disease is a more common cause of HTN in younger children.[239] Renal disorders (including vascular problems) accounted for 63% to 74% of children <6 years of age who were enrolled in 3 recent clinical trials of angiotensin receptor blockers (ARBs).[239,242–244] No increased frequency was seen in younger patients in a recent single-center case series, however.[101] It is appropriate to have a high index of suspicion for renal and renovascular disease in hypertensive pediatric patients, particularly in those <6 years of age.

5.3 Secondary Causes: Cardiac, Including Aortic Coarctation

Coarctation of the aorta is a congenital abnormality of the aortic arch characterized by discrete narrowing of the aortic arch, generally at the level of the aortic isthmus. It is usually associated with HTN and right arm BP that is 20 mm Hg (or more) greater than the lower extremity BP. Repair in infants is often surgical; adolescents may be treated with angioplasty or stenting. Long-segment narrowing of the abdominal aorta can also cause HTN and should be considered in children with refractory

Key Action Statement 11. Children and adolescents ≥6 years of age do not require an extensive evaluation for secondary causes of HTN if they have a positive family history of HTN, are overweight or obese, and/or do not have history or physical examination findings (Table 14) suggestive of a secondary cause of HTN (grade C, moderate recommendation).

Aggregate Evidence Quality	Grade C
Benefits	Avoidance of unnecessary diagnostic evaluation
Risks, harm, cost	Potential to miss some children with secondary HTN
Benefit–harm assessment	Benefit equals harm
Intentional vagueness	Not applicable
Role of patient preferences	Some families may want further testing performed
Exclusions	Hypertensive children <6 y of age
Strength	Moderate recommendation
Key references	16,129,235–240

HTN and a gradient between the upper and lower extremities in which the upper extremity SBP exceeds the lower extremity SBP by 20 mm Hg.[245] Of note, children with abdominal aortic obstruction may have neurofibromatosis, Williams syndrome, Alagille syndrome, or Takayasu arteritis.

Patients with coarctation can remain hypertensive or develop HTN even after early and successful repair, with reported prevalence varying from 17% to 77%.[112] HTN can be a manifestation of recoarctation. Recoarctation in repaired patients should be assessed for by using 4 extremity BP measurements and echocardiography. HTN can also occur without recoarctation.[246] The prevalence of HTN increases over time after successful coarctation repair.[112]

Routine office BP measurement alone is often insufficient for diagnosing HTN after coarctation repair.[113,246] Children who have undergone coarctation repair may have normal in-office BP but high BP out of the office, which is consistent with MH.[58,112] Of children with a history of aortic coarctation, ~45% have MH at ~1 to 14 years after coarctation repair.[58,113] Children with a history of repaired aortic coarctation and normal in-office BP are at risk for LVH,[58] HTN, and MH.[58,112]

ABPM has emerged as the gold standard for diagnosing HTN among individuals who have undergone coarctation repair, and it is likely more useful than casual BP.[58,245–247] Screening is recommended as a part of usual care on an annual basis beginning, at most, 12 years after coarctation repair. Earlier screening may be considered on the basis of risk factors and clinician discretion.

Key Action Statement 12

Children and adolescents who have undergone coarctation repair should undergo ABPM for the detection of HTN (including MH) (grade B, strong recommendation).

5.4 Secondary Causes: Endocrine HTN

HTN resulting from hormonal excess accounts for a relatively small proportion of children with secondary HTN. Although rare (with a prevalence ranging from 0.05% to 6% in children[101,237,239,240]), an accurate diagnosis of endocrine HTN provides the clinician with a unique treatment opportunity to render a surgical cure or achieve a dramatic response with pharmacologic therapy.[248] Known endocrine causes with associated molecular defects (when known) are summarized in Table 15.

5.5 Secondary Causes: Environmental Exposures

Several environmental exposures have been associated with higher childhood BP, although most studies are limited to small case series. Among the most prominent are lead, cadmium, mercury, and phthalates.

- Lead: Long-term exposure to lead in adults has been associated with higher BP in population studies[295,296] and in studies of industrial workers with high lead exposure,[297] although findings have not been consistent.[298] At least 1 cross-sectional study of 122 children demonstrated that children with higher blood lead concentrations had higher BP; lower socioeconomic status was also seen in this group, which may have confounded the BP results.[299] Furthermore, in a randomized study of lead-exposed children, those who received chelation with succimer did not have lower BP than in those who received a placebo.[300]
- Cadmium: Environmental cadmium exposure has been linked to higher BP levels and the development of HTN in adults, particularly among women.[296,301–303] Although cross-sectional studies have

Key Action Statement 12. Children and adolescents who have undergone coarctation repair should undergo ABPM for the detection of HTN (including MH) (grade B, strong recommendation).

Aggregate Evidence Quality	Grade B (Aggregate Level of Evidence Equals B, Given 3 Studies With Similar Findings)
Benefits	Early detection of HTN
Risks, harm, cost	Additional costs related to the placement of ABPM
Benefit–harm assessment	Benefits exceed harms
Intentional vagueness	Frequency of measurement. Because the development of HTN after coarctation repair is influenced by many factors, the ideal onset of screening for HTN (including MH) is unknown
Role of patient preferences	None
Exclusions	Individuals with a history of residual aortic arch obstruction
Strength	Strong recommendation
Key references	58,112,113

TABLE 14 Examples of Physical Examination Findings and History Suggestive of Secondary HTN or Related to End Organ Damage Secondary to HTN

Body System	Finding, History	Possible Etiology
Vital signs	Tachycardia	Hyperthyroidism PCC Neuroblastoma
	Decreased lower extremity pulses; drop in BP from upper to lower extremities	Coarctation of the aorta
Eyes	Proptosis	Hyperthyroidism
	Retinal changes[a]	Severe HTN, more likely to be associated with secondary HTN
Ear, nose, throat	Adenotonsillar hypertrophy	SDB
	History of snoring	Sleep apnea
Height, weight	Growth retardation	Chronic renal failure
	Obesity (high BMI)	Cushing syndrome
	Truncal obesity	Insulin resistance syndrome
Head, neck	Elfin facies	Williams syndrome
	Moon facies	Cushing syndrome
	Thyromegaly, goiter	Hyperthyroidism
	Webbed neck	Turner syndrome
Skin	Pallor, flushing, diaphoresis	PCC
	Acne, hirsutism, striae	Cushing syndrome Anabolic steroid abuse
	Café-au-lait spots	Neurofibromatosis
	Adenoma sebaceum	Tuberous sclerosis
	Malar rash	Systemic lupus
	Acanthosis nigricans	T2DM
Hematologic	Pallor	Renal disease
	Sickle cell anemia	
Chest, cardiac	Chest pain	Heart disease
	Palpitations	
	Exertional dyspnea	
	Widely spaced nipples	Turner syndrome
	Heart murmur	Coarctation of the aorta
	Friction rub	Systemic lupus (pericarditis) Collagen vascular disease
	Apical heave[a]	LVH
Abdomen	Abdominal mass	Wilms tumor Neuroblastoma PCC
	Epigastric, flank bruit	RAS
	Palpable kidneys	Polycystic kidney disease Hydronephrosis Multicystic dysplastic kidney
Genitourinary	Ambiguous or virilized genitalia	Congenital adrenal hyperplasia
	Urinary tract infection	Renal disease
	Vesicoureteral reflux	
	Hematuria, edema, fatigue	
	Abdominal trauma	
Extremities	Joint swelling	Systemic lupus Collagen vascular disease
	Muscle weakness	Hyperaldosteronism Liddle syndrome
Neurologic, metabolic	Hypokalemia, headache, dizziness, polyuria, nocturia	Reninoma
	Muscle weakness, hypokalemia	Monogenic HTN (Liddle syndrome, GRA, AME)

AME, apparent mineralocorticoid excess; GRA, glucocorticoid-remediable aldosteronism. Adapted from Flynn JT. Evaluation and management of hypertension in childhood. *Prog Pediatr Cardiol.* 2001;12(2):177–188; National High Blood Pressure Education Program Working Group on Hypertension Control in Children and Adolescents. The fourth report on the diagnosis, evaluation, and treatment of high blood pressure in children and adolescents. *Pediatrics.* 2004;114(2):555–576.
[a] Findings that may be indicative of end organ damage related to HTN.

confirmed potential nephrotoxicity of cadmium in children,[304] no definite effect on BP has been demonstrated.[304,305]

- Mercury: Mercury is a known nephrotoxin, particularly in its elemental form.[306,307] Severe mercury intoxication has been linked to acute HTN in children in several case reports; patients' symptoms may resemble those seen in patients with pheochromocytoma (PCC).[308–310]
- Phthalates: Antenatal and childhood exposure to phthalates has recently been associated with higher childhood BP[311–313] but not with the development of overt HTN. Specific metabolites of these ubiquitous chemicals may have differential effects on BP,[313] indicating that much more detailed study is needed to completely understand the effect of such exposure.

5.6 Secondary Causes: Neurofibromatosis

Neurofibromatosis type 1 (NF-1) (also known as Von Recklinghausen disease) is a rare autosomal dominant disorder characterized by distinct clinical examination findings. These include the following: cafe-au-lait macules, neurofibromas, Lisch nodules of the iris, axillary freckling, optic nerve gliomas, and distinctive bone lesions. Patients with NF-1 have several unique and potential secondary causes of HTN, most commonly renal artery stenosis (RAS); coarctation of the aorta, middle aortic syndrome, and PCC are also well described.[314–319]

Additionally, an increased incidence of idiopathic HTN has been documented in patients with NF-1, as high as 6.1% in a recent pediatric case series, which is a much greater incidence than in the general population.[320] PCC has also been well described in patients with NF-1, although exact incidences are difficult

TABLE 15 Endocrine Causes of HTN

Name of Disorder	Genetic Mutation	Mode of Inheritance	Clinical Feature(s)	Biochemical Mechanism and Notes	Ref No(s).
Catecholamine excess					
PCC, paraganglioma	VHL (49%)	De novo, AD	HTN	Diagnostic test: fractionated plasma[a] and/or urine metanephrines and normetanephrines	248–254
	SDHB (15%) SDHD (10%) RET		Palpitations, headache, sweating Abdominal mass Incidental radiographic finding Family screening		
Mineralocorticoid excess					
Specific etiologies addressed below		Screening test: ARR: PAC, PRA preferably obtained between 8:00 and 10:00 AM			255,256
Consider if: Early onset HTN Potassium level abnormalities Family history of primary aldosteronism Resistant HTN					
Congenital adrenal hyperplasia					
11β–hydroxylase deficiency	CYP11B1 (loss of function)	AR	HTN	Elevated levels of DOC, 11-deoxycortisol, androstenedione, testosterone, and DHEAS	257–259
			Hypokalemia Acne, hirsutism, and virilization in girls Pseudoprecocious puberty in boys 11% of congenital adrenal hyperplasia	Higher prevalence in Moroccan Jews	
17-α hydroxylase deficiency	CYP17 (loss of function)	AR	HTN and hypokalemia Low aldosterone and renin Undervirilized boys, sexual infantilism in girls <1% of congenital adrenal hyperplasia	Elevated DOC and corticosterone Decreased androstenedione, testosterone and DHEAS Prominent in Dutch Mennonites	260–262
Familial hyperaldosteronism					
Type 1	Hybrid CYP11B1 and CYP11B2 (11β-hydroxylase–aldosterone synthase, gain of function)	AD	Young subjects with PA Family history of young strokes	Excessive, ACTH-regulated aldosterone production Prescription with low-dose dexamethasone May add low-dose spironolactone, calcium channel blocker, or potassium supplementation	263,264
Type 2	Unknown, possibly 7p22	AD (prevalence varies from 1.2% to 6%)	PA in the patient with an affected first-degree relative Unresponsive to dexamethasone May have adrenal adenoma or bilateral adrenal hyperplasia	Excessive autonomous aldosterone production	265–267
Type 3	KCNJ5 G-protein potassium channel (loss of function)	AD	Early onset severe HTN in the first family described Milder phenotypes also seen	Mutation leads to loss of potassium+ sensitivity causing sodium+ influx that activates Ca^{++} channels, leading to aldosterone synthesis	268–270
Type 4	CACNA1D coding for calcium channel (gain of function)	AD	PA and HTN age <10 y Variable developmental abnormalities	Increased Ca^{++} channel sensitivity causing increased aldosterone synthesis	271,272
Other genetic causes					

TABLE 15 Continued

Name of Disorder	Genetic Mutation	Mode of Inheritance	Clinical Feature(s)	Biochemical Mechanism and Notes	Ref No(s).
Carney complex	PRKAR1A	AD	Skin pigmentation Pituitary and other tumors	Rare familial cause	273,274
McCune Albright syndrome	GNAS, α-subunit	Somatic	Cutaneous pigmentation Fibrous dysplasia	Tumors in the breast, thyroid, pituitary gland, or testicles may be present	275,276
Primary glucocorticoid resistance (Chrousos syndrome)	NR3C1 (loss of function glucocorticoid receptor)	AD	HTN Ambiguous genitalia Precocious puberty Androgen excess, menstrual abnormalities or infertility in women	Loss of function of glucocorticoid receptor	277–279
Apparent mineralocorticoid excess	HSD11B2 (loss of function)	AR	HTN Hypokalemia Low birth weight Failure to thrive Polyuria, polydipsia	Reduced or absent activity of 11 β-HSD2: cortisol gains access to MR Mimicked by licorice toxicity	280,281
Liddle syndrome	SCNN1B β-subunit–SCNN1G γ-subunit (activating mutation)		Severe HTN Hypokalemia Metabolic alkalosis Muscle weakness	Constitutive activation of the epithelial sodium channel causing salt retention and volume expansion	282,283
Geller syndrome	MCR (mineralocorticoid-d receptor, activating mutation)	AD	Onset of HTN <20 y Exacerbated by pregnancy	Constitutive activation of MR Also activated by progesterone	284
Pseudohypo-aldosteronism type 2 (Gordon syndrome)	WNK1,4; KLHL3; CUL3; SPAK (activating mutation)	AD	Short stature Hyperkalemic and hyperchloremic metabolic acidosis Borderline HTN	Increased activity of sodium chloride cotransporter causing salt retention and volume expansion	285–287
Glucocorticoid excess					
Cushing syndrome, adrenocortical carcinoma, iatrogenic excess	To be discovered	—	HTN Other signs of Cushing syndrome	Likely attributable to increased DOC, sensitivity to vasoconstriction, cardiac output, activation of RAS	288–290
Other endocrine abnormalities					
Hyperthyroidism	To be discovered	—	Tachycardia HTN Tremors Other signs of hyperthyroidism	Mechanism increased cardiac output, stroke volume, and decreased peripheral resistance Initial prescription with β blockers	291,292
Hyperparathyroidism	—	—	Hypercalcemia Other signs of hyperparathyroidism	Mechanism unknown, may not remit after treatment of hyperparathyroidism	293,294

ACTH, adrenocorticotropic hormone; AD, autosomal dominant; AR, autosomal recessive; DHEAS, dehydroepiandrosterone sulfate; DOC, deoxycortisol; MR, magnetic resonance; PA, primary hyperaldosteronism; PAC, plasma aldosterone concentration; RAS, renin angiotensin system; —, not applicable.

[a] influenced by posture, specialized center preferred.

to determine, and patients may not have classic symptoms of PCC.[321,322]

Vascular causes of HTN and PCC all require specific treatment and follow-up, so maintaining a high index of suspicion for these disorders is important in evaluating hypertensive children and adolescents with NF-1.

5.7 Secondary Causes: Medication Related

Many over-the-counter drugs, prescription medications, alternative therapies (ie, herbal and nutritional supplements), dietary products, and recreational drugs can increase BP. Common prescription medications associated with a rise in BP include oral contraceptives,[323–325] central nervous system stimulants,[326] and corticosteroids.[1,327] When a child has elevated BP measurements, the practitioner should inquire about the intake of pharmacologic agents (see Table 8).

Usually, the BP elevation is mild and reversible on discontinuation of the medication, but a significant increase in BP can occasionally occur with higher doses or as an idiosyncratic response. Over-the-counter cold medications that contain decongestants (eg, pseudoephedrine and phenylpropanolamine) may cause a mild increase in BP with the recommended dosing, but severe HTN has been observed as an idiosyncratic response with appropriate dosing as well as with excessive doses.

Nonsteroidal anti-inflammatory drugs may antagonize the BP-lowering effect of antihypertensive medications (specifically, angiotensin-converting enzyme [ACE] inhibitors) but do not appear to have an impact on BP in those without HTN. The commonly used supplement ephedra (ma haung) likely contains some amount of ephedrine and caffeine that can cause an unpredictable rise in BP. Recreational drugs associated with HTN include stimulants (eg, cocaine and amphetamine derivatives) and anabolic steroids.

5.8 Monogenic HTN

Monogenic forms of HTN are uncommon, although the exact incidence is unknown. In a study of select hypertensive children without a known etiology, genetic testing for familial hyperaldosteronism type I (FH-I), or glucocorticoid-remediable aldosteronism, confirmed responsible genetic mutations in 3% of the population.[263]

Other monogenic forms of HTN in children include Liddle syndrome, pseudohypoaldosteronism type II (Gordon syndrome), apparent mineralocorticoid excess, familial glucocorticoid resistance, mineralocorticoid receptor activating mutation, and congenital adrenal hyperplasia (see "Secondary Causes: Endocrine Causes of Hypertension").[328] All manifest as HTN with suppressed plasma renin activity (PRA) and increased sodium absorption in the distal tubule. Other features may include serum potassium abnormalities, metabolic acid-base disturbances, and abnormal plasma aldosterone concentrations, although the clinical presentations can be highly variable.[263,328,329] In the study of FH-I, all affected children had suppressed PRA and an aldosterone to renin ratio (ARR) (ng/dL and ng/M1 per hour, respectively) of >10; the authors suggest that an ARR >10 is an indication to perform genetic testing in a hypertensive child.[263] Monogenic forms of HTN should be suspected in hypertensive children with a suppressed PRA or elevated ARR, especially if there is a family history of early-onset HTN.

6. DIAGNOSTIC EVALUATION

6.1 Patient Evaluation

As with any medical condition, appropriate diagnostic evaluation is a critical component in the evaluation of a patient with suspected HTN. Evaluation focuses on determining possible causes of and/or comorbidities associated with HTN. Evaluation, as is detailed in the following sections, should include appropriate patient history, family history, physical examination, laboratory evaluation, and imaging.

6.2 History

The first step in the evaluation of the child or adolescent with elevated BP is to obtain a history. The various components of the history include the perinatal history, past medical history, nutritional history, activity history, and psychosocial history. Each is discussed in the following sections.

6.2a Perinatal History

As discussed, perinatal factors such as maternal HTN and low birth weight have been shown to influence later BP, even in childhood.[56,330] Additionally, a high incidence of preterm birth among hypertensive children has recently been reported in 1 large case series.[101] Thus, it is appropriate to obtain a history of pertinent prenatal information, including maternal pregnancy complications; gestational age; birth weight; and, if pertinent, complications occurring in the neonatal nursery and/or ICU. It is also appropriate to document pertinent procedures, such as umbilical catheter placement.

6.2b Nutritional History

High sodium intake has been linked to childhood HTN and increased LVMI and is the focus of several population health campaigns.[4,331] In NHANES 2003–2008, among children 8 to 18 years of age (n = 6235), higher sodium intake (as assessed by dietary recall) was associated with a twofold increase in the combined outcome of elevated BP or HTN. The effect was threefold among participants with obesity.[332] Limited data suggest the same effect is seen in younger children.[333] One study found that high intake of total fat and saturated fat, as well as adiposity and central obesity, were also predictors of SBP.[334–336]

Nutrition history is an important part of the patient assessment because it may identify dietary contributors to HTN and detect areas in which lifestyle modification may be appropriate. The important components to discuss include salt intake (including salt added in the kitchen and at the table and sodium hidden in processed and fast food), consumption of high-fat foods, and consumption of sugary beverages.[337,338] Infrequent consumption of fruits, vegetables, and low-fat dairy products should also be identified.

6.2c Physical Activity History

A detailed history of physical activity and inactivity is an integral part of the patient assessment, not only to understand contributors to the development of HTN but also to direct lifestyle modification counseling as an important part of management.[339–344]

6.2d Psychosocial History

Providers should obtain a psychosocial history in children and adolescents with suspected or confirmed HTN. Adverse experiences both prenatally[345] and during childhood (including maltreatment, early onset depression, and anxiety) are associated with adult-onset HTN.[346,347] The identification of stress may suggest a diagnosis of WCH. The psychosocial history should include questions about feelings of depression and anxiety, bullying, and body perceptions. The latter is particularly important for patients with overweight or obesity because ~70% of these children report having bullying and body perception concerns.[348] Starting at 11 years of age, the psychosocial history should include questions about smoking,[349,350] alcohol, and other drug use.[351]

6.2e Family History

Taking and updating the family history is a quick and easy way to risk-stratify pediatric patients with an increased risk for HTN. It is important to update the family history for HTN over the course of the pediatric patient's lifetime in the practice (typically until 18–21 years of age) because first- and second-degree relatives may develop HTN during this time. All too often, the diagnosis of HTN in the pediatric patient stimulates the collection of a detailed family history of HTN, sometimes even years after the pediatric patient has had elevated BP, instead of the other way around.[352]

6.3 Physical Examination

A complete physical examination may provide clues to potential secondary causes of HTN and assess possible hypertensive end organ damage. The child's height, weight, calculated BMI, and percentiles for age should be determined at the start of the physical examination. Poor growth may indicate an underlying chronic illness.

At the second visit with confirmed elevated BP or stage 1 HTN or the first visit with confirmed stage 2 HTN, BP should be measured in both arms and in a leg. Normally, BP is 10 to 20 mm Hg higher in the legs than the arms. If the leg BP is lower than the arm BP, or if femoral pulses are weak or absent, coarctation of the aorta may be present. Obesity alone is an insufficient explanation for diminished femoral pulses in the presence of high BP.

The remainder of the physical examination should pursue clues found in the history and should focus on body systems and findings that may indicate secondary HTN and/or end organ damage related to HTN. Table 14 lists important physical examination findings in hypertensive children.[353] These are examples of history and physical findings and do not represent all possible history and physical examination findings. The physical examination in hypertensive children is frequently normal except for the BP elevation.

Key Action Statement 13

In children and adolescents being evaluated for high BP, the provider should obtain a perinatal history, appropriate nutritional history, physical activity history, psychosocial history, and family history and perform a physical examination to identify findings suggestive of secondary causes of HTN (grade B, strong recommendation).

6.4 Laboratory Evaluation

The purpose of the laboratory evaluation is to identify underlying secondary causes of HTN (eg, renal or endocrine disease) that would require specific treatment guided by a subspecialist. In general, such testing includes a basic set of screening tests and additional, specific tests; the latter are selected on the basis of clues obtained from the history and physical examination and/or the results of the initial screening tests.[354] Table 10 provides a list of screening tests and the populations in which they should be performed.

6.5 Electrocardiography

Approximately one-half of adolescents with HTN have undergone electrocardiography at least once as an assessment for LVH.[355] Unlike echocardiography, electrocardiography takes little time and is a relatively low-cost test. Electrocardiography has high specificity but poor sensitivity for identifying children and adolescents with LVH.[356–358] The positive predictive value of electrocardiography to identify LVH is extremely low.[359]

Key Action Statement 14

Clinicians should not perform electrocardiography in hypertensive

Key Action Statement 13. In children and adolescents being evaluated for high BP, the provider should obtain a perinatal history, appropriate nutritional history, physical activity history, psychosocial history, and family history and perform a physical examination to identify findings suggestive of secondary causes of HTN (grade B, strong recommendation).

Aggregate Evidence Quality	Grade B
Benefits	Identify personal risk factors for HTN
Risks, harm, cost	None
Benefit–harm assessment	Identification of personal risk factors is useful in the assessment of childhood HTN
Intentional vagueness	None
Role of patient preferences	None
Exclusions	Children with normal BP
Strength	Strong recommendation
Key references	56,330

children and adolescents being evaluated for LVH (grade B, strong recommendation).

6.6 Imaging Evaluation, Echocardiography: Detection of Target Organ Damage

Echocardiography was identified in the Fourth Report as a tool to measure left ventricular (LV) target organ injury related to HTN in children.[1] The basis for this assessment is as follows: (1) the relationship of LV mass to BP,[361] (2) the independent and strong relationship of LVH to adverse CVD outcomes in adults,[362–364] and (3) that a significant percentage of children and adolescents with HTN demonstrate the degree of LVH associated with adverse outcomes in adults.[365–367] Antihypertensive treatment reduces LVH. Observational data suggest that the regression of LVH independently predicts outcomes in adults.[368]

The best-studied measures of LV target organ injury are measures of LV structure (LV mass and the relationship of LV wall thickness or mass to LV cavity volume) and systolic function (LV ejection fraction). LV structure is usually stratified into 4 groups on the basis of LV mass (normal or hypertrophied) and relative LV wall thickness (normal or increased). These 4 are as follows: (1) normal geometry with normal LV mass and wall thickness, (2) concentric geometry with normal LV mass and increased LV wall thickness, (3) eccentric LVH with increased LV mass and normal LV wall thickness, and (4) concentric LVH with both increased LV mass and increased relative wall thickness.[369,370]

Key Action Statement 14. Clinicians should not perform electrocardiography in hypertensive children and adolescents being evaluated for LVH (grade B, strong recommendation).

Aggregate Evidence Quality	Grade B (Aggregate of Level of Evidence Equals B Because of Multiple Level of Evidence C References With Similar Findings)
Benefits	Electrocardiography is less expensive than echocardiography or other imaging modalities for identifying LVH
Risks, harm, cost	Electrocardiography has a low sensitivity for detecting LVH
Benefit–harm assessment	The risk of concluding that a child with HTN does not have LVH on the basis of a normal electrocardiogram means that a diagnosis of end organ injury is potentially missed
Intentional vagueness	None
Role of patient preferences	Patients and families may prefer electrocardiography because of cost and convenience, but the sensitivity of the test is poor
Exclusions	None
Strength	Strong recommendation
Key references	1,355–360

The American Society of Echocardiography recommendations should be followed with regard to image acquisition and LV measurement for calculating LV ejection fraction, mass, and relative wall thickness.[369,371] LV ejection fraction may be significantly decreased in severe or acute onset HTN with associated congestive heart failure.[1] Rarely, LV ejection fraction may be mildly depressed in chronic HTN.

Because the heart increases in size in relation to body size, indexing LV mass is required.[361] Indexing LV mass is particularly important in infants and younger children because of their rapid growth.[372,373] Physical training increases LV mass in a healthful manner. Lean body mass is more strongly associated with LV mass than fat mass.[370] Because body composition is not routinely measured clinically, surrogate formulae for indexing are required. It is unclear whether expected values for LV mass should be derived from reference populations of normal weight and normotensive children or should include normotensive children who have overweight or obesity. The best method for indexing LV mass in children is an area of active investigation.

For this document, the following definitions for LV target organ injury have been chosen regarding hypertrophy, relative wall thickness, and ejection fraction. These definitions are based on published guidelines from the American Society of Echocardiography and associations of thresholds for indexed LV mass with adverse outcomes in adults[362,363,369]:

- LVH is defined as LV mass >51 g/m$^{2.7}$ or LV mass >115 g per body surface area (BSA) for boys and LV mass >95 g/BSA for girls. (Note that the values for LVH are well above the 95th percentile for distributions of LV mass in children and adolescents.[369] The clinical significance of values between the

95th percentile of a population-based distribution and these thresholds is uncertain[372]);

- An LV relative wall thickness >0.42 cm indicates concentric geometry. LV wall thickness >1.4 cm is abnormal[373]; and
- Decreased LV ejection fraction is a value <53%.

There are a number of additional evidence gaps related to the echocardiographic assessment of LV target organ injury. The value of LV mass assessment in risk reclassification independent of conventional risk assessment has not been established in adults.[364] The costs and benefits of incorporation of echocardiography into HTN care has not been assessed. Quality control regarding reproducibility of measurements across laboratories may be suboptimal.[374] The most accurate method to measure LV mass (M-mode; two-dimensional; or, in the near future, three-dimensional techniques) requires further research.

Key Action Statement 15

1. It is recommended that echocardiography be performed to assess for cardiac target organ damage (LV mass, geometry, and function) at the time of consideration of pharmacologic treatment of HTN;
2. LVH should be defined as LV mass >51 g/m$^{2.7}$ (boys and girls) for children and adolescents older than 8 years and defined by LV mass >115 g/BSA for boys and LV mass >95 g/BSA for girls;
3. Repeat echocardiography may be performed to monitor improvement or progression of target organ damage at 6- to 12-month intervals. Indications to repeat echocardiography include persistent HTN despite treatment, concentric LV hypertrophy, or reduced LV ejection fraction; and
4. In patients without LV target organ injury at initial echocardiographic assessment, repeat echocardiography at yearly intervals may be considered in those with stage 2 HTN, secondary HTN, or chronic stage 1 HTN incompletely treated (noncompliance or drug resistance) to assess for the development of worsening LV target organ injury (grade C, moderate recommendation).

TABLE 16 DASH Diet Recommendations

Food	Servings per Day
Fruits and vegetables	4–5
Low-fat milk products	≥2
Whole grains	6
Fish, poultry, and lean red meats	≤2
Legumes and nuts	1
Oils and fats	2–3
Added sugar and sweets (including sweetened beverages)	≤1
Dietary sodium	<2300 mg per d

Adapted from Barnes TL, Crandell JL, Bell RA, Mayer-Davis EJ, Dabelea D, Liese AD. Change in DASH diet score and cardiovascular risk factors in youth with type 1 and type 2 diabetes mellitus: the SEARCH for Diabetes in Youth study. *Nutr Diabetes.* 2013;3:e91; US Department of Health and Human Services, US Department of Agriculture. Appendix 7. Nutritional goals for age-sex groups based on dietary reference intakes and dietary guidelines recommendations. In: *2015-2020 Dietary Guidelines for Americans.* Washington, DC: US Department of Health and Human Services, US Department of Agriculture; 2015; and Expert Panel on Integrated Guidelines for Cardiovascular Health and Risk Reduction in Children and Adolescents; National Heart, Lung, and Blood Institute. Expert Panel on Integrated Guidelines for Cardiovascular Health and Risk Reduction in Children and Adolescents: Summary Report. *Pediatrics.* 2011;128 (suppl 5): S213–S256.

6.7 Vascular Structure and Function

Emerging data demonstrate an association of higher levels of BP in youth with adverse changes in measures of vascular structure and function, including ultrasonography of the cIMT, PWV, a robust measure of central arterial stiffness[66] that is related to hard CV events in adults

Key Action Statement 15. It is recommended that echocardiography be performed to assess for cardiac target organ damage (LV mass, geometry, and function) at the time of consideration of pharmacologic treatment of HTN;

LVH should be defined as LV mass >51 g/m2.7 (boys and girls) for children and adolescents older than 8 years and defined by LV mass >115 g/BSA for boys and LV mass >95 g/BSA for girls;

Repeat echocardiography may be performed to monitor improvement or progression of target organ damage at 6- to 12-month intervals. Indications to repeat echocardiography include persistent HTN despite treatment, concentric LV hypertrophy, or reduced LV ejection fraction; and

In patients without LV target organ injury at initial echocardiographic assessment, repeat echocardiography at yearly intervals may be considered in those with stage 2 HTN, secondary HTN, or chronic stage 1 HTN incompletely treated (noncompliance or drug resistance) to assess for the development of worsening LV target organ injury (grade C, moderate recommendation).

Aggregate Evidence Quality	Grade C
Benefits	Severe LV target organ damage can only be identified with LV imaging. May improve risk stratification
Risks, harm, cost	Adds cost; improvement in outcomes from incorporating echocardiography into clinical care is not established
Benefit–harm assessment	Benefits exceed harms
Intentional vagueness	None
Role of patient preferences	Patients may elect to not to have the study
Exclusions	None
Strength	Moderate recommendation
Key references	361,363,364,367–369

(eg, stroke, myocardial infarction, etc),[69] and FMD, which assesses endothelial function and describes the ability of the endothelium to release nitric oxide in response to stress.[375]

Although there are multiple large studies of PWV in youth,[376–381] they all suffer from notable limitations, primarily the lack of racial and ethnic diversity and differences in measurement devices and protocols. Researchers in the largest study of PWV in youth to date (N = 6576) only evaluated 10 and 11 year olds and measured only carotid-radial PWV across the arm; this measure has not been linked to CV events in adults.[382] Researchers in one large study of FMD performed in youth (N = 5809) only included 10- to 11-year-old children in England.[382] The largest set of data for cIMT included 1155 European youth who were 6 to 18 years of age.[383] No racial and ethnic breakdown was provided for this study. The wide heterogeneity in the methods for cIMT measurement hinders the pooling of data. For instance, researchers in the aforementioned article only measured common carotid,[383] although the bulb and internal carotid are the sites of earliest atherosclerotic disease.[384]

Many studies have had significant issues related to methodology. For example, carotid-femoral PWV is not measured identically with different devices and is not equivalent to other measures of PWV, such as brachial-femoral PWV.[385,386] No direct comparisons have been made between carotid-femoral and brachial-ankle PWV, methods in which brachial-ankle PWV provide values considerably higher than carotid-femoral PWV.[378] The brachial-ankle PWV measures stiffness along both a central elastic artery (aorta) and the medium muscular arteries of the leg.

Therefore, insufficient normative data are available to define clinically actionable cut-points between normal and abnormal for these vascular parameters. The routine measurement of vascular structure and function to stratify risk in hypertensive youth cannot be recommended at this time.

6.8 Imaging for Renovascular Disease

There are no evidence-based criteria for the identification of children and adolescents who may be more likely to have RAS. Some experts will do a more extensive evaluation for RAS in children and adolescents with stage 2 HTN, those with significant diastolic HTN (especially on ABPM), those with HTN and hypokalemia on screening laboratories, and those with a notable size discrepancy between the kidneys on standard ultrasound imaging. Bruits over the renal arteries are also suggestive of RAS but are not always present. Consultation with a subspecialist is recommended to help decide which patients warrant further investigation and to aid in the selection of the appropriate imaging modality.

6.8a Renal Ultrasonography

The utility of Doppler renal ultrasonography as a noninvasive screening study for the identification of RAS in children and adolescents has been examined in at least 2 recent case series; sensitivity has been reported to be 64% to 90%, with a specificity of 68% to 70%.[387,388] In another study that included both children and adults, sensitivity and specificity for the detection of renal artery stenoses was 75% and 89%, respectively.[389] Factors that may affect the accuracy of Doppler ultrasonography include patient cooperation, the technician's experience, the age of the child, and the child's BMI. Best results are obtained in older (≥8 years),[388] nonobese (BMI ≤85th percentile), cooperative children and adolescents who are examined in a facility with extensive pediatric vascular imaging experience. Doppler ultrasonography should probably not be obtained in patients who do not meet these criteria or in facilities that lack appropriate pediatric experience.

Key Action Statement 16

Doppler renal ultrasonography may be used as a noninvasive screening study for the evaluation of possible RAS in normal-weight children and adolescents ≥8 years of age who are suspected of having renovascular HTN and who will cooperate with the procedure (grade C, moderate recommendation).

6.8b Computed Tomographic Angiography, Magnetic Resonance Angiography, and Renography

Other noninvasive imaging studies that have been assessed for their ability to identify RAS include computed tomographic angiography (CTA), magnetic resonance angiography (MRA), and nuclear medicine studies. Each of these

Key Action Statement 16. Doppler renal ultrasonography may be used as a noninvasive screening study for the evaluation of possible RAS in normal-weight children and adolescents ≥8 years of age who are suspected of having renovascular HTN and who will cooperate with the procedure (grade C, moderate recommendation).

Aggregate Evidence Quality	Grade C
Benefits	Avoidance of complications of invasive procedure (angiography) or radiation from traditional or computed tomography angiography
Risks, harm, cost	Potential false-positive or false-negative results
Benefit–harm assessment	Potential for avoidance of an invasive procedure outweighs risk of false-negative or false-positive results
Intentional vagueness	None
Role of patient preferences	None
Exclusions	Children and adolescents without suspected renovascular HTN
Strength	Moderate recommendation
Key references	387–390

TABLE 17 Dosing Recommendations for the Initial Prescription of Antihypertensive Drugs for Outpatient Management of Chronic HTN

Drug	Age	Initial Dose	Maximal Dose	Dosing Interval	Formulations
ACE inhibitors					
Contraindications: pregnancy, angioedema					
Common adverse effects: cough, headache, dizziness, asthenia					
Severe adverse effects: hyperkalemia, acute kidney injury, angioedema, fetal toxicity					
Benazepril	≥6 y[a]	0.2 mg/kg per d (up to 10 mg per d)	0.6 mg/kg per d (up to 40 mg per d)	Daily	Tablet: 5, 10, 20, 40 mg (generic) Extemporaneous liquid: 2 mg/mL
Captopril	Infants	0.05 mg/kg per dose	6 mg/kg per d	Daily to 4 times a day	Tablet: 12.5, 25, 50, 100 mg (generic)
	Children	0.5 mg/kg per dose	6 mg/kg per d	Three times a day	Extemporaneous liquid: 1 mg/mL
Enalapril	≥1 mo[a]	0.08 mg/kg per d (up to 5 mg per d)	0.6 mg/kg per d (up to 40 mg per d)	Daily to twice a day	Tablet: 2.5, 5, 10, 20 mg (generic) Solution: 1 mg/mL
Fosinopril	≥6 y <50 kg	0.1 mg/kg per d (up to 5 mg per d)	40 mg per d	Daily	Tablet: 10, 20, 40 mg (generic)
	≥50 kg[a]	5 mg per d	40 mg per d		
Lisinopril	≥6 y[a]	0.07 mg/kg per d (up to 5 mg per d)	0.6 mg/kg per d (up to 40 mg per d)	Daily	Tablet: 2.5, 5, 10, 20, 30, 40 mg (generic) Solution: 1 mg/mL
Ramipril	—	1.6 mg/m^2 per d	6 mg/m^2 per d	Daily	Capsule: 1.25, 2.5, 5 10 mg (generic)
Quinapril	—	5 mg per d	80 mg per d	Daily	Tablet: 5, 10, 20, 40 mg (generic)
ARBs					
Contraindications: pregnancy					
Common adverse effects: headache, dizziness					
Severe adverse effects: hyperkalemia, acute kidney injury, fetal toxicity					
Candesartan	1–5 y[a]	0.02 mg/kg per d (up to 4 mg per d)	0.4 mg/kg per d (up to 16 mg per d)	Daily to twice a day	Tablet: 4, 8, 16, 32 mg
	≥6 y[a]				Extemporaneous liquid: 1 mg/mL
	<50 kg	4 mg per d	16 mg per d		
	≥50 kg	8 mg per d	32 mg per d		
Irbesartan	6–12 y	75 mg per d	150 mg per d	Daily	Tablet: 75, 150, 300 mg (generic)
	≥13	150 mg per d	300 mg per d		
Losartan	≥6 y[a]	0.7 mg/kg (up to 50 mg)	1.4 mg/kg (up to 100 mg)	Daily	Tablet: 25, 50 100 (generic) Extemporaneous liquid: 2.5 mg/mL
Olmesartan	≥6 y[a]	—	—	Daily	Tablet: 5, 20, 40 mg
	<35 kg	10 mg	20 mg		Extemporaneous liquid: 2 mg/mL
	≥35 kg	20 mg	40 mg		
Valsartan	≥6 y[a]	1.3 mg/kg (up to 40 mg)	2.7 mg/kg (up to 160 mg)	Daily	Tablet: 40, 80, 160, 320 mg (generic) Extemporaneous liquid: 4 mg/mL
Thiazide diuretics					
Contraindications: anuria					
Common adverse effects: dizziness, hypokalemia					
Severe adverse effects: cardiac dysrhythmias, cholestatic jaundice, new onset diabetes mellitus, pancreatitis					
Chlorthalidone	Child	0.3 mg/kg	2 mg/k per d (50 mg)	Daily	Tablet: 25, 50, 100 mg (generic)
Chlorothiazide	Child[a]	10 mg/kg per d	20 mg/kg per d (up to 375 mg per d)	Daily to twice a day	Tablet: 250, 500 mg (generic) Suspension: 250/5 mL Extemporaneous liquid: 1 mg/mL
Hydrochlorothiazide	Child[a]	1 mg/kg per d	2 mg/kg per d (up to 37.5 mg per d)	Daily to twice a day	Tablet: 12.5, 25, 50 mg

TABLE 17 Continued

Drug	Age	Initial Dose	Maximal Dose	Dosing Interval	Formulations
Calcium channel blockers					
Contraindications: hypersensitivity to CCBs					
Common adverse effects: flushing, peripheral edema, dizziness					
Severe adverse effects: angioedema					
Amlodipine	1–5 y	0.1 mg/kg	0.6 mg/kg (up to 5 mg per d)	Daily	Tablet: 2.5, 5,10 mg
	≥6 y[a]	2.5 mg	10 mg		Extemporaneous liquid: 1 mg/mL
Felodipine	≥6 y	2.5 mg	10 mg	Daily	Tablet (extended release): 2.5,5,10 mg (generic)
Isradipine	Child	0.05–0.1 mg/kg	0.6 mg/kg (up to 10 mg per d)	Capsule: twice daily to 3 times a day; extended-release tablet: daily	Capsule: 2.5, 5 mg Extended-release tablet: 5, 10 mg
Nifedipine extended release	Child	0.2–0.5 mg/kg per d	3 mg/kg/d (up to 120 mg per d)	Daily to twice a day	Tablet (extended-release): 30, 60, 90 mg (generic)

—, not applicable.
[a] FDA pediatric labeling.

has been compared with the gold standard, renal arteriography. CTA and MRA have generally been found to be acceptable as noninvasive imaging modalities for the identification of hemodynamically significant vascular stenosis. One study that included both pediatric and adult patients showed that the sensitivity and specificity for the detection of RAS was 94% and 93% for CTA and 90% and 94% for MRA, respectively.[389]

Unfortunately, studies of either technique that include only pediatric patients are limited at best for CTA and are nonexistent for MRA. Despite this, expert opinion holds that either modality may be used for noninvasive screening for suspected RAS, but neither is a substitute for angiography.[390] CTA typically involves significant radiation exposure, and MRA generally requires sedation or anesthesia in young children, which are factors that must be considered when deciding to use one of these modalities.

Nuclear renography is based on the principle that after the administration of an agent affecting the renin-angiotensin-aldosterone system (RAAS), there will be reduced blood flow to a kidney or kidney segment affected by hemodynamically significant RAS. Such reduced blood flow can be detected by a comparison of perfusion before and after the administration of the RAAS agent. Limited pediatric nuclear renography studies exist that show variable sensitivity and specificity, ranging from 48% to 85.7% and 73% to 92.3%, respectively.[391–393] The utility of nuclear renography may be less in children then adults because children with RAS often have more complicated vascular abnormalities than adults.[394] Given these issues, nuclear renography has generally been abandoned as a screening test for RAS in children and adolescents.[390]

Key Action Statement 17

In children and adolescents suspected of having RAS, either CTA or MRA may be performed as a noninvasive imaging study. Nuclear renography is less useful in pediatrics and should generally be avoided (grade D, weak recommendation).

6.9 Uric Acid

Cross-sectional data have suggested a relationship between elevated serum uric acid (UA) levels and HTN. Two recent studies of adolescents included in NHANES 1999–2000 and a small study conducted in Italy found that elevated UA levels were associated with higher BP.[395–397] In the Italian study and in another US study of youth with obesity and HTN,[397,398] elevated UA was also associated with other markers of CV risk. These findings suggest that the measurement of UA levels may best be viewed as 1 component of CV risk assessment, especially in those with obesity.

A causative role for elevated UA in the development of childhood HTN has not been definitively established, although recent studies suggest that it may be on the causal pathway. A longitudinal study in which researchers followed a group of children for an average of 12 years demonstrated that childhood UA levels were associated with adult BP levels even after controlling for baseline BP.[399] A few small, single-center clinical trials have also shown that lowering UA can decrease BP levels, and increased UA levels blunt the efficacy of lifestyle modifications on BP control.[400–404] No large-scale, multicenter study has yet been conducted to confirm these preliminary findings. Hence, there is currently not sufficient evidence to support the routine measurement of serum UA in the evaluation and management of children with elevated BP.

6.10 Microalbuminuria

Microalbuminuria (MA), which should be differentiated from proteinuria in CKD, has been shown to be a marker of HTN-related kidney injury and a predictor of CVD in adults.[405–408] MA has been shown to be effectively reduced via the use of ARBs and ACE inhibitors in adults. Lowering the degree of MA in adults has been associated with decreased CVD risk.

In contrast, data to support a clear relationship between HTN and MA in pediatric patients with primary HTN are limited.[408–410] A single, retrospective study of children with primary HTN and WCH found that 20% of the former had MA versus 0% of the latter.[411] MA appears to be a nonspecific finding in children that can occur in the absence of HTN; it can occur in children who have obesity, insulin resistance, diabetes, dyslipidemia, and even in those who have recently participated in vigorous physical activity.[412] The previously mentioned study by Seeman et al[411] did not control for these potential confounders.

Limited, single-center data suggest that a reduction in the degree of MA, more than a reduction in BMI or SBP, is associated with a decrease in LVMI. In particular, researchers in this single-center, nonrandomized, prospective study of 64 hypertensive children without kidney disease who were 11 to 19 years of age evaluated the children at baseline and after 12 months of combination ACE and hydrochlorothiazide ($N = 59$) or ACE, hydrochlorothiazide, and ARB therapy ($N = 5$). Results found that lowering MA in children is associated with a regression of LVH.[413] Given the single-center design and lack of a control group, however, the applicability of these findings to the general population of children with primary HTN is unknown.

Key Action Statement 18

Routine testing for MA is not recommended for children and adolescents with primary HTN (grade C, moderate recommendation).

7. TREATMENT

7.1 Overall Goals

The overall goals for the treatment of HTN in children and adolescents, including both primary and secondary HTN, include achieving a BP level that not only reduces the risk for target organ damage in childhood but also reduces the risk for HTN and related CVD in adulthood. Several studies have shown that currently available treatment options can even reverse target organ damage in hypertensive youth.[105,414,415]

The previous recommendations for HTN treatment target in children without CKD or diabetes were SBP and DBP <95th percentile. Since that recommendation was made, evidence has emerged that markers of target organ damage, such as increased LVMI, can be detected among some

Key Action Statement 17. In children and adolescents suspected of having RAS, either CTA or MRA may be performed as a noninvasive imaging study. Nuclear renography is less useful in pediatrics and should generally be avoided (grade D, weak recommendation).

Aggregate Evidence Quality	Grade D
Benefits	Avoidance of complications of an invasive procedure (angiography)
Risks, harm, cost	Potential false-positive or false-negative results
Benefit–harm assessment	Potential for avoidance of an invasive procedure outweighs risk of false-negative or false-positive results
Intentional vagueness	None
Role of patient preferences	None
Exclusions	Children and adolescents without suspected RAS
Strength	Weak recommendation; pediatric data are limited
Key references	389,390

Key Action Statement 18. Routine testing for MA is not recommended for children and adolescents with primary HTN (grade C, moderate recommendation).

Aggregate Evidence Quality	Grade C
Benefits	Avoid improper detection of MA in children with HTN. Detection of MA is strongly influenced by other factors, such as recent participation in rigorous physical activity, obesity, insulin resistance and diabetes. Hence, there is no clear benefit for testing for MA in the absence of other known comorbidities
Risks, harm, cost	No known risks given a lack of clear association between MA and primary HTN in children
Benefit–harm assessment	Limited data to support any real benefit for screening children for MA
Intentional vagueness	Screening of children with primary HTN versus screening of children with single kidney or CKD and HTN
Role of patient preferences	Unknown
Exclusions	None
Strength	Moderate recommendation
Key references	408,410,411,413

children with BP >90th percentile (or >120/80 mm Hg) but <95th percentile.[66,416,417] Longitudinal studies on BP from childhood to adulthood that include indirect measures of CV injury indicate that the risk for subsequent CVD in early adulthood increases as the BP level in adolescence exceeds 120/80 mm Hg.[11,103,418] In addition, there is some evidence that targeting a BP <90th percentile results in reductions in LVMI and prevalence of LVH.[104] Therefore, an optimal BP level to be achieved with treatment of childhood HTN is <90th percentile or <130/80 mm Hg, whichever is lower.

Treatment and management options are discussed below, including lifestyle modifications and pharmacologic therapy to achieve optimal BP levels in children and adolescents with HTN.

Key Action Statement 19

In children and adolescents diagnosed with HTN, the treatment goal with nonpharmacologic and pharmacologic therapy should be a reduction in SBP and DBP to <90th percentile and <130/80 mm Hg in adolescents ≥ 13 years old (grade C, moderate recommendation).

7.2 Lifestyle and Nonpharmacologic Interventions

Lifestyle interventions are recommended to lower BP. There is good evidence from studies in adults showing that nutritional interventions lower BP,[419] including clinical trials demonstrating that reducing dietary sodium results in lower BP and CV mortality,[338] and a diet high in olive oil polyphenols lowers BP.[420] Studies of hypertensive youth suggest that the relationship between diet, physical activity, and BP in childhood is similar to that observed in adults.

7.2a Diet

The Dietary Approaches to Stop Hypertension (DASH) approach and specific elements of that diet have been the primary dietary strategy tested in the literature. These elements include a diet that is high in fruits, vegetables, low-fat milk products, whole grains, fish, poultry, nuts, and lean red meats; it also includes a limited intake of sugar and sweets along with lower sodium intake (see Table 16). Cross-sectional studies demonstrate associations between elements of the DASH diet and BP. For example, population-based data from NHANES show correlations between dietary sodium and BP in childhood and elevated BP and HTN, particularly in people with excess weight.[332]

A high intake of fruits, vegetables, and legumes (ie, a plant-strong diet) is associated with lower BP.[421] A lack of fruit consumption in childhood has been linked to increases in cIMT in young adulthood in the Young Finns study.[422] Higher intake of low-fat dairy products has been associated with lower BP in childhood.[423]

Longitudinal, observational, and interventional data also support relationships between diet and BP in youth. The National Heart Lung and Blood Institute's Growth and Health Study, which followed 2185 girls over 10 years, demonstrated that consuming ≥2 servings of dairy and ≥3 servings of fruits and vegetables daily was associated with lower BP in childhood and a 36% lower risk of high BP by young adulthood.[424] Similar associations have been demonstrated in children and adolescents with diabetes.[425] Moreover, an improvement in diet

Key Action Statement 19. In children and adolescents diagnosed with HTN, the treatment goal with nonpharmacologic and pharmacologic therapy should be a reduction in SBP and DBP to <90th percentile and <130/80 mm Hg in adolescents ≥ 13 years old (grade C, moderate recommendation).

Aggregate Evidence Quality	Grade C
Benefits	Lower risk of childhood target organ damage, lower risk of adulthood HTN and CVD
Risk, harm, cost	Risk of drug adverse effects and polypharmacy
Benefit–harm assessment	Preponderance of benefit
Intentional vagueness	None
Role of patient preferences	Patient may have preference for nonpharmacologic or pharmacologic treatment
Exclusions	None
Strength	Moderate recommendation
Key references	11,66,103,104,416–418

led to lower BP in some studies of adolescents with elevated BP,[426] youth with overweight,[427] girls with metabolic syndrome,[428] and youth with T2DM.[429] However, consuming a healthier diet may increase costs.[430]

7.2b Physical Activity

Observational data support a relationship between physical activity and lower BP, although the data are scant.[339] Interventional data demonstrate increasing physical activity leads to lower BP. A review of 9 studies of physical activity interventions in children and adolescents with obesity suggested that 40 minutes of moderate to vigorous, aerobic physical activity at least 3 to 5 days per week improved SBP by an average of 6.6 mm Hg and prevented vascular dysfunction.[340] A number of subsequent, additional studies with small sample sizes support a benefit of physical activity on BP.[341] A more recent analysis of 12 randomized controlled trials including 1266 subjects found reductions of 1% and 3% for resting SBP and DBP, respectively. These results did not reach statistical significance, however, and the authors suggested that longer studies with larger sample sizes are needed.[344] Any type of exercise, whether it's aerobic training, resistance training, or combined training, appears to be beneficial[342] (see "HTN and the Athlete").

Programs that combine diet and physical activity can have a beneficial effect on SBP, as is shown in several studies designed to prevent childhood obesity and address cardiometabolic risk.[431]

Key Action Statement 20

At the time of diagnosis of elevated BP or HTN in a child or adolescent, clinicians should provide advice on the DASH diet and recommend moderate to vigorous physical activity at least 3 to 5 days per week (30–60 minutes per session) to help reduce BP (grade C, weak recommendation).

7.2c Weight Loss and Related CV Risk Factors

As is true for children and adolescents with isolated HTN, a DASH diet[426,432] and vigorous physical activity[431] are recommended in pediatric patients with multiple obesity-related risk factors as part of intensive weight-loss therapy.[433,434] Motivational interviewing (MI) is a tool recommended for pediatricians' use by the AAP Expert Committee Statement on Obesity.[435] MI may be a useful counseling tool to use in combination with other behavioral techniques to address overweight and obesity in children.[436] Studies in hypertensive adults support the use of MI to improve adherence to antihypertensive medications[437] and decrease SBP.[436] Although there are no trials investigating the use of MI in the care of hypertensive youth, a number of studies have shown that MI can be used successfully to address or prevent childhood obesity by promoting physical activity and dietary changes.[438–441] However, other studies have been less promising.[442,443] In addition to the standard lifestyle approaches, intensive weight-loss therapy

TABLE 18 OSAS Symptoms and Signs

History of frequent snoring (≥3 nights per week)
Labored breathing during sleep
Gasps, snorting noises, observed episodes of apnea
Sleep enuresis (especially secondary enuresis)
Sleeping in a seated position or with the neck hyperextended
Cyanosis
Headaches on awakening
Daytime sleepiness
Attention-deficit/hyperactivity disorder
Learning problems
Physical examination
Underweight or overweight
Tonsillar hypertrophy
Adenoidal facies
Micrognathia, retrognathia
High-arched palate
Failure to thrive
HTN

Adapted from Marcus CL, Brooks LJ, Draper KA, et al; American Academy of Pediatrics. Diagnosis and management of childhood obstructive sleep apnea syndrome. *Pediatrics*. 2012;130(3). Available at: www.pediatrics.org/cgi/content/full/130/3/e714.

Key Action Statement 20. At the time of diagnosis of elevated BP or HTN in a child or adolescent, clinicians should provide advice on the DASH diet and recommend moderate to vigorous physical activity at least 3 to 5 days per week (30–60 minutes per session) to help reduce BP (grade C, weak recommendation).

Aggregate Evidence Quality	Grade C
Benefits	Potential to reduce BP
Risk, harm, cost	No or low potential for harm. Following a healthier diet may increase costs to patients and families
Benefit–harm assessment	Potential benefit outweighs lack of harm and minimal cost
Intentional vagueness	None
Role of patient preferences	Level of caregiver and patient concern may influence adoption of the DASH diet and physical activity. Patients may also have preferences around the use of a medication. These factors may influence the efficacy of lifestyle change
Exclusions	None
Strength	Weak recommendation
Key references	332,339–342,424–431

involving regular patient and/or family contact and at least 1 hour of moderate to vigorous physical activity on a daily basis should be offered to children and adolescents with obesity and HTN.[444]

7.2d Stress Reduction

Complimentary medicine interventions have shown some promise in studies in normotensive children and adolescents and in those with elevated BP. Breathing-awareness meditation, a component of the Mindfulness-Based Stress Reduction Program at the University of Massachusetts Memorial Medical Center,[445] led to a reduction in daytime, nighttime, and 24-hour SBP (3–4 mm Hg) and DPB (1 mm Hg) in normotensive African American adolescents and African American adolescents with elevated BP.[446] Another study of transcendental meditation showed no significant BP effect but did lead to a decrease in LVM in African American adolescents with elevated BP.[447] Scant data suggest yoga may also be helpful.[448]

7.3 Pharmacologic Treatment

Children who remain hypertensive despite a trial of lifestyle modifications or who have symptomatic HTN, stage 2 HTN without a clearly modifiable factor (eg, obesity), or any stage of HTN associated with CKD or diabetes mellitus therapy should be initiated with a single medication at the low end of the dosing range (see Table 17). Depending on repeated BP measurements, the dose of the initial medication can be increased every 2 to 4 weeks until BP is controlled (eg, <90th percentile), the maximal dose is reached, or adverse effects occur. Although the dose can be titrated every 2 to 4 weeks using home BP measurements, the patient should be seen every 4 to 6 weeks until BP has normalized. If BP is not controlled with a single agent, a second agent can be added to the regimen and titrated as with the initial drug. Because of the salt and water retention that occurs with many antihypertensive medications, a thiazide diuretic is often the preferred second agent.

Lifestyle modifications should be continued in children requiring pharmacologic therapy. An ongoing emphasis on a healthy, plant-strong diet rich in fruits and vegetables; reduced sodium intake; and increased exercise can improve the effectiveness of antihypertensive medications. The use of a combination product as initial treatment has been studied only for bisoprolol and hydrochlorothiazide,[449] so the routine use of combination products to initiate treatment in children cannot be recommended. Once BP control has been achieved, a combination product can be considered as a means to improve adherence and reduce cost if the dose and formulation are appropriate.

7.3a Pharmacologic Treatment and Pediatric Exclusivity Studies

Studies completed in hypertensive children show that antihypertensive drugs decrease BP with few adverse effects.[173,202,242–244,450–467] There are few studies in children in which researchers compare different antihypertensive agents.[453] These studies do not show clinically significant differences in the degree of BP lowering between agents. There are no clinical trials in children that have CV end points as outcomes. Long-term studies on the safety of antihypertensive medications in children and their impact on future CVD are limited.[455]

Because of legislative acts that provide incentives and mandates for drug manufacturers to complete pediatric assessments,[468] most of the newer antihypertensive medications have undergone some degree of efficacy and safety evaluation. Antihypertensive drugs without patent protection have not been, and are unlikely to be, studied in children despite their continued widespread use.[238]

7.3b Pharmacologic Treatment: Choice of Agent

Pharmacologic treatment of HTN in children and adolescents should be initiated with an ACE inhibitor, ARB,[469] long-acting calcium channel blocker, or a thiazide diuretic. Because African American children may not have as robust a response to ACE inhibitors,[470,471] a higher initial dose for the ACE inhibitor may be considered; alternatively, therapy may be initiated with a thiazide diuretic or long-acting calcium channel blocker. In view of the expanded adverse effect profile and lack of association in adults with improved outcomes compared with other agents, β-blockers are not recommended as initial treatment in children. ACE inhibitors and ARBs are contraindicated in pregnancy because these agents can cause injury and death to the developing fetus. Adolescents of childbearing potential should be informed of the potential risks of these agents on the developing fetus; alternative medications (eg, calcium channel blocker, β-blocker) can be considered when appropriate.

In children with HTN and CKD, proteinuria, or diabetes mellitus, an ACE inhibitor or ARB is recommended as the initial antihypertensive agent unless there is an absolute contraindication. Other antihypertensive medications (eg, α-blockers, β-blockers, combination α- and β-blockers, centrally acting agents, potassium-sparing diuretics, and direct vasodilators) should be reserved for children who are not responsive to 2 or more of the preferred agents (see "Treatment in CKD").

Key Action Statement 21

In hypertensive children and adolescents who have failed lifestyle modifications (particularly those

TABLE 19 Oral and Intravenous Antihypertensive Medications for Acute Severe HTN

Drug	Class	Dose	Route	Comments
Useful for Severely Hypertensive Patients With Life-Threatening Symptoms				
Esmolol	β-adrenergic blocker	100–500 mcg/kg per min	Intravenous infusion	Short acting, constant infusion preferred. May cause profound bradycardia
Hydralazine	Direct vasodilator	0.1–0.2 mg/kg per dose up to 0.4 mg/kg per dose	Intravenous, intramuscular	Causes tachycardia Give every 4 h when given intravenous bolus
Labetalol	α- and β-adrenergic blocker	Bolus: 0.20–1.0 mg/kg per dose up to 40 mg per dose Infusion: 0.25–3.0 mg/kg per h	Intravenous bolus or infusion	Asthma and overt heart failure are relative contraindications
Nicardipine	Calcium channel blocker	Bolus: 30 mcg/kg up to 2 mg per dose Infusion: 0.5–4 mcg/kg per min	Intravenous bolus or infusion	May cause reflex tachycardia. Increases cyclosporine and tacrolimus levels
Sodium nitroprusside	Direct vasodilator	Starting: 0–3 mcg/kg per min Maximum: 10 mcg/kg per min	Intravenous infusion	Monitor cyanide levels with prolonged (>72 h) use or in renal failure; or coadminister with sodium thiosulfate
Useful for Severely Hypertensive Patients With Less Significant Symptoms				
Clonidine	Central α-agonist	2–5 mcg/kg per dose up to 10 mcg/kg per dose given every 6–8 h	Oral	Adverse effects include dry mouth and drowsiness
Fenoldopam	Dopamine receptor agonist	0.2–0.5 mcg/kg per min up to 0.8 mcg/kg per min	Intravenous infusion	Higher doses worsen tachycardia without further reducing BP
Hydralazine	Direct vasodilator	0.25 mg/kg per dose up to 25 mg per dose given every 6–8 h	Oral	Half-life varies with genetically determined acetylation rates
Isradipine	Calcium channel blocker	0.05–0.1 mg/kg per dose up to 5 mg per dose given every 6–8 h	Oral	Exaggerated decrease in BP can be seen in patients receiving azole antifungal agents
Minoxidil	Direct vasodilator	0.1–0.2 mg/kg per dose up to 10 mg per dose given Q 8–12 h	Oral	Most potent oral vasodilator, long acting

who have LV hypertrophy on echocardiography, symptomatic HTN, or stage 2 HTN without a clearly modifiable factor [eg, obesity]), clinicians should initiate pharmacologic treatment with an ACE inhibitor, ARB, long-acting calcium channel blocker, or thiazide diuretic (grade B, moderate recommendation).

7.3c Treatment: Follow-Up and Monitoring

Treatment of a child or adolescent with HTN requires ongoing monitoring because goal BP can be difficult to achieve.[472] If the decision has been made to initiate treatment with medication, the patient should be seen frequently (every 4–6 weeks) for dose adjustments and/or addition of a second or third agent until goal BP has been achieved (see the preceding section). After that, the frequency of visits can be extended to every 3 to 4 months.

If the decision has been made to proceed with lifestyle changes only, then follow-up visits can occur at longer intervals (every 3–6 months) so that adherence to lifestyle change can be reinforced and the need for initiation of medication can be reassessed.

In patients treated with antihypertensive medications, home BP measurement is frequently used to get a better assessment of BP control (see "At-Home Measurement"). Repeat ABPM may also be used to assess BP control and is especially important in patients with CKD (see "Treatment: Use of ABPM and Assessment").

At each follow-up visit, the patient should be assessed for adherence to prescribed therapy and for any adverse effects of the prescribed medication; such assessment may include laboratory testing depending on the medication (for example, electrolyte monitoring if the patient is on a diuretic). It is also important to continually reinforce adherence

Key Action Statement 21. In hypertensive children and adolescents who have failed lifestyle modifications (particularly those who have LV hypertrophy on echocardiography, symptomatic HTN, or stage 2 HTN without a clearly modifiable factor [eg, obesity]), clinicians should initiate pharmacologic treatment with an ACE inhibitor, ARB, long-acting calcium channel blocker, or thiazide diuretic (grade B, moderate recommendation).

Aggregate Evidence Quality	Grade B
Benefits	Potential prevention of progressive CVD; regression or avoidance of target organ damage; resolution of hypertensive symptoms; improved cognition; avoidance of worsening HTN; potential avoidance of stroke, heart failure, coronary artery disease, kidney failure
Risks, harm, cost	Potential for hypotension, financial cost, chronic medication treatment, adverse medication effects, impact on insurability (health and life)
Benefit–harm assessment	Preponderance of benefits over harms
Intentional vagueness	None
Role of patient preferences	The choice of which antihypertensive medication to use should be made in close discussion with the patient and parent regarding risk, benefits, and adverse effects
Exclusions	None
Strength	Moderate recommendation
Key references	452,455,467

to lifestyle changes because effective treatment will depend on the combination of effects from both medication and lifestyle measures. Finally, known hypertensive target organ damage (such as LVH) should be reassessed according to the recommendations in "Imaging Evaluation, Echocardiography: Coarctation of the Aorta and Detection of Target Organ Damage."

7.3d Treatment: Use of ABPM to Assess Treatment

ABPM can be an objective method to evaluate treatment effect during antihypertensive drug therapy. Data obtained in a multicenter, single-blind, crossover study in which hypertensive children received a placebo or no treatment demonstrated no change in ABPM after receiving the placebo.[473] A report from a single center found that among hypertensive children receiving antihypertensive drugs, BP data from ABPM resulted in medication changes in 63% of patients.[474] Another study of 38 hypertensive children used ABPM to evaluate the effectiveness of antihypertensive therapy (nonpharmacologic and pharmacologic). After 1 year of treatment, ABPM results indicated that treatment-goal BP was achieved in only one-third of children with HTN.[17]

Key Action Statement 22

ABPM may be used to assess treatment effectiveness in children and adolescents with HTN, especially when clinic and/or home BP measurements indicate insufficient BP response to treatment (grade B, moderate recommendation).

7.4 Treatment-Resistant HTN

Resistant HTN in adults is defined as persistently elevated BP despite treatment with 3 or more antihypertensive agents of different classes. All of these drugs should be prescribed at maximally effective doses, and at least 1 should be a diuretic. Key to the identification of patients with true resistant HTN is correct office BP measurement, confirmation of adherence to current therapy, and confirmation of treatment resistance by ABPM.

The treatment of patients with resistant HTN includes dietary sodium restriction, the elimination of substances known to elevate BP, the identification of previously undiagnosed secondary causes of HTN, the optimization of current therapy, and the addition of additional agents as needed.[475] Recent clinical trial data suggest that an aldosterone receptor antagonist (such as spironolactone) is the optimal additional agent in adults with resistant HTN; it helps address volume excess as well as untreated hyperaldosteronism, which is common in adult patients with true resistant HTN.[476,477]

At present, there are no data on whether true treatment-resistant HTN exists in pediatric patients. Evaluation and management strategies similar to those proven effective in adults with resistant HTN would be reasonable in children and adolescents who present with apparent treatment resistance.

Key Action Statement 22. ABPM may be used to assess treatment effectiveness in children and adolescents with HTN, especially when clinic and/or home BP measurements indicate insufficient BP response to treatment (grade B, moderate recommendation).

Aggregate Evidence Quality	Grade B
Benefits	ABPM results can guide adjustment in medication. ABPM can facilitate achieving treatment-goal BP levels
Risks, harm, cost	Inconvenience and patient annoyance in wearing an ABPM monitor. Cost of ABPM monitors
Benefit–harm assessment	Overall benefit
Intentional vagueness	None
Role of patient preferences	Patients may choose not to wear the ambulatory BP monitor repeatedly, which may necessitate alternative approaches to evaluate treatment efficacy
Exclusions	Uncomplicated HTN with satisfactory BP control
Strength	Moderate recommendation
Key references	17,474,475

8. TREATMENT IN SPECIAL POPULATIONS

8.1 Treatment in Patients With CKD and Proteinuria

8.1a CKD

Children and adolescents with CKD often present with or develop HTN.[478] HTN is a known risk factor for the progression of kidney disease in adults and children.[173,479,480] Evidence suggests that the treatment of HTN in children with CKD might slow the progression of or reverse end organ damage.[173,415] When evaluated by 24-hour ABPM, children and adolescents with CKD often have poor BP control even if BP measured in the clinic appears to be normal.[48] MH is associated with end organ damage, such as LVH.[203,481] Threshold values that define HTN are not different in children with CKD, although there is some evidence that lower treatment goals might improve outcomes.

In the European Effect of Strict Blood Pressure Control and ACE-Inhibition on Progression of Chronic Renal Failure in Pediatric Patients study, researchers randomly assigned children with CKD to standard antihypertensive therapy (with a treatment goal of 24-hour MAP <90th percentile by ABPM) or to intensive BP control (24-hour MAP <50th percentile by ABPM). The study demonstrated fewer composite CKD outcomes in children with the lower BP target.[173] Recent adult data from the Systolic Blood Pressure Intervention Trial suggest lower BP targets may be beneficial in preventing other, adverse CV outcomes as well.[482]

Key Action Statement 23

1. Children and adolescents with CKD should be evaluated for HTN at each medical encounter;
2. Children or adolescents with both CKD and HTN should be treated to lower 24-hour MAP to <50th percentile by ABPM; and
3. Regardless of apparent control of BP with office measures, children and adolescents with CKD and a history of HTN should have BP assessed by ABPM at least yearly to screen for MH (grade B; strong recommendation).

8.1b Proteinuria

Proteinuric renal disease is often associated with HTN and a rapid decline in glomerular filtration.[483] Studies in both adults and children have indicated that both BP control and a reduction in proteinuria are beneficial for preserving renal function. Researchers in multiple studies have evaluated the utility of RAAS blockade therapy in patients with CKD and HTN.[452,464,465,484–487] These medications have been shown to benefit both BP and proteinuria.

The benefit of such therapies may not be sustained, however.[173,488] The Effect of Strict Blood Pressure Control and ACE-Inhibition on Progression of Chronic Renal Failure in Pediatric Patients study demonstrated an initial 50% reduction in proteinuria in children with CKD after treatment with ramipril but with a rebound effect after 36 months.[450,464,488] This study also showed that BP reduction with a ramipril-based antihypertensive regimen improved renal outcomes. In children with HTN related to underlying CKD, the assessment of proteinuria and institution of RAAS blockade therapy appears to have important prognostic implications.

Key Action Statement 24

Children and adolescents with CKD and HTN should be evaluated for proteinuria (grade B, strong recommendation).

Key Action Statement 25

Children and adolescents with CKD, HTN, and proteinuria should be treated with an ACE inhibitor or ARB (grade B, strong recommendation).

Key Action Statement 23. Children and adolescents with CKD should be evaluated for HTN at each medical encounter;

Children or adolescents with both CKD and HTN should be treated to lower 24-hour MAP to <50th percentile by ABPM; and

Regardless of apparent control of BP with office measures, children and adolescents with CKD and a history of HTN should have BP assessed by ABPM at least yearly to screen for MH (grade B; strong recommendation).

Aggregate Evidence Quality	Grade B
Benefits	Control of BP in children and adolescents with CKD has been shown to decrease CKD progression and lead to resolution of LVH
Risks, harm, cost	Cost of ABPM and BP control, both financial and nonfinancial
Benefit–harm assessment	Benefits of BP control in patients with CKD outweigh treatment risks
Intentional vagueness	Threshold
Role of patient preferences	Patients may not want to wear the ambulatory BP monitor repeatedly, which should lead to detailed counseling regarding the benefits of this procedure in CKD
Exclusions	None
Strength	Strong recommendation
Key references	47,173,203,415,480–483

8.2. Treatment in Patients With Diabetes

Based on the Fourth Report criteria for the diagnosis of HTN,[1] between 4% and 16% of children and adolescents with T1DM are found to have HTN.[14,489–491] In the SEARCH study of 3691 youth between the ages of 3 and 17 years, elevated BP was documented in 6% of children with T1DM, with the highest prevalence in Asian Pacific Islander and American Indian children followed by African American and Hispanic children and those with higher glycosylated hemoglobin A1c levels.[14] An office-based study in Australia found much higher rates (16%) and a positive correlation with BMI.[490] BP >130/90 mm Hg has been associated with a more-than-fourfold increase in the relative risk of coronary artery disease and mortality at 10-year follow-up of individuals with T1DM.[492]

The prevalence of HTN is higher in youth with T2DM compared with T1DM, ranging from 12% at baseline (*N* = 699) in the Treatment Options for Type 2 Diabetes in Adolescents and Youth study[493] to 31% (*N* = 598) in the Pediatric Diabetes Consortium Type 2 Diabetes Clinic Registry.[494] BP and arterial stiffness in cohort studies have correlated with BMI, male sex, African American race, and age of onset of diabetes.[14,494,495] Unlike T1DM, HTN in T2DM is not correlated with glycosylated hemoglobin A1c levels or glycemic failure, and it develops early in the course of the disease.[496] It is also associated with rapid onset of adverse cardiac changes[111,497] and may not respond to diet changes.[425] The concurrence of obesity and T2DM compounds the risks for target end organ damage.[111,498]

Empirical evidence shows a poor awareness of HTN in youth with T1DM and T2DM.[14] Additionally, only a fraction of children with HTN and diabetes were found to be on pharmacologic therapy[14,490,498,499] despite treatment recommendations from the American Diabetes Association,[499] the International Society for Pediatric and Adolescent Diabetes,[500] AHA,[110] and the National Heart, Lung, and Blood Institute.[501]

Key Action Statement 26

Children and adolescents with T1DM or T2DM should be evaluated for HTN at each medical encounter and treated if BP is ≥95th percentile or >130/80 mm Hg in adolescents ≥13 years of age (grade C, moderate recommendation).

9. COMORBIDITIES

9.1 Comorbidities: Dyslipidemia

Children and adolescents with HTN are at increased risk for lipid disorders attributable to the "common soil" phenomenon,[502] in which poor diet, inactivity, and obesity contribute to both disorders. Some observational pediatric data confirm this association.[503–506] Furthermore, both HTN and dyslipidemias are associated with subclinical atherosclerosis[206] and are risk factors for future CVD.[503] Screening is recommended to identify those at increased risk for early atherosclerosis.[503] Treatment of lipid disorders identified in the setting of HTN should follow existing pediatric lipid guidelines with lifestyle advice, including weight loss and pharmacotherapy, as necessary.[503]

9.2 Comorbidities: OSAS

Children with snoring, daytime sleepiness (in adolescents), or hyperactivity (in younger children) may have OSAS and consequent HTN.[507] The more severe the OSAS, the more likely a child is to have elevated BP[44,45] (see Table 18). Children with moderate to severe OSAS are at increased risk for HTN. However, it is not known whether OSAS treatment with continuous positive airway pressure results in improved BP in all children.[44] Furthermore, adenotonsillectomy may not result in BP improvement in all children with OSAS. In particular, children who have obesity and OSAS may be less likely to experience a lowering of BP after an adenotonsillectomy.[508]

Therefore, children with signs of OSAS (eg, daytime fatigue, snoring, hyperactivity, etc) should undergo evaluation for elevated BP regardless of treatment status. Given that both nighttime and daytime BP is affected by OSAS, the use of ABPM is the recommended method for assessing the BP of children with suspected OSAS.

9.3 Comorbidities: Cognitive Impairment

Data from studies conducted in adults suggest that the central nervous system is a target organ that can be affected by HTN.[419] Preliminary studies suggest that this is true in children as well. Hypertensive children score lower on tests of neurocognition and on parental reports of executive function compared with normotensive controls.[509,510] Adams et al[511] found an increased prevalence of learning disabilities in children with primary HTN compared with normotensive controls. The postulated mechanism for these findings is impaired cerebrovascular reactivity.[512–515] At the present time, these findings do not have specific clinical implications with respect to the diagnostic evaluation of childhood HTN, although they underscore the importance of early detection and treatment.

Key Action Statement 24. Children and adolescents with CKD and HTN should be evaluated for proteinuria (grade B, strong recommendation).

Aggregate Evidence Quality	Grade B
Benefits	Detection of proteinuria among children with CKD and HTN may foster early detection and treatment of children at risk for more advanced renal disease
Risks, harm, cost	Additional testing
Benefit–harm assessment	Benefit of detection of a higher-risk group exceeds the risk of testing
Intentional vagueness	Whether to screen children with HTN without CKD for proteinuria
Role of patient preferences	None
Exclusions	Children without CKD
Strength	Strong recommendation
Key references	47,484

Key Action Statement 25. Children and adolescents with CKD, HTN, and proteinuria should be treated with an ACE inhibitor or ARB (grade B, strong recommendation).

Aggregate Evidence Quality	Grade B
Benefits	ACE inhibitor and ARB therapy has been shown in the short-term to be effective in reducing urine proteinuria
Risks, harm, cost	Positive effect on urine protein concentrations after the receipt of an ACE inhibitor may not be sustained over time
Benefit–harm assessment	Treatment with an ACE inhibitor or ARB may lower the rate of progression of renal disease even if the effect is not sustained in the long-term
Intentional vagueness	Whether to aggressively treat the BP so that it is <90th percentile
Role of patient preferences	Patients may have concerns about the choice of medication, which should be addressed
Exclusions	Children without CKD
Strength	Strong recommendation
Key references	173,464,465,485,487,488

Key Action Statement 26. Children and adolescents with T1DM or T2DM should be evaluated for HTN at each medical encounter and treated if BP is ≥95th percentile or >130/80 mm Hg in adolescents ≥13 years of age (grade C, moderate recommendation).

Aggregate Evidence Quality	Grade C
Benefits	Early detection and treatment of HTN in children with T1DM and T2DM may reduce future CV and kidney disease
Risks, harm, cost	Risk of drug adverse effects and polypharmacy
Benefit–harm assessment	Preponderance of benefit
Intentional vagueness	None
Role of patient preferences	Family concerns about additional testing and/or medication may need to be addressed
Exclusions	None
Strength	Weak to moderate recommendation
Key references	14,110,111,494

10. SEX, RACIAL, AND ETHNIC DIFFERENCES IN BP AND MEDICATION CHOICE

BP differences between various ethnic groups are well described in the adult population.[216,516] Large, cross-sectional studies have demonstrated that, per capita, minority ethnic groups have both a higher prevalence of HTN and more significant end organ damage and outcomes.[517,518] Although a growing body of evidence indicates that racial and ethnic differences in BP appear during adolescence,[519–521] the cause of these differences and when they develop in childhood are yet to be fully determined. The risk of HTN correlates more with obesity status than with ethnicity or race, although there may be some interaction.[216] At this time, although limited data suggest that there may be a racial difference in response to ACE inhibitors in the pediatric age group,[471] the strength of available evidence is insufficient to recommend using racial, sex, or ethnic factors to inform the evaluation or management of HTN in children.

11. SPECIAL POPULATIONS AND SITUATIONS

11.1 Acute Severe HTN

There is a lack of robust evidence to guide the evaluation and management of children and adolescents with acute presentations of severe HTN. Thus, much of what is known is derived from studies conducted in adults, including medication choice.[522] The evidence base has been enhanced somewhat over the past decade by the publication of several pediatric clinical trials and case series of antihypertensive agents that can be used to treat such patients.[465,523–530]

Although children and adolescents can become symptomatic from HTN at lesser degrees of BP elevation, in general, patients who present with acute severe HTN will have BP elevation well above the stage 2 HTN threshold. In a study of 55 children presenting to a pediatric ED in Taiwan with hypertensive crisis, 96% had SBP greater than that of stage 2 HTN, and 76% had DBP greater than that of stage 2 HTN.[531] The major clinical issue in such children is that this level of BP elevation may produce acute target organ effects, including encephalopathy, acute kidney injury, and congestive heart failure. Clinicians should be concerned about the development of these complications when a child's BP increases 30 mm Hg or more above the 95th percentile.

Although a few children with primary HTN may present with features of acute severe HTN,[532] the vast majority will have an underlying secondary cause of HTN.[532,533] Thus, for patients who present with acute severe HTN, an evaluation for secondary causes is appropriate and should be conducted expediently. Additionally, target organ effects should be assessed with renal function, echocardiography, and central nervous system imaging, among others.

Given the potential for the development of potentially life-threatening complications, expert opinion holds that children and adolescents who present with acute severe HTN require immediate treatment with short-acting antihypertensive medications that may abort such sequelae.[533,534] Treatment may be initiated with oral agents if the patient is able to tolerate oral therapy and if

TABLE 20 Comparison of HTN Screening Strategies

Dimension	Option A (Clinic BP Alone)	Option B (Clinic BP Confirmed by ABPM)	Option C (ABPM Only)	Preferred Option	Assumptions Made
Population: 170 cardiology, nephrology referred patients; analyzed at single-patient level	Auscultatory or oscillatory BP >95%	Auscultatory or oscillatory BP >90% then ABPM	Patients referred to provider who only used ABPM	—	—
Operational factors					
Percent adherence to care (goal of 80%)	Assumes 100%	Assumes 100%	Assumes 100%	—	—
Care delivery team effects	Baseline	Additional work to arrange or interpret confirmatory ABPM	Additional work to arrange and interpret ABPM for all patients	—	Assumes ABPM can be arranged and interpreted correctly
Patient, family effects	Baseline	Less desirable to have more visits; more desirable to have better accuracy		Family opinion depends on family's values	—
Benefits					
Clinical significance	Baseline	If HTN, treatment improves long-term outcome	If HTN, treatment improves long-term outcome	C	WCH estimated at 35%, ABPM results in fewer false-positive screening results
Cost of options					
Visit, diagnosis costs (annual estimated cost for 1 patient)	$1860 for visits and laboratory tests	$1330 for visits, ABPM, and laboratory tests	$1880 for visits, ABPM, and laboratory tests	B	—
Costs from complications, adverse events, nonoptimal treatment					
Likelihood of nonoptimal treatment	60% undiagnosed patients; 35% of those diagnosed with WCH	30% undiagnosed patients	All patients correctly diagnosed; fewer complications	C	Assumes treatment benefit for correctly diagnosed HTN has no complications
Costs of nonoptimal treatment	Increased mortality for not treating undiagnosed HTN; inconvenience of treatment of patients with WCH	Increased mortality for not treating undiagnosed HTN	All patients correctly diagnosed who are treated	C	—

—, none.

life-threatening complications have not yet developed. Intravenous agents are indicated when oral therapy is not possible because of the patient's clinical status or when a severe complication has developed (such as congestive heart failure) that warrants a more controlled BP reduction. In such situations, the BP should be reduced by no more than 25% of the planned reduction over the first 8 hours, with the remainder of the planned reduction over the next 12 to 24 hours.[533,534] The ultimate short-term BP goal in such patients should generally be around the 95th percentile. Table 19 lists suggested doses for oral and intravenous antihypertensive medications that may be used to treat patients with acute severe HTN.

Key Action Statement 27

In children and adolescents with acute severe HTN and life-threatening symptoms, immediate treatment with short-acting antihypertensive medication should be initiated, and BP should be reduced by no more than 25% of the planned reduction over the first 8 hours (grade expert opinion D, weak recommendation).

11.2 HTN and the Athlete

Sports participation and increased physical activity should be encouraged in children with HTN. In adults, physical fitness is associated with lower all-cause mortality.[536] Although meta-analyses and randomized controlled trials consistently show lower BP after exercise training in adults,[535] the results are less robust in children.[340] On the basis of this evidence, sports participation should improve BP over time. Additionally, there is evidence that exercise itself has a beneficial effect on cardiac structure in adolescents.[537]

The athlete interested in participating in competitive sports and/or intense training presents a special circumstance. Existing guidelines present conflicting recommendations.[1,538] Although increased LV wall dimension may be a consequence of athletic training,[360] recommendations from AHA and ACC include the following: (1) limiting competitive athletic participation among athletes with LVH beyond that seen with athlete's heart until BP is normalized by appropriate antihypertensive drug therapy, and (2) restricting athletes with stage 2 HTN (even among those without evidence of target organ injury) from participating in high-static sports (eg, weight lifting, boxing, and wrestling) until HTN is controlled with either lifestyle modification or drug therapy.[539]

The AAP policy statement "Athletic Participation by Children and Adolescents Who Have Systemic Hypertension" recommends that children with stage 2 HTN be restricted from high-static sports (classes IIIA to IIIC) in the absence of end organ damage, including LVH or concomitant heart disease, until their BP is in the normal range after lifestyle modification and/or drug therapy.[538] It is further recommended that athletes be promptly referred and evaluated by a qualified pediatric medical subspecialist within 1 week if they are asymptomatic or immediately if they are symptomatic. The subcommittee agrees with these recommendations.

It should be acknowledged that there are no data linking the presence of HTN to sudden death related to sports participation in children, although many cases of sudden death are of unknown etiology. That said, athletes identified as hypertensive (eg, during preparticipation sports screening) should undergo appropriate evaluation as outlined above. For athletes with more severe HTN (stage 2 or greater), treatment should be initiated before sports participation.

Key Action Statement 28

Children and adolescents with HTN may participate in competitive sports once hypertensive target organ effects and risk have been assessed (grade C, moderate recommendation).

Key Action Statement 29

Children and adolescents with HTN should receive treatment to lower BP below stage 2 thresholds before participating in competitive sports (grade C, weak recommendation).

11.3 HTN and the Posttransplant Patient

HTN is common in children after solid-organ transplants, with prevalence rates ranging from 50% to 90%.[179,180,540,541] Contributing factors include the use of steroids, calcineurin inhibitors, and mTOR (mammalian target of rapamycin) inhibitors. In patients with renal transplants, the presence of native kidneys, CKD, and transplant glomerulopathy are additional risk factors for HTN. HTN rates are higher by 24-hour ABPM compared with clinic BP measurements because these populations commonly have MH and nocturnal HTN.[179–183,542] Control of HTN in renal-transplant patients has been improved with the use of annual ABPM.[184,185] Therefore, ABPM should be used to identify and monitor nocturnal BP abnormalities and MH in pediatric kidney and heart-transplant recipients. The use of home BP assessment may provide a comparable alternative to ABPM for BP assessment after transplant as well.[186]

The management of identified HTN in the pediatric transplant patient can be challenging. Rates of control of HTN in renal-transplant patients generally range from 33% to 55%.[180,187] In studies by Seeman et al,[188] intensified antihypertensive treatment in pediatric renal-transplant recipients improved nocturnal SBP and significantly reduced proteinuria.[543] Children in these studies who achieved normotension had stable graft function, whereas those who remained hypertensive at 2 years had a progression of renal disease.[544]

Antihypertensive medications have rarely been systematically studied in this population. There is limited evidence that ACE inhibitors and ARBs may be superior to other agents in achieving BP control and improving long-term graft survival in renal-transplant patients.[185,543,544] However, the combination of ACE inhibitors and ARBs in renal-transplant patients has been associated with acidosis and hyperkalemia and is not recommended.[545]

Key Action Statement 27. In children and adolescents with acute severe HTN and life-threatening symptoms, immediate treatment with short-acting antihypertensive medication should be initiated, and BP should be reduced by no more than 25% of the planned reduction over the first 8 hours (grade expert opinion D, weak recommendation).

Aggregate Evidence Quality	Expert Opinion, D
Benefits	Avoidance of complications caused by rapid BP reduction
Risks, harm, cost	Severe BP elevation may persist
Benefit–harm assessment	Benefit outweighs harm
Intentional vagueness	None
Role of patient preferences	None
Exclusions	Patients without acute severe HTN and life-threatening symptoms
Strength	Weak recommendation because of expert opinion
Key references	240,533,535

12. LIFETIME HTN TREATMENT AND TRANSITION TO ADULTHOOD

For adolescents with HTN requiring ongoing treatment, the

Key Action Statement 28. Children and adolescents with HTN may participate in competitive sports once hypertensive target organ effects and risk have been assessed (grade C, moderate recommendation).

Aggregate Evidence Quality	Grade C
Benefits	Aerobic exercise improves CVD risk factors in children and adolescents with HTN
Risks, harm, cost	Unknown, but theoretical risk related to a rise in BP with strenuous exercise may exist
Benefit–harm assessment	The benefits of exercise likely outweigh the potential risk in the vast majority of children and adolescents with HTN
Intentional vagueness	None
Role of patient preferences	Families may have different opinions about sports participation in children with HTN
Exclusions	None
Strength	Moderate recommendation
Key references	341,360,538,540,541

Key Action Statement 29. Children and adolescents with HTN should receive treatment to lower BP below stage 2 thresholds before participating in competitive sports (grade C, weak recommendation).

Aggregate Evidence Quality	Grade C
Benefits	Aerobic exercise improves CVD risk factors in children and adolescents with HTN
Risks, harm, cost	Unknown, but theoretical risk related to a rise in BP with strenuous exercise may exist
Benefit–harm assessment	The benefits of exercise likely outweigh the potential risk in the vast majority of children and adolescents with HTN
Intentional vagueness	None
Role of patient preferences	None
Exclusions	None
Strength	Weak recommendation
Key references	341,360,538,540,541

transition from pediatric care to an adult provider is essential.[546] HTN definition and treatment recommendations in this guideline are generally consistent with the forthcoming adult HTN treatment guideline, so diagnosis and treatment should not typically change with transition.

Key Action Statement 30

Adolescents with elevated BP or HTN (whether they are receiving antihypertensive treatment) should typically have their care transitioned to an appropriate adult care provider by 22 years of age (recognizing that there may be individual cases in which this upper age limit is exceeded, particularly in the case of youth with special health care needs). There should be a transfer of information regarding HTN etiology and past manifestations and complications of the patient's HTN (grade X, strong recommendation).

13. PREVENTION OF HTN

13.1 Importance of Preventing HTN

BP levels tend to increase with time even after adult height is reached. The rate of progression to frank HTN in a study of more than 12 000 Japanese adults (20–35 years of age at baseline, followed for 9 years) was 36.5% and was greater with higher baseline BP category.[548] The rate of progression may also be accelerated in African American individuals. Similarly, both the Bogalusa Heart[63] and Fels Longitudinal[60] studies have clearly demonstrated that the risk of HTN in early adulthood is dependent on childhood BP, with greater numbers of elevated BP measurements in childhood conferring an increased risk of adult HTN.

Because the tracking of BP levels in children has also been well documented,[10] it is not surprising that analyses of the National Childhood BP database found 7% of adolescents with elevated BP per year progressed to true hypertensive BP levels. Of note, initial BMI and change in BMI were major determinants of the development of HTN.[22] Therefore, in both children and adults, efforts (discussed below) should be made to prevent progression to sustained HTN and to avoid the development of hypertensive CV diseases.

13.2 Strategies for Prevention

One of the largest trials of preventing progression to HTN in adults, the Trial of Preventing Hypertension study, proved that 2 years of treatment with candesartan reduced the number of subjects with elevated BP from developing stage 1 HTN even after the drug was withdrawn.[547] However, no similar study has been conducted in youth; for this reason, prevention efforts to date have focused on lifestyle modification, especially dietary intervention,[426] exercise,[549] and treatment of obesity.[550] The best evidence for the potential of such prevention strategies comes from epidemiologic evidence for risk factors for the development of HTN or from studies focused on the treatment of established HTN. These risk factors include positive family history, obesity, a high-sodium diet, the absence of a DASH-type diet, larger amounts of

Key Action Statement 30. Adolescents with elevated BP or HTN (whether they are receiving antihypertensive treatment) should typically have their care transitioned to an appropriate adult care provider by 22 years of age (recognizing that there may be individual cases in which this upper age limit is exceeded, particularly in the case of youth with special health care needs). There should be a transfer of information regarding HTN etiology and past manifestations and complications of the patient's HTN (grade X, strong recommendation).

Aggregate Evidence Quality	Grade X
Benefits	Provides continuity of care for patients
Risks, harm, cost	None
Benefit–harm assessment	No risk
Intentional vagueness	None
Role of patient preferences	Patient can pick adult care provider
Exclusions	None
Strength	Strong recommendation
Key references	547

sedentary time, and possibly other dietary factors.[551–553]

Because family history is immutable, it is difficult to build a preventive strategy around it. However, a positive family history of HTN should suggest the need for closer BP monitoring to detect HTN if it occurs.

Appropriate energy balance with calories eaten balanced by calories expended in physical activity is important. This is the best strategy to maintain an appropriate BMI percentile for age and sex and to avoid the development of obesity.[554] From a broader dietary perspective, a DASH-type diet (ie, high in fruits, vegetables, whole grains, and low-fat dairy, with decreased intake of foods high in saturated fat or sugar) may be beneficial (see Table 16).[423,427] Avoiding high-sodium foods may prove helpful in preventing HTN, particularly for individuals who are more sensitive to dietary sodium intake.[555]

Adhering to recommendations for 60 minutes a day of moderate to vigorous physical activity can be important to maintaining an appropriate weight and may be independently helpful to maintaining a lower BP.[344] The achievement of normal sleep habits and avoidance of tobacco products are also reasonable strategies to reduce CV risk.

These preventive strategies can be implemented as part of routine primary health care for children and adolescents.

14. CHALLENGES IN THE IMPLEMENTATION OF PEDIATRIC HTN GUIDELINES

Many studies have shown that physicians fail to meet benchmarks with respect to screening, especially universal screening for high BP in children.[7,115] Although the reasons for this failure likely vary from practice to practice, a number of common challenges can be identified.

The first challenge is determining how to identify every child in a clinic who merits a BP measurement. This could be accomplished through flags in an EHR, documentation rules for specific patients, and/or clinic protocols.

The second challenge is establishing a local clinic protocol for measuring BP correctly on the basis of the algorithms in this guideline. It is important to determine the optimal approach on the basis of the available equipment, the skills of clinic personnel, and the clinic's throughput needs.

The third challenge is for clinic personnel to be aware of what to do with high BP measurements when they occur. Knowing when to counsel patients, order tests or laboratory work, and reach out for help is essential. Making this part of standard practice so every child follows the prescribed pathway may be challenging.

The final diagnosis of HTN also relies on a number of sequential visits. Ensuring that patients return for all of these visits and are not lost to follow-up may require new clinic processes or mechanisms. Information technology may help remind providers to schedule these visits and remind patients to attend these visits; even with that assistance, however, completing all the visits may be difficult for some patients.

In addition, family medicine physicians and general pediatricians may face challenges in having normative pediatric BP values available for use at all times. Although adult BP cutoffs are easy to memorize, pediatric BP percentile cutoffs are greatly dependent on age and height. The BP tables in this guideline provide cutoffs to use for the proper diagnosis of HTN; their availability will simplify the recognition of abnormal BP values.

The AAP Education in Quality Improvement for Pediatric Practice module on HTN identification and management[556] and its accompanying implementation guide[557] should be of assistance to practitioners who wish to improve their approach to identifying and managing childhood HTN. This module is currently being updated to incorporate the new recommendations in this guideline.

15. OTHER TOPICS

15.1 Economic Impact of BP Management

Researchers in a small number of studies have examined the potential economic impacts related to pediatric BP management.[208,558,559] Wang et al[558] estimated both the effectiveness and cost-effectiveness of 3 screening strategies and interventions to normalize pediatric BP based on the literature and through a simulation of children (n = 4 017 821). The 3 screening strategies included the following: (1) no screening; (2) selected screening and treatment, as well as "treating everyone" (ie, with population-wide interventions, such as targeted programs for overweight adolescents [eg, weight-loss programs, exercise programs, and salt-reduction programs]); and (3) nontargeted programs for exercise and salt reduction.

The simulation suggested that these various strategies could reduce mortality, with a modest expected survival benefit of 0.5 to 8.6 days. The researchers also examined quality-adjusted life-years (QALYs) and the cost per QALY. Only 1 intervention, a nontargeted salt-reduction campaign, had a negative cost per QALY. This intervention and the other 2 described in that article support the concept that population-wide interventions may be the most cost-effective way to improve CV health. The article has serious limitations, however, including the fact that population-wide interventions for exercise and the reduction of sodium intake have not, thus far, been effective.

The accurate determination of those who actually have HTN (as opposed to WCH) is fundamental to providing sound care to patients. Researchers in two studies examined the effects of using ABPM in the diagnosis of HTN.[208,559] Davis et al[559] compared 3 HTN screening strategies; these options are summarized in the following value-analysis framework (see Table 20).[560] It appears that the implementation of ABPM for all patients is not ensured. The next best option, screening clinic BP with ABPM, is most likely to be implementable and has significant clinical benefit given the high prevalence of WCH.

Swartz et al[208] conducted a retrospective review of 267 children with elevated clinic BP measurements referred for ABPM. Of the 126 patients who received ABPM, 46% had WCH, 49% had stage 1 HTN, and 5% had stage 2 HTN. This is consistent with the concept that screening with clinic BP alone results in high numbers of false-positive results for HTN. The diagnosis of HTN in this study resulted in an additional $3420 for evaluation (includes clinic visit, facility fee, laboratory testing, renal ultrasound, and echocardiography) vs $1265 (includes clinic visit, facility fee, and ABPM). This suggests that ABPM is cost-effective because of the reduction of unnecessary testing in patients with WCH.

When examining these costs, the availability of ABPM, and the availability of practitioners who are skilled in pediatric interpretation, the most cost-effective and implementable screening solution is to measure clinic BP and confirm elevated readings by ABPM.

15.2 Patient Perspective and Pediatric HTN

Children and adolescents are not just patients; they are active participants in their health management. If children and adolescents lack a clear understanding of what is happening inside their bodies, they will not be able to make informed choices in their daily activities. Better choices lead to better decisions executed in self-care. For clear judgments to be made, there needs to be open communication between physicians and families, a provision of appropriate education on optimal HTN management, and a strong partnership assembled within a multidisciplinary health care team including physicians, advanced practice providers, dietitians, nurses, and medical and clinical assistants.

It is important for physicians to be mindful that children and adolescents want, and need, to be involved in their medical care. Pediatric HTN patients are likely to feel excluded when clinicians or other providers speak to their parents instead of including them in the conversation. When patients are neither included in the discussion nor encouraged to ask questions, their anxiety can increase, thus worsening their HTN. Keeping an open line of communication is important and is best done by using a team approach consisting of the patient, the family, health care support staff, and physicians. With practical education on HTN management provided in easily understandable terms, the patients will be more likely to apply the concepts presented to them. Education is important and should be given in a way that is appropriate for young children and their families to understand. Education should consist of suitable medication dosing, a proper diet and level of activity, the identification of symptoms, and appropriate BP monitoring (including cuff size).

15.3 Parental Perspective and Pediatric HTN

Parents play a key role in the management and care of their children's health. Parents and physicians should act as a cohesive unit to foster the best results. It is vital for physicians to provide concise information in plain language and do so using a team approach. This will facilitate parents having a clear understanding of the required tests, medications, follow-ups, and outcomes.

> Patient Perspective, by Matthew Goodwin
>
> "I am not just a 13 year old, I am a teenager who has lived with hypertension, renal disease, and midaortic syndrome since I was 4 years old. I have experienced surgeries, extended hospitalizations, daily medications, procedures, tests, continued blood pressure monitoring, lifestyle changes, and dietary restrictions. Hypertension is a part of my everyday life. It will always be a component of me. I had to learn the effects of hypertension at a young age. I knew what would happen to me if I ate too much salt or did not fully hydrate, thus I became watchful. I did this so I could efficiently communicate with my physicians any changes I physically felt or any symptoms that were new or different regarding my illness. This has allowed me, my family, and my doctors to work effectively as one unit. I am grateful for my doctors listening to me as a person and not as a kid."

Parents of children with hypertensive issues can encounter 1 or more specialists in addition to their pediatric clinician. This can prove to be overwhelming, frightening, and may fill the parent with anxiety. Taking these things into account and creating unified partners, built with the physician and family, will encourage the family to be more involved in the patient's health management. Plain language in a team approach will yield the most positive outcomes for the patient.

Understanding the family and patient's perception of HTN and any underlying disease that may be contributing to it is important to resolve any misconceptions and encourage adherence to the physician's recommendations. To attain therapeutic goals, proper education must be provided to the family as a whole. This education should include proper medication dosages, recommended sodium intake, any dietary changes, exercise expectations, and any other behavioral changes. It is equally important to stress to the family the short- and long-term effects of HTN if it is not properly managed. Parents with younger children will carry the ultimate burden of daily decisions as it applies to medications, food choices, and activity. Parents of older adolescents will partner with the children to encourage the right choices. Education as a family unit is important for everyone involved to understand the consequences.

A family-based approach is important for all pediatric diseases but plays a particular role in conditions that are substantially influenced by lifestyle behaviors. This has been shown in several pediatric populations, including those with T2DM and obesity.[561–565]

16. EVIDENCE GAPS AND PROPOSED FUTURE DIRECTIONS

In general, the pediatric HTN literature is not as robust as the adult HTN literature. The reasons for this are many, but the 2 most important are as follows: (1) the lower prevalence of HTN in childhood compared with adults, and (2) the lack of adverse CV events (myocardial infarction, stroke, and death) attributable to HTN in young patients. These factors make it difficult to conduct the types of clinical trials that are needed to produce high-quality evidence. For example, no large pediatric cohort has ever been assembled to answer the question of whether routine BP measurement in childhood is useful to prevent adult CVD.[566] Given this, other types of evidence, such as from cross-sectional and observational cohort studies, must be examined to guide practice.[567]

From the standpoint of the primary care provider, the most significant evidence gaps relate to whether diagnosing elevated BP and HTN in children and adolescents truly has long-term health consequences, whether antihypertensive medications should be used in a child or adolescent with elevated BP, and what medications should be preferentially used. These evidence gaps have been alluded to previously in this document.

Other important evidence gaps should be highlighted, including the following:

- Is there a specific BP level in childhood that predicts adverse outcomes, and can a single number (or numbers) be used to define HTN, as in adults?
- Can and should ABPM ever replace auscultation in the diagnosis of childhood HTN?
- Are the currently used, normative standards for ABPM appropriate, or are new normative data needed?[568]
- What is the best diagnostic evaluation to confidently exclude secondary causes of HTN?
- Are other assessments of hypertensive target organ damage (such as urine MA or vascular studies) better than echocardiography?
- How confident can we be that a child or teenager with elevated BP

will have HTN and/or CVD disease as an adult?

Some of these questions may eventually be answered by research that is currently in progress, such as further analysis of the International Childhood Cardiovascular Cohort Consortium[569] and the promising Adult Hypertension Onset in Youth study, which seeks to better define the level of BP in childhood that predicts the development of hypertensive target organ damage.[570] Other studies will need to be performed in children and adolescents to fill in the remaining gaps, including more rigorous validation studies of automated BP devices in the pediatric population, expanded trials of lifestyle interventions, further comparative trials of antihypertensive medications, and studies of the clinical applicability of hypertensive target organ assessments.

Furthermore, and perhaps more crucially, there needs to be prospective assessment of the recommendations made in this document with regular updates based on new evidence as it is generated (generally, per AAP policy, these occur approximately every 5 years). With such ongoing reassessment and revision, it is hoped that this document and its future revisions will come to be viewed as an effective guide to practice and will improve the care of the young patients who are entrusted to us.

Implementation tools for this guideline are available on the AAP Web site (https://www.aap.org/en-us/about-the-aap/Committees-Councils-Sections/coqips/Pages/Implementation-Guide.aspx).

AUTHORS

Joseph T. Flynn, MD, MS, FAAP
David C. Kaelber, MD, PhD, MPH, FAAP, FACP, FACMI
Carissa M. Baker-Smith, MD, MS, MPH, FAAP, FAHA
Douglas Blowey, MD
Aaron E. Carroll, MD, MS, FAAP
Stephen R. Daniels, MD, PhD, FAAP
Sarah D. de Ferranti, MD, MPH, FAAP
Janis M. Dionne, MD, FRCPC
Susan K. Flinn, MA
Bonita Falkner, MD
Samuel S. Gidding, MD
Celeste Goodwin
Michael G. Leu, MD, MS, MHS, FAAP
Makia E. Powers, MD, MPH, FAAP
Corinna Rea, MD, MPH, FAAP
Joshua Samuels, MD, MPH, FAAP
Madeline Simasek, MD, MSCP, FAAP
Vidhu V. Thaker, MD, FAAP
Elaine M. Urbina, MD, MS, FAAP

SUBCOMMITTEE ON SCREENING AND MANAGEMENT OF HIGH BLOOD PRESSURE IN CHILDREN (OVERSIGHT BY THE COUNCIL ON QUALITY IMPROVEMENT AND PATIENT SAFETY)†

Joseph T. Flynn, MD, MS, FAAP, Co-chair, Section on Nephrology
David Kaelber, MD, MPH, PhD, FAAP, Co-chair, Section on Medicine-Pediatrcs, Council on Clinical Information Technology
Carissa M. Baker-Smith, MD, MS, MPH, Epidemiologist and Methodologist
Aaron Carroll, MD, MS, FAAP, Partnership for Policy Implementation
Stephen R. Daniels, MD, PhD, FAAP, Committee on Nutrition
Sarah D. de Ferranti, MD, MPH, FAAP, Committee on Cardiology and Cardiac Surgery
Michael G. Leu, MD, MS, MHS, FAAP, Council on Quality Improvement and Patient Safety
Makia Powers, MD, MPH, FAAP, Committee on Adolescence
Corinna Rea, MD, MPH, FAAP, Section on Early Career Physicians
Joshua Samuels, MD, MPH, FAAP, Section on Nephrology
Madeline Simasek, MD, FAAP, Quality Improvement Innovation Networks
Vidhu Thaker, MD, FAAP, Section on Obesity

LIAISONS

Douglas Blowey, MD, *American Society of Pediatric Nephrology*
Janis Dionne, MD, FRCPC, *Canadian Association of Paediatric Nephrologists*
Bonita Falkner, MD, *International Pediatric Hypertension Association*
Samuel Gidding, MD, *American College of Cardiology, American Heart Association*
Celeste Goodwin, *National Pediatric Blood Pressure Awareness Foundation*
Elaine Urbina, MD, FAAP, *American Heart Association AHOY Committee*

MEDICAL WRITER

Susan K. Flinn, MA

STAFF

Kymika Okechukwu, MPA, Manager, Evidence-Based Practice Initiatives

ABBREVIATIONS

AAP: American Academy of Pediatrics
ABPM: ambulatory blood pressure monitoring
ACC: American College of Cardiology
ACE: angiotensin-converting enzyme
AHA: American Heart Association
ARB: angiotensin receptor blocker
ARR: aldosterone to renin ratio
BP: blood pressure
BSA: body surface area
cIMT: carotid intimamedia thickness
CKD: chronic kidney disease
CTA: computed tomographic angiography
CV: cardiovascular
CVD: cardiovascular disease
DASH: Dietary Approaches to Stop Hypertension
DBP: diastolic blood pressure
ED: emergency department
EHR: electronic health record
FMD: flow-mediated dilation
HTN: hypertension
LVH: left ventricular hypertrophy
LVMI: left ventricular mass index
MA: microalbuminuria
MAP: mean arterial pressure
MH: masked hypertension
MI: motivational interviewing
MRA: magnetic resonance angiography
NF-1: neurofibromatosis type 1
OSAS: obstructive sleep apnea syndrome
PCC: pheochromocytoma
PICOT: Patient, Intervention/Indicator, Comparison, Outcome, and Time
PRA: plasma renin activity
PWV: pulse wave velocity
QALY: quality-adjusted life-year
RAAS: renin-angiotensin-aldosterone system
RAS: renal artery stenosis
SBP: systolic blood pressure
SDB: sleep-disordered breathing
T1DM: type 1 diabetes mellitus
T2DM: type 2 diabetes mellitus
UA: uric acid
WCH: white coat hypertension

Seattle, Washington; [n]Department of Pediatrics, School of Medicine, Morehouse College, Atlanta, Georgia; [o]Associate Director, General Academic Pediatric Fellowship, Staff Physician, Boston's Children's Hospital Primary Care at Longwood, Instructor, Harvard Medical School, Boston, Massachusetts; Departments of [p]Pediatrics and Internal Medicine, McGovern Medical School, University of Texas, Houston, Texas; [q]Pediatric Education, University of Pittsburgh Medical Center Shadyside Family Medicine Residency, Clinical Associate Professor of Pediatrics, Children's Hospital of Pittsburgh of University of Pittsburgh Medical Center, and School of Medicine, University of Pittsburgh, Pittsburgh, Pennsylvania; [r]Division of Molecular Genetics, Department of Pediatrics, Columbia University Medical Center, New York, New York; and [s]Preventive Cardiology, Cincinnati Children's Hospital Medical Center, Department of Pediatrics, University of Cincinnati, Cincinnati, Ohio

Drs Flynn and Kaelber served as the specialty and primary care chairs of the Subcommittee and had lead roles in developing the framework for the guidelines and coordinating the overall guideline development; Dr Baker-Smith served as the epidemiologist and led the evidence review and synthesis; Ms. Flinn compiled the first draft of the manuscript and coordinated manuscript revisions; All other authors were significantly involved in all aspects of the guideline creation including initial scoping, literature review and synthesis, draft manuscript creation and manuscript review; and all authors approved the final manuscript as submitted.

This document is copyrighted and is property of the American Academy of Pediatrics and its Board of Directors. All authors have filed conflict of interest statements with the American Academy of Pediatrics. Any conflicts have been resolved through a process approved by the Board of Directors. The American Academy of Pediatrics has neither solicited nor accepted any commercial involvement in the development of the content of this publication.

The guidance in this report does not indicate an exclusive course of treatment or serve as a standard of medical care. Variations, taking into account individual circumstances, may be appropriate.

All clinical practice guidelines from the American Academy of Pediatrics automatically expire 5 years after publication unless reaffirmed, revised, or retired at or before that time.

Endorsed by the American Heart Association.

DOI: https://doi.org/10.1542/peds.2017-1904

Address correspondence to Joseph T Flynn. Email: joseph.flynn@seattlechildrens.org

PEDIATRICS (ISSN Numbers: Print, 0031-4005; Online, 1098-4275).

Copyright © 2017 by the American Academy of Pediatrics

FINANCIAL DISCLOSURE: The authors have indicated that they have no financial relationships relevant to this article to disclose.

FUNDING: The American Academy of Pediatrics provided funding to cover travel costs for subcommittee members to attend subcommittee meetings, to pay for the epidemiologist (Dr Baker-Smith) and consultant (Susan Flynn), and to produce the revised normative blood pressure tables.

POTENTIAL CONFLICT OF INTEREST: The authors have indicated that they have no potential conflicts of interest to disclose.

REFERENCES

1. National High Blood Pressure Education Program Working Group on High Blood Pressure in Children and Adolescents. The fourth report on the diagnosis, evaluation, and treatment of high blood pressure in children and adolescents. *Pediatrics*. 2004;114(2, suppl 4th Report):555–576
2. Institute of Medicine, Committee on Standards for Systematic Reviews of Comparative Effectiveness Research. In: Eden J, Levit L, Berg A, Morton S, eds. *Finding What Works in Health Care: Standards for Systematic Reviews*. Washington, DC: National Academies Press; 2011
3. American Academy of Pediatrics Steering Committee on Quality Improvement and Management. Classifying recommendations for clinical practice guidelines. *Pediatrics*. 2004;114(3):874–877
4. Rosner B, Cook NR, Daniels S, Falkner B. Childhood blood pressure trends and risk factors for high blood pressure: the NHANES experience 1988-2008. *Hypertension*. 2013;62(2):247–254
5. Din-Dzietham R, Liu Y, Bielo MV, Shamsa F. High blood pressure trends in children and adolescents in national surveys, 1963 to 2002. *Circulation*. 2007;116(13):1488–1496
6. Kit BK, Kuklina E, Carroll MD, Ostchega Y, Freedman DS, Ogden CL. Prevalence of and trends in dyslipidemia and blood pressure among US children and adolescents, 1999-2012. *JAMA Pediatr*. 2015;169(3):272–279
7. Hansen ML, Gunn PW, Kaelber DC. Underdiagnosis of hypertension in children and adolescents. *JAMA*. 2007;298(8):874–879
8. McNiece KL, Poffenbarger TS, Turner JL, Franco KD, Sorof JM, Portman RJ. Prevalence of hypertension and pre-hypertension among adolescents. *J Pediatr*. 2007;150(6):640–644, 644.e1
9. Chiolero A, Cachat F, Burnier M, Paccaud F, Bovet P. Prevalence of hypertension in schoolchildren based on repeated measurements and association with overweight. *J Hypertens*. 2007;25(11):2209–2217
10. Chen X, Wang Y. Tracking of blood pressure from childhood to adulthood: a systematic review and meta-regression analysis. *Circulation*. 2008;117(25):3171–3180
11. Theodore RF, Broadbent J, Nagin D, et al. Childhood to early-midlife systolic blood pressure trajectories: early-life predictors, effect modifiers, and adult cardiovascular outcomes. *Hypertension*. 2015;66(6):1108–1115
12. Mozaffarian D, Benjamin EJ, Go AS, et al; Writing Group Members; American Heart Association Statistics Committee; Stroke Statistics Subcommittee. Executive summary: heart disease and stroke statistics—2016 update: a report from the American Heart Association. *Circulation*. 2016;133(4):447–454
13. Liberman JN, Berger JE, Lewis M. Prevalence of antihypertensive, antidiabetic, and dyslipidemic prescription medication use among children and adolescents. *Arch Pediatr Adolesc Med*. 2009;163(4):357–364
14. Rodriguez BL, Dabelea D, Liese AD, et al; SEARCH Study Group. Prevalence and correlates of elevated blood pressure in youth with diabetes mellitus: the

SEARCH for diabetes in youth study. *J Pediatr.* 2010;157(2):245–251.e1

15. Willi SM, Hirst K, Jago R, et al; HEALTHY Study Group. Cardiovascular risk factors in multi-ethnic middle school students: the HEALTHY primary prevention trial. *Pediatr Obes.* 2012;7(3):230–239

16. DiPietro A, Kees-Folts D, DesHarnais S, Camacho F, Wassner SJ. Primary hypertension at a single center: treatment, time to control, and extended follow-up. *Pediatr Nephrol.* 2009;24(12):2421–2428

17. Seeman T, Gilík J. Long-term control of ambulatory hypertension in children: improving with time but still not achieving new blood pressure goals. *Am J Hypertens.* 2013;26(7):939–945

18. Foglia CF, von Vigier RO, Fossali E, et al. A simplified antihypertensive drug regimen does not ameliorate control of childhood hypertension. *J Hum Hypertens.* 2005;19(8):653–654

19. Sorof J, Daniels S. Obesity hypertension in children: a problem of epidemic proportions. *Hypertension.* 2002;40(4):441–447

20. Sorof JM, Lai D, Turner J, Poffenbarger T, Portman RJ. Overweight, ethnicity, and the prevalence of hypertension in school-aged children. *Pediatrics.* 2004;113(3, pt 1):475–482

21. Koebnick C, Black MH, Wu J, et al. High blood pressure in overweight and obese youth: implications for screening. *J Clin Hypertens (Greenwich).* 2013;15(11):793–805

22. Falkner B, Gidding SS, Ramirez-Garnica G, Wiltrout SA, West D, Rappaport EB. The relationship of body mass index and blood pressure in primary care pediatric patients. *J Pediatr.* 2006;148(2):195–200

23. Lurbe E, Invitti C, Torro I, et al. The impact of the degree of obesity on the discrepancies between office and ambulatory blood pressure values in youth [published correction appears in *J Hypertens.* 2007;25(1):258]. *J Hypertens.* 2006;24(8):1557–1564

24. Skinner AC, Perrin EM, Moss LA, Skelton JA. Cardiometabolic risks and severity of obesity in children and young adults. *N Engl J Med.* 2015;373(14):1307–1317

25. Zhang T, Zhang H, Li S, et al. Impact of adiposity on incident hypertension is modified by insulin resistance in adults: longitudinal observation from the Bogalusa Heart Study. *Hypertension.* 2016;67(1):56–62

26. So H-K, Yip GW-K, Choi K-C, et al; Hong Kong ABP Working Group. Association between waist circumference and childhood-masked hypertension: a community-based study. *J Paediatr Child Health.* 2016;52(4):385–390

27. Friedemann C, Heneghan C, Mahtani K, Thompson M, Perera R, Ward AM. Cardiovascular disease risk in healthy children and its association with body mass index: systematic review and meta-analysis. *BMJ.* 2012;345:e4759

28. Kelishadi R, Mirmoghtadaee P, Najafi H, Keikha M. Systematic review on the association of abdominal obesity in children and adolescents with cardio-metabolic risk factors. *J Res Med Sci.* 2015;20(3):294–307

29. Török K, Pálfi A, Szelényi Z, Molnár D. Circadian variability of blood pressure in obese children. *Nutr Metab Cardiovasc Dis.* 2008;18(6):429–435

30. Framme J, Dangardt F, Mårild S, Osika W, Währborg P, Friberg P. 24-h systolic blood pressure and heart rate recordings in lean and obese adolescents. *Clin Physiol Funct Imaging.* 2006;26(4):235–239

31. Westerståhl M, Marcus C. Association between nocturnal blood pressure dipping and insulin metabolism in obese adolescents. *Int J Obes.* 2010;34(3):472–477

32. Westerståhl M, Hedvall Kallerman P, Hagman E, Ek AE, Rössner SM, Marcus C. Nocturnal blood pressure non-dipping is prevalent in severely obese, prepubertal and early pubertal children. *Acta Paediatr.* 2014;103(2):225–230

33. Macumber IR, Weiss NS, Halbach SM, Hanevold CD, Flynn JT. The association of pediatric obesity with nocturnal non-dipping on 24-hour ambulatory blood pressure monitoring. *Am J Hypertens.* 2016;29(5):647–652

34. Perng W, Rifas-Shiman SL, Kramer MS, et al. Early weight gain, linear growth, and mid-childhood blood pressure: a prospective study in project viva. *Hypertension.* 2016;67(2):301–308

35. Parker ED, Sinaiko AR, Kharbanda EO, et al. Change in weight status and development of hypertension. *Pediatrics.* 2016;137(3):e20151662

36. Yip J, Facchini FS, Reaven GM. Resistance to insulin-mediated glucose disposal as a predictor of cardiovascular disease. *J Clin Endocrinol Metab.* 1998;83(8):2773–2776

37. Kashyap SR, Defronzo RA. The insulin resistance syndrome: physiological considerations. *Diab Vasc Dis Res.* 2007;4(1):13–19

38. Lurbe E, Torro I, Aguilar F, et al. Added impact of obesity and insulin resistance in nocturnal blood pressure elevation in children and adolescents. *Hypertension.* 2008;51(3):635–641

39. Chinali M, de Simone G, Roman MJ, et al. Cardiac markers of pre-clinical disease in adolescents with the metabolic syndrome: the strong heart study. *J Am Coll Cardiol.* 2008;52(11):932–938

40. Archbold KH, Vasquez MM, Goodwin JL, Quan SF. Effects of sleep patterns and obesity on increases in blood pressure in a 5-year period: report from the Tucson Children's Assessment of Sleep Apnea Study. *J Pediatr.* 2012;161(1):26–30

41. Javaheri S, Storfer-Isser A, Rosen CL, Redline S. Sleep quality and elevated blood pressure in adolescents. *Circulation.* 2008;118(10):1034–1040

42. Hartzell K, Avis K, Lozano D, Feig D. Obstructive sleep apnea and periodic limb movement disorder in a population of children with hypertension and/or nocturnal nondipping blood pressures. *J Am Soc Hypertens.* 2016;10(2):101–107

43. Au CT, Ho CK, Wing YK, Lam HS, Li AM. Acute and chronic effects of sleep duration on blood pressure. *Pediatrics.* 2014;133(1). Available at: www.pediatrics.org/cgi/content/full/133/1/e64

44. Li AM, Au CT, Ng C, Lam HS, Ho CKW, Wing YK. A 4-year prospective follow-up study of childhood OSA

and its association with BP. *Chest.* 2014;145(6):1255–1263

45. Li AM, Au CT, Sung RY, et al. Ambulatory blood pressure in children with obstructive sleep apnoea: a community based study. *Thorax.* 2008;63(9):803–809

46. Flynn JT, Mitsnefes M, Pierce C, et al; Chronic Kidney Disease in Children Study Group. Blood pressure in children with chronic kidney disease: a report from the Chronic Kidney Disease in Children study. *Hypertension.* 2008;52(4):631–637

47. Samuels J, Ng D, Flynn JT, et al; Chronic Kidney Disease in Children Study Group. Ambulatory blood pressure patterns in children with chronic kidney disease. *Hypertension.* 2012;60(1):43–50

48. Shatat IF, Flynn JT. Hypertension in children with chronic kidney disease. *Adv Chronic Kidney Dis.* 2005;12(4):378–384

49. Chavers BM, Solid CA, Daniels FX, et al. Hypertension in pediatric long-term hemodialysis patients in the United States. *Clin J Am Soc Nephrol.* 2009;4(8):1363–1369

50. Seeman T. Hypertension after renal transplantation. *Pediatr Nephrol.* 2009;24(5):959–972

51. Tkaczyk M, Nowicki M, Bałasz-Chmielewska I, et al. Hypertension in dialysed children: the prevalence and therapeutic approach in Poland–a nationwide survey. *Nephrol Dial Transplant.* 2006;21(3):736–742

52. Kramer AM, van Stralen KJ, Jager KJ, et al. Demographics of blood pressure and hypertension in children on renal replacement therapy in Europe. *Kidney Int.* 2011;80(10):1092–1098

53. Halbach SM, Martz K, Mattoo T, Flynn J. Predictors of blood pressure and its control in pediatric patients receiving dialysis. *J Pediatr.* 2012;160(4):621–625.e1

54. Kaelber DC. IBM explorys cohort discovery tool. Available at: www.ibm.com/watson/health/explorys. Accessed February 3, 2017

55. Barker DJ. The fetal and infant origins of adult disease. *BMJ.* 1990;301(6761):1111

56. Edvardsson VO, Steinthorsdottir SD, Eliasdottir SB, Indridason OS, Palsson R. Birth weight and childhood blood pressure. *Curr Hypertens Rep.* 2012;14(6):596–602

57. Mhanna MJ, Iqbal AM, Kaelber DC. Weight gain and hypertension at three years of age and older in extremely low birth weight infants. *J Neonatal Perinatal Med.* 2015;8(4):363–369

58. Di Salvo G, Castaldi B, Baldini L, et al. Masked hypertension in young patients after successful aortic coarctation repair: impact on left ventricular geometry and function. *J Hum Hypertens.* 2011;25(12):739–745

59. Bayrakci US, Schaefer F, Duzova A, Yigit S, Bakkaloglu A. Abnormal circadian blood pressure regulation in children born preterm. *J Pediatr.* 2007;151(4):399–403

60. Sun SS, Grave GD, Siervogel RM, Pickoff AA, Arslanian SS, Daniels SR. Systolic blood pressure in childhood predicts hypertension and metabolic syndrome later in life. *Pediatrics.* 2007;119(2):237–246

61. Juhola J, Oikonen M, Magnussen CG, et al. Childhood physical, environmental, and genetic predictors of adult hypertension: the cardiovascular risk in young Finns study. *Circulation.* 2012;126(4):402–409

62. Juhola J, Magnussen CG, Viikari JS, et al. Tracking of serum lipid levels, blood pressure, and body mass index from childhood to adulthood: the Cardiovascular Risk in Young Finns Study. *J Pediatr.* 2011;159(4):584–590

63. Bao W, Threefoot SA, Srinivasan SR, Berenson GS. Essential hypertension predicted by tracking of elevated blood pressure from childhood to adulthood: the Bogalusa Heart Study. *Am J Hypertens.* 1995;8(7):657–665

64. Falkner B, Gidding SS, Portman R, Rosner B. Blood pressure variability and classification of prehypertension and hypertension in adolescence. *Pediatrics.* 2008;122(2):238–242

65. Tracy RE, Newman WP III, Wattigney WA, Srinivasan SR, Strong JP, Berenson GS. Histologic features of atherosclerosis and hypertension from autopsies of young individuals in a defined geographic population: the Bogalusa Heart Study. *Atherosclerosis.* 1995;116(2):163–179

66. Urbina EM, Khoury PR, McCoy C, Daniels SR, Kimball TR, Dolan LM. Cardiac and vascular consequences of pre-hypertension in youth. *J Clin Hypertens (Greenwich).* 2011;13(5):332–342

67. de Simone G, Devereux RB, Daniels SR, Koren MJ, Meyer RA, Laragh JH. Effect of growth on variability of left ventricular mass: assessment of allometric signals in adults and children and their capacity to predict cardiovascular risk. *J Am Coll Cardiol.* 1995;25(5):1056–1062

68. O'Leary DH, Polak JF, Kronmal RA, Manolio TA, Burke GL, Wolfson SK Jr; Cardiovascular Health Study Collaborative Research Group. Carotid-artery intima and media thickness as a risk factor for myocardial infarction and stroke in older adults. *N Engl J Med.* 1999;340(1):14–22

69. Mitchell GF, Hwang SJ, Vasan RS, et al. Arterial stiffness and cardiovascular events: the Framingham Heart Study. *Circulation.* 2010;121(4):505–511

70. Lloyd-Jones DM, Hong Y, Labarthe D, et al; American Heart Association Strategic Planning Task Force and Statistics Committee. Defining and setting national goals for cardiovascular health promotion and disease reduction: the American Heart Association's strategic impact goal through 2020 and beyond. *Circulation.* 2010;121(4):586–613

71. Ning H, Labarthe DR, Shay CM, et al. Status of cardiovascular health in US children up to 11 years of age: the National Health and Nutrition Examination Surveys 2003-2010. *Circ Cardiovasc Qual Outcomes.* 2015;8(2):164–171

72. Steinberger J, Daniels SR, Hagberg N, et al; American Heart Association Atherosclerosis, Hypertension, and Obesity in the Young Committee of the Council on Cardiovascular Disease in the Young; Council on Cardiovascular and Stroke Nursing; Council on Epidemiology and Prevention; Council on Functional Genomics and Translational Biology; Stroke Council. Cardiovascular health promotion in children: challenges and opportunities for 2020 and beyond: a

scientific statement from the American Heart Association. *Circulation*. 2016;134(12):e236–e255

73. Ogden CL, Carroll MD, Lawman HG, et al. Trends in obesity prevalence among children and adolescents in the United States, 1988-1994 through 2013-2014. *JAMA*. 2016;315(21):2292–2299

74. Skinner AC, Perrin EM, Skelton JA. Prevalence of obesity and severe obesity in US children, 1999-2014. *Obesity (Silver Spring)*. 2016;24(5):1116–1123

75. Skinner AC, Skelton JA. Prevalence and trends in obesity and severe obesity among children in the United States, 1999-2012. *JAMA Pediatr*. 2014;168(6):561–566

76. Shay CM, Ning H, Daniels SR, Rooks CR, Gidding SS, Lloyd-Jones DM. Status of cardiovascular health in US adolescents: prevalence estimates from the National Health and Nutrition Examination Surveys (NHANES) 2005-2010. *Circulation*. 2013;127(13):1369–1376

77. Rosner B, Cook N, Portman R, Daniels S, Falkner B. Determination of blood pressure percentiles in normal-weight children: some methodological issues. *Am J Epidemiol*. 2008;167(6):653–666

78. Kaelber DC, Pickett F. Simple table to identify children and adolescents needing further evaluation of blood pressure. *Pediatrics*. 2009;123(6). Available at: www.pediatrics.org/cgi/content/full/123/6/e972

79. Dionne JM, Abitbol CL, Flynn JT. Hypertension in infancy: diagnosis, management and outcome [published correction appears in *Pediatr Nephrol*. 2012;27(1):159-60]. *Pediatr Nephrol*. 2012;27(1):17–32

80. Kent AL, Chaudhari T. Determinants of neonatal blood pressure. *Curr Hypertens Rep*. 2013;15(5):426–432

81. Report of the second task force on blood pressure control in children–1987. Task force on blood pressure control in children. National Heart, Lung, and Blood Institute, Bethesda, Maryland. *Pediatrics*. 1987;79(1):1–25

82. Savoca MR, MacKey ML, Evans CD, Wilson M, Ludwig DA, Harshfield GA. Association of ambulatory blood pressure and dietary caffeine in adolescents. *Am J Hypertens*. 2005;18(1):116–120

83. Pickering TG, Hall JE, Appel LJ, et al. Recommendations for blood pressure measurement in humans and experimental animals: part 1: blood pressure measurement in humans: a statement for professionals from the Subcommittee of Professional and Public Education of the American Heart Association Council on High Blood Pressure Research. *Circulation*. 2005;111(5):697–716

84. Becton LJ, Egan BM, Hailpern SM, Shatat IF. Blood pressure reclassification in adolescents based on repeat clinic blood pressure measurements. *J Clin Hypertens (Greenwich)*. 2013;15(10):717–722

85. Daley MF, Sinaiko AR, Reifler LM, et al. Patterns of care and persistence after incident elevated blood pressure. *Pediatrics*. 2013;132(2). Available at: www.pediatrics.org/cgi/content/full/132/2/e349

86. Ostchega Y, Prineas RJ, Nwankwo T, Zipf G. Assessing blood pressure accuracy of an aneroid sphygmomanometer in a national survey environment. *Am J Hypertens*. 2011;24(3):322–327

87. Ma Y, Temprosa M, Fowler S, et al; Diabetes Prevention Program Research Group. Evaluating the accuracy of an aneroid sphygmomanometer in a clinical trial setting. *Am J Hypertens*. 2009;22(3):263–266

88. Podoll A, Grenier M, Croix B, Feig DI. Inaccuracy in pediatric outpatient blood pressure measurement. *Pediatrics*. 2007;119(3). Available at: www.pediatrics.org/cgi/content/full/119/3/e538

89. Mourad A, Carney S. Arm position and blood pressure: an audit. *Intern Med J*. 2004;34(5):290–291

90. Mourad A, Carney S, Gillies A, Jones B, Nanra R, Trevillian P. Arm position and blood pressure: a risk factor for hypertension? *J Hum Hypertens*. 2003;17(6):389–395

91. Zaheer S, Watson L, Webb NJ. Unmet needs in the measurement of blood pressure in primary care. *Arch Dis Child*. 2014;99(5):463–464

92. Veiga EV, Arcuri EAM, Cloutier L, Santos JL. Blood pressure measurement: arm circumference and cuff size availability. *Rev Lat Am Enfermagem*. 2009;17(4):455–461

93. Thomas M, Radford T, Dasgupta I. Unvalidated blood pressure devices with small cuffs are being used in hospitals. *BMJ*. 2001;323(7309):398

94. Burke MJ, Towers HM, O'Malley K, Fitzgerald DJ, O'Brien ET. Sphygmomanometers in hospital and family practice: problems and recommendations. *Br Med J (Clin Res Ed)*. 1982;285(6340):469–471

95. Centers for Disease Control and Prevention. National Health and Nutrition Examination Survey (NHANES) Anthropometry Procedures Manual. Available at: https://www.cdc.gov/nchs/data/nhanes/nhanes_07_08/manual_an.pdf. Published January 2013. Accessed May 9, 2016

96. Prineas RJ, Ostchega Y, Carroll M, Dillon C, McDowell M. US demographic trends in mid-arm circumference and recommended blood pressure cuffs for children and adolescents: data from the National Health and Nutrition Examination Survey 1988-2004. *Blood Press Monit*. 2007;12(2):75–80

97. Kimble KJ, Darnall RA Jr, Yelderman M, Ariagno RL, Ream AK. An automated oscillometric technique for estimating mean arterial pressure in critically ill newborns. *Anesthesiology*. 1981;54(5):423–425

98. Sonesson SE, Broberger U. Arterial blood pressure in the very low birthweight neonate. Evaluation of an automatic oscillometric technique. *Acta Paediatr Scand*. 1987;76(2):338–341

99. Duncan AF, Rosenfeld CR, Morgan JS, Ahmad N, Heyne RJ. Interrater reliability and effect of state on blood pressure measurements in infants 1 to 3 years of age. *Pediatrics*. 2008;122(3). Available at: www.pediatrics.org/cgi/content/full/122/3/e590

100. Nwankwo MU, Lorenz JM, Gardiner JC. A standard protocol for blood pressure measurement in the newborn. *Pediatrics*. 1997;99(6). Available at: www.pediatrics.org/cgi/content/full/99/6/e10

101. Gupta-Malhotra M, Banker A, Shete S, et al. Essential hypertension vs. secondary hypertension among children. *Am J Hypertens.* 2015;28(1):73–80

102. Kelly RK, Thomson R, Smith KJ, Dwyer T, Venn A, Magnussen CG. Factors affecting tracking of blood pressure from childhood to adulthood: the Childhood Determinants of Adult Health Study. *J Pediatr.* 2015;167(6):1422–1428.e2

103. Juhola J, Magnussen CG, Berenson GS, et al. Combined effects of child and adult elevated blood pressure on subclinical atherosclerosis: the International Childhood Cardiovascular Cohort Consortium. *Circulation.* 2013;128(3):217–224

104. Sladowska-Kozłowska J, Litwin M, Niemirska A, Wierzbicka A, Wawer ZT, Janas R. Change in left ventricular geometry during antihypertensive treatment in children with primary hypertension. *Pediatr Nephrol.* 2011;26(12):2201–2209

105. Litwin M, Niemirska A, Sladowska-Kozlowska J, et al. Regression of target organ damage in children and adolescents with primary hypertension. *Pediatr Nephrol.* 2010;25(12):2489–2499

106. Meyer AA, Kundt G, Lenschow U, Schuff-Werner P, Kienast W. Improvement of early vascular changes and cardiovascular risk factors in obese children after a six-month exercise program. *J Am Coll Cardiol.* 2006;48(9):1865–1870

107. Juonala M, Magnussen CG, Berenson GS, et al. Childhood adiposity, adult adiposity, and cardiovascular risk factors. *N Engl J Med.* 2011;365(20):1876–1885

108. Lo JC, Chandra M, Sinaiko A, et al. Severe obesity in children: prevalence, persistence and relation to hypertension. *Int J Pediatr Endocrinol.* 2014;2014(1):3

109. Rademacher ER, Jacobs DR Jr, Moran A, Steinberger J, Prineas RJ, Sinaiko A. Relation of blood pressure and body mass index during childhood to cardiovascular risk factor levels in young adults. *J Hypertens.* 2009;27(9):1766–1774

110. Maahs DM, Daniels SR, de Ferranti SD, et al; American Heart Association Atherosclerosis, Hypertension and Obesity in Youth Committee of the Council on Cardiovascular Disease in the Young; Council on Clinical Cardiology; Council on Cardiovascular and Stroke Nursing; Council for High Blood Pressure Research; Council on Lifestyle and Cardiometabolic Health. Cardiovascular disease risk factors in youth with diabetes mellitus: a scientific statement from the American Heart Association. *Circulation.* 2014;130(17):1532–1558

111. Levitt Katz L, Gidding SS, Bacha F, et al; TODAY Study Group. Alterations in left ventricular, left atrial, and right ventricular structure and function to cardiovascular risk factors in adolescents with type 2 diabetes participating in the TODAY clinical trial. *Pediatr Diabetes.* 2015;16(1):39–47

112. Hager A, Kanz S, Kaemmerer H, Schreiber C, Hess J. Coarctation Long-term Assessment (COALA): significance of arterial hypertension in a cohort of 404 patients up to 27 years after surgical repair of isolated coarctation of the aorta, even in the absence of restenosis and prosthetic material. *J Thorac Cardiovasc Surg.* 2007;134(3):738–745

113. O'Sullivan JJ, Derrick G, Darnell R. Prevalence of hypertension in children after early repair of coarctation of the aorta: a cohort study using casual and 24 hour blood pressure measurement. *Heart.* 2002;88(2):163–166

114. Becker AM, Goldberg JH, Henson M, et al. Blood pressure abnormalities in children with sickle cell anemia. *Pediatr Blood Cancer.* 2014;61(3):518–522

115. Brady TM, Solomon BS, Neu AM, Siberry GK, Parekh RS. Patient-, provider-, and clinic-level predictors of unrecognized elevated blood pressure in children. *Pediatrics.* 2010;125(6). Available at: www.pediatrics.org/cgi/content/full/125/6/e1286

116. Stabouli S, Sideras L, Vareta G, et al. Hypertension screening during healthcare pediatric visits. *J Hypertens.* 2015;33(5):1064–1068

117. Shapiro DJ, Hersh AL, Cabana MD, Sutherland SM, Patel AI. Hypertension screening during ambulatory pediatric visits in the United States, 2000-2009. *Pediatrics.* 2012;130(4):604–610

118. Bijlsma MW, Blufpand HN, Key Action Statementpers GJ, Bökenkamp A. Why pediatricians fail to diagnose hypertension: a multicenter survey. *J Pediatr.* 2014;164(1):173–177.e7

119. Chaudhry B, Wang J, Wu S, et al. Systematic review: impact of health information technology on quality, efficiency, and costs of medical care. *Ann Intern Med.* 2006;144(10):742–752

120. Shojania KG, Jennings A, Mayhew A, Ramsay CR, Eccles MP, Grimshaw J. The effects of on-screen, point of care computer reminders on processes and outcomes of care. *Cochrane Database Syst Rev.* 2009;(3):CD001096

121. Garg AX, Adhikari NKJ, McDonald H, et al. Effects of computerized clinical decision support systems on practitioner performance and patient outcomes: a systematic review. *JAMA.* 2005;293(10):1223–1238

122. Hicks LS, Sequist TD, Ayanian JZ, et al. Impact of computerized decision support on blood pressure management and control: a randomized controlled trial. *J Gen Intern Med.* 2008;23(4):429–441

123. Samal L, Linder JA, Lipsitz SR, Hicks LS. Electronic health records, clinical decision support, and blood pressure control. *Am J Manag Care.* 2011;17(9):626–632

124. Heymann AD, Hoch I, Valinsky L, Shalev V, Silber H, Kokia E. Mandatory computer field for blood pressure measurement improves screening. *Fam Pract.* 2005;22(2):168–169

125. Brady TM, Neu AM, Miller ER III, Appel LJ, Siberry GK, Solomon BS. Real-time electronic medical record alerts increase high blood pressure recognition in children. *Clin Pediatr (Phila).* 2015;54(7):667–675

126. Romano MJ, Stafford RS. Electronic health records and clinical decision support systems: impact on national ambulatory care quality. *Arch Intern Med.* 2011;171(10):897–903

127. Alpert BS, Quinn D, Gallick D. Oscillometric blood pressure: a review for clinicians. *J Am Soc Hypertens.* 2014;8(12):930–938

128. Alpert BS. Oscillometric blood pressure values are algorithm-specific. *Am J Cardiol.* 2010;106(10):1524–1525, author reply 1524–1525

129. Flynn JT, Pierce CB, Miller ER III, et al; Chronic Kidney Disease in Children Study Group. Reliability of resting blood pressure measurement and classification using an oscillometric device in children with chronic kidney disease. *J Pediatr.* 2012;160(3):434–440.e1

130. Kamath N, Goud BR, Phadke KD, Iyengar A. Use of oscillometric devices for the measurement of blood pressure-comparison with the gold standard. *Indian J Pediatr.* 2012;79(9):1230–1232

131. Chiolero A, Bovet P, Stergiou GS. Automated oscillometric blood pressure measurement in children. *J Clin Hypertens (Greenwich).* 2014;16(6):468

132. Chiolero A, Paradis G, Lambert M. Accuracy of oscillometric devices in children and adults. *Blood Press.* 2010;19(4):254–259

133. Chio SS, Urbina EM, Lapointe J, Tsai J, Berenson GS. Korotkoff sound versus oscillometric cuff sphygmomanometers: comparison between auscultatory and DynaPulse blood pressure measurements. *J Am Soc Hypertens.* 2011;5(1):12–20

134. Eliasdottir SB, Steinthorsdottir SD, Indridason OS, Palsson R, Edvardsson VO. Comparison of aneroid and oscillometric blood pressure measurements in children. *J Clin Hypertens (Greenwich).* 2013;15(11):776–783

135. Urbina EM, Khoury PR, McCoy CE, Daniels SR, Dolan LM, Kimball TR. Comparison of mercury sphygmomanometry blood pressure readings with oscillometric and central blood pressure in predicting target organ damage in youth. *Blood Press Monit.* 2015;20(3):150–156

136. Negroni-Balasquide X, Bell CS, Samuel J, Samuels JA. Is one measurement enough to evaluate blood pressure among adolescents? A blood pressure screening experience in more than 9000 children with a subset comparison of auscultatory to mercury measurements. *J Am Soc Hypertens.* 2016;10(2):95–100

137. Leblanc M-É, Croteau S, Ferland A, et al. Blood pressure assessment in severe obesity: validation of a forearm approach. *Obesity (Silver Spring).* 2013;21(12):E533–E541

138. Altunkan S, Genç Y, Altunkan E. A comparative study of an ambulatory blood pressure measuring device and a wrist blood pressure monitor with a position sensor versus a mercury sphygmomanometer. *Eur J Intern Med.* 2007;18(2):118–123

139. Uen S, Fimmers R, Brieger M, Nickenig G, Mengden T. Reproducibility of wrist home blood pressure measurement with position sensor and automatic data storage. *BMC Cardiovasc Disord.* 2009;9:20

140. Fania C, Benetti E, Palatini P. Validation of the A&D BP UB-543 wrist device for home blood pressure measurement according to the European Society of Hypertension International Protocol revision 2010. *Blood Press Monit.* 2015;20(4):237–240

141. Kang Y-Y, Chen Q, Li Y, Wang JG. Validation of the SCIAN LD-735 wrist blood pressure monitor for home blood pressure monitoring according to the European Society of Hypertension International Protocol revision 2010. *Blood Press Monit.* 2016;21(4):255–258

142. Xie P, Wang Y, Xu X, Huang F, Pan J. Validation of the Pangao PG-800A11 wrist device assessed according to the European Society of Hypertension and the British Hypertension Society protocols. *Blood Press Monit.* 2015;20(2):108–111

143. Zweiker R, Schumacher M, Fruhwald FM, Watzinger N, Klein W. Comparison of wrist blood pressure measurement with conventional sphygmomanometry at a cardiology outpatient clinic. *J Hypertens.* 2000;18(8):1013–1018

144. Altunkan S, Yildiz S, Azer S. Wrist blood pressure-measuring devices: a comparative study of accuracy with a standard auscultatory method using a mercury manometer. *Blood Press Monit.* 2002;7(5):281–284

145. Palatini P, Longo D, Toffanin G, Bertolo O, Zaetta V, Pessina AC. Wrist blood pressure overestimates blood pressure measured at the upper arm. *Blood Press Monit.* 2004;9(2):77–81

146. Stergiou GS, Christodoulakis GR, Nasothimiou EG, Giovas PP, Kalogeropoulos PG. Can validated wrist devices with position sensors replace arm devices for self-home blood pressure monitoring? A randomized crossover trial using ambulatory monitoring as reference. *Am J Hypertens.* 2008;21(7):753–758

147. Khoshdel AR, Carney S, Gillies A. The impact of arm position and pulse pressure on the validation of a wrist-cuff blood pressure measurement device in a high risk population. *Int J Gen Med.* 2010;3:119–125

148. Kikuya M, Chonan K, Imai Y, Goto E, Ishii M; Research Group to Assess the Validity of Automated Blood Pressure Measurement Devices in Japan. Accuracy and reliability of wrist-cuff devices for self-measurement of blood pressure. *J Hypertens.* 2002;20(4):629–638

149. Westhoff TH, Schmidt S, Meissner R, Zidek W, van der Giet M. The impact of pulse pressure on the accuracy of wrist blood pressure measurement. *J Hum Hypertens.* 2009;23(6):391–395

150. Deutsch C, Krüger R, Saito K, et al. Comparison of the Omron RS6 wrist blood pressure monitor with the positioning sensor on or off with a standard mercury sphygmomanometer. *Blood Press Monit.* 2014;19(5):306–313

151. Yarows SA. Comparison of the Omron HEM-637 wrist monitor to the auscultation method with the wrist position sensor on or disabled. *Am J Hypertens.* 2004;17(1):54–58

152. Menezes AMB, Dumith SC, Noal RB, et al. Validity of a wrist digital monitor for blood pressure measurement in comparison to a mercury sphygmomanometer. *Arq Bras Cardiol.* 2010;94(3):345–349, 365–370

153. Wankum PC, Thurman TL, Holt SJ, Hall RA, Simpson PM, Heulitt MJ. Validation of a noninvasive blood pressure

monitoring device in normotensive and hypertensive pediatric intensive care patients. *J Clin Monit Comput.* 2004;18(4):253–263

154. Cua CL, Thomas K, Zurakowski D, Laussen PC. A comparison of the Vasotrac with invasive arterial blood pressure monitoring in children after pediatric cardiac surgery. *Anesth Analg.* 2005;100(5): 1289–1294

155. Flynn JT, Daniels SR, Hayman LL, et al; American Heart Association Atherosclerosis, Hypertension and Obesity in Youth Committee of the Council on Cardiovascular Disease in the Young. Update: ambulatory blood pressure monitoring in children and adolescents: a scientific statement from the American Heart Association. *Hypertension.* 2014;63(5): 1116–1135

156. Siu AL; U.S. Preventive Services Task Force. Screening for high blood pressure in adults: U.S. Preventive Services Task Force recommendation statement. *Ann Intern Med.* 2015;163(10):778–786

157. Díaz LN, Garin EH. Comparison of ambulatory blood pressure and Task Force criteria to identify pediatric hypertension. *Pediatr Nephrol.* 2007;22(4):554–558

158. Salice P, Ardissino G, Zanchetti A, et al. Age-dependent differences in office (OBP) vs ambulatory blood pressure monitoring (ABPM) in hypertensive children and adolescents: 8C.03. *J Hypertens.* 2010;28:e423–e424

159. Stergiou GS, Alamara CV, Salgami EV, Vaindirlis IN, Dacou-Voutetakis C, Mountokalakis TD. Reproducibility of home and ambulatory blood pressure in children and adolescents. *Blood Press Monit.* 2005;10(3):143–147

160. Li Z, Snieder H, Harshfield GA, Treiber FA, Wang X. A 15-year longitudinal study on ambulatory blood pressure tracking from childhood to early adulthood. *Hypertens Res.* 2009;32(5):404–410

161. Seeman T, Palyzová D, Dusek J, Janda J. Reduced nocturnal blood pressure dip and sustained nighttime hypertension are specific markers of secondary hypertension. *J Pediatr.* 2005;147(3):366–371

162. Bjelakovic B, Jaddoe VW, Vukomanovic V, et al. The relationship between currently recommended ambulatory systolic blood pressure measures and left ventricular mass index in pediatric hypertension. *Curr Hypertens Rep.* 2015;17(4):534

163. Brady TM, Fivush B, Flynn JT, Parekh R. Ability of blood pressure to predict left ventricular hypertrophy in children with primary hypertension. *J Pediatr.* 2008;152(1):73–78, 78.e1

164. McNiece KL, Gupta-Malhotra M, Samuels J, et al; National High Blood Pressure Education Program Working Group. Left ventricular hypertrophy in hypertensive adolescents: analysis of risk by 2004 National High Blood Pressure Education Program Working Group staging criteria. *Hypertension.* 2007;50(2):392–395

165. Richey PA, Disessa TG, Hastings MC, Somes GW, Alpert BS, Jones DP. Ambulatory blood pressure and increased left ventricular mass in children at risk for hypertension. *J Pediatr.* 2008;152(3):343–348

166. Conkar S, Yılmaz E, Hacıkara Ş, Bozabalı S, Mir S. Is daytime systolic load an important risk factor for target organ damage in pediatric hypertension? *J Clin Hypertens (Greenwich).* 2015;17(10):760–766

167. Flynn JT. Differentiation between primary and secondary hypertension in children using ambulatory blood pressure monitoring. *Pediatrics.* 2002;110(1, pt 1):89–93

168. Dursun H, Bayazit AK, Cengiz N, et al. Ambulatory blood pressure monitoring and renal functions in children with a solitary kidney. *Pediatr Nephrol.* 2007;22(4):559–564

169. Patzer L, Seeman T, Luck C, Wühl E, Janda J, Misselwitz J. Day- and night-time blood pressure elevation in children with higher grades of renal scarring. *J Pediatr.* 2003;142(2):117–122

170. Fidan K, Kandur Y, Buyukkaragoz B, Akdemir UO, Soylemezoglu O. Hypertension in pediatric patients with renal scarring in association with vesicoureteral reflux. *Urology.* 2013;81(1):173–177

171. Basiratnia M, Esteghamati M, Ajami GH, et al. Blood pressure profile in renal transplant recipients and its relation to diastolic function: tissue Doppler echocardiographic study. *Pediatr Nephrol.* 2011;26(3):449–457

172. Chaudhuri A, Sutherland SM, Begin B, et al. Role of twenty-four-hour ambulatory blood pressure monitoring in children on dialysis. *Clin J Am Soc Nephrol.* 2011;6(4):870–876

173. Wühl E, Trivelli A, Picca S, et al; ESCAPE Trial Group. Strict blood-pressure control and progression of renal failure in children. *N Engl J Med.* 2009;361(17):1639–1650

174. Chatterjee M, Speiser PW, Pellizzarri M, et al. Poor glycemic control is associated with abnormal changes in 24-hour ambulatory blood pressure in children and adolescents with type 1 diabetes mellitus. *J Pediatr Endocrinol Metab.* 2009;22(11):1061–1067

175. Darcan S, Goksen D, Mir S, et al. Alterations of blood pressure in type 1 diabetic children and adolescents. *Pediatr Nephrol.* 2006;21(5):672–676

176. Dost A, Klinkert C, Kapellen T, et al; DPV Science Initiative. Arterial hypertension determined by ambulatory blood pressure profiles: contribution to microalbuminuria risk in a multicenter investigation in 2,105 children and adolescents with type 1 diabetes. *Diabetes Care.* 2008;31(4):720–725

177. Ettinger LM, Freeman K, DiMartino-Nardi JR, Flynn JT. Microalbuminuria and abnormal ambulatory blood pressure in adolescents with type 2 diabetes mellitus. *J Pediatr.* 2005;147(1):67–73

178. Lurbe E, Redon J, Kesani A, et al. Increase in nocturnal blood pressure and progression to microalbuminuria in type 1 diabetes. *N Engl J Med.* 2002;347(11):797–805

179. Nagasako SS, Nogueira PC, Machado PG, Pestana JO. Risk factors for hypertension 3 years after renal transplantation in children. *Pediatr Nephrol.* 2007;22(9):1363–1368

180. Roche SL, Kaufmann J, Dipchand AI, Kantor PF. Hypertension after pediatric heart transplantation is primarily associated with immunosuppressive

regimen. *J Heart Lung Transplant.* 2008;27(5):501–507

181. Paripovic D, Kostic M, Spasojevic B, Kruscic D, Peco-Antic A. Masked hypertension and hidden uncontrolled hypertension after renal transplantation. *Pediatr Nephrol.* 2010;25(9):1719–1724

182. Ferraris JR, Ghezzi L, Waisman G, Krmar RT. ABPM vs office blood pressure to define blood pressure control in treated hypertensive paediatric renal transplant recipients. *Pediatr Transplant.* 2007;11(1):24–30

183. McGlothan KR, Wyatt RJ, Ault BH, et al. Predominance of nocturnal hypertension in pediatric renal allograft recipients. *Pediatr Transplant.* 2006;10(5):558–564

184. Balzano R, Lindblad YT, Vavilis G, Jogestrand T, Berg UB, Krmar RT. Use of annual ABPM, and repeated carotid scan and echocardiography to monitor cardiovascular health over nine yr in pediatric and young adult renal transplant recipients. *Pediatr Transplant.* 2011;15(6):635–641

185. Krmar RT, Berg UB. Blood pressure control in hypertensive pediatric renal transplants: role of repeated ABPM following transplantation. *Am J Hypertens.* 2008;21(10):1093–1099

186. Ambrosi P, Kreitmann B, Habib G. Home blood pressure monitoring in heart transplant recipients: comparison with ambulatory blood pressure monitoring. *Transplantation.* 2014;97(3):363–367

187. Seeman T, Simková E, Kreisinger J, et al. Reduction of proteinuria during intensified antihypertensive therapy in children after renal transplantation. *Transplant Proc.* 2007;39(10):3150–3152

188. Seeman T, Simková E, Kreisinger J, et al. Improved control of hypertension in children after renal transplantation: results of a two-yr interventional trial. *Pediatr Transplant.* 2007;11(5):491–497

189. Lurbe E, Alvarez V, Liao Y, et al. The impact of obesity and body fat distribution on ambulatory blood pressure in children and adolescents. *Am J Hypertens.* 1998;11(4, pt 1):418–424

190. Lurbe E, Alvarez V, Redon J. Obesity, body fat distribution, and ambulatory blood pressure in children and adolescents. *J Clin Hypertens (Greenwich).* 2001;3(6):362–367

191. Marcovecchio ML, Patricelli L, Zito M, et al. Ambulatory blood pressure monitoring in obese children: role of insulin resistance. *J Hypertens.* 2006;24(12):2431–2436

192. Shatat IF, Freeman KD, Vuguin PM, Dimartino-Nardi JR, Flynn JT. Relationship between adiponectin and ambulatory blood pressure in obese adolescents. *Pediatr Res.* 2009;65(6):691–695

193. Amin RS, Carroll JL, Jeffries JL, et al. Twenty-four-hour ambulatory blood pressure in children with sleep-disordered breathing. *Am J Respir Crit Care Med.* 2004;169(8):950–956

194. Leung LC, Ng DK, Lau MW, et al. Twenty-four-hour ambulatory BP in snoring children with obstructive sleep apnea syndrome. *Chest.* 2006;130(4):1009–1017

195. Akyürek N, Atabek ME, Eklioglu BS, Alp H. Ambulatory blood pressure and subclinical cardiovascular disease in children with turner syndrome. *Pediatr Cardiol.* 2014;35(1):57–62

196. Salgado CM, Jardim PC, Teles FB, Nunes MC. Low birth weight as a marker of changes in ambulatory blood pressure monitoring. *Arq Bras Cardiol.* 2009;92(2):107–121

197. Gimpel C, Wühl E, Arbeiter K, et al; ESCAPE Trial Group. Superior consistency of ambulatory blood pressure monitoring in children: implications for clinical trials. *J Hypertens.* 2009;27(8):1568–1574

198. Suláková T, Feber J. Should mean arterial pressure be included in the definition of ambulatory hypertension in children? *Pediatr Nephrol.* 2013;28(7):1105–1112

199. Lurbe E, Torro I, Alvarez V, et al. Prevalence, persistence, and clinical significance of masked hypertension in youth. *Hypertension.* 2005;45(4):493–498

200. Stabouli S, Kotsis V, Toumanidis S, Papamichael C, Constantopoulos A, Zakopoulos N. White-coat and masked hypertension in children: association with target-organ damage. *Pediatr Nephrol.* 2005;20(8):1151–1155

201. Furusawa ÉA, Filho UD, Junior DM, Koch VH. Home and ambulatory blood pressure to identify white coat and masked hypertension in the pediatric patient. *Am J Hypertens.* 2011;24(8):893–897

202. Wells TG, Portman R, Norman P, Haertter S, Davidai G, Fei Wang. Safety, efficacy, and pharmacokinetics of telmisartan in pediatric patients with hypertension. *Clin Pediatr (Phila).* 2010;49(10):938–946

203. Mitsnefes M, Flynn J, Cohn S, et al; CKiD Study Group. Masked hypertension associates with left ventricular hypertrophy in children with CKD. *J Am Soc Nephrol.* 2010;21(1):137–144

204. Lurbe E, Redon J. Discrepancies in office and ambulatory blood pressure in adolescents: help or hindrance? *Pediatr Nephrol.* 2008;23(3):341–345

205. Pogue V, Rahman M, Lipkowitz M, et al; African American Study of Kidney Disease and Hypertension Collaborative Research Group. Disparate estimates of hypertension control from ambulatory and clinic blood pressure measurements in hypertensive kidney disease. *Hypertension.* 2009;53(1):20–27

206. Urbina EM, Williams RV, Alpert BS, et al; American Heart Association Atherosclerosis, Hypertension, and Obesity in Youth Committee of the Council on Cardiovascular Disease in the Young. Noninvasive assessment of subclinical atherosclerosis in children and adolescents: recommendations for standard assessment for clinical research: a scientific statement from the American Heart Association. *Hypertension.* 2009;54(5):919–950

207. Kavey RE, Kveselis DA, Atallah N, Smith FC. White coat hypertension in childhood: evidence for end-organ effect. *J Pediatr.* 2007;150(5):491–497

208. Swartz SJ, Srivaths PR, Croix B, Feig DI. Cost-effectiveness of ambulatory blood pressure monitoring in the initial evaluation of hypertension in children. *Pediatrics.* 2008;122(6):1177–1181

209. Briasoulis A, Androulakis E, Palla M, Papageorgiou N, Tousoulis D. White-coat hypertension and cardiovascular events: a meta-analysis. *J Hypertens.* 2016;34(4):593–599

210. Valent-Morić B, Zigman T, Zaja-Franulović O, Malenica M, Cuk M. The importance of ambulatory blood pressure monitoring in children and adolescents. *Acta Clin Croat.* 2012;51(1):59–64

211. Palatini P, Parati G. Blood pressure measurement in very obese patients: a challenging problem. *J Hypertens.* 2011;29(3):425–429

212. Halm MA. Arm circumference, shape, and length: how interplaying variables affect blood pressure measurement in obese persons. *Am J Crit Care.* 2014;23(2):166–170

213. Ostchega Y, Hughes JP, Prineas RJ, Zhang G, Nwankwo T, Chiappa MM. Mid-arm circumference and recommended blood pressure cuffs for children and adolescents aged between 3 and 19 years: data from the National Health and Nutrition Examination Survey, 1999-2010. *Blood Press Monit.* 2014;19(1):26–31

214. Bonso E, Saladini F, Zanier A, Benetti E, Dorigatti F, Palatini P. Accuracy of a single rigid conical cuff with standard-size bladder coupled to an automatic oscillometric device over a wide range of arm circumferences. *Hypertens Res.* 2010;33(11):1186–1191

215. Palatini P, Benetti E, Fania C, Malipiero G, Saladini F. Rectangular cuffs may overestimate blood pressure in individuals with large conical arms. *J Hypertens.* 2012;30(3):530–536

216. Aguilar A, Ostrow V, De Luca F, Suarez E. Elevated ambulatory blood pressure in a multi-ethnic population of obese children and adolescents. *J Pediatr.* 2010;156(6):930–935

217. Ostrow V, Wu S, Aguilar A, Bonner R Jr, Suarez E, De Luca F. Association between oxidative stress and masked hypertension in a multi-ethnic population of obese children and adolescents. *J Pediatr.* 2011;158(4):628–633.e1

218. Woroniecki RP, Flynn JT. How are hypertensive children evaluated and managed? A survey of North American pediatric nephrologists. *Pediatr Nephrol.* 2005;20(6):791–797

219. Mengden T, Hernandez Medina RM, Beltran B, Alvarez E, Kraft K, Vetter H. Reliability of reporting self-measured blood pressure values by hypertensive patients. *Am J Hypertens.* 1998;11(12):1413–1417

220. Palatini P, Frick GN. Techniques for self-measurement of blood pressure: limitations and needs for future research. *J Clin Hypertens (Greenwich).* 2012;14(3):139–143

221. Stergiou GS, Karpettas N, Kapoyiannis A, Stefanidis CJ, Vazeou A. Home blood pressure monitoring in children and adolescents: a systematic review. *J Hypertens.* 2009;27(10):1941–1947

222. Stergiou GS, Nasothimiou E, Giovas P, Kapoyiannis A, Vazeou A. Diagnosis of hypertension in children and adolescents based on home versus ambulatory blood pressure monitoring. *J Hypertens.* 2008;26(8):1556–1562

223. Furusawa EA, Filho UD, Koch VH. Home blood pressure monitoring in paediatric chronic hypertension. *J Hum Hypertens.* 2009;23(7):464–469

224. Stergiou GS, Nasothimiou EG, Giovas PP, Rarra VC. Long-term reproducibility of home vs. office blood pressure in children and adolescents: the Arsakeion school study. *Hypertens Res.* 2009;32(4):311–315

225. Wühl E, Hadtstein C, Mehls O, Schaefer F; Escape Trial Group. Home, clinic, and ambulatory blood pressure monitoring in children with chronic renal failure. *Pediatr Res.* 2004;55(3):492–497

226. Stergiou GS, Karpettas N, Panagiotakos DB, Vazeou A. Comparison of office, ambulatory and home blood pressure in children and adolescents on the basis of normalcy tables. *J Hum Hypertens.* 2011;25(4):218–223

227. Stergiou GS, Alamara CV, Kalkana CB, et al. Out-of-office blood pressure in children and adolescents: disparate findings by using home or ambulatory monitoring. *Am J Hypertens.* 2004;17(10):869–875

228. Stergiou GS, Rarra VC, Yiannes NG. Changing relationship between home and office blood pressure with increasing age in children: the Arsakeion School study. *Am J Hypertens.* 2008;21(1):41–46

229. Salgado CM, Jardim PC, Viana JK, Jardim TS, Velasquez PP. Home blood pressure in children and adolescents: a comparison with office and ambulatory blood pressure measurements. *Acta Paediatr.* 2011;100(10):e163–e168

230. Stergiou GS, Ntineri A, Kollias A, Destounis A, Nasothimiou E, Roussias L. Changing relationship among clinic, home, and ambulatory blood pressure with increasing age. *J Am Soc Hypertens.* 2015;9(7):544–552

231. Stergiou GS, Yiannes NG, Rarra VC, Panagiotakos DB. Home blood pressure normalcy in children and adolescents: the Arsakeion School study. *J Hypertens.* 2007;25(7):1375–1379

232. Sorof JM, Turner J, Franco K, Portman RJ. Characteristics of hypertensive children identified by primary care referral compared with school-based screening. *J Pediatr.* 2004;144(4):485–489

233. King CA, Meadows BB, Engelke MK, Swanson M. Prevalence of elevated body mass index and blood pressure in a rural school-aged population: implications for school nurses. *J Sch Health.* 2006;76(4):145–149

234. Underwood SM, Averhart L, Dean A, et al. Clinical evaluation and follow-up of body mass and blood pressure in pre-elementary school children: program review. *J Natl Black Nurses Assoc.* 2012;23(1):8–15

235. Kapur G, Ahmed M, Pan C, Mitsnefes M, Chiang M, Mattoo TK. Secondary hypertension in overweight and stage 1 hypertensive children: a Midwest Pediatric Nephrology Consortium report. *J Clin Hypertens (Greenwich).* 2010;12(1):34–39

236. Flynn JT, Alderman MH. Characteristics of children with primary hypertension seen at a referral center. *Pediatr Nephrol.* 2005;20(7):961–966

237. Gomes RS, Quirino IG, Pereira RM, et al. Primary versus secondary

hypertension in children followed up at an outpatient tertiary unit. *Pediatr Nephrol.* 2011;26(3):441–447

238. Welch WP, Yang W, Taylor-Zapata P, Flynn JT. Antihypertensive drug use by children: are the drugs labeled and indicated? *J Clin Hypertens (Greenwich).* 2012;14(6):388–395

239. Flynn J, Zhang Y, Solar-Yohay S, Shi V. Clinical and demographic characteristics of children with hypertension. *Hypertension.* 2012;60(4):1047–1054

240. Baracco R, Kapur G, Mattoo T, et al. Prediction of primary vs secondary hypertension in children. *J Clin Hypertens (Greenwich).* 2012;14(5):316–321

241. Silverstein DM, Champoux E, Aviles DH, Vehaskari VM. Treatment of primary and secondary hypertension in children. *Pediatr Nephrol.* 2006;21(6):820–827

242. Flynn JT, Meyers KEC, Neto JP, et al; Pediatric Valsartan Study Group. Efficacy and safety of the angiotensin receptor blocker valsartan in children with hypertension aged 1 to 5 years. *Hypertension.* 2008;52(2):222–228

243. Schaefer F, van de Walle J, Zurowska A, et al; Candesartan in Children with Hypertension Investigators. Efficacy, safety and pharmacokinetics of candesartan cilexetil in hypertensive children from 1 to less than 6 years of age. *J Hypertens.* 2010;28(5):1083–1090

244. Webb NJ, Wells TG, Shahinfar S, et al. A randomized, open-label, dose-response study of losartan in hypertensive children. *Clin J Am Soc Nephrol.* 2014;9(8):1441–1448

245. Coleman DM, Eliason JL, Ohye RG, Stanley JC. Long-segment thoracoabdominal aortic occlusions in childhood. *J Vasc Surg.* 2012;56(2):482–485

246. Lee MG, Kowalski R, Galati JC, et al. Twenty-four-hour ambulatory blood pressure monitoring detects a high prevalence of hypertension late after coarctation repair in patients with hypoplastic arches. *J Thorac Cardiovasc Surg.* 2012;144(5):1110–1116

247. Agnoletti G, Bonnet C, Bonnet D, Sidi D, Aggoun Y. Mid-term effects of implanting stents for relief of aortic recoarctation on systemic hypertension, carotid mechanical properties, intimal medial thickness and reflection of the pulse wave. *Cardiol Young.* 2005;15(3):245–250

248. Young WF. Endocrine hypertension. In: Melmed S, Polonsky KS, Larsen R, Kronenberg HM, eds. *Williams Textbook of Endocrinology.* 13th ed. Philadelphia, PA: Elsevier Inc; 2016:556–588

249. Bausch B, Wellner U, Bausch D, et al. Long-term prognosis of patients with pediatric pheochromocytoma. *Endocr Relat Cancer.* 2013;21(1):17–25

250. Waguespack SG, Rich T, Grubbs E, et al. A current review of the etiology, diagnosis, and treatment of pediatric pheochromocytoma and paraganglioma. *J Clin Endocrinol Metab.* 2010;95(5):2023–2037

251. Fishbein L, Merrill S, Fraker DL, Cohen DL, Nathanson KL. Inherited mutations in pheochromocytoma and paraganglioma: why all patients should be offered genetic testing. *Ann Surg Oncol.* 2013;20(5):1444–1450

252. Barontini M, Levin G, Sanso G. Characteristics of pheochromocytoma in a 4- to 20-year-old population. *Ann N Y Acad Sci.* 2006;1073:30–37

253. Welander J, Söderkvist P, Gimm O. Genetics and clinical characteristics of hereditary pheochromocytomas and paragangliomas. *Endocr Relat Cancer.* 2011;18(6):R253–R276

254. Eisenhofer G, Peitzsch M. Laboratory evaluation of pheochromocytoma and paraganglioma. *Clin Chem.* 2014;60(12):1486–1499

255. Funder JW, Carey RM, Mantero F, et al. The management of primary aldosteronism: case detection, diagnosis, and treatment: an Endocrine Society clinical practice guideline. *J Clin Endocrinol Metab.* 2016;101(5):1889–1916

256. Stowasser M, Gordon RD. Monogenic mineralocorticoid hypertension. *Best Pract Res Clin Endocrinol Metab.* 2006;20(3):401–420

257. White PC, Dupont J, New MI, Leiberman E, Hochberg Z, Rösler A. A mutation in CYP11B1 (Arg-448-—His) associated with steroid 11 beta-hydroxylase deficiency in Jews of Moroccan origin. *J Clin Invest.* 1991;87(5):1664–1667

258. Parsa AA, New MI. Low-renin hypertension of childhood. *Endocrinol Metab Clin North Am.* 2011;40(2): 369–377, viii

259. Parajes S, Loidi L, Reisch N, et al. Functional consequences of seven novel mutations in the CYP11B1 gene: four mutations associated with nonclassic and three mutations causing classic 11beta-hydroxylase deficiency. *J Clin Endocrinol Metab.* 2010;95(2):779–788

260. New MI, Geller DS, Fallo F, Wilson RC. Monogenic low renin hypertension. *Trends Endocrinol Metab.* 2005;16(3):92–97

261. Imai T, Yanase T, Waterman MR, Simpson ER, Pratt JJ. Canadian Mennonites and individuals residing in the Friesland region of The Netherlands share the same molecular basis of 17 alpha-hydroxylase deficiency. *Hum Genet.* 1992;89(1):95–96

262. Dhir V, Reisch N, Bleicken CM, et al. Steroid 17alpha-hydroxylase deficiency: functional characterization of four mutations (A174E, V178D, R440C, L465P) in the CYP17A1 gene. *J Clin Endocrinol Metab.* 2009;94(8):3058–3064

263. Aglony M, Martínez-Aguayo A, Carvajal CA, et al. Frequency of familial hyperaldosteronism type 1 in a hypertensive pediatric population: clinical and biochemical presentation. *Hypertension.* 2011;57(6):1117–1121

264. Speiser PW, White PC. Congenital adrenal hyperplasia. *N Engl J Med.* 2003;349(8):776–788

265. Funder JW. Genetic disorders in primary aldosteronism — familial and somatic. *J Steroid Biochem Mol Biol.* 2017;165(pt A):154–157

266. Carss KJ, Stowasser M, Gordon RD, O'Shaughnessy KM. Further study of chromosome 7p22 to identify the molecular basis of familial hyperaldosteronism type II. *J Hum Hypertens.* 2011;25(9):560–564

267. So A, Duffy DL, Gordon RD, et al. Familial hyperaldosteronism type II is linked to the chromosome 7p22 region but also shows predicted heterogeneity. *J Hypertens.* 2005;23(8):1477–1484

268. Geller DS, Zhang J, Wisgerhof MV, Shackleton C, Key Action Statementhgarian M, Lifton RP. A novel form of human mendelian hypertension featuring nonglucocorticoid-remediable aldosteronism. *J Clin Endocrinol Metab.* 2008;93(8):3117–3123

269. Boulkroun S, Beuschlein F, Rossi GP, et al. Prevalence, clinical, and molecular correlates of KCNJ5 mutations in primary aldosteronism. *Hypertension.* 2012;59(3):592–598

270. Scholl UI, Nelson-Williams C, Yue P, et al. Hypertension with or without adrenal hyperplasia due to different inherited mutations in the potassium channel KCNJ5. *Proc Natl Acad Sci USA.* 2012;109(7):2533–2538

271. Scholl UI, Goh G, Stölting G, et al. Somatic and germline CACNA1D calcium channel mutations in aldosterone-producing adenomas and primary aldosteronism. *Nat Genet.* 2013;45(9):1050–1054

272. Scholl UI, Stölting G, Nelson-Williams C, et al. Recurrent gain of function mutation in calcium channel CACNA1H causes early-onset hypertension with primary aldosteronism. *Elife.* 2015;4:e06315

273. Rothenbuhler A, Stratakis CA. Clinical and molecular genetics of Carney complex. *Best Pract Res Clin Endocrinol Metab.* 2010;24(3):389–399

274. Stratakis CA, Salpea P, Raygada M. *Carney Complex.* Seattle, WA: University of Washington; 2015

275. Lietman SA, Schwindinger WF, Levine MA. Genetic and molecular aspects of McCune-Albright syndrome. *Pediatr Endocrinol Rev.* 2007;4(suppl 4):380–385

276. Lumbroso S, Paris F, Sultan C. McCune-Albright syndrome: molecular genetics. *J Pediatr Endocrinol Metab.* 2002;15(suppl 3):875–882

277. Malchoff CD, Javier EC, Malchoff DM, et al. Primary cortisol resistance presenting as isosexual precocity. *J Clin Endocrinol Metab.* 1990;70(2):503–507

278. Nicolaides NC, Charmandari E. Chrousos syndrome: from molecular pathogenesis to therapeutic management. *Eur J Clin Invest.* 2015;45(5):504–514

279. Malchoff DM, Brufsky A, Reardon G, et al. A mutation of the glucocorticoid receptor in primary cortisol resistance. *J Clin Invest.* 1993;91(5):1918–1925

280. Ferrari P. The role of 11β-hydroxysteroid dehydrogenase type 2 in human hypertension. *Biochim Biophys Acta.* 2010;1802(12):1178–1187

281. Morineau G, Sulmont V, Salomon R, et al. Apparent mineralocorticoid excess: report of six new cases and extensive personal experience. *J Am Soc Nephrol.* 2006;17(11):3176–3184

282. Nesterov V, Krueger B, Bertog M, Dahlmann A, Palmisano R, Korbmacher C. In Liddle syndrome, epithelial sodium channel is hyperactive mainly in the early part of the aldosterone-sensitive distal nephron. *Hypertension.* 2016;67(6):1256–1262

283. Hanukoglu I, Hanukoglu A. Epithelial sodium channel (ENaC) family: Phylogeny, structure-function, tissue distribution, and associated inherited diseases. *Gene.* 2016;579(2):95–132

284. Geller DS, Farhi A, Pinkerton N, et al. Activating mineralocorticoid receptor mutation in hypertension exacerbated by pregnancy. *Science.* 2000;289(5476):119–123

285. Wilson FH, Disse-Nicodème S, Choate KA, et al. Human hypertension caused by mutations in WNK kinases. *Science.* 2001;293(5532):1107–1112

286. Boyden LM, Choi M, Choate KA, et al. Mutations in kelch-like 3 and cullin 3 cause hypertension and electrolyte abnormalities. *Nature.* 2012;482(7383):98–102

287. Stowasser M, Pimenta E, Gordon RD. Familial or genetic primary aldosteronism and Gordon syndrome. *Endocrinol Metab Clin North Am.* 2011;40(2):343–368, viii

288. Sacerdote A, Weiss K, Tran T, Rokeya Noor B, McFarlane SI. Hypertension in patients with Cushing's disease: pathophysiology, diagnosis, and management. *Curr Hypertens Rep.* 2005;7(3):212–218

289. Baid S, Nieman LK. Glucocorticoid excess and hypertension. *Curr Hypertens Rep.* 2004;6(6):493–499

290. Michalkiewicz E, Sandrini R, Figueiredo B, et al. Clinical and outcome characteristics of children with adrenocortical tumors: a report from the International Pediatric Adrenocortical Tumor Registry. *J Clin Oncol.* 2004;22(5):838–845

291. Danzi S, Klein I. Thyroid hormone and blood pressure regulation. *Curr Hypertens Rep.* 2003;5(6):513–520

292. Bahn RS, Burch HB, Cooper DS, et al; American Thyroid Association; American Association of Clinical Endocrinologists. Hyperthyroidism and other causes of thyrotoxicosis: management guidelines of the American Thyroid Association and American Association of Clinical Endocrinologists. *Endocr Pract.* 2011;17(3):456–520

293. Heyliger A, Tangpricha V, Weber C, Sharma J. Parathyroidectomy decreases systolic and diastolic blood pressure in hypertensive patients with primary hyperparathyroidism. *Surgery.* 2009;146(6):1042–1047

294. Rydberg E, Birgander M, Bondeson AG, Bondeson L, Willenheimer R. Effect of successful parathyroidectomy on 24-hour ambulatory blood pressure in patients with primary hyperparathyroidism. *Int J Cardiol.* 2010;142(1):15–21

295. Gambelunghe A, Sallsten G, Borné Y, et al. Low-level exposure to lead, blood pressure, and hypertension in a population-based cohort. *Environ Res.* 2016;149:157–163

296. Lee BK, Ahn J, Kim NS, Lee CB, Park J, Kim Y. Association of blood pressure with exposure to lead and cadmium: analysis of data from the 2008-2013 Korean National Health and Nutrition Examination Survey. *Biol Trace Elem Res.* 2016;174(1):40–51

297. Rapisarda V, Ledda C, Ferrante M, et al. Blood pressure and occupational

exposure to noise and lead (Pb): a cross-sectional study. *Toxicol Ind Health.* 2016;32(10):1729–1736

298. Hara A, Thijs L, Asayama K, et al. Blood pressure in relation to environmental lead exposure in the national health and nutrition examination survey 2003 to 2010. *Hypertension.* 2015;65(1):62–69

299. Gump BB, Reihman J, Stewart P, Lonky E, Darvill T, Matthews KA. Blood lead (Pb) levels: a potential environmental mechanism explaining the relation between socioeconomic status and cardiovascular reactivity in children. *Health Psychol.* 2007;26(3):296–304

300. Chen A, Rhoads GG, Cai B, Salganik M, Rogan WJ. The effect of chelation on blood pressure in lead-exposed children: a randomized study. *Environ Health Perspect.* 2006;114(4):579–583

301. Chen X, Zhu G, Lei L, Jin T. The association between blood pressure and blood cadmium in a Chinese population living in cadmium polluted area. *Environ Toxicol Pharmacol.* 2013;36(2):595–599

302. Tellez-Plaza M, Navas-Acien A, Crainiceanu CM, Guallar E. Cadmium exposure and hypertension in the 1999-2004 National Health and Nutrition Examination Survey (NHANES). *Environ Health Perspect.* 2008;116(1):51–56

303. Gallagher CM, Meliker JR. Blood and urine cadmium, blood pressure, and hypertension: a systematic review and meta-analysis. *Environ Health Perspect.* 2010;118(12):1676–1684

304. Swaddiwudhipong W, Mahasakpan P, Jeekeeree W, et al. Renal and blood pressure effects from environmental cadmium exposure in Thai children. *Environ Res.* 2015;136:82–87

305. Cao Y, Chen A, Radcliffe J, et al. Postnatal cadmium exposure, neurodevelopment, and blood pressure in children at 2, 5, and 7 years of age. *Environ Health Perspect.* 2009;117(10):1580–1586

306. Park JD, Zheng W. Human exposure and health effects of inorganic and elemental mercury. *J Prev Med Public Health.* 2012;45(6):344–352

307. Weidemann DK, Weaver VM, Fadrowski JJ. Toxic environmental exposures and kidney health in children. *Pediatr Nephrol.* 2016;31(11):2043–2054

308. Torres AD, Rai AN, Hardiek ML. Mercury intoxication and arterial hypertension: report of two patients and review of the literature. *Pediatrics.* 2000;105(3). Available at: www.pediatrics.org/cgi/content/full/105/3/e34

309. Brannan EH, Su S, Alverson BK. Elemental mercury poisoning presenting as hypertension in a young child. *Pediatr Emerg Care.* 2012;28(8):812–814

310. Mercer JJ, Bercovitch L, Muglia JJ. Acrodynia and hypertension in a young girl secondary to elemental mercury toxicity acquired in the home. *Pediatr Dermatol.* 2012;29(2):199–201

311. Valvi D, Casas M, Romaguera D, et al. Prenatal phthalate exposure and childhood growth and blood pressure: evidence from the Spanish INMA-Sabadell Birth Cohort Study. *Environ Health Perspect.* 2015;123(10):1022–1029

312. Trasande L, Sathyanarayana S, Spanier AJ, Trachtman H, Attina TM, Urbina EM. Urinary phthalates are associated with higher blood pressure in childhood. *J Pediatr.* 2013;163(3):747–753.e1

313. Trasande L, Attina TM. Association of exposure to di-2-ethylhexylphthalate replacements with increased blood pressure in children and adolescents. *Hypertension.* 2015;66(2):301–308

314. Saif I, Seriki D, Moore R, Woywodt A. Midaortic syndrome in neurofibromatosis type 1 resulting in bilateral renal artery stenosis. *Am J Kidney Dis.* 2010;56(6):1197–1201

315. Kimura M, Kakizaki S, Kawano K, Sato S, Kure S. Neurofibromatosis type 1 complicated by atypical coarctation of the thoracic aorta. *Case Rep Pediatr.* 2013;2013:458543

316. Malav IC, Kothari SS. Renal artery stenosis due to neurofibromatosis. *Ann Pediatr Cardiol.* 2009;2(2):167–169

317. Mavani G, Kesar V, Devita MV, Rosenstock JL, Michelis MF, Schwimmer JA. Neurofibromatosis type 1-associated hypertension secondary to coarctation of the thoracic aorta. *Clin Kidney J.* 2014;7(4):394–395

318. Duan L, Feng K, Tong A, Liang Z. Renal artery stenosis due to neurofibromatosis type 1: case report and literature review. *Eur J Med Res.* 2014;19:17

319. Srinivasan A, Krishnamurthy G, Fontalvo-Herazo L, et al. Spectrum of renal findings in pediatric fibromuscular dysplasia and neurofibromatosis type 1. *Pediatr Radiol.* 2011;41(3):308–316

320. Dubov T, Toledano-Alhadef H, Chernin G, Constantini S, Cleper R, Ben-Shachar S. High prevalence of elevated blood pressure among children with neurofibromatosis type 1. *Pediatr Nephrol.* 2016;31(1):131–136

321. Erem C, Onder Ersöz H, Ukinç K, et al. Neurofibromatosis type 1 associated with pheochromocytoma: a case report and a review of the literature. *J Endocrinol Invest.* 2007;30(1):59–64

322. Zinnamosca L, Petramala L, Cotesta D, et al. Neurofibromatosis type 1 (NF1) and pheochromocytoma: prevalence, clinical and cardiovascular aspects. *Arch Dermatol Res.* 2011;303(5):317–325

323. Nawrot TS, Den Hond E, Fagard RH, Hoppenbrouwers K, Staessen JA. Blood pressure, serum total cholesterol and contraceptive pill use in 17-year-old girls. *Eur J Cardiovasc Prev Rehabil.* 2003;10(6):438–442

324. Le-Ha C, Beilin LJ, Burrows S, et al. Oral contraceptive use in girls and alcohol consumption in boys are associated with increased blood pressure in late adolescence. *Eur J Prev Cardiol.* 2013;20(6):947–955

325. Du Y, Rosner BM, Knopf H, Schwarz S, Dören M, Scheidt-Nave C. Hormonal contraceptive use among adolescent girls in Germany in relation to health behavior and biological cardiovascular risk factors. *J Adolesc Health.* 2011;48(4):331–337

326. Samuels JA, Franco K, Wan F, Sorof JM. Effect of stimulants on 24-h ambulatory blood pressure in children with ADHD: a double-blind, randomized, cross-over trial. *Pediatr Nephrol.* 2006;21(1):92–95

327. Covar RA, Leung DY, McCormick D, Steelman J, Zeitler P, Spahn JD. Risk

factors associated with glucocorticoid-induced adverse effects in children with severe asthma. *J Allergy Clin Immunol.* 2000;106(4):651–659

328. Vehaskari VM. Heritable forms of hypertension. *Pediatr Nephrol.* 2009;24(10):1929–1937

329. Halperin F, Dluhy RG. Glucocorticoid-remediable aldosteronism. *Endocrinol Metab Clin North Am.* 2011;40(2):333–341, viii

330. Staley JR, Bradley J, Silverwood RJ, et al. Associations of blood pressure in pregnancy with offspring blood pressure trajectories during childhood and adolescence: findings from a prospective study. *J Am Heart Assoc.* 2015;4(5):e001422

331. Daniels SD, Meyer RA, Loggie JM. Determinants of cardiac involvement in children and adolescents with essential hypertension. *Circulation.* 1990;82(4):1243–1248

332. Yang Q, Zhang Z, Kuklina EV, et al. Sodium intake and blood pressure among US children and adolescents. *Pediatrics.* 2012;130(4):611–619

333. He FJ, MacGregor GA. Importance of salt in determining blood pressure in children: meta-analysis of controlled trials. *Hypertension.* 2006;48(5):861–869

334. Aeberli I, Spinas GA, Lehmann R, l'Allemand D, Molinari L, Zimmermann MB. Diet determines features of the metabolic syndrome in 6- to 14-year-old children. *Int J Vitam Nutr Res.* 2009;79(1):14–23

335. Colín-Ramírez E, Castillo-Martínez L, Orea-Tejeda A, Villa Romero AR, Vergara Castañeda A, Asensio Lafuente E. Waist circumference and fat intake are associated with high blood pressure in Mexican children aged 8 to 10 years. *J Am Diet Assoc.* 2009;109(6):996–1003

336. Niinikoski H, Jula A, Viikari J, et al. Blood pressure is lower in children and adolescents with a low-saturated-fat diet since infancy: the special turku coronary risk factor intervention project. *Hypertension.* 2009;53(6):918–924

337. Institute of Medicine. *Strategies to Reduce Sodium Intake in the United States.* Washington, DC: National Academies Press; 2010

338. Adler AJ, Taylor F, Martin N, Gottlieb S, Taylor RS, Ebrahim S. Reduced dietary salt for the prevention of cardiovascular disease. *Cochrane Database Syst Rev.* 2014;(12):CD009217

339. Rebholz CM, Gu D, Chen J, et al; GenSalt Collaborative Research Group. Physical activity reduces salt sensitivity of blood pressure: the Genetic Epidemiology Network of Salt Sensitivity study. *Am J Epidemiol.* 2012;176(suppl 7):S106–S113

340. Torrance B, McGuire KA, Lewanczuk R, McGavock J. Overweight, physical activity and high blood pressure in children: a review of the literature. *Vasc Health Risk Manag.* 2007;3(1):139–149

341. Chen HH, Chen YL, Huang CY, Lee SD, Chen SC, Kuo CH. Effects of one-year swimming training on blood pressure and insulin sensitivity in mild hypertensive young patients. *Chin J Physiol.* 2010;53(3):185–189

342. Farpour-Lambert NJ, Aggoun Y, Marchand LM, Martin XE, Herrmann FR, Beghetti M. Physical activity reduces systemic blood pressure and improves early markers of atherosclerosis in pre-pubertal obese children. *J Am Coll Cardiol.* 2009;54(25):2396–2406

343. Cai L, Wu Y, Cheskin LJ, Wilson RF, Wang Y. Effect of childhood obesity prevention programmes on blood lipids: a systematic review and meta-analysis. *Obes Rev.* 2014;15(12):933–944

344. Kelley GA, Kelley KS, Tran ZV. The effects of exercise on resting blood pressure in children and adolescents: a meta-analysis of randomized controlled trials. *Prev Cardiol.* 2003;6(1):8–16

345. van Dijk AE, van Eijsden M, Stronks K, Gemke RJ, Vrijkotte TG. The association between prenatal psychosocial stress and blood pressure in the child at age 5-7 years. *PLoS One.* 2012;7(8):e43548

346. Stein DJ, Scott K, Haro Abad JM, et al. Early childhood adversity and later hypertension: data from the World Mental Health Survey. *Ann Clin Psychiatry.* 2010;22(1):19–28

347. Halonen JI, Stenholm S, Pentti J, et al. Childhood psychosocial adversity and adult neighborhood disadvantage as predictors of cardiovascular disease: a cohort study. *Circulation.* 2015;132(5):371–379

348. Maggio AB, Martin XE, Saunders Gasser C, et al. Medical and non-medical complications among children and adolescents with excessive body weight. *BMC Pediatr.* 2014;14:232

349. Yun M, Li S, Sun D, et al. Tobacco smoking strengthens the association of elevated blood pressure with arterial stiffness: the Bogalusa Heart Study. *J Hypertens.* 2015;33(2):266–274

350. Priest JR, Nead KT, Wehner MR, Cooke JP, Leeper NJ. Self-reported history of childhood smoking is associated with an increased risk for peripheral arterial disease independent of lifetime smoking burden. *PLoS One.* 2014;9(2):e88972

351. Hagan JFSJ, Duncan PM. *Bright Futures: Guidelines for Health Supervision of Infants, Children, and Adolescents.* 3rd ed. Elk Grove Village, IL: American Academy of Pediatrics; 2008

352. Benson L, Baer HJ, Greco PJ, Kaelber DC. When is family history obtained? - Lack of timely documentation of family history among overweight and hypertensive paediatric patients. *J Paediatr Child Health.* 2010;46(10):600–605

353. Flynn JT. Evaluation and management of hypertension in childhood. *Prog Pediatr Cardiol.* 2001;12(2):177–188

354. Wiesen J, Adkins M, Fortune S, et al. Evaluation of pediatric patients with mild-to-moderate hypertension: yield of diagnostic testing. *Pediatrics.* 2008;122(5). Available at: www.pediatrics.org/cgi/content/full/122/5/e988

355. Yoon EY, Cohn L, Rocchini A, et al. Use of diagnostic tests in adolescents with essential hypertension. *Arch Pediatr Adolesc Med.* 2012;166(9):857–862

356. Killian L, Simpson JM, Savis A, Rawlins D, Sinha MD. Electrocardiography is a poor screening test to detect left ventricular hypertrophy in children. *Arch Dis Child.* 2010;95(10):832–836

357. Ramaswamy P, Patel E, Fahey M, Mahgerefteh J, Lytrivi ID, Kupferman JC. Electrocardiographic predictors of left ventricular hypertrophy in pediatric hypertension. *J Pediatr.* 2009;154(1):106–110

358. Rijnbeek PR, van Herpen G, Kapusta L, Ten Harkel AD, Witsenburg M, Kors JA. Electrocardiographic criteria for left ventricular hypertrophy in children. *Pediatr Cardiol.* 2008;29(5):923–928

359. Grossman A, Prokupetz A, Koren-Morag N, Grossman E, Shamiss A. Comparison of usefulness of Sokolow and Cornell criteria for left ventricular hypertrophy in subjects aged <20 years versus >30 years. *Am J Cardiol.* 2012;110(3):440–444

360. Caselli S, Maron MS, Urbano-Moral JA, Pandian NG, Maron BJ, Pelliccia A. Differentiating left ventricular hypertrophy in athletes from that in patients with hypertrophic cardiomyopathy. *Am J Cardiol.* 2014;114(9):1383–1389

361. Urbina EM, Gidding SS, Bao W, Pickoff AS, Berdusis K, Berenson GS. Effect of body size, ponderosity, and blood pressure on left ventricular growth in children and young adults in the Bogalusa Heart Study. *Circulation.* 1995;91(9):2400–2406

362. Kuznetsova T, Haddad F, Tikhonoff V, et al; European Project On Genes in Hypertension (EPOGH) Investigators. Impact and pitfalls of scaling of left ventricular and atrial structure in population-based studies. *J Hypertens.* 2016;34(6):1186–1194

363. Armstrong AC, Gidding S, Gjesdal O, Wu C, Bluemke DA, Lima JA. LV mass assessed by echocardiography and CMR, cardiovascular outcomes, and medical practice. *JACC Cardiovasc Imaging.* 2012;5(8):837–848

364. Armstrong AC, Jacobs DR Jr, Gidding SS, et al. Framingham score and LV mass predict events in young adults: CARDIA study. *Int J Cardiol.* 2014;172(2):350–355

365. Gidding SS, Palermo RA, DeLoach SS, Keith SW, Falkner B. Associations of cardiac structure with obesity, blood pressure, inflammation, and insulin resistance in African-American adolescents. *Pediatr Cardiol.* 2014;35(2):307–314

366. Hanevold C, Waller J, Daniels S, Portman R, Sorof J; International Pediatric Hypertension Association. The effects of obesity, gender, and ethnic group on left ventricular hypertrophy and geometry in hypertensive children: a collaborative study of the International Pediatric Hypertension Association. *Pediatrics.* 2004;113(2):328–333

367. Daniels SR, Loggie JM, Khoury P, Kimball TR. Left ventricular geometry and severe left ventricular hypertrophy in children and adolescents with essential hypertension. *Circulation.* 1998;97(19):1907–1911

368. Devereux RB, Wachtell K, Gerdts E, et al. Prognostic significance of left ventricular mass change during treatment of hypertension. *JAMA.* 2004;292(19):2350–2356

369. Lang RM, Badano LP, Mor-Avi V, et al. Recommendations for cardiac chamber quantification by echocardiography in adults: an update from the American Society of Echocardiography and the European Association of Cardiovascular Imaging.*J Am Soc Echocardiogr.* 2015;28(1):1–39.e14

370. Daniels SR, Kimball TR, Morrison JA, Khoury P, Witt S, Meyer RA. Effect of lean body mass, fat mass, blood pressure, and sexual maturation on left ventricular mass in children and adolescents. Statistical, biological, and clinical significance. *Circulation.* 1995;92(11):3249–3254

371. Lopez L, Colan SD, Frommelt PC, et al. Recommendations for quantification methods during the performance of a pediatric echocardiogram: a report from the Pediatric Measurements Writing Group of the American Society of Echocardiography Pediatric and Congenital Heart Disease Council. *J Am Soc Echocardiogr.* 2010;23(5):465–495, quiz 576–577

372. Foster BJ, Khoury PR, Kimball TR, Mackie AS, Mitsnefes M. New reference centiles for left ventricular mass relative to lean body mass in children. *J Am Soc Echocardiogr.* 2016;29(5):441–447.e2

373. Khoury PR, Mitsnefes M, Daniels SR, Kimball TR. Age-specific reference intervals for indexed left ventricular mass in children. *J Am Soc Echocardiogr.* 2009;22(6):709–714

374. Lipshultz SE, Easley KA, Orav EJ, et al. Reliability of multicenter pediatric echocardiographic measurements of left ventricular structure and function: the prospective P(2)C(2) HIV study. *Circulation.* 2001;104(3):310–316

375. Urbina EM. Abnormalities of vascular structure and function in pediatric hypertension. *Pediatr Nephrol.* 2016;31(7):1061–1070

376. Elmenhorst J, Hulpke-Wette M, Barta C, Dalla Pozza R, Springer S, Oberhoffer R. Percentiles for central blood pressure and pulse wave velocity in children and adolescents recorded with an oscillometric device. *Atherosclerosis.* 2015;238(1):9–16

377. Hidvégi EV, Illyés M, Benczúr B, et al. Reference values of aortic pulse wave velocity in a large healthy population aged between 3 and 18 years. *J Hypertens.* 2012;30(12):2314–2321

378. Miyai N, Utsumi M, Gowa Y, et al. Age-specific nomogram of brachial-ankle pulse wave velocity in Japanese adolescents. *Clin Exp Hypertens.* 2013;35(2):95–101

379. Urbina EM, Khoury PR, McCoy CE, Dolan LM, Daniels SR, Kimball TR. Triglyceride to HDL-C ratio and increased arterial stiffness in children, adolescents, and young adults [published correction appears in *Pediatrics.* 2013;132(4):780]. *Pediatrics.* 2013;131(4). Available at: www.pediatrics.org/cgi/content/full/131/4/e1082

380. Lurbe E, Torro I, Garcia-Vicent C, Alvarez J, Fernández-Fornoso JA, Redon J. Blood pressure and obesity exert independent influences on pulse wave velocity in youth. *Hypertension.* 2012;60(2):550–555

381. Zhu H, Yan W, Ge D, et al. Relationships of cardiovascular phenotypes with healthy weight, at risk of overweight, and overweight in US youths. *Pediatrics.* 2008;121(1):115–122

382. Charakida M, Jones A, Falaschetti E, et al. Childhood obesity and vascular

phenotypes: a population study. *J Am Coll Cardiol.* 2012;60(25):2643–2650

383. Doyon A, Kracht D, Bayazit AK, et al; 4C Study Consortium. Carotid artery intima-media thickness and distensibility in children and adolescents: reference values and role of body dimensions. *Hypertension.* 2013;62(3):550–556

384. Urbina EM, Kimball TR, McCoy CE, Khoury PR, Daniels SR, Dolan LM. Youth with obesity and obesity-related type 2 diabetes mellitus demonstrate abnormalities in carotid structure and function. *Circulation.* 2009;119(22):2913–2919

385. Keehn L, Milne L, McNeill K, Chowienczyk P, Sinha MD. Measurement of pulse wave velocity in children: comparison of volumetric and tonometric sensors, brachial-femoral and carotid-femoral pathways. *J Hypertens.* 2014;32(7):1464–1469, discussion 1469

386. Kis E, Cseprekál O, Kerti A, et al. Measurement of pulse wave velocity in children and young adults: a comparative study using three different devices. *Hypertens Res.* 2011;34(11):1197–1202

387. Chhadia S, Cohn RA, Vural G, Donaldson JS. Renal Doppler evaluation in the child with hypertension: a reasonable screening discriminator? *Pediatr Radiol.* 2013;43(12):1549–1556

388. Castelli PK, Dillman JR, Kershaw DB, Khalatbari S, Stanley JC, Smith EA. Renal sonography with Doppler for detecting suspected pediatric renin-mediated hypertension - is it adequate? *Pediatr Radiol.* 2014;44(1):42–49

389. Rountas C, Vlychou M, Vassiou K, et al. Imaging modalities for renal artery stenosis in suspected renovascular hypertension: prospective intraindividual comparison of color Doppler US, CT angiography, GD-enhanced MR angiography, and digital substraction angiography. *Ren Fail.* 2007;29(3):295–302

390. Marks SD, Tullus K. Update on imaging for suspected renovascular hypertension in children and adolescents. *Curr Hypertens Rep.* 2012;14(6):591–595

391. Lagomarsino E, Orellana P, Muñoz J, Velásquez C, Cavagnaro F, Valdés F. Captopril scintigraphy in the study of arterial hypertension in pediatrics. *Pediatr Nephrol.* 2004;19(1):66–70

392. Abdulsamea S, Anderson P, Biassoni L, et al. Pre- and postcaptopril renal scintigraphy as a screening test for renovascular hypertension in children. *Pediatr Nephrol.* 2010;25(2):317–322

393. Günay EC, Oztürk MH, Ergün EL, et al. Losartan renography for the detection of renal artery stenosis: comparison with captopril renography and evaluation of dose and timing. *Eur J Nucl Med Mol Imaging.* 2005;32(9):1064–1074

394. Reusz GS, Kis E, Cseprekál O, Szabó AJ, Kis E. Captopril-enhanced renal scintigraphy in the diagnosis of pediatric hypertension. *Pediatr Nephrol.* 2010;25(2):185–189

395. Loeffler LF, Navas-Acien A, Brady TM, Miller ER III, Fadrowski JJ. Uric acid level and elevated blood pressure in US adolescents: National Health and Nutrition Examination Survey, 1999-2006. *Hypertension.* 2012;59(4): 811–817

396. Shatat IF, Abdallah RT, Sas DJ, Hailpern SM. Serum uric acid in U.S. adolescents: distribution and relationship to demographic characteristics and cardiovascular risk factors. *Pediatr Res.* 2012;72(1):95–100

397. Viazzi F, Antolini L, Giussani M, et al. Serum uric acid and blood pressure in children at cardiovascular risk. *Pediatrics.* 2013;132(1). Available at: www.pediatrics.org/cgi/content/full/132/1/e93

398. Reschke LD, Miller ER III, Fadrowski JJ, et al. Elevated uric acid and obesity-related cardiovascular disease risk factors among hypertensive youth. *Pediatr Nephrol.* 2015;30(12):2169–2176

399. Alper AB Jr, Chen W, Yau L, Srinivasan SR, Berenson GS, Hamm LL. Childhood uric acid predicts adult blood pressure: the Bogalusa Heart Study. *Hypertension.* 2005;45(1):34–38

400. Soletsky B, Feig DI. Uric acid reduction rectifies prehypertension in obese adolescents. *Hypertension.* 2012;60(5):1148–1156

401. Feig DI, Soletsky B, Johnson RJ. Effect of allopurinol on blood pressure of adolescents with newly diagnosed essential hypertension: a randomized trial. *JAMA.* 2008;300(8):924–932

402. Assadi F. Allopurinol enhances the blood pressure lowering effect of enalapril in children with hyperuricemic essential hypertension. *J Nephrol.* 2014;27(1):51–56

403. Feig DI, Nakagawa T, Karumanchi SA, et al. Hypothesis: uric acid, nephron number, and the pathogenesis of essential hypertension. *Kidney Int.* 2004;66(1):281–287

404. Viazzi F, Rebora P, Giussani M, et al. Increased serum uric acid levels blunt the antihypertensive efficacy of lifestyle modifications in children at cardiovascular risk. *Hypertension.* 2016;67(5):934–940

405. Klausen K, Borch-Johnsen K, Feldt-Rasmussen B, et al. Very low levels of microalbuminuria are associated with increased risk of coronary heart disease and death independently of renal function, hypertension, and diabetes. *Circulation.* 2004;110(1):32–35

406. Bigazzi R, Bianchi S, Baldari D, Campese VM. Microalbuminuria predicts cardiovascular events and renal insufficiency in patients with essential hypertension. *J Hypertens.* 1998;16(9):1325–1333

407. Chugh A, Bakris GL. Microalbuminuria: what is it? Why is it important? What should be done about it? An update. *J Clin Hypertens (Greenwich).* 2007;9(3):196–200

408. Flynn JT. Microalbuminuria in children with primary hypertension. *J Clin Hypertens (Greenwich).* 2016;18(10):962–965

409. Radhakishun NN, van Vliet M, von Rosenstiel IA, Beijnen JH, Diamant M. Limited value of routine microalbuminuria assessment in multi-ethnic obese children. *Pediatr Nephrol.* 2013;28(7):1145–1149

410. Tsioufis C, Mazaraki A, Dimitriadis K, Stefanidis CJ, Stefanadis C. Microalbuminuria in the paediatric age: current knowledge and

emerging questions. *Acta Paediatr.* 2011;100(9):1180–1184

411. Seeman T, Pohl M, Palyzova D, John U. Microalbuminuria in children with primary and white-coat hypertension. *Pediatr Nephrol.* 2012;27(3):461–467

412. Sanad M, Gharib A. Evaluation of microalbuminuria in obese children and its relation to metabolic syndrome. *Pediatr Nephrol.* 2011;26(12):2193–2199

413. Assadi F. Effect of microalbuminuria lowering on regression of left ventricular hypertrophy in children and adolescents with essential hypertension. *Pediatr Cardiol.* 2007;28(1):27–33

414. Niemirska A, Litwin M, Feber J, Jurkiewicz E. Blood pressure rhythmicity and visceral fat in children with hypertension. *Hypertension.* 2013;62(4):782–788

415. Kupferman JC, Paterno K, Mahgerefteh J, et al. Improvement of left ventricular mass with antihypertensive therapy in children with hypertension. *Pediatr Nephrol.* 2010;25(8):1513–1518

416. Falkner B, DeLoach S, Keith SW, Gidding SS. High risk blood pressure and obesity increase the risk for left ventricular hypertrophy in African-American adolescents. *J Pediatr.* 2013;162(1):94–100

417. Stabouli S, Kotsis V, Rizos Z, et al. Left ventricular mass in normotensive, prehypertensive and hypertensive children and adolescents. *Pediatr Nephrol.* 2009;24(8):1545–1551

418. Tirosh A, Afek A, Rudich A, et al. Progression of normotensive adolescents to hypertensive adults: a study of 26,980 teenagers. *Hypertension.* 2010;56(2):203–209

419. Chobanian AV, Bakris GL, Black HR; National Heart, Lung, and Blood Institute Joint National Committee on Prevention, Detection, Evaluation, and Treatment of High Blood Pressure; National High Blood Pressure Education Program Coordinating Committee. The seventh report of the Joint National Committee on prevention, detection, evaluation, and treatment of high blood pressure: the JNC 7 report [published correction appears in *JAMA.* 2003;290(2):197]. *JAMA.* 2003;289(19):2560–2571

420. Moreno-Luna R, Muñoz-Hernandez R, Miranda ML, et al. Olive oil polyphenols decrease blood pressure and improve endothelial function in young women with mild hypertension. *Am J Hypertens.* 2012;25(12):1299–1304

421. Damasceno MM, de Araújo MF, de Freitas RW, de Almeida PC, Zanetti ML. The association between blood pressure in adolescents and the consumption of fruits, vegetables and fruit juice--an exploratory study. *J Clin Nurs.* 2011;20(11–12):1553–1560

422. Juonala M, Viikari JS, Kähönen M, et al. Life-time risk factors and progression of carotid atherosclerosis in young adults: the Cardiovascular Risk in Young Finns study. *Eur Heart J.* 2010;31(14):1745–1751

423. Yuan WL, Kakinami L, Gray-Donald K, Czernichow S, Lambert M, Paradis G. Influence of dairy product consumption on children's blood pressure: results from the QUALITY cohort. *J Acad Nutr Diet.* 2013;113(7):936–941

424. Moore LL, Bradlee ML, Singer MR, Qureshi MM, Buendia JR, Daniels SR. Dietary approaches to stop hypertension (DASH) eating pattern and risk of elevated blood pressure in adolescent girls. *Br J Nutr.* 2012;108(9):1678–1685

425. Günther AL, Liese AD, Bell RA, et al. Association between the dietary approaches to hypertension diet and hypertension in youth with diabetes mellitus. *Hypertension.* 2009;53(1):6–12

426. Couch SC, Saelens BE, Levin L, Dart K, Falciglia G, Daniels SR. The efficacy of a clinic-based behavioral nutrition intervention emphasizing a DASH-type diet for adolescents with elevated blood pressure. *J Pediatr.* 2008;152(4):494–501

427. Davis JN, Ventura EE, Cook LT, Gyllenhammer LE, Gatto NMLA. LA Sprouts: a gardening, nutrition, and cooking intervention for Latino youth improves diet and reduces obesity. *J Am Diet Assoc.* 2011;111(8):1224–1230

428. Saneei P, Hashemipour M, Kelishadi R, Rajaei S, Esmaillzadeh A. Effects of recommendations to follow the dietary approaches to stop hypertension (DASH) diet v. usual dietary advice on childhood metabolic syndrome: a randomised cross-over clinical trial. *Br J Nutr.* 2013;110(12):2250–2259

429. Barnes TL, Crandell JL, Bell RA, Mayer-Davis EJ, Dabelea D, Liese AD. Change in DASH diet score and cardiovascular risk factors in youth with type 1 and type 2 diabetes mellitus: the SEARCH for Diabetes in Youth study. *Nutr Diabetes.* 2013;3:e91

430. Rao M, Afshin A, Singh G, Mozaffarian D. Do healthier foods and diet patterns cost more than less healthy options? A systematic review and meta-analysis. *BMJ Open.* 2013;3(12):e004277

431. Monzavi R, Dreimane D, Geffner ME, et al. Improvement in risk factors for metabolic syndrome and insulin resistance in overweight youth who are treated with lifestyle intervention. *Pediatrics.* 2006;117(6). Available at: www.pediatrics.org/cgi/content/full/117/6/e1111

432. Asghari G, Yuzbashian E, Mirmiran P, Hooshmand F, Najafi R, Azizi F. Dietary approaches to stop hypertension (DASH) dietary pattern is associated with reduced incidence of metabolic syndrome in children and adolescents. *J Pediatr.* 2016;174:178–184.e1

433. Pacifico L, Anania C, Martino F, et al. Management of metabolic syndrome in children and adolescents. *Nutr Metab Cardiovasc Dis.* 2011;21(6):455–466

434. Puri M, Flynn JT. Management of hypertension in children and adolescents with the metabolic syndrome. *J Cardiometab Syndr.* 2006;1(4):259–268

435. Davis MM, Gance-Cleveland B, Hassink S, Johnson R, Paradis G, Resnicow K. Recommendations for prevention of childhood obesity. *Pediatrics.* 2007;120(suppl 4):S229–S253

436. Ogedegbe G, Chaplin W, Schoenthaler A, et al. A practice-based trial of motivational interviewing and adherence in hypertensive African Americans. *Am J Hypertens.* 2008;21(10):1137–1143

437. Bosworth HB, Olsen MK, Neary A, et al. Take Control of Your Blood Pressure (TCYB) study: a multifactorial tailored behavioral and educational intervention for achieving blood pressure control. *Patient Educ Couns.* 2008;70(3):338–347

438. Resnicow K, McMaster F, Bocian A, et al. Motivational interviewing and dietary counseling for obesity in primary care: an RCT. *Pediatrics.* 2015;135(4):649–657

439. Davoli AM, Broccoli S, Bonvicini L, et al. Pediatrician-led motivational interviewing to treat overweight children: an RCT. *Pediatrics.* 2013;132(5). Available at: www.pediatrics.org/cgi/content/full/132/5/e1236

440. Broccoli S, Davoli AM, Bonvicini L, et al. Motivational interviewing to treat overweight children: 24-month follow-up of a randomized controlled trial. *Pediatrics.* 2016;137(1):e20151979

441. Flattum C, Friend S, Neumark-Sztainer D, Story M. Motivational interviewing as a component of a school-based obesity prevention program for adolescent girls. *J Am Diet Assoc.* 2009;109(1):91–94

442. Schwartz RP, Hamre R, Dietz WH, et al. Office-based motivational interviewing to prevent childhood obesity: a feasibility study. *Arch Pediatr Adolesc Med.* 2007;161(5):495–501

443. Döring N, Ghaderi A, Bohman B, et al. Motivational interviewing to prevent childhood obesity: a cluster RCT. *Pediatrics.* 2016;137(5):1–10

444. Spear BA, Barlow SE, Ervin C, et al. Recommendations for treatment of child and adolescent overweight and obesity. *Pediatrics.* 2007;120(4, suppl 4):S254–S288

445. Kabat-Zinn J, Hanh TN. *Full Catastrophe Living: Using the Wisdom of Your Body and Mind to Face Stress, Pain, and Illness.* New York, NY: Delta; 1990

446. Gregoski MJ, Barnes VA, Tingen MS, Harshfield GA, Treiber FA. Breathing awareness meditation and LifeSkills Training programs influence upon ambulatory blood pressure and sodium excretion among African American adolescents. *J Adolesc Health.* 2011;48(1):59–64

447. Barnes VA, Kapuku GK, Treiber FA. Impact of transcendental meditation on left ventricular mass in African American adolescents. *Evid Based Complement Alternat Med.* 2012;2012:923153

448. Sieverdes JC, Mueller M, Gregoski MJ, et al. Effects of Hatha yoga on blood pressure, salivary α-amylase, and cortisol function among normotensive and prehypertensive youth. *J Altern Complement Med.* 2014;20(4):241–250

449. Sorof JM, Cargo P, Graepel J, et al. β-blocker/thiazide combination for treatment of hypertensive children: a randomized double-blind, placebo-controlled trial. *Pediatr Nephrol.* 2002;17(5):345–350

450. Trachtman H, Hainer JW, Sugg J, Teng R, Sorof JM, Radcliffe J; Candesartan in Children with Hypertension (CINCH) Investigators. Efficacy, safety, and pharmacokinetics of candesartan cilexetil in hypertensive children aged 6 to 17 years. *J Clin Hypertens (Greenwich).* 2008;10(10):743–750

451. Herder SD, Weber E, Winkemann A, Herder C, Morck H. Efficacy and safety of angiotensin II receptor type 1 antagonists in children and adolescents. *Pediatr Nephrol.* 2010;25(5):801–811

452. Schaefer F, Litwin M, Zachwieja J, et al. Efficacy and safety of valsartan compared to enalapril in hypertensive children: a 12-week, randomized, double-blind, parallel-group study. *J Hypertens.* 2011;29(12):2484–2490

453. Gartenmann AC, Fossali E, von Vigier RO, et al. Better renoprotective effect of angiotensin II antagonist compared to dihydropyridine calcium channel blocker in childhood. *Kidney Int.* 2003;64(4):1450–1454

454. Chaturvedi S, Lipszyc DH, Licht C, Craig JC, Parekh R. Pharmacological interventions for hypertension in children. *Evid Based Child Health.* 2014;9(3):498–580

455. Flynn JT. Efficacy and safety of prolonged amlodipine treatment in hypertensive children. *Pediatr Nephrol.* 2005;20(5):631–635

456. Schaefer F, Coppo R, Bagga A, et al. Efficacy and safety of valsartan in hypertensive children 6 months to 5 years of age. *J Hypertens.* 2013;31(5):993–1000

457. Batisky DL, Sorof JM, Sugg J, et al; Toprol-XL Pediatric Hypertension Investigators. Efficacy and safety of extended release metoprolol succinate in hypertensive children 6 to 16 years of age: a clinical trial experience. *J Pediatr.* 2007;150(2):134–139, 139.e1

458. Wells T, Blumer J, Meyers KE, et al; Valsartan Pediatric Hypertension Study Group. Effectiveness and safety of valsartan in children aged 6 to 16 years with hypertension. *J Clin Hypertens (Greenwich).* 2011;13(5):357–365

459. Trachtman H, Frank R, Mahan JD, et al. Clinical trial of extended-release felodipine in pediatric essential hypertension. *Pediatr Nephrol.* 2003;18(6):548–553

460. Shahinfar S, Cano F, Soffer BA, et al. A double-blind, dose-response study of losartan in hypertensive children. *Am J Hypertens.* 2005;18(2, pt 1):183–190

461. Hazan L, Hernández Rodriguez OA, Bhorat AE, Miyazaki K, Tao B, Heyrman R; Assessment of Efficacy and Safety of Olmesartan in Pediatric Hypertension Study Group. A double-blind, dose-response study of the efficacy and safety of olmesartan medoxomil in children and adolescents with hypertension. *Hypertension.* 2010;55(6):1323–1330

462. Flynn JT, Newburger JW, Daniels SR, et al; PATH-1 Investigators. A randomized, placebo-controlled trial of amlodipine in children with hypertension. *J Pediatr.* 2004;145(3):353–359

463. Simonetti GD, Rizzi M, Donadini R, Bianchetti MG. Effects of antihypertensive drugs on blood pressure and proteinuria in childhood. *J Hypertens.* 2007;25(12):2370–2376

464. Seeman T, Dusek J, Vondrák K, Flögelová H, Geier P, Janda J. Ramipril in the treatment of hypertension and proteinuria in children with chronic kidney diseases. *Am J Hypertens.* 2004;17(5, pt 1):415–420

465. Hammer GB, Verghese ST, Drover DR, Yaster M, Tobin JR. Pharmacokinetics and pharmacodynamics of fenoldopam mesylate for blood pressure control

in pediatric patients. *BMC Anesthesiol.* 2008;8:6

466. Blowey DL. Update on the pharmacologic treatment of hypertension in pediatrics. *J Clin Hypertens (Greenwich).* 2012;14(6):383–387

467. Li JS, Flynn JT, Portman R, et al. The efficacy and safety of the novel aldosterone antagonist eplerenone in children with hypertension: a randomized, double-blind, dose-response study. *J Pediatr.* 2010;157(2):282–287

468. U.S. Food and Drug Administration. Pediatric product development. Available at: www.fda.gov/Drugs/DevelopmentApprovalProcess/DevelopmentResources/ucm049867.htm. Accessed February 6, 2017

469. Croxtall JD. Valsartan: in children and adolescents with hypertension. *Paediatr Drugs.* 2012;14(3):201–207

470. Menon S, Berezny KY, Kilaru R, et al. Racial differences are seen in blood pressure response to fosinopril in hypertensive children. *Am Heart J.* 2006;152(2):394–399

471. Li JS, Baker-Smith CM, Smith PB, et al. Racial differences in blood pressure response to angiotensin-converting enzyme inhibitors in children: a meta-analysis. *Clin Pharmacol Ther.* 2008;84(3):315–319

472. Seeman T, Dostálek L, Gilík J. Control of hypertension in treated children and its association with target organ damage. *Am J Hypertens.* 2012;25(3):389–395

473. Redwine K, Howard L, Simpson P, et al; Network of Pediatric Pharmacology Research Units. Effect of placebo on ambulatory blood pressure monitoring in children. *Pediatr Nephrol.* 2012;27(10):1937–1942

474. Halbach SM, Hamman R, Yonekawa K, Hanevold C. Utility of ambulatory blood pressure monitoring in the evaluation of elevated clinic blood pressures in children. *J Am Soc Hypertens.* 2016;10(5):406–412

475. White WB, Turner JR, Sica DA, et al. Detection, evaluation, and treatment of severe and resistant hypertension: proceedings from an American Society of Hypertension Interactive forum held in Bethesda, MD, U.S.A., October 10th, 2013. *J Am Soc Hypertens.* 2014;8(10):743–757

476. Narayan H, Webb DJ. New evidence supporting the use of mineralocorticoid receptor blockers in drug-resistant hypertension. *Curr Hypertens Rep.* 2016;18(5):34

477. Williams B, MacDonald TM, Morant S, et al; British Hypertension Society's PATHWAY Studies Group. Spironolactone versus placebo, bisoprolol, and doxazosin to determine the optimal treatment for drug-resistant hypertension (PATHWAY-2): a randomised, double-blind, crossover trial. *Lancet.* 2015;386(10008):2059–2068

478. Mitsnefes M, Ho PL, McEnery PT. Hypertension and progression of chronic renal insufficiency in children: a report of the North American Pediatric Renal Transplant Cooperative Study (NAPRTCS). *J Am Soc Nephrol.* 2003;14(10):2618–2622

479. Dionne JM. Evidence-based guidelines for the management of hypertension in children with chronic kidney disease. *Pediatr Nephrol.* 2015;30(11):1919–1927

480. VanDeVoorde RG, Mitsnefes MM. Hypertension and CKD. *Adv Chronic Kidney Dis.* 2011;18(5):355–361

481. Mitsnefes MM, Kimball TR, Kartal J, et al. Progression of left ventricular hypertrophy in children with early chronic kidney disease: 2-year follow-up study. *J Pediatr.* 2006;149(5):671–675

482. Wright JT Jr, Williamson JD, Whelton PK, et al; SPRINT Research Group. A randomized trial of intensive versus standard blood-pressure control. *N Engl J Med.* 2015;373(22):2103–2116

483. Wong H, Mylrea K, Feber J, Drukker A, Filler G. Prevalence of complications in children with chronic kidney disease according to KDOQI. *Kidney Int.* 2006;70(3):585–590

484. Simonetti GD, von Vigier RO, Konrad M, Rizzi M, Fossali E, Bianchetti MG. Candesartan cilexetil in children with hypertension or proteinuria: preliminary data. *Pediatr Nephrol.* 2006;21(10):1480–1482

485. White CT, Macpherson CF, Hurley RM, Matsell DG. Antiproteinuric effects of enalapril and losartan: a pilot study. *Pediatr Nephrol.* 2003;18(10):1038–1043

486. Webb NJ, Lam C, Loeys T, et al. Randomized, double-blind, controlled study of losartan in children with proteinuria. *Clin J Am Soc Nephrol.* 2010;5(3):417–424

487. Webb NJ, Shahinfar S, Wells TG, et al. Losartan and enalapril are comparable in reducing proteinuria in children. *Kidney Int.* 2012;82(7):819–826

488. Wühl E, Mehls O, Schaefer F; ESCAPE Trial Group. Antihypertensive and antiproteinuric efficacy of ramipril in children with chronic renal failure. *Kidney Int.* 2004;66(2):768–776

489. Eppens MC, Craig ME, Cusumano J, et al. Prevalence of diabetes complications in adolescents with type 2 compared with type 1 diabetes. *Diabetes Care.* 2006;29(6):1300–1306

490. Mayer-Davis EJ, Ma B, Lawson A, et al; SEARCH for Diabetes in Youth Study Group. Cardiovascular disease risk factors in youth with type 1 and type 2 diabetes: implications of a factor analysis of clustering. *Metab Syndr Relat Disord.* 2009;7(2):89–95

491. Margeirsdottir HD, Larsen JR, Brunborg C, Overby NC, Dahl-Jørgensen K; Norwegian Study Group for Childhood Diabetes. High prevalence of cardiovascular risk factors in children and adolescents with type 1 diabetes: a population-based study. *Diabetologia.* 2008;51(4):554–561

492. Orchard TJ, Forrest KY, Kuller LH, Becker DJ; Pittsburgh Epidemiology of Diabetes Complications Study. Lipid and blood pressure treatment goals for type 1 diabetes: 10-year incidence data from the Pittsburgh Epidemiology of Diabetes Complications Study. *Diabetes Care.* 2001;24(6):1053–1059

493. Copeland KC, Zeitler P, Geffner M, et al; TODAY Study Group. Characteristics of adolescents and youth with recent-onset type 2 diabetes: the TODAY cohort at baseline. *J Clin Endocrinol Metab.* 2011;96(1):159–167

494. Klingensmith GJ, Connor CG, Ruedy KJ, et al; Pediatric Diabetes Consortium. Presentation of youth with type 2

diabetes in the Pediatric Diabetes Consortium. *Pediatr Diabetes.* 2016;17(4):266–273

495. Shah AS, Dolan LM, Gao Z, Kimball TR, Urbina EM. Racial differences in arterial stiffness among adolescents and young adults with type 2 diabetes. *Pediatr Diabetes.* 2012;13(2):170–175

496. TODAY Study Group. Rapid rise in hypertension and nephropathy in youth with type 2 diabetes: the TODAY clinical trial. *Diabetes Care.* 2013;36(6):1735–1741

497. Shah AS, Khoury PR, Dolan LM, et al. The effects of obesity and type 2 diabetes mellitus on cardiac structure and function in adolescents and young adults. *Diabetologia.* 2011;54(4):722–730

498. Nambam B, DuBose SN, Nathan BM, et al; T1D Exchange Clinic Network. Therapeutic inertia: underdiagnosed and undertreated hypertension in children participating in the T1D Exchange Clinic Registry. *Pediatr Diabetes.* 2016;17(1):15–20

499. American Diabetes Association. Supplemental issue: standards of medical care in diabetes - 2016. *Diabetes Care.* 2016;39(suppl 1):S1–S2

500. Donaghue KC, Chiarelli F, Trotta D, Allgrove J, Dahl-Jorgensen K. Microvascular and macrovascular complications associated with diabetes in children and adolescents. *Pediatr Diabetes.* 2009;10(suppl 12): 195–203

501. Expert Panel on Integrated Guidelines for Cardiovascular Health and Risk Reduction in Children and Adolescents; National Heart, Lung, and Blood Institute. Expert panel on integrated guidelines for cardiovascular health and risk reduction in children and adolescents: summary report. *Pediatrics.* 2011;128(suppl 5):S213–S256

502. Stern MP. Diabetes and cardiovascular disease. The "common soil" hypothesis. *Diabetes.* 1995;44(4):369–374

503. Martino F, Puddu PE, Pannarale G, et al. Hypertension in children and adolescents attending a lipid clinic. *Eur J Pediatr.* 2013;172(12):1573–1579

504. Rodríguez-Morán M, Guerrero-Romero F, Aradillas-García C, et al. Atherogenic indices and prehypertension in obese and non-obese children. *Diab Vasc Dis Res.* 2013;10(1):17–24

505. Li J, Motsko SP, Goehring EL Jr, Vendiola R, Maneno M, Jones JK. Longitudinal study on pediatric dyslipidemia in population-based claims database. *Pharmacoepidemiol Drug Saf.* 2010;19(1):90–98

506. Liao CC, Su TC, Chien KL, et al. Elevated blood pressure, obesity, and hyperlipidemia.*J Pediatr.* 2009;155(1):79–83, 83.e1

507. Marcus CL, Brooks LJ, Draper KA, et al; American Academy of Pediatrics. Diagnosis and management of childhood obstructive sleep apnea syndrome. *Pediatrics.* 2012;130(3). Available at: www.pediatrics.org/cgi/content/full/130/3/e714

508. Kuo YL, Kang KT, Chiu SN, Weng WC, Lee PL, Hsu WC. Blood pressure after surgery among obese and nonobese children with obstructive sleep apnea. *Otolaryngol Head Neck Surg.* 2015;152(5):931–940

509. Lande MB, Adams HR, Kupferman JC, Hooper SR, Szilagyi PG, Batisky DL. A multicenter study of neurocognition in children with hypertension: methods, challenges, and solutions. *J Am Soc Hypertens.* 2013;7(5):353–362

510. Lande MB, Adams H, Falkner B, et al. Parental assessments of internalizing and externalizing behavior and executive function in children with primary hypertension. *J Pediatr.* 2009;154(2):207–212

511. Adams HR, Szilagyi PG, Gebhardt L, Lande MB. Learning and attention problems among children with pediatric primary hypertension. *Pediatrics.* 2010;126(6). Available at: www.pediatrics.org/cgi/content/full/126/6/e1425

512. Settakis G, Páll D, Molnár C, Katona E, Bereczki D, Fülesdi B. Hyperventilation-induced cerebrovascular reactivity among hypertensive and healthy adolescents. *Kidney Blood Press Res.* 2006;29(5):306–311

513. Wong LJ, Kupferman JC, Prohovnik I, et al. Hypertension impairs vascular reactivity in the pediatric brain. *Stroke.* 2011;42(7):1834–1838

514. Lande MB, Kupferman JC, Adams HR. Neurocognitive alterations in hypertensive children and adolescents. *J Clin Hypertens (Greenwich).* 2012;14(6):353–359

515. Ostrovskaya MA, Rojas M, Kupferman JC, et al. Executive function and cerebrovascular reactivity in pediatric hypertension. *J Child Neurol.* 2015;30(5):543–546

516. Ong KL, Cheung BM, Man YB, Lau CP, Lam KS. Prevalence, awareness, treatment, and control of hypertension among United States adults 1999-2004. *Hypertension.* 2007;49(1):69–75

517. Guo F, He D, Zhang W, Walton RG. Trends in prevalence, awareness, management, and control of hypertension among United States adults, 1999 to 2010. *J Am Coll Cardiol.* 2012;60(7):599–606

518. Hajjar I, Kotchen TA. Trends in prevalence, awareness, treatment, and control of hypertension in the United States, 1988-2000. *JAMA.* 2003;290(2):199–206

519. Daniels SR, McMahon RP, Obarzanek E, et al. Longitudinal correlates of change in blood pressure in adolescent girls. *Hypertension.* 1998;31(1):97–103

520. Wang X, Poole JC, Treiber FA, Harshfield GA, Hanevold CD, Snieder H. Ethnic and gender differences in ambulatory blood pressure trajectories: results from a 15-year longitudinal study in youth and young adults. *Circulation.* 2006;114(25):2780–2787

521. Rosner B, Cook N, Portman R, Daniels S, Falkner B. Blood pressure differences by ethnic group among United States children and adolescents. *Hypertension.* 2009;54(3):502–508

522. Peacock WF IV, Hilleman DE, Levy PD, Rhoney DH, Varon J. A systematic review of nicardipine vs labetalol for the management of hypertensive crises. *Am J Emerg Med.* 2012;30(6):981–993

523. Wiest DB, Garner SS, Uber WE, Sade RM. Esmolol for the management of pediatric hypertension after cardiac operations. *J Thorac Cardiovasc Surg.* 1998;115(4):890–897

524. Flynn JT, Mottes TA, Brophy PD, Kershaw DB, Smoyer WE, Bunchman TE. Intravenous nicardipine for treatment of severe hypertension in children. *J Pediatr.* 2001;139(1):38–43

525. Tabbutt S, Nicolson SC, Adamson PC, et al. The safety, efficacy, and pharmacokinetics of esmolol for blood pressure control immediately after repair of coarctation of the aorta in infants and children: a multicenter, double-blind, randomized trial. *J Thorac Cardiovasc Surg.* 2008;136(2):321–328

526. Miyashita Y, Peterson D, Rees JM, Flynn JT. Isradipine for treatment of acute hypertension in hospitalized children and adolescents. *J Clin Hypertens (Greenwich).* 2010;12(11):850–855

527. Thomas CA, Moffett BS, Wagner JL, Mott AR, Feig DI. Safety and efficacy of intravenous labetalol for hypertensive crisis in infants and small children. *Pediatr Crit Care Med.* 2011;12(1):28–32

528. Kako H, Gable A, Martin D, et al. A prospective, open-label trial of clevidipine for controlled hypotension during posterior spinal fusion. *J Pediatr Pharmacol Ther.* 2015;20(1):54–60

529. Hammer GB, Lewandowski A, Drover DR, et al. Safety and efficacy of sodium nitroprusside during prolonged infusion in pediatric patients. *Pediatr Crit Care Med.* 2015;16(5):397–403

530. Flynn JT, Bradford MC, Harvey EM. Intravenous hydralazine in hospitalized children and adolescents with hypertension. *J Pediatr.* 2016;168:88–92

531. Yang WC, Zhao LL, Chen CY, Wu YK, Chang YJ, Wu HP. First-attack pediatric hypertensive crisis presenting to the pediatric emergency department. *BMC Pediatr.* 2012;12:200

532. Baracco R, Mattoo TK. Pediatric hypertensive emergencies. *Curr Hypertens Rep.* 2014;16(8):456

533. Flynn JT, Tullus K. Severe hypertension in children and adolescents: pathophysiology and treatment [published correction appears in *Pediatr Nephrol.* 2012;27(3):503–504]. *Pediatr Nephrol.* 2009;24(6):1101–1112

534. Patel NH, Romero SK, Kaelber DC. Evaluation and management of pediatric hypertensive crises: hypertensive urgency and hypertensive emergencies. *Open Access Emerg Med.* 2012;4:85–92

535. Chen YL, Liu YF, Huang CY, et al. Normalization effect of sports training on blood pressure in hypertensives. *J Sports Sci.* 2010;28(4):361–367

536. Hupin D, Roche F, Gremeaux V, et al. Even a low-dose of moderate-to-vigorous physical activity reduces mortality by 22% in adults aged ≥60 years: a systematic review and meta-analysis. *Br J Sports Med.* 2015;49(19):1262–1267

537. Di Paolo FM, Schmied C, Zerguini YA, et al. The athlete's heart in adolescent Africans: an electrocardiographic and echocardiographic study. *J Am Coll Cardiol.* 2012;59(11):1029–1036

538. McCambridge TM, Benjamin HJ, Brenner JS, et al; Council on Sports Medicine and Fitness. Athletic participation by children and adolescents who have systemic hypertension. *Pediatrics.* 2010;125(6):1287–1294

539. Black HR, Sica D, Ferdinand K, White WB. Eligibility and disqualification recommendations for competitive athletes with cardiovascular abnormalities: Task Force 6: hypertension: a scientific statement from the American Heart Association and the American College of Cardiology. *J Am Coll Cardiol.* 2015;66(21):2393–2397

540. Tainio J, Qvist E, Miettinen J, et al. Blood pressure profiles 5 to 10 years after transplant in pediatric solid organ recipients. *J Clin Hypertens (Greenwich).* 2015;17(2):154–161

541. Seeman T, Simková E, Kreisinger J, et al. Control of hypertension in children after renal transplantation. *Pediatr Transplant.* 2006;10(3):316–322

542. Gülhan B, Topaloğlu R, Karabulut E, et al. Post-transplant hypertension in pediatric kidney transplant recipients. *Pediatr Nephrol.* 2014;29(6):1075–1080

543. Arbeiter K, Pichler A, Stemberger R, et al. ACE inhibition in the treatment of children after renal transplantation. *Pediatr Nephrol.* 2004;19(2):222–226

544. Suszynski TM, Rizzari MD, Gillingham KJ, et al. Antihypertensive pharmacotherapy and long-term outcomes in pediatric kidney transplantation. *Clin Transplant.* 2013;27(3):472–480

545. Sakallı H, Baskın E, Bayrakcı US, Moray G, Haberal M. Acidosis and hyperkalemia caused by losartan and enalapril in pediatric kidney transplant recipients. *Exp Clin Transplant.* 2014;12(4):310–313

546. Cooley WC, Sagerman PJ; American Academy of Pediatrics; American Academy of Family Physicians; American College of Physicians; Transitions Clinical Report Authoring Group. Supporting the health care transition from adolescence to adulthood in the medical home. *Pediatrics.* 2011;128(1):182–200

547. Julius S, Nesbitt SD, Egan BM, et al; Trial of Preventing Hypertension (TROPHY) Study Investigators. Feasibility of treating prehypertension with an angiotensin-receptor blocker. *N Engl J Med.* 2006;354(16):1685–1697

548. Kurioka S, Horie S, Inoue A, Mafune K, Tsuda Y, Otsuji Y. Risk of progression to hypertension in nonhypertensive Japanese workers aged 20-64 years. *J Hypertens.* 2014;32(2):236–244

549. Stabouli S, Papakatsika S, Kotsis V. The role of obesity, salt and exercise on blood pressure in children and adolescents. *Expert Rev Cardiovasc Ther.* 2011;9(6):753–761

550. Holm JC, Gamborg M, Neland M, et al. Longitudinal changes in blood pressure during weight loss and regain of weight in obese boys and girls. *J Hypertens.* 2012;30(2):368–374

551. Gillman MW, Ellison RC. Childhood prevention of essential hypertension. *Pediatr Clin North Am.* 1993;40(1):179–194

552. Krousel-Wood MA, Muntner P, He J, Whelton PK. Primary prevention of essential hypertension. *Med Clin North Am.* 2004;88(1):223–238

553. Whelton PK, He J, Appel LJ, et al; National High Blood Pressure Education Program Coordinating Committee. Primary prevention of

hypertension: clinical and public health advisory from the National High Blood Pressure Education Program. *JAMA*. 2002;288(15):1882–1888

554. Kim N, Seo DC, King MH, Lederer AM, Sovinski D. Long-term predictors of blood pressure among adolescents during an 18-month school-based obesity prevention intervention. *J Adolesc Health*. 2014;55(4):521–527

555. Aburto NJ, Ziolkovska A, Hooper L, Elliott P, Cappuccio FP, Meerpohl JJ. Effect of lower sodium intake on health: systematic review and meta-analyses. *BMJ*. 2013;346:f1326

556. American Academy of Pediatrics. EQIPP: hypertension recognition and management. Available at: http://shop.aap.org/eqipp-hypertension-identification-and-management. Accessed February 6, 2017

557. American Academy of Pediatrics, Council on Quality Improvement and Patient Safety. Implementation guide. Available at: https://www.aap.org/en-us/about-the-aap/Committees-Councils-Sections/coqips/Pages/Implementation-Guide.aspx. Accessed July 28, 2017

558. Wang YC, Cheung AM, Bibbins-Domingo K, et al. Effectiveness and cost-effectiveness of blood pressure screening in adolescents in the United States. *J Pediatr*. 2011;158(2):257–264.e1–e7

559. Davis ML, Ferguson MA, Zachariah JP. Clinical predictors and impact of ambulatory blood pressure monitoring in pediatric hypertension referrals. *J Am Soc Hypertens*. 2014;8(9):660–667

560. Leu MG, Austin E, Foti JL, et al. A framework for evaluating value of new clinical recommendations. *Hosp Pediatr*. 2016;6(10):578–586

561. Bradshaw B. The role of the family in managing therapy in minority children with type 2 diabetes mellitus. *J Pediatr Endocrinol Metab*. 2002;15(suppl 1):547–551

562. Pinhas-Hamiel O, Standiford D, Hamiel D, Dolan LM, Cohen R, Zeitler PS. The type 2 family: a setting for development and treatment of adolescent type 2 diabetes mellitus. *Arch Pediatr Adolesc Med*. 1999;153(10):1063–1067

563. Mulvaney SA, Schlundt DG, Mudasiru E, et al. Parent perceptions of caring for adolescents with type 2 diabetes. *Diabetes Care*. 2006;29(5):993–997

564. Summerbell CD, Ashton V, Campbell KJ, Edmunds L, Kelly S, Waters E. Interventions for treating obesity in children. *Cochrane Database Syst Rev*. 2003;(3):CD001872

565. Skinner AC, Weinberger M, Mulvaney S, Schlundt D, Rothman RL. Accuracy of perceptions of overweight and relation to self-care behaviors among adolescents with type 2 diabetes and their parents. *Diabetes Care*. 2008;31(2):227–229

566. Thompson M, Dana T, Bougatsos C, Blazina I, Norris SL. Screening for hypertension in children and adolescents to prevent cardiovascular disease. *Pediatrics*. 2013;131(3):490–525

567. Urbina EM, de Ferranti S, Steinberger J. Observational studies may be more important than randomized clinical trials: weaknesses in US Preventive Services Task Force recommendation on blood pressure screening in youth. *Hypertension*. 2014;63(4):638–640

568. Flynn JT. Ambulatory blood pressure monitoring in children: imperfect yet essential. *Pediatr Nephrol*. 2011;26(12):2089–2094

569. Juonala M, Magnussen CG, Venn A, et al. Influence of age on associations between childhood risk factors and carotid intima-media thickness in adulthood: the Cardiovascular Risk in Young Finns Study, the Childhood Determinants of Adult Health Study, the Bogalusa Heart Study, and the Muscatine Study for the International Childhood Cardiovascular Cohort (i3C) Consortium. *Circulation*. 2010;122(24):2514–2520

570. Muntner P, Becker RC, Calhoun D, et al. Introduction to the American Heart Association's hypertension strategically focused research network. *Hypertension*. 2016;67(4):674–680

High Blood Pressure Clinical Practice Guideline Quick Reference Tools

- Action Statement Summary
  — Clinical Practice Guideline for Screening and Management of High Blood Pressure in Children and Adolescents
- *ICD-10-CM* Coding Quick Reference for High Blood Pressure

Action Statement Summary

Clinical Practice Guideline for Screening and Management of High Blood Pressure in Children and Adolescents

Key Action Statement 1

BP should be measured annually in children and adolescents ≥3 years of age (grade C, moderate recommendation).

Key Action Statement 2

BP should be checked in all children and adolescents ≥3 years of age at every health care encounter if they have obesity, are taking medications known to increase BP, have renal disease, a history of aortic arch obstruction or coarctation, or diabetes (grade C, moderate recommendation).

Key Action Statement 3

Trained health care professionals in the office setting should make a diagnosis of HTN if a child or adolescent has auscultatory-confirmed BP readings ≥95th percentile on 3 different visits (grade C, moderate recommendation).

Key Action Statement 4

Organizations with EHRs used in an office setting should consider including flags for abnormal BP values both when the values are being entered and when they are being viewed (grade C, weak recommendation).

Key Action Statement 5

Oscillometric devices may be used for BP screening in children and adolescents. When doing so, providers should use a device that has been validated in the pediatric age group. If elevated BP is suspected on the basis of oscillometric readings, confirmatory measurements should be obtained by auscultation (grade B, strong recommendation).

Key Action Statement 6

ABPM should be performed for the confirmation of HTN in children and adolescents with office BP measurements in the elevated BP category for 1 year or more or with stage 1 HTN over 3 clinic visits (grade C, moderate recommendation).

Key Action Statement 7

The routine performance of ABPM should be strongly considered in children and adolescents with high-risk conditions to assess HTN severity and determine if abnormal circadian BP patterns are present, which may indicate increased risk for target organ damage (grade B, moderate recommendation).

Key Action Statement 8

ABPM should be performed by using a standardized approach with monitors that have been validated in a pediatric population, and studies should be interpreted by using pediatric normative data (grade C, moderate recommendation).

Key Action Statement 9

Children and adolescents with suspected WCH should undergo ABPM. Diagnosis is based on the presence of mean SBP and DBP <95th percentile and SBP and DBP load <25% (grade B, strong recommendation).

Key Action Statement 10

Home BP monitoring should not be used to diagnose HTN, MH, or WCH but may be a useful adjunct to office and ambulatory BP measurement after HTN has been diagnosed (grade C, moderate recommendation).

Key Action Statement 11

Children and adolescents ≥6 years of age do not require an extensive evaluation for secondary causes of HTN if they have a positive family history of HTN, are overweight or obese, and/or do not have history or physical examination findings suggestive of a secondary cause of HTN (grade C, moderate recommendation).

Key Action Statement 12

Children and adolescents who have undergone coarctation repair should undergo ABPM for the detection of HTN (including MH) (grade B, strong recommendation).

Key Action Statement 13

In children and adolescents being evaluated for high BP, the provider should obtain a perinatal history, appropriate nutritional history, physical activity history, psychosocial history, and family history and perform a physical examination to identify findings suggestive of secondary causes of HTN (grade B, strong recommendation).

Key Action Statement 14

Clinicians should not perform electrocardiography in hypertensive children and adolescents being evaluated for LVH (grade B, strong recommendation).

Key Action Statement 15

1. It is recommended that echocardiography be performed to assess for cardiac target organ damage (LV mass, geometry, and function) at the time of consideration of pharmacologic treatment of HTN;
2. LVH should be defined as LV mass >51 g/m$^{2.7}$ (boys and girls) for children and adolescents older than 8 years and defined by LV mass >115 g/BSA for boys and LV mass >95 g/BSA for girls;
3. Repeat echocardiography may be performed to monitor improvement or progression of target organ damage at 6- to 12-month intervals. Indications to repeat echocardiography include persistent HTN despite treatment, concentric LV hypertrophy, or reduced LV ejection fraction; and
4. In patients without LV target organ injury at initial echocardiographic assessment, repeat echocardiography at yearly intervals may be considered in those with stage 2 HTN, secondary HTN, or chronic stage 1 HTN incompletely treated (noncompliance or drug resistance) to assess for the development of worsening LV target organ injury (grade C, moderate recommendation).

Key Action Statement 16

Doppler renal ultrasonography may be used as a noninvasive screening study for the evaluation of possible RAS in normal-weight children and adolescents ≥8 years of age who are suspected of having renovascular HTN and who will cooperate with the procedure (grade C, moderate recommendation).

Key Action Statement 17

In children and adolescents suspected of having RAS, either CTA or MRA may be performed as a noninvasive imaging study. Nuclear renography is less useful in pediatrics and should generally be avoided (grade D, weak recommendation).

Key Action Statement 18

Routine testing for MA is not recommended for children and adolescents with primary HTN (grade C, moderate recommendation).

Key Action Statement 19

In children and adolescents diagnosed with HTN, the treatment goal with nonpharmacologic and pharmacologic therapy should be a reduction in SBP and DBP to <90th percentile and <130/80 mm Hg in adolescents ≥13 years of age (grade C, moderate recommendation).

Key Action Statement 20

At the time of diagnosis of elevated BP or HTN in a child or adolescent, clinicians should provide advice on the DASH diet and recommend moderate to vigorous physical activity at least 3 to 5 days per week (30–60 minutes per session) to help reduce BP (grade C, weak recommendation).

Key Action Statement 21

In hypertensive children and adolescents who have failed lifestyle modifications (particularly those who have LV hypertrophy on echocardiography, symptomatic HTN, or stage 2 HTN without a clearly modifiable factor [eg, obesity]), clinicians should initiate pharmacologic treatment with an ACE inhibitor, ARB, long-acting calcium channel blocker, or thiazide diuretic (grade B, moderate recommendation).

Key Action Statement 22

ABPM may be used to assess treatment effectiveness in children and adolescents with HTN, especially when clinic and/or home BP measurements indicate insufficient BP response to treatment (grade B, moderate recommendation).

Key Action Statement 23

1. Children and adolescents with CKD should be evaluated for HTN at each medical encounter;
2. Children or adolescents with both CKD and HTN should be treated to lower 24-hour MAP to <50th percentile by ABPM; and
3. Regardless of apparent control of BP with office measures, children and adolescents with CKD and a history of HTN should have BP assessed by ABPM at least yearly to screen for MH (grade B, strong recommendation).

Key Action Statement 24

Children and adolescents with CKD and HTN should be evaluated for proteinuria (grade B, strong recommendation).

Key Action Statement 25

Children and adolescents with CKD, HTN, and proteinuria should be treated with an ACE inhibitor or ARB (grade B, strong recommendation).

Key Action Statement 26

Children and adolescents with T1DM or T2DM should be evaluated for HTN at each medical encounter and treated if BP is ≥95th percentile or >130/80 mm Hg in adolescents ≥13 years of age (grade C, moderate recommendation).

Key Action Statement 27

In children and adolescents with acute severe HTN and life-threatening symptoms, immediate treatment with short-acting antihypertensive medication should be initiated, and BP should be reduced by no more than 25% of the planned reduction over the first 8 hours (grade expert opinion D, weak recommendation).

Key Action Statement 28

Children and adolescents with HTN may participate in competitive sports once hypertensive target organ effects and risk have been assessed (grade C, moderate recommendation).

Key Action Statement 29

Children and adolescents with HTN should receive treatment to lower BP below stage 2 thresholds before participating in competitive sports (grade C, weak recommendation).

Key Action Statement 30

Adolescents with elevated BP or HTN (whether they are receiving antihypertensive treatment) should typically have their care transitioned to an appropriate adult care provider by 22 years of age (recognizing that there may be individual cases in which this upper age limit is exceeded, particularly in the case of youth with special health care needs). There should be a transfer of information regarding HTN etiology and past manifestations and complications of the patient's HTN (grade X, strong recommendation).

Coding Quick Reference for High Blood Pressure

ICD-10-CM		
I10	**Essential (primary) hypertension**	
I11.9	Hypertensive heart disease without heart failure	
I12.0	Hypertensive chronic kidney disease with stage 5 chronic kidney disease or end stage renal disease*	
I12.9	Hypertensive chronic kidney disease with stage 1 through stage 4 chronic kidney disease, or unspecified chronic kidney disease*	
I15.0 **I15.1** **I15.2** **I15.8** **I15.9**	Renovascular hypertension [secondary] Hypertension secondary to other renal disorders Hypertension secondary to endocrine disorders Other secondary hypertension Secondary hypertension, unspecified	Underlying cause coded in addition*
R03.0	Elevated blood-pressure reading, without diagnosis of hypertension	
P29.2	Neonatal hypertension	
***Underlying Causes**		
E25.0	Congenital adrenogenital disorders associated with enzyme deficiency	
E26.02	Glucocorticoid-remediable aldosteronism	
N18.1	Chronic kidney disease, stage 1	
N18.2	Chronic kidney disease, stage 2 (mild)	
N18.3	Chronic kidney disease, stage 3 (moderate)	
N18.4	Chronic kidney disease, stage 4 (severe)	
N18.5	Chronic kidney disease, stage 5	
N18.9	Chronic kidney disease, unspecified	
Q25.1	Coarctation of aorta	
Q25.71	Coarctation of pulmonary artery	
Q27.1	Congenital renal artery stenosis	
Q85.00	Neurofibromatosis, unspecified	
Q85.01	Neurofibromatosis, type 1	
Z83.49	Family history of other endocrine, nutritional and metabolic diseases [hyperaldosteronism]	
Z87.74	Personal history of (corrected) congenital malformations of heart and circulatory system [coarctation repair]	

Coding Quick Reference for High Blood Pressure, continued	
Z77.011	Contact with and (suspected) exposure to lead
Z77.018	Contact with and (suspected) exposure to other hazardous metals
Z79.3	Long term (current) use of hormonal contraceptives
Z79.51	Long term (current) use of inhaled steroids
Z79.52	Long term (current) use of systemic steroids
Z79.899	Other long term (current) drug therapy [CNS stimulant]

Management of Hyperbilirubinemia in the Newborn Infant 35 or More Weeks of Gestation

- *Clinical Practice Guideline*

AMERICAN ACADEMY OF PEDIATRICS

CLINICAL PRACTICE GUIDELINE

Subcommittee on Hyperbilirubinemia

Management of Hyperbilirubinemia in the Newborn Infant 35 or More Weeks of Gestation

ABSTRACT. Jaundice occurs in most newborn infants. Most jaundice is benign, but because of the potential toxicity of bilirubin, newborn infants must be monitored to identify those who might develop severe hyperbilirubinemia and, in rare cases, acute bilirubin encephalopathy or kernicterus. The focus of this guideline is to reduce the incidence of severe hyperbilirubinemia and bilirubin encephalopathy while minimizing the risks of unintended harm such as maternal anxiety, decreased breastfeeding, and unnecessary costs or treatment. Although kernicterus should almost always be preventable, cases continue to occur. These guidelines provide a framework for the prevention and management of hyperbilirubinemia in newborn infants of 35 or more weeks of gestation. In every infant, we recommend that clinicians 1) promote and support successful breastfeeding; 2) perform a systematic assessment before discharge for the risk of severe hyperbilirubinemia; 3) provide early and focused follow-up based on the risk assessment; and 4) when indicated, treat newborns with phototherapy or exchange transfusion to prevent the development of severe hyperbilirubinemia and, possibly, bilirubin encephalopathy (kernicterus). ***Pediatrics*** **2004; 114:297–316;** ***hyperbilirubinemia, newborn, kernicterus, bilirubin encephalopathy, phototherapy.***

ABBREVIATIONS. AAP, American Academy of Pediatrics; TSB, total serum bilirubin; TcB, transcutaneous bilirubin; G6PD, glucose-6-phosphate dehydrogenase; $ETCO_c$, end-tidal carbon monoxide corrected for ambient carbon monoxide; B/A, bilirubin/albumin; UB, unbound bilirubin.

BACKGROUND

In October 1994, the Provisional Committee for Quality Improvement and Subcommittee on Hyperbilirubinemia of the American Academy of Pediatrics (AAP) produced a practice parameter dealing with the management of hyperbilirubinemia in the healthy term newborn.[1] The current guideline represents a consensus of the committee charged by the AAP with reviewing and updating the existing guideline and is based on a careful review of the evidence, including a comprehensive literature review by the New England Medical Center Evidence-Based Practice Center.[2] (See "An Evidence-Based Review of Important Issues Concerning Neonatal Hyperbilirubinemia"[3] for a description of the methodology, questions addressed, and conclusions of this report.) This guideline is intended for use by hospitals and pediatricians, neonatologists, family physicians, physician assistants, and advanced practice nurses who treat newborn infants in the hospital and as outpatients. A list of frequently asked questions and answers for parents is available in English and Spanish at www.aap.org/family/jaundicefaq.htm.

The recommendations in this guideline do not indicate an exclusive course of treatment or serve as a standard of medical care. Variations, taking into account individual circumstances, may be appropriate.

PEDIATRICS (ISSN 0031 4005). Copyright © 2004 by the American Academy of Pediatrics.

DEFINITION OF RECOMMENDATIONS

The evidence-based approach to guideline development requires that the evidence in support of a policy be identified, appraised, and summarized and that an explicit link between evidence and recommendations be defined. Evidence-based recommendations are based on the quality of evidence and the balance of benefits and harms that is anticipated when the recommendation is followed. This guideline uses the definitions for quality of evidence and balance of benefits and harms established by the AAP Steering Committee on Quality Improvement Management.[4] See Appendix 1 for these definitions.

The draft practice guideline underwent extensive peer review by committees and sections within the AAP, outside organizations, and other individuals identified by the subcommittee as experts in the field. Liaison representatives to the subcommittee were invited to distribute the draft to other representatives and committees within their specialty organizations. The resulting comments were reviewed by the subcommittee and, when appropriate, incorporated into the guideline.

BILIRUBIN ENCEPHALOPATHY AND KERNICTERUS

Although originally a pathologic diagnosis characterized by bilirubin staining of the brainstem nuclei and cerebellum, the term "kernicterus" has come to be used interchangeably with both the acute and chronic findings of bilirubin encephalopathy. Bilirubin encephalopathy describes the clinical central nervous system findings caused by bilirubin toxicity to the basal ganglia and various brainstem nuclei. To avoid confusion and encourage greater consistency in the literature, the committee recommends that in infants the term "acute bilirubin encephalopathy" be used to describe the acute manifestations of bilirubin toxicity seen in the first weeks after birth and that the term "kernicterus" be reserved for the chronic and permanent clinical sequelae of bilirubin toxicity.

See Appendix 1 for the clinical manifestations of acute bilirubin encephalopathy and kernicterus.

FOCUS OF GUIDELINE

The overall aim of this guideline is to promote an approach that will reduce the frequency of severe neonatal hyperbilirubinemia and bilirubin encephalopathy and minimize the risk of unintended harm such as increased anxiety, decreased breastfeeding, or unnecessary treatment for the general population and excessive cost and waste. Recent reports of kernicterus indicate that this condition, although rare, is still occurring.[2,5–10]

Analysis of these reported cases of kernicterus suggests that if health care personnel follow the recommendations listed in this guideline, kernicterus would be largely preventable.

These guidelines emphasize the importance of universal systematic assessment for the risk of severe hyperbilirubinemia, close follow-up, and prompt intervention when indicated. The recommendations apply to the care of infants at 35 or more weeks of gestation. These recommendations seek to further the aims defined by the Institute of Medicine as appropriate for health care:[11] safety, effectiveness, efficiency, timeliness, patient-centeredness, and equity. They specifically emphasize the principles of patient safety and the key role of timeliness of interventions to prevent adverse outcomes resulting from neonatal hyperbilirubinemia.

The following are the key elements of the recommendations provided by this guideline. Clinicians should:

1. Promote and support successful breastfeeding.
2. Establish nursery protocols for the identification and evaluation of hyperbilirubinemia.
3. Measure the total serum bilirubin (TSB) or transcutaneous bilirubin (TcB) level on infants jaundiced in the first 24 hours.
4. Recognize that visual estimation of the degree of jaundice can lead to errors, particularly in darkly pigmented infants.
5. Interpret all bilirubin levels according to the infant's age in hours.
6. Recognize that infants at less than 38 weeks' gestation, particularly those who are breastfed, are at higher risk of developing hyperbilirubinemia and require closer surveillance and monitoring.
7. Perform a systematic assessment on all infants before discharge for the risk of severe hyperbilirubinemia.
8. Provide parents with written and verbal information about newborn jaundice.
9. Provide appropriate follow-up based on the time of discharge and the risk assessment.
10. Treat newborns, when indicated, with phototherapy or exchange transfusion.

PRIMARY PREVENTION

In numerous policy statements, the AAP recommends breastfeeding for all healthy term and near-term newborns. This guideline strongly supports this general recommendation.

RECOMMENDATION 1.0: Clinicians should advise mothers to nurse their infants at least 8 to 12 times per day for the first several days[12] (evidence quality C: benefits exceed harms).

Poor caloric intake and/or dehydration associated with inadequate breastfeeding may contribute to the development of hyperbilirubinemia.[6,13,14] Increasing the frequency of nursing decreases the likelihood of subsequent significant hyperbilirubinemia in breastfed infants.[15–17] Providing appropriate support and advice to breastfeeding mothers increases the likelihood that breastfeeding will be successful.

Additional information on how to assess the adequacy of intake in a breastfed newborn is provided in Appendix 1.

RECOMMENDATION 1.1: The AAP recommends against routine supplementation of nondehydrated breastfed infants with water or dextrose water (evidence quality B and C: harms exceed benefits).

Supplementation with water or dextrose water will not prevent hyperbilirubinemia or decrease TSB levels.[18,19]

SECONDARY PREVENTION

RECOMMENDATION 2.0: Clinicians should perform ongoing systematic assessments during the neonatal period for the risk of an infant developing severe hyperbilirubinemia.

Blood Typing

RECOMMENDATION 2.1: All pregnant women should be tested for ABO and Rh (D) blood types and have a serum screen for unusual isoimmune antibodies (evidence quality B: benefits exceed harms).

RECOMMENDATION 2.1.1: If a mother has not had prenatal blood grouping or is Rh-negative, a direct antibody test (or Coombs' test), blood type, and an Rh (D) type on the infant's (cord) blood are strongly recommended (evidence quality B: benefits exceed harms).

RECOMMENDATION 2.1.2: If the maternal blood is group O, Rh-positive, it is an option to test the cord blood for the infant's blood type and direct antibody test, but it is not required provided that there is appropriate surveillance, risk assessment before discharge, and follow-up[20] (evidence quality C: benefits exceed harms).

Clinical Assessment

RECOMMENDATION 2.2: Clinicians should ensure that all infants are routinely monitored for the development of jaundice, and nurseries should have established protocols for the assessment of jaundice. Jaundice should be assessed whenever the infant's vital signs are measured but no less than every 8 to 12 hours (evidence quality D: benefits versus harms exceptional).

In newborn infants, jaundice can be detected by blanching the skin with digital pressure, revealing the underlying color of the skin and subcutaneous tissue. The assessment of jaundice must be per-

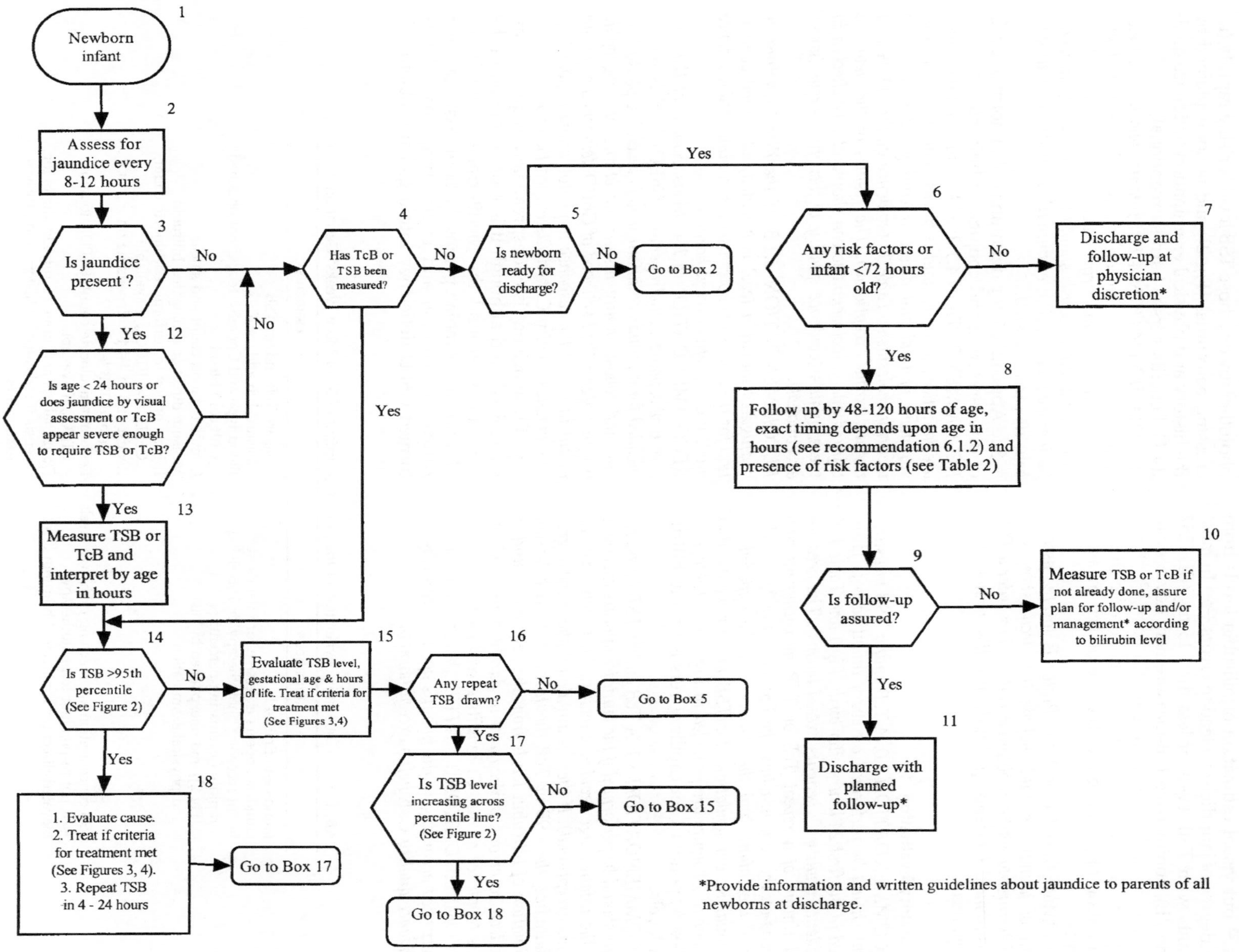

Fig 1. Algorithm for the management of jaundice in the newborn nursery.

formed in a well-lit room or, preferably, in daylight at a window. Jaundice is usually seen first in the face and progresses caudally to the trunk and extremities,[21] but visual estimation of bilirubin levels from the degree of jaundice can lead to errors.[22–24] In most infants with TSB levels of less than 15 mg/dL (257 μmol/L), noninvasive TcB-measurement devices can provide a valid estimate of the TSB level.[2,25–29] See Appendix 1 for additional information on the clinical evaluation of jaundice and the use of TcB measurements.

RECOMMENDATION 2.2.1: Protocols for the assessment of jaundice should include the circumstances in which nursing staff can obtain a TcB level or order a TSB measurement (evidence quality D: benefits versus harms exceptional).

Laboratory Evaluation

RECOMMENDATION 3.0: A TcB and/or TSB measurement should be performed on every infant who is jaundiced in the first 24 hours after birth (Fig 1 and Table 1)[30] (evidence quality C: benefits exceed harms). The need for and timing of a repeat TcB or TSB measurement will depend on the zone in which the TSB falls (Fig 2),[25,31] the age of the infant, and the evolution of the hyperbilirubinemia. Recommendations for TSB measurements after the age of 24 hours are provided in Fig 1 and Table 1.

See Appendix 1 for capillary versus venous bilirubin levels.

RECOMMENDATION 3.1: A TcB and/or TSB measurement should be performed if the jaundice appears excessive for the infant's age (evidence quality D: benefits versus harms exceptional). If there is any doubt about the degree of jaundice, the TSB or TcB should be measured. Visual estimation of bilirubin levels from the degree of jaundice can lead to errors, particularly in darkly pigmented infants (evidence quality C: benefits exceed harms).

RECOMMENDATION 3.2: All bilirubin levels should be interpreted according to the infant's age in hours (Fig 2) (evidence quality C: benefits exceed harms).

Cause of Jaundice

RECOMMENDATION 4.1: The possible cause of jaundice should be sought in an infant receiving phototherapy or whose TSB level is rising rapidly (ie, crossing percentiles [Fig 2]) and is not explained by the history and physical examination (evidence quality D: benefits versus harms exceptional).

RECOMMENDATION 4.1.1: Infants who have an elevation of direct-reacting or conjugated bilirubin should have a urinalysis and urine culture.[32] Additional laboratory evaluation for sepsis should be performed if indicated by history and physical examination (evidence quality C: benefits exceed harms).

See Appendix 1 for definitions of abnormal levels of direct-reacting and conjugated bilirubin.

RECOMMENDATION 4.1.2: Sick infants and those who are jaundiced at or beyond 3 weeks should have a measurement of total and direct or conjugated bilirubin to identify cholestasis (Table 1) (evidence quality D: benefit versus harms exceptional). The results of the newborn thyroid and galactosemia screen should also be checked in these infants (evidence quality D: benefits versus harms exceptional).

RECOMMENDATION 4.1.3: If the direct-reacting or conjugated bilirubin level is elevated, additional evaluation for the causes of cholestasis is recommended (evidence quality C: benefits exceed harms).

RECOMMENDATION 4.1.4: Measurement of the glucose-6-phosphate dehydrogenase (G6PD) level is recommended for a jaundiced infant who is receiving phototherapy and whose family history or ethnic or geographic origin suggest the likelihood of G6PD deficiency or for an infant in whom the response to phototherapy is poor (Fig 3) (evidence quality C: benefits exceed harms).

G6PD deficiency is widespread and frequently unrecognized, and although it is more common in the populations around the Mediterranean and in the Middle East, Arabian peninsula, Southeast Asia, and Africa, immigration and intermarriage have transformed G6PD deficiency into a global problem.[33,34]

TABLE 1. Laboratory Evaluation of the Jaundiced Infant of 35 or More Weeks' Gestation

Indications	Assessments
Jaundice in first 24 h	Measure TcB and/or TSB
Jaundice appears excessive for infant's age	Measure TcB and/or TSB
Infant receiving phototherapy or TSB rising rapidly (ie, crossing percentiles [Fig 2]) and unexplained by history and physical examination	Blood type and Coombs' test, if not obtained with cord blood Complete blood count and smear Measure direct or conjugated bilirubin It is an option to perform reticulocyte count, G6PD, and $ETCO_c$, if available Repeat TSB in 4–24 h depending on infant's age and TSB level
TSB concentration approaching exchange levels or not responding to phototherapy	Perform reticulocyte count, G6PD, albumin, $ETCO_c$, if available
Elevated direct (or conjugated) bilirubin level	Do urinalysis and urine culture. Evaluate for sepsis if indicated by history and physical examination
Jaundice present at or beyond age 3 wk, or sick infant	Total and direct (or conjugated) bilirubin level If direct bilirubin elevated, evaluate for causes of cholestasis Check results of newborn thyroid and galactosemia screen, and evaluate infant for signs or symptoms of hypothyroidism

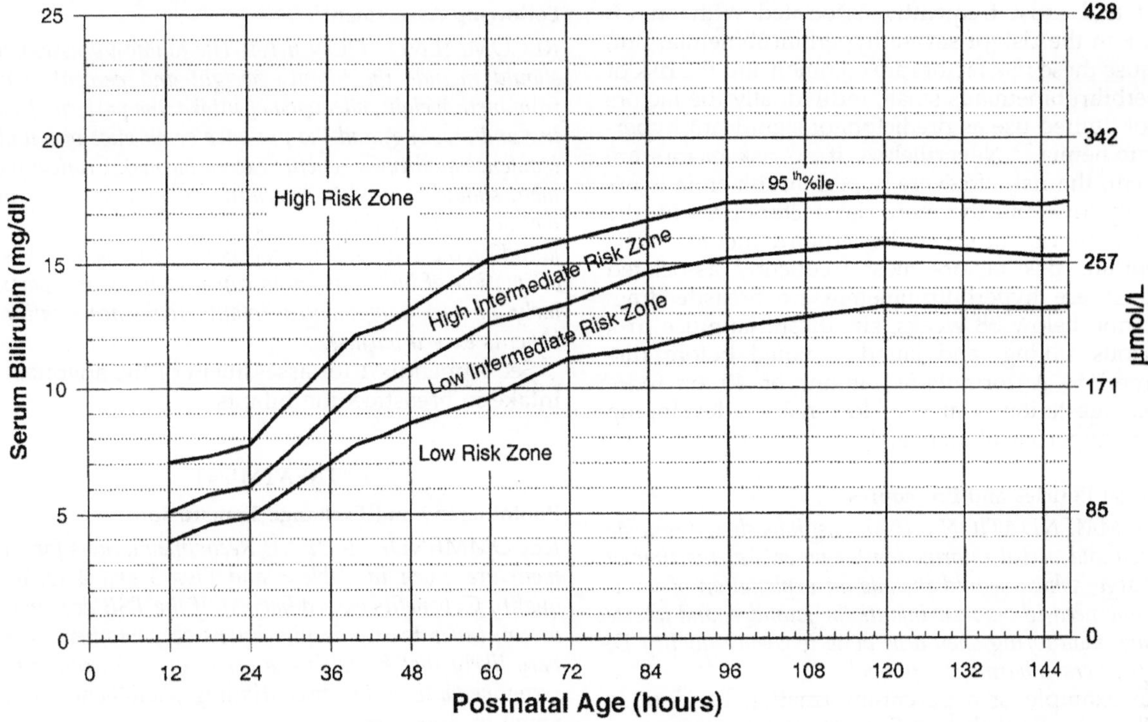

Fig 2. Nomogram for designation of risk in 2840 well newborns at 36 or more weeks' gestational age with birth weight of 2000 g or more or 35 or more weeks' gestational age and birth weight of 2500 g or more based on the hour-specific serum bilirubin values. The serum bilirubin level was obtained before discharge, and the zone in which the value fell predicted the likelihood of a subsequent bilirubin level exceeding the 95th percentile (high-risk zone) as shown in Appendix 1, Table 4. Used with permission from Bhutani et al.[31] See Appendix 1 for additional information about this nomogram, which should not be used to represent the natural history of neonatal hyperbilirubinemia.

Furthermore, G6PD deficiency occurs in 11% to 13% of African Americans, and kernicterus has occurred in some of these infants.[5,33] In a recent report, G6PD deficiency was considered to be the cause of hyperbilirubinemia in 19 of 61 (31.5%) infants who developed kernicterus.[5] (See Appendix 1 for additional information on G6PD deficiency.)

Risk Assessment Before Discharge

RECOMMENDATION 5.1: Before discharge, every newborn should be assessed for the risk of developing severe hyperbilirubinemia, and all nurseries should establish protocols for assessing this risk. Such assessment is particularly important in infants who are discharged before the age of 72 hours (evidence quality C: benefits exceed harms).

RECOMMENDATION 5.1.1: The AAP recommends 2 clinical options used individually or in combination for the systematic assessment of risk: predischarge measurement of the bilirubin level using TSB or TcB and/or assessment of clinical risk factors. Whether either or both options are used, appropriate follow-up after discharge is essential (evidence quality C: benefits exceed harms).

The best documented method for assessing the risk of subsequent hyperbilirubinemia is to measure the TSB or TcB level[25,31,35–38] and plot the results on a nomogram (Fig 2). A TSB level can be obtained at the time of the routine metabolic screen, thus obviating the need for an additional blood sample. Some authors have suggested that a TSB measurement should be part of the routine screening of all newborns.[5,31] An infant whose predischarge TSB is in the low-risk zone (Fig 2) is at very low risk of developing severe hyperbilirubinemia.[5,38]

Table 2 lists those factors that are clinically signif-

TABLE 2. Risk Factors for Development of Severe Hyperbilirubinemia in Infants of 35 or More Weeks' Gestation (in Approximate Order of Importance)

Major risk factors
Predischarge TSB or TcB level in the high-risk zone (Fig 2)[25,31]
Jaundice observed in the first 24 h[30]
Blood group incompatibility with positive direct antiglobulin test, other known hemolytic disease (eg, G6PD deficiency), elevated $ETCO_c$
Gestational age 35–36 wk[39,40]
Previous sibling received phototherapy[40,41]
Cephalohematoma or significant bruising[39]
Exclusive breastfeeding, particularly if nursing is not going well and weight loss is excessive[39,40]
East Asian race[39]*
Minor risk factors
Predischarge TSB or TcB level in the high intermediate-risk zone[25,31]
Gestational age 37–38 wk[39,40]
Jaundice observed before discharge[40]
Previous sibling with jaundice[40,41]
Macrosomic infant of a diabetic mother[42,43]
Maternal age ≥25 y[39]
Male gender[39,40]
Decreased risk (these factors are associated with decreased risk of significant jaundice, listed in order of decreasing importance)
TSB or TcB level in the low-risk zone (Fig 2)[25,31]
Gestational age ≥41 wk[39]
Exclusive bottle feeding[39,40]
Black race[38]*
Discharge from hospital after 72 h[40,44]

* Race as defined by mother's description.

icant and most frequently associated with an increase in the risk of severe hyperbilirubinemia. But, because these risk factors are common and the risk of hyperbilirubinemia is small, individually the factors are of limited use as predictors of significant hyperbilirubinemia.[39] Nevertheless, if no risk factors are present, the risk of severe hyperbilirubinemia is extremely low, and the more risk factors present, the greater the risk of severe hyperbilirubinemia.[39] The important risk factors most frequently associated with severe hyperbilirubinemia are breastfeeding, gestation below 38 weeks, significant jaundice in a previous sibling, and jaundice noted before discharge.[39,40] A formula-fed infant of 40 or more weeks' gestation is at very low risk of developing severe hyperbilirubinemia.[39]

Hospital Policies and Procedures

RECOMMENDATION 6.1: All hospitals should provide written and verbal information for parents at the time of discharge, which should include an explanation of jaundice, the need to monitor infants for jaundice, and advice on how monitoring should be done (evidence quality D: benefits versus harms exceptional).

An example of a parent-information handout is available in English and Spanish at www.aap.org/family/jaundicefaq.htm.

Follow-up

RECOMMENDATION 6.1.1: All infants should be examined by a qualified health care professional in the first few days after discharge to assess infant well-being and the presence or absence of jaundice. The timing and location of this assessment will be determined by the length of stay in the nursery, presence or absence of risk factors for hyperbilirubinemia (Table 2 and Fig 2), and risk of other neonatal problems (evidence quality C: benefits exceed harms).

Timing of Follow-up

RECOMMENDATION 6.1.2: Follow-up should be provided as follows:

Infant Discharged	Should Be Seen by Age
Before age 24 h	72 h
Between 24 and 47.9 h	96 h
Between 48 and 72 h	120 h

For some newborns discharged before 48 hours, 2 follow-up visits may be required, the first visit between 24 and 72 hours and the second between 72 and 120 hours. Clinical judgment should be used in determining follow-up. Earlier or more frequent follow-up should be provided for those who have risk factors for hyperbilirubinemia (Table 2), whereas those discharged with few or no risk factors can be seen after longer intervals (evidence quality C: benefits exceed harms).

RECOMMENDATION 6.1.3: If appropriate follow-up cannot be ensured in the presence of elevated risk for developing severe hyperbilirubinemia, it may be necessary to delay discharge either until appropriate follow-up can be ensured or the period of greatest risk has passed (72-96 hours) (evidence quality D: benefits versus harms exceptional).

Follow-up Assessment

RECOMMENDATION 6.1.4: The follow-up assessment should include the infant's weight and percent change from birth weight, adequacy of intake, the pattern of voiding and stooling, and the presence or absence of jaundice (evidence quality C: benefits exceed harms). Clinical judgment should be used to determine the need for a bilirubin measurement. If there is any doubt about the degree of jaundice, the TSB or TcB level should be measured. Visual estimation of bilirubin levels can lead to errors, particularly in darkly pigmented infants (evidence quality C: benefits exceed harms).

See Appendix 1 for assessment of the adequacy of intake in breastfeeding infants.

TREATMENT

Phototherapy and Exchange Transfusion

RECOMMENDATION 7.1: Recommendations for treatment are given in Table 3 and Figs 3 and 4 (evidence quality C: benefits exceed harms). If the TSB does not fall or continues to rise despite intensive phototherapy, it is very likely that hemolysis is occurring. The committee's recommendations for discontinuing phototherapy can be found in Appendix 2.

RECOMMENDATION 7.1.1: In using the guidelines for phototherapy and exchange transfusion (Figs 3 and 4), the direct-reacting (or conjugated) bilirubin level should not be subtracted from the total (evidence quality D: benefits versus harms exceptional).

In unusual situations in which the direct bilirubin level is 50% or more of the total bilirubin, there are no good data to provide guidance for therapy, and consultation with an expert in the field is recommended.

RECOMMENDATION 7.1.2: If the TSB is at a level at which exchange transfusion is recommended (Fig 4) or if the TSB level is 25 mg/dL (428 μmol/L) or higher at any time, it is a medical emergency and the infant should be admitted immediately and directly to a hospital pediatric service for intensive phototherapy. These infants should not be referred to the emergency department, because it delays the initiation of treatment[54] (evidence quality C: benefits exceed harms).

RECOMMENDATION 7.1.3: Exchange transfusions should be performed only by trained personnel in a neonatal intensive care unit with full monitoring and resuscitation capabilities (evidence quality D: benefits versus harms exceptional).

RECOMMENDATION 7.1.4: In isoimmune hemolytic disease, administration of intravenous γ-globulin (0.5-1 g/kg over 2 hours) is recommended if the TSB is rising despite intensive phototherapy or the TSB level is within 2 to 3 mg/dL (34-51 μmol/L) of the exchange level (Fig 4).[55] If necessary, this dose can be repeated in 12 hours (evidence quality B: benefits exceed harms).

Intravenous γ-globulin has been shown to reduce the need for exchange transfusions in Rh and ABO hemolytic disease.[55–58] Although data are limited, it is reasonable to assume that intravenous γ-globulin will also be helpful in the other types of Rh hemolytic disease such as anti-C and anti-E.

TABLE 3. Example of a Clinical Pathway for Management of the Newborn Infant Readmitted for Phototherapy or Exchange Transfusion

Treatment
- Use intensive phototherapy and/or exchange transfusion as indicated in Figs 3 and 4 (see Appendix 2 for details of phototherapy use)

Laboratory tests
- TSB and direct bilirubin levels
- Blood type (ABO, Rh)
- Direct antibody test (Coombs')
- Serum albumin
- Complete blood cell count with differential and smear for red cell morphology
- Reticulocyte count
- $ETCO_c$ (if available)
- G6PD if suggested by ethnic or geographic origin or if poor response to phototherapy
- Urine for reducing substances
- If history and/or presentation suggest sepsis, perform blood culture, urine culture, and cerebrospinal fluid for protein, glucose, cell count, and culture

Interventions
- If TSB ≥25 mg/dL (428 μmol/L) or ≥20 mg/dL (342 μmol/L) in a sick infant or infant <38 wk gestation, obtain a type and crossmatch, and request blood in case an exchange transfusion is necessary
- In infants with isoimmune hemolytic disease and TSB level rising in spite of intensive phototherapy or within 2–3 mg/dL (34–51 μmol/L) of exchange level (Fig 4), administer intravenous immunoglobulin 0.5–1 g/kg over 2 h and repeat in 12 h if necessary
- If infant's weight loss from birth is >12% or there is clinical or biochemical evidence of dehydration, recommend formula or expressed breast milk. If oral intake is in question, give intravenous fluids.

For infants receiving intensive phototherapy
- Breastfeed or bottle-feed (formula or expressed breast milk) every 2–3 h
- If TSB ≥25 mg/dL (428 μmol/L), repeat TSB within 2–3 h
- If TSB 20–25 mg/dL (342–428 μmol/L), repeat within 3–4 h. If TSB <20 mg/dL (342 μmol/L), repeat in 4–6 h. If TSB continues to fall, repeat in 8–12 h
- If TSB is not decreasing or is moving closer to level for exchange transfusion or the TSB/albumin ratio exceeds levels shown in Fig 4, consider exchange transfusion (see Fig 4 for exchange transfusion recommendations)
- When TSB is <13–14 mg/dL (239 μmol/L), discontinue phototherapy
- Depending on the cause of the hyperbilirubinemia, it is an option to measure TSB 24 h after discharge to check for rebound

Serum Albumin Levels and the Bilirubin/Albumin Ratio

RECOMMENDATION 7.1.5: It is an option to measure the serum albumin level and consider an albumin level of less than 3.0 g/dL as one risk factor for lowering the threshold for phototherapy use (see Fig 3) (evidence quality D: benefits versus risks exceptional.).

RECOMMENDATION 7.1.6: If an exchange transfusion is being considered, the serum albumin level should be measured and the bilirubin/albumin (B/A) ratio used in conjunction with the TSB level and other factors in determining the need for exchange transfusion (see Fig 4) (evidence quality D: benefits versus harms exceptional).

The recommendations shown above for treating hyperbilirubinemia are based primarily on TSB levels and other factors that affect the risk of bilirubin encephalopathy. This risk might be increased by a prolonged (rather than a brief) exposure to a certain TSB level.[59,60] Because the published data that address this issue are limited, however, it is not possible to provide specific recommendations for intervention based on the duration of hyperbilirubinemia.

See Appendix 1 for the basis for recommendations 7.1 through 7.1.6 and for the recommendations provided in Figs 3 and 4. Appendix 1 also contains a discussion of the risks of exchange transfusion and the use of B/A binding.

Acute Bilirubin Encephalopathy

RECOMMENDATION 7.1.7: Immediate exchange transfusion is recommended in any infant who is jaundiced and manifests the signs of the intermediate to advanced stages of acute bilirubin encephalopathy[61,62] (hypertonia, arching, retrocollis, opisthotonos, fever, high-pitched cry) even if the TSB is falling (evidence quality D: benefits versus risks exceptional).

Phototherapy

RECOMMENDATION 7.2: All nurseries and services treating infants should have the necessary equipment to provide intensive phototherapy (see Appendix 2) (evidence quality D: benefits exceed risks).

Outpatient Management of the Jaundiced Breastfed Infant

RECOMMENDATION 7.3: In breastfed infants who require phototherapy (Fig 3), the AAP recommends that, if possible, breastfeeding should be continued (evidence quality C: benefits exceed harms). It is also an option to interrupt temporarily breastfeeding and substitute formula. This can reduce bilirubin levels and/or enhance the efficacy of phototherapy[63–65] (evidence quality B: benefits exceed harms). In breastfed infants receiving phototherapy, supplementation with expressed breast milk or formula is appropriate if the infant's intake seems inadequate, weight loss is excessive, or the infant seems dehydrated.

IMPLEMENTATION STRATEGIES

The Institute of Medicine[11] recommends a dramatic change in the way the US health care system

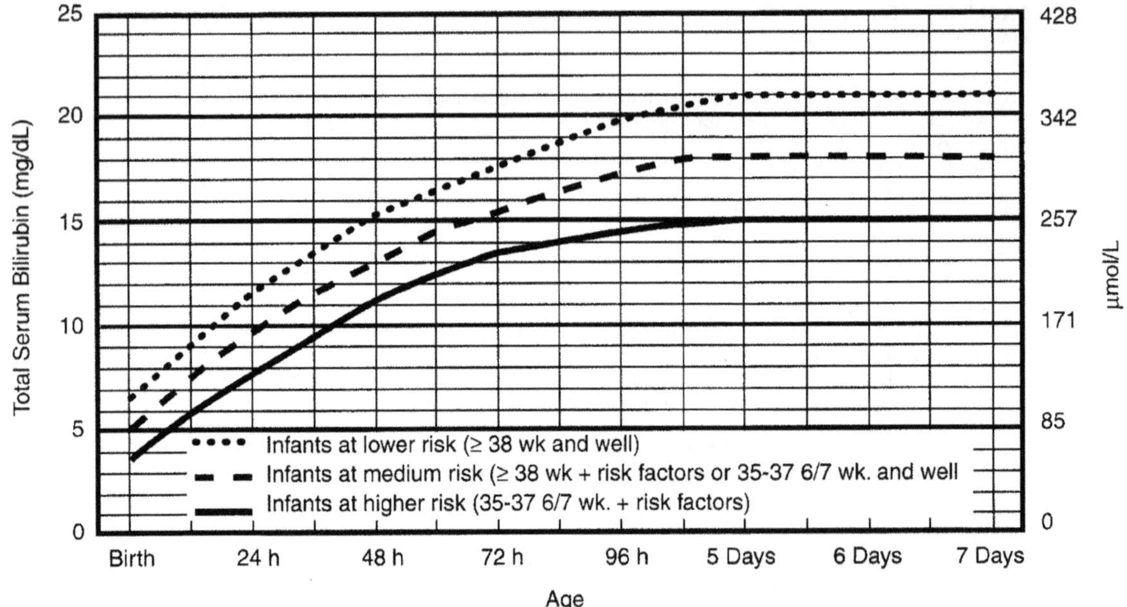

- Use total bilirubin. Do not subtract direct reacting or conjugated bilirubin.
- Risk factors = isoimmune hemolytic disease, G6PD deficiency, asphyxia, significant lethargy, temperature instability, sepsis, acidosis, or albumin < 3.0g/dL (if measured)
- For well infants 35-37 6/7 wk can adjust TSB levels for intervention around the medium risk line. It is an option to intervene at lower TSB levels for infants closer to 35 wks and at higher TSB levels for those closer to 37 6/7 wk.
- It is an option to provide conventional phototherapy in hospital or at home at TSB levels 2-3 mg/dL (35-50mmol/L) below those shown but home phototherapy should not be used in any infant with risk factors.

Fig 3. Guidelines for phototherapy in hospitalized infants of 35 or more weeks' gestation.

Note: These guidelines are based on limited evidence and the levels shown are approximations. The guidelines refer to the use of intensive phototherapy which should be used when the TSB exceeds the line indicated for each category. Infants are designated as "higher risk" because of the potential negative effects of the conditions listed on albumin binding of bilirubin,[45–47] the blood-brain barrier,[48] and the susceptibility of the brain cells to damage by bilirubin.[48]

"Intensive phototherapy" implies irradiance in the blue-green spectrum (wavelengths of approximately 430–490 nm) of at least 30 $\mu W/cm^2$ per nm (measured at the infant's skin directly below the center of the phototherapy unit) and delivered to as much of the infant's surface area as possible. Note that irradiance measured below the center of the light source is much greater than that measured at the periphery. Measurements should be made with a radiometer specified by the manufacturer of the phototherapy system.

See Appendix 2 for additional information on measuring the dose of phototherapy, a description of intensive phototherapy, and of light sources used. If total serum bilirubin levels approach or exceed the exchange transfusion line (Fig 4), the sides of the bassinet, incubator, or warmer should be lined with aluminum foil or white material.[50] This will increase the surface area of the infant exposed and increase the efficacy of phototherapy.[51]

If the total serum bilirubin does not decrease or continues to rise in an infant who is receiving intensive phototherapy, this strongly suggests the presence of hemolysis.

Infants who receive phototherapy and have an elevated direct-reacting or conjugated bilirubin level (cholestatic jaundice) may develop the bronze-baby syndrome. See Appendix 2 for the use of phototherapy in these infants.

ensures the safety of patients. The perspective of safety as a purely individual responsibility must be replaced by the concept of safety as a property of systems. Safe systems are characterized by a shared knowledge of the goal, a culture emphasizing safety, the ability of each person within the system to act in a manner that promotes safety, minimizing the use of memory, and emphasizing the use of standard procedures (such as checklists), and the involvement of patients/families as partners in the process of care.

These principles can be applied to the challenge of preventing severe hyperbilirubinemia and kernicterus. A systematic approach to the implementation of these guidelines should result in greater safety. Such approaches might include

- The establishment of standing protocols for nursing assessment of jaundice, including testing TcB and TSB levels, without requiring physician orders.
- Checklists or reminders associated with risk factors, age at discharge, and laboratory test results that provide guidance for appropriate follow-up.
- Explicit educational materials for parents (a key component of all AAP guidelines) concerning the identification of newborns with jaundice.

FUTURE RESEARCH

Epidemiology of Bilirubin-Induced Central Nervous System Damage

There is a need for appropriate epidemiologic data to document the incidence of kernicterus in the newborn population, the incidence of other adverse effects attributable to hyperbilirubinemia and its management, and the number of infants whose TSB levels exceed 25 or 30 mg/dL (428-513 μmol/L). Organizations such as the Centers for Disease Control and Prevention should implement strategies for appropriate data gathering to identify the number of

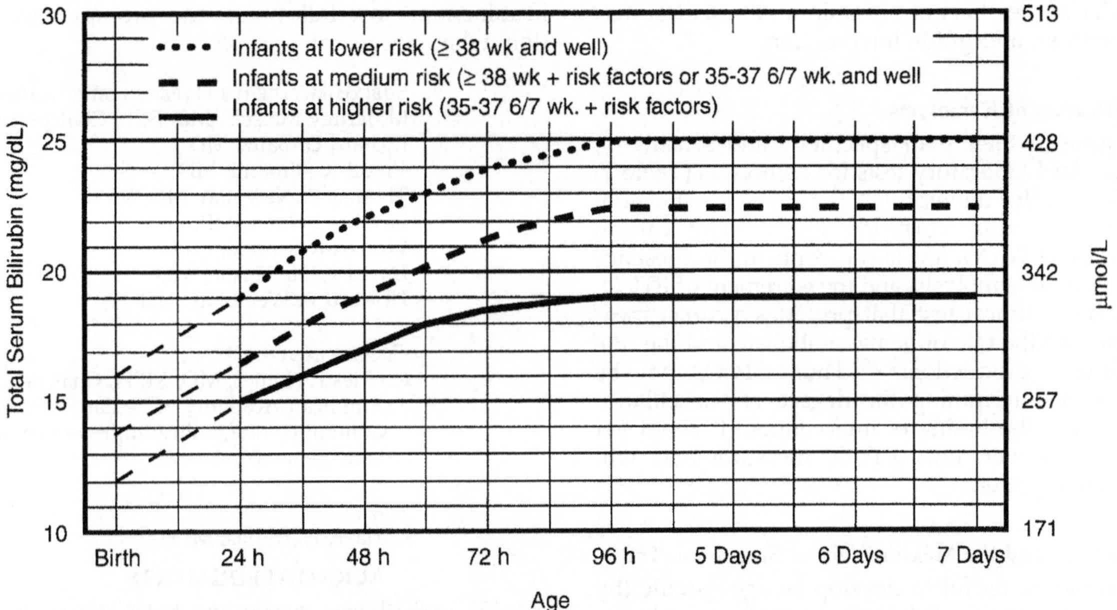

- The dashed lines for the first 24 hours indicate uncertainty due to a wide range of clinical circumstances and a range of responses to phototherapy.
- Immediate exchange transfusion is recommended if infant shows signs of acute bilirubin encephalopathy (hypertonia, arching, retrocollis, opisthotonos, fever, high pitched cry) or if TSB is ≥5 mg/dL (85 µmol/L) above these lines.
- Risk factors - isoimmune hemolytic disease, G6PD deficiency, asphyxia, significant lethargy, temperature instability, sepsis, acidosis.
- Measure serum albumin and calculate B/A ratio (See legend)
- Use total bilirubin. Do not subtract direct reacting or conjugated bilirubin
- If infant is well and 35-37 6/7 wk (median risk) can individualize TSB levels for exchange based on actual gestational age.

Fig 4. Guidelines for exchange transfusion in infants 35 or more weeks' gestation.

Note that these suggested levels represent a consensus of most of the committee but are based on limited evidence, and the levels shown are approximations. See ref. 3 for risks and complications of exchange transfusion. During birth hospitalization, exchange transfusion is recommended if the TSB rises to these levels despite intensive phototherapy. For readmitted infants, if the TSB level is above the exchange level, repeat TSB measurement every 2 to 3 hours and consider exchange if the TSB remains above the levels indicated after intensive phototherapy for 6 hours.

The following B/A ratios can be used together with but in not in lieu of the TSB level as an additional factor in determining the need for exchange transfusion[52]:

Risk Category	B/A Ratio at Which Exchange Transfusion Should be Considered	
	TSB mg/dL/Alb, g/dL	TSB µmol/L/Alb, µmol/L
Infants ≥38 0/7 wk	8.0	0.94
Infants 35 0/7–36 6/7 wk and well or ≥38 0/7 wk if higher risk or isoimmune hemolytic disease or G6PD deficiency	7.2	0.84
Infants 35 0/7–37 6/7 wk if higher risk or isoimmune hemolytic disease or G6PD deficiency	6.8	0.80

If the TSB is at or approaching the exchange level, send blood for immediate type and crossmatch. Blood for exchange transfusion is modified whole blood (red cells and plasma) crossmatched against the mother and compatible with the infant.[53]

infants who develop serum bilirubin levels above 25 or 30 mg/dL (428-513 µmol/L) and those who develop acute and chronic bilirubin encephalopathy. This information will help to identify the magnitude of the problem; the number of infants who need to be screened and treated to prevent 1 case of kernicterus; and the risks, costs, and benefits of different strategies for prevention and treatment of hyperbilirubinemia. In the absence of these data, recommendations for intervention cannot be considered definitive.

Effect of Bilirubin on the Central Nervous System

The serum bilirubin level by itself, except when it is extremely high and associated with bilirubin encephalopathy, is an imprecise indicator of long-term neurodevelopmental outcome.[2] Additional studies are needed on the relationship between central nervous system damage and the duration of hyperbilirubinemia, the binding of bilirubin to albumin, and changes seen in the brainstem auditory evoked response. These studies could help to better identify risk, clarify the effect of bilirubin on the central nervous system, and guide intervention.

Identification of Hemolysis

Because of their poor specificity and sensitivity, the standard laboratory tests for hemolysis (Table 1) are frequently unhelpful.[66,67] However, end-tidal carbon monoxide, corrected for ambient carbon monoxide ($ETCO_c$), levels can confirm the presence or absence of hemolysis, and measurement of $ETCO_c$ is the only clinical test that provides a direct measurement of the rate of heme catabolism and the rate of bilirubin production.[68,69] Thus, $ETCO_c$ may be helpful in determining the degree of surveillance needed and the timing of intervention. It is not yet known, however, how $ETCO_c$ measurements will affect management.

Nomograms and the Measurement of Serum and TcB

It would be useful to develop an age-specific (by hour) nomogram for TSB in populations of newborns that differ with regard to risk factors for hyperbilirubinemia. There is also an urgent need to improve the precision and accuracy of the measurement of TSB in the clinical laboratory.[70,71] Additional studies are also needed to develop and validate noninvasive (transcutaneous) measurements of serum bilirubin and to understand the factors that affect these measurements. These studies should also assess the cost-effectiveness and reproducibility of TcB measurements in clinical practice.[2]

Pharmacologic Therapy

There is now evidence that hyperbilirubinemia can be effectively prevented or treated with tin-mesoporphyrin,[72–75] a drug that inhibits the production of heme oxygenase. Tin-mesoporphyrin is not approved by the US Food and Drug Administration. If approved, tin-mesoporphyrin could find immediate application in preventing the need for exchange transfusion in infants who are not responding to phototherapy.[75]

Dissemination and Monitoring

Research should be directed toward methods for disseminating the information contained in this guideline to increase awareness on the part of physicians, residents, nurses, and parents concerning the issues of neonatal hyperbilirubinemia and strategies for its management. In addition, monitoring systems should be established to identify the impact of these guidelines on the incidence of acute bilirubin encephalopathy and kernicterus and the use of phototherapy and exchange transfusions.

CONCLUSIONS

Kernicterus is still occurring but should be largely preventable if health care personnel follow the recommendations listed in this guideline. These recommendations emphasize the importance of universal, systematic assessment for the risk of severe hyperbilirubinemia, close follow-up, and prompt intervention, when necessary.

Subcommittee on Hyperbilirubinemia
M. Jeffrey Maisels, MB, BCh, Chairperson
Richard D. Baltz, MD
Vinod K. Bhutani, MD
Thomas B. Newman, MD, MPH
Heather Palmer, MB, BCh
Warren Rosenfeld, MD
David K. Stevenson, MD
Howard B. Weinblatt, MD

Consultant
Charles J. Homer, MD, MPH, Chairperson
American Academy of Pediatrics Steering Committee on Quality Improvement and Management

Staff
Carla T. Herrerias, MPH

ACKNOWLEDGMENTS

M.J.M. received grant support from Natus Medical, Inc, for multinational study of ambient carbon monoxide; WellSpring Pharmaceutical Corporation for study of Stannsoporfin (tin-mesoporphyrin); and Minolta, Inc, for study of the Minolta/Hill-Rom Air-Shields transcutaneous jaundice meter model JM-103. V.K.B. received grant support from WellSpring Pharmaceutical Corporation for study of Stannsoporfin (tin-mesoporphyrin) and Natus Medical, Inc, for multinational study of ambient carbon monoxide and is a consultant (volunteer) to SpectrX (BiliChek transcutaneous bilirubinometer). D.K.S. is a consultant to and holds stock options through Natus Medical, Inc.

The American Academy of Pediatrics Subcommittee on Hyperbilirubinemia gratefully acknowledges the help of the following organizations, committees, and individuals who reviewed drafts of this guideline and provided valuable criticisms and commentary: American Academy of Pediatrics Committee on Nutrition; American Academy of Pediatrics Committee on Practice and Ambulatory Medicine; American Academy of Pediatrics Committee on Child Health Financing; American Academy of Pediatrics Committee on Medical Liability; American Academy of Pediatrics Committee on Fetus and Newborn; American Academy of Pediatrics Section on Perinatal Pediatrics; Centers for Disease Control and Prevention; Parents of Infants and Children With Kernicterus (PICK); Charles Ahlfors, MD; Daniel Batton, MD; Thomas Bojko, MD; Sarah Clune, MD; Sudhakar Ezhuthachan, MD; Lawrence Gartner, MD; Cathy Hammerman, MD; Thor Hansen, MD; Lois Johnson, MD; Michael Kaplan, MB, ChB; Tony McDonagh, PhD; Gerald Merenstein, MD; Mary O'Shea, MD; Max Perlman, MD; Ronald Poland, MD; Alex Robertson, MD; Firmino Rubaltelli, MD; Steven Shapiro, MD; Stanford Singer, MD; Ann Stark, MD; Gautham Suresh, MD; Margot VandeBor, MD; Hank Vreman, PhD; Philip Walson, MD; Jon Watchko, MD; Richard Wennberg, MD; and Chap-Yung Yeung, MD.

REFERENCES

1. American Academy of Pediatrics, Provisional Committee for Quality Improvement and Subcommittee on Hyperbilirubinemia. Practice parameter: management of hyperbilirubinemia in the healthy term newborn. *Pediatrics.* 1994;94:558–562
2. Ip S, Glicken S, Kulig J, Obrien R, Sege R, Lau J. *Management of Neonatal Hyperbilirubinemia.* Rockville, MD: US Department of Health and Human Services, Agency for Healthcare Research and Quality; 2003. AHRQ Publication 03-E011
3. Ip S, Chung M, Kulig J. et al. An evidence-based review of important issues concerning neonatal hyperbilirubinemia. *Pediatrics.* 2004;113(6). Available at: www.pediatrics.org/cgi/content/full/113/6/e644
4. American Academy of Pediatrics, Steering Committee on Quality Improvement and Management. A taxonomy of recommendations. *Pediatrics.* 2004; In press
5. Johnson LH, Bhutani VK, Brown AK. System-based approach to management of neonatal jaundice and prevention of kernicterus. *J Pediatr.* 2002;140:396–403

6. Maisels MJ, Newman TB. Kernicterus in otherwise healthy, breast-fed term newborns. *Pediatrics.* 1995;96:730–733
7. MacDonald M. Hidden risks: early discharge and bilirubin toxicity due to glucose-6-phosphate dehydrogenase deficiency. *Pediatrics.* 1995;96: 734–738
8. Penn AA, Enzman DR, Hahn JS, Stevenson DK. Kernicterus in a full term infant. *Pediatrics.* 1994;93:1003–1006
9. Washington EC, Ector W, Abboud M, Ohning B, Holden K. Hemolytic jaundice due to G6PD deficiency causing kernicterus in a female newborn. *South Med J.* 1995;88:776–779
10. Ebbesen F. Recurrence of kernicterus in term and near-term infants in Denmark. *Acta Paediatr.* 2000;89:1213–1217
11. Institue of Medicine. *Crossing the Quality Chasm: A New Health System for the 21st Century.* Washington, DC: National Academy Press; 2001
12. American Academy of Pediatrics, American College of Obstetricians and Gynecologists. *Guidelines for Perinatal Care.* 5th ed. Elk Grove Village, IL: American Academy of Pediatrics; 2002:220–224
13. Bertini G, Dani C, Trochin M, Rubaltelli F. Is breastfeeding really favoring early neonatal jaundice? *Pediatrics.* 2001;107(3). Available at: www.pediatrics.org/cgi/content/full/107/3/e41
14. Maisels MJ, Gifford K. Normal serum bilirubin levels in the newborn and the effect of breast-feeding. *Pediatrics.* 1986;78:837–843
15. Yamauchi Y, Yamanouchi I. Breast-feeding frequency during the first 24 hours after birth in full-term neonates. *Pediatrics.* 1990;86:171–175
16. De Carvalho M, Klaus MH, Merkatz RB. Frequency of breastfeeding and serum bilirubin concentration. *Am J Dis Child.* 1982;136:737–738
17. Varimo P, Similä S, Wendt L, Kolvisto M. Frequency of breast feeding and hyperbilirubinemia [letter]. *Clin Pediatr (Phila).* 1986;25:112
18. De Carvalho M, Holl M, Harvey D. Effects of water supplementation on physiological jaundice in breast-fed babies. *Arch Dis Child.* 1981;56: 568–569
19. Nicoll A, Ginsburg R, Tripp JH. Supplementary feeding and jaundice in newborns. *Acta Paediatr Scand.* 1982;71:759–761
20. Madlon-Kay DJ. Identifying ABO incompatibility in newborns: selective vs automatic testing. *J Fam Pract.* 1992;35:278–280
21. Kramer LI. Advancement of dermal icterus in the jaundiced newborn. *Am J Dis Child.* 1969;118:454–458
22. Moyer VA, Ahn C, Sneed S. Accuracy of clinical judgment in neonatal jaundice. *Arch Pediatr Adolesc Med.* 2000;154:391–394
23. Davidson LT, Merritt KK, Weech AA. Hyperbilirubinemia in the newborn. *Am J Dis Child.* 1941;61:958–980
24. Tayaba R, Gribetz D, Gribetz I, Holzman IR. Noninvasive estimation of serum bilirubin. *Pediatrics.* 1998;102(3). Available at: www.pediatrics.org/cgi/content/full/102/3/e28
25. Bhutani V, Gourley GR, Adler S, Kreamer B, Dalman C, Johnson LH. Noninvasive measurement of total serum bilirubin in a multiracial predischarge newborn population to assess the risk of severe hyperbilirubinemia. *Pediatrics.* 2000;106(2). Available at: www.pediatrics.org/cgi/content/full/106/2/e17
26. Yasuda S, Itoh S, Isobe K, et al. New transcutaneous jaundice device with two optical paths. *J Perinat Med.* 2003;31:81–88
27. Maisels MJ, Ostrea EJ Jr, Touch S, et al. Evaluation of a new transcutaneous bilirubinometer. *Pediatrics.* 2004;113:1638–1645
28. Ebbesen F, Rasmussen LM, Wimberley PD. A new transcutaneous bilirubinometer, bilicheck, used in the neonatal intensive care unit and the maternity ward. *Acta Paediatr.* 2002;91:203–211
29. Rubaltelli FF, Gourley GR, Loskamp N, et al. Transcutaneous bilirubin measurement: a multicenter evaluation of a new device. *Pediatrics.* 2001;107:1264–1271
30. Newman TB, Liljestrand P, Escobar GJ. Jaundice noted in the first 24 hours after birth in a managed care organization. *Arch Pediatr Adolesc Med.* 2002;156:1244–1250
31. Bhutani VK, Johnson L, Sivieri EM. Predictive ability of a predischarge hour-specific serum bilirubin for subsequent significant hyperbilirubinemia in healthy term and near-term newborns. *Pediatrics.* 1999;103: 6–14
32. Garcia FJ, Nager AL. Jaundice as an early diagnostic sign of urinary tract infection in infancy. *Pediatrics.* 2002;109:846–851
33. Kaplan M, Hammerman C. Severe neonatal hyperbilirubinemia: a potential complication of glucose-6-phosphate dehydrogenase deficiency. *Clin Perinatol.* 1998;25:575–590
34. Valaes T. Severe neonatal jaundice associated with glucose-6-phosphate dehydrogenase deficiency: pathogenesis and global epidemiology. *Acta Paediatr Suppl.* 1994;394:58–76
35. Alpay F, Sarici S, Tosuncuk HD, Serdar MA, Inanç N, Gökçay E. The value of first-day bilirubin measurement in predicting the development of significant hyperbilirubinemia in healthy term newborns. *Pediatrics.* 2000;106(2). Available at: www.pediatrics.org/cgi/content/full/106/2/e16
36. Carbonell X, Botet F, Figueras J, Riu-Godo A. Prediction of hyperbilirubinaemia in the healthy term newborn. *Acta Paediatr.* 2001;90:166–170
37. Kaplan M, Hammerman C, Feldman R, Brisk R. Predischarge bilirubin screening in glucose-6-phosphate dehydrogenase-deficient neonates. *Pediatrics.* 2000;105:533–537
38. Stevenson DK, Fanaroff AA, Maisels MJ, et al. Prediction of hyperbilirubinemia in near-term and term infants. *Pediatrics.* 2001;108:31–39
39. Newman TB, Xiong B, Gonzales VM, Escobar GJ. Prediction and prevention of extreme neonatal hyperbilirubinemia in a mature health maintenance organization. *Arch Pediatr Adolesc Med.* 2000;154:1140–1147
40. Maisels MJ, Kring EA. Length of stay, jaundice, and hospital readmission. *Pediatrics.* 1998;101:995–998
41. Gale R, Seidman DS, Dollberg S, Stevenson DK. Epidemiology of neonatal jaundice in the Jerusalem population. *J Pediatr Gastroenterol Nutr.* 1990;10:82–86
42. Berk MA, Mimouni F, Miodovnik M, Hertzberg V, Valuck J. Macrosomia in infants of insulin-dependent diabetic mothers. *Pediatrics.* 1989; 83:1029–1034
43. Peevy KJ, Landaw SA, Gross SJ. Hyperbilirubinemia in infants of diabetic mothers. *Pediatrics.* 1980;66:417–419
44. Soskolne El, Schumacher R, Fyock C, Young ML, Schork A. The effect of early discharge and other factors on readmission rates of newborns. *Arch Pediatr Adolesc Med.* 1996;150:373–379
45. Ebbesen F, Brodersen R. Risk of bilirubin acid precipitation in preterm infants with respiratory distress syndrome: considerations of blood/brain bilirubin transfer equilibrium. *Early Hum Dev.* 1982;6:341–355
46. Cashore WJ, Oh W, Brodersen R. Reserve albumin and bilirubin toxicity index in infant serum. *Acta Paediatr Scand.* 1983;72:415–419
47. Cashore WJ. Free bilirubin concentrations and bilirubin-binding affinity in term and preterm infants. *J Pediatr.* 1980;96:521–527
48. Bratlid D. How bilirubin gets into the brain. *Clin Perinatol.* 1990;17: 449–465
49. Wennberg RP. Cellular basis of bilirubin toxicity. *N Y State J Med.* 1991;91:493–496
50. Eggert P, Stick C, Schroder H. On the distribution of irradiation intensity in phototherapy. Measurements of effective irradiance in an incubator. *Eur J Pediatr.* 1984;142:58–61
51. Maisels MJ. Why use homeopathic doses of phototherapy? *Pediatrics.* 1996;98:283–287
52. Ahlfors CE. Criteria for exchange transfusion in jaundiced newborns. *Pediatrics.* 1994;93:488–494
53. American Association of Blood Banks Technical Manual Committee. Perinatal issues in transfusion practice. In: Brecher M, ed. *Technical Manual.* Bethesda, MD: American Association of Blood Banks; 2002: 497–515
54. Garland JS, Alex C, Deacon JS, Raab K. Treatment of infants with indirect hyperbilirubinemia. Readmission to birth hospital vs nonbirth hospital. *Arch Pediatr Adolesc Med.* 1994;148:1317–1321
55. Gottstein R, Cooke R. Systematic review of intravenous immunoglobulin in haemolytic disease of the newborn. *Arch Dis Child Fetal Neonatal Ed.* 2003;88:F6–F10
56. Sato K, Hara T, Kondo T, Iwao H, Honda S, Ueda K. High-dose intravenous gammaglobulin therapy for neonatal immune haemolytic jaundice due to blood group incompatibility. *Acta Paediatr Scand.* 1991; 80:163–166
57. Rubo J, Albrecht K, Lasch P, et al. High-dose intravenous immune globulin therapy for hyperbilirubinemia caused by Rh hemolytic disease. *J Pediatr.* 1992;121:93–97
58. Hammerman C, Kaplan M, Vreman HJ, Stevenson DK. Intravenous immune globulin in neonatal ABO isoimmunization: factors associated with clinical efficacy. *Biol Neonate.* 1996;70:69–74
59. Johnson L, Boggs TR. Bilirubin-dependent brain damage: incidence and indications for treatment. In: Odell GB, Schaffer R, Simopoulos AP, eds. *Phototherapy in the Newborn: An Overview.* Washington, DC: National Academy of Sciences; 1974:122–149
60. Ozmert E, Erdem G, Topcu M. Long-term follow-up of indirect hyperbilirubinemia in full-term Turkish infants. *Acta Paediatr.* 1996;85: 1440–1444
61. Volpe JJ. *Neurology of the Newborn.* 4th ed. Philadelphia, PA: W. B. Saunders; 2001
62. Harris M, Bernbaum J, Polin J, Zimmerman R, Polin RA. Developmental follow-up of breastfed term and near-term infants with marked hyperbilirubinemia. *Pediatrics.* 2001;107:1075–1080
63. Osborn LM, Bolus R. Breast feeding and jaundice in the first week of life. *J Fam Pract.* 1985;20:475–480

64. Martinez JC, Maisels MJ, Otheguy L, et al. Hyperbilirubinemia in the breast-fed newborn: a controlled trial of four interventions. *Pediatrics.* 1993;91:470–473
65. Amato M, Howald H, von Muralt G. Interruption of breast-feeding versus phototherapy as treatment of hyperbilirubinemia in full-term infants. *Helv Paediatr Acta.* 1985;40:127–131
66. Maisels MJ, Gifford K, Antle CE, Leib GR. Jaundice in the healthy newborn infant: a new approach to an old problem. *Pediatrics.* 1988;81:505–511
67. Newman TB, Easterling MJ. Yield of reticulocyte counts and blood smears in term infants. *Clin Pediatr (Phila).* 1994;33:71–76
68. Herschel M, Karrison T, Wen M, Caldarelli L, Baron B. Evaluation of the direct antiglobulin (Coombs') test for identifying newborns at risk for hemolysis as determined by end-tidal carbon monoxide concentration (ETCOc); and comparison of the Coombs' test with ETCOc for detecting significant jaundice. *J Perinatol.* 2002;22:341–347
69. Stevenson DK, Vreman HJ. Carbon monoxide and bilirubin production in neonates. *Pediatrics.* 1997;100:252–254
70. Vreman HJ, Verter J, Oh W, et al. Interlaboratory variability of bilirubin measurements. *Clin Chem.* 1996;42:869–873
71. Lo S, Doumas BT, Ashwood E. Performance of bilirubin determinations in US laboratories—revisited. *Clin Chem.* 2004;50:190–194
72. Kappas A, Drummond GS, Henschke C, Valaes T. Direct comparison of Sn-mesoporphyrin, an inhibitor of bilirubin production, and phototherapy in controlling hyperbilirubinemia in term and near-term newborns. *Pediatrics.* 1995;95:468–474
73. Martinez JC, Garcia HO, Otheguy L, Drummond GS, Kappas A. Control of severe hyperbilirubinemia in full-term newborns with the inhibitor of bilirubin production Sn-mesoporphyrin. *Pediatrics.* 1999;103:1–5
74. Suresh G, Martin CL, Soll R. Metalloporphyrins for treatment of unconjugated hyperbilirubinemia in neonates. *Cochrane Database Syst Rev.* 2003;2:CD004207
75. Kappas A, Drummond GS, Munson DP, Marshall JR. Sn-mesoporphyrin interdiction of severe hyperbilirubinemia in Jehovah's Witness newborns as an alternative to exchange transfusion. *Pediatrics.* 2001;108:1374–1377

APPENDIX 1: Additional Notes

Definitions of Quality of Evidence and Balance of Benefits and Harms

The Steering Committee on Quality Improvement and Management categorizes evidence quality in 4 levels:

1. Well-designed, randomized, controlled trials or diagnostic studies on relevant populations
2. Randomized, controlled trials or diagnostic studies with minor limitations; overwhelming, consistent evidence from observational studies
3. Observational studies (case-control and cohort design)
4. Expert opinion, case reports, reasoning from first principles

The AAP defines evidence-based recommendations as follows:[1]

- Strong recommendation: the committee believes that the benefits of the recommended approach clearly exceed the harms of that approach and that the quality of the supporting evidence is either excellent or impossible to obtain. Clinicians should follow these recommendations unless a clear and compelling rationale for an alternative approach is present.
- Recommendation: the committee believes that the benefits exceed the harms, but the quality of evidence on which this recommendation is based is not as strong. Clinicians should also generally follow these recommendations but should be alert to new information and sensitive to patient preferences. In this guideline, the term "should" implies a recommendation by the committee.
- Option: either the quality of the evidence that exists is suspect or well-performed studies have shown little clear advantage to one approach over another. Patient preference should have a substantial role in influencing clinical decision-making when a policy is described as an option.
- No recommendation: there is a lack of pertinent evidence and the anticipated balance of benefits and harms is unclear.

Anticipated Balance Between Benefits and Harms

The presence of clear benefits or harms supports stronger statements for or against a course of action. In some cases, however, recommendations are made when analysis of the balance of benefits and harms provides an exceptional dysequilibrium and it would be unethical or impossible to perform clinical trials to "prove" the point. In these cases the balance of benefit and harm is termed "exceptional."

Clinical Manifestations of Acute Bilirubin Encephalopathy and Kernicterus

Acute Bilirubin Encephalopathy

In the early phase of acute bilirubin encephalopathy, severely jaundiced infants become lethargic and hypotonic and suck poorly.[2,3] The intermediate phase is characterized by moderate stupor, irritability, and hypertonia. The infant may develop a fever and high-pitched cry, which may alternate with drowsiness and hypotonia. The hypertonia is manifested by backward arching of the neck (retrocollis) and trunk (opisthotonos). There is anecdotal evidence that an emergent exchange transfusion at this stage, in some cases, might reverse the central nervous system changes.[4] The advanced phase, in which central nervous system damage is probably irreversible, is characterized by pronounced retrocollis-opisthotonos, shrill cry, no feeding, apnea, fever, deep stupor to coma, sometimes seizures, and death.[2,3,5]

Kernicterus

In the chronic form of bilirubin encephalopathy, surviving infants may develop a severe form of athetoid cerebral palsy, auditory dysfunction, dental-enamel dysplasia, paralysis of upward gaze, and, less often, intellectual and other handicaps. Most infants who develop kernicterus have manifested some or all of the signs listed above in the acute phase of bilirubin encephalopathy. However, occasionally there are infants who have developed very high bilirubin levels and, subsequently, the signs of kernicterus but have exhibited few, if any, antecedent clinical signs of acute bilirubin encephalopathy.[3,5,6]

Clinical Evaluation of Jaundice and TcB Measurements

Jaundice is usually seen in the face first and progresses caudally to the trunk and extremities,[7] but because visual estimation of bilirubin levels from the degree of jaundice can lead to errors,[8–10] a low threshold should be used for measuring the TSB.

Devices that provide a noninvasive TcB measurement have proven very useful as screening tools,[11] and newer instruments give measurements that provide a valid estimate of the TSB level.[12–17] Studies using the new TcB-measurement instruments are limited, but the data published thus far suggest that in most newborn populations, these instruments generally provide measurements within 2 to 3 mg/dL (34–51 μmol/L) of the TSB and can replace a measurement of serum bilirubin in many circumstances, particularly for TSB levels less than 15 mg/dL (257 μmol/L).[12–17] Because phototherapy "bleaches" the skin, both visual assessment of jaundice and TcB measurements in infants undergoing phototherapy are not reliable. In addition, the ability of transcutaneous instruments to provide accurate measurements in different racial groups requires additional study.[18,19] The limitations of the accuracy and reproducibility of TSB measurements in the clinical laboratory[20–22] must also be recognized and are discussed in the technical report.[23]

Capillary Versus Venous Serum Bilirubin Measurement

Almost all published data regarding the relationship of TSB levels to kernicterus or developmental outcome are based on capillary blood TSB levels. Data regarding the differences between capillary and venous TSB levels are conflicting.[24,25] In 1 study the capillary TSB levels were higher, but in another they were lower than venous TSB levels.[24,25] Thus, obtaining a venous sample to "confirm" an elevated capillary TSB level is not recommended, because it will delay the initiation of treatment.

Direct-Reacting and Conjugated Bilirubin

Although commonly used interchangeably, direct-reacting bilirubin is not the same as conjugated bilirubin. Direct-reacting bilirubin is the bilirubin that reacts directly (without the addition of an accelerating agent) with diazotized sulfanilic acid. Conjugated bilirubin is bilirubin made water soluble by binding with glucuronic acid in the liver. Depending on the technique used, the clinical laboratory will report total and direct-reacting or unconjugated and conjugated bilirubin levels. In this guideline and for clinical purposes, the terms may be used interchangeably.

Abnormal Direct and Conjugated Bilirubin Levels

Laboratory measurement of direct bilirubin is not precise,[26] and values between laboratories can vary widely. If the TSB is at or below 5 mg/dL (85 μmol/L), a direct or conjugated bilirubin of more than 1.0 mg/dL (17.1 μmol/L) is generally considered abnormal. For TSB values higher than 5 mg/dL (85 μmol/L), a direct bilirubin of more than 20% of the TSB is considered abnormal. If the hospital laboratory measures conjugated bilirubin using the Vitros (formerly Ektachem) system (Ortho-Clinical Diagnostics, Raritan, NJ), any value higher than 1 mg/dL is considered abnormal.

Assessment of Adequacy of Intake in Breastfeeding Infants

The data from a number of studies[27–34] indicate that unsupplemented, breastfed infants experience their maximum weight loss by day 3 and, on average, lose 6.1% ± 2.5% (SD) of their birth weight. Thus, ~5% to 10% of fully breastfed infants lose 10% or more of their birth weight by day 3, suggesting that adequacy of intake should be evaluated and the infant monitored if weight loss is more than 10%.[35] Evidence of adequate intake in breastfed infants also includes 4 to 6 thoroughly wet diapers in 24 hours and the passage of 3 to 4 stools per day by the fourth day. By the third to fourth day, the stools in adequately breastfed infants should have changed from meconium to a mustard yellow, mushy stool.[36] The above assessment will also help to identify breastfed infants who are at risk for dehydration because of inadequate intake.

Nomogram for Designation of Risk

Note that this nomogram (Fig 2) does not describe the natural history of neonatal hyperbilirubinemia, particularly after 48 to 72 hours, for which, because of sampling bias, the lower zones are spuriously elevated.[37] This bias, however, will have much less effect on the high-risk zone (95th percentile in the study).[38]

G6PD Dehydrogenase Deficiency

It is important to look for G6PD deficiency in infants with significant hyperbilirubinemia, because some may develop a sudden increase in the TSB. In addition, G6PD-deficient infants require intervention at lower TSB levels (Figs 3 and 4). It should be noted also that in the presence of hemolysis, G6PD levels can be elevated, which may obscure the diagnosis in the newborn period so that a normal level in a hemolyzing neonate does not rule out G6PD deficiency.[39] If G6PD deficiency is strongly suspected, a repeat level should be measured when the infant is 3 months old. It is also recognized that immediate laboratory determination of G6PD is generally not available in most US hospitals, and thus translating the above information into clinical practice is cur-

TABLE 4. Risk Zone as a Predictor of Hyperbilirubinemia[39]

TSB Before Discharge	Newborns (Total = 2840), *n* (%)	Newborns Who Subsequently Developed a TSB Level >95th Percentile, *n* (%)
High-risk zone (>95th percentile)	172 (6.0)	68 (39.5)
High intermediate-risk zone	356 (12.5)	46 (12.9)
Low intermediate-risk zone	556 (19.6)	12 (2.26)
Low-risk zone	1756 (61.8)	0

rently difficult. Nevertheless, practitioners are reminded to consider the diagnosis of G6PD deficiency in infants with severe hyperbilirubinemia, particularly if they belong to the population groups in which this condition is prevalent. This is important in the African American population, because these infants, as a group, have much lower TSB levels than white or Asian infants.[40,41] Thus, severe hyperbilirubinemia in an African American infant should always raise the possibility of G6PD deficiency.

Basis for the Recommendations 7.1.1 Through 7.1.6 and Provided in Figs 3 and 4

Ideally, recommendations for when to implement phototherapy and exchange transfusions should be based on estimates of when the benefits of these interventions exceed their risks and cost. The evidence for these estimates should come from randomized trials or systematic observational studies. Unfortunately, there is little such evidence on which to base these recommendations. As a result, treatment guidelines must necessarily rely on more uncertain estimates and extrapolations. For a detailed discussion of this question, please see "An Evidence-Based Review of Important Issues Concerning Neonatal Hyperbilirubinemia."[23]

The recommendations for phototherapy and exchange transfusion are based on the following principles:

- The main demonstrated value of phototherapy is that it reduces the risk that TSB levels will reach a level at which exchange transfusion is recommended.[42–44] Approximately 5 to 10 infants with TSB levels between 15 and 20 mg/dL (257–342 μmol/L) will receive phototherapy to prevent the TSB in 1 infant from reaching 20 mg/dL (the number needed to treat).[12] Thus, 8 to 9 of every 10 infants with these TSB levels will not reach 20 mg/dL (342 μmol/L) even if they are not treated. Phototherapy has proven to be a generally safe procedure, although rare complications can occur (see Appendix 2).
- Recommended TSB levels for exchange transfusion (Fig 4) are based largely on the goal of keeping TSB levels below those at which kernicterus has been reported.[12,45–48] In almost all cases, exchange transfusion is recommended only after phototherapy has failed to keep the TSB level below the exchange transfusion level (Fig 4).
- The recommendations to use phototherapy and exchange transfusion at lower TSB levels for infants of lower gestation and those who are sick are based on limited observations suggesting that sick infants (particularly those with the risk factors listed in Figs 3 and 4)[49–51] and those of lower gestation[51–54] are at greater risk for developing kernicterus at lower bilirubin levels than are well infants of more than 38 6/7 weeks' gestation. Nevertheless, other studies have not confirmed all of these associations.[52,55,56] There is no doubt, however, that infants at 35 to 37 6/7 weeks' gestation are at a much greater risk of developing very high TSB levels.[57,58] Intervention for these infants is based on this risk as well as extrapolations from more premature, lower birth-weight infants who do have a higher risk of bilirubin toxicity.[52,53]
- For all newborns, treatment is recommended at lower TSB levels at younger ages because one of the primary goals of treatment is to prevent additional increases in the TSB level.

Subtle Neurologic Abnormalities Associated With Hyperbilirubinemia

There are several studies demonstrating measurable transient changes in brainstem-evoked potentials, behavioral patterns, and the infant's cry[59–63] associated with TSB levels of 15 to 25 mg/dL (257–428 μmol/L). In these studies, the abnormalities identified were transient and disappeared when the serum bilirubin levels returned to normal with or without treatment.[59,60,62,63]

A few cohort studies have found an association between hyperbilirubinemia and long-term adverse neurodevelopmental effects that are more subtle than kernicterus.[64–67] Current studies, however, suggest that although phototherapy lowers the TSB levels, it has no effect on these long-term neurodevelopmental outcomes.[68–70]

Risks of Exchange Transfusion

Because exchange transfusions are now rarely performed, the risks of morbidity and mortality associated with the procedure are difficult to quantify. In addition, the complication rates listed below may not be generalizable to the current era if, like most procedures, frequency of performance is an important determinant of risk. Death associated with exchange transfusion has been reported in approximately 3 in 1000 procedures,[71,72] although in otherwise well infants of 35 or more weeks' gestation, the risk is probably much lower.[71–73] Significant morbidity (apnea, bradycardia, cyanosis, vasospasm, thrombosis, necrotizing enterocolitis) occurs in as many as 5% of exchange transfusions,[71] and the risks associated with the use of blood products must always be considered.[74] Hypoxic-ischemic encephalopathy and acquired immunodeficiency syndrome have occurred in otherwise healthy infants receiving exchange transfusions.[73,75]

Serum Albumin Levels and the B/A Ratio

The legends to Figs 3 and 4 and recommendations 7.1.5 and 7.1.6 contain references to the serum albumin level and the B/A ratio as factors that can be considered in the decision to initiate phototherapy (Fig 3) or perform an exchange transfusion (Fig 4). Bilirubin is transported in the plasma tightly bound to albumin, and the portion that is unbound or loosely bound can more readily leave the intravascular space and cross the intact blood-brain barrier.[76] Elevations of unbound bilirubin (UB) have been associated with kernicterus in sick preterm newborns.[77,78] In addition, elevated UB concentrations are more closely associated than TSB levels with transient abnormalities in the audiometric brainstem response in term[79] and preterm[80] infants. Long-term studies relating B/A binding in infants to developmental outcome are limited and conflicting.[69,81,82] In addition, clinical laboratory measurement of UB is not currently available in the United States.

The ratio of bilirubin (mg/dL) to albumin (g/dL) does correlate with measured UB in newborns[83] and can be used as an approximate surrogate for the measurement of UB. It must be recognized, however, that both albumin levels and the ability of albumin to bind bilirubin vary significantly between newborns.[83,84] Albumin binding of bilirubin is impaired in sick infants,[84–86] and some studies show an increase in binding with increasing gestational[86,87] and postnatal[87,88] age, but others have not found a significant effect of gestational age on binding.[89] Furthermore, the risk of bilirubin encephalopathy is unlikely to be a simple function of the TSB level or the concentration of UB but is more likely a combination of both (ie, the total amount of bilirubin available [the miscible pool of bilirubin] as well as the tendency of bilirubin to enter the tissues [the UB concentration]).[83] An additional factor is the possible susceptibility of the cells of the central nervous system to damage by bilirubin.[90] It is therefore a clinical option to use the B/A ratio together with, but not in lieu of, the TSB level as an additional factor in determining the need for exchange transfusion[83] (Fig 4).

REFERENCES

1. American Academy of Pediatrics, Steering Committee on Quality Improvement and Management. Classification of recommendations for clinical practice guidelines. *Pediatrics.* 2004; In press
2. Johnson LH, Bhutani VK, Brown AK. System-based approach to management of neonatal jaundice and prevention of kernicterus. *J Pediatr.* 2002;140:396–403
3. Volpe JJ. *Neurology of the Newborn.* 4th ed. Philadelphia, PA: W. B. Saunders; 2001
4. Harris M, Bernbaum J, Polin J, Zimmerman R, Polin RA. Developmental follow-up of breastfed term and near-term infants with marked hyperbilirubinemia. *Pediatrics.* 2001;107:1075–1080
5. Van Praagh R. Diagnosis of kernicterus in the neonatal period. *Pediatrics.* 1961;28:870–876
6. Jones MH, Sands R, Hyman CB, Sturgeon P, Koch FP. Longitudinal study of incidence of central nervous system damage following erythroblastosis fetalis. *Pediatrics.* 1954;14:346–350
7. Kramer LI. Advancement of dermal icterus in the jaundiced newborn. *Am J Dis Child.* 1969;118:454–458
8. Moyer VA, Ahn C, Sneed S. Accuracy of clinical judgment in neonatal jaundice. *Arch Pediatr Adolesc Med.* 2000;154:391–394
9. Davidson LT, Merritt KK, Weech AA. Hyperbilirubinemia in the newborn. *Am J Dis Child.* 1941;61:958–980
10. Tayaba R, Gribetz D, Gribetz I, Holzman IR. Noninvasive estimation of serum bilirubin. *Pediatrics.* 1998;102(3). Available at: www.pediatrics.org/cgi/content/full/102/3/e28
11. Maisels MJ, Kring E. Transcutaneous bilirubinometry decreases the need for serum bilirubin measurements and saves money. *Pediatrics.* 1997;99:599–601
12. Ip S, Glicken S, Kulig J, Obrien R, Sege R, Lau J. *Management of Neonatal Hyperbilirubinemia.* Rockville, MD: US Department of Health and Human Services, Agency for Healthcare Research and Quality; 2003. AHRQ Publication 03-E011
13. Bhutani V, Gourley GR, Adler S, Kreamer B, Dalman C, Johnson LH. Noninvasive measurement of total serum bilirubin in a multiracial predischarge newborn population to assess the risk of severe hyperbilirubinemia. *Pediatrics.* 2000;106(2). Available at: www.pediatrics.org/cgi/content/full/106/2/e17
14. Yasuda S, Itoh S, Isobe K, et al. New transcutaneous jaundice device with two optical paths. *J Perinat Med.* 2003;31:81–88
15. Maisels MJ, Ostrea EJ Jr, Touch S, et al. Evaluation of a new transcutaneous bilirubinometer. *Pediatrics.* 2004;113:1638–1645
16. Ebbesen F, Rasmussen LM, Wimberley PD. A new transcutaneous bilirubinometer, bilicheck, used in the neonatal intensive care unit and the maternity ward. *Acta Paediatr.* 2002;91:203–211
17. Rubaltelli FF, Gourley GR, Loskamp N, et al. Transcutaneous bilirubin measurement: a multicenter evaluation of a new device. *Pediatrics.* 2001;107:1264–1271
18. Engle WD, Jackson GL, Sendelbach D, Manning D, Frawley W. Assessment of a transcutaneous device in the evaluation of neonatal hyperbilirubinemia in a primarily Hispanic population. *Pediatrics.* 2002;110: 61–67
19. Schumacher R. Transcutaneous bilirubinometry and diagnostic tests: "the right job for the tool." *Pediatrics.* 2002;110:407–408
20. Vreman HJ, Verter J, Oh W, et al. Interlaboratory variability of bilirubin measurements. *Clin Chem.* 1996;42:869–873
21. Doumas BT, Eckfeldt JH. Errors in measurement of total bilirubin: a perennial problem. *Clin Chem.* 1996;42:845–848
22. Lo S, Doumas BT, Ashwood E. Performance of bilirubin determinations in US laboratories—revisited. *Clin Chem.* 2004;50:190–194
23. Ip S, Chung M, Kulig J. et al. An evidence-based review of important issues concerning neonatal hyperbilirubinemia. *Pediatrics.* 2004;113(6). Available at: www.pediatrics.org/cgi/content/full/113/6/e644
24. Leslie GI, Philips JB, Cassady G. Capillary and venous bilirubin values: are they really different? *Am J Dis Child.* 1987;141:1199–1200
25. Eidelman AI, Schimmel MS, Algur N, Eylath U. Capillary and venous bilirubin values: they are different—and how [letter]! *Am J Dis Child.* 1989;143:642
26. Watkinson LR, St John A, Penberthy LA. Investigation into paediatric bilirubin analyses in Australia and New Zealand. *J Clin Pathol.* 1982;35: 52–58
27. Bertini G, Dani C, Trochin M, Rubaltelli F. Is breastfeeding really favoring early neonatal jaundice? *Pediatrics.* 2001;107(3). Available at: www.pediatrics.org/cgi/content/full/107/3/e41
28. De Carvalho M, Klaus MH, Merkatz RB. Frequency of breastfeeding and serum bilirubin concentration. *Am J Dis Child.* 1982;136:737–738
29. De Carvalho M, Holl M, Harvey D. Effects of water supplementation on physiological jaundice in breast-fed babies. *Arch Dis Child.* 1981;56: 568–569
30. Nicoll A, Ginsburg R, Tripp JH. Supplementary feeding and jaundice in newborns. *Acta Paediatr Scand.* 1982;71:759–761
31. Butler DA, MacMillan JP. Relationship of breast feeding and weight loss to jaundice in the newborn period: review of the literature and results of a study. *Cleve Clin Q.* 1983;50:263–268
32. De Carvalho M, Robertson S, Klaus M. Fecal bilirubin excretion and serum bilirubin concentration in breast-fed and bottle-fed infants. *J Pediatr.* 1985;107:786–790
33. Gourley GR, Kreamer B, Arend R. The effect of diet on feces and jaundice during the first three weeks of life. *Gastroenterology.* 1992;103: 660–667
34. Maisels MJ, Gifford K. Breast-feeding, weight loss, and jaundice. *J Pediatr.* 1983;102:117–118
35. Laing IA, Wong CM. Hypernatraemia in the first few days: is the incidence rising? *Arch Dis Child Fetal Neonatal Ed.* 2002;87:F158–F162
36. Lawrence RA. Management of the mother-infant nursing couple. In: *A Breastfeeding Guide for the Medical Profession.* 4th ed. St Louis, MO: Mosby-Year Book, Inc; 1994:215-277
37. Maisels MJ, Newman TB. Predicting hyperbilirubinemia in newborns: the importance of timing. *Pediatrics.* 1999;103:493–495
38. Bhutani VK, Johnson L, Sivieri EM. Predictive ability of a predischarge hour-specific serum bilirubin for subsequent significant hyperbilirubinemia in healthy term and near-term newborns. *Pediatrics.* 1999;103: 6–14
39. Beutler E. Glucose-6-phosphate dehydrogenase deficiency. *Blood.* 1994; 84:3613–3636
40. Linn S, Schoenbaum SC, Monson RR, Rosner B, Stubblefield PG, Ryan KJ. Epidemiology of neonatal hyperbilirubinemia. *Pediatrics.* 1985;75: 770–774
41. Newman TB, Easterling MJ, Goldman ES, Stevenson DK. Laboratory evaluation of jaundiced newborns: frequency, cost and yield. *Am J Dis Child.* 1990;144:364–368
42. Martinez JC, Maisels MJ, Otheguy L, et al. Hyperbilirubinemia in the breast-fed newborn: a controlled trial of four interventions. *Pediatrics.* 1993;91:470–473
43. Maisels MJ. Phototherapy—traditional and nontraditional. *J Perinatol.* 2001;21(suppl 1):S93–S97
44. Brown AK, Kim MH, Wu PY, Bryla DA. Efficacy of phototherapy in prevention and management of neonatal hyperbilirubinemia. *Pediatrics.* 1985;75:393–400

45. Armitage P, Mollison PL. Further analysis of controlled trials of treatment of hemolytic disease of the newborn. *J Obstet Gynaecol Br Emp.* 1953;60:602–605
46. Mollison PL, Walker W. Controlled trials of the treatment of haemolytic disease of the newborn. *Lancet.* 1952;1:429–433
47. Hsia DYY, Allen FH, Gellis SS, Diamond LK. Erythroblastosis fetalis. VIII. Studies of serum bilirubin in relation to kernicterus. *N Engl J Med.* 1952;247:668–671
48. Newman TB, Maisels MJ. Does hyperbilirubinemia damage the brain of healthy full-term infants? *Clin Perinatol.* 1990;17:331–358
49. Ozmert E, Erdem G, Topcu M. Long-term follow-up of indirect hyperbilirubinemia in full-term Turkish infants. *Acta Paediatr.* 1996;85: 1440–1444
50. Perlman JM, Rogers B, Burns D. Kernicterus findings at autopsy in 2 sick near-term infants. *Pediatrics.* 1997;99:612–615
51. Gartner LM, Snyder RN, Chabon RS, Bernstein J. Kernicterus: high incidence in premature infants with low serum bilirubin concentration. *Pediatrics.* 1970;45:906–917
52. Watchko JF, Oski FA. Kernicterus in preterm newborns: past, present, and future. *Pediatrics.* 1992;90:707–715
53. Watchko J, Claassen D. Kernicterus in premature infants: current prevalence and relationship to NICHD Phototherapy Study exchange criteria. *Pediatrics.* 1994;93(6 Pt 1):996–999
54. Stern L, Denton RL. Kernicterus in small, premature infants. *Pediatrics.* 1965;35:486–485
55. Turkel SB, Guttenberg ME, Moynes DR, Hodgman JE. Lack of identifiable risk factors for kernicterus. *Pediatrics.* 1980;66:502–506
56. Kim MH, Yoon JJ, Sher J, Brown AK. Lack of predictive indices in kernicterus. A comparison of clinical and pathologic factors in infants with or without kernicterus. *Pediatrics.* 1980;66:852–858
57. Newman TB, Xiong B, Gonzales VM, Escobar GJ. Prediction and prevention of extreme neonatal hyperbilirubinemia in a mature health maintenance organization. *Arch Pediatr Adolesc Med.* 2000;154:1140–1147
58. Newman TB, Escobar GJ, Gonzales VM, Armstrong MA, Gardner MN, Folck BF. Frequency of neonatal bilirubin testing and hyperbilirubinemia in a large health maintenance organization. *Pediatrics.* 1999;104: 1198–1203
59. Vohr BR. New approaches to assessing the risks of hyperbilirubinemia. *Clin Perinatol.* 1990;17:293–306
60. Perlman M, Fainmesser P, Sohmer H, Tamari H, Wax Y, Pevsmer B. Auditory nerve-brainstem evoked responses in hyperbilirubinemic neonates. *Pediatrics.* 1983;72:658–664
61. Nakamura H, Takada S, Shimabuku R, Matsuo M, Matsuo T, Negishi H. Auditory and brainstem responses in newborn infants with hyperbilirubinemia. *Pediatrics.* 1985;75:703–708
62. Nwaesei CG, Van Aerde J, Boyden M, Perlman M. Changes in auditory brainstem responses in hyperbilirubinemic infants before and after exchange transfusion. *Pediatrics.* 1984;74:800–803
63. Wennberg RP, Ahlfors CE, Bickers R, McMurtry CA, Shetter JL. Abnormal auditory brainstem response in a newborn infant with hyperbilirubinemia: improvement with exchange transfusion. *J Pediatr.* 1982;100:624–626
64. Soorani-Lunsing I, Woltil H, Hadders-Algra M. Are moderate degrees of hyperbilirubinemia in healthy term neonates really safe for the brain? *Pediatr Res.* 2001;50:701–705
65. Grimmer I, Berger-Jones K, Buhrer C, Brandl U, Obladen M. Late neurological sequelae of non-hemolytic hyperbilirubinemia of healthy term neonates. *Acta Paediatr.* 1999;88:661–663
66. Seidman DS, Paz I, Stevenson DK, Laor A, Danon YL, Gale R. Neonatal hyperbilirubinemia and physical and cognitive performance at 17 years of age. *Pediatrics.* 1991;88:828–833
67. Newman TB, Klebanoff MA. Neonatal hyperbilirubinemia and long-term outcome: another look at the collaborative perinatal project. *Pediatrics.* 1993;92:651–657
68. Scheidt PC, Bryla DA, Nelson KB, Hirtz DG, Hoffman HJ. Phototherapy for neonatal hyperbilirubinemia: six-year follow-up of the National Institute of Child Health and Human Development clinical trial. *Pediatrics.* 1990;85:455–463
69. Scheidt PC, Graubard BI, Nelson KB, et al. Intelligence at six years in relation to neonatal bilirubin levels: follow-up of the National Institute of Child Health and Human Development Clinical Trial of Phototherapy. *Pediatrics.* 1991;87:797–805
70. Seidman DS, Paz I, Stevenson DK, Laor A, Danon YL, Gale R. Effect of phototherapy for neonatal jaundice on cognitive performance. *J Perinatol.* 1994;14:23–28
71. Keenan WJ, Novak KK, Sutherland JM, Bryla DA, Fetterly KL. Morbidity and mortality associated with exchange transfusion. *Pediatrics.* 1985; 75:417–421
72. Hovi L, Siimes MA. Exchange transfusion with fresh heparinized blood is a safe procedure: Experiences from 1069 newborns. *Acta Paediatr Scand.* 1985;74:360–365
73. Jackson JC. Adverse events associated with exchange transfusion in healthy and ill newborns. *Pediatrics.* 1997;99(5):e7. Available at: www.pediatrics.org/cgi/content/full/99/5/e7
74. Schreiber GB, Busch MP, Kleinman SH, Korelitz JJ. The risk of transfusion-transmitted viral infections. *N Engl J Med.* 1996;334:1685–1690
75. Maisels MJ, Newman TB. Kernicterus in otherwise healthy, breast-fed term newborns. *Pediatrics.* 1995;96:730–733
76. Bratlid D. How bilirubin gets into the brain. *Clin Perinatol.* 1990;17: 449–465
77. Cashore WJ, Oh W. Unbound bilirubin and kernicterus in low-birth-weight infants. *Pediatrics.* 1982;69:481–485
78. Nakamura H, Yonetani M, Uetani Y, Funato M, Lee Y. Determination of serum unbound bilirubin for prediction of kernicterus in low birth-weight infants. *Acta Paediatr Jpn.* 1992;34:642–647
79. Funato M, Tamai H, Shimada S, Nakamura H. Vigintiphobia, unbound bilirubin, and auditory brainstem responses. *Pediatrics.* 1994;93:50–53
80. Amin SB, Ahlfors CE, Orlando MS, Dalzell LE, Merle KS, Guillet R. Bilirubin and serial auditory brainstem responses in premature infants. *Pediatrics.* 2001;107:664–670
81. Johnson L, Boggs TR. Bilirubin-dependent brain damage: incidence and indications for treatment. In: Odell GB, Schaffer R, Simopoulos AP, eds. *Phototherapy in the Newborn: An Overview.* Washington, DC: National Academy of Sciences; 1974:122–149
82. Odell GB, Storey GNB, Rosenberg LA. Studies in kernicterus. 3. The saturation of serum proteins with bilirubin during neonatal life and its relationship to brain damage at five years. *J Pediatr.* 1970;76:12–21
83. Ahlfors CE. Criteria for exchange transfusion in jaundiced newborns. *Pediatrics.* 1994;93:488–494
84. Cashore WJ. Free bilirubin concentrations and bilirubin-binding affinity in term and preterm infants. *J Pediatr.* 1980;96:521–527
85. Ebbesen F, Brodersen R. Risk of bilirubin acid precipitation in preterm infants with respiratory distress syndrome: considerations of blood/ brain bilirubin transfer equilibrium. *Early Hum Dev.* 1982;6:341–355
86. Cashore WJ, Oh W, Brodersen R. Reserve albumin and bilirubin toxicity index in infant serum. *Acta Paediatr Scand.* 1983;72:415–419
87. Ebbesen F, Nyboe J. Postnatal changes in the ability of plasma albumin to bind bilirubin. *Acta Paediatr Scand.* 1983;72:665–670
88. Esbjorner E. Albumin binding properties in relation to bilirubin and albumin concentrations during the first week of life. *Acta Paediatr Scand.* 1991;80:400–405
89. Robertson A, Sharp C, Karp W. The relationship of gestational age to reserve albumin concentration for binding of bilirubin. *J Perinatol.* 1988; 8:17–18
90. Wennberg RP. Cellular basis of bilirubin toxicity. *N Y State J Med.* 1991;91:493–496

APPENDIX 2: Phototherapy

There is no standardized method for delivering phototherapy. Phototherapy units vary widely, as do the types of lamps used in the units. The efficacy of phototherapy depends on the dose of phototherapy administered as well as a number of clinical factors (Table 5).[1]

Measuring the Dose of Phototherapy

Table 5 shows the radiometric quantities used in measuring the phototherapy dose. The quantity most commonly reported in the literature is the spectral irradiance. In the nursery, spectral irradiance can be measured by using commercially available radiometers. These instruments take a single measurement across a band of wavelengths, typically 425 to 475 or 400 to 480 nm. Unfortunately, there is no standardized method for reporting phototherapy dosages in the clinical literature, so it is difficult to compare published studies on the efficacy of phototherapy and manufacturers' data for the irradiance produced by different systems.[2] Measurements of irradiance from the same system, using different radiometers,

TABLE 5. Factors That Affect the Dose and Efficacy of Phototherapy

Factor	Mechanism/Clinical Relevance	Implementation and Rationale	Clinical Application
Spectrum of light emitted	Blue-green spectrum is most effective. At these wavelengths, light penetrates skin well and is absorbed maximally by bilirubin.	Special blue fluorescent tubes or other light sources that have most output in the blue-green spectrum and are most effective in lowering TSB.	Use special blue tubes or LED light source with output in blue-green spectrum for intensive PT.
Spectral irradiance (irradiance in certain wavelength band) delivered to surface of infant	↑ irradiance → ↑ rate of decline in TSB	Irradiance is measured with a radiometer as μW/cm² per nm. Standard PT units deliver 8–10 μW/cm² per nm (Fig 6). Intensive PT requires >30 μW/cm² per nm.	If special blue fluorescent tubes are used, bring tubes as close to infant as possible to increase irradiance (Fig 6). Note: This cannot be done with halogen lamps because of the danger of burn. Special blue tubes 10–15 cm above the infant will produce an irradiance of at least 35 μW/cm² per nm.
Spectral power (average spectral irradiance across surface area)	↑ surface area exposed → ↑ rate of decline in TSB	For intensive PT, expose maximum surface area of infant to PT.	Place lights above and fiber-optic pad or special blue fluorescent tubes* below the infant. For maximum exposure, line sides of bassinet, warmer bed, or incubator with aluminum foil.
Cause of jaundice	PT is likely to be less effective if jaundice is due to hemolysis or if cholestasis is present. (↑ direct bilirubin)		When hemolysis is present, start PT at lower TSB levels. Use intensive PT. Failure of PT suggests that hemolysis is the cause of jaundice. If ↑ direct bilirubin, watch for bronze baby syndrome or blistering.
TSB level at start of PT	The higher the TSB, the more rapid the decline in TSB with PT.		Use intensive PT for higher TSB levels. Anticipate a more rapid decrease in TSB when TSB >20 mg/dL (342 μmol/L).

PT indicates phototherapy; LED, light-emitting diode.
* Available in the Olympic BiliBassinet (Olympic Medical, Seattle, WA).

can also produce significantly different results. The width of the phototherapy lamp's emissions spectrum (narrow versus broad) will affect the measured irradiance. Measurements under lights with a very focused emission spectrum (eg, blue light-emitting diode) will vary significantly from one radiometer to another, because the response spectra of the radiometers vary from manufacturer to manufacturer. Broader-spectrum lights (fluorescent and halogen) have fewer variations among radiometers. Manufacturers of phototherapy systems generally recommend the specific radiometer to be used in measuring the dose of phototherapy when their system is used.

It is important also to recognize that the measured irradiance will vary widely depending on where the measurement is taken. Irradiance measured below the center of the light source can be more than double that measured at the periphery, and this dropoff at the periphery will vary with different phototherapy units. Ideally, irradiance should be measured at multiple sites under the area illuminated by the unit and the measurements averaged. The International Electrotechnical Commission[3] defines the "effective surface area" as the intended treatment surface that is illuminated by the phototherapy light. The commission uses 60 × 30 cm as the standard-sized surface.

Is It Necessary to Measure Phototherapy Doses Routinely?

Although it is not necessary to measure spectral irradiance before each use of phototherapy, it is important to perform periodic checks of phototherapy units to make sure that an adequate irradiance is being delivered.

The Dose-Response Relationship of Phototherapy

Figure 5 shows that there is a direct relationship between the irradiance used and the rate at which the serum bilirubin declines under phototherapy.[4] The data in Fig 5 suggest that there is a saturation point beyond which an increase in the irradiance produces no added efficacy. We do not know, however, that a saturation point exists. Because the conversion of bilirubin to excretable photoproducts is partly irreversible and follows first-order kinetics, there may not be a saturation point, so we do not know the maximum effective dose of phototherapy.

Effect on Irradiance of the Light Spectrum and the Distance Between the Infant and the Light Source

Figure 6 shows that as the distance between the light source and the infant decreases, there is a corresponding increase in the spectral irradiance.[5] Fig 6 also demonstrates the dramatic difference in irradi-

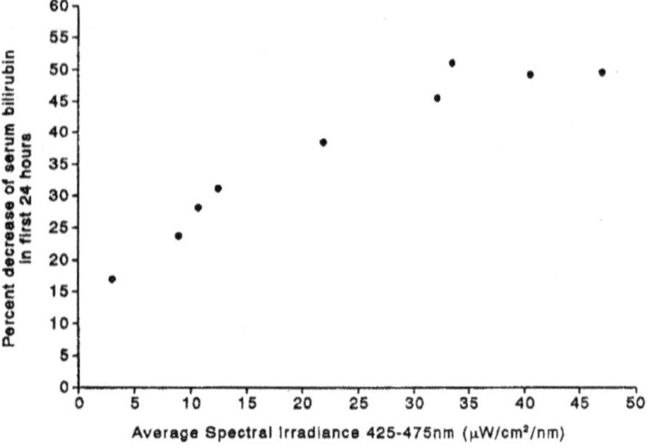

Fig 5. Relationship between average spectral irradiance and decrease in serum bilirubin concentration. Term infants with nonhemolytic hyperbilirubinemia were exposed to special blue lights (Phillips TL 52/20W) of different intensities. Spectral irradiance was measured as the average of readings at the head, trunk, and knees. Drawn from the data of Tan.[4] Source: *Pediatrics*. 1996;98: 283-287.

ance produced within the important 425- to 475-nm band by different types of fluorescent tubes.

What is Intensive Phototherapy?

Intensive phototherapy implies the use of high levels of irradiance in the 430- to 490-nm band (usually 30 μW/cm^2 per nm or higher) delivered to as much of the infant's surface area as possible. How this can be achieved is described below.

Using Phototherapy Effectively

Light Source

The spectrum of light delivered by a phototherapy unit is determined by the type of light source and any filters used. Commonly used phototherapy units contain daylight, cool white, blue, or "special blue" fluorescent tubes. Other units use tungsten-halogen lamps in different configurations, either free-standing or as part of a radiant warming device. Recently, a system using high-intensity gallium nitride light-emitting diodes has been introduced.[6] Fiber-optic systems deliver light from a high-intensity lamp to a fiber-optic blanket. Most of these devices deliver enough output in the blue-green region of the visible spectrum to be effective for standard phototherapy use. However, when bilirubin levels approach the range at which intensive phototherapy is recommended, maximal efficiency must be sought. The most effective light sources currently commercially available for phototherapy are those that use special blue fluorescent tubes[7] or a specially designed light-emitting diode light (Natus Inc, San Carlos, CA).[6] The special blue fluorescent tubes are labeled F20T12/BB (General Electric, Westinghouse, Sylvania) or TL52/20W (Phillips, Eindhoven, The Netherlands). It is important to note that special blue tubes provide much greater irradiance than regular blue tubes (labeled F20T12/B) (Fig 6). Special blue tubes are most effective because they provide light predominantly in the blue-green spectrum. At these wavelengths, light penetrates skin well and is absorbed maximally by bilirubin.[7]

There is a common misconception that ultraviolet light is used for phototherapy. The light systems used do not emit significant ultraviolet radiation, and the small amount of ultraviolet light that is emitted by fluorescent tubes and halogen bulbs is in longer wavelengths than those that cause erythema. In addition, almost all ultraviolet light is absorbed by the glass wall of the fluorescent tube and the Plexiglas cover of the phototherapy unit.

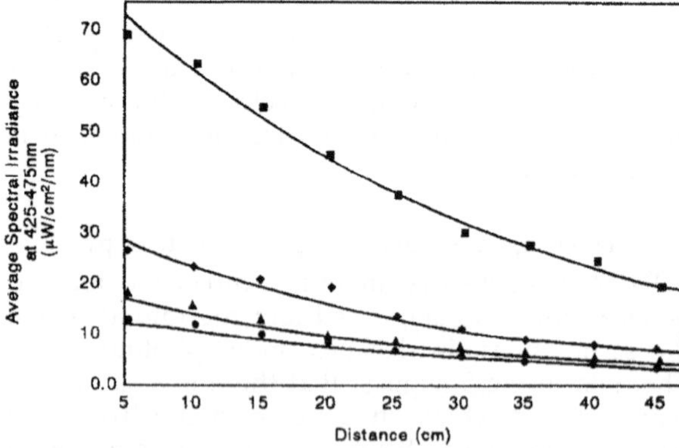

Fig 6. Effect of light source and distance from the light source to the infant on average spectral irradiance. Measurements were made across the 425- to 475-nm band by using a commercial radiometer (Olympic Bilimeter Mark II) and are the average of measurements taken at different locations at each distance (irradiance at the center of the light is much higher than at the periphery). The phototherapy unit was fitted with eight 24-in fluorescent tubes. ■ indicates special blue, General Electric 20-W F20T12/BB tube; ◆, blue, General Electric 20-W F20T12/B tube; ▲, daylight blue, 4 General Electric 20-W F20T12/B blue tubes and 4 Sylvania 20-W F20T12/D daylight tubes; •, daylight, Sylvania 20-W F20T12/D daylight tube. Curves were plotted by using linear curve fitting (True Epistat, Epistat Services, Richardson, TX). The best fit is described by the equation $y = Ae^{Bx}$. Source: *Pediatrics*. 1996;98:283-287.

Distance From the Light

As can be seen in Fig 6, the distance of the light source from the infant has a dramatic effect on the spectral irradiance, and this effect is most significant when special blue tubes are used. To take advantage of this effect, the fluorescent tubes should be placed as close to the infant as possible. To do this, the infant should be in a bassinet, not an incubator, because the top of the incubator prevents the light from being brought sufficiently close to the infant. In a bassinet, it is possible to bring the fluorescent tubes within approximately 10 cm of the infant. Naked term infants do not become overheated under these lights. It is important to note, however, that the halogen spot phototherapy lamps cannot be positioned closer to the infant than recommended by the manufacturers without incurring the risk of a burn. When halogen lamps are used, manufacturers recommendations should be followed. The reflectors, light source, and transparent light filters (if any) should be kept clean.

Surface Area

A number of systems have been developed to provide phototherapy above and below the infant.[8,9] One commercially available system that does this is the BiliBassinet (Olympic Medical, Seattle, WA). This unit provides special blue fluorescent tubes above and below the infant. An alternative is to place fiber-optic pads below an infant with phototherapy lamps above. One disadvantage of fiber-optic pads is that they cover a relatively small surface area so that 2 or 3 pads may be needed.[5] When bilirubin levels are extremely high and must be lowered as rapidly as possible, it is essential to expose as much of the infant's surface area to phototherapy as possible. In these situations, additional surface-area exposure can be achieved by lining the sides of the bassinet with aluminum foil or a white cloth.[10]

In most circumstances, it is not necessary to remove the infant's diaper, but when bilirubin levels approach the exchange transfusion range, the diaper should be removed until there is clear evidence of a significant decline in the bilirubin level.

What Decline in the Serum Bilirubin Can You Expect?

The rate at which the bilirubin declines depends on the factors listed in Table 5, and different responses can be expected depending on the clinical circumstances. When bilirubin levels are extremely high (more than 30 mg/dL [513 μmol/L]), and intensive phototherapy is used, a decline of as much as 10 mg/dL (171 μmol/L) can occur within a few hours,[11] and a decrease of at least 0.5 to 1 mg/dL per hour can be expected in the first 4 to 8 hours.[12] On average, for infants of more than 35 weeks' gestation readmitted for phototherapy, intensive phototherapy can produce a decrement of 30% to 40% in the initial bilirubin level by 24 hours after initiation of phototherapy.[13] The most significant decline will occur in the first 4 to 6 hours. With standard phototherapy systems, a decrease of 6% to 20% of the initial bilirubin level can be expected in the first 24 hours.[8,14]

Intermittent Versus Continuous Phototherapy

Clinical studies comparing intermittent with continuous phototherapy have produced conflicting results.[15–17] Because all light exposure increases bilirubin excretion (compared with darkness), no plausible scientific rationale exists for using intermittent phototherapy. In most circumstances, however, phototherapy does not need to be continuous. Phototherapy may be interrupted during feeding or brief parental visits. Individual judgment should be exercised. If the infant's bilirubin level is approaching the exchange transfusion zone (Fig 4), phototherapy should be administered continuously until a satisfactory decline in the serum bilirubin level occurs or exchange transfusion is initiated.

Hydration

There is no evidence that excessive fluid administration affects the serum bilirubin concentration. Some infants who are admitted with high bilirubin levels are also mildly dehydrated and may need supplemental fluid intake to correct their dehydration. Because these infants are almost always breastfed, the best fluid to use in these circumstances is a milk-based formula, because it inhibits the enterohepatic circulation of bilirubin and should help to lower the serum bilirubin level. Because the photoproducts responsible for the decline in serum bilirubin are excreted in urine and bile,[18] maintaining adequate hydration and good urine output should help to improve the efficacy of phototherapy. Unless there is evidence of dehydration, however, routine intravenous fluid or other supplementation (eg, with dextrose water) of term and near-term infants receiving phototherapy is not necessary.

When Should Phototherapy Be Stopped?

There is no standard for discontinuing phototherapy. The TSB level for discontinuing phototherapy depends on the age at which phototherapy is initiated and the cause of the hyperbilirubinemia.[13] For infants who are readmitted after their birth hospitalization (usually for TSB levels of 18 mg/dL [308 μmol/L] or higher), phototherapy may be discontinued when the serum bilirubin level falls below 13 to 14 mg/dL (239-239 μmol/L). Discharge from the hospital need not be delayed to observe the infant for rebound.[13,19,20] If phototherapy is used for infants with hemolytic diseases or is initiated early and discontinued before the infant is 3 to 4 days old, a follow-up bilirubin measurement within 24 hours after discharge is recommended.[13] For infants who are readmitted with hyperbilirubinemia and then discharged, significant rebound is rare, but a repeat TSB measurement or clinical follow-up 24 hours after discharge is a clinical option.[13]

Home Phototherapy

Because the devices available for home phototherapy may not provide the same degree of irradiance or surface-area exposure as those available in the hospital, home phototherapy should be used only in infants whose bilirubin levels are in the "optional phototherapy" range (Fig 3); it is not appropriate for infants with higher bilirubin concentrations. As with hospitalized infants, it is essential that serum bilirubin levels be monitored regularly.

Sunlight Exposure

In their original description of phototherapy, Cremer et al[21] demonstrated that exposure of newborns to sunlight would lower the serum bilirubin level. Although sunlight provides sufficient irradiance in the 425- to 475-nm band to provide phototherapy, the practical difficulties involved in safely exposing a naked newborn to the sun either inside or outside (and avoiding sunburn) preclude the use of sunlight as a reliable therapeutic tool, and it therefore is not recommended.

Complications

Phototherapy has been used in millions of infants for more than 30 years, and reports of significant toxicity are exceptionally rare. Nevertheless, phototherapy in hospital separates mother and infant, and eye patching is disturbing to parents. The most important, but uncommon, clinical complication occurs in infants with cholestatic jaundice. When these infants are exposed to phototherapy, they may develop a dark, grayish-brown discoloration of the skin, serum, and urine (the bronze infant syndrome).[22] The pathogenesis of this syndrome is unknown, but it may be related to an accumulation of porphyrins and other metabolites in the plasma of infants who develop cholestasis.[22,23] Although it occurs exclusively in infants with cholestasis, not all infants with cholestatic jaundice develop the syndrome.

This syndrome generally has had few deleterious consequences, and if there is a need for phototherapy, the presence of direct hyperbilirubinemia should not be considered a contraindication to its use. This is particularly important in sick neonates. Because the products of phototherapy are excreted in the bile, the presence of cholestasis will decrease the efficacy of phototherapy. Nevertheless, infants with direct hyperbilirubinemia often show some response to phototherapy. In infants receiving phototherapy who develop the bronze infant syndrome, exchange transfusion should be considered if the TSB is in the intensive phototherapy range and phototherapy does not promptly lower the TSB. Because of the paucity of data, firm recommendations cannot be made. Note, however, that the direct serum bilirubin should not be subtracted from the TSB concentration in making decisions about exchange transfusions (see Fig 4).

Rarely, purpura and bullous eruptions have been described in infants with severe cholestatic jaundice receiving phototherapy,[24,25] and severe blistering and photosensitivity during phototherapy have occurred in infants with congenital erythropoietic porphyria.[26,27] Congenital porphyria or a family history of porphyria is an absolute contraindication to the use of phototherapy, as is the concomitant use of drugs or agents that are photosensitizers.[28]

REFERENCES

1. Maisels MJ. Phototherapy—traditional and nontraditional. *J Perinatol.* 2001;21(suppl 1):S93–S97
2. Fiberoptic phototherapy systems. *Health Devices.* 1995;24:132–153
3. International Electrotechnical Commission. Medical electrical equipment—part 2-50: particular requirements for the safety of infant phototherapy equipment. 2000. IEC 60601-2-50. Available at www.iec.ch. Accessed June 7, 2004
4. Tan KL. The pattern of bilirubin response to phototherapy for neonatal hyperbilirubinemia. *Pediatr Res.* 1982;16:670–674
5. Maisels MJ. Why use homeopathic doses of phototherapy? *Pediatrics.* 1996;98:283–287
6. Seidman DS, Moise J, Ergaz Z, et al. A new blue light-emitting phototherapy device: a prospective randomized controlled study. *J Pediatr.* 2000;136:771–774
7. Ennever JF. Blue light, green light, white light, more light: treatment of neonatal jaundice. *Clin Perinatol.* 1990;17:467–481
8. Garg AK, Prasad RS, Hifzi IA. A controlled trial of high-intensity double-surface phototherapy on a fluid bed versus conventional phototherapy in neonatal jaundice. *Pediatrics.* 1995;95:914–916
9. Tan KL. Phototherapy for neonatal jaundice. *Clin Perinatol.* 1991;18: 423–439
10. Eggert P, Stick C, Schroder H. On the distribution of irradiation intensity in phototherapy. Measurements of effective irradiance in an incubator. *Eur J Pediatr.* 1984;142:58–61
11. Hansen TW. Acute management of extreme neonatal jaundice—the potential benefits of intensified phototherapy and interruption of enterohepatic bilirubin circulation. *Acta Paediatr.* 1997;86:843–846
12. Newman TB, Liljestrand P, Escobar GJ. Infants with bilirubin levels of 30 mg/dL or more in a large managed care organization. *Pediatrics.* 2003;111(6 Pt 1):1303–1311
13. Maisels MJ, Kring E. Bilirubin rebound following intensive phototherapy. *Arch Pediatr Adolesc Med.* 2002;156:669–672
14. Tan KL. Comparison of the efficacy of fiberoptic and conventional phototherapy for neonatal hyperbilirubinemia. *J Pediatr.* 1994;125: 607–612
15. Rubaltelli FF, Zanardo V, Granati B. Effect of various phototherapy regimens on bilirubin decrement. *Pediatrics.* 1978;61:838–841
16. Maurer HM, Shumway CN, Draper DA, Hossaini AA. Controlled trial comparing agar, intermittent phototherapy, and continuous phototherapy for reducing neonatal hyperbilirubinemia. *J Pediatr.* 1973;82:73–76
17. Lau SP, Fung KP. Serum bilirubin kinetics in intermittent phototherapy of physiological jaundice. *Arch Dis Child.* 1984;59:892–894
18. McDonagh AF, Lightner DA. 'Like a shrivelled blood orange'—bilirubin, jaundice, and phototherapy. *Pediatrics.* 1985;75:443–455
19. Yetman RJ, Parks DK, Huseby V, Mistry K, Garcia J. Rebound bilirubin levels in infants receiving phototherapy. *J Pediatr.* 1998;133:705–707
20. Lazar L, Litwin A, Merlob P. Phototherapy for neonatal nonhemolytic hyperbilirubinemia. Analysis of rebound and indications for discontinuing therapy. *Clin Pediatr (Phila).* 1993;32:264–267
21. Cremer RJ, Perryman PW, Richards DH. Influence of light on the hyperbilirubinemia of infants. *Lancet.* 1958;1(7030):1094–1097
22. Rubaltelli FF, Jori G, Reddi E. Bronze baby syndrome: a new porphyrin-related disorder. *Pediatr Res.* 1983;17:327–330
23. Meisel P, Jahrig D, Theel L, Ordt A, Jahrig K. The bronze baby syndrome: consequence of impaired excretion of photobilirubin? *Photobiochem Photobiophys.* 1982;3:345–352
24. Mallon E, Wojnarowska F, Hope P, Elder G. Neonatal bullous eruption as a result of transient porphyrinemia in a premature infant with hemolytic disease of the newborn. *J Am Acad Dermatol.* 1995;33:333–336
25. Paller AS, Eramo LR, Farrell EE, Millard DD, Honig PJ, Cunningham BB. Purpuric phototherapy-induced eruption in transfused neonates: relation to transient porphyrinemia. *Pediatrics.* 1997;100:360–364
26. Tonz O, Vogt J, Filippini L, Simmler F, Wachsmuth ED, Winterhalter KH. Severe light dermatosis following phototherapy in a newborn infant with congenital erythropoietic urophyria [in German]. *Helv Paediatr Acta.* 1975;30:47–56
27. Soylu A, Kavukcu S, Turkmen M. Phototherapy sequela in a child with congenital erythropoietic porphyria. *Eur J Pediatr.* 1999;158:526–527
28. Kearns GL, Williams BJ, Timmons OD. Fluorescein phototoxicity in a premature infant. *J Pediatr.* 1985;107:796–798

All clinical practice guidelines from the American Academy of Pediatrics automatically expire 5 years after publication unless reaffirmed, revised, or retired at or before that time.

ERRATUM

Two errors appeared in the American Academy of Pediatrics clinical practice guideline, titled "Management of Hyperbilirubinemia in the Newborn Infant 35 or More Weeks of Gestation," that was published in the July 2004 issue of *Pediatrics* (2004;114:297–316). On page 107, Background section, first paragraph, the second sentence should read: "The current guideline represents a consensus of the committee charged by the AAP with reviewing and updating the existing guideline and is based on a careful review of the evidence, including a comprehensive literature review by the Agency for Healthcare Research and Quality and the New England Medical Center Evidence-Based Practice Center.[2]" On page 118, Appendix 1, first paragraph, the 4 levels of evidence quality should have been labeled A, B, C, and D rather than 1, 2, 3, and 4, respectively. The American Academy of Pediatrics regrets these errors.

Hyperbilirubinemia Clinical Practice Guideline Quick Reference Tools

- Recommendation Summary
  — Management of Hyperbilirubinemia in the Newborn Infant 35 or More Weeks of Gestation
- *ICD-10-CM* Coding Quick Reference for Hyperbilirubinemia
- AAP Patient Education Handout
  — *Jaundice and Your Newborn*

Recommendation Summary

Management of Hyperbilirubinemia in the Newborn Infant 35 or More Weeks of Gestation

The following are the key elements of the recommendations provided by this guideline. Clinicians should:

1. Promote and support successful breastfeeding.
2. Establish nursery protocols for the identification and evaluation of hyperbilirubinemia.
3. Measure the total serum bilirubin (TSB) or transcutaneous bilirubin (TcB) level on infants jaundiced in the first 24 hours.
4. Recognize that visual estimation of the degree of jaundice can lead to errors, particularly in darkly pigmented infants.
5. Interpret all bilirubin levels according to the infant's age in hours.
6. Recognize that infants at less than 38 weeks' gestation, particularly those who are breastfed, are at higher risk of developing hyperbilirubinemia and require closer surveillance and monitoring.
7. Perform a systematic assessment on all infants before discharge for the risk of severe hyperbilirubinemia.
8. Provide parents with written and verbal information about newborn jaundice.
9. Provide appropriate follow-up based on the time of discharge and the risk assessment.
10. Treat newborns, when indicated, with phototherapy or exchange transfusion.

Coding Quick Reference for Hyperbilirubinemia	
ICD-10-CM	
P59.0	Neonatal jaundice associated with preterm delivery
P59.3	Neonatal jaundice from breast milk inhibitor
P59.9	Neonatal jaundice, unspecified
R17	Unspecified jaundice

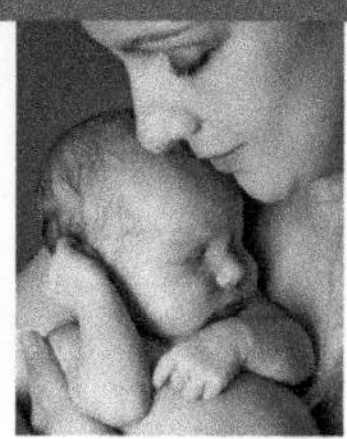

Jaundice and Your Newborn

Congratulations on the birth of your new baby!

To make sure your baby's first week is safe and healthy, it is important that

1. **You find a primary care provider, such as a pediatrician you are comfortable with, for your baby's ongoing care.**
2. **Your baby is checked for jaundice in the hospital.**
3. **If you are breastfeeding, you get the help you need to make sure it is going well.**
4. **You make sure your baby is seen by a doctor or nurse at 3 to 5 days of age.**
5. **If your baby is discharged before age 72 hours, your baby should be seen by a doctor or nurse within 2 days of discharge from the hospital.**

Q: What is jaundice?

A: Jaundice is the yellow color seen in the skin of many newborns. It happens when a chemical called *bilirubin* builds up in the baby's blood. Jaundice can occur in babies of any race or color.

Q: Why is jaundice common in newborns?

A: Everyone's blood contains bilirubin, which comes from red blood cells and is removed by the liver. Before birth, the mother's liver does this for the baby. Most babies develop jaundice in the first few days after birth because it takes a few days for the baby's liver to get better at removing bilirubin.

Q: How can I tell if my baby is jaundiced?

A: The skin of a baby with jaundice usually appears yellow. The best way to see jaundice is in good light, such as daylight or under fluorescent lights. Jaundice usually appears first in the face and then moves to the chest, abdomen, arms, and legs as the bilirubin level increases. The whites of the eyes may also be yellow. Jaundice may be harder to see in babies with darker skin color.

Q: Can jaundice hurt my baby?

A: Most babies have mild jaundice that is harmless, but in unusual situations the bilirubin level can get very high and might cause brain damage. This is why newborns should be checked carefully for jaundice and treated to prevent a high bilirubin level.

Q: How should my baby be checked for jaundice?

A: If your baby looks jaundiced in the first few days after birth, your baby's doctor or nurse may use a skin or blood test to check your baby's bilirubin level. However, because estimating the bilirubin level based on the baby's appearance can be difficult, most experts recommend that a skin or blood test be done in the first 2 days even if your baby does not appear jaundiced. A bilirubin level is always needed if jaundice develops before the baby is 24 hours old. Whether a test is needed after that depends on the baby's age, the amount of jaundice, and whether the baby has other factors that make jaundice more likely or harder to see.

Q: Does breastfeeding affect jaundice?

A: Breast milk (human milk) is the ideal food for your baby. Jaundice is more common in babies who are breastfed than babies who are formula-fed. However, this occurs more often in newborns who are not getting enough breast milk because their mothers are not producing enough milk (especially if the milk comes in late) or if breastfeeding is not going well, such as babies not latching on properly.

For the first 24 hours after birth, normal breastfed newborns receive only about 1 teaspoon of milk with each feeding. The amount of breast milk provided increases with each day. If you are breastfeeding, you should breastfeed your baby at least 8 to 12 times a day for the first few days. This will help you produce enough milk and will help keep the baby's bilirubin level down. If you are having trouble breastfeeding, ask your baby's doctor or nurse or a lactation specialist for help.

Q: When should my baby get checked after leaving the hospital?

A: It is important for your baby to be seen by a nurse or doctor when the baby is between 3 and 5 days old, because this is usually when a baby's bilirubin level is highest. This is why, if your baby is discharged before age 72 hours, your baby should be seen within 2 days of discharge. The timing of this visit may vary depending on your baby's age when released from the hospital and other factors.

Q: Why do some babies need an earlier follow-up visit after leaving the hospital?

A: Some babies have a greater risk for high levels of bilirubin and may need to be seen sooner after discharge from the hospital. Ask your doctor about an early follow-up visit if your baby has any of the following symptoms:

- A high bilirubin level before leaving the hospital
- Early birth (more than 2 weeks before the due date)
- Jaundice in the first 24 hours after birth
- Breastfeeding that is not going well
- A lot of bruising or bleeding under the scalp related to labor and delivery
- A parent, brother, or sister who had a high bilirubin level and received light therapy

Q: When should I call my baby's doctor?

A: Call your baby's doctor if

- Your baby's skin turns more yellow.
- Your baby's abdomen, arms, or legs are yellow.
- The whites of your baby's eyes are yellow.
- Your baby is jaundiced and is hard to wake, fussy, or not nursing or taking formula well.

Q: How is harmful jaundice prevented?

A: Most jaundice requires no treatment. When treatment is necessary, placing your baby under special lights while he or she is undressed will lower the bilirubin level. Depending on your baby's bilirubin level, this can be done in the hospital or at home. Jaundice is treated at levels that are much lower than those at which brain damage is a concern. In some babies, supplementing breast milk with formula can also help to lower the bilirubin level and prevent the need for phototherapy. Treatment can prevent the harmful effects of jaundice.

> **Note:** Exposing your baby to sunlight through a window might help lower the bilirubin level, but this will only work if the baby is undressed. Make sure the temperature in your home is comfortable and not too cold for your baby. Newborns should never be put in direct sunlight outside because they might get sunburned.

Q: When does jaundice go away?

A: In breastfed babies, it is common for jaundice to last 1 month or occasionally longer. In formula-fed babies, most jaundice goes away by 2 weeks. However, if your baby is jaundiced for more than 3 weeks, see your baby's doctor.

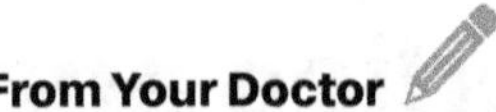

American Academy of Pediatrics
DEDICATED TO THE HEALTH OF ALL CHILDREN®

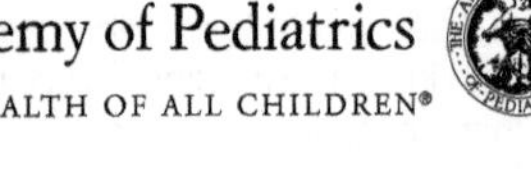

The American Academy of Pediatrics (AAP) is an organization of 66,000 primary care pediatricians, pediatric medical subspecialists, and pediatric surgical specialists dedicated to the health, safety, and well-being of infants, children, adolescents, and young adults.

The information contained in this publication should not be used as a substitute for the medical care and advice of your pediatrician. There may be variations in treatment that your pediatrician may recommend based on individual facts and circumstances. The persons whose photographs are depicted in this publication are professional models. They have no relation to the issues discussed. Any characters they are portraying are fictional.

© 2006 American Academy of Pediatrics, Updated 12/2016. All rights reserved.

Clinical Practice Guideline for the Management of Infantile Hemangiomas

- *Clinical Practice Guideline*

CLINICAL PRACTICE GUIDELINE Guidance for the Clinician in Rendering Pediatric Care

American Academy of Pediatrics

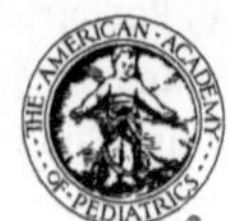

DEDICATED TO THE HEALTH OF ALL CHILDREN™

Clinical Practice Guideline for the Management of Infantile Hemangiomas

Daniel P. Krowchuk, MD, FAAP,[a] Ilona J. Frieden, MD, FAAP,[b] Anthony J. Mancini, MD, FAAP,[c] David H. Darrow, MD, DDS, FAAP,[d] Francine Blei, MD, MBA, FAAP,[e] Arin K. Greene, MD, FAAP,[f] Aparna Annam, DO, FAAP,[g] Cynthia N. Baker, MD, FAAP,[h] Peter C. Frommelt, MD, FAAP,[i] Amy Hodak, CPMSM,[j] Brian M. Pate, MD, FHM, FAAP,[k] Janice L. Pelletier, MD, FAAP,[l] Deborah Sandrock, MD, FAAP,[m] Stuart T. Weinberg, MD, FAAP,[n] Mary Anne Whelan, MD, PhD, FAAP,[o] SUBCOMMITTEE ON THE MANAGEMENT OF INFANTILE HEMANGIOMAS

abstract

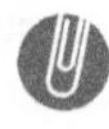

Infantile hemangiomas (IHs) occur in as many as 5% of infants, making them the most common benign tumor of infancy. Most IHs are small, innocuous, self-resolving, and require no treatment. However, because of their size or location, a significant minority of IHs are potentially problematic. These include IHs that may cause permanent scarring and disfigurement (eg, facial IHs), hepatic or airway IHs, and IHs with the potential for functional impairment (eg, periorbital IHs), ulceration (that may cause pain or scarring), and associated underlying abnormalities (eg, intracranial and aortic arch vascular abnormalities accompanying a large facial IH). This clinical practice guideline for the management of IHs emphasizes several key concepts. It defines those IHs that are potentially higher risk and should prompt concern, and emphasizes increased vigilance, consideration of active treatment and, when appropriate, specialty consultation. It discusses the specific growth characteristics of IHs, that is, that the most rapid and significant growth occurs between 1 and 3 months of age and that growth is completed by 5 months of age in most cases. Because many IHs leave behind permanent skin changes, there is a window of opportunity to treat higher-risk IHs and optimize outcomes. Early intervention and/or referral (ideally by 1 month of age) is recommended for infants who have potentially problematic IHs. When systemic treatment is indicated, propranolol is the drug of choice at a dose of 2 to 3 mg/kg per day. Treatment typically is continued for at least 6 months and often is maintained until 12 months of age (occasionally longer). Topical timolol may be used to treat select small, thin, superficial IHs. Surgery and/or laser treatment are most useful for the treatment of residual skin changes after involution and, less commonly, may be considered earlier to treat some IHs.

Departments of [a]Pediatrics and Dermatology, Wake Forest School of Medicine, Winston-Salem, North Carolina; Departments of [b]Dermatology and Pediatrics, School of Medicine, University of California, San Francisco, San Francisco, California; Departments of [c]Pediatrics and Dermatology, Feinberg School of Medicine, Northwestern University and Ann and Robert H. Lurie Children's Hospital of Chicago, Chicago, Illinois; Departments of [d]Otolaryngology and Pediatrics, Eastern Virginia Medical School and Children's Hospital of the King's Daughters, Norfolk, Virginia; [e]Donald and Barbara Zucker School of Medicine, Northwell Health, New York City, New York; [f]Department of Plastic and Oral Surgery, Boston Children's Hospital and Harvard Medical School, Harvard University, Boston, Massachusetts; [g]Department of Radiology, University of Colorado School of Medicine, Children's Hospital Colorado, Aurora, Colorado; [h]Department of Pediatrics, Kaiser Permanente Medical Center, Los Angeles, California; [i]Department of Pediatrics, Cardiology, Medical College of Wisconsin and Children's Hospital of Wisconsin, Milwaukee, Wisconsin; [j]American Board of Pediatrics, Chapel Hill, North Carolina; [k]Department of Pediatrics, University of Kansas School of Medicine-Wichita, Wichita, Kansas; [l]Department of Pediatrics, Northern Light Health, Bangor, Maine; [m]St Christopher's Hospital for Children and College of Medicine, Drexel University, Philadelphia, Pennsylvania; Departments of [n]Biomedical Informatics and Pediatrics, School of Medicine, Vanderbilt University, Nashville, Tennessee; and [o]College of Physicians and Surgeons, Columbia University, New York City, New York

This document is copyrighted and is property of the American Academy of Pediatrics and its Board of Directors. All authors have filed conflict of interest statements with the American Academy of Pediatrics. Any conflicts have been resolved through a process approved by the Board of Directors. The American Academy of Pediatrics has neither solicited nor accepted any commercial involvement in the development of the content of this publication.

To cite: Krowchuk DP, Frieden IJ, Mancini AJ, et al. Clinical Practice Guideline for the Management of Infantile Hemangiomas. *Pediatrics.* 2019;143(1):e20183475

INTRODUCTION

This is the first clinical practice guideline (CPG) from the American Academy of Pediatrics (AAP) regarding the management of infantile hemangiomas (IHs). Similar consensus statements have been published by European[1] and Australasian expert groups.[2] In addition, a recent AAP clinical report provided a comprehensive review of the pathogenesis, clinical features, and treatment of IH; it is available at http://pediatrics.aappublications.org/content/136/4/e1060.[3]

IHs occur in approximately 4% to 5% of infants, making them the most common benign tumor of childhood. They are more common in girls, twins, infants born preterm or with low birth weight (up to 30% of infants born weighing <1 kg are affected), and white neonates. The pathogenesis of IHs has yet to be fully defined. A leading hypothesis is that circulating endothelial progenitor cells migrate to locations in which conditions (eg, hypoxia and developmental field disturbances) are favorable for growth.[3]

Knowledge about IHs has advanced dramatically in the past decade, particularly regarding the unique timing and nature of proliferation and involution, risks of sequelae, and newer treatment options. As a result, pediatric providers have an opportunity to improve care and reduce morbidity in infants with IHs by promptly recognizing which IHs are potentially high risk and when intervention is needed.

In the broadest sense, the goal of this CPG from the AAP is to enhance primary care providers' ability to confidently evaluate, triage, and manage IHs, employing an evidence-based approach. Specifically, the CPG will:

- provide an approach to risk stratification and recognition of potentially problematic IHs;
- emphasize that early and frequent monitoring in the first few weeks and months of life is crucial in identifying those IHs that require intervention because IHs may change rapidly during this time period;
- review the role of imaging in patients who have IHs; and
- offer evidence-based guidance for the management of IHs, including indications for consultation, referral and possible intervention, pharmacologic options for therapy, the role of surgical modalities, and ongoing management and monitoring (including parent education).

This CPG is intended for pediatricians and other primary care providers who (1) manage IHs collaboratively with a hemangioma specialist (defined below), (2) care for children with IHs being managed primarily by a hemangioma specialist, or (3) manage IHs independently on the basis of their knowledge and expertise. It does not address the management of vascular malformations, congenital hemangiomas, or other vascular tumors. The CPG encourages enhanced communication between primary care clinicians and hemangioma specialists to ensure early assessment and treatment of infants in whom active intervention is indicated, to improve patient outcomes, and to enhance anticipatory guidance. It is not intended to be a sole source of guidance in the management of children with IHs, to replace clinical judgment, or to establish a protocol for all infants with IHs. Rather, it provides a framework for clinical decision-making.

METHODS

The methods of this CPG are discussed in detail in the Methods section of the Supplemental Information. Briefly, a comparative effectiveness review of potential benefits and harms of diagnostic modalities and pharmacologic and surgical treatments was conducted on behalf of the Agency for Healthcare Research and Quality (AHRQ). The literature search strategy employed Medline via the PubMed interface, the Cumulative Index to Nursing and Allied Health Literature (CINAHL), and Excerpta Medica Database (Embase). Searches were limited to the English language and to studies published from 1982 to June

TABLE 1 Highlights of This CPG

- IH growth characteristics are different than once taught.
  - Most rapid IH growth occurs between 1 and 3 months of age.
  - Although IHs involute, this process may be incomplete, leaving permanent skin changes that may be life altering. This is especially true for IHs that are thick.
  - There is a window of opportunity to treat problematic IHs. Consult early (by 1 month of age) for lesions that are potentially high risk because of the following associations (Table 3):
    - potential for disfigurement (the most common reason treatment is needed);
    - life-threatening complications;
    - functional impairment;
    - ulceration; and
    - underlying abnormalities.
- Oral propranolol is the treatment of choice for problematic IHs that require systemic therapy.
- Topical timolol may be used to treat some thin and/or superficial IHs.
- Surgery and/or laser treatment are most useful for the treatment of residual skin changes after involution. They may be used earlier to treat selected IHs.

TABLE 2 Definitions

Hemangioma specialist:	Unlike many diseases, management of IHs is not limited to 1 medical or surgical specialty. A hemangioma specialist may have expertise in dermatology, hematologyoncology, pediatrics, facial plastic and reconstructive surgery, ophthalmology, otolaryngology, pediatric surgery, and/or plastic surgery, and his or her practice is often focused primarily or exclusively on the pediatric age group.
Hemangioma specialists should:	• understand the time-sensitive nature of IHs during the growth phase and be able to accommodate requests for urgent evaluation; • have experience with accurate risk stratification and potential complications associated with IHs; • be able to provide recommendations for various management options, including observation, medical therapies, and surgical or laser procedures, and provide counseling regarding the potential risks and benefits of these interventions for specific patients; and • have a thorough knowledge of past and emerging medical literature regarding IHs. • Such specialists often have 1 or more of the following characteristics: o participated in a vascular anomalies program during previous medical training; o devotes a significant part of his or her clinical practice to IHs; o is a member of or collaborates with a multidisciplinary vascular anomalies center; o maintains membership in professional organizations or groups with a special interest in IHs; o participates in research studies in the field of IHs; or o publishes medical literature in the field of IHs.
IHs: infantile hemangiomas	Benign vascular tumors of infancy and childhood with unique clinical and histopathologic characteristics that distinguish them from other vascular tumors (eg, congenital hemangiomas) or malformations. These characteristics include development during the first weeks or months of life, a typical natural history of rapid growth followed by gradual involution, and immunohistochemical staining of biopsy specimens with erythrocyte-type glucose transporter protein and other unique markers not present on other benign vascular tumors. Many other entities are also called hemangiomas. Some are true vascular tumors, and others are vascular malformations. Therefore, it is important to use the adjective "infantile" when referring to true IHs. IHs are classified on the basis of soft-tissue depth and the pattern of anatomic involvement (see Supplemental Figs 5–10 for photographic examples).
Soft-tissue depth:	• Superficial: red with little or no evidence of a subcutaneous component (formerly called strawberry" hemangiomas); • Deep: blue and located below the skin surface (formerly called "cavernous" hemangiomas); and • Combined (mixed): both superficial and deep components are present.
Anatomic appearance:	• Localized: well-defined focal lesions (appearing to arise from a central point); • Segmental: IH involving an anatomic region that is often plaque-like and often measuring at >5 cm in diameter; • Indeterminate (undetermined): neither clearly localized or segmental (often called partial segmental); and • Multifocal: multiple discrete IHs at disparate sites.

2015. Because the therapy of IHs has been evolving rapidly, the CPG subcommittee performed an updated literature review for the period of July 2015 to January 2017 to augment the original search. This most recent search employed only Medline because previously, virtually all relevant articles had been accessed via this database. The search was concentrated on pharmacologic interventions, including topical timolol (an emerging therapeutic alternative for which limited data were available at the time of the original search). The original methodology and report, including the evidence search and review, are available in their entirety and as an executive summary at www.effectivehealthcare.ahrq.gov/reports/final.cfm.[4]

DEVELOPMENT OF THE CLINICAL PRACTICE GUIDELINE

In December 2016, the AAP convened a multidisciplinary subcommittee composed of IH experts in the fields of dermatology, cardiology, hematology-oncology, otolaryngology(head and neck surgery), plastic surgery, and radiology. The subcommittee also included general pediatricians, a parent representative, an implementation scientist, a representative from the Partnership for Policy Implementation (https://www.aap.org/en-us/professional-resources/quality-improvement/Pages/Partnership-for-Policy-Implementation.aspx), and an epidemiologist and methodologist. All panel members declared potential conflicts on the basis of the AAP policy on Conflict of Interest and Voluntary Disclosure. Subcommittee members repeated this process at the time of the publication of the guideline. All potential conflicts of interest are listed at the end of this document. The project was funded by the AAP.

The final recommendations were based on articles identified in the AHRQ and updated systematic reviews. Decisions and the strength of recommendations were based on a systematic grading of the quality of evidence by independent reviewers. Expert consensus was used when definitive data were not available. Key action statements (KASs), summarized in Table 4, were generated by subcommittee members authoring individual components of the CPG using

TABLE 3 High-Risk IHs

IH Clinical Findings	IH Risk
Life-threatening	
"Beard-area" IH	Obstructive airway hemangiomas
≥5 cutaneous IHs	Liver hemangiomas, cardiac failure, hypothyroidism
Functional impairment	
Periocular IH (>1 cm)	Astigmatism, anisometropia, proptosis, amblyopia
IH involving lip or oral cavity	Feeding impairment
Ulceration	
Segmental IH: IH of any size involving any of the following sites: lips, columella, superior helix of ear, gluteal cleft and/or perineum, perianal skin, and other intertriginous areas (eg, neck, axillae, inguinal region)	Increased risk of ulceration
Associated structural anomalies	
Segmental IH of face or scalp	PHACE syndrome
Segmental IH of lumbosacral and/or perineal area	LUMBAR syndrome
Disfigurement	
Segmental IH, especially of face and scalp	High risk of scarring and/or permanent disfigurement
Facial IH (measurements refer to size during infancy): nasal tip or lip (any size) or any facial location ≥2 cm (>1 cm if ≤3 mo of age)	Risk of disfigurement via distortion of anatomic landmarks and/or scarring and/or permanent skin changes
Scalp IH >2 cm	Permanent alopecia (especially if the hemangioma becomes thick or bulky); profuse bleeding if ulceration develops (typically more bleeding than at other anatomic sites)
Neck, trunk, or extremity IH >2 cm, especially in growth phase or if abrupt transition from normal to affected skin (ie, ledge effect); thick superficial IH (eg, ≥2 mm thickness)	Greater risk of leaving permanent scarring and/or permanent skin changes depending on anatomic location
Breast IH (female infants)	Permanent changes in breast development (eg, breast asymmetry) or nipple contour

Categorization of IH as high risk is based on published literature (including the AHRQ review and hemangioma severity scores) and consensus of CPG subcommittee members. Given the wide variation in IH location, size, and age at presentation, the subcommittee acknowledges that there may be situations in which an IH meets high-risk criteria and, therefore, merits consultation or referral, but the practitioner and parents do not believe this is necessary or practical. Clinical judgment is always involved in such decisions, and any plan of action needs to be individualized on the basis of a number of factors, including location of the lesion, age of child, family preferences, and geographic access to care.

the results of the literature review. These sections were reviewed and refined by the subcommittee chairperson and co-chairperson and ultimately by all subcommittee members.

Evidence-based guideline recommendations from the AAP may be graded as strong, moderate, weak on the basis of low-quality evidence, or weak on the basis of balance between benefits and harms. Strong and moderate recommendations usually are associated with "should" and "should not" recommendation statements, whereas some moderate and all weak recommendations may be recognized by use of "may" or "need not," signifying that moderate recommendations are based on a range of evidence strengths within the boundaries of the definition (Table 5, Fig 1).

The CPG underwent a comprehensive review by stakeholders (including AAP councils, committees, and sections), selected outside organizations, and individuals identified by the subcommittee as experts in the field before formal approval by the AAP. All comments were reviewed by the subcommittee and incorporated into the final guideline when appropriate.

RISK STRATIFICATION, TRIAGE, AND REFERRAL

Key Action Statement 1A (Table 6)

Clinicians should classify an IH as high risk if there is evidence of or potential for the following: (1) life-threatening complications, (2) functional impairment or ulceration, (3) structural anomalies (eg, in PHACE syndrome or LUMBAR syndrome), or (4) permanent disfigurement (grade X, strong recommendation).

The purpose of this statement is to ensure timely identification of IHs that may require early intervention. Clinicians in the primary care setting caring for infants with IH face 2 major challenges: disease heterogeneity and the unique growth characteristics of IHs.[24] For example, because IHs involute spontaneously, many that are small, are superficial, occur in areas covered by clothing, and/or are unlikely to cause disfigurement do not require hemangioma specialist evaluation or treatment. However, some IHs may be considered high risk, and depending on the clinician's comfort level and local access to specialty care, require a higher level of experience and expertise to determine if additional intervention is indicated. These high-risk IHs and their associated clinical findings are summarized in Table 3 and illustrated in Figs 2–4, Supplemental Table 22, and Supplemental Fig 11. Of particular note and as discussed later, segmental hemangiomas, those that cover an anatomic territory arising from 1 or more developmental units, confer a higher risk of morbidity and life-threatening complications than those that are localized, that is, seeming to arise from a central focal point.[5] At the same time, smaller IHs in particular anatomic locations, such as the cheek, tip of the

TABLE 4 Summary of Key Action Statements (KASs) for the Management of IHs

In Managing IH, Recommendations for Clinicians	Evidence Quality; Strength of Recommendation
1. Risk stratification	
1A. Classify an IH as high risk if there is evidence of or potential for the following: (1) life-threatening complications, (2) functional impairment or ulceration, (3) structural anomalies (eg, in PHACE syndrome or LUMBAR syndrome), or (4) permanent disfigurement	X; strong
1B. After identifying an IH as high risk, facilitate evaluation by a hemangioma specialist as soon possible	X; strong
2. Imaging	
2A. Do not perform imaging unless the diagnosis of IH is uncertain, there are ≥5 cutaneous IHs, or associated anatomic abnormalities are suspected	B; moderate
2B. Perform ultrasonography as the initial imaging modality when the diagnosis of IH is uncertain	C; weak
2C. Perform MRI when concerned about associated structural abnormalities (eg, PHACE syndrome or LUMBAR syndrome)	B; moderate
3. Pharmacotherapy	
3A. Use oral propranolol as the first-line agent for IHs requiring systemic treatment	A; strong
3B. Dose propranolol between 2 and 3 mg/kg per d unless there are comorbidities (eg, PHACE syndrome) or adverse effects (eg, sleep disturbance) that necessitate a lower dose	A; moderate
3C. Counsel that propranolol be administered with or after feeding and that doses be held at times of diminished oral intake or vomiting to reduce the risk of hypoglycemia	X; strong
3D. Evaluate patients for and educate caregivers about potential adverse effects of propranolol, including sleep disturbances, bronchial irritation, and clinically symptomatic bradycardia and hypotension	X; strong
3E. May prescribe oral prednisolone or prednisone to treat IHs if there are contraindications or an inadequate response to oral propranolol	B; moderate
3F. May recommend intralesional injection of triamcinolone and/or betamethasone to treat focal, bulky IHs during proliferation or in certain critical anatomic locations (eg, the lip)	B; moderate
3G. May prescribe topical timolol maleate as a therapy for thin and/or superficial IHs	B; moderate
4. Surgical management	
4. May recommend surgery and laser therapy as treatment options in managing selected IHs	C; moderate
5. Parent education	
5. Educate caregivers of infants with an IH about the condition, including the expected natural history and its potential for causing complications or disfigurement	X; strong

TABLE 5 Guideline Definitions for Key Action Statements

Statement	Definition	Implication
Strong recommendation	A particular action is favored because anticipated benefits clearly exceed harms (or vice versa), and quality of evidence is excellent or unobtainable.	Clinicians should follow a strong recommendation unless a clear and compelling rationale for an alternative approach is present.
Moderate recommendation	A particular action is favored because anticipated benefits clearly exceed harms (or vice versa), and the quality of evidence is good but not excellent (or is unobtainable).	Clinicians would be prudent to follow a moderate recommendation but should remain alert to new information and sensitive to patient preferences.
Weak recommendation (based on low-quality evidence)	A particular action is favored because anticipated benefits clearly exceed harms (or vice versa), but the quality of evidence is weak.	Clinicians would be prudent to follow a weak recommendation but should remain alert to new information and sensitive to patient preferences.
Weak recommendation (based on balance of benefits and harms)	A weak recommendation is provided when the aggregate database shows evidence of both benefit and harm that appears to be similar in magnitude for any available courses of action.	Clinicians should consider the options in their decision-making, but patient preference may have a substantial role.

PHACE indicates posterior fossa defects, hemangiomas, cerebrovascular arterial anomalies, cardiovascular anomalies including coarctation of the aorta, and eye anomalies; LUMBAR, lower body IH and other cutaneous defects, urogenital anomalies and ulceration, myelopathy, bony deformities, anorectal malformations, and arterial anomalies and renal anomalies.

nose, and perioral and periocular skin, can confer a high risk of complications as well (see discussion below).

There are 5 major indications for consideration of early treatment or need for further evaluation of IHs:

1. life-threatening complications;
2. functional impairment or risk thereof;
3. ulceration or risk thereof;
4. evaluation to identify important associated structural anomalies; and
5. risk of leaving permanent scarring or distortion of anatomic landmarks

Life-threatening Complications

Life-threatening lesions include obstructing IHs of the airway, liver IHs associated with high-output congestive heart failure and severe hypothyroidism, and, rarely, profuse bleeding from an ulcerated IH. Obstructing IHs of the airway typically involve the subglottis,

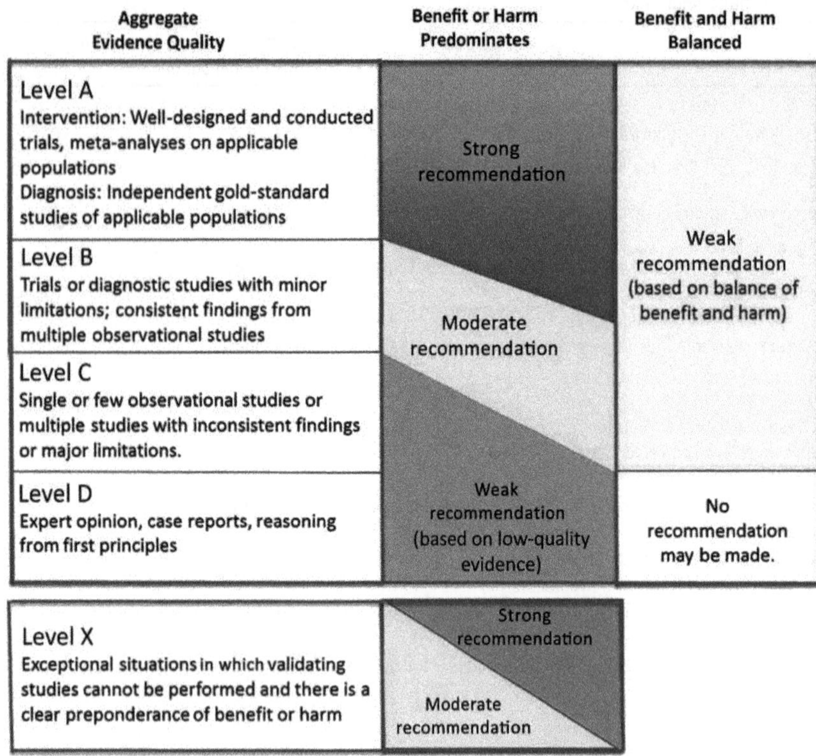

FIGURE 1
AAP rating of evidence and recommendations.

TABLE 6 Key Action Statement 1A: Clinicians should classify an IH as high risk if there is evidence of or potential for the following: (1) life-threatening complications, (2) functional impairment or ulceration, (3) structural anomalies (eg, in PHACE syndrome or LUMBAR syndrome), or (4) permanent disfigurement (grade X, strong recommendation).

Aggregate Evidence Quality	Grade X
Benefits	Early recognition of high-risk, potentially problematic IHs facilitates early specialist evaluation and management and potential avoidance of complications
Risks, harm, cost	Unnecessary parental concern regarding lesions inappropriately characterized as high-risk IHs
Benefit-harm assessment	The benefits of identifying high-risk IHs outweigh the harm
Intentional vagueness	None
Role of patient preference	None
Exclusions	Vascular lesions that are not true IHs
Strength	Strong recommendation
Key references	5–23

further compromising the narrowest portion of the pediatric airway. Although the mean age at the time of diagnosis is about 4 months, symptoms usually present much earlier but are often mistaken as infectious or inflammatory croup or reactive airway disease.[25–27] Most children who are affected develop biphasic stridor and barky cough as the IH enlarges. Approximately half of infants in whom an airway IH is diagnosed also will have a cutaneous IH. Segmental IH of the lower face ("beard distribution") or anterior neck and oral and/or pharyngeal mucosal IHs are the greatest risk factors for an airway IH.[6,27–29]

Hepatic hemangiomas have been characterized as occurring in 3 patterns: focal, multifocal, and diffuse; the latter 2 are attributable to IHs, whereas focal lesions more often represent congenital hemangiomas.[7,8] Most multifocal hepatic IHs are asymptomatic and do not require treatment. However, a minority of these lesions are associated with macrovascular shunting, causing high flow that can, in rare cases, result in high-output cardiac failure. So-called "diffuse" hepatic IHs are another rare subset that confers an even greater risk for morbidity and mortality. Infants who are affected typically present before 4 months of age with severe hepatomegaly, which can lead to potentially lethal abdominal compartment syndrome attributable to compromised ventilation, renal failure attributable to renal vein compression, or compromised inferior vena cava blood flow to the heart.[7,8] A consumptive form of hypothyroidism caused by the inactivation of thyroid hormones by type 3 iodothyronine deiodinase present in IH tissue can also be a complication of multifocal or diffuse hepatic IHs.[9] Although liver IHs can occasionally be seen in infants with 1 or no IH of the skin, the greatest risk for liver IHs is in infants who have 5 or more cutaneous IHs,[10] for whom screening ultrasonography is recommended (see KAS 2A).[11,30] Other sites of extracutaneous hemangiomas can occur, including the gastrointestinal tract, brain, and other organs. However, such involvement is rare and occurs mostly in association with large segmental IHs, and screening for these extracutaneous hemangiomas is not recommended unless signs or symptoms are present.[31,32] Severe bleeding, although often feared by parents, is an extremely rare complication of ulcerated IHs (see discussion of ulceration). Another potentially life-threatening complication is severe coarctation of the aorta not attributable to IHs but rather to structural anomalies seen in association with IHs in PHACE syndrome.

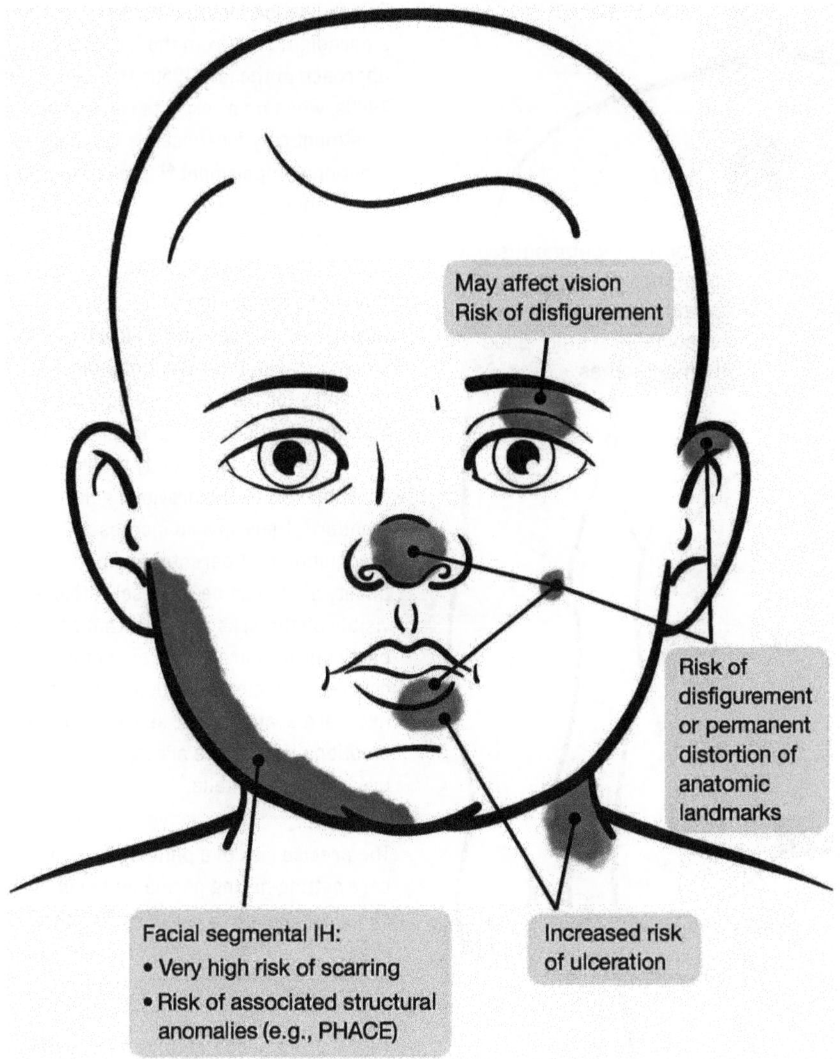

FIGURE 2
High-risk IHs involving the face and neck.

Functional Impairment

Examples of functional impairment include visual disturbance and interference with feeding because of IH involvement of the lips or mouth. IHs occurring in the periocular region have the potential to cause mechanical ptosis, strabismus, anisometropia, or astigmatism, which can quickly lead to the development of amblyopia.[12,13,33] Specific characteristics that place an infant at a higher risk for amblyopia include an IH size of >1 cm, upper eyelid involvement, associated ptosis, eyelid margin changes, medial location, and segmental morphology or displacement of the globe.[13,34,35] Feeding impairment can occur in infants with IHs involving either the perioral region or the airway. Infants with ulcerated lip IHs may have feeding difficulties secondary to severe pain.[36] Airway IHs may complicate breathing and swallowing, leading also to impaired feeding.[37]

Ulceration

Skin or mucosal ulceration of the IH surface occurs with an estimated incidence of 5% to 21% in referral populations.[14,38] Ulceration can lead to significant pain, bleeding, and secondary infection and virtually always results in scarring. Depending on the anatomic site of involvement, it can result in disfigurement. Ulceration occurs most frequently in infants younger than 4 months, during the period of active IH proliferation. Certain types of IHs are at higher risk, including superficial and mixed types, segmental IHs, and those involving the scalp, neck, and perioral, perineal, perianal, and intertriginous sites, the latter likely caused by maceration and friction. In addition, protuberant IHs can ulcerate as a result of trauma. Although concern for potential bleeding in IHs is common among caregivers and providers, most IH bleeding is minor and easily controllable with pressure. In rare cases, particularly IHs involving the scalp or with deep ulceration, bleeding can be more profuse, even life-threatening.[14,15]

Associated Structural Anomalies

A small subset of children with IHs have associated congenital anomalies. The best known phenomenon is PHACE syndrome (OMIM 606519).[39] The acronym "PHACES" is sometimes used instead to include potential ventral midline defects, specifically sternal cleft and/or supraumbilical raphe. Cerebrovascular anomalies, present in more than 90% of patients with PHACE syndrome, are the most common extracutaneous feature of the syndrome, followed by cardiac anomalies (67%) and structural brain anomalies (52%). The hallmark of PHACE syndrome is a large (often >5 cm in diameter) segmental IH that typically involves the face, scalp, and/or neck, although in rare cases, the face or scalp are spared, with a segmental IH located on the torso and upper extremity instead.[5,16] The risk of PHACE syndrome in an infant presenting with a large segmental IH of the head or neck is approximately 30%.[5] Revised consensus criteria for the diagnosis of PHACE syndrome and the care of infants who are affected have recently been published.[16]

LUMBAR syndrome may best be viewed as the "lower half of the body" equivalent of PHACE syndrome.[17] IHs in LUMBAR syndrome are almost invariably segmental, involving the

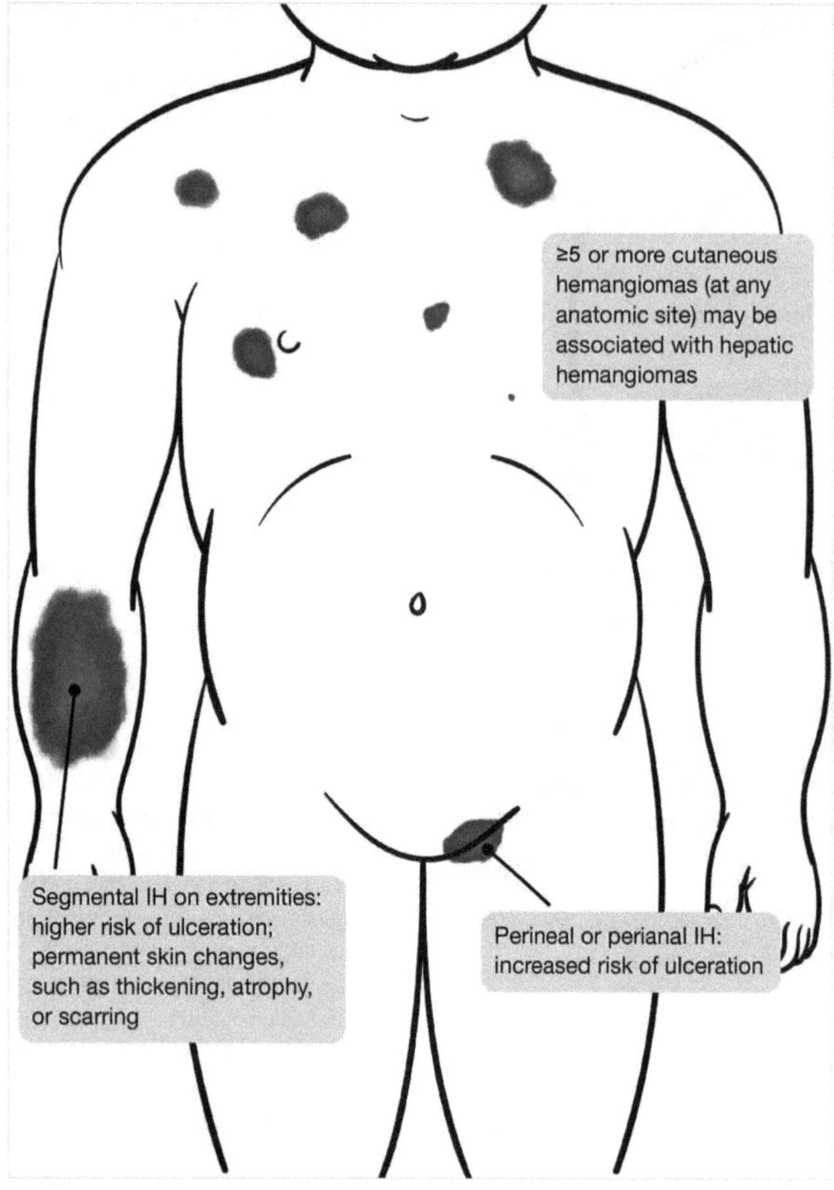

FIGURE 3
High-risk IHs involving the trunk, extremities, and perineum.

lumbosacral or perineal skin and often extending onto 1 leg. Many IHs in LUMBAR syndrome are minimally proliferative morphologically, with telangiectatic vascular stains predominating over bulkier superficial hemangiomas. In such cases, ulceration can be an early clue to the diagnosis.[17] Rarely, undergrowth or overgrowth of an affected limb may be present. Like PHACE syndrome, the cutaneous IH and underlying anomalies in LUMBAR syndrome reveal regional correlation. Myelopathy, particularly spinal dysraphism, is the most common extracutaneous anomaly.[17]

Disfigurement

IHs can lead to permanent disfigurement either via scarring of the skin or distortion of anatomic landmarks (see Table 3 for specific information). The risk of disfigurement is much higher than the risk of functional or life-threatening consequences. The majority of infants who receive treatment of IHs do so to prevent uncontrolled growth leading to permanent disfigurement.[1,18,40]

This indication for treatment represents a paradigm shift from the hands-off approach of the late 1950s through 1980s, when many experts recommended treatment only for those IHs causing functional impairment.[41] One reason for this change is an increased recognition that although IHs involute, they often leave behind permanent skin changes that, although not life or function threatening, are potentially life altering.[19,20] Moreover, with the advent of β-blocker therapies for IHs, there are now better treatment options with greater efficacy and lower potential toxicity than oral corticosteroids, the previous gold standard. There is also increased recognition that parental and patient quality of life can be adversely affected by visible birthmarks and resultant scarring, particularly in areas that cannot be easily covered with clothing, such as the face, neck, arms, and hands, as well as other emotionally sensitive areas, such as the breasts and genitalia.[42–44]

The precise risk of a patient in a primary care setting having permanent skin changes from an IH is not known, but in a referral setting, such changes are seen in 55% to 69% of those with untreated IHs.[19,20] This risk is greatest in IHs with a prominent and thick superficial (strawberry) component, especially when there is a steep step-off (ie, ledge effect) from affected to surrounding normal skin. However, the degree of superficial thickening may be difficult to predict in early infancy. Thus, even in IHs that do not initially appear to be high risk, it is prudent to serially follow lesion growth and establish a means for prompt evaluation if ongoing or rapid growth is observed because this could alter management.

Key Action Statement 1B (Table 7)

After identifying an IH as high risk, clinicians should facilitate an evaluation by a hemangioma specialist as soon as possible (grade X, strong recommendation).

The purpose of this statement is to ensure timely evaluation by a

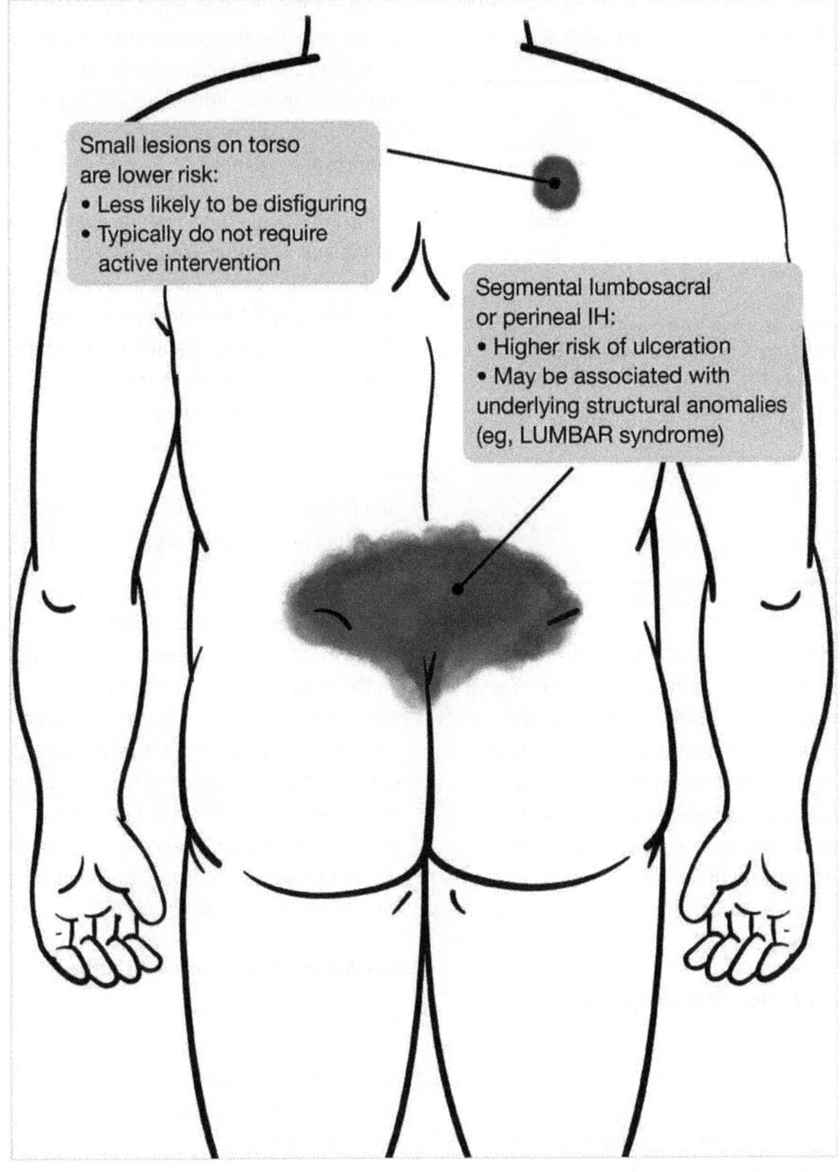

FIGURE 4
IHs involving the posterior trunk.

hemangioma specialist of an IH identified as high risk. IH is a disease with a window of opportunity in which to intervene and prevent poorer outcomes, and this critical time frame for optimizing outcomes can be missed if there are delays in referral or treatment. Recent literature suggests that the presence and growth of IHs is apparent much earlier than originally thought.[21,22] Premonitory findings appear in the skin during early infancy, including localized blanching or macular telangiectatic erythema.[21] As endothelial cell proliferation continues, the IH enlarges, becomes more elevated, and develops a rubbery consistency. IHs typically have their clinical onset before 4 weeks of age.[21,22]

Several studies have helped to better characterize the proliferative phase of IHs. Although IHs proliferate for variable periods of time and to varying degrees, the most rapid growth of superficial IHs typically occurs between 1 and 3 months' chronological age.[21] IHs reach 80% of their ultimate size by 3 months of age, and the large majority of IHs have completed growth by 5 months of age.[22] In a study in which parents' photographs were used, early IH growth was found to be nonlinear, with an accelerated period of rapid growth between 5 and 7 weeks of age, and the optimal time for referral or initiation of treatment was 1 month of age, a time far earlier than the time most infants with IHs are typically referred to (or seen by) hemangioma specialists.[21,22]

These observations regarding growth are helpful, but their impact in individual case management is limited by the tremendous degree of disease heterogeneity of IHs. Even for the most experienced clinicians, it can be difficult to predict the degree of IH growth until several weeks to months after the lesion is first noticed. By that time, damage to the dermis and subcutaneous tissues as well as permanent distortion of important anatomic landmarks, such as the nose or lips, may already have occurred.[19,20,44] Hence, decisions regarding intervention must be based on risk stratification, including the age of the child (in anticipation of possible IH growth), health considerations (like prematurity), anatomic site, the size of the IH, any actual or potential complications, and parental preferences. In high-risk IHs, a wait-and-see approach can result in a missed window of opportunity to prevent adverse outcomes.

The rate of growth and ultimate size of an IH can vary dramatically from patient to patient. Predicting the growth of a particular IH is, therefore, difficult and made even more challenging by the minority of lesions that do not exhibit the typical pattern of proliferation followed by slow involution.[23,45] Differences in growth can even be evident when comparing 1 IH to another on the same patient. For example, in patients who have 2 or more IHs, 1 lesion may become large and problematic, and others may barely grow. A subset of IHs known as infantile hemangiomas with minimal or arrested growth (IH-MAGs) typically present as a patch of fine or coarsely reticulated

TABLE 7 Key Action Statement 1B: After identifying an IH as high risk, clinicians should facilitate an evaluation by a hemangioma specialist as soon as possible (grade X, strong recommendation).

Aggregate Evidence Quality	Grade X
Benefits	Potential for early intervention for IH at a high risk of causing complications
Risks, harm, cost	Potential for delay in intervention if specialist evaluation cannot be arranged promptly or is unavailable in the geographic region; costs associated with specialist evaluation for IH incorrectly identified as high risk
Benefit-harm assessment	The benefits of specialist evaluation outweigh harms and costs
Intentional vagueness	The subcommittee recognizes the multidisciplinary nature of IH management and the diverse level of expertise among individuals in this field. As a result, the definition of a specialist with expertise in vascular birthmarks is vague. The subcommittee also recognizes that the time frame "as soon as possible" is vague.
Role of patient preference	Parental preference should be considered in the decision to see a specialist and in the choice of specialist
Exclusions	IHs not considered high risk
Strength	Strong recommendation
Key references	19–23

telangiectasias, often within a zone of vasoconstriction.[23] They may be mistaken for a port-wine stain or other vascular birthmark. Although they lack the robust proliferative phase characteristic of many IHs, IH-MAGs may be associated with complications, such as ulceration or, if segmental, structural anomalies. The growth trajectory of deeper IHs or those with deeper soft-tissue components also differs from that of localized superficial IHs, often presenting at a later age (eg, 1–2 months and, occasionally, even later).[22]

On the basis of this information, the consensus recommendation of the subcommittee is that patients with IHs identified as high risk have expedited consultation and/or referral to a hemangioma specialist (Supplemental Table 22, Supplemental Fig 11). The type of hemangioma specialist may depend on the specific concern (eg, a hemangioma specialist experienced in airway management will be needed if concern exists for a subglottic hemangioma). Because the time to appointment with a hemangioma specialist may exceed the window of opportunity during which evaluation and possible treatment would be of maximum benefit, those who care for infants with IHs should have mechanisms in place to expedite such appointments, including the education of office staff to give young infants with high-risk IHs priority appointments. In-person consultation may not always be possible or mandatory. Clinicians may also use telemedicine (either live interactive or store and forward of photographs taken in the office) to assist with triage, evaluation, and management.

Key Action Statement 2A (Table 8)

Clinicians should not perform imaging unless the diagnosis of IH is uncertain, there are 5 or more cutaneous IHs, or associated anatomic abnormalities are suspected (grade B, moderate recommendation).

The purpose of this statement is to provide guidance to clinicians regarding the indications for imaging of IHs. Most IHs can be diagnosed clinically. Therefore, imaging of IHs is not indicated for diagnostic purposes unless the lesion has an atypical appearance (ie, the diagnosis is uncertain) or it behaves in a manner that is inconsistent with the expected proliferative growth and involution phases within the expected time frame.[46,47] Noninvasive imaging may be used to monitor response to treatment but typically is not required.[47] Occasionally, differentiating an IH from a highly vascularized malignant tumor may be difficult. Clinical history, response to therapy, and imaging characteristics considered together are extremely important in this differentiation. In rare cases, a tissue biopsy may be needed to confirm the diagnosis.

Clinicians should use imaging, specifically abdominal ultrasonography, if 5 or more cutaneous IHs are present to screen for hepatic IH.[30] Ultrasonography has a sensitivity of 95% for detection of hepatic hemangiomas and avoids the need for sedation and exposure to ionizing radiation.[46] Early detection of these lesions may lead to improved monitoring and initiation of appropriate treatment, resulting in decreased morbidity and mortality.[8,46,49]

Imaging also is indicated if concern exists for structural anomalies, as would be the case in infants at risk for PHACE syndrome or LUMBAR syndrome. These infants would typically have large (eg, >5 cm in diameter) segmental facial or scalp IHs or segmental IHs of the perineum, gluteal cleft, or lumbosacral area, with or without lower extremity IHs (see KAS 2C for further discussion).[16,17,47,48]

Key Action Statement 2B (Table 9)

Clinicians should perform ultrasonography as the initial imaging modality when the diagnosis of IH is uncertain (grade C, weak recommendation).

Ultrasonography (with Doppler imaging) is the initial imaging modality of choice when the diagnosis of IH is uncertain. The study can be performed without sedation and does not necessitate exposure to ionizing radiation, which can be risky, particularly in young infants. On ultrasonography, most IHs appear as a well-defined mass with high-flow vascular characteristics and no arteriovenous shunting (an exception to the latter is that hepatic IHs may exhibit arteriovenous shunting). This may change as the IH involutes and has a more fatty appearance with decreased vascularity.[47,50] Doppler ultrasonography is also the modality of choice when screening for hepatic IHs and can be used to monitor

TABLE 8 Key Action Statement 2A: Clinicians should not perform imaging unless the diagnosis of IH is uncertain, there are 5 or more cutaneous IHs, or associated anatomic abnormalities are suspected (grade B, moderate recommendation).

Aggregate Evidence Quality	Grade B
Benefits	Avoid the cost, risk of sedation, and radiation associated with unnecessary imaging
Risks, harm, cost	Potential misdiagnosis if imaging is not performed
Benefit-harm assessment	Benefits outweigh harm
Intentional vagueness	None
Role of patient preference	Minimal; when parental anxiety is significant, ultrasonography is a low-cost and low-risk means of confirming the diagnosis
Exclusions	None
Strength	Moderate recommendation
Key references	8,46–48

TABLE 9 Key Action Statement 2B: Clinicians should perform ultrasonography as the initial imaging modality when the diagnosis of IH is uncertain (grade C, weak recommendation).

Aggregate Evidence Quality	Grade C
Benefits	Select the appropriate imaging study to aid in diagnosis and identify associated abnormalities; avoid ionizing radiation and sedation
Risks, harm, cost	Risk that ultrasonography may not be sufficiently diagnostic or may result in the misdiagnosis of a lesion believed to represent an IH
Benefit-harm assessment	Benefits outweigh harms
Intentional vagueness	None
Role of patient preference	Minimal
Exclusions	None
Strength	Weak recommendation
Key references	47,50

progression of disease and response to treatment.[47]

Key Action Statement 2C (Table 10)

Clinicians should perform MRI when concerned about associated structural abnormalities (eg, PHACE syndrome or LUMBAR syndrome) (grade B, moderate recommendation).

Imaging for associated structural anomalies is indicated in infants at risk for PHACE syndrome or LUMBAR syndrome. For example, an infant with a large (eg, >5 cm in diameter) segmental facial or scalp IH is at risk for PHACE syndrome, and further evaluation with MRI and/or magnetic resonance angiography (MRA) of the head and neck (including the aortic arch and brachiocephalic origins) and echocardiography is advisable.[16,47]

For patients with segmental IHs of the perineum, gluteal cleft, or lumbosacral area (with or without lower extremity IHs), imaging for LUMBAR syndrome should be considered.[17,48] If there is uncertainty about whether there is a risk of associated structural anomalies, consultation with a hemangioma specialist or other appropriate expert (eg, pediatric neurologist, neurosurgeon, or radiologist) can be helpful to determine if imaging is required and which studies should be performed.

MRI is the optimal imaging modality to define underlying structural abnormalities, and contrast is needed to assess vascular components.[46] MRA can illustrate the vascular anatomy. Thus, MRI and MRA, with and without contrast of the head and neck, are the best studies to detect PHACE syndrome. MRI does not use ionizing radiation but may require sedation given the duration of the examination.[51,52] The duration of imaging is important because it has been theorized that prolonged (>3 hours) or repeated exposures to general anesthetic and sedative drugs in children younger than 3 years may negatively affect brain development.[53,54] Single, brief exposures are unlikely to have similar effects. As more rapid MRI scanning protocols are developed, the need for sedation may diminish. As an alternative to sedation, young infants fed immediately before an MRI and swaddled may sleep through the procedure. Discussion between the radiologist, ordering clinician, and sedation team is critical to determine the optimal imaging and sedation protocols.[55]

In patients in whom there is a risk of LUMBAR syndrome, spinal ultrasonography (for those with a corrected age of less than 6 months) and Doppler ultrasonography of the abdomen and pelvis can be used as an initial screen for abnormalities.[56–58] Ultimately, however, MRI likely will be required to provide greater definition. For example, if a high suspicion for spinal abnormalities remains despite normal ultrasonography (ie, there are associated markers of dysraphism [eg, sacral dimple, skin appendage, tuft of hair, and lipoma]), MRI is a more sensitive diagnostic modality.[47]

Computed tomography is not the modality of choice for imaging IHs because it involves ionizing radiation, which should be avoided in children, particularly young infants, unless absolutely necessary. Advantages of computed tomography are that it can be rapidly performed and may not require sedation.

MANAGEMENT: PHARMACOTHERAPY

Key Action Statement 3A (Table 11)

Clinicians should use oral propranolol as the first-line agent for IHs requiring

TABLE 10 Key Action Statement 2C: Clinicians should perform MRI when concerned about associated structural abnormalities (eg, PHACE syndrome or LUMBAR syndrome) (grade B, moderate recommendation).

Aggregate Evidence Quality	Grade B
Benefits	Select the appropriate imaging study to aid in diagnosis and identify associated abnormalities; avoid ionizing radiation and sedation
Risks, harm, cost	Risk of sedation or general anesthesia Cost of MRI (but offers greater diagnostic sensitivity)
Benefit-harm assessment	Benefits outweigh harms
Intentional vagueness	None
Role of patient preference	Minimal
Exclusions	None
Strength	Moderate recommendation
Key references	46,51–55

TABLE 11 Key Action Statement 3A: Clinicians should use oral propranolol as the first-line agent for IHs requiring systemic treatment (grade A, strong recommendation).

Aggregate Evidence Quality	Grade A
Benefits	Improve IH treatment; avoid adverse effects associated with oral steroid therapy
Risks, harm, cost	Occurrence of adverse effects associated with propranolol use (see KAS 3D); medication cost and cost of hospitalization if drug is initiated while infant is an inpatient
Benefit-harm assessment	Benefits outweigh harms
Intentional vagueness	None
Role of patient preference	Parents should be involved in shared decision-making regarding treatment.
Exclusions	Caution (but not exclusion) in infants <5 wk of age, postconceptional age of <48 wk; potential exclusions that require appropriate subspecialty evaluation and/or clearance; evidence of cardiogenic shock or heart failure; sinus bradycardia; heart block greater than first degree; known or suspected PHACE syndrome, including presence or risk of coarctation of the aorta and cerebrovascular anomalies; known asthma and/or reactive airway disease; known hypersensitivity to propranolol
Strength	Strong recommendation
Key references	3,46,59–61

systemic treatment (grade A, strong recommendation).

The purpose of this statement is to advise clinicians that oral propranolol is the current treatment of choice for IHs requiring systemic therapy. After the serendipitous observation of its utility in treating IHs,[59] propranolol, a nonselective antagonist of both β-1 and β-2 adrenergic receptors, has evolved to become the treatment of choice for IHs.[1,3,60] The precise mechanisms of action of propranolol on IHs are unclear but have been hypothesized to be attributable to vasoconstriction, angiogenesis inhibition, induction of apoptosis, inhibition of nitric oxide production, and regulation of the renin-angiotensin system.[61–69] Oral propranolol hydrochloride (Hemangeol) was approved by the US Food and Drug Administration (FDA) in March 2014 for use in proliferating IHs requiring systemic therapy. This therapy has now replaced the previous gold standard therapy for threatening IHs, systemic or intralesional corticosteroids.[70]

In the AHRQ review, 18 studies were included in a network meta-analysis of the effectiveness and harms of corticosteroids and β-blockers. The mean estimate of expected clearance for oral propranolol was 95%, which was superior to other interventions.[46] Ten studies compared propranolol versus another modality, including steroids, pulsed-dye laser (PDL), bleomycin, or other treatments (Table 12). Propranolol was more effective in 3 studies, effectiveness did not differ significantly in 2 other studies, and studies comparing propranolol versus steroids to reduce IH size had conflicting results. Harms are discussed in subsequent KASs, but in the AHRQ analysis, propranolol's superior safety profile is confirmed.

The subcommittee's additional review yielded another 19 studies, 4 of which met inclusion criteria for benefits of interventions (and 9 of which met inclusion criteria for harms of interventions). These 4 studies evaluated propranolol versus placebo or observation. Propranolol was associated with significantly greater clearance of IH compared with the control group in all studies. The strength of evidence (SOE) was considered high for greater effectiveness of propranolol versus placebo or observation. The review also confirmed the superiority of oral propranolol over a variety of comparators. Propranolol was superior to ibuprofen and paracetamol in treating ulcerated hemangiomas[71] and to oral captopril in patients with problematic IHs.[72] In a randomized controlled trial (RCT) of oral propranolol compared with observation for IHs, the overall efficacy of propranolol (defined as excellent, good, or medium response) was 98.97%, compared with 31.25% in the observation group ($P < .05$).[73] Last, Aly et al[74] compared oral propranolol alone versus oral propranolol combined with 2 weeks of "priming" with oral prednisolone. Those in the prednisolone-primed propranolol group showed a statistically superior reduction in IH size at weeks 2, 4, and 8 compared with the propranolol group, but the 6-month response was equivocal for both groups regarding all assessed variables.[74]

TABLE 12 AHRQ Summary of Comparative Efficacy of Various Treatments for IHs

Drug	Mean Estimate of Expected Clearance, %	95% Bayesian Credible Interval, %
Propranolol	95	88–99
Topical timolol	62	39–83
Intralesional triamcinolone	58	21–93
Oral steroid	43	21–66
Control	6	1–11

Limited data exist on the utility of β-blockers other than propranolol or different delivery mechanisms for propranolol. The AHRQ review included 3 small studies comparing propranolol versus nadolol or atenolol and 1 study comparing oral, intralesional, and topical propranolol. Atenolol and nadolol each demonstrated effectiveness on lesion size, with little difference in efficacy between propranolol and atenolol and greater efficacy of nadolol in 1 small study. The review did not find differences in response with propranolol, nadolol, or atenolol, but the SOE in comparing these was low.[46] The subcommittee's additional review yielded 1 article on oral atenolol for IH, which did not meet the AHRQ inclusion criteria for comparative effectiveness but revealed an excellent treatment response in 56.5% of patients.[75]

Key Action Statement 3B (Table 13)

Clinicians should dose propranolol between 2 and 3 mg/kg per day unless there are comorbidities (eg, PHACE syndrome) or adverse effects (eg, sleep disturbance) that necessitate a lower dose (grade A, moderate recommendation).

The purpose of this statement is to provide clinicians guidance in dosing oral propranolol for IHs. To date, authors of most studies favor dosing at 2 to 3 mg/kg per day. An RCT of 456 infants compared a placebo versus 1 of 4 propranolol regimens (1 mg/kg per day or 3 mg/kg per day for 3 or 6 months duration). The regimen of 3 mg/kg per day for 6 months was superior, with complete or nearly complete resolution in 60% of patients, compared with 4% of patients in the placebo arm ($P < .0001$).[76] The FDA approval of propranolol hydrochloride oral solution (4.28 mg/mL) recommends a starting dose of 0.6 mg/kg twice daily, with a gradual increase over 2 weeks to a maintenance dose of 1.7 mg/kg twice daily (3.4 mg/kg per day based on expression as the hydrochloride salt of propranolol). As noted in the AHRQ review, other studies typically reported dosing of 2 to 2.5 mg/kg per day,[46] and a multidisciplinary, multiinstitutional expert panel and a European expert consensus group[1,61] support a starting dose of 1 mg/kg per day and a target dose of 2 to 3 mg/kg per day. Data comparing 2 and 3 mg/kg per day are lacking.

Similarly, available data do not permit evidence-based recommendations on dosing frequency (twice daily versus 3 times daily), but both the FDA and the European Medicine Evaluation Agency labeling is for twice-daily dosing. The site for initiation of propranolol (outpatient versus inpatient) is evolving as more evidence accumulates that cardiovascular and other acute toxicities occur rarely. Although in both the aforementioned consensus articles, initiation in an inpatient setting is favored for infants younger than 8 weeks, those with cardiovascular or respiratory comorbidities, and those with poor social support, FDA labeling sanctions initiation in an outpatient setting for infants >5 weeks' corrected gestational age.

A duration of 6 months of therapy was shown to be superior to 3 months in the large RCT conducted by Léauté-Labrèze et al.[76] In the AHRQ review, the duration of propranolol treatment ranged from 3 to 13 months.[46] Rebound growth during tapering or after stopping the medication may occur in 10% to 25% of patients and can occur even after 6 months of therapy.[18,76] A large multicenter retrospective cohort study found the greatest risk of rebound occurred in those in whom therapy was discontinued at <12 months of age (and especially before 9 months), and the lowest risk was in those in whom treatment was discontinued between 12 and 15 months of age.[18] Risk factors for rebound growth noted in this study were the presence of mixed or deep morphology and female sex. These observations have led many experts to recommend continuing therapy until at least 1 year of age.

Dosing may need to be modified in certain situations. Patients with PHACE syndrome may have an increased risk of stroke, and this risk may be greater if certain neurovascular anomalies are present.[16] In patients who merit systemic IH therapy, the benefits and risks must be carefully weighed. Evaluation with MRI and/or MRA of the head and neck and echocardiography should be performed before or shortly after the initiation of therapy.[61] If patients who are at high risk require treatment with propranolol, it is advisable to use the lowest effective dose, slowly titrate the dose, and administer the drug 3 times daily (to minimize abrupt changes in blood pressure); comanagement with a pediatric neurologist is recommended.[1,16,61,77] Other patients who may require lower propranolol doses include those with progressive IH ulceration while receiving therapy and those who experience adverse effects (such as sleep disturbances).

Key Action Statement 3C (Table 14)

Clinicians should counsel that propranolol be administered with or after feeding and that doses be held at times of diminished oral intake or vomiting to reduce the risk of hypoglycemia (grade X, strong recommendation).

TABLE 13 Key Action Statement 3B: Clinicians should dose propranolol between 2 and 3 mg/kg per day unless there are comorbidities (eg, PHACE syndrome) or adverse effects (eg, sleep disturbance) that necessitate a lower dose (grade A, moderate recommendation).

Aggregate Evidence Quality	Grade A
Benefits	The recommended doses have been associated with high clearance rates of IH
Risks, harm, cost	Response rates for higher or lower doses have not been well studied
Benefit-harm assessment	Benefits outweigh harms
Intentional vagueness	None
Role of patient preference	Parents will be involved in the decision about dosing in the setting of PHACE syndrome or the occurrence of adverse effects
Exclusions	See KAS 3A; dosing may be modified if comorbidities exist
Strength	Moderate recommendation
Key references	1,46,61,76

TABLE 14 Key Action Statement 3C: Clinicians should counsel that propranolol be administered with or after feeding and that doses be held at times of diminished oral intake or vomiting to reduce the risk of hypoglycemia (grade X, strong recommendation).

Aggregate Evidence Quality	Grade X
Benefits	Reduce the likelihood of adverse reactions
Risks, harm, cost	Risk that parents will decline therapy because of concerns about potential medication adverse effects
Benefit-harm assessment	Benefits outweigh harms
Intentional vagueness	None
Role of patient preference	None
Exclusions	None
Strength	Strong recommendation
Key references	46,60,61,76,78–80

The purpose of this statement is to reinforce the importance of administering oral propranolol with feeds and of holding therapy at times of restricted oral intake to prevent hypoglycemia and hypoglycemia-induced seizures. The association between hypoglycemia and propranolol in infants and children is well established and is related to effects on glycogenolysis and gluconeogenesis.[78] β-blockade by propranolol can affect these processes, and infants and children may be particularly susceptible to this effect.[78,79] Early clinical features of hypoglycemia in infants, which may be masqueraded by β-adrenergic blockade, include sweating, tachycardia, shakiness, and anxious appearance, whereas later manifestations (signs of neuroglycopenia) may include lethargy, poor feeding, apnea, seizures, stupor, and loss of consciousness.[79]

The AHRQ review identified 24 comparative studies (4 good quality) and 56 case series (4 good quality) that reported harms data of β-blockers for IHs. Rates of clinically important harms (hypoglycemia, hypotension, bradycardia, and bronchospasm) varied widely, and the authors assigned a moderate SOE for the association of propranolol with both clinically important and minor harms (with high study limitations).[46] Harms overall did not cause treatment discontinuation.

The subcommittee's additional review yielded 8 reports that met inclusion criteria for harms regarding oral propranolol for treatment of IHs. These reports provided more detailed information about the occurrence of hypoglycemia. Three of the 8 articles reported hypoglycemia; these articles included 1021 patients, 10 of whom experienced hypoglycemia (3 of these suffered hypoglycemic seizures in the setting of viral gastroenteritis and poor oral intake).[80–82]

In a large meta-analysis of oral propranolol for IHs not included in the AHRQ review, adverse events were reported for 1945 of 5862 patients who were treated.[60] The investigators identified 24 cases of hypoglycemia and 2 cases of hypoglycemic seizures among 3766 patients who were treated with propranolol from their literature review (some of whom are included in aforementioned studies). Of the 14 events with resolution details, 9 led to dose adjustment or temporary discontinuation of propranolol, and 1 led to permanent discontinuation of treatment. The authors mention that 1 case of hypoglycemic seizure was related to overdose, and the other was associated with diminished oral intake because of infection.[60]

Although the risk of hypoglycemia must be considered when prescribing oral propranolol for IHs, routine glucose screening is not indicated.[1,61] Hypoglycemia occurs infrequently and can be minimized with appropriate education of caregivers on the importance of administering propranolol during or immediately after a feeding and of temporarily withdrawing therapy during periods of fasting (including poor oral intake because of illness or before general anesthesia) or vomiting.[60] Prolonged fasting should be avoided, and parents should be advised that hypoglycemia becomes more likely after ≥8 hours of fasting in infants and young children.[83,84]

Key Action Statement 3D (Table 15)

Clinicians should evaluate patients for and educate caregivers about potential adverse effects of propranolol, including sleep disturbances, bronchial irritation, and clinically symptomatic bradycardia and hypotension (grade X, strong recommendation).

The purpose of this statement is to increase awareness of potential propranolol-associated adverse effects other than hypoglycemia for clinicians and caregivers of patients receiving this medical therapy for IHs. Propranolol has been used in pediatric patients for decades, primarily in an off-label fashion. In young infants, is has been used primarily for cardiac disorders and for the treatment of thyrotoxicosis at doses up to 6 to 8 mg/kg per day. Despite this use, many pediatricians will be unfamiliar with the drug, and reviewing its possible adverse effects is warranted.

As noted in the discussion of KAS 3C, the AHRQ review identified a number of adverse effects during propranolol treatment. Adverse effects most frequently reported included sleep disturbances, cold extremities, gastrointestinal symptoms, bronchial irritation (classified as hyperreactivity, bronchospasm, bronchiolitis, and cold-induced wheezing), and a decrease in heart rate or blood pressure. Rates of clinically important harms (hypoglycemia, hypotension, bradycardia, and bronchospasm) varied widely across the studies, and the authors assigned a moderate SOE for the association of propranolol with both clinically important and minor harms (with high study limitations).[46] Overall, harms did not cause treatment discontinuation.

Our additional review yielded 8 reports that met inclusion criteria for harms of interventions. Sleep disturbance, sleeping disorders, agitation during the night, and nightmares or night terrors were mentioned in 6 of 8 reports and occurred in 2% to 18.5% of patients who were treated.[80,82,85,86,89,90] In 3 of these 6 reports, propranolol treatment was modified (reduction in dosage, earlier-evening dosing, and early discontinuation of therapy) in response to these effects.[80,82,85]

In 4 reports, possible respiratory adverse effects were mentioned, including labored breathing in 0.9%,[86] breathing-related problems in 11.5%,[89] respiratory disorders in 3.4%,[80] and wheezing or bronchiolitis in 12.9%.[82] In 3 of these series treatment modifications in response to the respiratory events were mentioned, including temporary discontinuation of therapy[80,82] and decreased dosage of propranolol.[89]

TABLE 15 Key Action Statement 3D: Clinicians should evaluate patients for and educate caregivers about potential adverse effects of propranolol, including sleep disturbances, bronchial irritation, and clinically symptomatic bradycardia and hypotension (grade X, strong recommendation).

Aggregate Evidence Quality	Grade X
Benefits	Recognition of adverse effects of propranolol treatment
Risks, harm, cost	Risk of caregivers declining medical therapy because of concern about potential adverse effects
Benefit-harm assessment	Benefits outweigh harms
Intentional vagueness	None
Role of patient preference	None
Exclusions	None
Strength	Strong recommendation
Key references	3,46,61,76,80,85–88

Although bradycardia and hypotension are known to accompany propranolol-associated β-receptor blockade, both tend to be mild and asymptomatic in children treated for IHs who have no preexisting cardiac comorbidities.[3,84,87,88,91–93] In the subcommittee's review, only 1 of the 8 reports mentioned hypotension or bradycardia as an adverse event, with 1 of 906 patients (0.1%) exhibiting bradycardia and 2 of 906 exhibiting asymptomatic hypotension.[80] The use of pretreatment electrocardiography (ECG) is controversial. Although this initially was advocated by some, several studies have revealed no actionable findings with continuous ECG monitoring, and researchers have questioned its value.[61,91] FDA guidelines for patient monitoring do not include routine ECG.[61] In their consensus recommendations, Drolet et al[61] suggest ECG screening only (1) in infants with a baseline heart rate below normal for age, (2) in infants with a family history of congenital heart conditions or arrhythmias or with a maternal history of connective tissue disease, or (3) when there is a history of arrhythmia or one is auscultated during examination. Currently, the FDA-approved administration guidelines mirror those used in the pivotal clinical trial, with a recommendation for in-office intermittent heart rate and blood pressure monitoring for 2 hours after the first dose of propranolol or for increasing the dose for infants 5 weeks' adjusted gestational age or older.[76] Monitoring for those who are younger or for those with other comorbidities should be individualized and may require brief hospitalization for medication initiation. These recommendations may change over time as more information becomes available now that the medication is in widespread use.

Theoretical concerns about adverse effects of propranolol on brain development have been raised. As a highly lipophilic β-blocker, propranolol has the ability to cross the blood brain barrier.[94] Adult studies have revealed impairments in short- and long-term memory, psychomotor function, and mood, and prenatal β-blockade has been associated with long-term cognitive impairment,[95,96] leading some to question the potential central nervous system effects of this agent when used to treat young children with IHs.[97,98] In the large prospective randomized propranolol trial conducted by Léauté-Labrèze et al,[76] no appreciable neurodevelopmental differences were noted between the propranolol-treated groups and the placebo group at week 96. Four other studies addressing development in infants treated with propranolol for

IHs have yielded conflicting results. In 2 case series (with a total of 272 patients), gross motor delay was reported in 4.8% to 6.9%.[99,100] In contrast, a case series of 141 patients found psychomotor delay in only 1 child, and a controlled trial of 82 children found no increase in the rate of developmental concerns as assessed by the Ages and Stages Questionnaire.[101,102] Although these latter studies are reassuring, further prospective psychometric studies of children treated with oral propranolol for IHs may be warranted.

Key Action Statement 3E (Table 16)

Clinicians may prescribe oral prednisolone or prednisone to treat IHs if there are contraindications or an inadequate response to oral propranolol (grade B, moderate recommendation).

The purpose of this statement is to highlight the utility of systemic corticosteroid therapy for IHs in certain settings, such as for patients in whom β-blocker therapy is contraindicated, poorly tolerated, or ineffective. Systemic therapy with corticosteroids was considered the standard of care for several decades before being supplanted by oral propranolol.

In the AHRQ review, oral steroids had a mean estimate of expected clearance of 43% (Table 12).[46,103] The AHRQ report identified 24 studies (3 RCTs, 1 cohort study, and 20 case series) reporting outcomes and/or harms after corticosteroid use in children with IHs. One RCT was judged as good, 1 as fair, and 1 as poor quality, and the cohort study was judged as fair quality (all case series were judged as poor quality for harms reporting). The steroids studied varied in terms of dose, type, route of administration, and patient ages. Children in steroid treatment arms typically had modest improvement in lesion size, but outcomes were difficult to compare given differences in scales. The optimal dosing of systemic corticosteroids for IHs remains unclear. Dose ranges of prednisone or prednisolone reported most frequently in the literature are between 2 and 5 mg/kg per day,[3,70,104–106] and most consider optimal dosing to be 2 to 3 mg/kg per day. Typical protocols include treating at full dose for 4 to 12 weeks followed by a gradual taper and completion of therapy by 9 to 12 months of age.[3,70,105,106] Some have advocated for shorter treatment durations (1–6 weeks), with multiple intermittent courses as needed.[107]

In the AHRQ review, steroids were consistently associated with clinically important harms, including Cushingoid appearance, infection, growth retardation, hypertension, and mood changes. The authors considered the SOE to be moderate for the association of steroids with clinically important harms.[46]

Key Action Statement 3F (Table 17)

Clinicians may recommend intralesional injection of triamcinolone and/or betamethasone to treat focal, bulky IHs during proliferation or in certain critical anatomic locations (eg, the lip) (grade B, moderate recommendation).

The purpose of this statement is to highlight the utility of intralesional corticosteroid injection for certain IH subsets. Numerous studies have reported success in the use of steroid injections for IHs, demonstrating it to be safe and effective.[108–114] This modality is most often reserved for IHs that are relatively small and well localized where proliferation is resulting in increased bulk and threatening anatomic landmarks (eg, the lip or nose). Larger or more extensive lesions are poorer candidates for this treatment modality given the larger volume of steroids necessary (and the inherent systemic risks), the difficulty of obtaining even distribution throughout the tumor, and the potential for local complications in lesions that are mostly flat or superficial.[3] Most studies have used triamcinolone either alone or in conjunction with betamethasone, with injections given on average every 4 to 6 weeks (but with wide variability). Repeat injections are often administered, with the number used ranging in most reports from 1 to 7.[109–112]

The AHRQ review found that intralesional triamcinolone had a mean estimate of expected clearance of 58% (Table 12).[46,103] Overall, the SOE was low for intralesional steroids having a modest effect relative to control, with wide confidence bounds.[46] The subcommittee's additional search yielded 1 report that met inclusion criteria for benefits of interventions as a comparative study. This was a retrospective review of patients with periocular IHs treated with oral propranolol, who were compared with a cohort treated with intralesional corticosteroid injection. Both groups showed a reduction in astigmatism over 12 months, and neither experienced significant adverse effects necessitating dose reduction or treatment cessation.[115] The authors concluded that oral propranolol (given its efficacy and safety profiles) has emerged as the treatment of choice for periocular IHs requiring therapy.[115]

Steroids (oral and intralesional forms were grouped together in the AHRQ harms analysis) were consistently associated with clinically important harms, including Cushingoid appearance, infection, growth retardation, hypertension, and mood changes. The authors considered the SOE to be moderate for the association of steroids with clinically important harms. The most commonly reported complications associated with intralesional steroid injection for IHs are transient Cushingoid features, failure to thrive, and local skin complications.[109–112] Local complications may include fat and/or dermal atrophy and pigmentary changes.[108–110] Adrenal suppression is infrequently reported in association with intralesional steroid injections but has been observed when large doses (eg, >4 mg/kg) have been administered.[116,117] There have been rare reports of central retinal artery embolization, usually after injection into IHs of the upper eyelid, likely related to high injection pressures and/or volumes.[118–121]

TABLE 16 Key Action Statement 3E: Clinicians may prescribe oral prednisolone or prednisone to treat IHs if there are contraindications or an inadequate response to oral propranolol (grade B, moderate recommendation).

Aggregate Evidence Quality	Grade B
Benefits	Modest benefit in IH clearance; medication cost is low
Risks, harm, cost	Clinically important harms; cost associated with the evaluation and treatment of adverse effects
Intentional vagueness	None
Benefit-harm assessment	Benefits outweigh harms
Role of patient preference	Shared decision-making regarding treatment
Exclusions	None
Strength	Moderate recommendation
Key references	46,70,103

TABLE 17 Key Action Statement 3F: Clinicians may recommend intralesional injection of triamcinolone and/or betamethasone to treat focal, bulky IHs during proliferation or in certain critical anatomic locations (eg, the lip) (grade B, moderate recommendation).

Aggregate Evidence Quality	Grade B
Benefits	Modest benefit in IH clearance
Risks, harm, cost	Clinically important harms; cost of medication, visits for injection; risk of anesthesia if used
Benefit-harm assessment	Benefits outweigh harms in selected clinical situations
Intentional vagueness	None
Role of patient preference	Shared decision-making regarding route of drug delivery
Exclusions	None
Strength	Moderate recommendation
Key references	3,46,103,108–112

Key Action Statement 3G (Table 18)

Clinicians may prescribe topical timolol maleate as a therapy for thin and/or superficial IHs (grade B, moderate recommendation).

The purpose of this statement is to highlight the potential utility of topical timolol in treating thin and/or superficial IHs. Topical timolol maleate, a nonselective β-adrenergic receptor inhibitor, has been used in the treatment of pediatric glaucoma as a first-line agent for several decades.[122,127,128] Treatment of IHs with ophthalmic timolol maleate was initially reported in 2010, and since that time, there have been many reports (including some with hundreds of patients), as well as an RCT, with positive findings.[40,122–125,129–134] On the basis of these reports showing efficacy with minimal adverse effects, timolol is increasingly being used for thin and superficial IHs, and many centers report that their use of timolol exceeds that of oral β-blockers.[135]

In the AHRQ review, 2 RCTs and 4 cohort studies were included. Topical timolol had a mean estimate of expected clearance of 62% (Table 12).[46,103] Timolol was significantly more effective than observation or a placebo in 3 studies; 1 study comparing topical imiquimod with timolol did not demonstrate superiority of either agent but was found to have insufficient SOE.[46] Our subsequent review found 3 further reports meeting criteria for efficacy, including 1study comparing timolol to an ultrapotent corticosteroid and 2 other studies of timolol alone.[40,133,134] In the largest of these, a multicenter retrospective cohort study of 731 patients, most infants were treated with the 0.5% gel-forming solution. The study reveal improvement in nearly 70% of patients treated for 1 to 3 months and in 92.3% of patients who received 6 to 9 months of therapy. The greatest improvement was in color; however, with a longer duration of treatment, improvement in size, extent, and volume were also observed. Best responses were observed in thinner superficial IHs (ie, <1 mm thick) versus mixed or deep IHs. The large majority of infants studied were 6 months or younger at time of initiation of treatment, and 41% were ≤3 months of age. This suggests that early topical timolol treatment may also inhibit IH growth. Only 7% of infants required subsequent treatment with a systemic β-blocker.[40]

Although pharmacokinetic data are limited, evidence suggests that timolol maleate can be detected in the blood or urine of at least some infants treated topically.[126,136] Additional pharmacokinetic studies are needed given occasional reports of systemic toxicity.[137–139] It should be noted that timolol is significantly more potent than propranolol, and topical application avoids first-pass liver metabolism, as would occur with an oral β-blocker.[127] Pending the results of ongoing studies, these factors should lead to caution when using timolol, especially if prescribing more than 1 drop twice daily or when treating preterm or young infants.

The AHRQ report emphasized that there were far more reports of harms with oral β-blockers than with timolol but did note 1 report of shortness of breath and insomnia.[46] Subsequent to that report, tolerability data have been reassuring overall, but some adverse events have been reported.[40,122,124,125,131–134,140] In the large cohort study of 731 patients conducted by Püttgen et al,[40] adverse events were noted in 3.4% of patients and included local irritation (nearly half of the adverse events) and bronchospasm (in 3 patients); no cardiovascular events were reported. No adverse events were significant enough to necessitate drug discontinuation.[40] In a retrospective case series of 30 children with ulcerated IHs treated with topical timolol maleate 0.5% gel-forming solution and evaluating for

TABLE 18 Key Action Statement 3G: Clinicians may prescribe topical timolol maleate as a therapy for thin and/or superficial IHs (grade B, moderate recommendation).

Aggregate Evidence Quality	Grade B
Benefit	Modest benefit in IH clearance
Harm	Low but possible risk of local irritation, sleep disturbance, cold extremities, bronchospasm, and bradycardia, with more caution needed in preterm infants and those without intact skin (ie, ulceration)
Cost	Cost of medication
Benefits-harm assessment	Benefits outweigh harms
Value judgments	None
Role of patient preference	Parents have a significant role in decision-making regarding the desire to treat small superficial lesions for which timolol may be effective
Intentional vagueness	None
Exclusions	Lesions that are large size, significantly elevated, or life-threatening
Strength	Moderate recommendation
Key references	40,46,85,122–126

adverse events, sleep disturbance was observed in 1 infant (who was treated simultaneously with oral propranolol and topical timolol) and a single episode of cold extremities was reported in another. The remainder had no reported adverse events.[141] Bradycardia, both symptomatic and asymptomatic, was reported in 4 of 22 young and preterm infants given timolol for IHs. Two infants had bradycardia that was mild and asymptomatic, but in 2 (both of whom were born preterm and weighed less than 2500 g at initiation of therapy) there were associated symptoms.[126] To address concerns regarding potential percutaneous absorption and toxicity, many authors have advocated using limited amounts of medication (eg, 1 drop 2–3 times per day),[40] and some have cautioned against application to ulcerated lesions.[127]

SURGICAL MANAGEMENT

Key Action Statement 4 (Table 19)

Clinicians may recommend surgery and laser therapy as treatment options in managing selected IHs (grade C, moderate recommendation).

The purpose of this statement is to support surgery and laser therapy as treatment options for selected IHs, although it is recommended that decisions regarding their use should be made in consultation with a hemangioma specialist, especially in young infants. With the advent of β-blocker therapy, surgical and laser approaches are used less frequently.

In general, surgical interventions are not performed in infancy. During this time, anesthetic risks are of greater concern, and the tumor is highly vascular, posing a higher risk of blood loss, iatrogenic injury, and an inferior outcome.[142,143,145]

In certain locations, such as the lip and nasal tip, the final cosmetic result is superior when growth of the lesion has ceased and the number of surgical interventions can be kept to a minimum. Furthermore, there is no psychosocial urgency to improve a deformity caused by IHs in this age group because long-term memory and self-esteem are not established until later in childhood.[143,146–148] There are certain clinical situations, however, in which early surgery can be an important treatment option. These include IHs that ulcerate, obstruct or deform vital structures (such as the airway or orbit), or involve aesthetically sensitive areas. In these circumstances, surgery may be indicated when (1) the lesion has failed to improve with local wound care and/or pharmacotherapy; (2) the lesion is well localized, and early surgery will simplify later reconstruction (eg, a prominent IH involving the ear or eyelid [causing ptosis]); (3) the lesion is well localized in an anatomically favorable area; or (4) resection is likely to be necessary in the future, and the resultant scar would be the same.[142,143,145] The decision to undertake surgery during infancy should take into consideration current knowledge of the risks of general anesthesia in this age group.[53–55]

Surgery also is an important treatment option for IHs that, despite involution, have left residual skin changes (eg, thinned skin, scar, fibrofatty tissue, telangiectasias, and/or anatomic deformities in areas such as the nose, ear, or lip).[19,20,143] In most cases, deferring surgery until the child is 3 to 5 years of age is reasonable because: (1) the lesion may resolve significantly without leaving a deformity that necessitates intervention; (2) the tumor is smaller than it was during infancy, and thus, the operation is often easier, and the resultant scar may be smaller; and (3) the IH primarily is adipose tissue instead of blood vessels, and thus, the operation is safer.[142,143,145] However, it is usually unnecessary to wait longer than 3 to 5 years of age because the previously accepted adage that 50% of IHs complete involution by 5 years of age, 70% by 7 years of age, and 90% by 9 years of age has proven to be incorrect.[19,143,149] In fact, most IHs do not improve significantly after 3 to 4 years of age.[20,143] Moreover, performing surgery at this earlier age can be beneficial in minimizing stigma and impact on a child's self-esteem.[143] There is less urgency to correct a residual deformity in an area that is concealed by clothing (eg, a lesion on the trunk). Some parents may elect to wait until the child is older and able to help in decision-making, especially if the reason for surgery is the management of less disfiguring skin changes.[143]

Laser Management

PDL has been used for several decades to treat IHs. The AHRQ review noted that most studies that were reviewed

TABLE 19 Key Action Statement 4: Clinicians may recommend surgery and laser therapy as treatment options in managing selected IHs (grade C, moderate recommendation).

Aggregate Evidence Quality	Grade C
Benefits	Early surgical intervention after infancy corrects residual deformities before the child's self-esteem develops
Risks, harm, cost	Risk of surgical complications and general anesthesia; costs associated with operative intervention, anesthesia, and postoperative care
Benefits-harm assessment	Preponderance of benefit
Intentional vagueness	None
Role of patient preference	Significant
Exclusions	Children with a nonproblematic IH
Strength	Moderate recommendation
Key references	20,142–144

evaluated PDL (as opposed to other lasers) and examined heterogeneous end points (the latter factor limiting the ability to draw conclusions). However, there is low SOE that PDL is more effective in reducing IH size when compared with observation.[46] There is evidence that PDL is superior to other lasers. In contrast, there is wide recognition that PDL is effective and safe in removing residual macular erythema and superficial telangiectasias in involuting or involuted IHs, but it often requires several treatments to achieve optimal results.[1,142] Other lasers, such as erbium-yttrium-aluminum-garnet, have been reportedly effective in ameliorating textural changes in small case series.[150] Harms associated with laser therapy that were identified in the AHRQ review included skin atrophy, bleeding, scarring, ulceration, purpura, and pigmentation changes.[46] The AHRQ review also noted that most studies of lasers reviewed evaluated lasers as a first-line treatment, a practice that is less common since the advent of β-blocker treatment.

There is controversy regarding whether PDL should be used to treat IHs early in infancy (ie, during the proliferative phase). Several case reports and case series have revealed an increased risk of ulceration, scarring, and hypopigmentation when PDL is used during this period.[1,144,151] Moreover, PDL penetrates only into the superficial dermis, and thus, although redness may be diminished, deeper elements of the IH (that increase the risk of residual skin changes) are not affected.[144,152,153]

Some authors advocate for using PDL as a treatment of ulceration. However, evidence supporting the use of PDL for this indication comes from case reports and small case series. Propranolol has been associated with faster healing of ulceration when compared with laser therapy and antibiotics.[46]

PARENT EDUCATION

Key Action Statement 5 (Table 20)

Clinicians should educate parents of infants with an IH about the condition, including the expected natural history, and its potential for causing complications or disfigurement (grade X, strong recommendation).

The purpose of this statement is to ensure that parents are knowledgeable about their child's IH and to provide clinicians with a framework for educating those parents about IHs. The information provided by clinicians should be as specific to the patient's IH as possible (eg, indicating whether and why an IH is low risk and, thus, likely to cause no problems or sequelae or is potentially high risk and requires urgent evaluation or treatment; Table 3, illustrated in Figs 2–4, Supplemental Table 22, and Supplemental Fig 11).

IHs That Do Not Raise Concern

In a primary care setting, the majority of IHs are not problematic and require no active intervention (ie, are low risk; Supplemental Table 22, Supplemental Fig 11). However, given their appearance, even nonproblematic (that is, low-risk) IHs may cause significant parental anxiety and concern. These emotions may be amplified by information gleaned from Internet searches that show photographs emphasizing the more severe end of the disease spectrum as well as public reactions to the child's IH if the lesion is located at a site not easily covered by clothing.[42,155,156] Formal educational efforts can reduce parental anxiety and enhance comfort with a plan to observe the IH for any unexpected or worrisome changes.[154]

Parents should be educated about the natural history of IHs. Specifically, they may be advised that, although growth characteristics vary from case to case, most superficial IHs have a maximum growth potential between 1 and 3 months of age[3,21,157] and that the majority of growth is complete by 5 months of age.[22] Deeper IHs may have a slightly later onset and a more prolonged duration of growth. During the period of growth, clinicians should encourage parents to call, schedule an office visit, or share photographs of the IH with them to reassess if concerns exist about the lesion's appearance, unexpectedly rapid growth, ulceration, bleeding, or pain, all findings that indicate that a lesion is no longer low risk.

Parents should be advised that by age 5 to 12 months, most IHs have stopped growing and are beginning to involute. For IHs with a superficial component, this appears as a gradual change in color from red to milky-white or gray. Lesions gradually flatten and shrink from the center outward. Involution proceeds more slowly than growth. Newer studies have demonstrated that 90% of IH involution is complete by 4 years of age.[20,143] This is in contrast to traditional teaching that involution proceeds at 10% per year (ie, 50% of IHs resolve by 5 years of age and 90% by 9 years of age). Parents should be advised that even after involution, residual changes, such as telangiectasias, redundant skin, or a scar,[3,19] may be left. It is usually possible to tell whether such changes are going to persist by 4 years of age, and if concerning, consultation for management of these skin changes, particularly laser or surgical treatment, may be pursued.

A collection of serial photographs can be useful to demonstrate to parents the natural history of IHs and the process of spontaneous involution.[154] Such photos are available on the Hemangioma Investigator Group (https://hemangiomaeducation.org/) and Yale Dermatology (http://medicine.yale.edu/dermatology/patient/conditions/hemangioma.aspx) Web sites. Information sheets (ie, handouts) are available from the Society for Pediatric Dermatology Web site (http://pedsderm.net/) under the "For Patients and Families" tab, and adapted versions of their hemangioma patient information and propranolol sheets are included in the What Are Hemangiomas? Propranolol for Hemangiomas, and Medication Information sections of the Supplemental Information. A video for parents is also available on the Society for Pediatric Dermatology Web site (https://pedsderm.net/for-patients-families/patient-education-videos/#InfantileHemangiomas). Information also is available from the AHRQ (https://effectivehealthcare.ahrq.gov/topics/infantile-hemangioma/consumer/),[158] and answers to frequently asked questions are available on the Hemangioma Investigator Group and Yale Dermatology Web sites.

IHs That May Be Problematic

When confronted with a potentially problematic IH (ie, high risk; Table 3; illustrated in Figs 2–4, Supplemental Table 22, and Supplemental Fig 11), primary care clinicians are encouraged to consult promptly with a hemangioma specialist unless they have the experience and knowledge to manage such patients independently. Because IH proliferation may occur early and be unpredictable and because there is a window of opportunity for optimal treatment, caregivers can be advised that consultation should take place in a timely manner. Unfortunately, this does not always occur. Although caregivers first notice lesions by 1 month of age (on average, at 2 weeks) and the ideal time for consultation may be 4 weeks of age, 1 study found that the mean age at presentation to a dermatologist was 5 months, by which time most growth is complete.[21,22]

Recognizing that it may be difficult to obtain an appointment with a hemangioma specialist in a timely manner, caregivers and clinicians may need to advocate on behalf of the infant. In settings where a hemangioma specialist is not readily available, telemedicine triage or consultation, using photographs taken by caregivers or the clinician, can be helpful. In 1 academic center in Spain, teledermatology triage reduced the age at first evaluation of an infant with an IH from 5.9 to 3.5 months.[159]

Once the hemangioma specialist has an opportunity to meet with parents and evaluate the infant, a discussion about management can take place. If medical treatment is recommended, the specialist will educate parents about the medication and its dosing, its possible adverse effects, and the expected duration of treatment. If the medication selected is propranolol, as often is the case, a patient information sheet (such as that developed by the Society for Pediatric Dermatology or that provided in the What Are Hemangiomas? and Propranolol for Hemangiomas sections of the Supplemental Information) or information from the article by Martin et al[160] may be provided. For families unable to travel to see a hemangioma specialist, collaborative care may be considered. The hemangioma specialist can evaluate serial photographs and provide the primary care clinician with guidance on treatment. In this case, the primary care clinician will assume a more active role in parent education.

TABLE 20 Key Action Statement 5: Clinicians should educate parents of infants with an IH about the condition, including the expected natural history, and its potential for causing complications or disfigurement (grade X, strong recommendation).

Aggregate Evidence Quality	Grade X
Benefits	Promotes parent satisfaction and understanding, may reduce medication errors, may improve clinical outcomes
Risks, harm, cost	May increase parental anxiety because of the need to administer medication; time spent in education, may increase health care costs because of the need for follow-up visits
Benefit-harm assessment	Benefits outweigh harms
Intentional vagueness	None
Role of parental preferences	Essential; shared decision-making regarding the need for treatment is vital
Exclusions	None
Strength	Strong recommendation
Key references	21,22,154

CHALLENGES TO IMPLEMENTING THIS CPG

Several potential challenges exist to implementing this CPG. The first is the dynamic nature of individual IHs with a period of rapid growth, the degree of which can be difficult to predict, particularly in young infants. There are no surrogate markers or imaging studies that have been shown to reliably predict growth. Hence, frequent in-person visits or a review of parental photos may be needed, especially in infants younger than 3 to 4 months. However, this may be complicated by the frequency and timing of well-child visits during this period. After the first-week visit, an infant who is well, has regained birth weight, and has parents who are experienced caregivers may not be seen again until 2 months of age. As noted by Tollefson and Frieden,[21] most superficial IHs have accelerated growth between 5 and 7 weeks of age, and 4 weeks of age may be the ideal time for referral if high-risk features are present. Thus, the most dramatic IH growth (and potentially permanent skin changes) may occur during a time when an infant is not scheduled to see a health care provider. Although awareness of this issue does not justify altering the interval of well-child visits for all infants, it heightens the need for more frequent monitoring in those with possible or definite IHs. Prompt evaluation, either in-person or via photographs, is warranted for any infant reported by parents to have a changing birthmark during the first 2 months of life.

A second challenge is the wide heterogeneity of IHs in terms of size, location, patterns of distribution (ie, segmental versus localized), and depth (ie, superficial, mixed, or deep). This heterogeneity, particularly when combined with the unpredictable growth of any given IH, may lead to uncertainty in management (ie, whether to treat or observe). Although this CPG provides guidance regarding risk stratification and growth characteristics, there is no one-size-fits-all approach. If uncertainty exists, consultation with a hemangioma specialist (whether by an in-person visit or photographic triage) can be helpful.

A third challenge is the long-held tenet that IHs are benign and go away. Because of this myth, parents and caregivers are often reassured that the lesion will disappear, and this is accurate in the vast majority of cases. However, there is ample evidence that false reassurance can be given even in high-risk cases; indeed, all hemangioma specialists have seen examples of lost opportunities to intervene and prevent poor outcomes because of lack of or delayed referral. The availability of highly effective treatments for IHs makes it critical that this myth is debunked and that practitioners become more comfortable with the concept of identifying high-risk IHs that require close observation or prompt intervention.

Last, some geographical locations lack access to prompt specialty care from hemangioma specialists. Lack of access can also result in delays in referrals or prompt appointments. Possible solutions could include establishing resources for the photographic triage of cases in which risk stratification is uncertain or in which triage to hasten referral can be augmented by this methodology.

EVIDENCE GAPS AND PROPOSED FUTURE DIRECTIONS

The proportion of IHs in primary care settings that are truly high risk is not known. Even in a referral setting, the proportions needing active intervention vary depending on referral patterns.[3,161] This information would be useful to pediatricians and other primary care providers and should be the subject of future research.

Scoring systems for IH severity have been proposed, and one in particular, the Hemangioma Severity Score, has gained some favor as a triage tool.[162–164] However, more research is needed to ensure that it can accurately be interpreted by primary care physicians and to find scores that capture the vast majority of high-risk IHs requiring specialty care without overreferring.

Other important evidence gaps should be highlighted, including the following:

- How safe is topical timolol as a treatment during early infancy, and which patients being treated with the drug need referral versus which can be observed without referral by the pediatrician?
- Is outpatient in-office cardiovascular monitoring for propranolol truly needed in healthy infants 5 weeks or older? Is blood pressure monitoring necessary, or is measuring heart rate sufficient?
- What is the role of the pediatrician in managing infants placed on β-blocker therapies (both topical and systemic), and are there specific time frames for specialty reevaluation?
- How accurate are primary care physicians in identifying high-risk IHs using parameters such as those outlined in this CPG?
- Are pediatric trainees receiving adequate training in risk stratification and management of IHs?

Some of these questions may be answered by research that is currently underway. Other studies will be needed to identify and remedy remaining gaps. Moreover, because there has been a tremendous accrual of information about IH management, there will need to be periodic updates as new information becomes available (and possibly sooner than the 5 years typical for CPGs). With such ongoing reassessment and revision, the subcommittee hopes this CPG will be viewed as an effective guide to IH triage and management and to minimize poor outcomes from higher-risk IHs. One barrier to a better understanding of IHs and to answering the questions posed here is the imprecision of current diagnostic codes. For example, the *International Classification of Diseases, 10th Revision* code for "hemangioma of the skin and subcutaneous tissues" is not specific to IHs and can include other entities (eg, congenital hemangioma and verrucous hemangioma) that are not IHs. In addition, current diagnostic codes do not contain sufficient detail to permit appreciation of higher-risk features, such as location or multifocality. Advocacy for the creation of a unique and exclusive *International*

Classification of Diseases, 10th Revision code (and appropriate modifiers) for IHs would be an appropriate step in addressing this issue.

Implementation tools for this guideline are available on the AAP Web site at https://www.aap.org/en-us/professional-resources/quality-improvement/Pages/default.aspx (this may leave or stay depending on the Digital Transformation Initiative). A useful resource for clinicians is the AAP Web page, "Diagnosis and Management of Infantile Hemangiomas" (https://www.aap.org/en-us/advocacy-and-policy/aap-health-initiatives/Infantile-Hemangiomas/Pages/default.aspx).

LEAD AUTHORS

Daniel P. Krowchuk, MD, FAAP
Ilona J. Frieden, MD, FAAP
Anthony J. Mancini MD, FAAP
David H. Darrow, MD, DDS, FAAP
Francine Blei, MD, MBA, FAAP
Arin K. Greene, MD, FAAP
Aparna Annam, DO, FAAP
Cynthia N. Baker, MD, FAAP
Peter C. Frommelt, MD
Amy Hodak, CPMSM
Brian M. Pate, MD, FHM, FAAP
Janice L. Pelletier, MD, FAAP
Deborah Sandrock, MD, FAAP
Stuart T. Weinberg, MD, FAAP
Mary Anne Whelan, MD, PhD, FAAP

SUBCOMMITTEE ON THE MANAGEMENT OF INFANTILE HEMANGIOMAS (OVERSIGHT BY THE COUNCIL ON QUALITY IMPROVEMENT AND PATIENT SAFETY)

Daniel P. Krowchuk, MD, FAAP, Chairperson, General Pediatrics and Adolescent Medicine
Ilona Frieden, MD, FAAP, Vice Chairperson, Pediatric Dermatology
Aparna Annam, DO, FAAP, Pediatric Radiology
Cynthia N. Baker, MD, FAAP, General Pediatrics
Francine Blei, MD, MBA, FAAP, Pediatric Hematology-Oncology
David H. Darrow, MD, DDS, FAAP, Otolaryngology Head and Neck Surgery
Peter C. Frommelt, MD, Pediatric Cardiology
Arin K. Greene, MD, FAAP, Plastic Surgery
Amy Hodak, CPMSM, Family Representative
Anthony J. Mancini, MD, FAAP, Pediatric Dermatology
Brian M. Pate, MD, FHM, FAAP, Implementation Scientist
Janice L. Pelletier, MD, FAAP, General Pediatrics
Deborah Sandrock, MD, FAAP, General Pediatrics
Stuart T. Weinberg, MD, FAAP, Partnership for Policy Implementation Representative
Mary Anne Whelan, MD, PhD, FAAP, Epidemiologist and Methodologist

STAFF

Kymika Okechukwu, MPA, Senior Manager, Evidence-Based Medicine Initiatives

ABBREVIATIONS

AAP: American Academy of Pediatrics
AHRQ: Agency for Healthcare Research and Quality
CPG: clinical practice guideline
ECG: electrocardiography
FDA: Food and Drug Administration
IH: infantile hemangioma
IH-MAG: infantile hemangioma with minimal or arrested growth
KAS: key action statement
LUMBAR: lower body infantile hemangiomas and other cutaneous defects, urogenital anomalies and ulceration, myelopathy, bony deformities, anorectal malformations, and arterial anomalies and renal anomalies
MRA: magnetic resonance angiography
PDL: pulsed-dye laser
PHACE: posterior fossa defects, hemangiomas, cerebrovascular arterial anomalies, cardiovascular anomalies (including coarctation of the aorta), and eye anomalies
RCT: randomized controlled trial
SOE: strength of evidence

The guidance in this report does not indicate an exclusive course of treatment or serve as a standard of medical care. Variations, taking into account individual circumstances, may be appropriate.

All clinical practice guidelines from the American Academy of Pediatrics automatically expire 5 years after publication unless reaffirmed, revised, or retired at or before that time.

DOI: https://doi.org/10.1542/peds.2018-3475

Address correspondence to Daniel P. Krowchuk, MD, FAAP. E-mail: krowchuk@wakehealth.edu

PEDIATRICS (ISSN Numbers: Print, 0031-4005; Online, 1098-4275).

Copyright © 2019 by the American Academy of Pediatrics

FINANCIAL DISCLOSURE: Dr Frieden is a member of the Data Monitoring Safety Board for Pfizer and the Scientific Advisory Board for Venthera/Bridge Bio; Dr Mancini has indicated that he has advisory board relationships with Verrica, Valeant, and Pfizer; the other authors have indicated they have no financial relationships relevant to this article to disclose.

FUNDING: No external funding.

POTENTIAL CONFLICT OF INTEREST: The authors have indicated they have no potential conflicts of interest to disclose.

REFERENCES

1. Hoeger PH, Harper JI, Baselga E, et al. Treatment of infantile haemangiomas: recommendations of a European expert group. *Eur J Pediatr.* 2015;174(7):855–865
2. Smithson SL, Rademaker M, Adams S, et al. Consensus statement for the treatment of infantile haemangiomas with propranolol. *Australas J Dermatol.* 2017;58(2):155–159
3. Darrow DH, Greene AK, Mancini AJ, Nopper AJ; Section on Dermatology; Section on Otolaryngology–Head and Neck Surgery; Section on Plastic Surgery. Diagnosis and management of infantile hemangioma. *Pediatrics.* 2015;136(4). Available at: www.pediatrics.org/cgi/content/full/136/4/e1060
4. Agency for Healthcare Research and Quality. Effective health care program.

Available at: www.effectivehealthcare.ahrq.gov/reports/final.cfm. Accessed February 6, 2018

5. Haggstrom AN, Garzon MC, Baselga E, et al. Risk for PHACE syndrome in infants with large facial hemangiomas. *Pediatrics.* 2010;126(2). Available at: www.pediatrics.org/cgi/content/full/126/2/e418
6. Orlow SJ, Isakoff MS, Blei F. Increased risk of symptomatic hemangiomas of the airway in association with cutaneous hemangiomas in a "beard" distribution. *J Pediatr.* 1997;131(4):643–646
7. Kulungowski AM, Alomari AI, Chawla A, Christison-Lagay ER, Fishman SJ. Lessons from a liver hemangioma registry: subtype classification. *J Pediatr Surg.* 2012;47(1):165–170
8. Rialon KL, Murillo R, Fevurly RD, et al. Risk factors for mortality in patients with multifocal and diffuse hepatic hemangiomas. *J Pediatr Surg.* 2015;50(5):837–841
9. Huang SA, Tu HM, Harney JW, et al. Severe hypothyroidism caused by type 3 iodothyronine deiodinase in infantile hemangiomas. *N Engl J Med.* 2000;343(3):185–189
10. Horii KA, Drolet BA, Frieden IJ, et al; Hemangioma Investigator Group. Prospective study of the frequency of hepatic hemangiomas in infants with multiple cutaneous infantile hemangiomas. *Pediatr Dermatol.* 2011;28(3):245–253
11. Rialon KL, Murillo R, Fevurly RD, et al. Impact of screening for hepatic hemangiomas in patients with multiple cutaneous infantile hemangiomas. *Pediatr Dermatol.* 2015;32(6):808–812
12. Jockin YM, Friedlander SF. Periocular infantile hemangioma. *Int Ophthalmol Clin.* 2010;50(4):15–25
13. Schwartz SR, Blei F, Ceisler E, Steele M, Furlan L, Kodsi S. Risk factors for amblyopia in children with capillary hemangiomas of the eyelids and orbit. *J AAPOS.* 2006;10(3):262–268
14. Chamlin SL, Haggstrom AN, Drolet BA, et al. Multicenter prospective study of ulcerated hemangiomas [published correction appears in *J Pediatr.* 2008;152(4):597]. *J Pediatr.* 2007;151(6):684–689, 689.e1
15. Connelly EA, Viera M, Price C, Waner M. Segmental hemangioma of infancy complicated by life-threatening arterial bleed. *Pediatr Dermatol.* 2009;26(4):469–472
16. Garzon MC, Epstein LG, Heyer GL, et al. PHACE syndrome: consensus-derived diagnosis and care recommendations. *J Pediatr.* 2016;178:24–33.e2
17. Iacobas I, Burrows PE, Frieden IJ, et al. LUMBAR: association between cutaneous infantile hemangiomas of the lower body and regional congenital anomalies. *J Pediatr.* 2010;157(5):795–801.e1–e7
18. Shah SD, Baselga E, McCuaig C, et al. Rebound growth of infantile hemangiomas after propranolol therapy. *Pediatrics.* 2016;137(4):e20151754
19. Bauland CG, Lüning TH, Smit JM, Zeebregts CJ, Spauwen PH. Untreated hemangiomas: growth pattern and residual lesions. *Plast Reconstr Surg.* 2011;127(4):1643–1648
20. Baselga E, Roe E, Coulie J, et al. Risk factors for degree and type of sequelae after involution of untreated hemangiomas of infancy. *JAMA Dermatol.* 2016;152(11):1239–1243
21. Tollefson MM, Frieden IJ. Early growth of infantile hemangiomas: what parents' photographs tell us. *Pediatrics.* 2012;130(2). Available at: www.pediatrics.org/cgi/content/full/130/2/e314
22. Chang LC, Haggstrom AN, Drolet BA, et al; Hemangioma Investigator Group. Growth characteristics of infantile hemangiomas: implications for management. *Pediatrics.* 2008;122(2):360–367
23. Suh KY, Frieden IJ. Infantile hemangiomas with minimal or arrested growth: a retrospective case series. *Arch Dermatol.* 2010;146(9):971–976
24. Luu M, Frieden IJ. Haemangioma: clinical course, complications and management. *Br J Dermatol.* 2013;169(1):20–30
25. Shikhani AH, Jones MM, Marsh BR, Holliday MJ. Infantile subglottic hemangiomas. An update. *Ann Otol Rhinol Laryngol.* 1986;95(4, pt 1):336–347
26. Bitar MA, Moukarbel RV, Zalzal GH. Management of congenital subglottic hemangioma: trends and success over the past 17 years. *Otolaryngol Head Neck Surg.* 2005;132(2):226–231
27. Uthurriague C, Boccara O, Catteau B, et al. Skin patterns associated with upper airway infantile haemangiomas: a retrospective multicentre study. *Acta Derm Venereol.* 2016;96(7):963–966
28. Sherrington CA, Sim DK, Freezer NJ, Robertson CF. Subglottic haemangioma. *Arch Dis Child.* 1997;76(5):458–459
29. Sie KC, McGill T, Healy GB. Subglottic hemangioma: ten years' experience with the carbon dioxide laser. *Ann Otol Rhinol Laryngol.* 1994;103(3):167–172
30. Horii KA, Drolet BA, Baselga E, et al; Hemangioma Investigator Group. Risk of hepatic hemangiomas in infants with large hemangiomas. *Arch Dermatol.* 2010;146(2):201–203
31. Drolet BA, Pope E, Juern AM, et al. Gastrointestinal bleeding in infantile hemangioma: a complication of segmental, rather than multifocal, infantile hemangiomas. *J Pediatr.* 2012;160(6):1021–1026.e3
32. Viswanathan V, Smith ER, Mulliken JB, et al. Infantile hemangiomas involving the neuraxis: clinical and imaging findings. *AJNR Am J Neuroradiol.* 2009;30(5):1005–1013
33. von Noorden GK. Application of basic research data to clinical amblyopia. *Ophthalmology.* 1978;85(5):496–504
34. Dubois J, Milot J, Jaeger BI, McCuaig C, Rousseau E, Powell J. Orbit and eyelid hemangiomas: is there a relationship between location and ocular problems? *J Am Acad Dermatol.* 2006;55(4):614–619
35. Frank RC, Cowan BJ, Harrop AR, Astle WF, McPhalen DF. Visual development in infants: visual complications of periocular haemangiomas. *J Plast Reconstr Aesthet Surg.* 2010;63(1):1–8
36. Yan AC. Pain management for ulcerated hemangiomas. *Pediatr Dermatol.* 2008;25(6):586–589
37. Thomas MW, Burkhart CN, Vaghani SP, Morrell DS, Wagner AM. Failure to thrive in infants with complicated facial hemangiomas. *Pediatr Dermatol.* 2012;29(1):49–52

38. Shin HT, Orlow SJ, Chang MW. Ulcerated haemangioma of infancy: a retrospective review of 47 patients. *Br J Dermatol.* 2007;156(5):1050–1052

39. Frieden IJ, Reese V, Cohen D. PHACE syndrome. The association of posterior fossa brain malformations, hemangiomas, arterial anomalies, coarctation of the aorta and cardiac defects, and eye abnormalities. *Arch Dermatol.* 1996;132(3):307–311

40. Püttgen K, Lucky A, Adams D, et al; Hemangioma Investigator Group. Topical timolol maleate treatment of infantile hemangiomas. *Pediatrics.* 2016;138(3):e20160355

41. Jacobs AH. Strawberry hemangiomas; the natural history of the untreated lesion. *Calif Med.* 1957;86(1):8–10

42. Tanner JL, Dechert MP, Frieden IJ. Growing up with a facial hemangioma: parent and child coping and adaptation. *Pediatrics.* 1998;101 (3, pt 1):446–452

43. Fay A, Nguyen J, Waner M. Conceptual approach to the management of infantile hemangiomas. *J Pediatr.* 2010;157(6):881–888.e1–e5

44. O TM, Scheuermann-Poley C, Tan M, Waner M. Distribution, clinical characteristics, and surgical treatment of lip infantile hemangiomas. *JAMA Facial Plast Surg.* 2013;15(4):292–304

45. Ma EH, Robertson SJ, Chow CW, Bekhor PS. Infantile hemangioma with minimal or arrested growth: further observations on clinical and histopathologic findings of this unique but underrecognized entity. *Pediatr Dermatol.* 2017;34(1):64–71

46. Chinnadurai S, Snyder K, Sathe N, et al. *Diagnosis and Management of Infantile Hemangioma.* Rockville, MD: Agency for Healthcare Research and Quality; 2016

47. Menapace D, Mitkov M, Towbin R, Hogeling M. The changing face of complicated infantile hemangioma treatment. *Pediatr Radiol.* 2016;46(11):1494–1506

48. Bessis D, Bigorre M, Labrèze C. Reticular infantile hemangiomas with minimal or arrested growth associated with lipoatrophy. *J Am Acad Dermatol.* 2015;72(5):828–833

49. Dickie B, Dasgupta R, Nair R, et al. Spectrum of hepatic hemangiomas: management and outcome. *J Pediatr Surg.* 2009;44(1):125–133

50. Rotter A, Samorano LP, de Oliveira Labinas GH, et al. Ultrasonography as an objective tool for assessment of infantile hemangioma treatment with propranolol. *Int J Dermatol.* 2017;56(2):190–194

51. Mamlouk MD, Hess CP. Arterial spin-labeled perfusion for vascular anomalies in the pediatric head and neck. *Clin Imaging.* 2016;40(5):1040–1046

52. Aggarwal N, Tekes A, Bosemani T. Infantile hepatic hemangioma: role of dynamic contrast-enhanced magnetic resonance angiography. *J Pediatr.* 2015;167(4):940–940.e1

53. US Food and Drug Administration. FDA drug safety communications: FDA review results in new warnings about using general anesthetics and sedation drugs in young children and pregnant women. 2016. Available at: www.fda.gov/downloads/Drugs/DrugSafety/UCM533197.pdf. Accessed September 10, 2018

54. American Society of Anesthesiologists. ASA response to the FDA med watch warning - December 16, 2016. 2016. Available at: https://www.asahq.org/advocacy-and-asapac/fda-and-washington-alerts/washington-alerts/2016/12/asa-response-to-the-fda-med-watch. Accessed September 10, 2018

55. Practice advisory on anesthetic care for magnetic resonance imaging: an updated report by the American Society of Anesthesiologists Task Force on Anesthetic Care for Magnetic Resonance Imaging. *Anesthesiology.* 2015;122(3):495–520

56. Drolet BA, Chamlin SL, Garzon MC, et al. Prospective study of spinal anomalies in children with infantile hemangiomas of the lumbosacral skin. *J Pediatr.* 2010;157(5):789–794

57. Schumacher WE, Drolet BA, Maheshwari M, et al. Spinal dysraphism associated with the cutaneous lumbosacral infantile hemangioma: a neuroradiological review. *Pediatr Radiol.* 2012;42(3):315–320

58. Yu J, Maheshwari M, Foy AB, Calkins CM, Drolet BA. Neonatal lumbosacral ulceration masking lumbosacral and intraspinal hemangiomas associated with occult spinal dysraphism. *J Pediatr.* 2016;175:211–215

59. Léauté-Labrèze C, Dumas de la Roque E, Hubiche T, Boralevi F, Thambo JB, Taïeb A. Propranolol for severe hemangiomas of infancy. *N Engl J Med.* 2008;358(24):2649–2651

60. Léaute-Labrèze C, Boccara O, Degrugillier-Chopinet C, et al. Safety of oral propranolol for the treatment of infantile hemangioma: a systematic review. *Pediatrics.* 2016;138(4):e20160353

61. Drolet BA, Frommelt PC, Chamlin SL, et al. Initiation and use of propranolol for infantile hemangioma: report of a consensus conference. *Pediatrics.* 2013;131(1):128–140

62. Itinteang T, Withers AH, Davis PF, Tan ST. Biology of infantile hemangioma. *Front Surg.* 2014;1:38

63. Dai Y, Hou F, Buckmiller L, et al. Decreased eNOS protein expression in involuting and propranolol-treated hemangiomas. *Arch Otolaryngol Head Neck Surg.* 2012;138(2):177–182

64. Greenberger S, Bischoff J. Infantile hemangioma-mechanism(s) of drug action on a vascular tumor. *Cold Spring Harb Perspect Med.* 2011;1(1):a006460

65. Storch CH, Hoeger PH. Propranolol for infantile haemangiomas: insights into the molecular mechanisms of action. *Br J Dermatol.* 2010;163(2): 269–274

66. Sans V, de la Roque ED, Berge J, et al. Propranolol for severe infantile hemangiomas: follow-up report. *Pediatrics.* 2009;124(3). Available at: www.pediatrics.org/cgi/content/full/124/3/e423

67. Pan WK, Li P, Guo ZT, Huang Q, Gao Y. Propranolol induces regression of hemangioma cells via the down-regulation of the PI3K/Akt/eNOS/VEGF pathway. *Pediatr Blood Cancer.* 2015;62(8):1414–1420

68. Sharifpanah F, Saliu F, Bekhite MM, Wartenberg M, Sauer H. β-adrenergic receptor antagonists inhibit vasculogenesis of embryonic stem cells by downregulation of nitric oxide generation and interference

with VEGF signalling. *Cell Tissue Res.* 2014;358(2):443–452

69. Ji Y, Chen S, Xu C, Li L, Xiang B. The use of propranolol in the treatment of infantile haemangiomas: an update on potential mechanisms of action. *Br J Dermatol.* 2015;172(1):24–32
70. Greene AK, Couto RA. Oral prednisolone for infantile hemangioma: efficacy and safety using a standardized treatment protocol. *Plast Reconstr Surg.* 2011;128(3):743–752
71. Tiwari P, Pandey V, Gangopadhyay AN, Sharma SP, Gupta DK. Role of propranolol in ulcerated haemangioma of head and neck: a prospective comparative study. *Oral Maxillofac Surg.* 2016;20(1):73–77
72. Zaher H, Rasheed H, El-Komy MM, et al. Propranolol versus captopril in the treatment of infantile hemangioma (IH): a randomized controlled trial. *J Am Acad Dermatol.* 2016;74(3):499–505
73. Wu S, Wang B, Chen L, et al. Clinical efficacy of propranolol in the treatment of hemangioma and changes in serum VEGF, bFGF and MMP-9. *Exp Ther Med.* 2015;10(3):1079–1083
74. Aly MM, Hamza AF, Abdel Kader HM, Saafan HA, Ghazy MS, Ragab IA. Therapeutic superiority of combined propranolol with short steroids course over propranolol monotherapy in infantile hemangioma. *Eur J Pediatr.* 2015;174(11):1503–1509
75. Ji Y, Wang Q, Chen S, et al. Oral atenolol therapy for proliferating infantile hemangioma: a prospective study. *Medicine (Baltimore).* 2016;95(24):e3908
76. Léauté-Labrèze C, Hoeger P, Mazereeuw-Hautier J, et al. A randomized, controlled trial of oral propranolol in infantile hemangioma. *N Engl J Med.* 2015;372(8):735–746
77. Siegel DH, Tefft KA, Kelly T, et al. Stroke in children with posterior fossa brain malformations, hemangiomas, arterial anomalies, coarctation of the aorta and cardiac defects, and eye abnormalities (PHACE) syndrome: a systematic review of the literature. *Stroke.* 2012;43(6):1672–1674
78. Breur JM, de Graaf M, Breugem CC, Pasmans SG. Hypoglycemia as a result of propranolol during treatment of infantile hemangioma: a case report. *Pediatr Dermatol.* 2011;28(2):169–171
79. Holland KE, Frieden IJ, Frommelt PC, Mancini AJ, Wyatt D, Drolet BA. Hypoglycemia in children taking propranolol for the treatment of infantile hemangioma. *Arch Dermatol.* 2010;146(7):775–778
80. Prey S, Voisard JJ, Delarue A, et al. Safety of propranolol therapy for severe infantile hemangioma. *JAMA.* 2016;315(4):413–415
81. Techasatian L, Komwilaisak P, Panombualert S, Uppala R, Jetsrisuparb C. Propranolol was effective in treating cutaneous infantile haemangiomas in Thai children. *Acta Paediatr.* 2016;105(6):e257–e262
82. Stringari G, Barbato G, Zanzucchi M, et al. Propranolol treatment for infantile hemangioma: a case series of sixty-two patients. *Pediatr Med Chir.* 2016;38(2):113
83. Sreekantam S, Preece MA, Vijay S, Raiman J, Santra S. How to use a controlled fast to investigate hypoglycaemia. *Arch Dis Child Educ Pract Ed.* 2017;102(1):28–36
84. Cushing SL, Boucek RJ, Manning SC, Sidbury R, Perkins JA. Initial experience with a multidisciplinary strategy for initiation of propranolol therapy for infantile hemangiomas. *Otolaryngol Head Neck Surg.* 2011;144(1):78–84
85. Ng M, Knuth C, Weisbrod C, Murthy A. Propranolol therapy for problematic infantile hemangioma. *Ann Plast Surg.* 2016;76(3):306–310
86. Chang L, Ye X, Qiu Y, et al. Is propranolol safe and effective for outpatient use for infantile hemangioma? A prospective study of 679 cases from one center in China. *Ann Plast Surg.* 2016;76(5):559–563
87. Liu LS, Sokoloff D, Antaya RJ. Twenty-four-hour hospitalization for patients initiating systemic propranolol therapy for infantile hemangiomas—is it indicated? *Pediatr Dermatol.* 2013;30(5):554–560
88. El Ezzi O, Hohlfeld J, de Buys Roessingh A. Propranolol in infantile haemangioma: simplifying pretreatment monitoring. *Swiss Med Wkly.* 2014;144:w13943
89. Tang LY, Hing JW, Tang JY, et al. Predicting complications with pretreatment testing in infantile haemangioma treated with oral propranolol. *Br J Ophthalmol.* 2016;100(7):902–906
90. Ge J, Zheng J, Zhang L, Yuan W, Zhao H. Oral propranolol combined with topical timolol for compound infantile hemangiomas: a retrospective study. *Sci Rep.* 2016;6:19765
91. Raphael MF, Breugem CC, Vlasveld FA, et al. Is cardiovascular evaluation necessary prior to and during beta-blocker therapy for infantile hemangiomas?: a cohort study. *J Am Acad Dermatol.* 2015;72(3):465–472
92. de Graaf M, Breur JMPJ, Raphaël MF, Vos M, Breugem CC, Pasmans SGMA. Adverse effects of propranolol when used in the treatment of hemangiomas: a case series of 28 infants. *J Am Acad Dermatol.* 2011;65(2):320–327
93. Xu DP, Cao RY, Xue L, Sun NN, Tong S, Wang XK. Treatment of severe infantile hemangiomas with propranolol: an evaluation of the efficacy and effects of cardiovascular parameters in 25 consecutive patients. *J Oral Maxillofac Surg.* 2015;73(3):430–436
94. Street JA, Hemsworth BA, Roach AG, Day MD. Tissue levels of several radiolabelled beta-adrenoceptor antagonists after intravenous administration in rats. *Arch Int Pharmacodyn Ther.* 1979;237(2):180–190
95. Feenstra MG. Functional neuroteratology of drugs acting on adrenergic receptors. *Neurotoxicology.* 1992;13(1):55–63
96. Pitzer M, Schmidt MH, Esser G, Laucht M. Child development after maternal tocolysis with beta-sympathomimetic drugs. *Child Psychiatry Hum Dev.* 2001;31(3):165–182
97. Langley A, Pope E. Propranolol and central nervous system function: potential implications for paediatric patients with infantile haemangiomas. *Br J Dermatol.* 2015;172(1):13–23

98. Bryan BA. Reconsidering the use of propranolol in the treatment of cosmetic infantile hemangiomas. *Angiology: Open Access.* 2013;1:e101

99. Phillips RJ, Penington AJ, Bekhor PS, Crock CM. Use of propranolol for treatment of infantile haemangiomas in an outpatient setting. *J Paediatr Child Health.* 2012;48(10):902–906

100. Gonski K, Wargon O. Retrospective follow up of gross motor development in children using propranolol for treatment of infantile haemangioma at Sydney Children's Hospital. *Australas J Dermatol.* 2014;55(3):209–211

101. Moyakine AV, Hermans DJ, Fuijkschot J, van der Vleuten CJ. Propranolol treatment of infantile hemangiomas does not negatively affect psychomotor development. *J Am Acad Dermatol.* 2015;73(2):341–342

102. Moyakine AV, Kerstjens JM, Spillekom-van Koulil S, van der Vleuten CJ. Propranolol treatment of infantile hemangioma (IH) is not associated with developmental risk or growth impairment at age 4 years. *J Am Acad Dermatol.* 2016;75(1):59–63.e1

103. Chinnadurai S, Fonnesbeck C, Snyder KM, et al. Pharmacologic interventions for infantile hemangioma: a meta-analysis. *Pediatrics.* 2016;137(2):e20153896

104. Frieden IJ, Eichenfield LF, Esterly NB, Geronemus R, Mallory SB; American Academy of Dermatology Guidelines Outcomes Committee. Guidelines of care for hemangiomas of infancy. *J Am Acad Dermatol.* 1997;37(4):631–637

105. Sadan N, Wolach B. Treatment of hemangiomas of infants with high doses of prednisone. *J Pediatr.* 1996;128(1):141–146

106. Bennett ML, Fleischer AB Jr, Chamlin SL, Frieden IJ. Oral corticosteroid use is effective for cutaneous hemangiomas: an evidence-based evaluation. *Arch Dermatol.* 2001;137(9):1208–1213

107. Nieuwenhuis K, de Laat PC, Janmohamed SR, Madern GC, Oranje AP. Infantile hemangioma: treatment with short course systemic corticosteroid therapy as an alternative for propranolol. *Pediatr Dermatol.* 2013;30(1):64–70

108. Sloan GM, Reinisch JF, Nichter LS, Saber WL, Lew K, Morwood DT. Intralesional corticosteroid therapy for infantile hemangiomas. *Plast Reconstr Surg.* 1989;83(3):459–467

109. Chowdri NA, Darzi MA, Fazili Z, Iqbal S. Intralesional corticosteroid therapy for childhood cutaneous hemangiomas. *Ann Plast Surg.* 1994;33(1):46–51

110. Chen MT, Yeong EK, Horng SY. Intralesional corticosteroid therapy in proliferating head and neck hemangiomas: a review of 155 cases. *J Pediatr Surg.* 2000;35(3):420–423

111. Buckmiller LM, Francis CL, Glade RS. Intralesional steroid injection for proliferative parotid hemangiomas. *Int J Pediatr Otorhinolaryngol.* 2008;72(1):81–87

112. Prasetyono TO, Djoenaedi I. Efficacy of intralesional steroid injection in head and neck hemangioma: a systematic review. *Ann Plast Surg.* 2011;66(1):98–106

113. Zarem HA, Edgerton MT. Induced resolution of cavernous hemangiomas following prednisolone therapy. *Plast Reconstr Surg.* 1967;39(1):76–83

114. Kushner BJ. The treatment of periorbital infantile hemangioma with intralesional corticosteroid. *Plast Reconstr Surg.* 1985;76(4):517–526

115. Herlihy EP, Kelly JP, Sidbury R, Perkins JA, Weiss AH. Visual acuity and astigmatism in periocular infantile hemangiomas treated with oral beta-blocker versus intralesional corticosteroid injection. *J AAPOS.* 2016;20(1):30–33

116. Goyal R, Watts P, Lane CM, Beck L, Gregory JW. Adrenal suppression and failure to thrive after steroid injections for periocular hemangioma. *Ophthalmology.* 2004;111(2):389–395

117. Weiss AH. Adrenal suppression after corticosteroid injection of periocular hemangiomas. *Am J Ophthalmol.* 1989;107(5):518–522

118. Shorr N, Seiff SR. Central retinal artery occlusion associated with periocular corticosteroid injection for juvenile hemangioma. *Ophthalmic Surg.* 1986;17(4):229–231

119. Ruttum MS, Abrams GW, Harris GJ, Ellis MK. Bilateral retinal embolization associated with intralesional corticosteroid injection for capillary hemangioma of infancy. *J Pediatr Ophthalmol Strabismus.* 1993;30(1):4–7

120. Egbert JE, Schwartz GS, Walsh AW. Diagnosis and treatment of an ophthalmic artery occlusion during an intralesional injection of corticosteroid into an eyelid capillary hemangioma. *Am J Ophthalmol.* 1996;121(6):638–642

121. Egbert JE, Paul S, Engel WK, Summers CG. High injection pressure during intralesional injection of corticosteroids into capillary hemangiomas. *Arch Ophthalmol.* 2001;119(5):677–683

122. Chan H, McKay C, Adams S, Wargon O. RCT of timolol maleate gel for superficial infantile hemangiomas in 5- to 24-week-olds. *Pediatrics.* 2013;131(6). Available at: www.pediatrics.org/cgi/content/full/131/6/e1739

123. Pope E, Chakkittakandiyil A. Topical timolol gel for infantile hemangiomas: a pilot study. *Arch Dermatol.* 2010;146(5):564–565

124. Chakkittakandiyil A, Phillips R, Frieden IJ, et al. Timolol maleate 0.5% or 0.1% gel-forming solution for infantile hemangiomas: a retrospective, multicenter, cohort study. *Pediatr Dermatol.* 2012;29(1):28–31

125. Chambers CB, Katowitz WR, Katowitz JA, Binenbaum G. A controlled study of topical 0.25% timolol maleate gel for the treatment of cutaneous infantile capillary hemangiomas. *Ophthal Plast Reconstr Surg.* 2012;28(2):103–106

126. Frommelt P, Juern A, Siegel D, et al. Adverse events in young and preterm infants receiving topical timolol for infantile hemangioma. *Pediatr Dermatol.* 2016;33(4):405–414

127. McMahon P, Oza V, Frieden IJ. Topical timolol for infantile hemangiomas: putting a note of caution in "cautiously optimistic". *Pediatr Dermatol.* 2012;29(1):127–130

128. Coppens G, Stalmans I, Zeyen T, Casteels I. The safety and efficacy of glaucoma medication in the pediatric

population. *J Pediatr Ophthalmol Strabismus.* 2009;46(1):12–18

129. Guo S, Ni N. Topical treatment for capillary hemangioma of the eyelid using beta-blocker solution. *Arch Ophthalmol.* 2010;128(2):255–256

130. Ni N, Langer P, Wagner R, Guo S. Topical timolol for periocular hemangioma: report of further study. *Arch Ophthalmol.* 2011;129(3):377–379

131. Moehrle M, Léauté-Labrèze C, Schmidt V, Röcken M, Poets CF, Goelz R. Topical timolol for small hemangiomas of infancy. *Pediatr Dermatol.* 2013;30(2):245–249

132. Yu L, Li S, Su B, et al. Treatment of superficial infantile hemangiomas with timolol: evaluation of short-term efficacy and safety in infants. *Exp Ther Med.* 2013;6(2):388–390

133. Danarti R, Ariwibowo L, Radiono S, Budiyanto A. Topical timolol maleate 0.5% for infantile hemangioma: its effectiveness compared to ultrapotent topical corticosteroids - a single-center experience of 278 cases. *Dermatology.* 2016;232(5):566–571

134. Oranje AP, Janmohamed SR, Madern GC, de Laat PC. Treatment of small superficial haemangioma with timolol 0.5% ophthalmic solution: a series of 20 cases. *Dermatology.* 2011;223(4):330–334

135. Gomulka J, Siegel DH, Drolet BA. Dramatic shift in the infantile hemangioma treatment paradigm at a single institution. *Pediatr Dermatol.* 2013;30(6):751–752

136. Weibel L, Barysch MJ, Scheer HS, et al. Topical timolol for infantile hemangiomas: evidence for efficacy and degree of systemic absorption. *Pediatr Dermatol.* 2016;33(2): 184–190

137. Olson RJ, Bromberg BB, Zimmerman TJ. Apneic spells associated with timolol therapy in a neonate. *Am J Ophthalmol.* 1979;88(1):120–122

138. Burnstine RA, Felton JL, Ginther WH. Cardiorespiratory reaction to timolol maleate in a pediatric patient: a case report. *Ann Ophthalmol.* 1982;14(10):905–906

139. Kiryazov K, Stefova M, Iotova V. Can ophthalmic drops cause central nervous system depression and cardiogenic shock in infants? *Pediatr Emerg Care.* 2013; 29(11):1207–1209

140. Semkova K, Kazandjieva J. Topical timolol maleate for treatment of infantile haemangiomas: preliminary results of a prospective study. *Clin Exp Dermatol.* 2013;38(2):143–146

141. Boos MD, Castelo-Soccio L. Experience with topical timolol maleate for the treatment of ulcerated infantile hemangiomas (IH). *J Am Acad Dermatol.* 2016;74(3):567–570

142. Greene AK. Management of hemangiomas and other vascular tumors. *Clin Plast Surg.* 2011;38(1):45–63

143. Couto RA, Maclellan RA, Zurakowski D, Greene AK. Infantile hemangioma: clinical assessment of the involuting phase and implications for management. *Plast Reconstr Surg.* 2012;130(3):619–624

144. Batta K, Goodyear HM, Moss C, Williams HC, Hiller L, Waters R. Randomised controlled study of early pulsed dye laser treatment of uncomplicated childhood haemangiomas: results of a 1-year analysis. *Lancet.* 2002;360(9332):521–527

145. Mulliken JB, Fishman SJ, Burrows PE. Vascular anomalies. *Curr Probl Surg.* 2000;37(8):517–584

146. Charlesworth R. The toddler: affective development. In: *Understanding Child Development.* 6th ed. Delmar Learning; 1994:304

147. Santrock JW. The self and identity. In: *Child Development.* 7th ed. McGraw-Hill; 1996:378–385

148. Neisser U. Memory development: new questions and old. *Dev Rev.* 2004;24(1):154–158

149. Bowers RE, Graham EA, Tomlinson KM. The natural history of the strawberry nevus. *Arch Dermatol.* 1960;82(5):667–680

150. Laubach HJ, Anderson RR, Luger T, Manstein D. Fractional photothermolysis for involuted infantile hemangioma. *Arch Dermatol.* 2009;145(7):748–750

151. Witman PM, Wagner AM, Scherer K, Waner M, Frieden IJ. Complications following pulsed dye laser treatment of superficial hemangiomas. *Lasers Surg Med.* 2006;38(2):116–123

152. Scheepers JH, Quaba AA. Does the pulsed tunable dye laser have a role in the management of infantile hemangiomas? Observations based on 3 years' experience. *Plast Reconstr Surg.* 1995;95(2):305–312

153. Kessels JP, Hamers ET, Ostertag JU. Superficial hemangioma: pulsed dye laser versus wait-and-see. *Dermatol Surg.* 2013;39(3, pt 1):414–421

154. Liu LS, Sowa A, Antaya RJ. Educating caregivers about the natural history of infantile hemangiomas. *Acta Paediatr.* 2015;104(1):9–11

155. Zweegers J, van der Vleuten CJ. The psychosocial impact of an infantile haemangioma on children and their parents. *Arch Dis Child.* 2012;97(10):922–926

156. Minzer-Conzetti K, Garzon MC, Haggstrom AN, et al. Information about infantile hemangiomas on the Internet: how accurate is it? *J Am Acad Dermatol.* 2007;57(6):998–1004

157. Takahashi K, Mulliken JB, Kozakewich HP, Rogers RA, Folkman J, Ezekowitz RA. Cellular markers that distinguish the phases of hemangioma during infancy and childhood. *J Clin Invest.* 1994;93(6):2357–2364

158. Agency for Healthcare Research and Quality. Treating infantile hemangiomas in children. Available at: https://effectivehealthcare.ahrq.gov/topics/infantile-hemangioma/consumer. Accessed November 27, 2018

159. Bernabeu-Wittel J, Pereyra J, Corb R, Ruiz-Canela J, Tarilonte A M, Conejo-Mir J. Teledermatology for infantile hemangiomas. Comment on: Chang LC, Haggstrom AN, Drolet BA, et al for the Hemangioma Investigator Group. Growth characteristics of infantile hemangiomas: implications for management. Pediatrics. 2008;122:360-367. Available at: http://pediatrics.aappublications.org/content/122/2/360.comments

160. Martin K, Blei F, Chamlin SL, et al. Propranolol treatment of infantile hemangiomas: anticipatory guidance for parents and caretakers [published correction appears in *Pediatr*

Dermatol. 2013;30(2):280]. *Pediatr Dermatol.* 2013;30(1):155–159

161. Munden A, Butschek R, Tom WL, et al. Prospective study of infantile haemangiomas: incidence, clinical characteristics and association with placental anomalies. *Br J Dermatol.* 2014;170(4):907–913

162. Moyakine AV, Herwegen B, van der Vleuten CJM. Use of the Hemangioma Severity Scale to facilitate treatment decisions for infantile hemangiomas. *J Am Acad Dermatol.* 2017;77(5): 868–873

163. Mull JL, Chamlin SL, Lai JS, et al. Utility of the Hemangioma Severity Scale as a triage tool and predictor of need for treatment. *Pediatr Dermatol.* 2017;34(1):78–83

164. Haggstrom AN, Beaumont JL, Lai JS, et al. Measuring the severity of infantile hemangiomas: instrument development and reliability. *Arch Dermatol.* 2012;148(2):197–202

Infantile Hemangiomas Clinical Practice Guideline Quick Reference Tools

- Action Statement Summary
  — Clinical Practice Guideline for the Management of Infantile Hemangiomas
- *ICD-10-CM* Coding Quick Reference for Infantile Hemangiomas

Action Statement Summary

Clinical Practice Guideline for the Management of Infantile Hemangiomas

Key Action Statement 1

Risk stratification

Key Action Statement 1A

Clinicians should classify an IH as high risk if there is evidence of or potential for the following: (1) life-threatening complications, (2) functional impairment or ulceration, (3) structural anomalies (eg, in PHACE syndrome or LUMBAR syndrome), or (4) permanent disfigurement (grade X, strong recommendation).

Key Action Statement 1B

After identifying an IH as high risk, clinicians should facilitate an evaluation by a hemangioma specialist as soon as possible (grade X, strong recommendation).

Key Action Statement 2

Imaging

Key Action Statement 2A

Clinicians should not perform imaging unless the diagnosis of IH is uncertain, there are 5 or more cutaneous IHs, or associated anatomic abnormalities are suspected (grade B, moderate recommendation).

Key Action Statement 2B

Clinicians should perform ultrasonography as the initial imaging modality when the diagnosis of IH is uncertain (grade C, weak recommendation).

Key Action Statement 2C

Clinicians should perform MRI when concerned about associated structural abnormalities (eg, PHACE syndrome or LUMBAR syndrome) (grade B, moderate recommendation).

Key Action Statement 3

Pharmacotherapy

Key Action Statement 3A

Clinicians should use oral propranolol as the first-line agent for IHs requiring systemic treatment (grade A, strong recommendation).

Key Action Statement 3B

Clinicians should dose propranolol between 2 and 3 mg/kg per day unless there are comorbidities (eg, PHACE syndrome) or adverse effects (eg, sleep disturbance) that necessitate a lower dose (grade A, moderate recommendation).

Key Action Statement 3C

Clinicians should counsel that propranolol be administered with or after feeding and that doses be held at times of diminished oral intake or vomiting to reduce the risk of hypoglycemia (grade X, strong recommendation).

Key Action Statement 3D

Clinicians should evaluate patients for and educate caregivers about potential adverse effects of propranolol, including sleep disturbances, bronchial irritation, and clinically symptomatic bradycardia and hypotension (grade X, strong recommendation).

Key Action Statement 3E

Clinicians may prescribe oral prednisolone or prednisone to treat IHs if there are contraindications or an inadequate response to oral propranolol (grade B, moderate recommendation).

Key Action Statement 3F

Clinicians may recommend intralesional injection of triamcinolone and/or betamethasone to treat focal, bulky IHs during proliferation or in certain critical anatomic locations (eg, the lip) (grade B, moderate recommendation).

Key Action Statement 3G

Clinicians may prescribe topical timolol maleate as a therapy for thin and/or superficial IHs (grade B, moderate recommendation).

Key Action Statement 4

Clinicians may recommend surgery and laser therapy as treatment options in managing selected IHs (grade C, moderate recommendation).

Key Action Statement 5

Clinicians should educate parents of infants with an IH about the condition, including the expected natural history, and its potential for causing complications or disfigurement (grade X, strong recommendation).

Coding Quick Reference for Infantile Hemangiomas
ICD-10-CM
D18.00 Hemangioma unspecified site
D18.01 Hemangioma of skin and subcutaneous tissue
D18.02 Hemangioma of intracranial structures
D18.03 Hemangioma of intra-abdominal structures
D18.09 Hemangioma of other sites

Clinical Practice Guideline: Maintenance Intravenous Fluids in Children

- *Clinical Practice Guideline*

CLINICAL PRACTICE GUIDELINE Guidance for the Clinician in Rendering Pediatric Care

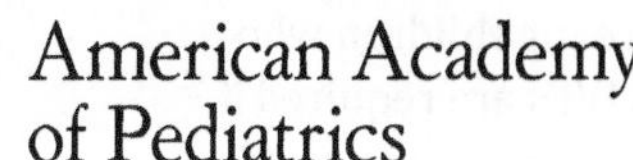

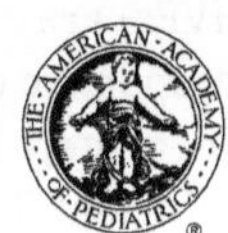

DEDICATED TO THE HEALTH OF ALL CHILDREN™

Clinical Practice Guideline: Maintenance Intravenous Fluids in Children

Leonard G. Feld, MD, PhD, MMM, FAAP,[a] Daniel R. Neuspiel, MD, MPH, FAAP,[b] Byron A. Foster, MD, MPH, FAAP,[c] Michael G. Leu, MD, MS, MHS, FAAP,[d] Matthew D. Garber, MD, FHM, FAAP,[e] Kelly Austin, MD, MS, FAAP, FACS,[f] Rajit K. Basu, MD, MS, FCCM,[g,h] Edward E. Conway Jr, MD, MS, FAAP,[i] James J. Fehr, MD, FAAP,[j] Clare Hawkins, MD,[k] Ron L. Kaplan, MD, FAAP,[l] Echo V. Rowe, MD, FAAP,[m] Muhammad Waseem, MD, MS, FAAP, FACEP,[n] Michael L. Moritz, MD, FAAP,[o] SUBCOMMITTEE ON FLUID AND ELECTROLYTE THERAPY

abstract

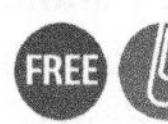

Maintenance intravenous fluids (IVFs) are used to provide critical supportive care for children who are acutely ill. IVFs are required if sufficient fluids cannot be provided by using enteral administration for reasons such as gastrointestinal illness, respiratory compromise, neurologic impairment, a perioperative state, or being moribund from an acute or chronic illness. Despite the common use of maintenance IVFs, there is high variability in fluid prescribing practices and a lack of guidelines for fluid composition administration and electrolyte monitoring. The administration of hypotonic IVFs has been the standard in pediatrics. Concerns have been raised that this approach results in a high incidence of hyponatremia and that isotonic IVFs could prevent the development of hyponatremia. Our goal in this guideline is to provide an evidence-based approach for choosing the tonicity of maintenance IVFs in most patients from 28 days to 18 years of age who require maintenance IVFs. This guideline applies to children in surgical (postoperative) and medical acute-care settings, including critical care and the general inpatient ward. Patients with neurosurgical disorders, congenital or acquired cardiac disease, hepatic disease, cancer, renal dysfunction, diabetes insipidus, voluminous watery diarrhea, or severe burns; neonates who are younger than 28 days old or in the NICU; and adolescents older than 18 years old are excluded. We specifically address the tonicity of maintenance IVFs in children.

The Key Action Statement of the subcommittee is as follows:

1A: The American Academy of Pediatrics recommends that patients 28 days to 18 years of age requiring maintenance IVFs should receive isotonic solutions with appropriate potassium chloride and dextrose because they significantly decrease the risk of developing hyponatremia (evidence quality: A; recommendation strength: strong)

[a]Retired, Nicklaus Children's Health System, Miami, Florida; [b]Retired, Levine Children's Hospital, Charlotte, North Carolina; [c]Oregon Health and Science University, Portland, Oregon; [l]Department of Pediatric Emergency Medicine, [d]School of Medicine, University of Washington and Seattle Children's Hospital, Seattle, Washington; [e]Department of Pediatrics, College of Medicine – Jacksonville, University of Florida, Jacksonville, Florida; Departments of [f]Surgery and [o]Pediatrics, University of Pittsburgh School of Medicine, Children's Hospital of Pittsburgh, Pittsburgh, Pennsylvania; [g]Division of Critical Care Medicine, Children's Healthcare of Atlanta, Atlanta, Georgia; [h]Department of Pediatrics, School of Medicine, Emory University, Atlanta, Georgia; [i]Division of Pediatric Critical Care Medicine, Department of Pediatrics, Jacobi Medical Center, Bronx, New York; Departments of [j]Anesthesiology and Pediatrics, Washington University in St Louis, St Louis, Missouri; [k]Department of Family Medicine, Houston Methodist Hospital, Houston, Texas; [m]Department of Anesthesia, Stanford University School of Medicine, Stanford, California; and [n]Lincoln Medical Center, Bronx, New York

This document is copyrighted and is property of the American Academy of Pediatrics and its Board of Directors. All authors have filed conflict of interest statements with the American Academy of Pediatrics. Any conflicts have been resolved through a process approved by the Board of Directors. The American Academy of Pediatrics has neither solicited nor accepted any commercial involvement in the development of the content of this publication.

The guidance in this report does not indicate an exclusive course of treatment or serve as a standard of medical care. Variations, taking into account individual circumstances, may be appropriate.

To cite: Feld LG, Neuspiel DR, Foster BA, et al. Clinical Practice Guideline: Maintenance Intravenous Fluids in Children. *Pediatrics.* 2018;142(6):e20183083

INTRODUCTION

Maintenance intravenous fluids (IVFs) are used to provide critical supportive care for children who are acutely ill. IVFs are required if sufficient fluids cannot be provided by using enteral administration for reasons such as gastrointestinal illness, respiratory compromise, neurologic impairment, a perioperative state, or being moribund from an acute or chronic illness. For the purposes of this document, specifying appropriate maintenance IVFs includes the composition of IVF needed to preserve a child's extracellular volume while simultaneously minimizing the risk of developing volume depletion, fluid overload, or electrolyte disturbances, such as hyponatremia or hypernatremia. Because maintenance IVFs may have both potential benefits and harms, they should only be administered when clinically indicated. The administration of hypotonic IVF has been the standard in pediatrics. Concerns have been raised that this approach results in a high incidence of hyponatremia and that isotonic IVF could prevent the development of hyponatremia. Guidelines for maintenance IVF therapy in children have primarily been opinion based, and evidence-based consensus guidelines are lacking.

OBJECTIVE

Despite the common use of maintenance IVFs, there is high variability in fluid prescribing practices and a lack of guidelines for fluid composition and electrolyte monitoring.[1–4] Our goal in this guideline is to provide an evidence-based approach for choosing the tonicity of maintenance IVFs in most patients from 28 days to 18 years of age who require maintenance IVFs. These recommendations do not apply to patients with neurosurgical disorders, congenital or acquired cardiac disease, hepatic disease, cancer, renal dysfunction, diabetes insipidus, voluminous watery diarrhea, or severe burns; neonates who are younger than 28 days old or in the NICU; or adolescents older than 18 years old.

BACKGROUND

Phases of Fluid Therapy

Recent literature has emerged in which researchers describe the context-dependent use of IVFs, which should be prescribed, ordered, dosed, and delivered like any other drug.[5–7] Four distinct physiology-driven time periods exist for children requiring IVFs. The resuscitative phase is the acute presentation window, when IVFs are needed to restore adequate tissue perfusion and prevent or mitigate end-organ injury. The titration phase is the time when IVFs are transitioned from boluses to maintenance; this is a critical window to determine what intravascular repletion has been achieved and the trajectory of fluid gains versus losses in children who are acutely ill. The maintenance phase accounts for fluids administered during the previous 2 stabilization phases and is a time when fluids should be supplied to achieve a precise homeostatic balance between needs and losses. Finally, the convalescent phase reflects the period when exogenous fluid administration is stopped, and the patient returns to intrinsic fluid regulation. The dose of fluid during these 4 phases of fluid therapy needs to be adjusted on the basis of the unique physiologic needs of each patient, and a specific protocoled dose is not able to be applied to all patients.[8,9]

A variety of IVFs are commercially available for use in infants and children. These solutions principally vary by their specific electrolyte composition, the addition of a buffer, and whether they contain glucose (Table 1).[10] The buffer in plasma is bicarbonate, but buffers in commercially available solutions include various concentrations of lactate, acetate, and gluconate. Multiple balanced salt solutions can be compared with normal saline (0.9% saline), which has the same sodium concentration as plasma but has a supraphysiologic chloride concentration.

Effect of Dextrose on Tonicity

Tonicity is used to describe the net vector of force on cells relative to a semipermeable membrane when in solution. Physiologic relevance occurs with tonicity studied in vivo (eg, as IVF is infused intravascularly). Infused isotonic fluids do not result in osmotic shifts; the cells stay the same size. Cellular expansion occurs during immersion in hypotonic fluids as free water, in higher relative abundance in the extracellular environment, and crosses the semipermeable membrane. The converse happens in hypertonic fluid immersion: free water shifts out of the cells, leading to cellular contraction. A distinct but related concept is the concept of osmolality. Osmolality is measured as osmoles of solute per kilogram of solvent. Serum osmolality can be estimated by the following formula:

$$2 \times \text{Na}(\text{mEq}/L) + \text{BUN}(\text{mg/dL})/2.8 + \text{glucose}(\text{mg/dL})/18$$

Osmolality is distinct from tonicity (effective osmolality) in that tonicity relates to both the effect on a cell of a fluid (dependent on the selective permeability of the membrane) and the osmolality of the fluid. In the plasma, urea affects osmolality but not tonicity because urea moves freely across cell membranes with no effect on tonicity. The tonicity of IVF is primarily affected by the sodium and potassium concentration.

Dextrose (D-glucose) can be added to IVFs (Table 1). Although dextrose affects the osmolarity of IVFs, it is not a significant contributor to the plasma osmotic pressure or tonicity

TABLE 1 Composition of Commonly Used Maintenance IVFs

Fluid	Glucose, g/dL	Sodium	Chloride	Potassium, mEq/L	Calcium	Magnesium	Buffer	Osmolarity,[a] mOsm/L
Human plasma	0.07–0.11	135–145	95–105	3.5–5.3	4.4–5.2	1.6–2.4	23–30 bicarbonate	308[b]
Hypotonic solutions								
D_5 0.2% NaCl	5	34	34	0	0	0	0	78
D_5 0.45% NaCl	5	77	77	0	0	0	0	154
Isotonic and/or near-isotonic solutions								
D_5 0.9% NaCl	5	154	154	0	0	0	0	308
D_5 lactated Ringer	5	130	109	4	3	0	28 lactate	273
PlasmaLyte[c,d]	0	140	98	5	0	3	27 acetate and 23 gluconate	294

[a] The osmolarity calculation excludes the dextrose in the solution because dextrose is rapidly metabolized on infusion.
[b] The osmolality for plasma is 275–295 mOsm/kg.
[c] Multiple electrolytes injection, type 1 *United States Pharmacopeia*, is the generic name for PlasmaLyte.
[d] PlasmaLyte with 5% dextrose is not available in the United States from Baxter Healthcare Corporation in Deerfield, Illinois.

in the absence of uncontrolled diabetes because it is rapidly metabolized after entering the blood stream. Thus, although dextrose will affect the osmolarity of solutions, for patients in whom maintenance IVFs are needed, the dextrose component generally is not believed to affect the tonicity of solutions.

Historical Maintenance IVF Practice and Hyponatremia

Hyponatremia (serum sodium concentration <135 mEq/L) is the most common electrolyte abnormality in patients who are hospitalized, affecting approximately 15% to 30% of children and adults.[11,12] Patients who are acutely ill frequently have disease states associated with arginine vasopressin (AVP) excess that can impair free-water excretion and place the patient at risk for developing hyponatremia when a source of electrolyte-free water is supplied, as in hypotonic fluids.[10] Nonosmotic stimuli of AVP release include pain, nausea, stress, a postoperative state, hypovolemia, medications, and pulmonary and central nervous system (CNS) disorders, including common childhood conditions such as pneumonia and meningitis.[13–15] These conditions can lead to the syndrome of inappropriate antidiuresis (SIAD) or SIAD-like states, which lead to water retention followed by a physiologic natriuresis in which fluid balance is maintained at the expense of plasma sodium.

Children have historically been administered hypotonic maintenance IVFs.[3,4] This practice is based on theoretical calculations from the 1950s.[16] The water requirement was based on the energy expenditure of healthy children, with 1 mL of fluid provided for each kilocalorie (kcal) expended, or 1500 mL/m^2 per day. The resting energy expenditure in healthy children is vastly different in those with an acute disease and/or illness or after surgery. When using calorimetric methods, energy expenditure in these patients is closer to the basal metabolic rate proposed by Talbot,[17] which averages 50 to 60 kcal/kg per day.[18] The electrolyte concentration of IVFs was estimated to reflect the composition of human and cow milk. The final composition consisted of 3 mEq of sodium and 2 mEq of potassium per 100 kcal metabolized.[16]

Most hyponatremia in patients who are hospitalized is hospital acquired and related to the administration of hypotonic IVFs in the setting of elevated AVP concentrations.[10,11] Studies in which researchers evaluated hospital-acquired hyponatremia have revealed a relationship with the administration of hypotonic IVFs.[11,19,20] The most serious complication of hospital-acquired hyponatremia is hyponatremic encephalopathy, which is a medical emergency that can be fatal or lead to irreversible brain injury if inadequately treated.[21–24] The reports of hospital-acquired hyponatremic encephalopathy have occurred primarily in otherwise healthy children who were receiving hypotonic IVFs, in many cases after minor surgical procedures.[21,23] Patients with hospital-acquired hyponatremia are at particular risk for hyponatremic encephalopathy, which usually develops acutely in less than 48 hours, leaving little time for the brain to adapt. Children are at particularly high risk of developing symptomatic hyponatremia because of their larger brain/skull size ratio.[24] Symptoms of hyponatremia can be nonspecific, including fussiness, headache, nausea, vomiting, confusion, lethargy, and muscle cramps, making prompt diagnosis difficult.

After reports of severe hyponatremia and associated neurologic injury were reported in 1992, a significant debate emerged regarding the appropriateness of administering hypotonic maintenance IVFs to children.[21] In 2003, it was recommended that isotonic fluids be administered to children who are acutely ill and require maintenance IVFs to prevent the development of hyponatremia.[24] Since then, the Institute for Safe Medical Practices of both the United States[25] and Canada[26] released reports on deaths from severe hyponatremia in patients who were hospitalized and received hypotonic IVFs. The United Kingdom released a national safety alert reporting 4 deaths and 1 near miss from hospital-acquired hyponatremia,[27] and 50 cases of serious injury or child death from hypotonic IVFs were reported in the international literature.[22]

After the recognition of hospital-acquired hyponatremia in patients receiving hypotonic IVFs and recommendations for avoiding them,[24] the use of 0.2% saline has declined with an increase in the use of 0.45% and 0.9% saline.[3,28] There have been concerns raised about the safety of the proposed use of isotonic maintenance IVFs in children who are acutely ill for the prevention of hospital-acquired hyponatremia.[18] Some believe that this approach could lead to complications such as hypernatremia, fluid overload with edema and hypertension, and hyperchloremic acidosis.[29] In the past 15 years, there have been a multitude of clinical trials and systematic reviews in which researchers have attempted to address this debate.[30–35] Authors of textbooks and review articles in the United States continue to recommend hypotonic fluids.[36–38] Conversely, the National Clinical Guideline Centre in the United Kingdom published evidence-based guidelines for IVF therapy in children younger than 16 years old and recommended isotonic IVFs.[34]

METHODS

In April 2016, the American Academy of Pediatrics (AAP) convened a multidisciplinary subcommittee composed of primary care clinicians and experts in the fields of general pediatrics, hospital medicine, emergency medicine, critical care medicine, nephrology, anesthesiology, surgery, and quality improvement. The subcommittee also included a guideline methodologist and/or informatician and an epidemiologist who were skilled in systematic reviews. All panel members declared potential conflicts on the basis of the AAP policy on conflicts of interest and voluntary disclosure. Subcommittee members repeated this process annually and on publication of the guideline. All potential conflicts of interest are listed at the end of this document. The project was funded by the AAP.

The subcommittee initiated its literature review by combining the search strategies in 7 recent systematic reviews of clinical trials of maintenance IVFs in children and adolescents, which consisted of 11 clinical trials involving 1139 patients.[9,33,34,39–42] The subcommittee then used this combined search strategy to discover 7 additional clinical trials of maintenance IVFs involving 1316 children and adolescents (ages 28 days to 18 years) published since 2013 (the last year included in the previous 6 systematic reviews) in the PubMed, Cumulative Index to Nursing and Allied Health Literature, and Cochrane Library databases. All articles that were initially identified were back searched for other relevant publications. Studies published as of March 15, 2016, were included. Three independent reviewers from the subcommittee then critically appraised the full text of each identified article (n = 17) using a structured data collection form that was based on published guidelines for evaluating medical literature.[43,44] These reviews were integrated into an evidence table by the subcommittee epidemiologist (Supplemental Table 3). Forest plots for all included randomized controlled trials (RCTs) in which researchers used random-effects models and Mantel-Haenzel (M-H) statistics with the outcome of hyponatremia are shown in Supplemental Figs 2–4.

To appraise the methodology of the included studies, a risk-of-bias assessment was completed by using the *Cochrane Handbook* risk of bias assessment framework.[45] Using this framework, raters placed a value of low, high, or unclear risk of bias for each article in the areas of selection bias (both random-sequence generation and allocation concealment), performance bias, detection bias, attrition bias, and reporting bias. Two authors independently reviewed each study identified in the systematic review and made an independent judgment. Differences in assessment were resolved via discussion.

The resulting systematic review was used to develop the guideline recommendations by following the Policy Statement from the AAP Steering Committee on Quality Improvement and Management, "Classifying Recommendations for Clinical Practice Guidelines."[46] Decisions and the strength of recommendations were based on a systematic grading of the quality of evidence from the updated literature review by the subcommittee with guidance by the epidemiologist. Expert consensus was used when definitive data were not available. If committee members disagreed with the consensus, they were encouraged to voice their concerns until full agreement was reached. Full agreement was reached on the clinical recommendations below.

Clinical recommendations were entered into Bridge-Wiz 2.1 for AAP software (Building Recommendations in a Developers Guideline Editor), an interactive software tool that is used to lead guideline development

TABLE 2 Key Action Statement 1A

Aggregate Evidence Quality	Grade A
Benefits	More physiologic fluid, less hyponatremia
Risks, harm, cost	Potential harms of hypernatremia, fluid overload, hypertension, hyperchloremic metabolic acidosis, and acute kidney injury have not been found to be of increased risk with isotonic maintenance fluids.
Benefit-harm assessment	Decreased risk of hyponatremia
Intentional vagueness	None
Role of patient preferences	None
Exclusions	Patients with neurosurgical disorders, congenital or acquired cardiac disease, hepatic disease, cancer, renal dysfunction, diabetes insipidus, voluminous watery diarrhea, or severe burns; neonates who are <28 d old or in the NICU; or adolescents >18 y old
Strength	Strong recommendation
Key references	9,33,39–42

teams through a series of questions that are intended to create clear, transparent, and actionable Key Action Statements.[47] The committee was actively involved while the software was used and solicited the inputs of this program, which included strength of evidence and balance of benefits versus harms, and chose which sentences recommended by the program to use as part of the guideline. Bridge-Wiz also integrates the quality of available evidence and a benefit-harm assessment into the final determination of the strength of each recommendation per the guidance in Fig 1.

Before formal approval by the AAP, this guideline underwent a comprehensive review by stakeholders, including AAP councils, committees, and sections; selected outside stakeholder organizations; and individuals who were identified by the subcommittee as experts in the field. All comments were reviewed by the subcommittee and incorporated into the final guideline when appropriate.

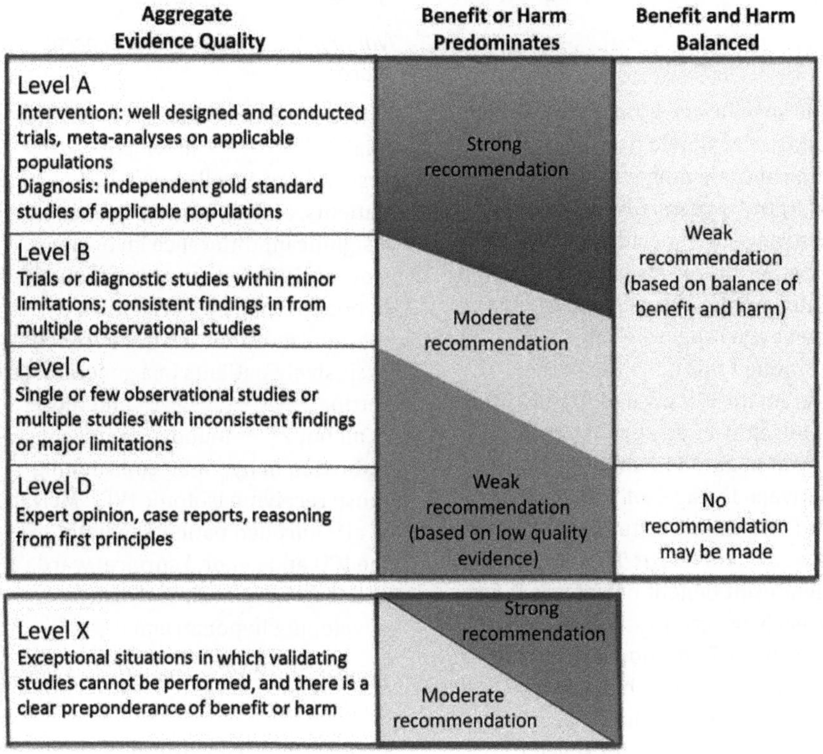

Aggregate Evidence Quality | Benefit or Harm Predominates | Benefit and Harm Balanced

Level A
Intervention: well designed and conducted trials, meta-analyses on applicable populations
Diagnosis: independent gold standard studies of applicable populations

Level B
Trials or diagnostic studies within minor limitations; consistent findings in from multiple observational studies

Level C
Single or few observational studies or multiple studies with inconsistent findings or major limitations

Level D
Expert opinion, case reports, reasoning from first principles

Strong recommendation

Moderate recommendation

Weak recommendation (based on low quality evidence)

Weak recommendation (based on balance of benefit and harm)

No recommendation may be made

Level X
Exceptional situations in which validating studies cannot be performed, and there is a clear preponderance of benefit or harm

Strong recommendation

Moderate recommendation

FIGURE 1
AAP rating of evidence and recommendations.

On the basis of the reviewed literature, this guideline applies to children 28 days to 18 years of age in surgical (postoperative) and medical acute-care settings, including critical care and the general inpatient ward. This guideline DOES NOT apply to children with neurosurgical disorders, congenital or acquired cardiac disease, hepatic disease, cancer, renal dysfunction, diabetes insipidus, voluminous watery diarrhea, or severe burns; neonates who are younger than 28 days old or in the NICU; or adolescents older than 18 years old because the majority of the researchers in the prospective studies reviewed in this guideline excluded these subsets of patients or did not include patients with these specific high-risk diagnoses.

RESULTS

Key Action Statement

The Key Action Statement is as follows:

1. Composition of Maintenance IVFs

1A: The AAP recommends that patients 28 days to 18 years of age requiring maintenance IVFs should receive isotonic solutions with appropriate potassium chloride (KCl) and dextrose because they significantly decrease the risk of developing hyponatremia (evidence quality: A; recommendation strength: strong; Table 2).

Isotonic Solutions Versus Hypotonic Solutions

Isotonic fluid has a sodium concentration similar to plasma (135–144 mEq/L). Plasma is approximately 93% aqueous and 7% anhydrous with a sodium concentration in the aqueous phase of plasma of 154 mEq/L and osmolarity of 308 mOsm/L, similar to that of 0.9% sodium chloride (NaCl). Conversely, hypotonic fluid has a sodium concentration lower than that of the aqueous phase of plasma. In the studies evaluated in the formulation of these guidelines, there is some heterogeneity in both the isotonic and hypotonic fluids used. The sodium concentration of isotonic fluids ranged from 131 to 154 mEq/L. Hartmann solution (sodium concentration 131 mEq/L; osmolality 279 mOsm/L) was used in only 46 patients.[48,49] PlasmaLyte (sodium concentration 140 mEq/L; osmolarity 294 mOsm/L) was used in 346 patients.[35] Researchers in the majority of the studies used either 0.9% NaCl (sodium concentration 154 mEq/L; osmolarity 308 mOsm/L) or a fluid of equivalent tonicity. Hypotonic fluids ranged from 30 to 100 mEq/L.[33] Lactated Ringer solution (sodium concentration 130 mEq/L; osmolarity 273 mOsm/L), a slightly hypotonic solution, was not involved in any of the clinical trials. For the purposes of this guideline, isotonic solutions have a sodium concentration similar to PlasmaLyte, or 0.9% NaCl. Recommendations are not made regarding the safety of lactated Ringer solution. Researchers in the majority of studies added dextrose (2.5%–5%) to the intravenous (IV) solution.

The search revealed 17 randomized clinical trials[20,31,32,35,48–60] that met the search criteria, including a total 2455 patients (2313 patients had primary outcome data for analysis in Supplemental Figs 2–4), to help evaluate the question of whether isotonic or hypotonic fluids should be used in children who are hospitalized. Sixteen of the studies revealed that isotonic fluids were superior to hypotonic fluids in preventing hyponatremia. There have also been 7 systematic reviews over the past 11 years in which researchers have synthesized various combinations of the above RCTs.[9,33,34,39–42] The number needed to treat with isotonic fluids to prevent hyponatremia (sodium <135 mEq/L) was 7.5 across all included studies and 27.8 for moderate hyponatremia (sodium <130 mEq/L).

Study appraisal for risk of bias (Supplemental Table 4) revealed the reviewed studies in total to be methodologically sound. Most types of bias were found to be of low risk in all but 2 studies. There was 1 study with 2 bias types of potentially high risk and 11 studies with 1 or more unclear bias areas.

Inclusion and Exclusion Criteria: Rationale for Specific Subgroups

Age

The specific age groups from which data are available from randomized clinical trials range from 1 day (1 trial) to 18 years. Given this broad age range, we specifically evaluated whether there was variability in the outcomes by age, particularly for the lower age range. McNab et al[33] examined this question in their systematic review and found 100 children studied at younger than 1 year of age, 243 children studied between the ages of 1 and 5 years, and 465 children studied at older than 5 years of age. They showed a significant benefit of isotonic IVFs in each age group stratum. There have been 7 additional studies in which researchers have also included children younger than 1 year old, although there are not specific outcome data reported for this age group.[31,32,35,50,51,55,58]

Surgical (Postoperative Patients)

Surgical or postoperative patients have been specifically studied in 7 studies[20,48,49,51,54,56,57] that included 529 patients. McNab[30] showed a pooled risk ratio of 0.48 (95% confidence interval [CI], 0.38–0.60) for the outcome of hyponatremia in favor of isotonic fluids.

Medical (Nonsurgical Patients)

Medical patients are defined here as children who are hospitalized in an acute-care setting with no indication for a surgical operation and no immediate history of a surgical operation. For these patients, there are 4 randomized clinical trials[32,52,55,58] in which researchers enrolled only medical patients and 6 randomized clinical trials[50,51,53,56,57,59] in which researchers enrolled both medical and surgical patients. Some of the mixed studies in which researchers looked at both medical and surgical patients include outcomes for only medical patients, whereas most include combined outcomes for both groups.

Varying Acuity (ICU Versus General Ward)

There are 6 randomized clinical trials[31,49,50,53,56,59] in which researchers enrolled only ICU patients, and all but one[50] revealed a significant difference favoring isotonic IVFs for the prevention of hyponatremia. Researchers in 8 randomized clinical trials enrolled exclusively patients in a general ward setting,[32,51,52,54,55,57,58,60] and those in all but 2[32,57] found a significant reduction in hyponatremia among those receiving isotonic IVFs. McNab et al[35] enrolled patients in both the ICU and general surgical ward, and they were at similar risk for developing hyponatremia.

Exclusion of Specific Populations Not Studied

Patients with neurosurgical disorders, congenital or acquired cardiac disease, hepatic disease, cancer, renal dysfunction, diabetes insipidus, voluminous watery diarrhea, or severe burns; neonates who were younger than 28 days old or in the NICU (researchers in the majority of prospective studies reviewed in this guideline excluded this subset of patients); and adolescents older than 18 years old were excluded. Patients with congenital or acquired heart disease have been either explicitly excluded from every study listed previously or were not described, so no conclusions may be drawn related to this specific population. Similarly, patients with known liver or renal disease or adrenal insufficiency have also been excluded from most of the studies listed, limiting any conclusions for these patients as well. Neurosurgical patients and those with traumatic brain injury were excluded from most studies. Oncology patients have been included in some of the randomized trials, but no specific subanalysis for them has been completed, and data are not available separately to conduct one. Many patients receiving chemotherapy receive high volumes of fluids to prevent renal injury, and there are reports of clinically significant hyponatremia, which is possibly associated with the fluid type.[61] Further study is needed to evaluate the fluid type, rate, and risk of renal injury and hyponatremia for this population. The committee did not specifically review literature for those with the following care needs: patients with significant renal concentrating defects, such as nephrogenic diabetes insipidus, and patients with voluminous diarrhea or severe burns who may have significant ongoing free-water losses.

Complications

Hyponatremia

The reviewed studies revealed the relative risk of developing mild and moderate hyponatremia (defined as a serum sodium concentration <135 mEq/L and <130 mEq/L, respectively) to be >2 and >5, respectively. The risk related to hyponatremia persisted regardless of age, medical versus surgical status, and intensive care versus general pediatric ward setting. These data strongly reveal an increased risk of hyponatremia when children receive hypotonic versus isotonic IVFs. This association is reinforced by the observations that increased hyponatremia occurs in (1) children with normal sodium at baseline (hospital-acquired hyponatremia) and (2) children who have a low sodium concentration at baseline (hospital-aggravated hyponatremia). This association has been found when using both 0.2% saline (sodium 34 mEq/L) and 0.45% saline (sodium 77 mEq/L). The risk for hyponatremia with hypotonic fluids persisted in the subgroup of patients who received fluids at a restricted rate.[49,54,58,59] A sensitivity analysis in which the Shamim et al[58] study was excluded given the anomalous number of events in both arms revealed no change in the overall estimated relative risk (0.43; 95% CI, 0.35–0.53) compared with that of all the studies included (0.46; 95% CI, 0.37–0.57; Supplemental Fig 2). In the clinical trials in which researchers assessed the possible mechanism for this finding, elevated antidiuretic hormone (ADH) concentration was found to play a putative role.[54]

There is heterogeneity in the design of the above studies in the types of patients enrolled, IVF rate and type, frequency of plasma sodium monitoring, and study duration. Despite this heterogeneity, the increased risk of hyponatremia with hypotonic IVFs is consistent. Some may argue that mild hyponatremia (plasma sodium 130–134 mEq/L) and moderate hyponatremia (plasma sodium 125–129 mEq/L) may not be clinically significant or constitute harm. However, the studies in which researchers evaluated moderate hyponatremia revealed benefits of isotonic versus hypotonic IVFs (Supplemental Figs 2 and 4). Furthermore, hypotonic solutions have been associated with a larger decrease in serum sodium. Also, the true effects of hypotonic IVFs may have been underestimated because many of the studies also included rigorous monitoring of sodium, during which patients were removed from the study if mild hyponatremia developed. Numerous studies of adults have revealed that mild and asymptomatic hyponatremia is associated with deleterious consequences, is an independent risk factor for mortality,[62,63] and leads to increased length of hospitalization and increases in costs of hospitalization.[64,65] Thus, the subcommittee believes that hyponatremia is an appropriate indicator of potential harm.

Hypernatremia

One of the concerns when providing a higher level of sodium in IVFs is the development of hypernatremia (serum sodium >145 mEq/L). This was evaluated in the most recently published systematic review.[33] Those authors identified that there was no evidence of an increased risk of hypernatremia associated with the administration of isotonic fluids, although the quality of evidence was judged to be low, primarily given the low incidence of hypernatremia in the studies included. To be clear, there was not evidence of no risk; the risk is unclear from the meta-analysis results. The estimated risk ratio from that meta-analysis was 1.24 (95% CI, 0.65–2.38), drawn from 9 studies with 937 patients, although 3 studies had no events and did not contribute to the estimate. Researchers in 2 large studies published since the meta-analysis did not find evidence of an increased risk of hypernatremia with isotonic IVFs. In the study by Friedman et al,[32] there was 1 patient in each randomized group ($N = 110$)

who developed hypernatremia, and in the study by McNab et al,[35] the incidence of hypernatremia was 4% in the isotonic IVF group and 6% in the hypotonic IVF group, with no significant difference noted between the 2 groups ($N = 641$ with data for analysis). The available data among the meta-analysis discussed above and subsequent large RCTs were unable to be used to demonstrate an increased risk of hypernatremia associated with the use of isotonic IVFs.

Acidosis

A hyperchloremic metabolic acidosis has been associated with 0.9% NaCl when it is used as a resuscitation fluid. Researchers in the majority of studies reviewed in this series did not specifically evaluate the development of acidosis or report on it as a complication. Researchers in 4 studies involving 496 patients evaluated the effect of IVF composition on acid and/or base status,[31,49,54,58] and the majority were not able to demonstrate that 0.9% NaCl resulted in acidosis. Two studies in which researchers compared 0.9% NaCl to 0.45% NaCl involving 357 children found no effect on the development of acidosis based on the change in total carbon dioxide (Tco_2), a measure of plasma bicarbonate, with a low Tco_2 being a surrogate marker for acidosis rather than a low pH.[31,54] Researchers in 1 study compared Hartman solution, which has a base equivalent to 0.45% NaCl, involving 79 patients and found no effect on the development of acidosis based on a change in Tco_2.[49] Researchers in 1 study involving 60 patients compared 0.9% NaCl to 0.18% NaCl and demonstrated a decrease in pH from 7.36 to 7.32 in the 0.9% NaCl group compared with an increase in pH from 7.36 to 7.38 in the 0.18% NaCl group ($P = .01$), but the effect on Tco_2 was not reported.[58]

Fluid Overload

Children receiving IVFs are at risk for fluid accumulation leading to a positive fluid balance or volume overload. A combination of excessive fluid and sodium can synergistically increase retained volume, a condition that is exacerbated in children with chronic comorbidities (such as systolic cardiac dysfunction [congestive heart failure (CHF)], cirrhotic hepatic failure, chronic kidney disease, and hepatorenal syndrome) and metabolic disturbances (such as hyperaldosteronism and long-term steroid use). Researchers in recent literature, most notably in the critically ill population (adults and children), have attempted to delineate the causative and outcome associations with significant positive fluid accumulation, termed "fluid overload."[66] In the non-ICU population, researchers in only a handful of studies mention an association between fluid tonicity and volume overload (or "weight gain").[20,59,60] Choong et al[20] reported on "overhydration" as estimated by using total weight gain, finding no significant difference between isotonic and hypotonic IVF administration. In the meta-analyses that encompass 12 different RCTs and more than 750 children, neither weight nor net fluid balance is discussed. Increasing scrutiny is being given to fluid management in the critically ill population.[33] To determine any association in patients who are noncritically ill, more evidence is required.

Specific Groups That May Be at Higher Risk for Developing Hyponatremia

Researchers in the RCTs reviewed for this statement excluded many groups of patients who are at particularly high risk for hyponatremia, such as those with congenital or acquired heart disease, liver disease, renal failure or dysfunction, or adrenal insufficiency; neurosurgical patients; and patients taking medication known to impair free-water excretion, such as desmopressin. Data on the efficacy of isotonic fluids to prevent hyponatremia and the potential complications related to isotonic fluids in these patients are lacking. Further studies in which researchers evaluate optimal fluid management in these groups of patients are necessary. Patients with edematous states, such as CHF, cirrhosis, and nephrotic syndrome, have an impaired ability to excrete both free water and sodium and are at risk for both volume overload and hyponatremia. Administering isotonic saline at typical maintenance rates will likely be excessive and risk volume overload, and IVFs should be restricted with close monitoring. Renal diseases can have multiple effects on sodium and water homeostasis; patients with glomerulonephritis may avidly reabsorb sodium, whereas those with tubulopathies may have obligatory urinary sodium losses. Patients with renal failure have a relative inability to excrete free water because of the reduced glomerular filtration rate and simultaneously are unable to produce maximally concentrated urine. Patients with adrenal insufficiency can have renal salt wasting and an impaired ability to excrete free water. Patients with CNS disorders can have multiple conditions that impair water excretion, including SIAD and cerebral salt wasting. Patients receiving certain medications are at particularly high risk for developing hyponatremia, such as desmopressin administered perioperatively for Von Willebrand disease, antiepileptic medications (such as carbamazepine), and chemotherapeutic agents (such as IV cyclophosphamide and vincristine). Isotonic IVFs may be the preferred fluid composition for these disease states, but care is needed in dosing the quantity of fluids, and close monitoring of both the volume status and electrolytes is required.

Limitations

The subcommittee's recommendation to use isotonic fluids when maintenance IVFs are required does not mean that there are no indications for administering hypotonic fluids or that isotonic fluids will be safe in all patients. Patients with significant renal concentrating defects, such as nephrogenic diabetes insipidus, could develop hypernatremia if they are administered isotonic fluids. Patients with voluminous diarrhea or severe burns may require a hypotonic fluid to keep up with ongoing free-water losses. Hypotonic fluids may also be required to correct hypernatremia. However, for the vast majority of patients, isotonic fluids are the most appropriate maintenance IVF and are the least likely to result in a disorder in serum sodium.

CONCLUSIONS

For the past 60 years, the prescription for maintenance IVFs for infants and children has been a hypotonic fluid. These recommendations were made on theoretical grounds and were not based on clinical trials. Despite this accepted dogma, over the past decade and longer, there have been increasing reports of the deleterious effect of hyponatremia in the acute care setting with the use of the prevailing hypotonic maintenance solutions. Using an evidence-based approach, recommendations for optimal sodium composition of maintenance IVFs are provided to prevent hyponatremia and acute or permanent neurologic impairment related to it. Recommendations are not made regarding the use of an isotonic buffered crystalloid solution versus saline, the optimal rate of fluid therapy, or the need for providing potassium in maintenance fluids. The use of this guideline differentiates the applicability to 2 subgroups of children: (1) The guideline applies to surgical (postoperative) medical patients in a critical care setting and the general inpatient ward. (2) The guideline does not apply to patients with neurosurgical disorders, congenital or acquired cardiac disease, hepatic disease, cancer, renal dysfunction, diabetes insipidus, voluminous watery diarrhea, or severe burns; neonates who are younger than 28 days old or in the NICU; or adolescents older than 18 years of age (Supplemental Fig 5).

This guideline is intended for use primarily by clinicians providing acute care for children and adolescents who require maintenance IVFs. It may be of interest to parents and payers, but it is not intended to be used for reimbursement or to determine insurance coverage. This guideline is not intended to be the sole source of guidance in the use of maintenance IVFs but rather is intended to assist clinicians by providing a framework for clinical decision-making.

The Key Action Statement is as follows:

1A: The AAP recommends that patients 28 days to 18 years of age requiring maintenance IVFs should receive isotonic solutions with appropriate KCl and dextrose because they significantly decrease the risk of developing hyponatremia (evidence quality: A; recommendation strength: strong).

BIOCHEMICAL LABORATORY MONITORING

Although the frequency for biochemical laboratory monitoring was not specifically addressed in the 17 RCTs included in the meta-analysis, researchers in most of the studies obtained serial plasma sodium values, with the first plasma sodium being measured between 6 hours and 12 hours. The incidence of hyponatremia in patients receiving isotonic fluids ranged from 0% to 23%, whereas that of hypotonic fluids ranged from 5% to 100%. This large variability was likely related to the different study designs. Many patients who were hospitalized and received isotonic IVFs will be at risk for hyponatremia if they are receiving IV medications containing free water or are consuming additional free water via the enteral route. For these reasons, clinicians should be aware that even patients receiving isotonic maintenance IVFs are at sufficient risk for developing hyponatremia. If an electrolyte abnormality is discovered, this could provide useful information to adjust maintenance fluid therapy. If patients receiving isotonic maintenance IVFs develop hyponatremia, they should be evaluated to determine if they are receiving other sources of free water or if they may have SIAD and/or an adrenal insufficiency. If hypernatremia develops (plasma sodium >144 mEq/L), patients should be evaluated for renal dysfunction or extrarenal free-water losses.

In patients at high risk for developing electrolyte abnormalities, such as those who have undergone major surgery, those in the ICU, or those with large gastrointestinal losses or receiving diuretics, frequent laboratory monitoring may be necessary. If neurologic symptoms that could be consistent with hyponatremic encephalopathy are present, such as unexplained nausea, vomiting, headache, confusion, or lethargy, electrolytes should be measured.

FUTURE QUALITY-IMPROVEMENT QUESTIONS

Future questions are as follows:

1. How frequently is plasma sodium concentration abnormal, and

is this abnormality clinically significant?

2. Will the widespread use of isotonic maintenance IVFs in the acute-care setting significantly reduce or eliminate hyponatremia- and hyponatremia-related neurologic events?
3. Will the widespread use of 0.9% saline for maintenance IVFs in the acute care setting increase clinically significant metabolic acidosis?
4. Are isotonic-balanced solutions superior to 0.9% saline for the maintenance IVF in the acute-care setting?
5. How frequently should clinicians monitor the serum sodium concentrations when a patient is receiving maintenance IVFs and for patients who are at high risk of sodium abnormalities?

SUBCOMMITTEE ON FLUID AND ELECTROLYTE THERAPY

Leonard G. Feld, MD, PhD, MMM, FAAP – *Chair, Pediatric Nephrology*
Daniel R. Neuspiel, MD, MPH, FAAP – *Pediatric Epidemiologist*
Byron Alexander Foster, MD, MPH, FAAP – *Pediatric Hospitalist*
Matthew D. Garber, MD, FHM, FAAP – *Pediatric Hospitalist; Implementation Scientist*
Michael G. Leu, MD, MS, MHS, FAAP – *Partnership for Policy Implementation*
Rajit K. Basu, MD, MS, FCCM – *Society of Critical Care Medicine, Pediatric Section*
Kelly Austin, MD, MS, FAAP, FACS – *American Pediatric Surgical Association*
Edward E. Conway, Jr, MD, MS, FAAP – *Pediatric Critical Care*
James J. Fehr, MD, FAAP – *Society for Pediatric Anesthesia*
Clare Hawkins, MD – *American Academy of Family Physicians*
Ron L. Kaplan, MD, FAAP – *Pediatric Emergency Medicine*
Echo V. Rowe, MD, FAAP – *Pediatric Anesthesiology and Pain Medicine*
Muhammad Waseem, MD, MS, FAAP, FACEP – *American College of Emergency Physicians*
Michael L. Moritz, MD, FAAP – *Pediatric Nephrology*

STAFF

Kymika Okechukwu, MPA – *Senior Manager, Evidence-Based Medicine Initiatives*

ABBREVIATIONS

AAP: American Academy of Pediatrics
ADH: antidiuretic hormone
AVP: arginine vasopressin
CHF: congestive heart failure
CI: confidence interval
CNS: central nervous system
IV: intravenous
IVF: intravenous fluid
kcal: kilocalorie
KCl: potassium chloride
M-H: Mantel-Haenzel
NaCl: sodium chloride
RCT: randomized controlled trial
SIAD: syndrome of inappropriate antidiuresis
Tco_2: total carbon dioxide

All clinical practice guidelines from the American Academy of Pediatrics automatically expire 5 years after publication unless reaffirmed, revised, or retired at or before that time.

DOI: https://doi.org/10.1542/peds.2018-3083

Address correspondence to Leonard G. Feld, MD, PhD, MMM, FAAP. E-mail: feldllc@gmail.com

PEDIATRICS (ISSN Numbers: Print, 0031-4005; Online, 1098-4275).

Copyright © 2018 by the American Academy of Pediatrics

FINANCIAL DISCLOSURE: The authors have indicated they have no financial relationships relevant to this article to disclose.

FUNDING: No external funding.

POTENTIAL CONFLICT OF INTEREST: The authors have indicated they have no potential conflicts of interest to disclose.

REFERENCES

1. Chawla G, Drummond GB. Textbook coverage of a common topic: fluid management of patients after surgery. *Med Educ.* 2008;42(6):613–618
2. Davies P, Hall T, Ali T, Lakhoo K. Intravenous postoperative fluid prescriptions for children: a survey of practice. *BMC Surg.* 2008;8:10
3. Freeman MA, Ayus JC, Moritz ML. Maintenance intravenous fluid prescribing practices among paediatric residents. *Acta Paediatr.* 2012;101(10):e465–e468
4. Lee JM, Jung Y, Lee SE, et al. Intravenous fluid prescription practices among pediatric residents in Korea. *Korean J Pediatr.* 2013;56(7):282–285
5. Goldstein SL. Fluid management in acute kidney injury. *J Intensive Care Med.* 2014;29(4):183–189
6. Hoste EA, Maitland K, Brudney CS, et al; ADQI XII Investigators Group. Four phases of intravenous fluid therapy: a conceptual model. *Br J Anaesth.* 2014;113(5): 740–747
7. McDermid RC, Raghunathan K, Romanovsky A, Shaw AD, Bagshaw SM. Controversies in fluid therapy: type, dose and toxicity. *World J Crit Care Med.* 2014;3(1):24–33
8. Jackson J, Bolte RG. Risks of intravenous administration of hypotonic fluids for pediatric patients in ED and prehospital settings: let's remove the handle from the pump. *Am J Emerg Med.* 2000;18(3):269–270
9. Wang J, Xu E, Xiao Y. Isotonic versus hypotonic maintenance IV fluids in hospitalized children: a meta-analysis. *Pediatrics.* 2014;133(1):105–113
10. Moritz ML, Ayus JC. Maintenance intravenous fluids in acutely ill patients. *N Engl J Med.* 2015;373(14):1350–1360
11. Carandang F, Anglemyer A, Longhurst CA, et al. Association between

maintenance fluid tonicity and hospital-acquired hyponatremia. *J Pediatr*. 2013;163(6):1646–1651

12. Upadhyay A, Jaber BL, Madias NE. Incidence and prevalence of hyponatremia. *Am J Med*. 2006;119 (7, suppl 1):S30–S35
13. Moritz ML, Ayus JC. Disorders of water metabolism in children: hyponatremia and hypernatremia. *Pediatr Rev*. 2002;23(11):371–380
14. Gerigk M, Gnehm HE, Rascher W. Arginine vasopressin and renin in acutely ill children: implication for fluid therapy. *Acta Paediatr*. 1996;85(5):550–553
15. Judd BA, Haycock GB, Dalton RN, Chantler C. Antidiuretic hormone following surgery in children. *Acta Paediatr Scand*. 1990;79(4):461–466
16. Holliday MA, Segar WE. The maintenance need for water in parenteral fluid therapy. *Pediatrics*. 1957;19(5):823–832
17. Talbot FB. Basal metabolism standards for children. *Am J Dis Child*. 1938;55(3):455–459
18. Hatherill M. Rubbing salt in the wound. *Arch Dis Child*. 2004;89(5):414–418
19. Hoorn EJ, Geary D, Robb M, Halperin ML, Bohn D. Acute hyponatremia related to intravenous fluid administration in hospitalized children: an observational study. *Pediatrics*. 2004;113(5):1279–1284
20. Choong K, Arora S, Cheng J, et al. Hypotonic versus isotonic maintenance fluids after surgery for children: a randomized controlled trial. *Pediatrics*. 2011;128(5):857–866
21. Arieff AI, Ayus JC, Fraser CL. Hyponatraemia and death or permanent brain damage in healthy children. *BMJ*. 1992;304(6836):1218–1222
22. Moritz ML, Ayus JC. Preventing neurological complications from dysnatremias in children. *Pediatr Nephrol*. 2005;20(12):1687–1700
23. Halberthal M, Halperin ML, Bohn D. Lesson of the week: acute hyponatraemia in children admitted to hospital: retrospective analysis of factors contributing to its development and resolution. *BMJ*. 2001;322(7289):780–782
24. Moritz ML, Ayus JC. Prevention of hospital-acquired hyponatremia: a case for using isotonic saline. *Pediatrics*. 2003;111(2):227–230
25. ISMP. Medication safety alert. Plain D5W or hypotonic saline solutions post-op could result in acute hyponatremia and death in healthy children. Available at: ismp.org. Accessed August 14, 2009
26. ISMP Canada. Hospital-acquired acute hyponatremia: two reports of pediatric deaths.*ISMP Canada Saf Bul*. 2009;9(7). Available at: http://www.ismp-canada.org/download/safetyBulletins/ISMPCSB2009-7-HospitalAcquiredAcuteHyponatremia.pdf. Accessed July 26, 2018
27. National Patient Safety Agency. Reducing the risk of hyponatraemia when administering intravenous infusions to children. 2007. Available at: www.npsa.nhs.uk/health/alerts. Accessed July 6, 2018
28. Drysdale SB, Coulson T, Cronin N, et al. The impact of the National Patient Safety Agency intravenous fluid alert on iatrogenic hyponatraemia in children. *Eur J Pediatr*. 2010;169(7):813–817
29. Holliday MA, Ray PE, Friedman AL. Fluid therapy for children: facts, fashions and questions. *Arch Dis Child*. 2007;92(6):546–550
30. McNab S. Isotonic vs hypotonic intravenous fluids for hospitalized children. *JAMA*. 2015;314(7):720–721
31. Almeida HI, Mascarenhas MI, Loureiro HC, et al. The effect of NaCl 0.9% and NaCl 0.45% on sodium, chloride, and acid-base balance in a PICU population. *J Pediatr (Rio J)*. 2015;91(5):499–505
32. Friedman JN, Beck CE, DeGroot J, Geary DF, Sklansky DJ, Freedman SB. Comparison of isotonic and hypotonic intravenous maintenance fluids: a randomized clinical trial. *JAMA Pediatr*. 2015;169(5):445–451
33. McNab S, Ware RS, Neville KA, et al. Isotonic versus hypotonic solutions for maintenance intravenous fluid administration in children. *Cochrane Database Syst Rev*. 2014;(12):CD009457
34. National Clinical Guideline Centre (UK). *IV Fluids in Children: Intravenous Fluid Therapy in Children and Young People in Hospital*. London, United Kingdom: National Clinical Guideline Centre; 2015. Available at: www.ncbi.nlm.nih.gov/pubmed/26741016. Accessed July 6, 2018
35. McNab S, Duke T, South M, et al. 140 mmol/L of sodium versus 77 mmol/L of sodium in maintenance intravenous fluid therapy for children in hospital (PIMS): a randomised controlled double-blind trial. *Lancet*. 2015;385(9974):1190–1197. Published online December 1, 2014
36. Siegel NJ, ed. Fluids, electrolytes and acid-base. In: *Rudolph's Pediatrics*. 21st ed. New York, NY: McGraw Hill; 2003:1653–1655
37. Greenbaum LA, ed. Pathophysiology of body fluids and fluid therapy. In: *Nelson's Textbook of Pediatrics*. 17th ed. Philadelphia, PA: WB Saunders; 2004:242–245
38. Powers KS. Dehydration: isonatremic, hyponatremic, and hypernatremic recognition and management. *Pediatr Rev*. 2015;36(7):274–283; quiz 284–285
39. Foster BA, Tom D, Hill V. Hypotonic versus isotonic fluids in hospitalized children: a systematic review and meta-analysis. *J Pediatr*. 2014;165(1):163–169.e2
40. Padua AP, Macaraya JR, Dans LF, Anacleto FE Jr. Isotonic versus hypotonic saline solution for maintenance intravenous fluid therapy in children: a systematic review. *Pediatr Nephrol*. 2015;30(7):1163–1172
41. Yang G, Jiang W, Wang X, Liu W. The efficacy of isotonic and hypotonic intravenous maintenance fluid for pediatric patients: a meta-analysis of randomized controlled trials. *Pediatr Emerg Care*. 2015;31(2):122–126
42. Choong K, Kho ME, Menon K, Bohn D. Hypotonic versus isotonic saline in hospitalised children: a systematic review. *Arch Dis Child*. 2006;91(10):828–835
43. Guyatt GH, Sackett DL, Cook DJ. Users' guides to the medical literature. II. How to use an article about therapy or prevention. A. Are the results of the study valid? Evidence-Based Medicine Working Group. *JAMA*. 1993;270(21):2598–2601
44. Guyatt GH, Sackett DL, Cook DJ. Users' guides to the medical literature. II.

How to use an article about therapy or prevention. B. What were the results and will they help me in caring for my patients? Evidence-Based Medicine Working Group. *JAMA.* 1994;271(1):59–63

45. Higgins JP, Green S, eds. *Cochrane Handbook for Systematic Reviews of Interventions. Version 5.1.0. Updated March 2011.* London, United Kingdom: The Cochrane Collaboration; 2011. Available at: http://handbook-5-1.cochrane.org/. Accessed July 6, 2018
46. American Academy of Pediatrics Steering Committee on Quality Improvement and Management. Classifying recommendations for clinical practice guidelines. *Pediatrics.* 2004;114(3):874–877
47. Bridge-Wiz. Guideline quality appraisal. Available at: http://gem.med.yale.edu/BRIDGE-Wiz/BridgeWiz_2.1_AAP.zip. Accessed April 12, 2016
48. Brazel PW, McPhee IB. Inappropriate secretion of antidiuretic hormone in postoperative scoliosis patients: the role of fluid management. *Spine.* 1996;21(6):724–727
49. Coulthard MG, Long DA, Ullman AJ, Ware RS. A randomised controlled trial of Hartmann's solution versus half normal saline in postoperative paediatric spinal instrumentation and craniotomy patients. *Arch Dis Child.* 2012;97(6):491–496
50. Jorro Barón FA, Meregalli CN, Rombola VA, et al. Hypotonic versus isotonic maintenance fluids in critically ill pediatric patients: a randomized controlled trial [in English and Spanish]. *Arch Argent Pediatr.* 2013;111(4):281–287
51. Flores Robles CM, Cuello García CA. A prospective trial comparing isotonic with hypotonic maintenance fluids for prevention of hospital-acquired hyponatraemia. *Paediatr Int Child Health.* 2016;36(3):168–174
52. Kannan L, Lodha R, Vivekanandhan S, Bagga A, Kabra SK, Kabra M. Intravenous fluid regimen and hyponatraemia among children: a randomized controlled trial. *Pediatr Nephrol.* 2010;25(11):2303–2309
53. Montañana PA, Modesto i Alapont V, Ocón AP, López PO, López Prats JL, Toledo Parreño JD. The use of isotonic fluid as maintenance therapy prevents iatrogenic hyponatremia in pediatrics: a randomized, controlled open study. *Pediatr Crit Care Med.* 2008;9(6):589–597
54. Neville KA, Sandeman DJ, Rubinstein A, et al. Prevention of hyponatremia during maintenance intravenous fluid administration: a prospective randomized study of fluid type versus fluid rate. *J Pediatr.* 2010;156(2):313–319.e1–e2
55. Ramanathan S, Kumar P, Mishra K, Dutta AK. Isotonic versus hypotonic parenteral maintenance fluids in very severe pneumonia. *Indian J Pediatr.* 2016;83(1):27–32
56. Rey C, Los-Arcos M, Hernández A, Sánchez A, Díaz JJ, López-Herce J. Hypotonic versus isotonic maintenance fluids in critically ill children: a multicenter prospective randomized study. *Acta Paediatr.* 2011;100(8):1138–1143
57. Saba TG, Fairbairn J, Houghton F, Laforte D, Foster BJ. A randomized controlled trial of isotonic versus hypotonic maintenance intravenous fluids in hospitalized children. *BMC Pediatr.* 2011;11:82
58. Shamim A, Afzal K, Ali SM. Safety and efficacy of isotonic (0.9%) vs. hypotonic (0.18%) saline as maintenance intravenous fluids in children: a randomized controlled trial. *Indian Pediatr.* 2014;51(12):969–974
59. Yung M, Keeley S. Randomised controlled trial of intravenous maintenance fluids. *J Paediatr Child Health.* 2009;45(1–2):9–14
60. Valadão MC S, Piva JP, Santana JC, Garcia PC. Comparison of two maintenance electrolyte solutions in children in the postoperative appendectomy period: a randomized, controlled trial. *J Pediatr (Rio J).* 2015;91(5):428–434
61. Duke T, Kinney S, Waters K. Hyponatraemia and seizures in oncology patients associated with hypotonic intravenous fluids. *J Paediatr Child Health.* 2005;41(12):685–686
62. Gankam-Kengne F, Ayers C, Khera A, de Lemos J, Maalouf NM. Mild hyponatremia is associated with an increased risk of death in an ambulatory setting. *Kidney Int.* 2013;83(4):700–706
63. Holland-Bill L, Christiansen CF, Heide-Jørgensen U, et al. Hyponatremia and mortality risk: a Danish cohort study of 279508 acutely hospitalized patients. *Eur J Endocrinol.* 2015;173(1):71–81
64. Amin A, Deitelzweig S, Christian R, et al. Evaluation of incremental healthcare resource burden and readmission rates associated with hospitalized hyponatremic patients in the US. *J Hosp Med.* 2012;7(8):634–639
65. Corona G, Giuliani C, Parenti G, et al. The economic burden of hyponatremia: systematic review and meta-analysis. *Am J Med.* 2016;129(8):823–835.e4
66. Alobaidi R, Morgan C, Basu RK, et al. Associations between fluid balance and outcomes in critically ill children: a protocol for a systematic review and meta-analysis. *Can J Kidney Health Dis.* 2017;4:2054358117692560
67. Pemde HK, Dutta AK, Sodani R, Mishra K. Isotonic intravenous maintenance fluid reduces hospital acquired hyponatremia in young children with central nervous system infections. *Indian J Pediatr.* 2015;82(1):13–18

Intravenous Fluids Clinical Practice Guideline Quick Reference Tools

- Action Statement Summary
  - Clinical Practice Guideline: Maintenance Intravenous Fluids in Children
- *ICD-10-CM* Coding Quick Reference for Maintenance Intravenous Fluids

Action Statement Summary

Clinical Practice Guideline: Maintenance Intravenous Fluids in Children

Key Action Statement 1

Composition of Maintenance IVFs

Key Action Statement 1A

The AAP recommends that patients 28 days to 18 years of age requiring maintenance IVFs should receive isotonic solutions with appropriate potassium chloride (KCl) and dextrose because they significantly decrease the risk of developing hyponatremia (evidence quality: A; recommendation strength: strong).

Coding Quick Reference for Maintenance Intravenous Fluids
ICD-10-CM
E86.0 Dehydration

The Diagnosis and Management of Acute Otitis Media

- *Clinical Practice Guideline*

CLINICAL PRACTICE GUIDELINE

The Diagnosis and Management of Acute Otitis Media

abstract

This evidence-based clinical practice guideline is a revision of the 2004 acute otitis media (AOM) guideline from the American Academy of Pediatrics (AAP) and American Academy of Family Physicians. It provides recommendations to primary care clinicians for the management of children from 6 months through 12 years of age with uncomplicated AOM.

In 2009, the AAP convened a committee composed of primary care physicians and experts in the fields of pediatrics, family practice, otolaryngology, epidemiology, infectious disease, emergency medicine, and guideline methodology. The subcommittee partnered with the Agency for Healthcare Research and Quality and the Southern California Evidence-Based Practice Center to develop a comprehensive review of the new literature related to AOM since the initial evidence report of 2000. The resulting evidence report and other sources of data were used to formulate the practice guideline recommendations.

The focus of this practice guideline is the appropriate diagnosis and initial treatment of a child presenting with AOM. The guideline provides a specific, stringent definition of AOM. It addresses pain management, initial observation versus antibiotic treatment, appropriate choices of antibiotic agents, and preventive measures. It also addresses recurrent AOM, which was not included in the 2004 guideline. Decisions were made on the basis of a systematic grading of the quality of evidence and benefit-harm relationships.

The practice guideline underwent comprehensive peer review before formal approval by the AAP.

This clinical practice guideline is not intended as a sole source of guidance in the management of children with AOM. Rather, it is intended to assist primary care clinicians by providing a framework for clinical decision-making. It is not intended to replace clinical judgment or establish a protocol for all children with this condition. These recommendations may not provide the only appropriate approach to the management of this problem. *Pediatrics* 2013;131:e964–e999

Allan S. Lieberthal, MD, FAAP, Aaron E. Carroll, MD, MS, FAAP, Tasnee Chonmaitree, MD, FAAP, Theodore G. Ganiats, MD, Alejandro Hoberman, MD, FAAP, Mary Anne Jackson, MD, FAAP, Mark D. Joffe, MD, FAAP, Donald T. Miller, MD, MPH, FAAP, Richard M. Rosenfeld, MD, MPH, FAAP, Xavier D. Sevilla, MD, FAAP, Richard H. Schwartz, MD, FAAP, Pauline A. Thomas, MD, FAAP, and David E. Tunkel, MD, FAAP, FACS

KEY WORDS

acute otitis media, otitis media, otoscopy, otitis media with effusion, watchful waiting, antibiotics, antibiotic prophylaxis, tympanostomy tube insertion, immunization, breastfeeding

ABBREVIATIONS

AAFP—American Academy of Family Physicians
AAP—American Academy of Pediatrics
AHRQ—Agency for Healthcare Research and Quality
AOM—acute otitis media
CI—confidence interval
FDA—US Food and Drug Administration
LAIV—live-attenuated intranasal influenza vaccine
MEE—middle ear effusion
MIC—minimum inhibitory concentration
NNT—number needed to treat
OM—otitis media
OME—otitis media with effusion
OR—odds ratio
PCV7—heptavalent pneumococcal conjugate vaccine
PCV13—13-valent pneumococcal conjugate vaccine
RD—rate difference
SNAP—safety-net antibiotic prescription
TIV—trivalent inactivated influenza vaccine
TM—tympanic membrane
WASP—wait-and-see prescription

This document is copyrighted and is property of the American Academy of Pediatrics and its Board of Directors. All authors have filed conflict of interest statements with the American Academy of Pediatrics. Any conflicts have been resolved through a process approved by the Board of Directors. The American Academy of Pediatrics has neither solicited nor accepted any commercial involvement in the development of the content of this publication.

The recommendations in this report do not indicate an exclusive course of treatment or serve as a standard of medical care. Variations, taking into account individual circumstances, may be appropriate.

(Continued on last page)

Key Action Statement 1A: Clinicians should diagnose acute otitis media (AOM) in children who present with moderate to severe bulging of the tympanic membrane (TM) *or* new onset of otorrhea not due to acute otitis externa. Evidence Quality: Grade B. Strength: Recommendation.

Key Action Statement 1B: Clinicians should diagnose AOM in children who present with mild bulging of the TM *and* recent (less than 48 hours) onset of ear pain (holding, tugging, rubbing of the ear in a nonverbal child) or intense erythema of the TM. Evidence Quality: Grade C. Strength: Recommendation.

Key Action Statement 1C: Clinicians should not diagnose AOM in children who do not have middle ear effusion (MEE) (based on pneumatic otoscopy and/or tympanometry). Evidence Quality: Grade B. Strength: Recommendation.

Key Action Statement 2: The management of AOM should include an assessment of pain. If pain is present, the clinician should recommend treatment to reduce pain. Evidence Quality: Grade B. Strength: Strong Recommendation.

Key Action Statement 3A: Severe AOM: The clinician should prescribe antibiotic therapy for AOM (bilateral or unilateral) in children 6 months and older with severe signs or symptoms (ie, moderate or severe otalgia or otalgia for at least 48 hours or temperature 39°C [102.2°F] or higher). Evidence Quality: Grade B. Strength: Strong Recommendation.

Key Action Statement 3B: Nonsevere bilateral AOM in young children: The clinician should prescribe antibiotic therapy for bilateral AOM in children 6 months through 23 months of age without severe signs or symptoms (ie, mild otalgia for less than 48 hours and temperature less than 39°C [102.2°F]). Evidence Quality: Grade B. Strength: Recommendation.

Key Action Statement 3C: Nonsevere unilateral AOM in young children: The clinician should either prescribe antibiotic therapy *or* offer observation with close follow-up based on joint decision-making with the parent(s)/caregiver for unilateral AOM in children 6 months to 23 months of age without severe signs or symptoms (ie, mild otalgia for less than 48 hours and temperature less than 39°C [102.2°F]). When observation is used, a mechanism must be in place to ensure follow-up and begin antibiotic therapy if the child worsens or fails to improve within 48 to 72 hours of onset of symptoms. Evidence Quality: Grade B. Strength: Recommendation.

Key Action Statement 3D: Nonsevere AOM in older children: The clinician should either prescribe antibiotic therapy *or* offer observation with close follow-up based on joint decision-making with the parent(s)/caregiver for AOM (bilateral or unilateral) in children 24 months or older without severe signs or symptoms (ie, mild otalgia for less than 48 hours and temperature less than 39°C [102.2°F]). When observation is used, a mechanism must be in place to ensure follow-up and begin antibiotic therapy if the child worsens or fails to improve within 48 to 72 hours of onset of symptoms. Evidence Quality: Grade B. Strength: Recommendation.

Key Action Statement 4A: Clinicians should prescribe amoxicillin for AOM when a decision to treat with antibiotics has been made *and* the child has not received amoxicillin in the past 30 days *or* the child does not have concurrent purulent conjunctivitis *or* the child is not allergic to penicillin. Evidence Quality: Grade B. Strength: Recommendation.

Key Action Statement 4B: Clinicians should prescribe an antibiotic with additional β-lactamase coverage for AOM when a decision to treat with antibiotics has been made, *and* the child has received amoxicillin in the last 30 days *or* has concurrent purulent conjunctivitis, *or* has a history of recurrent AOM unresponsive to amoxicillin. Evidence Quality: Grade C. Strength: Recommendation.

Key Action Statement 4C: Clinicians should reassess the patient if the caregiver reports that the child's symptoms have worsened or failed to respond to the initial antibiotic treatment within 48 to 72 hours and determine whether a change in therapy is needed. Evidence Quality: Grade B. Strength: Recommendation.

Key Action Statement 5A: Clinicians should not prescribe prophylactic antibiotics to reduce the frequency of episodes of AOM in children with recurrent AOM. Evidence Quality: Grade B. Strength: Recommendation.

Key Action Statement 5B: Clinicians may offer tympanostomy tubes for recurrent AOM (3 episodes in 6 months or 4 episodes in 1 year with 1 episode in the preceding 6 months). Evidence Quality: Grade B. Strength: Option.

Key Action Statement 6A: Clinicians should recommend pneumococcal conjugate vaccine to all children according to the schedule of the Advisory Committee on Immunization Practices of the Centers for Disease Control and Prevention, American Academy of Pediatrics (AAP), and American Academy of Family Physicians (AAFP). Evidence Quality: Grade B. Strength: Strong Recommendation.

Key Action Statement 6B: Clinicians should recommend annual influenza vaccine to all children according to the schedule of the Advisory Committee on Immunization Practices, AAP, and AAFP. Evidence Quality: Grade B. Strength: Recommendation.

2Key Action Statement 6C: Clinicians should encourage exclusive breastfeeding for at least 6 months. Evidence Quality: Grade B. Strength: Recommendation.

Key Action Statement 6D: Clinicians should encourage avoidance of tobacco smoke exposure. Evidence Quality: Grade C. Strength: Recommendation.

INTRODUCTION

In May 2004, the AAP and AAFP published the "Clinical Practice Guideline: Diagnosis and Management of Acute Otitis Media".[1] The guideline offered 8 recommendations ranked according to level of evidence and benefit-harm relationship. Three of the recommendations—diagnostic criteria, observation, and choice of antibiotics—led to significant discussion, especially among experts in the field of otitis media (OM). Also, at the time the guideline was written, information regarding the heptavalent pneumococcal conjugate vaccine (PCV7) was not yet published. Since completion of the guideline in November 2003 and its publication in May 2004, there has been a significant body of additional literature on AOM.

Although OM remains the most common condition for which antibacterial agents are prescribed for children in the United States[2,3] clinician visits for OM decreased from 950 per 1000 children in 1995–1996 to 634 per 1000 children in 2005–2006. There has been a proportional decrease in antibiotic prescriptions for OM from 760 per 1000 in 1995–1996 to 484 per 1000 in 2005–2006. The percentage of OM visits resulting in antibiotic prescriptions remained relatively stable (80% in 1995–1996; 76% in 2005–2006).[2] Many factors may have contributed to the decrease in visits for OM, including financial issues relating to insurance, such as copayments, that may limit doctor visits, public education campaigns regarding the viral nature of most infectious diseases, use of the PCV7 pneumococcal vaccine, and increased use of the influenza vaccine. Clinicians may also be more attentive to differentiating AOM from OM with effusion (OME), resulting in fewer visits coded for AOM and fewer antibiotic prescriptions written.

Despite significant publicity and awareness of the 2004 AOM guideline, evidence shows that clinicians are hesitant to follow the guideline recommendations. Vernacchio et al[4] surveyed 489 primary care physicians as to their management of 4 AOM scenarios addressed in the 2004 guideline. No significant changes in practice were noted on this survey, compared with a survey administered before the 2004 AOM guideline. Coco[5] used the National Ambulatory Medical Care Survey from 2002 through 2006 to determine the frequency of AOM visits without antibiotics before and after publication of the 2004 guideline. There was no difference in prescribing rates. A similar response to otitis guidelines was found in Italy as in the United States.[6,7] These findings parallel results of other investigations regarding clinician awareness and adherence to guideline recommendations in all specialties, including pediatrics.[8] Clearly, for clinical practice guidelines to be effective, more must be done to improve their dissemination and implementation.

This revision and update of the AAP/AAFP 2004 AOM guideline[1] will evaluate published evidence on the diagnosis and management of uncomplicated AOM and make recommendations based on that evidence. The guideline is intended for primary care clinicians including pediatricians and family physicians, emergency department physicians, otolaryngologists, physician assistants, and nurse practitioners. The scope of the guideline is the diagnosis and management of AOM, including recurrent AOM, in children 6 months through 12 years of age. It applies only to an otherwise healthy child without underlying conditions that may alter the natural course of AOM, including but not limited to the presence of tympanostomy tubes; anatomic abnormalities, including cleft palate; genetic conditions with craniofacial abnormalities, such as Down syndrome; immune deficiencies; and the presence of cochlear implants. Children with OME without AOM are also excluded.

Glossary of Terms

AOM—the rapid onset of signs and symptoms of inflammation in the middle ear[9,10]

Uncomplicated AOM—AOM without otorrhea[1]

Severe AOM—AOM with the presence of moderate to severe otalgia *or* fever equal to or higher than 39°C[9,10]

Nonsevere AOM—AOM with the presence of mild otalgia and a temperature below 39°C[9,10]

Recurrent AOM—3 or more well-documented and separate AOM episodes in the preceding 6 months *or* 4 or more episodes in the preceding 12 months with at least 1 episode in the past 6 months[11,12]

OME—inflammation of the middle ear with liquid collected in the middle ear; the signs and symptoms of acute infection are absent[9]

MEE—liquid in the middle ear without reference to etiology, pathogenesis, pathology, or duration[9]

Otorrhea—discharge from the ear, originating at 1 or more of the following sites: the external auditory canal, middle ear, mastoid, inner ear, or intracranial cavity

Otitis externa—an infection of the external auditory canal

Tympanometry—measuring acoustic immittance (transfer of acoustic energy) of the ear as a function of ear canal air pressure[13,14]

Number needed to treat (NNT)—the number of patients who need to be treated to prevent 1 additional bad outcome[15]

Initial antibiotic therapy—treatment of AOM with antibiotics that are prescribed at the time of diagnosis with the intent of starting antibiotic therapy as soon as possible after the encounter

Initial observation—initial management of AOM limited to symptomatic relief, with commencement of antibiotic therapy only if the child's condition worsens at any time or does not show clinical improvement within 48 to 72 hours of diagnosis; a mechanism must be in place to ensure follow-up and initiation of antibiotics if the child fails observation

METHODS

Guideline development using an evidence-based approach requires that all evidence related to the guideline is gathered in a systematic fashion, objectively assessed, and then described so readers can easily see the links between the evidence and recommendations made. An evidence-based approach leads to recommendations that are guided by both the quality of the available evidence and the benefit-to-harm ratio that results from following the recommendation. Figure 1 shows the relationship of evidence quality and benefit-harm balance in determining the level of recommendation. Table 1 presents the AAP definitions and implications of different levels of evidence-based recommendations.[16]

In preparing for the 2004 AAP guidelines, the Agency for Healthcare Research and Quality (AHRQ) funded and conducted an exhaustive review of the literature on diagnosis and management of AOM.[17–19] In 2008, the AHRQ and the Southern California Evidence-Based Practice Center began a similar process of reviewing the literature published since the 2001 AHRQ report. The AAP again partnered with AHRQ and the Southern California Evidence-Based Practice Center to develop the evidence report, which served as a major source of data for these practice guideline recommendations.[20,21] New key questions were determined by a technical expert panel. The scope of the new report went beyond the 2001 AHRQ report to include recurrent AOM.

The key questions addressed by AHRQ in the 2010 report were as follows:

1. Diagnosis of AOM: What are the operating characteristics (sensitivity, specificity, and likelihood ratios) of clinical symptoms and otoscopic findings (such as bulging TM) to diagnose uncomplicated AOM and to distinguish it from OME?
2. What has been the effect of the use of heptavalent PCV7 on AOM microbial epidemiology, what organisms (bacterial and viral) are associated with AOM since the introduction of PCV7, and what are the patterns of antimicrobial resistance in AOM since the introduction of PCV7?
3. What is the comparative effectiveness of various treatment options for treating uncomplicated AOM in average risk children?
4. What is the comparative effectiveness of different management options for recurrent OM (uncomplicated) and persistent OM or relapse of AOM?
5. Do treatment outcomes in Questions 3 and 4 differ by characteristics of the condition (AOM), patient, environment, and/or health care delivery system?
6. What adverse effects have been observed for treatments for which outcomes are addressed in Questions 3 and 4?

For the 2010 review, searches of PubMed and the Cochrane Database of Systematic Reviews, Cochrane Central Register of Controlled Trials, and Education Resources Information Center were conducted by using the same search strategies used for the 2001 report for publications from 1998 through June 2010. Additional terms or conditions not considered in the 2001 review (recurrent OM, new drugs, and heptavalent pneumococcal vaccine) were also included. The Web of Science was also used to search for citations of the 2001 report and its peer-reviewed publications. Titles were screened independently by 2

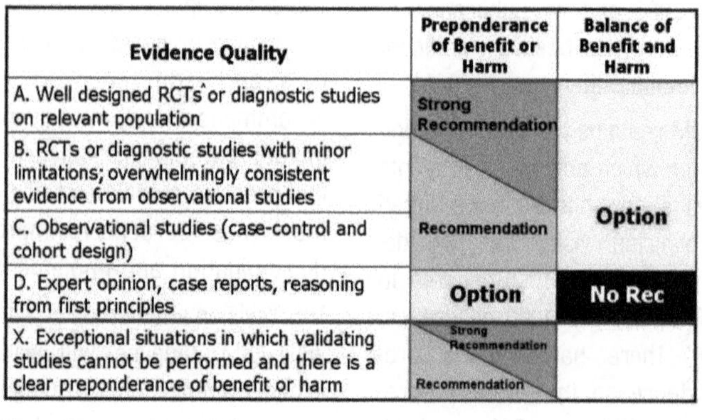

Evidence Quality	Preponderance of Benefit or Harm	Balance of Benefit and Harm
A. Well designed RCTs or diagnostic studies on relevant population	Strong Recommendation	Option
B. RCTs or diagnostic studies with minor limitations; overwhelmingly consistent evidence from observational studies		
C. Observational studies (case-control and cohort design)	Recommendation	
D. Expert opinion, case reports, reasoning from first principles	Option	No Rec
X. Exceptional situations in which validating studies cannot be performed and there is a clear preponderance of benefit or harm	Strong Recommendation / Recommendation	

FIGURE 1

Relationship of evidence quality and benefit-harm balance in determining the level of recommendation. RCT, randomized controlled trial.

TABLE 1 Guideline Definitions for Evidence-Based Statements

Statement	Definition	Implication
Strong Recommendation	A strong recommendation in favor of a particular action is made when the anticipated benefits of the recommended intervention clearly exceed the harms (as a strong recommendation against an action is made when the anticipated harms clearly exceed the benefits) and the quality of the supporting evidence is excellent. In some clearly identified circumstances, strong recommendations may be made when high-quality evidence is impossible to obtain and the anticipated benefits strongly outweigh the harms.	Clinicians should follow a strong recommendation unless a clear and compelling rationale for an alternative approach is present.
Recommendation	A recommendation in favor of a particular action is made when the anticipated benefits exceed the harms, but the quality of evidence is not as strong. Again, in some clearly identified circumstances, recommendations may be made when high-quality evidence is impossible to obtain but the anticipated benefits outweigh the harms.	Clinicians would be prudent to follow a recommendation but should remain alert to new information and sensitive to patient preferences.
Option	Options define courses that may be taken when either the quality of evidence is suspect or carefully performed studies have shown little clear advantage to 1 approach over another.	Clinicians should consider the option in their decision-making, and patient preference may have a substantial role.
No Recommendation	No recommendation indicates that there is a lack of pertinent published evidence and that the anticipated balance of benefits and harms is presently unclear.	Clinicians should be alert to new published evidence that clarifies the balance of benefit versus harm.

pediatricians with experience in conducting systematic reviews.

For the question pertaining to diagnosis, efficacy, and safety, the search was primarily for clinical trials. For the question pertaining to the effect of PCV7 on epidemiology and microbiology, the group searched for trials that compared microbiology in the same populations before and after introduction of the vaccine or observational studies that compared microbiology across vaccinated and unvaccinated populations.

In total, the reviewers examined 7646 titles, of which 686 titles were identified for further review. Of those, 72 articles that met the predetermined inclusion and exclusion criteria were reviewed in detail. Investigators abstracted data into standard evidence tables, with accuracy checked by a second investigator. Studies were quality-rated by 2 investigators by using established criteria. For randomized controlled trials, the Jadad criteria were used.[22] QUADAS criteria[23] were used to evaluate the studies that pertained to diagnosis. GRADE criteria were applied to pooled analyses.[24] Data abstracted included parameters necessary to define study groups, inclusion/exclusion criteria, influencing factors, and outcome measures. Some of the data for analysis were abstracted by a biostatistician and checked by a physician reviewer. A sequential resolution strategy was used to match and resolve the screening and review results of the 2 pediatrician reviewers.

For the assessment of treatment efficacy, pooled analyses were performed for comparisons for which 3 or more trials could be identified. Studies eligible for analyses of questions pertaining to treatment efficacy were grouped for comparisons by treatment options. Each comparison consisted of studies that were considered homogeneous across clinical practice. Because some of the key questions were addressed in the 2001 evidence report,[17] studies identified in that report were included with newly identified articles in the 2010 evidence report.[20]

Decisions were made on the basis of a systematic grading of the quality of evidence and strength of recommendations as well as expert consensus when definitive data were not available. Results of the literature review were presented in evidence tables and published in the final evidence report.[20]

In June 2009, the AAP convened a new subcommittee to review and revise the May 2004 AOM guideline.[1] The subcommittee comprised primary care physicians and experts in the fields of pediatrics, family practice, otolaryngology, epidemiology, infectious disease, emergency medicine, and guideline methodology. All panel members reviewed the AAP policy on conflict of interest and voluntary disclosure and were given an opportunity to present any potential conflicts with the subcommittee's work. All potential conflicts of interest are listed at the end of this document. The project was funded by the AAP. New literature on OM is continually being published. Although the systematic review performed by AHRQ could not be replicated with new literature, members of the Subcommittee on Diagnosis and Management of Acute Otitis Media reviewed additional articles. PubMed was searched by using the single search term "acute otitis media," approximately every 6 months from June 2009 through October 2011 to obtain new articles. Subcommittee members evaluated pertinent articles for quality of methodology and importance of results. Selected articles used in the AHRQ review were also reevaluated for their quality. Conclusions were based on the consensus of the subcommittee after the review of newer literature and reevaluation of the AHRQ evidence. Key action statements were generated using BRIDGE-Wiz (Building Recommendations in a Developers Guideline Editor), an interactive software tool that leads guideline development through a series of questions that are intended to create a more actionable set of key action statements.[25] BRIDGE-Wiz also incorporates the quality of available evidence into the final determination of the strength of each recommendation.

After thorough review by the subcommittee for this guideline, a draft was reviewed by other AAP committees and sections, selected outside organizations, and individuals identified by the subcommittee as experts in the field. Additionally, members of the subcommittee were encouraged to distribute the draft to interested parties in their respective specialties. All comments were reviewed by the writing group and incorporated into the final guideline when appropriate.

This clinical practice guideline is not intended as a sole source of guidance in the management of children with AOM. Rather, it is intended to assist clinicians in decision-making. It is not intended to replace clinical judgment or establish a protocol for the care of all children with this condition. These recommendations may not provide the only appropriate approach to the management of children with AOM.

It is AAP policy to review and update evidence-based guidelines every 5 years.

KEY ACTION STATEMENTS

Key Action Statement 1A

Clinicians should diagnose AOM in children who present with moderate to severe bulging of the TM *or* new onset of otorrhea not due to acute otitis externa. (Evidence Quality: Grade B, Rec. Strength: Recommendation)

Key Action Statement Profile: KAS 1A

Aggregate evidence quality	Grade B
Benefits	• Identify a population of children most likely to benefit from intervention. • Avoid unnecessary treatment of those without highly certain AOM. • Promote consistency in diagnosis.
Risks, harms, cost	May miss AOM that presents with a combination of mild bulging, intense erythema, or otalgia that may not necessarily represent less severe disease and may also benefit from intervention.
Benefits-harms assessment	Preponderance of benefit.
Value judgments	Identification of a population of children with highly certain AOM is beneficial. Accurate, specific diagnosis is helpful to the individual patient. Modification of current behavior of overdiagnosis is a goal. Increased specificity is preferred even as sensitivity is lowered.
Intentional vagueness	By using stringent diagnostic criteria, the TM appearance of less severe illness that might be early AOM has not been addressed.
Role of patient preferences	None
Exclusions	None
Strength	**Recommendation**
Notes	Tympanocentesis studies confirm that using these diagnostic findings leads to high levels of isolation of pathogenic bacteria. Evidence is extrapolated from treatment studies that included tympanocentesis.

Key Action Statement 1B

Clinicians should diagnose AOM in children who present with mild bulging of the TM *and* recent (less than 48 hours) onset of ear pain (holding, tugging, rubbing of the ear in a nonverbal child) or intense erythema of the TM. (Evidence Quality: Grade C, Rec. Strength: Recommendation)

Key Action Statement Profile: KAS 1B

Aggregate evidence quality	Grade C
Benefits	Identify AOM in children when the diagnosis is not highly certain.
Risks, harms, cost	Overdiagnosis of AOM. Reduced precision in diagnosis.
Benefits-harms assessment	Benefits greater than harms.
Value judgments	None.
Intentional vagueness	Criteria may be more subjective.
Role of patient preferences	None
Exclusions	None
Strength	**Recommendation**
Notes	Recent onset of ear pain means within the past 48 hours.

Key Action Statement 1C

Clinicians should not diagnose AOM in children who do not have MEE (based on pneumatic otoscopy and/or tympanometry). (Evidence Quality: Grade B, Rec. Strength: Recommendation)

Key Action Statement Profile: KAS 1C

Aggregate evidence quality	Grade B
Benefits	Reduces overdiagnosis and unnecessary treatment. Increases correct diagnosis of other conditions with symptoms that otherwise might be attributed to AOM. Promotes the use of pneumatic otoscopy and tympanometry to improve diagnostic accuracy.
Risks, harms, cost	Cost of tympanometry. Need to acquire or reacquire skills in pneumatic otoscopy and tympanometry for some clinicians.
Benefits-harms assessment	Preponderance of benefit.
Value judgments	AOM is overdiagnosed, often without adequate visualization of the TM. Early AOM without effusion occurs, but the risk of overdiagnosis supersedes that concern.
Intentional vagueness	None
Role of patient preferences	None
Exclusions	Early AOM evidenced by intense erythema of the TM.
Strength	**Recommendation**

Purpose of This Section

There is no gold standard for the diagnosis of AOM. In fact, AOM has a spectrum of signs as the disease develops.[26] Therefore, the purpose of this section is to provide clinicians and researchers with a working clinical definition of AOM and to differentiate AOM from OME. The criteria were chosen to achieve high specificity recognizing that the resulting decreased sensitivity may exclude less severe presentations of AOM.

Changes From AAP/AAFP 2004 AOM Guideline

Accurate diagnosis of AOM is critical to sound clinical decision-making and high-quality research. The 2004 "Clinical Practice Guideline: Diagnosis and Management of AOM"[1] used a 3-part definition for AOM: (1) acute onset of symptoms, (2) presence of MEE, and (3) signs of acute middle ear inflammation. This definition generated extensive discussion and reanalysis of the AOM diagnostic evidence. The 2004 definition lacked precision to exclude cases of OME, and diagnoses of AOM could be made in children with acute onset of symptoms, including severe otalgia and MEE, without other otoscopic findings of inflammation.[27] Furthermore, the use of "uncertain diagnosis" in the 2004 AOM guideline may have permitted diagnoses of AOM without clear visualization of the TM. Earlier studies may have enrolled children who had OME rather than AOM, resulting in the possible classification of such children as improved because their nonspecific symptoms would have abated regardless of therapy.[28–30] Two studies, published in 2011, used stringent diagnostic criteria for diagnosing AOM with much less risk of conclusions based on data from mixed patients.[31,32]

Since publication of the 2004 AOM guideline, a number of studies have been conducted evaluating scales for the presence of symptoms. These studies did not show a consistent correlation of symptoms with the initial diagnosis of AOM, especially in preverbal children.[33–35]

Recent research has used precisely stated stringent criteria of AOM for purposes of the studies.[31,32] The current guideline endorses stringent otoscopic diagnostic criteria as a basis for management decisions (described later). As clinicians use the proposed stringent criteria to diagnose AOM, they should be aware that children with AOM may also present with recent onset of ear pain and intense erythema of the TM as the only otoscopic finding.

Symptoms

Older children with AOM usually present with a history of rapid onset of ear pain. However, in young preverbal children, otalgia as suggested by tugging/rubbing/holding of the ear, excessive crying, fever, or changes in the child's sleep or behavior pattern as noted by the parent are often relatively nonspecific symptoms. A number of studies have attempted to correlate symptom scores with diagnoses of AOM.

A systematic review[36] identified 4 articles that evaluated the accuracy of symptoms.[37–40] Ear pain appeared useful in diagnosing AOM (combined positive likelihood ratio 3.0–7.3, negative likelihood ratio 0.4–0.6); however, it was only present in 50% to 60% of children with AOM. Conclusions from these studies may be limited, because they (1) enrolled children seen by specialists, not likely to represent the whole spectrum of severity of illness; (2) used a clinical diagnosis of AOM based more on symptomatology rather than on tympanocentesis; and (3) included relatively older children.[37,40]

Laine et al[34] used a questionnaire administered to 469 parents who suspected their children, aged 6 to 35 months, had AOM. Of the children, 237 had AOM using strict otoscopic criteria, and 232 had upper respiratory tract infection without AOM. Restless sleep, ear rubbing, fever, and nonspecific respiratory or gastrointestinal tract symptoms did not differentiate children with or without AOM.

McCormick et al[30] used 2 symptom scores—a 3-item score (OM-3), consisting of symptoms of physical suffering such as ear pain or fever, emotional distress (irritability, poor appetite), and limitation in activity; and a 5-item score (Ear Treatment Group Symptom Questionnaire, 5 Items [ETG-5]), including fever, earache, irritability, decreased appetite, and sleep disturbance—to assess AOM symptoms at the time of diagnosis and daily during the 10-day treatment or observation period. They found both to be a responsive measure of changes in clinical symptoms. The same group[35] also tested a visual scale, Acute Otitis Media-Faces Scale (AOM-FS), with faces similar to the Wong-Baker pain scale.[41] None of the scales were adequately sensitive for making the diagnosis of AOM based on symptoms. The AOM-FS combined with an otoscopy score, OS-8,[30] were presented as a double-sided pocket card. The combination of AOM-FS and OS-8 was more responsive to change than either instrument alone.

Shaikh et al[33,42] validated a 7-item parent-reported symptom score (Acute Otitis Media Severity of Symptom Scale [AOM-SOS]) for children with AOM, following stringent guidance of the US Food and Drug Administration (FDA) on the development of patient-reported outcome scales. Symptoms included ear tugging/rubbing/holding, excessive crying, irritability, difficulty sleeping, decreased activity or appetite, and fever. AOM-SOS was correlated with otoscopic diagnoses (AOM, OME, and normal middle ear status). AOM-SOS changed appropriately in response to clinical change. Its day-to-day responsiveness supports its usefulness in following AOM symptoms over time.

Signs of AOM

Few studies have evaluated the relationship of otoscopic findings in AOM and tympanocentesis. A study by Karma et al[43] is often cited as the best single study of otoscopic findings in AOM. However, the study uses only a symptom-based diagnosis of AOM plus the presence of MEE. Thus, children with acute upper respiratory tract infection symptoms and OME would have been considered to have AOM. There also were significant differences in findings at the 2 centers that participated in the study.

The investigators correlated TM color, mobility, and position with the presence of middle ear fluid obtained by tympanocentesis. At 2 sites in Finland (Tampere and Oulu), 2911 children were followed from 6 months to 2.5 years of age. A single otolaryngologist at Tampere and a single pediatrician at Oulu examined subjects. Color, position, and mobility were recorded. Myringotomy and aspiration were performed if MEE was suspected. AOM was diagnosed if MEE was found and the child had fever, earache, irritability, ear rubbing or tugging, simultaneous other acute respiratory tract symptoms, vomiting, or diarrhea. The presence or absence of MEE was noted, but no analyses of the fluid, including culture, were performed. Pneumatic otoscopic findings were classified as follows: color—hemorrhagic, strongly red, moderately red, cloudy or dull, slightly red, or normal; position—bulging, retracted, or normal; and mobility—distinctly impaired, slightly impaired, or normal.

For this analysis, 11 804 visits were available. For visits with acute symptoms, MEE was found in 84.9% and 81.8% at the 2 sites at which the study was performed. There were significant differences among the results at the 2 centers involved in the study. Table 2 shows specific data for each finding.

The combination of a "cloudy," bulging TM with impaired mobility was the best predictor of AOM using the symptom-based diagnosis in this study. Impaired mobility had the highest sensitivity and specificity (approximately 95% and 85%, respectively). Cloudiness had the next best combination of high sensitivity (~74%) and high specificity (~93%) in this study. Bulging had high specificity (~97%) but lower sensitivity (~51%). A TM that was hemorrhagic, strongly red, or moderately red also correlated with the presence of AOM, and a TM that was only "slightly red" was not helpful diagnostically.

McCormick et al reported that a bulging TM was highly associated with the presence of a bacterial pathogen, with or without a concomitant viral pathogen.[44] In a small study, 31 children (40 ears) underwent myringotomy.[45] Bulging TMs had positive bacterial cultures 75% of the time. The percentage of positive cultures for a pathogen increased to 80% if the color of the TM was yellow. The conclusion is that moderate to severe bulging of the TM represents the most important characteristic in the diagnosis of AOM—a finding that has

TABLE 2 Otoscopic Findings in Children With Acute Symptoms and MEE[a]

TM Finding in Acute Visits With MEE	Group I (Tampere, Finland), %	Group II (Oulo, Finland), %
Color		
Distinctly red	69.8	65.6
Hemorrhagic	81.3	62.9
Strongly red	87.7	68.1
Moderately red	59.8	66.0
Slightly red	39.4	16.7
Cloudy	95.7	80.0
Normal	1.7	4.9
Position		
Bulging	96.0	89
Retracted	46.8	48.6
Normal	32.1	22.2
Mobility		
Distinctly impaired	94.0	78.5
Slightly impaired	59.7	32.8
Normal	2.7	4.8

[a] Totals are greater than 100%, because each ear may have had different findings.[43]

implications for clinical care, research, and education.

The committee recognized that there is a progression from the presence of MEE to the bulging of the TM, and it is often difficult to differentiate this equivocal appearance from the highly certain AOM criteria advocated in this guideline.[26] As such, there is a role for individualized diagnosis and management decisions. Examples of normal, mild bulging, moderate bulging, and severe bulging can be seen in Fig 2.

Distinguishing AOM From OME

OME may occur either as the aftermath of an episode of AOM or as a consequence of eustachian tube dysfunction attributable to an upper respiratory tract infection.[46] However, OME may also precede and predispose to the development of AOM. These 2 forms of OM may be considered segments of a disease continuum.[47] However, because OME does not represent an acute infectious process that benefits from antibiotics, it is of utmost importance for clinicians to become proficient in distinguishing normal middle ear status from OME or AOM. Doing so will avoid unnecessary use of antibiotics, which leads to increased adverse effects of medication and facilitates the development of antimicrobial resistance.

Examination of the TM

Accurate diagnosis of AOM in infants and young children may be difficult. Symptoms may be mild or overlap with those of an upper respiratory tract illness. The TM may be obscured by cerumen, and subtle changes in the TM may be difficult to discern. Additional factors complicating diagnosis may include lack of cooperation from the child; less than optimal diagnostic equipment, including lack of a pneumatic bulb; inadequate instruments for clearing cerumen from the external auditory canal; inadequate assistance for restraining the child; and lack of experience in removing cerumen and performing pneumatic otoscopy.

The pneumatic otoscope is the standard tool used in diagnosing OM. Valuable also is a surgical head, which greatly facilitates cleaning cerumen from an infant's external auditory canal. Cerumen may be removed by using a curette, gentle suction, or irrigation.[48] The pneumatic otoscope should have a light source of sufficient brightness and an air-tight seal that permits application of positive and negative pressure. In general, nondisposable specula achieve a better seal with less pain because of a thicker, smoother edge and better light transmission properties. The speculum size should be chosen to gently seal at the outer portion of the external auditory canal.

Pneumatic otoscopy permits assessment of the contour of the TM (normal, retracted, full, bulging), its color (gray, yellow, pink, amber, white, red, blue), its translucency (translucent, semiopaque, opaque), and its mobility (normal, increased, decreased, absent). The normal TM is translucent, pearly gray, and has a ground-glass appearance (Fig 2A). Specific landmarks can be visualized. They include the short process and the manubrium of the malleus and the pars flaccida, located superiorly. These are easily observed and help to identify the position of the TM. Inward movement of the TM on positive pressure in the external canal and outward movement on negative pressure should occur, especially in the superior posterior quadrant. When the TM is retracted, the short process of the malleus becomes more prominent, and the manubrium appears shortened because of its change in position within the middle ear. Inward motion occurring with positive pressure is restricted or absent, because the TM is frequently as far inward as its range of motion allows. However, outward mobility can be visualized when negative pressure is applied. If the TM does not move perceptibly with applications of gentle positive or negative pressure, MEE is likely. Sometimes, the application of pressure will make an air-fluid interface behind the TM (which is diagnostic of MEE) more evident.[49]

Instruction in the proper evaluation of the child's middle ear status should begin with the first pediatric rotation in medical school and continue throughout postgraduate training.[50]

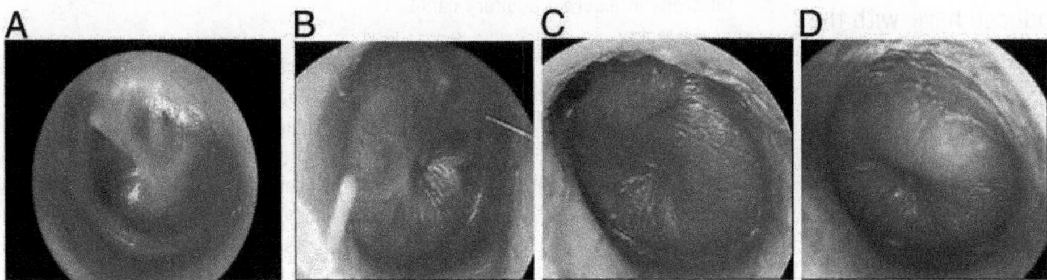

FIGURE 2
A, Normal TM. B, TM with mild bulging. C, TM with moderate bulging. D, TM with severe bulging. Courtesy of Alejandro Hoberman, MD.

Continuing medical education should reinforce the importance of, and retrain the clinician in, the use of pneumatic otoscopy.[51] Training tools include the use of a video-otoscope in residency programs, the use of Web-based educational resources,[49,52] as well as simultaneous or sequential examination of TMs with an expert otoscopist to validate findings by using a double headed or video otoscope. Tools for learning the ear examination can be found in a CD distributed by the Johns Hopkins University School of Medicine and the Institute for Johns Hopkins Nursing,[53] also available at http://www2.aap.org/sections/infectdis/video.cfm,[54] and through a Web-based program, ePROM: Enhancing Proficiency in Otitis Media.[52]

Key Action Statement 2

The management of AOM should include an assessment of pain. If pain is present, the clinician should recommend treatment to reduce pain. (Evidence Quality: Grade B, Rec. Strength: Strong Recommendation)

Key Action Statement Profile: KAS 2

Aggregate evidence quality	Grade B
Benefits	Relieves the major symptom of AOM.
Risks, harms, cost	Potential medication adverse effects. Variable efficacy of some modes of treatment.
Benefits-harms assessment	Preponderance of benefit.
Value judgments	Treating pain is essential whether or not antibiotics are prescribed.
Intentional vagueness	Choice of analgesic is not specified.
Role of patient preferences	Parents may assist in the decision as to what means of pain relief they prefer.
Exclusions	Topical analgesics in the presence of a perforated TM.
Strength	**Strong Recommendation**

Purpose of This Section

Pain is the major symptom of AOM. This section addresses and updates the literature on treating otalgia.

Changes From AAP/AAFP 2004 AOM Guideline

Only 2 new articles directly address the treatment of otalgia. Both address topical treatment. The 2 new articles are consistent with the 2004 guideline statement. The text of the 2004 guideline is, therefore, reproduced here, with the addition of discussion of the 2 new articles. Table 3 has been updated to include the new references.

Treatment of Otalgia

Many episodes of AOM are associated with pain.[55] Some children with OME also have ear pain. Although pain is a common symptom in these illnesses, clinicians often see otalgia as a peripheral concern not requiring direct attention.[56] Pain associated with AOM can be substantial in the first few days of illness and often persists longer in young children.[57] Antibiotic therapy of AOM does not provide symptomatic relief in the first 24 hours[58–61] and even after 3 to 7 days, there may be persistent pain, fever, or both in 30% of children younger than 2 years.[62] In contrast, analgesics do relieve pain associated with AOM within 24 hours[63] and should be used whether antibiotic therapy is or is not prescribed; they should be continued as long as needed. The AAP published the policy statement "The Assessment and Management of Acute Pain in Infants, Children, and Adolescents"[64] to assist the clinician in addressing pain in the context of illness. The management of pain, especially during the first 24 hours of an episode of AOM, should be addressed regardless of the use of antibiotics.

Various treatments of otalgia have been used, but none has been well studied. The clinician should select a treatment on the basis of a consideration of benefits and risks and, wherever possible, incorporate parent/caregiver and patient preference (Table 3).

TABLE 3 Treatments for Otalgia in AOM

Treatment Modality	Comments
Acetaminophen, ibuprofen[63]	Effective analgesia for mild to moderate pain. Readily available. Mainstay of pain management for AOM.
Home remedies (no controlled studies that directly address effectiveness)	May have limited effectiveness.
Distraction	
External application of heat or cold	
Oil drops in external auditory canal	
Topical agents	
Benzocaine, procaine, lidocaine[65,67,70]	Additional, but brief, benefit over acetaminophen in patients older than 5 y.
Naturopathic agents[68]	Comparable to amethocaine/phenazone drops in patients older than 6 y.
Homeopathic agents[71,72]	No controlled studies that directly address pain.
Narcotic analgesia with codeine or analogs	Effective for moderate or severe pain. Requires prescription; risk of respiratory depression, altered mental status, gastrointestinal tract upset, and constipation.
Tympanostomy/myringotomy[73]	Requires skill and entails potential risk.

Since the 2004 guideline was published, there have been only 2 significant new articles.

Bolt et al reported in 2008 on a double-blind placebo-controlled trial at the Australia Children's Hospital emergency department conducted in 2003–2004.[65] They used a convenience sample of children 3 to 17 years of age diagnosed with AOM in the ED. They excluded children with perforation of the TM, pressure-equalizing tube, allergy to local anesthetic or paracetamol, epilepsy, or liver, renal, or cardiac disease. Sixty-three eligible children were randomized to receive aqueous lidocaine or normal saline ear drops up to 3 times in 24 hours. They demonstrated a statistically significant 50% reduction in reported pain at 10 and 30 minutes but not at 20 minutes after application of topical lidocaine, compared with normal saline. Complications were minimal: 3 children reported some dizziness the next day, and none reported tinnitus. A limitation was that some children had received oral acetaminophen before administration of ear drops.

A Cochrane review of topical analgesia for AOM[66] searched the Cochrane register of controlled trials, randomized controlled trials, or quasi-randomized controlled trials that compared otic preparations to placebo or that compared 2 otic preparations. It included studies of adults and children, without TM perforation. It identified 5 trials in children 3 to 18 years of age. Two (including Bolt et al,[65] discussed above) compared anesthetic drops and placebo at diagnosis of AOM. In both studies, some children also received oral analgesics. Three studies compared anesthetic ear drops with naturopathic herbal drops. Naturopathic drops were favored 15 to 30 minutes after installation, and 1 to 3 days after diagnosis, but the difference was not statistically significant. The Cochrane group concluded that there is limited evidence that ear drops are effective at 30 minutes and unclear if results from these studies are a result of the natural course of illness, placebo effect of receiving treatment, soothing effect of any liquid in the ear, or the drops themselves. Three of the studies included in this review were cited in the 2004 AAP guideline[67–69] and the 1 new paper by Bolt et al.[65]

Key Action Statement 3A

Severe AOM

The clinician should prescribe antibiotic therapy for AOM (bilateral or unilateral) in children 6 months and older with severe signs or symptoms (ie, moderate or severe otalgia or otalgia for at least 48 hours, or temperature 39°C [102.2°F] or higher). (Evidence Quality: Grade B, Rec. Strength: Strong Recommendation)

Key Action Statement Profile: KAS 3A

Aggregate evidence quality	Grade B
Benefits	Increased likelihood of more rapid resolution of symptoms. Increased likelihood of resolution of AOM.
Risks, harms, cost	Adverse events attributable to antibiotics, such as diarrhea, diaper dermatitis, and allergic reactions. Overuse of antibiotics leads to increased bacterial resistance. Cost of antibiotics.
Benefits-harms assessment	Preponderance of benefit over harm.
Value judgments	None
Role of patient preference	None
Intentional vagueness	None
Exclusions	None
Strength	**Strong Recommendation**

Key Action Statement 3B

Nonsevere Bilateral AOM in Young Children

The clinician should prescribe antibiotic therapy for bilateral AOM in children younger than 24 months without severe signs or symptoms (ie, mild otalgia for less than 48 hours, temperature less than 39°C [102.2°F]). (Evidence Quality: Grade B, Rec. Strength: Recommendation)

Key Action Statement Profile: KAS 3B

Aggregate evidence quality	Grade B
Benefits	Increased likelihood of more rapid resolution of symptoms. Increased likelihood of resolution of AOM.
Risks, harms, cost	Adverse events attributable to antibiotics, such as diarrhea, diaper dermatitis, and allergic reactions. Overuse of antibiotics leads to increased bacterial resistance. Cost of antibiotics.
Benefits-harms assessment	Preponderance of benefit over harm.
Value judgments	None
Role of patient preference	None
Intentional vagueness	None
Exclusions	None
Strength	**Recommendation**

Key Action Statement 3C

Nonsevere Unilateral AOM in Young Children

The clinician should either prescribe antibiotic therapy *or* offer observation with close follow-up based on joint decision-making with the parent(s)/caregiver for unilateral AOM in children 6 months to 23 months of age without severe signs or symptoms (ie, mild otalgia for less than 48 hours, temperature less than 39°C [102.2°F]). When observation is used, a mechanism must be in place to ensure

follow-up and begin antibiotic therapy if the child worsens or fails to improve within 48 to 72 hours of onset of symptoms. (Evidence Quality: Grade B, Rec. Strength: Recommendation)

Key Action Statement Profile: KAS 3C

Aggregate evidence quality	Grade B
Benefits	Moderately increased likelihood of more rapid resolution of symptoms with initial antibiotics. Moderately increased likelihood of resolution of AOM with initial antibiotics.
Risks, harms, cost	Adverse events attributable to antibiotics, such as diarrhea, diaper dermatitis, and allergic reactions. Overuse of antibiotics leads to increased bacterial resistance. Cost of antibiotics.
Benefits-harms assessment	Moderate degree of benefit over harm.
Value judgments	Observation becomes an alternative as the benefits and harms approach balance.
Role of patient preference	Joint decision-making with the family is essential before choosing observation.
Intentional vagueness	Joint decision-making is highly variable from family to family
Exclusions	None
Strength	**Recommendation**
Note	In the judgment of 1 Subcommittee member (AH), antimicrobial treatment of these children is preferred because of a preponderance of benefit over harm. AH did not endorse Key Action Statement 3C

Key Action Statement 3D

Nonsevere AOM in Older Children

The clinician should either prescribe antibiotic therapy *or* offer observation with close follow-up based on joint decision-making with the parent(s)/caregiver for AOM (bilateral or unilateral) in children 24 months or older without severe signs or symptoms (ie, mild otalgia for less than 48 hours, temperature less than 39°C [102.2°F]). When observation is used, a mechanism must be in place to ensure follow-up and begin antibiotic therapy if the child worsens or fails to improve within 48 to 72 hours of onset of symptoms. (Evidence Quality: Grade B, Rec Strength: Recommendation)

Key Action Statement Profile: KAS 3D

Aggregate evidence quality	Grade B
Benefits	*Initial antibiotic treatment*: Slightly increased likelihood of more rapid resolution of symptoms; slightly increased likelihood of resolution of AOM. *Initial observation*: Decreased use of antibiotics; decreased adverse effects of antibiotics; decreased potential for development of bacterial resistance.
Risks, harms, cost	*Initial antibiotic treatment*: Adverse events attributable to antibiotics such as diarrhea, rashes, and allergic reactions. Overuse of antibiotics leads to increased bacterial resistance. *Initial observation*: Possibility of needing to start antibiotics in 48 to 72 h if the patient continues to have symptoms. Minimal risk of adverse consequences of delayed antibiotic treatment. Potential increased phone calls and doctor visits.
Benefits-harms assessment	Slight degree of benefit of initial antibiotics over harm.
Value judgments	Observation is an option as the benefits and harms approach balance.
Role of patient preference	Joint decision-making with the family is essential before choosing observation.
Intentional vagueness	Joint decision-making is highly variable from family to family.
Exclusions	None
Strength	**Recommendation.**

Purpose of This Section

The purpose of this section is to offer guidance on the initial management of AOM by helping clinicians choose between the following 2 strategies:

1. *Initial antibiotic therapy*, defined as treatment of AOM with antibiotics that are prescribed at the time of diagnosis with the intent of starting antibiotic therapy as soon as possible after the encounter.
2. *Initial observation*, defined as initial management of AOM limited to symptomatic relief, with commencement of antibiotic therapy only if the child's condition worsens at any time or does not show clinical improvement within 48 to 72 hours of diagnosis. A mechanism must be in place to ensure follow-up and initiation of antibiotics if the child fails observation.

This section assumes that the clinician has made an accurate diagnosis of AOM by using the criteria and strategies outlined earlier in this guideline. Another assumption is that a clear distinction is made between the role of analgesics and antibiotics in providing symptomatic relief for children with AOM.

Changes From Previous AOM Guideline

The AOM guideline published by the AAP and AAFP in 2004 proposed, for the first time in North America, an "observation option" for selected children with AOM, building on successful implementation of a similar policy in the state of New York[74] and the use of a similar paradigm in many countries in Europe. A common feature of both approaches was to prioritize initial antibiotic therapy according to diagnostic certainty, with greater reliance on observation when the diagnosis was uncertain. In response to criticism that allowing an "uncertain diagnosis" might condone incomplete visualization of the TM or allow inappropriate antibiotic use, this category has been eliminated with greater emphasis now placed on maximizing diagnostic accuracy for AOM.

Since the earlier AOM guideline was published, there has been substantial new research on initial management of AOM, including randomized controlled trials of antibiotic therapy versus placebo or no therapy,[31,32,75] immediate versus delayed antibiotic therapy,[30,76,77] or delayed antibiotic with or without a concurrent prescription.[78] The Hoberman and Tähtinen articles are especially important as they used stringent criteria for diagnosing AOM.[31,32] Systematic reviews have been published on delayed antibiotic therapy,[79] the natural history of AOM in untreated children,[57] predictive factors for antibiotic benefits,[62] and the effect of antibiotics on asymptomatic MEE after therapy.[80] Observational studies provide additional data on outcomes of initial observation with delayed antibiotic therapy, if needed,[81] and on the relationship of previous antibiotic therapy for AOM to subsequent acute mastoiditis.[82,83]

In contrast to the earlier AOM guideline,[1] which recommended antibiotic therapy for all children 6 months to 2 years of age with a certain diagnosis, the current guideline indicates a choice between initial antibiotic therapy or initial observation in this age group for children with unilateral AOM and mild symptoms but only after joint decision-making with the parent(s)/caregiver (Table 4). This change is supported by evidence on the safety of observation or delayed prescribing in young children.[30,31,32,75,76,81] A mechanism must be in place to ensure follow-up and begin antibiotics if the child fails observation.

Importance of Accurate Diagnosis

The recommendations for management of AOM assume an accurate diagnosis on the basis of criteria outlined in the diagnosis section of this guideline. Many of the studies since the 2004 AAP/AAFP AOM guideline[1] used more stringent and well-defined AOM diagnostic definitions than were previously used. Bulging of the TM was required for diagnosis of AOM for most of the children enrolled in the most recent studies.[31,32] By using the criteria in this guideline, clinicians will more accurately distinguish AOM from OME. The management of OME can be found in guidelines written by the AAP, AAFP, and American Academy of Otolaryngology-Head and Neck Surgery.[84,85]

TABLE 4 Recommendations for Initial Management for Uncomplicated AOM[a]

Age	Otorrhea With AOM[a]	Unilateral or Bilateral AOM[a] With Severe Symptoms[b]	Bilateral AOM[a] Without Otorrhea	Unilateral AOM[a] Without Otorrhea
6 mo to 2 y	Antibiotic therapy	Antibiotic therapy	Antibiotic therapy	Antibiotic therapy or additional observation
≥2 y	Antibiotic therapy	Antibiotic therapy	Antibiotic therapy or additional observation	Antibiotic therapy or additional observation[c]

[a] Applies only to children with well-documented AOM with high certainty of diagnosis (see Diagnosis section).
[b] A toxic-appearing child, persistent otalgia more than 48 h, temperature ≥39°C (102.2°F) in the past 48 h, or if there is uncertain access to follow-up after the visit.
[c] This plan of initial management provides an opportunity for shared decision-making with the child's family for those categories appropriate for additional observation. If observation is offered, a mechanism must be in place to ensure follow-up and begin antibiotics if the child worsens or fails to improve within 48 to 72 h of AOM onset.

Age, Severity of Symptoms, Otorrhea, and Laterality

Rovers et al[62] performed a systematic search for AOM trials that (1) used random allocation of children, (2) included children 0 to 12 years of age with AOM, (3) compared antibiotics with placebo or no treatment, and (4) had pain or fever as an outcome. The original investigators were asked for their original data.

Primary outcome was pain and/or fever (>38°C) at 3 to 7 days. The adverse effects of antibiotics were also analyzed. Baseline predictors were age <2 years versus ≥2 years, bilateral AOM versus unilateral AOM, and the presence versus absence of otorrhea. Statistical methods were used to assess heterogeneity and to analyze the data.

Of the 10 eligible studies, the investigators of 6 studies[30,75,86–89] provided the original data requested, and 4 did not. A total of 1642 patients were included in the 6 studies from which data were obtained. Of the cases submitted, the average age was 3 to 4 years, with 35% of children younger than 2 years. Bilateral AOM was present in 34% of children, and 42% of children had a bulging TM. Otorrhea was present in 21% of children. The antibiotic and control groups were comparable for all characteristics.

The rate difference (RD) for pain, fever, or both between antibiotic and control groups was 13% (NNT = 8). For children younger than 2 years, the RD was 15% (NNT = 7); for those ≥2 years, RD was 11% (NNT = 10). For unilateral AOM, the RD was 6% (NNT = 17); for bilateral AOM, the RD was 20% (NNT = 5). When unilateral AOM was broken into age groups, among those younger than 2 years, the RD was 5% (NNT = 20), and among those ≥2 years, the RD was 7% (NNT = 15). For bilateral AOM in children younger than 2 years, the RD was 25% (NNT = 4); for bilateral AOM in children ≥2 years, the RD was 12% (NNT = 9). For otorrhea, the RD was 36% (NNT = 3). One child in the control group who developed meningitis had received antibiotics beginning on day 2 because of worsening status. There were no cases of mastoiditis.

In a Cochrane Review, Sanders et al[59] identified 10 studies that met the following criteria: (1) randomized controlled trial, (2) compared antibiotic versus placebo or antibiotic versus observation, (3) age 1 month to 15 years, (4) reported severity and duration of pain, (5) reported adverse events, and (6) reported serious complications of AOM, recurrent attacks, and hearing problems. Studies were analyzed for risk of bias and assessment of heterogeneity. The studies were the same as analyzed by Rovers et al[62] but included the 4 studies for which primary data were not available to Rovers.[60,61,90,91]

The authors' conclusions were that antibiotics produced a small reduction in the number of children with pain 2 to 7 days after diagnosis. They also concluded that most cases spontaneously remitted with no complications (NNT = 16). Antibiotics were most beneficial in children younger than 2 years with bilateral AOM and in children with otorrhea.

Two recent studies only included children younger than 3 years[32] or younger than 2 years.[31] Both included only subjects in whom the diagnosis of AOM was certain. Both studies used improvement of symptoms and improvement in the appearance of the TM in their definitions of clinical success or failure.

Hoberman et al[31] conducted a randomized, double-blind, placebo-controlled study of the efficacy of antimicrobial treatment on AOM. The criteria for AOM were acute symptoms with a score of at least 3 on the AOM-SOS, a validated symptom scale[33,92]; MEE; and moderate or marked bulging of the TM or slight bulging accompanied by either otalgia or marked erythema of the TM. They chose to use high-dose amoxicillin-clavulanate (90 mg/kg/day) as active treatment, because it has the best oral antibiotic coverage for organisms causing AOM. Included in the study were 291 patients 6 to 23 months of age: 144 in the antibiotic group and 147 in the placebo group. The primary outcome measures were the time to resolution of symptoms and the symptom burden over time. The initial resolution of symptoms (ie, the first recording of an AOM-SOS score of 0 or 1) was recorded among the children who received amoxicillin-clavulanate in 35% by day 2, 61% by day 4, and 80% by day 7. Among children who received placebo, an AOM-SOS score of 0 or 1 was recorded in 28% by day 2, 54% by day 4, and 74% by day 7 (P = .14 for the overall comparison). For sustained resolution of symptoms (ie, the time to the second of 2 successive recordings of an AOM-SOS score of 0 or 1), the corresponding values were 20% at day 2, 41% at day 4, and 67% at day 7 with amoxicillin-clavulanate, compared with 14%, 36%, and 53% with placebo (P = .04 for the overall comparison). The symptom burden (ie, mean AOM-SOS scores) over the first 7 days were lower for the children treated with amoxicillin-clavulanate than for those who received placebo (P = .02). Clinical failure at or before the 4- to 5-day visit was defined as "either a lack of substantial improvement in symptoms, a worsening of signs on otoscopic examination, or both," and clinical failure at the 10- to 12-day visit was defined as "the failure to achieve complete or nearly complete resolution of symptoms and of otoscopic signs, without regard to the persistence or resolution of middle ear effusion." Treatment failure occurred by day 4 to 5 in 4% of the antimicrobial treatment group versus 23% in the placebo group ($P < .001$) and at day 10 to 12 in 16% of the antimicrobial treatment group versus 51% in the placebo group (NNT = 2.9, $P < .001$). In a comparison of outcome in unilateral versus bilateral AOM, clinical failure rates by day 10 to 12 in children with unilateral AOM were 9% in those treated with amoxicillin-clavulanate versus 41% in those treated with placebo (RD, 32%; NNT = 3) and 23% vs 60% (RD, 37%; NNT = 3) in those with bilateral AOM. Most common adverse events were diarrhea (25% vs 15% in the treatment versus placebo groups, respectively; P = .05) and diaper dermatitis (51% vs 35% in the treatment versus placebo groups, respectively; P = .008). One placebo recipient developed mastoiditis. According to these results, antimicrobial treatment of AOM was more beneficial than in previous studies that used less stringent diagnostic criteria.

Tähtinen et al[32] conducted a randomized, double-blind, placebo-controlled, intention-to-treat study of amoxicillin-clavulanate (40 mg/kg/day) versus placebo. Three hundred nineteen patients from 6 to 35 months of age were studied: 161 in the antibiotic group and 158 in the placebo group. AOM definition was the presence of MEE, distinct erythema over a bulging or yellow TM, and acute symptoms such as ear pain, fever, or respiratory symptoms. Compliance was measured by using daily patient diaries and number of capsules remaining at the end of the study. Primary outcome was time to treatment failure defined as a composite of 6 independent components: no improvement in overall condition by day 3, worsening of the child's condition at any time, no improvement in otoscopic signs by day 8, perforation of the TM, development of severe infection (eg, pneumonia, mastoiditis), and any other reason for stopping the study drug/placebo.

Groups were comparable on multiple parameters. In the treatment group, 135 of 161 patients (84%) were younger than 24 months, and in the placebo group, 124 of 158 patients (78%) were younger than 24 months. Treatment failure occurred in 18.6% of the treatment group and 44.9% in the placebo group (NNT = 3.8, $P < .001$). Rescue treatment was needed in 6.8% of the treatment group and 33.5% of placebo patients ($P < .001$). Contralateral AOM developed in 8.2% and 18.6% of treatment and placebo groups, respectively ($P = .007$). There was no significant difference in use of analgesic or antipyretic medicine, which was used in 84.2% of the amoxicillin-clavulanate group and 85.9% of the placebo group.

Parents of child care attendees on placebo missed more days of work ($P = .005$). Clinical failure rates in children with unilateral AOM were 17.2% in those treated with amoxicillin-clavulanate versus 42.7% in those treated with placebo; for bilateral AOM, clinical failure rates were 21.7% for those treated with amoxicillin-clavulanate versus 46.3% in the placebo group. Reported rates of treatment failure by day 8 were 17.2% in the amoxicillin-clavulanate group versus 42.7% in the placebo group in children with unilateral AOM and 21.7% vs 46.3% among those with bilateral disease.

Adverse events, primarily diarrhea and/or rash, occurred in 52.8% of the treatment group and 36.1% of the placebo group ($P = .003$). Overall condition as evaluated by the parents and otoscopic appearance of the TM showed a benefit of antibiotics over placebo at the end of treatment visit ($P < .001$). Two placebo recipients developed a severe infection; 1 developed pneumococcal bacteremia, and 1 developed radiographically confirmed pneumonia.

Most studies have excluded children with severe illness and all exclude those with bacterial disease other than AOM (pneumonia, mastoiditis, meningitis, streptococcal pharyngitis). Kaleida et al[91] compared myringotomy alone with myringotomy plus antibiotics. Severe AOM was defined as temperature >39°C (102.2°F) or the presence of severe otalgia. Patients with severe AOM in the group that received only myringotomy (without initial antibiotics) had much worse outcomes.

Initial Antibiotic Therapy

The rationale for antibiotic therapy in children with AOM is based on a high prevalence of bacteria in the accompanying MEE.[93] Bacterial and viral cultures of middle ear fluid collected by tympanocentesis from children with AOM showed 55% with bacteria only and 15% with bacteria and viruses. A beneficial effect of antibiotics on AOM was first demonstrated in 1968,[94] followed by additional randomized trials and a meta-analysis[95] showing a 14% increase in absolute rates of clinical improvement. Systematic reviews of the literature published before 2011[21,59,62] revealed increases of clinical improvement with initial antibiotics of 6% to 12%.

Randomized clinical trials using stringent diagnostic criteria for AOM in young children[31,32] show differences in clinical improvement of 26% to 35% favoring initial antibiotic treatment as compared with placebo. Greater benefit of immediate antibiotic therapy was observed for bilateral AOM[62,96] or AOM associated with otorrhea.[62] In most randomized trials,[30,75,77,88,89] antibiotic therapy also decreased the duration of pain, analgesic use, or school absence and parent days missed from work.

Children younger than 2 years with AOM may take longer to improve clinically than older children,[57] and although they are more likely to benefit from antibiotics,[31,32] AOM in many children will resolve without antibiotics.[62] A clinically significant benefit of immediate antibiotic therapy is observed for bilateral AOM,[62,96] *Streptococcus pneumoniae* infection, or AOM associated with otorrhea.[62]

Initial Observation for AOM

In systematic reviews of studies that compare antibiotic therapy for AOM with placebo, a consistent finding has been the overall favorable natural history in control groups (NNT = 8–16).[12,59,62,95] However, randomized trials in these reviews had varying diagnostic criteria that would have permitted inclusion of some children with OME, viral upper respiratory infections, or myringitis, thereby limiting the ability to apply these findings to children with a highly certain AOM diagnosis. In more recent AOM studies[31,32] using stringent diagnostic criteria, approximately half of young children (younger than 2–3 years) experienced clinical success when given placebo, but the effect of antibiotic therapy was substantially greater than suggested by studies without precise diagnosis (NNT = 3–4).

Observation as initial management for AOM in properly selected children does not increase suppurative complications, provided that follow-up is ensured and a rescue antibiotic is given for persistent or worsening symptoms.[17] In contrast, withholding of antibiotics in all children with AOM, regardless of clinical course, would risk a return to the suppurative complications observed in the preantibiotic era. At the population level, antibiotics halve the risk of mastoiditis after AOM, but the high NNT of approximately 4800 patients to prevent 1 case of mastoiditis precludes a strategy of universal antibiotic therapy as a means to prevent mastoiditis.[83]

The favorable natural history of AOM makes it difficult to demonstrate significant differences in efficacy between antibiotic and placebo when a successful outcome is defined by relief or improvement of presenting signs and symptoms. In contrast, when otoscopic improvement (resolution of TM bulging, intense erythema, or both) is also required for a positive outcome,[31,32] the NNT is 3 to 4, compared with 8 to 16 for symptom improvement alone in older studies that used less precise diagnostic criteria. MEE, however, may persist for weeks or months after an AOM episode and is not a criterion for otoscopic failure.

National guidelines for initial observation of AOM in select children were first implemented in the Netherlands[97] and subsequently in Sweden,[98] Scotland,[99] the United States,[1] the United Kingdom,[100] and Italy.[101] All included observation as an initial treatment option under specified circumstances.

In numerous studies, only approximately one-third of children initially observed received a rescue antibiotic for persistent or worsening AOM,[30,32,76,81,89,102] suggesting that antibiotic use could potentially be reduced by 65% in eligible children. Given the high incidence of AOM, this reduction could help substantially in curtailing antibiotic-related adverse events.

McCormick et al[30] reported on 233 patients randomly assigned to receive immediate antibiotics (amoxicillin, 90 mg/kg/day) or to undergo watchful waiting. Criteria for inclusion were symptoms of ear infection, otoscopic evidence of AOM, and nonsevere AOM based on a 3-item symptom score (OM-3) and TM appearance based on an 8-item scale (OS-8). Primary outcomes were parent satisfaction with AOM care, resolution of AOM symptoms after initial treatment, AOM failure and recurrence, and nasopharyngeal carriage of *S pneumoniae* strains resistant to antibiotics after treatment. The study was confounded by including patients who had received antibiotics in the previous 30 days.

In the watchful waiting group, 66% of children completed the study without antibiotics. There was no difference in parent satisfaction scores at day 12. A 5-item symptom score (ETG-5) was assessed at days 0 to 10 by using patient diaries. Subjects receiving immediate antibiotics resolved their symptoms faster than did subjects who underwent watchful waiting (P = .004). For children younger than 2 years, the difference was greater (P = .008). Otoscopic and tympanogram scores were also lower in the antibiotic group as opposed to the watchful waiting group (P = .02 for otoscopic score, P = .004 for tympanogram). Combining all ages, failure and recurrence rates were lower for the antibiotic group (5%) than for the watchful waiting group (21%) at 12 days. By day 30, there was no difference in failure or recurrence for the antibiotic and watchful waiting groups (23% and 24%, respectively). The association between clinical outcome and intervention group was not significantly different between age groups. Immediate antibiotics resulted in eradication of *S pneumoniae* carriage in the majority of children, but *S pneumoniae* strains cultured from children in the antibiotic group at day 12 were more likely to be multidrug resistant than were strains cultured from children in the watchful waiting group.

The decision not to give initial antibiotic treatment and observe should be a joint decision of the clinician and the parents. In such cases, a system for close follow-up and a means of beginning antibiotics must be in place if symptoms worsen or no improvement is seen in 48 to 72 hours.

Initial observation of AOM should be part of a larger management strategy that includes analgesics, parent information, and provisions for a rescue antibiotic. Education of parents should include an explanation about the self-limited nature of most episodes of AOM, especially in children 2 years and older; the importance of pain management early in the course; and the potential adverse effects of antibiotics. Such an approach can substantially reduce prescription fill rates for rescue antibiotics.[103]

A critical component of any strategy involving initial observation for AOM is the ability to provide a rescue antibiotic if needed. This is often done by using a "safety net" or a "wait-and-see prescription,"[76,102] in which the parent/caregiver is given an antibiotic prescription during the clinical encounter but is instructed to fill the prescription only if the child fails to improve within 2 to 3 days or if symptoms worsen at any time. An alternative approach is not to provide a written prescription but to instruct the parent/caregiver to call or return if the child fails to improve within 2 to 3 days or if symptoms worsen.

In one of the first major studies of observation with a safety-net antibiotic prescription (SNAP), Siegel et al[102] enrolled 194 patients with protocol defined AOM, of whom 175 completed the study. Eligible patients were given a SNAP with instructions to fill the prescription only if symptoms worsened or did not improve in 48 hours. The SNAP was valid for 5 days. Pain medicine was recommended to be taken as needed. A phone interview was conducted 5 to 10 days after diagnosis.

One hundred twenty of 175 families did not fill the prescription. Reasons for filling the prescription (more than 1 reason per patient was acceptable) were as follows: continued pain, 23%; continued fever, 11%; sleep disruption, 6%; missed days of work, 3%; missed days of child care, 3%; and no reason given, 5%. One 16-month-old boy completed observation successfully but 6 weeks later developed AOM in the opposite ear, was treated with antibiotics, and developed postauricular cellulitis.

In a similar study of a "wait-and-see prescription" (WASP) in the emergency department, Spiro et al[76] randomly assigned 283 patients to either a WASP or standard prescription. Clinicians were educated on the 2004 AAP diagnostic criteria and initial treatment options for AOM; however, diagnosis was made at the discretion of the clinician. Patients were excluded if they did not qualify for observation per the 2004 guidelines. The primary outcome was whether the prescription was filled within 3 days of diagnosis. Prescriptions were not filled for 62% and 13% of the WASP and standard prescription patients, respectively ($P < .001$). Reasons for filling the prescription in the WASP group were fever (60%), ear pain (34%), or fussy behavior (6%). No serious adverse events were reported.

Strategies to observe children with AOM who are likely to improve on their own without initial antibiotic therapy reduces common adverse effects of antibiotics, such as diarrhea and diaper dermatitis. In 2 trials, antibiotic therapy significantly increased the absolute rates of diarrhea by 10% to 20% and of diaper rash or dermatitis by 6% to 16%.[31,32] Reduced antibiotic use may also reduce the prevalence of resistant bacterial pathogens. Multidrug-resistant *S pneumoniae* continues to be a significant concern for AOM, despite universal immunization of children in the United States with heptavalent pneumococcal conjugate vaccine.[104,105] In contrast, countries with low antibiotic use for AOM have a low prevalence of resistant nasopharyngeal pathogens in children.[106]

Key Action Statement 4A

Clinicians should prescribe amoxicillin for AOM when a decision to treat with antibiotics has been made *and* the child has not received amoxicillin in the past 30 days *or* the child does not have concurrent purulent conjunctivitis *or* the child is not allergic to penicillin. (Evidence Quality: Grade B, Rec. Strength: Recommendation)

Key Action Statement Profile: KAS 4A

Aggregate evidence quality	Grade B
Benefits	Effective antibiotic for most children with AOM. Inexpensive, safe, acceptable taste, narrow antimicrobial spectrum.
Risks, harms, cost	Ineffective against β-lactamase–producing organisms. Adverse effects of amoxicillin.
Benefits-harms assessment	Preponderance of benefit.
Value judgments	Better to use a drug that has reasonable cost, has an acceptable taste, and has a narrow antibacterial spectrum.
Intentional vagueness	The clinician must determine whether the patient is truly penicillin allergic.
Role of patient preferences	Should be considered if previous bad experience with amoxicillin.
Exclusions	Patients with known penicillin allergy.
Strength	**Recommendation.**

Key Action Statement 4B

Clinicians should prescribe an antibiotic with additional β-lactamase coverage for AOM when a decision to treat with antibiotics has been made *and* the child has received amoxicillin in the past 30 days *or* has concurrent purulent conjunctivitis *or* has a history of recurrent AOM unresponsive to amoxicillin. (Evidence Quality: Grade C, Rec. Strength: Recommendation)

Key Action Statement Profile: KAS 4B

Aggregate evidence quality	Grade C
Benefits	Successful treatment of β-lactamase–producing organisms.
Risks, harms, cost	Cost of antibiotic. Increased adverse effects.
Benefits-harms assessment	Preponderance of benefit.
Value judgments	Efficacy is more important than taste.
Intentional vagueness	None.
Role of patient preferences	Concern regarding side effects and taste.
Exclusions	Patients with known penicillin allergy.
Strength	**Recommendation**

Key Action Statement 4C

Clinicians should reassess the patient if the caregiver reports that the child's symptoms have worsened or failed to respond to the initial antibiotic treatment within 48 to 72 hours and determine whether a change in therapy is needed. (Evidence Quality: Grade B, Rec. Strength: Recommendation)

Key Action Statement Profile: KAS 4C

Aggregate evidence quality	Grade B
Benefits	Identify children who may have AOM caused by pathogens resistant to previous antibiotics.
Risks, harms, cost	Cost. Time for patient and clinician to make change. Potential need for parenteral medication.
Benefit-harm assessment	Preponderance of benefit.
Value judgments	None.
Intentional vagueness	"Reassess" is not defined. The clinician may determine the method of assessment.
Role of patient preferences	Limited.
Exclusions	Appearance of TM improved.
Strength	**Recommendation**

Purpose of This Section

If an antibiotic will be used for treatment of a child with AOM, whether as initial management or after a period of observation, the clinician must choose an antibiotic that will have a high likelihood of being effective against the most likely etiologic bacterial pathogens with considerations of cost, taste, convenience, and adverse effects. This section proposes first- and second-line antibiotics that best meet these criteria while balancing potential benefits and harms.

Changes From AAP/AAFP 2004 AOM Guideline

Despite new data on the effect of PCV7 and updated data on the in vitro susceptibility of bacterial pathogens most likely to cause AOM, the recommendations for the first-line antibiotic remains unchanged from 2004. The current guideline contains revised recommendations regarding penicillin allergy based on new data. The increase of multidrug-resistant strains of pneumococci is noted.

Microbiology

Microorganisms detected in the middle ear during AOM include pathogenic bacteria, as well as respiratory viruses.[107–110] AOM occurs most frequently as a consequence of viral upper respiratory tract infection,[111–113] which leads to eustachian tube inflammation/dysfunction, negative middle ear pressure, and movement of secretions containing the upper respiratory tract infection causative virus and pathogenic bacteria in the nasopharynx into the middle ear cleft. By using comprehensive and sensitive microbiologic testing, bacteria and/or viruses can be detected in the middle ear fluid in up to 96% of AOM cases (eg, 66% bacteria and viruses together, 27% bacteria alone, and 4% virus alone).[114] Studies using less sensitive or less comprehensive microbiologic assays have yielded less positive results for bacteria and much less positive results for viruses.[115–117] The 3 most common bacterial pathogens in AOM are *S pneumoniae*, nontypeable *Haemophilus influenzae*, and *Moraxella catarrhalis*.[111] *Streptococcus pyogenes* (group A β-hemolytic streptococci) accounts for less than 5% of AOM cases. The proportion of AOM cases with pathogenic bacteria isolated from the middle ear fluids varies depending on bacteriologic techniques, transport issues, and stringency of AOM definition. In series of reports from the United States and Europe from 1952–1981 and 1985–1992, the mean percentage of cases with bacterial pathogens isolated from the middle ear fluids was 69% and 72%, respectively.[118] A large series from the University of Pittsburgh Otitis Media Study Group reported bacterial pathogens in 84% of the middle ear fluids from 2807 cases of AOM.[118] Studies that applied more stringent otoscopic criteria and/or use of bedside specimen plating on solid agar in addition to liquid transport media have a reported rate of recovery of pathogenic bacteria from middle ear exudates ranging from 85% to 90%.[119–121] When using appropriate stringent diagnostic criteria, careful specimen handling, and sensitive microbiologic techniques, the vast majority of cases of AOM will involve pathogenic bacteria either alone or in concert with viral pathogens.

Among AOM bacterial pathogens, *S pneumoniae* was the most frequently cultured in earlier reports. Since the debut and routine use of PCV7 in 2000, the ordinal frequency of these 3 major middle ear pathogens has evolved.[105] In the first few years after PCV7 introduction, *H influenzae* became the most frequently isolated middle ear pathogen, replacing *S pneumoniae*.[122,123] Shortly thereafter, a shift to non-PCV7 serotypes of *S pneumoniae* was described.[124] Pichichero et al[104] later reported that 44% of 212 AOM cases seen in 2003–2006 were caused by *H influenzae*, and 28% were caused by *S pneumoniae*, with a high proportion of highly resistant *S pneumoniae*. In that study, a majority (77%) of cases involved recurrent disease or initial treatment failure. A later report[125] with data from 2007 to 2009, 6 to 8 years after the introduction of PCV7 in the United States, showed that PCV7 strains of *S pneumoniae* virtually disappeared from the middle ear fluid of children with AOM who had been vaccinated. However, the frequency of isolation of non-PCV7 serotypes of *S pneumoniae* from the middle ear fluid overall was increased; this has made isolation of *S pneumoniae* and *H influenzae* of children with AOM nearly equal.

In a study of tympanocentesis over 4 respiratory tract illness seasons in a private practice, the percentage of

S pneumoniae initially decreased relative to *H influenzae*. In 2005–2006 (*N* = 33), 48% of bacteria were *S pneumoniae*, and 42% were *H influenzae*. For 2006–2007 (*N* = 37), the percentages were equal at 41%. In 2007–2008 (*N* = 34), 35% were *S pneumoniae*, and 59% were *H influenzae*. In 2008–2009 (*N* = 24), the percentages were 54% and 38%, respectively, with an increase in intermediate and nonsusceptible *S pneumoniae*.[126] Data on nasopharyngeal colonization from PCV7-immunized children with AOM have shown continued presence of *S pneumoniae* colonization. Revai et al[127] showed no difference in *S pneumoniae* colonization rate among children with AOM who have been unimmunized, underimmunized, or fully immunized with PCV7. In a study during a viral upper respiratory tract infection, including mostly PCV7-immunized children (6 months to 3 years of age), *S pneumoniae* was detected in 45.5% of 968 nasopharyngeal swabs, *H influenzae* was detected in 32.4%, and *M catarrhalis* was detected in 63.1%.[128] Data show that nasopharyngeal colonization of children vaccinated with PCV7 increasingly is caused by *S pneumoniae* serotypes not contained in the vaccine.[129–132] With the use of the recently licensed 13-valent pneumococcal conjugate vaccine (PCV13),[133] the patterns of nasopharyngeal colonization and infection with these common AOM bacterial pathogens will continue to evolve.

Investigators have attempted to predict the type of AOM pathogenic bacteria on the basis of clinical severity, but results have not been promising. *S pyogenes* has been shown to occur more commonly in older children[134] and to cause a greater degree of inflammation of the middle ear and TM, a greater frequency of spontaneous rupture of the TM, and more frequent progression to acute mastoiditis compared with other bacterial pathogens.[134–136] As for clinical findings in cases with *S pneumoniae* and nontypeable *H influenzae*, some studies suggest that signs and symptoms of AOM caused by *S pneumoniae* may be more severe (fever, severe earache, bulging TM) than those caused by other pathogens.[44,121,137] These findings were refuted by results of the studies that found AOM caused by nontypeable *H influenzae* to be associated with bilateral AOM and more severe inflammation of the TM.[96,138] Leibovitz et al[139] concluded, in a study of 372 children with AOM caused by *H influenzae* (*N* = 138), *S pneumoniae* (*N* = 64), and mixed *H influenzae* and *S pneumoniae* (*N* = 64), that clinical/otologic scores could not discriminate among various bacterial etiologies of AOM. However, there were significantly different clinical/otologic scores between bacterial culture negative and culture positive cases. A study of middle ear exudates of 82 cases of bullous myringitis has shown a 97% bacteria positive rate, primarily *S pneumoniae*. In contrast to the previous belief, mycoplasma is rarely the causative agent in this condition.[140] Accurate prediction of the bacterial cause of AOM on the basis of clinical presentation, without bacterial culture of the middle ear exudates, is not possible, but specific etiologies may be predicted in some situations. Published evidence has suggested that AOM associated with conjunctivitis (otitis-conjunctivitis syndrome) is more likely caused by nontypeable *H influenzae* than by other bacteria.[141–143]

Bacterial Susceptibility to Antibiotics

Selection of antibiotic to treat AOM is based on the suspected type of bacteria and antibiotic susceptibility pattern, although clinical pharmacology and clinical and microbiologic results and predicted compliance with the drug are also taken into account. Early studies of AOM patients show that 19% of children with *S pneumoniae* and 48% with *H influenzae* cultured on initial tympanocentesis who were not treated with antibiotic cleared the bacteria at the time of a second tympanocentesis 2 to 7 days later.[144] Approximately 75% of children infected with *M catarrhalis* experienced bacteriologic cure even after treatment with amoxicillin, an antibiotic to which it is not susceptible.[145,146]

Antibiotic susceptibility of major AOM bacterial pathogens continues to change, but data on middle ear pathogens have become scanty because tympanocentesis is not generally performed in studies of children with uncomplicated AOM. Most available data come from cases of persistent or recurrent AOM. Current US data from a number of centers indicates that approximately 83% and 87% of isolates of *S pneumoniae* from all age groups are susceptible to regular (40 mg/kg/day) and high-dose amoxicillin (80–90 mg/kg/day divided twice daily), respectively.[130,147–150] Pediatric isolates are smaller in number and include mostly ear isolates collected from recurrent and persistent AOM cases with a high percentage of multidrug-resistant *S pneumoniae*, most frequently nonvaccine serotypes that have recently increased in frequency and importance.[104]

High-dose amoxicillin will yield middle ear fluid levels that exceed the minimum inhibitory concentration (MIC) of all *S pneumoniae* serotypes that are intermediately resistant to penicillin (penicillin MICs, 0.12–1.0 μg/mL), and many but not all highly resistant serotypes (penicillin MICs, ≥2 μg/mL) for a longer period of the dosing interval and has been shown to improve bacteriologic and clinical efficacy compared with the regular dose.[151–153] Hoberman et al[154] reported superior efficacy of high-dose amoxicillin-clavulanate in eradication of *S pneumoniae* (96%) from the middle ear at days 4 to 6 of therapy compared with azithromycin.

The antibiotic susceptibility pattern for *S pneumoniae* is expected to continue to evolve with the use of PCV13, a conjugate vaccine containing 13 serotypes of *S pneumoniae*.[133,155,156] Widespread use of PCV13 could potentially reduce diseases caused by multidrug-resistant pneumococcal serotypes and diminish the need for the use of higher dose of amoxicillin or amoxicillin-clavulanate for AOM.

Some *H influenzae* isolates produce β-lactamase enzyme, causing the isolate to become resistant to penicillins. Current data from different studies with non-AOM sources and geographic locations that may not be comparable show that 58% to 82% of *H influenzae* isolates are susceptible to regular- and high-dose amoxicillin.[130,147,148,157,158] These data represented a significant decrease in β-lactamase–producing *H influenzae*, compared with data reported in the 2004 AOM guideline.

Nationwide data suggest that 100% of *M catarrhalis* derived from the upper respiratory tract are β-lactamase–positive but remain susceptible to amoxicillin-clavulanate.[159] However, the high rate of spontaneous clinical resolution occurring in children with AOM attributable to *M catarrhalis* treated with amoxicillin reduces the concern for the first-line coverage for this microorganism.[145,146] AOM attributable to *M catarrhalis* rarely progresses to acute mastoiditis or intracranial infections.[102,160,161]

Antibiotic Therapy

High-dose amoxicillin is recommended as the first-line treatment in most patients, although there are a number of medications that are clinically effective (Table 5). The justification for the use of amoxicillin relates to its effectiveness against common AOM bacterial pathogens as well as its safety, low cost, acceptable taste, and narrow microbiologic spectrum.[145,151] In children who have taken amoxicillin in the previous 30 days, those with concurrent conjunctivitis, or those for whom coverage for β-lactamase–positive *H influenzae* and *M catarrhalis* is desired, therapy should be initiated with high-dose amoxicillin-clavulanate (90 mg/kg/day of amoxicillin, with 6.4 mg/kg/day of clavulanate, a ratio of amoxicillin to clavulanate of 14:1, given in 2 divided doses, which is less likely to cause diarrhea than other amoxicillin-clavulanate preparations).[162]

Alternative initial antibiotics include cefdinir (14 mg/kg per day in 1 or 2 doses), cefuroxime (30 mg/kg per day in 2 divided doses), cefpodoxime (10 mg/kg per day in 2 divided doses), or ceftriaxone (50 mg/kg, administered intramuscularly). It is important to note that alternative antibiotics vary in their efficacy against AOM pathogens. For example, recent US data on in vitro susceptibility of *S pneumoniae* to cefdinir and cefuroxime are 70% to 80%, compared with 84% to 92% amoxicillin efficacy.[130,147–149] In vitro efficacy of cefdinir and cefuroxime against *H influenzae* is approximately 98%, compared with 58% efficacy of amoxicillin and nearly 100% efficacy of amoxicillin-clavulanate.[158] A multicenter double tympanocentesis open-label study of

TABLE 5 Recommended Antibiotics for (Initial or Delayed) Treatment and for Patients Who Have Failed Initial Antibiotic Treatment

Initial Immediate or Delayed Antibiotic Treatment		Antibiotic Treatment After 48–72 h of Failure of Initial Antibiotic Treatment	
Recommended First-line Treatment	Alternative Treatment (if Penicillin Allergy)	Recommended First-line Treatment	Alternative Treatment
Amoxicillin (80–90 mg/ kg per day in 2 divided doses)	Cefdinir (14 mg/kg per day in 1 or 2 doses)	Amoxicillin-clavulanate[a] (90 mg/kg per day of amoxicillin, with 6.4 mg/kg per day of clavulanate in 2 divided doses)	Ceftriaxone, 3 d Clindamycin (30–40 mg/kg per day in 3 divided doses), with or without third-generation cephalosporin
or	Cefuroxime (30 mg/kg per day in 2 divided doses)	or	Failure of second antibiotic
Amoxicillin-clavulanate[a] (90 mg/kg per day of amoxicillin, with 6.4 mg/kg per day of clavulanate [amoxicillin to clavulanate ratio, 14:1] in 2 divided doses)	Cefpodoxime (10 mg/kg per day in 2 divided doses)	Ceftriaxone (50 mg IM or IV for 3 d)	Clindamycin (30–40 mg/kg per day in 3 divided doses) plus third-generation cephalosporin
			Tympanocentesis[b]
	Ceftriaxone (50 mg IM or IV per day for 1 or 3 d)		Consult specialist[b]

IM, intramuscular; IV, intravenous.

[a] May be considered in patients who have received amoxicillin in the previous 30 d or who have the otitis-conjunctivitis syndrome.

[b] Perform tympanocentesis/drainage if skilled in the procedure, or seek a consultation from an otolaryngologist for tympanocentesis/drainage. If the tympanocentesis reveals multidrug-resistant bacteria, seek an infectious disease specialist consultation.

[c] Cefdinir, cefuroxime, cefpodoxime, and ceftriaxone are highly unlikely to be associated with cross-reactivity with penicillin allergy on the basis of their distinct chemical structures. See text for more information.

cefdinir in recurrent AOM attributable to *H influenzae* showed eradication of the organism in 72% of patients.[163]

For penicillin-allergic children, recent data suggest that cross-reactivity among penicillins and cephalosporins is lower than historically reported.[164–167] The previously cited rate of cross-sensitivity to cephalosporins among penicillin-allergic patients (approximately 10%) is likely an overestimate. The rate was based on data collected and reviewed during the 1960s and 1970s. A study analyzing pooled data of 23 studies, including 2400 patients with reported history of penicillin allergy and 39 000 with no penicillin allergic history concluded that many patients who present with a history of penicillin allergy do not have an immunologic reaction to penicillin.[166] The chemical structure of the cephalosporin determines the risk of cross-reactivity between specific agents.[165,168] The degree of cross-reactivity is higher between penicillins and first-generation cephalosporins but is negligible with the second- and third-generation cephalosporins. Because of the differences in the chemical structures, cefdinir, cefuroxime, cefpodoxime, and ceftriaxone are highly unlikely to be associated with cross-reactivity with penicillin.[165] Despite this, the Joint Task Force on Practice Parameters; American Academy of Allergy, Asthma and Immunology; American College of Allergy, Asthma and Immunology; and Joint Council of Allergy, Asthma and Immunology[169] stated that "cephalosporin treatment of patients with a history of penicillin allergy, selecting out those with severe reaction histories, show a reaction rate of 0.1%." They recommend a cephalosporin in cases without severe and/or recent penicillin allergy reaction history when skin test is not available.

Macrolides, such as erythromycin and azithromycin, have limited efficacy against both *H influenzae* and *S pneumoniae*.[130,147–149] Clindamycin lacks efficacy against *H influenzae*. Clindamycin alone (30–40 mg/kg per day in 3 divided doses) may be used for suspected penicillin-resistant *S pneumoniae*; however, the drug will likely not be effective for the multidrug-resistant serotypes.[130,158,166]

Several of these choices of antibiotic suspensions are barely palatable or frankly offensive and may lead to avoidance behaviors or active rejection by spitting out the suspension. Palatability of antibiotic suspensions has been compared in many studies.[170–172] Specific antibiotic suspensions such as cefuroxime, cefpodoxime, and clindamycin may benefit from adding taste-masking products, such as chocolate or strawberry flavoring agents, to obscure the initial bitter taste and the unpleasant aftertaste.[172,173] In the patient who is persistently vomiting or cannot otherwise tolerate oral medication, even when the taste is masked, ceftriaxone (50 mg/kg, administered intramuscularly in 1 or 2 sites in the anterior thigh, or intravenously) has been demonstrated to be effective for the initial or repeat antibiotic treatment of AOM.[174,175] Although a single injection of ceftriaxone is approved by the US FDA for the treatment of AOM, results of a double tympanocentesis study (before and 3 days after single dose ceftriaxone) by Leibovitz et al[175] suggest that more than 1 ceftriaxone dose may be required to prevent recurrence of the middle ear infection within 5 to 7 days after the initial dose.

Initial Antibiotic Treatment Failure

When antibiotics are prescribed for AOM, clinical improvement should be noted within 48 to 72 hours. During the 24 hours after the diagnosis of AOM, the child's symptoms may worsen slightly. In the next 24 hours, the patient's symptoms should begin to improve. If initially febrile, the temperature should decline within 48 to 72 hours. Irritability and fussiness should lessen or disappear, and sleeping and drinking patterns should normalize.[176,177] If the patient is not improved by 48 to 72 hours, another disease or concomitant viral infection may be present, or the causative bacteria may be resistant to the chosen therapy.

Some children with AOM and persistent symptoms after 48 to 72 hours of initial antibacterial treatment may have combined bacterial and viral infection, which would explain the persistence of ongoing symptoms despite appropriate antibiotic therapy.[109,178,179] Literature is conflicting on the correlation between clinical and bacteriologic outcomes. Some studies report good correlation ranging from 86% to 91%,[180,181] suggesting continued presence of bacteria in the middle ear in a high proportion of cases with persistent symptoms. Others report that middle ear fluid from children with AOM in whom symptoms are persistent is sterile in 42% to 49% of cases.[123,182] A change in antibiotic may not be required in some children with mild persistent symptoms.

In children with persistent, severe symptoms of AOM and unimproved otologic findings after initial treatment, the clinician may consider changing the antibiotic (Table 5). If the child was initially treated with amoxicillin and failed to improve, amoxicillin-clavulanate should be used. Patients who were given amoxicillin-clavulanate or oral third-generation cephalosporins may receive intramuscular ceftriaxone (50 mg/kg). In the treatment of AOM unresponsive to initial antibiotics, a 3-day course of ceftriaxone has been shown to be better than a 1-day regimen.[175]

Although trimethoprim-sulfamethoxazole and erythromycin-sulfisoxazole had been useful as therapy for patients with AOM, pneumococcal surveillance studies have indicated that resistance to these 2 combination agents is substantial.[130,149,183] Therefore, when patients fail to improve while receiving amoxicillin, neither trimethoprim-sulfamethoxazole[184] nor erythromycin-sulfisoxazole is appropriate therapy.

Tympanocentesis should be considered, and culture of middle ear fluid should be performed for bacteriologic diagnosis and susceptibility testing when a series of antibiotic drugs have failed to improve the clinical condition. If tympanocentesis is not available, a course of clindamycin may be used, with or without an antibiotic that covers nontypeable *H influenzae* and *M catarrhalis*, such as cefdinir, cefixime, or cefuroxime.

Because *S pneumoniae* serotype 19A is usually multidrug-resistant and may not be responsive to clindamycin,[104,149] newer antibiotics that are not approved by the FDA for treatment of AOM, such as levofloxacin or linezolid, may be indicated.[185–187] Levofloxacin is a quinolone antibiotic that is not approved by the FDA for use in children. Linezolid is effective against resistant Gram-positive bacteria. It is not approved by the FDA for AOM treatment and is expensive. In children with repeated treatment failures, every effort should be made for bacteriologic diagnosis by tympanocentesis with Gram stain, culture, and antibiotic susceptibility testing of the organism (s) present. The clinician may consider consulting with pediatric medical subspecialists, such as an otolaryngologist for possible tympanocentesis, drainage, and culture and an infectious disease expert, before use of unconventional drugs such as levofloxacin or linezolid.

When tympanocentesis is not available, 1 possible way to obtain information on the middle ear pathogens and their antimicrobial susceptibility is to obtain a nasopharyngeal specimen for bacterial culture. Almost all middle ear pathogens derive from the pathogens colonizing the nasopharynx, but not all nasopharyngeal pathogens enter the middle ear to cause AOM. The positive predictive value of nasopharyngeal culture during AOM (likelihood that bacteria cultured from the nasopharynx is the middle ear pathogen) ranges from 22% to 44% for *S pneumoniae*, 50% to 71% for nontypeable *H influenzae*, and 17% to 19% for *M catarrhalis*. The negative predictive value (likelihood that bacteria not found in the nasopharynx are not AOM pathogens) ranges from 95% to 99% for all 3 bacteria.[188,189] Therefore, if nasopharyngeal culture is negative for specific bacteria, that organism is likely not the AOM pathogen. A negative culture for *S pneumoniae*, for example, will help eliminate the concern for multidrug-resistant bacteria and the need for unconventional therapies, such as levofloxacin or linezolid. On the other hand, if *S pneumoniae* is cultured from the nasopharynx, the antimicrobial susceptibility pattern can help guide treatment.

Duration of Therapy

The optimal duration of therapy for patients with AOM is uncertain; the usual 10-day course of therapy was derived from the duration of treatment of streptococcal pharyngotonsillitis. Several studies favor standard 10-day therapy over shorter courses for children younger than 2 years.[162,190–194] Thus, for children younger than 2 years and children with severe symptoms, a standard 10-day course is recommended. A 7-day course of oral antibiotic appears to be equally effective in children 2 to 5 years of age with mild or moderate AOM. For children 6 years and older with mild to moderate symptoms, a 5- to 7-day course is adequate treatment.

Follow-up of the Patient With AOM

Once the child has shown clinical improvement, follow-up is based on the usual clinical course of AOM. There is little scientific evidence for a routine 10- to 14-day reevaluation visit for all children with an episode of AOM. The physician may choose to reassess some children, such as young children with severe symptoms or recurrent AOM or when specifically requested by the child's parent.

Persistent MEE is common and can be detected by pneumatic otoscopy (with or without verification by tympanometry) after resolution of acute symptoms. Two weeks after successful antibiotic treatment of AOM, 60% to 70% of children have MEE, decreasing to 40% at 1 month and 10% to 25% at 3 months after successful antibiotic treatment.[177,195] The presence of MEE without clinical symptoms is defined as OME. OME must be differentiated clinically from AOM and requires infrequent additional monitoring but not antibiotic therapy. Assurance that OME resolves is particularly important for parents of children with cognitive or developmental delays that may be affected adversely by transient hearing loss associated with MEE. Detailed recommendations for the management of the child with OME can be found in the evidence-based guideline from the AAP/AAFP/American Academy of Otolaryngology-Head and Neck Surgery published in 2004.[84,85]

Key Action Statement 5A

Clinicians should *NOT* prescribe prophylactic antibiotics to reduce the frequency of episodes of AOM in children with recurrent AOM. (Evidence Quality: Grade B, Rec. Strength: Recommendation)

Key Action Statement Profile: KAS 5A

Aggregate evidence quality	Grade B
Benefits	No adverse effects from antibiotic. Reduces potential for development of bacterial resistance. Reduced costs.
Risks, harms, cost	Small increase in episodes of AOM.
Benefit-harm assessment	Preponderance of benefit.
Value judgments	Potential harm outweighs the potential benefit.
Intentional vagueness	None.
Role of patient preferences	Limited.
Exclusions	Young children whose only alternative would be tympanostomy tubes.
Strength	**Recommendation**

Key Action Statement 5B

Clinicians may offer tympanostomy tubes for recurrent AOM (3 episodes in 6 months or 4 episodes in 1 year, with 1 episode in the preceding 6 months). (Evidence Quality: Grade B, Rec. Strength: Option)

Key Action Statement Profile: KAS 5B

Aggregate evidence quality	**Grade B**
Benefits	Decreased frequency of AOM. Ability to treat AOM with topical antibiotic therapy.
Risks, harms, cost	Risks of anesthesia or surgery. Cost. Scarring of TM, chronic perforation, cholesteatoma. Otorrhea.
Benefits-harms assessment	Equilibrium of benefit and harm.
Value judgments	None.
Intentional vagueness	Option based on limited evidence.
Role of patient preferences	Joint decision of parent and clinician.
Exclusions	Any contraindication to anesthesia and surgery.
Strength	**Option**

Purpose of This Section

Recurrent AOM has been defined as the occurrence of 3 or more episodes of AOM in a 6-month period or the occurrence of 4 or more episodes of AOM in a 12-month period that includes at least 1 episode in the preceding 6 months.[20] These episodes should be well documented and separate acute infections.[11]

Winter season, male gender, and passive exposure to smoking have been associated with an increased likelihood of recurrence. Half of children younger than 2 years treated for AOM will experience a recurrence within 6 months. Symptoms that last more than 10 days may also predict recurrence.[196]

Changes From AAP/AAFP 2004 AOM Guideline

Recurrent AOM was not addressed in the 2004 AOM guideline. This section addresses the literature on recurrent AOM.

Antibiotic Prophylaxis

Long-term, low-dose antibiotic use, referred to as antibiotic prophylaxis or chemoprophylaxis, has been used to treat children with recurrent AOM to prevent subsequent episodes.[85] A 2006 Cochrane review analyzed 16 studies of long-term antibiotic use for AOM and found such use prevented 1.5 episodes of AOM per year, reducing in half the number of AOM episodes during the period of treatment.[197] Randomized placebo-controlled trials of prophylaxis reported a decrease of 0.09 episodes per month in the frequency of AOM attributable to therapy (approximately 0.5 to 1.5 AOM episodes per year for 95% of children). An estimated 5 children would need to be treated for 1 year to prevent 1 episode of OM. The effect may be more substantial for children with 6 or more AOM episodes in the preceding year.[12]

This decrease in episodes of AOM occurred only while the prophylactic antibiotic was being given. The modest benefit afforded by a 6-month course of antibiotic prophylaxis does not have longer-lasting benefit after cessation of therapy. Teele showed no differences between children who received prophylactic antibiotics compared with those who received placebo in AOM recurrences or persistence of OME.[198]

Antibiotic prophylaxis is not appropriate for children with long-term MEE or for children with infrequent episodes of AOM. The small reduction in frequency of AOM with long-term antibiotic prophylaxis must be weighed against the cost of such therapy; the potential adverse effects of antibiotics, principally allergic reaction and gastrointestinal tract consequences, such as diarrhea; and their contribution to the emergence of bacterial resistance.

Surgery for Recurrent AOM

The use of tympanostomy tubes for treatment of ear disease in general, and for AOM in particular, has been controversial.[199] Most published studies of surgical intervention for OM focus on children with persistent MEE with or without AOM. The literature on surgery for recurrent AOM as defined here is scant. A lack of consensus among otolaryngologists regarding the role of surgery for recurrent AOM was reported in a survey of Canadian otolaryngologists in which 40% reported they would "never," 30% reported they would "sometimes," and 30% reported they would "often or always" place tympanostomy tubes for a hypothetical 2-year-old child with frequent OM without persistent MEE or hearing loss.[200]

Tympanostomy tubes, however, remain widely used in clinical practice for both OME and recurrent OM.[201] Recurrent

AOM remains a common indication for referral to an otolaryngologist.

Three randomized controlled trials have compared the number of episodes of AOM after tympanostomy tube placement or no surgery.[202] Two found significant improvement in mean number of AOM episodes after tympanostomy tubes during a 6-month follow-up period.[203,204] One study randomly assigned children with recurrent AOM to groups receiving placebo, amoxicillin prophylaxis, or tympanostomy tubes and followed them for 2 years.[205] Although prophylactic antibiotics reduced the rate of AOM, no difference in number of episodes of AOM was noted between the tympanostomy tube group and the placebo group over 2 years. A Cochrane review of studies of tympanostomy tubes for recurrent AOM analyzed 2 studies[204,206] that met inclusion criteria and found that tympanostomy tubes reduced the number of episodes of AOM by 1.5 episodes in the 6 months after surgery.[207] Tympanostomy tube insertion has been shown to improve disease-specific quality-of-life measures in children with OM.[208] One multicenter, nonrandomized observational study showed large improvements in a disease-specific quality-of-life instrument that measured psychosocial domains of physical suffering, hearing loss, speech impairment, emotional distress, activity limitations, and caregiver concerns that are associated with ear infections.[209] These benefits of tympanostomy tubes have been demonstrated in mixed populations of children that include children with OME as well as recurrent AOM.

Beyond the cost, insertion of tympanostomy tubes is associated with a small but finite surgical and anesthetic risk. A recent review looking at protocols to minimize operative risk reported no major complications, such as sensorineural hearing loss, vascular injury, or ossicular chain disruption, in 10 000 tube insertions performed primarily by residents, although minor complications such as TM tears or displaced tubes in the middle ear were seen in 0.016% of ears.[210] Long-term sequelae of tympanostomy tubes include TM structural changes including focal atrophy, tympanosclerosis, retraction pockets, and chronic perforation. One meta-analysis found tympanosclerosis in 32% of patients after placement of tympanostomy tubes and chronic perforations in 2.2% of patients who had short-term tubes and 16.6% of patients with long-term tubes.[211]

Adenoidectomy, without myringotomy and/or tympanostomy tubes, did not reduce the number of episodes of AOM when compared with chemoprophylaxis or placebo.[212] Adenoidectomy alone should not be used for prevention of AOM but may have benefit when performed with placement of tympanostomy tubes or in children with previous tympanostomy tube placement in OME.[213]

Prevention of AOM: Key Action Statement 6A

Pneumococcal Vaccine

Clinicians should recommend pneumococcal conjugate vaccine to all children according to the schedule of the Advisory Committee on Immunization Practices, AAP, and AAFP. (Evidence Quality: Grade B, Rec. Strength: Strong Recommendation)

Key Action Statement Profile: KAS 6A

Aggregate evidence quality	Grade B
Benefits	Reduced frequency of AOM attributable to vaccine serotypes. Reduced risk of serious pneumococcal systemic disease.
Risks, harms, cost	Potential vaccine side effects. Cost of vaccine.
Benefits-harms assessment	Preponderance of benefit.
Value judgments	Potential vaccine adverse effects are minimal.
Intentional vagueness	None.
Role of patient preferences	Some parents may choose to refuse the vaccine.
Exclusions	Severe allergic reaction (eg, anaphylaxis) to any component of pneumococcal vaccine or any diphtheria toxoid-containing vaccine.
Strength	**Strong Recommendation**

Key Action Statement 6B

Influenza Vaccine: Clinicians should recommend annual influenza vaccine to all children according to the schedule of the Advisory Committee on Immunization Practices, AAP, and AAFP. (Evidence Quality: Grade B, Rec. Strength: Recommendation)

Key Action Statement Profile: KAS 6B

Aggregate evidence quality	Grade B
Benefits	Reduced risk of influenza infection. Reduction in frequency of AOM associated with influenza.
Risks, harms, cost	Potential vaccine adverse effects. Cost of vaccine. Requires annual immunization.
Benefits-harms assessment	Preponderance of benefit.
Value judgments	Potential vaccine adverse effects are minimal.
Intentional vagueness	None
Role of patient preferences	Some parents may choose to refuse the vaccine.
Exclusions	See CDC guideline on contraindications (http://www.cdc.gov/flu/professionals/acip/shouldnot.htm).
Strength	**Recommendation**

Key Action Statement 6C

Breastfeeding: Clinicians should encourage exclusive breastfeeding for at least 6 months. (Evidence Quality: Grade B, Rec. Strength: Recommendation)

Key Action Statement Profile: KAS 6C

Aggregate evidence quality	Grade B
Benefits	May reduce the risk of early AOM. Multiple benefits of breastfeeding unrelated to AOM.
Risk, harm, cost	None
Benefit-harm assessment	Preponderance of benefit.
Value judgments	The intervention has value unrelated to AOM prevention.
Intentional vagueness	None
Role of patient preferences	Some parents choose to feed formula.
Exclusions	None
Strength	**Recommendation**

Key Action Statement 6D

Clinicians should encourage avoidance of tobacco smoke exposure. (Evidence Quality: Grade C, Rec. Strength: Recommendation)

Key Action Statement Profile: KAS 6D

Aggregate evidence quality	Grade C
Benefits	May reduce the risk of AOM.
Risks, harms, cost	None
Benefits-harms assessment	Preponderance of benefit.
Value judgments	Avoidance of tobacco exposure has inherent value unrelated to AOM.
Intentional vagueness	None
Role of patient preferences	Many parents/caregivers choose not to stop smoking. Some also remain addicted, and are unable to quit smoking.
Exclusions	None
Strength	**Recommendation**

Purpose of This Section

The 2004 AOM guideline noted data on immunizations, breastfeeding, and lifestyle changes that would reduce the risk of acquiring AOM. This section addresses new data published since 2004.

Changes From AAP/AAFP 2004 AOM Guideline

PCV7 has been in use in the United States since 2000. PCV13 was introduced in the United States in 2010. The 10-valent pneumococcal nontypeable *H influenzae* protein D-conjugate vaccine was recently licensed in Europe for prevention of diseases attributable to *S pneumoniae* and nontypeable *H influenzae*. Annual influenza immunization is now recommended for all children 6 months of age and older in the United States.[214,215] Updated information regarding these vaccines and their effect on the incidence of AOM is reviewed.

The AAP issued a new breastfeeding policy statement in February 2012.[216] This guideline also includes a recommendation regarding tobacco smoke exposure. Bottle propping, pacifier use, and child care are discussed, but no recommendations are made because of limited evidence. The use of xylitol, a possible adjunct to AOM prevention, is discussed; however, no recommendations are made.

Pneumococcal Vaccine

Pneumococcal conjugate vaccines have proven effective in preventing OM caused by pneumococcal serotypes contained in the vaccines. A meta-analysis of 5 studies with AOM as an outcome determined that there is a 29% reduction in AOM caused by all pneumococcal serotypes among children who received PCV7 before 24 months of age.[217] Although the overall benefit seen in clinical trials for all causes of AOM is small (6%–7%),[218–221] observational studies have shown that medical office visits for otitis were reduced by up to 40% comparing years before and after introduction of PCV7.[222–224] Grijvala[223] reported no effect, however, among children first vaccinated at older ages. Poehling et al[225] reported reductions of frequent AOM and PE tube use after introduction of PCV7. The observations by some of greater benefit observed in the community than in clinical trials is not fully understood but may be related to effects of herd immunity or may be attributed to secular trends or changes in AOM diagnosis patterns over time.[223,226–229] In a 2009 Cochrane review,[221] Jansen et al found that the overall reduction in AOM incidence may only be 6% to 7% but noted that even that small rate may have public health relevance. O'Brien et al concurred and noted in addition the potential for cost savings.[230] There is evidence that serotype replacement may reduce the long-term efficacy of pneumococcal conjugate vaccines against AOM,[231] but it is possible that new pneumococcal conjugate vaccines may demonstrate an increased effect on reduction in AOM.[232–234] Data on AOM reduction secondary to the PCV13 licensed in the United States in 2010 are not yet available.

The *H influenzae* protein D-conjugate vaccine recently licensed in Europe has potential benefit of protection against 10 serotypes of *S pneumoniae* and nontypeable *H influenzae*.[221,234]

Influenza Vaccine

Most cases of AOM follow upper respiratory tract infections caused by viruses, including influenza viruses. As many as two-thirds of young children with influenza may have AOM.[235] Investigators have studied the efficacy of trivalent inactivated influenza vaccine (TIV) and live-attenuated intranasal influenza vaccine (LAIV) in preventing AOM. Many studies have demonstrated 30% to 55% efficacy of influenza vaccine in prevention of AOM during the respiratory illness season.[6,235–239] One study reported no benefit of TIV in reducing AOM burden; however, 1 of the 2 respiratory illness seasons during which this study was conducted had a relatively low influenza activity. A pooled analysis[240] of 8 studies comparing LAIV versus TIV or placebo[241–248] showed a higher efficacy of LAIV compared with both placebo and with TIV. Influenza vaccination is now recommended for all children 6 months of age and older in the United States.[214,215]

Breastfeeding

Multiple studies provide evidence that breastfeeding for at least 4 to 6 months reduces episodes of AOM and recurrent AOM.[249–253] Two cohort studies, 1 retrospective study[250] and 1 prospective study,[253] suggest a dose response, with some protection from partial breastfeeding and the greatest protection from exclusive breastfeeding through 6 months of age. In multivariate analysis controlling for exposure to child care settings, the risk of nonrecurrent otitis is 0.61 (95% confidence interval [CI]: 0.4–0.92) comparing exclusive breastfeeding through 6 months of age with no breastfeeding or breastfeeding less than 4 months. In a prospective cohort, Scariatti[253] found a significant dose-response effect. In this study, OM was self-reported by parents. In a systematic review, McNiel et al[254] found that when exclusive breastfeeding was set as the normative standard, the recalculated odds ratios (ORs) revealed the risks of any formula use. For example, any formula use in the first 6 months of age was significantly associated with increased incidence of OM (OR: 1.78; 95% CI: 1.19–2.70; OR: 4.55; 95% CI: 1.64–12.50 in the available studies; pooled OR for any formula in the first 3 months of age, 2.00; 95% CI: 1.40–2.78). A number of studies[255–259] addressed the association of AOM and other infectious illness in infants with duration and exclusivity of breastfeeding, but all had limitations and none had a randomized controlled design. However, taken together, they continue to show a protective effect of exclusive breastfeeding. In all studies, there has been a predominance of white subjects, and child care attendance and smoking exposure may not have been completely controlled. Also, feeding methods were self-reported.

The consistent finding of a lower incidence of AOM and recurrent AOM with increased breastfeeding supports the AAP recommendation to encourage exclusive breastfeeding for the first 6 months of life and to continue for at least the first year and beyond for as long as mutually desired by mother and child.[216]

Lifestyle Changes

In addition to its many other benefits,[260] eliminating exposure to passive tobacco smoke has been postulated to reduce the incidence of AOM in infancy.[252,261–264] Bottles and pacifiers have been associated with AOM. Avoiding supine bottle feeding ("bottle propping") and reducing or eliminating pacifier use in the second 6 months of life may reduce AOM incidence.[265–267] In a recent cohort study, pacifier use was associated with AOM recurrence.[268]

During infancy and early childhood, reducing the incidence of upper respiratory tract infections by altering child care-center attendance patterns can reduce the incidence of recurrent AOM significantly.[249,269]

Xylitol

Xylitol, or birch sugar, is chemically a pentitol or 5-carbon polyol sugar alcohol. It is available as chewing gum, syrup, or lozenges. A 2011 Cochrane review[270] examined the evidence for the use of xylitol in preventing recurrent AOM. A statistically significant 25% reduction in the risk of occurrence of AOM among healthy children at child care centers in the xylitol group compared with the control group (relative risk: 0.75; 95% CI: 0.65 to 0.88; RD: –0.07; 95% CI: –0.12 to –0.03) in the 4 studies met criteria for analysis.[271–274] Chewing gum and lozenges containing xylitol appeared to be more effective than syrup. Children younger than 2 years, those at the greatest risk of having AOM, cannot safely use lozenges or chewing gum. Also, xylitol needs to be given 3 to 5 times a day to be effective. It is not effective for treating AOM and it must be taken daily throughout the respiratory illness season to have an effect. Sporadic or as-needed use is not effective.

Future Research

Despite advances in research partially stimulated by the 2004 AOM guideline, there are still many unanswered clinical questions in the field. Following are possible clinical research questions that still need to be resolved.

Diagnosis

There will probably never be a gold standard for diagnosis of AOM because of the continuum from OME to AOM. Conceivably, new techniques that could be used on the small amount of fluid obtained during tympanocentesis could identify inflammatory markers in addition to the presence of bacteria or viruses. However, performing tympanocentesis studies on children with uncomplicated otitis is likely not feasible because of ethical and other considerations.

Devices that more accurately identify the presence of MEE and bulging that are easier to use than tympanometry during office visits would be welcome, especially in the difficult-to-examine infant. Additional development of inexpensive, easy-to-use video pneumatic otoscopes is still a goal.

Initial Treatment

The recent studies of Hoberman[31] and Tähtinen[32] have addressed clinical and TM appearance by using stringent diagnostic criteria of AOM. However, the outcomes for less stringent diagnostic criteria, a combination of symptoms, MEE, and TM appearance not completely consistent with OME can only be inferred from earlier studies that used less stringent criteria but did not specify outcomes for various grades of findings. Randomized controlled trials on these less certain TM appearances using scales similar to the OS-8 scale[35] could clarify the benefit of initial antibiotics and initial observation for these less certain diagnoses. Such studies must also specify severity of illness, laterality, and otorrhea.

Appropriate end points must be established. Specifically is the appearance of the TM in patients without clinical symptoms at the end of a study significant for relapse, recurrence, or persistent MEE. Such a study would require randomization of patients with unimproved TM appearance to continued observation and antibiotic groups.

The most efficient and acceptable methods of initial observation should continue to be studied balancing the convenience and benefits with the potential risks to the patient.

Antibiotics

Amoxicillin-clavulanate has a broader spectrum than amoxicillin and may be a better initial antibiotic. However, because of cost and adverse effects, the subcommittee has chosen amoxicillin as first-line AOM treatment. Randomized controlled trials comparing the 2 with adequate power to differentiate clinical efficacy would clarify this choice. Stringent diagnostic criteria should be the standard for these studies. Antibiotic comparisons for AOM should now include an observation arm for patients with nonsevere illness to ensure a clinical benefit over placebo. Studies should also have enough patients to show small but meaningful differences.

Although there have been studies on the likelihood of resistant *S pneumoniae* or *H influenzae* in children in child care settings and with siblings younger than 5 years, studies are still needed to determine whether these and other risk factors would indicate a need for different initial treatment than noted in the guideline.

New antibiotics that are safe and effective are needed for use in AOM because of the development of multidrug-resistant organisms. Such new antibiotics must be tested against the currently available medications.

Randomized controlled trials using different durations of antibiotic therapy in different age groups are needed to optimize therapy with the possibility of decreasing duration of antibiotic use. These would need to be performed initially with amoxicillin and amoxicillin-clavulanate but should also be performed for any antibiotic used in AOM. Again, an observation arm should be included in nonsevere illness.

Recurrent AOM

There have been adequate studies regarding prophylactic antibiotic use in recurrent AOM. More and better controlled studies of tympanostomy tube placement would help determine its benefit versus harm.

Prevention

There should be additional development of vaccines targeted at common organisms associated with AOM.[275] Focused epidemiologic studies on the benefit of breastfeeding, specifically addressing AOM prevention, including duration of breastfeeding and partial versus exclusive breastfeeding, would clarify what is now a more general database. Likewise, more focused studies of the effects of lifestyle changes would help clarify their effect on AOM.

Complementary and Alternative Medicine

There are no well-designed randomized controlled trials of the usefulness of complementary and alternative medicine in AOM, yet a large number of families turn to these methods. Although most alternative therapies are relatively inexpensive, some may be costly. Such studies should compare the alternative therapy to observation rather than antibiotics and only use an antibiotic arm if the alternative therapy is shown to be better than observation. Such studies should focus on children with less stringent criteria of AOM but using the same descriptive criteria for the patients as noted above.

DISSEMINATION OF GUIDELINES

An Institute of Medicine Report notes that "Effective multifaceted implementation strategies targeting both individuals and healthcare systems should be employed by implementers to promote adherence to trustworthy [clinical practice guidelines]."[230]

Many studies of the effect of clinical practice guidelines have been performed. In general, the studies show little overt change in practice after a guideline is published. However, as was seen after the 2004 AOM guideline, the number of visits for AOM and the number of prescriptions for antibiotics for AOM had decreased publication. Studies of educational and dissemination methods both at the practicing physician level and especially at the resident level need to be examined.

SUBCOMMITTEE ON DIAGNOSIS AND MANAGEMENT OF ACUTE OTITIS MEDIA

Allan S. Lieberthal, MD, FAAP (Chair, general pediatrician, no conflicts)

Aaron E. Carroll, MD, MS, FAAP (Partnership for Policy Implementation [PPI] Informatician, general academic pediatrician, no conflicts)

Tasnee Chonmaitree, MD, FAAP (pediatric infectious disease physician, no financial conflicts; published research related to AOM)

Theodore G. Ganiats, MD (family physician, American Academy of Family Physicians, no conflicts)

Alejandro Hoberman, MD, FAAP (general academic pediatrician, no financial conflicts; published research related to AOM)

Mary Anne Jackson, MD, FAAP (pediatric infectious disease physician, AAP Committee on Infectious Disease, no conflicts)

Mark D. Joffe, MD, FAAP (pediatric emergency medicine physician, AAP Committee/Section on Pediatric Emergency Medicine, no conflicts)

Donald T. Miller, MD, MPH, FAAP (general pediatrician, no conflicts)

Richard M. Rosenfeld, MD, MPH, FAAP (otolaryngologist, AAP Section on Otolaryngology, Head and Neck Surgery, American Academy of Otolaryngology-Head and Neck Surgery, no financial conflicts; published research related to AOM)

Xavier D. Sevilla, MD, FAAP (general pediatrics, Quality Improvement Innovation Network, no conflicts)

Richard H. Schwartz, MD, FAAP (general pediatrician, no financial conflicts; published research related to AOM)

Pauline A. Thomas, MD, FAAP (epidemiologist, general pediatrician, no conflicts)

David E. Tunkel, MD, FAAP, FACS (otolaryngologist, AAP Section on Otolaryngology, Head and Neck Surgery, periodic consultant to Medtronic ENT)

CONSULTANT

Richard N. Shiffman, MD, FAAP, FACMI (informatician, guideline methodologist, general academic pediatrician, no conflicts)

STAFF

Caryn Davidson, MA

Oversight by the Steering Committee on Quality Improvement and Management, 2009–2012

REFERENCES

1. American Academy of Pediatrics Subcommittee on Management of Acute Otitis Media. Diagnosis and management of acute otitis media. *Pediatrics*. 2004;113(5):1451–1465
2. Grijalva CG, Nuorti JP, Griffin MR. Antibiotic prescription rates for acute respiratory tract infections in US ambulatory settings. *JAMA*. 2009;302(7):758–766
3. McCaig LF, Besser RE, Hughes JM. Trends in antimicrobial prescribing rates for children and adolescents. *JAMA*. 2002;287(23):3096–3102
4. Vernacchio L, Vezina RM, Mitchell AA. Management of acute otitis media by primary care physicians: trends since the release of the 2004 American Academy of Pediatrics/American Academy of Family Physicians clinical practice guideline. *Pediatrics*. 2007;120(2):281–287
5. Coco A, Vernacchio L, Horst M, Anderson A. Management of acute otitis media after publication of the 2004 AAP and AAFP clinical practice guideline. *Pediatrics*. 2010;125(2):214–220
6. Marchisio P, Mira E, Klersy C, et al. Medical education and attitudes about acute otitis media guidelines: a survey of Italian pediatricians and otolaryngologists. *Pediatr Infect Dis J*. 2009;28(1):1–4
7. Arkins ER, Koehler JM. Use of the observation option and compliance with guidelines in treatment of acute otitis media. *Ann Pharmacother*. 2008;42(5):726–727
8. Flores G, Lee M, Bauchner H, Kastner B. Pediatricians' attitudes, beliefs, and practices regarding clinical practice guidelines: a national survey. *Pediatrics*. 2000;105(3 pt 1):496–501
9. Bluestone CD. Definitions, terminology, and classification. In: Rosenfeld RM, Bluestone CD, eds. *Evidence-Based Otitis Media*. Hamilton, Canada: BC Decker; 2003:120–135
10. Bluestone CD, Klein JO. Definitions, terminology, and classification. In: Bluestone CD, Klein JO, eds. *Otitis Media in Infants and Children*. 4th ed. Hamilton, Canada: BC Decker; 2007:1–19
11. Dowell SF, Marcy MS, Phillips WR, et al. Otitis media: principles of judicious use of antimicrobial agents. *Pediatrics*. 1998;101(suppl):165–171
12. Rosenfeld RM. Clinical pathway for acute otitis media. In: Rosenfeld RM, Bluestone CD, eds. *Evidence-Based Otitis Media*. 2nd ed. Hamilton, Canada: BC Decker; 2003:280–302
13. Carlson LH, Carlson RD. Diagnosis. In: Rosenfeld RM, Bluestone CD, eds. *Evidence-Based Otitis Media*. Hamilton, Canada: BC Decker; 2003: 136–146
14. Bluestone CD, Klein JO. Diagnosis. In: *Otitis Media in Infants and Children*. 4th ed. Hamilton, Canada: BC Decker; 2007:147–212
15. University of Oxford, Centre for Evidence Based Medicine. Available at: www.cebm.net/index.aspx?o=1044. Accessed July 17, 2012
16. American Academy of Pediatrics Steering Committee on Quality Improvement and Management. Classifying recommendations for clinical practice guidelines. *Pediatrics*. 2004;114(3):874–877
17. Marcy M, Takata G, Shekelle P, et al. *Management of Acute Otitis Media*. Evidence Report/Technology Assessment No. 15. Rockville, MD: Agency for Healthcare Research and Quality; 2000

18. Chan LS, Takata GS, Shekelle P, Morton SC, Mason W, Marcy SM. Evidence assessment of management of acute otitis media: II. Research gaps and priorities for future research. *Pediatrics.* 2001;108(2):248–254

19. Takata GS, Chan LS, Shekelle P, Morton SC, Mason W, Marcy SM. Evidence assessment of management of acute otitis media: I. The role of antibiotics in treatment of uncomplicated acute otitis media. *Pediatrics.* 2001;108(2):239–247

20. Shekelle PG, Takata G, Newberry SJ, et al. *Management of Acute Otitis Media: Update.* Evidence Report/Technology Assessment No. 198. Rockville, MD: Agency for Healthcare Research and Quality; 2010

21. Coker TR, Chan LS, Newberry SJ, et al. Diagnosis, microbial epidemiology, and antibiotic treatment of acute otitis media in children: a systematic review. *JAMA.* 2010;304(19):2161–2169

22. Jadad AR, Moore RA, Carroll D, et al. Assessing the quality of reports of randomized clinical trials: is blinding necessary? *Control Clin Trials.* 1996;17(1):1–12

23. Whiting P, Rutjes AW, Reitsma JB, Bossuyt PM, Kleijnen J. The development of QUADAS: a tool for the quality assessment of studies of diagnostic accuracy included in systematic reviews. *BMC Med Res Methodol.* 2003;3:25

24. Guyatt GH, Oxman AD, Vist GE, et al; GRADE Working Group. GRADE: an emerging consensus on rating quality of evidence and strength of recommendations. *BMJ.* 2008;336(7650):924–926

25. Hoffman RN, Michel G, Rosenfeld RM, Davidson C. Building better guidelines with BRIDGE-Wiz: development and evaluation of a software assistant to promote clarity, transparency, and implementability. *J Am Med Inform Assoc.* 2012;19(1):94–101

26. Kalu SU, Ataya RS, McCormick DP, Patel JA, Revai K, Chonmaitree T. Clinical spectrum of acute otitis media complicating upper respiratory tract viral infection. *Pediatr Infect Dis J.* 2011;30(2):95–99

27. Block SL, Harrison CJ. *Diagnosis and Management of Acute Otitis Media.* 3rd ed. Caddo, OK: Professional Communications; 2005:48–50

28. Wald ER. Acute otitis media: more trouble with the evidence. *Pediatr Infect Dis J.* 2003;22(2):103–104

29. Paradise JL, Rockette HE, Colborn DK, et al. Otitis media in 2253 Pittsburgh-area infants: prevalence and risk factors during the first two years of life. *Pediatrics.* 1997;99(3):318–333

30. McCormick DP, Chonmaitree T, Pittman C, et al. Nonsevere acute otitis media: a clinical trial comparing outcomes of watchful waiting versus immediate antibiotic treatment. *Pediatrics.* 2005;115(6):1455–1465

31. Hoberman A, Paradise JL, Rockette HE, et al. Treatment of acute otitis media in children under 2 years of age. *N Engl J Med.* 2011;364(2):105–115

32. Tähtinen PA, Laine MK, Huovinen P, Jalava J, Ruuskanen O, Ruohola A. A placebo-controlled trial of antimicrobial treatment for acute otitis media. *N Engl J Med.* 2011;364(2):116–126

33. Shaikh N, Hoberman A, Paradise JL, et al. Development and preliminary evaluation of a parent-reported outcome instrument for clinical trials in acute otitis media. *Pediatr Infect Dis J.* 2009;28(1):5–8

34. Laine MK, Tähtinen PA, Ruuskanen O, Huovinen P, Ruohola A. Symptoms or symptom-based scores cannot predict acute otitis media at otitis-prone age. *Pediatrics.* 2010;125(5). Available at: www.pediatrics.org/cgi/content/full/125/5/e1154

35. Friedman NR, McCormick DP, Pittman C, et al. Development of a practical tool for assessing the severity of acute otitis media. *Pediatr Infect Dis J.* 2006;25(2):101–107

36. Rothman R, Owens T, Simel DL. Does this child have acute otitis media? *JAMA.* 2003;290(12):1633–1640

37. Niemela M, Uhari M, Jounio-Ervasti K, Luotonen J, Alho OP, Vierimaa E. Lack of specific symptomatology in children with acute otitis media. *Pediatr Infect Dis J.* 1994;13(9):765–768

38. Heikkinen T, Ruuskanen O. Signs and symptoms predicting acute otitis media. *Arch Pediatr Adolesc Med.* 1995;149(1):26–29

39. Ingvarsson L. Acute otalgia in children—findings and diagnosis. *Acta Paediatr Scand.* 1982;71(5):705–710

40. Kontiokari T, Koivunen P, Niemelä M, Pokka T, Uhari M. Symptoms of acute otitis media. *Pediatr Infect Dis J.* 1998;17(8):676–679

41. Wong DL, Baker CM. Pain in children: comparison of assessment scales. *Pediatr Nurs.* 1988;14(1):9–17

42. Shaikh N, Hoberman A, Paradise JL, et al. Responsiveness and construct validity of a symptom scale for acute otitis media. *Pediatr Infect Dis J.* 2009;28(1):9–12

43. Karma PH, Penttilä MA, Sipilä MM, Kataja MJ. Otoscopic diagnosis of middle ear effusion in acute and non-acute otitis media. I. The value of different otoscopic findings. *Int J Pediatr Otorhinolaryngol.* 1989;17(1):37–49

44. McCormick DP, Lim-Melia E, Saeed K, Baldwin CD, Chonmaitree T. Otitis media: can clinical findings predict bacterial or viral etiology? *Pediatr Infect Dis J.* 2000;19(3):256–258

45. Schwartz RH, Stool SE, Rodriguez WJ, Grundfast KM. Acute otitis media: toward a more precise definition. *Clin Pediatr (Phila).* 1981;20(9):549–554

46. Rosenfeld RM. Antibiotic prophylaxis for recurrent acute otitis media. In: Alper CM, Bluestone CD, eds. *Advanced Therapy of Otitis Media.* Hamilton, Canada: BC Decker; 2004

47. Paradise J, Bernard B, Colborn D, Smith C, Rockette H; Pittsburgh-area Child Development/Otitis Media Study Group. Otitis media with effusion: highly prevalent and often the forerunner of acute otitis media during the first year of life [abstract]. *Pediatr Res.* 1993;33:121A

48. Roland PS, Smith TL, Schwartz SR, et al. Clinical practice guideline: cerumen impaction. *Otolaryngol Head Neck Surg.* 2008;139(3 suppl 2):S1–S21

49. Shaikh N, Hoberman A, Kaleida PH, Ploof DL, Paradise JL. Videos in clinical medicine. Diagnosing otitis media—otoscopy and cerumen removal. *N Engl J Med.* 2010;362(20):e62

50. Pichichero ME. Diagnostic accuracy, tympanocentesis training performance, and antibiotic selection by pediatric residents in management of otitis media. *Pediatrics.* 2002;110(6):1064–1070

51. Kaleida PH, Ploof DL, Kurs-Lasky M, et al. Mastering diagnostic skills: Enhancing Proficiency in Otitis Media, a model for diagnostic skills training. *Pediatrics.* 2009;124(4). Available at: www.pediatrics.org/cgi/content/full/124/4/e714

52. Kaleida PH, Ploof D. ePROM: Enhancing Proficiency in Otitis Media. Pittsburgh, PA: University of Pittsburgh School of Medicine. Available at: http://pedsed.pitt.edu. Accessed December 31, 2011

53. Innovative Medical Education. *A View Through the Otoscope: Distinguishing Acute Otitis Media from Otitis Media with Effusion.* Paramus, NJ: Innovative Medical Education; 2000

54. American Academy of Pediatrics. Section on Infectious Diseases. A view through the otoscope: distinguishing acute otitis media from otitis media with effusion [video]. Available at: http://www2.aap.org/sections/infectdis/video.cfm. Accessed January 20, 2012

55. Hayden GF, Schwartz RH. Characteristics of earache among children with acute

otitis media. *Am J Dis Child.* 1985;139(7): 721–723

56. Schechter NL. Management of pain associated with acute medical illness. In: Schechter NL, Berde CB, Yaster M, eds. *Pain in Infants, Children, and Adolescents.* Baltimore, MD: Williams & Wilkins; 1993: 537–538
57. Rovers MM, Glasziou P, Appelman CL, et al. Predictors of pain and/or fever at 3 to 7 days for children with acute otitis media not treated initially with antibiotics: a meta-analysis of individual patient data. *Pediatrics.* 2007;119(3):579–585
58. Burke P, Bain J, Robinson D, Dunleavey J. Acute red ear in children: controlled trial of nonantibiotic treatment in children: controlled trial of nonantibiotic treatment in general practice. *BMJ.* 1991;303(6802): 558–562
59. Sanders S, Glasziou PP, DelMar C, Rovers M. Antibiotics for acute otitis media in children [review]. *Cochrane Database Syst Rev.* 2009;(2):1–43
60. van Buchem FL, Dunk JH, van't Hof MA. Therapy of acute otitis media: myringotomy, antibiotics, or neither? A double-blind study in children. *Lancet.* 1981;2(8252): 883–887
61. Thalin A, Densert O, Larsson A, et al. Is penicillin necessary in the treatment of acute otitis media? In: *Proceedings of the International Conference on Acute and Secretory Otitis Media. Part 1.* Amsterdam, Netherlands: Kugler Publications; 1986:441–446
62. Rovers MM, Glasziou P, Appelman CL, et al. Antibiotics for acute otitis media: an individual patient data meta-analysis. *Lancet.* 2006;368(9545):1429–1435
63. Bertin L, Pons G, d'Athis P, et al. A randomized, double-blind, multicentre controlled trial of ibuprofen versus acetaminophen and placebo for symptoms of acute otitis media in children. *Fundam Clin Pharmacol.* 1996;10(4):387–392
64. American Academy of Pediatrics. Committee on Psychosocial Aspects of Child and Family Health; Task Force on Pain in Infants, Children, and Adolescents. The assessment and management of acute pain in infants, children, and adolescents. *Pediatrics.* 2001;108(3): 793–797
65. Bolt P, Barnett P, Babl FE, Sharwood LN. Topical lignocaine for pain relief in acute otitis media: results of a double-blind placebo-controlled randomised trial. *Arch Dis Child.* 2008;93(1):40–44
66. Foxlee R, Johansson AC, Wejfalk J, Dawkins J, Dooley L, Del Mar C. Topical analgesia for acute otitis media. *Cochrane Database Syst Rev.* 2006;(3):CD005657
67. Hoberman A, Paradise JL, Reynolds EA, Urkin J. Efficacy of Auralgan for treating ear pain in children with acute otitis media. *Arch Pediatr Adolesc Med.* 1997; 151(7):675–678
68. Sarrell EM, Mandelberg A, Cohen HA. Efficacy of naturopathic extracts in the management of ear pain associated with acute otitis media. *Arch Pediatr Adolesc Med.* 2001;155(7):796–799
69. Sarrell EM, Cohen HA, Kahan E. Naturopathic treatment for ear pain in children. *Pediatrics.* 2003;111(5 pt 1):e574–e579
70. Adam D, Federspil P, Lukes M, Petrowicz O. Therapeutic properties and tolerance of procaine and phenazone containing ear drops in infants and very young children. *Arzneimittelforschung.* 2009;59(10):504–512
71. Barnett ED, Levatin JL, Chapman EH, et al. Challenges of evaluating homeopathic treatment of acute otitis media. *Pediatr Infect Dis J.* 2000;19(4):273–275
72. Jacobs J, Springer DA, Crothers D. Homeopathic treatment of acute otitis media in children: a preliminary randomized placebo-controlled trial. *Pediatr Infect Dis J.* 2001;20(2):177–183
73. Rosenfeld RM, Bluestone CD. Clinical efficacy of surgical therapy. In: Rosenfeld RM, Bluestone CD, eds. *Evidence-Based Otitis Media. 2003.* Hamilton, Canada: BC Decker; 2003:227–240
74. Rosenfeld RM. Observation option toolkit for acute otitis media. *Int J Pediatr Otorhinolaryngol.* 2001;58(1):1–8
75. Le Saux N, Gaboury I, Baird M, et al. A randomized, double-blind, placebo-controlled noninferiority trial of amoxicillin for clinically diagnosed acute otitis media in children 6 months to 5 years of age. *CMAJ.* 2005;172(3):335–341
76. Spiro DM, Tay KY, Arnold DH, Dziura JD, Baker MD, Shapiro ED. Wait-and-see prescription for the treatment of acute otitis media: a randomized controlled trial. *JAMA.* 2006;296(10):1235–1241
77. Neumark T, Mölstad S, Rosén C, et al. Evaluation of phenoxymethylpenicillin treatment of acute otitis media in children aged 2–16. *Scand J Prim Health Care.* 2007;25(3):166–171
78. Chao JH, Kunkov S, Reyes LB, Lichten S, Crain EF. Comparison of two approaches to observation therapy for acute otitis media in the emergency department. *Pediatrics.* 2008;121(5). Available at: www.pediatrics.org/cgi/content/full/121/5/e1352
79. Spurling GK, Del Mar CB, Dooley L, Foxlee R. Delayed antibiotics for respiratory infections. *Cochrane Database Syst Rev.* 2007;(3):CD004417
80. Koopman L, Hoes AW, Glasziou PP, et al. Antibiotic therapy to prevent the development of asymptomatic middle ear effusion in children with acute otitis media: a meta-analysis of individual patient data. *Arch Otolaryngol Head Neck Surg.* 2008;134(2):128–132
81. Marchetti F, Ronfani L, Nibali SC, Tamburlini G; Italian Study Group on Acute Otitis Media. Delayed prescription may reduce the use of antibiotics for acute otitis media: a prospective observational study in primary care. *Arch Pediatr Adolesc Med.* 2005; 159(7):679–684
82. Ho D, Rotenberg BW, Berkowitz RG. The relationship between acute mastoiditis and antibiotic use for acute otitis media in children. *Arch Otolaryngol Head Neck Surg.* 2008;34(1):45–48
83. Thompson PL, Gilbert RE, Long PF, Saxena S, Sharland M, Wong IC. Effect of antibiotics for otitis media on mastoiditis in children: a retrospective cohort study using the United Kingdom general practice research database. *Pediatrics.* 2009; 123(2):424–430
84. American Academy of Family Physicians; American Academy of Otolaryngology-Head and Neck Surgery; American Academy of Pediatrics Subcommittee on Otitis Media With Effusion. Otitis media with effusion. *Pediatrics.* 2004;113(5):1412–1429
85. Rosenfeld RM, Culpepper L, Doyle KJ, et al; American Academy of Pediatrics Subcommittee on Otitis Media with Effusion; American Academy of Family Physicians; American Academy of Otolaryngology—Head and Neck Surgery. Clinical practice guideline: otitis media with effusion. *Otolaryngol Head Neck Surg.* 2004;130(suppl 5): S95–S118
86. Appelman CL, Claessen JQ, Touw-Otten FW, Hordijk GJ, de Melker RA. Co-amoxiclav in recurrent acute otitis media: placebo controlled study. *BMJ.* 1991;303(6815): 1450–1452
87. Burke P, Bain J, Robinson D, Dunleavey J. Acute red ear in children: controlled trial of nonantibiotic treatment in children: controlled trial of nonantibiotic treatment in general practice. *BMJ.* 1991;303(6802): 558–562
88. van Balen FA, Hoes AW, Verheij TJ, de Melker RA. Primary care based randomized, double blind trial of amoxicillin versus placebo in children aged under 2 years. *BMJ.* 2000;320(7231):350–354

89. Little P, Gould C, Williamson I, Moore M, Warner G, Dunleavey J. Pragmatic randomised controlled trial of two prescribing strategies for childhood acute otitis media. *BMJ*. 2001;322(7282):336–342

90. Mygind N, Meistrup-Larsen K-I, Thomsen J, Thomsen VF, Josefsson K, Sørensen H. Penicillin in acute otitis media: a double-blind placebo-controlled trial. *Clin Otolaryngol Allied Sci*. 1981;6(1):5–13

91. Kaleida PH, Casselbrant ML, Rockette HE, et al. Amoxicillin or myringotomy or both for acute otitis media: results of a randomized clinical trial. *Pediatrics*. 1991;87(4):466–474

92. Shaikh N, Hoberman A, Paradise JL, et al. Responsiveness and construct validity of a symptom scale for acute otitis media. *Pediatr Infect Dis J*. 2009;28(1):9–12

93. Heikkinen T, Chonmaitree T. Importance of respiratory viruses in acute otitis media. *Clin Microbiol Rev*. 2003;16(2):230–241

94. Halsted C, Lepow ML, Balassanian N, Emmerich J, Wolinsky E. Otitis media. Clinical observations, microbiology, and evaluation of therapy. *Am J Dis Child*. 1968;115(5):542–551

95. Rosenfeld RM, Vertrees J, Carr J, et al. Clinical efficacy of antimicrobials for acute otitis media: meta-analysis of 5,400 children from 33 randomized trials. *J Pediatr*. 1994;124(3):355–367

96. McCormick DP, Chandler SM, Chonmaitree T. Laterality of acute otitis media: different clinical and microbiologic characteristics. *Pediatr Infect Dis J*. 2007;26(7):583–588

97. Appelman CLM, Bossen PC, Dunk JHM, Lisdonk EH, de Melker RA, van Weert HCPM. NHG Standard Otitis Media Acuta (Guideline on acute otitis media of the Dutch College of General Practitioners). *Huisarts Wet*. 1990;33:242–245

98. Swedish Medical Research Council. Treatment for acute inflammation of the middle ear: consensus statement. Stockholm, Sweden: Swedish Medical Research Council; 2000. Available at: http://soapimg.icecube.snowfall.se/strama/Konsensut_ora_eng.pdf. Accessed July 18, 2012

99. Scottish Intercollegiate Guideline Network. Diagnosis and management of childhood otitis media in primary care. Edinburgh, Scotland: Scottish Intercollegiate Guideline Network; 2000. Available at: www.sign.ac.uk/guidelines/fulltext/66/index.html. Accessed July 18, 2012

100. National Institute for Health and Clinical Excellence, Centre for Clinical Practice. Respiratory tract infections—antibiotic prescribing: prescribing of antibiotics for self-limiting respiratory tract infections in adults and children in primary care. NICE Clinical Guideline 69. London, United Kingdom: National Institute for Health and Clinical Excellence; July 2008. Available at: www.nice.org.uk/CG069. Accessed July 18, 2012

101. Marchisio P, Bellussi L, Di Mauro G, et al. Acute otitis media: from diagnosis to prevention. Summary of the Italian guideline. *Int J Pediatr Otorhinolaryngol*. 2010;74(11):1209–1216

102. Siegel RM, Kiely M, Bien JP, et al. Treatment of otitis media with observation and a safety-net antibiotic prescription. *Pediatrics*. 2003;112(3 pt 1):527–531

103. Pshetizky Y, Naimer S, Shvartzman P. Acute otitis media—a brief explanation to parents and antibiotic use. *Fam Pract*. 2003;20(4):417–419

104. Pichichero ME, Casey JR. Emergence of a multiresistant serotype 19A pneumococcal strain not included in the 7-valent conjugate vaccine as an otopathogen in children. *JAMA*. 2007;298(15):1772–1778

105. Pichichero ME, Casey JR. Evolving microbiology and molecular epidemiology of acute otitis media in the pneumococcal conjugate vaccine era. *Pediatr Infect Dis J*. 2007;26(suppl 10):S12–S16

106. Nielsen HUK, Konradsen HB, Lous J, Frimodt-Møller N. Nasopharyngeal pathogens in children with acute otitis media in a low-antibiotic use country. *Int J Pediatr Otorhinolaryngol*. 2004;68(9):1149–1155

107. Pitkäranta A, Virolainen A, Jero J, Arruda E, Hayden FG. Detection of rhinovirus, respiratory syncytial virus, and coronavirus infections in acute otitis media by reverse transcriptase polymerase chain reaction. *Pediatrics*. 1998;102(2 pt 1):291–295

108. Heikkinen T, Thint M, Chonmaitree T. Prevalence of various respiratory viruses in the middle ear during acute otitis media. *N Engl J Med*. 1999;340(4):260–264

109. Chonmaitree T. Acute otitis media is not a pure bacterial disease. *Clin Infect Dis*. 2006;43(11):1423–1425

110. Williams JV, Tollefson SJ, Nair S, Chonmaitree T. Association of human metapneumovirus with acute otitis media. *Int J Pediatr Otorhinolaryngol*. 2006;70(7):1189–1193

111. Chonmaitree T, Heikkinen T. Role of viruses in middle-ear disease. *Ann N Y Acad Sci*. 1997;830:143–157

112. Klein JO, Bluestone CD. Otitis media. In: Feigin RD, Cherry JD, Demmler-Harrison GJ, Kaplan SL, eds. *Textbook of Pediatric Infectious Diseases*. 6th ed. Philadelphia, PA: Saunders; 2009:216–237

113. Chonmaitree T, Revai K, Grady JJ, et al. Viral upper respiratory tract infection and otitis media complication in young children. *Clin Infect Dis*. 2008;46(6):815–823

114. Ruohola A, Meurman O, Nikkari S, et al. Microbiology of acute otitis media in children with tympanostomy tubes: prevalences of bacteria and viruses. *Clin Infect Dis*. 2006;43(11):1417–1422

115. Ruuskanen O, Arola M, Heikkinen T, Ziegler T. Viruses in acute otitis media: increasing evidence for clinical significance. *Pediatr Infect Dis J*. 1991;10(6):425–427

116. Chonmaitree T. Viral and bacterial interaction in acute otitis media. *Pediatr Infect Dis J*. 2000;19(suppl 5):S24–S30

117. Nokso-Koivisto J, Räty R, Blomqvist S, et al. Presence of specific viruses in the middle ear fluids and respiratory secretions of young children with acute otitis media. *J Med Virol*. 2004;72(2):241–248

118. Bluestone CD, Klein JO. Microbiology. In: Bluestone CD, Klein JO, eds. *Otitis Media in Infants and Children*. 4th ed. Hamilton, Canada: BC Decker; 2007:101–126

119. Del Beccaro MA, Mendelman PM, Inglis AF, et al. Bacteriology of acute otitis media: a new perspective. *J Pediatr*. 1992;120(1):81–84

120. Block SL, Harrison CJ, Hedrick JA, et al. Penicillin-resistant *Streptococcus pneumoniae* in acute otitis media: risk factors, susceptibility patterns and antimicrobial management. *Pediatr Infect Dis J*. 1995;14(9):751–759

121. Rodriguez WJ, Schwartz RH. *Streptococcus pneumoniae* causes otitis media with higher fever and more redness of tympanic membranes than *Haemophilus influenzae* or *Moraxella catarrhalis*. *Pediatr Infect Dis J*. 1999;18(10):942–944

122. Block SL, Hedrick J, Harrison CJ, et al. Community-wide vaccination with the heptavalent pneumococcal conjugate significantly alters the microbiology of acute otitis media. *Pediatr Infect Dis J*. 2004;23(9):829–833

123. Casey JR, Pichichero ME. Changes in frequency and pathogens causing acute otitis media in 1995–2003. *Pediatr Infect Dis J*. 2004;23(9):824–828

124. McEllistrem MC, Adams JM, Patel K, et al. Acute otitis media due to penicillin-nonsusceptible *Streptococcus pneumoniae* before and after the introduction of the pneumococcal conjugate vaccine. *Clin Infect Dis*. 2005;40(12):1738–1744

125. Casey JR, Adlowitz DG, Pichichero ME. New patterns in the otopathogens causing acute otitis media six to eight years after introduction of pneumococcal conjugate vaccine. *Pediatr Infect Dis J*. 2010;29(4):304–309

126. Grubb MS, Spaugh DC. Microbiology of acute otitis media, Puget Sound region, 2005–2009. *Clin Pediatr (Phila)*. 2010;49(8):727–730
127. Revai K, McCormick DP, Patel J, Grady JJ, Saeed K, Chonmaitree T. Effect of pneumococcal conjugate vaccine on nasopharyngeal bacterial colonization during acute otitis media. *Pediatrics*. 2006;117(5):1823–1829
128. Pettigrew MM, Gent JF, Revai K, Patel JA, Chonmaitree T. Microbial interactions during upper respiratory tract infections. *Emerg Infect Dis*. 2008;14(10):1584–1591
129. O'Brien KL, Millar EV, Zell ER, et al. Effect of pneumococcal conjugate vaccine on nasopharyngeal colonization among immunized and unimmunized children in a community-randomized trial. *J Infect Dis*. 2007;196(8):1211–1220
130. Jacobs MR, Bajaksouzian S, Windau A, Good C. Continued emergence of nonvaccine serotypes of *Streptococcus pneumoniae* in Cleveland. *Proceedings of the 49th Interscience Conference on Antimicrobial Agents and Chemotherapy*, 2009:G1-G1556
131. Hoberman A, Paradise JL, Shaikh N, et al. Pneumococcal resistance and serotype 19A in Pittsburgh-area children with acute otitis media before and after introduction of 7-valent pneumococcal polysaccharide vaccine. *Clin Pediatr (Phila)*. 2011;50(2):114–120
132. Huang SS, Hinrichsen VL, Stevenson AE, et al. Continued impact of pneumococcal conjugate vaccine on carriage in young children. *Pediatrics*. 2009;124(1). Available at: www.pediatrics.org/cgi/content/full/124/1/e1
133. Centers for Disease Control and Prevention (CDC). Licensure of a 13-valent pneumococcal conjugate vaccine (PCV13) and recommendations for use among children—Advisory Committee on Immunization Practices (ACIP), 2010. *MMWR Morb Mortal Wkly Rep*. 2010;59(9):258–261
134. Segal N, Givon-Lavi N, Leibovitz E, Yagupsky P, Leiberman A, Dagan R. Acute otitis media caused by *Streptococcus pyogenes* in children. *Clin Infect Dis*. 2005;41(1):35–41
135. Luntz M, Brodsky A, Nusem S, et al. Acute mastoiditis—the antibiotic era: a multicenter study. *Int J Pediatr Otorhinolaryngol*. 2001;57(1):1–9
136. Nielsen JC. *Studies on the Aetiology of Acute Otitis Media*. Copenhagen, Denmark: Ejnar Mundsgaard Forlag; 1945
137. Palmu AA, Herva E, Savolainen H, Karma P, Mäkelä PH, Kilpi TM. Association of clinical signs and symptoms with bacterial findings in acute otitis media. *Clin Infect Dis*. 2004;38(2):234–242
138. Leibovitz E, Asher E, Piglansky L, et al. Is bilateral acute otitis media clinically different than unilateral acute otitis media? *Pediatr Infect Dis J*. 2007;26(7):589–592
139. Leibovitz E, Satran R, Piglansky L, et al. Can acute otitis media caused by *Haemophilus influenzae* be distinguished from that caused by *Streptococcus pneumoniae*? *Pediatr Infect Dis J*. 2003;22(6):509–515
140. Palmu AA, Kotikoski MJ, Kaijalainen TH, Puhakka HJ. Bacterial etiology of acute myringitis in children less than two years of age. *Pediatr Infect Dis J*. 2001;20(6):607–611
141. Bodor FF. Systemic antibiotics for treatment of the conjunctivitis-otitis media syndrome. *Pediatr Infect Dis J*. 1989;8(5):287–290
142. Bingen E, Cohen R, Jourenkova N, Gehanno P. Epidemiologic study of conjunctivitis-otitis syndrome. *Pediatr Infect Dis J*. 2005;24(8):731–732
143. Barkai G, Leibovitz E, Givon-Lavi N, Dagan R. Potential contribution by nontypable *Haemophilus influenzae* in protracted and recurrent acute otitis media. *Pediatr Infect Dis J*. 2009;28(6):466–471
144. Howie VM, Ploussard JH. Efficacy of fixed combination antibiotics versus separate components in otitis media. Effectiveness of erythromycin estrolate, triple sulfonamide, ampicillin, erythromycin estolate-triple sulfonamide, and placebo in 280 patients with acute otitis media under two and one-half years of age. *Clin Pediatr (Phila)*. 1972;11(4):205–214
145. Klein JO. Microbiologic efficacy of antibacterial drugs for acute otitis media. *Pediatr Infect Dis J*. 1993;12(12):973–975
146. Barnett ED, Klein JO. The problem of resistant bacteria for the management of acute otitis media. *Pediatr Clin North Am*. 1995;42(3):509–517
147. Tristram S, Jacobs MR, Appelbaum PC. Antimicrobial resistance in *Haemophilus influenzae*. *Clin Microbiol Rev*. 2007;20(2):368–389
148. Critchley IA, Jacobs MR, Brown SD, Traczewski MM, Tillotson GS, Janjic N. Prevalence of serotype 19A *Streptococcus pneumoniae* among isolates from U.S. children in 2005≠2006 and activity of faropenem. *Antimicrob Agents Chemother*. 2008;52(7):2639–2643
149. Jacobs MR, Good CE, Windau AR, et al. Activity of ceftaroline against emerging serotypes of Streptococcus pneumoniae. *Antimicrob Agents Chemother*. 2010;54(6):2716–2719
150. Jacobs MR. Antimicrobial-resistant *Streptococcus pneumoniae:* trends and management. *Expert Rev Anti Infect Ther*. 2008;6(5):619–635
151. Piglansky L, Leibovitz E, Raiz S, et al. Bacteriologic and clinical efficacy of high dose amoxicillin for therapy of acute otitis media in children. *Pediatr Infect Dis J*. 2003;22(5):405–413
152. Dagan R, Johnson CE, McLinn S, et al. Bacteriologic and clinical efficacy of amoxicillin/clavulanate vs. azithromycin in acute otitis media. *Pediatr Infect Dis J*. 2000;19(2):95–104
153. Dagan R, Hoberman A, Johnson C, et al. Bacteriologic and clinical efficacy of high dose amoxicillin/clavulanate in children with acute otitis media. *Pediatr Infect Dis J*. 2001;20(9):829–837
154. Hoberman A, Dagan R, Leibovitz E, et al. Large dosage amoxicillin/clavulanate, compared with azithromycin, for the treatment of bacterial acute otitis media in children. *Pediatr Infect Dis J*. 2005;24(6):525–532
155. De Wals P, Erickson L, Poirier B, Pépin J, Pichichero ME. How to compare the efficacy of conjugate vaccines to prevent acute otitis media? *Vaccine*. 2009;27(21):2877–2883
156. Shouval DS, Greenberg D, Givon-Lavi N, Porat N, Dagan R. Serotype coverage of invasive and mucosal pneumococcal disease in Israeli children younger than 3 years by various pneumococcal conjugate vaccines. *Pediatr Infect Dis J*. 2009;28(4):277–282
157. Jones RN, Farrell DJ, Mendes RE, Sader HS. Comparative ceftaroline activity tested against pathogens associated with community-acquired pneumonia: results from an international surveillance study. *J Antimicrob Chemother*. 2011;66(suppl 3):iii69–iii80
158. Harrison CJ, Woods C, Stout G, Martin B, Selvarangan R. Susceptibilities of Haemophilus influenzae, Streptococcus pneumoniae, including serotype 19A, and Moraxella catarrhalis paediatric isolates from 2005 to 2007 to commonly used antibiotics. *J Antimicrob Chemother*. 2009;63(3):511–519
159. Doern GV, Jones RN, Pfaller MA, Kugler K. *Haemophilus influenzae* and *Moraxella catarrhalis* from patients with community-acquired respiratory tract infections: antimicrobial susceptibility patterns from the SENTRY antimicrobial Surveillance Program (United States and Canada, 1997).

Antimicrob Agents Chemother. 1999;43(2): 385–389

160. Nussinovitch M, Yoeli R, Elishkevitz K, Varsano I. Acute mastoiditis in children: epidemiologic, clinical, microbiologic, and therapeutic aspects over past years. *Clin Pediatr (Phila).* 2004;43(3):261–267
161. Roddy MG, Glazier SS, Agrawal D. Pediatric mastoiditis in the pneumococcal conjugate vaccine era: symptom duration guides empiric antimicrobial therapy. *Pediatr Emerg Care.* 2007;23(11):779–784
162. Hoberman A, Paradise JL, Burch DJ, et al. Equivalent efficacy and reduced occurrence of diarrhea from a new formulation of amoxicillin/clavulanate potassium (Augmentin) for treatment of acute otitis media in children. *Pediatr Infect Dis J.* 1997;16(5):463–470
163. Arguedas A, Dagan R, Leibovitz E, Hoberman A, Pichichero M, Paris M. A multicenter, open label, double tympanocentesis study of high dose cefdinir in children with acute otitis media at high risk of persistent or recurrent infection. *Pediatr Infect Dis J.* 2006;25(3):211–218
164. Atanasković-Marković M, Velicković TC, Gavrović-Jankulović M, Vucković O, Nestorović B. Immediate allergic reactions to cephalosporins and penicillins and their cross-reactivity in children. *Pediatr Allergy Immunol.* 2005;16(4):341–347
165. Pichichero ME. Use of selected cephalosporins in penicillin-allergic patients: a paradigm shift. *Diagn Microbiol Infect Dis.* 2007;57(suppl 3):13S–18S
166. Pichichero ME, Casey JR. Safe use of selected cephalosporins in penicillin-allergic patients: a meta-analysis. *Otolaryngol Head Neck Surg.* 2007;136(3):340–347
167. DePestel DD, Benninger MS, Danziger L, et al. Cephalosporin use in treatment of patients with penicillin allergies. *J Am Pharm Assoc (2003).* 2008;48(4):530–540
168. Fonacier L, Hirschberg R, Gerson S. Adverse drug reactions to a cephalosporins in hospitalized patients with a history of penicillin allergy. *Allergy Asthma Proc.* 2005;26(2):135–141
169. Joint Task Force on Practice Parameters; American Academy of Allergy, Asthma and Immunology; American College of Allergy, Asthma and Immunology; Joint Council of Allergy, Asthma and Immunology. Drug allergy: an updated practice parameter. *Ann Allergy Asthma Immunol.* 2010;105(4): 259–273
170. Powers JL, Gooch WM, III, Oddo LP. Comparison of the palatability of the oral suspension of cefdinir vs. amoxicillin/clavulanate potassium, cefprozil and azithromycin in pediatric patients. *Pediatr Infect Dis J.* 2000; 19(suppl 12):S174–S180
171. Steele RW, Thomas MP, Bégué RE. Compliance issues related to the selection of antibiotic suspensions for children. *Pediatr Infect Dis J.* 2001;20(1):1–5
172. Steele RW, Russo TM, Thomas MP. Adherence issues related to the selection of antistaphylococcal or antifungal antibiotic suspensions for children. *Clin Pediatr (Phila).* 2006;45(3):245–250
173. Schwartz RH. Enhancing children's satisfaction with antibiotic therapy: a taste study of several antibiotic suspensions. *Curr Ther Res.* 2000;61(8):570–581
174. Green SM, Rothrock SG. Single-dose intramuscular ceftriaxone for acute otitis media in children. *Pediatrics.* 1993;91(1): 23–30
175. Leibovitz E, Piglansky L, Raiz S, Press J, Leiberman A, Dagan R. Bacteriologic and clinical efficacy of one day vs. three day intramuscular ceftriaxone for treatment of nonresponsive acute otitis media in children. *Pediatr Infect Dis J.* 2000;19(11): 1040–1045
176. Rosenfeld RM, Kay D. Natural history of untreated otitis media. *Laryngoscope.* 2003;113(10):1645–1657
177. Rosenfeld RM, Kay D. Natural history of untreated otitis media. In: Rosenfeld RM, Bluestone CD, eds. *Evidence-Based Otitis Media.* 2nd ed. Hamilton, Canada: BC Decker; 2003:180–198
178. Arola M, Ziegler T, Ruuskanen O. Respiratory virus infection as a cause of prolonged symptoms in acute otitis media. *J Pediatr.* 1990;116(5):697–701
179. Chonmaitree T, Owen MJ, Howie VM. Respiratory viruses interfere with bacteriologic response to antibiotic in children with acute otitis media. *J Infect Dis.* 1990; 162(2):546–549
180. Dagan R, Leibovitz E, Greenberg D, Yagupsky P, Fliss DM, Leiberman A. Early eradication of pathogens from middle ear fluid during antibiotic treatment of acute otitis media is associated with improved clinical outcome. *Pediatr Infect Dis J.* 1998;17(9):776–782
181. Carlin SA, Marchant CD, Shurin PA, Johnson CE, Super DM, Rehmus JM. Host factors and early therapeutic response in acute otitis media. *J Pediatr.* 1991;118(2):178–183
182. Teele DW, Pelton SI, Klein JO. Bacteriology of acute otitis media unresponsive to initial antimicrobial therapy. *J Pediatr.* 1981; 98(4):537–539
183. Doern GV, Pfaller MA, Kugler K, Freeman J, Jones RN. Prevalence of antimicrobial resistance among respiratory tract isolates of *Streptococcus pneumoniae* in North America: 1997 results from the SENTRY antimicrobial surveillance program. *Clin Infect Dis.* 1998;27(4):764–770
184. Leiberman A, Leibovitz E, Piglansky L, et al. Bacteriologic and clinical efficacy of trimethoprim-sulfamethoxazole for treatment of acute otitis media. *Pediatr Infect Dis J.* 2001;20(3):260–264
185. Humphrey WR, Shattuck MH, Zielinski RJ, et al. Pharmacokinetics and efficacy of linezolid in a gerbil model of *Streptococcus pneumoniae*-induced acute otitis media. *Antimicrob Agents Chemother.* 2003; 47(4):1355–1363
186. Arguedas A, Dagan R, Pichichero M, et al. An open-label, double tympanocentesis study of levofloxacin therapy in children with, or at high risk for, recurrent or persistent acute otitis media. *Pediatr Infect Dis J.* 2006;25(12):1102–1109
187. Noel GJ, Blumer JL, Pichichero ME, et al. A randomized comparative study of levofloxacin versus amoxicillin/clavulanate for treatment of infants and young children with recurrent or persistent acute otitis media. *Pediatr Infect Dis J.* 2008;27(6): 483–489
188. Howie VM, Ploussard JH. Simultaneous nasopharyngeal and middle ear exudate culture in otitis media. *Pediatr Digest.* 1971;13:31–35
189. Gehanno P, Lenoir G, Barry B, Bons J, Boucot I, Berche P. Evaluation of nasopharyngeal cultures for bacteriologic assessment of acute otitis media in children. *Pediatr Infect Dis J.* 1996;15(4): 329–332
190. Cohen R, Levy C, Boucherat M, Langue J, de La Rocque F. A multicenter, randomized, double-blind trial of 5 versus 10 days of antibiotic therapy for acute otitis media in young children. *J Pediatr.* 1998;133(5): 634–639
191. Pessey JJ, Gehanno P, Thoroddsen E, et al. Short course therapy with cefuroxime axetil for acute otitis media: results of a randomized multicenter comparison with amoxicillin/clavulanate. *Pediatr Infect Dis J.* 1999;18(10):854–859
192. Cohen R, Levy C, Boucherat M, et al. Five vs. ten days of antibiotic therapy for acute otitis media in young children. *Pediatr Infect Dis J.* 2000;19(5):458–463
193. Pichichero ME, Marsocci SM, Murphy ML, Hoeger W, Francis AB, Green JL. A prospective observational study of 5-, 7-, and 10-day antibiotic treatment for acute otitis media. *Otolaryngol Head Neck Surg.* 2001; 124(4):381–387

194. Kozyrskyj AL, Klassen TP, Moffatt M, Harvey K. Short-course antibiotics for acute otitis media. *Cochrane Database Syst Rev.* 2010;(9):CD001095
195. Shurin PA, Pelton SI, Donner A, Klein JO. Persistence of middle-ear effusion after acute otitis media in children. *N Engl J Med.* 1979;300(20):1121–1123
196. Damoiseaux RA, Rovers MM, Van Balen FA, Hoes AW, de Melker RA. Long-term prognosis of acute otitis media in infancy: determinants of recurrent acute otitis media and persistent middle ear effusion. *Fam Pract.* 2006;23(1):40–45
197. Leach AJ, Morris PS. Antibiotics for the prevention of acute and chronic suppurative otitis media in children. *Cochrane Database Syst Rev.* 2006;(4):CD004401
198. Teele DW, Klein JO, Word BM, et al; Greater Boston Otitis Media Study Group. Antimicrobial prophylaxis for infants at risk for recurrent acute otitis media. *Vaccine.* 2000;19(suppl 1):S140–S143
199. Paradise JL. On tympanostomy tubes: rationale, results, reservations, and recommendations. *Pediatrics.* 1977;60(1):86–90
200. McIsaac WJ, Coyte PC, Croxford R, Asche CV, Friedberg J, Feldman W. Otolaryngologists' perceptions of the indications for tympanostomy tube insertion in children. *CMAJ.* 2000;162(9):1285–1288
201. Casselbrandt ML. Ventilation tubes for recurrent acute otitis media. In: Alper CM, Bluestone CD, eds. *Advanced Therapy of Otitis Media.* Hamilton, Canada: BC Decker; 2004:113–115
202. Shin JJ, Stinnett SS, Hartnick CJ. Pediatric recurrent acute otitis media. In: Shin JJ, Hartnick CJ, Randolph GW, eds. *Evidence-Based Otolaryngology.* New York, NY: Springer; 2008:91–95
203. Gonzalez C, Arnold JE, Woody EA, et al. Prevention of recurrent acute otitis media: chemoprophylaxis versus tympanostomy tubes. *Laryngoscope.* 1986;96(12):1330–1334
204. Gebhart DE. Tympanostomy tubes in the otitis media prone child. *Laryngoscope.* 1981;91(6):849–866
205. Casselbrant ML, Kaleida PH, Rockette HE, et al. Efficacy of antimicrobial prophylaxis and of tympanostomy tube insertion for prevention of recurrent acute otitis media: results of a randomized clinical trial. *Pediatr Infect Dis J.* 1992;11(4):278–286
206. El-Sayed Y. Treatment of recurrent acute otitis media chemoprophylaxis versus ventilation tubes. *Aust J Otolaryngol.* 1996;2(4):352–355
207. McDonald S, Langton Hewer CD, Nunez DA. Grommets (ventilation tubes) for recurrent acute otitis media in children. *Cochrane Database Syst Rev.* 2008;(4):CD004741
208. Rosenfeld RM, Bhaya MH, Bower CM, et al. Impact of tympanostomy tubes on child quality of life. *Arch Otolaryngol Head Neck Surg.* 2000;126(5):585–592
209. Witsell DL, Stewart MG, Monsell EM, et al. The Cooperative Outcomes Group for ENT: a multicenter prospective cohort study on the outcomes of tympanostomy tubes for children with otitis media. *Otolaryngol Head Neck Surg.* 2005;132(2):180–188
210. Isaacson G. Six Sigma tympanostomy tube insertion: achieving the highest safety levels during residency training. *Otolaryngol Head Neck Surg.* 2008;139(3):353–357
211. Kay DJ, Nelson M, Rosenfeld RM. Meta-analysis of tympanostomy tube sequelae. *Otolaryngol Head Neck Surg.* 2001;124(4):374–380
212. Koivunen P, Uhari M, Luotonen J, et al. Adenoidectomy versus chemoprophylaxis and placebo for recurrent acute otitis media in children aged under 2 years: randomised controlled trial. *BMJ.* 2004;328(7438):487
213. Rosenfeld RM. Surgical prevention of otitis media. *Vaccine.* 2000;19(suppl 1):S134–S139
214. Centers for Disease Control and Prevention (CDC). Prevention and control of influenza with vaccines: recommendations of the Advisory Committee on Immunization Practices (ACIP), 2011. *MMWR Morb Mortal Wkly Rep.* 2011;60(33):1128–1132
215. American Academy of Pediatrics Committee on Infectious Diseases. Recommendations for prevention and control of influenza in children, 2011–2012. *Pediatrics.* 2011;128(4):813–825
216. Section on Breastfeeding. Breastfeeding and the use of human milk. *Pediatrics.* 2012;129(3). Available at: www.pediatrics.org/cgi/content/full/129/3/e827
217. Pavia M, Bianco A, Nobile CG, Marinelli P, Angelillo IF. Efficacy of pneumococcal vaccination in children younger than 24 months: a meta-analysis. *Pediatrics.* 2009;123(6). Available at: www.pediatrics.org/cgi/content/full/123/6/e1103
218. Eskola J, Kilpi T, Palmu A, et al; Finnish Otitis Media Study Group. Efficacy of a pneumococcal conjugate vaccine against acute otitis media. *N Engl J Med.* 2001;344(6):403–409
219. Black S, Shinefield H, Fireman B, et al; Northern California Kaiser Permanente Vaccine Study Center Group. Efficacy, safety and immunogenicity of heptavalent pneumococcal conjugate vaccine in children. *Pediatr Infect Dis J.* 2000;19(3):187–195
220. Jacobs MR. Prevention of otitis media: role of pneumococcal conjugate vaccines in reducing incidence and antibiotic resistance. *J Pediatr.* 2002;141(2):287–293
221. Jansen AG, Hak E, Veenhoven RH, Damoiseaux RA, Schilder AG, Sanders EA. Pneumococcal conjugate vaccines for preventing otitis media. *Cochrane Database Syst Rev.* 2009;(2):CD001480
222. Fireman B, Black SB, Shinefield HR, Lee J, Lewis E, Ray P. Impact of the pneumococcal conjugate vaccine on otitis media. *Pediatr Infect Dis J.* 2003;22(1):10–16
223. Grijalva CG, Poehling KA, Nuorti JP, et al. National impact of universal childhood immunization with pneumococcal conjugate vaccine on otitis media. *Pediatr Infect Dis J.* 2006;118(3):865–873
224. Zhou F, Shefer A, Kong Y, Nuorti JP. Trends in acute otitis media-related health care utilization by privately insured young children in the United States, 1997–2004. *Pediatrics.* 2008;121(2):253–260
225. Poehling KA, Szilagyi PG, Grijalva CG, et al. Reduction of frequent otitis media and pressure-equalizing tube insertions in children after introduction of pneumococcal conjugate vaccine. *Pediatrics.* 2007;119(4):707–715
226. Pelton SI. Prospects for prevention of otitis media. *Pediatr Infect Dis J.* 2007;26(suppl 10):S20–S22
227. Pelton SI, Leibovitz E. Recent advances in otitis media. *Pediatr Infect Dis J.* 2009;28(suppl 10):S133–S137
228. De Wals P, Erickson L, Poirier B, Pépin J, Pichichero ME. How to compare the efficacy of conjugate vaccines to prevent acute otitis media? *Vaccine.* 2009;27(21):2877–2883
229. Plasschaert AI, Rovers MM, Schilder AG, Verheij TJ, Hak E. Trends in doctor consultations, antibiotic prescription, and specialist referrals for otitis media in children: 1995–2003. *Pediatrics.* 2006;117(6):1879–1886
230. O'Brien MA, Prosser LA, Paradise JL, et al. New vaccines against otitis media: projected benefits and cost-effectiveness. *Pediatrics.* 2009;123(6):1452–1463
231. Hanage WP, Auranen K, Syrjänen R, et al. Ability of pneumococcal serotypes and clones to cause acute otitis media: implications for the prevention of otitis media by conjugate vaccines. *Infect Immun.* 2004;72(1):76–81
232. Prymula R, Peeters P, Chrobok V, et al. Pneumococcal capsular polysaccharides

conjugated to protein D for prevention of acute otitis media caused by both Streptococcus pneumoniae and non-typable *Haemophilus influenzae*: a randomised double-blind efficacy study. *Lancet*. 2006; 367(9512):740–748

233. Prymula R, Schuerman L. 10-valent pneumococcal nontypeable *Haemophilus influenzae* PD conjugate vaccine: Synflorix. *Expert Rev Vaccines*. 2009;8(11):1479–1500
234. Schuerman L, Borys D, Hoet B, Forsgren A, Prymula R. Prevention of otitis media: now a reality? *Vaccine*. 2009;27(42):5748–5754
235. Heikkinen T, Ruuskanen O, Waris M, Ziegler T, Arola M, Halonen P. Influenza vaccination in the prevention of acute otitis media in children. *Am J Dis Child*. 1991;145(4):445–448
236. Clements DA, Langdon L, Bland C, Walter E. Influenza A vaccine decreases the incidence of otitis media in 6- to 30-month-old children in day care. *Arch Pediatr Adolesc Med*. 1995;149(10):1113–1117
237. Belshe RB, Gruber WC. Prevention of otitis media in children with live attenuated influenza vaccine given intranasally. *Pediatr Infect Dis J*. 2000;19(suppl 5):S66–S71
238. Marchisio P, Cavagna R, Maspes B, et al. Efficacy of intranasal virosomal influenza vaccine in the prevention of recurrent acute otitis media in children. *Clin Infect Dis*. 2002;35(2):168–174
239. Ozgur SK, Beyazova U, Kemaloglu YK, et al. Effectiveness of inactivated influenza vaccine for prevention of otitis media in children. *Pediatr Infect Dis J*. 2006;25(5): 401–404
240. Block SL, Heikkinen T, Toback SL, Zheng W, Ambrose CS. The efficacy of live attenuated influenza vaccine against influenza-associated acute otitis media in children. *Pediatr Infect Dis J*. 2011;30(3):203–207
241. Ashkenazi S, Vertruyen A, Arístegui J, et al; CAIV-T Study Group. Superior relative efficacy of live attenuated influenza vaccine compared with inactivated influenza vaccine in young children with recurrent respiratory tract infections. *Pediatr Infect Dis J*. 2006;25(10):870–879
242. Belshe RB, Edwards KM, Vesikari T, et al; CAIV-T Comparative Efficacy Study Group. Live attenuated versus inactivated influenza vaccine in infants and young children [published correction appears in *N Engl J Med*. 2007;356(12):1283]. *N Engl J Med*. 2007;356(7):685–696
243. Bracco Neto H, Farhat CK, Tregnaghi MW, et al; D153-P504 LAIV Study Group. Efficacy and safety of 1 and 2 doses of live attenuated influenza vaccine in vaccine-naive children. *Pediatr Infect Dis J*. 2009;28(5): 365–371
244. Tam JS, Capeding MR, Lum LC, et al; Pan-Asian CAIV-T Pediatric Efficacy Trial Network. Efficacy and safety of a live attenuated, cold-adapted influenza vaccine, trivalent against culture-confirmed influenza in young children in Asia. *Pediatr Infect Dis J*. 2007;26(7):619–628
245. Vesikari T, Fleming DM, Aristegui JF, et al; CAIV-T Pediatric Day Care Clinical Trial Network. Safety, efficacy, and effectiveness of cold-adapted influenza vaccine-trivalent against community-acquired, culture-confirmed influenza in young children attending day care. *Pediatrics*. 2006;118(6):2298–2312
246. Forrest BD, Pride MW, Dunning AJ, et al. Correlation of cellular immune responses with protection against culture-confirmed influenza virus in young children. *Clin Vaccine Immunol*. 2008;15(7): 1042–1053
247. Lum LC, Borja-Tabora CF, Breiman RF, et al. Influenza vaccine concurrently administered with a combination measles, mumps, and rubella vaccine to young children. *Vaccine*. 2010;28(6):1566–1574
248. Belshe RB, Mendelman PM, Treanor J, et al. The efficacy of live attenuated, cold-adapted, trivalent, intranasal influenzavirus vaccine in children. *N Engl J Med*. 1998;338(20): 1405–1412
249. Daly KA, Giebink GS. Clinical epidemiology of otitis media. *Pediatr Infect Dis J*. 2000; 19(suppl 5):S31–S36
250. Duncan B, Ey J, Holberg CJ, Wright AL, Martinez FD, Taussig LM. Exclusive breast-feeding for at least 4 months protects against otitis media. *Pediatrics*. 1993;91(5): 867–872
251. Duffy LC, Faden H, Wasielewski R, Wolf J, Krystofik D. Exclusive breastfeeding protects against bacterial colonization and day care exposure to otitis media. *Pediatrics*. 1997;100(4). Available at: www.pediatrics.org/cgi/content/full/100/4/e7
252. Paradise JL. Short-course antimicrobial treatment for acute otitis media: not best for infants and young children. *JAMA*. 1997;278(20):1640–1642
253. Scariati PD, Grummer-Strawn LM, Fein SB. A longitudinal analysis of infant morbidity and the extent of breastfeeding in the United States. *Pediatrics*. 1997;99(6). Available at: www.pediatrics.org/cgi/content/full/99/6/e5
254. McNiel ME, Labbok MH, Abrahams SW. What are the risks associated with formula feeding? A re-analysis and review. *Breastfeed Rev*. 2010;18(2):25–32
255. Chantry CJ, Howard CR, Auinger P. Full breastfeeding duration and associated decrease in respiratory tract infection in US children. *Pediatrics*. 2006;117(2):425–432
256. Hatakka K, Piirainen L, Pohjavuori S, Poussa T, Savilahti E, Korpela R. Factors associated with acute respiratory illness in day care children. *Scand J Infect Dis*. 2010;42(9):704–711
257. Ladomenou F, Kafatos A, Tselentis Y, Galanakis E. Predisposing factors for acute otitis media in infancy. *J Infect*. 2010;61(1):49–53
258. Ladomenou F, Moschandreas J, Kafatos A, Tselentis Y, Galanakis E. Protective effect of exclusive breastfeeding against infections during infancy: a prospective study. *Arch Dis Child*. 2010;95(12):1004–1008
259. Duijts L, Jaddoe VW, Hofman A, Moll HA. Prolonged and exclusive breastfeeding reduces the risk of infectious diseases in infancy. *Pediatrics*. 2010;126(1). Available at: www.pediatrics.org/cgi/content/full/126/1/e18
260. Best D; Committee on Environmental Health; Committee on Native American Child Health; Committee on Adolescence. From the American Academy of Pediatrics: technical report—secondhand and prenatal tobacco smoke exposure. *Pediatrics*. 2009;124(5). Available at: www.pediatrics.org/cgi/content/full/124/5/e1017
261. Etzel RA, Pattishall EN, Haley NJ, Fletcher RH, Henderson FW. Passive smoking and middle ear effusion among children in day care. *Pediatrics*. 1992;90(2 pt 1): 228–232
262. Ilicali OC, Keleş N, Değer K, Savaş I. Relationship of passive cigarette smoking to otitis media. *Arch Otolaryngol Head Neck Surg*. 1999;125(7):758–762
263. Wellington M, Hall CB. Pacifier as a risk factor for acute otitis media [letter]. *Pediatrics*. 2002;109(2):351–352, author reply 353
264. Kerstein R. Otitis media: prevention instead of prescription. *Br J Gen Pract*. 2008;58(550):364–365
265. Brown CE, Magnuson B. On the physics of the infant feeding bottle and middle ear sequela: ear disease in infants can be associated with bottle feeding. *Int J Pediatr Otorhinolaryngol*. 2000;54(1):13–20
266. Niemelä M, Pihakari O, Pokka T, Uhari M. Pacifier as a risk factor for acute otitis media: a randomized, controlled trial of parental counseling. *Pediatrics*. 2000;106(3): 483–488

267. Tully SB, Bar-Haim Y, Bradley RL. Abnormal tympanography after supine bottle feeding. *J Pediatr.* 1995;126(6):S105–S111

268. Rovers MM, Numans ME, Langenbach E, Grobbee DE, Verheij TJ, Schilder AG. Is pacifier use a risk factor for acute otitis media? A dynamic cohort study. *Fam Pract.* 2008;25(4):233–236

269. Adderson EE. Preventing otitis media: medical approaches. *Pediatr Ann.* 1998;27(2):101–107

270. Azarpazhooh A, Limeback H, Lawrence HP, Shah PS. Xylitol for preventing acute otitis media in children up to 12 years of age. *Cochrane Database Syst Rev.* 2011;(11):CD007095

271. Hautalahti O, Renko M, Tapiainen T, Kontiokari T, Pokka T, Uhari M. Failure of xylitol given three times a day for preventing acute otitis media. *Pediatr Infect Dis J.* 2007;26(5):423–427

272. Tapiainen T, Luotonen L, Kontiokari T, Renko M, Uhari M. Xylitol administered only during respiratory infections failed to prevent acute otitis media. *Pediatrics.* 2002;109(2). Available at: www.pediatrics.org/cgi/content/full/109/2/e19

273. Uhari M, Kontiokari T, Koskela M, Niemelä M. Xylitol chewing gum in prevention of acute otitis media: double blind randomised trial. *BMJ.* 1996;313(7066):1180–1184

274. Uhari M, Kontiokari T, Niemelä M. A novel use of xylitol sugar in preventing acute otitis media. *Pediatrics.* 1998;102(4 pt 1):879–884

275. O'Brien MA, Prosser LA, Paradise JL, et al. New vaccines against otitis media: projected benefits and cost-effectiveness. *Pediatrics.* 2009;123(6):1452–1463

(Continued from first page)

All clinical practice guidelines from the American Academy of Pediatrics automatically expire 5 years after publication unless reaffirmed, revised, or retired at or before that time.

www.pediatrics.org/cgi/doi/10.1542/peds.2012-3488

doi:10.1542/peds.2012-3488

PEDIATRICS (ISSN Numbers: Print, 0031-4005; Online, 1098-4275).

Copyright © 2013 by the American Academy of Pediatrics

Otitis Media With Effusion

- *Clinical Practice Guideline*

AMERICAN ACADEMY OF PEDIATRICS

Clinical Practice Guideline

American Academy of Family Physicians, American Academy of Otolaryngology-Head and Neck Surgery, and American Academy of Pediatrics Subcommittee on Otitis Media With Effusion

Otitis Media With Effusion

ABSTRACT. The clinical practice guideline on otitis media with effusion (OME) provides evidence-based recommendations on diagnosing and managing OME in children. This is an update of the 1994 clinical practice guideline "Otitis Media With Effusion in Young Children," which was developed by the Agency for Healthcare Policy and Research (now the Agency for Healthcare Research and Quality). In contrast to the earlier guideline, which was limited to children 1 to 3 years old with no craniofacial or neurologic abnormalities or sensory deficits, the updated guideline applies to children aged 2 months through 12 years with or without developmental disabilities or underlying conditions that predispose to OME and its sequelae. The American Academy of Pediatrics, American Academy of Family Physicians, and American Academy of Otolaryngology-Head and Neck Surgery selected a subcommittee composed of experts in the fields of primary care, otolaryngology, infectious diseases, epidemiology, hearing, speech and language, and advanced-practice nursing to revise the OME guideline.

The subcommittee made a strong recommendation that clinicians use pneumatic otoscopy as the primary diagnostic method and distinguish OME from acute otitis media.

The subcommittee made recommendations that clinicians should 1) document the laterality, duration of effusion, and presence and severity of associated symptoms at each assessment of the child with OME, 2) distinguish the child with OME who is at risk for speech, language, or learning problems from other children with OME and more promptly evaluate hearing, speech, language, and need for intervention in children at risk, and 3) manage the child with OME who is not at risk with watchful waiting for 3 months from the date of effusion onset (if known) or diagnosis (if onset is unknown).

The subcommittee also made recommendations that 4) hearing testing be conducted when OME persists for 3 months or longer or at any time that language delay, learning problems, or a significant hearing loss is suspected in a child with OME, 5) children with persistent OME who are not at risk should be reexamined at 3- to 6-month intervals until the effusion is no longer present, significant hearing loss is identified, or structural abnormalities of the eardrum or middle ear are suspected, and 6) when a child becomes a surgical candidate (tympanostomy tube insertion is the preferred initial procedure). Adenoidectomy should not be performed unless a distinct indication exists (nasal obstruction, chronic adenoiditis); repeat surgery consists of adenoidectomy plus myringotomy with or without tubeinsertion. Tonsillectomy alone or myringotomy alone should not be used to treat OME.

The subcommittee made negative recommendations that 1) population-based screening programs for OME not be performed in healthy, asymptomatic children, and 2) because antihistamines and decongestants are ineffective for OME, they should not be used for treatment; antimicrobials and corticosteroids do not have long-term efficacy and should not be used for routine management.

The subcommittee gave as options that 1) tympanometry can be used to confirm the diagnosis of OME and 2) when children with OME are referred by the primary clinician for evaluation by an otolaryngologist, audiologist, or speech-language pathologist, the referring clinician should document the effusion duration and specific reason for referral (evaluation, surgery) and provide additional relevant information such as history of acute otitis media and developmental status of the child. The subcommittee made no recommendations for 1) complementary and alternative medicine as a treatment for OME, based on a lack of scientific evidence documenting efficacy, or 2) allergy management as a treatment for OME, based on insufficient evidence of therapeutic efficacy or a causal relationship between allergy and OME. Last, the panel compiled a list of research needs based on limitations of the evidence reviewed.

The purpose of this guideline is to inform clinicians of evidence-based methods to identify, monitor, and manage OME in children aged 2 months through 12 years. The guideline may not apply to children more than 12 years old, because OME is uncommon and the natural history is likely to differ from younger children who experience rapid developmental change. The target population includes children with or without developmental disabilities or underlying conditions that predispose to OME and its sequelae. The guideline is intended for use by providers of health care to children, including primary care and specialist physicians, nurses and nurse practitioners, physician assistants, audiologists, speech-language pathologists, and child-development specialists. The guideline is applicable to any setting in which children with OME would be identified, monitored, or managed.

This guideline is not intended as a sole source of guidance in evaluating children with OME. Rather, it is designed to assist primary care and other clinicians by providing an evidence-based framework for decision-making strategies. It is not intended to replace clinical judgment or establish a protocol for all children with this condition and may not provide the only appropriate approach to diagnosing and managing this problem. *Pediatrics* 2004;113:1412–1429; *acute otitis media, antibacterial, antibiotic.*

This document was approved by the American Academy of Otolaryngology–Head and Neck Surgery Foundation, Inc and the American Academy of Pediatrics, and is published in the May 2004 issue of *Otolaryngology-Head and Neck Surgery* and the May 2004 issue of *Pediatrics*.
PEDIATRICS (ISSN 0031 4005). Copyright © 2004 by the American Academy of Otolaryngology–Head and Neck Surgery Foundation, Inc and the American Academy of Pediatrics.

ABBREVIATIONS. OME, otitis media with effusion; AOM, acute otitis media; AAP, American Academy of Pediatrics; AHRQ, Agency for Healthcare Research and Quality; EPC, Southern California Evidence-Based Practice Center; CAM, complementary and alternative medicine; HL, hearing level.

Otitis media with effusion (OME) as discussed in this guideline is defined as the presence of fluid in the middle ear without signs or symptoms of acute ear infection.[1,2] OME is considered distinct from acute otitis media (AOM), which is defined as a history of acute onset of signs and symptoms, the presence of middle-ear effusion, and signs and symptoms of middle-ear inflammation. Persistent middle-ear fluid from OME results in decreased mobility of the tympanic membrane and serves as a barrier to sound conduction.[3] Approximately 2.2 million diagnosed episodes of OME occur annually in the United States, yielding a combined direct and indirect annual cost estimate of $4.0 billion.[2]

OME may occur spontaneously because of poor eustachian tube function or as an inflammatory response following AOM. Approximately 90% of children (80% of individual ears) have OME at some time before school age,[4] most often between ages 6 months and 4 years.[5] In the first year of life, >50% of children will experience OME, increasing to >60% by 2 years.[6] Many episodes resolve spontaneously within 3 months, but ~30% to 40% of children have recurrent OME, and 5% to 10% of episodes last 1 year or longer.[1,4,7]

The primary outcomes considered in the guideline include hearing loss; effects on speech, language, and learning; physiologic sequelae; health care utilization (medical, surgical); and quality of life.[1,2] The high prevalence of OME, difficulties in diagnosis and assessing duration, increased risk of conductive hearing loss, potential impact on language and cognition, and significant practice variations in management[8] make OME an important condition for the use of up-to-date evidence-based practice guidelines.

METHODS

General Methods and Literature Search

In developing an evidence-based clinical practice guideline on managing OME, the American Academy of Pediatrics (AAP), American Academy of Family Physicians, and American Academy of Otolaryngology-Head and Neck Surgery worked with the Agency for Healthcare Research and Quality (AHRQ) and other organizations. This effort included representatives from each partnering organization along with liaisons from audiology, speech-language pathology, informatics, and advanced-practice nursing. The most current literature on managing children with OME was reviewed, and research questions were developed to guide the evidence-review process.

The AHRQ report on OME from the Southern California Evidence-Based Practice Center (EPC) focused on key questions of natural history, diagnostic methods, and long-term speech, language, and hearing outcomes.[2] Searches were conducted through January 2000 in Medline, Embase, and the Cochrane Library. Additional articles were identified by review of reference listings in proceedings, reports, and other guidelines. The EPC accepted 970 articles for full review after screening 3200 abstracts. The EPC reviewed articles by using established quality criteria[9,10] and included randomized trials, prospective cohorts, and validations of diagnostic tests (validating cohort studies).

The AAP subcommittee on OME updated the AHRQ review with articles identified by an electronic Medline search through April 2003 and with additional material identified manually by subcommittee members. Copies of relevant articles were distributed to the subcommittee for consideration. A specific search for articles relevant to complementary and alternative medicine (CAM) was performed by using Medline and the Allied and Complementary Medicine Database through April 2003. Articles relevant to allergy and OME were identified by using Medline through April 2003. The subcommittee met 3 times over a 1-year period, ending in May 2003, with interval electronic review and feedback on each guideline draft to ensure accuracy of content and consistency with standardized criteria for reporting clinical practice guidelines.[11]

In May 2003, the Guidelines Review Group of the Yale Center for Medical Informatics used the Guideline Elements Model[12] to categorize content of the present draft guideline. Policy statements were parsed into component decision variables and actions and then assessed for decidability and executability. Quality appraisal using established criteria[13] was performed with Guideline Elements Model-Q Online.[14,15] Implementation issues were predicted by using the Implementability Rating Profile, an instrument under development by the Yale Guidelines Review Group (R. Shiffman, MD, written communication, May 2003). OME subcommittee members received summary results and modified an advanced draft of the guideline.

The final draft practice guideline underwent extensive peer review by numerous entities identified by the subcommittee. Comments were compiled and reviewed by the subcommittee cochairpersons. The recommendations contained in the practice guideline are based on the best available published data through April 2003. Where data are lacking, a combination of clinical experience and expert consensus was used. A scheduled review process will occur 5 years from publication or sooner if new compelling evidence warrants earlier consideration.

Classification of Evidence-Based Statements

Guidelines are intended to reduce inappropriate variations in clinical care, produce optimal health outcomes for patients, and minimize harm. The evidence-based approach to guideline development requires that the evidence supporting a policy be identified, appraised, and summarized and that an explicit link between evidence and statements be defined. Evidence-based statements reflect the quality of evidence and the balance of benefit and harm that is anticipated when the statement is followed. The AAP definitions for evidence-based statements[16] are listed in Tables 1 and 2.

Guidelines are never intended to overrule professional judgment; rather, they may be viewed as a relative constraint on individual clinician discretion in a particular clinical circumstance. Less frequent variation in practice is expected for a strong recommendation than might be expected with a recommendation. Options offer the most opportunity for practice variability.[17] All clinicians should always act and decide in a way that they believe will best serve their patients' interests and needs regardless of guideline recommendations. Guidelines represent the best judgment of a team of experienced clinicians and methodologists addressing the scientific evidence for a particular topic.[16]

Making recommendations about health practices involves value judgments on the desirability of various outcomes associated with management options. Value judgments applied by the OME subcommittee were made in an effort to minimize harm and diminish unnecessary therapy. Emphasis was placed on promptly identifying and managing children at risk for speech, language, or learning problems to maximize opportunities for beneficial outcomes. Direct costs also were considered in the statements concerning diagnosis and screening and to a lesser extent in other statements.

1A. PNEUMATIC OTOSCOPY: CLINICIANS SHOULD USE PNEUMATIC OTOSCOPY AS THE PRIMARY DIAGNOSTIC METHOD FOR OME, AND OME SHOULD BE DISTINGUISHED FROM AOM

This is a strong recommendation based on systematic review of cohort studies and the preponderance of benefit over harm.

TABLE 1. Guideline Definitions for Evidence-Based Statements

Statement	Definition	Implication
Strong Recommendation	A strong recommendation means that the subcommittee believes that the benefits of the recommended approach clearly exceed the harms (or that the harms clearly exceed the benefits in the case of a strong negative recommendation) and that the quality of the supporting evidence is excellent (grade A or B).* In some clearly identified circumstances, strong recommendations may be made based on lesser evidence when high-quality evidence is impossible to obtain and the anticipated benefits strongly outweigh the harms.	Clinicians should follow a strong recommendation unless a clear and compelling rationale for an alternative approach is present.
Recommendation	A recommendation means that the subcommittee believes that the benefits exceed the harms (or that the harms exceed the benefits in the case of a negative recommendation), but the quality of evidence is not as strong (grade B or C).* In some clearly identified circumstances, recommendations may be made based on lesser evidence when high-quality evidence is impossible to obtain and the anticipated benefits outweigh the harms.	Clinicians also should generally follow a recommendation but should remain alert to new information and sensitive to patient preferences.
Option	An option means that either the quality of evidence that exists is suspect (grade D)* or that well-done studies (grade A, B, or C)* show little clear advantage to one approach versus another.	Clinicians should be flexible in their decision-making regarding appropriate practice, although they may set boundaries on alternatives; patient preference should have a substantial influencing role.
No Recommendation	No recommendation means that there is both a lack of pertinent evidence (grade D)* and an unclear balance between benefits and harms.	Clinicians should feel little constraint in their decision-making and be alert to new published evidence that clarifies the balance of benefit versus harm; patient preference should have a substantial influencing role.

* See Table 2 for the definitions of evidence grades.

TABLE 2. Evidence Quality for Grades of Evidence

Grade	Evidence Quality
A	Well-designed, randomized, controlled trials or diagnostic studies performed on a population similar to the guideline's target population
B	Randomized, controlled trials or diagnostic studies with minor limitations; overwhelmingly consistent evidence from observational studies
C	Observational studies (case-control and cohort design)
D	Expert opinion, case reports, or reasoning from first principles (bench research or animal studies)

1B. TYMPANOMETRY: TYMPANOMETRY CAN BE USED TO CONFIRM THE DIAGNOSIS OF OME

This option is based on cohort studies and a balance of benefit and harm.

Diagnosing OME correctly is fundamental to proper management. Moreover, OME must be differentiated from AOM to avoid unnecessary antimicrobial use.[18,19]

OME is defined as fluid in the middle ear without signs or symptoms of acute ear infection.[2] The tympanic membrane is often cloudy with distinctly impaired mobility,[20] and an air-fluid level or bubble may be visible in the middle ear. Conversely, diagnosing AOM requires a history of acute onset of signs and symptoms, the presence of middle-ear effusion, and signs and symptoms of middle-ear inflammation. The critical distinguishing feature is that only AOM has acute signs and symptoms. Distinct redness of the tympanic membrane should not be a criterion for prescribing antibiotics, because it has poor predictive value for AOM and is present in ~5% of ears with OME.[20]

The AHRQ evidence report[2] systematically reviewed the sensitivity, specificity, and predictive values of 9 diagnostic methods for OME. Pneumatic otoscopy had the best balance of sensitivity and specificity, consistent with the 1994 guideline.[1] Meta-analysis revealed a pooled sensitivity of 94% (95% confidence interval: 91%–96%) and specificity of 80% (95% confidence interval: 75%–86%) for validated observers using pneumatic otoscopy versus myringotomy as the gold standard. Pneumatic otoscopy therefore should remain the primary method of OME diagnosis, because the instrument is readily available in practice settings, cost-effective, and accurate in experienced hands. Non–pneumatic otoscopy is not advised for primary diagnosis.

The accuracy of pneumatic otoscopy in routine clinical practice may be less than that shown in published results, because clinicians have varying training and experience.[21,22] When the diagnosis of OME is uncertain, tympanometry or acoustic reflectometry should be considered as an adjunct to pneumatic otoscopy. Tympanometry with a standard 226-Hz probe tone is reliable for infants 4 months old or older and has good interobserver agreement of curve patterns in routine clinical practice.[23,24] Younger infants require specialized equipment with a higher probe tone frequency. Tympanometry generates costs related to instrument purchase, annual calibration, and test administration. Acoustic reflectometry with spectral gradient analysis is a low-cost alternative to tympanometry that does not require an airtight seal in the ear canal; however, validation studies primarily have used children 2 years old or older with a high prevalence of OME.[25–27]

Although no research studies have examined whether pneumatic otoscopy causes discomfort, expert consensus suggests that the procedure does not have to be painful, especially when symptoms of acute infection (AOM) are absent. A nontraumatic examination is facilitated by using a gentle touch, restraining the child properly when necessary, and inserting the speculum only into the outer one third (cartilaginous portion) of the ear canal.[28] The pneumatic bulb should be compressed slightly before insertion, because OME often is associated with a negative middle-ear pressure, which can be assessed more accurately by releasing the already compressed bulb. The otoscope must be fully charged, the bulb (halogen or xenon) bright and luminescent,[29] and the insufflator bulb attached tightly to the head to avoid the loss of an air seal. The window must also be sealed.

Evidence Profile: Pneumatic Otoscopy

- Aggregate evidence quality: A, diagnostic studies in relevant populations.
- Benefit: improved diagnostic accuracy; inexpensive equipment.
- Harm: cost of training clinicians in pneumatic otoscopy.
- Benefits-harms assessment: preponderance of benefit over harm.
- Policy level: strong recommendation.

Evidence Profile: Tympanometry

- Aggregate evidence quality: B, diagnostic studies with minor limitations.
- Benefit: increased diagnostic accuracy beyond pneumatic otoscopy; documentation.
- Harm: acquisition cost, administrative burden, and recalibration.
- Benefits-harms assessment: balance of benefit and harm.
- Policy level: option.

1C. SCREENING: POPULATION-BASED SCREENING PROGRAMS FOR OME ARE NOT RECOMMENDED IN HEALTHY, ASYMPTOMATIC CHILDREN

This recommendation is based on randomized, controlled trials and cohort studies, with a preponderance of harm over benefit.

This recommendation concerns population-based screening programs of all children in a community or a school without regard to any preexisting symptoms or history of disease. This recommendation does not address hearing screening or monitoring of specific children with previous or recurrent OME.

OME is highly prevalent in young children. Screening surveys of healthy children ranging in age from infancy to 5 years old show a 15% to 40% point prevalence of middle-ear effusion.[5,7,30–36] Among children examined at regular intervals for a year, ~50% to 60% of child care center attendees[32] and 25% of school-aged children[37] were found to have a middle-ear effusion at some time during the examination period, with peak incidence during the winter months.

Population-based screening has not been found to influence short-term language outcomes,[33] and its long-term effects have not been evaluated in a randomized, clinical trial. Therefore, the recommendation against screening is based not only on the ability to identify OME but more importantly on a lack of demonstrable benefits from treating children so identified that exceed the favorable natural history of the disease. The New Zealand Health Technology Assessment[38] could not determine whether preschool screening for OME was effective. More recently, the Canadian Task Force on Preventive Health Care[39] reported that insufficient evidence was available to recommend including or excluding routine early screening for OME. Although screening for OME is not inherently harmful, potential risks include inaccurate diagnoses, overtreating self-limited disease, parental anxiety, and the costs of screening and unnecessary treatment.

Population-based screening is appropriate for conditions that are common, can be detected by a sensitive and specific test, and benefit from early detection and treatment.[40] The first 2 requirements are fulfilled by OME, which affects up to 80% of children by school entry[2,5,7] and can be screened easily with tympanometry (see recommendation 1B). Early detection and treatment of OME identified by screening, however, have not been shown to improve intelligence, receptive language, or expressive language.[2,39,41,42] Therefore, population-based screening for early detection of OME in asymptomatic children has not been shown to improve outcomes and is not recommended.

Evidence Profile: Screening

- Aggregate evidence quality: B, randomized, controlled trials with minor limitations and consistent evidence from observational studies.
- Benefit: potentially improved developmental outcomes, which have not been demonstrated in the best current evidence.

- Harm: inaccurate diagnosis (false-positive or false-negative), overtreating self-limited disease, parental anxiety, cost of screening, and/or unnecessary treatment.
- Benefits-harms assessment: preponderance of harm over benefit.
- Policy level: recommendation against.

2. DOCUMENTATION: CLINICIANS SHOULD DOCUMENT THE LATERALITY, DURATION OF EFFUSION, AND PRESENCE AND SEVERITY OF ASSOCIATED SYMPTOMS AT EACH ASSESSMENT OF THE CHILD WITH OME

This recommendation is based on observational studies and strong preponderance of benefit over harm.

Documentation in the medical record facilitates diagnosis and treatment and communicates pertinent information to other clinicians to ensure patient safety and reduce medical errors.[43] Management decisions in children with OME depend on effusion duration and laterality plus the nature and severity of associated symptoms. Therefore, these features should be documented at every medical encounter for OME. Although no studies have addressed documentation for OME specifically, there is room for improvement in documentation of ambulatory care medical records.[44]

Ideally, the time of onset and laterality of OME can be defined through diagnosis of an antecedent AOM, a history of acute onset of signs or symptoms directly referable to fluid in the middle ear, or the presence of an abnormal audiogram or tympanogram closely after a previously normal test. Unfortunately, these conditions are often lacking, and the clinician is forced to speculate on the onset and duration of fluid in the middle ear(s) in a child found to have OME at a routine office visit or school screening audiometry.

In ~40% to 50% of cases of OME, neither the affected children nor their parents or caregivers describe significant complaints referable to a middle-ear effusion.[45,46] In some children, however, OME may have associated signs and symptoms caused by inflammation or the presence of effusion (not acute infection) that should be documented, such as

- Mild intermittent ear pain, fullness, or "popping"
- Secondary manifestations of ear pain in infants, which may include ear rubbing, excessive irritability, and sleep disturbances
- Failure of infants to respond appropriately to voices or environmental sounds, such as not turning accurately toward the sound source
- Hearing loss, even when not specifically described by the child, suggested by seeming lack of attentiveness, behavioral changes, failure to respond to normal conversational-level speech, or the need for excessively high sound levels when using audio equipment or viewing television
- Recurrent episodes of AOM with persistent OME between episodes
- Problems with school performance
- Balance problems, unexplained clumsiness, or delayed gross motor development[47–50]
- Delayed speech or language development

The laterality (unilateral versus bilateral), duration of effusion, and presence and severity of associated symptoms should be documented in the medical record at each assessment of the child with OME. When OME duration is uncertain, the clinician must take whatever evidence is at hand and make a reasonable estimate.

Evidence Profile: Documentation

- Aggregate evidence quality: C, observational studies.
- Benefits: defines severity, duration has prognostic value, facilitates future communication with other clinicians, supports appropriate timing of intervention, and, if consistently unilateral, may identify a problem with specific ear other than OME (eg, retraction pocket or cholesteatoma).
- Harm: administrative burden.
- Benefits-harms assessment: preponderance of benefit over harm.
- Policy level: recommendation.

3. CHILD AT RISK: CLINICIANS SHOULD DISTINGUISH THE CHILD WITH OME WHO IS AT RISK FOR SPEECH, LANGUAGE, OR LEARNING PROBLEMS FROM OTHER CHILDREN WITH OME AND SHOULD EVALUATE HEARING, SPEECH, LANGUAGE, AND NEED FOR INTERVENTION MORE PROMPTLY

This recommendation is based on case series, the preponderance of benefit over harm, and ethical limitations in studying children with OME who are at risk.

The panel defines the child at risk as one who is at increased risk for developmental difficulties (delay or disorder) because of sensory, physical, cognitive, or behavioral factors listed in Table 3. These factors are not caused by OME but can make the child less tolerant of hearing loss or vestibular problems secondary to middle-ear effusion. In contrast the child with OME who is not at risk is otherwise healthy and does not have any of the factors shown in Table 3.

Earlier guidelines for managing OME have applied only to young children who are healthy and exhibit no developmental delays.[1] Studies of the relationship between OME and hearing loss or speech/language development typically exclude children with craniofacial anomalies, genetic syndromes, and other developmental disorders. Therefore, the available literature mainly applies to otherwise healthy children who meet inclusion criteria for randomized,

TABLE 3. Risk Factors for Developmental Difficulties*

Permanent hearing loss independent of OME
Suspected or diagnosed speech and language delay or disorder
Autism-spectrum disorder and other pervasive developmental disorders
Syndromes (eg, Down) or craniofacial disorders that include cognitive, speech, and language delays
Blindness or uncorrectable visual impairment
Cleft palate with or without associated syndrome
Developmental delay

* Sensory, physical, cognitive, or behavioral factors that place children who have OME at an increased risk for developmental difficulties (delay or disorder).

controlled trials. Few, if any, existing studies dealing with developmental sequelae caused by hearing loss from OME can be generalized to children who are at risk.

Children who are at risk for speech or language delay would likely be affected additionally by hearing problems from OME,[51] although definitive studies are lacking. For example, small comparative studies of children or adolescents with Down syndrome[52] or cerebral palsy[53] show poorer articulation and receptive language associated with a history of early otitis media. Large studies are unlikely to be forthcoming because of methodologic and ethical difficulties inherent in studying children who are delayed or at risk for further delays. Therefore, clinicians who manage children with OME should determine whether other conditions coexist that put a child at risk for developmental delay (Table 3) and then take these conditions into consideration when planning assessment and management.

Children with craniofacial anomalies (eg, cleft palate; Down syndrome; Robin sequence; coloboma, heart defect, choanal atresia, retarded growth and development, genital anomaly, and ear defect with deafness [CHARGE] association) have a higher prevalence of chronic OME, hearing loss (conductive and sensorineural), and speech or language delay than do children without these anomalies.[54–57] Other children may not be more prone to OME but are likely to have speech and language disorders, such as those children with permanent hearing loss independent of OME,[58,59] specific language impairment,[60] autism-spectrum disorders,[61] or syndromes that adversely affect cognitive and linguistic development. Some retrospective studies[52,62,63] have found that hearing loss caused by OME in children with cognitive delays, such as Down syndrome, has been associated with lower language levels. Children with language delays or disorders with OME histories perform more poorly on speech-perception tasks than do children with OME histories alone.[64,65]

Children with severe visual impairments may be more susceptible to the effects of OME, because they depend on hearing more than children with normal vision.[51] Any decrease in their most important remaining sensory input for language (hearing) may significantly compromise language development and their ability to interact and communicate with others. All children with severe visual impairments should be considered more vulnerable to OME sequelae, especially in the areas of balance, sound localization, and communication.

Management of the child with OME who is at increased risk for developmental delays should include hearing testing and speech and language evaluation and may include speech and language therapy concurrent with managing OME, hearing aids or other amplification devices for hearing loss independent of OME, tympanostomy tube insertion,[54,63,66,67] and hearing testing after OME resolves to document improvement, because OME can mask a permanent underlying hearing loss and delay detection.[59,68,69]

Evidence Profile: Child at Risk

- Aggregate evidence quality: C, observational studies of children at risk; D, expert opinion on the ability of prompt assessment and management to alter outcomes.
- Benefits: optimizing conditions for hearing, speech, and language; enabling children with special needs to reach their potential; avoiding limitations on the benefits of educational interventions because of hearing problems from OME.
- Harm: cost, time, and specific risks of medications or surgery.
- Benefits-harms assessment: exceptional preponderance of benefits over harm based on subcommittee consensus because of circumstances to date precluding randomized trials.
- Policy level: recommendation.

4. WATCHFUL WAITING: CLINICIANS SHOULD MANAGE THE CHILD WITH OME WHO IS NOT AT RISK WITH WATCHFUL WAITING FOR 3 MONTHS FROM THE DATE OF EFFUSION ONSET (IF KNOWN) OR DIAGNOSIS (IF ONSET IS UNKNOWN)

This recommendation is based on systematic review of cohort studies and the preponderance of benefit over harm.

This recommendation is based on the self-limited nature of most OME, which has been well documented in cohort studies and in control groups of randomized trials.[2,70]

The likelihood of spontaneous resolution of OME is determined by the cause and duration of effusion.[70] For example, ~75% to 90% of residual OME after an AOM episode resolves spontaneously by 3 months.[71–73] Similar outcomes of defined onset during a period of surveillance in a cohort study are observed for OME.[32,37] Another favorable situation involves improvement (not resolution) of newly detected OME defined as change in tympanogram from type B (flat curve) to non-B (anything other than a flat curve). Approximately 55% of children so defined improve by 3 months,[70] but one third will have OME relapse within the next 3 months.[4] Although a type B tympanogram is an imperfect measure of OME (81% sensitivity and 74% specificity versus myringotomy), it is the most widely reported measure suitable for deriving pooled resolution rates.[2,70]

Approximately 25% of newly detected OME of unknown prior duration in children 2 to 4 years old resolves by 3 months when resolution is defined as a change in tympanogram from type B to type A/C1 (peak pressure >200 daPa).[2,70,74–77] Resolution rates may be higher for infants and young children in whom the preexisting duration of effusion is generally shorter, and particularly for those observed prospectively in studies or in the course of well-child care. Documented bilateral OME of 3 months' duration or longer resolves spontaneously after 6 to 12 months in ~30% of children primarily 2 years old or older, with only marginal benefits if observed longer.[70]

Any intervention for OME (medical or surgical) other than observation carries some inherent harm. There is little harm associated with a specified period of observation in the child who is not at risk for speech, language, or learning problems. When observing children with OME, clinicians should inform the parent or caregiver that the child may experience reduced hearing until the effusion resolves, especially if it is bilateral. Clinicians may discuss strategies for optimizing the listening and learning environment until the effusion resolves. These strategies include speaking in close proximity to the child, facing the child and speaking clearly, repeating phrases when misunderstood, and providing preferential classroom seating.[78,79]

The recommendation for a 3-month period of observation is based on a clear preponderance of benefit over harm and is consistent with the original OME guideline intent of avoiding unnecessary surgery.[1] At the discretion of the clinician, this 3-month period of watchful waiting may include interval visits at which OME is monitored by using pneumatic otoscopy, tympanometry, or both. Factors to consider in determining the optimal interval(s) for follow-up include clinical judgment, parental comfort level, unique characteristics of the child and/or his environment, access to a health care system, and hearing levels (HLs) if known.

After documented resolution of OME in all affected ears, additional follow-up is unnecessary.

Evidence Profile: Watchful Waiting

- Aggregate evidence quality: B, systematic review of cohort studies.
- Benefit: avoid unnecessary interventions, take advantage of favorable natural history, and avoid unnecessary referrals and evaluations.
- Harm: delays in therapy for OME that will not resolve with observation; prolongation of hearing loss.
- Benefits-harms assessment: preponderance of benefit over harm.
- Policy level: recommendation.

5. MEDICATION: ANTIHISTAMINES AND DECONGESTANTS ARE INEFFECTIVE FOR OME AND ARE NOT RECOMMENDED FOR TREATMENT; ANTIMICROBIALS AND CORTICOSTEROIDS DO NOT HAVE LONG-TERM EFFICACY AND ARE NOT RECOMMENDED FOR ROUTINE MANAGEMENT

This recommendation is based on systematic review of randomized, controlled trials and the preponderance of harm over benefit.

Therapy for OME is appropriate only if persistent and clinically significant benefits can be achieved beyond spontaneous resolution. Although statistically significant benefits have been demonstrated for some medications, they are short-term and relatively small in magnitude. Moreover, significant adverse events may occur with all medical therapies.

The prior OME guideline[1] found no data supporting antihistamine-decongestant combinations in treating OME. Meta-analysis of 4 randomized trials showed no significant benefit for antihistamines or decongestants versus placebo. No additional studies have been published since 1994 to change this recommendation. Adverse effects of antihistamines and decongestants include insomnia, hyperactivity, drowsiness, behavioral change, and blood-pressure variability.

Long-term benefits of antimicrobial therapy for OME are unproved despite a modest short-term benefit for 2 to 8 weeks in randomized trials.[1,80,81] Initial benefits, however, can become nonsignificant within 2 weeks of stopping the medication.[82] Moreover, ~7 children would need to be treated with antimicrobials to achieve one short-term response.[1] Adverse effects of antimicrobials are significant and may include rashes, vomiting, diarrhea, allergic reactions, alteration of the child's nasopharyngeal flora, development of bacterial resistance,[83] and cost. Societal consequences include direct transmission of resistant bacterial pathogens in homes and child care centers.[84]

The prior OME guideline[1] did not recommend oral steroids for treating OME in children. A later meta-analysis[85] showed no benefit for oral steroid versus placebo within 2 weeks but did show a short-term benefit for oral steroid plus antimicrobial versus antimicrobial alone in 1 of 3 children treated. This benefit became nonsignificant after several weeks in a prior meta-analysis[1] and in a large, randomized trial.[86] Oral steroids can produce behavioral changes, increased appetite, and weight gain.[1] Additional adverse effects may include adrenal suppression, fatal varicella infection, and avascular necrosis of the femoral head.[3] Although intranasal steroids have fewer adverse effects, one randomized trial[87] showed statistically equivalent outcomes at 12 weeks for intranasal beclomethasone plus antimicrobials versus antimicrobials alone for OME.

Antimicrobial therapy with or without steroids has not been demonstrated to be effective in long-term resolution of OME, but in some cases this therapy can be considered an option because of short-term benefit in randomized trials, when the parent or caregiver expresses a strong aversion to impending surgery. In this circumstance, a single course of therapy for 10 to 14 days may be used. The likelihood that the OME will resolve long-term with these regimens is small, and prolonged or repetitive courses of antimicrobials or steroids are strongly not recommended.

Other nonsurgical therapies that are discussed in the OME literature include autoinflation of the eustachian tube, oral or intratympanic use of mucolytics, and systemic use of pharmacologic agents other than antimicrobials, steroids, and antihistamine-decongestants. Insufficient data exist for any of these therapies to be recommended in treating OME.[3]

Evidence Profile: Medication

- Aggregate evidence quality: A, systematic review of well-designed, randomized, controlled trials.

- Benefit: avoid side effects and reduce cost by not administering medications; avoid delays in definitive therapy caused by short-term improvement then relapse.
- Harm: adverse effects of specific medications as listed previously; societal impact of antimicrobial therapy on bacterial resistance and transmission of resistant pathogens.
- Benefits-harms assessment: preponderance of harm over benefit.
- Policy level: recommendation against.

6. HEARING AND LANGUAGE: HEARING TESTING IS RECOMMENDED WHEN OME PERSISTS FOR 3 MONTHS OR LONGER OR AT ANY TIME THAT LANGUAGE DELAY, LEARNING PROBLEMS, OR A SIGNIFICANT HEARING LOSS IS SUSPECTED IN A CHILD WITH OME; LANGUAGE TESTING SHOULD BE CONDUCTED FOR CHILDREN WITH HEARING LOSS

This recommendation is based on cohort studies and the preponderance of benefit over risk.

Hearing Testing

Hearing testing is recommended when OME persists for 3 months or longer or at any time that language delay, learning problems, or a significant hearing loss is suspected. Conductive hearing loss often accompanies OME[1,88] and may adversely affect binaural processing,[89] sound localization,[90] and speech perception in noise.[91–94] Hearing loss caused by OME may impair early language acquisition,[95–97] but the child's home environment has a greater impact on outcomes[98]; recent randomized trials[41,99,100] suggest no impact on children with OME who are not at risk as identified by screening or surveillance.

Studies examining hearing sensitivity in children with OME report that average pure-tone hearing loss at 4 frequencies (500, 1000, 2000, and 4000 Hz) ranges from normal hearing to moderate hearing loss (0–55 dB). The 50th percentile is an ~25-dB HL, and ~20% of ears exceed 35-dB HL.[101,102] Unilateral OME with hearing loss results in overall poorer binaural hearing than in infants with normal middle-ear function bilaterally.[103,104] However, based on limited research, there is evidence that children experiencing the greatest conductive hearing loss for the longest periods may be more likely to exhibit developmental and academic sequelae.[1,95,105]

Initial hearing testing for children 4 years old or older can be done in the primary care setting.[106] Testing should be performed in a quiet environment, preferably in a separate closed or sound-proofed area set aside specifically for that purpose. Conventional audiometry with earphones is performed with a fail criterion of more than 20-dB HL at 1 or more frequencies (500, 1000, 2000, and 4000 Hz) in either ear.[106,107] Methods not recommended as substitutes for primary care hearing testing include tympanometry and pneumatic otoscopy,[102] caregiver judgment regarding hearing loss,[108,109] speech audiometry, and tuning forks, acoustic reflectometry, and behavioral observation.[1]

Comprehensive audiologic evaluation is recommended for children who fail primary care testing, are less than 4 years old, or cannot be tested in the primary care setting. Audiologic assessment includes evaluating air-conduction and bone-conduction thresholds for pure tones, speech-detection or speech-recognition thresholds,[102] and measuring speech understanding if possible.[94] The method of assessment depends on the developmental age of the child and might include visual reinforcement or conditioned orienting-response audiometry for infants 6 to 24 months old, play audiometry for children 24 to 48 months old, or conventional screening audiometry for children 4 years old and older.[106] The auditory brainstem response and otoacoustic emission are tests of auditory pathway structural integrity, not hearing, and should not substitute for behavioral pure-tone audiometry.[106]

Language Testing

Language testing should be conducted for children with hearing loss (pure-tone average more than 20-dB HL on comprehensive audiometric evaluation). Testing for language delays is important, because communication is integral to all aspects of human functioning. Young children with speech and language delays during the preschool years are at risk for continued communication problems and later delays in reading and writing.[110–112] In one study, 6% to 8% of children 3 years old and 2% to 13% of kindergartners had language impairment.[113] Language intervention can improve communication and other functional outcomes for children with histories of OME.[114]

Children who experience repeated and persistent episodes of OME and associated hearing loss during early childhood may be at a disadvantage for learning speech and language.[79,115] Although Shekelle et al[2] concluded that there was no evidence to support the concern that OME during the first 3 years of life was related to later receptive or expressive language, this meta-analysis should be interpreted cautiously, because it did not examine specific language domains such as vocabulary and the independent variable was OME and not hearing loss. Other meta-analyses[79,115] have suggested at most a small negative association of OME and hearing loss on children's receptive and expressive language through the elementary school years. The clinical significance of these effects for language and learning is unclear for the child not at risk. For example, in one randomized trial,[100] prompt insertion of tympanostomy tubes for OME did not improve developmental outcomes at 3 years old regardless of baseline hearing. In another randomized trial,[116] however, prompt tube insertion achieved small benefits for children with bilateral OME and hearing loss.

Clinicians should ask the parent or caregiver about specific concerns regarding their child's language development. Children's speech and language can be tested at ages 6 to 36 months by direct engagement of a child and interviewing the parent using the Early Language Milestone Scale.[117] Other approaches require interviewing only the child's parent or caregiver, such as the MacArthur Communicative Development Inventory[118] and the Language Development Survey.[119] For older children, the Denver Developmental Screening Test II[120] can be used to screen general development including speech and language. Comprehensive speech and language evaluation is recommended for children who fail testing or whenever the child's parent or caregiver expresses concern.[121]

Evidence Profile: Hearing and Language

- Aggregate evidence quality: B, diagnostic studies with minor limitations; C, observational studies.
- Benefit: to detect hearing loss and language delay and identify strategies or interventions to improve developmental outcomes.
- Harm: parental anxiety, direct and indirect costs of assessment, and/or false-positive results.
- Balance of benefit and harm: preponderance of benefit over harm.
- Policy level: recommendation.

7. SURVEILLANCE: CHILDREN WITH PERSISTENT OME WHO ARE NOT AT RISK SHOULD BE REEXAMINED AT 3- TO 6-MONTH INTERVALS UNTIL THE EFFUSION IS NO LONGER PRESENT, SIGNIFICANT HEARING LOSS IS IDENTIFIED, OR STRUCTURAL ABNORMALITIES OF THE EARDRUM OR MIDDLE EAR ARE SUSPECTED

This recommendation is based on randomized, controlled trials and observational studies with a preponderance of benefit over harm.

If OME is asymptomatic and is likely to resolve spontaneously, intervention is unnecessary even if OME persists for more than 3 months. The clinician should determine whether risk factors exist that would predispose the child to undesirable sequelae or predict nonresolution of the effusion. As long as OME persists, the child is at risk for sequelae and must be reevaluated periodically for factors that would prompt intervention.

The 1994 OME guideline[1] recommended surgery for OME persisting 4 to 6 months with hearing loss but requires reconsideration because of later data on tubes and developmental sequelae.[122] For example, selecting surgical candidates using duration-based criteria (eg, OME >3 months or exceeding a cumulative threshold) does not improve developmental outcomes in infants and toddlers who are not at risk.[41,42,99,100] Additionally, the 1994 OME guideline did not specifically address managing effusion without significant hearing loss persisting more than 6 months.

Asymptomatic OME usually resolves spontaneously, but resolution rates decrease the longer the effusion has been present,[36,76,77] and relapse is common.[123] Risk factors that make spontaneous resolution less likely include[124,125]:

- Onset of OME in the summer or fall season
- Hearing loss more than 30-dB HL in the better-hearing ear
- History of prior tympanostomy tubes
- Not having had an adenoidectomy

Children with chronic OME are at risk for structural damage of the tympanic membrane[126] because the effusion contains leukotrienes, prostaglandins, and arachidonic acid metabolites that invoke a local inflammatory response.[127] Reactive changes may occur in the adjacent tympanic membrane and mucosal linings. A relative underventilation of the middle ear produces a negative pressure that predisposes to focal retraction pockets, generalized atelectasis of the tympanic membrane, and cholesteatoma.

Structural integrity is assessed by carefully examining the entire tympanic membrane, which, in many cases, can be accomplished by the primary care clinician using a handheld pneumatic otoscope. A search should be made for retraction pockets, ossicular erosion, and areas of atelectasis or atrophy. If there is any uncertainty that all observed structures are normal, the patient should be examined by using an otomicroscope. All children with these tympanic membrane conditions, regardless of OME duration, should have a comprehensive audiologic evaluation.

Conditions of the tympanic membrane that generally mandate inserting a tympanostomy tube are posterosuperior retraction pockets, ossicular erosion, adhesive atelectasis, and retraction pockets that accumulate keratin debris. Ongoing surveillance is mandatory, because the incidence of structural damage increases with effusion duration.[128]

As noted in recommendation 6, children with persistent OME for 3 months or longer should have their hearing tested. Based on these results, clinicians can identify 3 levels of action based on HLs obtained for the better-hearing ear using earphones or in sound field using speakers if the child is too young for ear-specific testing.

1. HLs of ≥40 dB (at least a moderate hearing loss): A comprehensive audiologic evaluation is indicated if not previously performed. If moderate hearing loss is documented and persists at this level, surgery is recommended, because persistent hearing loss of this magnitude that is permanent in nature has been shown to impact speech, language, and academic performance.[129–131]
2. HLs of 21 to 39 dB (mild hearing loss): A comprehensive audiologic evaluation is indicated if not previously performed. Mild sensorineural hearing loss has been associated with difficulties in speech, language, and academic performance in school,[129,132] and persistent mild conductive hearing loss from OME may have a similar impact. Further management should be individualized based on effusion duration, severity of hearing loss, and parent or caregiver preference and may include strategies to optimize the listening and learning environment (Table 4) or surgery. Repeat hearing testing should be performed in 3 to 6 months if OME persists at follow-up evaluation or tympanostomy tubes have not been placed.
3. HLs of ≤20 dB (normal hearing): A repeat hearing test should be performed in 3 to 6 months if OME persists at follow-up evaluation.

TABLE 4. Strategies for Optimizing the Listening-Learning Environment for Children With OME and Hearing Loss*

Get within 3 feet of the child before speaking.
Turn off competing audio signals such as unnecessary music and television in the background.
Face the child and speak clearly, using visual clues (hands, pictures) in addition to speech.
Slow the rate, raise the level, and enunciate speech directed at the child.
Read to or with the child, explaining pictures and asking questions.
Repeat words, phrases, and questions when misunderstood.
Assign preferential seating in the classroom near the teacher.
Use a frequency-modulated personal- or sound-field-amplification system in the classroom.

* Modified with permission from Roberts et al.[78,79]

In addition to hearing loss and speech or language delay, other factors may influence the decision to intervene for persistent OME. Roberts et al[98,133] showed that the caregiving environment is more strongly related to school outcome than was OME or hearing loss. Risk factors for delays in speech and language development caused by a poor caregiving environment included low maternal educational level, unfavorable child care environment, and low socioeconomic status. In such cases, these factors may be additive to the hearing loss in affecting lower school performance and classroom behavior problems.

Persistent OME may be associated with physical or behavioral symptoms including hyperactivity, poor attention, and behavioral problems in some studies[134–136] and reduced child quality of life.[46] Conversely, young children randomized to early versus late tube insertion for persistent OME showed no behavioral benefits from early surgery.[41,100] Children with chronic OME also have significantly poorer vestibular function and gross motor proficiency when compared with non-OME controls.[48–50] Moreover, vestibular function, behavior, and quality of life can improve after tympanostomy tube insertion.[47,137,138] Other physical symptoms of OME that, if present and persistent, may warrant surgery include otalgia, unexplained sleep disturbance, and coexisting recurrent AOM. Tubes reduce the absolute incidence of recurrent AOM by ~1 episode per child per year, but the relative risk reduction is 56%.[139]

The risks of continued observation of children with OME must be balanced against the risks of surgery. Children with persistent OME examined regularly at 3- to 6-month intervals, or sooner if OME-related symptoms develop, are most likely at low risk for physical, behavioral, or developmental sequelae of OME. Conversely, prolonged watchful waiting of OME is not appropriate when regular surveillance is impossible or when the child is at risk for developmental sequelae of OME because of comorbidities (Table 3). For these children, the risks of anesthesia and surgery (see recommendation 9) may be less than those of continued observation.

Evidence Profile: Surveillance

- Aggregate evidence quality: C, observational studies and some randomized trials.
- Benefit: avoiding interventions that do not improve outcomes.
- Harm: allowing structural abnormalities to develop in the tympanic membrane, underestimating the impact of hearing loss on a child, and/or failing to detect significant signs or symptoms that require intervention.
- Balance of benefit and harm: preponderance of benefit over harm.
- Policy level: recommendation.

8. REFERRAL: WHEN CHILDREN WITH OME ARE REFERRED BY THE PRIMARY CARE CLINICIAN FOR EVALUATION BY AN OTOLARYNGOLOGIST, AUDIOLOGIST, OR SPEECH-LANGUAGE PATHOLOGIST, THE REFERRING CLINICIAN SHOULD DOCUMENT THE EFFUSION DURATION AND SPECIFIC REASON FOR REFERRAL (EVALUATION, SURGERY) AND PROVIDE ADDITIONAL RELEVANT INFORMATION SUCH AS HISTORY OF AOM AND DEVELOPMENTAL STATUS OF THE CHILD

This option is based on panel consensus and a preponderance of benefit over harm.

This recommendation emphasizes the importance of communication between the referring primary care clinician and the otolaryngologist, audiologist, and speech-language pathologist. Parents and caregivers may be confused and frustrated when a recommendation for surgery is made for their child because of conflicting information about alternative management strategies. Choosing among management options is facilitated when primary care physicians and advanced-practice nurses who best know the patient's history of ear problems and general medical status provide the specialist with accurate information. Although there are no studies showing improved outcomes from better documentation of OME histories, there is a clear need for better mechanisms to convey information and expectations from primary care clinicians to consultants and subspecialists.[140–142]

When referring a child for evaluation to an otolaryngologist, the primary care physician should explain the following to the parent or caregiver of the patient:

- Reason for referral: Explain that the child is seeing an otolaryngologist for evaluation, which is likely to include ear examination and audiologic testing, and not necessarily simply to be scheduled for surgery.
- What to expect: Explain that surgery may be recommended, and let the parent know that the otolaryngologist will explain the options, benefits, and risks further.
- Decision-making process: Explain that there are many alternatives for management and that surgical decisions are elective; the parent or caregiver should be encouraged to express to the surgeonany concerns he or she may have about the recommendations made.

When referring a child to an otolaryngologist, audiologist, or speech-language pathologist, the minimum information that should be conveyed in writing includes:

- Duration of OME: State how long fluid has been present.
- Laterality of OME: State whether one or both ears have been affected.
- Results of prior hearing testing or tympanometry.
- Suspected speech or language problems: State whether there had been a delay in speech and language development or whether the parent or a caregiver has expressed concerns about the child's communication abilities, school achievement, or attentiveness.
- Conditions that might exacerbate the deleterious effects of OME: State whether the child has conditions such as permanent hearing loss, impaired cognition, developmental delays, cleft lip or palate, or an unstable or nonsupportive family or home environment.
- AOM history: State whether the child has a history of recurrent AOM.

Additional medical information that should be provided to the otolaryngologist by the primary care clinician includes:

- Parental attitude toward surgery: State whether the parents have expressed a strong preference for or against surgery as a management option.
- Related conditions that might require concomitant surgery: State whether there have been other conditions that might warrant surgery if the child is going to have general anesthesia (eg, nasal obstruction and snoring that might be an indication for adenoidectomy or obstructive breathing during sleep that might mean tonsillectomy is indicated).
- General health status: State whether there are any conditions that might present problems for surgery or administering general anesthesia, such as congenital heart abnormality, bleeding disorder, asthma or reactive airway disease, or family history of malignant hyperthermia.

After evaluating the child, the otolaryngologist, audiologist, or speech-language pathologist should inform the referring physician regarding his or her diagnostic impression, plans for additional assessment, and recommendations for ongoing monitoring and management.

Evidence Profile: Referral

- Aggregate evidence quality: C, observational studies.
- Benefit: better communication and improved decision-making.
- Harm: confidentiality concerns, administrative burden, and/or increased parent or caregiver anxiety.
- Benefits-harms assessment: balance of benefit and harm.
- Policy level: option.

9. SURGERY: WHEN A CHILD BECOMES A SURGICAL CANDIDATE, TYMPANOSTOMY TUBE INSERTION IS THE PREFERRED INITIAL PROCEDURE; ADENOIDECTOMY SHOULD NOT BE PERFORMED UNLESS A DISTINCT INDICATION EXISTS (NASAL OBSTRUCTION, CHRONIC ADENOIDITIS). REPEAT SURGERY CONSISTS OF ADENOIDECTOMY PLUS MYRINGOTOMY, WITH OR WITHOUT TUBE INSERTION. TONSILLECTOMY ALONE OR MYRINGOTOMY ALONE SHOULD NOT BE USED TO TREAT OME

This recommendation is based on randomized, controlled trials with a preponderance of benefit over harm.

Surgical candidacy for OME largely depends on hearing status, associated symptoms, the child's developmental risk (Table 3), and the anticipated chance of timely spontaneous resolution of the effusion. Candidates for surgery include children with OME lasting 4 months or longer with persistent hearing loss or other signs and symptoms, recurrent or persistent OME in children at risk regardless of hearing status, and OME and structural damage to the tympanic membrane or middle ear. Ultimately, the recommendation for surgery must be individualized based on consensus between the primary care physician, otolaryngologist, and parent or caregiver that a particular child would benefit from intervention. Children with OME of any duration who are at risk are candidates for earlier surgery.

Tympanostomy tubes are recommended for initial surgery because randomized trials show a mean 62% relative decrease in effusion prevalence and an absolute decrease of 128 effusion days per child during the next year.[139,143–145] HLs improve by a mean of 6 to 12 dB while the tubes remain patent.[146,147] Adenoidectomy plus myringotomy (without tube insertion) has comparable efficacy in children 4 years old or older[143] but is more invasive, with additional surgical and anesthetic risks. Similarly, the added risk of adenoidectomy outweighs the limited, short-term benefit for children 3 years old or older without prior tubes.[148] Consequently, adenoidectomy is not recommended for initial OME surgery unless a distinct indication exists, such as adenoiditis, postnasal obstruction, or chronic sinusitis.

Approximately 20% to 50% of children who have had tympanostomy tubes have OME relapse after tube extrusion that may require additional surgery.[144,145,149] When a child needs repeat surgery for OME, adenoidectomy is recommended (unless the child has an overt or submucous cleft palate), because it confers a 50% reduction in the need for future operations.[143,150,151] The benefit of adenoidectomy is apparent at 2 years old,[150] greatest for children 3 years old or older, and independent of adenoid size.[143,151,152] Myringotomy is performed concurrent with adenoidectomy. Myringotomy plus adenoidectomy is effective for children 4 years old or older,[143] but tube insertion is advised for younger children, when potential relapse of effusion must be minimized (eg, children at risk) or pronounced inflammation of the tympanic membrane and middle-ear mucosa is present.

Tonsillectomy or myringotomy alone (without adenoidectomy) is not recommended to treat OME. Although tonsillectomy is either ineffective[152] or of limited efficacy,[148,150] the risks of hemorrhage (~2%) and additional hospitalization outweigh any potential benefits unless a distinct indication for tonsillectomy exists. Myringotomy alone, without tube placement or adenoidectomy, is ineffective for chronic OME,[144,145] because the incision closes within several days. Laser-assisted myringotomy extends the ventilation period several weeks,[153] but randomized trials with concurrent controls have not been conducted to establish efficacy. In contrast, tympanostomy tubes ventilate the middle ear for an average of 12 to 14 months.[144,145]

Anesthesia mortality has been reported to be ~1: 50 000 for ambulatory surgery,[154] but the current fatality rate may be lower.[155] Laryngospasm and bronchospasm occur more often in children receiving anesthesia than adults. Tympanostomy tube sequelae are common[156] but are generally transient (otorrhea) or do not affect function (tympanosclerosis, focal atrophy, or shallow retraction pocket). Tympanic membrane perforations, which may require repair, are seen in 2% of children after placement of short-term (grommet-type) tubes and 17% after long-term tubes.[156] Adenoidectomy has a 0.2% to 0.5% incidence of hemorrhage[150,157] and 2% incidence of transient velopharyngeal insufficiency.[148] Other potential risks of adenoidectomy, such as nasopharyngeal stenosis and persistent velopharyngeal insufficiency, can be minimized with appropriate patient selection and surgical technique.

There is a clear preponderance of benefit over harm when considering the impact of surgery for OME on effusion prevalence, HLs, subsequent incidence of AOM, and the need for reoperation after adenoidectomy. Information about adenoidectomy in children less than 4 years old, however, remains limited. Although the cost of surgery and anesthesia is nontrivial, it is offset by reduced OME and AOM after tube placement and by reduced need for reoperation after adenoidectomy. Approximately 8 adenoidectomies are needed to avoid a single instance of tube reinsertion; however, each avoided surgery probably represents a larger reduction in the number of AOM and OME episodes, including those in children who did not require additional surgery.[150]

Evidence Profile: Surgery

- Aggregate evidence quality: B, randomized, controlled trials with minor limitations.
- Benefit: improved hearing, reduced prevalence of OME, reduced incidence of AOM, and less need for additional tube insertion (after adenoidectomy).
- Harm: risks of anesthesia and specific surgical procedures; sequelae of tympanostomy tubes.
- Benefits-harms assessment: preponderance of benefit over harm.
- Policy level: recommendation.

10. CAM: NO RECOMMENDATION IS MADE REGARDING CAM AS A TREATMENT FOR OME

There is no recommendation based on lack of scientific evidence documenting efficacy and an uncertain balance of harm and benefit.

The 1994 OME guideline[1] made no recommendation regarding CAM as a treatment for OME, and no subsequent controlled studies have been published to change this conclusion. The current statement of "no recommendation" is based on the lack of scientific evidence documenting efficacy plus the balance of benefit and harm.

Evidence concerning CAM is insufficient to determine whether the outcomes achieved for OME differ from those achieved by watchful waiting and spontaneous resolution. There are no randomized, controlled trials with adequate sample sizes on the efficacy of CAM for OME. Although many case reports and subjective reviews on CAM treatment of AOM were found, little is published on OME treatment or prevention. Homeopathy[158] and chiropractic treatments[159] were assessed in pilot studies with small numbers of patients that failed to show clinically or statistically significant benefits. Consequently, there is no research base on which to develop a recommendation concerning CAM for OME.

The natural history of OME in childhood (discussed previously) is such that almost any intervention can be "shown" to have helped in an anecdotal, uncontrolled report or case series. The efficacy of CAM or any other intervention for OME can only be shown with parallel-group, randomized, controlled trials with valid diagnostic methods and adequate sample sizes. Unproved modalities that have been claimed to provide benefit in middle-ear disease include osteopathic and chiropractic manipulation, dietary exclusions (such as dairy), herbal and other dietary supplements, acupuncture, traditional Chinese medicine, and homeopathy. None of these modalities, however, have been subjected yet to a published, peer-reviewed, clinical trial.

The absence of any published clinical trials also means that all reports of CAM adverse effects are anecdotal. A systematic review of recent evidence[160] found significant serious adverse effects of unconventional therapies for children, most of which were associated with inadequately regulated herbal medicines. One report on malpractice liability associated with CAM therapies[161] did not address childhood issues specifically. Allergic reactions to echinacea occur but seem to be rare in children.[162] A general concern about herbal products is the lack of any governmental oversight into product quality or purity.[160,163,164] Additionally, herbal products may alter blood levels of allopathic medications, including anticoagulants. A possible concern with homeopathy is the worsening of symptoms, which is viewed as a positive, early sign of homeopathic efficacy. The adverse effects of manipulative therapies (such as chiropractic treatments and osteopathy) in children are difficult to assess because of scant evidence, but a case series of 332 children treated for AOM or OME with chiropractic manipulation did not mention any side effects.[165] Quadriplegia has been reported, however, after spinal manipulation in an infant with torticollis.[166]

Evidence Profile: CAM

- Aggregate evidence quality: D, case series without controls.
- Benefit: not established.
- Harm: potentially significant depending on the intervention.
- Benefits-harms assessment: uncertain balance of benefit and harm.
- Policy level: no recommendation.

11. ALLERGY MANAGEMENT: NO RECOMMENDATION IS MADE REGARDING ALLERGY MANAGEMENT AS A TREATMENT FOR OME

There is no recommendation based on insufficient evidence of therapeutic efficacy or a causal relationship between allergy and OME.

The 1994 OME guideline[1] made no recommendation regarding allergy management as a treatment for OME, and no subsequent controlled studies have been published to change this conclusion. The current statement of "no recommendation" is based on insufficient evidence of therapeutic efficacy or a causal relationship between allergy and OME plus the balance of benefit and harm.

A linkage between allergy and OME has long been speculated but to date remains unquantified. The prevalence of allergy among OME patients has been reported to range from less than 10% to more than 80%.[167] Allergy has long been postulated to cause OME through its contribution to eustachian tube dysfunction.[168] The cellular response of respiratory mucosa to allergens has been well studied. Therefore, similar to other parts of respiratory mucosa, the mucosa lining the middle-ear cleft is capable of an allergic response.[169,170] Sensitivity to allergens varies among individuals, and atopy may involve neutrophils in type I allergic reactions that enhance the inflammatory response.[171]

The correlation between OME and allergy has been widely reported, but no prospective studies have examined the effects of immunotherapy compared with observation alone or other management options. Reports of OME cure after immunotherapy or food-elimination diets[172] are impossible to interpret without concurrent control groups because of the favorable natural history of most untreated OME. The documentation of allergy in published reports has been defined inconsistently (medical history, physical examination, skin-prick testing, nasal smears, serum immunoglobulin E and eosinophil counts, inflammatory mediators in effusions). Study groups have been drawn primarily from specialist offices, likely lack heterogeneity, and are not representative of general medical practice.

Evidence Profile: Allergy Management

- Aggregate evidence quality: D, case series without controls.
- Benefit: not established.
- Harm: adverse effects and cost of medication, physician evaluation, elimination diets, and desensitization.
- Benefits-harms assessment: balance of benefit and harm.
- Policy level: no recommendation.

RESEARCH NEEDS

Diagnosis

- Further standardize the definition of OME.
- Assess the performance characteristics of pneumatic otoscopy as a diagnostic test for OME when performed by primary care physicians and advanced-practice nurses in the routine office setting.
- Determine the optimal methods for teaching pneumatic otoscopy to residents and clinicians.
- Develop a brief, reliable, objective method for diagnosing OME.
- Develop a classification method for identifying the presence of OME for practical use by clinicians that is based on quantifiable tympanometric characteristics.
- Assess the usefulness of algorithms combining pneumatic otoscopy and tympanometry for detecting OME in clinical practice.
- Conduct additional validating cohort studies of acoustic reflectometry as a diagnostic method for OME, particularly in children less than 2 years old.

Child At Risk

- Better define the child with OME who is at risk for speech, language, and learning problems.
- Conduct large, multicenter, observational cohort studies to identify the child at risk who is most susceptible to potential adverse sequelae of OME.
- Conduct large, multicenter, observational cohort studies to analyze outcomes achieved with alternative management strategies for OME in children at risk.

Watchful Waiting

- Define the spontaneous resolution of OME in infants and young children (existing data are limited primarily to children 2 years old or older).
- Conduct large-scale, prospective cohort studies to obtain current data on the spontaneous resolution of newly diagnosed OME of unknown prior duration (existing data are primarily from the late 1970s and early 1980s).
- Develop prognostic indicators to identify the best candidates for watchful waiting.
- Determine whether the lack of impact from prompt insertion of tympanostomy tubes on speech and language outcomes seen in asymptomatic young children with OME identified by screening or intense surveillance can be generalized to older children with OME or to symptomatic children with OME referred for evaluation.

Medication

- Clarify which children, if any, should receive antimicrobials, steroids, or both for OME.
- Conduct a randomized, placebo-controlled trial on the efficacy of antimicrobial therapy, with or without concurrent oral steroid, in avoiding surgery in children with OME who are surgical candidates and have not received recent antimicrobials.
- Investigate the role of mucosal surface biofilms in refractory or recurrent OME and develop targeted interventions.

Hearing and Language

- Conduct longitudinal studies on the natural history of hearing loss accompanying OME.
- Develop improved methods for describing and quantifying the fluctuations in hearing of children with OME over time.
- Conduct prospective controlled studies on the relation of hearing loss associated with OME to later auditory, speech, language, behavioral, and academic sequelae.
- Develop reliable, brief, objective methods for estimating hearing loss associated with OME.
- Develop reliable, brief, objective methods for estimating speech or language delay associated with OME.
- Evaluate the benefits and administrative burden of language testing by primary care clinicians.
- Agree on the aspects of language that are vulnerable to or affected by hearing loss caused by OME, and reach a consensus on the best tools for measurement.
- Determine whether OME and associated hearing loss place children from special populations at greater risk for speech and language delays.

Surveillance

- Develop better tools for monitoring children with OME that are suitable for routine clinical care.
- Assess the value of new strategies for monitoring OME, such as acoustic reflectometry performed at home by the parent or caregiver, in optimizing surveillance.
- Improve our ability to identify children who would benefit from early surgery instead of prolonged surveillance.
- Promote early detection of structural abnormalities in the tympanic membrane associated with OME that may require surgery to prevent complications.
- Clarify and quantify the role of parent or caregiver education, socioeconomic status, and quality of the caregiving environment as modifiers of OME developmental outcomes.
- Develop methods for minimizing loss to follow-up during OME surveillance.

Surgery

- Define the role of adenoidectomy in children 3 years old or younger as a specific OME therapy.
- Conduct controlled trials on the efficacy of tympanostomy tubes for developmental outcomes in children with hearing loss, other symptoms, or speech and language delay.
- Conduct randomized, controlled trials of surgery versus no surgery that emphasize patient-based outcome measures (quality of life, functional health status) in addition to objective measures (effusion prevalence, HLs, AOM incidence, reoperation).
- Identify the optimal ways to incorporate parent or caregiver preference into surgical decision-making.

CAM

- Conduct randomized, controlled trials on the efficacy of CAM modalities for OME.
- Develop strategies to identify parents or caregivers who use CAM therapies for their child's OME, and encourage surveillance by the primary care clinician.

Allergy Management

- Evaluate the causal role of atopy in OME.
- Conduct randomized, controlled trials on the efficacy of allergy therapy for OME that are generalizable to the primary care setting.

CONCLUSIONS

This evidence-based practice guideline offers recommendations for identifying, monitoring, and managing the child with OME. The guideline emphasizes appropriate diagnosis and provides options for various management strategies including observation, medical intervention, and referral for surgical intervention. These recommendations should provide primary care physicians and other health care providers with assistance in managing children with OME.

SUBCOMMITTEE ON OTITIS MEDIA WITH EFFUSION
Richard M. Rosenfeld, MD, MPH, Cochairperson
American Academy of Pediatrics
American Academy of Otolaryngology-Head and Neck Surgery
Larry Culpepper, MD, MPH, Cochairperson
American Academy of Family Physicians
Karen J. Doyle, MD, PhD
American Academy of Otolaryngology-Head and Neck Surgery
Kenneth M. Grundfast, MD
American Academy of Otolaryngology-Head and Neck Surgery
Alejandro Hoberman, MD
American Academy of Pediatrics
Margaret A. Kenna, MD
American Academy of Otolaryngology-Head and Neck Surgery
Allan S. Lieberthal, MD
American Academy of Pediatrics
Martin Mahoney, MD, PhD
American Academy of Family Physicians
Richard A. Wahl, MD
American Academy of Pediatrics
Charles R. Woods, Jr, MD, MS
American Academy of Pediatrics

Barbara Yawn, MD, MSc
American Academy of Family Physicians

CONSULTANTS
S. Michael Marcy, MD
Richard N. Shiffman, MD

LIAISONS
Linda Carlson, MS, CPNP
National Association of Pediatric Nurse Practitioners
Judith Gravel, PhD
American Academy of Audiology
Joanne Roberts, PhD
American Speech-Language-Hearing Association
STAFF
Maureen Hannley, PhD
American Academy of Otolaryngology-Head and Neck Surgery
Carla T. Herrerias, MPH
American Academy of Pediatrics
Bellinda K. Schoof, MHA, CPHQ
American Academy of Family Physicians

ACKNOWLEDGMENTS

Dr Marcy serves as a consultant to Abbott Laboratories GlaxoSmithKline (vaccines).

REFERENCES

1. Stool SE, Berg AO, Berman S, et al. *Otitis Media With Effusion in Young Children. Clinical Practice Guideline, Number 12.* AHCPR Publication No. 94-0622. Rockville, MD: Agency for Health Care Policy and Research, Public Health Service, US Department of Health and Human Services; 1994
2. Shekelle P, Takata G, Chan LS, et al. *Diagnosis, Natural History, and Late Effects of Otitis Media With Effusion. Evidence Report/Technology Assessment No. 55.* AHRQ Publication No. 03-E023. Rockville, MD: Agency for Healthcare Research and Quality; 2003
3. Williamson I. Otitis media with effusion. *Clin Evid.* 2002;7:469–476
4. Tos M. Epidemiology and natural history of secretory otitis. *Am J Otol.* 1984;5:459–462
5. Paradise JL, Rockette HE, Colborn DK, et al. Otitis media in 2253 Pittsburgh area infants: prevalence and risk factors during the first two years of life. *Pediatrics.* 1997;99:318–333
6. Casselbrant ML, Mandel EM. Epidemiology. In: Rosenfeld RM, Bluestone CD, eds. *Evidence-Based Otitis Media.* 2nd ed. Hamilton, Ontario: BC Decker; 2003:147–162
7. Williamson IG, Dunleavy J, Baine J, Robinson D. The natural history of otitis media with effusion—a three-year study of the incidence and prevalence of abnormal tympanograms in four South West Hampshire infant and first schools. *J Laryngol Otol.* 1994;108:930–934
8. Coyte PC, Croxford R, Asche CV, To T, Feldman W, Friedberg J. Physician and population determinants of rates of middle-ear surgery in Ontario. *JAMA.* 2001;286:2128–2135
9. Tugwell P. How to read clinical journals: III. To learn the clinical course and prognosis of disease. *Can Med Assoc J.* 1981;124:869–872
10. Jaeschke R, Guyatt G, Sackett DL. Users' guides to the medical literature. III. How to use an article about a diagnostic test. A. Are the results of the study valid? Evidence-Based Medicine Working Group. *JAMA.* 1994;271:389–391
11. Shiffman RN, Shekelle P, Overhage JM, Slutsky J, Grimshaw J, Deshpande AM. Standardized reporting of clinical practice guidelines: a proposal from the Conference on Guideline Standardization. *Ann Intern Med.* 2003;139:493–498
12. Shiffman RN, Karras BT, Agrawal A, Chen R, Marenco L, Nath S. GEM: a proposal for a more comprehensive guideline document model using XML. *J Am Med Inform Assoc.* 2000;7:488–498
13. Shaneyfelt TM, Mayo-Smith MF, Rothwangl J. Are guidelines following guidelines? The methodological quality of clinical practice guidelines in the peer-reviewed medical literature. *JAMA.* 1999;281:1900–1905
14. Agrawal A, Shiffman RN. Evaluation of guideline quality using GEM-Q. *Medinfo.* 2001;10:1097–1101
15. Yale Center for Medical Informatics. GEM: The Guideline Elements Model. Available at: http://ycmi.med.yale.edu/GEM/. Accessed December 8, 2003
16. American Academy of Pediatrics, Steering Committee on Quality Improvement and Management. A taxonomy of recommendations for clinical practice guidelines. *Pediatrics.* 2004; In press
17. Eddy DM. *A Manual for Assessing Health Practices and Designing Practice Policies: The Explicit Approach.* Philadelphia, PA: American College of Physicians; 1992
18. Dowell SF, Marcy MS, Phillips WR, Gerber MA, Schwartz B. Otitis media—principles of judicious use of antimicrobial agents. *Pediatrics.* 1998;101:165–171
19. Dowell SF, Butler JC, Giebink GS, et al. Acute otitis media: management and surveillance in an era of pneumococcal resistance—a report from the Drug-Resistant *Streptococcus pneumoniae* Therapeutic Working Group. *Pediatr Infect Dis J.* 1999;18:1–9
20. Karma PH, Penttila MA, Sipila MM, Kataja MJ. Otoscopic diagnosis of middle ear effusion in acute and non-acute otitis media. I. The value of different otoscopic findings. *Int J Pediatr Otorhinolaryngol.* 1989;17:37–49
21. Pichichero ME, Poole MD. Assessing diagnostic accuracy and tympanocentesis skills in the management of otitis media. *Arch Pediatr Adolesc Med.* 2001;155:1137–1142
22. Steinbach WJ, Sectish TC. Pediatric resident training in the diagnosis and treatment of acute otitis media. *Pediatrics.* 2002;109:404–408
23. Palmu A, Puhakka H, Rahko T, Takala AK. Diagnostic value of tympanometry in infants in clinical practice. *Int J Pediatr Otorhinolaryngol.* 1999;49:207–213
24. van Balen FA, Aarts AM, De Melker RA. Tympanometry by general practitioners: reliable? *Int J Pediatr Otorhinolaryngol.* 1999;48:117–123
25. Block SL, Mandel E, McLinn S, et al. Spectral gradient acoustic reflectometry for the detection of middle ear effusion by pediatricians and parents. *Pediatr Infect Dis J.* 1998;17:560–564, 580
26. Barnett ED, Klein JO, Hawkins KA, Cabral HJ, Kenna M, Healy G. Comparison of spectral gradient acoustic reflectometry and other diagnostic techniques for detection of middle ear effusion in children with middle ear disease. *Pediatr Infect Dis J.* 1998;17:556–559, 580
27. Block SL, Pichichero ME, McLinn S, Aronovitz G, Kimball S. Spectral gradient acoustic reflectometry: detection of middle ear effusion by pediatricians in suppurative acute otitis media. *Pediatr Infect Dis J.* 1999;18:741–744
28. Schwartz RH. A practical approach to the otitis prone child. *Contemp Pediatr.* 1987;4:30–54
29. Barriga F, Schwartz RH, Hayden GF. Adequate illumination for otoscopy. Variations due to power source, bulb, and head and speculum design. *Am J Dis Child.* 1986;140:1237–1240
30. Sorenson CH, Jensen SH, Tos M. The post-winter prevalence of middle-ear effusion in four-year-old children, judged by tympanometry. *Int J Pediatr Otorhinolaryngol.* 1981;3:119–128
31. Fiellau-Nikolajsen M. Epidemiology of secretory otitis media. A descriptive cohort study. *Ann Otol Rhinol Laryngol.* 1983;92:172–177
32. Casselbrant ML, Brostoff LM, Cantekin EI, et al. Otitis media with effusion in preschool children. *Laryngoscope.* 1985;95:428–436
33. Zielhuis GA, Rach GH, van den Broek P. Screening for otitis media with effusion in preschool children. *Lancet.* 1989;1:311–314
34. Poulsen G, Tos M. Repetitive tympanometric screenings of two-year-old children. *Scand Audiol.* 1980;9:21–28
35. Tos M, Holm-Jensen S, Sorensen CH. Changes in prevalence of secretory otitis from summer to winter in four-year-old children. *Am J Otol.* 1981;2:324–327
36. Thomsen J, Tos M. Spontaneous improvement of secretory otitis. A long-term study. *Acta Otolaryngol.* 1981;92:493–499
37. Lous J, Fiellau-Nikolajsen M. Epidemiology of middle ear effusion and tubal dysfunction. A one-year prospective study comprising monthly tympanometry in 387 non-selected seven-year-old children. *Int J Pediatr Otorhinolaryngol.* 1981;3:303–317
38. New Zealand Health Technology Assessment. *Screening Programmes for the Detection of Otitis Media With Effusion and Conductive Hearing Loss in Pre-School and New Entrant School Children: A Critical Appraisal of the Literature.* Christchurch, New Zealand: New Zealand Health Technology Assessment; 1998:61
39. Canadian Task Force on Preventive Health Care. Screening for otitis media with effusion: recommendation statement from the Canadian Task Force on Preventive Health Care. *CMAJ.* 2001;165:1092–1093
40. US Preventive Services Task Force. *Guide to Clinical Preventive Services.* 2nd ed. Baltimore, MD: Williams & Wilkins; 1995
41. Paradise JL, Feldman HM, Campbell TF, et al. Effect of early or delayed insertion of tympanostomy tubes for persistent otitis media on

developmental outcomes at the age of three years. *N Engl J Med.* 2001;344:1179–1187
42. Rovers MM, Krabble PF, Straatman H, Ingels K, van der Wilt GJ, Zielhuis GA. Randomized controlled trial of the effect of ventilation tubes (grommets) on quality of life at age 1–2 years. *Arch Dis Child.* 2001;84:45–49
43. Wood DL. Documentation guidelines: evolution, future direction, and compliance. *Am J Med.* 2001;110:332–334
44. Soto CM, Kleinman KP, Simon SR. Quality and correlates of medical record documentation in the ambulatory care setting. *BMC Health Serv Res.* 2002;2:22–35
45. Marchant CD, Shurin PA, Turczyk VA, Wasikowski DE, Tutihasi MA, Kinney SE. Course and outcome of otitis media in early infancy: a prospective study. *J Pediatr.* 1984;104:826–831
46. Rosenfeld RM, Goldsmith AJ, Tetlus L, Balzano A. Quality of life for children with otitis media. *Arch Otolaryngol Head Neck Surg.* 1997;123: 1049–1054
47. Casselbrant ML, Furman JM, Rubenstein E, Mandel EM. Effect of otitis media on the vestibular system in children. *Ann Otol Rhinol Laryngol.* 1995;104:620–624
48. Orlin MN, Effgen SK, Handler SD. Effect of otitis media with effusion on gross motor ability in preschool-aged children: preliminary findings. *Pediatrics.* 1997;99:334–337
49. Golz A, Angel-Yeger B, Parush S. Evaluation of balance disturbances in children with middle ear effusion. *Int J Pediatr Otorhinolaryngol.* 1998;43:21–26
50. Casselbrant ML, Redfern MS, Furman JM, Fall PA, Mandel EM. Visual-induced postural sway in children with and without otitis media. *Ann Otol Rhinol Laryngol.* 1998;107:401–405
51. Ruben R. Host susceptibility to otitis media sequelae. In: Rosenfeld RM, Bluestone CD, eds. *Evidence-Based Otitis Media.* 2nd ed. Hamilton, ON, Canada: BC Decker; 2003:505–514
52. Whiteman BC, Simpson GB, Compton WC. Relationship of otitis media and language impairment on adolescents with Down syndrome. *Ment Retard.* 1986;24:353–356
53. van der Vyver M, van der Merwe A, Tesner HE. The effects of otitis media on articulation in children with cerebral palsy. *Int J Rehabil Res.* 1988;11:386–389
54. Paradise JL, Bluestone CD. Early treatment of the universal otitis media of infants with cleft palate. *Pediatrics.* 1974;53:48–54
55. Schwartz DM, Schwartz RH. Acoustic impedance and otoscopic findings in young children with Down's syndrome. *Arch Otolaryngol.* 1978; 104:652–656
56. Corey JP, Caldarelli DD, Gould HJ. Otopathology in cranial facial dysostosis. *Am J Otol.* 1987;8:14–17
57. Schonweiler R, Schonweiler B, Schmelzeisen R. Hearing capacity and speech production in 417 children with facial cleft abnormalities [in German]. *HNO.* 1994;42:691–696
58. Ruben RJ, Math R. Serous otitis media associated with sensorineural hearing loss in children. *Laryngoscope.* 1978;88:1139–1154
59. Brookhouser PE, Worthington DW, Kelly WJ. Middle ear disease in young children with sensorineural hearing loss. *Laryngoscope.* 1993;103: 371–378
60. Rice ML. Specific language impairments: in search of diagnostic markers and genetic contributions. *Ment Retard Dev Disabil Res Rev.* 1997;3: 350–357
61. Rosenhall U, Nordin V, Sandstrom M, Ahlsen G, Gillberg C. Autism and hearing loss. *J Autism Dev Disord.* 1999;29:349–357
62. Cunningham C, McArthur K. Hearing loss and treatment in young Down's syndrome children. *Child Care Health Dev.* 1981;7:357–374
63. Shott SR, Joseph A, Heithaus D. Hearing loss in children with Down syndrome. *Int J Pediatr Otorhinolaryngol.* 2001;61:199–205
64. Clarkson RL, Eimas PD, Marean GC. Speech perception in children with histories of recurrent otitis media. *J Acoust Soc Am.* 1989;85: 926–933
65. Groenen P, Crul T, Maassen B, van Bon W. Perception of voicing cues by children with early otitis media with and without language impairment. *J Speech Hear Res.* 1996;39:43–54
66. Hubbard TW, Paradise JL, McWilliams BJ, Elster BA, Taylor FH. Consequences of unremitting middle-ear disease in early life. Otologic, audiologic, and developmental findings in children with cleft palate. *N Engl J Med.* 1985;312:1529–1534
67. Nunn DR, Derkay CS, Darrow DH, Magee W, Strasnick B. The effect of very early cleft palate closure on the need for ventilation tubes in the first years of life. *Laryngoscope.* 1995;105:905–908
68. Pappas DG, Flexer C, Shackelford L. Otological and habilitative management of children with Down syndrome. *Laryngoscope.* 1994;104: 1065–1070
69. Vartiainen E. Otitis media with effusion in children with congenital or early-onset hearing impairment. *J Otolaryngol.* 2000;29:221–223
70. Rosenfeld RM, Kay D. Natural history of untreated otitis media. *Laryngoscope.* 2003;113:1645–1657
71. Teele DW, Klein JO, Rosner BA. Epidemiology of otitis media in children. *Ann Otol Rhinol Laryngol Suppl.* 1980;89:5–6
72. Mygind N, Meistrup-Larsen KI, Thomsen J, Thomsen VF, Josefsson K, Sorensen H. Penicillin in acute otitis media: a double-blind, placebo-controlled trial. *Clin Otolaryngol.* 1981;6:5–13
73. Burke P, Bain J, Robinson D, Dunleavey J. Acute red ear in children: controlled trial of nonantibiotic treatment in general practice. *BMJ.* 1991;303:558–562
74. Fiellau-Nikolajsen M, Lous J. Prospective tympanometry in 3-year-old children. A study of the spontaneous course of tympanometry types in a nonselected population. *Arch Otolaryngol.* 1979;105:461–466
75. Fiellau-Nikolajsen M. Tympanometry in 3-year-old children. Type of care as an epidemiological factor in secretory otitis media and tubal dysfunction in unselected populations of 3-year-old children. *ORL J Otorhinolaryngol Relat Spec.* 1979;41:193–205
76. Tos M. Spontaneous improvement of secretory otitis and impedance screening. *Arch Otolaryngol.* 1980;106:345–349
77. Tos M, Holm-Jensen S, Sorensen CH, Mogensen C. Spontaneous course and frequency of secretory otitis in 4-year-old children. *Arch Otolaryngol.* 1982;108:4–10
78. Roberts JE, Zeisel SA. *Ear Infections and Language Development.* Rockville, MD: American Speech-Language-Hearing Association and the National Center for Early Development and Learning; 2000
79. Roberts JE, Rosenfeld RM, Zeisel SA. Otitis media and speech and language: a meta-analysis of prospective studies. *Pediatrics.* 2004; 113(3). Available at: www.pediatrics.org/cgi/content/full/113/3/e238
80. Williams RL, Chalmers TC, Stange KC, Chalmers FT, Bowlin SJ. Use of antibiotics in preventing recurrent otitis media and in treating otitis media with effusion. A meta-analytic attempt to resolve the brouhaha. *JAMA.* 1993;270:1344–1351
81. Rosenfeld RM, Post JC. Meta-analysis of antibiotics for the treatment of otitis media with effusion. *Otolaryngol Head Neck Surg.* 1992;106: 378–386
82. Mandel EM, Rockette HE, Bluestone CD, Paradise JL, Nozza RJ. Efficacy of amoxicillin with and without decongestant-antihistamine for otitis media with effusion in children. Results of a double-blind, randomized trial. *N Engl J Med.* 1987;316:432–437
83. McCormick AW, Whitney CG, Farley MM, et al. Geographic diversity and temporal trends of antimicrobial resistance in *Streptococcus pneumoniae* in the United States. *Nat Med.* 2003;9:424–430
84. Levy SB. *The Antibiotic Paradox. How the Misuse of Antibiotic Destroys Their Curative Powers.* Cambridge, MA: Perseus Publishing; 2002
85. Butler CC, van der Voort JH. Oral or topical nasal steroids for hearing loss associated with otitis media with effusion in children. *Cochrane Database Syst Rev.* 2002;4:CD001935
86. Mandel EM, Casselbrant ML, Rockette HE, Fireman P, Kurs-Lasky M, Bluestone CD. Systemic steroid for chronic otitis media with effusion in children. *Pediatrics.* 2002;110:1071–1080
87. Tracy JM, Demain JG, Hoffman KM, Goetz DW. Intranasal beclomethasone as an adjunct to treatment of chronic middle ear effusion. *Ann Allergy Asthma Immunol.* 1998;80:198–206
88. Joint Committee on Infant Hearing. Year 2000 position statement: principles and guidelines for early hearing detection and intervention programs. *Am J Audiol.* 2000;9:9–29
89. Pillsbury HC, Grose JH, Hall JW III. Otitis media with effusion in children. Binaural hearing before and after corrective surgery. *Arch Otolaryngol Head Neck Surg.* 1991;117:718–723
90. Besing J, Koehnke J A test of virtual auditory localization. *Ear Hear.* 1995;16:220–229
91. Jerger S, Jerger J, Alford BR, Abrams S. Development of speech intelligibility in children with recurrent otitis media. *Ear Hear.* 1983;4: 138–145
92. Gravel JS, Wallace IF. Listening and language at 4 years of age: effects of early otitis media. *J Speech Hear Res.* 1992;35:588–595
93. Schilder AG, Snik AF, Straatman H, van den Broek P. The effect of otitis media with effusion at preschool age on some aspects of auditory perception at school age. *Ear Hear.* 1994;15:224–231
94. Rosenfeld RM, Madell JR, McMahon A. Auditory function in normal-hearing children with middle ear effusion. In: Lim DJ, Bluestone CD, Casselbrant M, Klein JO, Ogra PL, eds. *Recent Advances in Otitis Media: Proceedings of the 6th International Symposium.* Hamilton, ON, Canada: BC Decker; 1996:354–356

95. Friel-Patti S, Finitzo T. Language learning in a prospective study of otitis media with effusion in the first two years of life. *J Speech Hear Res.* 1990;33:188–194
96. Wallace IF, Gravel JS, McCarton CM, Stapells DR, Bernstein RS, Ruben RJ. Otitis media, auditory sensitivity, and language outcomes at one year. *Laryngoscope.* 1988;98:64–70
97. Roberts JE, Burchinal MR, Medley LP, et al. Otitis media, hearing sensitivity, and maternal responsiveness in relation to language during infancy. *J Pediatr.* 1995;126:481–489
98. Roberts JE, Burchinal MR, Zeisel SA. Otitis media in early childhood in relation to children's school-age language and academic skills. *Pediatrics.* 2002;110:696–706
99. Rovers MM, Straatman H, Ingels K, van der Wilt GJ, van den Broek P, Zielhuis GA. The effect of ventilation tubes on language development in infants with otitis media with effusion: a randomized trial. *Pediatrics.* 2000;106(3). Available at: www.pediatrics.org/cgi/content/full/106/3/e42
100. Paradise JL, Feldman HM, Campbell TF, et al. Early versus delayed insertion of tympanostomy tubes for persistent otitis media: developmental outcomes at the age of three years in relation to prerandomization illness patterns and hearing levels. *Pediatr Infect Dis J.* 2003;22:309–314
101. Kokko E. Chronic secretory otitis media in children. A clinical study. *Acta Otolaryngol Suppl.* 1974;327:1–44
102. Fria TJ, Cantekin EI, Eichler JA. Hearing acuity of children with otitis media with effusion. *Arch Otolaryngol.* 1985;111:10–16
103. Gravel JS, Wallace IF. Effects of otitis media with effusion on hearing in the first three years of life. *J Speech Lang Hear Res.* 2000;43:631–644
104. Roberts JE, Burchinal MR, Zeisel S, et al. Otitis media, the caregiving environment, and language and cognitive outcomes at 2 years. *Pediatrics.* 1998;102:346–354
105. Gravel JS, Wallace IF, Ruben RJ. Early otitis media and later educational risk. *Acta Otolaryngol.* 1995;115:279–281
106. Cunningham M, Cox EO; American Academy of Pediatrics, Committee on Practice and Ambulatory Medicine, Section on Otolaryngology and Bronchoesophagology. Hearing assessment in infants and children: recommendations beyond neonatal screening. *Pediatrics.* 2003;111:436–440
107. American Speech-Language-Hearing Association Panel on Audiologic Assessment. *Guidelines for Audiologic Screening*. Rockville, MD: American Speech-Language-Hearing Association; 1996
108. Rosenfeld RM, Goldsmith AJ, Madell JR. How accurate is parent rating of hearing for children with otitis media? *Arch Otolaryngol Head Neck Surg.* 1998;124:989–992
109. Brody R, Rosenfeld RM, Goldsmith AJ, Madell JR. Parents cannot detect mild hearing loss in children. *Otolaryngol Head Neck Surg.* 1999;121:681–686
110. Catts HW, Fey ME, Zhang X, Tomblin JB. Language basis of reading and reading disabilities: evidence from a longitudinal investigation. *Sci Stud Read.* 1999;3:331–362
111. Johnson CJ, Beitchman JH, Young A, et al. Fourteen-year follow-up of children with and without speech/language impairments: speech/language stability and outcomes. *J Speech Lang Hear Res.* 1999;42:744–760
112. Scarborough H, Dobrich W. Development of children with early language delay. *J Speech Hear Res.* 1990;33:70–83
113. Tomblin JB, Records NL, Buckwalter P, Zhang X, Smith E, O'Brien M. Prevalence of specific language impairment in kindergarten children. *J Speech Lang Hear Res.* 1997;40:1245–1260
114. Glade MJ. *Diagnostic and Therapeutic Technology Assessment: Speech Therapy in Patients With a Prior History of Recurrent Acute or Chronic Otitis Media With Effusion*. Chicago, IL: American Medical Association; 1996:1–14
115. Casby MW. Otitis media and language development: a meta-analysis. *Am J Speech Lang Pathol.* 2001;10:65–80
116. Maw R, Wilks J, Harvey I, Peters TJ, Golding J. Early surgery compared with watchful waiting for glue ear and effect on language development in preschool children: a randomised trial. *Lancet.* 1999;353:960–963
117. Coplan J. *Early Language Milestone Scale*. 2nd ed. Austin, TX: PRO-ED; 1983
118. Fenson L, Dale PS, Reznick JS, et al. *MacArthur Communicative Development Inventories. User's Guide and Technical Manual*. San Diego, CA: Singular Publishing Group; 1993
119. Rescoria L. The Language Development Survey: a screening tool for delayed language in toddlers. *J Speech Hear Dis.* 1989;54:587–599
120. Frankenburg WK, Dodds JA, Faucal A, et al. *Denver Developmental Screening Test II*. Denver, CO: University of Colorado Press; 1990
121. Klee T, Pearce K, Carson DK. Improving the positive predictive value of screening for developmental language disorder. *J Speech Lang Hear Res.* 2000;43:821–833
122. Shekelle PG, Ortiz E, Rhodes S, et al. Validity of the Agency for Healthcare Research and Quality clinical practice guidelines: how quickly do guidelines become outdated? *JAMA.* 2001;286:1461–1467
123. Zielhuis GA, Straatman H, Rach GH, van den Broek P. Analysis and presentation of data on the natural course of otitis media with effusion in children. *Int J Epidemiol.* 1990;19:1037–1044
124. MRC Multi-centre Otitis Media Study Group. Risk factors for persistence of bilateral otitis media with effusion. *Clin Otolaryngol.* 2001;26:147–156
125. van Balen FA, De Melker RA. Persistent otitis media with effusion: can it be predicted? A family practice follow-up study in children aged 6 months to 6 years. *J Fam Pract.* 2000;49:605–611
126. Sano S, Kamide Y, Schachern PA, Paparella MM. Micropathologic changes of pars tensa in children with otitis media with effusion. *Arch Otolaryngol Head Neck Surg.* 1994;120:815–819
127. Yellon RF, Doyle WJ, Whiteside TL, Diven WF, March AR, Fireman P. Cytokines, immunoglobulins, and bacterial pathogens in middle ear effusions. *Arch Otolaryngol Head Neck Surg.* 1995;121:865–869
128. Maw RA, Bawden R. Tympanic membrane atrophy, scarring, atelectasis and attic retraction in persistent, untreated otitis media with effusion and following ventilation tube insertion. *Int J Pediatr Otorhinolaryngol.* 1994;30:189–204
129. Davis JM, Elfenbein J, Schum R, Bentler RA. Effects of mild and moderate hearing impairment on language, educational, and psychosocial behavior of children. *J Speech Hear Disord.* 1986;51:53–62
130. Carney AE, Moeller MP. Treatment efficacy: hearing loss in children. *J Speech Lang Hear Res.* 1998;41:S61–S84
131. Karchmer MA, Allen TE. The functional assessment of deaf and hard of hearing students. *Am Ann Deaf.* 1999;144:68–77
132. Bess FH, Dodd-Murphy J, Parker RA. Children with minimal sensorineural hearing loss: prevalence, educational performance, and functional status. *Ear Hear.* 1998;19:339–354
133. Roberts JE, Burchinal MR, Jackson SC, et al. Otitis media in early childhood in relation to preschool language and school readiness skills among black children. *Pediatrics.* 2000;106:725–735
134. Haggard MP, Birkin JA, Browning GG, Gatehouse S, Lewis S. Behavior problems in otitis media. *Pediatr Infect Dis J.* 1994;13:S43–S50
135. Bennett KE, Haggard MP. Behaviour and cognitive outcomes from middle ear disease. *Arch Dis Child.* 1999;80:28–35
136. Bennett KE, Haggard MP, Silva PA, Stewart IA. Behaviour and developmental effects of otitis media with effusion into the teens. *Arch Dis Child.* 2001;85:91–95
137. Wilks J, Maw R, Peters TJ, Harvey I, Golding J. Randomised controlled trial of early surgery versus watchful waiting for glue ear: the effect on behavioural problems in pre-school children. *Clin Otolaryngol.* 2000;25:209–214
138. Rosenfeld RM, Bhaya MH, Bower CM, et al. Impact of tympanostomy tubes on child quality of life. *Arch Otolaryngol Head Neck Surg.* 2000;126:585–592
139. Rosenfeld RM, Bluestone CD. Clinical efficacy of surgical therapy. In: Rosenfeld RM, Bluestone CD, eds. *Evidence-Based Otitis Media*. 2nd ed. Hamilton, ON, Canada: BC Decker; 2003:227–240
140. Kuyvenhoven MM, De Melker RA. Referrals to specialists. An exploratory investigation of referrals by 13 general practitioners to medical and surgical departments. *Scand J Prim Health Care.* 1990;8:53–57
141. Haldis TA, Blankenship JC. Telephone reporting in the consultant-generalist relationship. *J Eval Clin Pract.* 2002;8:31–35
142. Reichman S. The generalist's patient and the subspecialist. *Am J Manag Care.* 2002;8:79–82
143. Gates GA, Avery CA, Prihoda TJ, Cooper JC Jr. Effectiveness of adenoidectomy and tympanostomy tubes in the treatment of chronic otitis media with effusion. *N Engl J Med.* 1987;317:1444–1451
144. Mandel EM, Rockette HE, Bluestone CD, Paradise JL, Nozza RJ. Myringotomy with and without tympanostomy tubes for chronic otitis media with effusion. *Arch Otolaryngol Head Neck Surg.* 1989;115:1217–1224
145. Mandel EM, Rockette HE, Bluestone CD, Paradise JL, Nozza RJ. Efficacy of myringotomy with and without tympanostomy tubes for chronic otitis media with effusion. *Pediatr Infect Dis J.* 1992;11:270–277
146. University of York Centre for Reviews and Dissemination. The treatment of persistent glue ear in children. *Eff Health Care.* 1992;4:1–16
147. Rovers MM, Straatman H, Ingels K, van der Wilt GJ, van den Broek P, Zielhuis GA. The effect of short-term ventilation tubes versus watchful waiting on hearing in young children with persistent otitis media with effusion: a randomized trial. *Ear Hear.* 2001;22:191–199

148. Paradise JL, Bluestone CD, Colborn DK, et al. Adenoidectomy and adenotonsillectomy for recurrent acute otitis media: parallel randomized clinical trials in children not previously treated with tympanostomy tubes. *JAMA.* 1999;282:945–953
149. Boston M, McCook J, Burke B, Derkay C. Incidence of and risk factors for additional tympanostomy tube insertion in children. *Arch Otolaryngol Head Neck Surg.* 2003;129:293–296
150. Coyte PC, Croxford R, McIsaac W, Feldman W, Friedberg J. The role of adjuvant adenoidectomy and tonsillectomy in the outcome of insertion of tympanostomy tubes. *N Engl J Med.* 2001;344:1188–1195
151. Paradise JL, Bluestone CD, Rogers KD, et al. Efficacy of adenoidectomy for recurrent otitis media in children previously treated with tympanostomy-tube placement. Results of parallel randomized and nonrandomized trials. *JAMA.* 1990;263:2066–2073
152. Maw AR. Chronic otitis media with effusion (glue ear) and adenotonsillectomy: prospective randomised controlled study. *Br Med J (Clin Res Ed).* 1983;287:1586–1588
153. Cohen D, Schechter Y, Slatkine M, Gatt N, Perez R. Laser myringotomy in different age groups. *Arch Otolaryngol Head Neck Surg.* 2001;127: 260–264
154. Holzman RS. Morbidity and mortality in pediatric anesthesia. *Pediatr Clin North Am.* 1994;41:239–256
155. Cottrell JE, Golden S. *Under the Mask: A Guide to Feeling Secure and Comfortable During Anesthesia and Surgery.* New Brunswick, NJ: Rutgers University Press; 2001
156. Kay DJ, Nelson M, Rosenfeld RM. Meta-analysis of tympanostomy tube sequelae. *Otolaryngol Head Neck Surg.* 2001;124:374–380
157. Crysdale WS, Russel D. Complications of tonsillectomy and adenoidectomy in 9409 children observed overnight. *CMAJ.* 1986;135: 1139–1142
158. Harrison H, Fixsen A, Vickers A. A randomized comparison of homeopathic and standard care for the treatment of glue ear in children. *Complement Ther Med.* 1999;7:132–135
159. Sawyer CE, Evans RL, Boline PD, Branson R, Spicer A. A feasibility study of chiropractic spinal manipulation versus sham spinal manipulation for chronic otitis media with effusion in children. *J Manipulative Physiol Ther.* 1999;22:292–298
160. Ernst E. Serious adverse effects of unconventional therapies for children and adolescents: a systematic review of recent evidence. *Eur J Pediatr.* 2003;162:72–80
161. Cohen MH, Eisenberg DM. Potential physician malpractice liability associated with complementary and integrative medical therapies. *Ann Intern Med.* 2002;136:596–603
162. Mullins RJ, Heddle R. Adverse reactions associated with echinacea: the Australian experience. *Ann Allergy Asthma Immunol.* 2002;88:42–51
163. Miller LG, Hume A, Harris IM, et al. White paper on herbal products. American College of Clinical Pharmacy. *Pharmacotherapy.* 2000;20: 877–891
164. Angell M, Kassirer JP. Alternative medicine—the risks of untested and unregulated remedies. *N Engl J Med.* 1998;339:839–841
165. Fallon JM. The role of chiropractic adjustment in the care and treatment of 332 children with otitis media. *J Clin Chiropractic Pediatr.* 1997;2:167–183
166. Shafrir Y, Kaufman BA. Quadriplegia after chiropractic manipulation in an infant with congenital torticollis caused by a spinal cord astrocytoma. *J Pediatr.* 1992;120:266–269
167. Corey JP, Adham RE, Abbass AH, Seligman I. The role of IgE-mediated hypersensitivity in otitis media with effusion. *Am J Otolaryngol.* 1994;15:138–144
168. Bernstein JM. Role of allergy in eustachian tube blockage and otitis media with effusion: a review. *Otolaryngol Head Neck Surg.* 1996;114: 562–568
169. Ishii TM, Toriyama M, Suzuki JI. Histopathological study of otitis media with effusion. *Ann Otol Rhinol Laryngol.* 1980;89(suppl):83–86
170. Hurst DS, Venge P. Evidence of eosinophil, neutrophil, and mast-cell mediators in the effusion of OME patients with and without atopy. *Allergy.* 2000;55:435–441
171. Hurst DS, Venge P. The impact of atopy on neutrophil activity in middle ear effusion from children and adults with chronic otitis media. *Arch Otolaryngol Head Neck Surg.* 2002;128:561–566
172. Hurst DS. Allergy management of refractory serous otitis media. *Otolaryngol Head Neck Surg.* 1990;102:664–669

Otitis Media Clinical Practice Guidelines Quick Reference Tools

- Action Statement Summary
  - —The Diagnosis and Management of Acute Otitis Media
  - —Otitis Media With Effusion
- *ICD-10-CM* Coding Quick Reference for Otitis Media
- Bonus Feature
  - —Continuum Model for Otitis Media
- AAP Patient Education Handouts
  - —*Acute Ear Infections and Your Child*
  - —*Middle Ear Fluid and Your Child*

Action Statement Summary

The Diagnosis and Management of Acute Otitis Media

Key Action Statement 1A

Clinicians should diagnose acute otitis media (AOM) in children who present with moderate to severe bulging of the tympanic membrane (TM) *or* new onset of otorrhea not due to acute otitis externa. Evidence Quality: Grade B. Strength: Recommendation.

Key Action Statement 1B

Clinicians should diagnose AOM in children who present with mild bulging of the TM *and* recent (less than 48 hours) onset of ear pain (holding, tugging, rubbing of the ear in a nonverbal child) or intense erythema of the TM. Evidence Quality: Grade C. Strength: Recommendation.

Key Action Statement 1C

Clinicians should not diagnose AOM in children who do not have middle ear effusion (MEE) (based on pneumatic otoscopy and/or tympanometry). Evidence Quality: Grade B. Strength: Recommendation.

Key Action Statement 2

The management of AOM should include an assessment of pain. If pain is present, the clinician should recommend treatment to reduce pain. Evidence Quality: Grade B. Strength: Strong Recommendation.

Key Action Statement 3A

Severe AOM: The clinician should prescribe antibiotic therapy for AOM (bilateral or unilateral) in children 6 months and older with severe signs or symptoms (ie, moderate or severe otalgia or otalgia for at least 48 hours or temperature 39°C [102.2°F] or higher). Evidence Quality: Grade B. Strength: Strong Recommendation.

Key Action Statement 3B

Nonsevere bilateral AOM in young children: The clinician should prescribe antibiotic therapy for bilateral AOM in children 6 months through 23 months of age without severe signs or symptoms (ie, mild otalgia for less than 48 hours and temperature less than 39°C [102.2°F]). Evidence Quality: Grade B. Strength: Recommendation.

Key Action Statement 3C

Nonsevere unilateral AOM in young children: The clinician should either prescribe antibiotic therapy *or* offer observation with close follow-up based on joint decision-making with the parent(s)/caregiver for unilateral AOM in children 6 months to 23 months of age without severe signs or symptoms (ie, mild otalgia for less than 48 hours and temperature less than 39°C [102.2°F]). When observation is used, a mechanism must be in place to ensure follow-up and begin antibiotic therapy if the child worsens or fails to improve within 48 to 72 hours of onset of symptoms. Evidence Quality: Grade B. Strength: Recommendation.

Key Action Statement 3D

Nonsevere AOM in older children: The clinician should either prescribe antibiotic therapy *or* offer observation with close follow-up based on joint decision-making with the parent(s)/caregiver for AOM (bilateral or unilateral) in children 24 months or older without severe signs or symptoms (ie, mild otalgia for less than 48 hours and temperature less than 39°C [102.2°F]). When observation is used, a mechanism must be in place to ensure follow-up and begin antibiotic therapy if the child worsens or fails to improve within 48 to 72 hours of onset of symptoms. Evidence Quality: Grade B. Strength: Recommendation.

Key Action Statement 4A

Clinicians should prescribe amoxicillin for AOM when a decision to treat with antibiotics has been made *and* the child has not received amoxicillin in the past 30 days *or* the child does not have concurrent purulent conjunctivitis *or* the child is not allergic to penicillin. Evidence Quality: Grade B. Strength: Recommendation.

Key Action Statement 4B

Clinicians should prescribe an antibiotic with additional β-lactamase coverage for AOM when a decision to treat with antibiotics has been made, *and* the child has received amoxicillin in the last 30 days *or* has concurrent purulent conjunctivitis, *or* has a history of recurrent AOM unresponsive to amoxicillin. Evidence Quality: Grade C. Strength: Recommendation.

Key Action Statement 4C

Clinicians should reassess the patient if the caregiver reports that the child's symptoms have worsened or failed to respond to the initial antibiotic treatment within 48 to 72 hours and determine whether a change in therapy is needed. Evidence Quality: Grade B. Strength: Recommendation.

Key Action Statement 5A
Clinicians should not prescribe prophylactic antibiotics to reduce the frequency of episodes of AOM in children with recurrent AOM. Evidence Quality: Grade B. Strength: Recommendation.

Key Action Statement 5B
Clinicians may offer tympanostomy tubes for recurrent AOM (3 episodes in 6 months or 4 episodes in 1 year with 1 episode in the preceding 6 months). Evidence Quality: Grade B. Strength: Option.

Key Action Statement 6A
Clinicians should recommend pneumococcal conjugate vaccine to all children according to the schedule of the Advisory Committee on Immunization Practices of the Centers for Disease Control and prevention, American Academy of Pediatrics (AAP), and American Academy of Family Physicians (AAFP). Evidence Quality: Grade B. Strength: Strong Recommendation.

Otitis Media With Effusion

1A. Pneumatic Otoscopy
Clinicians should use pneumatic otoscopy as the primary diagnostic method for OME, and OME should be distinguished from AOM.

This is a strong recommendation based on systematic review of cohort studies and the preponderance of benefit over harm.

1B. Tympanometry
Tympanometry can be used to confirm the diagnosis a of OME.

This option is based on cohort studies and a balance of benefit and harm.

1C. Screening
Population-based screening programs for OME are not recommended in healthy, asymptomatic children.

This recommendation is based on randomized, controlled trials and cohort studies, with a preponderance of harm over benefit.

2. Documentation
Clinicians should document the laterality, duration of effusion, and presence and severity of associated symptoms at each assessment of the child with OME.

This recommendation is based on observational studies and strong preponderance of benefit over harm.

3. Child at Risk
Clinicians should distinguish the child with OME who is at risk for speech, language, or learning problems from other children with OME and should evaluate hearing, speech, language, and need for intervention more promptly.

This recommendation is based on case series, the preponderance of benefit over harm, and ethical limitations in studying children with OME who are at risk.

4. Watchful Waiting
Clinicians should manage the child with OME who is not at risk with watchful waiting for 3 months from the date of effusion onset (if known) or diagnosis (if onset is unknown).

This recommendation is based on systematic review of cohort studies and the preponderance of benefit over harm.

5. Medication
Antihistamines and decongestants are ineffective for OME and are not recommended for treatment; antimicrobials and corticosteroids do not have long-term efficacy and are not recommended for routine management.

This recommendation is based on systematic review of randomized, controlled trials and the preponderance of harm over benefit.

6. Hearing and Language
Hearing testing is recommended when OME persists for 3 months or longer or at any time that language delay, learning problems, or a significant hearing loss is suspected in a child with OME; language testing should be conducted for children with hearing loss.

This recommendation is based on cohort studies and the preponderance of benefit over risk.

7. Surveillance
Children with persistent OME who are not at risk should be reexamined at 3- to 6-month intervals until the effusion is no longer present, significant hearing loss is identified, or structural abnormalities of the eardrum or middle ear are suspected.

This recommendation is based on randomized, controlled trials and observational studies with a preponderance of benefit over harm.

8. Referral
When children with OME are referred by the primary care clinician for evaluation by an otolaryngologist, audiologist, or speech-language pathologist, the referring clinician should document the effusion duration and specific reason for referral (evaluation, surgery) and provide additional relevant information such as history of AOM and developmental status of the child.

This option is based on panel consensus and a preponderance of benefit over harm.

9. Surgery
When a child becomes a surgical candidate, tympanostomy tube insertion is the preferred initial procedure; adenoidectomy should not be performed unless a distinct indication exists (nasal obstruction, chronic adenoiditis). Repeat surgery consists of adenoidectomy plus myringotomy, with or without tube insertion. tonsillectomy alone or myringotomy alone should not be used to treat OME.

This recommendation is based on randomized, controlled trials with a preponderance of benefit over harm.

10. CAM
No recommendation is made regarding CAM as a treatment for OME.

There is no recommendation based on lack of scientific evidence documenting efficacy and an uncertain balance of harm and benefit.

11. Allergy Management
No recommendation is made regarding allergy management as a treatment for OME.

There is no recommendation based on insufficient evidence of therapeutic efficacy or a causal relationship between allergy and OME.

Coding Quick Reference for Otitis Media

ICD-10-CM	
H65.01	Acute serous otitis media, right ear
H65.02	Left ear
H65.03	Bilateral
H65.04	Recurrent, right ear
H65.05	Recurrent, left ear
H65.06	Recurrent, bilateral
H65.21	Chronic serous otitis media, right ear
H65.22	Left ear
H65.23	Bilateral
H65.91	Unspecified nonsuppurative otitis media, right ear
H65.92	Left ear
H65.93	Bilateral
H66.001	Acute suppurative otitis media without spontaneous rupture of ear drum, right ear
H66.002	Left ear
H66.003	Bilateral
H66.004	Recurrent, right ear
H66.005	Recurrent, left ear
H66.006	Recurrent, bilateral
H66.011	Acute suppurative otitis media with spontaneous rupture of ear drum, right ear
H66.012	Left ear
H66.013	Bilateral
H66.014	Recurrent, right ear
H66.015	Recurrent, left ear
H66.016	Recurrent, bilateral
H67.1	Otitis media in diseases classified elsewhere, right ear
H67.2	Left ear
H67.3	Bilateral
H66.3X1	Other chronic suppurative otitis media, right ear
H66.3X2	Left ear
H66.3X3	Bilateral

Continuum Model for Otitis Media

The following continuum model from *Coding for Pediatrics 2020* has been devised to express the various levels of service for otitis media. This model demonstrates the cumulative effect of the key criteria for each level of service using a single diagnosis as the common denominator. It also shows the importance of other variables, such as patient age, duration and severity of illness, social contexts, and comorbid conditions, that often have key roles in pediatric cases.

Quick Reference for Codes Used in Continuum for Otitis Media—Established Patients

E/M Code Level	History	Examination	MDM	Time
99211[a]	NA	NA	NA	5 min
99212	Problem-focused	Problem-focused	Straightforward	10 min
99213	Problem-focused	Expanded problem-focused	Low	15 min
99214	Detailed	Detailed	Moderate	25 min
99215	Detailed	Detailed	High	40 min

Abbreviations: E/M, evaluation and management; MDM; medical decision-making; NA, not applicable.

[a] Low level E/M service that may not require the presence of a physician.

Adapted from American Academy of Pediatrics. *Coding for Pediatrics 2020: A Manual for Pediatric Documentation and Payment.* 25th ed. Itasca, IL: American Academy of Pediatrics; 2020.

CPT® copyright 2019 American Medical Association. All rights reserved.

Continuum Model for Otitis Media

Code selection at any level above 99211 may be based on time when documentation states that more than 50% of the total face-to-face time of the encounter is spent in counseling and/or coordination of care. Select the code with the typical time closest to the total face-to-face time.

CPT® Code Vignette	History	Physical Examination (systems)	Medical Decision-making (diagnoses, data, risk)
99211 Clinical staff evaluations Follow-up on serous fluid or hearing loss with tympanogram (Be sure to code tympanogram [**92567**] and/or audiogram [**92551** series] in addition to **99211**.)	No specific key components required. Must indicate continuation of physician's plan of care, medical necessity, assessment, and/or education provided. CC: Follow-up on serous fluid OR on hearing loss. HPI: Mom reports medication completed and previous symptoms resolved. Assessment: Problem resolved. Follow-up with physician for recommended preventive service.		
99212 Follow-up otitis media, uncomplicated	**Problem focused** CC: Follow-up otitis media HPI: History of treatment, difficulties with medication, hearing status	**Problem focused** 1. ENMT	**Straightforward** 1. One established problem, improved 2. No tests ordered/data reviewed 3. Risk: No need for further follow-up
99213 2-year-old presents with tugging at her right ear. Afebrile. Mild otitis media.	**Problem focused** CC: Tugging at right ear HPI: Duration, associated signs/symptoms, and home management, including over-the-counter medications, and response ROS: Constitutional, eyes, ENMT, gastrointestinal, genitourinary	**Expanded problem focused** 1. ENMT 2. Conjunctiva 3. Overall appearance	**Low complexity** 1. Minor problem 2. No tests ordered/data reviewed 3. Risk: Observation and nonprescription analgesics
99214 Infant presents for suspected third episode of otitis media within 3 months. Infant presents with fever and cough.	**Detailed** CC: Fever and cough, suspected otitis media HPI: Duration, severity of fever, other symptoms, modifying factor (medication) ROS: Constitutional, eyes, ENMT, respiratory, gastrointestinal, urinary PSFH: Allergies, frequency of similar infection in past and response to treatment, environmental factors (eg, tobacco exposure, child care), immunization status	**Detailed** 1. Constitutional 2. Eyes 3. ENMT 4. Lungs 5. Skin	**Moderate complexity** 1. Established problem, not responding to management 2. Hearing evaluation planned 3. Risk: Prescription drug management
99215 3-month-old presents with high fever, vomiting, irritability.	**Detailed** CC: Fever, vomiting, irritability HPI: Severity of fever, quality of irritability, duration of symptoms, and modifying factors ROS: Constitutional, eyes, ENMT, respiratory, gastrointestinal, genitourinary PFSH: Medications, allergies, frequency of similar infection in past and response to treatment, environmental factors (eg, tobacco exposure, child care)	**Comprehensive** 1. Overall appearance, hydration status 2. Head 3. Eyes 4. ENMT 5. Neck 6. Cardiovascular 7. Respiratory 8. Skin	**High complexity** 1. New problem with additional work-up planned. 2. Tests ordered: Complete blood cell count with differential, blood culture, blood urea nitrogen, creatinine, electrolytes, urinalysis with culture, chest radiograph, and possible lumbar puncture. 3. Risk: Consider admission to NICU.

Continuum Model for Otitis Media (*continued*)

Code selection at any level above **99211** may be based on time when documentation states that more than 50% of the total face-to-face time of the encounter is spent in counseling and/or coordination of care. Select the code with the typical time closest to the total face-to-face time.

CPT® Code Vignette	History	Physical Examination (systems)	Medical Decision-making (diagnoses, data, risk)
99214 or **99215** **NOTE:** Depending on the variables (ie, time), this example could be reported as **99214** or **99215**. Extended evaluation of child with chronic or recurrent otitis media	Documentation of total face-to-face time and >50% of time spent in extensive discussion of treatment options, including, but not limited to 1. Continued episodic treatment with antibiotics 2. Myringotomy and tube placement 3. Adenoidectomy 4. Allergy evaluation 5. Steroid therapy with weighing of risk to benefit ratio of various therapies **NOTE:** Time is the key factor when counseling and/or coordination of care are more than 50% of the face-to-face time with the patient. For **99214**, the total visit time would be 25 minutes; for **99215**, the total time is 40 minutes. You must document time spent on counseling and/or coordination of care and include the areas discussed.		

Abbreviations: CC, chief complaint; CPT, Current Procedural Terminology; ENMT, ears, nose, throat, mouth; HPI, history of present illness; PFSH, past, family, and social history; ROS, review of systems.

Acute Ear Infections and Your Child

Next to the common cold, an ear infection is the most common childhood illness. In fact, most children have at least one ear infection by the time they are 3 years old. Many ear infections clear up without causing any lasting problems.

The following is information from the American Academy of Pediatrics about the symptoms, treatments, and possible complications of acute *otitis media*, a common infection of the middle ear.

How do ear infections develop?

The ear has 3 parts—the outer ear, middle ear, and inner ear. A narrow channel (eustachian tube) connects the middle ear to the back of the nose. When a child has a cold, nose or throat infection, or allergy, the mucus and fluid can enter the eustachian tube causing a buildup of fluid in the middle ear. If bacteria or a virus infects this fluid, it can cause swelling and pain in the ear. This type of ear infection is called *acute otitis media* (*middle ear inflammation*).

Often after the symptoms of acute otitis media clear up, fluid remains in the ear, creating another kind of ear problem called *otitis media with effusion* (*middle ear fluid*). This condition is harder to detect than acute otitis media because except for the fluid and usually some mild hearing loss, there is often no pain or other symptoms present. This fluid may last several months and, in most cases, disappears on its own. The child's hearing then returns to normal.

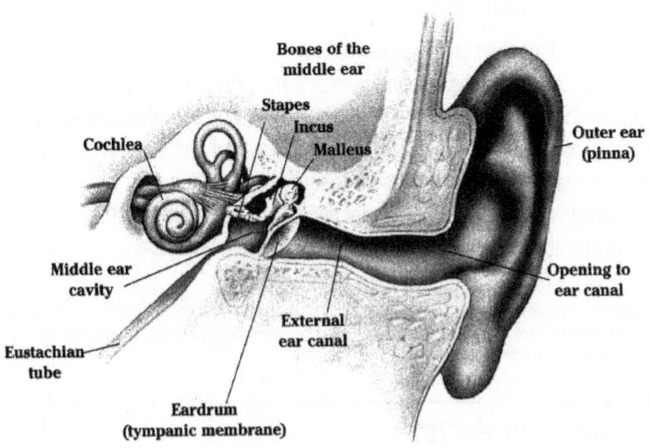

Cross-Section of the Ear

Is my child at risk for developing an ear infection?

Risk factors for developing childhood ear infections include

- **Age.** Infants and young children are more likely to get ear infections than older children. The size and shape of an infant's eustachian tube makes it easier for an infection to develop. Ear infections occur most often in children between 6 months and 3 years of age. Also, the younger a child is at the time of the first ear infection, the greater the chance he will have repeated infections.
- **Family history.** Ear infections can run in families. Children are more likely to have repeated middle ear infections if a parent or sibling also had repeated ear infections.
- **Colds.** Colds often lead to ear infections. Children in group child care settings have a higher chance of passing their colds to each other because they are exposed to more viruses from the other children.
- **Tobacco smoke.** Children who breathe in someone else's tobacco smoke have a higher risk of developing health problems, including ear infections.

How can I reduce the risk of an ear infection?

Some things you can do to help reduce your child's risk of getting an ear infection are

- Breastfeed instead of bottle-feed. Breastfeeding may decrease the risk of frequent colds and ear infections.
- Keep your child away from tobacco smoke, especially in your home or car.
- Throw away pacifiers or limit to daytime use, *if your child is older than 1 year.*
- Keep vaccinations up to date. Vaccines against bacteria (such as pneumococcal vaccine) and viruses (such as influenza vaccine) reduce the number of ear infections in children with frequent infections.

What are the symptoms of an ear infection?

Your child may have many symptoms during an ear infection. Talk with your pediatrician about the best way to treat your child's symptoms.

- **Pain.** The most common symptom of an ear infection is pain. Older children can tell you that their ears hurt. Younger children may only seem irritable and cry. You may notice this more during feedings because sucking and swallowing may cause painful pressure changes in the middle ear.
- **Loss of appetite.** Your child may have less of an appetite because of the ear pain.
- **Trouble sleeping.** Your child may have trouble sleeping because of the ear pain.
- **Fever.** Your child may have a temperature ranging from 100°F (normal) to 104°F.

- **Ear drainage.** You might notice yellow or white fluid, possibly blood-tinged, draining from your child's ear. The fluid may have a foul odor and will look different from normal earwax (which is orange-yellow or reddish-brown). Pain and pressure often decrease after this drainage begins, but this doesn't always mean that the infection is going away. If this happens it's not an emergency, but your child will need to see your pediatrician.
- **Trouble hearing.** During and after an ear infection, your child may have trouble hearing for several weeks. This occurs because the fluid behind the eardrum gets in the way of sound transmission. This is usually temporary and clears up after the fluid from the middle ear drains away.

Important: Your doctor *cannot* diagnose an ear infection over the phone; your child's eardrum must be examined by your doctor to confirm fluid buildup and signs of inflammation.

What causes ear pain?

There are other reasons why your child's ears may hurt besides an ear infection. The following can cause ear pain:

- An infection of the skin of the ear canal, often called "swimmer's ear"
- Reduced pressure in the middle ear from colds or allergies
- A sore throat
- Teething or sore gums
- Inflammation of the eardrum alone during a cold (without fluid buildup)

How are ear infections treated?

Because pain is often the first and most uncomfortable symptom of an ear infection, it's important to help comfort your child by giving her pain medicine. Acetaminophen and ibuprofen are over-the-counter (OTC) pain medicines that may help decrease much of the pain. Be sure to use the right dosage for your child's age and size. *Don't give aspirin to your child.* It has been associated with Reye syndrome, a disease that affects the liver and brain. There are also ear drops that may relieve ear pain for a short time. Ask your pediatrician whether these drops should be used. There is no need to use OTC cold medicines (decongestants and antihistamines), because they don't help clear up ear infections.

Not all ear infections require antibiotics. Some children who don't have a high fever and aren't severely ill may be observed without antibiotics. In most cases, pain and fever will improve in the first 1 to 2 days.

If your child is younger than 2 years, has drainage from the ear, has a fever higher than 102.5°F, seems to be in a lot of pain, is unable to sleep, isn't eating, or is acting ill, it's important to call your pediatrician. If your child is older than 2 years and your child's symptoms are mild, you may wait a couple of days to see if she improves.

Your child's ear pain and fever should improve or go away within 3 days of their onset. If your child's condition doesn't improve within 3 days, or worsens at any time, call your pediatrician. Your pediatrician may wish to see your child and may prescribe an antibiotic to take by mouth, if one wasn't given initially. If an antibiotic was already started, your child may need a different antibiotic. Be sure to follow your pediatrician's instructions closely.

If an antibiotic was prescribed, make sure your child finishes the entire prescription. If you stop the medicine too soon, some of the bacteria that caused the ear infection may still be present and cause an infection to start all over again.

As the infection starts to clear up, your child might feel a "popping" in the ears. This is a normal sign of healing. Children with ear infections don't need to stay home if they are feeling well, as long as a child care provider or someone at school can give them their medicine properly, if needed. If your child needs to travel in an airplane, or wants to swim, contact your pediatrician for specific instructions.

What are signs of hearing problems?

Because your child can have trouble hearing without other symptoms of an ear infection, watch for the following changes in behavior (especially during or after a cold):

- Talking more loudly or softly than usual
- Saying "huh?" or "what?" more than usual
- Not responding to sounds
- Having trouble understanding speech in noisy rooms
- Listening with the TV or radio turned up louder than usual

If you think your child may have difficulty hearing, call your pediatrician. Being able to hear and listen to others talk helps a child learn speech and language. This is especially important during the first few years of life.

Are there complications from ear infections?

Although it's very rare, complications from ear infections can develop, including the following:

- An infection of the inner ear that causes dizziness and imbalance (labyrinthitis)
- An infection of the skull behind the ear (mastoiditis)
- Scarring or thickening of the eardrum
- Loss of feeling or movement in the face (facial paralysis)
- Permanent hearing loss

It's normal for children to have several ear infections when they are young—even as many as 2 separate infections within a few months. Most ear infections that develop in children are minor. Recurring ear infections may be a nuisance, but they usually clear up without any lasting problems. With proper care and treatment, ear infections can usually be managed successfully. But, if your child has one ear infection after another for several months, you may want to talk about other treatment options with your pediatrician.

The information contained in this publication should not be used as a substitute for the medical care and advice of your pediatrician. There may be variations in treatment that your pediatrician may recommend based on individual facts and circumstances.

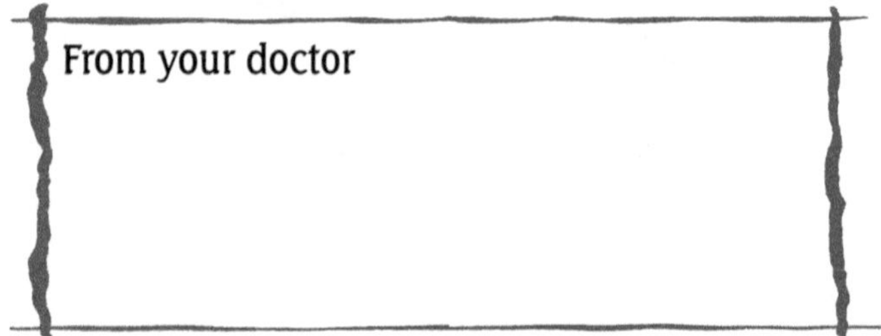

American Academy of Pediatrics

DEDICATED TO THE HEALTH OF ALL CHILDREN™

The American Academy of Pediatrics is an organization of 66,000 primary care pediatricians, pediatric medical subspecialists, and pediatric surgical specialists dedicated to the health, safety, and well-being of infants, children, adolescents, and young adults.

American Academy of Pediatrics
Web site—www.HealthyChildren.org

© 2010 American Academy of Pediatrics, Reaffirmed 10/2017. All rights reserved.

Middle Ear Fluid and Your Child

The *middle* ear is the space behind the eardrum that is usually filled with air. When a child has middle ear fluid (otitis media with effusion), it means that a watery or mucus-like fluid has collected in the middle ear. *Otitis media* means *middle ear inflammation*, and *effusion* means *fluid*.

Middle ear fluid is **not** the same as an ear infection. An ear infection occurs when middle ear fluid is infected with viruses, bacteria, or both, often during a cold. Children with middle ear fluid have no signs or symptoms of infection. Most children don't have fever or severe pain, but may have mild discomfort or trouble hearing. About 90% of children get middle ear fluid at some time before age 5.

The following is information from the American Academy of Pediatrics about the causes, symptoms, risk reduction, testing, and treatments for middle ear fluid, as well as how middle ear fluid may affect your child's learning.

What causes middle ear fluid?

There is no one cause for middle ear fluid. Often your child's doctor may not know the cause. Middle ear fluid could be caused by

- A past ear infection
- A cold or flu
- Blockage of the eustachian tube (a narrow channel that connects the middle ear to the back of the nose)

What are the symptoms of middle ear fluid?

Many healthy children with middle ear fluid have little or no problems. They usually get better on their own. Often middle ear fluid is found at a regular checkup. Ear discomfort, if present, is usually mild. Your child may be irritable, rub his ears, or have trouble sleeping. Other symptoms include hearing loss, irritability, sleep problems, clumsiness, speech or language problems, and poor school performance. You may notice your child sitting closer to the TV or turning the sound up louder than usual. Sometimes it may seem like your child isn't paying attention to you, especially when at the playground or in a noisy environment.

Talk with your child's doctor if you are concerned about your child's hearing. Keep a record of your child's ear problems. Write down your child's name, child's doctor's name and number, date and type of ear problem or infection, treatment, and results. This may help your child's doctor find the cause of the middle ear fluid.

Can middle ear fluid affect my child's learning?

Some children with middle ear fluid are at risk for delays in speaking or may have problems with learning or schoolwork, especially children with

- Permanent hearing loss not caused by middle ear fluid
- Speech and language delays or disorders
- Developmental delay of social and communication skills disorders (for example, autism spectrum disorders)
- Syndromes that affect cognitive, speech, and language delays (for example, Down syndrome)
- Craniofacial disorders that affect cognitive, speech, and language delays (for example, cleft palate)
- Blindness or visual loss that can't be corrected

If your child is at risk and has ongoing middle ear fluid, her hearing, speech, and language should be checked.

How can I reduce the risk of middle ear fluid?

Children who live with smokers, attend group child care, or use pacifiers have more ear infections. Because some children who have middle ear infections later get middle ear fluid, you may want to

- Keep your child away from tobacco smoke.
- Keep your child away from children who are sick.
- Throw away pacifiers or limit to daytime use, *if your child is older than 1 year.*

Are there special tests to check for middle ear fluid?

Two tests that can check for middle ear fluid are *pneumatic otoscopy* and *tympanometry*. A pneumatic otoscope is the recommended test for middle ear fluid. With this tool, the doctor looks at the eardrum and uses air to see how well the eardrum moves. Tympanometry is another test for middle ear fluid that uses sound to see how well the eardrum moves. An eardrum with fluid behind it doesn't move as well as a normal eardrum. Your child must sit still for both tests; the tests are painless.

Because these tests don't check hearing level, a hearing test may be given, if needed. Hearing tests measure how well your child hears. Although hearing tests don't test for middle ear fluid, they can measure if the fluid is affecting your child's hearing level. The type of hearing test given depends on your child's age and ability to participate.

How can middle ear fluid be treated?

Middle ear fluid can be treated in several ways. Treatment options include observation and tube surgery or adenoid surgery. Because a treatment that works for one child may not work for another, your child's doctor can help you decide which treatment is best for your child and when you should see an ear, nose, and throat (ENT) specialist. If one treatment doesn't work, another treatment can be tried. Ask your child's doctor or ENT specialist about the costs, advantages, and disadvantages of each treatment.

When should middle ear fluid be treated?

Your child is more likely to need treatment for middle ear fluid if she has any of the following:

- Conditions placing her at risk for developmental delays (see "Can middle ear fluid affect my child's learning?")
- Fluid in both ears, especially if present more than 3 months
- Hearing loss or other significant symptoms (see "What are the symptoms of middle ear fluid?")

What treatments are not recommended?

A number of treatments are **not** recommended for young children with middle ear fluid.

- **Medicines** not recommended include antibiotics, decongestants, antihistamines, and steroids (by mouth or in nasal sprays). All of these have side effects and do not cure middle ear fluid.
- **Surgical treatments** not recommended include myringotomy (draining of fluid without placing a tube) and tonsillectomy (removal of the tonsils). If your child's doctor or ENT specialist suggests one of these surgeries, it may be for another medical reason. Ask your doctor why your child needs the surgery.

What about other treatment options?

There is no evidence that complementary and alternative medicine treatments or that treatment for allergies works to decrease middle ear fluid. Some of these treatments may be harmful and many are expensive.

The information contained in this publication should not be used as a substitute for the medical care and advice of your pediatrician. There may be variations in treatment that your pediatrician may recommend based on individual facts and circumstances.

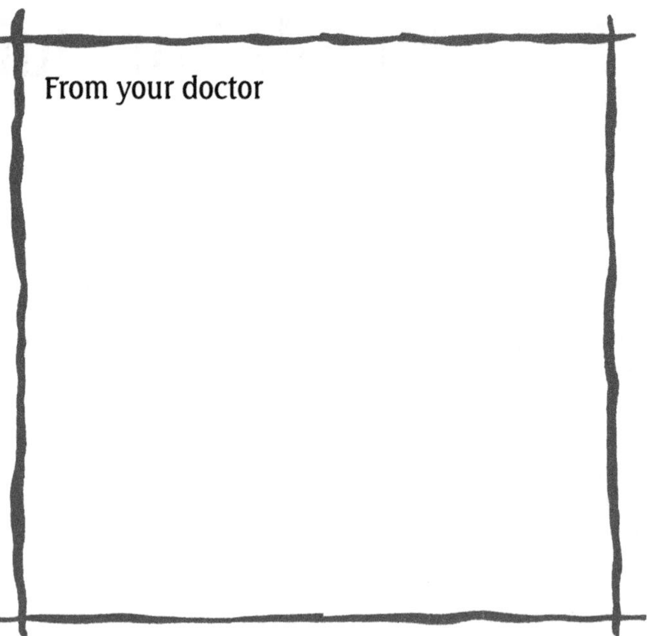

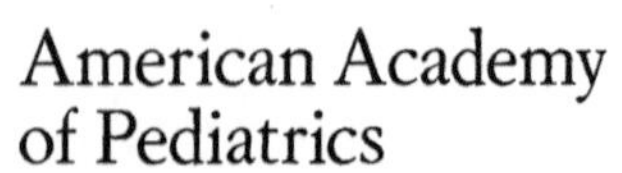

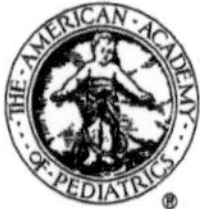

DEDICATED TO THE HEALTH OF ALL CHILDREN™

The American Academy of Pediatrics is an organization of 66,000 primary care pediatricians, pediatric medical subspecialists, and pediatric surgical specialists dedicated to the health, safety, and well-being of infants, children, adolescents, and young adults.

American Academy of Pediatrics
Web site—www.HealthyChildren.org

© 2010 American Academy of Pediatrics, Reaffirmed 10/2017. All rights reserved.

Clinical Practice Guideline for the Diagnosis and Management of Acute Bacterial Sinusitis in Children Aged 1 to 18 Years

- *Clinical Practice Guideline*
  - *PPI: AAP Partnership for Policy Implementation See Appendix 1 for more information.*

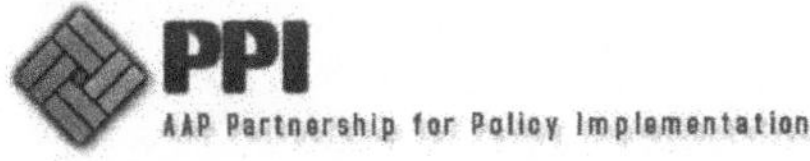

CLINICAL PRACTICE GUIDELINE

Clinical Practice Guideline for the Diagnosis and Management of Acute Bacterial Sinusitis in Children Aged 1 to 18 Years

abstract

OBJECTIVE: To update the American Academy of Pediatrics clinical practice guideline regarding the diagnosis and management of acute bacterial sinusitis in children and adolescents.

METHODS: Analysis of the medical literature published since the last version of the guideline (2001).

RESULTS: The diagnosis of acute bacterial sinusitis is made when a child with an acute upper respiratory tract infection (URI) presents with (1) persistent illness (nasal discharge [of any quality] or daytime cough or both lasting more than 10 days without improvement), (2) a worsening course (worsening or new onset of nasal discharge, daytime cough, or fever after initial improvement), or (3) severe onset (concurrent fever [temperature ≥39°C/102.2°F] and purulent nasal discharge for at least 3 consecutive days). Clinicians should not obtain imaging studies of any kind to distinguish acute bacterial sinusitis from viral URI, because they do not contribute to the diagnosis; however, a contrast-enhanced computed tomography scan of the paranasal sinuses should be obtained whenever a child is suspected of having orbital or central nervous system complications. The clinician should prescribe antibiotic therapy for acute bacterial sinusitis in children with severe onset or worsening course. The clinician should either prescribe antibiotic therapy or offer additional observation for 3 days to children with persistent illness. Amoxicillin with or without clavulanate is the first-line treatment of acute bacterial sinusitis. Clinicians should reassess initial management if there is either a caregiver report of worsening (progression of initial signs/symptoms or appearance of new signs/symptoms) or failure to improve within 72 hours of initial management. If the diagnosis of acute bacterial sinusitis is confirmed in a child with worsening symptoms or failure to improve, then clinicians may change the antibiotic therapy for the child initially managed with antibiotic or initiate antibiotic treatment of the child initially managed with observation.

CONCLUSIONS: Changes in this revision include the addition of a clinical presentation designated as "worsening course," an option to treat immediately or observe children with persistent symptoms for 3 days before treating, and a review of evidence indicating that imaging is not necessary in children with uncomplicated acute bacterial sinusitis. *Pediatrics* 2013;132:e262–e280

Ellen R. Wald, MD, FAAP, Kimberly E. Applegate, MD, MS, FAAP, Clay Bordley, MD, FAAP, David H. Darrow, MD, DDS, FAAP, Mary P. Glode, MD, FAAP, S. Michael Marcy, MD, FAAP, Carrie E. Nelson, MD, MS, Richard M. Rosenfeld, MD, FAAP, Nader Shaikh, MD, MPH, FAAP, Michael J. Smith, MD, MSCE, FAAP, Paul V. Williams, MD, FAAP, and Stuart T. Weinberg, MD, FAAP

KEY WORDS

acute bacterial sinusitis, sinusitis, antibiotics, imaging, sinus aspiration

ABBREVIATIONS

AAP—American Academy of Pediatrics
AOM—acute otitis media
CT—computed tomography
PCV-13—13-valent pneumococcal conjugate vaccine
RABS—recurrent acute bacterial sinusitis
RCT—randomized controlled trial
URI—upper respiratory tract infection

This document is copyrighted and is property of the American Academy of Pediatrics and its Board of Directors. All authors have filed conflict of interest statements with the American Academy of Pediatrics. Any conflicts have been resolved through a process approved by the Board of Directors. The American Academy of Pediatrics has neither solicited nor accepted any commercial involvement in the development of the content of this publication.

The recommendations in this report do not indicate an exclusive course of treatment or serve as a standard of medical care. Variations, taking into account individual circumstances, may be appropriate.

www.pediatrics.org/cgi/doi/10.1542/peds.2013-1071

doi:10.1542/peds.2013-1071

PEDIATRICS (ISSN Numbers: Print, 0031-4005; Online, 1098-4275).

Copyright © 2013 by the American Academy of Pediatrics

INTRODUCTION

Acute bacterial sinusitis is a common complication of viral upper respiratory infection (URI) or allergic inflammation. Using stringent criteria to define acute sinusitis, it has been observed that between 6% and 7% of children seeking care for respiratory symptoms has an illness consistent with this definition.[1–4]

This clinical practice guideline is a revision of the clinical practice guideline published by the American Academy of Pediatrics (AAP) in 2001.[5] It has been developed by a subcommittee of the Steering Committee on Quality Improvement and Management that included physicians with expertise in the fields of primary care pediatrics, academic general pediatrics, family practice, allergy, epidemiology and informatics, pediatric infectious diseases, pediatric otolaryngology, radiology, and pediatric emergency medicine. None of the participants had financial conflicts of interest, and only money from the AAP was used to fund the development of the guideline. The guideline will be reviewed in 5 years unless new evidence emerges that warrants revision sooner.

The guideline is intended for use in a variety of clinical settings (eg, office, emergency department, hospital) by clinicians who treat pediatric patients. The data on which the recommendations are based are included in a companion technical report, published in the electronic pages.[6] The Partnership for Policy Implementation has developed a series of definitions using accepted health information technology standards to assist in the implementation of this guideline in computer systems and quality measurement efforts. This document is available at: http://www2.aap.org/informatics/PPI.html.

This revision focuses on the diagnosis and management of acute sinusitis in children between 1 and 18 years of age. It does not apply to children with subacute or chronic sinusitis. Similar to the previous guideline, this document does not consider neonates and children younger than 1 year or children with anatomic abnormalities of the sinuses, immunodeficiencies, cystic fibrosis, or primary ciliary dyskinesia. The most significant areas of change from the 2001 guideline are in the addition of a clinical presentation designated as "worsening course," inclusion of new data on the effectiveness of antibiotics in children with acute sinusitis,[4] and a review of evidence indicating that imaging is not necessary to identify those children who will benefit from antimicrobial therapy.

METHODS

The Subcommittee on Management of Sinusitis met in June 2009 to identify research questions relevant to guideline revision. The primary goal was to update the 2001 report by identifying and reviewing additional studies of pediatric acute sinusitis that have been performed over the past decade.

Searches of PubMed were performed by using the same search term as in the 2001 report. All searches were limited to English-language and human studies. Three separate searches were performed to maximize retrieval of the most recent and highest-quality evidence for pediatric sinusitis. The first limited results to all randomized controlled trials (RCTs) from 1966 to 2009, the second to all meta-analyses from 1966 to 2009, and the third to all pediatric studies (limited to ages <18 years) published since the last technical report (1999–2009). Additionally, the Web of Science was queried to identify studies that cited the original AAP guidelines. This literature search was replicated in July 2010

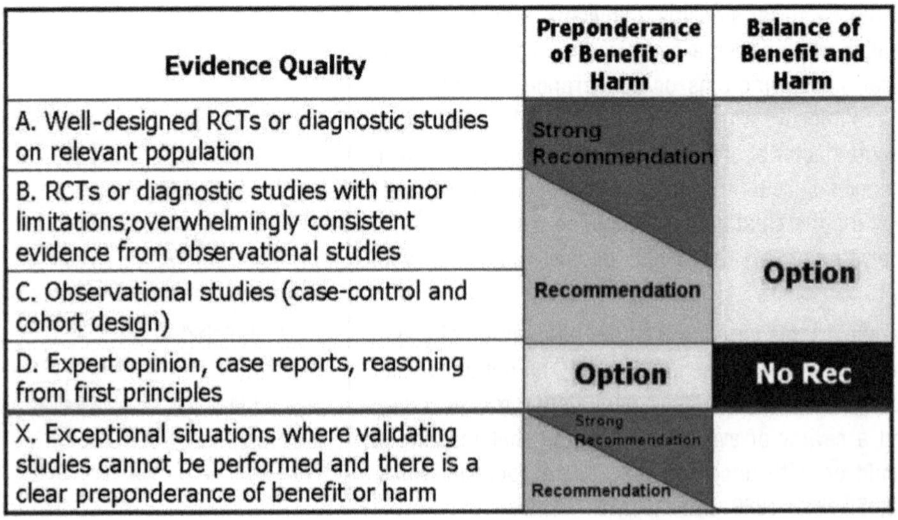

Evidence Quality	Preponderance of Benefit or Harm	Balance of Benefit and Harm
A. Well-designed RCTs or diagnostic studies on relevant population	Strong Recommendation	Option
B. RCTs or diagnostic studies with minor limitations;overwhelmingly consistent evidence from observational studies		
C. Observational studies (case-control and cohort design)	Recommendation	
D. Expert opinion, case reports, reasoning from first principles	Option	No Rec
X. Exceptional situations where validating studies cannot be performed and there is a clear preponderance of benefit or harm	Strong Recommendation / Recommendation	

FIGURE 1
Levels of recommendations. Rec, recommendation.

and November 2012 to capture recently published studies. The complete results of the literature review are published separately in the technical report.[6] In summary, 17 randomized studies of sinusitis in children were identified and reviewed. Only 3 trials met inclusion criteria. Because of significant heterogeneity among these studies, formal meta-analyses were not pursued.

The results from the literature review were used to guide development of the key action statements included in this document. These action statements were generated by using BRIDGE-Wiz (Building Recommendations in a Developers Guideline Editor, Yale School of Medicine, New Haven, CT), an interactive software tool that leads guideline development through a series of questions that are intended to create a more actionable set of key action statements.[7] BRIDGE-Wiz also incorporates the quality of available evidence into the final determination of the strength of each recommendation.

The AAP policy statement "Classifying Recommendations for Clinical Practice Guidelines" was followed in designating levels of recommendations (Fig 1).[8] Definitions of evidence-based statements are provided in Table 1. This guideline was reviewed by multiple groups in the AAP and 2 external organizations. Comments were compiled and reviewed by the subcommittee, and relevant changes were incorporated into the guideline.

KEY ACTION STATEMENTS

Key Action Statement 1

Clinicians should make a presumptive diagnosis of acute bacterial sinusitis when a child with an acute URI presents with the following:

- **Persistent illness, ie, nasal discharge (of any quality) or daytime cough or both lasting more than 10 days without improvement;**

OR

- **Worsening course, ie, worsening or new onset of nasal discharge, daytime cough, or fever after initial improvement;**

OR

- **Severe onset, ie, concurrent fever (temperature ≥39°C/102.2°F) and purulent nasal discharge for at least 3 consecutive days (Evidence Quality: B; Recommendation).**

KAS Profile 1

Aggregate evidence quality: B	
Benefit	Diagnosis allows decisions regarding management to be made. Children likely to benefit from antimicrobial therapy will be identified.
Harm	Inappropriate diagnosis may lead to unnecessary treatment. A missed diagnosis may lead to persistent infection or complications
Cost	Inappropriate diagnosis may lead to unnecessary cost of antibiotics. A missed diagnosis leads to cost of persistent illness (loss of time from school and work) or cost of caring for complications.
Benefits-harm assessment	Preponderance of benefit.
Value judgments	None.
Role of patient preference	Limited.
Intentional vagueness	None.
Exclusions	Children aged <1 year or older than 18 years and with underlying conditions.
Strength	Recommendation.

TABLE 1 Guideline Definitions for Evidence-Based Statements

Statement	Definition	Implication
Strong recommendation	A strong recommendation in favor of a particular action is made when the anticipated benefits of the recommended intervention clearly exceed the harms (as a strong recommendation against an action is made when the anticipated harms clearly exceed the benefits) and the quality of the supporting evidence is excellent. In some clearly identified circumstances, strong recommendations may be made when high-quality evidence is impossible to obtain and the anticipated benefits strongly outweigh the harms.	Clinicians should follow a strong recommendation unless a clear and compelling rationale for an alternative approach is present.
Recommendation	A recommendation in favor of a particular action is made when the anticipated benefits exceed the harms but the quality of evidence is not as strong. Again, in some clearly identified circumstances, recommendations may be made when high-quality evidence is impossible to obtain but the anticipated benefits outweigh the harms.	Clinicians would be prudent to follow a recommendation, but should remain alert to new information and sensitive to patient preferences.
Option	Options define courses that may be taken when either the quality of evidence is suspect or carefully performed studies have shown little clear advantage to one approach over another.	Clinicians should consider the option in their decision-making, and patient preference may have a substantial role.
No recommendation	No recommendation indicates that there is a lack of pertinent published evidence and that the anticipated balance of benefits and harms is presently unclear.	Clinicians should be alert to new published evidence that clarifies the balance of benefit versus harm.

The purpose of this action statement is to guide the practitioner in making a diagnosis of acute bacterial sinusitis on the basis of stringent clinical criteria. To develop criteria to be used in distinguishing episodes of acute bacterial sinusitis from other common respiratory infections, it is helpful to describe the features of an uncomplicated viral URI. Viral URIs are usually characterized by nasal symptoms (discharge and congestion/obstruction) or cough or both. Most often, the nasal discharge begins as clear and watery. Often, however, the quality of nasal discharge changes during the course of the illness. Typically, the nasal discharge becomes thicker and more mucoid and may become purulent (thick, colored, and opaque) for several days. Then the situation reverses, with the purulent discharge becoming mucoid and then clear again or simply resolving. The transition from clear to purulent to clear again occurs in uncomplicated viral URIs without the use of antimicrobial therapy.

Fever, when present in uncomplicated viral URI, tends to occur early in the illness, often in concert with other constitutional symptoms such as headache and myalgias. Typically, the fever and constitutional symptoms disappear in the first 24 to 48 hours, and the respiratory symptoms become more prominent (Fig 2).

The course of most uncomplicated viral URIs is 5 to 7 days.[9–12] As shown in Fig 2, respiratory symptoms usually peak in severity by days 3 to 6 and then begin to improve; however, resolving symptoms and signs may persist in some patients after day 10.[9,10]

Symptoms of acute bacterial sinusitis and uncomplicated viral URI overlap considerably, and therefore it is their persistence without improvement that suggests a diagnosis of acute sinusitis.[9,10,13] Such symptoms include nasal discharge (of any quality: thick or thin, serous, mucoid, or purulent) or daytime cough (which may be worse at night) or both. Bad breath, fatigue, headache, and decreased appetite, although common, are not specific indicators of acute sinusitis.[14] Physical examination findings are also not particularly helpful in distinguishing sinusitis from uncomplicated URIs. Erythema and swelling of the nasal turbinates are nonspecific findings.[14] Percussion of the sinuses is not useful. Transillumination of the sinuses is difficult to perform correctly in children and has been shown to be unreliable.[15,16] Nasopharyngeal cultures do not reliably predict the etiology of acute bacterial sinusitis.[14,16]

Only a minority (~6%–7%) of children presenting with symptoms of URI will meet criteria for persistence.[3,4,11] As a result, before diagnosing acute bacterial sinusitis, it is important for the practitioner to attempt to (1) differentiate between sequential episodes of uncomplicated viral URI (which may seem to coalesce in the mind of the patient or parent) from the onset of acute bacterial sinusitis with persistent symptoms and (2) establish whether the symptoms are clearly not improving.

A worsening course of signs and symptoms, termed "double sickening," in the context of a viral URI is another presentation of acute bacterial sinusitis.[13,17] Affected children experience substantial and acute worsening of respiratory symptoms (nasal discharge or nasal congestion or daytime cough) or a new fever, often on the sixth or seventh day of illness, after initial signs of recovery from an uncomplicated viral URI. Support for this definition comes from studies in children and adults, for whom antibiotic treatment of worsening symptoms after a period of apparent improvement was associated with better outcomes.[4]

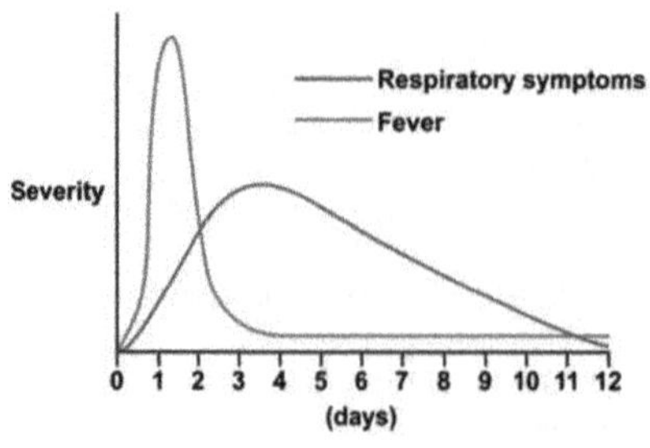

FIGURE 2
Uncomplicated viral URI.

Finally, some children with acute bacterial sinusitis may present with severe onset, ie, concurrent high fever (temperature >39°C) and purulent nasal discharge. These children usually are ill appearing and need to be distinguished from children with uncomplicated viral infections that are unusually severe. If fever is present in uncomplicated viral URIs, it tends to be present early in the illness, usually accompanied by other constitutional symptoms, such as headache and myalgia.[9,13,18] Generally, the constitutional symptoms resolve in the first 48 hours and then the respiratory symptoms become prominent. In most uncomplicated viral infections, including influenza, purulent nasal discharge does not appear for several days. Accordingly, it is the concurrent presentation of high fever and purulent nasal discharge for the first 3 to 4 days of an acute URI that helps to define the severe onset of acute bacterial sinusitis.[13,16,18] This presentation in children is the corollary to acute onset of headache, fever, and facial pain in adults with acute sinusitis.

Allergic and nonallergic rhinitis are predisposing causes of some cases of acute bacterial sinusitis in childhood. In addition, at their onset, these conditions may be mistaken for acute bacterial sinusitis. A family history of atopic conditions, seasonal occurrences, or occurrences with exposure to common allergens and other allergic diatheses in the index patient (eczema, atopic dermatitis, asthma) may suggest the presence of non-infectious rhinitis. The patient may have complaints of pruritic eyes and nasal mucosa, which will provide a clue to the likely etiology of the condition. On physical examination, there may be a prominent nasal crease, allergic shiners, cobblestoning of the conjunctiva or pharyngeal wall, or pale nasal mucosa as other indicators of the diagnosis.

Key Action Statement 2A

Clinicians should not obtain imaging studies (plain films, contrast-enhanced computed tomography [CT], MRI, or ultrasonography) to distinguish acute bacterial sinusitis from viral URI (Evidence Quality: B; Strong Recommendation).

KAS Profile 2A

Aggregate evidence quality: B; overwhelmingly consistent evidence from observational studies.	
Benefit	Avoids exposure to radiation and costs of studies. Avoids unnecessary therapy for false-positive diagnoses.
Harm	None.
Cost	Avoids cost of imaging.
Benefits-harm assessment	Exclusive benefit.
Value judgments	Concern for unnecessary radiation and costs.
Role of patient preference	Limited. Parents may value a negative study and avoidance of antibiotics as worthy of radiation but panel disagrees.
Intentional vagueness	None.
Exclusions	Patients with complications of sinusitis.
Strength	Strong recommendation.

The purpose of this key action statement is to discourage the practitioner from obtaining imaging studies in children with uncomplicated acute bacterial sinusitis. As emphasized in Key Action Statement 1, acute bacterial sinusitis in children is a diagnosis that is made on the basis of stringent clinical criteria that describe signs, symptoms, and temporal patterns of a URI. Although historically imaging has been used as a confirmatory or diagnostic modality in children suspected to have acute bacterial sinusitis, it is no longer recommended.

The membranes that line the nose are continuous with the membranes (mucosa) that line the sinus cavities, the middle ear, the nasopharynx, and the oropharynx. When an individual experiences a viral URI, there is inflammation of the nasal mucosa and, often, the mucosa of the middle ear and paranasal sinuses as well. The continuity of the mucosa of the upper respiratory tract is responsible for the controversy regarding the usefulness of images of the paranasal sinuses in contributing to a diagnosis of acute bacterial sinusitis.

As early as the 1940s, observations were made regarding the frequency of abnormal sinus radiographs in healthy children without signs or symptoms of current respiratory disease.[19] In addition, several investigators in the 1970s and 1980s observed that children with uncomplicated viral URI had frequent abnormalities of the paranasal sinuses on plain radiographs.[20–22] These abnormalities were the same as those considered to be diagnostic of acute bacterial sinusitis (diffuse opacification, mucosal swelling of at least 4 mm, or an air-fluid level).[16]

As technology advanced and CT scanning of the central nervous system and skull became prevalent, several studies reported on incidental abnormalities of the paranasal sinuses that were observed in children.[23,24] Gwaltney et al[25] showed striking abnormalities (including air-fluid levels) in sinus CT scans of young adults with uncomplicated colds. Manning et al[26] evaluated children undergoing either CT or MRI of the head for indications other than respiratory complaints or suspected sinusitis. Each patient underwent rhinoscopy and otoscopy before imaging and each patient's parent was asked to fill out a questionnaire regarding recent symptoms of URI. Sixty-two percent of patients overall had physical findings or history consistent with an upper respiratory inflammatory process, and 55% of the total group showed some abnormalities on sinus imaging; 33% showed pronounced mucosal thickening or an air-fluid level. Gordts et al[27] made similar observations in children undergoing MRI. Finally, Kristo et al[28] performed MRI in children with URIs and confirmed the high frequency (68%) of major abnormalities seen in the paranasal sinuses.

In summary, when the paranasal sinuses are imaged, either with plain radiographs, contrast-enhanced CT, or MRI in children with uncomplicated URI, the majority of studies will be significantly abnormal with the same kind of findings that are associated with bacterial infection of the sinuses. Accordingly, although normal radiographs or CT or MRI results can ensure that a patient with respiratory symptoms does not have acute bacterial sinusitis, an abnormal image cannot confirm the diagnosis. Therefore, it is not necessary to perform imaging in children with uncomplicated episodes of clinical sinusitis. Similarly, the high likelihood of an abnormal imaging result in a child with an uncomplicated URI indicates that radiographic studies not be performed in an attempt to eliminate the diagnosis of sinusitis.

Key Action Statement 2B

Clinicians should obtain a contrast-enhanced CT scan of the paranasal sinuses and/or an MRI with contrast whenever a child is suspected of having orbital or central nervous system complications of acute bacterial sinusitis (Evidence Quality: B; Strong Recommendation).

KAS Profile 2B

Aggregate evidence quality: B; overwhelmingly consistent evidence from observational studies.	
Benefit	Determine presence of abscesses, which may require surgical intervention; avoid sequelae because of appropriate aggressive management.
Harm	Exposure to ionizing radiation for CT scans; need for sedation for MRI.
Cost	Direct cost of studies.
Benefits-harm assessment	Preponderance of benefit.
Value judgments	Concern for significant complication that may be unrecognized and, therefore, not treated appropriately.
Role of patient preference	Limited.
Intentional vagueness	None.
Exclusions	None.
Strength	Strong recommendation.

The purpose of this key action statement is to have the clinician obtain contrast-enhanced CT images when children are suspected of having serious complications of acute bacterial sinusitis. The most common complication of acute sinusitis involves the orbit in children with ethmoid sinusitis who are younger than 5 years.[29–31] Orbital complications should be suspected when the child presents with a swollen eye, especially if accompanied by proptosis or impaired function of the extraocular muscles. Orbital complications of acute sinusitis have been divided into 5 categories: sympathetic effusion, subperiosteal abscess, orbital cellulitis, orbital abscess, and cavernous sinus thrombosis.[32] Although sympathetic effusion (inflammatory edema) is categorized as an orbital complication, the site of infection remains confined to the sinus cavities; eye swelling is attributable to the impedance of venous drainage secondary to congestion within the ethmoid sinuses. Alternative terms for sympathetic effusion (inflammatory edema) are preseptal or periorbital cellulitis. The remaining "true" orbital complications are best visualized by contrast-enhanced CT scanning.

Intracranial complications of acute sinusitis, which are substantially less common than orbital complications, are more serious, with higher morbidity and mortality than those involving the orbit. Intracranial complications should be suspected in the patient who presents with a very severe headache, photophobia, seizures, or other focal neurologic findings. Intracranial complications include subdural empyema, epidural empyema, venous thrombosis, brain abscess, and meningitis.[29] Typically, patients with intracranial complications of acute bacterial sinusitis are previously healthy adolescent males with frontal sinusitis.[33,34]

There have been no head-to-head comparisons of the diagnostic accuracy of contrast-enhanced CT scanning to MRI with contrast in the evaluation of orbital and intracranial complications of sinusitis in children. In general, the contrast-enhanced CT scan has been the preferred imaging study when complications of sinusitis are suspected.[35,36] However, there are documented cases in which a contrast-enhanced CT scan has not revealed the abnormality responsible for the clinical presentation and the MRI with contrast has, especially for intracranial complications and rarely for orbital complications.[37,38] Accordingly, the most recent appropriateness criteria from the American College of Radiology endorse both MRI with contrast and contrast-enhanced CT as complementary examinations when evaluating potential complications of sinusitis.[35] The availability and speed of obtaining the contrast-enhanced CT are desirable; however, there is increasing concern regarding exposure to radiation. The MRI, although very sensitive, takes longer than the contrast-enhanced CT and often requires sedation in young children (which carries its own risks). In older children and adolescents who may not require sedation, MRI with contrast, if available, may be preferred when intracranial complications are likely. Furthermore, MRI with contrast should be performed when there is persistent clinical concern or incomplete information has been provided by the contrast-enhanced CT scan.

Key Action Statement 3

Initial Management of Acute Bacterial Sinusitis

3A: "Severe onset and worsening course" acute bacterial sinusitis. The clinician should prescribe antibiotic therapy for acute bacterial sinusitis in children with severe onset or worsening course (signs, symptoms, or both) (Evidence Quality: B; Strong Recommendation).

KAS Profile 3A

Aggregate evidence quality: B; randomized controlled trials with limitations.	
Benefit	Increase clinical cures, shorten illness duration, and may prevent suppurative complications in a high-risk patient population.
Harm	Adverse effects of antibiotics.
Cost	Direct cost of therapy.
Benefits-harm assessment	Preponderance of benefit.
Value judgments	Concern for morbidity and possible complications if untreated.
Role of patient preference	Limited.
Intentional vagueness	None.
Exclusions	None.
Strength	Strong recommendation.

3B: "Persistent illness." The clinician should either prescribe antibiotic therapy OR offer additional outpatient observation for 3 days to children with persistent illness (nasal discharge of any quality or cough or both for at least 10 days without evidence of improvement) (Evidence Quality: B; Recommendation).

The purpose of this section is to offer guidance on initial management of persistent illness sinusitis by helping clinicians choose between the following 2 strategies:

1. Antibiotic therapy, defined as initial treatment of acute bacterial sinusitis with antibiotics, with the intent of starting antibiotic therapy as soon as possible after the encounter.
2. Additional outpatient observation, defined as initial management of acute bacterial sinusitis limited to continued observation for 3 days, with commencement of antibiotic therapy if either the child does not improve clinically within several days of diagnosis or if there is clinical worsening of the child's condition at any time.

In contrast to the 2001 AAP guideline,[5] which recommended antibiotic therapy for all children diagnosed with acute bacterial sinusitis, this guideline allows for additional observation of children presenting with persistent illness (nasal discharge of any quality or daytime cough or both for at least 10 days without evidence of improvement). In both guidelines, however, children presenting with severe or worsening illness (which was not defined explicitly in the 2001 guideline[5]) are to receive antibiotic therapy. The rationale for this approach (Table 2) is discussed below.

KAS Profile 3B

Aggregate evidence quality: B; randomized controlled trials with limitations.	
Benefit	Antibiotics increase the chance of improvement or cure at 10 to 14 days (number needed to treat, 3–5); additional observation may avoid the use of antibiotics with attendant cost and adverse effects.
Harm	Antibiotics have adverse effects (number needed to harm, 3) and may increase bacterial resistance. Observation may prolong illness and delay start of needed antibiotic therapy.
Cost	Direct cost of antibiotics as well as cost of adverse reactions; indirect costs of delayed recovery when observation is used.
Benefits-harm assessment	Preponderance of benefit (because both antibiotic therapy and additional observation with rescue antibiotic, if needed, are appropriate management).
Value judgments	Role for additional brief observation period for selected children with persistent illness sinusitis, similar to what is recommended for acute otitis media, despite the lack of randomized trials specifically comparing additional observation with immediate antibiotic therapy and longer duration of illness before presentation.
Role of patient preference	Substantial role in shared decision-making that should incorporate illness severity, child's quality of life, and caregiver values and concerns.
Intentional vagueness	None.
Exclusions	Children who are excluded from randomized clinical trials of acute bacterial sinusitis, as defined in the text.
Strength	Recommendation.

Antibiotic Therapy for Acute Bacterial Sinusitis

In the United States, antibiotics are prescribed for 82% of children with acute sinusitis.[39] The rationale for antibiotic therapy of acute bacterial sinusitis is based on the recovery of bacteria in high density ($\geq 10^4$ colony-forming units/mL) in 70% of maxillary sinus aspirates obtained from children with a clinical syndrome characterized by persistent nasal discharge, daytime cough, or both.[16,40] Children who present with severe-onset acute bacterial sinusitis are presumed to have bacterial infection, because a temperature of at least 39°C/102.2°F coexisting for at least 3 consecutive days with purulent nasal discharge is not consistent with the well-documented pattern of acute viral URI. Similarly, children with worsening-course acute bacterial sinusitis have a clinical course that is also not consistent with the steady improvement that characterizes an uncomplicated viral URI.[9,10]

Three RCTs have compared antibiotic therapy with placebo for the initial management of acute bacterial sinusitis in children. Two trials by Wald et al[4,41] found an increase in cure or improvement after antibiotic therapy compared with placebo with a number needed to treat of 3 to 5 children. Most children in these studies had persistent acute bacterial sinusitis, but children with severe or worsening illness were also included. Conversely, Garbutt et al,[42] who studied only children with persistent acute bacterial sinusitis, found no difference in outcomes for antibiotic versus placebo. Another RCT by Kristo et al,[43] often cited as showing no benefit from antibiotics for acute bacterial sinusitis, will not be considered further because of methodologic flaws, including weak entry criteria and inadequate dosing of antibiotic treatment.

The guideline recommends antibiotic therapy for severe or worsening acute bacterial sinusitis because of the benefits revealed in RCTs[4,41] and a theoretically higher risk of suppurative complications than for children who present with persistent symptoms. Orbital and intracranial complications of acute bacterial sinusitis have not been observed in RCTs, even when placebo was administered; however, sample sizes have inadequate power to preclude an increased risk. This risk, however, has caused some investigators to exclude children with severe acute bacterial sinusitis from trial entry.[42]

Additional Observation for Persistent Onset Acute Bacterial Sinusitis

The guideline recommends either antibiotic therapy or an additional brief period of observation as initial management strategies for children with persistent acute bacterial sinusitis because, although there are benefits to antibiotic therapy (number needed to treat, 3–5), some children improve on their own, and the risk of suppurative complications is low.[4,41] Symptoms of persistent acute bacterial sinusitis may be mild and have varying effects on a given child's quality of life, ranging from slight (mild cough, nasal discharge) to significant (sleep disturbance, behavioral changes, school or child care absenteeism). The benefits of antibiotic therapy in some trials[4,41] must also be balanced against an increased risk of adverse events (number need to harm, 3), most often self-limited diarrhea, but also including occasional rash.[4]

Choosing between antibiotic therapy or additional observation for initial management of persistent illness sinusitis presents an opportunity for shared decision-making with families (Table 2). Factors that might influence this decision include symptom severity, the child's quality of life, recent antibiotic use, previous experience or outcomes with acute bacterial sinusitis, cost of antibiotics, ease of administration, caregiver concerns about potential adverse effects of antibiotics, persistence of respiratory symptoms, or development of complications. Values and preferences expressed by the caregiver should be taken into consideration (Table 3).

Children with persistent acute bacterial sinusitis who received antibiotic therapy in the previous 4 weeks, those with concurrent bacterial infection (eg, pneumonia, suppurative cervical adenitis, group A streptococcal pharyngitis, or acute otitis media), those with actual or suspected complications of acute bacterial sinusitis, or those with underlying conditions should generally be managed with antibiotic therapy. The latter group includes children with asthma, cystic fibrosis, immunodeficiency, previous sinus surgery, or anatomic abnormalities of the upper respiratory tract.

Limiting antibiotic use in children with persistent acute bacterial sinusitis who may improve on their own reduces common antibiotic-related adverse events, such as diarrhea, diaper dermatitis, and skin rash. The most recent RCT of acute bacterial sinusitis in children[4] found adverse events of 44% with antibiotic and 14% with placebo.

Limiting antibiotics may also reduce the prevalence of resistant bacterial pathogens. Although this is always a desirable goal, no increase in resistant bacterial species was observed within the group of children treated with a single course of antimicrobial agents (compared with those receiving placebo) in 2 recent large studies of antibiotic versus placebo for children with acute otitis media.[44,45]

Key Action Statement 4

Clinicians should prescribe amoxicillin with or without clavulanate as first-line treatment when a decision has been made to initiate antibiotic treatment of acute bacterial sinusitis (Evidence Quality: B; Recommendation).

KAS Profile 4

Aggregate evidence quality: B; randomized controlled trials with limitations.

Benefit	Increase clinical cures with narrowest spectrum drug; stepwise increase in broadening spectrum as risk factors for resistance increase.
Harm	Adverse effects of antibiotics including development of hypersensitivity.
Cost	Direct cost of antibiotic therapy.
Benefits-harm assessment	Preponderance of benefit.
Value judgments	Concerns for not encouraging resistance if possible.
Role of patient preference	Potential for shared decision-making that should incorporate the caregiver's experiences and values.
Intentional vagueness	None.
Exclusions	May include allergy or intolerance.
Strength	Recommendation.

TABLE 2 Recommendations for Initial Use of Antibiotics for Acute Bacterial Sinusitis

Clinical Presentation	Severe Acute Bacterial Sinusitis[a]	Worsening Acute Bacterial Sinusitis[b]	Persistent Acute Bacterial Sinusitis[c]
Uncomplicated acute bacterial sinusitis without coexisting illness	Antibiotic therapy	Antibiotic therapy	Antibiotic therapy or additional observation for 3 days[d]
Acute bacterial sinusitis with orbital or intracranial complications	Antibiotic therapy	Antibiotic therapy	Antibiotic therapy
Acute bacterial sinusitis with coexisting acute otitis media, pneumonia, adenitis, or streptococcal pharyngitis	Antibiotic therapy	Antibiotic therapy	Antibiotic therapy

[a] Defined as temperature ≥39°C and purulent (thick, colored, and opaque) nasal discharge present concurrently for at least 3 consecutive days.
[b] Defined as nasal discharge or daytime cough with sudden worsening of symptoms (manifested by new-onset fever ≥38° C/100.4°F or substantial increase in nasal discharge or cough) after having experienced transient improvement of symptoms.
[c] Defined as nasal discharge (of any quality), daytime cough (which may be worse at night), or both, persisting for >10 days without improvement.
[d] Opportunity for shared decision-making with the child's family; if observation is offered, a mechanism must be in place to ensure follow-up and begin antibiotics if the child worsens at any time or fails to improve within 3 days of observation.

The purpose of this key action statement is to guide the selection of antimicrobial therapy once the diagnosis of acute bacterial sinusitis has been made. The microbiology of acute bacterial sinusitis was determined nearly 30 years ago through direct maxillary sinus aspiration in children with compatible signs and symptoms. The major bacterial pathogens recovered at that time were *Streptococcus pneumoniae* in approximately 30% of children and nontypeable *Haemophilus influenzae* and *Moraxella catarrhalis* in approximately 20% each.[16,40] Aspirates from the remaining 25% to 30% of children were sterile.

Maxillary sinus aspiration is rarely performed at the present time unless the course of the infection is unusually prolonged or severe. Although some authorities have recommended obtaining cultures from the middle meatus to determine the cause of a maxillary sinus infection, there are no data in children with acute bacterial sinusitis that have compared such cultures with cultures of a maxillary sinus aspirate. Furthermore, there are data indicating that the middle meatus in healthy children is commonly colonized with *S pneumoniae*, *H influenzae*, and *M catarrhalis*.[46]

Recent estimates of the microbiology of acute sinusitis have, of necessity, been based primarily on that of acute otitis media (AOM), a condition with relatively easy access to infective fluid through performance of tympanocentesis and one with a similar pathogenesis to acute bacterial sinusitis.[47,48] The 3 most common bacterial pathogens recovered from the middle ear fluid of children with AOM are the same as those that have been associated with acute bacterial sinusitis: *S pneumoniae*, nontypeable *H influenzae*, and *M catarrhalis*.[49] The proportion of each has varied from study to study depending on criteria used for diagnosis of AOM, patient characteristics, and bacteriologic techniques. Recommendations since the year 2000 for the routine use in infants of 7-valent and, more recently, 13-valent pneumococcal conjugate vaccine (PCV-13) have been associated with a decrease in recovery of *S pneumoniae* from ear fluid of children with AOM and a relative increase in the incidence of infections attributable to *H influenzae*.[50] Thus, on the basis of the proportions of bacteria found in middle ear infections, it is estimated that *S pneumoniae* and *H influenzae* are currently each responsible for approximately 30% of cases of acute bacterial sinusitis in children, and *M catarrhalis* is responsible for approximately 10%. These percentages are contingent on the assumption that approximately one-quarter of aspirates of maxillary sinusitis would still be sterile, as reported in earlier studies. *Staphylococcus aureus* is rarely isolated from sinus aspirates in children with acute bacterial sinusitis, and with the exception of acute maxillary sinusitis associated with infections of dental origin,[51] respiratory anaerobes are also rarely recovered.[40,52] Although *S aureus* is a very infrequent cause of acute bacterial sinusitis in children, it is a significant pathogen in the orbital and intracranial complications of sinusitis. The reasons for this discrepancy are unknown.

Antimicrobial susceptibility patterns for *S pneumoniae* vary considerably from community to community. Isolates obtained from surveillance centers nationwide indicate that, at the present time, 10% to 15% of upper respiratory tract isolates of *S pneumoniae* are nonsusceptible to penicillin[53,54]; however, values for penicillin nonsusceptibility as high as 50% to 60% have been reported in some areas.[55,56] Of the organisms that are resistant, approximately half are highly resistant to penicillin and the remaining half are intermediate in resistance.[53,54,56–59] Between 10% and 42% of *H influenzae*[56–59] and close to 100% of *M catarrhalis* are likely to be β-lactamase positive and nonsusceptible to amoxicillin. Because of dramatic geographic variability in the prevalence of β-lactamase–positive *H influenzae*, it is extremely desirable for the practitioner to be familiar with local patterns of susceptibility. Risk factors for the presence of organisms likely to be resistant to amoxicillin include attendance at child care, receipt of antimicrobial treatment within the previous 30 days, and age younger than 2 years.[50,55,60]

Amoxicillin remains the antimicrobial agent of choice for first-line treatment of uncomplicated acute bacterial sinusitis in situations in which antimicrobial resistance is not suspected. This recommendation is based on amoxicillin's effectiveness, safety, acceptable taste, low cost, and relatively narrow microbiologic spectrum. For children aged 2 years or older with uncomplicated acute bacterial sinusitis that is mild to moderate in degree of severity who do not attend child care and who have not been treated with an antimicrobial agent within the last 4 weeks, amoxicillin is recommended at a standard dose of 45 mg/kg per day in 2 divided doses. In communities with a high prevalence of nonsusceptible *S pneumoniae* (>10%, including intermediate- and high-level resistance), treatment may be initiated at 80 to 90 mg/kg per day in 2 divided doses, with a maximum of 2 g per dose.[55] This high-dose amoxicillin therapy is likely to achieve sinus fluid concentrations that are adequate to overcome the resistance of *S pneumoniae*, which is attributable to alteration in penicillin-binding proteins on the basis of data derived from patients with AOM.[61] If, within the next several years after licensure of PCV-13, a continuing decrease in isolates of *S pneumoniae* (including a decrease in isolates of nonsusceptible *S pneumoniae)* and an increase in β-lactamase–producing *H influenzae* are observed, standard-dose amoxicillin-clavulanate (45 mg/kg per day) may be most appropriate.

Patients presenting with moderate to severe illness as well as those younger than 2 years, attending child care, or who have recently been treated with an antimicrobial may receive high-dose amoxicillin-clavulanate (80–90 mg/kg per day of the amoxicillin component with 6.4 mg/kg per day of clavulanate in 2 divided doses with a maximum of 2 g per dose). The potassium clavulanate levels are adequate to inhibit all β-lactamase–producing *H influenzae* and *M catarrhalis*.[56,59]

A single 50-mg/kg dose of ceftriaxone, given either intravenously or intramuscularly, can be used for children who are vomiting, unable to tolerate oral medication, or unlikely to be adherent to the initial doses of antibiotic.[62–64] The 3 major bacterial pathogens involved in acute bacterial sinusitis are susceptible to ceftriaxone in 95% to 100% of cases.[56,58,59] If clinical improvement is observed at 24 hours, an oral antibiotic can be substituted to complete the course of therapy. Children who are still significantly febrile or symptomatic at 24 hours may require additional parenteral doses before switching to oral therapy.

The treatment of patients with presumed allergy to penicillin has been controversial. However, recent publications indicate that the risk of a serious allergic reaction to second- and third-generation cephalosporins in patients with penicillin or amoxicillin allergy appears to be almost nil and no greater than the risk among patients without such allergy.[65–67] Thus, patients allergic to amoxicillin with a non–type 1 (late or delayed, >72 hours) hypersensitivity reaction can safely be treated with cefdinir, cefuroxime, or cefpodoxime.[66–68] Patients with a history of a serious type 1 immediate or accelerated (anaphylactoid) reaction to amoxicillin can also safely be treated with cefdinir, cefuroxime, or cefpodoxime. In both circumstances, clinicians may wish to determine individual tolerance by referral to an allergist for penicillin and/or cephalosporin skin-testing before initiation of therapy.[66–68] The susceptibility of *S pneumoniae* to cefdinir, cefpodoxime, and cefuroxime varies from 60% to 75%,[56–59] and the susceptibility of *H influenzae* to these agents varies from 85% to 100%.[56,58] In young children (<2 years) with a serious type 1 hypersensitivity to penicillin and moderate or more severe sinusitis, it may be prudent to use a combination of clindamycin (or linezolid) and cefixime to achieve the most comprehensive coverage against both resistant *S pneumoniae* and *H influenzae*. Linezolid has excellent activity against all *S pneumoniae*, including penicillin-resistant strains, but lacks activity against *H influenzae* and *M catarrhalis*. Alternatively, a quinolone, such as levofloxacin, which has a high level of activity against both *S pneumoniae* and *H influenzae*, may be prescribed.[57,58] Although the use of quinolones is usually restricted because of concerns for toxicity, cost, and emerging resistance, their use in this circumstance can be justified.

Pneumococcal and *H influenzae* surveillance studies have indicated that resistance of these organisms to trimethoprim-sulfamethoxazole and azithromycin is sufficient to preclude their use for treatment of acute bacterial sinusitis in patients with penicillin hypersensitivity.[56,58,59,69]

The optimal duration of antimicrobial therapy for patients with acute bacterial sinusitis has not received systematic study. Recommendations based on clinical observations have varied widely, from 10 to 28 days of treatment. An alternative suggestion has been made that antibiotic therapy be continued for 7 days after the patient becomes free of signs and symptoms.[5] This strategy has the advantage of individualizing the treatment of each patient, results in a minimum course of 10 days, and avoids prolonged antimicrobial therapy in patients who are asymptomatic and therefore unlikely to adhere to the full course of treatment.[5]

Patients who are acutely ill and appear toxic when first seen (see below) can be managed with 1 of 2 options. Consultation can be requested from an otolaryngologist for consideration of maxillary sinus aspiration (with appropriate analgesia/anesthesia) to obtain a sample of sinus secretions for Gram stain, culture, and susceptibility testing so that antimicrobial therapy can be adjusted precisely. Alternatively, inpatient therapy can be initiated with intravenous cefotaxime or ceftriaxone, with referral to an otolaryngologist if the patient's condition worsens or fails to show improvement within 48 hours. If a complication is suspected, management will differ depending on the site and severity.

A recent guideline was published by the Infectious Diseases Society of America for acute bacterial rhinosinusitis in children and adults.[70] Their recommendation for initial empirical antimicrobial therapy for acute bacterial sinusitis in children was amoxicillin-clavulanate based on the concern that there is an increasing prevalence of *H influenzae* as a cause of sinusitis since introduction of the pneumococcal conjugate vaccines and an increasing prevalence of β-lactamase production among these strains. In contrast, this guideline from the AAP allows either amoxicillin or amoxicillin-clavulanate as first-line empirical therapy and is therefore inclusive of the Infectious Diseases Society of America's recommendation. Unfortunately, there are scant data available regarding the precise microbiology of acute bacterial sinusitis in the post–PCV-13 era. Prospective surveillance of nasopharyngeal cultures may be helpful in completely aligning these recommendations in the future.

Key Action Statement 5A

Clinicians should reassess initial management if there is either a caregiver report of worsening (progression of initial signs/symptoms or appearance of new signs/symptoms) OR failure to improve (lack of reduction in all presenting signs/symptoms) within 72 hours of initial management (Evidence Quality: C; Recommendation).

KAS Profile 5A

Aggregate evidence quality: C; observational studies	
Benefits	Identification of patients who may have been misdiagnosed, those at risk of complications, and those who require a change in management.
Harm	Delay of up to 72 hours in changing therapy if patient fails to improve.
Cost	Additional provider and caregiver time and resources.
Benefits-harm assessment	Preponderance of benefit.
Value judgments	Use of 72 hours to assess progress may result in excessive classification as treatment failures if premature; emphasis on importance of worsening illness in defining treatment failures.
Role of patient preferences	Caregivers determine whether the severity of the patient's illness justifies the report to clinician of the patient's worsening or failure to improve.
Intentional vagueness	None.
Exclusions	Patients with severe illness, poor general health, complicated sinusitis, immune deficiency, previous sinus surgery, or coexisting bacterial illness.
Strength	Recommendation.

The purpose of this key action statement is to ensure that patients with acute bacterial sinusitis who fail to improve symptomatically after initial management are reassessed to be certain that they have been correctly diagnosed and to consider initiation of alternate therapy to hasten resolution of symptoms and avoid complications. "Worsening" is defined as progression of presenting signs or symptoms of acute bacterial sinusitis or onset of new signs or symptoms. "Failure to improve" is lack of reduction in presenting signs or symptoms of acute bacterial sinusitis by 72 hours after diagnosis and initial management; patients with persistent but improving symptoms do not meet this definition.

The rationale for using 72 hours as the time to assess treatment failure for acute bacterial sinusitis is based on clinical outcomes in RCTs. Wald et al[41] found that 18 of 35 patients (51%) receiving placebo demonstrated symptomatic improvement within 3 days of initiation of treatment; only an additional 3 patients receiving placebo (9%) improved between days 3 and 10. In the same study, 48 of 58 patients (83%) receiving antibiotics were cured or improved within 3 days; at 10 days, the overall rate of improvement was 79%, suggesting that no additional patients improved between days 3 and 10. In a more recent study, 17 of 19 children who ultimately failed initial therapy with either antibiotic or placebo demonstrated failure to improve within 72 hours.[4] Although Garbutt et al[42] did not report the percentage of patients who improved by day 3, they did demonstrate that the majority of improvement in symptoms occurred within the first 3 days of study entry whether they received active treatment or placebo.

Reporting of either worsening or failure to improve implies a shared responsibility between clinician and caregiver. Although the clinician should educate the caregiver regarding the anticipated reduction in symptoms within 3 days, it is incumbent on the caregiver to appropriately notify the clinician of concerns regarding worsening or failure to improve. Clinicians should emphasize the importance of reassessing those children whose symptoms are worsening whether or not antibiotic therapy was prescribed. Reassessment may be indicated before the 72-hour mark if the patient is substantially worse, because it may indicate the development of complications or a need for parenteral therapy. Conversely, in some cases, caregivers may think that symptoms are not severe enough to justify a change to an antibiotic with a less desirable safety profile or even the time, effort, and resources required for reassessment. Accordingly, the circumstances under which caregivers report back to the clinician and the process by which such reporting occurs should be discussed at the time the initial management strategy is determined.

Key Action Statement 5B

If the diagnosis of acute bacterial sinusitis is confirmed in a child with worsening symptoms or failure to improve in 72 hours, then clinicians may change the antibiotic therapy for the child initially managed with antibiotic OR initiate antibiotic treatment of the child initially managed with observation (Evidence Quality: D; Option based on expert opinion, case reports, and reasoning from first principles).

KAS Profile 5B

Aggregate evidence quality: D; expert opinion and reasoning from first principles.	
Benefit	Prevention of complications, administration of effective therapy.
Harm	Adverse effects of secondary antibiotic therapy.
Cost	Direct cost of medications, often substantial for second-line agents.
Benefits-harm assessment	Preponderance of benefit.
Value judgments	Clinician must determine whether cost and adverse effects associated with change in antibiotic is justified given the severity of illness.
Role of patient preferences	Limited in patients whose symptoms are severe or worsening, but caregivers of mildly affected children who are failing to improve may reasonably defer change in antibiotic.
Intentional vagueness	None.
Exclusions	None.
Strength	Option.

The purpose of this key action statement is to ensure optimal antimicrobial treatment of children with acute bacterial sinusitis whose symptoms worsen or fail to respond to the initial intervention to prevent complications and reduce symptom severity and duration (see Table 4).

Clinicians who are notified by a caregiver that a child's symptoms are worsening or failing to improve should confirm that the clinical diagnosis of acute bacterial sinusitis corresponds to the patient's pattern of illness, as defined in Key Action Statement 1. If caregivers report worsening of symptoms at any time in a patient for whom observation was the initial intervention, the clinician should begin treatment as discussed in Key Action Statement 4. For patients whose symptoms are mild and who have failed to improve but have not worsened, initiation of antimicrobial agents or continued observation (for up to 3 days) is reasonable.

If caregivers report worsening of symptoms after 3 days in a patient initially treated with antimicrobial agents, current signs and symptoms should be reviewed to determine whether acute bacterial sinusitis is still the best diagnosis. If sinusitis is still the best diagnosis, infection with drug-resistant bacteria is probable, and an alternate antimicrobial agent may be administered. Face-to-face reevaluation of the patient is desirable. Once the decision is made to change medications, the clinician should consider the limitations of the initial antibiotic coverage, the anticipated susceptibility of residual bacterial pathogens, and the ability of antibiotics to adequately penetrate the site of infection. Cultures of sinus or nasopharyngeal secretions in patients with initial antibiotic failure have identified a large percentage of bacteria with resistance to the original antibiotic.[71,72] Furthermore, multidrug-resistant *S pneumoniae* and β-lactamase–positive *H influenzae* and *M catarrhalis* are more commonly isolated after previous antibiotic exposure.[73–78] Unfortunately, there are no studies in children that have investigated the microbiology of treatment failure in acute bacterial sinusitis or cure rates using second-line antimicrobial agents. As a result, the likelihood of adequate antibiotic coverage for resistant organisms must be addressed by extrapolations from studies of acute otitis media in children and sinusitis in adults and by using the results of data generated in vitro. A general guide to management of the child who worsens in 72 hours is shown in Table 4.

NO RECOMMENDATION

Adjuvant Therapy

Potential adjuvant therapy for acute sinusitis might include intranasal corticosteroids, saline nasal irrigation or lavage, topical or oral decongestants, mucolytics, and topical or oral antihistamines. A recent Cochrane review on decongestants, antihistamines, and nasal irrigation for acute sinusitis in children found no appropriately designed studies to determine the effectiveness of these interventions.[79]

Intranasal Steroids

The rationale for the use of intranasal corticosteroids in acute bacterial sinusitis is that an antiinflammatory agent may reduce the swelling around the sinus ostia and encourage drainage, thereby hastening recovery. However, there are limited data on how much inflammation is present, whether the inflammation is responsive to steroids, and whether there are differences in responsivity according to age. Nonetheless, there are several RCTs in adolescents and adults, most of which do show significant differences compared with placebo or active comparator that favor intranasal steroids in the reduction of symptoms and the patient's global assessment of overall improvement.[80–85] Several studies in adults with acute bacterial sinusitis provide data supporting the use of intranasal steroids as either monotherapy or adjuvant therapy to antibiotics.[81,86] Only one study did not show efficacy.[85]

There have been 2 trials of intranasal steroids performed exclusively in children: one comparing intranasal corticosteroids versus an oral decongestant[87] and the other comparing intranasal corticosteroids with placebo.[88] These studies showed a greater rate of complete resolution[87] or greater reduction in symptoms in patients receiving the steroid preparation, although the effects were modest.[88] It is important to note that nearly all of these studies (both those reported in children and adults) suffered from substantial methodologic problems. Examples of these methodologic problems are as follows: (1) variable inclusion criteria for sinusitis, (2) mixed populations of allergic and nonallergic subjects, and (3) different outcome criteria. All of these factors make deriving a clear conclusion difficult. Furthermore, the lack of stringent criteria in selecting the subject population increases the chance that the subjects had viral URIs or even persistent allergies rather than acute bacterial sinusitis.

The intranasal steroids studied to date include budesonide, flunisolide, fluticasone, and mometasone. There is no reason to believe that one steroid would be more effective than another, provided equivalent doses are used.

Potential harm in using nasal steroids in children with acute sinusitis includes the increased cost of therapy, difficulty in effectively administering nasal sprays in young children, nasal irritation and epistaxis, and potential systemic adverse effects of steroid use. Fortunately, no clinically significant steroid adverse effects have been discovered in studies in children.[89–96]

Saline Irrigation

Saline nasal irrigation or lavage (not saline nasal spray) has been used to remove debris from the nasal cavity and temporarily reduce tissue edema (hypertonic saline) to promote drainage from the sinuses. There have been very few RCTs using saline nasal irrigation or lavage in acute sinusitis, and these have had mixed results.[97,98] The 1 study in children showed greater improvement in nasal airflow and quality of life as well as a better rate of improvement in total symptom score when compared with placebo in patients treated with antibiotics and decongestants.[98] There are 2 Cochrane reviews published on the use of saline nasal irrigation in acute sinusitis in adults that showed variable results. One review published in 2007[99] concluded that it is a beneficial adjunct, but the other, published in 2010,[100] concluded that most trials were too small or contained too high a risk of bias to be confident about benefits.

Nasal Decongestants, Mucolytics, and Antihistamines

Data are insufficient to make any recommendations about the use of oral or topical nasal decongestants, mucolytics, or oral or nasal spray antihistamines as adjuvant therapy for acute bacterial sinusitis in children.[79] It is the opinion of the expert panel that antihistamines should not be used for the primary indication of acute bacterial sinusitis in any child, although such therapy might be helpful in reducing typical allergic symptoms in patients with atopy who also have acute sinusitis.

OTHER RELATED CONDITIONS

Recurrence of Acute Bacterial Sinusitis

Recurrent acute bacterial sinusitis (RABS) is an uncommon occurrence in healthy children and must be distinguished from recurrent URIs, exacerbations of allergic rhinitis, and chronic sinusitis. The former is defined by episodes of bacterial infection of the paranasal sinuses lasting fewer than 30 days and separated by intervals of

TABLE 3 Parent Information Regarding Initial Management of Acute Bacterial Sinusitis

How common are sinus infections in children?	Thick, colored, or cloudy mucus from your child's nose frequently occurs with a common cold or viral infection and does not by itself mean your child has sinusitis. In fact, fewer than 1 in 15 children get a true bacterial sinus infection during or after a common cold.
How can I tell if my child has bacterial sinusitis or simply a common cold?	Most colds have a runny nose with mucus that typically starts out clear, becomes cloudy or colored, and improves by about 10 d. Some colds will also include fever (temperature >38°C [100.4°F]) for 1 to 2 days. In contrast, acute bacterial sinusitis is likely when the pattern of illness is persistent, severe, or worsening. 1. *Persistent* sinusitis is the most common type, defined as runny nose (of any quality), daytime cough (which may be worse at night), or both for at least 10 days without improvement. 2. *Severe* sinusitis is present when fever (temperature ≥39°C [102.2°F]) lasts for at least 3 days in a row and is accompanied by nasal mucus that is thick, colored, or cloudy. 3. *Worsening* sinusitis starts with a viral cold, which begins to improve but then worsens when bacteria take over and cause new-onset fever (temperature ≥38°C [100.4°F]) or a substantial increase in daytime cough or runny nose.
If my child has sinusitis, should he or she take an antibiotic?	Children with *persistent* sinusitis may be managed with either an antibiotic or with an additional brief period of observation, allowing the child up to another 3 days to fight the infection and improve on his or her own. The choice to treat or observe should be discussed with your doctor and may be based on your child's quality of life and how much of a problem the sinusitis is causing. In contrast, all children diagnosed with *severe* or *worsening* sinusitis should start antibiotic treatment to help them recover faster and more often.
Why not give all children with acute bacterial sinusitis an immediate antibiotic?	Some episodes of *persistent* sinusitis include relatively mild symptoms that may improve on their own in a few days. In addition, antibiotics can have adverse effects, which may include vomiting, diarrhea, upset stomach, skin rash, allergic reactions, yeast infections, and development of resistant bacteria (that make future infections more difficult to treat).

at least 10 days during which the patient is asymptomatic. Some experts require at least 4 episodes in a calendar year to fulfill the criteria for this condition. Chronic sinusitis is manifest as 90 or more uninterrupted days of respiratory symptoms, such as cough, nasal discharge, or nasal obstruction.

Children with RABS should be evaluated for underlying allergies, particularly allergic rhinitis; quantitative and functional immunologic defect(s), chiefly immunoglobulin A and immunoglobulin G deficiency; cystic fibrosis; gastroesophageal reflux disease; or dysmotile cilia syndrome.[101] Anatomic abnormalities obstructing one or more sinus ostia may be present. These include septal deviation, nasal polyps, or concha bullosa (pneumatization of the middle turbinate); atypical ethmoid cells with compromised drainage; a lateralized middle turbinate; and intrinsic ostiomeatal anomalies.[102] Contrast-enhanced CT, MRI, or endoscopy or all 3 should be performed for detection of obstructive conditions, particularly in children with genetic or acquired craniofacial abnormalities.

The microbiology of RABS is similar to that of isolated episodes of acute bacterial sinusitis and warrants the same treatment.[72] It should be recognized that closely spaced sequential courses of antimicrobial therapy may foster the emergence of antibiotic-resistant bacterial species as the causative agent in recurrent episodes. There are no systematically evaluated options for prevention of RABS in children. In general, the use of prolonged prophylactic antimicrobial therapy should be avoided and is not usually recommended for children with recurrent acute otitis media. However, when there are no recognizable predisposing conditions to remedy in children with RABS, prophylactic antimicrobial agents may be used for several months during the respiratory season. Enthusiasm for this strategy is tempered by concerns regarding the encouragement of bacterial resistance. Accordingly, prophylaxis should only be considered in carefully selected children whose infections have been thoroughly documented.

Influenza vaccine should be administered annually, and PCV-13 should be administered at the recommended ages for all children, including those with RABS. Intranasal steroids and nonsedating antihistamines can be helpful for children with allergic rhinitis, as can antireflux medications for those with gastroesophageal reflux disease. Children with anatomic abnormalities may require endoscopic surgery for removal of or reduction in ostiomeatal obstruction.

The pathogenesis of chronic sinusitis is poorly understood and appears to be multifactorial; however, many of the conditions associated with RABS

TABLE 4 Management of Worsening or Lack of Improvement at 72 Hours

Initial Management	Worse in 72 Hours	Lack of Improvement in 72 Hours
Observation	Initiate amoxicillin with or without clavulanate	Additional observation or initiate antibiotic based on shared decision-making
Amoxicillin	High-dose amoxicillin-clavulanate	Additional observation or high-dose amoxicillin-clavulanate based on shared decision-making
High-dose amoxicillin-clavulanate	Clindamycin[a] and cefixime OR linezolid and cefixime OR levofloxacin	Continued high-dose amoxicillin-clavulanate OR clindamycin[a] and cefixime OR linezolid and cefixime OR levofloxacin

[a] Clindamycin is recommended to cover penicillin-resistant *S pneumoniae*. Some communities have high levels of clindamycin-resistant *S pneumoniae*. In these communities, linezolid is preferred.

have also been implicated in chronic sinusitis, and it is clear that there is an overlap between the 2 syndromes.[101,102] In some cases, there may be episodes of acute bacterial sinusitis superimposed on a chronic sinusitis, warranting antimicrobial therapy to hasten resolution of the acute infection.

Complications of Acute Bacterial Sinusitis

Complications of acute bacterial sinusitis should be diagnosed when the patient develops signs or symptoms of orbital and/or central nervous system (intracranial) involvement. Rarely, complicated acute bacterial sinusitis can result in permanent blindness, other neurologic sequelae, or death if not treated promptly and appropriately. Orbital complications have been classified by Chandler et al.[32] Intracranial complications include epidural or subdural abscess, brain abscess, venous thrombosis, and meningitis.

Periorbital and intraorbital inflammation and infection are the most common complications of acute sinusitis and most often are secondary to acute ethmoiditis in otherwise healthy young children. These disorders are commonly classified in relation to the orbital septum; periorbital or preseptal inflammation involves only the eyelid, whereas postseptal (intraorbital) inflammation involves structures of the orbit. Mild cases of preseptal cellulitis (eyelid <50% closed) may be treated on an outpatient basis with appropriate oral antibiotic therapy (high-dose amoxicillin-clavulanate for comprehensive coverage) for acute bacterial sinusitis and daily follow-up until definite improvement is noted. If the patient does not improve within 24 to 48 hours or if the infection is progressive, it is appropriate to admit the patient to the hospital for antimicrobial therapy. Similarly, if proptosis, impaired visual acuity, or impaired and/or painful extraocular mobility is present on examination, the patient should be hospitalized, and a contrast-enhanced CT should be performed. Consultation with an otolaryngologist, an ophthalmologist, and an infectious disease expert is appropriate for guidance regarding the need for surgical intervention and the selection of antimicrobial agents.

Intracranial complications are most frequently encountered in previously healthy adolescent males with frontal sinusitis.[33,34] In patients with altered mental status, severe headache, or Pott's puffy tumor (osteomyelitis of the frontal bone), neurosurgical consultation should be obtained. A contrast-enhanced CT scan (preferably coronal thin cut) of the head, orbits, and sinuses is essential to confirm intracranial or intraorbital suppurative complications; in such cases, intravenous antibiotics should be started immediately. Alternatively, an MRI may also be desirable in some cases of intracranial abnormality. Appropriate antimicrobial therapy for intraorbital complications include vancomycin (to cover possible methicillin-resistant *S aureus* or penicillin-resistant *S pneumoniae*) and either ceftriaxone, ampicillin-sulbactam, or piperacillin-tazobactam.[103] Given the polymicrobial nature of sinogenic abscesses, coverage for anaerobes (ie, metronidazole) should also be considered for intraorbital complications and should be started in all cases of intracranial complications if ceftriaxone is prescribed.

Patients with small orbital, subperiosteal, or epidural abscesses and minimal ocular and neurologic abnormalities may be managed with intravenous antibiotic treatment for 24 to 48 hours while performing frequent visual and mental status checks.[104] In patients who develop progressive signs and symptoms, such as impaired visual acuity, ophthalmoplegia, elevated intraocular pressure (>20 mm), severe proptosis (>5 mm), altered mental status, headache, or vomiting, as well as those who fail to improve within 24 to 48 hours while receiving antibiotics, prompt surgical intervention and drainage of the abscess should be undertaken.[104] Antibiotics can be tailored to the results of culture and sensitivity studies when they become available.

AREAS FOR FUTURE RESEARCH

Since the publication of the original guideline in 2001, only a small number of high-quality studies of the diagnosis and treatment of acute bacterial sinusitis in children have been published.[5] Ironically, the number of published guidelines on the topic (5) exceeds the number of prospective, placebo-controlled clinical trials of either antibiotics or ancillary treatments of acute bacterial sinusitis. Thus, as was the case in 2001, there are scant data on which to base recommendations. Accordingly, areas for future research include the following:

Etiology

1. Reexamine the microbiology of acute sinusitis in children in the postpneumococcal conjugate vaccine era and determine the value of using newer polymerase chain reaction–based respiratory testing to document viral, bacterial, and polymicrobial disease.
2. Correlate cultures obtained from the middle meatus of the maxillary sinus of infected children with cultures obtained from the maxillary sinus by puncture of the antrum.
3. Conduct more and larger studies to more clearly define and correlate the clinical findings with the various available diagnostic criteria of acute bacterial sinusitis (eg, sinus aspiration and treatment outcome).
4. Develop noninvasive strategies to accurately diagnose acute bacterial sinusitis in children.
5. Develop imaging technology that differentiates bacterial infection from viral infection or allergic inflammation, preferably without radiation.

Treatment

1. Determine the optimal duration of antimicrobial therapy for children with acute bacterial sinusitis.
2. Evaluate a "wait-and-see prescription" strategy for children with persistent symptom presentation of acute sinusitis.
3. Determine the optimal antimicrobial agent for children with acute bacterial sinusitis, balancing the incentives of choosing narrow-spectrum agents against the known microbiology of the disease and resistance patterns of likely pathogens.
4. Determine the causes and treatment of subacute, recurrent acute, and chronic bacterial sinusitis.
5. Determine the efficacy of prophylaxis with antimicrobial agents to prevent RABS.
6. Determine the effects of bacterial resistance among *S pneumoniae*, *H influenzae*, and *M catarrhalis* on outcome of treatment with antibiotics by the performance of randomized, double-blind, placebo-controlled studies in well-defined populations of patients.
7. Determine the role of adjuvant therapies (antihistamines, nasal corticosteroids, mucolytics, decongestants, nasal irrigation, etc) in patients with acute bacterial sinusitis by the performance of prospective, randomized clinical trials.
8. Determine whether early treatment of acute bacterial sinusitis prevents orbital or central nervous system complications.
9. Determine the role of complementary and alternative medicine strategies in patients with acute bacterial sinusitis by performing systematic, prospective, randomized clinical trials.
10. Develop new bacterial and viral vaccines to reduce the incidence of acute bacterial sinusitis.

SUBCOMMITTEE ON ACUTE SINUSITIS

Ellen R. Wald, MD, FAAP (Chair, Pediatric Infectious Disease Physician: no financial conflicts; published research related to sinusitis)
Kimberly E. Applegate, MD, MS, FAAP (Radiologist, AAP Section on Radiology: no conflicts)
Clay Bordley, MD, MPH, FAAP (Pediatric Emergency and Hospitalist Medicine physician: no conflicts)
David H. Darrow, MD, FAAP (Otolaryngologist, AAP Section on Otolaryngology–Head and Neck Surgery: no conflicts)
Mary P. Glode, MD, FAAP (Pediatric Infectious Disease Physician, AAP Committee on Infectious Disease: no conflicts)
S. Michael Marcy, MD, FAAP (General Pediatrician with Infectious Disease Expertise, AAP Section on Infectious Diseases: no conflicts)
Nader Shaikh, MD, FAAP (General Academic Pediatrician: no financial conflicts; published research related to sinusitis)
Michael J. Smith, MD, MSCE, FAAP (Epidemiologist, Pediatric Infectious Disease Physician: research funding for vaccine clinical trials from Sanofi Pasteur and Novartis)
Paul V. Williams, MD, FAAP (Allergist, AAP Section on Allergy, Asthma, and Immunology: no conflicts)
Stuart T. Weinberg, MD, FAAP (PPI Informatician, General Academic Pediatrician: no conflicts)
Carrie E. Nelson, MD, MS (Family Physician, American Academy of Family Physicians: employed by McKesson Health Solutions)
Richard M. Rosenfeld, MD, MPH, FAAP (Otolaryngologist, AAP Section on Otolaryngology–Head and Neck Surgery, American Academy of Otolaryngology–Head and Neck Surgery: no financial conflicts; published research related to sinusitis)

CONSULTANT

Richard N. Shiffman, MD, FAAP (Informatician, Guideline Methodologist, General Academic Pediatrician: no conflicts)

STAFF

Caryn Davidson, MA

REFERENCES

1. Aitken M, Taylor JA. Prevalence of clinical sinusitis in young children followed up by primary care pediatricians. *Arch Pediatr Adolesc Med.* 1998;152(3):244–248
2. Kakish KS, Mahafza T, Batieha A, Ekteish F, Daoud A. Clinical sinusitis in children attending primary care centers. *Pediatr Infect Dis J.* 2000;19(11):1071–1074
3. Ueda D, Yoto Y. The ten-day mark as a practical diagnostic approach for acute paranasal sinusitis in children. *Pediatr Infect Dis J.* 1996;15(7):576–579

4. Wald ER, Nash D, Eickhoff J. Effectiveness of amoxicillin/clavulanate potassium in the treatment of acute bacterial sinusitis in children. *Pediatrics.* 2009;124(1):9–15

5. American Academy of Pediatrics, Subcommittee on Management of Sinusitis and Committee on Quality Improvement. Clinical practice guideline: management of sinusitis. *Pediatrics.* 2001;108(3):798–808

6. Smith MJ. AAP technical report: evidence for the diagnosis and treatment of acute uncomplicated sinusitis in children: a systematic review. 2013, In press.

7. Shiffman RN, Michel G, Rosenfeld RM, Davidson C. Building better guidelines with BRIDGE-Wiz: development and evaluation of a software assistant to promote clarity, transparency, and implementability. *J Am Med Inform Assoc.* 2012;19(1):94–101

8. American Academy of Pediatrics, Steering Committee on Quality Improvement and Management. Classifying recommendations for clinical practice guidelines. *Pediatrics.* 2004;114(3):874–877

9. Gwaltney JM, Jr, Hendley JO, Simon G, Jordan WS Jr. Rhinovirus infections in an industrial population. II. Characteristics of illness and antibody response. *JAMA.* 1967;202(6):494–500

10. Pappas DE, Hendley JO, Hayden FG, Winther B. Symptom profile of common colds in school-aged children. *Pediatr Infect Dis J.* 2008;27(1):8–11

11. Wald ER, Guerra N, Byers C. Frequency and severity of infections in day care: three-year follow-up. *J Pediatr.* 1991;118(4 pt 1):509–514

12. Wald ER, Guerra N, Byers C. Upper respiratory tract infections in young children: duration of and frequency of complications. *Pediatrics.* 1991;87(2):129–133

13. Meltzer EO, Hamilos DL, Hadley JA, et al. Rhinosinusitis: establishing definitions for clinical research and patient care. *J Allergy Clin Immunol.* 2004;114(6 suppl):155–212

14. Shaikh N, Wald ER. Signs and symptoms of acute sinusitis in children. *Pediatr Infect Dis J.* 2013; in press

15. Wald ER. The diagnosis and management of sinusitis in children: diagnostic considerations. *Pediatr Infect Dis.* 1985;4(6 suppl):S61–S64

16. Wald ER, Milmoe GJ, Bowen A, Ledesma-Medina J, Salamon N, Bluestone CD. Acute maxillary sinusitis in children. *N Engl J Med.* 1981;304(13):749–754

17. Lindbaek M, Hjortdahl P, Johnsen UL. Use of symptoms, signs, and blood tests to diagnose acute sinus infections in primary care: comparison with computed tomography. *Fam Med.* 1996;28(3):183–188

18. Wald ER. Beginning antibiotics for acute rhinosinusitis and choosing the right treatment. *Clin Rev Allergy Immunol.* 2006;30(3):143–152

19. Maresh MM, Washburn AH. Paranasal sinuses from birth to late adolescence. II. Clinical and roentgenographic evidence of infection. *Am J Dis Child.* 1940;60:841–861

20. Glasier CM, Mallory GB, Jr, Steele RW. Significance of opacification of the maxillary and ethmoid sinuses in infants. *J Pediatr.* 1989;114(1):45–50

21. Kovatch AL, Wald ER, Ledesma-Medina J, Chiponis DM, Bedingfield B. Maxillary sinus radiographs in children with nonrespiratory complaints. *Pediatrics.* 1984;73(3):306–308

22. Shopfner CE, Rossi JO. Roentgen evaluation of the paranasal sinuses in children. *Am J Roentgenol Radium Ther Nucl Med.* 1973;118(1):176–186

23. Diament MJ, Senac MO, Jr, Gilsanz V, Baker S, Gillespie T, Larsson S. Prevalence of incidental paranasal sinuses opacification in pediatric patients: a CT study. *J Comput Assist Tomogr.* 1987;11(3):426–431

24. Glasier CM, Ascher DP, Williams KD. Incidental paranasal sinus abnormalities on CT of children: clinical correlation. *AJNR Am J Neuroradiol.* 1986;7(5):861–864

25. Gwaltney JM, Jr, Phillips CD, Miller RD, Riker DK. Computed tomographic study of the common cold. *N Engl J Med.* 1994;330(1):25–30

26. Manning SC, Biavati MJ, Phillips DL. Correlation of clinical sinusitis signs and symptoms to imaging findings in pediatric patients. *Int J Pediatr Otorhinolaryngol.* 1996;37(1):65–74

27. Gordts F, Clement PA, Destryker A, Desprechins B, Kaufman L. Prevalence of sinusitis signs on MRI in a non-ENT paediatric population. *Rhinology.* 1997;35(4):154–157

28. Kristo A, Uhari M, Luotonen J, et al. Paranasal sinus findings in children during respiratory infection evaluated with magnetic resonance imaging. *Pediatrics.* 2003;111(5 pt 1):e586–e589

29. Brook I. Microbiology and antimicrobial treatment of orbital and intracranial complications of sinusitis in children and their management. *Int J Pediatr Otorhinolaryngol.* 2009;73(9):1183–1186

30. Sultesz M, Csakanyi Z, Majoros T, Farkas Z, Katona G. Acute bacterial rhinosinusitis and its complications in our pediatric otolaryngological department between 1997 and 2006. *Int J Pediatr Otorhinolaryngol.* 2009;73(11):1507–1512

31. Wald ER. Periorbital and orbital infections. *Infect Dis Clin North Am.* 2007;21(2):393–408

32. Chandler JR, Langenbrunner DJ, Stevens ER. The pathogenesis of orbital complications in acute sinusitis. *Laryngoscope.* 1970;80(9):1414–1428

33. Kombogiorgas D, Seth R, Modha J, Singh J. Suppurative intracranial complications of sinusitis in adolescence. Single institute experience and review of the literature. *Br J Neurosurg.* 2007;21(6):603–609

34. Rosenfeld EA, Rowley AH. Infectious intracranial complications of sinusitis, other than meningitis in children: 12 year review. *Clin Infect Dis.* 1994;18(5):750–754

35. American College of Radiology. Appropriateness criteria for sinonasal disease. 2009. Available at: www.acr.org/~/media/8172B4DE503149248E64856857674BB5.pdf. Accessed November 6, 2012

36. Triulzi F, Zirpoli S. Imaging techniques in the diagnosis and management of rhinosinusitis in children. *Pediatr Allergy Immunol.* 2007;18(suppl 18):46–49

37. McIntosh D, Mahadevan M. Failure of contrast enhanced computed tomography scans to identify an orbital abscess. The benefit of magnetic resonance imaging. *J Laryngol Otol.* 2008;122(6):639–640

38. Younis RT, Anand VK, Davidson B. The role of computed tomography and magnetic resonance imaging in patients with sinusitis with complications. *Laryngoscope.* 2002;112(2):224–229

39. Shapiro DJ, Gonzales R, Cabana MD, Hersh AL. National trends in visit rates and antibiotic prescribing for children with acute sinusitis. *Pediatrics.* 2011;127(1):28–34

40. Wald ER, Reilly JS, Casselbrant M, et al. Treatment of acute maxillary sinusitis in childhood: a comparative study of amoxicillin and cefaclor. *J Pediatr.* 1984;104(2):297–302

41. Wald ER, Chiponis D, Ledesma-Medina J. Comparative effectiveness of amoxicillin and amoxicillin-clavulanate potassium in acute paranasal sinus infections in children: a double-blind, placebo-controlled trial. *Pediatrics.* 1986;77(6):795–800

42. Garbutt JM, Goldstein M, Gellman E, Shannon W, Littenberg B. A randomized, placebo-controlled trial of antimicrobial treatment for children with clinically diagnosed acute sinusitis. *Pediatrics.* 2001;107(4):619–625

43. Kristo A, Uhari M, Luotonen J, Ilkko E, Koivunen P, Alho OP. Cefuroxime axetil versus placebo for children with acute respiratory infection and imaging evidence of sinusitis: a randomized, controlled trial. *Acta Paediatr.* 2005;94(9):1208–1213
44. Hoberman A, Paradise JL, Rockette HE, et al. Treatment of acute otitis media in children under 2 years of age. *N Engl J Med.* 2011;364(2):105–115
45. Tahtinen PA, Laine MK, Huovinen P, Jalava J, Ruuskanen O, Ruohola A. A placebo-controlled trial of antimicrobial treatment for acute otitis media. *N Engl J Med.* 2011;364(2):116–126
46. Gordts F, Abu Nasser I, Clement PA, Pierard D, Kaufman L. Bacteriology of the middle meatus in children. *Int J Pediatr Otorhinolaryngol.* 1999;48(2):163–167
47. Parsons DS, Wald ER. Otitis media and sinusitis: similar diseases. *Otolaryngol Clin North Am.* 1996;29(1):11–25
48. Revai K, Dobbs LA, Nair S, Patel JA, Grady JJ, Chonmaitree T. Incidence of acute otitis media and sinusitis complicating upper respiratory tract infection: the effect of age. *Pediatrics.* 2007;119(6). Available at: www.pediatrics.org/cgi/content/full/119/6/e1408
49. Klein JO, Bluestone CD. *Textbook of Pediatric Infectious Diseases.* 6th ed. Philadelphia, PA: Saunders; 2009
50. Casey JR, Adlowitz DG, Pichichero ME. New patterns in the otopathogens causing acute otitis media six to eight years after introduction of pneumococcal conjugate vaccine. *Pediatr Infect Dis J.* 2010;29(4):304–309
51. Brook I, Gober AE. Frequency of recovery of pathogens from the nasopharynx of children with acute maxillary sinusitis before and after the introduction of vaccination with the 7-valent pneumococcal vaccine. *Int J Pediatr Otorhinolaryngol.* 2007;71(4):575–579
52. Wald ER. Microbiology of acute and chronic sinusitis in children. *J Allergy Clin Immunol.* 1992;90(3 pt 2):452–456
53. Centers for Disease Control and Prevention. Effects of new penicillin susceptibility breakpoints for *Streptococcus pneumoniae*—United States, 2006-2007. *MMWR Morb Mortal Wkly Rep.* 2008;57(50):1353–1355
54. Centers for Disease Control and Prevention. Active Bacterial Core Surveillance (ABCs): Emerging Infections Program Network. 2011. Available at: www.cdc.gov/abcs/reports-findings/survreports/spneu09.html. Accessed November 6, 2012
55. Garbutt J, St Geme JW, III, May A, Storch GA, Shackelford PG. Developing community-specific recommendations for first-line treatment of acute otitis media: is high-dose amoxicillin necessary? *Pediatrics.* 2004;114(2):342–347
56. Harrison CJ, Woods C, Stout G, Martin B, Selvarangan R. Susceptibilities of *Haemophilus influenzae, Streptococcus pneumoniae,* including serotype 19A, and *Moraxella catarrhalis* paediatric isolates from 2005 to 2007 to commonly used antibiotics. *J Antimicrob Chemother.* 2009;63(3):511–519
57. Critchley IA, Jacobs MR, Brown SD, Traczewski MM, Tillotson GS, Janjic N. Prevalence of serotype 19A Streptococcus pneumoniae among isolates from U.S. children in 2005-2006 and activity of faropenem. *Antimicrob Agents Chemother.* 2008;52(7):2639–2643
58. Jacobs MR, Good CE, Windau AR, et al. Activity of ceftaroline against recent emerging serotypes of *Streptococcus pneumoniae* in the United States. *Antimicrob Agents Chemother.* 2010;54(6):2716–2719
59. Tristram S, Jacobs MR, Appelbaum PC. Antimicrobial resistance in *Haemophilus influenzae. Clin Microbiol Rev.* 2007;20(2):368–389
60. Levine OS, Farley M, Harrison LH, Lefkowitz L, McGeer A, Schwartz B. Risk factors for invasive pneumococcal disease in children: a population-based case-control study in North America. *Pediatrics.* 1999;103(3). Available at: www.pediatrics.org/cgi/content/full/103/3/e28
61. Seikel K, Shelton S, McCracken GH Jr. Middle ear fluid concentrations of amoxicillin after large dosages in children with acute otitis media. *Pediatr Infect Dis J.* 1997;16(7):710–711
62. Cohen R, Navel M, Grunberg J, et al. One dose ceftriaxone vs. ten days of amoxicillin/clavulanate therapy for acute otitis media: clinical efficacy and change in nasopharyngeal flora. *Pediatr Infect Dis J.* 1999;18(5):403–409
63. Green SM, Rothrock SG. Single-dose intramuscular ceftriaxone for acute otitis media in children. *Pediatrics.* 1993;91(1):23–30
64. Leibovitz E, Piglansky L, Raiz S, Press J, Leiberman A, Dagan R. Bacteriologic and clinical efficacy of one day vs. three day intramuscular ceftriaxone for treatment of nonresponsive acute otitis media in children. *Pediatr Infect Dis J.* 2000;19(11):1040–1045
65. DePestel DD, Benninger MS, Danziger L, et al. Cephalosporin use in treatment of patients with penicillin allergies. *J Am Pharm Assoc.* 2008;48(4):530–540
66. Pichichero ME. A review of evidence supporting the American Academy of Pediatrics recommendation for prescribing cephalosporin antibiotics for penicillin-allergic patients. *Pediatrics.* 2005;115(4):1048–1057
67. Pichichero ME, Casey JR. Safe use of selected cephalosporins in penicillin-allergic patients: a meta-analysis. *Otolaryngol Head Neck Surg.* 2007;136(3):340–347
68. Park MA, Koch CA, Klemawesch P, Joshi A, Li JT. Increased adverse drug reactions to cephalosporins in penicillin allergy patients with positive penicillin skin test. *Int Arch Allergy Immunol.* 2010;153(3):268–273
69. Jacobs MR. Antimicrobial-resistant Streptococcus pneumoniae: trends and management. *Expert Rev Anti Infect Ther.* 2008;6(5):619–635
70. Chow AW, Benninger MS, Brook I, et al; Infectious Diseases Society of America. IDSA clinical practice guideline for acute bacterial rhinosinusitis in children and adults. *Clin Infect Dis.* 2012;54(8):e72–e112
71. Brook I, Gober AE. Resistance to antimicrobials used for therapy of otitis media and sinusitis: effect of previous antimicrobial therapy and smoking. *Ann Otol Rhinol Laryngol.* 1999;108(7 pt 1):645–647
72. Brook I, Gober AE. Antimicrobial resistance in the nasopharyngeal flora of children with acute maxillary sinusitis and maxillary sinusitis recurring after amoxicillin therapy. *J Antimicrob Chemother.* 2004;53(2):399–402
73. Dohar J, Canton R, Cohen R, Farrell DJ, Felmingham D. Activity of telithromycin and comparators against bacterial pathogens isolated from 1,336 patients with clinically diagnosed acute sinusitis. *Ann Clin Microbiol Antimicrob.* 2004;3(3):15–21
74. Jacobs MR, Bajaksouzian S, Zilles A, Lin G, Pankuch GA, Appelbaum PC. Susceptibilities of *Streptococcus pneumoniae* and *Haemophilus influenzae* to 10 oral antimicrobial agents based on pharmacodynamic parameters: 1997 U.S. surveillance study. *Antimicrob Agents Chemother.* 1999;43(8):1901–1908
75. Jacobs MR, Felmingham D, Appelbaum PC, Gruneberg RN. The Alexander Project 1998-2000: susceptibility of pathogens isolated from community-acquired respiratory tract infection to commonly used antimicrobial agents. *J Antimicrob Chemother.* 2003;52(2):229–246

76. Lynch JP, III, Zhanel GG. *Streptococcus pneumoniae*: epidemiology and risk factors, evolution of antimicrobial resistance, and impact of vaccines. *Curr Opin Pulm Med*. 2010;16(3):217–225
77. Sahm DF, Jones ME, Hickey ML, Diakun DR, Mani SV, Thornsberry C. Resistance surveillance of *Streptococcus pneumoniae, Haemophilus influenzae* and *Moraxella catarrhalis* isolated in Asia and Europe, 1997-1998. *J Antimicrob Chemother*. 2000; 45(4):457–466
78. Sokol W. Epidemiology of sinusitis in the primary care setting: results from the 1999-2000 respiratory surveillance program. *Am J Med*. 2001;111(suppl 9A):19S–24S
79. Shaikh N, Wald ER, Pi M. Decongestants, antihistamines and nasal irrigation for acute sinusitis in children. *Cochrane Database Syst Rev*. 2010;(12):CD007909
80. Dolor RJ, Witsell DL, Hellkamp AS, Williams JW, Jr, Califf RM, Simel DL. Comparison of cefuroxime with or without intranasal fluticasone for the treatment of rhinosinusitis. The CAFFS Trial: a randomized controlled trial. *JAMA*. 2001;286(24):3097–3105
81. Meltzer EO, Bachert C, Staudinger H. Treating acute rhinosinusitis: comparing efficacy and safety of mometasone furoate nasal spray, amoxicillin, and placebo. *J Allergy Clin Immunol*. 2005;116(6):1289–1295
82. Meltzer EO, Charous BL, Busse WW, Zinreich SJ, Lorber RR, Danzig MR. Added relief in the treatment of acute recurrent sinusitis with adjunctive mometasone furoate nasal spray. The Nasonex Sinusitis Group. *J Allergy Clin Immunol*. 2000;106 (4):630–637
83. Meltzer EO, Orgel HA, Backhaus JW, et al. Intranasal flunisolide spray as an adjunct to oral antibiotic therapy for sinusitis. *J Allergy Clin Immunol*. 1993;92(6):812–823
84. Nayak AS, Settipane GA, Pedinoff A, et al. Effective dose range of mometasone furoate nasal spray in the treatment of acute rhinosinusitis. *Ann Allergy Asthma Immunol*. 2002;89(3):271–278
85. Williamson IG, Rumsby K, Benge S, et al. Antibiotics and topical nasal steroid for treatment of acute maxillary sinusitis: a randomized controlled trial. *JAMA*. 2007; 298(21):2487–2496
86. Zalmanovici A, Yaphe J. Intranasal steroids for acute sinusitis. *Cochrane Database Syst Rev*. 2009;(4):CD005149
87. Yilmaz G, Varan B, Yilmaz T, Gurakan B. Intranasal budesonide spray as an adjunct to oral antibiotic therapy for acute sinusitis in children. *Eur Arch Otorhinolaryngol*. 2000;257(5):256–259
88. Barlan IB, Erkan E, Bakir M, Berrak S, Basaran MM. Intranasal budesonide spray as an adjunct to oral antibiotic therapy for acute sinusitis in children. *Ann Allergy Asthma Immunol*. 1997;78(6):598–601
89. Bruni FM, De Luca G, Venturoli V, Boner AL. Intranasal corticosteroids and adrenal suppression. *Neuroimmunomodulation*. 2009;16 (5):353–362
90. Kim KT, Rabinovitch N, Uryniak T, Simpson B, O'Dowd L, Casty F. Effect of budesonide aqueous nasal spray on hypothalamic-pituitary-adrenal axis function in children with allergic rhinitis. *Ann Allergy Asthma Immunol*. 2004;93(1):61–67
91. Meltzer EO, Tripathy I, Maspero JF, Wu W, Philpot E. Safety and tolerability of fluticasone furoate nasal spray once daily in paediatric patients aged 6-11 years with allergic rhinitis: subanalysis of three randomized, double-blind, placebo-controlled, multicentre studies. *Clin Drug Investig*. 2009;29(2):79–86
92. Murphy K, Uryniak T, Simpson B, O'Dowd L. Growth velocity in children with perennial allergic rhinitis treated with budesonide aqueous nasal spray. *Ann Allergy Asthma Immunol*. 2006;96(5):723–730
93. Ratner PH, Meltzer EO, Teper A. Mometasone furoate nasal spray is safe and effective for 1-year treatment of children with perennial allergic rhinitis. *Int J Pediatr Otorhinolaryngol*. 2009;73(5):651–657
94. Skoner DP, Gentile DA, Doyle WJ. Effect on growth of long-term treatment with intranasal triamcinolone acetonide aqueous in children with allergic rhinitis. *Ann Allergy Asthma Immunol*. 2008;101(4): 431–436
95. Weinstein S, Qaqundah P, Georges G, Nayak A. Efficacy and safety of triamcinolone acetonide aqueous nasal spray in children aged 2 to 5 years with perennial allergic rhinitis: a randomized, double-blind, placebo-controlled study with an open-label extension. *Ann Allergy Asthma Immunol*. 2009;102(4):339–347
96. Zitt M, Kosoglou T, Hubbell J. Mometasone furoate nasal spray: a review of safety and systemic effects. *Drug Saf*. 2007;30(4): 317–326
97. Adam P, Stiffman M, Blake RL Jr. A clinical trial of hypertonic saline nasal spray in subjects with the common cold or rhinosinusitis. *Arch Fam Med*. 1998;7(1):39–43
98. Wang YH, Yang CP, Ku MS, Sun HL, Lue KH. Efficacy of nasal irrigation in the treatment of acute sinusitis in children. *Int J Pediatr Otorhinolaryngol*. 2009;73(12): 1696–1701
99. Harvey R, Hannan SA, Badia L, Scadding G. Nasal saline irrigations for the symptoms of chronic rhinosinusitis. *Cochrane Database Syst Rev*. 2007;(3):CD006394
100. Kassel JC, King D, Spurling GK. Saline nasal irrigation for acute upper respiratory tract infections. *Cochrane Database Syst Rev*. 2010;(3):CD006821
101. Shapiro GG, Virant FS, Furukawa CT, Pierson WE, Bierman CW. Immunologic defects in patients with refractory sinusitis. *Pediatrics*. 1991;87(3):311–316
102. Wood AJ, Douglas RG. Pathogenesis and treatment of chronic rhinosinusitis. *Postgrad Med J*. 2010;86(1016):359–364
103. Liao S, Durand ML, Cunningham MJ. Sinogenic orbital and subperiosteal abscesses: microbiology and methicillin-resistant Staphylococcus aureus incidence. *Otolaryngol Head Neck Surg*. 2010;143(3):392–396
104. Oxford LE, McClay J. Medical and surgical management of subperiosteal orbital abscess secondary to acute sinusitis in children. *Int J Pediatr Otorhinolaryngol*. 2006;70(11):1853–1861

Sinusitis Clinical Practice Guideline Quick Reference Tools

- Action Statement Summary
  — Clinical Practice Guideline for the Diagnosis and Management of Acute Bacterial Sinusitis in Children Aged 1 to 18 Years
- *ICD-10-CM* Coding Quick Reference for Sinusitis
- AAP Patient Education Handout
  — *Sinusitis and Your Child*

Action Statement Summary

Clinical Practice Guideline for the Diagnosis and Management of Acute Bacterial Sinusitis in Children Aged 1 to 18 Years

Key Action Statement 1

Clinicians should make a presumptive diagnosis of acute bacterial sinusitis when a child with an acute URI presents with the following:

- Persistent illness, ie, nasal discharge (of any quality) or daytime cough or both lasting more than 10 days without improvement;

OR

- Worsening course, ie, worsening or new onset of nasal discharge, daytime cough, or fever after initial improvement;

OR

- Severe onset, ie, concurrent fever (temperature ≥39°C/102.2°F) and purulent nasal discharge for at least 3 consecutive days (Evidence Quality: B; Recommendation).

Key Action Statement 2A

Clinicians should not obtain imaging studies (plain films, contrast-enhanced computed tomography [CT], MRI, or ultrasonography) to distinguish acute bacterial sinusitis from viral URI (Evidence Quality: B; Strong Recommendation).

Key Action Statement 2B

Clinicians should obtain a contrast-enhanced CT scan of the paranasal sinuses and/or an MRI with contrast whenever a child is suspected of having orbital or central nervous system complications of acute bacterial sinusitis (Evidence Quality: B; Strong Recommendation).

Key Action Statement 3

Initial Management of Acute Bacterial Sinusitis

3A: "Severe onset and worsening course" acute bacterial sinusitis. The clinician should prescribe antibiotic therapy for acute bacterial sinusitis in children with severe onset or worsening course (signs, symptoms, or both) (Evidence Quality: B; Strong Recommendation).

3B: "Persistent illness." The clinician should either prescribe antibiotic therapy OR offer additional outpatient observation for 3 days to children with persistent illness (nasal discharge of any quality or cough or both for at least 10 days without evidence of improvement) (Evidence Quality: B; Recommendation).

Key Action Statement 4

Clinicians should prescribe amoxicillin with or without clavulanate as first-line treatment when a decision has been made to initiate antibiotic treatment of acute bacterial sinusitis (Evidence Quality: B; Recommendation).

Key Action Statement 5A

Clinicians should reassess initial management if there is either a caregiver report of worsening (progression of initial signs/symptoms or appearance of new signs/symptoms) OR failure to improve (lack of reduction in all presenting signs/symptoms) within 72 hours of initial management (Evidence Quality: C; Recommendation).

Key Action Statement 5B

If the diagnosis of acute bacterial sinusitis is confirmed in a child with worsening symptoms or failure to improve in 72 hours, then clinicians may change the antibiotic therapy for the child initially managed with antibiotic OR initiate antibiotic treatment of the child initially managed with observation (Evidence Quality: D; Option based on expert opinion, case reports, and reasoning from first principles).

Coding Quick Reference for Sinusitis
ICD-10-CM
J01.00 Acute maxillary sinusitis, unspecified
J01.01 Acute recurrent maxillary sinusitis
J01.10 Acute frontal sinusitis, unspecified
J01.11 Acute recurrent frontal sinusitis
J01.21 Acute recurrent ethmoidal sinusitis
J01.30 Acute sphenoidal sinusitis, unspecified
J01.31 Acute recurrent sphenoidal sinusitis
J01.40 Acute pansinusitis, unspecified
J01.41 Acute recurrent pansinusitis
J01.80 Other acute sinusitis
J01.81 Other acute recurrent sinusitis
J01.90 Acute sinusitis, unspecified
J01.91 Acute recurrent sinusitis, unspecified
J32.9 Sinusitis NOS

Sinusitis and Your Child

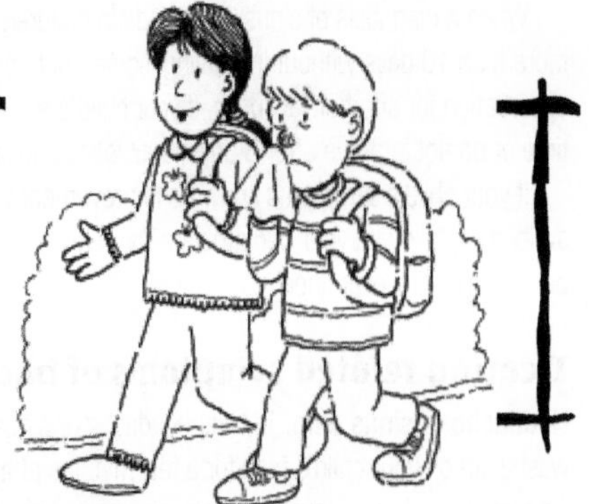

Sinusitis is an inflammation of the lining of the nose and sinuses. It is a very common infection in children.

Viral sinusitis usually accompanies a cold. Allergic sinusitis may accompany allergies such as hay fever. Bacterial sinusitis is a secondary infection caused by the trapping of bacteria in the sinuses during the course of a cold or allergy.

Fluid inside the sinuses

When your child has a viral cold or hay fever, the linings of the nose and sinus cavities swell up and produce more fluid than usual. This is why the nose gets congested and is "runny" during a cold.

Most of the time the swelling disappears by itself as the cold or allergy goes away. However, if the swelling does not go away, the openings that normally allow the sinuses to drain into the back of the nose get blocked and the sinuses fill with fluid. Because the sinuses are blocked and cannot drain properly, bacteria are trapped inside and grow there, causing a secondary infection. Although nose blowing and sniffing may be natural responses to this blockage, when excessive they can make the situation worse by pushing bacteria from the back of the nose into the sinuses.

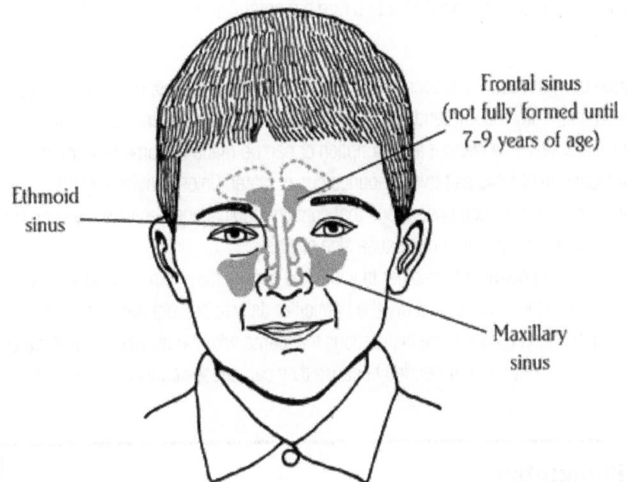

The linings of the sinuses and the nose always produce some fluid (secretions). This fluid keeps the nose and sinus cavities from becoming too dry and adds moisture to the air that you breathe.

Is it a cold or bacterial sinusitis?

It is often difficult to tell if an illness is just a viral cold or if it is complicated by a bacterial infection of the sinuses.

Generally viral colds have the following characteristics:

- Colds usually last only 5 to 10 days.
- Colds typically start with clear, watery nasal discharge. After a day or 2, it is normal for the nasal discharge to become thicker and white, yellow, or green. After several days, the discharge becomes clear again and dries.
- Colds include a daytime cough that often gets worse at night.
- If a fever is present, it is usually at the beginning of the cold and is generally low grade, lasting for 1 or 2 days.
- Cold symptoms usually peak in severity at 3 or 5 days, then improve and disappear over the next 7 to 10 days.

Signs and symptoms that your child may have bacterial sinusitis include:

- Cold symptoms (nasal discharge, daytime cough, or both) lasting more than 10 days *without improving*
- Thick yellow nasal discharge *and* a fever for at least 3 or 4 days in a row
- A severe headache behind or around the eyes that gets worse when bending over
- Swelling and dark circles around the eyes, especially in the morning
- Persistent bad breath along with cold symptoms (However, this also could be from a sore throat or a sign that your child is not brushing his teeth!)

In very rare cases, a bacterial sinus infection may spread to the eye or the central nervous system (the brain). If your child has the following symptoms, call your pediatrician immediately:

- Swelling and/or redness around the eyes, not just in the morning but all day
- Severe headache and/or pain in the back of the neck
- Persistent vomiting
- Sensitivity to light
- Increasing irritability

Diagnosing bacterial sinusitis

It may be difficult to tell a sinus infection from an uncomplicated cold, especially in the first few days of the illness. Your pediatrician will most likely be able to tell if your child has bacterial sinusitis after examining your child and hearing about the progression of symptoms. In older children, when the diagnosis is uncertain, your pediatrician may order computed tomographic (CT) scans to confirm the diagnosis.

Treating bacterial sinusitis

If your child has bacterial sinusitis, your pediatrician may prescribe an antibiotic for at least 10 days. Once your child is on the medication, symptoms should start to go away over the next 2 to 3 days—the nasal discharge will clear and the cough will improve. *Even though your child may seem better, continue to give the antibiotics for the prescribed length of time. Ending the medications too early could cause the infection to return.*

When a diagnosis of sinusitis is made in children with cold symptoms lasting more than 10 days without improving, some doctors may choose to continue observation for another few days. If your child's symptoms worsen during this time or do not improve after 3 days, antibiotics should be started.

If your child's symptoms show no improvement 2 to 3 days after starting the antibiotics, talk with your pediatrician. Your child might need a different medication or need to be re-examined.

Treating related symptoms of bacterial sinusitis

Headache or sinus pain. To treat headache or sinus pain, try placing a warm washcloth on your child's face for a few minutes at a time. Pain medications such as acetaminophen or ibuprofen may also help. (However, do not give your child aspirin. It has been associated with a rare but potentially fatal disease called Reye syndrome.)

Nasal congestion. If the secretions in your child's nose are especially thick, your pediatrician may recommend that you help drain them with saline nose drops. These are available without a prescription or can be made at home by adding 1⁄4 teaspoon of table salt to an 8-ounce cup of water. Unless advised by your pediatrician, do not use nose drops that contain medications because they can be absorbed in amounts that can cause side effects.

Placing a cool-mist humidifier in your child's room may help keep your child more comfortable. Clean and dry the humidifier daily to prevent bacteria or mold from growing in it (follow the instructions that came with the humidifier). Hot water vaporizers are not recommended because they can cause scalds or burns.

Remember

If your child has symptoms of a bacterial sinus infection, see your pediatrician. Your pediatrician can properly diagnose and treat the infection and recommend ways to help alleviate the discomfort from some of the symptoms.

The information contained in this publication should not be used as a substitute for the medical care and advice of your pediatrician. There may be variations in treatment that your pediatrician may recommend based on individual facts and circumstances.

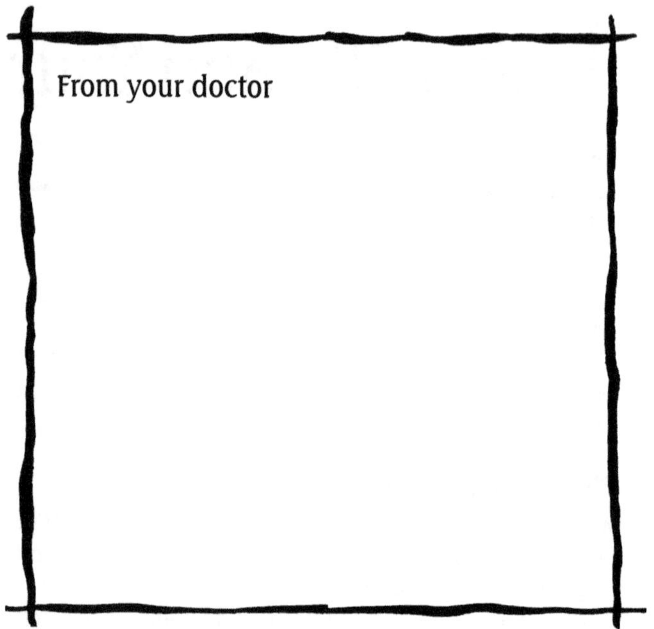

American Academy of Pediatrics

DEDICATED TO THE HEALTH OF ALL CHILDREN™

The American Academy of Pediatrics is an organization of 60,000 primary care pediatricians, pediatric medical subspecialists, and pediatric surgical specialists dedicated to the health, safety, and well-being of infants, children, adolescents, and young adults.

American Academy of Pediatrics
Web site—www.HealthyChildren.org

Copyright © 2003
American Academy of Pediatrics, Updated 07/2013
All Rights Reserved

Diagnosis and Management of Childhood Obstructive Sleep Apnea Syndrome

- *Clinical Practice Guideline*

CLINICAL PRACTICE GUIDELINE

Diagnosis and Management of Childhood Obstructive Sleep Apnea Syndrome

abstract

OBJECTIVES: This revised clinical practice guideline, intended for use by primary care clinicians, provides recommendations for the diagnosis and management of the obstructive sleep apnea syndrome (OSAS) in children and adolescents. This practice guideline focuses on uncomplicated childhood OSAS, that is, OSAS associated with adenotonsillar hypertrophy and/or obesity in an otherwise healthy child who is being treated in the primary care setting.

METHODS: Of 3166 articles from 1999–2010, 350 provided relevant data. Most articles were level II–IV. The resulting evidence report was used to formulate recommendations.

RESULTS AND CONCLUSIONS: The following recommendations are made. (1) All children/adolescents should be screened for snoring. (2) Polysomnography should be performed in children/adolescents with snoring and symptoms/signs of OSAS; if polysomnography is not available, then alternative diagnostic tests or referral to a specialist for more extensive evaluation may be considered. (3) Adenotonsillectomy is recommended as the first-line treatment of patients with adenotonsillar hypertrophy. (4) High-risk patients should be monitored as inpatients postoperatively. (5) Patients should be reevaluated postoperatively to determine whether further treatment is required. Objective testing should be performed in patients who are high risk or have persistent symptoms/signs of OSAS after therapy. (6) Continuous positive airway pressure is recommended as treatment if adenotonsillectomy is not performed or if OSAS persists postoperatively. (7) Weight loss is recommended in addition to other therapy in patients who are overweight or obese. (8) Intranasal corticosteroids are an option for children with mild OSAS in whom adenotonsillectomy is contraindicated or for mild postoperative OSAS. *Pediatrics* 2012;130:576–584

Carole L. Marcus, MBBCh, Lee Jay Brooks, MD, Kari A. Draper, MD, David Gozal, MD, Ann Carol Halbower, MD, Jacqueline Jones, MD, Michael S. Schechter, MD, MPH, Stephen Howard Sheldon, DO, Karen Spruyt, PhD, Sally Davidson Ward, MD, Christopher Lehmann, MD, Richard N. Shiffman, MD

KEY WORDS

snoring, sleep-disordered breathing, adenotonsillectomy, continuous positive airway pressure

ABBREVIATIONS

AAP—American Academy of Pediatrics
AHI—apnea hypopnea index
CPAP—continuous positive airway pressure
OSAS—obstructive sleep apnea syndrome

This document is copyrighted and is property of the American Academy of Pediatrics and its Board of Directors. All authors have filed conflict of interest statements with the American Academy of Pediatrics. Any conflicts have been resolved through a process approved by the Board of Directors. The American Academy of Pediatrics has neither solicited nor accepted any commercial involvement in the development of the content of this publication.

The recommendations in this report do not indicate an exclusive course of treatment or serve as a standard of medical care. Variations, taking into account individual circumstances, may be appropriate.

All clinical practice guidelines from the American Academy of Pediatrics automatically expire 5 years after publication unless reaffirmed, revised, or retired at or before that time.

www.pediatrics.org/cgi/doi/10.1542/peds.2012-1671

doi:10.1542/peds.2012-1671

PEDIATRICS (ISSN Numbers: Print, 0031-4005; Online, 1098-4275).

Copyright © 2012 by the American Academy of Pediatrics

INTRODUCTION

Obstructive sleep apnea syndrome (OSAS) is a common condition in childhood and can result in severe complications if left untreated. In 2002, the American Academy of Pediatrics (AAP) published a practice guideline for the diagnosis and management of childhood OSAS.[1] Since that time, there has been a considerable increase in publications and research on the topic; thus, the guidelines have been revised.

The purposes of this revised clinical practice guideline are to (1) increase the recognition of OSAS by primary care clinicians to minimize delay in diagnosis and avoid serious sequelae of OSAS; (2) evaluate diagnostic techniques; (3) describe treatment options; (4) provide guidelines for follow-up; and (5) discuss areas requiring further research. The recommendations in this statement do not indicate an exclusive course of treatment. Variations, taking into account individual circumstances, may be appropriate.

This practice guideline focuses on uncomplicated childhood OSAS—that is, the OSAS associated with adenotonsillar hypertrophy and/or obesity in an otherwise healthy child who is being treated in the primary care setting. This guideline specifically excludes infants younger than 1 year of age, patients with central apnea or hypoventilation syndromes, and patients with OSAS associated with other medical disorders, including but not limited to Down syndrome, craniofacial anomalies, neuromuscular disease (including cerebral palsy), chronic lung disease, sickle cell disease, metabolic disease, or laryngomalacia. These important patient populations are too complex to discuss within the scope of this article and require consultation with a pediatric subspecialist.

Additional information providing justification for the key action statements and a detailed review of the literature are provided in the accompanying technical report available online.[2]

METHODS OF GUIDELINE DEVELOPMENT

Details of the methods of guideline development are included in the accompanying technical report.[2] The AAP selected a subcommittee composed of pediatricians and other experts in the fields of sleep medicine, pulmonology, and otolaryngology, as well as experts from epidemiology and pediatric practice to develop an evidence base of literature on this topic. The committee included liaison members from the AAP Section on Otolaryngology-Head and Neck Surgery, American Thoracic Society, American Academy of Sleep Medicine, American College of Chest Physicians, and the National Sleep Foundation. Committee members signed forms disclosing conflicts of interest.

An automated search of the literature on childhood OSAS from 1999 to 2008 was performed by using 5 scientific literature search engines.[2] The medical subject heading terms that were used in all fields were snoring, apnea, sleep-disordered breathing, sleep-related breathing disorders, upper airway resistance, polysomnography, sleep study, adenoidectomy, tonsillectomy, continuous positive airway pressure, obesity, adiposity, hypopnea, hypoventilation, cognition, behavior, and neuropsychology. Reviews, case reports, letters to the editor, and abstracts were not included. Non–English-language articles, animal studies, and studies relating to infants younger than 1 year and to special populations (eg, children with craniofacial anomalies or sickle cell disease) were excluded. In several steps, a total of 3166 hits was reduced to 350 articles, which underwent detailed review.[2] Committee members selectively updated this literature search for articles published from 2008 to 2011 specific to guideline categories. Details of the literature grading system are available in the accompanying technical report.

Since publication of the previous guidelines, there has been an improvement in the quality of OSAS studies in the literature; however, there remain few randomized, blinded, controlled studies. Most studies were questionnaire or polysomnography based. Many studies used standard definitions for pediatric polysomnography scoring, but the interpretation of polysomnography (eg, the apnea hypopnea index [AHI] criterion used for diagnosis or to determine treatment) varied widely. The guideline notes the quality of evidence for each key action statement. Additional details are available in the technical report.

The evidence-based approach to guideline development requires that the evidence in support of each key action statement be identified, appraised, and summarized and that an explicit link between evidence and recommendations be defined. Evidence-based recommendations reflect the quality of evidence and the balance of benefit and harm that is anticipated when the recommendation is followed. The AAP policy statement, "Classifying Recommendations for Clinical Practice Guidelines,"[3] was followed in designating levels of recommendation (see Fig 1 and Table 1).

DEFINITION

This guideline defines OSAS in children as a "disorder of breathing during sleep characterized by prolonged partial upper airway obstruction and/or intermittent complete obstruction (obstructive apnea) that disrupts normal ventilation during sleep and normal sleep patterns,"[4] accompanied by symptoms or signs, as listed in Table 2. Prevalence rates based on level I and II studies range from 1.2% to 5.7%.[5–7] Symptoms include habitual snoring (often with intermittent pauses, snorts, or gasps), disturbed sleep, and daytime neurobehavioral problems. Daytime sleepiness may occur, but is uncommon in young children. OSAS is associated with neurocognitive impairment, behavioral problems, failure to thrive, hypertension, cardiac dysfunction, and systemic inflammation. Risk factors include adenotonsillar hypertrophy, obesity, craniofacial anomalies, and neuromuscular disorders. Only the first 2 risk factors are

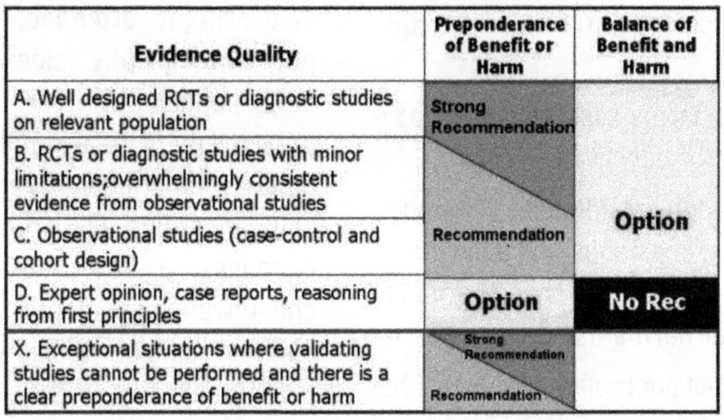

Evidence Quality	Preponderance of Benefit or Harm	Balance of Benefit and Harm
A. Well designed RCTs or diagnostic studies on relevant population	Strong Recommendation	Option
B. RCTs or diagnostic studies with minor limitations;overwhelmingly consistent evidence from observational studies		
C. Observational studies (case-control and cohort design)	Recommendation	
D. Expert opinion, case reports, reasoning from first principles	Option	No Rec
X. Exceptional situations where validating studies cannot be performed and there is a clear preponderance of benefit or harm	Strong Recommendation / Recommendation	

FIGURE 1

Evidence quality. Integrating evidence quality appraisal with an assessment of the anticipated balance between benefits and harms if a policy is carried out leads to designation of a policy as a strong recommendation, recommendation, option, or no recommendation. RCT, randomized controlled trial; Rec, recommendation.

discussed in this guideline. In this guideline, obesity is defined as a BMI >95th percentile for age and gender.[8]

KEY ACTION STATEMENTS

Key Action Statement 1: Screening for OSAS

As part of routine health maintenance visits, clinicians should inquire whether the child or adolescent snores. If the answer is affirmative or if a child or adolescent presents with signs or symptoms of OSAS (Table 2), clinicians should perform a more focused evaluation. (Evidence Quality: Grade B, Recommendation Strength: Recommendation.)

Evidence Profile KAS 1

- Aggregate evidence quality: B
- Benefit: Early identification of OSAS is desirable, because it is a high-prevalence condition, and identification and treatment can result in alleviation of current symptoms, improved quality of life, prevention of sequelae, education of parents, and decreased health care utilization.
- Harm: Provider time, patient and parent time.
- Benefits-harms assessment: Preponderance of benefit over harm.
- Value judgments: Panelists believe that identification of a serious medical condition outweighs the time expenditure necessary for screening.
- Role of patient preferences: None.
- Exclusions: None.
- Intentional vagueness: None.
- Strength: Recommendation.

Almost all children with OSAS snore,[9–11] although caregivers frequently do not volunteer this information at medical visits.[12] Thus, asking about snoring at each health maintenance visit (as well as at other appropriate times, such as when evaluating for tonsillitis) is a sensitive, albeit nonspecific, screening measure that is quick and easy to perform. Snoring is common in children and adolescents; however, OSAS is less common. Therefore, an affirmative answer should be followed by a detailed history and examination to determine whether further evaluation for OSAS is needed (Table 2); this clinical evaluation alone

TABLE 1 Definitions and Recommendation Implications

Statement	Definition	Implication
Strong recommendation	A strong recommendation in favor of a particular action is made when the anticipated benefits of the recommended intervention clearly exceed the harms (as a strong recommendation against an action is made when the anticipated harms clearly exceed the benefits) and the quality of the supporting evidence is excellent. In some clearly identified circumstances, strong recommendations may be made when high-quality evidence is impossible to obtain and the anticipated benefits strongly outweigh the harms.	Clinicians should follow a strong recommendation unless a clear and compelling rationale for an alternative approach is present.
Recommendation	A recommendation in favor of a particular action is made when the anticipated benefits exceed the harms but the quality of evidence is not as strong. Again, in some clearly identified circumstances, recommendations may be made when high-quality evidence is impossible to obtain but the anticipated benefits outweigh the harms.	It would be prudent for clinicians to follow a recommendation, but they should remain alert to new information and sensitive to patient preferences.
Option	Options define courses that may be taken when either the quality of evidence is suspect or carefully performed studies have shown little clear advantage to one approach over another.	Clinicians should consider the option in their decision-making, and patient preference may have a substantial role.
No recommendation	No recommendation indicates that there is a lack of pertinent published evidence and that the anticipated balance of benefits and harms is presently unclear.	Clinicians should be alert to new published evidence that clarifies the balance of benefit versus harm.

TABLE 2 Symptoms and Signs of OSAS

History
Frequent snoring (≥3 nights/wk)
Labored breathing during sleep
Gasps/snorting noises/observed episodes of apnea
Sleep enuresis (especially secondary enuresis)[a]
Sleeping in a seated position or with the neck hyperextended
Cyanosis
Headaches on awakening
Daytime sleepiness
Attention-deficit/hyperactivity disorder
Learning problems
Physical examination
Underweight or overweight
Tonsillar hypertrophy
Adenoidal facies
Micrognathia/retrognathia
High-arched palate
Failure to thrive
Hypertension

[a] Enuresis after at least 6 mo of continence.

does not establish the diagnosis (see technical report). Occasional snoring, for example, with an upper respiratory tract infection, is less of a concern than snoring that occurs at least 3 times a week and is associated with any of the symptoms or signs listed in Table 2.

Key Action Statement 2A: Polysomnography

If a child or adolescent snores on a regular basis and has any of the complaints or findings shown in Table 2, clinicians should either (1) obtain a polysomnogram (Evidence Quality A, Key Action strength: Recommendation) OR (2) refer the patient to a sleep specialist or otolaryngologist for a more extensive evaluation (Evidence quality D, Key Action strength: Option). (Evidence Quality: Grade A for polysomnography; Grade D for specialist referral, Recommendation Strength: Recommendation.)

Evidence Profile KAS 2A: Polysomnography

- Aggregate evidence quality: A
- Benefits: Establish diagnosis and determine severity of OSAS.
- Harm: Expense, time, anxiety/discomfort.
- Benefits-harms assessment: Preponderance of benefit over harm.
- Value judgments: Panelists weighed the value of establishing a diagnosis as more important than the minor potential harms listed.
- Role of patient preferences: Small because of preponderance of evidence that polysomnography is the most accurate way to make a diagnosis.
- Exclusions: See Key Action Statement 2B regarding lack of availability.
- Intentional vagueness: None.
- Strength: Recommendation.

Evidence Profile KAS 2A: Referral

- Aggregate evidence quality: D
- Benefits: Subspecialist may be better able to establish diagnosis and determine severity of OSAS.
- Harm: Expense, time, anxiety/discomfort.
- Benefits-harms assessment: Preponderance of benefit over harm.
- Value judgments: Panelists weighed the value of establishing a diagnosis as more important than the minor potential harms listed.
- Role of patient preferences: Large.
- Exclusions: None.
- Intentional vagueness: None.
- Strength: Option.

Although history and physical examination are useful to screen patients and determine which patients need further investigation for OSAS, the sensitivity and specificity of the history and physical examination are poor (see accompanying technical report). Physical examination when the child is awake may be normal, and the size of the tonsils cannot be used to predict the presence of OSAS in an individual child. Thus, objective testing is required. The gold standard test is overnight, attended, in-laboratory polysomnography (sleep study). This is a noninvasive test involving the measurement of a number of physiologic functions overnight, typically including EEG; pulse oximetry; oronasal airflow, abdominal and chest wall movements, partial pressure of carbon dioxide (P_{CO_2}); and video recording.[13] Specific pediatric measuring and scoring criteria should be used.[13] Polysomnography will demonstrate the presence or absence of OSAS. Polysomnography also demonstrates the severity of OSAS, which is helpful in planning treatment and in postoperative short- and long-term management.

Key Action Statement 2B: Alternative Testing

If polysomnography is not available, then clinicians may order alternative diagnostic tests, such as nocturnal video recording, nocturnal oximetry, daytime nap polysomnography, or ambulatory polysomnography. (Evidence Quality: Grade C, Recommendation Strength: Option.)

Evidence Profile KAS 2B

- Aggregate evidence quality: C
- Benefit: Varying positive and negative predictive values for establishing diagnosis.
- Harm: False-negative and false-positive results may underestimate or overestimate severity, expense, time, anxiety/discomfort.
- Benefits-harms assessment: Equilibrium of benefits and harms.
- Value judgments: Opinion of the panel that some objective testing is better than none. Pragmatic decision based on current shortage of pediatric polysomnography facilities (this may change over time).
- Role of patient preferences: Small, if choices are limited by availability;

families may choose to travel to centers where more extensive facilities are available.

- Exclusions: None.
- Intentional vagueness: None.
- Strength: Option.

Although polysomnography is the gold standard for diagnosis of OSAS, there is a shortage of sleep laboratories with pediatric expertise. Hence, polysomnography may not be readily available in certain regions of the country. Alternative diagnostic tests have been shown to have weaker positive and negative predictive values than polysomnography, but nevertheless, objective testing is preferable to clinical evaluation alone. If an alternative test fails to demonstrate OSAS in a patient with a high pretest probability, full polysomnography should be sought.

Key Action Statement 3: Adenotonsillectomy

If a child is determined to have OSAS, has a clinical examination consistent with adenotonsillar hypertrophy, and does not have a contraindication to surgery (see Table 3), the clinician should recommend adenotonsillectomy as the first line of treatment. If the child has OSAS but does not have adenotonsillar hypertrophy, other treatment should be considered (see Key Action Statement 6). Clinical judgment is required to determine the benefits of adenotonsillectomy compared with other treatments in obese children with varying degrees of adenotonsillar hypertrophy. (Evidence Quality: Grade B, Recommendation Strength: Recommendation.)

Evidence Profile KAS 3

- Aggregate evidence quality: B
- Benefit: Improve OSAS and accompanying symptoms and sequelae.
- Harm: Pain, anxiety, dehydration, anesthetic complications, hemorrhage, infection, postoperative respiratory difficulties, velopharyngeal incompetence, nasopharyngeal stenosis, death.
- Benefits-harms assessment: Preponderance of benefit over harm.
- Value judgments: The panel sees the benefits of treating OSAS as more beneficial than the low risk of serious consequences.
- Role of patient preferences: Low; continuous positive airway pressure (CPAP) is an option but involves prolonged, long-term treatment as compared with a single, relatively low-risk surgical procedure.
- Exclusions: See Table 3.
- Intentional vagueness: None.
- Strength: Recommendation.

Adenotonsillectomy is very effective in treating OSAS. Adenoidectomy or tonsillectomy alone may not be sufficient, because residual lymphoid tissue may contribute to persistent obstruction. In otherwise healthy children with adenotonsillar hypertrophy, adenotonsillectomy is associated with improvements in symptoms and sequelae of OSAS. Postoperative polysomnography typically shows a major decrease in the number of obstructive events, although some obstructions may still be present. Although obese children may have less satisfactory results, many will be adequately treated with adenotonsillectomy; however, further research is needed to determine which obese children are most likely to benefit from surgery. In this population, the benefits of a 1-time surgical procedure, with a small but real risk of complications, need to be weighed against long-term treatment with CPAP, which is associated with discomfort, disruption of family lifestyle, and risks of poor adherence. Potential complications of adenotonsillectomy are shown in Table 4. Although serious complications (including death) may occur, the rate of these complications is low, and the risks of complications need to be weighed against the consequences of untreated OSAS. In general, a 1-time only procedure with a relatively low morbidity is preferable to lifelong treatment with CPAP; furthermore, the efficacy of CPAP is limited by generally suboptimal adherence. Other treatment options, such as anti-inflammatory medications, weight loss, or tracheostomy, are less effective, are difficult to achieve, or have higher morbidity, respectively.

TABLE 3 Contraindications for Adenotonsillectomy

Absolute contraindications
No adenotonsillar tissue (tissue has been surgically removed)
Relative contraindications
Very small tonsils/adenoid
Morbid obesity and small tonsils/adenoid
Bleeding disorder refractory to treatment
Submucus cleft palate
Other medical conditions making patient medically unstable for surgery

Key Action Statement 4: High-Risk Patients Undergoing Adenotonsillectomy

Clinicians should monitor high-risk patients (Table 5) undergoing adenotonsillectomy as inpatients postoperatively. (Evidence Quality: Grade B, Recommendation Strength: Recommendation.)

TABLE 4 Risks of Adenotonsillectomy

Minor
Pain
Dehydration attributable to postoperative nausea/vomiting and poor oral intake
Major
Anesthetic complications
Acute upper airway obstruction during induction or emergence from anesthesia
Postoperative respiratory compromise
Hemorrhage
Velopharyngeal incompetence
Nasopharyngeal stenosis
Death

TABLE 5 Risk Factors for Postoperative Respiratory Complications in Children With OSAS Undergoing Adenotonsillectomy

Younger than 3 y of age
Severe OSAS on polysomnography[a]
Cardiac complications of OSAS
Failure to thrive
Obesity
Craniofacial anomalies[b]
Neuromuscular disorders[b]
Current respiratory infection

[a] It is difficult to provide exact polysomnographic criteria for severity, because these criteria will vary depending on the age of the child; additional comorbidities, such as obesity, asthma, or cardiac complications of OSAS; and other polysomnographic criteria that have not been evaluated in the literature, such as the level of hypercapnia and the frequency of desaturation (as compared with lowest oxygen saturation). Nevertheless, on the basis of published studies (primarily Level III, see Technical Report), it is recommended that all patients with a lowest oxygen saturation <80% (either on preoperative polysomnography or during observation in the recovery room postoperatively) or an AHI ≥24/h be observed as inpatients postoperatively as they are at increased risk for postoperative respiratory compromise. Additionally, on the basis of expert consensus, it is recommended that patients with significant hypercapnia on polysomnography (peak P_{CO_2} ≥60 mm Hg) be admitted postoperatively. The committee noted that that most published studies were retrospective and not comprehensive, and therefore these recommendations may change if higher-level studies are published. Clinicians may decide to admit patients with less severe polysomnographic abnormalities based on a constellation of risk factors (age, comorbidities, and additional polysomnographic factors) for a particular individual.

[b] Not discussed in these guidelines.

Evidence Profile KAS 4

- Aggregate evidence quality: B
- Benefit: Effectively manage severe respiratory compromise and avoid death.
- Harm: Expense, time, anxiety.
- Benefits-harms assessment: Preponderance of benefit over harm.
- Value judgments: The panel believes that early recognition of any serious adverse events is critically important.
- Role of patient preferences: Minimal; this is an important safety issue.
- Exclusions: None.
- Intentional vagueness: None.
- Strength: Recommendation.

Patients with OSAS may develop respiratory complications, such as worsening of OSAS or pulmonary edema, in the immediate postoperative period. Death attributable to respiratory complications in the immediate postoperative period has been reported in patients with severe OSAS. Identified risk factors are shown in Table 5. High-risk patients should undergo surgery in a center capable of treating complex pediatric patients. They should be hospitalized overnight for close monitoring postoperatively. Children with an acute respiratory infection on the day of surgery, as documented by fever, cough, and/or wheezing, are at increased risk of postoperative complications and, therefore, should be rescheduled or monitored closely postoperatively. Clinicians should decide on an individual basis whether these patients should be rescheduled, taking into consideration the severity of OSAS in the particular patient and keeping in mind that many children with adenotonsillar hypertrophy have chronic rhinorrhea and nasal congestion, even in the absence of viral infections.

Key Action Statement 5: Reevaluation

Clinicians should clinically reassess all patients with OSAS for persisting signs and symptoms after therapy to determine whether further treatment is required. (Evidence Quality: Grade B, Recommendation Strength: Recommendation.)

Evidence Profile KAS 5A

- Aggregate evidence quality: B
- Benefit: Determine effects of treatment.
- Harm: Expense, time.
- Benefits-harms assessment: Preponderance of benefit over harm.
- Value judgments: Data show that a significant proportion of children continue to have abnormalities postoperatively; therefore, the panel determined that the benefits of follow-up outweigh the minor inconveniences.
- Role of patient preferences: Minimal; follow-up is good clinical practice.
- Exclusions: None.
- Intentional vagueness: None.
- Strength: Recommendation.

Clinicians should reassess OSAS-related symptoms and signs (Table 2) after 6 to 8 weeks of therapy to determine whether further evaluation and treatment are indicated. Objective data regarding the timing of the postoperative evaluation are not available. Most clinicians recommend reevaluation 6 to 8 weeks after treatment to allow for healing of the operative site and to allow time for upper airway, cardiac, and central nervous system recovery. Patients who remain symptomatic should undergo objective testing (see Key Action Statement 2) or be referred to a sleep specialist for further evaluation.

Key Action Statement 5B: Reevaluation of High-Risk Patients

Clinicians should reevaluate high-risk patients for persistent OSAS after adenotonsillectomy, including those who had a significantly abnormal baseline polysomnogram, have sequelae of OSAS, are obese, or remain symptomatic after treatment, with an objective test (see Key Action Statement 2) or refer such patients to a sleep specialist. (Evidence Quality: Grade B, Recommendation Strength: Recommendation.)

Evidence Profile KAS 5B

- Aggregate evidence quality: B
- Benefit: Determine effects of treatment.
- Harm: Expense, time, anxiety/discomfort.
- Benefits-harms assessment: Preponderance of benefit over harm.

- Value judgments: Given the panel's concerns about the consequences of OSAS and the frequency of postoperative persistence in high-risk groups, the panel believes that the follow-up costs are outweighed by benefits of recognition of persistent OSAS. A minority of panelists believed that all children with OSAS should have follow-up polysomnography because of the high prevalence of persistent postoperative abnormalities on polysomnography, but most panelists believed that persistent polysomnographic abnormalities in uncomplicated children with mild OSAS were usually mild in patients who were asymptomatic after surgery.
- Role of patient preferences: Minimal. Further evaluation is needed to determine the need for further treatment.
- Exclusions: None.
- Intentional vagueness: None.
- Strength: Recommendation.

Numerous studies have shown that a large proportion of children at high risk continue to have some degree of OSAS postoperatively[10,13,14]; thus, objective evidence is required to determine whether further treatment is necessary.

Key Action Statement 6: CPAP

Clinicians should refer patients for CPAP management if symptoms/signs (Table 2) or objective evidence of OSAS persists after adenotonsillectomy or if adenotonsillectomy is not performed. (Evidence Quality: Grade B, Recommendation Strength: Recommendation.)

Evidence Profile KAS 6

- Aggregate evidence quality: B
- Benefit: Improve OSAS and accompanying symptoms and sequelae.
- Harm: Expense, time, anxiety; parental sleep disruption; nasal and skin adverse effects; possible midface remodeling; extremely rare serious pressure-related complications, such as pneumothorax; poor adherence.
- Benefits-harms assessment: Preponderance of benefit over harm.
- Value judgments: Panelists believe that CPAP is the most effective treatment of OSAS that persists postoperatively and that the benefits of treatment outweigh the adverse effects. Other treatments (eg, rapid maxillary expansion) may be effective in specially selected patients.
- Role of patient preferences: Other treatments may be effective in specially selected patients.
- Exclusions: Rare patients at increased risk of severe pressure complications.
- Intentional vagueness: None.
- Policy level: Recommendation.

CPAP therapy is delivered by using an electronic device that delivers air at positive pressure via a nasal mask, leading to mechanical stenting of the airway and improved functional residual capacity in the lungs. There is no clear advantage of using bilevel pressure over CPAP.[15] CPAP should be managed by an experienced and skilled clinician with expertise in its use in children. CPAP pressure requirements vary among individuals and change over time; thus, CPAP must be titrated in the sleep laboratory before prescribing the device and periodically readjusted thereafter. Behavioral modification therapy may be required, especially for young children or those with developmental delays. Objective monitoring of adherence, by using the equipment software, is important. If adherence is suboptimal, the clinician should institute measures to improve adherence (such as behavioral modification, or treating side effects of CPAP) and institute alternative treatments if these measures are ineffective.

Key Action Statement 7: Weight Loss

Clinicians should recommend weight loss in addition to other therapy if a child/adolescent with OSAS is overweight or obese. (Evidence Quality: Grade C, Recommendation Strength: Recommendation.)

Evidence Profile KAS 7

- Aggregate evidence quality: C
- Benefit: Improve OSAS and accompanying symptoms and sequelae; non–OSAS-related benefits of weight loss.
- Harm: Hard to achieve and maintain weight loss.
- Benefits-harms assessment: Preponderance of benefit over harm.
- Value judgments: The panel agreed that weight loss is beneficial for both OSAS and other health issues, but clinical experience suggests that weight loss is difficult to achieve and maintain, and even effective weight loss regimens take time; therefore, additional treatment is required in the interim.
- Role of patient preferences: Strong role for patient and family preference regarding nutrition and exercise.
- Exclusions: None.
- Intentional vagueness: None.
- Strength: Recommendation.

Weight loss has been shown to improve OSAS,[16,17] although the degree of weight loss required has not been determined. Because weight loss is a slow and unreliable process, other treatment modalities (such as adenotonsillectomy or CPAP therapy) should be instituted until sufficient weight loss has been achieved and maintained.

Key Action Statement 8: Intranasal Corticosteroids

Clinicians may prescribe topical intranasal corticosteroids for children with mild OSAS in whom adenotonsillectomy is contraindicated or for children with mild postoperative OSAS. (Evidence Quality: Grade B, Recommendation Strength: Option.)

Evidence Profile KAS 8

- Aggregate evidence quality: B
- Benefit: Improves mild OSAS and accompanying symptoms and sequelae.
- Harm: Some subjects may not have an adequate response. It is not known whether therapeutic effect persists long-term; therefore, long-term observation is required. Low risk of steroid-related adverse effects.
- Benefits-harms assessment: Preponderance of benefit over harm.
- Value judgments: The panel agreed that intranasal steroids provide a less invasive treatment than surgery or CPAP and, therefore, may be preferred in some cases despite lower efficacy and lack of data on long-term efficacy.
- Role of patient preferences: Moderate role for patient and family preference if OSAS is mild.
- Exclusions: None.
- Intentional vagueness: None.
- Strength: Option.

Mild OSAS is defined, for this indication, as an AHI <5 per hour, on the basis of studies on intranasal corticosteroids described in the accompanying technical report.[2] Several studies have shown that the use of intranasal steroids decreases the degree of OSAS; however, although OSAS improves, residual OSAS may remain. Furthermore, there is individual variability in response to treatment, and long-term studies have not been performed to determine the duration of improvement. Therefore, nasal steroids are not recommended as a first-line therapy. The response to treatment should be measured objectively after a course of treatment of approximately 6 weeks. Because the long-term effect of this treatment is unknown, the clinician should continue to observe the patient for symptoms of recurrence and adverse effects of corticosteroids.

AREAS FOR FUTURE RESEARCH

A detailed list of research recommendations is provided in the accompanying technical report.[2] There is a great need for further research into the prevalence of OSAS, sequelae of OSAS, best treatment methods, and the role of obesity. In particular, well-controlled, blinded studies, including randomized controlled trials of treatment, are needed to determine the best care for children and adolescents with OSAS.

SUBCOMMITTEE ON OBSTRUCTIVE SLEEP APNEA SYNDROME*

Carole L. Marcus, MBBCh, Chairperson (Sleep Medicine, Pediatric Pulmonologist; Liaison, American Academy of Sleep Medicine; Research Support from Philips Respironics; Affiliated with an academic sleep center; Published research related to OSAS)

Lee J. Brooks, MD (Sleep Medicine, Pediatric Pulmonologist; Liaison, American College of Chest Physicians; No financial conflicts; Affiliated with an academic sleep center; Published research related to OSAS)

Sally Davidson Ward, MD (Sleep Medicine, Pediatric Pulmonologist; No financial conflicts; Affiliated with an academic sleep center; Published research related to OSAS)

Kari A. Draper, MD (General Pediatrician; No conflicts)

David Gozal, MD (Sleep Medicine, Pediatric Pulmonologist; Research support from AstraZeneca; Speaker for Merck Company; Affiliated with an academic sleep center; Published research related to OSAS)

Ann C. Halbower, MD (Sleep Medicine, Pediatric Pulmonologist; Liaison, American Thoracic Society; Research Funding from Resmed; Affiliated with an academic sleep center; Published research related to OSAS)

Jacqueline Jones, MD (Pediatric Otolaryngologist; AAP Section on Otolaryngology-Head and Neck Surgery; Liaison, American Academy of Otolaryngology-Head and Neck Surgery; No financial conflicts; Affiliated with an academic otolaryngologic practice)

Christopher Lehman, MD (Neonatologist, Informatician; No conflicts)

Michael S. Schechter, MD, MPH (Pediatric Pulmonologist; AAP Section on Pediatric Pulmonology; Consultant to Genentech, Inc and Gilead, Inc, not related to Obstructive Sleep Apnea; Research Support from Mpex Pharmaceuticals, Inc, Vertex Pharmaceuticals Incorporated, PTC Therapeutics, Bayer Healthcare, not related to Obstructive Sleep Apnea)

Stephen Sheldon, MD (Sleep Medicine, General Pediatrician; Liaison, National Sleep Foundation; No financial conflicts; Affiliated with an academic sleep center; Published research related to OSAS)

Richard N. Shiffman, MD, MCIS (General pediatrics, Informatician; No conflicts)

Karen Spruyt, PhD (Clinical Psychologist, Child Neuropsychologist, and Biostatistician/Epidemiologist; No financial conflicts; Affiliated with an academic sleep center)

Oversight from the Steering Committee on Quality Improvement and Management, 2009–2012

STAFF

Caryn Davidson, MA

*Areas of expertise are shown in parentheses after each name.

ACKNOWLEDGMENTS

The committee thanks Jason Caboot, June Chan, Mary Currie, Fiona Healy, Maureen Josephson, Sofia Konstantinopoulou, H. Madan Kumar, Roberta Leu, Darius Loghmanee, Rajeev Bhatia, Argyri Petrocheilou, Harsha Vardhan, and Colleen Walsh for assisting with evidence extraction.

REFERENCES

1. Section on Pediatric Pulmonology, Subcommittee on Obstructive Sleep Apnea Syndrome. American Academy of Pediatrics. Clinical practice guideline: diagnosis and management of childhood obstructive sleep apnea syndrome. *Pediatrics*. 2002;109(4):704–712
2. Marcus CL, Brooks LJ, Davidson C, et al; American Academy of Pediatrics, Subcommittee on Obstructive Sleep Apnea

Syndrome. Technical report: diagnosis and management of childhood obstructive sleep apnea syndrome. *Pediatrics.* 2012; 130(3):In press

3. American Academy of Pediatrics Steering Committee on Quality Improvement and Management. Classifying recommendations for clinical practice guidelines. *Pediatrics.* 2004;114(3):874–877
4. American Thoracic Society. Standards and indications for cardiopulmonary sleep studies in children. *Am J Respir Crit Care Med.* 1996;153(2):866–878
5. Bixler EO, Vgontzas AN, Lin HM, et al. Sleep disordered breathing in children in a general population sample: prevalence and risk factors. *Sleep.* 2009;32(6):731–736
6. Li AM, So HK, Au CT, et al. Epidemiology of obstructive sleep apnoea syndrome in Chinese children: a two-phase community study. *Thorax.* 2010;65(11):991–997
7. O'Brien LM, Holbrook CR, Mervis CB, et al. Sleep and neurobehavioral characteristics of 5- to 7-year-old children with parentally reported symptoms of attention-deficit/hyperactivity disorder. *Pediatrics.* 2003; 111(3):554–563
8. Himes JH, Dietz WH; The Expert Committee on Clinical Guidelines for Overweight in Adolescent Preventive Services. Guidelines for overweight in adolescent preventive services: recommendations from an expert committee. *Am J Clin Nutr.* 1994;59(2):307–316
9. Mitchell RB. Adenotonsillectomy for obstructive sleep apnea in children: outcome evaluated by pre- and postoperative polysomnography. *Laryngoscope.* 2007;117(10):1844–1854
10. Suen JS, Arnold JE, Brooks LJ. Adenotonsillectomy for treatment of obstructive sleep apnea in children. *Arch Otolaryngol Head Neck Surg.* 1995;121(5):525–530
11. Nieminen P, Tolonen U, Löppönen H. Snoring and obstructive sleep apnea in children: a 6-month follow-up study. *Arch Otolaryngol Head Neck Surg.* 2000;126(4):481–486
12. Blunden S, Lushington K, Lorenzen B, Wong J, Balendran R, Kennedy D. Symptoms of sleep breathing disorders in children are underreported by parents at general practice visits. *Sleep Breath.* 2003;7(4):167–176
13. Apostolidou MT, Alexopoulos EI, Chaidas K, et al. Obesity and persisting sleep apnea after adenotonsillectomy in Greek children. *Chest.* 2008;134(6):1149–1155
14. Mitchell RB, Kelly J. Outcome of adenotonsillectomy for severe obstructive sleep apnea in children. *Int J Pediatr Otorhinolaryngol.* 2004;68(11):1375–1379
15. Marcus CL, Rosen G, Ward SL, et al. Adherence to and effectiveness of positive airway pressure therapy in children with obstructive sleep apnea. *Pediatrics.* 2006; 117(3). Available at: www.pediatrics.org/cgi/content/full/117/3/e442
16. Verhulst SL, Franckx H, Van Gaal L, De Backer W, Desager K. The effect of weight loss on sleep-disordered breathing in obese teenagers. *Obesity (Silver Spring).* 2009;17(6):1178–1183
17. Kalra M, Inge T. Effect of bariatric surgery on obstructive sleep apnoea in adolescents. *Paediatr Respir Rev.* 2006;7(4):260–267

Sleep Apnea Clinical Practice Guideline Quick Reference Tools

- Action Statement Summary
  — Diagnosis and Management of Childhood Obstructive Sleep Apnea Syndrome
- *ICD-10-CM* Coding Quick Reference for Sleep Apnea
- AAP Patient Education Handout
  — *Sleep Apnea and Your Child*

Action Statement Summary

Diagnosis and Management of Childhood Obstructive Sleep Apnea Syndrome

Key Action Statement 1: Screening for OSAS

As part of routine health maintenance visits, clinicians should inquire whether the child or adolescent snores. If the answer is affirmative or if a child or adolescent presents with signs or symptoms of OSAS (Table 2), clinicians should perform a more focused evaluation. (Evidence Quality: Grade B, Recommendation Strength: Recommendation.)

Key Action Statement 2A: Polysomnography

If a child or adolescent snores on a regular basis and has any of the complaints or findings shown in Table 2, clinicians should either (1) obtain a polysomnogram (Evidence Quality A, Key Action strength: Recommendation) OR (2) refer the patient to a sleep specialist or otolaryngologist for a more extensive evaluation (Evidence quality D, Key Action strength: Option). (Evidence Quality: Grade A for polysomnography; Grade D for specialist referral, Recommendation Strength: Recommendation.)

Key Action Statement 2B: Alternative Testing

If polysomnography is not available, then clinicians may order alternative diagnostic tests, such as nocturnal video recording, nocturnal oximetry, daytime nap polysomnography, or ambulatory polysomnography. (Evidence Quality: Grade C, Recommendation Strength: Option.)

Key Action Statement 3: Adenotonsillectomy

If a child is determined to have OSAS, has a clinical examination consistent with adenotonsillar hypertrophy, and does not have a contraindication to surgery (see Table 3), the clinician should recommend adenotonsillectomy as the first line of treatment. If the child has OSAS but does not have adenotonsillar hypertrophy, other treatment should be considered (see Key Action Statement 6). Clinical judgment is required to determine the benefits of adenotonsillectomy compared with other treatments in obese children with varying degrees of adenotonsillar hypertrophy. (Evidence Quality: Grade B, Recommendation Strength: Recommendation.)

Key Action Statement 4: High-Risk Patients Undergoing Adenotonsillectomy

Clinicians should monitor high-risk patients (Table 5) undergoing adenotonsillectomy as inpatients postoperatively. (Evidence Quality: Grade B, Recommendation Strength: Recommendation.)

Key Action Statement 5: Reevaluation

Clinicians should clinically reassess all patients with OSAS for persisting signs and symptoms after therapy to determine whether further treatment is required. (Evidence Quality: Grade B, Recommendation Strength: Recommendation.)

Key Action Statement 5B: Reevaluation of High-Risk Patients

Clinicians should reevaluate high-risk patients for persistent OSAS after adenotonsillectomy, including those who had a significantly abnormal baseline polysomnogram, have sequelae of OSAS, are obese, or remain symptomatic after treatment, with an objective test (see Key Action Statement 2) or refer such patients to a sleep specialist. (Evidence Quality: Grade B, Recommendation Strength: Recommendation.)

Key Action Statement 6: CPAP

Clinicians should refer patients for CPAP management if symptoms/signs (Table 2) or objective evidence of OSAS persists after adenotonsillectomy or if adenotonsillectomy is not performed. (Evidence Quality: Grade B, Recommendation Strength: Recommendation.)

Key Action Statement 7: Weight Loss

Clinicians should recommend weight loss in addition to other therapy if a child/adolescent with OSAS is overweight or obese. (Evidence Quality: Grade C, Recommendation Strength: Recommendation.)

Key Action Statement 8: Intranasal Corticosteroids

Clinicians may prescribe topical intranasal corticosteroids for children with mild OSAS in whom adenotonsillectomy is contraindicated or for children with mild postoperative OSAS. (Evidence Quality: Grade B, Recommendation Strength: Option.)

Coding Quick Reference for Sleep Apnea	
ICD-10-CM	
G47.30	Sleep apnea, unspecified
G47.31	Primary central sleep apnea
G47.33 _______	Obstructive sleep apnea (adult) (pediatric) (Code additional underlying conditions.)
J35.3	Hypertrophy of tonsils with hypertrophy of adenoids
E66.01	Morbid (severe) obesity due to excess calories
E66.09	Other obesity due to excess calories
E66.3	Overweight
E66.8	Other obesity
E66.9	Obesity, unspecified

Sleep Apnea and Your Child

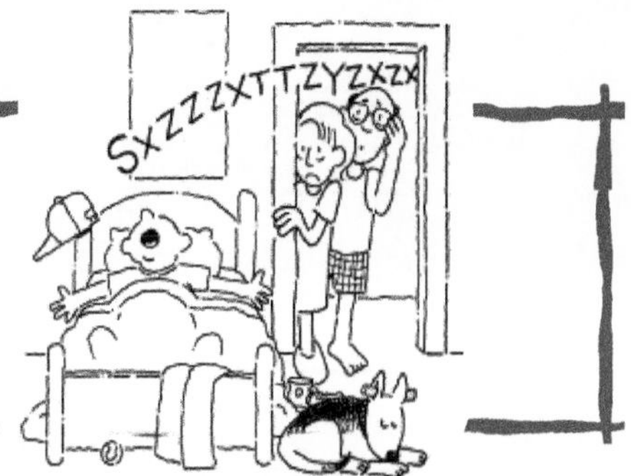

Does your child snore a lot? Does he sleep restlessly? Does he have difficulty breathing, or does he gasp or choke, while he sleeps?

If your child has these symptoms, he may have a condition known as sleep apnea.

Sleep apnea is a common problem that affects an estimated 2% of all children, including many who are undiagnosed.

If not treated, sleep apnea can lead to a variety of problems. These include heart, behavior, learning, and growth problems.

How do I know if my child has sleep apnea?

Symptoms of sleep apnea include

- Frequent snoring
- Problems breathing during the night
- Sleepiness during the day
- Difficulty paying attention
- Behavior problems

If you notice any of these symptoms, let your pediatrician know as soon as possible. Your pediatrician may recommend an overnight sleep study called a *polysomnogram.* Overnight polysomnograms are conducted at hospitals and major medical centers. During the study, medical staff will watch your child sleep. Several sensors will be attached to your child to monitor breathing, oxygenation, and brain waves. An electroencephalogram (EEG) is a test that measures brain waves.

The results of the study will show whether your child suffers from sleep apnea. Other specialists, such as pediatric pulmonologists, otolaryngologists, neurologists, and pediatricians with specialty training in sleep disorders, may help your pediatrician make the diagnosis.

What causes sleep apnea?

Many children with sleep apnea have larger tonsils and adenoids.

Tonsils are the round, reddish masses on each side of your child's throat. They help fight infections in the body. You can only see the adenoid with an x-ray or special mirror. It lies in the space between the nose and throat.

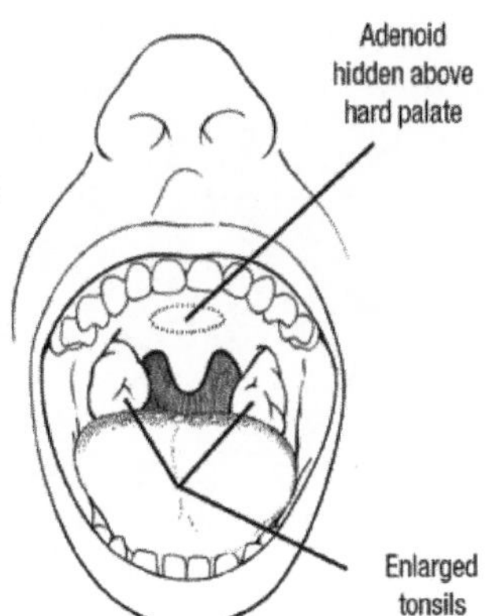

Large tonsils and adenoid may block a child's airway while she sleeps. This causes her to snore and wake up often during the night. However, not every child with large tonsils and adenoid has sleep apnea. A sleep study can tell your doctor whether your child has sleep apnea or if she is simply snoring.

Children born with other medical conditions, such as Down syndrome, cerebral palsy, or craniofacial (skull and face) abnormalities, are at higher risk for sleep apnea. Overweight children are also more likely to suffer from sleep apnea.

How is sleep apnea treated?

The most common way to treat sleep apnea is to remove your child's tonsils and adenoid. This surgery is called a tonsillectomy and adenoidectomy. It is highly effective in treating sleep apnea.

Another effective treatment is nasal continuous positive airway pressure (CPAP), which requires the child to wear a mask while he sleeps. The mask delivers steady air pressure through the child's nose, allowing him to breathe comfortably. Continuous positive airway pressure is usually used in children who do not improve after tonsillectomy and adenoidectomy, or who are not candidates for tonsillectomy and adenoidectomy.

Children who may need additional treatment include children who are overweight or suffering from another complicating condition. Overweight children will improve if they lose weight, but may need to use CPAP until the weight is lost.

Remember

A good night's sleep is important to good health. If your child suffers from the symptoms of sleep apnea, talk with your pediatrician. A proper diagnosis and treatment can mean restful nights and restful days for your child and your family.

The information contained in this publication should not be used as a substitute for the medical care and advice of your pediatrician. There may be variations in treatment that your pediatrician may recommend based on individual facts and circumstances.

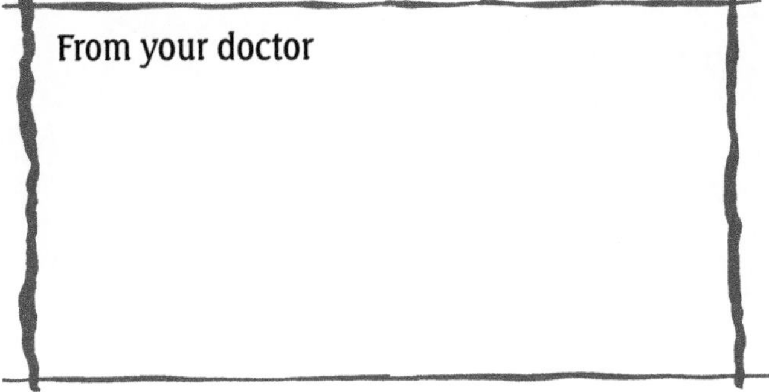

American Academy of Pediatrics

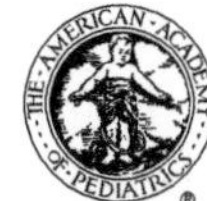

DEDICATED TO THE HEALTH OF ALL CHILDREN™

The American Academy of Pediatrics is an organization of 60,000 primary care pediatricians, pediatric medical subspecialists, and pediatric surgical specialists dedicated to the health, safety, and well-being of infants, children, adolescents, and young adults.

American Academy of Pediatrics
Web site—www.HealthyChildren.org

Copyright © 2003
American Academy of Pediatrics, Updated 10/2012
All rights reserved.

Reaffirmation of AAP Clinical Practice Guideline: The Diagnosis and Management of the Initial Urinary Tract Infection in Febrile Infants and Young Children 2–24 Months of Age

- *Reaffirmation of AAP Clinical Practice Guideline*
- *Clinical Practice Guideline*
  - *PPI: AAP Partnership for Policy Implementation See Appendix 1 for more information.*

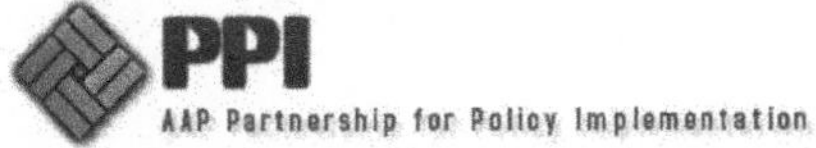

CLINICAL PRACTICE GUIDELINE Guidance for the Clinician in Rendering Pediatric Care

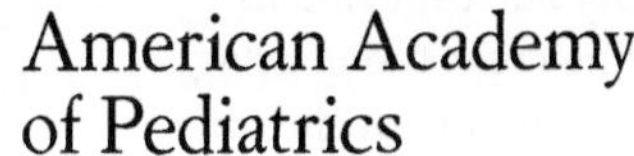

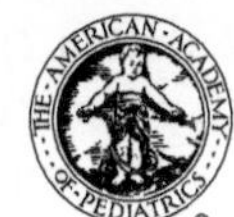

DEDICATED TO THE HEALTH OF ALL CHILDREN™

Reaffirmation of AAP Clinical Practice Guideline: The Diagnosis and Management of the Initial Urinary Tract Infection in Febrile Infants and Young Children 2–24 Months of Age

SUBCOMMITTEE ON URINARY TRACT INFECTION

It is the policy of the American Academy of Pediatrics to reassess clinical practice guidelines (CPGs) every 5 years and retire, revise, or reaffirm them. The members of the urinary tract infection (UTI) subcommittee who developed the 2011 UTI CPG[1] have reviewed the literature published since 2011 along with unpublished manuscripts and the status of some clinical trials still in progress. With this article, we reaffirm the 2011 UTI CPG and provide an updated review of the supporting evidence. For the convenience of the reader, we reiterate the 7 Key Action Statements here to obviate the need to consult the 2011 UTI CPG, although interested readers may want to review the text of the guideline[1] and/or its accompanying technical report.[2]

This document is copyrighted and is property of the American Academy of Pediatrics and its Board of Directors. All authors have filed conflict of interest statements with the American Academy of Pediatrics. Any conflicts have been resolved through a process approved by the Board of Directors. The American Academy of Pediatrics has neither solicited nor accepted any commercial involvement in the development of the content of this publication.

The recommendations in this practice guideline do not indicate an exclusive course of treatment or serve as a standard of medical care. Variations, taking into account individual circumstances, may be appropriate.

All clinical practice guidelines from the American Academy of Pediatrics automatically expire 5 years after publication unless reaffirmed, revised, or retired at or before that time.

DOI: 10.1542/peds.2016-3026

PEDIATRICS (ISSN Numbers: Print, 0031-4005; Online, 1098-4275).

Copyright © 2016 by the American Academy of Pediatrics

FINANCIAL DISCLOSURE: The authors have indicated they do not have a financial relationship relevant to this article to disclose.

FUNDING: No external funding.

POTENTIAL CONFLICT OF INTEREST: The authors have indicated they have no potential conflicts of interest to disclose.

To cite: AAP SUBCOMMITTEE ON URINARY TRACT INFECTION. Reaffirmation of AAP Clinical Practice Guideline: The Diagnosis and Management of the Initial Urinary Tract Infection in Febrile Infants and Young Children 2–24 Months of Age. *Pediatrics.* 2016;138(6):e20163026

ACTION STATEMENT 1

If a clinician decides that a febrile infant with no apparent source for the fever requires antimicrobial therapy to be administered because of ill appearance or another pressing reason, the clinician should ensure that a urine specimen is obtained for both culture and urinalysis before an antimicrobial is administered; the specimen needs to be obtained through catheterization or suprapubic aspiration (SPA), because the diagnosis of UTI cannot be established reliably through culture of urine collected in a bag (evidence quality: A; strong recommendation).

Comment

A key to an accurate diagnosis of UTI is obtaining a sample of urine for culture with minimal contamination before starting antimicrobial agents. Urine collected in a bag or via a clean catch method is suitable for urinalysis (see Action Statement 2, Option 2), but such specimens (especially urine collected in a bag) are less appropriate for culture. If a culture obtained by bag is positive, the likelihood of a false positive is extremely high, so the result must be confirmed by culturing urine obtained by a more reliable method; if an antimicrobial agent is present in the urine, the opportunity for confirmation is likely to be lost.

Although samples of urine obtained by transurethral catheterization may be contaminated by urethral flora, meticulous technique can reduce this possibility. To avoid contamination, 2 practical steps should be implemented: (1) the first few milliliters obtained by catheter should be discarded (allowed to fall outside of the sterile collecting vessel) and only the subsequent urine cultured; and (2) if the attempt at catheterization is unsuccessful, a new, clean catheter should be used (aided, in girls, by leaving the initial catheter in place as a marker).

ACTION STATEMENT 2

If a clinician assesses a febrile infant with no apparent source for the fever as not being so ill as to require immediate antimicrobial therapy, then the clinician should assess the likelihood of UTI.

Action Statement 2a. If the clinician determines the febrile infant to have a low likelihood of UTI (see text), then clinical follow-up monitoring without testing is sufficient (evidence quality: A; strong recommendation).

Action Statement 2b. If the clinician determines that the febrile infant is not in a low-risk group (see below), then there are 2 choices (evidence quality: A; strong recommendation).

Option 1 is to obtain a urine specimen through catheterization or SPA for culture and urinalysis.

Option 2 is to obtain a urine specimen through the most convenient means and to perform a urinalysis. If the urinalysis results suggest a UTI (positive leukocyte esterase test results or nitrite test or microscopic analysis results for leukocytes or bacteria), then a urine specimen should be obtained through catheterization or SPA and cultured; if urinalysis of fresh (less than 1 hour since void) urine yields negative leukocyte esterase and nitrite results, then it is reasonable to monitor the clinical course without initiating antimicrobial therapy, recognizing that a negative urinalysis does not rule out a UTI with certainty.

Comment

When the patient's degree of illness does not warrant immediate antimicrobial treatment and the risk of UTI is extremely low, the patient may be observed without assessing the urine. (The risk assessment tables in the 2011 UTI CPG have been simplified into algorithm form.[3]) If there is a low but real risk of infection, then either the best possible specimen should be obtained for urinalysis and culture, or a sample of urine obtained by a convenient method and a judgment made about culturing the urine dependent on the findings of the urinalysis or dipstick. A positive urinalysis provides sufficient concern to mandate a properly obtained urine specimen. This 2-step process (Option 2) is not only suitable for office practice but has been demonstrated to be feasible and beneficial in a busy pediatric emergency department, with the catheterization rate decreasing from 63% to fewer than 30% without increasing length of stay or missing UTIs.[4]

ACTION STATEMENT 3

To establish the diagnosis of UTI, clinicians should require both urinalysis results that suggest infection (pyuria and/or bacteriuria) and the presence of at least 50 000 colony-forming units (cfu) per milliliter of a uropathogen cultured from a urine specimen obtained through transurethral catheterization or SPA (evidence quality: C; recommendation).

Comment

The thrust of this key action statement is that the diagnosis of UTI in febrile infants is signaled by the presence of both bacteriuria and pyuria. In general, pyuria without bacteriuria is insufficient to make a diagnosis of UTI because it is nonspecific and occurs in the absence of infection (eg, Kawasaki disease, chemical urethritis, streptococcal infections). Likewise, bacteriuria, without pyuria is attributable to external contamination, asymptomatic bacteriuria, or, rarely, very early infection (before the onset of inflammation). Non–*Escherichia coli* isolates are less frequently associated with pyuria than *E coli*,[5] but the significance of this association is not clear at present. Non–*E coli* uropathogens are of concern because they are more likely to result in scarring than *E coli*,[6] but animal studies demonstrate the host inflammatory response to be what causes scarring rather than the presence of organisms.[7] Moreover, the rate of asymptomatic bacteriuria is sufficient to account for the lack of association with pyuria.

The remaining question is what constitutes "significant" bacteriuria and "significant" pyuria. In 1994, by using single versus multiple organisms to distinguish true UTI from contamination, 50 000 cfu/mL was proposed as the appropriate threshold for specimens obtained by catheterization,[8] recommended in the 2011 UTI CPG and implemented in the Randomized Intervention for Children with Vesicoureteral Reflux (RIVUR) trial.[9] Lower colony counts are sufficient if the urine specimen is obtained by SPA and, thus, less likely to be contaminated, but most (80%) cases of UTI documented with urine obtained by SPA have 10^5 cfu/mL or more. Colony counts lower than 50 000 cfu/mL are currently being considered for the diagnosis of UTI.[10] If 10 000 cfu/mL coupled with symptoms (eg, fever) and evidence of inflammation (pyuria) proves both sensitive and specific, this threshold would be of particular assistance to clinicians who use laboratories that do not specify colony counts between 10 000 and 100 000 cfu/mL and, thereby, make the criterion of 50 000 cfu/mL difficult to use.

Significant pyuria is ≥10 white blood cells/mm^3 on an "enhanced urinalysis" or ≥5 white blood cells per high power field on a centrifuged specimen of urine or any leukocyte esterase on a dipstick.

ACTION STATEMENT 4

Action Statement 4a. When initiating treatment, the clinician should base the choice of route of administration on practical considerations: initiating treatment orally or parenterally is equally efficacious. The clinician should base the choice of agent on local antimicrobial sensitivity patterns (if available) and should adjust the choice according to sensitivity testing of the isolated uropathogen (evidence quality: A; strong recommendation).

Action Statement 4b. The clinician should choose 7 to 14 days as the duration of antimicrobial therapy (evidence quality B; recommendation).

Comment

Basing the choice of an initial antimicrobial agent on local sensitivity patterns can be difficult because applicable information may not be available. Whether the child has received antimicrobial therapy in the recent past should be considered. This exposure constitutes a risk factor for resistance to the recently prescribed antimicrobial. Further delineation of treatment duration has not been forthcoming, but a randomized controlled trial is currently under way comparing the effectiveness of 5 days versus 10 days of treatment.[11]

Note: The dose of ceftriaxone in Table 2 should be 50 mg/kg, every 24 h.

ACTION STATEMENT 5

Febrile infants with UTIs should undergo renal and bladder ultrasonography (RBUS) (evidence quality: C; recommendation).

Comment

As noted in the 2011 CPG, it is important that the study be a renal and bladder ultrasonogram, not a limited renal ultrasonogram. Ideally, the patient should be well-hydrated for the examination and the bladder should be evaluated while distended. Concern has been raised that RBUS is not effective to detect vesicoureteral reflux (VUR), as it is frequently normal in infants with low-grade VUR and even in some who have high-grade VUR. Moreover, nonspecific RBUS findings, such as mild renal pelvic or ureteral distention, are common and are not necessarily associated with reflux. However, low-grade VUR is generally not considered of concern for renal damage, and most studies (other than the RIVUR trial[9]) have demonstrated continuous antimicrobial prophylaxis (CAP) to lack benefit in this group.[1,2] Although RBUS is not invariably abnormal in infants with grades IV and V VUR, it does identify most, and, of particular importance, an abnormal RBUS is a major risk factor for scarring.[6]

ACTION STATEMENT 6

Action Statement 6a. Voiding cystourethrography (VCUG) should not be performed routinely after the first febrile UTI; VCUG is indicated if RBUS reveals hydronephrosis, scarring, or other findings that would suggest either high-grade VUR or obstructive uropathy, as well as in other atypical or complex clinical circumstances (evidence quality B; recommendation).

Action Statement 6b. Further evaluation should be conducted if there is a recurrence of febrile UTI (evidence quality: X; recommendation).

Comment

For decades, UTIs in infants were considered harbingers of underlying anatomic and/or physiologic abnormalities, so RBUS and VCUG were recommended to be performed routinely. VUR was a particular concern; CAP was assumed to be effective in preventing UTI and became standard practice when VUR was discovered. In the years leading up to the 2011 guideline, randomized controlled trials of CAP were performed. Authors of the 6 studies published in 2006-2010 graciously provided data to the guideline committee, permitting a meta-analysis of data specifically targeting febrile infants 2 to 24 months of age. CAP was not demonstrated to be effective, so the need to identify VUR by routine voiding cystourethrography was discouraged.[1,2] A recent large trial in the United States, the RIVUR trial, concluded that CAP was of benefit, but, to prevent 1 UTI recurrence required 5840 doses of antimicrobial and did not reduce the rate of renal scarring.[9]

Since the publication of the 2011 guideline, multiple studies have demonstrated that abnormalities are missed by the selective imaging recommended in the guideline; however, there is no evidence that identifying these missed abnormalities is of sufficient clinical benefit to offset the cost, discomfort, and radiation.[12] Compared with performing the full array of imaging tests, the radiation burden incurred with the application of the guideline has been calculated to be reduced by 93%.[13] Moreover, in population studies, the significance of VUR and the value of treating VUR have been questioned.[14,15]

The authors of the RIVUR trial and its companion study, Careful Urinary Tract Infection Evaluation, have called attention to bowel/bladder dysfunction (BBD) as a major risk factor for UTI recurrences and recognize that, in children who have a UTI recurrence, evaluation for BBD (ie, constipation), rather than for VUR, can be performed by nonspecialists and does not incur high cost, cause discomfort, or require radiation.[16] BBD has long been underappreciated and deserves greater consideration.

ACTION STATEMENT 7

After confirmation of UTI, the clinician should instruct parents or guardians to seek prompt medical evaluation (ideally within 48 hours) for future febrile illnesses to ensure that recurrent infections can be detected and treated promptly (evidence quality: C; recommendation).

Comment

Prompt treatment is of clinical benefit to the child with the acute infection. What has been controversial is the definition of "prompt" and the relationship to renal scarring. A recent study identified that the median time to treatment was shorter in infants who did not incur a scar than in those who did (48 vs 72 hours). The study also noted that the rate of scarring increased minimally between days 1 and 2 and between days 2 and 3 but was much higher thereafter.[17]

SUBCOMMITTEE ON URINARY TRACT INFECTION, 2009-2011

Kenneth B. Roberts, MD, FAAP Chair
Stephen M. Downs, MD, MS, FAAP
S. Maria E. Finnell, MD, MS, FAAP
*Stanley Hellerstein, MD (deceased)
Linda D. Shortliffe, MD
Ellen R. Wald, MD, FAAP, Vice-Chair
J. Michael Zerin, MD

STAFF

Kymika Okechukwu, MPA, Manager, Evidence-Based Practice Initiatives

ABBREVIATIONS

BBD: bowel/bladder dysfunction
CAP: continuous antimicrobial prophylaxis
cfu: colony-forming units
CPG: clinical practice guideline
RBUS: renal and bladder ultrasonography
RIVUR: Randomized Intervention for Children with Vesicoureteral Reflux
SPA: suprapubic aspiration
UTI: urinary tract infection
VCUG: voiding cystourethrography
VUR: vesicoureteral reflux

REFERENCES

1. Roberts KB; Subcommittee on Urinary Tract Infection, Steering Committee on Quality Improvement and Management. Urinary tract infection: clinical practice guideline for the diagnosis and management of the initial UTI in febrile infants and children 2 to 24 months. *Pediatrics.* 2011;128(3):595–610
2. Finnell SM, Carroll AE, Downs SM; Subcommittee on Urinary Tract Infection. Technical report—Diagnosis and management of an initial UTI in febrile infants and young children. *Pediatrics.* 2011;128(3). Available at: www.pediatrics.org/cgi/content/full/128/3/e749 PubMed
3. Roberts KB. Revised AAP Guideline on UTI in Febrile Infants and Young Children. *Am Fam Physician.* 2012;86(10):940–946
4. Lavelle JM, Blackstone MM, Funari MK, et al. Two-step process for ED UTI screening in febrile young children: reducing catheterization rates. *Pediatrics.* 2016;138(1):e20153023
5. Shaikh N, Shope TR, Hoberman A, Vigliotti A, Kurs-Lasky M, Martin JM. Association between uropathogen and pyuria. *Pediatrics.* 2016;138(1):e20160087
6. Shaikh N, Craig JC, Rovers MM, et al. Identification of children and adolescents at risk for renal scarring after a first urinary tract infection: a meta-analysis with individual patient data. *JAMA Pediatr.* 2014;168(10):893–900
7. Glauser MP, Meylan P, Bille J. The inflammatory response and tissue damage. The example of renal scars following acute renal infection. *Pediatr Nephrol.* 1987;1(4):615–622
8. Hoberman A, Wald ER, Reynolds EA, Penchansky L, Charron M. Pyuria and bacteriuria in urine specimens obtained by catheter from young children with fever. *J Pediatr.* 1994;124(4):513–519
9. Hoberman A, Greenfield SP, Mattoo TK, et al; RIVUR Trial Investigators. Antimicrobial prophylaxis for children with vesicoureteral reflux. *N Engl J Med.* 2014;370(25):2367–2376
10. Tullus K. Low urinary bacterial counts: do they count? *Pediatr Nephrol.* 2016;31(2):171–174
11. Hoberman A. The SCOUT study: short course therapy for urinary tract infections in children. Available at: https://clinicaltrials.gov/ct2/show/

NCT01595529. Accessed October 14, 2016

12. Narchi H, Marah M, Khan AA, et al Renal tract abnormalities missed in a historical cohort of your children with UTI if the NICE and AAP imaging guidelines were applied. *J Pediatr Urol.* 2015;11(5):252.e1–7
13. La Scola C, De Mutiis C, Hewitt IK, et al. Different guidelines for imaging after first UTI in febrile infants: yield, cost, and radiation. *Pediatrics.* 2013;131(3). Available at: www.pediatrics.org/cgi/content/full/131/3/e665 PubMed
14. Salo J, Ikäheimo R, Tapiainen T, Uhari M. Childhood urinary tract infections as a cause of chronic kidney disease. *Pediatrics.* 2011;128(5):840–847
15. Craig JC, Williams GJ. Denominators do matter: it's a myth—urinary tract infection does not cause chronic kidney disease. *Pediatrics.* 2011;128(5):984–985
16. Shaikh N, Hoberman A, Keren R, et al. Recurrent urinary tract infections in children with bladder and bowel dysfunction. *Pediatrics.* 2016;137(1):e20152982
17. Shaikh N, Mattoo TK, Keren R, et al. Early antibiotic treatment for pediatric febrile urinary tract infection and renal scarring. *JAMA Pediatr.* 2016;170(9):848–854

CLINICAL PRACTICE GUIDELINE

Urinary Tract Infection: Clinical Practice Guideline for the Diagnosis and Management of the Initial UTI in Febrile Infants and Children 2 to 24 Months

SUBCOMMITTEE ON URINARY TRACT INFECTION, STEERING COMMITTEE ON QUALITY IMPROVEMENT AND MANAGEMENT

KEY WORDS
urinary tract infection, infants, children, vesicoureteral reflux, voiding cystourethrography

ABBREVIATIONS
SPA—suprapubic aspiration
AAP—American Academy of Pediatrics
UTI—urinary tract infection
RCT—randomized controlled trial
CFU—colony-forming unit
VUR—vesicoureteral reflux
WBC—white blood cell
RBUS—renal and bladder ultrasonography
VCUG—voiding cystourethrography

This document is copyrighted and is property of the American Academy of Pediatrics and its Board of Directors. All authors have filed conflict of interest statements with the American Academy of Pediatrics. Any conflicts have been resolved through a process approved by the Board of Directors. The American Academy of Pediatrics has neither solicited nor accepted any commercial involvement in the development of the content of this publication.

The recommendations in this report do not indicate an exclusive course of treatment or serve as a standard of medical care. Variations, taking into account individual circumstances, may be appropriate.

All clinical practice guidelines from the American Academy of Pediatrics automatically expire 5 years after publication unless reaffirmed, revised, or retired at or before that time.

www.pediatrics.org/cgi/doi/10.1542/peds.2011-1330

doi:10.1542/peds.2011-1330

PEDIATRICS (ISSN Numbers: Print, 0031-4005; Online, 1098-4275).

Copyright © 2011 by the American Academy of Pediatrics

COMPANION PAPERS: Companions to this article can be found on pages 572 and e749, and online at www.pediatrics.org/cgi/doi/10.1542/peds.2011-1818 and www.pediatrics.org/cgi/doi/10.1542/peds.2011-1332.

abstract

OBJECTIVE: To revise the American Academy of Pediatrics practice parameter regarding the diagnosis and management of initial urinary tract infections (UTIs) in febrile infants and young children.

METHODS: Analysis of the medical literature published since the last version of the guideline was supplemented by analysis of data provided by authors of recent publications. The strength of evidence supporting each recommendation and the strength of the recommendation were assessed and graded.

RESULTS: Diagnosis is made on the basis of the presence of both pyuria and at least 50 000 colonies per mL of a single uropathogenic organism in an appropriately collected specimen of urine. After 7 to 14 days of antimicrobial treatment, close clinical follow-up monitoring should be maintained to permit prompt diagnosis and treatment of recurrent infections. Ultrasonography of the kidneys and bladder should be performed to detect anatomic abnormalities. Data from the most recent 6 studies do not support the use of antimicrobial prophylaxis to prevent febrile recurrent UTI in infants without vesicoureteral reflux (VUR) or with grade I to IV VUR. Therefore, a voiding cystourethrography (VCUG) is not recommended routinely after the first UTI; VCUG is indicated if renal and bladder ultrasonography reveals hydronephrosis, scarring, or other findings that would suggest either high-grade VUR or obstructive uropathy and in other atypical or complex clinical circumstances. VCUG should also be performed if there is a recurrence of a febrile UTI. The recommendations in this guideline do not indicate an exclusive course of treatment or serve as a standard of care; variations may be appropriate. Recommendations about antimicrobial prophylaxis and implications for performance of VCUG are based on currently available evidence. As with all American Academy of Pediatrics clinical guidelines, the recommendations will be reviewed routinely and incorporate new evidence, such as data from the Randomized Intervention for Children With Vesicoureteral Reflux (RIVUR) study.

CONCLUSIONS: Changes in this revision include criteria for the diagnosis of UTI and recommendations for imaging. *Pediatrics* 2011;128:595–610

INTRODUCTION

Since the early 1970s, occult bacteremia has been the major focus of concern for clinicians evaluating febrile infants who have no recognizable source of infection. With the introduction of effective conjugate vaccines against *Haemophilus influenzae* type b and *Streptococcus pneumoniae* (which have resulted in dramatic decreases in bacteremia and meningitis), there has been increasing appreciation of the urinary tract as the most frequent site of occult and serious bacterial infections. Because the clinical presentation tends to be nonspecific in infants and reliable urine specimens for culture cannot be obtained without invasive methods (urethral catheterization or suprapubic aspiration [SPA]), diagnosis and treatment may be delayed. Most experimental and clinical data support the concept that delays in the institution of appropriate treatment of pyelonephritis increase the risk of renal damage.[1,2]

This clinical practice guideline is a revision of the practice parameter published by the American Academy of Pediatrics (AAP) in 1999.[3] It was developed by a subcommittee of the Steering Committee on Quality Improvement and Management that included physicians with expertise in the fields of academic general pediatrics, epidemiology and informatics, pediatric infectious diseases, pediatric nephrology, pediatric practice, pediatric radiology, and pediatric urology. The AAP funded the development of this guideline; none of the participants had any financial conflicts of interest. The guideline was reviewed by multiple groups within the AAP (7 committees, 1 council, and 9 sections) and 5 external organizations in the United States and Canada. The guideline will be reviewed and/or revised in 5 years, unless new evidence emerges that warrants revision sooner. The guideline is intended for use in a variety of clinical settings (eg, office, emergency department, or hospital) by clinicians who treat infants and young children. This text is a summary of the analysis. The data on which the recommendations are based are included in a companion technical report.[4]

Like the 1999 practice parameter, this revision focuses on the diagnosis and management of initial urinary tract infections (UTIs) in febrile infants and young children (2–24 months of age) who have no obvious neurologic or anatomic abnormalities known to be associated with recurrent UTI or renal damage. (For simplicity, in the remainder of this guideline the phrase "febrile infants" is used to indicate febrile infants and young children 2–24 months of age.) The lower and upper age limits were selected because studies on infants with unexplained fever generally have used these age limits and have documented that the prevalence of UTI is high (~5%) in this age group. In those studies, fever was defined as temperature of at least 38.0°C (≥100.4°F); accordingly, this definition of fever is used in this guideline. Neonates and infants less than 2 months of age are excluded, because there are special considerations in this age group that may limit the application of evidence derived from the studies of 2- to 24-month-old children. Data are insufficient to determine whether the evidence generated from studies of infants 2 to 24 months of age applies to children more than 24 months of age.

METHODS

To provide evidence for the guideline, 2 literature searches were conducted, that is, a surveillance of Medline-listed literature over the past 10 years for significant changes since the guideline was published and a systematic review of the literature on the effectiveness of prophylactic antimicrobial therapy to prevent recurrence of febrile UTI/pyelonephritis in children with vesicoureteral reflux (VUR). The latter was based on the new and growing body of evidence questioning the effectiveness of antimicrobial prophylaxis to prevent recurrent febrile UTI in children with VUR. To explore this particular issue, the literature search was expanded to include trials published since 1993 in which antimicrobial prophylaxis was compared with no treatment or placebo treatment for children with VUR. Because all except 1 of the recent randomized controlled trials (RCTs) of the effectiveness of prophylaxis included children more than 24 months of age and some did not provide specific data according to grade of VUR, the authors of the 6 RCTs were contacted; all provided raw data from their studies specifically addressing infants 2 to 24 months of age, according to grade of VUR. Meta-analysis of these data was performed.

Results from the literature searches and meta-analyses were provided to committee members. Issues were raised and discussed until consensus was reached regarding recommendations. The quality of evidence supporting each recommendation and the strength of the recommendation were assessed by the committee member most experienced in informatics and epidemiology and were graded according to AAP policy[5] (Fig 1).

The subcommittee formulated 7 recommendations, which are presented in the text in the order in which a clinician would use them when evaluating and treating a febrile infant, as well as in algorithm form in the Appendix. This clinical practice guideline is not intended to be a sole source of guidance for the treatment of febrile infants with UTIs. Rather, it is intended to assist clinicians in decision-making. It is not intended to replace clinical judgment or to

Evidence Quality	Preponderance of Benefit or Harm	Balance of Benefit and Harm
A. Well designed RCTs or diagnostic studies on relevant population	Strong Recommendation	
B. RCTs or diagnostic studies with minor limitations;overwhelmingly consistent evidence from observational studies		
C. Observational studies (case-control and cohort design)	Recommendation	Option
D. Expert opinion, case reports, reasoning from first principles	Option	No Rec
X. Exceptional situations where validating studies cannot be performed and there is a clear preponderance of benefit or harm	Strong Recommendation / Recommendation	

FIGURE 1
AAP evidence strengths.

establish an exclusive protocol for the care of all children with this condition.

DIAGNOSIS

Action Statement 1

If a clinician decides that a febrile infant with no apparent source for the fever requires antimicrobial therapy to be administered because of ill appearance or another pressing reason, the clinician should ensure that a urine specimen is obtained for both culture and urinalysis before an antimicrobial agent is administered; the specimen needs to be obtained through catheterization or SPA, because the diagnosis of UTI cannot be established reliably through culture of urine collected in a bag (evidence quality: A; strong recommendation).

When evaluating febrile infants, clinicians make a subjective assessment of the degree of illness or toxicity, in addition to seeking an explanation for the fever. This clinical assessment determines whether antimicrobial therapy should be initiated promptly and affects the diagnostic process regarding UTI. If the clinician determines that the degree of illness warrants immediate antimicrobial therapy, then a urine specimen suitable for culture should be obtained through catheterization or SPA before antimicrobial agents are administered, because the antimicrobial agents commonly prescribed in such situations would almost certainly obscure the diagnosis of UTI.

SPA has been considered the standard method for obtaining urine that is uncontaminated by perineal flora. Variable success rates for obtaining urine have been reported (23%–90%).[6–8] When ultrasonographic guidance is used, success rates improve.[9,10] The technique has limited risks, but technical expertise and experience are required, and many parents and physicians perceive the procedure as unacceptably invasive, compared with catheterization. However, there may be no acceptable alternative to SPA for boys with moderate or severe phimosis or girls with tight labial adhesions.

Urine obtained through catheterization for culture has a sensitivity of 95% and a specificity of 99%, compared with that obtained through SPA.[7,11,12] The techniques required for catheterization and SPA are well described.[13] When catheterization or SPA is being attempted, the clinician should have a sterile container ready to collect a urine specimen, because the preparation for the procedure may stimulate the child to void. Whether the urine is obtained through catheterization or is voided, the first few drops should be allowed to fall outside the sterile container, because they may be contaminated by bacteria in the distal urethra.

Cultures of urine specimens collected in a bag applied to the perineum have an unacceptably high false-positive rate and are valid only when they yield negative results.[6,14–16] With a prevalence of UTI of 5% and a high rate of false-positive results (specificity: ~63%), a "positive" culture result for urine collected in a bag would be a false-positive result 88% of the time. For febrile boys, with a prevalence of UTI of 2%, the rate of false-positive results is 95%; for circumcised boys, with a prevalence of UTI of 0.2%, the rate of false-positive results is 99%. Therefore, in cases in which antimicrobial therapy will be initiated, catheterization or SPA is required to establish the diagnosis of UTI.

- Aggregate quality of evidence: A (diagnostic studies on relevant populations).
- Benefits: A missed diagnosis of UTI can lead to renal scarring if left untreated; overdiagnosis of UTI can lead to overtreatment and unnecessary and expensive imaging. Once antimicrobial therapy is initiated, the opportunity to make a definitive diagnosis is lost; multiple studies of antimicrobial therapy have shown that the urine may be rapidly sterilized.
- Harms/risks/costs: Catheterization is invasive.
- Benefit-harms assessment: Preponderance of benefit over harm.
- Value judgments: Once antimicrobial therapy has begun, the opportunity to make a definitive diagnosis is lost. Therefore, it is important to have the most-accurate test for UTI performed initially.
- Role of patient preferences: There is no evidence regarding patient preferences for bag versus catheterized urine. However, bladder tap has

been shown to be more painful than urethral catheterization.

- Exclusions: None.
- Intentional vagueness: The basis of the determination that antimicrobial therapy is needed urgently is not specified, because variability in clinical judgment is expected; considerations for individual patients, such as availability of follow-up care, may enter into the decision, and the literature provides only general guidance.
- Policy level: Strong recommendation.

Individual Risk Factors: Girls
White race
Age < 12 mo
Temperature ≥ 39°C
Fever ≥ 2 d
Absence of another source of infection

Probability of UTI	No. of Factors Present
≤1%	No more than 1
≤2%	No more than 2

Individual Risk Factors: Boys
Nonblack race
Temperature ≥ 39°C
Fever > 24 h
Absence of another source of infection

Probability of UTI	No. of Factors Present	
	Uncircumcised	Circumcised
≤1%	a	No more than 2
≤2%	None	No more than 3

FIGURE 2

Probability of UTI Among Febrile Infant Girls[28] and Infant Boys[30] According to Number of Findings Present. [a]Probability of UTI exceeds 1% even with no risk factors other than being uncircumcised.

Action Statement 2

If a clinician assesses a febrile infant with no apparent source for the fever as not being so ill as to require immediate antimicrobial therapy, then the clinician should assess the likelihood of UTI (see below for how to assess likelihood).

Action Statement 2a

If the clinician determines the febrile infant to have a low likelihood of UTI (see text), then clinical follow-up monitoring without testing is sufficient (evidence quality: A; strong recommendation).

Action Statement 2b

If the clinician determines that the febrile infant is not in a low-risk group (see below), then there are 2 choices (evidence quality: A; strong recommendation). Option 1 is to obtain a urine specimen through catheterization or SPA for culture and urinalysis. Option 2 is to obtain a urine specimen through the most convenient means and to perform a urinalysis. If the urinalysis results suggest a UTI (positive leukocyte esterase test results or nitrite test or microscopic analysis results positive for leukocytes or bacteria), then a urine specimen should be obtained through catheterization or SPA and cultured; if urinalysis of fresh (<1 hour since void) urine yields negative leukocyte esterase and nitrite test results, then it is reasonable to monitor the clinical course without initiating antimicrobial therapy, recognizing that negative urinalysis results do not rule out a UTI with certainty.

If the clinician determines that the degree of illness does not require immediate antimicrobial therapy, then the likelihood of UTI should be assessed. As noted previously, the overall prevalence of UTI in febrile infants who have no source for their fever evident on the basis of history or physical examination results is approximately 5%,[17,18] but it is possible to identify groups with higher-than-average likelihood and some with lower-than-average likelihood. The prevalence of UTI among febrile infant girls is more than twice that among febrile infant boys (relative risk: 2.27). The rate for uncircumcised boys is 4 to 20 times higher than that for circumcised boys, whose rate of UTI is only 0.2% to 0.4%.[19–24] The presence of another, clinically obvious source of infection reduces the likelihood of UTI by one-half.[25]

In a survey asking, "What yield is required to warrant urine culture in febrile infants?," the threshold was less than 1% for 10.4% of academicians and 11.7% for practitioners[26]; when the threshold was increased to 1% to 3%, 67.5% of academicians and 45.7% of practitioners considered the yield sufficiently high to warrant urine culture. Therefore, attempting to operationalize "low likelihood" (ie, below a threshold that warrants a urine culture) does not produce an absolute percentage; clinicians will choose a threshold depending on factors such as their confidence that contact will be maintained through the illness (so that a specimen can be obtained at a later time) and comfort with diagnostic uncertainty. Fig 2 indicates the number of risk factors associated with threshold probabilities of UTI of at least 1% and at least 2%.

In a series of studies, Gorelick, Shaw, and colleagues[27–29] derived and validated a prediction rule for febrile infant girls on the basis of 5 risk factors, namely, white race, age less than 12 months, temperature of at least 39°C, fever for at least 2 days, and absence of another source of infection. This prediction rule, with sensitivity of 88% and specificity of 30%, permits some infant girls to be considered in a low-likelihood group (Fig 2). For example, of girls with no identifiable source of infection, those who are nonwhite and more than 12 months of age with a recent onset (<2 days) of low-grade fever (<39°C) have less than a 1% probability of UTI; each additional risk factor increases the probability. It should be noted, however, that some of the factors (eg, duration of fever) may change during the course of the illness, excluding the infant from a low-likelihood designation and prompting testing as described in action statement 2a.

As demonstrated in Fig 2, the major risk factor for febrile infant boys is whether they are circumcised. The probability of UTI can be estimated on the basis of 4 risk factors, namely, nonblack race, temperature of at least 39°C, fever for more than 24 hours, and absence of another source of infection.[4,30]

If the clinician determines that the infant does not require immediate antimicrobial therapy and a urine specimen is desired, then often a urine collection bag affixed to the perineum is used. Many clinicians think that this collection technique has a low contamination rate under the following circumstances: the patient's perineum is properly cleansed and rinsed before application of the collection bag, the urine bag is removed promptly after urine is voided into the bag, and the specimen is refrigerated or processed immediately. Even if contamination from the perineal skin is minimized, however, there may be significant contamination from the vagina in girls or the prepuce in uncircumcised boys, the 2 groups at highest risk of UTI. A "positive" culture result from a specimen collected in a bag cannot be used to document a UTI; confirmation requires culture of a specimen collected through catheterization or SPA. Because there may be substantial delay waiting for the infant to void and a second specimen, obtained through catheterization, may be necessary if the urinalysis suggests the possibility of UTI, many clinicians prefer to obtain a definitive urine specimen through catheterization initially.

- Aggregate quality of evidence: A (diagnostic studies on relevant populations).
- Benefits: Accurate diagnosis of UTI can prevent the spread of infection and renal scarring; avoiding overdiagnosis of UTI can prevent overtreatment and unnecessary and expensive imaging.
- Harms/risks/costs: A small proportion of febrile infants, considered at low likelihood of UTI, will not receive timely identification and treatment of their UTIs.
- Benefit-harms assessment: Preponderance of benefit over harm.
- Value judgments: There is a risk of UTI sufficiently low to forestall further evaluation.
- Role of patient preferences: The choice of option 1 or option 2 and the threshold risk of UTI warranting obtaining a urine specimen may be influenced by parents' preference to avoid urethral catheterization (if a bag urine sample yields negative urinalysis results) versus timely evaluation (obtaining a definitive specimen through catheterization).
- Exclusions: Because it depends on a range of patient- and physician-specific considerations, the precise threshold risk of UTI warranting obtaining a urine specimen is left to the clinician but is below 3%.
- Intentional vagueness: None.
- Policy level: Strong recommendation.

TABLE 1 Sensitivity and Specificity of Components of Urinalysis, Alone and in Combination

Test	Sensitivity (Range), %	Specificity (Range), %
Leukocyte esterase test	83 (67–94)	78 (64–92)
Nitrite test	53 (15–82)	98 (90–100)
Leukocyte esterase or nitrite test positive	93 (90–100)	72 (58–91)
Microscopy, WBCs	73 (32–100)	81 (45–98)
Microscopy, bacteria	81 (16–99)	83 (11–100)
Leukocyte esterase test, nitrite test, or microscopy positive	99.8 (99–100)	70 (60–92)

Action Statement 3

To establish the diagnosis of UTI, clinicians should require *both* urinalysis results that suggest infection (pyuria and/or bacteriuria) *and* the presence of at least 50 000 colony-forming units (CFUs) per mL of a uropathogen cultured from a urine specimen obtained through catheterization or SPA (evidence quality: C; recommendation).

Urinalysis

General Considerations

Urinalysis cannot substitute for urine culture to document the presence of UTI but needs to be used in conjunction with culture. Because urine culture results are not available for at least 24 hours, there is considerable interest in tests that may predict the results of the urine culture and enable presumptive therapy to be initiated at the first encounter. Urinalysis can be performed on any specimen, including one collected from a bag applied to the perineum. However, the specimen must be fresh (<1 hour after voiding with maintenance at room temperature or <4 hours after voiding with refrigeration), to ensure sensitivity and specificity of the urinalysis. The tests that have received the most attention are biochemical analyses of leukocyte esterase and nitrite through a rapid dipstick method and urine microscopic examination for white blood cells (WBCs) and bacteria (Table 1).

Urine dipsticks are appealing, because they provide rapid results, do not require microscopy, and are eligible for a waiver under the Clinical Laboratory Improvement Amendments. They indicate the presence of leukocyte esterase (as a surrogate marker for pyuria) and urinary nitrite (which is converted from dietary nitrates in the presence of most Gram-negative enteric bacteria in the urine). The conversion of dietary nitrates to nitrites by bacteria requires approximately 4 hours in the bladder.[31] The performance characteristics of both leukocyte esterase and nitrite tests vary according to the definition used for positive urine culture results, the age and symptoms of the population being studied, and the method of urine collection.

Nitrite Test

A nitrite test is not a sensitive marker for children, particularly infants, who empty their bladders frequently. Therefore, negative nitrite test results have little value in ruling out UTI. Moreover, not all urinary pathogens reduce nitrate to nitrite. The test is helpful when the result is positive, however, because it is highly specific (ie, there are few false-positive results).[32]

Leukocyte Esterase Test

The sensitivity of the leukocyte esterase test is 94% when it used in the context of clinically suspected UTI. Overall, the reported sensitivity in various studies is lower (83%), because the results of leukocyte esterase tests were related to culture results without exclusion of individuals with asymptomatic bacteriuria. The absence of leukocyte esterase in the urine of individuals with asymptomatic bacteriuria is an advantage of the test, rather than a limitation, because it distinguishes individuals with asymptomatic bacteriuria from those with true UTI.

The specificity of the leukocyte esterase test (average: 72% [range: 64%–92%]) generally is not as good as the sensitivity, which reflects the nonspecificity of pyuria in general. Accordingly, positive leukocyte esterase test results should be interpreted with caution, because false-positive results are common. With numerous conditions other than UTI, including fever resulting from other conditions (eg, streptococcal infections or Kawasaki disease), and after vigorous exercise, WBCs may be found in the urine. Therefore, a finding of pyuria by no means confirms that an infection of the urinary tract is present.

The absence of pyuria in children with true UTIs is rare, however. It is theoretically possible if a febrile child is assessed before the inflammatory response has developed, but the inflammatory response to a UTI produces both fever and pyuria; therefore, children who are being evaluated because of fever should already have WBCs in their urine. More likely explanations for significant bacteriuria in culture in the absence of pyuria include contaminated specimens, insensitive criteria for pyuria, and asymptomatic bacteriuria. In most cases, when true UTI has been reported to occur in the absence of pyuria, the definition of pyuria has been at fault. The standard method of assessing pyuria has been centrifugation of the urine and microscopic analysis, with a threshold of 5 WBCs per high-power field (~25 WBCs per μL). If a counting chamber is used, however, the finding of at least 10 WBCs per μL in uncentrifuged urine has been demonstrated to be more sensitive[33] and performs well in clinical situations in which the standard method does not, such as with very young infants.[34]

An important cause of bacteriuria in the absence of pyuria is asymptomatic bacteriuria. Asymptomatic bacteriuria often is associated with school-aged and older girls,[35] but it can be present during infancy. In a study of infants 2 to 24 months of age, 0.7% of afebrile girls had 3 successive urine cultures with 10^5 CFUs per mL of a single uropathogen.[26] Asymptomatic bacteriuria can be easily confused with true UTI in a febrile infant but needs to be distinguished, because studies suggest that antimicrobial treatment may do more harm than good.[36] The key to distinguishing true UTI from asymptomatic bacteriuria is the presence of pyuria.

Microscopic Analysis for Bacteriuria

The presence of bacteria in a fresh, Gram-stained specimen of uncentrifuged urine correlates with 10^5 CFUs per mL in culture.[37] An "enhanced urinalysis," combining the counting chamber assessment of pyuria noted previously with Gram staining of drops of uncentrifuged urine, with a threshold of at least 1 Gram-negative rod in 10 oil immersion fields, has greater sensitivity, specificity, and positive predictive value than does the standard urinalysis[33] and is the preferred method of urinalysis when appropriate equipment and personnel are available.

Automated Urinalysis

Automated methods to perform urinalysis are now being used in many hospitals and laboratories. Image-based systems use flow imaging analysis technology and software to classify particles in uncentrifuged urine specimens rapidly.[38] Results correlate well with manual methods, especially for red blood cells, WBCs, and squamous epithelial cells. In the future, this may be the most common method by which urinalysis is performed in laboratories.

Culture

The diagnosis of UTI is made on the basis of quantitative urine culture results in addition to evidence of pyuria and/or bacteriuria. Urine specimens should be processed as expediently as possible. If the specimen is not processed promptly, then it should be refrigerated to prevent the growth of organisms that can occur in urine at room temperature; for the same reason, specimens that require transportation to another site for processing should be transported on ice. A properly collected urine specimen should be inoculated on culture medium that will allow identification of urinary tract pathogens.

Urine culture results are considered positive or negative on the basis of the number of CFUs that grow on the culture medium.[36] Definition of significant colony counts with regard to the method of collection considers that the distal urethra and periurethral area are commonly colonized by the same bacteria that may cause UTI; therefore, a low colony count may be present in a specimen obtained through voiding or catheterization when bacteria are not present in bladder urine. Definitions of positive and negative culture results are operational and not absolute. The time the urine resides in the bladder (bladder incubation time) is an important determinant of the magnitude of the colony count. The concept that more than 100 000 CFUs per mL indicates a UTI was based on morning collections of urine from adult women, with comparison of specimens from women without symptoms and women considered clinically to have pyelonephritis; the transition range, in which the proportion of women with pyelonephritis exceeded the proportion of women without symptoms, was 10 000 to 100 000 CFUs per mL.[39] In most instances, an appropriate threshold to consider bacteriuria "significant" in infants and children is the presence of at least 50 000 CFUs per mL of a single urinary pathogen.[40] (Organisms such as *Lactobacillus* spp, coagulase-negative staphylococci, and *Corynebacterium* spp are not considered clinically relevant urine isolates for otherwise healthy, 2- to 24-month-old children.) Reducing the threshold from 100 000 CFUs per mL to 50 000 CFUs per mL would seem to increase the sensitivity of culture at the expense of decreased specificity; however, because the proposed criteria for UTI now include evidence of pyuria in addition to positive culture results, infants with "positive" culture results alone will be recognized as having asymptomatic bacteriuria rather than a true UTI. Some laboratories report growth only in the following categories: 0 to 1000, 1000 to 10 000, 10 000 to 100 000, and more than 100 000 CFUs per mL. In such cases, results in the 10 000 to 100 000 CFUs per mL range need to be evaluated in context, such as whether the urinalysis findings support the diagnosis of UTI and whether the organism is a recognized uropathogen.

Alternative culture methods, such as dipslides, may have a place in the office setting; sensitivity is reported to be in the range of 87% to 100%, and specificity is reported to be 92% to 98%, but dipslides cannot specify the organism or antimicrobial sensitivities.[41] Practices that use dipslides should do so in collaboration with a certified laboratory for identification and sensitivity testing or, in the absence of such results, may need to perform "test of cure" cultures after 24 hours of treatment.

- Aggregate quality of evidence: C (observational studies).
- Benefits: Accurate diagnosis of UTI can prevent the spread of infection and renal scarring; avoiding overdiagnosis of UTI can prevent overtreatment and unnecessary and expensive imaging. These criteria reduce the likelihood of overdiagnosis of UTI in infants with asymptomatic bacteriuria or contaminated specimens.
- Harms/risks/costs: Stringent diagnostic criteria may miss a small number of UTIs.
- Benefit-harms assessment: Preponderance of benefit over harm.
- Value judgments: Treatment of asymptomatic bacteriuria may be harmful.
- Role of patient preferences: We assume that parents prefer no action in the absence of a UTI (avoiding false-positive results) over a very small chance of missing a UTI.
- Exclusions: None.
- Intentional vagueness: None.
- Policy level: Recommendation.

MANAGEMENT

Action Statement 4

Action Statement 4a

When initiating treatment, the clinician should base the choice of route of administration on practical considerations. Initiating treatment orally or parenterally is equally efficacious. The clinician should base the choice of agent on local antimicrobial sensitivity patterns (if available) and should adjust the choice according to sensitivity testing of the isolated uropathogen (evidence quality: A; strong recommendation).

Action Statement 4b

The clinician should choose 7 to 14 days as the duration of antimicrobial therapy (evidence quality: B; recommendation).

The goals of treatment of acute UTI are to eliminate the acute infection, to prevent complications, and to reduce the likelihood of renal damage. Most children can be treated orally.[42–44] Patients whom clinicians judge to be "toxic" or who are unable to retain oral intake (including medications) should receive an antimicrobial agent parenter-

TABLE 2 Some Empiric Antimicrobial Agents for Parenteral Treatment of UTI

Antimicrobial Agent	Dosage
Ceftriaxone	75 mg/kg, every 24 h
Cefotaxime	150 mg/kg per d, divided every 6–8 h
Ceftazidime	100–150 mg/kg per d, divided every 8 h
Gentamicin	7.5 mg/kg per d, divided every 8 h
Tobramycin	5 mg/kg per d, divided every 8 h
Piperacillin	300 mg/kg per d, divided every 6–8 h

TABLE 3 Some Empiric Antimicrobial Agents for Oral Treatment of UTI

Antimicrobial Agent	Dosage
Amoxicillin-clavulanate	20–40 mg/kg per d in 3 doses
Sulfonamide	
Trimethoprim-sulfamethoxazole	6–12 mg/kg trimethoprim and 30-60 mg/kg sulfamethoxazole per d in 2 doses
Sulfisoxazole	120–150 mg/kg per d in 4 doses
Cephalosporin	
Cefixime	8 mg/kg per d in 1 dose
Cefpodoxime	10 mg/kg per d in 2 doses
Cefprozil	30 mg/kg per d in 2 doses
Cefuroxime axetil	20–30 mg/kg per d in 2 doses
Cephalexin	50–100 mg/kg per d in 4 doses

ally (Table 2) until they exhibit clinical improvement, generally within 24 to 48 hours, and are able to retain orally administered fluids and medications. In a study of 309 febrile infants with UTIs, only 3 (1%) were deemed too ill to be assigned randomly to either parenteral or oral treatment.[42] Parenteral administration of an antimicrobial agent also should be considered when compliance with obtaining an antimicrobial agent and/or administering it orally is uncertain. The usual choices for oral treatment of UTIs include a cephalosporin, amoxicillin plus clavulanic acid, or trimethoprim-sulfamethoxazole (Table 3). It is essential to know local patterns of susceptibility of coliforms to antimicrobial agents, particularly trimethoprim-sulfamethoxazole and cephalexin, because there is substantial geographic variability that needs to be taken into account during selection of an antimicrobial agent before sensitivity results are available. Agents that are excreted in the urine but do not achieve therapeutic concentrations in the bloodstream, such as nitrofurantoin, should not be used to treat febrile infants with UTIs, because parenchymal and serum antimicrobial concentrations may be insufficient to treat pyelonephritis or urosepsis.

Whether the initial route of administration of the antimicrobial agent is oral or parenteral (then changed to oral), the total course of therapy should be 7 to 14 days. The committee attempted to identify a single, preferred, evidence-based duration, rather than a range, but data comparing 7, 10, and 14 days directly were not found. There is evidence that 1- to 3-day courses for febrile UTIs are inferior to courses in the recommended range; therefore, the minimal duration selected should be 7 days.

- Aggregate quality of evidence: A/B (RCTs).
- Benefits: Adequate treatment of UTI can prevent the spread of infection and renal scarring. Outcomes of short courses (1–3 d) are inferior to those of 7- to 14-d courses.
- Harms/risks/costs: There are minimal harm and minor cost effects of antimicrobial choice and duration of therapy.
- Benefit-harms assessment: Preponderance of benefit over harm.
- Value judgments: Adjusting antimicrobial choice on the basis of available data and treating according to best evidence will minimize cost and consequences of failed or unnecessary treatment.
- Role of patient preferences: It is assumed that parents prefer the most-effective treatment and the least amount of medication that ensures effective treatment.
- Exclusions: None.
- Intentional vagueness: No evidence distinguishes the benefit of treating 7 vs 10 vs 14 days, and the range is allowable.
- Policy level: Strong recommendation/recommendation.

Action Statement 5

Febrile infants with UTIs should undergo renal and bladder ultrasonography (RBUS) (evidence quality: C; recommendation).

The purpose of RBUS is to detect anatomic abnormalities that require further evaluation, such as additional imaging or urologic consultation. RBUS also provides an evaluation of the renal parenchyma and an assessment of renal size that can be used to monitor renal growth. The yield of actionable findings is relatively low.[45,46] Widespread application of prenatal ultrasonography clearly has reduced the prevalence of previously unsuspected obstructive uropathy in infants, but the consequences of prenatal screening with respect to the risk of renal abnormalities in infants with UTIs have not yet been well defined. There is considerable variability in the timing and quality of prenatal ultrasonograms, and the report of "normal" ultrasonographic results cannot necessarily be relied on to dismiss completely the possibility of a structural abnormality unless the study was a detailed anatomic survey (with measurements), was performed during the third trimester, and was performed and interpreted by qualified individuals.[47]

The timing of RBUS depends on the clinical situation. RBUS is recommended during the first 2 days of treatment to identify serious complications, such as renal or perirenal abscesses or pyonephrosis associated with obstructive uropathy when the clinical illness is unusually severe or substantial clinical improvement is not occurring. For febrile infants with UTIs who demonstrate substantial clinical improvement, however, imaging does not need to occur early during the acute infection and can even be misleading; animal studies demonstrate that *Escherichia coli* endotoxin can produce dilation during acute infection, which could be confused with hydronephrosis, pyonephrosis, or obstruction.[48] Changes in the size and shape of the kidneys and the echogenicity of renal parenchyma attributable to edema also are common during acute infection. The presence of these abnormalities makes it inappropriate to consider RBUS performed early during acute infection to be a true baseline study for later comparisons in the assessment of renal growth.

Nuclear scanning with technetium-labeled dimercaptosuccinic acid has greater sensitivity for detection of acute pyelonephritis and later scarring than does either RBUS or voiding cystourethrography (VCUG). The scanning is useful in research, because it ensures that all subjects in a study have pyelonephritis to start with and it permits assessment of later renal scarring as an outcome measure. The findings on nuclear scans rarely affect acute clinical management, however, and are not recommended as part of routine evaluation of infants with their first febrile UTI. The radiation dose to the patient during dimercaptosuccinic acid scanning is generally low (~1 mSv),[49] although it may be increased in children with reduced renal function. The radiation dose from dimercaptosuccinic acid is additive with that of VCUG when both studies are performed.[50] The radiation dose from VCUG depends on the equipment that is used (conventional versus pulsed digital fluoroscopy) and is related directly to the total fluoroscopy time. Moreover, the total exposure for the child will be increased when both acute and follow-up studies are obtained. The lack of exposure to radiation is a major advantage of RBUS, even with recognition of the limitations of this modality that were described previously.

- Aggregate quality of evidence: C (observational studies).
- Benefits: RBUS in this population will yield abnormal results in ~15% of cases, and 1% to 2% will have abnormalities that would lead to action (eg, additional evaluation, referral, or surgery).
- Harms/risks/costs: Between 2% and 3% will be false-positive results, leading to unnecessary and invasive evaluations.
- Benefit-harms assessment: Preponderance of benefit over harm.
- Value judgments: The seriousness of the potentially correctable abnormalities in 1% to 2%, coupled with the absence of physical harm, was judged sufficiently important to tip the scales in favor of testing.
- Role of patient preferences: Because ultrasonography is noninvasive and poses minimal risk, we assume that parents will prefer RBUS over taking even a small risk of missing a serious and correctable condition.
- Exclusions: None.
- Intentional vagueness: None.
- Policy level: Recommendation.

Action Statement 6

Action Statement 6a

VCUG should not be performed routinely after the first febrile UTI; VCUG is indicated if RBUS reveals hydronephrosis, scarring, or other findings that would suggest either high-grade VUR or obstructive uropathy, as well as in other atypical or complex clinical circumstances (evidence quality B; recommendation).

Action Statement 6b

Further evaluation should be conducted if there is a recurrence of febrile UTI (evidence quality: X; recommendation).

For the past 4 decades, the strategy to protect the kidneys from further damage after an initial UTI has been to detect childhood genitourinary abnormalities in which recurrent UTI could increase renal damage. The most common of these is VUR, and VCUG is used to detect this. Management included continuous antimicrobial administration as prophylaxis and surgical intervention if VUR was persistent or recurrences of infection were not prevented with an antimicrobial prophylaxis regimen; some have advocated surgical intervention to correct high-grade reflux even when infection has not recurred. However, it is clear that there are a significant number of infants who develop pyelonephritis in whom VUR cannot be demonstrated, and the effectiveness of antimicrobial prophylaxis for patients who have VUR has been challenged in the past decade. Several studies have suggested that prophylaxis does not confer the desired benefit of preventing recurrent febrile UTI.[51–55] If prophylaxis is, in fact, not beneficial and VUR is not required for development of pyelonephritis, then the rationale for performing VCUG routinely after an initial febrile UTI must be questioned.

TABLE 4 Recurrences of Febrile UTI/Pyelonephritis in Infants 2 to 24 Months of Age With and Without Antimicrobial Prophylaxis, According to Grade of VUR

Reflux Grade	Prophylaxis		No Prophylaxis		*P*
	No. of Recurrences	Total *N*	No. of Recurrences	Total *N*	
None	7	210	11	163	.15
I	2	37	2	35	1.00
II	11	133	10	124	.95
III	31	140	40	145	.29
IV	16	55	21	49	.14

RCTs of the effectiveness of prophylaxis performed to date generally included children more than 24 months of age, and some did not provide complete data according to grade of VUR. These 2 factors have compromised meta-analyses. To ensure direct comparisons, the committee contacted the 6 researchers who had conducted the most recent RCTs and requested raw data from their studies.[51–56] All complied, which permitted the creation of a data set with data for 1091 infants 2 to 24 months of age according to grade of VUR. A χ^2 analysis (2-tailed) and a formal meta-analysis did not detect a statistically significant benefit of prophylaxis in preventing recurrence of febrile UTI/pyelonephritis in infants without reflux or those with grades I, II, III, or IV VUR (Table 4 and Fig 3). Only 5 infants with grade V VUR were included in the RCTs; therefore, data for those infants are not included in Table 4 or Fig 3.

The proportion of infants with high-grade VUR among all infants with febrile UTIs is small. Data adapted from current studies (Table 5) indicate that, of a hypothetical cohort of 100 infants with febrile UTIs, only 1 has grade V VUR; 99 do not. With a practice of waiting for a second UTI to perform VCUG, only 10 of the 100 would need to undergo the procedure and the 1 with grade V VUR would be identified. (It also is possible that the 1 infant with grade V VUR might have been identified after the first UTI on the basis of abnormal RBUS results that prompted VCUG to be performed.) Data to quantify additional potential harm to an infant who is not revealed to have high-grade VUR until a second UTI are not precise but suggest that the increment is insufficient to justify routinely subjecting all infants with an initial febrile UTI to VCUG (Fig 4). To minimize any harm incurred by that infant, attempts have been made to identify, at the time of the initial UTI, those who have the greatest likelihood of having high-grade VUR. Unfortunately, there are no clinical or laboratory indicators that have been demonstrated to identify infants with high-grade VUR. Indications for VCUG have been proposed on the basis of consensus in the absence of data[57]; the predictive value of any of the indications for VCUG proposed in this manner is not known.

The level of evidence supporting routine imaging with VCUG was deemed insufficient at the time of the 1999 practice parameter to receive a recommendation, but the consensus of the subcommittee was to "strongly encourage" imaging studies. The position of the current subcommittee reflects the new evidence demonstrating antimicrobial prophylaxis not to be effective as presumed previously. Moreover, prompt diagnosis and effective treatment of a febrile UTI recurrence may be of greater importance regardless of whether VUR is present or the child is receiving antimicrobial prophylaxis. A national study (the Randomized Intervention for Children With Vesicoureteral Reflux study) is currently in progress to identify the effects of a prophylactic antimicrobial regimen for children 2 months to 6 years of age who have experienced a UTI, and it is anticipated to provide additional important data[58] (see Areas for Research).

Action Statement 6a

- Aggregate quality of evidence: B (RCTs).
- Benefits: This avoids, for the vast majority of febrile infants with UTIs, radiation exposure (of particular concern near the ovaries in girls), expense, and discomfort.
- Harms/risks/costs: Detection of a small number of cases of high-grade reflux and correctable abnormalities is delayed.
- Benefit-harms assessment: Preponderance of benefit over harm.
- Value judgments: The risks associated with radiation (plus the expense and discomfort of the procedure) for the vast majority of infants outweigh the risk of delaying the detection of the few with correctable abnormalities until their second UTI.
- Role of patient preferences: The judgment of parents may come into play, because VCUG is an uncomfortable procedure involving radiation exposure. In some cases, parents may prefer to subject their children to the procedure even when the chance of benefit is both small and uncertain. Antimicrobial prophylaxis seems to be ineffective in preventing recurrence of febrile UTI/pyelonephritis for the vast majority of infants. Some parents may want to avoid VCUG even after the second UTI. Because the benefit of identifying high-grade reflux is still in some doubt, these preferences should be considered. It is the judgment of the committee that VCUG is indicated after the second UTI.
- Exclusions: None.

A

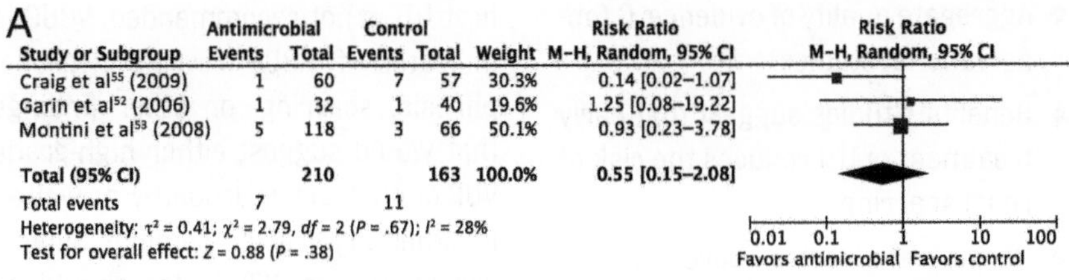

Study or Subgroup	Antimicrobial Events	Antimicrobial Total	Control Events	Control Total	Weight	Risk Ratio M-H, Random, 95% CI
Craig et al[55] (2009)	1	60	7	57	30.3%	0.14 [0.02–1.07]
Garin et al[52] (2006)	1	32	1	40	19.6%	1.25 [0.08–19.22]
Montini et al[53] (2008)	5	118	3	66	50.1%	0.93 [0.23–3.78]
Total (95% CI)		210		163	100.0%	0.55 [0.15–2.08]
Total events	7		11			

Heterogeneity: $\tau^2 = 0.41$; $\chi^2 = 2.79$, $df = 2$ ($P = .67$); $I^2 = 28\%$
Test for overall effect: $Z = 0.88$ ($P = .38$)

B

Study or Subgroup	Antimicrobial Events	Antimicrobial Total	Control Events	Control Total	Weight	Risk Ratio M-H, Random, 95% CI
Craig et al[55] (2009)	1	10	1	12	49.9%	1.20 [0.09–16.84]
Garin et al[52] (2006)	0	5	0	3		Not estimable
Montini et al[53] (2008)	1	15	1	8	50.1%	0.53 [0.04–7.44]
Roussey-Kesler et al[54] (2008)	0	7	0	12		Not estimable
Total (95% CI)		37		35	100.0%	0.80 [0.12–5.16]
Total events	2		2			

Heterogeneity: $\tau^2 = 0.00$; $\chi^2 = 0.18$, $df = 1$ ($P = .67$); $I^2 = 0\%$
Test for overall effect: $z = 0.24$ ($P = .81$)

0.01 0.1 1 10 100
Favors antimicrobial Favors control

C

Study or Subgroup	Antimicrobial Events	Antimicrobial Total	Control Events	Control Total	Weight	Risk Ratio M-H, Random, 95% CI
Craig et al[55] (2009)	0	27	1	23	6.3%	0.29 [0.01–6.69]
Garin et al[52] (2006)	1	12	0	10	6.5%	2.54 [0.11–56.25]
Montini et al[53] (2008)	3	31	2	18	21.7%	0.87 [0.16–4.73]
Pennesi et al[51] (2008)	1	11	0	10	6.5%	2.75 [0.12–60.70]
Roussey-Kesler et al[54] (2008)	6	52	7	63	59.0%	1.04 [0.37–2.90]
Total (95% CI)		133		124	100.0%	1.04 [0.47–2.29]
Total events	11		10			

Heterogeneity: $\tau^2 = 0.00$; $\chi^2 = 1.38$, $df = 4$ ($P = .85$); $I^2 = 0\%$
Test for overall effect: $z = 0.10$ ($P = .92$)

0.01 0.1 1 10 100
Favors antimicrobial Favors control

D

Study or Subgroup	Antimicrobial Events	Antimicrobial Total	Control Events	Control Total	Weight	Risk Ratio M-H, Random, 95% CI
Brandström et al[56] (2010)	5	41	14	43	20.9%	0.37 [0.15–0.95]
Craig et al[55] (2009)	1	24	4	29	7.1%	0.30 [0.04–2.53]
Garin et al[52] (2006)	4	8	0	12	4.5%	13.00 [0.79–212.80]
Montini et al[53] (2008)	6	22	6	13	21.5%	0.59 [0.24–1.45]
Pennesi et al[51] (2008)	9	22	7	24	23.6%	1.40 [0.63–3.12]
Roussey-Kesler et al[54] (2008)	6	23	9	24	22.3%	0.70 [0.29–1.64]
Total (95% CI)		140		145	100.0%	0.75 [0.40–1.40]
Total events	31		40			

Heterogeneity: $\tau^2 = 0.27$; $\chi^2 = 9.54$, $df = 5$ ($P = .09$); $I^2 = 48\%$
Test for overall effect: $z = 0.90$ ($P = .37$)

0.01 0.1 1 10 100
Favors antimicrobial Favors control

E

Study or Subgroup	Antimicrobial Events	Antimicrobial Total	Control Events	Control Total	Weight	Risk Ratio M-H, Random, 95% CI
Brandström et al[56] (2010)	5	28	11	25	35.0%	0.41 [0.16–1.01]
Craig et al[55] (2009)	3	10	2	8	14.8%	1.20 [0.26–5.53]
Pennesi et al[51] (2008)	8	17	8	16	50.2%	0.94 [0.47–1.90]
Total (95% CI)		55		49	100.0%	0.73 [0.39–1.35]
Total events	16		21			

Heterogeneity: $\tau^2 = 0.07$; $\chi^2 = 2.57$, $df = 2$ ($P = .28$); $I^2 = 22\%$
Test for overall effect: $z = 1.01$ ($P = .31$)

0.01 0.1 1 10 100
Favors antimicrobial Favors control

FIGURE 3

A, Recurrences of febrile UTI/pyelonephritis in 373 infants 2 to 24 months of age without VUR, with and without antimicrobial prophylaxis (based on 3 studies; data provided by Drs Craig, Garin, and Montini). B, Recurrences of febrile UTI/pyelonephritis in 72 infants 2 to 24 months of age with grade I VUR, with and without antimicrobial prophylaxis (based on 4 studies; data provided by Drs Craig, Garin, Montini, and Roussey-Kesler). C, Recurrences of febrile UTI/pyelonephritis in 257 infants 2 to 24 months of age with grade II VUR, with and without antimicrobial prophylaxis (based on 5 studies; data provided by Drs Craig, Garin, Montini, Pennesi, and Roussey-Kesler). D, Recurrences of febrile UTI/pyelonephritis in 285 infants 2 to 24 months of age with grade III VUR, with and without antimicrobial prophylaxis (based on 6 studies; data provided by Drs Brandström, Craig, Garin, Montini, Pennesi, and Roussey-Kesler). E, Recurrences of febrile UTI/pyelonephritis in 104 infants 2 to 24 months of age with grade IV VUR, with and without antimicrobial prophylaxis (based on 3 studies; data provided by Drs Brandström, Craig, and Pennesi). M-H indicates Mantel-Haenszel; CI, confidence interval.

TABLE 5 Rates of VUR According to Grade in Hypothetical Cohort of Infants After First UTI and After Recurrence

	Rate, %	
	After First UTI ($N = 100$)	After Recurrence ($N = 10$)
No VUR	65	26
Grades I–III VUR	29	56
Grade IV VUR	5	12
Grade V VUR	1	6

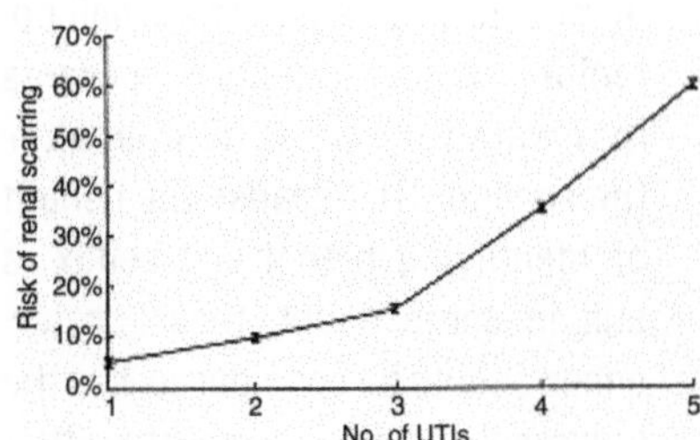

FIGURE 4

Relationship between renal scarring and number of bouts of pyelonephritis. Adapted from Jodal.[59]

- Intentional vagueness: None.
- Policy level: Recommendation.

Action Statement 6b

- Aggregate quality of evidence: X (exceptional situation).
- Benefits: VCUG after a second UTI should identify infants with very high-grade reflux.
- Harms/risks/costs: VCUG is an uncomfortable, costly procedure that involves radiation, including to the ovaries of girls.
- Benefit-harms assessment: Preponderance of benefit over harm.
- Value judgments: The committee judged that patients with high-grade reflux and other abnormalities may benefit from interventions to prevent further scarring. Further studies of treatment for grade V VUR are not underway and are unlikely in the near future, because the condition is uncommon and randomization of treatment in this group generally has been considered unethical.

- Role of patient preferences: As mentioned previously, the judgment of parents may come into play, because VCUG is an uncomfortable procedure involving radiation exposure. In some cases, parents may prefer to subject their children to the procedure even when the chance of benefit is both small and uncertain. The benefits of treatment of VUR remain unproven, but the point estimates suggest a small potential benefit. Similarly, parents may want to avoid VCUG even after the second UTI. Because the benefit of identifying high-grade reflux is still in some doubt, these preferences should be considered. It is the judgment of the committee that VCUG is indicated after the second UTI.
- Exclusions: None.
- Intentional vagueness: Further evaluation will likely start with VCUG but may entail additional studies depending on the findings. The details of further evaluation are beyond the scope of this guideline.
- Policy level: Recommendation.

Action Statement 7

After confirmation of UTI, the clinician should instruct parents or guardians to seek prompt medical evaluation (ideally within 48 hours) for future febrile illnesses, to ensure that recurrent infections can be detected and treated promptly (evidence quality: C; recommendation).

Early treatment limits renal damage better than late treatment,[1,2] and the risk of renal scarring increases as the number of recurrences increase (Fig 4).[59] For these reasons, all infants who have sustained a febrile UTI should have a urine specimen obtained at the onset of subsequent febrile illnesses, so that a UTI can be diagnosed and treated promptly.

- Aggregate quality of evidence: C (observational studies).
- Benefits: Studies suggest that early treatment of UTI reduces the risk of renal scarring.
- Harms/risks/costs: There may be additional costs and inconvenience to parents with more-frequent visits to the clinician for evaluation of fever.
- Benefit-harms assessment: Preponderance of benefit over harm.
- Value judgments: None.
- Role of patient preferences: Parents will ultimately make the judgment to seek medical care.
- Exclusions: None.
- Intentional vagueness: None.
- Policy level: Recommendation.

CONCLUSIONS

The committee formulated 7 key action statements for the diagnosis and treatment of infants and young children 2 to 24 months of age with UTI and unexplained fever. Strategies for diagnosis and treatment depend on whether the clinician determines that antimicrobial therapy is warranted immediately or can be delayed safely until urine culture and urinalysis results are available. Diagnosis is based on the presence of pyuria and at least 50 000 CFUs per mL of a single uropathogen in an appropriately collected specimen of urine; urinalysis alone does not provide a definitive diagnosis. After 7 to 14 days of antimicrobial treatment, close clinical follow-up monitoring should be maintained, with evaluation of the urine during subsequent febrile episodes to permit prompt diagnosis and treatment of recurrent infections. Ultrasonography of the kidneys and bladder should be performed to detect anatomic abnormalities that require further evaluation (eg, additional imaging or urologic consultation). Routine VCUG after the first UTI is not recommended; VCUG is indicated if RBUS reveals hydronephrosis, scarring, or other findings that would suggest either high-grade VUR or obstructive uropathy, as well as in other atypical or complex clinical circumstances. VCUG also should be performed if there is a recurrence of febrile UTI.

AREAS FOR RESEARCH

One of the major values of a comprehensive literature review is the identification of areas in which evidence is lacking. The following 8 areas are presented in an order that parallels the previous discussion.

1. The relationship between UTIs in infants and young children and reduced renal function in adults has been established but is not well characterized in quantitative terms. The ideal prospective cohort study from birth to 40 to 50 years of age has not been conducted and is unlikely to be conducted. Therefore, estimates of undesirable outcomes in adulthood, such as hypertension and end-stage renal disease, are based on the mathematical product of probabilities at several steps, each of which is subject to bias and error. Other attempts at decision analysis and thoughtful literature review have recognized the same limitations. Until recently, imaging tools available for assessment of the effects of UTIs have been insensitive. With the imaging techniques now available, it may be possible to identify the relationship of scarring to renal impairment and hypertension.
2. The development of techniques that would permit an alternative to invasive sampling and culture would be valuable for general use. Special attention should be given to infant girls and uncircumcised boys, because urethral catheterization may

be difficult and can produce contaminated specimens and SPA now is not commonly performed. Incubation time, which is inherent in the culture process, results in delayed treatment or presumptive treatment on the basis of tests that lack the desired sensitivity and specificity to replace culture.

3. The role of VUR (and therefore of VCUG) is incompletely understood. It is recognized that pyelonephritis (defined through cortical scintigraphy) can occur in the absence of VUR (defined through VCUG) and that progressive renal scarring (defined through cortical scintigraphy) can occur in the absence of demonstrated VUR.[52,53] The presumption that antimicrobial prophylaxis is of benefit for individuals with VUR to prevent recurrences of UTI or the development of renal scars is not supported by the aggregate of data from recent studies and currently is the subject of the Randomized Intervention for Children With Vesicoureteral Reflux study.[58]
4. Although the effectiveness of antimicrobial prophylaxis for the prevention of UTI has not been demonstrated, the concept has biological plausibility. Virtually all antimicrobial agents used to treat or to prevent infections of the urinary tract are excreted in the urine in high concentrations. Barriers to the effectiveness of antimicrobial prophylaxis are adherence to a daily regimen, adverse effects associated with the various agents, and the potential for emergence of antimicrobial resistance. To overcome these issues, evidence of effectiveness with a well-tolerated, safe product would be required, and parents would need sufficient education to understand the value and importance of adherence. A urinary antiseptic, rather than an antimicrobial agent, would be particularly desirable, because it could be taken indefinitely without concern that bacteria would develop resistance. Another possible strategy might be the use of probiotics.
5. Better understanding of the genome (human and bacterial) may provide insight into risk factors (VUR and others) that lead to increased scarring. Blood specimens will be retained from children enrolled in the Randomized Intervention for Children With Vesicoureteral Reflux study, for future examination of genetic determinants of VUR, recurrent UTI, and renal scarring.[58] VUR is recognized to "run in families,"[60,61] and multiple investigators are currently engaged in research to identify a genetic basis for VUR. Studies may also be able to distinguish the contribution of congenital dysplasia from acquired scarring attributable to UTI.
6. One of the factors used to assess the likelihood of UTI in febrile infants is race. Data regarding rates among Hispanic individuals are limited and would be useful for prediction rules.
7. This guideline is limited to the initial management of the first UTI in febrile infants 2 to 24 months of age. Some of the infants will have recurrent UTIs; some will be identified as having VUR or other abnormalities. Further research addressing the optimal course of management in specific situations would be valuable.
8. The optimal duration of antimicrobial treatment has not been determined. RCTs of head-to-head comparisons of various duration would be valuable, enabling clinicians to limit antimicrobial exposure to what is needed to eradicate the offending uropathogen.

LEAD AUTHOR

Kenneth B. Roberts, MD

SUBCOMMITTEE ON URINARY TRACT INFECTION, 2009–2011

Kenneth B. Roberts, MD, Chair
Stephen M. Downs, MD, MS
S. Maria E. Finnell, MD, MS
Stanley Hellerstein, MD
Linda D. Shortliffe, MD
Ellen R. Wald, MD
J. Michael Zerin, MD

OVERSIGHT BY THE STEERING COMMITTEE ON QUALITY IMPROVEMENT AND MANAGEMENT, 2009–2011

STAFF

Caryn Davidson, MA

ACKNOWLEDGMENTS

The committee gratefully acknowledges the generosity of the researchers who graciously shared their data to permit the data set with data for 1091 infants aged 2 to 24 months according to grade of VUR to be compiled, that is, Drs Per Brandström, Jonathan Craig, Eduardo Garin, Giovanni Montini, Marco Pennesi, and Gwenaelle Roussey-Kesler.

REFERENCES

1. Winter AL, Hardy BE, Alton DJ, Arbus GS, Churchill BM. Acquired renal scars in children. *J Urol.* 1983;129(6):1190–1194
2. Smellie JM, Poulton A, Prescod NP. Retrospective study of children with renal scarring associated with reflux and urinary infection. *BMJ.* 1994;308(6938):1193–1196
3. American Academy of Pediatrics, Committee on Quality Improvement, Subcommittee on Urinary Tract Infection. Practice parameter: the diagnosis, treatment, and evaluation of the initial urinary tract infection in febrile infants and young children. *Pediatrics.* 1999;103(4):843–852
4. Finnell SM, Carroll AE, Downs SM, et al. Technical report: diagnosis and management of an initial urinary tract infection in febrile infants and young children. *Pediatrics.* 2011;128(3):e749
5. American Academy of Pediatrics, Steering Committee on Quality Improvement and Management. Classifying recommenda-

tions for clinical practice guidelines. *Pediatrics.* 2004;114(3):874–877

6. Leong YY, Tan KW. Bladder aspiration for diagnosis of urinary tract infection in infants and young children. *J Singapore Paediatr Soc.* 1976;18(1):43–47
7. Pryles CV, Atkin MD, Morse TS, Welch KJ. Comparative bacteriologic study of urine obtained from children by percutaneous suprapubic aspiration of the bladder and by catheter. *Pediatrics.* 1959;24(6):983–991
8. Djojohadipringgo S, Abdul Hamid RH, Thahir S, Karim A, Darsono I. Bladder puncture in newborns: a bacteriological study. *Paediatr Indones.* 1976;16(11–12):527–534
9. Gochman RF, Karasic RB, Heller MB. Use of portable ultrasound to assist urine collection by suprapubic aspiration. *Ann Emerg Med.* 1991;20(6):631–635
10. Buys H, Pead L, Hallett R, Maskell R. Suprapubic aspiration under ultrasound guidance in children with fever of undiagnosed cause. *BMJ.* 1994;308(6930):690–692
11. Kramer MS, Tange SM, Drummond KN, Mills EL. Urine testing in young febrile children: a risk-benefit analysis. *J Pediatr.* 1994;125(1): 6–13
12. Bonadio WA. Urine culturing technique in febrile infants. *Pediatr Emerg Care.* 1987;3(2): 75–78
13. Lohr J. *Pediatric Outpatient Procedures.* Philadelphia, PA: Lippincott; 1991
14. Taylor CM, White RH. The feasibility of screening preschool children for urinary tract infection using dipslides. *Int J Pediatr Nephrol.* 1983;4(2):113–114
15. Sørensen K, Lose G, Nathan E. Urinary tract infections and diurnal incontinence in girls. *Eur J Pediatr.* 1988;148(2):146–147
16. Shannon F, Sepp E, Rose G. The diagnosis of bacteriuria by bladder puncture in infancy and childhood. *Aust Pediatr J.* 1969;5(2): 97–100
17. Hoberman A, Chao HP, Keller DM, Hickey R, Davis HW, Ellis D. Prevalence of urinary tract infection in febrile infants. *J Pediatr.* 1993; 123(1):17–23
18. Haddon RA, Barnett PL, Grimwood K, Hogg GG. Bacteraemia in febrile children presenting to a paediatric emergency department. *Med J Aust.* 1999;170(10):475–478
19. Wiswell TE, Roscelli JD. Corroborative evidence for the decreased incidence of urinary tract infections in circumcised male infants. *Pediatrics.* 1986;78(1):96–99
20. To T, Agha M, Dick PT, Feldman W. Cohort study on circumcision of newborn boys and subsequent risk of urinary-tract infection. *Lancet.* 1998;352(9143):1813–1816
21. Wiswell TE, Hachey WE. Urinary tract infections and the uncircumcised state: an update. *Clin Pediatr (Phila).* 1993;32(3): 130–134
22. Wiswell TE, Smith FR, Bass JW. Decreased incidence of urinary tract infections in circumcised male infants. *Pediatrics.* 1985; 75(5):901–903
23. Ginsburg CM, McCracken GH Jr. Urinary tract infections in young infants. *Pediatrics.* 1982;69(4):409–412
24. Craig JC, Knight JF, Sureshkumar P, Mantz E, Roy LP. Effect of circumcision on incidence of urinary tract infection in preschool boys. *J Pediatr.* 1996;128(1):23–27
25. Levine DA, Platt SL, Dayan PS, et al. Risk of serious bacterial infection in young febrile infants with respiratory syncytial virus infections. *Pediatrics.* 2004;113(6): 1728–1734
26. Roberts KB, Charney E, Sweren RJ, et al. Urinary tract infection in infants with unexplained fever: a collaborative study. *J Pediatr.* 1983;103(6):864–867
27. Gorelick MH, Hoberman A, Kearney D, Wald E, Shaw KN. Validation of a decision rule identifying febrile young girls at high risk for urinary tract infection. *Pediatr Emerg Care.* 2003;19(3):162–164
28. Gorelick MH, Shaw KN. Clinical decision rule to identify febrile young girls at risk for urinary tract infection. *Arch Pediatr Adolesc Med.* 2000;154(4):386–390
29. Shaw KN, Gorelick M, McGowan KL, Yakscoe NM, Schwartz JS. Prevalence of urinary tract infection in febrile young children in the emergency department. *Pediatrics.* 1998;102(2). Available at: www.pediatrics.org/cgi/content/full/102/2/e16
30. Shaikh N, Morone NE, Lopez J, et al. Does this child have a urinary tract infection? *JAMA.* 2007;298(24):2895–2904
31. Powell HR, McCredie DA, Ritchie MA. Urinary nitrite in symptomatic and asymptomatic urinary infection. *Arch Dis Child.* 1987;62(2): 138–140
32. Kunin CM, DeGroot JE. Sensitivity of a nitrite indicator strip method in detecting bacteriuria in preschool girls. *Pediatrics.* 1977; 60(2):244–245
33. Hoberman A, Wald ER, Reynolds EA, Penchansky L, Charron M. Is urine culture necessary to rule out urinary tract infection in young febrile children? *Pediatr Infect Dis J.* 1996;15(4):304–309
34. Herr SM, Wald ER, Pitetti RD, Choi SS. Enhanced urinalysis improves identification of febrile infants ages 60 days and younger at low risk for serious bacterial illness. *Pediatrics.* 2001;108(4):866–871
35. Kunin C. A ten-year study of bacteriuria in schoolgirls: final report of bacteriologic, urologic, and epidemiologic findings. *J Infect Dis.* 1970;122(5):382–393
36. Kemper K, Avner E. The case against screening urinalyses for asymptomatic bacteriuria in children. *Am J Dis Child.* 1992;146(3): 343–346
37. Wald E. Genitourinary tract infections: cystitis and pyelonephritis. In: Feigin R, Cherry JD, Demmler GJ, Kaplan SL, eds. *Textbook of Pediatric Infectious Diseases.* 5th ed. Philadelphia, PA: Saunders; 2004:541–555
38. Mayo S, Acevedo D, Quiñones-Torrelo C, Canós I, Sancho M. Clinical laboratory automated urinalysis: comparison among automated microscopy, flow cytometry, two test strips analyzers, and manual microscopic examination of the urine sediments. *J Clin Lab Anal.* 2008;22(4):262–270
39. Kass E. Asymptomatic infections of the urinary tract. *Trans Assoc Am Phys.* 1956;69: 56–64
40. Hoberman A, Wald ER, Reynolds EA, Penchansky L, Charron M. Pyuria and bacteriuria in urine specimens obtained by catheter from young children with fever. *J Pediatr.* 1994;124(4):513–519
41. Downs SM. Technical report: urinary tract infections in febrile infants and young children. *Pediatrics.* 1999;103(4). Available at: www.pediatrics.org/cgi/content/full/103/4/e54
42. Hoberman A, Wald ER, Hickey RW, et al. Oral versus initial intravenous therapy for urinary tract infections in young febrile children. *Pediatrics.* 1999;104(1):79–86
43. Hodson EM, Willis NS, Craig JC. Antibiotics for acute pyelonephritis in children. *Cochrane Database Syst Rev.* 2007;(4): CD003772
44. Bloomfield P, Hodson EM, Craig JC. Antibiotics for acute pyelonephritis in children. *Cochrane Database Syst Rev.* 2005;(1): CD003772
45. Hoberman A, Charron M, Hickey RW, Baskin M, Kearney DH, Wald ER. Imaging studies after a first febrile urinary tract infection in young children. *N Engl J Med.* 2003;348(3): 195–202
46. Jahnukainen T, Honkinen O, Ruuskanen O, Mertsola J. Ultrasonography after the first febrile urinary tract infection in children. *Eur J Pediatr.* 2006;165(8):556–559
47. Economou G, Egginton J, Brookfield D. The importance of late pregnancy scans for renal tract abnormalities. *Prenat Diagn.* 1994; 14(3):177–180
48. Roberts J. Experimental pyelonephritis in the monkey, part III: pathophysiology of ure-

teral malfunction induced by bacteria. *Invest Urol*. 1975;13(2):117–120

49. Smith T, Evans K, Lythgoe MF, Anderson PJ, Gordon I. Radiation dosimetry of technetium-99m-DMSA in children. *J Nucl Med*. 1996;37(8):1336–1342
50. Ward VL. Patient dose reduction during voiding cystourethrography. *Pediatr Radiol*. 2006;36(suppl 2):168–172
51. Pennesi M, Travan L, Peratoner L, et al. Is antibiotic prophylaxis in children with vesicoureteral reflux effective in preventing pyelonephritis and renal scars? A randomized, controlled trial. *Pediatrics*. 2008; 121(6). Available at: www.pediatrics.org/cgi/content/full/121/6/e1489
52. Garin EH, Olavarria F, Garcia Nieto V, Valenciano B, Campos A, Young L. Clinical significance of primary vesicoureteral reflux and urinary antibiotic prophylaxis after acute pyelonephritis: a multicenter, randomized, controlled study. *Pediatrics*. 2006;117(3): 626–632
53. Montini G, Rigon L, Zucchetta P, et al. Prophylaxis after first febrile urinary tract infection in children? A multicenter, randomized, controlled, noninferiority trial. *Pediatrics*. 2008;122(5):1064–1071
54. Roussey-Kesler G, Gadjos V, Idres N, et al. Antibiotic prophylaxis for the prevention of recurrent urinary tract infection in children with low grade vesicoureteral reflux: results from a prospective randomized study. *J Urol*. 2008;179(2):674–679
55. Craig J, Simpson J, Williams G. Antibiotic prophylaxis and recurrent urinary tract infection in children. *N Engl J Med*. 2009; 361(18):1748–1759
56. Brandström P, Esbjorner E, Herthelius M, Swerkersson S, Jodal U, Hansson S. The Swedish Reflux Trial in Children, part III: urinary tract infection pattern. *J Urol*. 2010; 184(1):286–291
57. National Institute for Health and Clinical Excellence. *Urinary Tract Infection in Children: Diagnosis, Treatment, and Long-term Management: NICE Clinical Guideline 54*. London, England: National Institute for Health and Clinical Excellence; 2007. Available at: www.nice.org.uk/nicemedia/live/11819/36032/36032.pdf. Accessed March 14, 2011
58. Keren R, Carpenter MA, Hoberman A, et al. Rationale and design issues of the Randomized Intervention for Children With Vesicoureteral Reflux (RIVUR) study. *Pediatrics*. 2008;122(suppl 5):S240–S250
59. Jodal U. The natural history of bacteriuria in childhood. *Infect Dis Clin North Am*. 1987; 1(4):713–729
60. Eccles MR, Bailey RR, Abbott GD, Sullivan MJ. Unravelling the genetics of vesicoureteric reflux: a common familial disorder. *Hum Mol Genet*. 1996;5(Spec No.):1425–1429
61. Scott JE, Swallow V, Coulthard MG, Lambert HJ, Lee RE. Screening of newborn babies for familial ureteric reflux. *Lancet*. 1997; 350(9075):396–400

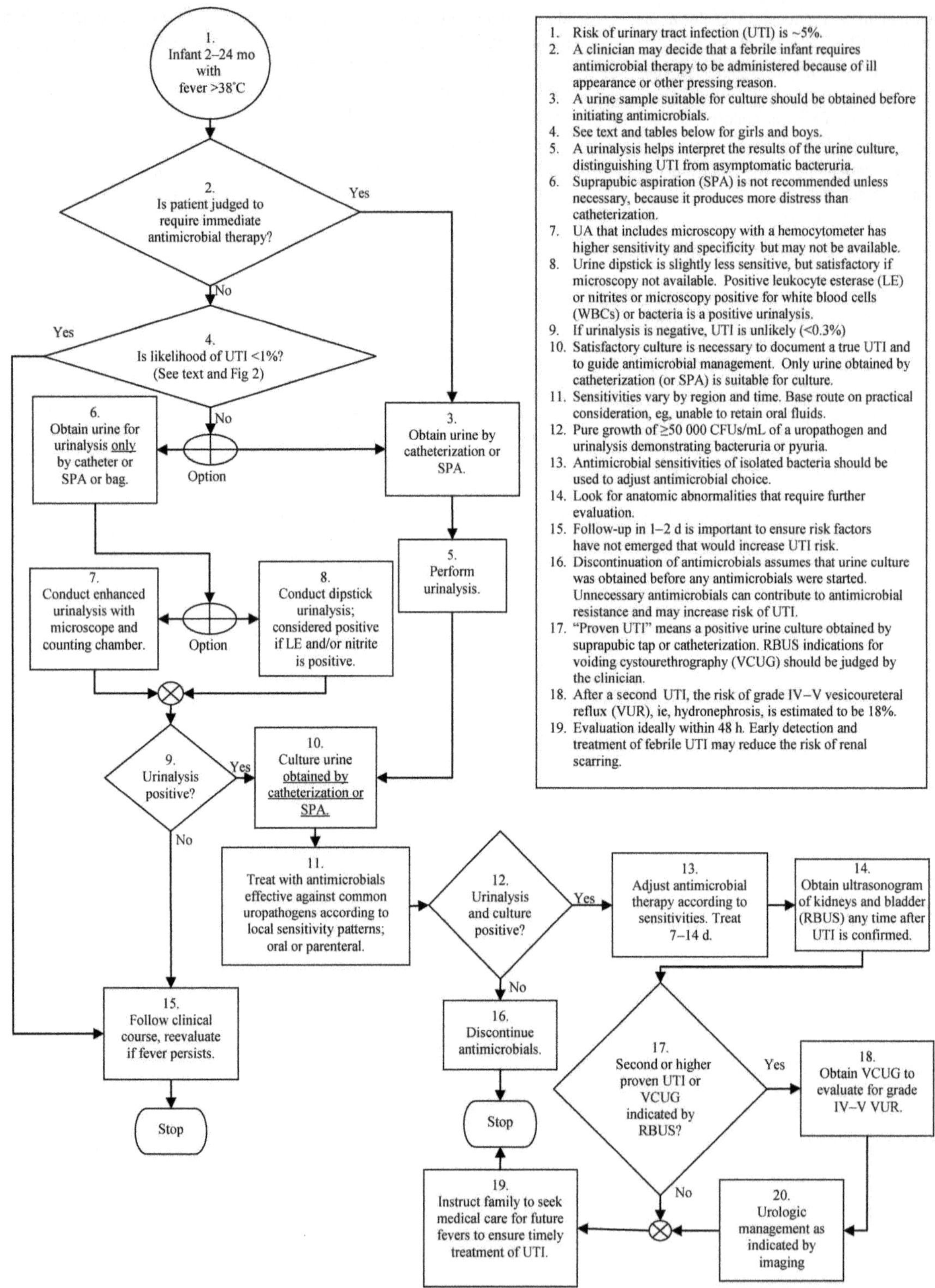

APPENDIX
Clinical practice guideline algorithm.

Urinary Tract Infection Clinical Practice Guideline Quick Reference Tools

- Action Statement Summary
  - Urinary Tract Infection: Clinical Practice Guideline for the Diagnosis and Management of the Initial UTI in Febrile Infants and Children 2 to 24 Months
- *ICD-10-CM* Coding Quick Reference for Urinary Tract Infection
- AAP Patient Education Handout
  - *Urinary Tract Infections in Young Children*

Action Statement Summary

Urinary Tract Infection: Clinical Practice Guideline for the Diagnosis and Management of the Initial UTI in Febrile Infants and Children 2 to 24 Months

Action Statement 1

If a clinician decides that a febrile infant with no apparent source for the fever requires antimicrobial therapy to be administered because of ill appearance or another pressing reason, the clinician should ensure that a urine specimen is obtained for both culture and urinalysis before an antimicrobial agent is administered; the specimen needs to be obtained through catheterization or SPA, because the diagnosis of UTI cannot be established reliably through culture of urine collected in a bag (evidence quality: A; strong recommendation).

Action Statement 2

If a clinician assesses a febrile infant with no apparent source for the fever as not being so ill as to require immediate antimicrobial therapy, then the clinician should assess the likelihood of UTI (see below for how to assess likelihood).

Action Statement 2a

If the clinician determines the febrile infant to have a low likelihood of UTI (see text), then clinical follow-up monitoring without testing is sufficient (evidence quality: A; strong recommendation).

Action Statement 2b

If the clinician determines that the febrile infant is not in a low-risk group (see below), then there are 2 choices (evidence quality: A; strong recommendation). Option 1 is to obtain a urine specimen through catheterization or SPA for culture and urinalysis. Option 2 is to obtain a urine specimen through the most convenient means and to perform a urinalysis. If the urinalysis results suggest a UTI (positive leukocyte esterase test results or nitrite test or microscopic analysis results positive for leukocytes or bacteria), then a urine specimen should be obtained through catheterization or SPA and cultured; if urinalysis of fresh (<1 hour since void) urine yields negative leukocyte esterase and nitrite test results, then it is reasonable to monitor the clinical course without initiating antimicrobial therapy, recognizing that negative urinalysis results do not rule out a UTI with certainty.

Action Statement 3

To establish the diagnosis of UTI, clinicians should require *both* urinalysis results that suggest infection (pyuria and/or bacteriuria) *and* the presence of at least 50 000 colony-forming units (CFUs) per mL of a uropathogen cultured from a urine specimen obtained through catheterization or SPA (evidence quality: C; recommendation).

Action Statement 4a

When initiating treatment, the clinician should base the choice of route of administration on practical considerations. Initiating treatment orally or parenterally is equally efficacious. The clinician should base the choice of agent on local antimicrobial sensitivity patterns (if available) and should adjust the choice according to sensitivity testing of the isolated uropathogen (evidence quality: A; strong recommendation).

Action Statement 4b

The clinician should choose 7 to 14 days as the duration of antimicrobial therapy (evidence quality: B; recommendation).

Action Statement 5

Febrile infants with UTIs should undergo renal and bladder ultrasonography (RBUS) (evidence quality: C; recommendation).

Action Statement 6a

VCUG should not be performed routinely after the first febrile UTI; VCUG is indicated if RBUS reveals hydronephrosis, scarring, or other findings that would suggest either high-grade VUR or obstructive uropathy, as well as in other atypical or complex clinical circumstances (evidence quality B; recommendation).

Action Statement 6b

Further evaluation should be conducted if there is a recurrence of febrile UTI (evidence quality: X; recommendation).

Action Statement 7

After confirmation of UTI, the clinician should instruct parents or guardians to seek prompt medical evaluation (ideally within 48 hours) for future febrile illnesses, to ensure that recurrent infections can be detected and treated promptly (evidence quality: C; recommendation).

Coding Quick Reference for Urinary Tract Infection
ICD-10-CM
N39.0 Urinary tract infection, site not specified
P39.3 Neonatal urinary tract infection

Urinary Tract Infections in Young Children

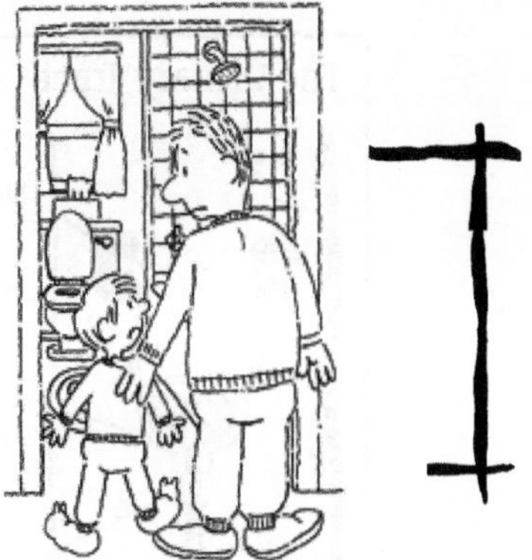

Urinary tract infections (UTIs) are common in young children. These infections can lead to serious health problems. UTIs may go untreated because the symptoms may not be obvious to the child or the parents. The following is information from the American Academy of Pediatrics about UTIs—what they are, how children get them, and how they are treated.

The urinary tract

The urinary tract makes and stores urine. It is made up of the kidneys, ureters, bladder, and urethra (see illustration on the next page). The kidneys produce urine. Urine travels from the kidneys down 2 narrow tubes called the ureters to the bladder. The bladder is a thin muscular bag that stores urine until it is time to empty urine out of the body. When it is time to empty the bladder, a muscle at the bottom of the bladder relaxes. Urine then flows out of the body through a tube called the urethra. The opening of the urethra is at the end of the penis in boys and above the vaginal opening in girls.

Urinary tract infections

Normal urine has no germs (bacteria). However, bacteria can get into the urinary tract from 2 sources: (1) the skin around the rectum and genitals and (2) the bloodstream from other parts of the body. Bacteria may cause infections in any or all parts of the urinary tract, including the following:

- Urethra (called urethritis)
- Bladder (called cystitis)
- Kidneys (called pyelonephritis)

UTIs are common in infants and young children. The frequency of UTIs in girls is much greater than in boys. About 3% of girls and 1% of boys will have a UTI by 11 years of age. A young child with a high fever and no other symptoms has a 1 in 20 chance of having a UTI. Uncircumcised boys have more UTIs than those who have been circumcised.

Symptoms

Symptoms of UTIs may include the following:

- Fever
- Pain or burning during urination
- Need to urinate more often, or difficulty getting urine out
- Urgent need to urinate, or wetting of underwear or bedding by a child who knows how to use the toilet
- Vomiting, refusal to eat
- Abdominal pain
- Side or back pain
- Foul-smelling urine
- Cloudy or bloody urine
- Unexplained and persistent irritability in an infant
- Poor growth in an infant

Diagnosis

If your child has symptoms of a UTI, your child's doctor will do the following:

- Ask about your child's symptoms.
- Ask about any family history of urinary tract problems.
- Ask about what your child has been eating and drinking.
- Examine your child.
- Get a urine sample from your child.

Your child's doctor will need to test your child's urine to see if there are bacteria or other abnormalities.

Ways urine is collected

Urine must be collected and analyzed to determine if there is a bacterial infection. Older children are asked to urinate into a container.

There are 3 ways to collect urine from a young child:

1. The preferred method is to place a small tube, called a catheter, through the urethra into the bladder. Urine flows through the tube into a special urine container.
2. Another method is to insert a needle through the skin of the lower abdomen to draw urine from the bladder. This is called needle aspiration.
3. If your child is very young or not yet toilet trained, the child's doctor may place a plastic bag over the genitals to collect the urine. Since bacteria on the skin can contaminate the urine and give a false test result, this method is used only to screen for infection. If an infection seems to be present, the doctor will need to collect urine through 1 of the first 2 methods in order to determine if bacteria are present.

Your child's doctor will discuss with you the best way to collect your child's urine.

Treatment

UTIs are treated with antibiotics. The way your child receives the antibiotic depends on the severity and type of infection. Antibiotics are usually given by mouth, as liquid or pills. If your child has a fever or is vomiting and is unable to keep fluids down, the antibiotics may be put directly into a vein or injected into a muscle.

UTIs need to be treated right away to

- Get rid of the infection.
- Prevent the spread of the infection outside of the urinary tract.
- Reduce the chances of kidney damage.

Infants and young children with UTIs usually need to take antibiotics for 7 to 14 days, sometimes longer. Make sure your child takes all the medicine your child's doctor prescribes. Do not stop giving your child the medicine until the child's doctor says the treatment is finished, even if your child feels better. UTIs can return if not fully treated.

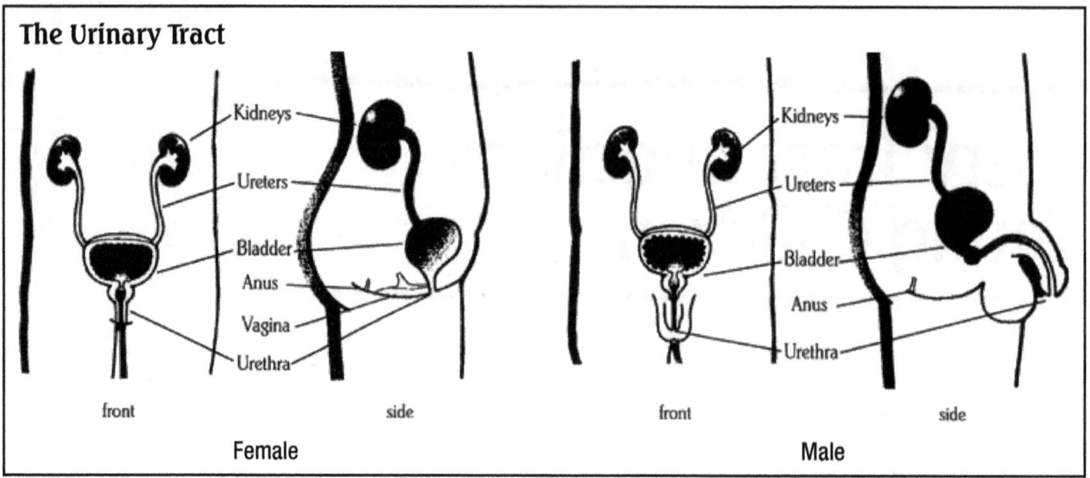

Follow-up

If the UTI occurs early in life, your child's doctor will probably want to make sure the urinary tract is normal with a kidney and bladder ultrasound. This test uses sound waves to examine the bladder and kidneys.

In addition, your child's doctor may want to make sure that the urinary tract is functioning normally and is free of any damage. Several tests are available to do this, including the following:

Voiding cystourethrogram (VCUG). A catheter is placed into the urethra and the bladder is filled with a liquid that can be seen on x-rays. This test shows whether the urine is flowing back from the bladder toward the kidneys instead of all of it coming out through the urethra as it should.

Nuclear scans. Radioactive material is injected into a vein to see if the kidneys are normal. There are many kinds of nuclear scans, each giving different information about the kidneys and bladder. The radioactive material gives no more radiation than any other kind of x-ray.

Remember

UTIs are common and most are easy to treat. Early diagnosis and prompt treatment are important because untreated or repeated infections can cause long-term medical problems. Children who have had one UTI are more likely to have another. Be sure to see your child's doctor early if your child has had a UTI in the past and has fever. Talk with your child's doctor if you suspect that your child might have a UTI.

The information contained in this publication should not be used as a substitute for the medical care and advice of your pediatrician. There may be variations in treatment that your pediatrician may recommend based on individual facts and circumstances.

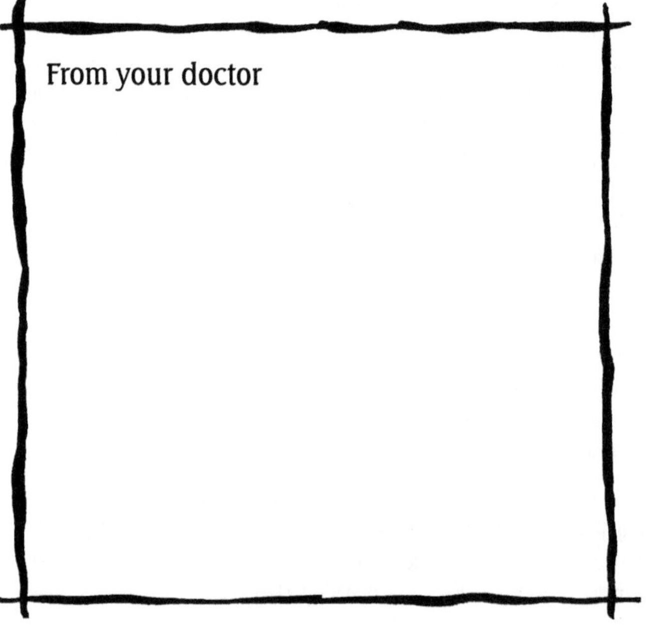

American Academy of Pediatrics

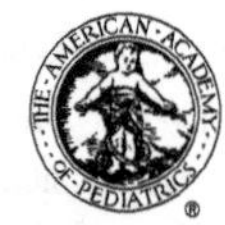

DEDICATED TO THE HEALTH OF ALL CHILDREN™

The American Academy of Pediatrics is an organization of 66,000 primary care pediatricians, pediatric medical subspecialists, and pediatric surgical specialists dedicated to the health, safety, and well-being of infants, children, adolescents, and young adults.

American Academy of Pediatrics
Web site—www.HealthyChildren.org

© 2010 American Academy of Pediatrics, Reaffirmed 01/2017.
All rights reserved.

SECTION 2

Endorsed Clinical Practice Guidelines

The American Academy of Pediatrics endorses and accepts as its policy the following guidelines from other organizations.

AUTISM SPECTRUM DISORDER

Screening and Diagnosis of Autism

Quality Standards Subcommittee of the American Academy of Neurology and the Child Neurology Society

ABSTRACT. Autism is a common disorder of childhood, affecting 1 in 500 children. Yet, it often remains unrecognized and undiagnosed until or after late preschool age because appropriate tools for routine developmental screening and screening specifically for autism have not been available. Early identification of children with autism and intensive, early intervention during the toddler and preschool years improves outcome for most young children with autism. This practice parameter reviews the available empirical evidence and gives specific recommendations for the identification of children with autism. This approach requires a dual process: (1) routine developmental surveillance and screening specifically for autism to be performed on all children to first identify those at risk for any type of atypical development, and to identify those specifically at risk for autism; and (2) to diagnose and evaluate autism, to differentiate autism from other developmental disorders. (8/00, reaffirmed 10/03, 7/06, 7/10, 8/14)

CARDIOVASCULAR HEALTH

Expert Panel on Integrated Guidelines for Cardiovascular Health and Risk Reduction in Children and Adolescents: Summary Report

National Heart, Lung, and Blood Institute

INTRODUCTION (EXCERPT). Atherosclerotic cardiovascular disease (CVD) remains the leading cause of death in North Americans, but manifest disease in childhood and adolescence is rare. By contrast, risk factors and risk behaviors that accelerate the development of atherosclerosis begin in childhood, and there is increasing evidence that risk reduction delays progression toward clinical disease. In response, the former director of the National Heart, Lung, and Blood Institute (NHLBI), Dr Elizabeth Nabel, initiated development of cardiovascular health guidelines for pediatric care providers based on a formal evidence review of the science with an integrated format addressing all the major cardiovascular risk factors simultaneously. An expert panel was appointed to develop the guidelines in the fall of 2006. (10/12)

CEREBRAL PALSY

Diagnostic Assessment of the Child With Cerebral Palsy

Quality Standards Subcommittee of the American Academy of Neurology and the Practice Committee of the Child Neurology Society

ABSTRACT. ***Objective.*** The Quality Standards Subcommittee of the American Academy of Neurology and the Practice Committee of the Child Neurology Society develop practice parameters as strategies for patient management based on analysis of evidence. For this parameter the authors reviewed available evidence on the assessment of a child suspected of having cerebral palsy (CP), a nonprogressive disorder of posture or movement due to a lesion of the developing brain.

Methods. Relevant literature was reviewed, abstracted, and classified. Recommendations were based on a four-tiered scheme of evidence classification.

Results. CP is a common problem, occurring in about 2 to 2.5 per 1,000 live births. In order to establish that a brain abnormality exists in children with CP that may, in turn, suggest an etiology and prognosis, neuroimaging is recommended with MRI preferred to CT (Level A). Metabolic and genetic studies should not be routinely obtained in the evaluation of the child with CP (Level B). If the clinical history or findings on neuroimaging do not determine a specific structural abnormality or if there are additional and atypical features in the history or clinical examination, metabolic and genetic testing should be considered (Level C). Detection of a brain malformation in a child with CP warrants consideration of an underlying genetic or metabolic etiology. Because the incidence of cerebral infarction is high in children with hemiplegic CP, diagnostic testing for coagulation disorders should be considered (Level B). However, there is insufficient evidence at present to be precise as to what studies should be ordered. An EEG is not recommended unless there are features suggestive of epilepsy or a specific epileptic syndrome (Level A). Because children with CP may have associated deficits of mental retardation, ophthalmologic and hearing impairments, speech and language disorders, and oral-motor dysfunction, screening for these conditions should be part of the initial assessment (Level A).

Conclusions. Neuroimaging results in children with CP are commonly abnormal and may help determine the etiology. Screening for associated conditions is warranted as part of the initial evaluation. (3/04, reaffirmed 7/07)

CERUMEN IMPACTION

Cerumen Impaction

American Academy of Otolaryngology—Head and Neck Surgery Foundation

ABSTRACT. This update of the 2008 American Academy of Otolaryngology—Head and Neck Surgery Foundation cerumen impaction clinical practice guideline provides evidence-based recommendations on managing cerumen impaction. Cerumen impaction is defined as an accumulation of cerumen that causes symptoms, prevents assessment of the ear, or both. Changes from the prior guideline include

- a consumer added to the development group;
- new evidence (3 guidelines, 5 systematic reviews, and 6 randomized controlled trials);
- enhanced information on patient education and counseling;
- a new algorithm to clarify action statement relationships;
- expanded action statement profiles to explicitly state quality improvement opportunities, confidence in the evidence, intentional vagueness, and differences of opinion;
- an enhanced external review process to include public comment and journal peer review; and
- new key action statements on managing cerumen impaction that focus on primary prevention, contraindicated intervention, and referral and coordination of care. (1/17)

CONGENITAL MUSCULAR DYSTROPHY

Evidence-based Guideline Summary: Evaluation, Diagnosis, and Management of Congenital Muscular Dystrophy. Report of the Guideline Development Subcommittee of the American Academy of Neurology and the Practice Issues Review Panel of the American Association of Neuromuscular & Electrodiagnostic Medicine

American Academy of Neurology and American Association of Neuromuscular & Electrodiagnostic Medicine

ABSTRACT. ***Objective.*** To delineate optimal diagnostic and therapeutic approaches to congenital muscular dystrophy (CMD) through a systematic review and analysis of the currently available literature.

Methods. Relevant, peer-reviewed research articles were identified using a literature search of the MEDLINE, EMBASE, and Scopus databases. Diagnostic and therapeutic data from these articles were extracted and analyzed in accordance with the American Academy of Neurology classification of evidence schemes for diagnostic, prognostic, and therapeutic studies. Recommendations were linked to the strength of the evidence, other related literature, and general principles of care.

Results. The geographic and ethnic backgrounds, clinical features, brain imaging studies, muscle imaging studies, and muscle biopsies of children with suspected CMD help predict subtype-specific diagnoses. Genetic testing can confirm some subtype-specific diagnoses, but not all causative genes for CMD have been described. Seizures and respiratory complications occur in specific subtypes. There is insufficient evidence to determine the efficacy of various treatment interventions to optimize respiratory, orthopedic, and nutritional outcomes, and more data are needed regarding complications.

Recommendations. Multidisciplinary care by experienced teams is important for diagnosing and promoting the health of children with CMD. Accurate assessment of clinical presentations and genetic data will help in identifying the correct subtype-specific diagnosis in many cases. Multiorgan system complications occur frequently; surveillance and prompt interventions are likely to be beneficial for affected children. More research is needed to fill gaps in knowledge regarding this category of muscular dystrophies. (3/15, reaffirmed 7/18)

DEPRESSION

Guidelines for Adolescent Depression in Primary Care (GLAD-PC): Part I. Practice Preparation, Identification, Assessment, and Initial Management

Rachel A. Zuckerbrot, MD; Amy Cheung, MD; Peter S. Jensen, MD; Ruth E.K. Stein, MD; Danielle Laraque, MD; and GLAD-PC Steering Group

ABSTRACT. ***Objectives.*** To update clinical practice guidelines to assist primary care (PC) clinicians in the management of adolescent depression. This part of the updated guidelines is used to address practice preparation, identification, assessment, and initial management of adolescent depression in PC settings.

Methods. By using a combination of evidence- and consensus-based methodologies, guidelines were developed by an expert steering committee in 2 phases as informed by (1) current scientific evidence (published and unpublished) and (2) draft revision and iteration among the steering committee, which included experts, clinicians, and youth and families with lived experience.

Results. Guidelines were updated for youth aged 10 to 21 years and correspond to initial phases of adolescent depression management in PC, including the identification of at-risk youth, assessment and diagnosis, and initial management. The strength of each recommendation and its evidence base are summarized. The practice preparation, identification, assessment, and initial management section of the guidelines include recommendations for (1) the preparation of the PC practice for improved care of adolescents with depression; (2) annual universal screening of youth 12 and over at health maintenance visits; (3) the identification of depression in youth who are at high risk; (4) systematic assessment procedures by using reliable depression scales, patient and caregiver interviews, and *Diagnostic and Statistical Manual of Mental Disorders, Fifth Edition* criteria; (5) patient and family psychoeducation; (6) the establishment of relevant links in the community; and (7) the establishment of a safety plan.

Conclusions. This part of the guidelines is intended to assist PC clinicians in the identification and initial management of adolescents with depression in an era of great clinical need and shortage of mental health specialists, but they cannot replace clinical judgment; these guidelines are not meant to be the sole source of guidance for depression management in adolescents. Additional research that addresses the identification and initial management of youth with depression in PC is needed, including empirical testing of these guidelines. (2/18)

Guidelines for Adolescent Depression in Primary Care (GLAD-PC): Part II. Treatment and Ongoing Management

Amy H. Cheung, MD; Rachel A. Zuckerbrot, MD; Peter S. Jensen, MD; Danielle Laraque, MD; Ruth E.K. Stein, MD; and GLAD-PC Steering Group

ABSTRACT. ***Objectives.*** To update clinical practice guidelines to assist primary care (PC) in the screening and assessment of depression. In this second part of the updated guidelines, we address treatment and ongoing management of adolescent depression in the PC setting.

Methods. By using a combination of evidence- and consensus-based methodologies, the guidelines were updated in 2 phases as informed by (1) current scientific evidence (published and unpublished) and (2) revision and iteration among the steering committee, including youth and families with lived experience.

Results. These updated guidelines are targeted for youth aged 10 to 21 years and offer recommendations for the management of adolescent depression in PC, including (1) active monitoring of mildly depressed youth, (2) treatment with evidence-based medication and psychotherapeutic approaches in cases of moderate and/or severe depression, (3) close monitoring of side effects, (4) consultation and comanagement of care with mental health specialists, (5) ongoing tracking of outcomes, and (6) specific steps to be taken in instances of partial or no improvement after an initial treatment has begun. The strength of each recommendation and the grade of its evidence base are summarized.

Conclusions. The Guidelines for Adolescent Depression in Primary Care cannot replace clinical judgment, and they should not be the sole source of guidance for adolescent depression management. Nonetheless, the guidelines may assist PC clinicians in the management of depressed adolescents in an era of great clinical need and a shortage of mental health specialists. Additional research concerning the management of depressed youth in PC is needed, including the usability, feasibility, and sustainability of guidelines, and determination of the extent to which the guidelines actually improve outcomes of depressed youth. (2/18)

DUCHENNE MUSCULAR DYSTROPHY

Practice Guideline Update Summary: Corticosteroid Treatment of Duchenne Muscular Dystrophy

David Gloss, MD, MPH&TM; Richard T. Moxley III, MD; Stephen Ashwal, MD; and Maryam Oskoui, MD, for the American Academy of Neurology Guideline Development Subcommittee

ABSTRACT. ***Objective.*** To update the 2005 American Academy of Neurology (AAN) guideline on corticosteroid treatment of Duchenne muscular dystrophy (DMD).

Methods. We systematically reviewed the literature from January 2004 to July 2014 using the AAN classification scheme for therapeutic articles and predicated recommendations on the strength of the evidence.

Results. Thirty-four studies met inclusion criteria.

Recommendations. In children with DMD, prednisone should be offered for improving strength (Level B) and pulmonary function (Level B). Prednisone may be offered for improving timed motor function (Level C), reducing the need for scoliosis surgery (Level C), and delaying cardiomyopathy onset by 18 years of age (Level C). Deflazacort may be offered for improving strength and timed motor function and delaying age at loss of ambulation by 1.4–2.5 years (Level C). Deflazacort may be offered for improving pulmonary function, reducing the need for scoliosis surgery, delaying cardiomyopathy onset, and increasing survival at 5–15 years of follow-up (Level C for each). Deflazacort and prednisone may be equivalent in improving motor function (Level C). Prednisone may be associated with greater weight gain in the first years of treatment than deflazacort (Level C).

Deflazacort may be associated with a greater risk of cataracts than prednisone (Level C). The preferred dosing regimen of prednisone is 0.75 mg/kg/d (Level B). Over 12 months, prednisone 10 mg/kg/weekend is equally effective (Level B), with no long-term data available. Prednisone 0.75 mg/kg/d is associated with significant risk of weight gain, hirsutism, and cushingoid appearance (Level B). *Neurology®* 2016;86:465–472 (2/16, reaffirmed 1/19)

DYSPLASIA OF THE HIP

Guideline on Detection and Nonoperative Management of Pediatric Developmental Dysplasia of the Hip in Infants up to Six Months of Age: Evidence-based Clinical Practice Guideline

American Academy of Orthopaedic Surgeons

OVERVIEW. This clinical practice guideline is based upon a systematic review of published articles related to the detection and early management of hip instability and dysplasia in typically developing children less than 6 months of age. This guideline provides practice recommendations for the early screening and detection of hip instability and dysplasia and also highlights gaps in the published literature that should stimulate additional research. This guideline is intended towards appropriately trained practitioners involved in the early examination and assessment of typically developing children for hip instability and dysplasia. (9/14)

FOOD ALLERGY

Guidelines for the Diagnosis and Management of Food Allergy in the United States: Report of the NIAID-Sponsored Expert Panel

National Institute of Allergy and Infectious Diseases

ABSTRACT. Food allergy is an important public health problem that affects children and adults and may be increasing in prevalence. Despite the risk of severe allergic reactions and even death, there is no current treatment for food allergy: the disease can only be managed by allergen avoidance or treatment of symptoms. The diagnosis and management of food allergy also may vary from one clinical practice setting to another. Finally, because patients frequently confuse nonallergic food reactions, such as food intolerance, with food allergies, there is an unfounded belief among the public that food allergy prevalence is higher than it truly is. In response to these concerns, the National Institute of Allergy and Infectious Diseases, working with 34 professional organizations, federal agencies, and patient advocacy groups, led the development of clinical guidelines for the diagnosis and management of food allergy. These Guidelines are intended for use by a wide variety of health care professionals, including family practice physicians, clinical specialists, and nurse practitioners. The Guidelines include a consensus definition for food allergy, discuss comorbid conditions often associated with food allergy, and focus on both IgE-mediated and non-IgE-mediated reactions to food. Topics addressed include the epidemiology, natural history, diagnosis, and management of food allergy, as well as the management of severe symptoms and anaphylaxis. These Guidelines provide 43 concise clinical recommendations and additional guidance on points of current controversy in patient management. They also identify gaps in the current scientific knowledge to be addressed through future research. (12/10)

HEMORRHAGE

An Evidence-based Prehospital Guideline for External Hemorrhage Control

American College of Surgeons Committee on Trauma

ABSTRACT. This report describes the development of an evidence-based guideline for external hemorrhage control in the prehospital setting. This project included a systematic review of the literature regarding the use of tourniquets and hemostatic agents for management of life-threatening extremity and junctional hemorrhage. Using the GRADE methodology to define the key clinical questions, an expert panel then reviewed the results of the literature review, established the quality of the evidence and made recommendations for EMS care. A clinical care guideline is proposed for adoption by EMS systems. (3/14)

HIV

Guidelines for the Prevention and Treatment of Opportunistic Infections in HIV-Exposed and HIV-Infected Children

US Department of Health and Human Services

SUMMARY. This report updates the last version of the Guidelines for the Prevention and Treatment of Opportunistic Infections (OIs) in HIV-Exposed and HIV-Infected Children, published in 2009. These guidelines are intended for use by clinicians and other health-care workers providing medical care for HIV-exposed and HIV-infected children in the United States. The guidelines discuss opportunistic pathogens that occur in the United States and ones that might be acquired during international travel, such as malaria. Topic areas covered for each OI include a brief description of the epidemiology, clinical presentation, and diagnosis of the OI in children; prevention of exposure; prevention of first episode of disease; discontinuation of primary prophylaxis after immune reconstitution; treatment of disease; monitoring for adverse effects during treatment, including immune reconstitution inflammatory syndrome (IRIS); management of treatment failure; prevention of disease recurrence; and discontinuation of secondary prophylaxis after immune reconstitution. A separate document providing recommendations for prevention and treatment of OIs among HIV-infected adults and post-pubertal adolescents (*Guidelines for the Prevention and Treatment of Opportunistic Infections in HIV-Infected Adults and Adolescents*) was prepared by a panel of adult HIV and infectious disease specialists (see http://aidsinfo.nih.gov/guidelines).

These guidelines were developed by a panel of specialists in pediatric HIV infection and infectious diseases (the Panel on Opportunistic Infections in HIV-Exposed and HIV-Infected Children) from the U.S. government and academic institutions. For each OI, one or more pediatric specialists with subject-matter expertise reviewed the literature for new information since the last guidelines were published and then proposed revised recommendations for review by the full Panel. After these reviews and discussions, the guidelines underwent further revision, with review and approval by the Panel, and final endorsement by the National Institutes of Health (NIH), Centers for Disease Control and Prevention (CDC), the HIV Medicine Association (HIVMA) of the Infectious Diseases Society of America (IDSA), the Pediatric Infectious Disease Society (PIDS), and the American Academy of Pediatrics (AAP). So that readers can ascertain how best to apply the recommendations in their practice environments, the recommendations are rated by a letter that indicates the strength of the recommendation, a Roman numeral that indicates the quality of the evidence supporting the recommendation, and where applicable, a * notation that signifies a hybrid of higher-quality adult study evidence and consistent but lower-quality pediatric study evidence.

More detailed methodologic considerations are listed in Appendix 1 (Important Guidelines Considerations), including a description of the make-up and organizational structure of the Panel, definition of financial disclosure and management of conflict of interest, funding sources for the guidelines, methods of collecting and synthesizing evidence and formulating recommendations, public commentary, and plans for updating the guidelines. The names and financial disclosures for each of the Panel members are listed in Appendices 2 and 3, respectively.

An important mode of childhood acquisition of OIs and HIV infection is from infected mothers. HIV-infected women may be more likely to have coinfections with opportunistic pathogens (e.g., hepatitis C) and more likely than women who are not HIV-infected to transmit these infections to their infants. In addition, HIV-infected women or HIV-infected family members coinfected with certain opportunistic pathogens may be more likely to transmit these infections horizontally to their children, resulting in increased likelihood of primary acquisition of such infections in young children. Furthermore, transplacental transfer of antibodies that protect infants against serious infections may be lower in HIV-infected women than in women who are HIV-uninfected. Therefore, infections with opportunistic pathogens may affect not just HIV-infected infants but also HIV-exposed, uninfected infants. These guidelines for treating OIs in children, therefore, consider treatment of infections in all children—HIV-infected and HIV-uninfected—born to HIV-infected women.

In addition, HIV infection increasingly is seen in adolescents with perinatal infection who are now surviving into their teens and in youth with behaviorally acquired HIV infection. Guidelines for postpubertal adolescents can be found in the adult OI guidelines, but drug pharmacokinetics (PK) and response to treatment may differ in younger prepubertal or pubertal adolescents. Therefore, these guidelines also apply to treatment of HIV-infected youth who have not yet completed pubertal development.

Major changes in the guidelines from the previous version in 2009 include:

- Greater emphasis on the importance of antiretroviral therapy (ART) for prevention and treatment of OIs, especially those OIs for which no specific therapy exists;
- Increased information about diagnosis and management of IRIS;
- Information about managing ART in children with OIs, including potential drug-drug interactions;
- Updated immunization recommendations for HIV-exposed and HIV-infected children, including pneumococcal, human papillomavirus, meningococcal, and rotavirus vaccines;
- Addition of sections on influenza, giardiasis, and isosporiasis;
- Elimination of sections on aspergillosis, bartonellosis, and HHV-6 and HHV-7 infections; and
- Updated recommendations on discontinuation of OI prophylaxis after immune reconstitution in children.

The most important recommendations are highlighted in boxed major recommendations preceding each section, and a table of dosing recommendations appears at the end of each section. The guidelines conclude with summary tables that display dosing recommendations for all of the conditions, drug toxicities and drug interactions, and 2 figures describing immunization recommendations for children aged 0 to 6 years and 7 to 18 years.

The terminology for describing use of antiretroviral (ARV) drugs for treatment of HIV infection has been standardized to ensure consistency within the sections of these guidelines and with the *Guidelines for the Use of Antiretroviral Agents in Pediatric HIV Infection.* Combination antiretroviral therapy (cART) indicates use of multiple (generally 3 or more) ARV drugs as part of an HIV treatment regimen that is designed to achieve virologic suppression; highly active antiretroviral therapy (HAART), synonymous with cART, is no longer used and has been replaced by cART; the term ART has been used when referring to use of ARV drugs for HIV treatment more generally, including (mostly historical) use of one- or two-agent ARV regimens that do not meet criteria for cART.

Because treatment of OIs is an evolving science, and availability of new agents or clinical data on existing agents may change therapeutic options and preferences, these recommendations will be periodically updated and will be available at http://AIDSinfo.nih.gov. (11/13, updated 11/18)

HYPOTENSION

The Management of Hypotension in the Very-Lowbirth-Weight Infant: Guideline for Practice

National Association of Neonatal Nurses

ABSTRACT. This guideline, released in 2011, focuses on the clinical management of systemic hypotension in the very-low-birth-weight (VLBW) infant during the first 3 days of postnatal life. (2011)

INFANTILE SPASMS

Evidence-based Guideline Update: Medical Treatment of Infantile Spasms

American Academy of Neurology and Child Neurology Society

ABSTRACT. ***Objective.*** To update the 2004 American Academy of Neurology/Child Neurology Society practice parameter on treatment of infantile spasms in children.

Methods. MEDLINE and EMBASE were searched from 2002 to 2011 and searches of reference lists of retrieved articles were performed. Sixty-eight articles were selected for detailed review; 26 were included in the analysis. Recommendations were based on a 4-tiered classification scheme combining pre-2002 evidence and more recent evidence.

Results. There is insufficient evidence to determine whether other forms of corticosteroids are as effective as adrenocorticotropic hormone (ACTH) for short-term treatment of infantile spasms. However, low-dose ACTH is probably as effective as high-dose ACTH. ACTH is more effective than vigabatrin (VGB) for short-term treatment of children with infantile spasms (excluding those with tuberous sclerosis complex). There is insufficient evidence to show that other agents and combination therapy are effective for short-term treatment of infantile spasms. Short lag time to treatment leads to better long-term developmental outcome. Successful short-term treatment of cryptogenic infantile spasms with ACTH or prednisolone leads to better long-term developmental outcome than treatment with VGB.

Recommendations. Low-dose ACTH should be considered for treatment of infantile spasms. ACTH or VGB may be useful for short-term treatment of infantile spasms, with ACTH considered preferentially over VGB. Hormonal therapy (ACTH or prednisolone) may be considered for use in preference to VGB in infants with cryptogenic infantile spasms, to possibly improve developmental outcome. A shorter lag time to treatment of infantile spasms with either hormonal therapy or VGB possibly improves long-term developmental outcomes. (6/12, reaffirmed 1/18)

INTRAVASCULAR CATHETER-RELATED INFECTIONS

Guidelines for the Prevention of Intravascular Catheter-Related Infections

Society of Critical Care Medicine, Infectious Diseases Society of America, Society for Healthcare Epidemiology of America, Surgical Infection Society, American College of Chest Physicians, American Thoracic Society, American Society of Critical Care Anesthesiologists, Association for Professionals in Infection Control and Epidemiology, Infusion Nurses Society, Oncology Nursing Society, Society of Cardiovascular and Interventional Radiology, American Academy of Pediatrics, and the Healthcare Infection Control Practices Advisory Committee of the Centers for Disease Control and Prevention

ABSTRACT. These guidelines have been developed for practitioners who insert catheters and for persons responsible for surveillance and control of infections in hospital, outpatient, and home health-care settings. This report was prepared by a working group comprising members from professional organizations representing the disciplines of critical care medicine, infectious diseases, health-care infection control, surgery, anesthesiology, interventional radiology, pulmonary medicine, pediatric medicine, and nursing. The working group was led by the Society of Critical Care Medicine (SCCM), in collaboration with the Infectious Disease Society of America (IDSA), Society for Healthcare Epidemiology of America (SHEA), Surgical Infection Society (SIS), American College of Chest Physicians (ACCP), American Thoracic Society (ATS), American Society of Critical Care Anesthesiologists (ASCCA), Association for Professionals in Infection Control and Epidemiology (APIC), Infusion Nurses Society (INS), Oncology Nursing Society (ONS), Society of Cardiovascular and Interventional Radiology (SCVIR), American Academy of Pediatrics (AAP), and the Healthcare Infection Control Practices Advisory Committee (HICPAC) of the Centers for Disease Control and Prevention (CDC) and is intended to replace the *Guideline for Prevention of Intravascular Device-Related Infections* published in 1996. These guidelines are intended to provide evidence-based recommendations for preventing catheter-related infections. Major areas of emphasis include (1) educating and training health-care providers who insert and maintain catheters; (2) using maximal sterile barrier precautions during central venous catheter insertion; (3) using a 2% chlorhexidine preparation for skin antisepsis; (4) avoiding routine replacement of central venous catheters as a strategy to prevent infection; and (5) using antiseptic/antibiotic impregnated short-term central venous catheters if the rate of infection is high despite adherence to other strategies (ie, education and training, maximal sterile barrier precautions, and 2% chlorhexidine for skin antisepsis). These guidelines also identify performance indicators that can be used locally by health-care institutions or organizations to monitor their success in implementing these evidence-based recommendations. (11/02)

MEDULLARY THYROID CARCINOMA

Revised American Thyroid Association Guidelines for the Management of Medullary Thyroid Carcinoma

American Thyroid Association Guidelines Task Force on Medullary Thyroid Carcinoma

ABSTRACT. ***Introduction.*** The American Thyroid Association appointed a Task Force of experts to revise the original Medullary Thyroid Carcinoma: Management Guidelines of the American Thyroid Association.

Methods. The Task Force identified relevant articles using a systematic PubMed search, supplemented with additional published materials, and then created evidence-based recommendations, which were set in categories using criteria adapted from the United States Preventive Services Task Force Agency for Healthcare Research and Quality. The original guidelines provided abundant source material and an excellent organizational structure that served as the basis for the current revised document.

Results. The revised guidelines are focused primarily on the diagnosis and treatment of patients with sporadic medullary thyroid carcinoma (MTC) and hereditary MTC.

Conclusions. The Task Force developed 67 evidence-based recommendations to assist clinicians in the care of patients with MTC. The Task Force considers the recommendations to represent current, rational, and optimal medical practice. (6/15)

MIGRAINE HEADACHE

Practice Guideline Update Summary: Acute Treatment of Migraine in Children and Adolescents. Report of the Guideline Development, Dissemination, and Implementation Subcommittee of the American Academy of Neurology and the American Headache Society

Maryam Oskoui, Tamara Pringsheim, Yolanda Holler-Managan, Sonja Potrebic, Lori Billinghurst, David Gloss, Andrew D. Hershey, Nicole Licking, Michael Sowell, M. Cristina Victorio, Elaine M. Gersz, Emily Leininger, Heather Zanitsch, Marcy Yonker, Kenneth Mack

ABSTRACT. ***Objective.*** To provide evidence-based recommendations for the acute symptomatic treatment of children and adolescents with migraine.

Methods. We performed a systematic review of the literature and rated risk of bias of included studies according to the American Academy of Neurology classification of evidence criteria. A multidisciplinary panel developed practice recommendations, integrating findings from the systematic review and following an Institute of Medicine–compliant process to ensure transparency and patient engagement. Recommendations were supported by structured rationales, integrating evidence from the systematic review, related evidence, principles of care, and inferences from evidence.

Results. There is evidence to support the efficacy of the use of ibuprofen, acetaminophen (in children and adolescents), and triptans (mainly in adolescents) for the relief of migraine pain, although confidence in the evidence varies between agents. There is high confidence in the evidence that adolescents receiving oral sumatriptan/naproxen and zolmitriptan nasal spray are more likely to be headache-free at 2 hours than those receiving placebo. No acute treatments were effective for migraine-related nausea or vomiting; some triptans were effective for migraine-related phonophobia and photophobia.

Recommendations. Recommendations for the treatment of acute migraine in children and adolescents focus on the importance of early treatment, choosing the route of administration best suited to the characteristics of the individual migraine attack, and providing counseling on lifestyle factors that can exacerbate migraine, including trigger avoidance and medication overuse. (8/19)

Practice Guideline Update Summary: Pharmacologic Treatment for Pediatric Migraine Prevention. Report of the Guideline Development, Dissemination, and Implementation Subcommittee of the American Academy of Neurology and the American Headache Society

Maryam Oskoui, Tamara Pringsheim, Lori Billinghurst, Sonja Potrebic, Elaine M. Gersz, David Gloss, Yolanda Holler-Managan, Emily Leininger, Nicole Licking, Kenneth Mack, Scott W. Powers, Michael Sowell, M. Cristina Victorio, Marcy Yonker, Heather Zanitsch, Andrew D. Hershey

ABSTRACT. ***Objective.*** To provide updated evidence-based recommendations for migraine prevention using pharmacologic treatment with or without cognitive behavioral therapy in the pediatric population.

Methods. The authors systematically reviewed literature from January 2003 to August 2017 and developed practice recommendations using the American Academy of Neurology 2011 process, as amended.

Results. Fifteen Class I–III studies on migraine prevention in children and adolescents met inclusion criteria. There is insufficient evidence to determine if children and adolescents receiving divalproex, onabotulinumtoxinA, amitriptyline, nimodipine, or flunarizine are more or less likely than those receiving placebo to have a reduction in headache frequency. Children with migraine receiving propranolol are possibly more likely than those receiving placebo to have an at least 50% reduction in headache frequency. Children and adolescents receiving topiramate and cinnarizine are probably more likely than those receiving placebo to have a decrease in headache frequency. Children with migraine receiving amitriptyline plus cognitive behavioral therapy are more likely than those receiving amitriptyline plus headache education to have a reduction in headache frequency.

Recommendations. The majority of randomized controlled trials studying the efficacy of preventive medications for pediatric migraine fail to demonstrate superiority to placebo. Recommendations for the prevention of migraine in children include counseling on lifestyle and behavioral factors that influence headache frequency and assessment and management of comorbid disorders associated with headache persistence. Clinicians should engage in shared decision-making with patients and caregivers regarding the use of preventive treatments for migraine, including discussion of the limitations in the evidence to support pharmacologic treatments. (8/19)

PALLIATIVE CARE

Clinical Practice Guidelines for Quality Palliative Care, 4th Edition
National Consensus Project for Quality Palliative Care (2018)

POSITIONAL PLAGIOCEPHALY

Systematic Review and Evidence-based Guidelines for the Management of Patients With Positional Plagiocephaly
Congress of Neurologic Surgeons

ABSTRACT. *Background.* Positional plagiocephaly is a common problem seen by pediatricians, pediatric neurologists, and pediatric neurosurgeons. Currently, there are no evidence-based guidelines on the management of positional plagiocephaly. The topics addressed in subsequent chapters of this guideline include: diagnosis, repositioning, physical therapy, and orthotic devices.

Objective. To evaluate topics relevant to the diagnosis and management of patients with positional plagiocephaly. The rigorous systematic process in which this guideline was created is presented in this chapter.

Methods. This guideline was prepared by the Plagiocephaly Guideline Task Force, a multidisciplinary team comprised of physician volunteers (clinical experts), medical librarians, and clinical guidelines specialists. The task force conducted a series of systematic literature searches of the National Library of Medicine and the Cochrane Library, according to standard protocols described below, for each topic addressed in subsequent chapters of this guideline.

Results. The systematic literature searches returned 396 abstracts relative to the 4 main topics addressed in this guideline. The results were analyzed and are described in detail in each subsequent chapter included in this guideline.

Conclusion. Evidence-based guidelines for the management of infants with positional plagiocephaly will help practitioners manage this common disorder. (11/16)

RHINOPLASTY

Improving Nasal Form and Function after Rhinoplasty
American Academy of Otolaryngology—Head and Neck Surgery Foundation

ABSTRACT. Rhinoplasty, a surgical procedure that alters the shape or appearance of the nose while preserving or enhancing the nasal airway, ranks among the most commonly performed cosmetic procedures in the United States, with >200,000 procedures reported in 2014. While it is difficult to calculate the exact economic burden incurred by rhinoplasty patients following surgery with or without complications, the average rhinoplasty procedure typically exceeds $4000. The costs incurred due to complications, infections, or revision surgery may include the cost of long-term antibiotics, hospitalization, or lost revenue from hours/days of missed work.

The resultant psychological impact of rhinoplasty can also be significant. Furthermore, the health care burden from psychological pressures of nasal deformities/aesthetic shortcomings, surgical infections, surgical pain, side effects from antibiotics, and nasal packing materials must also be considered for these patients. Prior to this guideline, limited literature existed on standard care considerations for pre- and postsurgical management and for standard surgical practice to ensure optimal outcomes for patients undergoing rhinoplasty. The impetus for this guideline is to utilize current evidence-based medicine practices and data to build unanimity regarding the peri- and postoperative strategies to maximize patient safety and to optimize surgical results for patients. (2/17)

SEIZURE

Treatment of the Child With a First Unprovoked Seizure
Quality Standards Subcommittee of the American Academy of Neurology and the Practice Committee of the Child Neurology Society

ABSTRACT. The Quality Standards Subcommittee of the American Academy of Neurology and the Practice Committee of the Child Neurology Society develop practice parameters as strategies for patient management based on analysis of evidence regarding risks and benefits. This parameter reviews published literature relevant to the decision to begin treatment after a child or adolescent experiences a first unprovoked seizure and presents evidence-based practice recommendations. Reasons why treatment may be considered are discussed. Evidence is reviewed concerning risk of recurrence as well as effect of treatment on prevention of recurrence and development of chronic epilepsy. Studies of side effects of anticonvulsants commonly used to treat seizures in children are also reviewed. Relevant articles are classified according to the Quality Standards Subcommittee classification scheme. Treatment after a first unprovoked seizure appears to decrease the risk of a second seizure, but there are few data from studies involving only children. There appears to be no benefit of treatment with regard to the prognosis for long-term seizure remission. Antiepileptic drugs (AED) carry risks of side effects that are particularly important in children. The decision as to whether or not to treat children and adolescents who have experienced a first unprovoked seizure must be based on a risk–benefit assessment that weighs the risk of having another seizure against the risk of chronic AED therapy. The decision should be individualized and take into account both medical issues and patient and family preference. (1/03, reaffirmed 7/06, 7/10, 7/13, 1/16, 10/18)

STATUS EPILEPTICUS

Diagnostic Assessment of the Child With Status Epilepticus (An Evidence-based Review)
Quality Standards Subcommittee of the American Academy of Neurology and the Practice Committee of the Child Neurology Society

ABSTRACT. ***Objective.*** To review evidence on the assessment of the child with status epilepticus (SE).

Methods. Relevant literature were reviewed, abstracted, and classified. When data were missing, a minimum diagnostic yield was calculated. Recommendations were based on a four-tiered scheme of evidence classification.

Results. Laboratory studies (Na^{++} or other electrolytes, Ca^{++}, glucose) were abnormal in approximately 6% and are generally ordered as routine practice. When blood or spinal fluid cultures were done on these children, blood cultures were abnormal in at least 2.5% and a CNS infection was found in at least 12.8%. When antiepileptic drug (AED) levels were ordered in known epileptic children already taking AEDs, the levels were low in 32%. A total of 3.6% of children had evidence of ingestion. When studies for inborn errors of metabolism were done, an abnormality was found in 4.2%. Epileptiform abnormalities occurred in 43% of EEGs of children with SE and helped determine the nature and location of precipitating electroconvulsive events (8% generalized, 16% focal, and 19% both). Abnormalities on neuroimaging studies that may explain the etiology of SE were found in at least 8% of children.

Recommendations. Although common clinical practice is that blood cultures and lumbar puncture are obtained if there is a clinical suspicion of a systemic or CNS infection, there are insufficient data to support or refute recommendations as to whether blood cultures or lumbar puncture should be done on a routine basis in children in whom there is no clinical suspicion of a systemic or CNS infection (Level U). AED levels should be considered when a child with treated epilepsy develops SE (Level B). Toxicology studies and metabolic studies for inborn errors of metabolism may be considered in children with SE when there are clinical indicators for concern or when the initial evaluation reveals no etiology (Level C). An EEG may be considered in a child with SE as it may be helpful in determining whether there are focal or generalized epileptiform abnormalities that may guide further testing for the etiology of SE, when there is a suspicion of pseudostatus epilepticus (nonepileptic SE), or nonconvulsive SE, and may guide treatment (Level C). Neuroimaging may be considered after the child with SE has been stabilized if there are clinical indications or if the etiology is unknown (Level C). There is insufficient evidence to support or refute routine neuroimaging in a child presenting with SE (Level U). (11/06, Reaffirmed 7/10, 7/13, 7/16, 1/19)

TELEHEALTH

Operating Procedures for Pediatric Telehealth

American Telemedicine Association

INTRODUCTION. Children represent one of our most vulnerable populations, and, as such, require special considerations when participating in telehealth encounters. Some services provided to adult patients by telehealth may not be easily adapted to or appropriate for pediatric patients due to physical factors (patient size), legal factors (consent, confidentiality), the ability to communicate and provide a history, developmental stage, unique pediatric conditions, and age-specific differences in both normal and disease states (AHRQ, n.d.; Alverson, 2008). These operating procedures for pediatric telehealth aim to improve the overall telehealth experience for pediatric patients, providers, and patient families. Telehealth holds particular promise in facilitating the management and coordination of care for medically complex children and those with chronic conditions, such as asthma, chronic lung disease, autism, diabetes, and behavioral health conditions.

Through the use of telehealth, providers can provide appointment flexibility, increase access, promote continuity of care, and improve quality, either as a part of or as a complement to care delivered through the patient-centered medical home (PCMH). Whether telehealth services are delivered through the PCMH or as a complement to it, telehealth providers **should** routinely communicate with a patient's primary care provider and any relevant specialists regarding a telehealth encounter. Telehealth providers **shall** have a standard mechanism in place to share secure documentation of the encounter with the PCMH (AAP, 2015) in a timely manner.

These operating procedures do reference general telehealth operating principles that apply beyond pediatrics and that warrant particular emphasis, but they are not meant to serve as a comprehensive stand-alone guide to the development and operation of a telemedicine service. ATA has developed and published core standards for telehealth operations that provide overarching guidance for clinical, technical and administrative standards (ATA, 2014a). The Pediatric Operating Procedures complement existing professional organization guidance from the American Academy of Pediatrics, the American Psychological Association, the American Association of Family Physicians and the Society of Adolescent Health and Medicine. (4/17)

THYROID NODULES AND DIFFERENTIATED THYROID CANCER

Management Guidelines for Children With Thyroid Nodules and Differentiated Thyroid Cancer

American Thyroid Association Guidelines Task Force on Pediatric Thyroid Cancer

ABSTRACT. ***Background.*** Previous guidelines for the management of thyroid nodules and cancers were geared toward adults. Compared with thyroid neoplasms in adults, however, those in the pediatric population exhibit differences in pathophysiology, clinical presentation, and long-term outcomes. Furthermore, therapy that may be recommended for an adult may not be appropriate for a child who is at low risk for death but at higher risk for long-term harm from overly aggressive treatment. For these reasons, unique guidelines for children and adolescents with thyroid tumors are needed.

Methods. A task force commissioned by the American Thyroid Association (ATA) developed a series of clinically relevant questions pertaining to the management of children with thyroid nodules and differentiated thyroid cancer (DTC). Using an extensive literature search, primarily focused on studies that included subjects ≤18 years of age, the task force identified and reviewed relevant articles through April 2014. Recommendations were made based upon scientific evidence and expert opinion and were graded using a modified schema from the United States Preventive Services Task Force.

Results. These inaugural guidelines provide recommendations for the evaluation and management of thyroid nodules in children and adolescents, including the role and interpretation of ultrasound, fine-needle aspiration cytology, and the management of benign nodules. Recommendations for the evaluation, treatment, and follow-up of children and adolescents with DTC are outlined and include preoperative staging, surgical management, postoperative staging, the role of radioactive iodine therapy, and goals for thyrotropin suppression. Management algorithms are proposed and separate recommendations for papillary and follicular thyroid cancers are provided.

Conclusions. In response to our charge as an independent task force appointed by the ATA, we developed recommendations based on scientific evidence and expert opinion for the management of thyroid nodules and DTC in children and adolescents. In our opinion, these represent the current optimal care for children and adolescents with these conditions. (7/15)

TOBACCO USE

Treating Tobacco Use and Dependence: 2008 Update

US Department of Health and Human Services

ABSTRACT. *Treating Tobacco Use and Dependence: 2008 Update,* a Public Health Service-sponsored Clinical Practice Guideline, is a product of the Tobacco Use and Dependence Guideline Panel ("the Panel"), consortium representatives, consultants, and staff.

These 37 individuals were charged with the responsibility of identifying effective, experimentally validated tobacco dependence treatments and practices. The updated Guideline was sponsored by a consortium of eight Federal Government and nonprofit organizations: the Agency for Healthcare Research and Quality (AHRQ); Centers for Disease Control and Prevention (CDC); National Cancer Institute (NCI); National Heart, Lung, and Blood Institute (NHLBI); National Institute on Drug Abuse (NIDA); American Legacy Foundation; Robert Wood Johnson Foundation (RWJF); and University of Wisconsin School of Medicine and Public Health's Center for Tobacco Research and Intervention (UW-CTRI). This Guideline is an updated version of the 2000 *Treating Tobacco Use and Dependence: Clinical Practice Guideline* that was sponsored by the U.S. Public Health Service, U. S. Department of Health and Human Services.

An impetus for this Guideline update was the expanding literature on tobacco dependence and its treatment. The original 1996 Guideline was based on some 3,000 articles on tobacco treatment published between 1975 and 1994. The 2000 Guideline entailed the collection and screening of an additional 3,000 articles published between 1995 and 1999. The 2008 Guideline update screened an additional 2,700 articles; thus, the present Guideline update reflects the distillation of a literature base of more than 8,700 research articles. Of course, this body of research was further reviewed to identify a much smaller group of articles that served as the basis for focused Guideline data analyses and review.

This Guideline contains strategies and recommendations designed to assist clinicians; tobacco dependence treatment specialists; and health care administrators, insurers, and purchasers in delivering and supporting effective treatments for tobacco use and dependence. The recommendations were made as a result of a systematic review and meta-analysis of 11 specific topics identified by the Panel (proactive quitlines; combining counseling and medication relative to either counseling or medication alone; varenicline; various medication combinations; long-term medications; cessation interventions for individuals with low socioeconomic status/limited formal education; cessation interventions for adolescent smokers; cessation interventions for pregnant smokers; cessation interventions for individuals with psychiatric disorders, including substance use disorders; providing cessation interventions as a health benefit; and systems interventions, including provider training and the combination of training and systems interventions). The strength of evidence that served as the basis for each recommendation is indicated clearly in the Guideline update. A draft of the Guideline update was peer reviewed prior to publication, and the input of 81 external reviewers was considered by the Panel prior to preparing the final document. In addition, the public had an opportunity to comment through a *Federal Register* review process. The key recommendations of the updated Guideline, *Treating Tobacco Use and Dependence: 2008 Update,* based on the literature review and expert Panel opinion, are as follows:

Ten Key Guideline Recommendations

The overarching goal of these recommendations is that clinicians strongly recommend the use of effective tobacco dependence counseling and medication treatments to their patients who use tobacco, and that health systems, insurers, and purchasers assist clinicians in making such effective treatments available.

1. Tobacco dependence is a chronic disease that often requires repeated intervention and multiple attempts to quit. Effective treatments exist, however, that can significantly increase rates of long-term abstinence.
2. It is essential that clinicians and health care delivery systems consistently identify and document tobacco use status and treat every tobacco user seen in a health care setting.
3. Tobacco dependence treatments are effective across a broad range of populations. Clinicians should encourage every patient willing to make a quit attempt to use the counseling treatments and medications recommended in this Guideline.
4. Brief tobacco dependence treatment is effective. Clinicians should offer every patient who uses tobacco at least the brief treatments shown to be effective in this Guideline.
5. Individual, group, and telephone counseling are effective, and their effectiveness increases with treatment intensity. Two components of counseling are especially effective, and clinicians should use these when counseling patients making a quit attempt:
   - Practical counseling (problem solving/skills training)
   - Social support delivered as part of treatment
6. Numerous effective medications are available for tobacco dependence, and clinicians should encourage their use by all patients attempting to quit smoking—except when medically contraindicated or with specific populations for which there is insufficient evidence of effectiveness (i.e., pregnant women, smokeless tobacco users, light smokers, and adolescents).
   - Seven first-line medications (5 nicotine and 2 non-nicotine) reliably increase long-term smoking abstinence rates:
     - Bupropion SR
     - Nicotine gum
     - Nicotine inhaler
     - Nicotine lozenge
     - Nicotine nasal spray
     - Nicotine patch
     - Varenicline
     - Clinicians also should consider the use of certain combinations of medications identified as effective in this Guideline.
7. Counseling and medication are effective when used by themselves for treating tobacco dependence. The combination of counseling and medication, however, is more effective than either alone. Thus, clinicians should encourage all individuals making a quit attempt to use both counseling and medication.
8. Telephone quitline counseling is effective with diverse populations and has broad reach. Therefore, both clinicians and health care delivery systems should ensure patient access to quitlines and promote quitline use.
9. If a tobacco user currently is unwilling to make a quit attempt, clinicians should use the motivational treatments shown in this Guideline to be effective in increasing future quit attempts.
10. Tobacco dependence treatments are both clinically effective and highly cost-effective relative to interventions for other clinical disorders. Providing coverage for these treatments increases quit rates. Insurers and purchasers should ensure that all insurance plans include the counseling and medication identified as effective in this Guideline as covered benefits.

The updated Guideline is divided into seven chapters that provide an overview, including methods (Chapter 1); information on the assessment of tobacco use (Chapter 2); clinical interventions, both for patients willing and unwilling to make a quit attempt at this time (Chapter 3); intensive interventions (Chapter 4); systems interventions for health care administrators, insurers, and purchasers (Chapter 5); the scientific evidence supporting the Guideline recommendations (Chapter 6); and information relevant to specific populations and other topics (Chapter 7).

A comparison of the findings of the updated Guideline with the 2000 Guideline reveals the considerable progress made in tobacco research over the brief period separating these two publications. Tobacco dependence increasingly is recognized as a chronic disease, one that typically requires ongoing assessment and repeated intervention. In addition, the updated Guideline offers the clinician many more effective treatment strategies than were identified in the original Guideline. There now are seven different first-line effective agents in the smoking cessation pharmacopoeia, allowing the clinician and patient many different medication options. In addition, recent evidence provides even stronger support for counseling (both when used alone and with other treatments) as an effective tobacco cessation strategy; counseling adds to the effectiveness of tobacco cessation medications, quitline counseling is an effective intervention with a broad reach, and counseling increases tobacco cessation among adolescent smokers.

Finally, there is increasing evidence that the success of any tobacco dependence treatment strategy cannot be divorced from the health care system in which it is embedded. The updated Guideline contains new evidence that health care policies significantly affect the likelihood that smokers will receive effective tobacco dependence treatment and successfully stop tobacco use. For instance, making tobacco dependence treatment a covered benefit of insurance plans increases the likelihood that a tobacco user will receive treatment and quit successfully. Data strongly indicate that effective tobacco interventions require coordinated interventions. Just as the clinician must intervene with his or her patient, so must the health care administrator, insurer, and purchaser foster and support tobacco intervention as an integral element of health care delivery. Health care administrators and insurers should ensure that clinicians have the training and support to deliver consistent, effective intervention to tobacco users.

One important conclusion of this Guideline update is that the most effective way to move clinicians to intervene is to provide them with information regarding multiple effective treatment options and to ensure that they have ample institutional support to use these options. Joint actions by clinicians, administrators, insurers, and purchasers can encourage a culture of health care in which failure to intervene with a tobacco user is inconsistent with standards of care. (5/08, last reviewed 9/19)

TURNER SYNDROME

Clinical Practice Guidelines for the Care of Girls and Women With Turner Syndrome: Proceedings From the 2016 Cincinnati International Turner Syndrome Meeting

Claus H. Gravholt; Niels H. Andersen; Gerard S. Conway; Olaf M. Dekkers; Mitchell E. Geffner; Karen O. Klein; Angela E. Lin; Nelly Mauras; Charmian A. Quigley; Karen Rubin; David E. Sandberg; Theo C. J. Sas; Michael Silberbach; Viveca Söderström-Anttila; Kirstine Stochholm; Janielle A. van Alfen-van derVelden; Joachim Woelfle; and Philippe F. Backeljauw (on behalf of the International Turner Syndrome Consensus Group)

ABSTRACT. Turner syndrome affects 25–50 per 100,000 females and can involve multiple organs through all stages of life, necessitating multidisciplinary approach to care. Previous guidelines have highlighted this, but numerous important advances have been noted recently. These advances cover all specialty fields involved in the care of girls and women with TS. This paper is based on an international effort that started with exploratory meetings in 2014 in both Europe and the USA, and culminated with a Consensus Meeting held in Cincinnati, Ohio, USA in July 2016. Prior to this meeting, five groups each addressed important areas in TS care: 1) diagnostic and genetic issues, 2) growth and development during childhood and adolescence, 3) congenital and acquired cardiovascular disease, 4) transition and adult care, and 5) other comorbidities and neurocognitive issues. These groups produced proposals for the present guidelines. Additionally, four pertinent questions were submitted for formal GRADE (Grading of Recommendations, Assessment, Development and Evaluation) evaluation with a separate systematic review of the literature. These four questions related to the efficacy and most optimal treatment of short stature, infertility, hypertension, and hormonal replacement therapy. The guidelines project was initiated by the European Society of Endocrinology and the Pediatric Endocrine Society, in collaboration with the European Society for Paediatric Endocrinology, the Endocrine Society, the European Society of Human Reproduction and Embryology, the American Heart Association, the Society for Endocrinology, and the European Society of Cardiology. The guideline has been formally endorsed by the European Society of Endocrinology, the Pediatric Endocrine Society, the European Society for Paediatric Endocrinology, the European Society of Human Reproduction and Embryology and the Endocrine Society. Advocacy groups appointed representatives who participated in pre-meeting discussions and in the consensus meeting. (9/17)

SECTION 3

2019 Policies

From the American Academy of Pediatrics

- *Policy Statements*
  ORGANIZATIONAL PRINCIPLES TO GUIDE AND DEFINE THE CHILD HEALTH CARE SYSTEM AND TO IMPROVE THE HEALTH OF ALL CHILDREN

- *Clinical Reports*
  GUIDANCE FOR THE CLINICIAN IN RENDERING PEDIATRIC CARE

- *Technical Reports*
  BACKGROUND INFORMATION TO SUPPORT AMERICAN ACADEMY OF PEDIATRICS POLICY

Includes policy statements, clinical reports, and technical reports published between January 1, 2019, and December 31, 2019

INTRODUCTION

This section of ***Pediatric Clinical Practice Guidelines & Policies: A Compendium of Evidence-based Research for Pediatric Practice*** is composed of policy statements, clinical reports, and technical reports issued by the American Academy of Pediatrics (AAP) and is designed as a quick reference tool for AAP members, AAP staff, and other interested parties. Section 3 includes the full text of all AAP policies published in 2019. Section 4 is a compilation of all active AAP policies (through December 31, 2019) arranged alphabetically, with abstracts where applicable. A subject index is also available. These materials should help answer questions that arise about the AAP position on child health care issues. **However, remember that AAP policy statements, clinical reports, and technical reports do not indicate an exclusive course of treatment or serve as a standard of medical care. Variations, taking into account individual circumstances, may be appropriate.**

Policy statements have been written by AAP committees, councils, task forces, or sections and approved by the AAP Board of Directors. Most of these statements have appeared previously in ***Pediatrics, AAP News,*** or ***News & Comments*** (the forerunner of ***AAP News***).

This section does not contain all AAP policies. It does not include
- Press releases.
- Motions and resolutions that were approved by the Board of Directors. These can be found in the Board of Directors' minutes.
- Policies in manuals, pamphlets, booklets, or other AAP publications. These items can be ordered through the AAP. To order, visit http://shop.aap.org/books or call 866/843-2271.
- Testimony before Congress or government agencies.

All policy statements, clinical reports, and technical reports from the American Academy of Pediatrics automatically expire 5 years after publication unless reaffirmed, revised, or retired at or before that time. Please check the American Academy of Pediatrics website at www.aap.org for up-to-date reaffirmations, revisions, and retirements.

2019 Recommendations for Preventive Pediatric Health Care

- *Policy Statement*

POLICY STATEMENT Organizational Principles to Guide and Define the Child Health Care System and/or Improve the Health of all Children

American Academy of Pediatrics

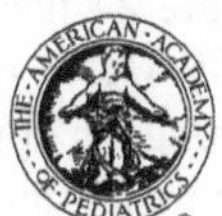

DEDICATED TO THE HEALTH OF ALL CHILDREN™

2019 Recommendations for Preventive Pediatric Health Care

COMMITTEE ON PRACTICE AND AMBULATORY MEDICINE, BRIGHT FUTURES PERIODICITY SCHEDULE WORKGROUP

The 2019 Recommendations for Preventive Pediatric Health Care (Periodicity Schedule) have been approved by the American Academy of Pediatrics (AAP) and represent a consensus of AAP and the Bright Futures Periodicity Schedule Workgroup. Each child and family is unique; therefore, these recommendations are designed for the care of children who are receiving competent parenting, have no manifestations of any important health problems, and are growing and developing in a satisfactory fashion. Developmental, psychosocial, and chronic disease issues for children and adolescents may require frequent counseling and treatment visits separate from preventive care visits. Additional visits also may become necessary if circumstances suggest variations from the normal.

The AAP continues to emphasize the great importance of continuity of care in comprehensive health supervision and the need to avoid fragmentation of care.[1]

The Periodicity Schedule will not be published in *Pediatrics*. Readers are referred to the AAP Web site (www.aap.org/periodicityschedule) for the most recent version of the Periodicity Schedule and the full set of footnotes. This process will ensure that health care professionals have the most current recommendations. The Periodicity Schedule will be reviewed and revised annually to reflect current recommendations.

Following are the changes made to the Periodicity Schedule since it was last published in April 2017.

BLOOD PRESSURE

Footnote 6 has been updated to read, "Screening should occur per 'Clinical Practice Guideline for Screening and Management of High Blood Pressure in Children and Adolescents' (http://pediatrics.aappublications.org/content/140/3/e20171904). Blood pressure measurement in infants and children with specific risk conditions should be performed at visits before age 3 years."

This document is copyrighted and is property of the American Academy of Pediatrics and its Board of Directors. All authors have filed conflict of interest statements with the American Academy of Pediatrics. Any conflicts have been resolved through a process approved by the Board of Directors. The American Academy of Pediatrics has neither solicited nor accepted any commercial involvement in the development of the content of this publication.

Policy statements from the American Academy of Pediatrics benefit from expertise and resources of liaisons and internal (AAP) and external reviewers. However, policy statements from the American Academy of Pediatrics may not reflect the views of the liaisons or the organizations or government agencies that they represent.

The guidance in this statement does not indicate an exclusive course of treatment or serve as a standard of medical care. Variations, taking into account individual circumstances, may be appropriate.

All policy statements from the American Academy of Pediatrics automatically expire 5 years after publication unless reaffirmed, revised, or retired at or before that time.

DOI: https://doi.org/10.1542/peds.2018-3971

PEDIATRICS (ISSN Numbers: Print, 0031-4005; Online, 1098-4275).

Copyright © 2019 by the American Academy of Pediatrics

FINANCIAL DISCLOSURE: The authors have indicated they have no financial relationships relevant to this article to disclose.

FUNDING: *No external funding.*

POTENTIAL CONFLICT OF INTEREST: *The authors have indicated they have no potential conflicts of interest to disclose.*

To cite: COMMITTEE ON PRACTICE AND AMBULATORY MEDICINE, AAP BRIGHT FUTURES PERIODICITY SCHEDULE WORKGROUP. 2019 Recommendations for Preventive Pediatric Health Care. *Pediatrics.* 2019;143(3):e20183971

ANEMIA

Footnote 24 has been updated to read, "Perform risk assessment or screening, as appropriate, per recommendations in the current edition of the AAP *Pediatric Nutrition: Policy of the American Academy of Pediatrics* (Iron chapter)."

LEAD

Footnote 25 has been updated to read, "For children at risk of lead exposure, see 'Prevention of Childhood Lead Toxicity' (http://pediatrics.aappublications.org/content/138/1/e20161493) and 'Low Level Lead Exposure Harms Children: A Renewed Call for Primary Prevention' (https://www.cdc.gov/nceh/lead/ACCLPP/Final_Document_030712.pdf)."

COMMITTEE ON PRACTICE AND AMBULATORY MEDICINE, 2018–2019

Julia E. Richerson, MD, FAAP, Chairperson
Joseph J. Abularrage, MD, MPH, MPhil, FAAP
Yvette M. Almendarez, MD, FAAP
Alexy D. Arauz Boudreau, MD, FAAP
Patricia E. Cantrell, MD, FAAP
Jesse M. Hackell, MD, FAAP
Amy P. Hardin, MD, FAAP
Scot B. Moore, MD, FAAP
Robin Warner, MD, FAAP

STAFF

Dana Bright, MSW

BRIGHT FUTURES PERIODICITY SCHEDULE WORKGROUP

Alexy D. Arauz Boudreau, MD, FAAP
Joseph F. Hagan Jr, MD, FAAP
Alex R. Kemper, MD, FAAP, Bright Futures Evidence Expert
Kelley E. Meade, MD, FAAP
Judith S. Shaw, EdD, MPH, RN, FAAP

STAFF

Jane B. Bassewitz, MA
Kathryn M. Janies

ABBREVIATION

AAP: American Academy of Pediatrics

REFERENCE

1. Hagan JF, Shaw JS, Duncan PM, eds. *Bright Futures: Guidelines for Health Supervision of Infants, Children, and Adolescents*. 4th ed. Elk Grove Village, IL: American Academy of Pediatrics; 2017

Achieving the Pediatric Mental Health Competencies

- *Technical Report*

TECHNICAL REPORT

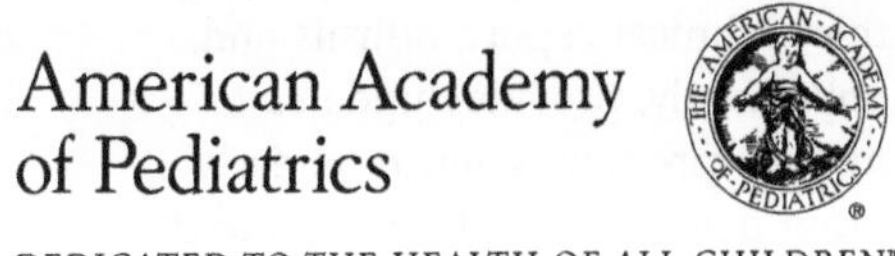

Achieving the Pediatric Mental Health Competencies

Cori M. Green, MD, MS, FAAP,[a] Jane Meschan Foy, MD, FAAP,[b] Marian F. Earls, MD, FAAP,[c] COMMITTEE ON PSYCHOSOCIAL ASPECTS OF CHILD AND FAMILY HEALTH, MENTAL HEALTH LEADERSHIP WORK GROUP

abstract

Mental health disorders affect 1 in 5 children; however, the majority of affected children do not receive appropriate services, leading to adverse adult outcomes. To meet the needs of children, pediatricians need to take on a larger role in addressing mental health problems. The accompanying policy statement, "Mental Health Competencies for Pediatric Practice," articulates mental health competencies pediatricians could achieve to improve the mental health care of children; yet, the majority of pediatricians do not feel prepared to do so. In this technical report, we summarize current initiatives and resources that exist for trainees and practicing pediatricians across the training continuum. We also identify gaps in mental health clinical experience and training and suggest areas in which education can be strengthened. With this report, we aim to stimulate efforts to address gaps by summarizing educational strategies that have been applied and could be applied to undergraduate medical education, residency and fellowship training, continuing medical education, maintenance of certification, and practice quality improvement activities to achieve the pediatric mental health competencies. In this report, we also articulate the research questions important to the future of pediatric mental health training and practice.

[a]Department of Pediatrics, Weill Cornell Medicine, Cornell University and New York–Presbyterian Hospital, New York, New York; [b]Department of Pediatrics, School of Medicine, Wake Forest University, Winston-Salem, North Carolina; and [c]Community Care of North Carolina, School of Medicine, University of North Carolina at Chapel Hill, Chapel Hill, North Carolina

All authors contributed to the drafting and revising of this manuscript and approved the final manuscript as submitted.

This document is copyrighted and is property of the American Academy of Pediatrics and its Board of Directors. All authors have filed conflict of interest statements with the American Academy of Pediatrics. Any conflicts have been resolved through a process approved by the Board of Directors. The American Academy of Pediatrics has neither solicited nor accepted any commercial involvement in the development of the content of this publication.

Technical reports from the American Academy of Pediatrics benefit from expertise and resources of liaisons and internal (AAP) and external reviewers. However, technical reports from the American Academy of Pediatrics may not reflect the views of the liaisons or the organizations or government agencies that they represent.

The guidance in this report does not indicate an exclusive course of treatment or serve as a standard of medical care. Variations, taking into account individual circumstances, may be appropriate.

All technical reports from the American Academy of Pediatrics automatically expire 5 years after publication unless reaffirmed, revised, or retired at or before that time.

DOI: https://doi.org/10.1542/peds.2019-2758

Address correspondence to Cori M. Green, MD, MS, FAAP. E-mail: cmg9004@med.cornell.edu

PEDIATRICS (ISSN Numbers: Print, 0031-4005; Online, 1098-4275).

Copyright © 2019 by the American Academy of Pediatrics

To cite: Green CM, Foy JM, Earls MF, AAP COMMITTEE ON PSYCHOSOCIAL ASPECTS OF CHILD AND FAMILY HEALTH, MENTAL HEALTH LEADERSHIP WORK GROUP. Achieving the Pediatric Mental Health Competencies. *Pediatrics.* 2019; 144(5):e20192758

INTRODUCTION

Mental health disorders have surpassed physical conditions as the most common reasons children have impairments and limitations.[1] Mental health disorders affect 1 in 5 children; however, a shortage of mental health specialists, stigma, cost, and other barriers prevent the majority of affected children from receiving appropriate services.[2–4] Pediatricians have unique opportunities and a growing sense of responsibility to promote healthy social-emotional development of children and to prevent and address their mental health and substance use problems. In 2009, the American Academy of Pediatrics (AAP) published a policy statement proposing mental health competencies for pediatric primary care and recommended steps toward achieving them.[5] The policy statement

"Mental Health Competencies for Pediatric Practice,"[6] accompanying this technical report, affirms and, importantly, provides updates to incorporate new science on early brain development, to articulate the pediatrician's role in addressing social determinants of health and trauma, and to consider mental health practice in subspecialty, as well as primary care, settings.

Currently, the majority of pediatricians do not feel prepared to achieve these mental health competencies.[7,8] Furthermore, more than half of pediatric program directors (PDs) surveyed in 2011 were unaware of the 2009 competencies, making it unlikely that training programs have enhanced their curriculum to prepare future pediatricians to achieve them.[9] With this technical report, we aim to stimulate efforts to address these gaps by summarizing educational strategies that have been applied and could be applied to undergraduate medical education, residency and fellowship training, continuing medical education (CME), maintenance of certification, and quality improvement activities to achieve the pediatric mental health competencies proposed in the accompanying policy statement. This report also articulates research questions important to the future of pediatric mental health training and practice.

HISTORY

Deficiencies in mental health training have been recognized for more than 4 decades, and in the 1980s, the AAP first called for improved education of pediatricians in the care of children with psychosocial and mental health problems.[10,11] Pediatric trainees and graduates since the 1980s report feeling less prepared to care for these children than they do children with other pediatric conditions.[12,13] Surveys over 3 decades have documented little change in their reported preparedness, despite the considerable efforts described below.[14–16]

In 1997, the Accreditation Council for Graduate Medical Education (ACGME) mandated that all pediatric residency programs include a 4-week developmental-behavioral pediatrics (DBP) rotation.[17] Completion of all 4 weeks of this rotation has had a positive effect on pediatricians' self-reported competence, practices, and willingness to accept responsibility for providing mental health care.[18,19] However, change in mental health practice has been modest, as measured by the AAP's periodic surveys of members, and mental health training is still not emphasized during residency and is considered to be suboptimal per PDs.[8,9,20,21] Advances in science have continued to demonstrate the interplay between the environment—particularly the child's social environment—and both physical and mental health; the pervasiveness of environmental influence makes it evident that mental health training needs to expand beyond a single rotation. Well-meaning efforts to address deficiencies in mental competencies by requiring DBP rotations and/or offering clinical rotations in psychiatry may have the unintended consequence of implying that mental health is primarily the domain of DBP subspecialists or child psychiatrists.[22] Ideally, mental health content and practice experiences would be integrated throughout the pediatric curriculum, during both inpatient and outpatient experiences, conveying the message that mental health competencies are integral to all aspects of pediatric practice.

AAP RESPONSES

In response to the needs of practicing pediatricians, the AAP Task Force on Mental Health (2004–2010) published a supplement to *Pediatrics*[23] describing the rationale for enhancing pediatric mental health care, offering community-level and practice-level strategies to support enhanced pediatric mental health care, and presenting algorithms for integrating mental health care into the flow of primary care pediatric practice. The task force also published *Addressing Mental Health Concerns in Primary Care: A Clinician's Toolkit*,[24] providing an array of pragmatic tools to assess a practice's capacity for providing mental health care, to build capacity when needed, and to operationalize the process laid out in the supplement. Also, within this toolkit, symptom "cluster" guidance offered a pragmatic clinical approach to addressing the common symptom constellations faced in pediatrics: anxiety, low mood, disruptive behavior and aggression, inattention and impulsivity, substance use, learning difficulty, and social-emotional symptoms in young children. This guidance has subsequently been incorporated into several publications of the AAP: *Signs and Symptoms in Pediatrics*,[25] *Textbook of Pediatric Care, Second Edition*,[26] *Pediatric Care Online*,[27] and *Mental Health Care of Children and Adolescents: A Guide for Primary Care Clinicians*.[28] The AAP has also published or endorsed clinical guidelines, reports, or statements guiding the assessment and management of attention-deficit/hyperactivity disorder (ADHD),[29] depression,[30,31] maladaptive aggression,[32,33] early social-emotional problems,[34] early childhood trauma and toxic stress,[35] and substance use.[36]

The AAP Mental Health Leadership Work Group (2011 to present), in collaboration with other AAP groups, has offered additional resources: a set of videos on using motivational interviewing (MI) to address mental health problems, e-mail notification about new publications relevant to pediatric mental health, Webinars, a curriculum and course for continuity clinic preceptors (see below), and a Web site with mental health resources.[37,38] Unfortunately, dissemination and evaluation of these approaches remain a challenge, and the mental health toolkit and other materials created to help pediatricians integrate mental health into their practice have not reached the majority of pediatricians.[39,40]

RESPONSES OF ACCREDITING BODIES

Improving training and competence in mental health care for future pediatricians—subspecialists as well as primary care pediatricians—has increasingly received national attention and is now a priority of the American Board of Pediatrics (ABP).[41,42] In 2013, the ACGME and ABP created the "Pediatric Milestones Project" to assess incremental achievement of pediatric competencies across the career span, from novice to expert.[43] Seventeen entrustable professional activities (EPAs)—professional units of work that define a specialty—were developed for general pediatrics.[44,45] A number of EPAs have implications for mental health care, and one—number 9—specifically states that the general pediatrician should be able to "assess and manage patients with common behavior/mental health problems."[45] This EPA lists the following functions expected of the pediatrician: (1) identify and manage common behavioral/mental health issues, (2) refer and/or comanage patients with appropriate specialist(s), (3) know mental health resources available in one's community, (4) know team member roles and/or monitor care, and (5) provide developmentally and culturally sensitive care. This EPA reinforces many of the mental health competencies from the 2009 AAP statement[5] and the accompanying policy statement "Mental Health Competencies for Pediatric Practice." Pediatric medical subspecialty practices are at times the de facto medical home for children with chronic conditions who are at a higher risk than their peers for mental health problems.[46,47] However, subspecialists often focus on their organ system, and studies have revealed that subspecialists are not routinely inquiring about psychosocial and mental health problems in children with chronic medical conditions or referring them for mental health care.[48,49] Promisingly, the majority of PDs agree that all trainees, regardless of future career plans, need to be competent in identifying, referring, and comanaging children with mental health problems. However, only half of PDs believe trainees going into a subspecialty should be responsible for mental health treatment.[42]

PURPOSE OF THIS REPORT

With this report, we identify gaps in mental health clinical experience and education across the training continuum and describe innovative strategies created and/or tested to improve pediatricians' ability to care for children with mental health problems. As reflected in the material below, efforts to date have been focused mainly on pediatric residency training programs and CME efforts.

PROMISING APPROACHES ACROSS THE EDUCATIONAL CONTINUUM

Undergraduate Medical Education

Currently, the Liaison Committee on Medical Education includes communication skills as 1 of the 9 mandated areas of content.[50] Although there are no specifications as to which skills should be taught and how, medical school curricula offer opportunities to enhance physician-patient communication and professionalism. The first step in addressing any mental health concern is to engage the family and build a therapeutic relationship by using communication skills such as MI and a "common-factors" approach, which builds on MI (see Discussion in accompanying policy statement[6]). These skills (eg, building hope, providing empathy, partnering with families, rolling with resistance, managing conflict) are necessary in all aspects of patient care and should be emphasized and taught throughout the continuum of medical education, starting with medical school.

It is essential that medical students choosing pediatrics be aware of and be prepared for their role in caring for pediatric mental health problems. The Council on Medical Student Education in Pediatrics does include pediatric behavior in its third-year competencies and objectives.[51] However, whether this is emphasized and whether preceptors model the provision of care to children with mental health problems during pediatric rotations is unknown. These questions should be addressed in further study.

Graduate Medical Education

As of 2013, 68% of practicing pediatricians reported receiving no training in MI during residency training, and more than half reported receiving no training in other interviewing techniques.[19] Until medical schools consistently provide this training, residency programs will need to provide it and ensure trainees' competence in these skills, and regardless of when it is introduced, preceptors will need to model and reinforce evidence-based communication skills.[21,42] Unfortunately, only 20% of PDs currently report that their residents receive optimal training in common-factors communication skills.[21]

It is promising that most residents believe they are responsible for identifying and referring children with mental health problems, yet few believe they are responsible for treating them.[52] In the unified theory of health behavior change, intention is what is most predictive of behavior,[53] yet for trainees and practicing pediatricians, perceived responsibility does not always lead to practicing in a way that is consistent with that perception.[18,54] This discrepancy between intent and practice is likely the result of a learning environment that does not provide the teaching and support needed to practice the requisite skills.[54,55] Trainees request experiential learning opportunities to care for children with mental health problems.[55] This request aligns with principles of andragogy (ie, to build self-efficacy, the clinical learning environment must provide opportunities to learn and practice skills guided by knowledgeable clinicians who can role model and demonstrate these skills).[56]

In response, educational interventions have included not only curriculum development but also a variety of instructional methods: role plays,[38] videos,[57,58] standardized patients (SPs),[59,60] and training alongside mental health professionals and trainees.[52,61,62] Successful interventions have used multimodal approaches, allowing trainees to gain knowledge and practice skills. Specifically, Fallucco et al[59] demonstrated that interns who received instruction using both didactics and SP trainings had increased knowledge and confidence in assessing for suicide compared with trainees who received only the lecture, those who received only the SP training, or controls who did not receive either of these experiences. Jee et al[60] had similar results combining case-based didactics with the use of SPs, leading to increased confidence among trainees in use of anxiety screening tools and later practices in performing a warm handoff (ie, an in-person, facilitated transfer of care from the trainee to another provider).

Additional examples highlight important caveats. One institution created a multimodal instructional approach using role plays, cases, and SPs on screening for substance use, brief intervention, and referral to treatment, which increased trainees' knowledge and confidence in the screening technique; however, these gains declined over time.[63] Another institution successfully implemented a multimodal curriculum for addressing substance use using screening, brief intervention, and referral to treatment while also creating an assessment tool to measure performance. Residents improved in patient-centered discussions and identifying motives and plans when practicing skills with SPs.[64] At another institution, the combination of computer modules and SPs to teach how to assess and diagnose depression improved trainees' interpersonal skills, diagnostic skills, and confidence in treatment of depression; however, gaps in history taking and assessment for comorbidities remained.[65] These findings reinforce the need for ongoing assessment of trainees' skills and, importantly, their practice of skills to supplement curricular efforts.

As an attempt to stimulate mental health training nationally, the AAP created a curriculum and training for pediatric continuity clinic preceptors and trainees in the common-factors approach.[38] This curriculum was created with various teaching modalities, including videos and role plays, with flexibility in implementation so that it can be adapted regardless of program characteristics. A faculty guide was included as an attempt to provide guidance for preceptors who may not have learned these concepts already. The curriculum has been disseminated by the AAP online and at national meetings as an attempt to train preceptors to deliver the modules. However, this curriculum has yet to be evaluated, and the majority of PDs are not familiar with the contents of the AAP curriculum.[40]

Trainees have stated that the most effective way they will learn to provide mental health care is for their own pediatric preceptors to model the mental health practices,[55] yet many pediatricians, including continuity preceptors, do not feel competent to serve as role models for mental health practice.[8,20,55] As an attempt to fill this gap, more than half of residency continuity clinics have an on-site developmental-behavioral pediatrician, social worker, child psychiatrist, psychologist, or other mental health specialist.[21,42] Although the role of these mental health specialists is not clear and likely varies between sites, PDs and residents trained in clinics with enhanced mental health services do report increased confidence and competence in systems-based practice and in coordinating and collaborating with mental health specialists.[9,52,61,62]

One study revealed that residents training on-site with mental health professionals were more likely to identify and refer patients with ADHD and reported that having the support of an on-site professional made them more comfortable to delve into their patients' problems.[52] However, as stated in the accompanying policy statement, pediatricians should be able to manage common mental health problems themselves, and having an on-site mental health provider has not been shown to increase trainees' practice of treating mental health problems. It is necessary to clarify the role of on-site mental health professionals as teachers rather than simply referral sources; their purpose is to increase the knowledge and skills of trainees and preceptors rather than offer them a way to avoid caring for mental health issues that are within pediatricians' scope of practice. Further study is needed to delineate how an on-site mental health professional can best impact practices because there are currently no financial structures to support them as preceptors without direct patient care responsibilities.

Study of successful integrated models has underscored the importance of preparing behavioral health providers to work within a primary care culture —for example, accommodating interruptions for consultation, participating in interdisciplinary meetings for peer-to-peer problem solving, and allowing unscheduled time for collaboration with other team members on unanticipated behavioral health issues.[66] Educational resources, including well-developed competencies, are available to guide mental health/ substance use professionals in serving as primary care team members, comanagers, or consultants.[67] Some psychiatry residency programs and a number of other mental health professional programs have started training licensed mental health trainees in integrated programs (ie, programs that combine mental health and primary care services in a single site).[68,69] One innovative program providing interdisciplinary training is the "buddy system," in which pediatric and mental health trainees were paired to teach skills in integration and collaboration; its premise is that interdisciplinary team meetings help clinicians from different backgrounds to develop and understand each other's work and services.[70] Impacts of this program are currently unknown, but it will likely lead to improved skills in collaboration between primary care pediatricians and mental health specialists. In 1 pediatric residency program, having pediatric and mental health trainees see patients in the same clinic has improved collaboration skills.[71]

The ACGME requires 6 months of individualized learning for pediatric residents; because subspecialty-bound residents are likely to focus on their future subspecialty during this time, this requirement may result in their receiving less training in caring for mental health problems.[72] Currently, the ACGME guidelines for subspecialty training in pediatrics do specify communication and interpersonal skills that are expected of all fellows, regardless of specialty, including working and collaborating as a team member, but there is no mention of providing fully integrated care that would include addressing psychosocial and mental health concerns.[73] Many pediatric subspecialty clinics incorporate a mental health professional as a team member, and there is likely some crossfertilization of the fellows and subspecialists who participate in these models; however, the mental health professional typically has a clinical rather than an educational role and is often stretched thin with inpatient duties.[49] Additional research is needed to address how best to prepare future specialists to integrate mental health care into their practice.

The need to improve pediatric graduates' training in mental health has been established, and the initiatives discussed above reveal promise. However, at this point, evaluation of educational interventions has mainly been limited to self-reported confidence, competence, and practices.[18,19,52] More assessment tools to measure competence are needed to evaluate the impact of educational innovations.[42] It will also be important to study actual practices and patient outcomes related to educational interventions.

Education of Experienced Clinicians

Educational efforts have successfully reached experienced pediatricians, building on skills they have developed over years of working with children and families. For instance, Wissow et al[74] have demonstrated that experienced primary care clinicians (PCCs) can acquire common-factors skills (described in the accompanying policy statement and above) and that the skills are helpful across a range of mental health conditions.[75,76] Children treated by PCCs trained in the common-factors techniques have shown modest but significant improvement in mental health functioning, and their parents have shown reduction in distress compared with children treated by clinicians who did not receive this training.[75,76]

Practicing pediatricians often feel that treating mental health problems is outside their scope of practice and often report that they do not have time to effectively implement psychosocial interventions.[8,18] Brief interventions that pediatricians can learn readily and implement in a short time period may offer a solution. See the accompanying policy statement for a full discussion.[6] Research will be necessary to develop and hone strategies for training residents and fellows in these approaches.

Several groups of mental health educators have successfully developed comprehensive training and CME programs to prepare mental health specialists and primary care professionals for their respective roles in collaborative practice.[77–79] The AAP is collecting information about such trainings on its Mental Health Initiatives Web site (https://www.aap.org/en-us/advocacy-and-policy/aap-health-initiatives/Mental-Health/Pages/Collaborative-Projects.aspx). The following are several examples:

The Resource for Advancing Children's Health Institute offers a 3-day mini-fellowship for primary care physicians using active learning methods to teach how to improve skills in recognition, diagnosis, and treatment of children with mental health disorders. This is followed by 6 months of biweekly case conferences. This program has changed physicians' practice patterns, as measured by an increase in the quality of referrals and a decrease in emergency department referrals, both of which can lead to decreased health care costs.[80] In New York, Project Training and Education for the Advancement of Children's Health uses the Resource for Advancing Children's Health mini-fellowship to train primary care physicians and offers a telepsychiatry consult line for support in diagnosis and management and to help find appropriate referrals. This program has trained more than 600 primary care physicians and consulted on over 8000 children and adolescents using telepsychiatry. Trained physicians felt more confident in addressing mental health problems with their patients and were motivated by the supportive and positive interactions with mental health specialists.[77,81]

In Massachusetts, a regional network of child psychiatrists offering real-time telephone consultation and referral to PCCs in Massachusetts enhanced the capacity of PCCs to care for children with diagnostic comorbidity, complicated ADHD, anxiety, and depression.[82–85] The Massachusetts Child Psychiatry Access Program has the resources to provide consultation and care coordination to 95% of the state's children, and in 2013, it had already served more than 10 500 children.[86] This program has been well received by pediatricians and now has expanded to offer support for mothers with depression.[87] At least 27 states have such consultation networks.[88] Congress authorized Pediatric Mental Health Care Access grants (§10002) that are modeled after the Massachusetts Child Psychiatry Access Program to support the development of new or improvement of existing pediatric mental health care telehealth access programs.[89]

Clinicians may also work toward enhancing mental health competence in maintenance of certification by using such quality improvement programs as Education in Quality Improvement for Pediatric Practice, AAP chapter-led quality improvement learning collaboratives, and development of relevant pay-for-performance and quality indicators for health plans. A growing number of educational resources developed by the AAP, the ABP, the American Academy of Family Physicians, the National Association of Pediatric Nurse Practitioners, the American Psychiatric Association, the National Association of Social Workers, the American Academy of Child and Adolescent Psychiatry, and the American Psychological Association are available on each organization's Web site.

Even when practicing pediatricians acquire the knowledge and skills needed to integrate mental health into primary care, time and other practice barriers (culture, processes) may impede intentions from becoming practices. Building Mental Wellness was a state initiative developed by the Ohio Chapter of the AAP as a way to engage practices and primary care physicians in integrating mental health.[90] This initiative successfully taught physicians skills in prevention, identification, and management of mental health problems using online educational sessions. Importantly, this program also addressed organizational climate, culture, and care processes. Study of uptake of this program revealed that practice organization and culture were associated with the uptake of interventions, suggesting that education alone will not transform pediatricians' practices, but focus on office processes, culture, and climate is needed as well.[91]

The American Medical Association has suggested 10 steps to improve office culture including first diagnosing team culture by using measurement tools and brainstorming improvements and creating processes to improve teamwork and communication to change a practice's culture.[92] As discussed in the policy statement, thinking of a mental health concern (eg, inattention and impulsivity) similarly to fever may help clarify processes: an initial visit to assess severity and offer symptomatic care (antipyretic for fever or brief common-elements intervention such as helping parents apply effective behavioral management techniques for inattention and impulsivity), follow-up visits and further assessment possibly using objective measures if symptoms persist (a complete blood cell count for fever or a rating scale such as the Vanderbilt to assess for ADHD), targeted treatment if a diagnosis is made (antibiotics for a pneumonia or stimulants and behavioral therapy for ADHD), and referral if first-line treatment fails and/or severity worsens (the emergency department for respiratory distress or mental health specialist for complicated ADHD).

The AAP mental health toolkit, as mentioned previously, offers tools to support mental health processes in practices. Other tools have been developed and studied, such as a brief intervention for anxiety using an anxiety action plan.[93] Study of this tool, which is comparable to an asthma action plan, has shown it to be feasibly implemented into primary care and helpful in reducing children's symptoms. Maternal depression screening was successfully implemented into practice in North Carolina by Community Care of North Carolina through a guided Maintenance of Certification Part 4 activity that reached over 100 PCCs (www.communitycarenc.org). Outreach by regional quality improvement coordinators in 14 regions across the state and "1-pagers" for practices resulted in high rates of implementation of perinatal depression screening (87% at all 1-month well visits, as of quarter 4, 2018). Technical assistance to practices included use of the screening tool, support resources for mothers, evidence-based dyadic therapies, referral, and follow-up. Similar progress has been seen with adolescent depression screening. Lastly, approaching mental health concerns through a stepwise approach as described through the AAP algorithm (see accompanying policy statement) can make it more feasible to implement in busy practices.

Expansion of the medical home team to include a mental health provider is financially feasible in some payment environments and clinically beneficial to patients and families.[94–97] In addition, it offers PCCs the benefit of crossdisciplinary learning through experiences such as collaborative care planning, clinical problem solving, and comanagement of patients with mental health morbidities and comorbidities.[98–100] These integrated models of care in which a licensed mental health specialist is on-site in a primary care practice have shown promise in improving access to mental health care for patients, improving patient functioning and productivity, and improving patient and provider satisfaction.[94,100–103] The majority of mental health care is provided during well-child visits and spans the continuum from promotion, to screening, to initiation of medications.[28] However, simply placing a mental health specialist on-site in pediatric practices may not necessarily enhance pediatricians' own mental health skills or practice; the roles of both the mental health specialist and pediatrician(s) must be well thought out and clear to avoid inappropriate referral to the on-site mental health specialist of patients ideally managed by the PCC.[104] In addition, there are barriers to sustaining integrated models of care in fee-for-service plans because productivity of the mental health professional is variable.[102,105] As mentioned in the accompanying policy statement, systems changes are needed for pediatricians to achieve the proposed mental health competencies.

For some subspecialties, guidelines have specified inclusion of a mental health professional as a team member. For example, the International Society for Pediatric and Adolescent Diabetes "Clinical Practice Consensus Guidelines 2014" for care of children and adolescents with type 1 diabetes mellitus state "Resources should be made available to include professionals with expertise in the mental health and behavioral health of children and adolescents within the interdisciplinary diabetes health care team. These mental health specialists should include psychologists, social workers, and psychiatrists."[106] A recent supplement to *Pediatric Blood and Cancer* outlined 15 evidence-based standards for the psychosocial care of children with hematologic and oncologic conditions and their families, including 1 on integrating a mental health team member.[107] Even when such standards exist, however, there is no assurance that an integrated model can be implemented or sustained in a given clinical setting.[108] Additional research is needed to assess whether these models of care better integrate mental health into the care of children with chronic physical conditions.

PROMISING DIRECTIONS

Achieving the proposed competencies will require new educational approaches and evaluation of their effectiveness, as well as significant enhancement in the interest and competence of pediatric faculty members who serve as teachers and role models. On the basis of experiences described above and the opinion of experts, the following strategies seem most promising and are offered here for the consideration of pediatric educators:

- prioritize training in common-factors communication skills for all pediatric faculty and for learners at all levels;
- incorporate the mental health competencies into curricular objectives, as described in the ABP EPA number 9, "assess and manage patients with common behavior/mental health problems,"[45] in accordance with the level of training;
- incorporate the promotion of healthy social-emotional development into the residency curriculum, including reinforcing strengths in the child and family and identifying risks to healthy social-emotional development and emerging symptoms to prevent or mitigate impairment from future mental health symptoms;
- prepare medical educators and preceptors to model, teach, and assess mental health competencies;
- consider including mental health specialists and/or developmental specialists as copreceptors and team members in teaching clinics (both general pediatric and subspecialty), inpatient rounds, and other clinical teaching settings, taking care to ensure that learners participate in mental health care, not just refer to specialists;
- consider incorporating trainees in psychology, social work, child psychiatry, DBP, and other specialties as team members in continuity and subspecialty clinics;
- consider addition of clinical experience(s) in child psychiatry to pediatric residency programs, either as a block rotation or, preferably, a longitudinal experience;
- monitor their learners' success in achieving the mental health

competencies and ensure ongoing opportunities to practice skills; and

- participate in and/or support research to answer such questions as:
- ○ What do medical students know about the role pediatricians play and will play in caring for children with mental health problems?
- ○ How much exposure is there during the pediatric clerkship to mental health promotion, primary and secondary prevention, and care of pediatric mental health problems?
- ○ What are the best educational strategies to change attitudes and encourage the pediatric community that mental health care is within their scope of practice?
- ○ What are the most effective ways to teach foundational communication skills to inexperienced as well as experienced clinicians?
- ○ How can common elements of evidence-based psychosocial treatments be most effectively adapted for pediatric practice? What impact do they have? How can they be incorporated into residency training and CME?
- ○ Which competencies are most relevant to subspecialty pediatric practice and therefore necessary to residency and/or fellowship training?
- ○ How can achievement of competence in providing mental health care be assessed within the context of residency and fellowship training?
- ○ How can practicing subspecialists be engaged in enhancing their mental health practice and improving coordination with PCCs and mental health specialists around the mental health needs of their patients?
- ○ Which collaborative models are most effective with respect to outcomes for children? Which are most effective for enhancing pediatricians' competence?
- ○ How can pediatricians not currently able or motivated to enhance their mental health competence or practice best be engaged?
- ○ Will better preparing pediatricians to care for mental health problems in their practice improve the mental health care of children and reduce the societal burden of untreated mental health problems?

CONCLUSIONS

Attainment of the mental health competencies proposed in the accompanying AAP policy statement will require innovative educational methods and research as described in this report. Significant enhancement in pediatric faculty competence, medical education, pediatric residency and fellowship training, and practicing pediatricians' own educational efforts will also be needed, along with effective assessment methods to document learners' progress toward achieving the competencies. These changes will continue to require investments by the AAP and its partner organizations, pediatric educators, and pediatricians working at both the community and practice levels.

AAP RESOURCES

Clinical Tools and/or Tool Kits

AAP clinical tools and/or tool kits include the following:

Addressing Mental Health Concerns in Primary Care: A Clinician's Toolkit;

Common Elements;

Hope, Empathy, Loyalty, Language, Permission, Partnership, Plan ("HELP") mnemonic;

Mental Health Algorithm; and

Mental Health Symptom Cluster Guidance.

Education, Training Materials, and/or Videos

AAP education, training materials, and/or videos include the following:

Mental Health Residency Curriculum; and

Implementing Mental Health Priorities in Practice video series.

PUBLICATIONS AND/OR BOOKS

AAP publications and/or books include the following:

Developmental Behavioral Pediatrics;

Mental Health Care of Children and Adolescents: A Guide for Primary Care Clinicians; and

Pediatric Psychopharmacology for Primary Care.

Reports

AAP reports include the report "Reducing Administrative and Financial Barriers."

Web Site

Web site resources include the AAP mental health Web site.

LEAD AUTHORS

Cori M. Green, MD, MS, FAAP

Jane Meschan Foy, MD, FAAP

Marian F. Earls, MD, FAAP

COMMITTEE ON PSYCHOSOCIAL ASPECTS OF CHILD AND FAMILY HEALTH, 2018–2019

Arthur Lavin, MD, FAAP, Chairperson

George LaMonte Askew, MD, FAAP

Rebecca Baum, MD, FAAP

Evelyn Berger-Jenkins, MD, FAAP

Thresia B. Gambon, MD, FAAP

Arwa Abdulhaq Nasir, MBBS, MSc, MPH, FAAP

Lawrence Sagin Wissow, MD, MPH, FAAP

FORMER COMMITTEE ON PSYCHOSOCIAL ASPECTS OF CHILD AND FAMILY HEALTH MEMBERS

Michael Yogman, MD, FAAP, Former Chairperson

Gerri Mattson, MD, FAAP

Jason Richard Rafferty, MD, MPH, EdM, FAAP

LIAISONS

Sharon Berry, PhD, ABPP, LP – *Society of Pediatric Psychology*

Edward R. Christophersen, PhD, FAAP – *Society of Pediatric Psychology*

Norah L. Johnson, PhD, RN, CPNP-BC – *National Association of Pediatric Nurse Practitioners*

Abigail Boden Schlesinger, MD – *American Academy of Child and Adolescent Psychiatry*

Rachel Shana Segal, MD – *Section on Pediatric Trainees*

Amy Starin, PhD – *National Association of Social Workers*

MENTAL HEALTH LEADERSHIP WORK GROUP, 2017–2018

Marian F. Earls, MD, FAAP, Chairperson

Cori M. Green, MD, MS, FAAP

Alain Joffe, MD, MPH, FAAP

STAFF

Linda Paul, MPH

ABBREVIATIONS

AAP: American Academy of Pediatrics
ABP: American Board of Pediatrics
ACGME: Accreditation Council for Graduate Medical Education
ADHD: attention-deficit/hyperactivity disorder
CME: continuing medical education
DBP: developmental-behavioral pediatrics
EPA: entrustable professional activity
MI: motivational interviewing
PCC: primary care clinician
PD: program director
SP: standardized patient

FINANCIAL DISCLOSURE: The authors have indicated they have no financial relationships relevant to this article to disclose.

FUNDING: No external funding.

POTENTIAL CONFLICT OF INTEREST: The authors have indicated they have no potential conflicts of interest to disclose.

REFERENCES

1. Halfon N, Houtrow A, Larson K, Newacheck PW. The changing landscape of disability in childhood. *Future Child.* 2012;22(1): 13–42
2. American Academy of Child and Adolescent Psychiatry, Committee on Health Care Access and Economics Task Force on Mental Health. Improving mental health services in primary care: reducing administrative and financial barriers to access and collaboration. *Pediatrics.* 2009;123(4): 1248–1251
3. Merikangas KR, He JP, Brody D, et al. Prevalence and treatment of mental disorders among US children in the 2001-2004 NHANES. *Pediatrics.* 2010; 125(1):75–81
4. Merikangas KR, He JP, Burstein M, et al. Service utilization for lifetime mental disorders in U.S. adolescents: results of the National Comorbidity Survey-Adolescent Supplement (NCS-A). *J Am Acad Child Adolesc Psychiatry.* 2011;50(1):32–45
5. Committee on Psychosocial Aspects of Child and Family Health; Task Force on Mental Health. Policy statement–the future of pediatrics: mental health competencies for pediatric primary care. *Pediatrics.* 2009;124(1):410–421
6. Foy JM, Green CM, Earls MF; Committee on Psychosocial Aspects of Child and Family Health; Mental Health Leadership Work Group. Mental health competencies for pediatric practice. *Pediatrics.* 2019;144(5):e20192757
7. Fox HB, McManus MA, Klein JD, et al. Adolescent medicine training in pediatric residency programs. *Pediatrics.* 2010;125(1):165–172
8. Horwitz SM, Storfer-Isser A, Kerker BD, et al. Barriers to the identification and management of psychosocial problems: changes from 2004 to 2013. *Acad Pediatr.* 2015;15(6):613–620
9. Green C, Hampton E, Ward MJ, Shao H, Bostwick S. The current and ideal state of mental health training: pediatric program director perspectives. *Acad Pediatr.* 2014;14(5): 526–532
10. Haggerty RJ. The changing role of the pediatrician in child health care. *Am J Dis Child.* 1974;127(4):545–549
11. Green M, Brazelton TB, Friedman DB, et al; American Academy of Pediatrics Committee on Psychosocial Aspects of Child and Family Health. Pediatrics and the psychosocial aspects of child and family health. *Pediatrics.* 1982;70(1): 126–127
12. Burns BJ, Scott JE, Burke JD Jr, Kessler LG. Mental health training of primary care residents: a review of recent literature (1974-1981). *Gen Hosp Psychiatry.* 1983;5(3):157–169
13. Dworkin PH, Shonkoff JP, Leviton A, Levine MD. Training in developmental pediatrics. How practitioners perceive the gap. *Am J Dis Child.* 1979;133(7): 709–712
14. Freed GL, Dunham KM, Switalski KE, Jones MD Jr, McGuinness GA; Research Advisory Committee of the American

Board of Pediatrics. Recently trained general pediatricians: perspectives on residency training and scope of practice. *Pediatrics*. 2009;123(suppl 1): S38–S43

15. Camp BW, Gitterman B, Headley R, Ball V. Pediatric residency as preparation for primary care practice. *Arch Pediatr Adolesc Med*. 1997;151(1):78–83
16. Rosenberg AA, Kamin C, Glicken AD, Jones MD Jr. Training gaps for pediatric residents planning a career in primary care: a qualitative and quantitative study. *J Grad Med Educ*. 2011;3(3): 309–314
17. Coury DL, Berger SP, Stancin T, Tanner JL. Curricular guidelines for residency training in developmental-behavioral pediatrics. *J Dev Behav Pediatr*. 1999; 20(suppl 2):S1–S38
18. Horwitz SM, Caspary G, Storfer-Isser A, et al. Is developmental and behavioral pediatrics training related to perceived responsibility for treating mental health problems? *Acad Pediatr*. 2010; 10(4):252–259
19. Stein RE, Storfer-Isser A, Kerker BD, et al. Does length of developmental behavioral pediatrics training matter? *Acad Pediatr*. 2017;17(1):61–67
20. Stein RE, Storfer-Isser A, Kerker BD, et al. Beyond ADHD: how well are we doing? *Acad Pediatr*. 2016;16(2):115–121
21. Shahidullah JD, Kettlewell PW, Palejwala MH, et al. Behavioral health training in pediatric residency programs: a national survey of training directors. *J Dev Behav Pediatr*. 2018;39(4):292–302
22. Stein RE. Are we on the right track? Examining the role of developmental behavioral pediatrics. *Pediatrics*. 2015; 135(4):589–591
23. Foy JM; American Academy of Pediatrics Task Force on Mental Health. Enhancing pediatric mental health care: algorithms for primary care. *Pediatrics*. 2010;125(suppl 3):S109–S125
24. American Academy of Pediatrics. *Addressing Mental Health Concerns in Primary Care: A Clinician's Toolkit*. Elk Grove Village, IL: American Academy of Pediatrics; 2010
25. Adam H, Foy J. *Signs and Symptoms in Pediatrics*. Elk Grove Village, IL: American Academy of Pediatrics; 2015
26. McInerny TK, Adam HM, Campbell DE, eds, et al. *Textbook of Pediatric Care*, 2nd ed. Elk Grove Village, IL: American Academy of Pediatrics; 2016
27. American Academy of Pediatrics. Pediatric care online. Available at: https://pediatriccare.solutions.aap.org/Pediatric-Care.aspx. Accessed November 3, 2018
28. Foy JM. *Mental Health Care of Children and Adolescents: A Guide for Primary Care Clinicians*. Itasca, IL: American Academy of Pediatrics; 2018
29. Wolraich ML, Hagan JF Jr., Allan C, et al; Subcommittee on Children and Adolescents With Attention-Deficit/Hyperactive Disorder. Clinical practice guideline for the diagnosis, evaluation, and treatment of attention-deficit/hyperactivity disorder in children and adolescents. *Pediatrics*. 2019;144(4): e20192528
30. Zuckerbrot RA, Cheung A, Jensen PS, Stein REK, Laraque D; GLAD-PC Steering Group. Guidelines for Adolescent Depression in Primary Care (GLAD-PC): part I. Practice preparation, identification, assessment, and initial management. *Pediatrics*. 2018;141(3): e20174081
31. Cheung AH, Zuckerbrot RA, Jensen PS, Laraque D, Stein REK; GLAD-PC Steering Group. Guidelines for Adolescent Depression in Primary Care (GLAD-PC): part II. Treatment and ongoing management. *Pediatrics*. 2018;141(3): e20174082
32. Knapp P, Chait A, Pappadopulos E, Crystal S, Jensen PS; T-MAY Steering Group. Treatment of maladaptive aggression in youth: CERT guidelines I. Engagement, assessment, and management. *Pediatrics*. 2012;129(6). Available at: www.pediatrics.org/cgi/content/full/129/6/e1562
33. Scotto Rosato N, Correll CU, Pappadopulos E, et al; Treatment of Maladaptive Aggressive in Youth Steering Committee. Treatment of maladaptive aggression in youth: CERT guidelines II. Treatments and ongoing management. *Pediatrics*. 2012;129(6). Available at: www.pediatrics.org/cgi/content/full/129/6/e1577
34. Gleason MM, Goldson E, Yogman MW; Council on Early Childhood; Committee on Psychosocial Aspects of Child and Family Health; Section on Developmental and Behavioral Pediatrics. Addressing early childhood emotional and behavioral problems. *Pediatrics*. 2016;138(6):e20163025
35. Garner AS, Shonkoff JP; Committee on Psychosocial Aspects of Child and Family Health; Committee on Early Childhood, Adoption, and Dependent Care; Section on Developmental and Behavioral Pediatrics. Early childhood adversity, toxic stress, and the role of the pediatrician: translating developmental science into lifelong health. *Pediatrics*. 2012;129(1). Available at: www.pediatrics.org/cgi/content/full/129/1/e224
36. Levy SJ, Williams JF; Committee on Substance Use and Prevention. Substance use screening, brief intervention, and referral to treatment. *Pediatrics*. 2016;138(1):e20161211
37. American Academy of Pediatrics. Mental health initiatives: implementing mental health priorities in practice. Available at: https://www.aap.org/en-us/advocacy-and-policy/aap-health-initiatives/Mental-Health/Pages/implementing_mental_health_priorities_in_practice.aspx. Accessed May 17, 2019
38. American Academy of Pediatrics. Mental health initiatives: residency curriculum. Available at: https://www.aap.org/en-us/advocacy-and-policy/aap-health-initiatives/Mental-Health/Pages/Residency-Curriculum.aspx. Accessed May 17, 2019
39. Garner AS, Storfer-Isser A, Szilagyi M, et al. Promoting early brain and child development: perceived barriers and the utilization of resources to address them. *Acad Pediatr*. 2017;17(7):697–705
40. Green C. Mental health initiatives. In: Association of Pediatric Program Directors 2017 Annual Spring Meeting Pre-Meeting Workshop: The Behavioral/Mental Health Crisis: Preparing Future Pediatricians to Meet the Challenge: April 5, 2017; Anaheim, CA. Available at: https://www.appd.org/home/pdf/ABP_APPD_Training_Behavioral_Mental_Health.pdf. Accessed September 27, 2019
41. McMillan JA, Land M Jr, Leslie LK. Pediatric residency education and the behavioral and mental health crisis:

a call to action. *Pediatrics*. 2017;139(1): e20162141

42. McMillan JA, Land ML Jr, Rodday AM, et al. Report of a joint association of pediatric program directors-American Board of Pediatrics workshop: preparing future pediatricians for the mental health crisis. *J Pediatr*. 2018; 201:285–291
43. Hicks PJ, Englander R, Schumacher DJ, et al. Pediatrics milestone project: next steps toward meaningful outcomes assessment. *J Grad Med Educ*. 2010; 2(4):577–584
44. Ten Cate O, Chen HC, Hoff RG, et al. Curriculum development for the workplace using Entrustable Professional Activities (EPAs): AMEE guide No. 99. *Med Teach*. 2015;37(11): 983–1002
45. American Board of Pediatrics. Entrustable professional activities for general pediatrics. 2016. Available at: https://www.abp.org/entrustable-professional-activities-epas. Accessed May 23, 2019
46. Boat TF, Land ML Jr, Leslie LK. Health care workforce development to enhance mental and behavioral health of children and youths. *JAMA Pediatr*. 2017;171(11):1031–1032
47. Perrin JM, Gnanasekaran S, Delahaye J. Psychological aspects of chronic health conditions. *Pediatr Rev*. 2012;33(3): 99–109
48. Green C, Stein REK, Storfer-Isser A, et al. Do subspecialists ask about and refer families with psychosocial concerns? A comparison with general pediatricians. *Matern Child Health J*. 2019;23(1):61–71
49. Samsel C, Ribeiro M, Ibeziako P, DeMaso DR. Integrated behavioral health care in pediatric subspecialty clinics. *Child Adolesc Psychiatr Clin N Am*. 2017;26(4): 785–794
50. Liaison Committee on Education. *Functions and Structure of a Medical School: Standards for Accreditation of Medical Education Programs Leading to the MD Degree*. Washington, DC: Association of American Medical Colleges and American Medical Association; 2018
51. Council on Medical Student Education in Pediatrics. Curricular competencies and objectives. 2017. Available at: https://www.comsep.org/curriculum-competencies-and-objectives/ Accessed September 27, 2019
52. Ragunanthan B, Frosch EJ, Solomon BS. On-site mental health professionals and pediatric residents in continuity clinic. *Clin Pediatr (Phila)*. 2017;56(13): 1219–1226
53. Guilamo-Ramos V, Jaccard J, Dittus P, Collins S. Parent-adolescent communication about sexual intercourse: an analysis of maternal reluctance to communicate. *Health Psychol*. 2008;27(6):760–769
54. Green C. How can we use education to improve the mental health of today's children? In: Association of Pediatric Program Directors 2017 Annual Spring Meeting Pre-Meeting Workshop: The Behavioral/Mental Health Crisis: Preparing Future Pediatricians to Meet the Challenge: April 5, 2017; Anaheim, CA. Available at: https://www.appd.org/home/pdf/ABP_APPD_Training_Behavioral_Mental_Health.pdf. Accessed September 27, 2019
55. Hampton E, Richardson JE, Bostwick S, Ward MJ, Green C. The current and ideal state of mental health training: pediatric resident perspectives. *Teach Learn Med*. 2015;27(2):147–154
56. Kaufman DM. Applying educational theory in practice. *BMJ*. 2003;326(7382): 213–216
57. Bauer NS, Sullivan PD, Hus AM, Downs SM. Promoting mental health competency in residency training. *Patient Educ Couns*. 2011;85(3): e260–e264
58. Kutner L, Olson CK, Schlozman S, et al. Training pediatric residents and pediatricians about adolescent mental health problems: a proof-of-concept pilot for a proposed national curriculum. *Acad Psychiatry*. 2008;32(5): 429–437
59. Fallucco EM, Hanson MD, Glowinski AL. Teaching pediatric residents to assess adolescent suicide risk with a standardized patient module. *Pediatrics*. 2010;125(5):953–959
60. Jee SH, Baldwin C, Dadiz R, Jones M, Alpert-Gillis L. Integrated mental health training for pediatric and psychology trainees using standardized patient encounters. *Acad Pediatr*. 2018;18(1): 119–121
61. Garfunkel LC, Pisani AR, leRoux P, Siegel DM. Educating residents in behavioral health care and collaboration: comparison of conventional and integrated training models. *Acad Med*. 2011;86(2):174–179
62. Bunik M, Talmi A, Stafford B, et al. Integrating mental health services in primary care continuity clinics: a national CORNET study. *Acad Pediatr*. 2013;13(6):551–557
63. Schram P, Harris SK, Van Hook S, et al. Implementing adolescent Screening, Brief Intervention, and Referral to Treatment (SBIRT) education in a pediatric residency curriculum. *Subst Abus*. 2015;36(3):332–338
64. Ryan S, Pantalon MV, Camenga D, Martel S, D'Onofrio G. Evaluation of a pediatric resident skills-based screening, brief intervention and referral to treatment (SBIRT) curriculum for substance use. *J Adolesc Health*. 2018;63(3):327–334
65. Lewy C, Sells CW, Gilhooly J, McKelvey R. Adolescent depression: evaluating pediatric residents' knowledge, confidence, and interpersonal skills using standardized patients. *Acad Psychiatry*. 2009;33(5):389–393
66. Cohen DJ, Davis MM, Hall JD, Gilchrist EC, Miller BF. *A Guidebook of Professional Practices for Behavioral Health and Primary Care Integration: Observations From Exemplary Sites*. Rockville, MD: Agency for Healthcare Research and Quality; 2015
67. Miller BF, Gilchrist EC, Ross KM, Wong SL, Blount A, Peek CJ. Core competencies for behavioral health providers working in primary care. 2016. Available at: http://farleyhealthpolicycenter.org/wp-content/uploads/2016/02/Core-Competencies-for-Behavioral-Health-Providers-Working-in-Primary-Care.pdf. Accessed May 17, 2019
68. Burkey MD, Kaye DL, Frosch E. Training in integrated mental health-primary care models: a national survey of child psychiatry program directors. *Acad Psychiatry*. 2014;38(4):485–488
69. Zomorodi M, de Saxe Zerden L, Alexander L, Nance-Floyd B; Healthcare

PROMISE team. Engaging students in the development of an interprofessional population health management course. *Nurse Educ.* 2017; 42(1):5–7

70. Moran M. Innovative 'buddy system' teaches collaboration. *Psychiatr News.* 2014;49(9). Available at: https://psychnews.psychiatryonline.org/doi/10.1176/appi.pn.2014.5a15/. Accessed May 17, 2019

71. Pisani AR, leRoux P, Siegel DM. Educating residents in behavioral health care and collaboration: integrated clinical training of pediatric residents and psychology fellows. *Acad Med.* 2011;86(2):166–173

72. Accreditation Council on Graduate Medical Education. ACGME core competencies. Available at: https://www.ecfmg.org/echo/acgme-core-competencies.html. Accessed March 9, 2018

73. Accreditation Council on Graduate Medical Education. ACGME program requirements for graduate medical education in the subspecialties of pediatrics. 2016. Available at: https://www.acgme.org/Portals/0/PFAssets/ProgramRequirements/CPRFellowship2019.pdf Accessed September 27, 2019

74. Wissow LS, Gadomski A, Roter D, et al. Improving child and parent mental health in primary care: a cluster-randomized trial of communication skills training. *Pediatrics.* 2008;121(2): 266–275

75. Wissow LS, Brown JD, Krupnick J. Therapeutic alliance in pediatric primary care: preliminary evidence for a relationship with physician communication style and mothers' satisfaction. *J Dev Behav Pediatr.* 2010; 31(2):83–91

76. Wissow L, Anthony B, Brown J, et al. A common factors approach to improving the mental health capacity of pediatric primary care. *Adm Policy Ment Health.* 2008;35(4):305–318

77. Gadomski AM, Wissow LS, Palinkas L, et al. Encouraging and sustaining integration of child mental health into primary care: interviews with primary care providers participating in Project TEACH (CAPES and CAP PC) in NY. *Gen Hosp Psychiatry.* 2014;36(6):555–562

78. Integrated Primary Care. The portal to information and tools for the integration of behavioral health and primary care. Available at: https://sites.google.com/view/integratedprimarycare2/training. Accessed September 27, 2019

79. The Resource for Advancing Children's Health Institute. Child and adolescent training institute in evidence-based psychotherapies (CATIE). Available at: www.thereachinstitute.org/services/for-healthcare-organizations/staff-training/child-adolescent-training-in-evidence-based-psychotherapies-catie-1. Accessed March 26, 2019

80. McCaffrey ESN, Chang S, Farrelly G, Rahman A, Cawthorpe D. Mental health literacy in primary care: Canadian Research and Education for the Advancement of Child Health (CanREACH). *Evid Based Med.* 2017; 22(4):123–131

81. Kaye DL, Fornari V, Scharf M, et al. Description of a multi-university education and collaborative care child psychiatry access program: New York State's CAP PC. *Gen Hosp Psychiatry.* 2017;48:32–36

82. Dvir Y, Wenz-Gross M, Jeffers-Terry M, Metz WP. An assessment of satisfaction with ambulatory child psychiatry consultation services to primary care providers by parents of children with emotional and behavioral needs: the Massachusetts Child Psychiatry Access Project University of Massachusetts parent satisfaction study. *Front Psychiatry.* 2012;3:7

83. Massachusetts Child Psychiatry Access Project. Available at: www.mcpap.org. Accessed March 26, 2019

84. Sarvet B, Gold J, Bostic JQ, et al. Improving access to mental health care for children: the Massachusetts Child Psychiatry Access Project. *Pediatrics.* 2010;126(6):1191–1200

85. Van Cleave J, Le TT, Perrin JM. Point-of-care child psychiatry expertise: the Massachusetts Child Psychiatry Access Project. *Pediatrics.* 2015;135(5):834–841

86. Straus JH, Sarvet B. Behavioral health care for children: the Massachusetts Child Psychiatry Access Project. *Health Aff (Millwood).* 2014;33(12):2153–2161

87. Byatt N, Biebel K, Moore Simas TA, et al. Improving perinatal depression care: the Massachusetts Child Psychiatry Access Project for Moms. *Gen Hosp Psychiatry.* 2016;40:12–17

88. National Network of Child Psychiatry Access Programs. Available at: http://web.jhu.edu/pedmentalhealth/nncpap_members.html. Accessed September 27, 2019

89. Health Resources and Services Administration. Pediatric Mental Health Care Access Program. Available at: https://www.hrsa.gov/grants/fundingopportunities/default.aspx?id=f1fe7b69-4d80-4a92-a3e8-aecee0fbbdee. Accessed March 26, 2019

90. American Academy of Pediatrics Ohio Chapter. Building mental wellness. Available at: http://ohioaap.org/projects/building-mental-wellness/. Accessed March 26, 2019

91. King MA, Wissow LS, Baum RA. The role of organizational context in the implementation of a statewide initiative to integrate mental health services into pediatric primary care. *Health Care Manage Rev.* 2018;43(3):206–217

92. Association Medical Association. Team culture: strengthen team cohesion and engagement. 2015. Available at: https://edhub.ama-assn.org/steps-forward/module/2702515. Accessed March 26, 2019

93. Ginsburg GS, Drake K, Winegrad H, Fothergill K, Wissow L. An open trial of the Anxiety Action Plan (*AxAP*): a brief pediatrician-delivered intervention for anxious youth. *Child Youth Care Forum.* 2016;45(1):19–32

94. Asarnow JR, Rozenman M, Wiblin J, Zeltzer L. Integrated medical-behavioral care compared with usual primary care for child and adolescent behavioral health: a meta-analysis. *JAMA Pediatr.* 2015;169(10):929–937

95. Richardson LP, McCarty CA, Radovic A, Suleiman AB. Research in the integration of behavioral health for adolescents and young adults in primary care settings: a systematic review. *J Adolesc Health.* 2017;60(3): 261–269

96. Kaplan-Sanoff M, Talmi A, Augustyn M. Infusing mental health services into primary care for very young children

and their families. *Zero Three.* 2012; 33(2):73–77

97. Talmi A, Fazio E. Commentary: promoting health and well-being in pediatric primary care settings: using health and behavior codes at routine well-child visits. *J Pediatr Psychol.* 2012; 37(5):496–502

98. Greene CA, Ford JD, Ward-Zimmerman B, Honigfeld L, Pidano AE. Strengthening the coordination of pediatric mental health and medical care: piloting a collaborative model for freestanding practices. *Child Youth Care Forum.* 2016;45(5):729–744

99. Pidano AE, Marcaly KH, Ihde KM, Kurowski EC, Whitcomb JM. Connecticut's enhanced care clinic initiative: early returns from pediatric-behavioral health partnerships. *Fam Syst Health.* 2011;29(2):138–143

100. Talmi A, Muther EF, Margolis K, et al. The scope of behavioral health integration in a pediatric primary care setting. *J Pediatr Psychol.* 2016;41(10): 1120–1132

101. Blount A, ed. *Integrated Primary Care: The Future of Medical and Mental Health Collaboration.* New York, NY: W. W. Norton and Company, Inc; 1998

102. Kolko DJ, Perrin E. The integration of behavioral health interventions in children's health care: services, science, and suggestions. *J Clin Child Adolesc Psychol.* 2014;43(2):216–228

103. Williams J, Shore SE, Foy JM. Co-location of mental health professionals in primary care settings: three North Carolina models. *Clin Pediatr (Phila).* 2006;45(6):537–543

104. Horwitz S, Storfer-Isser A, Kerker BD, et al. Do on-site mental health professionals change pediatricians' responses to children's mental health problems? *Acad Pediatr.* 2016;16(7):676–683

105. Ader J, Stille CJ, Keller D, et al. The medical home and integrated behavioral health: advancing the policy agenda. *Pediatrics.* 2015;135(5): 909–917

106. Delamater AM, de Wit M, McDarby V, Malik J, Acerini CL; International Society for Pediatric and Adolescent Diabetes. ISPAD Clinical Practice Consensus Guidelines 2014. Psychological care of children and adolescents with type 1 diabetes. *Pediatr Diabetes.* 2014; 15(suppl 20):232–244

107. Wiener L, Kazak AE, Noll RB, Patenaude AF, Kupst MJ. Standards for the psychosocial care of children with cancer and their families: an introduction to the special issue. *Pediatr Blood Cancer.* 2015;62(suppl 5): S419–S424

108. Freeman DS, Hudgins C, Hornberger J. Legislative and policy developments and imperatives for advancing the Primary Care Behavioral Health (PCBH) model. *J Clin Psychol Med Settings.* 2018;25(2):210–223

Alcohol Use by Youth

- *Policy Statement*

POLICY STATEMENT Organizational Principles to Guide and Define the Child Health Care System and/or Improve the Health of all Children

American Academy of Pediatrics

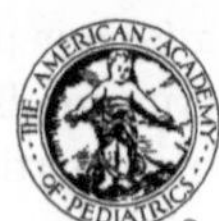

DEDICATED TO THE HEALTH OF ALL CHILDREN™

Alcohol Use by Youth

Joanna Quigley, MD, FAAP, COMMITTEE ON SUBSTANCE USE AND PREVENTION

abstract

Alcohol use continues to be problematic for youth and young adults in the United States. Understanding of neurobiology and neuroplasticity continues to highlight the potential adverse impact of underage drinking on the developing brain. This policy statement provides the position of the American Academy of Pediatrics on the issue of alcohol and is supported by an accompanying technical report.

Department of Psychiatry, University of Michigan, Ann Arbor, Michigan

Dr Quigley wrote and revised the manuscript with input from internal and external reviewers as well as the Board of Directors; and she approves of the final publication.

This document is copyrighted and is property of the American Academy of Pediatrics and its Board of Directors. All authors have filed conflict of interest statements with the American Academy of Pediatrics. Any conflicts have been resolved through a process approved by the Board of Directors. The American Academy of Pediatrics has neither solicited nor accepted any commercial involvement in the development of the content of this publication.

Policy statements from the American Academy of Pediatrics benefit from expertise and resources of liaisons and internal (AAP) and external reviewers. However, policy statements from the American Academy of Pediatrics may not reflect the views of the liaisons or the organizations or government agencies that they represent.

The guidance in this statement does not indicate an exclusive course of treatment or serve as a standard of medical care. Variations, taking into account individual circumstances, may be appropriate.

All policy statements from the American Academy of Pediatrics automatically expire 5 years after publication unless reaffirmed, revised, or retired at or before that time.

DOI: https://doi.org/10.1542/peds.2019-1356

Address correspondence to Joanna Quigley, MD, FAAP, Department of Psychiatry, University of Michigan, Ann Arbor, MI. E-mail: joannaq@med.umich.edu

PEDIATRICS (ISSN Numbers: Print, 0031-4005; Online, 1098-4275).

Copyright © 2019 by the American Academy of Pediatrics

FINANCIAL DISCLOSURE: The authors have indicated they have no financial relationships relevant to this article to disclose.

FUNDING: No external funding.

POTENTIAL CONFLICT OF INTEREST: The authors have indicated they have no potential conflicts of interest to disclose.

To cite: Quigley J, AAP COMMITTEE ON SUBSTANCE USE AND PREVENTION. Alcohol Use by Youth. *Pediatrics.* 2019;144(1): e20191356

Data from the 2018 Monitoring the Future study (national annual survey of eighth-, 10th-, and 12th-grade students regarding health behaviors and attitudes) indicate that overall alcohol use had been in decline for several years until 2017, when there were no significant changes found in any prevalence measures in any grade, but in 2018, the trend of declining rates resumed.[1] According to the 2018 Monitoring the Future data, by the end of 12th grade, 59% of students had "consumed more than a few sips" of alcohol, and 42.9% of 12th-graders "reported having been drunk at least once in their life."[1] The 2017 National Survey on Drug Use and Health revealed that 9.9% of those aged 12 to 17 years and 55.9% of those aged 18 to 25 years reported drinking alcohol during the past month.[2] This policy statement serves as an update to the previously published American Academy of Pediatrics (AAP) policy statement on alcohol use by adolescents[3] and is accompanied in this issue of *Pediatrics* by a technical report.[4]

Occasional or weekend use of alcohol is often dismissed as typical teenage behavior by adults, and its biological and functional implications are not recognized as being significant. Adolescent substance use frequently co-occurs with other psychiatric diagnoses, including anxiety, mood, psychotic, and disruptive disorders, and can increase the risk of behaviors such as suicide attempts and unplanned sexual encounters.[5–7] The younger youth initiate alcohol use, the greater their risk of developing an alcohol use disorder (AUD) later in life.[8,9] Pediatricians are uniquely positioned to reduce adolescent alcohol use and intervene with those at high risk.

Alcohol use among adolescents frequently involves binge drinking rather than more frequent consumption of fewer drinks on each occasion. Binge drinking is defined as 4 drinks for women and 5 drinks for men within a 2-hour period.[10] However, this criterion is thought to be too high, particularly for younger adolescents.[11] A detailed clinical report discussing binge drinking was published by the AAP in 2015.[12] The 2017 National Survey on Drug Use and Health data indicate that 5.3% of adolescents aged 12 to 17 years engaged in binge drinking, and 36.9% of those aged 18 to 25 years had engaged in binge drinking during the past month.[2] The 2017 national Youth Risk Behavior Surveillance study revealed that 13.5% of students in grades 9 through 12 reported binge drinking on at least 1 day during the 30 days before survey administration.[13] The financial and societal costs of binge drinking are significant.[14]

ALCOHOL USE AND AUDs

Accurately eliciting the frequency and consequences of alcohol use can be difficult for practitioners. Alcohol use among youth ranges from nondrinkers to those who meet criteria for severe AUD. Determining which youth may be at risk for the development of an AUD in the future can also be challenging. The *Diagnostic and Statistical Manual of Mental Disorders, Fifth Edition* was published in May 2013 and presents a new diagnostic categorization and labeling of substance use disorders and AUDs.[15] The *Diagnostic and Statistical Manual of Mental Disorders, Fifth Edition* describes substance-related disorders on a severity continuum (substance use disorder and substance-induced disorders). Discussion continues as to the applicability of these diagnostic criteria to youth.[16] Concern exists that use by a youth at risk may not hit threshold criteria for a diagnosable disorder, and the youth may not receive appropriate interventions, although that use may be problematic and pose significant consequences, medically and psychosocially.

HAZARDS ASSOCIATED WITH USE OF ALCOHOL

Despite legislation such as setting a minimum age for purchase of alcohol at 21 years, youth continue to access and consume alcohol readily. Because alcohol could impact ongoing brain development, the National Institute on Alcohol Abuse and Alcoholism recommends no alcohol use before the age of 21 years.[17] The majority of those diagnosed with an AUD began drinking by the age of 18 years.[18] Heavy drinking during adolescence is associated with heavy drinking during young adulthood.[19] Underage drinking is also associated with an increased risk of depression, anxiety, sleep disturbance, self-injuries, and suicidal behavior and greater involvement in other risky behaviors such as high-risk sexual behavior and criminal behavior.[14,18] Use of alcohol during adolescence can have a negative impact on school attendance and performance.[20]

Motor vehicle crashes remain the leading cause of death for youth 16 to 20 years of age.[21] In 2016, 39% of alcohol-impaired drivers involved in fatal motor vehicle collisions were 16 to 24 years of age.[22] Data from the 2017 national Youth Risk Behavior Surveillance of youth in grades 9 through 12 reveal that during the 30 days before survey administration, 16.5% of students had ridden in a vehicle at least once with a driver who had been drinking alcohol; of those students who drove a vehicle during the 30 days before survey administration, 5.5% drove when they had been consuming alcohol.[13]

Legislation targeting the legal age for the purchase of alcohol and graduated driving laws have had a positive impact on the morbidity associated with youth alcohol consumption. Since the establishment of 21 years as the minimum purchase age for alcohol in the United States, there has been a significant reduction in highway deaths.[23] Graduated driver licensing laws in the United States have resulted in reduced crash rates for those 16 to 17 years of age.[21] Examination of data from New Zealand after its 1999 decision to decrease the minimum purchase age for alcohol from 20 to 18 years reveals concerning shifts. These shifts include higher rates of drinking in 16- to 19-year-olds, increased quantities of alcohol consumption among 16- to 17-year-olds, and an increase in alcohol-related problems among 16-to 19-year-olds.[24] Examination of alcohol policy in the United States highlights an association between stricter policy and a reduction in alcohol-related motor vehicle crash mortality in youth.[25]

NEUROBIOLOGY OF ADOLESCENT DEVELOPMENT AND THE IMPACT OF ALCOHOL

The neurobiological and developmental hazards of alcohol use are significant. It is well established that brain development continues well into early adulthood.[26] The prefrontal cortex, which is important in executive decision-making and impulse control, is not fully developed until 21 to 25 years of age.[27] In comparison, the areas of the brain involved in reward and sensation seeking develop earlier. Of note, adolescents who display traits of novelty seeking and poor impulse control are at greater risk of developing substance use disorders.[28] The neuroadaptation associated with addiction also affects the developing prefrontal cortex and executive functioning processes.[28] Several studies suggest that exposure to alcohol may impair synaptic maturation in the adolescent brain.[29] Hippocampal volumes have been found to be smaller in teenagers reporting heavy alcohol use.[30] Neurocognitive deficits in the domains of attention, information processing, memory, and executive functioning have been identified in those adolescents using alcohol compared with controls not using substances.[31,32] Furthermore, adolescence is a time when signs and symptoms of mental illness may first emerge. It is important to note that many of these studies are correlational and that true causal relationships between alcohol and observed brain effects have not been fully established.

FACTORS THAT CONTRIBUTE TO HAZARDOUS USE

Genetics, epigenetics, and environmental and social factors are each cited as influencing an individual's behaviors concerning alcohol use. Early onset of drinking and heavy drinking in adolescence increase the risk of problematic drinking in adulthood; reasons for this vulnerability include genetic and neurobiological factors.[33] A study by Chorlian et al[34] revealed that variants in the cholinergic M2 receptor gene appear to increase the risk of developing an AUD 2 years after initiation of regular alcohol use (before the age of 16 years).

A youth's environment, particularly parental and peer modeling, can affect his or her alcohol use.[35,36] Alcohol use among vulnerable populations is of particular concern. Homeless youth are at higher risk for substance use.[37] Lesbian, gay, bisexual, and transgender adolescents, a population at greater risk of depression and suicidality,[38] are at increased risk for alcohol use.[39] Adolescents report drinking more when they are exposed to parents who appear tolerant of underage drinking.[40] However, environment can play a protective role for youth; for example, clear parental disapproval of underage alcohol consumption[41] and a teenager's close alliance to parents and family can be protective factors against adolescent alcohol use.[42] The youth's environment also includes his or her exposure to passive and active alcohol marketing on a variety of social media platforms, such as YouTube, Twitter, Instagram, and Facebook.[43,44] It is difficult to capture exact demographic data from social media platforms, and the presence of alcohol brand marketing has increased in these settings over the past several years.[45] These newer venues fall outside the purview of regulation by the Federal Trade Commission. Advertisement of alcohol products can significantly influence first use of alcohol and consumption patterns in adolescents.[46] Researchers have identified associations between ownership of alcohol-branded merchandise and alcohol use by adolescents.[46]

Newer types and formulations of alcohol-containing products are constantly being introduced into consumer markets. These products include but are not limited to alcoholic gelatin shots and pops; fruit-flavored alcohol beverages, such as fruit-flavored beers; caffeinated alcohol drinks; devices to vape alcohol; and powdered alcohol. Devices that allow for the vaping of alcohol can be ordered online, and do-it-yourself online video instructions are available as well. Alcohol is also contained in some of the e-liquids in e-cigarettes; some of these liquid products have contents modified to increase the amount of alcohol.[47] In March 2015, the Alcohol and Tobacco Tax and Trade Bureau approved the sale of powdered alcohol (eg, marketed by the brand name Palcohol). One packet of freeze-dried alcohol is designed to be added to 6 oz of liquid, making a drink that is 10% alcohol by volume.[48] State legislation has responded to the approval of powdered alcohol for sale. More than half of the states have preemptively banned the sale of powdered alcohol. Federal legislation has also been proposed to prohibit powdered alcohol nationwide (Senate bill S. 728, 114th Congress).

These newer forms of alcohol products are highly appealing to younger consumers and may lead to greater amounts of alcohol consumption. Studies have revealed that underage drinkers who consumed flavored alcoholic beverages, as well as those who consumed caffeinated alcoholic beverages, consumed more alcohol in one sitting, drank on more days each month, and were more likely to binge drink.[49,50]

ROLE OF THE PEDIATRICIAN

The pediatrician can play an important role in reducing the morbidity and mortality associated with adolescent alcohol use. Anticipatory guidance with regard to alcohol use is recommended as a routine part of care for youth and their families, as outlined in the AAP's *Bright Futures: Guidelines for Health Supervision of Infants, Children, and Adolescents*.[51]

The AAP published a policy statement and clinical report on the practice of substance use screening, brief intervention, and referral to treatment.[52,53] In addition, the AAP published a clinical report on binge drinking.[12] The Substance Abuse and Mental Health Services Administration devotes considerable resources to the promotion of screening, brief intervention, and referral to treatment as a standard for universal screening in the primary care setting.[54] Although the availability of treatment facilities for adolescents is limited, it is nonetheless vital to refer adolescents to treatment services for early intervention and treatment.

Pediatricians can continue to support advocacy efforts to strengthen policy that protects youth from both individual and societal impacts of alcohol use. It would be prudent for pediatricians to support continued research into the understanding of adolescent and brain developmental, the impact of alcohol use on adolescent health, and the role of comorbid mental illness and risk-taking behaviors. This research includes important national efforts such as the Longitudinal Study of Adolescent Brain and Cognitive Development, supported by the National Institutes of Health.[55]

RECOMMENDATIONS

The AAP supports the following:

1. Sending a clear message against the use of alcohol by adolescents and young adults under the age of 21 years.
2. Existing state laws that dictate a minimum purchase age of 21 years for alcohol.
3. Existing state laws granting graduated driver licensing over the course of adolescence, in addition to best practices for screening and intervention when there is concern for potential alcohol use by teenage drivers.
4. Advocacy for continued research on the impact of alcohol use on the developing brain.
5. Continued work for evidence-based policy to target social media in addition to traditional marketing of alcohol to youth.
6. Advocacy for taxes on alcohol products.
7. Continued support for the role of schools in providing general health education, community programming, and focused screening and education regarding alcohol use.
8. State legislation to ban the sale and distribution of powdered alcohol and upholding existing state legislation.
9. Continued awareness, knowledge, and skill development so that pediatricians screen for alcohol use, implement brief interventions targeting use, and provide education to adolescents and their families about hazards, consequences, and interventions around alcohol use.
10. Pediatricians' support for increased investment in treatment services for adolescents and young adults that target substance use disorders.

RESOURCES

Bright Futures: Guidelines for health supervision of infants, children, and adolescents. Available at: brightfutures.aap.org.

National Institute on Alcohol Abuse and Alcoholism. Alcohol screening and brief intervention for youth: a practitioner's guide. Available at: www.niaaa.nih.gov/YouthGuide.

Substance Abuse and Mental Health Service Administration. Talk. They hear you. Available at: www.samhsa.gov/underage-drinking.

American Academy of Pediatrics. Brief intervention to address substance use. Available at: www.aap.org/en-us/advocacy-and-policy/aap-health-initiatives/Mental-Health/Pages/substance-use.aspx.

The Guide to Community Preventive Services. Preventing excessive alcohol consumption. Available at: www.thecommunityguide.org/alcohol.

US Preventive Services Task Force. Alcohol misuse: screening and behavioral counseling interventions in primary care. Available at: www.uspreventiveservicestaskforce.org/uspstf/uspsdrin.htm.

National Institute on Alcohol Abuse and Alcoholism. Make a difference: talk to your child about alcohol. Available at: https://pubs.niaaa.nih.gov/publications/MakeADiff_HTML/makediff.htm.

HealthyChildren.org. Official consumer web site of the AAP. Substance use. Available at: www.healthychildren.org/English/ages-stages/teen/substance-abuse.

Substance Abuse and Mental Health Service Administration. National registry of evidence-based programs and practices. Available at: https://www.samhsa.gov/nrepp.

Substance Abuse and Mental Health Services Administration. Talking with your college-bound young adult about alcohol. Available at: https://store.samhsa.gov/shin/content/SMA15-4897/SMA15-4897.pdf.

American Academy of Pediatrics. Substance use coding fact sheep for primary care pediatrics. Available at: https://www.aap.org/en-us/Documents/coding_factsheet_substance_use.pdf.

LEAD AUTHOR

Joanna Quigley, MD, FAAP

COMMITTEE ON SUBSTANCE USE AND PREVENTION, 2018–2019

Sheryl A. Ryan, MD, FAAP, Chairperson
Deepa R. Camenga, MD, MHS, FAAP
Stephen W. Patrick, MD, MPH, MS, FAAP
Jennifer Plumb, MD, MPH, FAAP
Joanna Quigley, MD, FAAP
Leslie Walker-Harding, MD, FAAP

LIASIONS

Gregory Tau, MD, PhD – *American Academy of Child and Adolescent Psychiatry*

STAFF

Renee Jarrett, MPH

ABBREVIATIONS

AAP: American Academy of Pediatrics
AUD: alcohol use disorder

REFERENCES

1. Johnston LD, Miech RA, O'Malley PM, Bachman JG, Schulenberg JE, Patrick ME. *Monitoring the Future: National Survey Results on Drug Use, 1975-2018. Overview, Key Findings on Adolescent*

Drug Use. Ann Arbor, MI: Institute for Social Research, University of Michigan; 2019. Available at www.monitoringthefuture.org//pubs/monographs/mtf-overview2018.pdf. Accessed March 26, 2019

2. Center for Behavioral Health Statistics and Quality. *2017 National Survey on Drug Use and Health: Detailed Tables*. Rockville, MD: Substance Abuse and Mental Health Services Administration; 2018. Available at: https://www.samhsa.gov/data/sites/default/files/cbhsq-reports/NSDUHDetailedTabs2017/NSDUHDetailedTabs2017.pdf. Accessed March 26, 2019
3. Kokotailo P; Committee on Substance Abuse. Policy statement–alcohol use by youth and adolescents: a pediatric concern. *Pediatrics*. 2010;125(5):1078–1087
4. Ryan S, Kokotailo P; American Academy of Pediatrics, Committee on Substance Use Prevention. Technical report: alcohol use by youth. *Pediatrics*. 2019;144(1):e20191357
5. Simkin DR. Adolescent substance use disorders and comorbidity. *Pediatr Clin North Am*. 2002;49(2):463–477
6. Windle M. Suicidal behaviors and alcohol use among adolescents: a developmental psychopathology perspective. *Alcohol Clin Exp Res*. 2004;28(suppl 5):29S–37S
7. Hingson R, Heeren T, Winter MR, Wechsler H. Early age of first drunkenness as a factor in college students' unplanned and unprotected sex attributable to drinking. *Pediatrics*. 2003;111(1):34–41
8. Dawson DA, Goldstein RB, Chou SP, Ruan WJ, Grant BF. Age at first drink and the first incidence of adult-onset DSM-IV alcohol use disorders. *Alcohol Clin Exp Res*. 2008;32(12):2149–2160
9. DeWit DJ, Adlaf EM, Offord DR, Ogborne AC. Age at first alcohol use: a risk factor for the development of alcohol disorders. *Am J Psychiatry*. 2000;157(5):745–750
10. National Institute on Alcohol Abuse and Alcoholism. Drinking levels defined. Available at: www.niaaa.nih.gov/alcohol-health/overview-alcohol-consumption/moderate-binge-drinking. Accessed March 26, 2019
11. Donovan JE. Estimated blood alcohol concentrations for child and adolescent drinking and their implications for screening instruments. *Pediatrics*. 2009;123(6). Available at: www.pediatrics.org/cgi/content/full/123/6/e975
12. Siqueira L, Smith VC; Committee on Substance Abuse. Binge drinking. *Pediatrics*. 2015;136(3). Available at: www.pediatrics.org/cgi/content/full/136/3/e718
13. Kann L, McManus T, Harris WA, et al. Youth risk behavior surveillance - United States, 2017. *MMWR Surveill Summ*. 2018;67(8):1–114
14. Miller TR, Levy DT, Spicer RS, Taylor DM. Societal costs of underage drinking. *J Stud Alcohol*. 2006;67(4):519–528
15. American Psychiatric Association. *Diagnostic and Statistical Manual of Mental Disorders (DSM-5)*. 5th ed. Washington, DC: American Psychiatric Association; 2013
16. Kaminer Y, Winters KC. DSM-5 criteria for youth substance use disorders: lost in translation? *J Am Acad Child Adolesc Psychiatry*. 2015;54(5):350–351
17. National Institute on Alcohol Abuse and Alcoholism. Fact sheet: underage drinking. 2017. Available at: https://pubs.niaaa.nih.gov/publications/UnderageDrinking/UnderageFact.htm. Accessed March 26, 2019
18. Richter L, Pugh BS, Peters EA, Vaughan RD, Foster SE. Underage drinking: prevalence and correlates of risky drinking measures among youth aged 12-20. *Am J Drug Alcohol Abuse*. 2016;42(4):385–394
19. McCarty CA, Ebel BE, Garrison MM, DiGiuseppe DL, Christakis DA, Rivara FP. Continuity of binge and harmful drinking from late adolescence to early adulthood. *Pediatrics*. 2004;114(3):714–719
20. Engberg J, Morral AR. Reducing substance use improves adolescents' school attendance. *Addiction*. 2006;101(12):1741–1751
21. Romano E, Scherer M, Fell J, Taylor E. A comprehensive examination of U.S. laws enacted to reduce alcohol-related crashes among underage drivers. *J Safety Res*. 2015;55:213–221
22. National Highway Traffic Safety Administration, US Department of Transportation. Drunk driving: risk factors: age. Available at: https://www.nhtsa.gov/risky-driving/drunk-driving#age-5056. Accessed March 26, 2019
23. DeJong W, Blanchette J. Case closed: research evidence on the positive public health impact of the age 21 minimum legal drinking age in the United States. *J Stud Alcohol Drugs*. 2014;75(suppl 17):108–115
24. Gruenewald PJ, Treno AJ, Ponicki WR, Huckle T, Yeh LC, Casswell S. Impacts of New Zealand's lowered minimum purchase age on context-specific drinking and related risks. *Addiction*. 2015;110(11):1757–1766
25. Hadland SE, Xuan Z, Sarda V, et al. Alcohol policies and alcohol-related motor vehicle crash fatalities among young people in the US. *Pediatrics*. 2017;139(3):e20163037
26. Sowell ER, Thompson PM, Holmes CJ, Jernigan TL, Toga AW. In vivo evidence for post-adolescent brain maturation in frontal and striatal regions. *Nat Neurosci*. 1999;2(10):859–861
27. Giedd JN, Blumenthal J, Jeffries NO, et al. Brain development during childhood and adolescence: a longitudinal MRI study. *Nat Neurosci*. 1999;2(10):861–863
28. Volkow ND, Koob GF, McLellan AT. Neurobiologic advances from the brain disease model of addiction. *N Engl J Med*. 2016;374(4):363–371
29. Crews FT, Vetreno RP, Broadwater MA, Robinson DL. Adolescent alcohol exposure persistently impacts adult neurobiology and behavior. *Pharmacol Rev*. 2016;68(4):1074–1109
30. Nagel BJ, Schweinsburg AD, Phan V, Tapert SF. Reduced hippocampal volume among adolescents with alcohol use disorders without psychiatric comorbidity. *Psychiatry Res*. 2005;139(3):181–190
31. Brown SA, Tapert SF, Granholm E, Delis DC. Neurocognitive functioning of adolescents: effects of protracted alcohol use. *Alcohol Clin Exp Res*. 2000;24(2):164–171
32. Tapert SF, Granholm E, Leedy NG, Brown SA. Substance use and withdrawal:

neuropsychological functioning over 8 years in youth. *J Int Neuropsychol Soc.* 2002;8(7):873–883

33. Deutsch AR, Slutske WS, Richmond-Rakerd LS, Chernyavskiy P, Heath AC, Martin NG. Causal influence of age at first drink on alcohol involvement in adulthood and its moderation by familial context. *J Stud Alcohol Drugs.* 2013;74(5):703–713
34. Chorlian DB, Rangaswamy M, Manz N, et al. Genetic and neurophysiological correlates of the age of onset of alcohol use disorders in adolescents and young adults. *Behav Genet.* 2013;43(5):386–401
35. Foley KL, Altman D, Durant RH, Wolfson M. Adults' approval and adolescents' alcohol use. *J Adolesc Health.* 2004; 35(4):345.e17–345.e26
36. Wang C, Hipp JR, Butts CT, Jose R, Lakon CM. Alcohol use among adolescent youth: the role of friendship networks and family factors in multiple school studies. *PLoS One.* 2015;10(3):e0119965
37. Tompsett CJ, Domoff SE, Toro PA. Peer substance use and homelessness predicting substance abuse from adolescence through early adulthood. *Am J Community Psychol.* 2013;51(3–4): 520–529
38. Marshal MP, Dietz LJ, Friedman MS, et al. Suicidality and depression disparities between sexual minority and heterosexual youth: a meta-analytic review. *J Adolesc Health.* 2011;49(2): 115–123
39. Huebner DM, Thoma BC, Neilands TB. School victimization and substance use among lesbian, gay, bisexual, and transgender adolescents. *Prev Sci.* 2015;16(5):734–743
40. Komro KA, Maldonado-Molina MM, Tobler AL, Bonds JR, Muller KE. Effects of home access and availability of alcohol on young adolescents' alcohol use. *Addiction.* 2007;102(10):1597–1608
41. Nash SG, McQueen A, Bray JH. Pathways to adolescent alcohol use: family environment, peer influence, and parental expectations. *J Adolesc Health.* 2005;37(1):19–28
42. Resnick MD, Bearman PS, Blum RW, et al; Findings from the National Longitudinal Study on Adolescent Health. Protecting adolescents from harm. *JAMA.* 1997;278(10):823–832
43. Weaver ERN, Wright CJC, Dietze PM, Lim MSC. 'A drink that makes you feel happier, relaxed and loving': young people's perceptions of alcohol advertising on Facebook. *Alcohol Alcohol.* 2016;51(4):481–486
44. Cabrera-Nguyen EP, Cavazos-Rehg P, Krauss M, Bierut LJ, Moreno MA. Young adults' exposure to alcohol- and marijuana-related content on twitter. *J Stud Alcohol Drugs.* 2016;77(2): 349–353
45. Jernigan DH, Rushman AE. Measuring youth exposure to alcohol marketing on social networking sites: challenges and prospects. *J Public Health Policy.* 2014; 35(1):91–104
46. Jones SC. Alcohol-branded merchandise ownership and drinking. *Pediatrics.* 2016;137(5):e20153970
47. Valentine GW, Jatlow PI, Coffman M, Nadim H, Gueorguieva R, Sofuoglu M. The effects of alcohol-containing e-cigarettes on young adult smokers. *Drug Alcohol Depend.* 2016;159:272–276
48. Naimi TS, Mosher JF. Powdered alcohol products new challenge in an era in need of regulation. *JAMA.* 2015;314(2): 119–120
49. Albers AB, Siegel M, Ramirez RL, Ross C, DeJong W, Jernigan DH. Flavored alcoholic beverage use, risky drinking behaviors, and adverse outcomes among underage drinkers: results from the ABRAND Study. *Am J Public Health.* 2015;105(4):810–815
50. Kponee KZ, Siegel M, Jernigan DH. The use of caffeinated alcoholic beverages among underage drinkers: results of a national survey. *Addict Behav.* 2014; 39(1):253–258
51. Hagan JF, Shaw JS, Duncan PM, eds. *Bright Futures: Guidelines for Health Supervision of Infants, Children, and Adolescents.* 4th ed. Elk Grove Village, IL: American Academy of Pediatrics; 2017
52. Committee on Substance Use and Prevention. Substance use screening, brief intervention, and referral to treatment. *Pediatrics.* 2016;138(1): e20161210
53. Levy SJ, Williams JF; Committee on Substance Use and Prevention. Substance use screening, brief intervention, and referral to treatment. *Pediatrics.* 2016;138(1):e20161211
54. Substance Abuse and Mental Health Services Administration. Screening, brief intervention, and referral to treatment. Available at: www.samhsa.gov/sbirt. Accessed March 26, 2019
55. Adolescent Brain Cognitive Development Study. Available at: https://abcdstudy.org/about/. Accessed March 26, 2019

Alcohol Use by Youth

- *Technical Report*

TECHNICAL REPORT

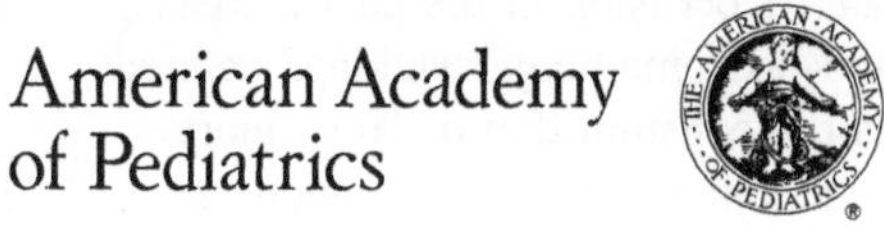

Alcohol Use by Youth

Sheryl A. Ryan, MD, FAAP,[a] Patricia Kokotailo, MD, MPH, FAAP,[b] COMMITTEE ON SUBSTANCE USE AND PREVENTION

abstract

Alcohol use continues to be a major concern from preadolescence through young adulthood in the United States. Results of recent neuroscience research have helped to elucidate neurobiological models of addiction, substantiated the deleterious effects of alcohol on adolescent brain development, and added additional evidence to support the call to prevent and reduce underage drinking. This technical report reviews the relevant literature and supports the accompanying policy statement in this issue of *Pediatrics*.

[a]Division of Adolescent Medicine, Department of Pediatrics, Penn State Health Milton S. Hershey Medical Center, Hershey, Pennsylvania; and [b]Department of Pediatrics, School of Medicine and Public Health, University of Wisconsin–Madison, Madison, Wisconsin

Drs Ryan and Kokotailo were directly involved in the planning, researching, and writing of this report; and both authors approved the final manuscript as submitted.

This document is copyrighted and is property of the American Academy of Pediatrics and its Board of Directors. All authors have filed conflict of interest statements with the American Academy of Pediatrics. Any conflicts have been resolved through a process approved by the Board of Directors. The American Academy of Pediatrics has neither solicited nor accepted any commercial involvement in the development of the content of this publication.

Technical reports from the American Academy of Pediatrics benefit from expertise and resources of liaisons and internal (AAP) and external reviewers. However, technical reports from the American Academy of Pediatrics may not reflect the views of the liaisons or the organizations or government agencies that they represent.

The guidance in this report does not indicate an exclusive course of treatment or serve as a standard of medical care. Variations, taking into account individual circumstances, may be appropriate.

All technical reports from the American Academy of Pediatrics automatically expire 5 years after publication unless reaffirmed, revised, or retired at or before that time.

DOI: https://doi.org/10.1542/peds.2019-1357

Address correspondence to Sheryl A. Ryan, MD, FAAP, Division of Adolescent Medicine, Department of Pediatrics, Penn State Health Milton S. Hershey Medical Center, Hershey, PA. E-mail: sryan4@pennstatehealth.psu.edu

PEDIATRICS (ISSN Numbers: Print, 0031-4005; Online, 1098-4275).

Copyright © 2019 by the American Academy of Pediatrics

FINANCIAL DISCLOSURE: The authors have indicated they have no financial relationships relevant to this article to disclose.

FUNDING: No external funding.

To cite: Ryan SA, Kokotailo P, AAP COMMITTEE ON SUBSTANCE USE AND PREVENTION. Alcohol Use by Youth. *Pediatrics*. 2019;144(1):e20191357

Alcohol is the substance most widely used by adolescents, often in large volumes, although the minimum legal drinking age across the United States is 21 years.[1] Some people may initiate harmful alcohol consumption in childhood. The prevalence of problematic alcohol use continues to escalate from adolescence into young adulthood. Heavy episodic drinking by students enrolled in college remains a major public health problem. In results of recent research, it has been indicated that brain development continues well into early adulthood[2] and that alcohol consumption can interfere with such development, underscoring concerns that alcohol use by youth is an even greater pediatric health concern than previously thought.[3,4] This technical report supports the accompanied policy statement that outlines recommendations from the American Academy of Pediatrics (AAP).[5]

EPIDEMIOLOGY

Alcohol, tobacco, and marijuana remain the substances most widely used by youth in the United States. There is both heartening and less heartening news about the use of alcohol by US youth, however. The 2018 Monitoring the Future Study, supported by the National Institute of Drug Abuse and conducted by the University of Michigan, is now in its 44th year of tracking the prevalence of alcohol, tobacco, and other drug use and youth perceptions of such use. A sample of more than 45 000 young people in eighth, 10th, and 12th grade in approximately 380 private and public secondary schools in the United States provides these data.[1] The data include use by youth in all 3 grades in their lifetime, in the past year (annual use), and in the 30 days preceding the survey as well as "binge" drinking, defined as the consumption of 5 or more drinks in a row on at least 1 occasion in the past 2 weeks, and "extreme binge drinking," defined as the consumption of 10 or more drinks in a row in the previous 2 weeks. The good news is that there has been a long, substantial decline in alcohol use in all of these categories from peaks in the 1990s. For example, in 1997, the highest number of youth reported using alcohol over the previous year (61%); by 2018, 36.1% of youth in the 3 grades surveyed reported use in the 12 months before the survey. Perhaps even more important, the percentage of young people in the 3 grades reporting binge drinking decreased by half or more from peaks in 1997. In 2017, rates of lifetime prevalence, annual prevalence, and 30-day prevalence of alcohol use in all 3 grades showed plateauing, which was interpreted as a sign that the trend of declining rates was at an end. In addition, in 2017, 4% of eighth-graders, 10% of 10th-graders, and 17% of 12th-graders still reported binge drinking in the past 2 weeks, all slightly increased from 2016.[1] However, in 2018, declines in rates of use continued: the 30-day prevalence rates for eighth, 10th, and 12th-graders was 8%, 19%, and 30%, respectively, and the prevalence of binge drinking in the previous 2 weeks in 10th- and 12th-graders declined to 9% and 14%, respectively, although it remained at 4% for eighth-graders. For the 3 grades combined, this survey documented the lowest levels of alcohol use and binge drinking that have been recorded to date.[1] The criterion used for binge drinking as 5 or more drinks in a row has been thought to be too high, especially for younger children and girls, with the literature suggesting that for 9- to 13-year-old children and 14- to 17-year-old girls, binge drinking should be defined as 3 or more drinks. For boys, binge drinking should be defined as 4 or more drinks for those 14 or 15 years old and 5 or more drinks for those 16 or 17 years old.[6]

To examine higher levels of consumption by 12th-graders, the Monitoring the Future study has more recently been tracking 2 levels of extreme binge drinking, defined as having 10 or more or 15 or more drinks in a row on at least 1 occasion in the preceding 2 weeks. These measures have also declined from 11% in 2005 (the first year of this category's measurement) to 4.6% for the 10 drinks in a row category and from 6% to 2.5% for 15 drinks in a row in 2018. Each of these measures increased slightly from 2016 to 2017 but resumed the decline in 2018.[1] Declines in perceived availability as well as increased peer disapproval of binge drinking may be some of the factors that are contributing to these lower prevalence numbers.[1] These epidemiologic statistics are corroborated by data from 2 other large surveys of youth alcohol use in the United States: the Youth Risk Behavior Survey, conducted biannually by the Centers for Disease Control and Prevention, and the National Survey on Drug Use and Health, conducted annually by the Substance Abuse and Mental Health Services Administration.[7,8]

Use of alcohol at an early age is particularly problematic and is associated with future alcohol-related problems.[9–11] Data from the National Longitudinal Alcohol Epidemiologic Study indicate that the prevalence of both lifetime alcohol dependence and alcohol abuse, as defined by the *Diagnostic and Statistical Manual of Mental Disorders, Fourth Edition* criteria, show a striking decrease with increasing age at the onset of alcohol use.[9] According to the National Longitudinal Alcohol Epidemiologic Study, for people 12 years or younger at first use, the prevalence of lifetime alcohol dependence was 40.6%. In contrast, for people who initiated alcohol consumption at 18 years of age, the prevalence was 16.6%, and for those who initiated drinking at 21 years, the prevalence was 10.6%. Similarly, the prevalence of lifetime alcohol abuse was 8.3% for those who initiated use at 12 years or younger, 7.8% for those who initiated at 18 years, and 4.8% for those who initiated at 21 years. The contribution of age at alcohol use initiation to the odds of lifetime dependence and abuse varied little across sex and racial subgroups in the study.[9] In analyses of data from subsequent surveys, researchers have also illustrated this relationship between early initiation of drinking and subsequent alcohol use disorder (AUD).[12–15]

ALCOHOL USE BY ADOLESCENTS

Adolescent alcohol exposure covers a spectrum, from primary abstinence to alcohol dependence. The *Diagnostic and Statistical Manual of Mental Disorders, Fifth Edition* (DSM-5)[16] defines AUD as follows:

A problematic pattern of alcohol use leading to clinically significant impairment or distress as manifested by 2 or more of the following, occurring during a 12-month period:

1. Alcohol is often taken in larger amounts or over a longer period than was intended.

2. There is a persistent desire or unsuccessful efforts to cut down or control alcohol use.

3. A great deal of time is spent in activities necessary to obtain alcohol, use alcohol, or recover from its effects.

4. Craving, or a strong desire or urge to use alcohol.

5. Recurrent alcohol use results in a failure to fulfill major role obligations at work, school, or home.

6. Continued alcohol use despite having persistent or recurrent social or interpersonal problems caused or exacerbated by the effects of alcohol.

7. Important social, occupational, or recreational activities are given up or reduced because of alcohol use.

8. Recurrent alcohol use in situations in which it is physically hazardous.

9. Alcohol use is continued despite knowledge of having a persistent or recurrent physical or psychological problem that is likely to have been caused or exacerbated by alcohol.

10. Tolerance, as defined by either of the following:

a. A need for markedly increased amounts of alcohol to achieve intoxication or desired effect.

b. A markedly diminished effect with continued use of the same amount of alcohol.

11. Withdrawal, as manifested by either of the following:

a. The characteristic withdrawal syndrome for alcohol.

b. Alcohol is taken to relieve or avoid withdrawal symptoms.

Reprinted with permission from the *Diagnostic and Statistical Manual of Mental Disorders, Fifth Edition* (Copyright 2013). American Psychiatric Association. All Rights Reserved.

The disorder is characterized as mild (2–3 symptoms), moderate (4–5 symptoms), or severe (6 or more symptoms). Because these diagnostic criteria were developed largely from research and clinical work with adults, there are limitations to applying these diagnostic criteria to classify alcohol use and associated risks to adolescents.[17–19] As defined by the DSM-5, an adolescent, especially a younger one, may not have had time to develop an AUD, yet the adolescent may be engaging in very risky behavior. Despite being viewed as an improvement in specificity for adolescents, the applicability of these revised criteria may still be limited in that several of the criteria, such as withdrawal, are not typically experienced by adolescents, and other criteria, such as tolerance, have low sensitivity for adolescents.[20] Tolerance can be anticipated as a developmental process that will occur over time in most adolescents who drink.[17] Thus, an adolescent may present with a subsyndromal level of alcohol use that may not meet the formal threshold for addiction or an AUD but that may still be associated with significant impairments in social functioning and well-being.[21] These limitations to applying a diagnostic algorithm designed for adults to children and youth are often cited as a reason for advocating for the development of more age-appropriate criteria.

Alcohol misuse, although not a formal diagnosis, can be defined as "alcohol-related disturbances of behavior, disease, or other consequences that are likely to cause an individual, his/her family, or society harm now or in the future."[22] Because the term "alcohol misuse" encompasses earlier stages of AUDs that do not meet diagnostic criteria, it may be a more useful concept clinically in pediatrics and when developing alcohol use primary prevention programs for youth.

HAZARDS OF ALCOHOL USE

Underage drinking is associated with wide range of negative consequences for adolescents, including adverse effects on normal brain development and cognitive functioning, risky sexual behavior, physical and sexual assaults, injuries, AUD, blackouts, alcohol overdose, and even death. When compared with use by adults, alcohol use by adolescents is much more likely to be episodic and in larger volumes (binge drinking), which makes alcohol use by those in this age group particularly dangerous. Rapid binge drinking puts the teenager at even higher risk of alcohol overdose or alcohol poisoning, in which suppression of the gag reflex and respiratory drive and hypoglycemia can be fatal. Binge drinking and its sequelae of elevated blood alcohol concentration (BAC) are especially dangerous for young people who, when compared with adults, may be less likely to be sedated and, therefore, more likely to engage in activities such as driving despite impairment in coordination and judgment.[23]

Alcohol use is a major contributor to the leading causes of adolescent death (ie, motor vehicle crashes, homicide, and suicide) in the United States. Motor vehicle crashes rank as the leading cause of death for US teenagers and young adults. Data from the 2017 Youth Risk Behavior Survey found that during the 30 days preceding the survey, 16.5% of high school students nationwide had ridden one or more times in a car or other vehicle driven by someone who had been drinking alcohol. Of the 62.6% of high school students reporting having driven in the 30 days preceding the survey, 5.5% of students had driven a car or other vehicle at least once when they had been drinking alcohol during this time.[7] These data represent a significant linear decline in reports of use while driving after alcohol use or riding with someone who had been drinking since 1991, when rates reported for riding with a drinking driver and driving oneself after drinking were 39.9% and 16.7%, respectively.[7] In further analysis of the Youth Risk Behavior Survey data, it was shown that in 2011, the prevalence of drinking and driving was more than 3 times higher among those youth who binge drank compared with those who reported current alcohol use but not binge drinking (32.1% vs 9.7%).[24]

The important relationship of alcohol use and motor vehicle crashes involving youth is also highlighted by the fact that after the legal drinking age was changed uniformly to 21 years across the United States, the number of motor vehicle fatalities in individuals younger than 21 years decreased significantly.[25] Since 1998, every state has enacted laws establishing a lower BAC for drivers younger than 21 years, referred to as "zero tolerance laws." These laws are important because young people who drive after consuming any amount of alcohol pose risk to themselves and others. These laws are also estimated to have reduced alcohol-involved fatal crashes among inexperienced drivers by 9% to 24%.[26] Data show that for each 0.02 increase in BAC, the relative risk of a 16- to 20-year-old driver dying in a motor vehicle crash is estimated to be more than double.[27] Graduated driver licensing (GDL) systems have now been adopted in all 50 states and the District of Columbia.[28] These laws indirectly affect drinking and driving by restricting nighttime driving and the transportation of young passengers in the early months after licensure. In a recent national study, it was shown that GDL nighttime driving restrictions were associated with a 13% reduction in fatal drinking driver crashes among drivers 16 to 17 years old compared with drivers 19 to 20 years old who were not under these restrictions.[29] In a Cochrane review, the implementation of GDL was shown to be effective in reducing the crash rates of young drivers and specifically alcohol-related crashes in most studies in the United States and internationally.[30]

Adolescents who report binge drinking violate GDL laws more frequently and engage in more high-risk driving behaviors, such as speeding and using a cell phone while driving. They also received more traffic tickets and reported having more crashes and near crashes.[31] The importance of the additive effect of alcohol with other illicit substances, particularly marijuana, in contributing to motor vehicle crashes should also not be underestimated. Researchers have suggested that the combination of marijuana and alcohol significantly increases the likelihood of a motor vehicle crash, particularly at levels of alcohol that are below legal limits. For example, Dubois et al[32] found that the odds of a motor vehicle crash increased from 66% to 117% with BACs at 0.05 and 0.08, respectively, to 81% and 128% when detectable levels of tetrahydrocannabinol (THC) were present at these same BACs.

Although legislation has greatly improved transportation safety, young people still are involved in a high proportion of fatal motor vehicle accidents involving alcohol. In 2016, the National Highway Traffic Safety Administration reported a 5.6% increase in traffic fatalities from 2015.[33] Although many factors were reported as responsible for this increase, 10 497 people were killed as a direct result of alcohol-impaired driving crashes, accounting for 28% of the total motor vehicle traffic fatalities (37 461 people) in the United States.[33] In fatal crashes in 2016, the second highest percentage of drivers with BACs of 0.08 or higher was for drivers 21 to 24 years old at 26%; the rate for drivers 16 to 20 years old was 15%.[34]

Underage alcohol use and AUD in adolescents are also associated with other mental and physical disorders. AUD is a risk factor for suicide attempts.[35] Miller et al[36] estimated that 9.1% of suicide attempts resulting in hospitalization by people younger than 21 years involved alcohol and that 72% of these cases were attributable to alcohol. Of note, higher minimum legal drinking ages in the United States have been associated with lower youth suicide rates.[37] Psychiatric conditions most likely to co-occur with AUD include mood disorders, particularly depression; anxiety disorders; attention-deficit/hyperactivity disorder; conduct disorders; bulimia; posttraumatic stress disorder; and schizophrenia.[38] Associated physical health problems include trauma sequelae,[39] sleep disturbance, modestly elevated serum liver enzyme concentrations, and dental and other oral abnormalities,[40] despite relatively few abnormalities being evident on physical examination.[40,41]

Early alcohol initiation, in particular, has been associated with greater involvement in a number of high-risk behaviors, such as sexual risk-taking (unprotected sexual intercourse, multiple partners, being drunk or high during sexual intercourse, and pregnancy), academic problems, other substance use, and delinquent behavior in mid to later adolescence.[18,19,38,42–45] By young adulthood, early alcohol use is associated with employment problems, other substance abuse, and criminal and violent behavior.[42]

FACTORS THAT CONTRIBUTE TO HARMFUL USE

Genetic, Familial, and Environmental Factors

Twin studies in adult populations have consistently demonstrated genetic influences on the use of alcohol,[46–48] but less research has examined genetic influences in the adolescent age range.[49–51] Through a sibling, twin, and adoption study of adolescents, Rhee et al[52] examined the relative contribution of genetics and environment on initiation, use, and problem use of substances. The results of this study demonstrated that for adolescents (compared with adult twin study findings), the magnitude of genetic influences was greater than the effect of shared environmental influences on problem alcohol or drug use. The reverse was true, however, for initiation of use, with shared environmental factors more important than genetic background. In a recent study, Chorlian et al[53] concluded that when alcohol is consumed regularly in the youngest age range, affecting a less-mature brain, the addiction-producing effects in those who have 2 copies of the genetic allele of the cholinergic M2 receptor gene are accelerated, which can lead to rapid transition from regular alcohol use to alcohol dependence. It has been suggested that gene and environmental effects may vary depending on developmental period of the individual and the stage of the problematic use or addiction.[54]

It has been suggested that the progression to heavy or compulsive alcohol or other drug use is strongly influenced by genetics.[54] Specific genetic studies have helped to elucidate the scientific basis for the relationship observed between early initiation of drinking and subsequent AUD.[12–15] A longitudinal study of the genetic and neurophysiologic correlates of AUD in adolescents and young adults has identified neurophysiological endophenotype differences and variants of the cholinergic M2 receptor gene in adolescent brains that have an age-specific influence on the age of onset of such a disorder.[53] The authors reported that among people who became regular users of alcohol before the age of 16 years, a majority of those who became alcohol dependent within 2 years had the risk genotype, whereas the majority of people who became alcohol dependent 4 or more years after the onset of regular drinking did not have the risk genotype.[53] Another study also found an association between a polymorphism of the μ-opioid receptor encoding gene and adolescent alcohol use.[55]

In a number of studies, researchers have demonstrated the importance of family and social factors on the initiation and early use of alcohol and other drugs. Independent of genetic risk, families play an important role in the development of alcohol and other drug problems in youth, and exposure to alcohol or other drug use disorders of parents predicts substance use disorders in children.[56] Generational transmission has been widely hypothesized as a factor shaping the alcohol use patterns of youth. Whether through genetics, social learning, or cultural values and community norms, researchers have repeatedly found a correlation between youth drinking and a number of family factors, such as the drinking practices of parents.[57,58] Results of these studies suggest that policies primarily affecting adult drinkers, such as pricing and taxation, hours of sale, and on-premises drink promotions, may also affect underage drinking. Foley et al[59] found in a national sample (n = 6245) of teenagers 16 to 20 years old whose parents provided alcohol to them and supervised their drinking were less likely to report being regular drinkers or binge drinkers than those who obtained alcohol through friends or nonparent relatives and participated in unsupervised drinking. They also found that teenagers who obtained alcohol from parents for parties that were unsupervised by those parents reported the highest rates of regular and binge drinking. Although the practice of parents buying alcohol for their teenagers and supervising their drinking cannot be recommended, this study highlights the role that parental behaviors toward alcohol can have on an adolescent's subsequent drinking behaviors. Parental monitoring of children's use, the convincing conveyance and consistent enforcement of household rules governing use, and perceived consequences of "getting caught" by parents after drinking all protected youth from drinking behaviors.[59–62]

In the United States, approximately 7.5 million children younger than 18 years (10.5% of all children) are reported to live with at least 1 parent who had an AUD in the past year.[63] These children are at increased risk of many behavioral and medical problems, including depression, anxiety disorders, problems with cognitive and verbal skills, and parental abuse or neglect.[64] Children who have a parent with an AUD are also estimated to be 4 times more likely than other children to develop alcohol problems themselves.[65] See the AAP clinical report "Families Affected by Parental Substance Use" for further information.[66]

Other Factors

Having friends who use alcohol, tobacco, or other substances is one of the strongest predictors of substance use by youth.[67] Social and physical settings for underage drinking also affect patterns of alcohol consumption. In a special data-analytic study conducted in 2012, the Substance Abuse and Mental Health Services Administration and the Center for Behavioral Health Statistics and Quality, using data from the National Survey on Drug Use and Health,[68,69] found that the usual number of drinks consumed by young people is substantially higher when 2 or more other people are present than when drinking by oneself or with 1 other person. Drinking in the presence of others is by far the most common setting for youth, with more than 80% of youth who had consumed alcohol in the past month reporting doing so when at least 2 others were present.[68,69] Most young people drink in social contexts that appear to promote heavy consumption. Private residences are the most common setting for youth alcohol consumption, and the majority of underage drinkers report drinking in either someone else's home or their own. The next most popular drinking locations reported are at a restaurant, bar, or club; at a park, on a beach, or in a parking lot; or in a car or other vehicle. Older youth in the 18- to 20-year-old age group are more likely than younger adolescents to report drinking in restaurants, bars, or clubs, although the absolute rates of such drinking are low compared with drinking in private residences. The data that demonstrate that underage drinking occurs primarily in social settings in groups at a private residence are consistent with previous research findings that underage drinking parties are high-risk settings for binge drinking and associated alcohol problems.[70] Similar findings exist for binge drinking by college students.[71]

Media influences on the use of alcohol by young people are substantial.[72,73] Exposure to alcohol marketing increases the likelihood to varying degrees that young people will initiate drinking and drink at higher levels.[74,75] Grenard et al[76] have recently demonstrated using prospective data that exposure to alcohol advertising and liking of those ads by adolescents in seventh grade has a significant influence on the severity of alcohol-related problems reported by 10th grade. In 2003, the US alcohol industry voluntarily agreed not to advertise products on television programs for which greater than 30% of the audience is reasonably expected to be younger than 21 years. The National Research Council of the Institute of Medicine (now the National Academy of Medicine) proposed in that same year that the industry standard should move toward a 15% threshold for alcohol advertising on television. A recent evaluation of adherence to these standards conducted in 25 of the largest US television markets revealed that the alcohol industry has not consistently met its self-regulatory standards, indicating the need for continued public health surveillance of youth exposure to alcohol advertising.[77] Young people can be influenced in their alcohol use by other media, including movies, the Internet, and social media. A 2014 study demonstrated that adolescents with exposure to friends' risky online displays are more likely to use alcohol themselves.[78]

ADOLESCENT DEVELOPMENTAL AND NEUROBIOLOGICAL FACTORS

Normal Adolescent Brain Development

Over the past decade, great strides have been made in understanding the neurobiological basis of addiction. Studies investigating normal brain development have also yielded information that elucidates the effects of alcohol and other drugs on the developing adolescent brain. As summarized by Sowell et al,[79] results of postmortem studies have shown that myelination, a cellular maturational process of the lipid and protein sheath of nerve fibers, begins near the end of the second trimester of fetal development and extends well into the third decade of life and beyond. Autopsy results have revealed both a temporal and spatial systematic sequence of myelination, which progresses from inferior to superior and posterior to anterior regions of the brain. This sequencing results in initial brain myelination occurring in the brainstem and cerebellar regions and myelination of the cerebral hemispheres and frontal lobes occurring last. Converging evidence from electrophysiological and cerebral glucose metabolism studies shows that frontal lobe maturation is a relatively late process, and neuropsychological studies have shown that performance of tasks involving the frontal lobes continues to improve into adolescence and young adulthood.

Sowell et al[79] documented reduction in gray matter in the regions of the frontal cortex between adolescence and adulthood, which probably reflects increased myelination in the peripheral regions of the cortex. Gray matter loss, with pruning and elimination of neural connections during normative adolescent development, reflects a sculpting process that progresses in a caudal-to-rostral direction. The prefrontal cortex is the last area to reach adult maturation, and this may not be completed until young adulthood.[80] These changes are thought to improve cognitive processing in adulthood, such as cognitive control (ie, the ability to discount rewards) and executive functioning in risk-reward decision-making.[80] Results of neuropsychological studies have shown that the prefrontal cortex areas are essential for functions such as response inhibition, emotional regulation, planning, and organization, all of which may continue to develop between adolescence and young adulthood. Conversely, parietal, temporal, and occipital lobes show little change in maturation between adolescence and adulthood. Parietal association cortices are involved in spatial relationships and sensory functions, and the lateral temporal lobes are associated with auditory and language processing; these functions are largely mature by adolescence. Hence, the observed patterns of brain maturational changes are consistent with cognitive development.[79] Connections are being fine-tuned in adolescence with the pruning of overabundant synapses and the strengthening of relevant connections with development and experience. It is likely that the further development of the prefrontal cortex aids in the filtering of information and suppression of inappropriate actions.[80]

Effect of Substances on Adolescent Brain Development

Our current understanding of the biology of brain development in the adolescent has lent support to several models that explain the vulnerability of the adolescent to AUDs. One of these models posits that because the subcortical systems that are important for incentive and reward mature earlier than the areas responsible for cognitive control, this results in an "imbalance." Thus, activation and reinforcement of those incentive and reward pathways in response to the substance used may occur. This leaves youth uniquely vulnerable to the motivational aspects of alcohol and other drugs and the development of problematic substance use.[21] Without the modulating effect of cognitive control, an adolescent may be less able to resist the short-term result of using substances, compared with long-term, goal-oriented behaviors, such as abstaining. Given that these maturation imbalances in the development of different brain systems is greatest during adolescence, it is not surprising that teenagers may not be able to regulate the emotional or motivational states experienced with the use of substances as adults.[3,21] Researchers studying the role of several neurotransmitters in the development and maintenance of substance use and dependence have elucidated the underlying effects of these neurotransmitters in key areas of the brain involved in substance dependence and addiction.

Alcohol interacts with a number of neurotransmitter systems throughout the brain, including the inhibitory neurotransmitters γ-aminobutyric acid and glutamate, that are responsible for the euphoric as well as sedating effects of alcohol intoxication. In addition, neurons that release the neurotransmitter dopamine are activated by all addictive substances, including alcohol. The activation of dopamine release in the nucleus accumbens subregion of the basal ganglia, the area involved in both reward experiences and motivation, results in the "rewarding effect" experienced by users of alcohol and other drugs. In addition, the brain's endogenous opioid system and the 3 opioid receptors (μ, κ, and δ) interact with the dopamine system and play a key role in the effect that substances such as alcohol have on "rewards" and incentives to continue use of a substance. Brain imaging studies have demonstrated that both the opioid and the dopamine neurotransmitter systems are activated during alcohol and other substance use. The reader is referred to the comprehensive discussion of this in the Surgeon General's 2016 report: "Facing Addiction in America: The Surgeon General's Report on Alcohol, Drugs, and Health."[81]

Determining the specific effect of alcohol exposure or dependence on brain function and structure is challenging given potential biological differences that are normative versus those reflective of recent or past use of substances other than alcohol or of comorbid psychiatric disorders. In several studies, researchers using animal models have demonstrated the inhibition of the growth of adolescent neural progenitor cells with acute alcohol ingestions; similar results were observed with binge alcohol ingestion.[82,83] Chronic alcohol ingestion in animal models also disrupts neurogenesis primarily in the hippocampus, an area of the brain especially important for memory.[84]

In adolescents, varying levels of alcohol ingestion ranging from binge-pattern drinking to AUDs have been correlated with both structural and functional brain changes.[21] For example, hippocampal asymmetry was increased and hippocampal volumes were decreased in adolescents with alcohol abuse or dependence patterns compared with both controls who did not use substances and those reporting both alcohol and cannabis use.[85] In another study, adolescents with AUDs had smaller overall and white matter prefrontal cortex volumes compared with nondrinking controls, with girls with AUDs having larger decreases than boys with AUDs.[86] In studies in which researchers used diffusion tensor imaging techniques, which are used to assess white matter architecture, adolescent binge drinking or alcohol use was correlated with reduced factional anisotropy, which is an index that measures neural fiber tract integrity and organization.[87–90] These changes in white matter tract integrity were seen in multiple brain pathways, including those in the corpus callosum as well as limbic, brainstem, and cortical projection fibers.[87–89] It is important to note, however, that all of these studies are correlational and that a true causal relationship between alcohol use in youth and subsequent brain changes has not been demonstrated with this research.

Deficits in neurocognitive function have also been found in adolescents using both alcohol and marijuana compared with controls using no substances. These include deficits in attention, visuospatial processing in teenagers experiencing alcohol withdrawal, poorer performance with verbal and nonverbal retention tasks in adolescents reporting protracted alcohol use, and reduced speed of information processing and overall memory and executive functioning in those reporting alcohol dependence.[4,91–93] These abnormalities are postulated to result, in part, from the morphologic and functional changes seen in specific brain areas involved in memory (hippocampus) and executive function and decision-making (prefrontal cortex). In addition, genetic predisposition, such as family history of alcoholism, may enhance the vulnerability of specific brain areas, such as the hippocampus, to the effects of alcohol use in adolescents.[94] These potential genetic factors and epigenetic contributors (the impact of environmental and social factors on gene expression) are areas of active study.[21] The Adolescent Brain and Cognitive Development study, supported by the National Institutes of Health and the National Institute on Drug Abuse, is a 10-year longitudinal study that started in 2015 designed to assess the environmental, social, genetic, and biological factors involved in adolescent brain and cognitive development. The initial year of recruitment and baseline assessment of 11 875 10-year-olds has been completed, and this study holds great promise in terms of informing scientists and clinicians of the effect of licit and illicit substances, among many factors being studied, on the trajectory of brain development and cognitive functioning over the course of adolescent and young adulthood.[95]

PREVENTION

Several recent Cochrane reviews have examined the prevention of substance abuse in young people through family-based prevention programs,[96] universal school-based prevention programs,[97] brief school-based interventions,[98] universal multicomponent prevention programs,[99] and mentoring programs.[100] Although there were variations in programs in all of these reviews and generally few high-quality studies, all of these prevention strategies showed some success. Family-based prevention programs typically take the form of supporting the development of parenting skills, including parental support, nurturing behaviors, establishing clear boundaries or rules, and parental monitoring. The development of social and peer resistance skills and the development of positive peer affiliations can also be addressed in these programs. The Cochrane systematic review found that "the effects of family-based prevention are small but generally consistent and persistent into the medium- to longer-term"[96] and are consistent with an earlier systematic review supporting the effectiveness of family-focused prevention programs.[101]

SCREENING AND BRIEF INTERVENTIONS

Recognition of the pervasive use of alcohol among young people, the hazards that may be encountered with even low-level use, and the association between early initiation of alcohol use and future alcohol problems underscores the need to integrate our approaches to alcohol and other drug use by youth into pediatric primary care. The AAP recommends that pediatricians screen and discuss substance use as part of anticipatory guidance and preventive care.[102–104] Screening, brief intervention, and referral to treatment (SBIRT) for youth is such an integrated approach that has grown in recent years to bridge the gap between universal prevention programs and specialty substance abuse treatment by pediatric primary care providers.[105,106] The reader is referred to the AAP clinical report on SBIRT for pediatricians.[104] The effectiveness of SBIRT is well supported for addressing hazardous use of alcohol by adults in medical settings, but there is less evidence for its effectiveness in adolescents.[107–115]

Several screening strategies have been validated and used to identify youth at risk for or involved in the use of alcohol and other substances that can be incorporated into general psychosocial screening efforts, such as interviewing strategies like HEADSS (home, education, activities, drugs and alcohol, sex, suicidality)[116] and SSHADESS (strengths, school, home, activities, drugs and alcohol, substance use, emotions and depression, sexuality, safety).[117] The CRAFFT is a tool developed for screening adolescents for alcohol and other substance use with 3 introductory questions followed by 6 questions using the CRAFFT mnemonic.[118] It has been well validated and is brief enough for use in busy clinical settings.[119] In 2011, the National Institute on Alcohol Abuse and Alcoholism (NIAAA) collaborated with the AAP to develop a brief screening tool to assist health care providers in identifying alcohol use, AUD, and risk for use in children and adolescents ages 9 to 18 years.[120] This tool includes brief 2-question screeners and support materials about brief intervention and referral to treatment and is designed to help surmount common obstacles to youth alcohol screening in primary care. The screen administration varies by age and grade and focuses on drinking frequency over the previous 12 months to determine level of risk.[121] This tool has been expanded to include tobacco and other substances and is sensitive and specific for identifying substance use disorders in a pediatric clinic population.[122] Although developed for use primarily in the primary care setting, Spirito et al[123] have demonstrated its usefulness in screening for AUDs in pediatric emergency settings.

In several studies, researchers have confirmed the validity of using a single question about the frequency of use of alcohol and other drugs over the previous 12 months to determine level of risk.[124] Studying a population of adolescents and young adults in rural Pennsylvania, Clark et al[124] compared a single question of past-year frequency of alcohol use versus comprehensive diagnostic interviews on the basis of DSM-5 criteria for AUD to determine the validity of this question in identifying problematic alcohol use. They found both high sensitivity and specificity for adolescents ages 12 to 17 years using 3 or more days with 1 or more drinks as a cutoff to identify AUDs. For young adults 18 to 20 years of age, using 12 or more days or 12 or more drinks over the previous year also had excellent ability to identify AUDs.[124] Levy et al[125] have also validated a single-question screen, referred to as the "S2BI": "In the past year, how many times have you used alcohol?" They have found that responses that include never, once or twice, monthly, weekly, almost daily, or daily can differentiate between those with mild, moderate, and severe AUDs, per DSM-5 criteria, and can indicate those individuals who would benefit from education versus brief intervention or more-specific substance abuse treatment.[125] This screening question has also been shown to identify problematic use of illicit drugs, over-the-counter medications, and tobacco. These screening tools, as well as the NIAAA screening tool, continue to be validated, and the results reported here are promising.

Questions often remain about how to incorporate parents into this screening process and how and when to provide confidentiality for a youth's report of underage alcohol use. The NIAAA 2-question screening tool recommends that screening begin as early as 9 to 11 years of age, and given that most preteens will be questioned in the presence of a parent or guardian, this offers an opportunity to discuss the parent's philosophy regarding alcohol use by minors, situations in which they might deem it appropriate (such as at holidays), and their own practices regarding their own drinking and consequences for their child's drinking. This screening can also be performed routinely for all adolescents during preventive care visits. For the older adolescent, whenever possible, it is preferable to include parents in any discussion with a youth who reports drinking; however, when this is seen by the youth as a major deterrent to his or her alliance with the provider and there are no "red flag" behaviors that are believed to be unsafe, such as the youth riding or driving after drinking, heavy binge drinking, or when an AUD is suspected, maintaining confidentiality and counseling the adolescent is often preferable because this maintains the alliance between the provider and the adolescent. There are no hard and fast rules as to when parents should be included in discussions about their adolescent's alcohol use; this can be a delicate matter and is generally a judgment call by the primary medical provider, unless the safety of the youth is put in jeopardy by drinking behaviors. Studies have shown that parents tend to underestimate the extent of their teenagers' drinking behaviors, and including parents in the discussions with their teenagers often serves to highlight a greater amount of use than what is anticipated by parents. Discussions about minimizing risk, such as contracting with the youth to call parents if they are concerned about friends drinking while driving, may also be helpful. Students Against Destructive Decisions is a youth-focused organization promoting healthy and safe decision-making, especially around driving behaviors. The Students Against Destructive Decisions Web site (https://www.sadd.org/what-we-care-about/) provides educational information as well as the "Contract for Life," which is a contract that teenagers sign along with their parents, promising to avoid alcohol and other substances when driving.

Once screening has been conducted and the level of risk has been determined, the provider can provide anticipatory guidance supporting abstinence, perform brief intervention strategies, or refer the adolescent for further evaluation or to a higher level of treatment. Brief intervention strategies are short, efficient, office-based techniques that health care providers who work with adolescents can use to detect alcohol use and intervene. On the basis of the principles of motivational interviewing, these procedures can be readily performed in the office setting, build on the individual's readiness to change drinking behaviors, and support the adolescent's need for involvement in one's own health care choices and decisions. Harris et al[105] have provided an excellent review of counseling strategies at different levels of risk behaviors of young people, and the NIAAA Alcohol Screening Practitioner Guide provides strategies for brief intervention at different ages.[120] D'Onofrio and colleagues[126] have developed a brief (5- to 7-minute) scripted intervention approach, the Brief Negotiation Interview (BNI), for use with adults reporting harmful and hazardous alcohol use in the emergency setting, and Ryan et al[127] have adapted this BNI for use in a pediatric residency training setting for use with adolescents in a primary care clinic. Pediatrics residents trained in the BNI reported that this intervention was easily learned and highly applicable in clinical settings with teens reporting alcohol and other illicit substance use.[127]

TREATMENT

The National Institute on Drug Abuse publication "Principles of Adolescent Substance Use Disorders Treatment: A Research Guide" is a comprehensive guide of evidence-based approaches to treating adolescent substance use disorders and emphasizes that treatment is not "one size fits all" but requires taking into consideration the needs of the individual, including his or her developmental stage; cognitive abilities; the influence of friends, family, and others; and mental and physical health conditions.[128] The AAP clinical report on SBIRT also includes a list of optimal standards for a substance use disorder treatment program.[66] Behavioral therapies are effective in treating alcohol and other substance use disorders as well as multiple substances and include individual therapy, such as cognitive-behavioral therapy and motivational enhancement therapy. Family-based approaches, including multidimensional family therapy and multisystemic therapy, have been proven to be effective.[129] Addiction medications for AUD include acamprosate, disulfiram, and naltrexone. Medication-assisted therapies are not commonly used to treat adolescent AUDs but may be used in specific circumstances. These medications are approved by the US Food and Drug Administration for treatment of people 18 years and older.

In most cases, the primary care pediatrician's initial role is to identify, through screening, teenagers in need of intervention and referral for further treatment. However, continued involvement by the primary pediatric provider with the teenager and the family, through regular follow-up and care coordination, is essential in any treatment plan after referral.

CONCLUSIONS

Although it is heartening that alcohol use among adolescents and youth has decreased over the last several years, researchers have even more clearly elucidated links between alcohol use and deleterious effects on adolescents' developing brains as well as other aspects of their physical and mental health. Pediatricians are in an excellent position to recognize risk factors for use and screen for hazardous use among youth. Pediatricians can also assess youth whose screening results are positive for alcohol use to determine the level of intervention needed. Brief intervention techniques used by pediatricians have been shown to be effective in a limited number of studies and may be especially helpful in aiding youth and their families to obtain appropriate treatment of AUDs. Pediatricians also have an important advocacy role in health systems' changes as well as legislative efforts, such as increasing alcohol taxes, resisting efforts to weaken minimum drinking age laws, and supporting GDL programs.[130,131]

LEAD AUTHORS

Sheryl A. Ryan, MD, FAAP
Patricia Kokotailo, MD, MPH, FAAP

COMMITTEE ON SUBSTANCE USE AND PREVENTION, 2018–2019

Sheryl A. Ryan, MD, FAAP, Chairperson
Deepa R. Camenga, MD, MHS, FAAP
Stephen W. Patrick, MD, MPH, MS, FAAP
Jennifer Plumb, MD, MPH, FAAP
Joanna Quigley, MD, FAAP
Leslie Walker-Harding, MD, FAAP

FORMER COMMITTEE MEMBER

Patricia Kokotailo, MD, MPH, FAAP

LIAISON

Gregory Tau, MD, PhD – *American Academy of Child and Adolescent Psychiatry*

STAFF

Renee Jarrett, MPH

ABBREVIATIONS

AAP: American Academy of Pediatrics
AUD: alcohol use disorder
BAC: blood alcohol concentration
BNI: Brief Negotiation Interview
DSM-5: *Diagnostic and Statistical Manual of Mental Disorders, Fifth Edition*
GDL: graduated driver licensing
NIAAA: National Institute on Alcohol Abuse and Alcoholism
SBIRT: screening, brief intervention, and referral to treatment

POTENTIAL CONFLICT OF INTEREST: The authors have indicated they have no potential conflicts of interest to disclose.

REFERENCES

1. Johnston LD, Miech RA, O'Malley PM, Bachman JG, Schulenberg JE, Patrick ME. *Monitoring the Future: National Survey Results on Drug Use, 1975-2018. Overview, Key Findings on Adolescent Drug Use*. Ann Arbor, MI: Institute for Social Research, University of Michigan; 2019. Available at: www.monitoringthefuture.org//pubs/monographs/mtf-overview2018.pdf. Accessed March 26, 2019
2. Giedd JN. The teen brain: insights from neuroimaging. *J Adolesc Health*. 2008; 42(4):335–343
3. Chambers RA, Taylor JR, Potenza MN. Developmental neurocircuitry of motivation in adolescence: a critical period of addiction vulnerability. *Am J Psychiatry*. 2003;160(6): 1041–1052
4. Brown SA, Tapert SF. Adolescence and the trajectory of alcohol use: basic to clinical studies. *Ann N Y Acad Sci*. 2004;1021:234–244
5. Quigley J; American Academy of Pediatrics, Committee on Substance Use Prevention. Policy statement: alcohol use by youth. *Pediatrics*. 2019; 144(1):e20191356
6. Donovan JE. Estimated blood alcohol concentrations for child and adolescent drinking and their implications for screening instruments. *Pediatrics*. 2009;123(6). Available at: www.pediatrics.org/cgi/content/full/123/6/e975
7. Kann L, McManus T, Harris WA, et al. Youth risk behavior surveillance - United States, 2017. *MMWR Surveill Summ*. 2018;67(8):1–114
8. Center for Behavioral Health Statistics and Quality. *2017 National Survey on Drug Use and Health: Detailed Tables*. Rockville, MD: Substance Abuse and Mental Health Services Administration; 2018. Available at: https://www.samhsa.gov/data/sites/default/files/cbhsq-reports/NSDUHDetailedTabs2017/NSDUHDetailedTabs2017.pdf. Accessed March 26, 2019
9. Grant BF, Dawson DA. Age at onset of alcohol use and its association with DSM-IV alcohol abuse and dependence: results from the National Longitudinal Alcohol Epidemiologic Survey. *J Subst Abuse*. 1997;9:103–110
10. Grant BF, Stinson FS, Harford TC. Age at onset of alcohol use and DSM-IV alcohol abuse and dependence: a 12-year

follow-up. *J Subst Abuse.* 2001;13(4): 493–504

11. DeWit DJ, Adlaf EM, Offord DR, Ogborne AC. Age at first alcohol use: a risk factor for the development of alcohol disorders. *Am J Psychiatry.* 2000;157(5): 745–750
12. Dawson DA, Goldstein RB, Chou SP, Ruan WJ, Grant BF. Age at first drink and the first incidence of adult-onset DSM-IV alcohol use disorders. *Alcohol Clin Exp Res.* 2008;32(12):2149–2160
13. Hingson RW, Heeren T, Winter MR. Age at drinking onset and alcohol dependence: age at onset, duration, and severity. *Arch Pediatr Adolesc Med.* 2006;160(7): 739–746
14. Heron J, Macleod J, Munafò MR, et al. Patterns of alcohol use in early adolescence predict problem use at age 16. *Alcohol Alcohol.* 2012;47(2):169–177
15. Lee LO, Young-Wolff KC, Kendler KS, Prescott CA. The effects of age at drinking onset and stressful life events on alcohol use in adulthood: a replication and extension using a population-based twin sample [published correction appears in *Alcohol Clin Exp Res.* 2012;36(6):1116]. *Alcohol Clin Exp Res.* 2012;36(4):693–704
16. American Psychiatric Association. Diagnostic and Statistical Manual of Mental Disorders *(DSM-5).* 5th ed. Arlington, VA: American Psychiatric Publishing; 2013
17. Martin CS, Winters KC. Diagnosis and assessment of alcohol use disorders among adolescents. *Alcohol Health Res World.* 1998;22(2):95–105
18. Clark DB. The natural history of adolescent alcohol use disorders. *Addiction.* 2004;99(suppl 2):5–22
19. Irons BL. Alcohol use disorders: a clinical update. *Adolesc Med Clin.* 2006;17(2):259–282
20. Winters KC, Martin CS, Chung T. Substance use disorders in DSM-V when applied to adolescents. *Addiction.* 2011;106(5):882–884; discussion 895–897
21. Hammond CJ, Mayes LC, Potenza MN. Neurobiology of adolescent substance use and addictive behaviors: treatment implications. *Adolesc Med State Art Rev.* 2014;25(1):15–32
22. Foxcroft DR, Ireland D, Lister-Sharp DJ, Lowe G, Breen R. Primary prevention for alcohol misuse in young people. *Cochrane Database Syst Rev.* 2002;(3): CD003024
23. Spear LP, Varlinskaya EI. Adolescence. Alcohol sensitivity, tolerance, and intake. *Recent Dev Alcohol.* 2005;17: 143–159
24. Shults RA; Centers for Disease Control and Prevention (CDC). Vital signs: drinking and driving among high school students aged ≥16 years - United States, 1991-2011. *MMWR Morb Mortal Wkly Rep.* 2012;61(39):796–800
25. Centers for Disease Control (CDC). Alcohol-related traffic fatalities among youth and young adults–United States, 1982-1989. *MMWR Morb Mortal Wkly Rep.* 1991;40(11):178–179, 185–187
26. Shults RA, Elder RW, Sleet DA, et al; Task Force on Community Preventive Services. Reviews of evidence regarding interventions to reduce alcohol-impaired driving. *Am J Prev Med.* 2001;21(suppl 4):66–88
27. Voas RB, Torres P, Romano E, Lacey JH. Alcohol-related risk of driver fatalities: an update using 2007 data. *J Stud Alcohol Drugs.* 2012;73(3):341–350
28. Insurance Institute for Highway Safety, Highway Loss Data Institute. Graduated driver licensing introduction. Available at: www.iihs.org/iihs/topics/laws/graduatedlicenseintro. Accessed March 26, 2019
29. Fell JC, Todd M, Voas RB. A national evaluation of the nighttime and passenger restriction components of graduated driver licensing. *J Safety Res.* 2011;42(4):283–290
30. Hartling L, Wiebe N, Russell K, Petruk J, Spinola C, Klassen TP. Graduated driver licensing for reducing motor vehicle crashes among young drivers. *Cochrane Database Syst Rev.* 2004;(2): CD003300
31. Marcotte TD, Bekman NM, Meyer RA, Brown SA. High-risk driving behaviors among adolescent binge drinkers. *Am J Drug Alcohol Abuse.* 2012;38(4): 322–327
32. Dubois S, Mullen N, Weaver B, Bédard M. The combined effects of alcohol and cannabis on driving: impact on crash risk. *Forensic Sci Int.* 2015;248:94–100
33. National Center for Statistics and Analysis. *2016 Fatal Motor Vehicle Crashes: Overview. Traffic Safety Facts Research Note.* Report No. DOT HS 812 456. Washington, DC: National Highway Traffic Safety Administration; 2017. Available at: https://crashstats.nhtsa.dot.gov/Api/Public/ViewPublication/812456. Accessed March 26, 2019
34. National Center for Statistics and Analysis. *Alcohol-Impaired Driving: 2016 Data. Traffic Safety Facts.* Report No. DOT HS 812 450. Washington, DC: National Highway Traffic Safety Administration; 2017. Available at: https://crashstats.nhtsa.dot.gov/Api/Public/ViewPublication/812450. Accessed March 26, 2019
35. Windle M. Suicidal behaviors and alcohol use among adolescents: a developmental psychopathology perspective. *Alcohol Clin Exp Res.* 2004; 28(suppl 5):29S–37S
36. Miller TR, Levy DT, Spicer RS, Taylor DM. Societal costs of underage drinking. *J Stud Alcohol.* 2006;67(4):519–528
37. Birckmayer J, Hemenway D. Minimum-age drinking laws and youth suicide, 1970-1990. *Am J Public Health.* 1999; 89(9):1365–1368
38. Simkin DR. Adolescent substance use disorders and comorbidity. *Pediatr Clin North Am.* 2002;49(2):463–477
39. Vitale S, van de Mheen D. Illicit drug use and injuries: a review of emergency room studies. *Drug Alcohol Depend.* 2006;82(1):1–9
40. Clark DB, Lynch KG, Donovan JE, Block GD. Health problems in adolescents with alcohol use disorders: self-report, liver injury, and physical examination findings and correlates. *Alcohol Clin Exp Res.* 2001;25(9):1350–1359
41. Arria AM, Dohey MA, Mezzich AC, Bukstein OG, Van Thiel DH. Self-reported health problems and physical symptomatology in adolescent alcohol abusers. *J Adolesc Health.* 1995;16(3): 226–231
42. Ellickson PL, Tucker JS, Klein DJ. Ten-year prospective study of public health problems associated with early drinking. *Pediatrics.* 2003;111(5 pt 1): 949–955

43. Champion HL, Foley KL, DuRant RH, Hensberry R, Altman D, Wolfson M. Adolescent sexual victimization, use of alcohol and other substances, and other health risk behaviors. *J Adolesc Health.* 2004;35(4):321–328

44. Miller JW, Naimi TS, Brewer RD, Jones SE. Binge drinking and associated health risk behaviors among high school students. *Pediatrics.* 2007; 119(1):76–85

45. Stueve A, O'Donnell LN. Early alcohol initiation and subsequent sexual and alcohol risk behaviors among urban youths. *Am J Public Health.* 2005;95(5): 887–893

46. Kaprio J, Koskenvuo M, Langinvainio H, Romanov K, Sarna S, Rose RJ. Genetic influences on use and abuse of alcohol: a study of 5638 adult Finnish twin brothers. *Alcohol Clin Exp Res.* 1987; 11(4):349–356

47. Kendler KS, Prescott CA, Neale MC, Pedersen NL. Temperance board registration for alcohol abuse in a national sample of Swedish male twins, born 1902 to 1949. *Arch Gen Psychiatry.* 1997;54(2):178–184

48. McGue M, Pickens RW, Svikis DS. Sex and age effects on the inheritance of alcohol problems: a twin study. *J Abnorm Psychol.* 1992;101(1):3–17

49. Han C, McGue MK, Iacono WG. Lifetime tobacco, alcohol and other substance use in adolescent Minnesota twins: univariate and multivariate behavioral genetic analyses. *Addiction.* 1999;94(7): 981–993

50. Maes HH, Woodard CE, Murrelle L, et al. Tobacco, alcohol and drug use in eight- to sixteen-year-old twins: the Virginia Twin Study of Adolescent Behavioral Development. *J Stud Alcohol.* 1999; 60(3):293–305

51. McGue M, Elkins I, Iacono WG. Genetic and environmental influences on adolescent substance use and abuse. *Am J Med Genet.* 2000;96(5):671–677

52. Rhee SH, Hewitt JK, Young SE, Corley RP, Crowley TJ, Stallings MC. Genetic and environmental influences on substance initiation, use, and problem use in adolescents. *Arch Gen Psychiatry.* 2003; 60(12):1256–1264

53. Chorlian DB, Rangaswamy M, Manz N, et al. Genetic and neurophysiological correlates of the age of onset of alcohol use disorders in adolescents and young adults. *Behav Genet.* 2013;43(5):386–401

54. Pagan JL, Rose RJ, Viken RJ, Pulkkinen L, Kaprio J, Dick DM. Genetic and environmental influences on stages of alcohol use across adolescence and into young adulthood. *Behav Genet.* 2006;36(4):483–497

55. Miranda R, Ray L, Justus A, et al. Initial evidence of an association between OPRM1 and adolescent alcohol misuse. *Alcohol Clin Exp Res.* 2010;34(1):112–122

56. Biederman J, Faraone SV, Monuteaux MC, Feighner JA. Patterns of alcohol and drug use in adolescents can be predicted by parental substance use disorders. *Pediatrics.* 2000;106(4): 792–797

57. Pemberton MR, Colliver JD, Robbins TM, Gfroerer JC. *Underage Alcohol Use: Findings from the 2002-2006 National Surveys on Drug Use and Health.* HHS Publication No. SMA08-4333, Analytic Series A-30. Rockville, MD: Substance Abuse and Mental Health Services Administration, Office of Applied Studies; 2008

58. Nelson DE, Naimi TS, Brewer RD, Nelson HA. State alcohol-use estimates among youth and adults, 1993-2005. *Am J Prev Med.* 2009;36(3):218–224

59. Foley KL, Altman D, Durant RH, Wolfson M. Adults' approval and adolescents' alcohol use. *J Adolesc Health.* 2004; 35(4):345.e17–345.e26

60. Jackson C, Henriksen L, Dickinson D. Alcohol-specific socialization, parenting behaviors and alcohol use by children. *J Stud Alcohol.* 1999;60(3):362–367

61. Yu J. The association between parental alcohol-related behaviors and children's drinking. *Drug Alcohol Depend.* 2003;69(3):253–262

62. Ryan SM, Jorm AF, Lubman DI. Parenting factors associated with reduced adolescent alcohol use: a systematic review of longitudinal studies. *Aust N Z J Psychiatry.* 2010;44(9):774–783

63. Lipari RN, Van Horn SL. Children living with parents who have a substance use disorder. *The CBHSQ Report.* August 24, 2017. Rockville, MD: Center for Behavioral Health Statistics and Quality, Substance Abuse and Mental Health Services Administration. Available at: https://www.samhsa.gov/data/sites/default/files/report_3223/ShortReport-3223.pdf. Accessed March 26, 2019

64. Lipari RN, Van Horn SL. Children living with parents who have a substance use disorder. The CBHSQ report: August 24, 2017. Center for Behavioral Health Statistics and Quality, SAMHSA, Rockville, MD. Available at: https://www.samhsa.gov/data/sites/default/files/report_3223/ShortReport-3223.pdf. Accessed May 20, 2019

65. Anda RF, Whitfield CL, Felitti VJ, et al. Adverse childhood experiences, alcoholic parents, and later risk of alcoholism and depression. *Psychiatr Serv.* 2002;53(8):1001–1009

66. Smith VC, Wilson CR; Committee on Substance Use and Prevention. Families affected by parental substance use. *Pediatrics.* 2016;138(2):e20161575

67. Cruz JE, Emery RE, Turkheimer E. Peer network drinking predicts increased alcohol use from adolescence to early adulthood after controlling for genetic and shared environmental selection. *Dev Psychol.* 2012;48(5):1390–1402

68. US Department of Health and Human Services. *Report to Congress on the Prevention and Reduction of Underage Drinking.* Rockville, MD: Substance Abuse and Mental Health Services Administration; 2013. Available at: https://www.nabca.org/sites/default/files/assets/files/Report-to-Congress-on-Prevention-Reduction-Underage-Drinking.pdf. Accessed July 9, 2018

69. Substance Abuse and Mental Health Services Administration. *Results from the 2011 National Survey on Drug Use and Health: Summary of National Findings.* NSDUH Series H- 44, HHS Publication No. SMA 12-4713. Rockville, MD: Substance Abuse and Mental Health Services Administration; 2012. Available at: https://www.samhsa.gov/data/sites/default/files/Revise d2k11NSDUHSummNatFindings/Revise d2k11NSDUHSummNatFindings/NSDUHresults2011.htm. Accessed March 26, 2019

70. Mayer RR, Forster JL, Murray DM, Wagenaar AC. Social settings and situations of underage drinking. *J Stud Alcohol.* 1998;59(2):207–215

71. Clapp JD, Shillington AM, Segars LB. Deconstructing contexts of binge

drinking among college students. *Am J Drug Alcohol Abuse*. 2000;26(1): 139–154

72. Council on Communications and Media. Media use in school-aged children and adolescents. *Pediatrics*. 2016;138(5): e20162592
73. Jernigan D, Noel J, Landon J, Thornton N, Lobstein T. Alcohol marketing and youth alcohol consumption: a systematic review of longitudinal studies published since 2008. *Addiction*. 2017;112(suppl 1):7–20
74. Anderson P, de Bruijn A, Angus K, Gordon R, Hastings G. Impact of alcohol advertising and media exposure on adolescent alcohol use: a systematic review of longitudinal studies. *Alcohol Alcohol*. 2009;44(3):229–243
75. Hanewinkel R, Sargent JD, Hunt K, et al. Portrayal of alcohol consumption in movies and drinking initiation in low-risk adolescents. *Pediatrics*. 2014; 133(6):973–982
76. Grenard JL, Dent CW, Stacy AW. Exposure to alcohol advertisements and teenage alcohol-related problems. *Pediatrics*. 2013;131(2). Available at: www.pediatrics.org/cgi/content/full/131/2/e369
77. Centers for Disease Control and Prevention (CDC). Youth exposure to alcohol advertising on television–25 markets, United States, 2010. *MMWR Morb Mortal Wkly Rep*. 2013;62(44): 877–880
78. Huang GC, Unger JB, Soto D, et al. Peer influences: the impact of online and offline friendship networks on adolescent smoking and alcohol use. *J Adolesc Health*. 2014;54(5):508–514
79. Sowell ER, Thompson PM, Holmes CJ, Jernigan TL, Toga AW. In vivo evidence for post-adolescent brain maturation in frontal and striatal regions. *Nat Neurosci*. 1999;2(10):859–861
80. Casey BJ, Tottenham N, Liston C, Durston S. Imaging the developing brain: what have we learned about cognitive development? *Trends Cogn Sci*. 2005;9(3):104–110
81. US Department of Health and Human Services, Office of the Surgeon General. *Facing Addiction in America: The Surgeon General's Report on Alcohol, Drugs, and Health*. Washington, DC: US Department of Health and Human Services; 2016
82. Crews FT, Mdzinarishvili A, Kim D, He J, Nixon K. Neurogenesis in adolescent brain is potently inhibited by ethanol. *Neuroscience*. 2006;137(2):437–445
83. Crews F, Nixon K, Kim D, et al. BHT blocks NF-kappaB activation and ethanol-induced brain damage. *Alcohol Clin Exp Res*. 2006;30(11):1938–1949
84. He J, Nixon K, Shetty AK, Crews FT. Chronic alcohol exposure reduces hippocampal neurogenesis and dendritic growth of newborn neurons. *Eur J Neurosci*. 2005;21(10):2711–2720
85. Medina KL, Schweinsburg AD, Cohen-Zion M, Nagel BJ, Tapert SF. Effects of alcohol and combined marijuana and alcohol use during adolescence on hippocampal volume and asymmetry. *Neurotoxicol Teratol*. 2007;29(1):141–152
86. Medina KL, McQueeny T, Nagel BJ, Hanson KL, Schweinsburg AD, Tapert SF. Prefrontal cortex volumes in adolescents with alcohol use disorders: unique gender effects. *Alcohol Clin Exp Res*. 2008;32(3):386–394
87. Roberts TP, Schwartz ES. Principles and implementation of diffusion-weighted and diffusion tensor imaging. *Pediatr Radiol*. 2007;37(8):739–748
88. McQueeny T, Schweinsburg BC, Schweinsburg AD, et al. Altered white matter integrity in adolescent binge drinkers. *Alcohol Clin Exp Res*. 2009; 33(7):1278–1285
89. Tapert SF, Theilmann RJ, Schweinsburg AD. Reduced fractional anisotropy in the splenium of adolescents with alcohol use disorders [abstract]. *Proc Int Soc Magn Reson Med*. 2003;11(8217):2241
90. Schmithorst VJ, Wilke M, Dardzinski BJ, Holland SK. Cognitive functions correlate with white matter architecture in a normal pediatric population: a diffusion tensor MRI study. *Hum Brain Mapp*. 2005;26(2): 139–147
91. Brown SA, Tapert SF, Granholm E, Delis DC. Neurocognitive functioning of adolescents: effects of protracted alcohol use. *Alcohol Clin Exp Res*. 2000; 24(2):164–171
92. Tapert SF, Brown SA. Substance dependence, family history of alcohol dependence and neuropsychological functioning in adolescence. *Addiction*. 2000;95(7):1043–1053
93. Tapert SF, Granholm E, Leedy NG, Brown SA. Substance use and withdrawal: neuropsychological functioning over 8 years in youth. *J Int Neuropsychol Soc*. 2002;8(7):873–883
94. Hanson KL, Medina KL, Nagel BJ, Spadoni AD, Gorlick A, Tapert SF. Hippocampal volumes in adolescents with and without a family history of alcoholism. *Am J Drug Alcohol Abuse*. 2010;36(3):161–167
95. Adolescent Brain Cognitive Development Study. The longitudinal adolescent brain cognitive development study. Available at: https://abcdstudy.org. Accessed July 24, 2018
96. Foxcroft DR, Tsertsvadze A. Universal family-based prevention programs for alcohol misuse in young people. *Cochrane Database Syst Rev*. 2011;(9): CD009308
97. Foxcroft DR, Tsertsvadze A. Universal school-based prevention programs for alcohol misuse in young people. *Cochrane Database Syst Rev*. 2011;(5): CD009113
98. Carney T, Myers BJ, Louw J, Okwundu CI. Brief school-based interventions and behavioural outcomes for substance-using adolescents. *Cochrane Database Syst Rev*. 2014;(2):CD008969
99. Foxcroft DR, Tsertsvadze A. Universal multi-component prevention programs for alcohol misuse in young people. *Cochrane Database Syst Rev*. 2011;(9): CD009307
100. Thomas RE, Lorenzetti D, Spragins W. Mentoring adolescents to prevent drug and alcohol use. *Cochrane Database Syst Rev*. 2011;(11):CD007381
101. Petrie J, Bunn F, Byrne G. Parenting programmes for preventing tobacco, alcohol or drugs misuse in children <18: a systematic review. *Health Educ Res*. 2007;22(2):177–191
102. Hagan JF, Shaw JS, Duncan PM, eds. *Bright Futures: Guidelines for Health Supervision of Infants, Children, and Adolescents*. 4th ed. Elk Grove Village, IL: American Academy of Pediatrics; 2017
103. Committee on Substance Use and Prevention. Substance use screening,

brief intervention, and referral to treatment. *Pediatrics*. 2016;138(1): e20161210

104. Levy SJ, Williams JF; Committee on Substance Use and Prevention. Substance use screening, brief intervention, and referral to treatment. *Pediatrics*. 2016;138(1):e20161211

105. Harris SK, Louis-Jacques J, Knight JR. Screening and brief intervention for alcohol and other abuse. *Adolesc Med State Art Rev*. 2014;25(1):126–156

106. Babor TF, McRee BG, Kassebaum PA, Grimaldi PL, Ahmed K, Bray J. Screening, Brief Intervention, and Referral to Treatment (SBIRT): toward a public health approach to the management of substance abuse. *Subst Abus*. 2007;28(3):7–30

107. Jonas DE, Garbutt JC, Amick HR, et al. Behavioral counseling after screening for alcohol misuse in primary care: a systematic review and meta-analysis for the U.S. Preventive Services Task Force. *Ann Intern Med*. 2012;157(9): 645–654

108. Kaner EF, Beyer F, Dickinson HO, et al. Effectiveness of brief alcohol interventions in primary care populations. *Cochrane Database Syst Rev*. 2007;18(2):CD004148

109. Bertholet N, Daeppen JB, Wietlisbach V, Fleming M, Burnand B. Reduction of alcohol consumption by brief alcohol intervention in primary care: systematic review and meta-analysis. *Arch Intern Med*. 2005;165(9):986–995

110. O'Donnell A, Anderson P, Newbury-Birch D, et al. The impact of brief alcohol interventions in primary healthcare: a systematic review of reviews. *Alcohol Alcohol*. 2014;49(1):66–78

111. Mitchell SG, Gryczynski J, Gonzales A, et al. Screening, brief intervention, and referral to treatment (SBIRT) for substance use in a school-based program: services and outcomes. *Am J Addict*. 2012;21(suppl 1):S5–S13

112. Mitchell SG, Gryczynski J, O'Grady KE, Schwartz RP. SBIRT for adolescent drug and alcohol use: current status and future directions. *J Subst Abuse Treat*. 2013;44(5):463–472

113. Yuma-Guerrero PJ, Lawson KA, Velasquez MM, von Sternberg K, Maxson T, Garcia N. Screening, brief intervention, and referral for alcohol use in adolescents: a systematic review. *Pediatrics*. 2012;130(1):115–122

114. Agerwala SM, McCance-Katz EF. Integrating screening, brief intervention, and referral to treatment (SBIRT) into clinical practice settings: a brief review. *J Psychoactive Drugs*. 2012;44(4):307–317

115. Curtis BL, McLellan AT, Gabellini BN. Translating SBIRT to public school settings: an initial test of feasibility. *J Subst Abuse Treat*. 2014;46(1):15–21

116. Goldenring J, Cohen G. Getting into adolescent heads. *Contemp Pediatr*. 1988;5(7):75–90

117. Ginsburg K. Viewing our adolescent patients through a positive lens. *Contemp Pediatr*. 2007;24(1):65–76

118. Center for Adolescent Substance Abuse Research, Children's Hospital Boston. The CRAFFT screening questions. Available at: https://www.integration.samhsa.gov/clinical-practice/sbirt/CRAFFT_Screening_interview.pdf. Accessed March 26, 2019

119. Knight JR, Shrier LA, Bravender TD, Farrell M, Vander Bilt J, Shaffer HJ. A new brief screen for adolescent substance abuse. *Arch Pediatr Adolesc Med*. 1999;153(6):591–596

120. National Institute on Alcohol Abuse and Alcoholism, American Academy of Pediatrics. *Alcohol Screening and Brief Intervention for Youth: A Practitioner's Guide*. Rockville, MD: National Institute on Alcohol Abuse and Alcoholism; 2011. Available at: www.niaaa.nih.gov/YouthGuide. Accessed March 26, 2019

121. Chung T, Smith GT, Donovan JE, et al. Drinking frequency as a brief screen for adolescent alcohol problems. *Pediatrics*. 2012;129(2):205–212

122. Kelly SM, Gryczynski J, Mitchell SG, Kirk A, O'Grady KE, Schwartz RP. Validity of brief screening instrument for adolescent tobacco, alcohol, and drug use. *Pediatrics*. 2014;133(5): 819–826

123. Spirito A, Bromberg JR, Casper TC, et al; Pediatric Emergency Care Applied Research Network. Reliability and validity of a two-question alcohol screen in the pediatric emergency department. *Pediatrics*. 2016;138(6):e20160691

124. Clark DB, Martin CS, Chung T, et al. Screening for underage drinking and Diagnostic and Statistical Manual of Mental Disorders, 5th Edition alcohol use disorder in rural primary care practice. *J Pediatr*. 2016;173:214–220

125. Levy S, Weiss R, Sherritt L, et al. An electronic screen for triaging adolescent substance use by risk levels. *JAMA Pediatr*. 2014;168(9): 822–828

126. D'Onofrio G, Pantalon MV, Degutis LC, Fiellin DA, O'connor PG. Development implementation and testing of an emergency physician-performed brief intervention for harmful and hazardous drinkers in the emergency department. *Acad Emerg Med*. 2005; 12(3):249–256

127. Ryan SA, Martel S, Pantalon M, et al. Screening, brief intervention, and referral to treatment (SBIRT) for alcohol and other drug use among adolescents: evaluation of a pediatric residency curriculum. *Subst Abus*. 2012; 33(3):251–260

128. National Institutes of Health, National Institute on Drug Abuse. *Principles of Adolescent Substance Use Disorder Treatment: A Research-based Guide*. Rockville, MD: National Institute on Drug Abuse; 2014. Available at: www.drugabuse.gov/sites/default/files/podata_1_17_14.pdf. Accessed March 26, 2019

129. Santisteban DA, Coatsworth JD, Perez-Vidal A, et al. Efficacy of brief strategic family therapy in modifying Hispanic adolescent behavior problems and substance use. *J Fam Psychol*. 2003; 17(1):121–133

130. Bonnie RJ, O'Connell ME, eds; National Research Council and Institute of Medicine; Division of Behavioral and Social Sciences and Education; Board on Children; Youth and Families; Committee on Developing a Strategy to Reduce and Prevent Underage Drinking. *Reducing Underage Drinking: A Collective Responsibility*. Washington, DC: National Academies Press; 2004

131. Alderman EA, Johnston BD; Committee on Adolescence; Council on Injury, Violence, and Poison Prevention. The teen driver. *Pediatrics*. 2018;142(4): e20182163

Aluminum Effects in Infants and Children

- *Technical Report*

TECHNICAL REPORT

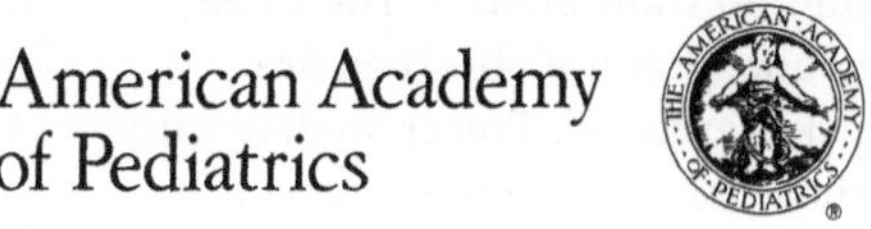

Aluminum Effects in Infants and Children

Mark R. Corkins, MD, FAAP, COMMITTEE ON NUTRITION

abstract

Aluminum has no known biological function; however, it is a contaminant present in most foods and medications. Aluminum is excreted by the renal system, and patients with renal diseases should avoid aluminum-containing medications. Studies demonstrating long-term toxicity from the aluminum content in parenteral nutrition components led the US Food and Drug Administration to implement rules for these solutions. Large-volume ingredients were required to reduce the aluminum concentration, and small-volume components were required to be labeled with the aluminum concentration. Despite these rules, the total aluminum concentration from some components continues to be above the recommended final concentration. The concerns about toxicity from the aluminum present in infant formulas and antiperspirants have not been substantiated but require more research. Aluminum is one of the most effective adjuvants used in vaccines, and a large number of studies have documented minimal adverse effects from this use. Long-term, high-concentration exposure to aluminum has been linked in meta-analyses with the development of Alzheimer disease.

INTRODUCTION

Aluminum is one of the most common metals on earth.[1] Aluminum is lightweight, strong, and easily sterilizable; therefore, it is used in a variety of packaging and manufacturing processes, such as milling and blending. These uses result in the presence of aluminum in our food, water supply, and medications. The aluminum present in the body normally enters via gastrointestinal ingestion. However, the gastrointestinal mucosa is exceptionally efficient in preventing absorption, and little to none of ingested aluminum appears to be absorbed.[1] One calculated fraction of aluminum absorption in adults was only 0.14%.[1] Data from an adult human study in which an aluminum isotope was used revealed the absorption to be 0.08%.[1] The Agency for Toxic Substances and Disease Registry of the US Department of Health and Human Services has set the minimum risk level for oral aluminum intake at 1 mg/kg per day.[2]

Division of Pediatric Gastroenterology, Hepatology, and Nutrition, Department of Pediatrics, The University of Tennessee Health Science Center, Memphis, Tennessee

Technical reports from the American Academy of Pediatrics benefit from expertise and resources of liaisons and internal (AAP) and external reviewers. However, technical reports from the American Academy of Pediatrics may not reflect the views of the liaisons or the organizations or government agencies that they represent.

Dr Corkins was responsible for all aspects of developing and revising the technical report and approved the final manuscript as submitted.

The guidance in this report does not indicate an exclusive course of treatment or serve as a standard of medical care. Variations, taking into account individual circumstances, may be appropriate.

All technical reports from the American Academy of Pediatrics automatically expire 5 years after publication unless reaffirmed, revised, or retired at or before that time.

This document is copyrighted and is property of the American Academy of Pediatrics and its Board of Directors. All authors have filed conflict of interest statements with the American Academy of Pediatrics. Any conflicts have been resolved through a process approved by the Board of Directors. The American Academy of Pediatrics has neither solicited nor accepted any commercial involvement in the development of the content of this publication.

DOI: https://doi.org/10.1542/peds.2019-3148

Address correspondence to Mark R. Corkins, MD, FAAP. E-mail: mcorkins@uthsc.edu

PEDIATRICS (ISSN Numbers: Print, 0031-4005; Online, 1098-4275).

Copyright © 2019 by the American Academy of Pediatrics

FINANCIAL DISCLOSURE: The author has indicated he has no financial relationships relevant to this article to disclose.

FUNDING: No external funding.

To cite: Corkins MR, AAP COMMITTEE ON NUTRITION. Aluminum Effects in Infants and Children. *Pediatrics.* 2019; 144(6):e20193148

The aluminum that does make it to the bloodstream is more than 80% bound to transferrin.[3,4] The small amounts that are absorbed are quickly excreted. Tracer studies with radioactive aluminum in human adults have revealed that only 0.5% of the total aluminum concentration is still in the bloodstream 24 hours after injection.[5,6] The great majority of aluminum that is in the bloodstream is cleared by the renal system.[1] In contrast to the wide variety of minerals that have been found to have a role in an enzymatic metalloproteins, only aluminum has not been found to have any biological role. In fact, in the presence of renal disease, when normal barriers are bypassed, aluminum has been shown to have some clearly associated toxicity.

Studies have revealed no biomarkers for aluminum levels in humans.[2] Because aluminum is poorly absorbed and rapidly excreted by the renal system, concentrations measured in blood or urine do not reflect exposures unless they are acute excessive amounts. A study in which researchers compared serum, plasma, and 24-hour urine aluminum concentrations among different reference laboratory tests revealed wide variations in the reported numbers.[7] The ranges used in these laboratory tests as normal were derived from small samples of normal individuals, often adults, and none that were age specific. The use of other tissues, such as hair, was found to be unreliable.[7]

RENAL DISEASES

The previous American Academy of Pediatrics policy statement on aluminum toxicity was focused on the aluminum effects observed in patients with renal disease.[8] At that time, the dialysates used for peritoneal dialysis had a high aluminum level and bypassed the normal protective epithelial barriers. Because the patients had decreased renal function, they could not excrete the aluminum. These patients developed symptoms of bone pain. Adults on long-term aluminum-containing dialysate had increased aluminum concentrations in the brain, with progressive dementia.[9] When the aluminum was removed from the dialysate, these issues resolved. Of ongoing concern was the use of aluminum-containing phosphate binders in pediatric patients with renal disease. Multiple case reports were published of patients who developed encephalopathy and had aluminum bone deposition.[8] The previous policy recommended discontinuing the use of aluminum-containing phosphate binders in patients with renal disease. Awareness regarding aluminum toxicity resulted in discontinued use of these agents. Patients with renal disease should also avoid aluminum-containing antacids and medications, such sucralfate.

PARENTERAL NUTRITION

Intravenous compounds containing high aluminum concentrations have a risk of resulting in aluminum toxicity because they bypass the protective gastrointestinal mucosa. As indicated previously, aluminum is normally cleared quickly by the renal system. There is greater concern with high levels of aluminum intake over longer periods of time. Parenteral nutrition solutions are the most chronic intravenous infusions used in patient care. Aluminum is present in all of the ingredients of parenteral nutrition, the highest levels being found in calcium gluconate, inorganic phosphates, and cysteine hydrochloride.[10]

Developmental Effects

The blood-brain barrier is efficient at blocking the passage of aluminum into the brain[3,11]; however, this barrier may not be as well developed in preterm infants. Because preterm infants are known to have immature renal function, Bishop et al[12] were concerned about aluminum toxicity in preterm infants receiving parenteral nutrition. They performed a study to compare 90 preterm infants randomly assigned to receive standard parenteral nutrition with 92 preterm infants randomly assigned to receive purposefully aluminum-depleted parenteral nutrition.[12] At a postterm age of 18 months, a subgroup of the infants had the Bayley Scales of Infant Development Mental Developmental Index performed. The index score for 39 infants who received the standard aluminum-containing parenteral nutrition was 92, compared with a score of 102 for the 41 infants who received the aluminum-depleted parenteral nutrition ($P = .02$). The study revealed a loss of 1 index point for each day infants received the standard aluminum-containing parenteral nutrition solution.[12]

Bone Effects

As indicated earlier, there is little accumulation of aluminum in the body. The skeleton is the only part of the body that appears to concentrate aluminum, with 54% of the body's total aluminum concentrated in bone.[13] When aluminum accumulates to a high enough level, bone formation is blocked and osteomalacia develops, increasing the risk of fracture.[1] An older study in which the authors evaluated preterm infants receiving parenteral nutrition revealed that aluminum deposited at the leading edge of bone mineralization.[14] The same infants studied by Bishop et al[12] were later examined for long-term bone effects. The researchers followed-up with these patients when they were 13 to 15 years of age with dual-energy radiograph absorptiometry scans for bone mineral content. Patients who had received the standard (higher) aluminum parenteral nutrition were found to have lower lumbar spine bone mineral content, and patients with the highest intakes had lower bone mineral content of their hips.[15]

Regulatory Response

In response to the studies cited here, the US Food and Drug Administration (FDA) became concerned about the aluminum content of intravenous solutions. In 1990, the FDA announced an intention to regulate the aluminum in parenteral solutions. In 2000, the final rule was published but did not take effect until July 26, 2004.[16] The rule requires the reduction of aluminum content in large-volume parenteral nutrition solutions to less than 25 μg/L and requires that small-volume parenteral nutrition solutions be labeled to indicate the maximum aluminum concentration present on their expiration date. The expiration date is important because the aluminum level increases with time as it leaches out of the glass in the containers. One of the key requirements of the FDA was to add a warning onto the label stating that in patients with impaired renal function, infusion of solutions with more than 5 μg/kg per day of aluminum may result in central nervous system and bone toxicity.[16] Because the labels on the components list the maximum aluminum concentration that could be present, when the actual final aluminum concentration of parenteral nutrition solutions has been measured, it has been less than the projected maximum value.[17] Despite the solutions having lower aluminum concentrations than the component labels project, when actually measured, none of the compounded neonatal or pediatric parenteral nutrition solutions had an aluminum concentration below the FDA-recommended 5 μg/kg per day.[17,18] When another group used the actual measured aluminum concentration in the components and formulated a parenteral nutrition solution with the lowest levels possible, the daily dose of aluminum was still greater than the recommended 5 μg/kg per day.[19] When plasma aluminum concentrations were measured in patients with intestinal failure who were receiving long-term parenteral nutrition, the average concentration was 8 times greater than that in healthy controls.[20] The aluminum concentrations present in small-volume parenteral nutrition solutions have not changed since the studies that revealed a developmental effect were published. Unfortunately, until new parenteral components with lower aluminum content are available, no matter how thoughtful the prescriber, parenteral nutrition solutions for most pediatric patients will contain aluminum concentrations above the recommended amount.

FORMULAS

Studies have documented significantly higher aluminum concentrations in infant formulas compared with human milk.[21,22] Despite this, there are no studies reporting any evidence of clinical aluminum toxicity related to formula feeding. Nonetheless, the disparity in the measured concentrations has resulted in some calls for an effort to reduce the aluminum content in infant formulas.[22] As indicated earlier, there is minimal absorption of aluminum via the gastrointestinal tract, so regulatory agencies have not responded to these calls. One study measured the plasma aluminum concentrations of infants fed human milk versus a variety of infant formulas and found no significant differences, except with hydrolysate formulas.[23] In this study, the hydrolysate formulas were all used in infants with a gastrointestinal illness; however, data on aluminum content in hydrolysate infant formulas are insufficient to make recommendations at this time. Studies are greatly needed on the potential health risks attributable to the aluminum in infant formulas, especially in populations such as preterm infants and those with gastrointestinal or renal diseases.

ANTIPERSPIRANTS

Skin is an excellent barrier against aluminum; however, claims have been made that the high levels of aluminum in antiperspirants lead to dermal absorption. This concern has been used to market antiperspirants low in aluminum. There are no published medical studies in which authors report large numbers of patients with toxicity attributable to transdermal aluminum absorption. The concern is that increased absorption may occur in skin that has been abraded by shaving. There is a single case report of an adult female patient who used a daily aluminum-containing antiperspirant, regularly shaved the skin under her arms, and had elevated aluminum concentrations.[24] In vitro studies in which researchers used skin biopsies in a diffusion cell revealed little absorption of an aluminum antiperspirant preparation.[25] However, when the skin was stripped by using adhesive tape, the uptake was significantly greater. The clinical relevance of this model to skin that has been shaved is difficult to extrapolate. A study in adults in which researchers used radiolabeled aluminum in an antiperspirant revealed absorption of only 0.012% of the tracer.[26] This study involved using tape to strip the previously shaved underarm area for skin samples. This would indicate that the absorption of aluminum from antiperspirants, even with skin that has been shaved, is apparently minimal. Mixed epidemiological data from population studies reveal no association[27] or a possible association[28] of aluminum-containing antiperspirants with breast cancer. Although there is no solid clinical evidence of toxicity, there are calls in the literature for reduction of the aluminum in antiperspirants.[29]

VACCINE ADJUVANTS

Aluminum is the predominant adjuvant used in human vaccines, although not all vaccines. The aluminum content of vaccines is limited by the Code of Federal Regulations to 1.25 mg per dose.[30] The regulations also stipulate that data are required to reveal that the amount of aluminum is safe and necessary to produce the intended effect. The Centers for Disease Control and Prevention has stated that the amount of aluminum exposure from following the recommended vaccine schedule is low and that the aluminum is not readily absorbed by the body.[31] The Centers for Disease Control and Prevention cited a study in which researchers calculated the aluminum exposure from vaccines during infancy and found the total to be far below the minimal risk levels established by the Agency for Toxic Substances and Disease Registry.[32] The aluminum-containing adjuvants are reported to have minimal adverse effects but are effective at improving the antibody response.[33] There are reports of a chronic local granulomatous inflammation known as macrophagic myofasciitis in a small number of patients after receiving intramuscular vaccines containing aluminum.[33,34] This condition allegedly results from a chronic inflammatory response to the residual adjuvant aluminum at the vaccination site that leads to a constellation of neurologic symptoms, including myalgia, arthralgia, chronic fatigue, weakness, and cognitive issues.[34] The number of patients reported to have the neurologic symptoms is low compared with the number of vaccinated individuals. The World Health Organization Global Advisory Committee of Vaccine Safety has not found that the data support an association between aluminum adjuvants and chronic neurologic diseases.[35] The aluminum content of vaccines has been blamed for autism spectrum disorders, but a large meta-analysis of cohort studies evaluating vaccination and the risk of autism revealed that in pooled data of 1 256 407 children, the odds ratio of developing autism after vaccination was 0.99, with a 95% confidence interval of 0.92 to 1.06.[36]

The aluminum adjuvants in the human papillomavirus vaccine have also been suggested as causing primary ovary insufficiency. However, the relationship suggested is based on a total of 6 case reports, most occurring years after vaccination, with only 1 patient having ovarian failure within several months of vaccination.[37] These cases reports come after more than 170 million doses of the human papillomavirus vaccine have been administered. The aluminum adjuvants in vaccines are also accused of potentially triggering an autoimmune process. The autoimmune syndrome induced by adjuvants was proposed in 2011.[38] The proposed criteria for this syndrome are extremely vague and general. Two of the major criteria are exposure to an external stimulus (infection, vaccine, silicone, or adjuvant) before symptoms occur and appearance of a long list of general somatic complaints. A review of the available literature for the purported autoimmune syndrome induced by adjuvants revealed that the human cases were so dissimilar in proposed triggers and clinical conditions that there was no evidence for a relationship between adjuvants and autoimmune conditions.[39]

ALUMINUM AND ALZHEIMER DISEASE

A long-standing hypothesis has been that aluminum is involved in the etiology of Alzheimer disease. This theory is based on the assumption that a long-term accumulation of aluminum in the brain could produce symptoms like dialysis-associated encephalopathy. The aluminum-induced neurofibrillary degeneration in animal studies also was similar to the pathology observed in human patients with Alzheimer disease.[40] A meta-analysis used to evaluate chronic aluminum-containing antacid use and the risk of Alzheimer disease revealed no association.[41] In another meta-analysis, researchers examined dietary patterns of food consumption high in aluminum and the risk of dementia (70% of dementia is attributable to Alzheimer disease).[42] This meta-analysis also included 1 study of aluminum in drinking water and 1 study of aluminum-containing dust inhalation. The meta-analysis revealed an increased relative risk of dementia of 2.24 with increased aluminum exposure ($P < .001$).[42] The largest meta-analysis of the association between aluminum and Alzheimer disease included a total of 8 studies and a total of 10 567 individuals.[43] The follow-up time from the cited studies ranged from 8 to 48 years, and the studies included drinking water (>100 μg/L aluminum concentration) and occupational exposures. Regarding the increased risk of Alzheimer disease, the authors of this meta-analysis reported a pooled odds ratio of 1.71, with a 95% confidence interval of 1.35 to 2.18.[43]

SUMMARY OF KEY POINTS

The 1996 American Academy of Pediatrics publication regarding aluminum toxicity was a policy statement. The primary concern in 1996 was renal dialysates, which has resolved. Currently, there are a variety of new issues concerning aluminum, the primary one being the aluminum concentration in parenteral nutrition components. However, there are no clinic alternatives for some of these components, and some of the other issues are still lacking the depth of data to support more definitive policy statements. Therefore, this updated document on aluminum toxicity was prepared as a technical review. A summary of the primary issues concerning aluminum is provided in the following points:

1. The greatest risk of aluminum exposure occurs in intravenous preparations for micronutrient delivery in parenteral nutrition. Aluminum exposure via parenteral nutrition has been shown to have long-term effects in preterm infants. Every effort should be made to minimize the aluminum content, although with the currently available products, the concentration will still be above the recommended amount.
2. Patients with renal disease should reduce aluminum exposure by avoiding aluminum-containing phosphate binders and other medications containing high amounts of aluminum to reduce aluminum exposure.
3. Despite having aluminum concentrations higher than those in human milk, infant formulas have not been documented to result in any long-term health concerns. Studies are needed to assess the potential health risks attributable to the aluminum content in infant formulas, especially in potentially vulnerable populations.
4. Antiperspirants have a high aluminum content, but there is not enough evidence to suggest long-term health concerns.
5. Aluminum adjuvants are extremely safe and effective at producing an immune response with rare adverse effects.
6. Meta-analyses have suggested an association between aluminum and Alzheimer disease with long-term high-concentration exposures.

LEAD AUTHOR

Mark R. Corkins, MD, FAAP

COMMITTEE ON NUTRITION, 2018–2019

Steven A. Abrams, MD, FAAP, Chairperson

George J. Fuchs III, MD, FAAP

Praveen S. Goday, MD, FAAP

Tamara S. Hannon, MD, FAAP

Jae H. Kim, MD, PhD, FAAP

C. Wesley Lindsey, MD, FAAP

Ellen S. Rome, MD, MPH, FAAP

PAST COMMITTEE MEMBERS

Mark R. Corkins, MD, FAAP

Stephen Daniels, MD, PhD, FAAP

Neville H. Golden, MD, FAAP

Sheela N. Magge, MD, MSCE, FAAP

Sarah Jane Schwarzenberg, MD, FAAP

LIAISONS

Andrea Lotze, MD, FAAP – *US Food and Drug Administration*

Catherine M. Pound, MD – *Canadian Pediatric Society*

Brian K. Kit, MD, FAAP – *National Institutes of Health*

Cria Perrine, PhD – *Centers for Disease Control and Prevention*

Valery Soto, MS, RD, LD – *US Department of Agriculture*

STAFF

Debra Burrowes, MHA

ABBREVIATION

FDA: US Food and Drug Administration

POTENTIAL CONFLICT OF INTEREST: The author has indicated he has no potential conflicts of interest to disclose.

REFERENCES

1. Priest ND. The biological behaviour and bioavailability of aluminium in man, with special reference to studies employing aluminium-26 as a tracer: review and study update. *J Environ Monit*. 2004;6(5): 375–403
2. Agency for Toxic Substances and Disease Registry. *Toxicological Profile for Aluminum*. Atlanta, GA: Agency for Toxic Substances and Disease Registry; 2008
3. Yokel RA, McNamara PJ. Aluminium toxicokinetics: an updated minireview. *Pharmacol Toxicol*. 2001;88(4): 159–167
4. Harris WR. Equilibrium model for speciation of aluminum in serum. *Clin Chem*. 1992;38(9):1809–1818
5. Priest ND, Newton D, Day JP, Talbot RJ, Warner AJ. Human metabolism of aluminium-26 and gallium-67 injected as citrates. *Hum Exp Toxicol*. 1995;14(3): 287–293
6. Priest ND, Newton D, Talbot RJ. *Metabolism of Aluminum-26 and Gallium-67 in a Volunteer Following Their Injection as Citrates*. Abingdon, United Kingdom: United Kingdom Atomic Energy Authority; 1991
7. Zeager M, Woolf AD, Goldman RH. Wide variation in reference values for aluminum levels in children. *Pediatrics*. 2012;129(1). Available at: www.pediatrics.org/cgi/content/full/129/1/e142
8. American Academy of Pediatrics, Committee on Nutrition. Aluminum toxicity in infants and children. *Pediatrics*. 1996;97(3):413–416
9. O'Hare JA, Callaghan NM, Murnaghan DJ. Dialysis encephalopathy. Clinical, electroencephalographic and interventional aspects. *Medicine (Baltimore)*. 1983;62(3):129–141

10. Hernández-Sánchez A, Tejada-González P, Arteta-Jiménez M. Aluminium in parenteral nutrition: a systematic review. *Eur J Clin Nutr.* 2013;67(3): 230–238

11. Yokel RA, Allen DD, Ackley DC. The distribution of aluminum into and out of the brain. *J Inorg Biochem.* 1999;76(2): 127–132

12. Bishop NJ, Morley R, Day JP, Lucas A. Aluminum neurotoxicity in preterm infants receiving intravenous-feeding solutions. *N Engl J Med.* 1997;336(22): 1557–1561

13. International Commission on Radiological Protection. *Report of Task Force on Reference Man.* Oxford, United Kingdom: Pergamon Press; 1975

14. Koo WW, Kaplan LA, Bendon R, et al. Response to aluminum in parenteral nutrition during infancy. *J Pediatr.* 1986; 109(5):877–883

15. Fewtrell MS, Bishop NJ, Edmonds CJ, Isaacs EB, Lucas A. Aluminum exposure from parenteral nutrition in preterm infants: bone health at 15-year follow-up. *Pediatrics.* 2009;124(5):1372–1379

16. US Food and Drug Administration. Aluminum in large and small volume parenterals used in total parenteral solutions. *Fed Regist.* 2000;65(17): 4103–4111

17. Speerhas RA, Seidner DL. Measured versus estimated aluminum content of parenteral nutrient solutions. *Am J Health Syst Pharm.* 2007;64(7):740–746

18. Hall AR, Arnold CJ, Miller GG, Zello GA. Infant parenteral nutrition remains a significant source for aluminum toxicity. *JPEN J Parenter Enteral Nutr.* 2017;41(7):1228–1233

19. Poole RL, Pieroni KP, Gaskari S, Dixon T, Kerner JA. Aluminum exposure in neonatal patients using the least contaminated parenteral nutrition solution products. *Nutrients.* 2012;4(11): 1566–1574

20. Courtney-Martin G, Kosar C, Campbell A, et al. Plasma aluminum concentrations in pediatric patients receiving long-term parenteral nutrition. *JPEN J Parenter Enteral Nutr.* 2015;39(5):578–585

21. Fernandez-Lorenzo JR, Cocho JA, Rey-Goldar ML, Couce M, Fraga JM. Aluminum contents of human milk, cow's milk, and infant formulas. *J Pediatr Gastroenterol Nutr.* 1999;28(3): 270–275

22. Chuchu N, Patel B, Sebastian B, Exley C. The aluminium content of infant formulas remains too high. *BMC Pediatr.* 2013;13:162

23. Hawkins NM, Coffey S, Lawson MS, Delves HT. Potential aluminium toxicity in infants fed special infant formula. *J Pediatr Gastroenterol Nutr.* 1994;19(4): 377–381

24. Guillard O, Fauconneau B, Olichon D, Dedieu G, Deloncle R. Hyperaluminemia in a woman using an aluminum-containing antiperspirant for 4 years. *Am J Med.* 2004;117(12):956–959

25. Pineau A, Guillard O, Favreau F, Marrauld A, Fauconneau B. In vitro study of percutaneous absorption of aluminum from antiperspirants through human skin in the Franz™ diffusion cell [published correction appears in *J Inorg Biochem.* 2012;116:228]. *J Inorg Biochem.* 2012;110:21–26

26. Flarend R, Bin T, Elmore D, Hem SL. A preliminary study of the dermal absorption of aluminium from antiperspirants using aluminium-26. *Food Chem Toxicol.* 2001;39(2):163–168

27. Mirick DK, Davis S, Thomas DB. Antiperspirant use and the risk of breast cancer. *J Natl Cancer Inst.* 2002; 94(20):1578–1580

28. McGrath KG. An earlier age of breast cancer diagnosis related to more frequent use of antiperspirants/deodorants and underarm shaving. *Eur J Cancer Prev.* 2003;12(6):479–485

29. Pineau A, Fauconneau B, Sappino AP, Deloncle R, Guillard O. If exposure to aluminium in antiperspirants presents health risks, its content should be reduced. *J Trace Elem Med Biol.* 2014; 28(2):147–150

30. Code of Federal Regulations Title 21 – Food and Drugs, 21 CFR §610.15 (2016)

31. Centers for Disease Control and Prevention. Adjuvants help vaccines work better. 2018. Available at: www.cdc.gov/vaccinesafety/concerns/adjuvants.html#alum. Accessed July 8, 2019

32. Mitkus RJ, King DB, Hess MA, Forshee RA, Walderhaug MO. Updated aluminum pharmacokinetics following infant exposures through diet and vaccination. *Vaccine.* 2011;29(51):9538–9543

33. Petrovsky N. Comparative safety of vaccine adjuvants: a summary of current evidence and future needs. *Drug Saf.* 2015;38(11):1059–1074

34. Shaw CA, Li D, Tomljenovic L. Are there negative CNS impacts of aluminum adjuvants used in vaccines and immunotherapy? *Immunotherapy.* 2014; 6(10):1055–1071

35. World Health Organization, Global Advisory Committee on Vaccine Safety. *Statement from the Global Advisory Committee on Vaccine Safety on Aluminum-Containing Vaccines.* Geneva, Switzerland: World Health Organization; 2008

36. Taylor LE, Swerdfeger AL, Eslick GD. Vaccines are not associated with autism: an evidence-based meta-analysis of case-control and cohort studies. *Vaccine.* 2014;32(29): 3623–3629

37. Hawkes D, Buttery JP. Human papillomavirus vaccination and primary ovarian insufficiency: an association based on ideology rather than evidence. *Curr Opin Obstet Gynecol.* 2016;28(1): 70–72

38. Shoenfeld Y, Agmon-Levin N. 'ASIA' - autoimmune/inflammatory syndrome induced by adjuvants. *J Autoimmun.* 2011;36(1):4–8

39. Hawkes D, Benhamu J, Sidwell T, Miles R, Dunlop RA. Revisiting adverse reactions to vaccines: a critical appraisal of Autoimmune Syndrome Induced by Adjuvants (ASIA). *J Autoimmun.* 2015;59: 77–84

40. Miu AC, Benga O. Aluminum and Alzheimer's disease: a new look. *J Alzheimers Dis.* 2006;10(2–3):179–201

41. Virk SA, Eslick GD. Brief Report: meta-analysis of antacid use and Alzheimer's disease: implications for the Aluminum Hypothesis. *Epidemiology.* 2015;26(5): 769–773

42. Cao L, Tan L, Wang HF, et al. Dietary patterns and risk of dementia: a systematic review and meta-analysis of cohort studies. *Mol Neurobiol.* 2016; 53(9):6144–6154

43. Wang Z, Wei X, Yang J, et al. Chronic exposure to aluminum and risk of Alzheimer's disease: a meta-analysis. *Neurosci Lett.* 2016;610:200–206

Comprehensive Health Evaluation of the Newly Adopted Child

• *Clinical Report*

CLINICAL REPORT Guidance for the Clinician in Rendering Pediatric Care

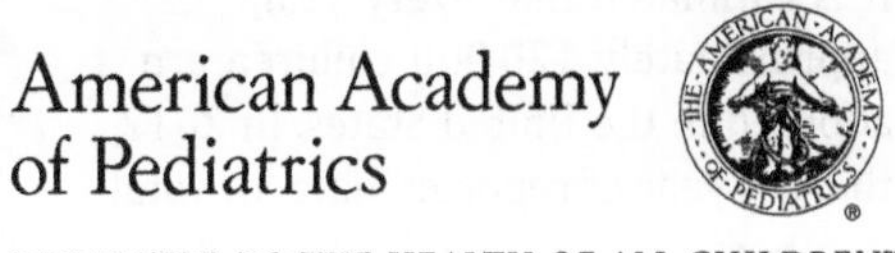

DEDICATED TO THE HEALTH OF ALL CHILDREN™

Comprehensive Health Evaluation of the Newly Adopted Child

Veronnie Faye Jones, MD, PhD, MSPH, FAAP,[a] Elaine E. Schulte, MD, MPH, FAAP,[b] COUNCIL ON FOSTER CARE, ADOPTION, AND KINSHIP CARE

abstract

Children who join families through the process of adoption, whether through a domestic or international route, often have multiple health care needs. Pediatricians and other health care personnel are in a unique position to guide families in achieving optimal health for the adopted children as families establish a medical home. Shortly after placement in an adoptive home, it is recommended that children have a timely comprehensive health evaluation to provide care for known medical needs and identify health issues that are unknown. It is important to begin this evaluation with a review of all available medical records and pertinent verbal history. A complete physical examination then follows. The evaluation should also include diagnostic testing based on findings from the history and physical examination as well as the risks presented by the child's previous living conditions. Age-appropriate screenings may include, but are not limited to, newborn screening panels and hearing, vision, dental, and formal behavioral and/or developmental screenings. The comprehensive assessment may occur at the time of the initial visit to the physician after adoptive placement or can take place over several visits. Adopted children can be referred to other medical specialists as deemed appropriate. The Council on Adoption, Foster Care, and Kinship Care is a resource within the American Academy of Pediatrics for physicians providing care for children who are being adopted.

[a]Division of General Pediatrics, Department of Pediatrics, School of Medicine, University of Louisville, Louisville, Kentucky; and [b]The Children's Hospital at Montefiore, Bronx, New York

Dr Jones conducted the literature review, conceptualized and designed the format of the manuscript, and revised the manuscript during each iteration; Dr Schulte conducted the literature review, conceptualized and designed the format of the manuscript, and revised the manuscript during each iteration; the members of the Council on Foster Care, Adoption, and Kinship Care reviewed and revised the manuscript; and all authors approved the final manuscript as submitted.

This document is copyrighted and is property of the American Academy of Pediatrics and its Board of Directors. All authors have filed conflict of interest statements with the American Academy of Pediatrics. Any conflicts have been resolved through a process approved by the Board of Directors. The American Academy of Pediatrics has neither solicited nor accepted any commercial involvement in the development of the content of this publication.

Clinical reports from the American Academy of Pediatrics benefit from expertise and resources of liaisons and internal (AAP) and external reviewers. However, clinical reports from the American Academy of Pediatrics may not reflect the views of the liaisons or the organizations or government agencies that they represent.

The guidance in this report does not indicate an exclusive course of treatment or serve as a standard of medical care. Variations, taking into account individual circumstances, may be appropriate.

All clinical reports from the American Academy of Pediatrics automatically expire 5 years after publication unless reaffirmed, revised, or retired at or before that time.

DOI: https://doi.org/10.1542/peds.2019-0657

Address correspondence to V. Faye Jones, MD, PhD. Email: vfjone01@louisville.edu

To cite: Jones VF, Schulte EE, AAP COUNCIL ON FOSTER CARE, ADOPTION, AND KINSHIP CARE. Comprehensive Health Evaluation of the Newly Adopted Child. *Pediatrics.* 2019; 143(5):e20190657

Pediatricians have played a significant role in the adoption process, in some cases providing counseling to parents during the preadoption phase and subsequently providing health care for these children. Special needs among adopted children need to be identified so they may be evaluated and treated appropriately. The pediatrician also needs to become knowledgeable about the resources available to help families integrate the new adoptee into the family unit. The purpose of this Clinical Report is to provide the general pediatrician with practical guidance that addresses the initial comprehensive health evaluation of adopted children.

CURRENT STATUS OF ADOPTION

It is estimated that every year, approximately 120 000 children are adopted in the United States. In 2012, the last year of reported data for total numbers of adoptions in the United States, 119 514 children joined families through adoption.[1] This number represents a 14% decrease from 2008 and a 15% decrease from 2001. Children may be adopted through the national public welfare system, through private agencies, through existing relationships, or internationally.

TRENDS IN DOMESTIC ADOPTION

Most domestic adoptions occur through the national public welfare system or independent agencies. According to data from the Adoption and Foster Care Analysis and Reporting System, the number of children adopted from the foster care system had remained flat until a slight increase was noted in 2015.[2] The number of adoptions had been approximately 50 000 to 52 000 between 2005 and 2014, except for 2008 and 2009, when the number reached a high of 57 200. The number of finalized adoptions leveled back to 50 800 in 2013 and 50 600 in 2014. In 2015, the number of adoptions from the foster care system increased to 53 500. A review of the data revealed a similar increase in the number of children within the foster care system since 2013 who were designated as waiting to be adopted and whose parents' rights had been terminated, which may be attributable to increased accountability by the states for permanency planning in compliance with the Adoption and Safe Families Act of 1997.[3]

An assessment of demographic data revealed the mean age at the time of adoption was 6.2 years, with male adoptees accounting for 51% of the population.[2] The mean time elapsed from termination of parental rights to adoption was 11.9 months.[2] White children accounted for 48% of adoptions. Twenty-two percent of children who were adopted were identified as Hispanic and/or Latino, and 18% were identified as black or African American. Children were adopted by foster parents in 52% of cases. Other relatives became adoptive parents for 34% of adoptees. Married couples and single women represented the majority of adoptive parents, accounting for 68% and 29%, respectively.[2]

A report from the Child Welfare Information Gateway stated that in 2012, approximately 49% of all adoptions in the United States were from sources other than the public child welfare system or intercountry sources.[1] Other sources include private agencies, American Indian and/or Alaskan native tribes, and facilitated, independent, or step-parent adoptions.[1,4] However, unlike adoptions through public child welfare and orphan visas for foreign-born children, for which there is federally mandated reporting, there is not a complementary system for domestic placements from other sources, which are typically governed by widely varying state laws, making it difficult to determine exact numbers.

TRENDS IN INTERNATIONAL ADOPTION

Primarily because of changes in internal policies of several countries, partnering countries' concerns about illegal or unethical practices by adoption service providers and the ability to appropriately monitor adoption service provider activities, and concerns about the unregulated custody transfer of adopted children, the number of international adoptions has been decreasing over recent years, with only 5372 immigrant visas issued to children adopted abroad or coming to the United States to be adopted by US citizens in 2016 (down from 7037 in 2015).[5] These numbers represent a decrease of nearly 77% from the high of 22 989 adoptions in 2004.[5] China accounted for the majority of international adoptees with 2231 adoptions (down 5% from 2015). The Democratic Republic of the Congo and Ukraine accounted for the second and third largest numbers of adoptions with 359 and 303 child adoptees, respectively.[5] Available data revealed that boys accounted for 51% of adoptions, which is a shift from previous years. Children 2 years or younger accounted for 18% of adoptees, children between the ages of 3 and 4 years accounted for 29% of adoptees, and children between the ages of 5 and 12 years accounted for 38% of adoptees. Only 13% of internationally adopted children were between the ages of 13 and 17 years, with young adults 18 years of age or older making up 2% of the population.[5]

Numerous studies have demonstrated that children in the foster care system, children adopted through private domestic agencies, and those adopted internationally all have an increased incidence of physical, developmental, and mental health concerns.[6–11] Children adopted through the international route may have additional concerns related to development and infectious diseases.[12–19] Early life experiences of adoptees that may account for the aforementioned health needs include poverty, inadequate prenatal care, malnutrition, prenatal and postnatal exposure to toxins and pathogens, inadequate developmental stimulation, child abuse, and exposure to extreme violence.[20,21] Children waiting for adoption are at high risk of having been exposed prenatally to illegal drugs and/or alcohol.[12,21–23] Before adoption, children may have been directly or indirectly exposed to physical, emotional, or sexual abuse.[12,24] Although these concerns may be addressed before adoption, many of these issues persist and continue to be significant or do not become apparent until after the time of placement in an adoptive home.

COMPONENTS OF THE INITIAL PLACEMENT EVALUATION

A comprehensive medical evaluation is best completed soon after placement in an adoptive home to confirm and clarify existing medical diagnoses; assess for any previously unrecognized medical issues, including oral health problems; discuss developmental and behavioral concerns; and make appropriate referrals.[12,25] This evaluation typically includes a thorough review of the medical history, incorporating an assessment of health risks, a developmental assessment, and a complete, unclothed physical examination.[12,13,18,21,25,26] The initial health evaluation of an adopted child needs to be comprehensive in nature, but it is not necessary for this to occur during only 1 medical visit. Several visits to the pediatrician may be necessary to complete the assessment of the child's history, review laboratory findings, and make referrals to medical, developmental, mental health, and dental specialists. Subsequent evaluations, including referrals and laboratory testing, can be undertaken to allow for comprehensive health planning.

THE PREADOPTION VISIT

The preadoption visit can be helpful for the adoptive family.[18,21,24,26–30] In an ideal situation, the future adoptive parents would present medical records of the child and/or biological parents to the pediatrician for review. Desired information includes general past medical history, including growth and development; immunization records; medications; allergies; chronic illness; dental problems; hospitalizations; and infectious disease exposures. Information about family history, pregnancy course, and childbirth may be relevant. Many children have faced adverse childhood experiences related to the combination of early life experiences and environmental influences, which have been shown to impact the genetic predisposition of the emerging brain architecture and can alter lifelong health outcomes.[26] The pediatrician can work closely with adoptive families to develop strategies to ameliorate some of the effects of the adverse childhood experiences on the prospective adoptees.

It is important to document environmental history and any childhood experiences, including developmental, mental, and educational history, as well as previous relationship histories.[24] If this information were available, the pediatrician would be able to use those records to help parents determine additional questions that could clarify a particular health issue and help parents clarify what special needs they would be prepared to accept. Unfortunately, in most cases, complete information is not obtainable, particularly with international adoption. However, using the available information, the pediatrician may be able to address specific issues in the medical records, including growth trends and a preliminary assessment of developmental progress, allowing for appropriate referral to services. The pediatrician may offer clarification of medical diagnoses, particularly in cases of international adoptions, because a particular diagnosis may be more prevalent in particular regions of the world.[18,27,29] In addition to medical records, parents may have other materials, such as photographs and videos, for review. Although these may be informative to confirm or refute what is written in the medical record, they do not provide a conclusive diagnosis.

The preadoption visit allows the pediatrician time to counsel families on other issues.[24] Closed versus open adoption can be discussed. Open adoption describes a continuum of communication between the birth parents and the adoptive family.[24,31] Pediatricians can discuss with adoptive families the extent of their comfort level with communication between them and the biological families and provide needed support by identifying potential and real benefits and drawbacks to the relationship. Special issues related to the nutrition of the children need to be addressed. Pediatricians need to be cognizant of short- and long-term problems related to malnutrition. This is particularly relevant for internationally adopted children, especially if a child has a previous history of residing in an institutional setting.[25,32] Some families may be interested in breastfeeding their infants, so the pediatrician needs to be familiar and supportive of the option and techniques of induced lactation.[33,34]

The preadoption visit may also allow the pediatrician to discuss other relevant issues related to the adoptive family. The immunization status of adoptive family members can be explored, and relevant information can be provided. It is recommended that unvaccinated household contacts or caregivers of adopted children with chronic hepatitis B virus (HBV) infection should receive a hepatitis B vaccine. If children are adopted internationally from a country with intermediate or high hepatitis A virus infection prevalence, administering a hepatitis A vaccine to household contacts or caregivers 2 or more weeks before the child's arrival is suggested.[18] Finally, providing information about available community support services may ease the transition for the expected family. For further assistance, the primary care physician can consult with the American Academy of Pediatrics (AAP) Council on Foster Care, Adoption, and Kinship Care (aap.org/cofcakc).

INITIAL HISTORY AND REVIEW OF MEDICAL RECORDS

When a child presents for an initial complete adoption evaluation, it is important to review the current and any available past medical history, with particular attention to any previous medical findings in the child's medical records. The electronic health record, using health information exchange standards, may eventually help facilitate the transfer of health information. A list of information to be sought from the child's history is provided in Table 1.

A complete medical history, including prenatal history obtained from the mother and genetic history obtained from both parents, is ideal but rarely available.[14,24,25] The adoption agency's social worker (who may be trained appropriately to do a skilled genetic, medical, and prenatal interview) may take an extensive history from the birth parent(s), if possible, and enter these data into the formal medical record for the future adoptive parent. It is important to review perinatal risks, which include lifestyle-related information about the birth parent(s) that may affect the fetus, neonate at birth, or child later in development.[28–30,36,37] Such information includes parental use of alcohol or drugs (licit and/or illicit use) and history of sexual practices that increase the risk of sexually transmitted infections both in the mother and her partner(s). Physicians and adoption agency social workers can be trained to obtain such information in a manner that is sensitive to the psychological and cultural needs of the families.[38]

Children being adopted from foster care most likely have had fragmented care and limited continuity of medical records. Health care before foster care placement may have been inadequate, with multiple unmet medical needs.[24,28,39] The AAP recommends a comprehensive health evaluation of all children at the time of entrance into foster care.[1,39–41] Adoptive parents may wish to review any available medical records from all previous health care providers, ideally before placement into an adoptive home and certainly before finalization of adoption from foster care. Incomplete or unavailable medical records should not prevent parents from scheduling timely initial comprehensive health evaluations. Parents, working in collaboration with their legal representative, their pediatrician, and local child welfare and adoption agencies, can continue to work to obtain the child's complete medical records, including (if possible) oral health history and developmental, educational, and mental health assessments.[24,25,42] For children being adopted from foster care, equal emphasis is placed on review of the medical history and the physical examination.[28,40,41]

With international placements, medical history may be sparse or inaccurate. The evaluation of a child who has been adopted internationally will depend, to a large degree, on a complete physical examination and comprehensive laboratory screening based on environmental, nutritional, ethnic, and infectious disease risks.[12,18,25,43,44] All internationally adopted children are required to have a medical evaluation performed by a panel physician who is a US Department of State–designated physician before departure from the country of origin. This examination is not considered a comprehensive examination; it is simply addressing legal requirements of screening for communicable diseases and serious physical or mental conditions that would prevent the issue of a permanent residency visa.[25] Therefore, all internationally adopted children need to undergo screening evaluations based on the risks presented by their previous life circumstances, including health risks specific to country of origin.[18,43–46]

INITIAL PHYSICAL EXAMINATION

The initial physical examination, as noted in Table 2, is comprehensive, with particular attention being given to the child's growth parameters and to systems that have been found to be more at risk for adopted children.[1,9,25,47] Care needs to be exercised when approaching the newly adopted child, particularly for older children (who may have had traumatic experiences with health care) and internationally adopted children (who may have never experienced a comprehensive examination). For older international adoptees, it is advisable to have an interpreter present, either in person or by telephone, to explain what is happening. For all children, one needs to proceed slowly, be sensitive to the children's cues, and provide reassurance.

Accurately measured growth parameters, including height, weight, and head circumference, are needed for all children. Racial- and ethnic-specific charts are no longer recommended to plot growth parameters; measurements can be plotted on standard Centers for Disease Control and Prevention (CDC) or World Health Organization growth charts as appropriate for age.[25,27,48] Although some controversy continues around the validity of these growth charts for varying ethnic groups, they allow for monitoring of the child's growth rates over time.[48–51] When possible, previous measurements should be obtained and plotted because trend data may provide a more objective assessment of the child's nutritional and medical status.[21,30]

Assessing nutritional status is an important component of the comprehensive examination. Children may present with low height for age (growth stunting), which may be attributable to inadequate nutrition as well as a result of chronic adversity. In contrast, children in

TABLE 1 Review of Medical History and/or Previous Records

- Birth record data
  - o Prenatal blood and urine test results of biological mother
  - o Exposure to medications, licit and/or illicit substances, alcohol, tobacco, marijuana
  - o Gestational age, birth wt, length, head size, Apgar scores
  - o Prenatal concerns, neonatal complications
  - o Newborn hearing screening results
  - o Newborn cardiac screening results
  - o Newborn metabolic screening results
- Previous growth points, including head circumference
- History of abuse: emotional, physical, and sexual; history of neglect
- Reason for placement into adoptive home
  - o Voluntary versus involuntary termination of parental rights
- Nutritional history, particularly with respect to iron, calcium, vitamin D, iodine, and other nutrients
  - o Assess history of food insecurity as well as current dietary habits
  - o Determine if the child has any sensory or oral motor eating difficulties
  - o Exercise history
- Developmental milestones, past and present
- Behavioral issues, particularly with respect to socialization, indiscriminate friendliness, response to stress
- Laboratory test results, radiographic studies, other studies
- Document immunization history
  - o School records may be sufficient, particularly for older children
  - o Review original international records with adequate timing of doses
  - o Children with no records or records that do not appear to be original or accurate are to be immunized according to standard Advisory Committee on Immunization Practices and/or AAP catch-up schedules[35]
- Document results (if known) of previous testing or treatment of tuberculosis
- Document chronic medical diagnoses
- Allergies (medication, food, environmental, latex, or insect stings)
- Medications (traditional and/or herbal, used acutely and chronically)
- Reports from previous specialists seen
  - o If available, have an original translation of records from other countries
- Family history (when available)
  - o Vision, hearing concerns
  - o Genetic diseases
  - o Concerns related to specific populations (eg, sickle cell anemia, thalassemia, Tay Sachs disease, or lactose intolerance)
  - o Mental health diagnoses
  - o Alcohol and/or substance use (licit and/or illicit use)
- Environmental risk factors
  - o Assessment of lead risks
  - o Document whether the child had experience with institutionalization
    - ■ If known, reason and timing of placement
    - ■ If known, feeding and sleeping schedule and environment where feeding and sleeping occurred
  - o Risks for previous physical, emotional, and sexual abuse
    - ■ Substandard housing, multiple changes in residence
    - ■ Family members using licit and/or illicit substances or alcohol, domestic violence
  - o Passive tobacco exposure, methamphetamine production products, other licit and/or illicit substances in the home environment
  - o Other environmental toxins, both in the home and surrounding community
- No. previous placements, quality of such care

Notes
- Children who have been adopted internationally may have neurologic, hematologic, cardiac, and metabolic disorders that were previously overdiagnosed, underdiagnosed, or undiagnosed.
- Medical records from other countries (if available) may be limited in information, inaccurate, or falsified.
- For children adopted domestically, there may be issues of confidentiality associated with obtaining records, particularly if a child's name was changed at the time of the adoption. In all cases, physicians can work with families and adoption workers to obtain complete medical records while also strictly adhering to laws regarding confidentiality of medical information.
- Relationship history
  - o Important ongoing relationships, including with biological family members, foster parents, and/or friends and important relationship losses

foster care may be classified as overweight or obese because of diets high in fat and sugar combined with being physically inactive secondary to their past environments.[52–54]

It is recommended that the child's general appearance be assessed and that any dysmorphic features that might be suggestive of a genetic disorder or syndrome (such as fetal alcohol syndrome) or congenital defects be noted. A thorough examination of the skin may lead to a diagnosis of an infectious disease or identification of lesions suggestive of previous abuse. It is necessary to perform a thorough but sensitive examination of the genital area to identify any abnormality suggestive of previous sexual abuse as well as documentation of female genital cutting.[55] The timing of this examination may need to be adjusted depending on the child. Children who have been traumatized in the past and are new to their adoptive homes may become anxious and overwhelmed. If the relationship with the adoptive parent is still new, the child may feel helpless without adequate support. As is expected for any new patient, a comprehensive neurologic examination can be performed.

REFERRAL FOR DIAGNOSTIC TESTING

It is recommended that diagnostic studies appropriate for the evaluation of the adopted child's risk factors be completed according to US recommendations, even for internationally adopted children who have received these tests outside of the United States (Table 3).[18,21] Children born outside of the United States should have all tests that were completed in the country of birth repeated, according to US recommendations.[18,21] Previous laboratory testing is often not verifiable, leaving concerns about the accuracy, appropriate reporting and interpretation, and timing of the tests.

TABLE 2 Components of the Comprehensive Physical Examination Pertinent to Adoption

- Vital signs (temperature, pulse, respiratory rate, and blood pressure)
- Growth points, including length or height, wt (unclothed), head circumference (on all children); plot data on WHO or CDC growth charts, along with comparison with any measurements previously obtained; BMI can be calculated and plotted
- Complete physical examination, with emphasis on the following areas
  - o Careful assessment for dysmorphic features suggestive of possible syndromes, including fetal alcohol spectrum disorders
  - o Careful eye examination, including red reflex and/or funduscopic examination and assessment of extraocular muscle functioning
  - o Skin examination
    - ■ Identify infectious diseases, rashes, or infestations, including scabies, lice, candidiasis, pediculosis, and impetigo
    - ■ Identify and document any congenital skin abnormalities, including hemangiomas, nevi, and blue macules of infancy (usually seen in children of Asian, African, or Hispanic ethnicity)
    - ■ Identify and document bruises or scars that may have resulted from previous abuse or immunization
  - o Perform a careful genitalia examination (including the anus) to identify any abnormality that may indicate previous sexual abuse or genital cutting
    - ■ If indicated, referral for full forensic evaluation may be needed
  - o Neurologic examination with emphasis on developmental and neurologic abnormalities; careful examination of the spine, including stigmata of spinal dysraphism

WHO, World Health Organization.

Recommendations are also available for children who have lived in foster care,[39] including the AAP Policy Statement and Technical Report, both titled, "Health Care Issues for Children and Adolescents in Foster Care and Kinship Care."[40,41]

Diagnostic testing may vary depending on whether the child was adopted through the domestic or international route. For children who lived in a foster home in the United States before finalization of adoption, verifiable diagnostic studies do not need to be repeated unless there has been additional risk of infectious disease or environmental exposures. Infants being adopted domestically shortly after birth need to have accurate verification of the biological mothers' prenatal laboratory test results, with testing being performed on the infants if the information is unavailable or if the accuracy of the records is unclear.

It is recommended that children adopted internationally be tested for tuberculosis, HIV, HBV, and sexually transmitted infections. For those adopted domestically, testing is recommended for children with definite or unknown exposure to and/or risk for tuberculosis, HIV, HBV, and sexually transmitted infections.[18,45,46,56,58] Other tests can be considered on an individual basis.[18,45,46,56,58] Consideration of individual risk factors is particularly relevant for internationally adopted children, for whom infectious diseases are among the most common medical diagnoses identified after arrival in the United States.[18,44,56] The latest edition of the AAP *Red Book*[18] and the CDC's *Health Information for International Travel* (commonly known as the *Yellow Book*)[44] should be consulted regarding follow-up for positive test results.

In many countries, perinatal screening for HBV is inconsistent, and administration of a hepatitis B vaccine at birth is unreliable. Prenatal screening for syphilis and HIV is also variable. In addition, according to the CDC *Yellow Book*,[44] many countries have a high prevalence of intestinal parasites and tuberculosis. Accordingly, all international adoptees should be screened for these infections after arrival in the United States. Other recommended screening tests for infectious diseases in international adoptees include *Trypanosoma cruzi* serological testing for children from countries where infection is endemic. In children with eosinophilia and negative stool ova and parasite examination results, testing for *Strongyloides* species, *Schistosoma* species, *Toxocara* species, and lymphatic filariasis can be considered depending on the children's country of origin. Other diseases, such as malaria, typhoid fever, leprosy, and melioidosis, are rare and not routinely tested for in internationally adopted children. However, if a child has findings such as unexplained fever, splenomegaly, anemia, or eosinophilia and is from a country where the disease is endemic, appropriate evaluation should be pursued.[18,56] For children with abnormal developmental screening results whose birth mother resided or spent time in a country with endemic Zika virus infection during pregnancy, current guidance is available from the CDC (www.cdc.gov/zika/index.html).[59]

Children, whether domestically or internationally adopted, may be at risk for iron, calcium, and vitamin D deficiency secondary to past dietary inadequacies.[25,54,56,60,61] Therefore, screening for anemia and rickets is suggested. Newly adopted children should also be screened for lead toxicity and thyroid function.[25] Screening for lipidemia may be indicated, according to guidelines, on the basis of known or unknown biologic family history.[35]

IMMUNIZATIONS

Immunization records should be reviewed carefully, particularly with respect to vaccines administered, the dates when vaccines were administered, intervals between vaccines, and the age of the child at the time the vaccines were administered.[18,47] Immunization records for children who have lived in several foster homes may be incomplete; children can be caught up using standard catch-up schedules.[62] Children who were immunized in an

TABLE 3 Diagnostic Testing

- Infectious diseases (for updates and further details on infectious disease screening, please consult the current AAP *Red Book*[18,56])
  - o Positive results for any infectious testing need to be treated according to standard guidelines[56]
  - o Hepatitis B surface antigen, hepatitis B surface antibody, and hepatitis B core antibody[a]
  - o Hepatitis C virus serological testing
  - o Hepatitis A (IgM and IgG)
  - o HIV 1 and 2 serological testing[a]
  - o Syphilis serological testing[a]
    - ■ Nontreponemal test (RPR or VDRL)
    - ■ Treponemal test (MHA-TP, FTA-ABS, or TPPA)
    - ■ For children adopted internationally, repeat all testing performed before adoption
    - ■ If sexual abuse is suspected or history is unknown, test the child for gonorrhea, *Chlamydia*, and other sexually transmitted infections; testing should include any suspected site of abuse, including the mouth and rectum
  - o Tuberculosis[a]
    - ■ TST or IGRA; TST is preferred. Although TST can be performed, IGRA may be preferred in children with previous exposure to Bacillus Calmette–Guérin vaccine and in people in whom follow-up with TST reading is questionable. For children adopted internationally, consider repeating this testing after 6 mo to rule out exposure just before leaving the country of origin.
  - o In children from countries with endemic infection, *T cruzi* serological testing (http://www.who.int/mediacentre/factsheets/fs340/en/)
  - o Stool screening for pathogens for any child who previously lived in inadequate housing, another country, or an institution or has diarrhea (diarrhea need not be present for children to have parasite infections)
    - ■ Ova and parasites: 3 tests collected on separate days for optimal screening with a specific request for *Giardia* intestinalis and *Cryptosporidium* species testing
    - ■ Stool testing by using culture or nonculture methods for *Salmonella*, *Shigella*, and *Campylobacter* if the child has diarrhea and *Escherichia coli* 0157:H7 and *Clostridium difficile* if bloody diarrhea or known or suspected history of prolonged antibiotic exposure
  - o Complete blood cell count with red cell indices
    - ■ Routine anemia screening for all children ≥6 mo old as well as all children adopted internationally
    - ■ In children with absolute eosinophil count exceeding 450 cells/mm^3 and negative stool ova and parasite examination results
      - *Strongyloides* species serological testing
      - *Schistosoma* species serological testing for children from sub-Saharan African, Southeast Asian, and certain Latin American countries
      - *Toxocara canis* species serological testing
      - Lymphatic filariasis serological testing for children >2 y old from countries with endemic infection (http://gamapserver.who.int/mapLibrary/Files/Maps/LF_2016.png)
  - o Screening for hemoglobinopathies and blood disorders in children of African, Asian, Hispanic, or Mediterranean ethnicities
    - ■ Sickle cell disease
    - ■ Thalassemia
    - ■ G6PD deficiency
  - o Blood lead concentration for children up to 6 y of age; older ages if indicated (ie, refugees, with history of institutional care, in at-risk cultural practices)
  - o Thyroid function ascertainment in all new international adoptees
  - o Newborn screening panel (young infants)
  - o Rickets screening (calcium, phosphorus, alkaline phosphatase) for children who were institutionalized, have growth delay, or had a history of poor vitamin D intake or limited sunlight
- It is recommended that children adopted internationally be retested for hepatitis B and HIV 6 mo after placement in the home.[44] Testing does not need to be repeated for children adopted from the US foster care system who recently had verifiable laboratory studies consistent with recommendations from the AAP.[57]

FTA-ABS, fluorescent treponemal antibody absorbed; G6PD, glucose-6-phosphate dehydrogenase; IgG, immunoglobulin G; IgM, immunoglobulin M; IGRA, interferon-γ release assay; MHA-TP, microhemagglutination assay for *Treponema pallidum* antibodies; RPR, rapid plasma reagin; TPPA, *Treponema pallidum* particle agglutination; TST, tuberculin skin test; VDRL, Venereal Disease Research Laboratory.

[a] For all children adopted internationally, it is recommended that they be tested for tuberculosis, HIV, hepatitis B, and sexually transmitted infections. Other tests can be considered on an individual basis.

institutional setting may have an inadequate immunologic response because of poor storage of vaccines or vaccines being used beyond the expiration date.[63] In addition, there may be no adult who can verify that the child actually received the vaccines written on the record. A recommended alternative is to reimmunize the child by using the appropriate AAP catch-up schedule.[56] If reimmunization is not acceptable, antibody concentrations may be measured to confirm immunity (see Table 4 for recommended antibody titers).[56] If antibody concentrations are to be obtained, it is important to interpret results in light of the dates of the last vaccine doses and possible persistence of maternal antibodies.[56]

CHRONIC HEALTH CONCERNS

During the health assessment of an adopted child, health concerns known and not previously diagnosed need to be identified. For many children, the availability of health information, including history of maternal and/or child drug use, previous hospitalizations, medications, and types of subspecialists the children have seen, may be incomplete or, when present, may need further exploration to define its significance. This scarcity of information may leave the family and the health care team uncertain of events that may affect the overall health of a child. Previous studies have confirmed that many adopted children have previous chronic illnesses or are at risk for the development of physical and mental health issues.[26,64–71] In 2014, a report from the Congressional Research Service found that 35% to 60% of children in the child welfare system had at least 1 chronic or acute physical health condition that needed treatment.[64] Some of the most common findings were growth failure, asthma, obesity, vision impairment, hearing loss, neurologic problems, sexually transmitted infections, and complex chronic

TABLE 4 Serological Testing to Assess Immunization Status of Adopted Children

- Diphtheria, tetanus
  - o In children >6 mo old with or without written documentation of immunization, serological testing to document antibodies to diphtheria and tetanus may be considered to determine if the child likely has received and responded to dose(s) of the vaccine.
- Pertussis, rotavirus
  - o No serological test is available to assess immunity to pertussis or rotavirus.
- Measles, mumps, rubella
  - o In children >12 mo old, measles, mumps, and rubella antibody concentrations could be measured to determine if the child is immune.
  - o Do not perform antibody testing in children <12 mo old because of the potential presence of maternal antibody.
  - o Measles antibody testing may be irrelevant if the child has not received mumps or rubella vaccines and will need the measles-mumps-rubella vaccine anyway.
- Varicella
  - o In children >12 mo old, varicella antibody concentrations could be measured to determine if the child is immune.
  - o Do not perform antibody testing in children <12 mo old because of the potential presence of maternal antibody.
  - o The documented receipt of 2 doses of the varicella vaccine is the best indication of immunity to varicella because commercially available varicella antibody tests are insensitive.
- Poliovirus
  - o Neutralizing antibody for types 1, 2, and 3 can confirm immunity to poliovirus.
- *Haemophilus influenzae* type B
  - o If no records are available, it may be prudent to reimmunize according to the routine catch-up schedule. If there are records of immunization available, it may be prudent to check titers to validate, but this does not convey full immunity. Use of the catch-up schedule may still be warranted.
  - o For immunocompetent children ≥5 y old, there is no need to perform serological testing because no dose is indicated, except certain high-risk older children may still require vaccination.
- Hepatitis B
  - o HBV infection is covered in Table 3. HBsAb can be tested to confirm immunity if the child has a record of vaccines administered with appropriate timing.
- Hepatitis A
  - o Serological tests for anti–hepatitis A virus (IgG and IgM) can be considered.
- Pneumococcus
  - o No serological test is available.

Information is taken from the AAP *Red Book*.[18,56] For non–US-born children, serological testing may be a strategy to determine if antibody concentrations are present for some vaccine-preventable diseases. However, serological testing is not available for all vaccine-preventable diseases, can be costly, and does not confirm whether the child is fully immunized. Therefore, it may be judicious to repeat the administration of all immunizations in question.[56] HBsAb, hepatitis B surface antibody; IgG, immunoglobulin G; IgM, immunoglobulin M.

illnesses. The report also noted that one-half to three-fourths of these children exhibit behavioral or social competency problems that necessitate care from health services. The findings confirmed that many of these problems persist even in children who are adopted.

Children with a history of foster care involvement have frequently experienced psychological trauma.[40,41] Studies have shown early experiences and environmental influences may have long-term sequelae on the emerging brain architecture, resulting in long-term health problems.[26] These children are more likely to report externalizing and internalizing psychiatric symptoms.[65–69] Common mental health diagnoses for children in foster care include disorders related to attention-deficit/hyperactivity disorder and oppositional defiant and conduct disorders. Other problems include anxiety disorders; eating disorders; elimination disorders; mood disorders, including major depression and mania; and disruptive behavioral symptoms. In addition, adolescents in foster care are at increased risk for having attempted suicide and having a drug dependency diagnosis within the preceding 12 months compared with their peers who had not been involved with the foster care system.[69,71]

The pediatrician plays a key role in coordinating the health care management of adopted children with special health care needs. After any acute and chronic illnesses have been identified, a review of any previous medical testing is appropriate to make referrals to pediatric medical subspecialists. Although referral is important, carefully prioritizing acute and chronic conditions is critical to promoting successful adjustment and encouraging the family to establish a medical home for ongoing continuity of care.

HEARING SCREENING

Assessment of hearing is recommended for all children (Table 5). Newborn hearing screening is recommended for all newborn infants in the United States. It is recommended to document the results and make them a part of the child's permanent medical record. For international adoptees, conductive and sensorineural hearing loss has been shown to occur at a higher rate compared with the general population, justifying the recommendation of a formal audiological examination for all adoptees.[25,57,72] Regardless of the route of adoption, if hearing loss is noted, the child is at risk for speech and language delay.

VISION SCREENING

Pediatricians should ask the parents about any history of vision problems. An eye examination needs to be performed on all children, as the AAP recommends in Bright Futures (Table 5).[73] Vision screening is particularly important for international adoptees. A study involving the Minnesota International Adoption Project survey reported approximately 30% of international adoptees screened had vision problems.[74] Diagnoses included myopia, hyperopia, astigmatism,

TABLE 5 Other Screening Evaluations

- Hearing
  - o Validate newborn screening when available
  - o Screen all children, particularly those with risk factors for hearing loss as well as developmental (speech) delays
- Vision
  - o Eye examination as appropriate for age
  - o Screening for refraction error at 3 y of age
  - o Funduscopic examination for children with birth wt <1500 g
- Dental
  - o Referral to dentist for all children ≥12 mo old
  - o Earlier referral if evidence of dental caries or abuse via the mouth
- Developmental screening, assessment, and/or interventions
  - o Timely identification of developmental delays is strongly recommended
  - o Risk factors include prematurity, licit and/or illicit drug and/or alcohol exposure, poor prenatal care, institutionalization
    - ■ Formal referral for all children adopted in the newborn period or beyond with risk factors as listed or other concerns
    - ■ Referral for all children adopted beyond the newborn period with risk factors or concerns about development when appropriate
    - ■ For children adopted internationally, a speech evaluation within a few weeks of arrival home by a speech therapist fluent in the child's native language is optimal to help reveal gaps in articulation and language processing skills
  - o Referrals may be made to an early intervention program for children from birth up to 36 mo of age
  - o Referrals through the school system for children ≥36 mo old with establishment of an IEP when appropriate
  - o Referral for speech and/or language, occupational, and physical therapy when indicated; children adopted internationally can be placed in an educational setting with flexible placement based on the child's developmental profile, not solely on the child's age

strabismus, and other abnormalities, including optic atrophy and abnormal tearing. Of note, international adoptees who were institutionalized are 10% to 25% more likely to have strabismus.[25] The red reflex should be documented in all newborn infants. A funduscopic examination of dilated eyes can be performed by an ophthalmologist for all children with a birth weight <1500 g.[75] It is recommended that older children be examined for strabismus and abnormalities of the fundus, eyelids, and extraocular muscles. Vision screening should be performed for all children 3 years and older.[73] For internationally adopted children, particularly if the history includes institutionalization, it is recommended that an ophthalmologist see the children within the first few months after arrival in the United States.[25]

DENTAL

A dental assessment should be performed on all children, and referral to a dentist is recommend on the basis of risk assessment (including abuse of the mouth) as early as 6 months of age, 6 months after the first tooth erupts, and no later than 12 months of age (Table 5).[73] Any previous dental diagnoses should be reviewed, including appropriate referrals to dental specialists, for the establishment of a dental home. Dental professionals should be informed about any previous medical illnesses and malnutrition as well as periods in which the child lived in an area of the world with no fluoride in the diet.

AGE DETERMINATION

For some international adoptees, accuracy of date of birth may be questionable. For children younger than 1 year, a difference of weeks or a few months will not be critical in the long-term.[27,47] For older children, age determination may be more important, especially with respect to placement in school and eligibility for special education services.[27,47] There are no accurate or reliable tests for age determination. Malnutrition and deprivation may affect assessments using standard measurements, including radiographic bone age and dental eruption. Onset of puberty may be advanced as a child's nutritional status rapidly improves. It is usually best to delay changing a birth date until at least 12 months after adoption to allow for catch-up growth as well as prolonged observation of a child's physical and emotional development.[42,47] Input from other providers and professionals interacting with the child is advisable to facilitate optimal outcomes for the child.

DEVELOPMENTAL SCREENING

Developmental screening should be performed by using validated screening tools; for the internationally adopted child, this may be a complicated issue (Table 5). Validated screening tools performed shortly after arrival often may be difficult to interpret. The child usually faces a language barrier, and his or her exposure to the types of materials used for testing may be limited. For these children, early scores may not be predictive of later functioning.[76] Several studies have demonstrated significant developmental delays in children as they enter foster care, particularly in speech and language.[6,9,68,77–79] Likewise, children adopted internationally nearly always demonstrate delays in at least 1 area of development, with nearly half having global delays.[17,80–82] Children adopted internationally may demonstrate delays in expressive and receptive language that are not solely related to acquisition of a new language.[17,21,83] Although catch-up development does occur, studies have shown that many children are at increased risk of long-term consequences of developmental delay depending on age at adoption and length of time spent in an institutional setting.[75,82] Therefore, it is recommended that pediatricians refer adopted children to an intervention program in a timely manner.

MENTAL HEALTH REVIEW

Children adopted from foster care and children adopted from institutions are at an increased risk of mental health disorders, including socioemotional problems.[8,82,83] Preplacement factors, such as prenatal stress, prenatal drug and alcohol exposure, prolonged institutionalization, multiple placements, and previous trauma, contribute significantly to the emotional problems of these children.[24,26,36,42,76,83–85] These early experiences, either singularly or in combination, may have a lifelong effect on the developing brain secondary to the body's physiologic responses or toxic stress reaction.[26] Children who have been exposed to high levels of stress because of life experiences may develop heightened activity of the stress system, resulting in problem behaviors later in life.

When available, it is recommended that pediatricians consider any history of mental health diagnoses in members of the birth family and manage a child or adolescent carefully with the use of validated screening tests, such as the Pediatric Symptom Checklist,[86] Brief Infant-Toddler Social and Emotional Assessment,[87] Ages and Stages Questionnaire: Social-Emotional,[88] Early Childhood Screening Assessment,[89] Strengths and Difficulties Questionnaire,[90] or Patient Health Questionnaire 2.[91] Appropriate referrals for evidence-based therapies[92–94] need to be made when such a risk presents itself. Although referrals may be performed at the time of placement for children with a history of abuse or neglect, screening for mental health disorders needs to be conducted at all medical visits, particularly at the time of regular health assessments (Table 6).

ISSUES OF ADJUSTMENT AND TRANSITIONS

It is important to address adjustment issues at the time of placement into the home. Many of these issues may be intensified by the many transitions that the adopted child may have experienced. Children may be withdrawn, have temper tantrums, be aggressive or defiant, cry inconsolably, or even have autisticlike behavior as they undergo changes in their family placement.[16] Some children may regress in previously obtained skills. Older internationally adopted children may encounter frustrating language barriers with their adoptive family.[16,21] Even if transitions into an adoptive home are gradual, most children experience grief with the change in their caregivers, peers, and home environment.[16,95,96] Sleep problems are also common.[16,95,96] Difficulties in timing, location, duration, and quality of sleep are typical.[16] Feeding problems may present after adoption. Feeding issues may include overeating, hoarding, or food refusal.[16] Pediatricians need to counsel families about potential adjustment issues and encourage them to look for cues that the children may be overwhelmed and help them to develop strategies to promote strong, healthy attachments within the family unit.[96] Parenting strategies to address overeating, food hoarding, and sleep struggles may need to be different from usual pediatric advice, addressing the child's need for extra security around food and sleep.

KINSHIP-SPECIFIC ISSUES

The Child Welfare League of America defines kinship care as "the full-time care, nurturing, and protection of children by relatives, members of their tribes or clans, godparents, step-parents, or any adult who has

TABLE 6 Behavioral and Mental Health Recommendations

- Review behavior, including past and present concerns
  - o Adjustment
  - o Fostering or positive relationships
  - o Aggressive behavior
  - o Disruptive behaviors (stealing and lying)
  - o Hyperactivity
  - o Impulsivity
  - o Internalizing behaviors (withdrawal and anxiety)
  - o Sleep issues
  - o Feeding issues, including overeating or hoarding food
  - o Enuresis and/or encopresis
  - o Selective mutism
  - o Habit disorders (trichotillomania and dermatillomania)
- Document psychiatric medications used currently or in the past
- Document any past psychiatric hospitalizations
- Previous violent behavior or animal cruelty
- Sexualizing behaviors
  - o Sexual promiscuity or acting out
  - o Excessive or inappropriate masturbation
- Substance use
  - o Tobacco, alcohol, and licit and/or illicit substances
- Suicide
  - o Suicidal ideology
  - o Previous suicide attempts
- Monitor for issues related to loss and grief, attachment disturbances, posttraumatic stress disorder
  - o Children may not admit to previous abuse or neglect until they are secure in a new family. This may be revealed months or years after placement.
  - o Even children placed as newborn infants may have struggles related to their history of adoption (ie, identity development) that do not necessarily rise to the level of mental health issues.

a kinship bond with a child."[97] The Annie E. Casey Foundation reports that 2.7 million (4%) US children are being raised by extended family members or family friends, with the majority being in an informal arrangement.[98] Only about 104 000 of these children have been placed in a formal kinship arrangement, accounting for one-fourth of all children who have been removed from their homes by the child welfare system and placed in state custody.[98]

Kinship care has been shown to add value for children in care.[98–102] Children in kinship care experience greater stability by having fewer placement changes and fewer school changes.[98–102] Children are more likely to live with their siblings and, if they reunify with birth parents after kinship care, are less likely to reenter foster care.[100–102] Children in kinship care report being more likely to have positive views of their living environment, feel more culturally connected, and have a feeling of being loved than children in nonkinship foster care.[101,102]

Although kinship care has many advantages for children, there are some notable potential concerns. Contact with biological parents, who may be responsible for the neglect or abuse of the child, may be unavoidable.[102,103] Caregivers are typically older and less economically stable.[102–104] Many families who are eligible for benefits fail to request and accept government assistance.[102,105] Children are also more likely to be in guardianship rather than being adopted.[101,102]

Children placed with kin need the same comprehensive evaluation as those living in nonrelative placements.[40,41,102] This recommendation applies even if the child has had no interruption in his or her medical home before or after placement. Studies have demonstrated that the incidence of chronic medical problems and mental health concerns in children living in kinship foster care are similar to those of children living in nonrelative foster care.[102,106–108]

SAFE HAVEN INFANTS

All states, including the District of Columbia and Puerto Rico, have enacted legislation to address infant abandonment and infanticide.[109] Infants can be safely placed anonymously in designated locations where they can be protected and given medical care until a permanent home can be found. Age limits for relinquishing infants through this program are state specific, ranging from no more than 72 hours to up to 1 month of age. Physician responsibility and legal accountability also differ by state.[109] Although the purpose of infant safety is enhanced, maternal and infant history may be deidentified, scarce, or unknown. Therefore, the same attention to care given to other adopted children needs to be given to these infants.

SPECIAL ISSUES IN THE EDUCATION ENVIRONMENT

Despite the route of adoption, children come to the educational system with their own unique needs secondary to their complex life experiences. Their physical and mental health, as well as their socioemotional responses, affect their ability to maximize learning. Pediatricians need to be aware of available resources within the educational system. For children younger than 3 years, there are early intervention programs available in every state and territory. After the third birthday, it is recommended that children who are at risk or have known developmental deficits or academic challenges be referred to the school system for evaluation and ongoing services. Important resources include the Individualized Educational Program (IEP) and the 504 Plan.[110] Pediatricians can be helpful in this process by providing detailed information concerning the children's chronic or complex health care needs on school forms (Table 7).

An IEP uses a multidisciplinary approach to establish a written educational program designed to meet a child's individual needs and how progress will be monitored. Typically, the IEP involves a psychological and educational assessment, review of the child's developmental and psychosocial histories, and an examination of medical data. For children who do not meet the criteria for an IEP, an option for support services is the 504 Plan. Many schools use the 504 Plan as a first step to provide services and then advance to an IEP. It is available to children who may have medical needs that affect learning even if they do not have a verified learning disorder or chronic disease.[110]

ROLE OF ADOPTION MEDICAL SPECIALISTS

Adoption and foster care medicine is an evolving subspecialty within the field of pediatrics that serves as a valuable resource for adoptive and foster families, especially families with international adoptees. Many international adoption specialists may review records electronically, thereby increasing the availability of this resource to families who may not live near an international adoption clinic. The AAP Council on Foster Care, Adoption, and Kinship Care is a resource for further training for physicians who care for children who have been adopted or are in foster or kinship care.

FINANCIAL CONSIDERATIONS

The comprehensive assessment of a newly adopted child requires extensive physician time and commitment. The initial evaluation visits are far more in-depth than simple well-child visits and can be billed as problem-based encounter

TABLE 7 Educational Resources

- 504 Plan
  - o Children who do not meet criteria for an IEP but still need classroom support services, including educational or speech and language services
- IEP
  - o A legal document detailing the child's learning needs and the school system's responsibility in providing the needed services to maximize student success and how it will be measured
  - o Plans typically include a psychological assessment, educational assessment, developmental history, psychosocial history, and medical data

visits. Coding of the problem-based encounter is then based on the complexity of the visit or time spent in counseling and/or coordination of care.[111,112] Services such as the preplacement consultation may not be covered by most insurance carriers, but the pediatrician may want to advise the adoptive parent to seek information from the parent's employer about benefits covered through an adoption subsidy plan or flexible-spending account. Children adopted through the foster care system may have continuation of their Medicaid benefits even after the adoption is finalized. Finally, families may be eligible for the federal adoption tax credit to offset some of the adoption-related costs.

ADDITIONAL RESOURCE

The CDC's *Yellow Book*[44] can serve as a useful resource for international travel and includes a chapter specifically for international adoption (https://wwwnc.cdc.gov/travel/yellowbook/2018/international-travel-with-infants-children/international-adoption).[113] It provides information on pretravel preparation of adoptive parents, discussion of the overseas medical examination, and the follow-up examination after arrival in the United States. There is also information on screening for infectious diseases and review of immunizations.

CONCLUSIONS

Children who are adopted are in need of a comprehensive health evaluation to fully address all their health and developmental needs. This comprehensive evaluation is best accomplished with the establishment of a medical home for adopted children. The comprehensive health evaluation should include a review of the child's medical history, complete physical examination, and necessary diagnostic testing. It is recommended that important consideration be given to risks in the child's past with full attention given to infectious diseases and environmental, nutritional, developmental, and mental health risks. Pediatricians play an important role in working with families to identify children's needs and providing emotional support to help families through the adoption process. Ongoing awareness of the adopted child's history through enhanced well-child care and follow-up visits will enable the pediatrician to identify other health issues that may develop and assist families in accessing resources that will help them in the long-term.

LEAD AUTHORS

Veronnie Faye Jones, MD, PhD, MSPH, FAAP
Elaine E. Schulte, MD, MPH, FAAP

COUNCIL ON FOSTER CARE, ADOPTION, AND KINSHIP CARE EXECUTIVE COMMITTEE, 2017–2018

Sarah Springer, MD, FAAP, Chairperson
Moira Ann Szilagyi, MD, PhD, FAAP, Immediate Past Chair
Heather Forkey, MD, FAAP
Mary V. Greiner, MD, MS, FAAP
David Harmon, MD, FAAP
Veronnie Faye Jones, MD, PhD, MSPH, FAAP
Paul Lee, MD, FAAP
Lisa Maxine Nalven, MD, MA, FAAP
Linda Davidson Sagor, MD, MPH, FAAP
Jonathan D. Thackery, MD, FAAP
Douglas Waite, MD, FAAP
Lisa W. Zetley, MD, FAAP

LIAISONS

George Alex Fouras, MD – *American Academy of Child and Adolescent Psychiatry*
Jeremy Harvey – *Foster Care Alumni of America*
Timothy D. Chow, MD – *American Academy of Pediatrics Section on Pediatric Trainees*

STAFF

Mary Crane, PhD, LSW

ABBREVIATIONS

AAP: American Academy of Pediatrics
CDC: Centers for Disease Control and Prevention
HBV: hepatitis B virus
IEP: Individualized Education Program

PEDIATRICS (ISSN Numbers: Print, 0031-4005; Online, 1098-4275).

Copyright © 2019 by the American Academy of Pediatrics

FINANCIAL DISCLOSURE: The authors have indicated they have no financial relationships relevant to this article to disclose.

FUNDING: No external funding.

POTENTIAL CONFLICT OF INTEREST: The authors have indicated they have no potential conflicts of interest to disclose.

REFERENCES

1. Child Welfare Information Gateway. Trends in U.S. adoptions: 2008–2012. 2016. Available at: www.childwelfare.gov. Accessed March 15, 2016
2. US Department of Health and Human Services, Administration for Children and Families, Administration on Children, Youth and Families, Children's Bureau. Trends in foster care and adoption: FY 2005–2014. Available at: www.acf.hhs.gov/programs/cb. Accessed March 16, 2016
3. Adoption and Safe Families Act of 1997, 42 USC §1305, Pub L No. 105-89
4. Willis CD, Norris DM. Custodial evaluations of Native American families: implications for forensic psychiatrists. *J Am Acad Psychiatry Law.* 2010;38(4):540–546
5. Department of the State. Intercountry adoption: adoption statistics. Available at: https://travel.state.gov/content/adoptionsabroad/en/about-us/statistics.html. Accessed March 17, 2018
6. Chernoff R, Combs-Orme T, Risley-Curtiss C, Heisler A. Assessing the health status of children entering foster care. *Pediatrics.* 1994;93(4):594–601
7. Simms MD, Dubowitz H, Szilagyi MA. Health care needs of children in the foster care system. *Pediatrics.* 2000;106(suppl 4):909–918
8. Juffer F, van Ijzendoorn MH. Behavior problems and mental health referrals of international adoptees: a meta-analysis. *JAMA.* 2005;293(20):2501–2515
9. Bramlett MD, Radel LF, Blumberg SJ. The health and well-being of adopted children. *Pediatrics.* 2007;119(suppl 1):S54–S60
10. Zill N, Bramlett MD. Health and well-being of children adopted from foster care. *Child Youth Serv Rev.* 2014;40:29–40
11. Harwood R, Feng X, Yu S. Preadoption adversities and postadoption mediators of mental health and school outcomes among international, foster, and private adoptees in the United States. *J Fam Psychol.* 2013;27(3):409–420
12. Dawood F, Serwint JR. International adoption. *Pediatr Rev.* 2008;29(8):292–294
13. Jenista JA, Chapman D. Medical problems of foreign-born adopted children. *Am J Dis Child.* 1987;141(3):298–302
14. Hostetter MK, Iverson S, Dole K, Johnson D. Unsuspected infectious diseases and other medical diagnoses in the evaluation of internationally adopted children. *Pediatrics.* 1989;83(4):559–564
15. Barnett ED. Immunizations and infectious disease screening for internationally adopted children. *Pediatr Clin North Am.* 2005;52(5):1287–1309, vi
16. Miller LC. Immediate behavioral and developmental considerations for internationally adopted children transitioning to families. *Pediatr Clin North Am.* 2005;52(5):1311–1330, vi–vii
17. Bolton MK, Day D. A systemic evidenced based literature review of medical and developmental issues of international adoptees with emphasis on the need for immediate and thorough medical attention post-adoption. In: Eichhorn DM, Kovar S, eds. *Proceedings: 3rd Annual Symposium: Graduate Research and Scholarly Projects.* Wichita, KS: Wichita State University; 2007:135–136
18. American Academy of Pediatrics. Medical evaluation for infectious diseases for internationally adopted, refugee, and immigrant children. In: Kimberlin DW, Brady MT, Jackson MA, Long SS, eds. *Red Book: 2018 Report of the Committee on Infectious Diseases.* 31st ed. Itasca, IL: American Academy of Pediatrics; 2018:176–185
19. Eckerle JK, Howard CR, John CC. Infections in internationally adopted children. *Pediatr Clin North Am.* 2013;60(2):487–505
20. Sperling R. The primary care physician's role in caring for internationally adopted children. *J Am Osteopath Assoc.* 2001;101(6):345–346
21. Bledsoe JM, Johnston BD. Preparing families for international adoption. *Pediatr Rev.* 2004;25(7):242–250
22. Davies JK, Bledsoe JM. Prenatal alcohol and drug exposures in adoption. *Pediatr Clin North Am.* 2005;52(5):1369–1393, vii
23. National Center on Substance Abuse and Child Welfare. Fact sheet 3—research studies on the prevalence of substance use disorders in the child welfare population. Available at: https://ncsacw.samhsa.gov/files/Research_Studies_Prevalence_Factsheets.pdf. Accessed March 1, 2016
24. American Academy of Pediatrics. Pre-adoption considerations for pediatricians. In: Mason P, Johnson DE, Prock LA, eds. *Adoption Medicine: Caring for Children and Families.* Elk Grove Village, IL: American Academy of Pediatrics; 2014:73–96
25. American Academy of Pediatrics. Postadoption evaluation for the health care professional. In: Mason P, Johnson DE, Prock LA, eds. *Adoption Medicine: Caring for Children and Families.* Elk Grove Village, IL: American Academy of Pediatrics; 2014:163–175
26. Garner AS, Shonkoff JP; Committee on Psychosocial Aspects of Child and Family Health; Committee on Early Childhood, Adoption, and Dependent Care; Section on Developmental and Behavioral Pediatrics. Early childhood adversity, toxic stress, and the role of the pediatrician: translating developmental science into lifelong health. *Pediatrics.* 2012;129(1). Available at: www.pediatrics.org/cgi/content/full/129/1/e224
27. Mitchell MA, Jenista JA. Health care of the internationally adopted child part 1. Before and at arrival into the adoptive home. *J Pediatr Health Care.* 1997;11(2):51–60
28. Jenista JA. Findings from foreign medical records. *Adoption/Medical News.* 1999;10:1–6
29. Jenista JA. Preadoption review of medical records. *Pediatr Ann.* 2000;29(4):212–215
30. Chambers J. Preadoption opportunities for pediatric providers. *Pediatr Clin North Am.* 2005;52(5):1247–1269, v–vi
31. Siegel DH. Open adoption of infants: adoptive parents' feelings seven years later. *Soc Work.* 2003;48(3):409–419

32. Gustafson KL, Eckerle JK, Howard CR, Andrews B, Polgreen LE. Prevalence of vitamin D deficiency in international adoptees within the first 6 months after adoption. *Clin Pediatr (Phila)*. 2013; 52(12):1149–1153

33. Bryant CA. Nursing the adopted infant. *J Am Board Fam Med*. 2006;19(4): 374–379

34. Wittig SL, Spatz DL. Induced lactation: gaining a better understanding. *MCN Am J Matern Child Nurs*. 2008;33(2): 76–81; quiz 82–83

35. Howard T, Grosel J. Updated guidelines for lipid screening in children and adolescents. *JAAPA*. 2015;28(3):30–36

36. American Academy of Pediatrics. Prenatal substance exposure: alcohol and other substances – implications for adoption. In: Mason P, Johnson DE, Prock LA, eds. *Adoption Medicine: Caring for Children and Families*. Elk Grove Village, IL: American Academy of Pediatrics; 2014:97–122

37. American Academy of Pediatrics. Relating genetics to psychiatric issues for children with a history of adoption. In: Mason P, Johnson DE, Prock LA, eds. *Adoption Medicine: Caring for Children and Families*. Elk Grove Village, IL: American Academy of Pediatrics; 2014: 123–137

38. Dominicé Dao M, Inglin S, Vilpert S, Hudelson P. The relevance of clinical ethnography: reflections on 10 years of a cultural consultation service. *BMC Health Serv Res*. 2018;18(1):19

39. American Academy of Pediatrics; District II, New York State Task Force on Health Care for Children in Foster Care. *Fostering Health: Health Care for Children and Adolescents in Foster Care*. 2nd ed. Elk Grove Village, IL: American Academy of Pediatrics, District II, New York State Task Force on Health Care for Children in Foster Care; 2005

40. Szilagyi MA, Rosen DS, Rubin D, Zlotnik S; Council on Foster Care, Adoption, and Kinship Care; Committee on Adolescence; Council on Early Childhood. Health care issues for children and adolescents in foster care and kinship care. *Pediatrics*. 2015; 136(4). Available at: www.pediatrics.org/cgi/content/full/136/4/e1142

41. Council on Foster Care; Adoption, and Kinship Care; Committee on Adolescence, and Council on Early Childhood. Health care issues for children and adolescents in foster care and kinship care. *Pediatrics*. 2015; 136(4). Available at: www.pediatrics.org/cgi/content/full/136/4/e1131

42. Szilagyi M. The pediatrician and the child in foster care. *Pediatr Rev*. 1998; 19(2):39–50

43. Aronson J. Medical evaluation and infectious considerations on arrival. *Pediatr Ann*. 2000;29(4):218–223

44. Centers for Disease Control and Prevention. Travelers' health. Available at: https://wwwnc.cdc.gov/travel/yellowbook/2018/table-of-contents. Accessed October 13, 2017

45. Obringer E, Walsh L. Infectious diseases and immunizations in international adoption. *Pediatr Ann*. 2017;46(2): e56–e60

46. Abdulla RY, Rice MA, Donauer S, Hicks KR, Poore D, Staat MA. Hepatitis A in internationally adopted children: screening for acute and previous infections. *Pediatrics*. 2010;126(5). Available at: www.pediatrics.org/cgi/content/full/126/5/e1039

47. Jenista JA. The immigrant, refugee, or internationally adopted child. *Pediatr Rev*. 2001;22(12):419–429

48. Grummer-Strawn LM, Reinold C, Krebs NF; Centers for Disease Control and Prevention (CDC). Use of World Health Organization and CDC growth charts for children aged 0-59 months in the United States. *MMWR Recomm Rep*. 2010;59 (RR-9):1–15

49. Garza C, de Onis M. Rationale for developing a new international growth reference. *Food Nutr Bull*. 2004;25 (suppl):S5–S14

50. Kuczmarski RJ, Ogden CL, Guo SS, et al. 2000 CDC Growth Charts for the United States: methods and development. *Vital Health Stat 11*. 2002;(246):1–190

51. Natale V, Rajagopalan A. Worldwide variation in human growth and the World Health Organization growth standards: a systematic review. *BMJ Open*. 2014;4(1):e003735

52. Hadfield SC, Preece PM. Obesity in looked after children: is foster care protective from the dangers of obesity? *Child Care Health Dev*. 2008;34(6): 710–712

53. Schneiderman JU, Smith C, Arnold-Clark JS, Fuentes J, Duan L, Palinkas LA. Overweight and obesity among Hispanic children entering foster care: a preliminary examination of polyvictimization. *Child Maltreat*. 2013; 18(4):264–273

54. Schneiderman JU, Smith C, Arnold-Clark JS, Fuentes J, Duan L. Weight changes in children in foster care for 1 year. *Child Abuse Negl*. 2013;37(10):832–840

55. Abdulcadir J, Catania L, Hindin MJ, Say L, Petignat P, Abdulcadir O. Female genital mutilation: a visual reference and learning tool for health care professionals. *Obstet Gynecol*. 2016; 128(5):958–963

56. American Academy of Pediatrics. Considerations for testing for infectious agents. In: Kimberlin DW, Brady MT, Jackson MA, Long SS, eds. *Red Book: 2018 Report of the Committee on Infectious Diseases*, 31st ed. Itasca, IL: American Academy of Pediatrics; 2018: 178–185

57. Harlor AD Jr, Bower C; Committee on Practice and Ambulatory Medicine; Section on Otolaryngology-Head and Neck Surgery. Hearing assessment in infants and children: recommendations beyond neonatal screening. *Pediatrics*. 2009;124(4):1252–1263

58. Young TL, Riggs M, Robinson JL. Childhood sexual abuse severity reconsidered: a factor structure of CSA characteristics. *J Child Sex Abuse*. 2011; 20(4):373–395

59. Centers for Disease Control and Prevention. Zika virus. Available at: www.cdc.gov/zika/index.html. Accessed March 12, 2019

60. Miller L, Chan W, Comfort K, Tirella L. Health of children adopted from Guatemala: comparison of orphanage and foster care. *Pediatrics*. 2005;115(6). Available at: www.pediatrics.org/cgi/content/full/115/6/e710

61. Fuglestad AJ, Kroupina MG, Johnson DE, Georgieff MK. Micronutrient status and neurodevelopment in internationally adopted children. *Acta Paediatr*. 2016; 105(2):e67–e76

62. Centers for Disease Control and Prevention. Immunization schedules. Available at: www.cdc.gov/vaccines/schedules/index.html. Accessed March 15, 2018

63. Miller LC, Comfort K, Kely N. Immunization status of internationally adopted children. *Pediatrics.* 2001; 108(4):1050–1051

64. Stoltzfus E, Baumrucker EP, Fernandes-Alcantara AL, Fernandez B. *Child Welfare: Health Care Needs of Children in Foster Care and Related Federal Issues.* Washington, DC: Congressional Research Service; 2014. Available at https://www.fas.org/sgp/crs/misc/R42378.pdf. Accessed March 15, 2018

65. McMillen JC, Zima BT, Scott LD Jr, et al. Prevalence of psychiatric disorders among older youths in the foster care system. *J Am Acad Child Adolesc Psychiatry.* 2005;44(1):88–95

66. Vanderwerker L, Akincigil A, Olfson M, Gerhard T, Neese-Todd S, Crystal S. Foster care, externalizing disorders, and antipsychotic use among Medicaid-enrolled youths. *Psychiatr Serv.* 2014; 65(10):1281–1284

67. Deutsch SA, Lynch A, Zlotnik S, Matone M, Kreider A, Noonan K. Mental health, behavioral and developmental issues for youth in foster care. *Curr Probl Pediatr Adolesc Health Care.* 2015; 45(10):292–297

68. Leslie LK, Gordon JN, Meneken L, Premji K, Michelmore KL, Ganger W. The physical, developmental, and mental health needs of young children in child welfare by initial placement type. *J Dev Behav Pediatr.* 2005;26(3):177–185

69. Pilowsky DJ, Wu LT. Psychiatric symptoms and substance use disorders in a nationally representative sample of American adolescents involved with foster care. *J Adolesc Health.* 2006; 38(4):351–358

70. Behnke M, Smith VC; Committee on Substance Abuse; Committee on Fetus and Newborn. Prenatal substance abuse: short- and long-term effects on the exposed fetus. *Pediatrics.* 2013; 131(3). Available at: www.pediatrics.org/cgi/content/full/131/3/e1009

71. National Institute on Drug Use. Is there a link between drug use and psychiatric disorders? Available at: https://www.drugabuse.gov/publications/research-reports/marijuana/there-link-between-marijuana-use-psychiatric-disorders. Accessed March 2, 2017

72. Johnson DE. Long-term medical issues in international adoptees. *Pediatr Ann.* 2000;29(4):234–241

73. Hagan JF, Shaw JS, Duncan PM, eds. *Bright Futures: Guidelines for Health Supervision of Infants, Children, and Adolescents.* 4th ed. Elk Grove Village, IL: American Academy of Pediatrics; 2017

74. Eckerle JK, Hill LK, Iverson S, Hellerstedt W, Gunnar M, Johnson DE. Vision and hearing deficits and associations with parent-reported behavioral and developmental problems in international adoptees. *Matern Child Health J.* 2014;18(3):575–583

75. Holmström G, Larsson E. Long-term follow-up of visual functions in prematurely born children-- a prospective population-based study up to 10 years of age. *J AAPOS.* 2008; 12(2):157–162

76. Rutter M; English and Romanian Adoptees (ERA) Study Team. Developmental catch-up, and deficit, following adoption after severe global early privation. *J Child Psychol Psychiatry.* 1998;39(4):465–476

77. Halfon N, Mendonca A, Berkowitz G. Health status of children in foster care. The experience of the Center for the Vulnerable Child. *Arch Pediatr Adolesc Med.* 1995;149(4):386–392

78. Takayama JI, Wolfe E, Coulter KP. Relationship between reason for placement and medical findings among children in foster care. *Pediatrics.* 1998; 101(2):201–207

79. Ringeisen H, Casanueva C, Urato M, Cross T. Special health care needs among children in the child welfare system. *Pediatrics.* 2008;122(1). Available at: www.pediatrics.org/cgi/content/full/122/1/e232

80. Miller LC, Kiernan MT, Mathers MI, Klein-Gitelman M. Developmental and nutritional status of internationally adopted children. *Arch Pediatr Adolesc Med.* 1995;149(1):40–44

81. Albers LH, Johnson DE, Hostetter MK, Iverson S, Miller LC. Health of children adopted from the former Soviet Union and Eastern Europe. Comparison with preadoptive medical records. *JAMA.* 1997;278(11):922–924

82. Weitzman C, Albers L. Long-term developmental, behavioral, and attachment outcomes after international adoption. *Pediatr Clin North Am.* 2005;52(5):1395–1419, viii

83. Miller LC. Initial assessment of growth, development, and the effects of institutionalization in internationally adopted children. *Pediatr Ann.* 2000; 29(4):224–232

84. Beijers R, Buitelaar JK, de Weenth C. Mechanisms underlying the effects of prenatal psychosocial stress on child outcomes: beyond the HPA axis. *Eur Child Adolesc Psychiatry.* 2014;23(10): 943–956

85. Kofman O. The role of prenatal stress in the etiology of developmental behavioural disorders. *Neurosci Biobehav Rev.* 2002;26(4):457–470

86. Jellinek MS, Murphy JM, Burns BJ. Brief psychosocial screening in outpatient pediatric practice. *J Pediatr.* 1986; 109(2):371–378

87. Briggs-Gowan MJ, Carter AS. Social-emotional screening status in early childhood predicts elementary school outcomes. *Pediatrics.* 2008;121(5): 957–962

88. Squires J, Bricker D, Twombly E, et al. *Ages and Stages Questionnaire: Social-Emotional ASQ:SE-2: A Parent-Completed Child Monitoring System for Socio-Emotional Behaviors.* 2nd ed. Baltimore, MD: Brookes Publishing Inc; 2015. Available at: www.brookespublishing.com/resource-center/screening-and-assessment/asq/asq-se-2/. Accessed June 8, 2016

89. Fallucco EM, Robertson Blackmore E, Bejarano CM, Wysocki T, Kozikowski CB, Gleason MM. Feasibility of screening for preschool behavioral and emotional problems in primary care using the Early Childhood Screening Assessment. *Clin Pediatr (Phila).* 2017;56(1):37–45

90. Theunissen MHC, Vogels AG, de Wolff MS, Reijneveld SA. Characteristics of the Strengths and Difficulties Questionnaire in preschool children. *Pediatrics.* 2013;131(2). Available at: www.pediatrics.org/cgi/content/full/131/2/e446

91. Kroenke K, Spitzer RL, Williams JB. The Patient Health Questionnaire-2: validity of a two-item depression screener. *Med Care*. 2003;41(11):1284–1292

92. Substance Abuse and Mental Health Services Administration. *Interventions for Disruptive Behavior Disorders: Evidence-Based and Promising Practices. HHS Publication No. SMA-11-4634*. Rockville, MD: Center for Mental Health Services, Substance Abuse and Mental Health Services Administration, US Department of Health and Human Services; 2011

93. National Child Traumatic Stress Network. Trauma-focused cognitive behavioral therapy. Available at: www.nctsn.org/sites/default/files/assets/pdfs/tfcbt_general.pdf. Accessed March 12, 2016

94. Lohr WD, Jones VF. Mental health issues in foster care. *Pediatr Ann*. 2016;45(10):e342–e348

95. Schulte EE, Springer SH. Health care in the first year after international adoption. *Pediatr Clin North Am*. 2005;52(5):1331–1349, vii

96. Jones VF, Schulte EE; Committee on Early Childhood; Council on Foster Care, Adoption, and Kinship Care. The pediatrician's role in supporting adoptive families. *Pediatrics*. 2012;130(4). Available at: www.pediatrics.org/cgi/content/full/130/4/e1040

97. Child Welfare League of America. Kinship care: Traditions of caring and collaborating model of practice. Available at: https://www.cwla.org/kinship-care/. Accessed March 12, 2019

98. The Annie E. Casey Foundation. Stepping up for kids: what government and communities should do to support kinship families. Available at: www.aecf.org/m/resourcedoc/AECF-SteppingUpForKids-2012.pdf. Accessed May, 2016

99. Generations United. In loving arms: the protective role of grandparents and other relatives in raising children exposed to trauma. The 2017 State of Grandfamilies in America Annual Report. Available at: https://www.gu.org/app/uploads/2018/05/Grandfamilies-Report-SOGF-2017.pdf. Accessed March 22, 2019

100. Conway T, Hutson RQ. Is kinship care good for kids? Available at: www.clasp.org/resources-and-publications/files/0347.pdf. Accessed March 31, 2016

101. Winokur M, Holtan A, Valentine D. Kinship care for the safety, permanency, and well-being of children removed from the home for maltreatment. *Campbell Syst Rev*. 2008;16:1–174

102. Rubin D, Springer SH, Zlotnik S, Kang-Yi CD; Council on Foster Care, Adoption, and Kinship Care. Needs of kinship care families and pediatric practice. *Pediatrics*. 2017;139(4):e20170099

103. Terling-Watt T. Permanency in kinship care: an exploration of disruption rates and factors associated with placement disruption. *Child Youth Serv Rev*. 2001;23(2):111–112

104. Harris MS. Kinship care for African American children: disproportionate and disadvantageous. *J Fam Issues*. 2008;29(8):1013–1030

105. Dubowitz H, Feigelman S, Zuravin S, Tepper V, Davidson N, Lichenstein R. The physical health of children in kinship care. *Am J Dis Child*. 1992;146(5):603–610

106. Dubowitz H, Zuravin S, Starr RH Jr, Feigelman S, Harrington D. Behavior problems of children in kinship care. *J Dev Behav Pediatr*. 1993;14(6):386–393

107. Feigelman S, Zuravin S, Dubowitz H, Harrington D, Starr RH Jr, Tepper V. Sources of health care and health needs among children in kinship care. *Arch Pediatr Adolesc Med*. 1995;149(8):882–886

108. Stein RE, Hurlburt MS, Heneghan AM, et al. Health status and type of out-of-home placement: informal kinship care in an investigated sample. *Acad Pediatr*. 2014;14(6):559–564

109. Child Welfare Information Gateway. Infant safe haven laws. Available at: https://www.childwelfare.gov/pubPDFs/safehaven.pdf. Accessed March 5, 2017

110. Kennedy K. IEPs vs. 504 plans: pediatrician's office often first stop for families navigating educational issues. AAP News. January 9, 2017. Available at: https://www.aappublications.org/news/2017/01/09/IEP010917. Accessed March 12, 2019

111. American Academy of Pediatrics, Committee on Coding. *Coding for Pediatrics 2016: A Manual for Pediatric Documentation and Payment*. 21st ed. Elk Grove Village, IL: American Academy of Pediatrics; 2015

112. Trauma Dissociation.com. Trauma and stressor-related disorders. Available at: http://traumadissociation.com/trauma-stressor. Accessed June 5, 2016

113. Centers for Disease Control and Prevention. Chapter 7: international travel with infants and children. Available at: https://wwwnc.cdc.gov/travel/yellowbook/2018/international-travel-with-infants-children/traveling-safely-with-infants-children. Accessed October 13, 2017

Dealing With the Caretaker Whose Judgment Is Impaired by Alcohol or Drugs: Legal and Ethical Considerations

- *Policy Statement*

CLINICAL REPORT Guidance for the Clinician in Rendering Pediatric Care

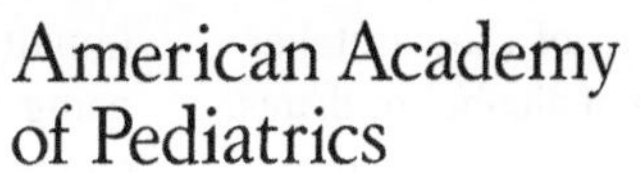
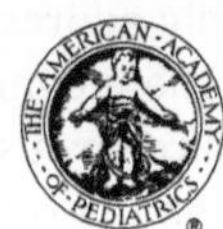

DEDICATED TO THE HEALTH OF ALL CHILDREN™

Dealing With the Caretaker Whose Judgment Is Impaired by Alcohol or Drugs: Legal and Ethical Considerations

Steven A. Bondi, JD, MD, FAAP,[a] James Scibilia, MD, FAAP,[b] COMMITTEE ON MEDICAL LIABILITY AND RISK MANAGEMENT

abstract

An estimated 8.7 million children live in a household with a substance-using parent or guardian. Substance-using caretakers may have impaired judgment that can negatively affect their child's well-being, including his or her ability to receive appropriate medical care. Although the physician-patient relationship exists between the pediatrician and the child, obligations related to safety and confidentiality should be considered as well. In managing encounters with impaired caretakers who may become disruptive or dangerous, pediatricians should be aware of their responsibilities before acting. In addition to fulfilling the duty involved with an established physician-patient relationship, the pediatrician should take reasonable care to safeguard patient confidentiality; protect the safety of their patient, other patients in the facility, visitors, and employees; and comply with reporting mandates. This clinical report identifies and discusses the legal and ethical concepts related to these circumstances. The report offers implementation suggestions when establishing anticipatory procedures and training programs for staff in such situations to maximize the patient's well-being and safety and minimize the liability of the pediatrician.

[a]Department of Pediatrics, School of Medicine and Dentistry, University of Rochester, Rochester, New York; and [b]Heritage Valley Pediatrics, Beaver, Pennsylvania

Dr Bondi conceptualized and conducted the literature search and wrote and revised the manuscript; Dr Scibilia conceptualized and revised the manuscript; and both authors considered input from all reviewers and the Board of Directors and approved the final manuscript as submitted.

Clinical reports from the American Academy of Pediatrics benefit from expertise and resources of liaisons and internal (AAP) and external reviewers. However, clinical reports from the American Academy of Pediatrics may not reflect the views of the liaisons or the organizations or government agencies that they represent.

The guidance in this report does not indicate an exclusive course of treatment or serve as a standard of medical care. Variations, taking into account individual circumstances, may be appropriate.

All clinical reports from the American Academy of Pediatrics automatically expire 5 years after publication unless reaffirmed, revised, or retired at or before that time.

The information contained in this clinical report is provided for educational purposes only and should not be used as a substitute for licensed legal advice.

This document is copyrighted and is property of the American Academy of Pediatrics and its Board of Directors. All authors have filed conflict of interest statements with the American Academy of Pediatrics. Any conflicts have been resolved through a process approved by the Board of Directors. The American Academy of Pediatrics has neither solicited nor accepted any commercial involvement in the development of the content of this publication.

DOI: https://doi.org/10.1542/peds.2019-3153

To cite: Bondi SA, Scibilia J, AAP COMMITTEE ON MEDICAL LIABILITY AND RISK MANAGEMENT. Dealing With the Caretaker Whose Judgment Is Impaired by Alcohol or Drugs: Legal and Ethical Considerations. *Pediatrics.* 2019; 144(6):e20193153

In the course of providing health care services to children, pediatricians may encounter situations in which a patient arrives at the office accompanied by a parent, guardian, or caretaker* who displays signs of judgment impairment. In these circumstances, pediatricians are challenged by an array of professional, ethical, and legal obligations, some of which may conflict. Pediatricians have sought guidance from the American Academy of Pediatrics (AAP) on how to respond to these potentially volatile and risk-laden scenarios. The purpose of this clinical report is to analyze the physician's potentially conflicting duties and suggest ways to interact with both the child and the judgment-impaired

* The term "caretaker" will be used throughout this report to represent a parent, guardian, or other adult who is accompanying a child and providing permission for treatment.

Downloaded from www.aappublications.org/news at American Academy of Pediatrics on January 23, 2020

adult in a situation fraught with legal complexity. This clinical report primarily addresses the situation in which the judgment of the caretaker is impaired by use of alcohol or drugs. However, the principles are also applicable to judgment impairment attributable to any cause, such as behavioral health issues, dementia, or an unstable medical condition.

SCOPE OF THE PROBLEM

The US Department of Health and Human Services estimates that 8.7 million children in the United States live in a household with a parent with a substance use disorder. Of those, 7.5 million children are currently living with a parent with an alcohol use disorder, and 2.1 million children are living with at least 1 parent with a drug use disorder.[1] Given the commonality of substance use disorders, it is likely that pediatricians will interact with caretakers under the influence of drugs or alcohol at some point in their careers. Encounters with children accompanied by an impaired caretaker may take place wherever pediatric services are delivered.

The impact of caretaker substance use on children is profound and has been described in the pediatric literature. Two AAP publications examine the pivotal role of the primary health care provider in addressing the health needs of children whose caretakers use drugs or alcohol.[2,3] An extensive discussion of the impact of parental substance use is better addressed by those resources and is beyond the scope of this report. Instead, the report outlines the immediate risks and legal considerations associated with managing a caretaker whose judgment is impaired for any reason during a medical encounter.

ETHICAL AND LEGAL CONSIDERATIONS

There are multiple ethical and legal issues involved when dealing with a caretaker whose judgment is impaired by any means, but most often, this involves alcohol or drugs. Impairment is defined as "the state of being diminished, weakened, or damaged, especially mentally or physically."[4] What constitutes a significant impairment is highly contextual. Consider that an airline pilot may not consume alcohol for 8 to 12 hours before flying, but adults are legally permitted to drive having just consumed an appropriate-sized alcoholic beverage. Given that the assessment of impairment can be subjective and influenced (perhaps unconsciously) by such factors as the caretaker's race, ethnicity, or socioeconomic status, it is critically important for the pediatrician to be aware of his or her own biases, including the possibility of unconscious bias, when making a determination of impairment. For example, in 1 study, given comparable levels of maternal drug use based on urine drug screens, women who were economically disadvantaged or from ethnic or racial minorities were more likely to be reported to child protective services compared with other women.[5] Staff training for the acknowledgment and recognition of bias can be helpful.

Pediatricians should consider how caretaker impairment might affect

- the physician-child, physician-family, and family-child relationships;
- the duty to act in the best interest and for the safety of the patient;
- the need to obtain informed permission from a competent legal guardian;
- the importance of safeguarding patient confidentiality;
- the mandated reporting of suspected child abuse and neglect; and
- the duty as an employer, business owner, or supervisor to protect the safety of employees and visitors in the office.

These obligations can be complex and nuanced and can appear to conflict. The general considerations in this report are provided to enable pediatricians to develop broad policies responsive to these situations. In translating this guidance into specific policy, pediatricians should seek advice from competent legal counsel so that policies accord with appropriate state law. The report serves as general guidance and, as such, should not be considered a specific course of action for any particular situation.

PHYSICIAN-PATIENT RELATIONSHIP

The parents, guardians, and other caretakers who accompany infants, children, and adolescents play an important role in pediatric encounters. For most children, the adult provides permission for treatment, furnishes pertinent historical information, is responsible for implementing the treatment plan, and is financially responsible for medical care. It is important to remember, however, that the physician-patient relationship exists between the pediatrician and the child. The pediatrician's first duty is to the best interests of the patient.[6]

The physician-patient relationship conveys many duties, the first of which is to prevent harm. When the pediatrician believes that the accompanying adult's impaired judgment substantially risks harming the patient, the caretaker himself, or others, the pediatrician should act. Confrontations should be avoided, if possible. For instance, all reasonable steps should be taken to keep an impaired caretaker from driving. Not only would the patient be in considerable danger if allowed to ride in a motor vehicle being driven by someone who is impaired, but the caretaker and the public would also be endangered. Depending on the circumstances, appropriate action could involve arranging alternate

Downloaded from www.aappublications.org/news at American Academy of Pediatrics on January 23, 2020

transportation (eg, calling a taxi, contacting another family member to intervene) or providing temporary emergency child care. In cases of immediate danger when discussion with the caretaker fails to result in a safe and satisfactory resolution, law enforcement should be called. In such circumstances, child protective services should also be contacted (see below, Mandated Reporting). Courts have generally not recognized a duty to protect a nonpatient from his or her own behavior, so it is unlikely that a physician would be held civilly liable for failure to protect the impaired caregiver. Failing to safeguard the child patient from the caregiver, however, could constitute negligence.

BEST INTEREST OF THE PATIENT

Parents and guardians are legally and morally required to act in the best interests of their children.[7,8] Caretakers exhibiting signs of alcohol or drug impairment may be incapable of caring for a child properly. Therefore, the pediatrician's actions should be guided by the child's best interest, especially when the caretaker's condition compromises his or her ability to share that interest.

PERMISSION FOR CARE

Permission for medical care can be complicated in pediatrics. The doctrine of informed consent has limited direct application in pediatrics because parents and other surrogates provide informed permission rather than informed consent for diagnosis and treatment of children. Ethical and legal considerations are articulated in a number of AAP publications.[9–12] A pediatrician should always use his or her judgment to determine if a parent, guardian, or medical proxy is capable of providing informed permission. Judgment-impaired caretakers may lack the capacity to provide informed permission for their child's medical treatment. In some situations, it may be apparent that the caretaker has recently used alcohol or drugs but may not be obviously impaired. Pediatricians should take care in these circumstances because the sufficiency of informed permission can be challenged after the fact. Accordingly, if the child, by virtue of age, medical condition, or legal status, cannot consent to his or her own treatment, and the caretaker's capacity to give permission is uncertain because of the impairment, it would be advisable to postpone routine, nonurgent medical care, including, but not limited to, routine physical examinations or immunizations. The provision of nonurgent care without appropriate consent or permission is unethical and risks allegations of unauthorized treatment and even battery.[13–15]

Hospital emergency departments are bound by the Emergency Medical Treatment and Active Labor Act.[16] Under this law, a physician in certain situations is mandated to perform a "medical screening examination" to assess for an emergent medical condition, regardless of consent. Additional care may need to be given in the absence of consent or permission if a delay would result in a threat of harm to the child's life or health. The Emergency Medical Treatment and Active Labor Act requirement for a medical screening examination generally does not apply to physician offices, unless located at the same facility as a hospital.

CONFIDENTIALITY AND PRIVACY

Caretakers have a reasonable expectation that information provided to the child's physician during a medical encounter will be considered confidential and protected by applicable laws. Physicians should take reasonable care to safeguard health information obtained from the caretaker concerning the family, such as health and social history. Additional safeguards may be needed for topics such as substance use or mental health concerns. These efforts should be reflected in the medical office's privacy and security policies for protecting patient records and other forms of identifiable health data according to any state and federal laws, including the Health Insurance Portability and Accountability Act of 1996.[17–19]

Although generally not protected by law, attempting to maintain the privacy of interactions with an impaired caretaker is appropriate. Discussions with caretakers, patients, and others concerning substance use or other impairing problems should be conducted in a manner that maximizes privacy and confidentiality. For example, if the receptionist notices that a caretaker appears to be intoxicated when checking in for an appointment, it might be prudent to direct the impaired person to an area where he or she may be spoken to discreetly. This would be preferable to a confrontation in the reception area in the presence of the caretaker's child and other patients. However, if the impaired individual is disruptive, quick action may be needed to contain the situation. In such instances, keeping the impaired person from harming others would take precedence over preserving his or her privacy. Office policy and staff training can be helpful in anticipating and appropriately dealing with these circumstances.

MANDATED REPORTING

Every state has enacted laws to mandate reporting of child abuse and neglect. Physicians and other mandated reporters are required to put the child's best interest above the privacy concerns of the caretaker.[19,20]

The standards used to determine when a mandatory reporter is

Downloaded from www.aappublications.org/news at American Academy of Pediatrics on January 23, 2020

required to notify authorities of abuse or neglect differ from state to state, including who is a mandated reporter, the level of knowledge or suspicion of abuse necessary to report, and what constitutes abuse.[21] Although definitions vary, generally, the pediatrician is required to report when he or she has a reasonable suspicion that a child has been abused or neglected. A child driven to the pediatrician's office by an intoxicated caretaker would clearly meet this threshold. In situations in which the caretaker is using a legal substance but is not actually intoxicated or in which there is a recent history of caretaker substance abuse, the decision to report is more challenging. In such circumstances, it is incumbent on the pediatrician to consider all available information in the decision to report, including but not limited to past medical and social history, conversations with the child and family, results of the medical examination, and any other relevant factors. Even interactions with the caretaker on social medial might be informative. It is important to remember that the threshold for reporting is generally low: a reasonable suspicion.

The US Department of Health and Human Services has compiled a summary of state and territory laws regarding mandated reporting.[21–23] State Web sites may offer additional guidance to health care providers on mandated reporting of child abuse. Health care providers are wise to understand the applicable law in their jurisdiction and to seek qualified legal advice interpreting the applicable laws and regulations as necessary. Forty-eight states, as well as the District of Columbia and a number of US territories, permit penalties on mandatory reporters who knowingly or willfully fail to report suspected abuse. Penalties vary from state to state but typically include monetary fines and/or jail time.[22] In addition, mandatory reporters expose themselves to civil lawsuits for failure to report. Should the patient subsequently be harmed as a consequence of the physician failing to act, the physician could be sued for medical negligence[24] or face possible sanctions from a state licensing board.[25] Reports made in good faith out of concern for the welfare of the child provide criminal and civil immunity to the reporter, but this immunity does not apply if there is willful misconduct or gross negligence by the reporter.[23,26] As of 2015, 29 states impose penalties for false reporting of abuse. These vary from state to state, range from misdemeanor to felony charges, and include monetary fines and potential jail time. False or negligent reporting also places the reporter at risk for a civil lawsuit.[22]

DUTY TO PROTECT EMPLOYEES AND VISITORS

In recent years, health care facilities have become targets of violence. Violence or threat of violence necessitates the involvement of law enforcement. There are no national standards specifically addressing workplace violence, although federal law requires that "each employer shall furnish to each of his employees employment and a place of employment, which are free from recognized hazards that are causing or are likely to cause death or serious physical harm to his employees."[27] This is referred to as the General Duty Clause, and specific recommendations are enumerated by the Occupational Safety and Health Administration (OSHA).[28] Helpful information in establishing step-by-step safety policies to protect health care employees from potentially violent visitors can be found on the OSHA Web site (https://www.osha.gov/SLTC/workplaceviolence/).[29] Certain "low-risk industries," including physicians' offices, are exempt from reporting injuries and illness to OSHA.[30] However, when a workplace incident results in a fatality or serious injury, including inpatient hospitalization, reporting is required.[31] State and local agencies may have broader regulatory and reporting requirements.

A safety audit can be performed to evaluate the workplace for various hazards, including workplace violence. Online resources are available for a self-performed audit, but a safety and security professional may provide a more-detailed and comprehensive analysis.

RECOMMENDATIONS

The following recommendations are intended to help pediatricians implement office policies and procedures that may minimize legal risks should a patient arrive at the medical office in the care of an adult whose judgment is impaired.

Safety

Physician practice owners and employers: conduct a safety audit of your facility, including procedures for management of judgment-impaired visitors. Establish an office policy and train staff to respond appropriately. Incorporate this policy into your OSHA compliance program. Review and update the policy periodically. If the procedure is implemented, document the incident, how it was handled, and any injuries that occurred and evaluate whether the safety policy needs to be revised as a result of this occurrence. Maintain these records in a secure area of the office. Contact your professional liability insurance company to determine if consulting services for developing such a loss-prevention program are available. Report any episodes of workplace violence to your insurance carrier, OSHA, and any state or local agencies as appropriate.

Physician employees: review facility safety policies and discuss procedures with your employer.

Downloaded from www.aappublications.org/news at American Academy of Pediatrics on January 23, 2020

Encourage the employer to conduct periodic safety audits of the premesis.

Confidentiality

Verify applicable confidentiality laws and align your office policies with these laws. Unless state law indicates otherwise, the physician's duty to the patient should take precedence over the caretaker's expectation of confidentiality.

Conversations regarding the caretaker's substance use can be challenging. The tension of this dialogue can be mitigated by

- having a supporting and safe environment;
- emphasizing that your purpose is the safety and well-being of the child as well as support for the caretaker;
- discussing your concerns regarding the risk to the child caused by the caretaker's impairment in a compassionate and nonjudgmental manner, using the benefit of your previous rapport and professional relationship; and
- assisting the individual in finding resources to address his or her substance use and its effect on the child, as appropriate. A recommendation for the individual to discuss options with their primary care physician can also be an effective means to medically address related issues.

Consent and Permission

An impaired caretaker may not be able to give permission to medical treatment of the child. Therefore, it would be prudent to postpone nonurgent pediatric care until a time at which permission can be obtained. If no care is delivered, it is suggested that the physician document in the medical record that "valid and sufficient consent or permission was not given by the caretaker for treatment today."

Mandated Reporting

Use your best clinical judgment to determine the specific risks that the caretaker's condition poses to the child. Take action accordingly. Be knowledgeable of your state's laws governing reporting child abuse, standards of abuse, and consequences of failing to report for mandated reporters. If you believe there is an acute risk to the child because of the caretaker's condition, contacting law enforcement and child protective agencies is an appropriate means to secure the child's safety and obtain appropriate treatment of the impaired caretaker. Should the child's custodial parent or guardian agree, it may be preferable to release the child to the care of a relative rather than have the child accompany the caretaker to the emergency department or police station. Child protective services may be in the best position to make such determinations.

LEAD AUTHORS

Steven A. Bondi, JD, MD, FAAP
James P. Scibilia, MD, FAAP

COMMITTEE ON MEDICAL LIABILITY AND RISK MANAGEMENT, 2017–2018

Jon Mark Fanaroff, MD, JD, FAAP, Chairperson
Robin L. Altman, MD, FAAP
Steven A. Bondi, JD, MD, FAAP
Sandeep K. Narang, MD, JD, FAAP
Richard L. Oken, MD, FAAP
John W. Rusher, MD, JD, FAAP
Karen A. Santucci, MD, FAAP
James P. Scibilia, MD, FAAP
Susan M. Scott, MD, JD, FAAP
Laura J. Sigman, MD, JD, FAAP

STAFF

Julie Kersten Ake

ABBREVIATIONS

AAP: American Academy of Pediatrics
OSHA: Occupational Safety and Health Administration

Address correspondence to Steven A. Bondi, JD, MD, FAAP, Department of Pediatrics, University of Rochester School of Medicine and Dentistry, Rochester, NY. E-mail: steven_bondi@urmc.rochester.edu

PEDIATRICS (ISSN Numbers: Print, 0031-4005; Online, 1098-4275).

Copyright © 2019 by the American Academy of Pediatrics

FINANCIAL DISCLOSURE: The authors have indicated they have no financial relationships relevant to this article to disclose.

FUNDING: No external funding.

POTENTIAL CONFLICT OF INTEREST: The authors have indicated they have no potential conflicts of interest to disclose.

REFERENCES

1. Lipari RN, Van Horn SL. *Children Living With Parents Who Have a Substance Use Disorder. The CBHSQ Report.* Rockville, MD: Center for Behavioral Health Statistics and Quality, Substance Abuse and Mental Health Services Administration; 2017
2. Smith VC, Wilson CR; Committee on Substance Use and Prevention. Families affected by parental substance use. *Pediatrics.* 2016;138(2):e20161575
3. Committee on Early Childhood, Adoption, and Dependent Care. The pediatrician's role in family support

Downloaded from www.aappublications.org/news at American Academy of Pediatrics on January 23, 2020

and family support programs. *Pediatrics.* 2011;128(6). Available at: www.pediatrics.org/cgi/content/full/128/6/e1680

4. Dictionary.com. Impairment. Available at: https://www.dictionary.com/browse/impairment. Accessed December 4, 2018
5. Chasnoff IJ, Landress HJ, Barrett ME. The prevalence of illicit-drug or alcohol use during pregnancy and discrepancies in mandatory reporting in Pinellas County, Florida. *N Engl J Med.* 1990;322(17):1202–1206
6. Lantos J. The patient-parent-pediatrician relationship: everyday ethics in the office. *Pediatr Rev.* 2015; 36(1):22–29; quiz 30
7. *Archer v Cassel*, 2015 WL 1500447 (Conn Sup, 2015)
8. United Nations. *Convention on the Rights of the Child.* New York, NY: United Nations Treaty Series; 1989
9. Committee on Bioethics. Informed consent in decision-making in pediatric practice. *Pediatrics.* 2016;138(2): e20161484
10. Committee on Pediatric Emergency Medicine and Committee on Bioethics. Consent for emergency medical services for children and adolescents. *Pediatrics.* 2011;128(2):427–433
11. Fanaroff JM; Committee on Medical Liability and Risk Management. Consent by proxy for nonurgent pediatric care. *Pediatrics.* 2017;139(2):e20163911
12. Committee on Bioethics. Conflicts between religious or spiritual beliefs and pediatric care: informed refusal, exemptions, and public funding. *Pediatrics.* 2013;132(5):962–965
13. *Hodge v Lafayette General Hospital*, 399 So 2d 744 (La App 3rd Cir 1981)
14. *Buie v Reynolds*, 571 P2d 1230 (Okla Ct App 1977)
15. McAbee GN, Donn SM, McDonnell WM. The evolving doctrine of informed consent in medical malpractice lawsuits: a reason for concern for neonatologists. *J Neonatal Perinatal Med.* 2011;4(4):303–307
16. Emergency Medical Treatment and Active Labor Act, 42 USC §1395dd (1986)
17. Health Insurance Portability and Accountability Act of 1996, Pub L No. 104-191, 110 Stat. 1936 (1996)
18. Modifications to the HIPAA privacy, security, enforcement, and breach notification rules under the health information technology for economic and clinical health act and the genetic information nondiscrimination act; other modifications to the HIPAA rules. *Fed Regist.* 2013;78(17):5565–5702
19. Committee on Child Abuse and Neglect. Policy statement–Child abuse, confidentiality, and the Health Insurance Portability and Accountability Act. *Pediatrics.* 2010;125(1):197–201
20. Committee on Injury, Violence, and Poison Prevention. Policy statement–Role of the pediatrician in youth violence prevention. *Pediatrics.* 2009;124(1):393–402
21. Child Welfare Information Gateway. *Definitions of Child Abuse and Neglect.* Washington, DC: US Department of Health and Human Services, Children's Bureau; 2016. Available at: https://www.childwelfare.gov/pubPDFs/define.pdf. Accessed November 3, 2018
22. Child Welfare Information Gateway. *Penalties for Failure to Report and False Reporting of Child Abuse and Neglect.* Washington, DC: US Department of Health and Human Services, Children's Bureau; 2016. Available at: https://www.childwelfare.gov/topics/systemwide/laws-policies/statutes/report/. Accessed November 3, 2018
23. Child Welfare Information Gateway. *Immunity for Reporters of Child Abuse and Neglect.* Washington, DC: US Department of Health and Human Services, Children's Bureau; 2016. Available at: https://www.childwelfare.gov/topics/systemwide/laws-policies/statutes/immunity/. Accessed November 3, 2018
24. *Landeros v Flood*, 17 Cal. 3d 399, 551 P.2d 389 (Cal Sup, 1976)
25. *Malur v Illinois Dept of Professional Regulation*, No. 11 MR 297 (Cir. Ct. Madison County, 2013)
26. Child Abuse Prevention and Treatment Act, 42 USC §5106a(b)(2)(B)vii (2010)
27. General Duty Clause of the OSH Act of 1970, 27 USC §654 5(a)1. Available at: https://www.osha.gov/laws-regs/oshact/section5-duties. Accessed December 4, 2018
28. US Occupational Safety and Health Administration. *Guidelines for Preventing Workplace Violence for Health Care and Social Service Workers.* Washington, DC: US Department of Labor; 2016. Available at: https://www.osha.gov/Publications/osha3148.pdf. Accessed November 3, 2018
29. US Occupational Safety and Health Administration. Workplace violence: enforcement. Available at: https://www.osha.gov/SLTC/workplaceviolence/standards.html. Accessed January 26, 2018
30. Partial exemption for establishments in certain industries. 29 CFR §1904.2 (2016). Available at: https://www.gpo.gov/fdsys/granule/CFR-2016-title29-vol5/CFR-2016-title29-vol5-sec1904-2. Accessed December 4, 2018
31. Reporting fatalities and multiple hospitalization incidents to OSHA. 29 CFR 1904.39 (2013). Available at: https://www.gpo.gov/fdsys/granule/CFR-2013-title29-vol5/CFR-2013-title29-vol5-sec1904-39. Accessed December 4, 2018

Downloaded from www.aappublications.org/news at American Academy of Pediatrics on January 23, 2020

E-Cigarettes and Similar Devices

- *Policy Statement*

POLICY STATEMENT Organizational Principles to Guide and Define the Child Health Care System and/or Improve the Health of all Children

American Academy of Pediatrics

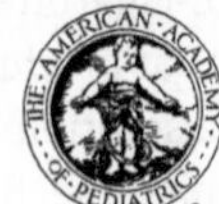

DEDICATED TO THE HEALTH OF ALL CHILDREN™

E-Cigarettes and Similar Devices

Brian P. Jenssen, MD, MSHP, FAAP,[a] Susan C. Walley, MD, FAAP,[b] SECTION ON TOBACCO CONTROL

abstract

Electronic cigarettes (e-cigarettes) are the most commonly used tobacco product among youth. The 2016 US Surgeon General's Report on e-cigarette use among youth and young adults concluded that e-cigarettes are unsafe for children and adolescents. Furthermore, strong and consistent evidence finds that children and adolescents who use e-cigarettes are significantly more likely to go on to use traditional cigarettes—a product that kills half its long-term users. E-cigarette manufacturers target children with enticing candy and fruit flavors and use marketing strategies that have been previously successful with traditional cigarettes to attract youth to these products. Numerous toxicants and carcinogens have been found in e-cigarette solutions. Nonusers are involuntarily exposed to the emissions of these devices with secondhand and thirdhand aerosol. To prevent children, adolescents, and young adults from transitioning from e-cigarettes to traditional cigarettes and minimize the potential public health harm from e-cigarette use, there is a critical need for e-cigarette regulation, legislative action, and counterpromotion to protect youth.

[a]*Department of Pediatrics, Perelman School of Medicine, University of Pennsylvania and PolicyLab, Center for Pediatric Clinical Effectiveness, Children's Hospital of Philadelphia, Philadelphia, Pennsylvania; and* [b]*Department of Pediatrics, The University of Alabama at Birmingham and Children's of Alabama, Birmingham, Alabama*

Drs Jenssen and Walley conceptualized the manuscript, drafted the initial manuscript, reviewed the final manuscript, and note substantial involvement and contribution to the manuscript; the members of the Section on Tobacco Control Executive Committee reviewed the manuscript, provided critical appraisal, and note substantial involvement and contribution to the manuscript; and all authors approved the final manuscript as submitted.

This document is copyrighted and is property of the American Academy of Pediatrics and its Board of Directors. All authors have filed conflict of interest statements with the American Academy of Pediatrics. Any conflicts have been resolved through a process approved by the Board of Directors. The American Academy of Pediatrics has neither solicited nor accepted any commercial involvement in the development of the content of this publication.

Policy statements from the American Academy of Pediatrics benefit from expertise and resources of liaisons and internal (AAP) and external reviewers. However, policy statements from the American Academy of Pediatrics may not reflect the views of the liaisons or the organizations or government agencies that they represent.

The guidance in this statement does not indicate an exclusive course of treatment or serve as a standard of medical care. Variations, taking into account individual circumstances, may be appropriate.

All policy statements from the American Academy of Pediatrics automatically expire 5 years after publication unless reaffirmed, revised, or retired at or before that time.

DOI: https://doi.org/10.1542/peds.2018-3652

Address correspondence to Brian P. Jenssen, MD, MSHP, FAAP. E-mail: jenssenb@email.chop.edu

PEDIATRICS (ISSN Numbers: Print, 0031-4005; Online, 1098-4275).

Copyright © 2019 by the American Academy of Pediatrics

To cite: Jenssen BP, Walley SC, AAP SECTION ON TOBACCO CONTROL. E-Cigarettes and Similar Devices. *Pediatrics.* 2019;143(2):e20183652

DEFINITIONS

- Electronic cigarette (e-cigarette): handheld devices that produce an aerosol from a solution typically containing nicotine, flavoring chemicals, and other additives for inhalation through a mouthpiece by the user (alternative names include "e-cigs, " electronic cigars [or "e-cigars"], electronic nicotine delivery systems, electronic hookah [or "e-hookah"], hookah sticks, personal vaporizers, mechanical mods, vape pens, pod systems, and vaping devices);
- secondhand aerosol: e-cigarette emissions that are discharged into the surrounding environment with e-cigarette use both directly from the e-cigarette and exhaled from the lungs of the user; and
- thirdhand aerosol: e-cigarette emissions that remain on surfaces and in dust after e-cigarette use.

BACKGROUND

E-cigarettes are handheld devices that produce an aerosol from a solution typically containing nicotine, flavoring chemicals, and other additives for inhalation through a mouthpiece by the user.[1] There is wide variability in e-cigarette terminology, product design, engineering, and solution components (ie, electronic liquid [e-liquid]).[2] For the purposes of this Policy Statement update,[3] the term "e-cigarettes" encompasses the wide variety of devices that are known as vapes, "mods," tanks, and pod systems, including currently popular brands, such as JUUL.[4] E-cigarettes were introduced to the US market in the mid-2000s, and the design of these products has evolved over time, varying considerably in price, quality, and design.[2,4,5] Early products initially resembled conventional cigarettes, with prefilled cartridges of e-liquid, but quickly developed into tank-style systems, with large refillable cartridges, adding variability in the amount and composition of the e-liquid and potential additives.[1,2] More recent e-cigarette products are more diverse in their design, sometimes resembling common items such as a pen, flashlight, or computer flash drive. In addition to product manufacturers referring to the product as "vaping devices," they are often known as "mods" because of the ability to modify the devices.[1,2] Although commonly referred to as a vapor, the emission from e-cigarettes is most accurately classified as an aerosol, which is a suspension of fine particles in a gas.[6] Nonusers can be exposed involuntarily to the emissions from the exhaled aerosol.[1]

EPIDEMIOLOGY OF YOUTH E-CIGARETTE USE

Use of e-cigarettes increased dramatically over the past decade, making them the most common tobacco product used among youth. Because of the shifting landscape in e-cigarette product design and terminology, combined with different survey definitions, various sources are used to capture data on e-cigarette use. Similar trends have been observed across 3 cross-sectional surveys with data on youth use: the National Youth Tobacco Survey, Monitoring the Future, and the Youth Risk Behavior Surveillance System.[7–9] For the latest data as of 2018, the National Youth Tobacco Survey reported 20.8% of high school students and 4.9% of middle school students currently used e-cigarettes (defined as use of an e-cigarette at least 1 day in the past 30 days)[10]; for 2017, Monitoring the Future reported 17% of 12th graders, 13% of 10th graders, and 7% of eighth graders currently used e-cigarettes[8]; while the Youth Risk Behavior Surveillance System reported 13.2% of high school students currently used e-cigarettes.[9] Current e-cigarette use increased considerably among middle and high school students during 2017-2018 (increasing by 78% from 11.7% to 20.8% among high school students),[10] increasing overall tobacco use and reversing a decline observed in recent years.[7–9] More than 3 million high school students and 570 000 middle school students currently use e-cigarettes.[10] E-cigarette use has been documented as highest among boys, non-Hispanic white youth, and Hispanic youth.[7,11] E-cigarette use is generally greatest among adolescents and young adults and decreases with age in adults. Adult e-cigarette users tend to be previous users of combustible tobacco products, such as traditional cigarettes.[2]

E-CIGARETTE MARKETING, ADVERTISING, AND SALES

E-cigarettes can be purchased in various retail outlets, including vendors that sell tobacco, vape shops, mall kiosks, gas stations, convenience stores, grocery stores, and pharmacies as well as through online/Internet vendors. E-cigarette companies market their products to children and adolescents by promoting flavors and using a wide variety of media channels, approaches used by the tobacco industry to successfully market conventional tobacco products to youth.[1] E-cigarette companies, many of which are owned by major tobacco companies, use promotional tactics including television advertisements targeted to stations with clear youth appeal[12]; advertisements at the point of sale at retail stores[13]; product Web sites and social media[14]; targeted advertisements through search engines and Web sites that are focused on music, entertainment, and sports[15]; celebrity endorsements; and sponsorships and free samples at youth-oriented events.[1] Many of these e-cigarette methods of advertising are illegal for conventional cigarettes precisely because such tactics promote youth initiation and progression to traditional tobacco product use.[16,17]

E-cigarette advertising has effectively reached youth and young adults and is associated with current e-cigarette use. In 2016, 78.2% of middle and high school students (20.5 million youth) were exposed to e-cigarette advertisements from at least 1 source.[18] Exposure to these advertisements increases intention to use e-cigarettes among adolescent nonusers.[19] It is associated with current e-cigarette use,[20] with increasing exposure being associated with increased odds of use.[21,22] The increased use of and exposure to e-cigarettes among youth, combined with dramatic increases in advertising,[23] have serious potential to undermine successful efforts to deglamorize, restrict, and decrease the use of tobacco products.

E-CIGARETTE SOLUTION AND HEALTH EFFECTS

Components of e-cigarette solutions generally include nicotine, flavoring chemicals, and other additives (including those unknown and/or unadvertised to the user).[1] Currently, there are no federal quality standards to ensure the accuracy of e-cigarette constituents as advertised or labeled. Refillable cartridges allow the user to deliver other psychoactive substances, including marijuana.[24] Numerous toxicants and carcinogens have been found in e-cigarette solutions, including aldehydes, tobacco-specific nitrosamines, metals, tobacco alkaloids, and polycyclic aromatic hydrocarbons.[25,26] E-cigarette solution has also been shown to be cytotoxic to human embryonic stem cells.[27]

Nicotine is the major psychoactive component of e-cigarette solution.[1] There are often wide discrepancies between the labeled amount and actual nicotine content within the solution.[2] Reported nicotine concentration in e-cigarette solution ranges widely[28,29] and, depending on how the product is used, can be comparable to or exceed the amount of nicotine in a single conventional cigarette.[30] Nicotine is a highly addictive drug that can have lasting damaging effects on adolescent brain development and has been linked to a variety of adverse health outcomes, especially for the developing fetus.[30,31] Nicotine has neurotoxic effects on the developing brain.[32,33] In early adolescence, executive function and neurocognitive processes in the brain have not fully developed or matured. Adolescents are more likely to engage in experimentation with substances such as cigarettes, and they are also physiologically more vulnerable to addiction.[34] The earlier in childhood an individual uses nicotine-containing products, the stronger the addiction and the more difficult it is to quit.[35] The vast majority of adult smokers initiated tobacco use by 18 years of age.[31]

E-cigarette solutions are often flavored, with thousands of unique flavors advertised.[36,37] Popular options include fruit, candy, and dessert flavors and are appealing to children and youth.[36,37] Availability of flavors is among the most prominently cited reasons for youth e-cigarette use.[38–40] Studies reveal that candy- or fruit-flavored e-cigarettes are more appealing than tobacco flavors to adolescents and young adults.[41,42] Furthermore, adolescents perceive that e-cigarettes with flavors are less harmful than those with tobacco flavors,[41] creating a potential misperception that e-cigarettes with flavors do not contain nicotine.[8] Many of the flavoring chemicals contain aldehydes, known respiratory irritants, in sufficient concentrations to be of toxicologic concern.[37] Flavorings (other than menthol) have been banned in conventional cigarettes since the Family Smoking Prevention and Tobacco Control Act of 2009 because flavoring encourages youth experimentation and regular use and results in addiction.[16,43,44]

Carrier solvents, such as propylene glycol or vegetable glycerin (glycerol), are used in e-cigarette solutions to produce an aerosol that, when heated, simulates conventional cigarette smoke.[1] Although these carrier solvents are used in other settings, there are insufficient data on the health effects of repeated long-term inhalation and exposure to these solvents.[45]

HEALTH EFFECTS OF E-CIGARETTE AEROSOL

The aerosol generated by e-cigarettes is inhaled and then exhaled by the user, and some of the generated aerosol may be discharged directly into the surrounding environment and deposited on surface areas. Bystanders are exposed to this secondhand and thirdhand aerosol in a manner similar to that of secondhand and thirdhand cigarette smoke. Known harmful toxicants and carcinogens have been found in e-cigarette emissions.[1,2] These include polycyclic aromatic hydrocarbons[46] as well as nicotine, volatile organic compounds, and fine and ultrafine particles.[47,48] Metal and silicate particles, some of which are at higher levels than in conventional cigarettes, have been detected in e-cigarette aerosol, resulting from degradation of the metal coil used to heat the solution.[49] There are limited data on the human health effects of e-cigarette emissions. Studies suggest adolescent e-cigarette users are at increased risk of cough, wheeze, and asthma exacerbations.[2]

POISONINGS AND INJURIES

Unintentional exposure to and poisoning from e-cigarette solutions containing nicotine have increased dramatically in the United States since 2011. Although symptoms of acute nicotine toxicity are generally mild and resolve within 12 hours with no treatment, large exposure can be fatal.[50] One child death caused by ingestion of liquid nicotine has been reported in the United States.[51] The Child Nicotine Poisoning Prevention Act of 2015, which was enacted nationally in January 2016, requires containers of liquid nicotine to be in child-resistant packaging; nonetheless, there continue to be thousands of reports of exposure to e-cigarette liquid nicotine yearly to the National Poison Data System.[52] In addition, the lithium-ion batteries used in e-cigarettes have exploded, leading to burns and fires.[2]

E-CIGARETTE USE AND PROGRESSION TO TRADITIONAL CIGARETTE USE

Studies of US youth who use e-cigarettes identify remarkably consistent findings: adolescents and young adults who use e-cigarettes, compared with those who do not, are at higher risk of transitioning to traditional cigarettes.[2,53] This finding is based on substantial evidence from several separate, well-designed, longitudinal studies.[54–61] Adolescents and young adults (14–30 years of age) who have used e-cigarettes are 3.6 times more likely to report using traditional cigarettes at follow-up compared with those who had not, according to a recent meta-analysis.[53] In addition, adolescents who use e-cigarettes appear to have fewer social and behavioral risk factors than conventional cigarette users.[56–58,60] These findings raise significant concern that e-cigarettes have the potential to addict a new generation to nicotine and tobacco, slowing or reversing the decline in adolescent cigarette smoking that has occurred over the past 20 years.

ROLE IN SMOKING CESSATION AMONG ESTABLISHED SMOKERS

Health claims that e-cigarettes are effective smoking cessation aids are not currently supported by scientific evidence. According to the National Academies of Sciences, Engineering, and Medicine, there is limited evidence regarding the ability of e-cigarettes to promote smoking cessation.[2] In particular, with a limited number of small, randomized-controlled trials, there is insufficient evidence on the effectiveness of e-cigarettes as a cessation aid compared with no treatment or Food and Drug Administration (FDA)–approved smoking-cessation treatments.[2] Studies in real-world clinical settings of smokers interested in quitting reveal that e-cigarette users have lower rates of successful quitting compared with those who never used e-cigarettes.[62] Given the current state of the science, smokers interested in quitting should seek and be referred to evidence-based, safe, and effective treatments, including nicotine replacement therapy, behavioral counseling, and additional pharmacotherapy.[63]

For established smokers, e-cigarettes may reduce health risks for the individual user compared with the risk of continued combustible tobacco use.[2] However, the nuance in this finding must be placed in a larger public health context. Tobacco, when used as intended, causes disease, disability, and death.[31] Operationally, even if e-cigarettes themselves pose less risk to the user than other tobacco products, they still represent a significant public health burden in need of further regulation, particularly if they cause more adolescents and adults to begin harmful combustible tobacco use or prevent fewer people from quitting tobacco use.[2]

FEDERAL, STATE, AND LOCAL E-CIGARETTE REGULATION

The federal government first regulated e-cigarettes in 2016 with the Child Nicotine Poisoning Prevention Act and the FDA Deeming Rule, which extended FDA regulatory authority to all tobacco products, including e-cigarettes.[64] FDA regulations of e-cigarettes now include banning sales to people younger than 18 years, requiring photo identification verification from consumers younger than 27 years, banning free samples and vending machine sales, and including a warning statement on e-cigarette packaging and advertising explaining that nicotine is addictive. Following the FDA Deeming Rule, e-cigarette manufacturers will be required to submit a "premarket review application," which will enable the FDA to assess the public health impact of these products to determine if they can continue to sell them to consumers.[65] However, in 2017, the FDA delayed implementation of the Deeming Rule, allowing e-cigarettes to remain on the market without premarket review until 2022.[66]

Although only the federal government can regulate the manufacture of tobacco products, states have the ability to regulate how tobacco products are sold and used. Many states and localities have enacted e-cigarette regulations, including applying excise taxes to the purchase price, incorporating e-cigarettes in smoke-free–air laws, implementing point-of-sale restrictions, and raising the minimum purchasing age to 21 years.[67] The State Tobacco Activities Tracking and Evaluation system of the Centers for Disease Control and Prevention tracks individual state laws related to e-cigarettes.[68]

Significant gaps remain in e-cigarette regulation. As of this publication date, federal laws and regulations do not appropriately restrict the advertising of e-cigarettes to youth. Furthermore, with no restrictions on flavored e-cigarettes in general, child-friendly flavors are still available and marketed to youth. In addition, the delayed implementation of the FDA Deeming Rule allows all e-cigarettes currently on the market to continue to be marketed and sold to consumers without FDA review through 2022. In 2018, the American Academy of Pediatrics (AAP) and 6 other health groups filed a lawsuit against the FDA,[69] noting that the agency's decision to delay product reviews leaves youth vulnerable to the use of these products and deprives the public of critical health information about e-cigarettes that are already on the market. In 2018, the FDA publicly acknowledged the "epidemic of e-cigarette use among teenagers" and proposed regulatory action[70] in response to data demonstrating rapid acceleration in use.[10] As these usage trends continue, with the rapid rise in popularity among youth of the latest generation of e-cigarettes,[71] the need for federal regulation becomes even more evident. As of this publication date, the FDA is considering policy actions that could protect youth from e-cigarettes, including newer systems like JUUL.[72]

ONGOING RESEARCH

As the e-cigarette market grows, there is continued need for research to inform regulatory standards and understand the effects of use and exposure across the life span.[2] Additional research is needed to understand the trajectory of addiction among youth and the progression to combustible tobacco products.[1] Studies are needed to determine if and how e-cigarettes may be effective for smoking cessation; these trials must be carefully designed and adequately powered.[2] Finally, research is needed to evaluate effective countermessaging and public health interventions.

Despite the need for ongoing research, the evidence base is sufficient to support immediate regulatory and public health actions. Lessons learned from tobacco control of combustible cigarettes along with available e-cigarette research can be used to build science-based regulations and interventions, including preventing youth access, banning flavors, incorporating e-cigarettes into smoke-free–air laws, regulating marketing practices, and implementing public education programs.[1] It is critical that pediatric health care providers; local, state, and federal governments; and the public health community act immediately to protect youth from these products.

RECOMMENDED ACTIONS FOR THE PEDIATRICIAN

I. Screen for e-cigarette use and exposure and provide prevention counseling in clinical practice.

II. Provide counseling that homes, cars, and places where children and adolescents live, learn, play, work, and visit should have comprehensive tobacco-free bans that include e-cigarettes as well as combustible tobacco products.

III. Do not recommend e-cigarettes as a tobacco-dependence treatment product.

PUBLIC POLICY RECOMMENDATIONS

I. Reduce youth access to e-cigarettes.

a. The FDA should act immediately to regulate e-cigarettes similar to how traditional cigarettes are regulated to protect public health.

b. Ban the sale of e-cigarettes to children and youth younger than 21 years.

c. Ban Internet sales of e-cigarettes and e-cigarette solution.

II. Reduce youth demand for e-cigarettes.

a. Ban all characterizing flavors, including menthol, in e-cigarettes.

b. Ban all e-cigarette product advertising and promotion in forms that are accessible to children and youth.

c. Tax e-cigarettes at comparable rates to those of conventional cigarettes.

III. Incorporate e-cigarettes into current tobacco-free laws and ordinances where children and adolescents live, learn, play, work, and visit.

For more information, including an e-cigarette fact sheet, please refer to the AAP Julius B. Richmond Center of Excellence e-cigarette Web page (https://www.aap.org/en-us/advocacy-and-policy/aap-health-initiatives/Richmond-Center/Pages/Electronic-Nicotine-Delivery-Systems.aspx).

For additional AAP clinical and policy recommendations to protect children from the harms of tobacco, see "Clinical Practice Policy to Protect Children From Tobacco, Nicotine, and Tobacco Smoke" (http://pediatrics.aappublications.org/content/early/2015/10/21/peds.2015-3108), and "Public Policy to Protect Children From Tobacco, Nicotine, and Tobacco Smoke" (http://pediatrics.aappublications.org/content/136/5/998).

CONCLUSIONS

E-cigarettes are the most common tobacco product used among youth. E-cigarettes are marketed and advertised by promoting flavors and using a wide variety of media channels and approaches previously used with success by the tobacco industry to market conventional tobacco products to youth. E-cigarette advertising has effectively reached youth and young adults and is associated with current e-cigarette use. Numerous toxicants and carcinogens have been found in e-cigarette solutions. Adolescents and young adults who use e-cigarettes are at high risk of transitioning to traditional cigarettes. The increasing use of e-cigarettes among youth threatens 5 decades of public health gains in successfully deglamorizing, restricting, and decreasing the use of tobacco products. To prevent children, adolescents, and young adults from transitioning from e-cigarettes to traditional cigarettes and to minimize the potential public health harm from e-cigarette use, there is a critical need for e-cigarette regulation, legislative action, and counterpromotion to help youth live tobacco-free lives.

ACKNOWLEDGMENT

The Section on Tobacco Control acknowledges Julie Gorzkowski, Director of the AAP Division of Tobacco Control, for her expertise and important contributions to this article.

LEAD AUTHORS

Brian P. Jenssen, MD, FAAP
Susan C. Walley, MD, FAAP

SECTION ON TOBACCO CONTROL, 2018–2019

Judith A. Groner, MD, FAAP
Maria Rahmandar, MD, FAAP
Rachel Boykan, MD, FAAP
Bryan Mih, MD, FAAP
Jyothi N. Marbin, MD, FAAP
Alice Little Caldwell, MD, FAAP

STAFF

Julie Gorzkowski, MSW
Nana Ama Bullock, MPH
Colleen Spatz, MSBA

ABBREVIATIONS

AAP: American Academy of Pediatrics
e-cigarette: electronic cigarette
e-liquid: electronic liquid
FDA: Food and Drug Administration

FINANCIAL DISCLOSURE: The authors have indicated they have no financial relationships relevant to this article to disclose.

FUNDING: No external funding.

POTENTIAL CONFLICT OF INTEREST: The authors have indicated they have no potential conflicts of interest to disclose.

REFERENCES

1. US Department of Health and Human Services. *E-Cigarette Use Among Youth and Young Adults. A Report of the Surgeon General.* Atlanta, GA: US Department of Health and Human Services, Centers for Disease Control and Prevention, National Center for Chronic Disease Prevention and Health Promotion, Office on Smoking and Health; 2016
2. National Academies of Sciences, Engineering, and Medicine. *Public Health Consequences of E-Cigarettes.* Washington, DC: The National Academies Press; 2018
3. Walley SC, Jenssen BP; Section on Tobacco Control. Electronic nicotine delivery systems. *Pediatrics.* 2015;136(5):1018–1026
4. Barrington-Trimis JL, Leventhal AM. Adolescents' Use of "Pod Mod" E-Cigarettes -- Urgent Concerns. *N Engl J Med.* 2018;379(12):1099–1102
5. Hsu G, Sun JY, Zhu SH. Evolution of electronic cigarette brands from 2013-2014 to 2016-2017: analysis of brand websites. *J Med Internet Res.* 2018;20(3):e80
6. Cheng T. Chemical evaluation of electronic cigarettes. *Tob Control.* 2014;23(suppl 2):ii11–ii17
7. Wang TW, Gentzke A, Sharapova S, Cullen KA, Ambrose BK, Jamal A. Tobacco product use among middle and high school students - United States, 2011-2017. *MMWR Morb Mortal Wkly Rep.* 2018;67(22):629–633
8. Johnston LD, Miech RA, O'Malley PM, Bachman JG, Schulenberg JE, Patrick ME. *Monitoring the Future National Survey Results on Drug Use: 1975-2017: Overview, Key Findings on Adolescent Drug Use.* Ann Arbor, MI: Institute for Social Research, University of Michigan; 2018
9. Kann L, McManus T, Harris WA, et al. Youth risk behavior surveillance - United States, 2017. *MMWR Surveill Summ.* 2018;67(8):1–114
10. Cullen KA, Ambrose BK, Gentzke AS, Apelberg BJ, Jamal A, King BA. Notes from the Field: Use of Electronic Cigarettes and Any Tobacco Product Among Middle and High School Students -- United States, 2011-2018. *MMWR Morb Mortal Wkly Rep.* 2018;67(45):1276–1277
11. Arrazola RA, Neff LJ, Kennedy SM, Holder-Hayes E, Jones CD; Centers for Disease Control and Prevention (CDC). Tobacco use among middle and high school students–United States, 2013. *MMWR Morb Mortal Wkly Rep.* 2014;63(45):1021–1026
12. Duke JC, Lee YO, Kim AE, et al. Exposure to electronic cigarette television advertisements among youth and young adults. *Pediatrics.* 2014;134(1). Available at: www.pediatrics.org/cgi/content/full/134/1/e29
13. Giovenco DP, Hammond D, Corey CG, Ambrose BK, Delnevo CD. E-cigarette market trends in traditional U.S. retail channels, 2012-2013. *Nicotine Tob Res.* 2015;17(10):1279–1283
14. Huang J, Kornfield R, Szczypka G, Emery SL. A cross-sectional examination of marketing of electronic cigarettes on Twitter. *Tob Control.* 2014;23(suppl 3):iii26–iii30
15. Richardson A, Ganz O, Vallone D. Tobacco on the web: surveillance and characterisation of online tobacco and e-cigarette advertising. *Tob Control.* 2015;24(4):341–347
16. National Center for Chronic Disease Prevention and Health Promotion, Office on Smoking and Health. *Preventing Tobacco Use Among Youth and Young Adults: A Report of the Surgeon General.* Atlanta, GA: Centers for Disease Control and Prevention; 2012
17. US Department of Health and Human Services. *Preventing Tobacco Use Among Youth and Young Adults: A Report of the Surgeon General.* Atlanta, GA: US Department of Health and Human Services, Centers for Disease Control and Prevention, Office on Smoking and Health; 2012
18. Marynak K, Gentzke A, Wang TW, Neff L, King BA. Exposure to electronic cigarette advertising among middle and high school students - United States, 2014-2016. *MMWR Morb Mortal Wkly Rep.* 2018;67(10):294–299
19. Farrelly MC, Duke JC, Crankshaw EC, et al. A randomized trial of the effect of e-cigarette TV advertisements on intentions to use e-cigarettes. *Am J Prev Med.* 2015;49(5):686–693
20. Hammig B, Daniel-Dobbs P, Blunt-Vinti H. Electronic cigarette initiation among minority youth in the United States. *Am J Drug Alcohol Abuse.* 2017;43(3):306–310
21. Singh T, Agaku IT, Arrazola RA, et al. Exposure to advertisements and

electronic cigarette use among US middle and high school students. *Pediatrics.* 2016;137(5):e20154155

22. Mantey DS, Cooper MR, Clendennen SL, Pasch KE, Perry CL. E-cigarette marketing exposure is associated with e-cigarette use among US youth. *J Adolesc Health.* 2016;58(6):686–690
23. Cantrell J, Emelle B, Ganz O, Hair EC, Vallone D. Rapid increase in e-cigarette advertising spending as Altria's MarkTen enters the marketplace. *Tob Control.* 2016;25(e1):e16–e18
24. Grana R, Benowitz N, Glantz SA. E-cigarettes: a scientific review. *Circulation.* 2014;129(19):1972–1986
25. Goniewicz ML, Knysak J, Gawron M, et al. Levels of selected carcinogens and toxicants in vapour from electronic cigarettes. *Tob Control.* 2014;23(2):133–139
26. Jensen RP, Luo W, Pankow JF, Strongin RM, Peyton DH. Hidden formaldehyde in e-cigarette aerosols. *N Engl J Med.* 2015;372(4):392–394
27. Bahl V, Lin S, Xu N, Davis B, Wang YH, Talbot P. Comparison of electronic cigarette refill fluid cytotoxicity using embryonic and adult models. *Reprod Toxicol.* 2012;34(4):529–537
28. Collaco JM, Drummond MB, McGrath-Morrow SA. Electronic cigarette use and exposure in the pediatric population. *JAMA Pediatr.* 2015;169(2):177–182
29. Grana RA, Ling PM. "Smoking revolution": a content analysis of electronic cigarette retail websites. *Am J Prev Med.* 2014;46(4):395–403
30. Soghoian S. Nicotine. In: Hoffman RS, Howland MA, Lewin NA, Nelson LS, Goldfrank LR, eds. *Goldfrank's Toxicologic Emergencies*, 10th ed. New York, NY: McGraw-Hill Education; 2015:1138–1143
31. US Department of Health and Human Services. *The Health Consequences of Smoking—50 Years of Progress: A Report of the Surgeon General.* Atlanta, GA: US Department of Health and Human Services, Centers for Disease Control and Prevention, National Center for Chronic Disease Prevention and Health Promotion, Office on Smoking and Health; 2014. Available at: www.surgeongeneral.gov/library/reports/50-years-of-progress/. Accessed February 11, 2016
32. Dwyer JB, McQuown SC, Leslie FM. The dynamic effects of nicotine on the developing brain. *Pharmacol Ther.* 2009;122(2):125–139
33. Schraufnagel DE. Electronic cigarettes: vulnerability of youth. *Pediatr Allergy Immunol Pulmonol.* 2015;28(1):2–6
34. Pentz MA, Shin H, Riggs N, Unger JB, Collison KL, Chou CP. Parent, peer, and executive function relationships to early adolescent e-cigarette use: a substance use pathway? *Addict Behav.* 2015;42:73–78
35. Siqueira LM; Committee on Substance Use and Prevention. Nicotine and tobacco as substances of abuse in children and adolescents. *Pediatrics.* 2017;139(1):e20163436
36. Zhu SH, Sun JY, Bonnevie E, et al. Four hundred and sixty brands of e-cigarettes and counting: implications for product regulation. *Tob Control.* 2014;23(suppl 3):iii3–iii9
37. Tierney PA, Karpinski CD, Brown JE, Luo W, Pankow JF. Flavour chemicals in electronic cigarette fluids. *Tob Control.* 2016;25(e1):e10–e15
38. Ambrose BK, Day HR, Rostron B, et al. Flavored tobacco product use among US youth aged 12-17 years, 2013-2014. *JAMA.* 2015;314(17):1871–1873
39. Patrick ME, Miech RA, Carlier C, O'Malley PM, Johnston LD, Schulenberg JE. Self-reported reasons for vaping among 8th, 10th, and 12th graders in the US: nationally-representative results. *Drug Alcohol Depend.* 2016;165:275–278
40. Tsai J, Walton K, Coleman BN, et al. Reasons for electronic cigarette use among middle and high school students - National Youth Tobacco Survey, United States, 2016. *MMWR Morb Mortal Wkly Rep.* 2018;67(6):196–200
41. Pepper JK, Ribisl KM, Brewer NT. Adolescents' interest in trying flavoured e-cigarettes. *Tob Control.* 2016;25(suppl 2):ii62–ii66
42. Harrell MB, Weaver SR, Loukas A, et al. Flavored e-cigarette use: characterizing youth, young adult, and adult users. *Prev Med Rep.* 2016;5:33–40
43. Deyton L, Sharfstein J, Hamburg M. Tobacco product regulation–a public health approach. *N Engl J Med.* 2010;362(19):1753–1756
44. Courtemanche CJ, Palmer MK, Pesko MF. Influence of the flavored cigarette ban on adolescent tobacco use. *Am J Prev Med.* 2017;52(5):e139–e146
45. Callahan-Lyon P. Electronic cigarettes: human health effects. *Tob Control.* 2014;23(suppl 2):ii36–ii40
46. Schober W, Szendrei K, Matzen W, et al. Use of electronic cigarettes (e-cigarettes) impairs indoor air quality and increases FeNO levels of e-cigarette consumers. *Int J Hyg Environ Health.* 2014;217(6):628–637
47. Schripp T, Markewitz D, Uhde E, Salthammer T. Does e-cigarette consumption cause passive vaping? *Indoor Air.* 2013;23(1):25–31
48. Czogala J, Goniewicz ML, Fidelus B, Zielinska-Danch W, Travers MJ, Sobczak A. Secondhand exposure to vapors from electronic cigarettes. *Nicotine Tob Res.* 2014;16(6):655–662
49. Williams M, Villarreal A, Bozhilov K, Lin S, Talbot P. Metal and silicate particles including nanoparticles are present in electronic cigarette cartomizer fluid and aerosol. *PLoS One.* 2013;8(3):e57987
50. Mayer B. How much nicotine kills a human? Tracing back the generally accepted lethal dose to dubious self-experiments in the nineteenth century. *Arch Toxicol.* 2014;88(1):5–7
51. Eggleston W, Nacca N, Stork CM, Marraffa JM. Pediatric death after unintentional exposure to liquid nicotine for an electronic cigarette. *Clin Toxicol (Phila).* 2016;54(9): 890–891
52. Govindarajan P, Spiller HA, Casavant MJ, Chounthirath T, Smith GA. E-cigarette and liquid nicotine exposures among young children. *Pediatrics.* 2018;141(5):e20173361
53. Soneji S, Barrington-Trimis JL, Wills TA, et al. Association between initial use of e-cigarettes and subsequent cigarette smoking among adolescents and young adults: a systematic review

and meta-analysis. *JAMA Pediatr.* 2017;171(8):788–797

54. Primack BA, Soneji S, Stoolmiller M, Fine MJ, Sargent JD. Progression to traditional cigarette smoking after electronic cigarette use among US adolescents and young adults. *JAMA Pediatr.* 2015;169(11):1018–1023

55. Miech R, Patrick ME, O'Malley PM, Johnston LD. E-cigarette use as a predictor of cigarette smoking: results from a 1-year follow-up of a national sample of 12th grade students. *Tob Control.* 2017;26(e2):e106–e111

56. Barrington-Trimis JL, Urman R, Berhane K, et al. E-cigarettes and future cigarette use. *Pediatrics.* 2016;138(1):e20160379

57. Leventhal AM, Strong DR, Kirkpatrick MG, et al. Association of electronic cigarette use with initiation of combustible tobacco product smoking in early adolescence. *JAMA.* 2015;314(7):700–707

58. Wills TA, Knight R, Sargent JD, Gibbons FX, Pagano I, Williams RJ. Longitudinal study of e-cigarette use and onset of cigarette smoking among high school students in Hawaii. *Tob Control.* 2017;26(1):34–39

59. Bold KW, Kong G, Camenga DR, et al. Trajectories of e-cigarette and conventional cigarette use among youth. *Pediatrics.* 2018;141(1):e20171832

60. Watkins SL, Glantz SA, Chaffee BW. Association of noncigarette tobacco product use with future cigarette smoking among youth in the population assessment of tobacco and health (PATH) study, 2013-2015. *JAMA Pediatr.* 2018;172(2):181–187

61. Chaffee BW, Watkins SL, Glantz SA. Electronic cigarette use and progression from experimentation to established smoking. *Pediatrics.* 2018;141(4):e20173594

62. Kalkhoran S, Glantz SA. E-cigarettes and smoking cessation in real-world and clinical settings: a systematic review and meta-analysis. *Lancet Respir Med.* 2016;4(2):116–128

63. Fiore MC, Jaén CR, Baker TB, et al. *Treating Tobacco Use and Dependence: 2008 Update. Clinical Practice Guideline.* Rockville, MD: US Department of Health and Human Services. Public Health Service; 2008

64. US Food and Drug Administration. FDA takes significant steps to protect Americans from dangers of tobacco through new regulation. Available at: www.fda.gov/NewsEvents/Newsroom/PressAnnouncements/ucm499234.htm. Accessed September 9, 2016

65. US Food and Drug Administration. The facts on the FDA's new tobacco rule. Available at: https://www.fda.gov/ForConsumers/ConsumerUpdates/ucm506676.htm. Accessed April 3, 2018

66. US Food and Drug Administration. Statement from FDA commissioner Scott Gottlieb, M.D., on pivotal public health step to dramatically reduce smoking rates by lowering nicotine in combustible cigarettes to minimally or non-addictive levels. Available at: https://www.fda.gov/NewsEvents/Newsroom/PressAnnouncements/ucm601039.htm. Accessed April 4, 2018

67. Marynak K, Kenemer B, King BA, Tynan MA, MacNeil A, Reimels E. State laws regarding indoor public use, retail sales, and prices of electronic cigarettes - U.S. states, Guam, Puerto Rico, and U.S. Virgin Islands, September 30, 2017. *MMWR Morb Mortal Wkly Rep.* 2017;66(49):1341–1346

68. Centers for Disease Control and Prevention. State Tobacco Activities Tracking and Evaluation (STATE) System. 2018. Available at: https://www.cdc.gov/statesystem/index.html. Accessed April 4, 2018

69. McGinley L. FDA sued for delaying e-cigarette, cigar regulations. *Washington Post.* March 27, 2018. Available at: https://www.washingtonpost.com/news/to-your-health/wp/2018/03/27/fda-sued-for-delaying-e-cigarette-cigar-regulations/. Accessed April 4, 2018

70. US Food and Drug Administration. Statement from FDA commissioner Scott Gottlieb, MD, on new steps to address epidemic of youth e-cigarette use. 2018. Available at: https://www.fda.gov/NewsEvents/Newsroom/PressAnnouncements/ucm620185.htm. Accessed October 30, 2018

71. King BA, Gammon DG, Marynak KL, Rogers T. Electronic Cigarette Sales in the United States, 2013-2017. *JAMA.* 2018;320(13):1379–1380

72. Office of the Commissioner C for TP. Press Announcements - Statement from FDA Commissioner Scott Gottlieb, M.D., on proposed new steps to protect youth by preventing access to flavored tobacco products and banning menthol in cigarettes. 2018. Available at: https://www.fda.gov/NewsEvents/Newsroom/PressAnnouncements/ucm625884.htm. Accessed November 28, 2018

The Effects of Early Nutritional Interventions on the Development of Atopic Disease in Infants and Children: The Role of Maternal Dietary Restriction, Breastfeeding, Hydrolyzed Formulas, and Timing of Introduction of Allergenic Complementary Foods

- *Clinical Report*

CLINICAL REPORT Guidance for the Clinician in Rendering Pediatric Care

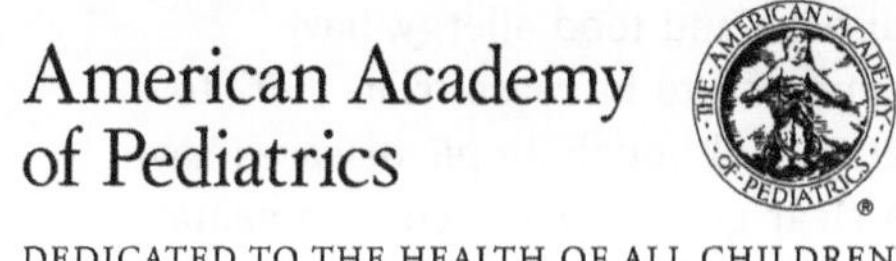

The Effects of Early Nutritional Interventions on the Development of Atopic Disease in Infants and Children: The Role of Maternal Dietary Restriction, Breastfeeding, Hydrolyzed Formulas, and Timing of Introduction of Allergenic Complementary Foods

Frank R. Greer, MD, FAAP,[a] Scott H. Sicherer, MD, FAAP,[b] A. Wesley Burks, MD, FAAP,[c] COMMITTEE ON NUTRITION, SECTION ON ALLERGY AND IMMUNOLOGY

abstract

This clinical report updates and replaces a 2008 clinical report from the American Academy of Pediatrics, which addressed the roles of maternal and early infant diet on the prevention of atopic disease, including atopic dermatitis, asthma, and food allergy. As with the previous report, the available data still limit the ability to draw firm conclusions about various aspects of atopy prevention through early dietary interventions. Current evidence does not support a role for maternal dietary restrictions during pregnancy or lactation. Although there is evidence that exclusive breastfeeding for 3 to 4 months decreases the incidence of eczema in the first 2 years of life, there are no short- or long-term advantages for exclusive breastfeeding beyond 3 to 4 months for prevention of atopic disease. The evidence now suggests that any duration of breastfeeding ≥3 to 4 months is protective against wheezing in the first 2 years of life, and some evidence suggests that longer duration of any breastfeeding protects against asthma even after 5 years of age. No conclusions can be made about the role of breastfeeding in either preventing or delaying the onset of specific food allergies. There is a lack of evidence that partially or extensively hydrolyzed formula prevents atopic disease. There is no evidence that delaying the introduction of allergenic foods, including peanuts, eggs, and fish, beyond 4 to 6 months prevents atopic disease. There is now evidence that early introduction of peanuts may prevent peanut allergy.

[a]Department of Pediatrics, School of Medicine and Public Health, University of Wisconsin-Madison, Madison, Wisconsin; [b]Jaffe Food Allergy Institute, Division of Allergy and Immunology, Department of Pediatrics, Icahn School of Medicine at Mount Sinai, New York, New York; and [c]Department of Pediatrics, School of Medicine, University of North Carolina at Chapel Hill, Chapel Hill, North Carolina

Drs Greer, Sicherer, and Burks contributed to identification, incorporation, and interpretation of the literature used to compose the report; assisted in drafting, reviewing, and editing the manuscript; and approved the final manuscript as submitted.

This document is copyrighted and is property of the American Academy of Pediatrics and its Board of Directors. All authors have filed conflict of interest statements with the American Academy of Pediatrics. Any conflicts have been resolved through a process approved by the Board of Directors. The American Academy of Pediatrics has neither solicited nor accepted any commercial involvement in the development of the content of this publication.

To cite: Greer FR, Sicherer SH, Burks AW, AAP COMMITTEE ON NUTRITION, AAP SECTION ON ALLERGY AND IMMUNOLOGY. The Effects of Early Nutritional Interventions on the Development of Atopic Disease in Infants and Children: The Role of Maternal Dietary Restriction, Breastfeeding, Hydrolyzed Formulas, and Timing of Introduction of Allergenic Complementary Foods. *Pediatrics.* 2019;143(4): e20190281

The incidence of pediatric atopic diseases, particularly allergic skin disease and food allergy, have appeared to increase from 1997 to 2011.[1] Although atopic diseases have a clear genetic basis, environmental factors, including early infant nutrition, have an important influence on their development. Thus, for pediatric health care providers, there is great interest in early nutritional strategies that may ameliorate or prevent this disease. This clinical report updates and replaces a 2008 clinical report from the American Academy of Pediatrics (AAP), which addressed the roles of maternal and early infant diet on the prevention of atopic disease, including atopic dermatitis, asthma, and food allergy.[2] The literature reviewed for this revised clinical report has largely been focused on new randomized controlled investigations, systematic reviews and meta-analyses, and recent recommendations from other professional groups. Of special note for this updated clinical report are the recently published investigations in which the relationship between the introduction (timing and amount) of complementary foods containing peanut and egg proteins and the development of food allergy is evaluated. On the other hand, information regarding the role of prebiotics and probiotics, vitamin D, and long-chain polyunsaturated fatty acids in the prevention of atopic disease is limited at this time and will not be discussed. This report is not directed at the treatment of atopic disease once an infant or child has developed specific atopic symptoms.

DEFINITIONS

The following definitions are used throughout this clinical report:

- allergy: a hypersensitivity reaction initiated by immunologic mechanisms[3];
- allergenic foods: 8 major groups of allergenic foods that account for approximately 90% of all food allergies and must be declared on labels for processed foods in the United States. These include cow milk, eggs, fish, crustacean shellfish, tree nuts, peanuts, wheat, and soybean.[4] More than 170 foods have been described to cause allergic reactions, and additional foods (eg, sesame) are included in labeling laws in other countries[4];
- atopy: a personal or familial tendency to produce immunoglobulin E (IgE) antibodies in response to low-dose allergens, confirmed by a positive skin-prick test result[3];
- atopic disease: a clinical disease characterized by atopy. Atopic disease typically refers to atopic dermatitis, asthma, allergic rhinitis, and food allergy. This report will be limited to the discussion of conditions for which substantial information is available in the medical literature[3];
- atopic dermatitis (eczema): a pruritic, chronic, inflammatory skin disease that commonly presents during early childhood and is often associated with a personal or family history of other atopic diseases[3];
- asthma: an allergic-mediated response in the bronchial airways that is verified by the variation in lung function (measured by spirometry), either spontaneously or after bronchodilating drugs[3];
- complementary foods: foods and/or beverages (liquids, semisolids, and solids) other than human milk, infant formula, and cow's milk (consumed in the first year of life) provided to an infant or young child to provide micro- and macronutrients, including energy[5];
- food allergy: an immunologically mediated hypersensitivity reaction to any food, including IgE-mediated and/or non–IgE-mediated allergic reactions[2];
- hypoallergenic: reduced allergenicity or reduced ability to stimulate an IgE response and induce IgE-mediated reactions[3]; and
- Infants at high risk for developing allergy: infants with at least 1 first-degree relative (parent or sibling) with documented allergic disease.[3] Some of the studies included in this report used different criteria for labeling infants high risk for developing atopic disease.

The following definitions are from various industry sources[2]:

- partially hydrolyzed formula: formula that contains reduced oligopeptides having a molecular weight of generally less than 5000 Da;
- extensively hydrolyzed formula: formula that contains only peptides that have a molecular weight of less than 3000 Da; and
- free amino acid-based formula: peptide-free formula that contains mixtures of essential and nonessential amino acids.

DIETARY RESTRICTIONS FOR PREGNANT AND LACTATING WOMEN

The earliest possible nutritional influence on atopic disease in an infant is the prenatal diet. However, studies have not supported a protective effect of a maternal exclusion diet (including the exclusion of cow's milk, eggs, and peanuts) during pregnancy or during lactation on the development of atopic disease in infants. The 2008 AAP report concluded that there was lack of evidence to support maternal dietary restrictions during pregnancy and lactation to prevent atopic disease.[2] There are no new clinical trials that would change this conclusion for the current report. This conclusion is affirmed in a 2014 a meta-analysis[6] and 2 new systematic reviews.[7,8] In 1 systematic review, the authors noted that maternal diets rich in fruits and vegetables, fish, and foods containing vitamin D and Mediterranean dietary patterns were among the few consistent associations with lower risk for allergic disease in their children. On the other hand, foods associated with higher risk included vegetable oils and margarine, nuts, and fast food.[8] However, further randomized controlled trials of maternal antigen avoidance with larger sample sizes and longer follow-up are needed.

EXTENT AND DURATION OF BREASTFEEDING ON THE DEVELOPMENT OF ATOPIC DISEASE

Since the 1930s, authors of many studies have examined the impact of breastfeeding on the development of atopic disease. It has been thought that the immunologic components of human milk may modify induction of immune tolerance and decrease the risk of allergic disease.
In general, these studies have been nonrandomized, retrospective, or observational in design and have included many cohort studies.

Duration of Exclusive Breastfeeding

The 2008 AAP report concluded that there were no short- or long-term advantages for exclusive breastfeeding beyond 3 to 4 months for prevention of atopic disease.[2] One new meta-analysis looking specifically at the question of duration of exclusive breastfeeding was published in 2012.[9] It included only 3 studies in which exclusive breastfeeding for 3 to 4 months was compared with exclusive breastfeeding for 6 months or longer.[10–12] Of these 3 studies, 1 was a cluster randomized trial with a 6.5 year follow-up.[11] In this meta-analysis, the authors concluded that there was no difference in atopic eczema, asthma, or other atopic outcomes between exclusive breastfeeding for 3 to 4 months versus exclusive breastfeeding for 6 months or longer.[9] Two other new meta-analyses in which exclusive breastfeeding and atopic disease are addressed have also have been published.[13,14] One of these meta-analyses showed that there was no evidence that exclusive breastfeeding (versus any duration of breastfeeding) offered any significant advantage for the prevention of asthma.[13] The second meta-analysis found no significant association between exclusive breastfeeding for ≥3 to 4 months versus breastfeeding for a shorter duration and asthma at 5 to 18 years of age (13 studies).[14] However, this study did find that exclusive breastfeeding for at least 3 to 4 months decreases the cumulative incidence of eczema in the first 2 years of life, with or without any additional breastfeeding.[14] This conclusion is unchanged from the 2008 AAP report.[2]

Breastfeeding and Asthma

Since the 2008 AAP report,[2] there have been at least 64 new studies on the relationship between asthma and breastfeeding. Descriptions of these studies can be found in 3 new systematic reviews of the relationship between asthma and breastfeeding.[13–15] All 3 reviews concluded that there were concerns about combining the results of these studies given the high degree of heterogeneity among the included studies, with Dogaru et al[13] reporting that the index of heterogeneity (I^2) among the studies was high, ranging from 71% to 92%.

In addition to the observation on exclusive breastfeeding and asthma as discussed above, the meta-analysis of Dogaru et al[13] found evidence that more breastfeeding (longer duration) as opposed to less breastfeeding (shorter duration) reduced the risk of asthma across all age groups. The greatest protective effect for duration of any breastfeeding, including exclusive breastfeeding (3–6 months), on the risk of asthma was for the first 2 years of life, during which time period wheezing is associated with childhood illness and not considered to be atopic asthma. There is also some evidence the longer duration was protective against childhood asthma until at least 3 to 6 years of age. This finding supports the rationale that wheezing conditions in infants, typically triggered by viral respiratory infections, may be protected by breastfeeding through reduction in the impact of the infections themselves.

The meta-analysis by Brew et al[15] looked at the relationship between any breastfeeding versus no breastfeeding or exclusive breastfeeding for at least 3 to 4 months versus exclusive breastfeeding for a shorter duration and wheezing in children 5 years of age or older. This study found no evidence that any duration of breastfeeding is protective against wheezing illness in children 5 years and older, emphasizing the differences in the asthma "phenotype," or early childhood wheezing versus wheezing beyond 5 years of age. On the other hand, Lodge et al[14] pooled the results of 29 studies that looked at more versus less of any category of breastfeeding (ever versus never [n = 8]; exclusive versus other [n = 13]; more versus less [n = 8]) and found that there was a reduced risk of asthma with longer versus shorter duration of any breastfeeding at 5 to 18 years of age (odds ratio [OR], 0.90; 95% confidence interval [CI], 0.84–0.97; I^2, 63%). Categorizing studies as "more versus less" breastfeeding allowed for inclusion of more studies and might have accounted for the difference in results in the Lodge et al[14] versus Brew et al[15] meta-analysis in older children. The Lodge et al[14] study also found a protective effect of ever breastfeeding versus never breastfeeding on asthma from 5 to 18 years of age when the estimates from 3 cohort studies and 10 cross-sectional studies were pooled (OR, 0.88; 95% CI, 0.82–0.95, I^2, 44%).

The 2008 AAP report concluded that exclusive breastfeeding for at least 3 months protects against wheezing early in life.[2] In addition, newer evidence now suggests that the protection of breastfeeding in early childhood (wheezing in the first 2 years) occurs because of duration of any breastfeeding, not just exclusive breastfeeding. Unlike in 2008, there is now evidence that longer duration of breastfeeding may protect against asthma after 5 years of age.

Breastfeeding and Eczema

Since publication of the 2008 AAP report, there have been 2 meta-analyses and approximately 7 new studies on the relationship between breastfeeding and childhood eczema (follow-up up to age 7 years). In a meta-analysis by Yang et al,[16] the authors concluded that there was no protective effect of breastfeeding for ≥3 months compared with breastfeeding for a shorter duration or infant formula feeding, even in children with a family history of allergy (OR, 0.78; 95% CI, 0.58–1.05). A second meta-analysis that included 15 cohort studies (7 of which were published since the 2008 AAP report) found no protection of the exposure for more versus less of any duration of breastfeeding and the risk of eczema up to 2 years of age (OR, 0.95; 95% CI, 0.85–1.07).[13] However, another analysis in this same study (pooling only 6 cohort studies in which exclusive breastfeeding for at least 3 to 4 months was compared with a shorter duration of breastfeeding) revealed a significantly reduced risk of eczema below the age of 2 years (OR, 0.74; 95% CI, 0.57–0.97).[13] No association was found between breastfeeding and eczema beyond 2 years of age in this study, again suggesting that protection afforded by breastfeeding may be limited to the infantile eczema phenotype. This study, limiting the analysis to only infants with a family history of atopic disease (7 studies), did not change the results for eczema.[13]

In summary, there is evidence that exclusive breastfeeding for at least 3 to 4 months decreases the cumulative incidence of atopic dermatitis in the first 2 years of life. This is similar to the results found in the Duration of Exclusive Breastfeeding section, noted earlier in this report. There is no evidence that longer duration of any breastfeeding affects the outcome.

Breastfeeding and Food Allergy

Data are insufficient regarding a direct relationship of breastfeeding on food allergy outcomes. It has been suggested that the early introduction of allergenic foods while breastfeeding might be protective against development of food allergy. However, there are no published trials directly comparing timing of introduction of allergenic foods in exclusively formula-fed versus exclusively breastfed infants on the development of food allergy. In the recent Enquiring About Tolerance (EAT) trial in infants who were breastfed, discussed in more detail elsewhere in this report, the goal was to determine if the early introduction of common allergenic foods at 3 months of age in infants who were exclusively breastfed in the general population would prevent food allergies, but the control group was both breastfed and formula fed.[17] Similarly, in the Learning Early About Peanut Allergy (LEAP) trial (described in more detail later), in which infants were randomly assigned to ingest or avoid peanuts, the subjects were mainly infants who were breastfed (92%), without sufficient controls to evaluate the effect of breastfeeding itself on peanut allergy outcomes.[18]

In summary, as in the 2008 report,[2] no conclusions can be made about the role of breastfeeding in either preventing or delaying the onset of specific food allergies.

THE ROLE OF HYDROLYZED FORMULAS ON THE DEVELOPMENT OF ATOPIC DISEASE

The role of partially hydrolyzed and extensively hydrolyzed formulas in the prevention of atopic disease has been the subject of many studies, and it has been suggested that if high-risk infants cannot be exclusively breastfed, use of such formulas will prevent atopic disease. Since the AAP report was published in 2008, 1 randomized trial of partially hydrolyzed formula and 1 meta-analysis of the effects of hydrolyzed formula on allergic disease were published.[19,20] There is also a new trial in which a partially hydrolyzed formula is compared with added prebiotics to a standard formula for the prevention of atopic disease.[21] In addition, for a study initially cited in the AAP 2008 report (the German Infant Nutritional Intervention study), there is now a 10-year follow-up of the effects of partially and extensively hydrolyzed infant formulas on atopic disease.[22] The overall results of these new studies have weakened previous conclusions that there was modest evidence that the use of either partially or extensively hydrolyzed formula prevents atopic dermatitis in high-risk infants who are formula fed or initially breastfed after birth.

In a study published in 2011 by Lowe et al,[19] 620 infants with a family history of allergic disease were randomly assigned to receive standard cow's milk formula, partially hydrolyzed formula, or soy formula after cessation of breastfeeding. Fifty percent of the infants were receiving their allotted formula by 4 months of age. The primary outcome was development of allergic manifestations (eczema and food reactions) measured 18 times in the first 2 years of life, with follow-up until 6 or 7 years of age. There was no evidence that infants allocated to partially hydrolyzed formula were at a lower risk for allergic manifestations in infancy compared with infants allocated to conventional formula (OR, 1.21; 95% CI, 0.81–1.80). Similarly, in the new trial of the combination of partially hydrolyzed protein and prebiotics in an infant formula, there was no impact on eczema at 12 months of age, compared with a standard formula in high-risk infants (OR, 0.99; 95% CI, 0.71–1.37).[21]

In the 10-year follow-up to the 2003 German Infant Nutritional Intervention study (cited in the 2008 report), the relative risk (RR) for the cumulative incidence of any allergic disease through 10 years of age in the intention-to-treat analysis (n = 2252) was 0.87 (95% CI, 0.77–0.99) for the partially hydrolyzed whey-based formula, 0.94 (95% CI, 0.83–1.07) for the extensively hydrolyzed whey-based formula, and 0.83 (95% CI, 0.72–0.95) for the extensively hydrolyzed casein-based formula, compared with standard cow's milk formula. The corresponding figures for atopic eczema and/or dermatitis were 0.82 (95% CI, 0.68–1.00) for partially hydrolyzed whey-based formula, 0.91 (95% CI, 0.76–1.10) for extensively hydrolyzed whey-based formula, and 0.72 (95% CI, 0.58–0.88) for extensively hydrolyzed casein-based formula, compared with standard cow's milk formula.[22] Although the prevalence of atopic dermatitis at 7 to 10 years of age was significantly reduced with extensively hydrolyzed casein-based formula, there was no preventive effect on asthma or allergic rhinitis. The study was weakened by the 37% drop-out rate at 10 years; thus, the authors concluded that there was insufficient evidence of ongoing preventive activity of hydrolyzed formulas between 7 and 10 years of age for prevention of atopic disease.

The 2016 meta-analysis by Boyle et al,[20] which included 37 studies, found no consistent evidence to support a protective role of partially or extensively hydrolyzed formula for reducing risk of allergic disease, even in high-risk infants. This review included studies of any hydrolyzed formula of cow's milk origin as the intervention of interest, compared with any nonhydrolyzed cow's milk formula or human milk. Also included were studies in which hydrolyzed formula was given as part of a multifaceted intervention. ORs for eczema at age 0 to 4 years, compared with standard cow milk formula, were 0.84 (95% CI, 0.67–1.07) for partially hydrolyzed formula, 0.55 (95% CI, 0.28–1.09) for extensively hydrolyzed casein-based formula, and 1.12 (95% CI, 0.88–1.42) for extensively hydrolyzed whey-based formula.

In summary, there is lack of evidence that partially or extensively hydrolyzed formula prevents atopic disease in infants and children, even in those at high risk for allergic disease. This point is a change from the 2008 AAP clinical report, which concluded that there was modest evidence that the use of either partially or exclusively hydrolyzed formula prevents atopic dermatitis in high-risk infants who are formula fed or initially breastfed after birth.

TIMING OF INTRODUCTION OF ALLERGENIC COMPLEMENTARY FOODS AND FOOD ALLERGY

Since the 2008 AAP report, there has been considerable new information published relative to the timing of introduction of allergenic complementary foods and the subsequent development of food allergy. There have been 7 new randomized controlled trials[17,23–28] and 1 new meta-analysis that includes these studies.[29] Egg allergy was evaluated in 6 trials,[17,24–28] and peanut allergy was evaluated in 2 trials.[17,23]

In the EAT study on the timing of introduction of allergenic complementary foods in infants who were breastfed, all infants in the early introduction group (n = 567) were exclusively breastfeeding at 3 months of age and still breastfeeding at 5 months.[17] Six different allergenic foods were introduced between 3 and 5 months of age (median age, 3.4 months): peanut (peanut butter), cooked egg (1 small hardboiled egg), cow's milk, sesame, whitefish, and wheat. In the standard introduction group (n = 595), the allergenic foods were not introduced before 5 months, at which time all infants were still breastfeeding but consuming up to 300 mL of formula per day. In the intention-to-treat analysis, food allergy developed in 5.6% of the subjects in the early introduction group (mostly breastfeeding) and in 7.1% of the subjects in the standard introduction group (mixed feeding), a difference that was not significant. However, only 43% of participants in the early introduction group could follow the protocol, presumably because many of the infants were not developmentally ready to accept complementary foods at 3 months of age or because parents observed avoidance behaviors, leading to their cessation (reverse causality). However, in the per-protocol analysis, the prevalence of any food allergy was lower in the early introduction group than in the standard introduction group (2.4% vs 7.3%; P = .01). For the prevalence of specific food allergies in the per-protocol analysis, there was a significant protective effect of early consumption of both peanuts (0% vs 2.5%; P = .003) and eggs (1.4% vs 5.5%; P = .009). This was not observed for any of the other allergenic foods introduced.[17] The data were analyzed according to allergy outcomes and mean weekly dose ingested; consumption of 2 g/week of peanut or egg-white protein was associated with a significantly lower prevalence of these allergies, respectively, compared with less consumption. This subgroup analysis suggests that in infants who are breastfed, prevention of peanut and egg allergy (see discussion below) may depend on the amount and duration of early exposure.

In the LEAP trial of the early introduction of peanut products, 640 infants who were severely atopic (severe eczema and/or egg allergy) 4 to 11 months of age were randomly assigned to consume 6 g of peanut protein per week (Bamba or cooked peanut product) or to avoid peanut protein until age 60 months.[23] Infants were given skin-prick tests for peanuts, and all infants randomly assigned to the early consumption group underwent an open-label food challenge to ensure tolerance before incorporating peanuts into the diet. The mean age at randomization was 7.8 ± 1.7 months, but only 18% (116 infants) of the total cohort was younger than 6 months at the time of the first peanut introduction. Ninety percent of the subjects had received formula at the time of randomization; 42% of the subjects were still breastfeeding at the time of randomization, and in these 268 infants, breastfeeding continued for an average of 4.8 ± 4.9 months after randomization. There were no differences between the intervention and control groups in breastfeeding characteristics. Among the 530 infants in the intention-to-treat population who initially had negative results on the skin-prick test, the prevalence of peanut allergy at 60 months (blinded food-challenge test) was 13.7% in the avoidance group and 1.9% in the early peanut consumption group, an 11.8 percentage point reduction (95% CI, 3.4–20.3; $P < .001$). This represents an 86% reduction in peanut allergy. Among infants who had an initial positive result on the skin-prick test (n = 98) who still participated in the protocol and underwent random assignment, the prevalence of peanut allergy was 35.3% in the avoidance group and 10.6% in the early consumption group (P = .004; 70% RR reduction). A follow-up study revealed that this approach was long-lasting, demonstrating induction of tolerance rather than transient desensitization.[30]

A meta-analysis of the LEAP and the EAT studies revealed that, for peanut allergy, early peanut introduction at 4 to 11 months of age was associated with a reduced risk of peanut allergy (RR, 0.29; 95% CI, 0.11–0.74; I^2 = 66%; P = .009).[29] Largely on the basis of the results of the LEAP trial, an expert panel recently advised peanut introduction as early as 4 to 6 months of age in infants at high risk (presence of severe eczema and/or egg allergy).[31] Given that the pathophysiology of protection is likely to be similar for infants at a lower risk and on the basis of additional studies in an unselected population, the guidelines based the timing of early peanut introduction on the degree of risk (see below).[31]

Egg allergy is a common early food allergy. Six new studies have been published since the 2008 AAP report regarding the early introduction of eggs for the prevention of egg allergy.[17,24–28] There are significant differences among all of these studies, including the risk characteristics of the population exposed, differences in dosing of eggs, and the formulation of the egg introduced.

Two recent studies using heated forms of egg showed a benefit of early egg introduction for prevention of egg allergy. In the first of these 2 studies, the EAT trial (discussed previously), authors concluded that, in a subgroup analysis of the 43% of the subjects who completed the protocol, the introduction of whole boiled eggs between 3 and 5 months of age significantly reduced the prevalence of egg allergy.[17] The poorest compliance rate for individual foods introduced was for eggs (43%), which may reflect the poor acceptance of the texture of hardboiled eggs by the infants or subtle infant avoidance behavior observed by parents. Only 3 infants in the early introduction group demonstrated egg allergy at baseline (oral food-challenge test) and were not exposed to additional egg protein.

In a second randomized controlled trial, Natsume et al[24] introduced infants to increasing amounts of heated whole-egg powder in a stepwise approach, beginning with 50 mg at 6 months of age and increasing to 250 mg at 9 months of age. The final outcome was an open oral food-challenge test at 12 months, assessed blindly by standardized methods by using the same product given for the intervention. In the primary analysis population, 5 (8%) of 60 participants had an egg allergy in the egg group, compared with 23 (38%) of 61 in the placebo group. This difference was highly significant ($P < .0002$; RR, 0.221; 95% CI, 0.09–0.543; P = .001). The 90% compliance rate was much higher than that in the EAT study.[17] Of note, the study was terminated early after an interim analysis of the first 100 patients revealed a significant difference between groups. In this study, the authors concluded that heated whole-egg powder introduced in a stepwise manner prevents egg allergy in high-risk infants.

In 2 studies, pasteurized, uncooked egg-white powder was used, with differing results.[25,26] In the Hen's Egg Allergy Prevention trial, a randomized placebo-controlled trial of early egg introduction in 383 infants between 4 and 6 months, the primary outcome was sensitization to hen eggs (increased serum IgE levels) by age 12 months. The secondary outcome was confirmation of hen egg allergy by clinical reaction to pasteurized hen eggs on an oral food-challenge test. The study was terminated early because of the increased sensitization rate in the early egg introduction (4–6 months) group at 12 months of age. The authors of the study concluded that there was no evidence that consumption of hen eggs in the amount of 1 egg per week in its most allergic form, starting at 4 to 6 months age, prevents hen egg sensitization in a general population.[25] However, the authors acknowledged that additional data were needed to determine if eggs introduced even earlier than 4 months or in a less allergic form may prevent egg food allergy. In a second randomized trial of egg-white power introduced between 4 and 6 months of age in 319 infants, the primary outcome was a positive result on the skin-prick test at 12 months of age.[26] Egg sensitization (skin prick) was significantly reduced at 12 months in the egg group (10.7%) compared with placebo group (20.5%), with an OR of 0.46 (95% CI, 0.22–0.95; P = .03).[26]

In 2 additional randomized studies from the same Australian investigators, pasteurized, raw whole-egg powder was used versus rice powder as the control.[27,28] In the smaller of these 2 studies, 86 infants at high risk with moderate to severe eczema were randomly assigned at 4 months of age and continued on daily egg or rice powder until 8 months of age. At 8 months of age, cooked egg was introduced to both groups.[27] The primary outcome was IgE-mediated egg allergy at 12 months of age on the basis of results of an observed pasteurized raw-egg challenge and skin-prick testing. At 12 months of age, a lower proportion of infants in the egg group (33%) were given a diagnosis of IgE-mediated egg allergy compared with controls (51%), but the results were not significant (RR, 0.65; 95% CI, 0.38–1.11; P = .11). Of note, this study was not sufficiently powered to rule out a significant difference, as acknowledged by the authors. In the second, much larger, study, more than 800 infants (without a diagnosis of eczema) were randomly assigned at 4 to 6 months of age to consume pasteurized, raw whole-egg powder (0.4 g) or rice powder daily until 10 months of age.[28] Cooked whole egg was then introduced to both groups. Again, the primary outcome was IgE-mediated egg allergy by a positive result on a pasteurized raw-egg challenge and egg sensitization at 12 months of age. However, the study revealed no evidence that raw-egg intake from 4 to 6 months of age significantly altered the risk of egg allergy by age 1 year (7.0% in the egg group versus 10.3% in the control group; RR, 0.75; 95% CI, 0.48–1.17; P = .20). The authors did note that 90% of infants who had a reaction to the pasteurized raw-egg challenge were tolerating cooked eggs in their diet at 12 months of age, which raises the question of how many infants would have had egg allergy diagnosed if whole cooked egg rather than raw egg was used for the oral food-challenge test.

In a 2016 meta-analysis that included 5[17,24–27] of these 6 studies, the authors concluded that there was moderate certainty of evidence from the 5 trials (1915 participants) that early egg introduction at 4 to 6 months of age was associated with reduced egg allergy risks (RR, 0.56; 95% CI, 0.36–0.87; I^2 = 36%; P = .009).[29] In a number of these studies, it was reported that many of the infants tested positive for the presence of an egg allergy (range, 5% to 31%) before random assignment at 4 to 6 months of age, suggesting that 4 months may be too late for the introduction of eggs to prevent egg allergy.[25–27] In addition, it is not clear from these studies that early introduction of cooked eggs, as opposed to more reactive raw eggs, may decrease the prevalence of egg allergy. These are questions that must be addressed in future studies. For egg introduction, thousands of additional trial participants would be needed to confirm with reasonable certainty that early egg introduction has an effect size of a 30% reduction.[32]

Since the publication of the LEAP and EAT trials, there have been revised recommendations from a number of groups regarding the early nutritional interventions for the prevention of atopic disease, specifically regarding food allergies.[31,33–36] In general, these groups have acknowledged that there is no need to delay the introduction of allergenic foods beyond 6 months of age and that they should not be introduced before 4 months of age. An expert panel from the National Institute of Allergy and Infectious Diseases has recommended a 3-pronged approach,[31] specifically for the introduction of infant-safe forms of peanuts to infants, on the basis of the level of risk for peanut allergy and the results of the LEAP trial.[23] The AAP has endorsed these guidelines.[37] These guidelines are detailed and resource intense, and evaluation of their implementation requires more study. The details of the guidelines are not reiterated here, but briefly, infants with severe eczema, egg allergy, or both (highest risk) should have peanuts introduced as early as between 4 and 6 months of age (peanut allergy testing before introduction is recommended). This highest-risk group is the only one for which testing for peanut allergy is recommended. For infants with mild to moderate eczema (less risk), peanuts should be introduced as early as 6 months of age. For infants with no history of eczema or food allergy (lowest risk), peanuts should be introduced when age appropriate and in accordance with family preferences and cultural practices (ie, 6 months and later for infants who are exclusively breastfed). The level of evidence for the recommendations for infants other than those in the highest-risk category is not based on randomized controlled trials, especially for those in the lowest risk group. It is hoped that the screening process for the infants at highest risk (specific IgE measurement, skin-prick test, and oral food-challenge test) will not be a deterrent or generate "screening creep" for infants not in the high-risk category. Furthermore, these guidelines may be difficult to follow in communities where there is no access to the medical care needed for their implementation. Information on how these guidelines are being adopted in clinical settings is needed. It is hoped that further research will provide more information on how to introduce peanuts to populations not at risk for peanut allergy.

In the 2008 clinical report, the AAP concluded that there was no convincing evidence of benefit for delaying the introduction allergenic foods beyond 4 to 6 months for the prevention of atopic disease, including peanuts, eggs, and fish.[2] This conclusion has not changed. However, there is now strong evidence from a randomized trial that purposeful early introduction of peanuts may prevent peanut allergies in high-risk infants, resulting in the recommendation to introduce peanut protein as early as between 4 and 6 months. As reviewed previously, the data supporting a beneficial effect of early introduction of eggs is less clear.

SUMMARY AND RECOMMENDATIONS

As with the previous 2008 AAP clinical report, the available data still limit the ability to draw firm conclusions about various aspects of atopy prevention through early dietary interventions. The statements below summarize the current evidence within the context of the limitations of the published reports.

1. There is lack of evidence to support maternal dietary restrictions either during pregnancy or during lactation to prevent atopic disease. This conclusion is unchanged from the 2008 report.
2. The evidence regarding the role of breastfeeding in the prevention of atopic disease can be summarized as follows:
   A. There is evidence that exclusive breastfeeding for the first 3 to 4 months decreases the cumulative incidence of eczema in the first 2 years of life. This conclusion is unchanged from the 2008 report;
   B. There are no short- or long-term advantages for exclusive breastfeeding beyond 3 to 4 months for prevention of atopic disease. This conclusion is unchanged from the 2008 report;
   C. The evidence now suggests that any duration of breastfeeding beyond 3 to 4 months is protective against wheezing in the first 2 years of life. This effect is irrespective of duration of exclusivity. This conclusion differs slightly from the 2008 report, which stated that exclusive breastfeeding for at least 3 months protects against wheezing early in life;
   D. unlike the 2008 report, there is now some evidence that longer duration of any breastfeeding, as opposed to less breastfeeding, protects against asthma, even after 5 years of age; and
   E. similar to the 2008 report, no conclusions can be made about the role of any duration of breastfeeding in either preventing or delaying the onset of specific food allergies.
3. There is lack of evidence that partially or extensively hydrolyzed formula prevents atopic disease in infants and children, even in those at high risk for allergic disease. This is a change from the 2008 report, in which the AAP concluded that there was modest evidence that hydrolyzed formulas delayed or prevented atopic dermatitis in infants who were formula fed or not exclusively breastfed for 3 to 4 months.[2]
4. The current evidence for the importance of the timing of introduction of allergenic foods and the prevention of atopic disease can be summarized as follows:
   A. There is no evidence that delaying the introduction of allergenic foods, including peanuts, eggs, and fish, beyond 4 to 6 months prevents atopic disease. This conclusion has not changed from the 2008 report[2];
   B. There is now evidence that the early introduction of infant-safe forms of peanuts reduces the risk for peanut allergies. Data are less clear for timing of introduction of eggs; and
   C. The new recommendations for the prevention of peanut allergy are based largely on the LEAP trial and are endorsed by the AAP.[37] An expert panel has advised peanut introduction as early as 4 to 6 months of age for infants at high risk for peanut allergy (presence of severe eczema and/or egg allergy). The recommendations contain details of implementation for high-risk infants, including appropriate use of testing (specific IgE measurement, skin-prick test, and oral food challenges) and introduction of peanut-containing foods in the health care provider's office versus the home setting, as well as amount and frequency.[31] For infants with mild to moderate eczema, the panel recommended introduction of peanut-containing foods at around 6 months of age, and

for infants at low risk for peanut allergy (no eczema or any food allergy), the panel recommended introduction of peanut-containing food when age appropriate and depending on family preferences and cultural practices (ie, after 6 months of age if exclusively breastfeeding).

5. This report describes means to prevent or delay atopic disease through early dietary intervention. For the child who has developed atopic disease, treatment may require specific identification and restriction of causal food proteins; this topic is not addressed in this report.

LEAD AUTHORS

Frank R. Greer, MD, FAAP
Scott H. Sicherer, MD, FAAP
A. Wesley Burks, MD, FAAP

COMMITTEE ON NUTRITION, 2017–2018

Steven A. Abrams, MD, FAAP, Chair
George J. Fuchs III, MD, FAAP
Jae H. Kim, MD, PhD, FAAP
C. Wesley Lindsey, MD, FAAP
Sheela N. Magge, MD, MSCE, FAAP
Ellen S. Rome, MD, FAAP
Sarah Jane Schwarzenberg, MD, FAAP

PAST COMMITTEE MEMBERS

Mark R. Corkins, MD, FAAP
Steven R. Daniels, MD, PhD, FAAP
Neville H. Golden, MD, FAAP

LIAISONS

Janet de Jesus, MS, RD – *National Institutes of Health*
Andrea Lotze, MD, FAAP – *Food and Drug Administration*
Cria Perrine, PhD – *Centers for Disease Control and Prevention*
Valery Soto, MS, RD, LD – *US Department of Agriculture*

STAFF

Debra Burrowes, MHA

SECTION ON ALLERGY AND IMMUNOLOGY EXECUTIVE COMMITTEE, 2017–2018

Elizabeth C. Matsui, MD, FAAP, Chair
John Andrew Bird, MD, FAAP
Carla McGuire Davis, MD, FAAP
Vivian Pilar Hernandez-Trujillo, MD, FAAP
Todd A. Mahr, MD, FAAP, Immediate Past Chair
Jordan S. Orange, MD, PhD, FAAP
Michael Pistiner, MD, FAAP
Julie Wang, MD, FAAP
Paul V. Williams, MD, FAAP, Liaison, *American Academy of Allergy, Asthma, and Immunology*

PAST EXECUTIVE COMMITTEE MEMBERS

Chitra Dinakar, MD, FAAP
Anne-Marie Irani, MD, FAAP
Jennifer S. Kim, MD, FAAP
Scott H. Sicherer, MD, FAAP

STAFF

Debra Burrowes, MHA

ABBREVIATIONS

AAP: American Academy of Pediatrics
CI: confidence interval
EAT: Enquiring About Tolerance
IgE: immunoglobulin E
LEAP: Learning Early About Peanut Allergy
OR: odds ratio
RR: relative risk

Clinical reports from the American Academy of Pediatrics benefit from expertise and resources of liaisons and internal (AAP) and external reviewers. However, clinical reports from the American Academy of Pediatrics may not reflect the views of the liaisons or the organizations or government agencies that they represent.

The guidance in this report does not indicate an exclusive course of treatment or serve as a standard of medical care. Variations, taking into account individual circumstances, may be appropriate.

All clinical reports from the American Academy of Pediatrics automatically expire 5 years after publication unless reaffirmed, revised, or retired at or before that time.

DOI: https://doi.org/10.1542/peds.2019-0281

Address correspondence to Frank R. Greer, MD, FAAP. E-mail: frgreer@pediatrics.wisc.edu

PEDIATRICS (ISSN Numbers: Print, 0031-4005; Online, 1098-4275).

Copyright © 2019 by the American Academy of Pediatrics

FINANCIAL DISCLOSURE: The authors have indicated they have no financial relationships relevant to this article to disclose.

FUNDING: No external funding.

POTENTIAL CONFLICT OF INTEREST: Dr Sicherer received royalties from UpToDate and Johns Hopkins University Press; grants to his institution from HAL Allergy Group, Food Allergy Research and Education, the Immune Tolerance Network, and the National Institute of Allergy and Infectious Diseases; and honoraria from the American Academy of Allergy, Asthma, and Immunology (as an associate editor) and is a medical advisor to the Food Allergy Fund and the International Association for Food Protein Enterocolitis. He was a member of the following sponsored expert panel: Guidelines for the Prevention of Peanut Allergy in the United States: Summary of the National Institute of Allergy and Infectious Diseases; and Drs Greer and Burks have indicated they have no potential conflicts of interest to disclose.

REFERENCES

1. Jackson KD, Howie LD, Akinbami LJ. Trends in allergic conditions among children: United States, 1997–2011. NCHS Data Brief, No 121. Hyattsville, MD: National Center for Health Statistics; 2013. Available at: https://www.cdc.gov/nchs/data/databriefs/db121.pdf. Accessed February 5, 2019
2. Greer FR, Sicherer SH, Burks AW; American Academy of Pediatrics Committee on Nutrition; American Academy of Pediatrics Section on Allergy and Immunology. Effects of early nutritional interventions on the development of atopic disease in infants and children: the role of maternal dietary restriction, breastfeeding, timing of introduction of complementary foods, and hydrolyzed formulas. *Pediatrics*. 2008;121(1): 183–191
3. Muraro A, Dreborg S, Halken S, et al. Dietary prevention of allergic diseases in infants and small children. Part II. Evaluation of methods in allergy prevention studies and sensitization markers. Definitions and diagnostic criteria of allergic diseases. *Pediatr Allergy Immunol*. 2004;15(3): 196–205
4. American Academy of Pediatrics Committee on Nutrition. Food allergy. In: Kleinman RE, Greer FR, eds. *Pediatric Nutrition*. 7th ed. Elk Grove Village, IL: American Academy of Pediatrics; 2014: 845–862
5. American Academy of Pediatrics Committee on Nutrition. Complementary feeding. In: Kleinman RE, Greer FR, eds. *Pediatric Nutrition*. 7th ed. Elk Grove Village, IL: American Academy of Pediatrics; 2014: 123–140
6. Kramer MS, Kakuma R. Maternal dietary antigen avoidance during pregnancy or lactation, or both, for preventing or treating atopic disease in the child. *Evid Based Child Health*. 2014;9(2): 447–483
7. de Silva D, Geromi M, Halken S, et al; EAACI Food Allergy and Anaphylaxis Guidelines Group. Primary prevention of food allergy in children and adults: systematic review. *Allergy*. 2014;69(5): 581–589
8. Netting MJ, Middleton PF, Makrides M. Does maternal diet during pregnancy and lactation affect outcomes in offspring? A systematic review of food-based approaches. *Nutrition*. 2014; 30(11–12):1225–1241
9. Kramer MS, Kakuma R. Optimal duration of exclusive breastfeeding. *Cochrane Database Syst Rev*. 2012;(8): CD003517
10. Kajosaari M, Saarinen UM. Prophylaxis of atopic disease by six months' total solid food elimination. Evaluation of 135 exclusively breast-fed infants of atopic families. *Acta Paediatr Scand*. 1983; 72(3):411–414
11. Kramer MS, Matush L, Vanilovich I, et al; Promotion of Breastfeeding Intervention Trial (PROBIT) Study Group. Effect of prolonged and exclusive breast feeding on risk of allergy and asthma: cluster randomised trial. *BMJ*. 2007; 335(7624):815
12. Oddy WH, Holt PG, Sly PD, et al. Association between breast feeding and asthma in 6 year old children: findings of a prospective birth cohort study. *BMJ*. 1999;319(7213):815–819
13. Dogaru CM, Nyffenegger D, Pescatore AM, Spycher BD, Kuehni CE. Breastfeeding and childhood asthma: systematic review and meta-analysis. *Am J Epidemiol*. 2014;179(10): 1153–1167
14. Lodge CJ, Tan DJ, Lau MX, et al. Breastfeeding and asthma and allergies: a systematic review and meta-analysis. *Acta Paediatr*. 2015; 104(467):38–53
15. Brew BK, Allen CW, Toelle BG, Marks GB. Systematic review and meta-analysis investigating breast feeding and childhood wheezing illness. *Paediatr Perinat Epidemiol*. 2011;25(6):507–518
16. Yang YW, Tsai CL, Lu CY. Exclusive breastfeeding and incident atopic dermatitis in childhood: a systematic review and meta-analysis of prospective cohort studies. *Br J Dermatol*. 2009;161(2):373–383
17. Perkin MR, Logan K, Tseng A, et al; EAT Study Team. Randomized trial of introduction of allergenic foods in breast-fed infants. *N Engl J Med*. 2016; 374(18):1733–1743
18. Du Toit G, Roberts G, Sayre PH, et al; Learning Early About Peanut Allergy (LEAP) Study Team. Identifying infants at high risk of peanut allergy: the Learning Early About Peanut Allergy (LEAP) screening study. *J Allergy Clin Immunol*. 2013;131(1):135–143.e1–143.e12
19. Lowe AJ, Hosking CS, Bennett CM, et al. Effect of a partially hydrolyzed whey infant formula at weaning on risk of allergic disease in high-risk children: a randomized controlled trial. *J Allergy Clin Immunol*. 2011;128(2): 360–365.e4
20. Boyle RJ, Ierodiakonou D, Khan T, et al. Hydrolysed formula and risk of allergic or autoimmune disease: systematic review and meta-analysis. *BMJ*. 2016; 352:i974
21. Boyle RJ, Tang ML, Chiang WC, et al; PATCH study investigators. Prebiotic-supplemented partially hydrolysed cow's milk formula for the prevention of eczema in high-risk infants: a randomized controlled trial. *Allergy*. 2016;71(5):701–710
22. von Berg A, Filipiak-Pittroff B, Krämer U, et al; GINIplus study group. Allergies in high-risk schoolchildren after early intervention with cow's milk protein hydrolysates: 10-year results from the German Infant Nutritional Intervention (GINI) study. *J Allergy Clin Immunol*. 2013;131(6):1565–1573
23. Du Toit G, Roberts G, Sayre PH, et al; LEAP Study Team. Randomized trial of peanut consumption in infants at risk for peanut allergy [published correction appears in *N Engl J Med*. 2016;375(4):398]. *N Engl J Med*. 2015; 372(9):803–813
24. Natsume O, Kabashima S, Nakazato J, et al; PETIT Study Team. Two-step egg introduction for prevention of egg allergy in high-risk infants with eczema (PETIT): a randomised, double-blind, placebo-controlled trial. *Lancet*. 2017; 389(10066):276–286
25. Bellach J, Schwarz V, Ahrens B, et al. Randomized placebo-controlled trial of hen's egg consumption for primary prevention in infants. *J Allergy Clin Immunol*. 2017;139(5): 1591–1599.e2

26. Wei-Liang Tan J, Valerio C, Barnes EH, et al; Beating Egg Allergy Trial (BEAT) Study Group. A randomized trial of egg introduction from 4 months of age in infants at risk for egg allergy. *J Allergy Clin Immunol.* 2017;139(5):1621–1628.e8

27. Palmer DJ, Metcalfe J, Makrides M, et al. Early regular egg exposure in infants with eczema: a randomized controlled trial. *J Allergy Clin Immunol.* 2013;132(2):387–392.e1

28. Palmer DJ, Sullivan TR, Gold MS, Prescott SL, Makrides M. Randomized controlled trial of early regular egg intake to prevent egg allergy. *J Allergy Clin Immunol.* 2017;139(5):1600–1607.e2

29. Ierodiakonou D, Garcia-Larsen V, Logan A, et al. Timing of allergenic food introduction to the infant diet and risk of allergic or autoimmune disease: a systematic review and meta-analysis. *JAMA.* 2016;316(11):1181–1192

30. Du Toit G, Sayre PH, Roberts G, et al; Immune Tolerance Network LEAP-On Study Team. Effect of avoidance on peanut allergy after early peanut consumption. *N Engl J Med.* 2016; 374(15):1435–1443

31. Togias A, Cooper SF, Acebal ML, et al. Addendum guidelines for the prevention of peanut allergy in the United States: report of the National Institute of Allergy and Infectious Diseases-Sponsored Expert Panel. *J Allergy Clin Immunol.* 2017;139(1): 29–44

32. Greenhawt M. Early allergen introduction for preventing development of food allergy. *JAMA.* 2016;316(11):1157–1159

33. Oria MP, Stallings VA, eds; National Academies of Sciences, Engineering, and Medicine; Health and Medicine Division; Food and Nutrition Board; Committee on Food Allergies: Global Burden, Causes, Treatment, Prevention, and Public Policy. *Finding a Path to Safety in Food Allergy: Assessment of the Global Burden, Causes, Prevention, Management, and Public Policy.* Washington, DC: The National Academies Press; 2017

34. Australasian Society of Clinical Immunology and Allergy. ASCIA guidelines - infant feeding and allergy prevention. 2016. Available at: https://www.allergy.org.au/patients/allergy-prevention/ascia-guidelines-for-infant-feeding-and-allergy-prevention. Accessed June 11, 2018

35. Healthy Eating Research. Feeding guidelines for infants and young toddlers: a responsive parenting approach. Guidelines for health professionals. Appendix 7. Food allergy considerations for infants and toddlers. Available at: https://healthyeatingresearch.org/wp-content/uploads/2017/02/her_feeding_guidelines_report_021416-1.pdf. Accessed February 5, 2019

36. Fewtrell M, Bronsky J, Campoy C, et al. Complementary feeding: a position paper by the European Society for Paediatric Gastroenterology, Hepatology, and Nutrition (ESPGHAN) Committee on Nutrition. *J Pediatr Gastroenterol Nutr.* 2017;64(1): 119–132

37. Sicherer SH. New guidelines detail use of 'infant-safe' peanut to prevent allergy. *AAP News.* January 5, 2017. Available at: http://www.aappublications.org/news/2017/01/05/PeanutAllergy010517. Accessed February 5, 2019

Electronic Communication of the Health Record and Information With Pediatric Patients and Their Guardians

- *Policy Statement*

POLICY STATEMENT Organizational Principles to Guide and Define the Child Health Care System and/or Improve the Health of all Children

American Academy of Pediatrics

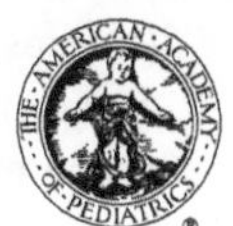

DEDICATED TO THE HEALTH OF ALL CHILDREN™

Electronic Communication of the Health Record and Information With Pediatric Patients and Their Guardians

Emily C. Webber, MD, FAAP, FAMIA,[a] David Brick, MD, FAAP,[b] James P. Scibilia, MD, FAAP,[c] Peter Dehnel, MD, FAAP,[d] COUNCIL ON CLINICAL INFORMATION TECHNOLOGY, COMMITTEE ON MEDICAL LIABILITY AND RISK MANAGEMENT, SECTION ON TELEHEALTH CARE

abstract

Communication of health data has evolved rapidly with the widespread adoption of electronic health records (EHRs) and communication technology. What used to be sent to patients via paper mail, fax, or e-mail may now be accessed by patients via their EHRs, and patients may also communicate securely with their medical team via certified technology. Although EHR technologies have great potential, their most effective applications and uses for communication between pediatric and adolescent patients, guardians, and medical teams has not been realized. There are wide variations in available technologies, guiding policies, and practices; some physicians and patients are successful in using certified tools but others are forced to limit their patients' access to e-health data and associated communication altogether. In general, pediatric and adolescent patients are less likely than adult patients to have electronic access and the ability to exchange health data. There are several reasons for these limitations, including inconsistent standards and recommendations regarding the recommended age for independent access, lack of routine EHR support for the ability to filter or proxy such access, and conflicting laws about patients' and physicians' rights to access EHRs and ability to communicate electronically. Effective, safe electronic exchange of health data requires active collaboration between physicians, patients, policy makers, and health information technology vendors. This policy statement addresses current best practices for these stakeholders and delineates the continued gaps and how to address them.

[a]Department of Pediatrics, School of Medicine, Indiana University and Riley Hospital for Children at Indiana University Health, Indianapolis, Indiana; [b]Department of Pediatrics, School of Medicine, New York University, New York, New York; [c]Heritage Valley Health System, Beaver, Pennsylvania; and [d]Abbott Northwestern Hospital and Children's Hospitals and Clinics of Minnesota, Minneapolis, Minnesota

Drs Webber and Brick participated in the initial concept and design, analysis, drafting, and revision of the manuscript. Drs Webber, Brick, Scibilia, and Dehnel all reviewed and revised the manuscript and approve it as submitted.

This document is copyrighted and is property of the American Academy of Pediatrics and its Board of Directors. All authors have filed conflict of interest statements with the American Academy of Pediatrics. Any conflicts have been resolved through a process approved by the Board of Directors. The American Academy of Pediatrics has neither solicited nor accepted any commercial involvement in the development of the content of this publication.

Policy statements from the American Academy of Pediatrics benefit from expertise and resources of liaisons and internal (AAP) and external reviewers. However, policy statements from the American Academy of Pediatrics may not reflect the views of the liaisons or the organizations or government agencies that they represent.

The guidance in this statement does not indicate an exclusive course of treatment or serve as a standard of medical care. Variations, taking into account individual circumstances, may be appropriate.

All policy statements from the American Academy of Pediatrics automatically expire 5 years after publication unless reaffirmed, revised, or retired at or before that time.

DOI: https://doi.org/10.1542/peds.2019-1359

To cite: Webber EC, Brick D, Scibilia JP, et al. AAP COUNCIL ON CLINICAL INFORMATION TECHNOLOGY, AAP COMMITTEE ON MEDICAL LIABILITY AND RISK MANAGEMENT, AAP SECTION ON TELEHEALTH CARE. Electronic Communication of the Health Record and Information With Pediatric Patients and Their Guardians. *Pediatrics.* 2019;144(1):e20191359

DEFINITIONS

In this document, the terms below are used with these definitions:

- Guardian: legal guardians, including parents, who have access to all or part of the child's medical record and/or patient portal.

- Health care team: includes physicians, nonphysician clinicians (nurses, pharmacists and others), and nonclinician personnel (eg, office managers, billing staff, etc).

BACKGROUND INFORMATION

The workflow, technologies, rules, and regulations regarding electronic communication of health data between health care teams and patients have evolved quickly over the last decade. As electronic health records (EHRs) have made medical data more rapidly accessible to patients and guardians, health care teams have struggled to sustain the traditional model of being the curator and guardian of a patient's health information.[1]

Although technology can facilitate more effective and timely care, it has been challenging to reach a consensus about the ideal uses of technology. Defining the most effective use requires aligning legislative policy, legal requirements, technology functionality, and clinical workflow and impact.[2,3] Although access to health data via electronic means is strongly recommended by professional medical organizations,[4–6] there has not been the accompanying change in legislative policy or practice to support consistent access, privacy, and electronic communication of clinical data in EHRs for patients (particularly for pediatric and adolescent patients). Health care teams, pediatric patients of all ages, and guardians need more guidance to effectively and safely use technology for electronic communication about health record information. In addition, successful adoption of existing guidance and future recommendations requires health care teams, policy makers, and EHR vendors to collaborate and optimize these technologies. This policy statement provides guidance for a broad audience; it includes recommendations for policy makers and EHR vendors on incorporating standards to improve electronic communication of health record information as well as health care teams for best use.

STATEMENT OF THE PROBLEM

Areas that present particular challenges for EHR communication include:

- Variable laws and regulations and rapidly changing non-EHR electronic communication;
- Variable definitions of a health record;
- Variable maturity of pediatric patients and guardianship roles as well as age of the majority;
- Limited pediatric functionality capabilities of EHRs and other health information technology (HIT)[5]; and
- Privacy and confidentiality needs of adolescent patients.

Variable Laws and Regulations and Rapidly Changing Non-EHR Electronic Communication

Most regulations regarding the communication of health record data have been focused on the requirements for "meaningful use," the federal regulations closely associated with use of a certified EHR and the Health Information Technology for Economic and Clinical Health Act in early 2009, which is now part of the Merit-Based Incentive Payment System. The operational requirements include the ability to exchange information with patients using a patient portal.[7] However, in addition to meaningful use, there is a broad range of federal and state rules, laws, statutes, and regulations that reference electronic communication of health record information between patients and guardians and health care teams,[8] particularly for adolescent patients.[9] These regulations can make it challenging to determine what practices are compliant and can result in restrictive policies for institutions and systems.

Although meaningful use regulations have stimulated the implementation of EHRs and patient portals, the regulations do not make recommendations regarding the best use of other modes of electronic communication of health record data, such as text messages and mobile applications, outside of portals attached to EHRs. This policy addresses electronic communication of the health record between health care teams and pediatric patients and their guardians.

Telehealth services are generally included in this non-EHR category. Telehealth has been expanded in definition by the federal government to include "the use of telecommunications and information technology to provide access to health assessment, diagnosis, intervention, consultation, supervision and information across distance."[10] The broad definition expands the notion of the health record to multiple access points and multiple new technologies, all of which require security, confidentiality, and accuracy. A summary of state definitions of telehealth can be found on the Web site of the Center for Connected Health Policy (https://www.cchpca.org/telehealth-policy/current-state-laws-and-reimbursement-policies).

The recommendations in this policy statement pertain to electronic communications not currently included in the telehealth summary, which are addressed in separate AAP policy statements.[11,12] Telehealth pertains to the delivery of health care; this policy speaks to electronic communication of the health record. Health care teams and patients communicating electronically to this point have not had widespread standards with regard to the technology they use.

Variable Definitions of a Health Record

The definition of what constitutes the "legal health record" may be brought into question when responding to requests for information, which is a form of communication. The American Health Information Management Association defines the legal health record as "the documentation of healthcare services provided to an individual during any aspect of healthcare delivery in any type of healthcare organization."[13]

In the United States, EHRs are certified on the basis of requirements for meaningful use. Although widely accepted, meaningful use legislation and regulations are not comprehensive in defining the components of EHRs deemed necessary by clinicians and their patients to promote clinical care. Communication, especially electronic communication by different members of the medical team, is 1 of those necessary features not yet clearly delineated. For example, if a physician, nurse, or other medical team member calls a patient's guardian or patient to share normal laboratory results, there are no widely accepted standards for whether and how the physician and medical team should capture this communication in the EHR. Similarly, if a radiology image is shared with the patient or guardian through the patient portal, there is no clear guidance as to whether the text of the report should be recorded in a note or if the image itself should be retained (because it may be stored in another system).

Variable Maturity and Guardianship of Pediatric Patients

As they mature, adolescents develop maturity and an increasing capacity to manage their own communications and health data over time. Accordingly, there need to be different types of communication of health record information supported by different types of technology for different levels of autonomy and maturity.

Sharing health information is part of teaching and empowering children and their guardians to assume responsibility for managing their illnesses and promoting their own health and occurs as a result of discussion between the patient, guardian, and physician. Children develop the ability to process information as they mature, and although general guidelines exist to predict readiness,[14] there are necessary exceptions and adaptions for individuals. This need to assess and support variable levels of autonomy existed before EHRs and electronic communication; however, EHR use has highlighted both the wide variation in patient capacity and readiness and the lack of granular functionality in EHRs to support best practices.

Pediatric patients may have individuals who serve as guardians who are not their parents. The rights to receive communications about care may also be different from the rights to authorize care.[15] The ability of technology to support different communications to multiple guardians of pediatric patients and the associated workflows involved in their validation are often limited.

Limited Ability of EHRs and Other HIT To Segment Information Access

Physicians and other clinical team members in clinical practice are able to both identify and control how to manage disclosure of information usually deemed "sensitive" (including but not limited to sexual health, mental health, and social history). This clinical practice pertains to patients of all ages but handling of sensitive information is particularly challenging for pediatric and adolescent patients and their guardians when sharing clinical information electronically.

There is no widely accepted or easily implemented set of standards defining exactly what data (documentation, clinical results, or other data) should be categorized consistently as sensitive information in the medical record.[16] For example, medications for sexually transmitted diseases or mental health may be appropriate for 1 patient and his or her guardian to share, but for another patient, that information would need to be segmented (filtered) to maintain privacy.

EHRs do not yet provide widely available features to allow for granular filtering by the physician and clinical team or the patient to preserve confidentiality in these nuanced and complex situations. There is also not a consistent, widely available way for pediatric and adolescent patients to control the content and method by which they share their EHR data.

These limitations have left many physicians and clinical team members with a "first, do no harm" approach to providing access to EHRs using the provided portal and access tools, leading to either extensive customization of the EHRs when being used for pediatric populations or exclusion of pediatric and adolescent patients from electronic access to their records.[17] Many EHRs have an all-or-nothing privacy and confidentiality approach that is typically used by EHRs for communicating health data such as demographics, problems, medications, and other data (eg, laboratory results, radiology results, and progress notes) and do not support the granular filtering needed to provide the types of protection needed by patients; this is especially true in the special case of pediatric records.[18]

Privacy and Confidentiality Needs of Adolescent Patients

Adolescent privacy and/or confidentiality is a special case of the limited segmenting of functionality capabilities in EHRs that is compounded by variations in state laws regarding adolescent health records. Health care teams may experience difficulty complying with state requirements and professional recommendations for adolescent privacy because of federal rules for disclosure. For example, 1 portion of care may be protected by law as confidential for which the patient consents independently, but other aspects of care may not be protected, turning a simple routine visit into a potential series of confidentiality challenges. As a result, meeting the requirements of broad federal mandates regarding the sharing of health data with patients is difficult to achieve. This challenge results in fewer pediatric patients enrolling in portals, thereby depriving of them of access to their own records. Adolescent access to their EHRs has been recommended by both the AAP and the Society of Adolescent Health and Medicine.[6,10]

All states have laws allowing minors to access medical care for certain types of medical conditions without consent of a guardian and with some expectation of privacy, although laws vary significantly by state.[19] EHR system access and data sharing can be multidirectional and used in a variety of ways, making it more challenging for the clinical teams as well as EHR vendors to maintain the privacy necessary to support confidentiality. Failure to maintain the confidentiality of this information can lead to fines or adverse licensure action against individual physician licenses. This may also result in civil litigation against health care teams and systems.[20–22]

As previously mentioned, managing and protecting sensitive clinical data is 1 challenge. Disclosure of other data, such as private health information through claims data and details of billing systems, can be automated in some EHRs and sent to guardians, which is another way in which confidentiality may be compromised. For example, testing for *Chlamydia* or other sexually transmitted infections may be noted on an itemized explanation of benefits. Sustaining an adolescent's privacy in this situation places additional burdens on the health care team.

The AAP policy statement "Standards for Health Information Technology to Ensure Adolescent Privacy"[6] contains recommended standards for EHR vendors, including the ability to filter data as previously mentioned, but most EHRs do not support these recommendations in a manner that is easy to adapt.[18] The Guttmacher Institute summarizes state laws aimed at remedying this problem in its report "Protecting confidentiality for individuals insured as dependents."[23] The problem is compounded when health record information is sent from EHRs to health information exchanges, as mandated by federal law, but a certified EHR does not routinely segment (ie, allow for filtering) confidential data to support adolescent privacy without completely blocking access to the entire record. This challenge results in fewer pediatric patients enrolling in portals, thereby depriving of them of the access recommended by multiple medical societies.[17]

CONCLUSIONS

It is important for physician-patient relationships to have clear expectations and safeguards for patients, guardians, and health care teams in electronic communication of health record information. Much of the published literature regarding this sharing pertains to adult patients leveraging patient portals, so there is little specification as to how shared access (eg, a "proxy" or "surrogate" relationship) of a guardian to a child's EHR is most effectively and appropriately established and governed unless using custom tools. The sharing of the clinical data in the EHR depends on the complex relationships that are rife with the variations previously detailed.

These factors have led to several examples of extensive customization of vendor EHRs and "homegrown" solutions that are difficult to scale outside of the hospital or system in which they were developed. Even with customization, EHRs may not comport with relevant federal and state laws, statutes, and regulations governing confidentiality. For example, the HIPAA Privacy Rule allows covered health care health care teams to communicate electronically, such as through e-mail, with their patients provided they apply reasonable safeguards when doing so; however, institutional policy makers and health care teams are left to determine those safeguards. Most health care teams are currently trying to adapt patient portals and other technologies designed for independent adults to children with diverse living situations, developing and changing levels of autonomy, and complex confidentiality needs.

The recommendations that follow are intended to address the challenges and pitfalls of using EHR and non-EHR electronic communication with patients and guardians regarding the child's or adolescent's health record.

RECOMMENDATIONS

These recommendations are suited for health care teams and health systems using electronic communication with their patients and guardians regarding a child's health record. Collaboration between health care teams, policy makers, and EHR and/or HIT developers is critical to implementation of the following recommendations.

Recommendations for Physicians and Health Care Teams

1. Health care teams should use secure platforms that protect communications with patients and guardians. Electronic communication of health record information should be incorporated directly into the standard EHR, making use of secured and certified technology

such as embedded secure messaging and portals to share clinical information and capture communication whenever appropriate.

2. Health care teams should provide a clear understanding of the limitations of electronic communication of health record information to guardians. Electronic communication should not be used in isolation to communicate or provide medical care unless there is confirmation of receipt and comprehension of the information (ie, "closed-loop communication"). For example, discussing changes in therapy or providing test results or a diagnosis may be more efficiently and safely accomplished in face-to-face or verbal communication because those methods provide a way to ask clarifying questions in real time. Electronic communication can provide appropriate support for many patients to seek guidance, ask questions, and provide feedback but may be asynchronous or more limited than face-to-face communication. Although electronic communication allows patients to receive and access their information differently, health care teams should continue clinical practices that best support patient care, including in-person counseling and assessments.
3. Health care teams should be aware of the risks of unsecured communication and take steps to minimize the risk to patients. EHR technology certified by the Office of the National Coordinator adheres to a consistent measure of security. EHR technology may be used for electronic communication as long as:
    - Adequate technology exists to allow adolescent patients privacy around protected laboratory results, diagnosis, medications, and other clinical data; and
    - There is adequate understanding for use of the electronic communication between the patient, the guardian, the physician, and the health care team.
4. Health care teams and patients using electronic communication that is not HIPAA compliant should be aware that this technology may not be secure. All parties should be aware of these security risks and use the appropriate technology to support their communication. Technology that is not HIPAA compliant may not be secure and exposes the physician and patient to the risk of breach of protected health information.

Recommendations for Institutional Policy Makers and Health Care Organizations

5. Institutional policies and practices for electronic communications should support clear expectations between medical teams and patients. Because EHRs and other technology can make health data directly available and accessible to the patient and/or guardian without the physician or medical team as the intermediary, clear expectations about what information should be shared with which users are needed to provide context and support for patients. Policies that support the development of skills in counseling and use for health care teams and staff are needed. As new technology tools become available, communication between patients and health care teams will evolve and, therefore, policies must evolve with them.
6. Institutional policy should include a communication agreement between health care teams and patients and/or guardians to support safe and effective electronic communication of health record information. This agreement could reflect but is not limited to the following aspects:
    - The consent of the patient and/or guardian to receive electronic communication and, when mandated by law, the guardian's consent for the minor patient to have electronic communication between physician and patient.
    - Respect for patients' privacy as well as their right to access their health information under the law while acknowledging the unique and changing needs of patients as they mature.
    - Expectations for both parties regarding the content of electronic communication, including appropriate requests and the timeliness of responses.
    - Circumstances appropriate for the use of unencrypted electronic communications such as unencrypted e-mails. For example, a reminder to get an influenza vaccination should not contain protected health information and does not necessarily require a private, secure electronic means of delivery. However, conveying specific results, such as laboratory or radiology tests, might require encryption.
7. Professional organizations and health institutions should have systems to ensure health care teams are aware of state and federal requirements and to assist them in complying with standards, rules, and regulations. These actions may include the following:
    - Establishing systems that promote patient and guardian awareness of the risks, benefits, and limitations of electronic communications.
    - Aligning consent for electronic communication with the general consent for care when possible.

- Defining standards for when a patient may confidentially and reliably communicate electronically directly with his or her physician. This standard should be applicable to any patient for whom guardianship is a consideration, regardless of the patient's age. In the absence of specific regulations, it is reasonable for the clinician, using their clinical assessment and judgement in collaboration with the patient and family, to determine when a patient has the ability, cognitive skills, and maturity needed to safely and effectively use independent electronic communication so that the clinician may provide appropriate expectations and support.

Recommendations for Federal Policy Makers and Health Information Technology Developers

8. Standard EHR functionality should include the capacity for health care teams and patients to segment or filter clinical data that can compromise confidentiality. Although this filtering ability contains risks because it allows for an incomplete record to be shared or viewed, it is necessary to uphold the dual requirements of patient privacy as well as patient access when access is shared. This filtering may be needed for any patients who are accessing or sharing their electronic communication but is especially needed for pediatric and adolescent patients establishing independent communication and decision-making with their medical teams.
9. EHR vendors should enable safeguards for medical teams to restrict electronic communication in cases of acute patient safety risk (eg, when guardianship of a patient changes because of risk to patient safety such as in cases of child abuse and neglect).

LEAD AUTHORS

Emily C. Webber, MD, FAAP
David Brick, MD, FAAP
James P. Scibilia, MD, FAAP
Peter Dehnel, MD, FAAP

COUNCIL ON CLINICAL INFORMATION TECHNOLOGY EXECUTIVE COMMITTEE, 2016–2017

Stuart T. Weinberg, MD, FAAP
Emily C. Webber, MD, FAAP
Gregg M. Alexander, DO
Eric L. Beyer, MD, FAAP
Alexander M. Hamling, MD, FAAP
Eric S. Kirkendall, MD, MBI, FAAP
Donald E. Lighter, MD, MBA, FAAP
Ann M. Mann, MD, FAAP
Stephen J. Morgan, MD, FAAP
Eric Shelov, MD, FAAP
Jeffrey A. Wright, MD, FAAP

LIAISONS

Dale C. Alverson, MD, FAAP (Section on Telehealth Care)
Francis D. Chan, MD, FAAP (Section on Advances in Therapeutics and Technology)
Melissa S. Van Cain, MD (Section on Pediatric Trainees)

STAFF

Lisa A. Krams, MAHS

COMMITTEE ON MEDICAL LIABILITY AND RISK MANAGEMENT, 2016–2017

Robin L. Altman, MD, FAAP
Steven A. Bondi, JD, MD, FAAP
Jonathan M. Fanaroff, MD, JD, FCLM, FAAP
Sandeep K. Narang, MD, JD, FAAP
Richard L. Oken, MD, FAAP
John W. Rusher, MD, JD, FAAP
Karen A. Santucci, MD, FAAP
James P. Scibilia, MD, FAAP
Susan M. Scott, MD, JD, FAAP

STAFF

Julie Kersten Ake

SECTION ON TELEHEALTH CARE EXECUTIVE COMMITTEE, 2017–2018

Joshua J. Alexander, MD, FAAP (chairperson)
Chelsea E.F. Bodnar, MD, FAAP
Alison Curfman, MD, FAAP
Neil E. Herendeen, MD, MS, FAAP
Joseph A. Kahn, MD, FAAP
Steven D. McSwain, MD, FAAP

LIAISON

Kelli M. Garber, PPCNP-BC

STAFF

Trisha M. Calabrese, MPH

ABBREVIATIONS

EHR: e-health record
HIPAA: Health Insurance Portability and Accountability Act
HIT: health information technology

Address correspondence to Emily C. Webber, MD, FAAP. E-mail: ewebber@iuhealth.org

PEDIATRICS (ISSN Numbers: Print, 0031-4005; Online, 1098-4275).

Copyright © 2019 by the American Academy of Pediatrics

FINANCIAL DISCLOSURE: The authors have indicated they have no financial relationships relevant to this article to disclose.

FUNDING: No external funding.

POTENTIAL CONFLICT OF INTEREST: The authors have indicated they have no potential conflicts of interest to disclose.

REFERENCES

1. Roscam Abbing HD. Medical confidentiality and electronic patient files. *Med Law.* 2000;19(1):107–112
2. Kruse CS, Bolton K, Freriks G. The effect of patient portals on quality outcomes and its implications to meaningful use: a systematic review. *J Med Internet Res.* 2015;17(2):e44
3. de Lusignan S, Mold F, Sheikh A, et al. Patients' online access to their electronic health records and linked online services: a systematic interpretative review. *BMJ Open.* 2014; 4(9):e006021
4. Thompson LA, Martinko T, Budd P, Mercado R, Schentrup AM. Meaningful use of a confidential adolescent patient portal. *J Adolesc Health.* 2016;58(2): 134–140
5. Lehmann CU; Council on Clinical Information Technology. Pediatric aspects of inpatient health information technology systems. *Pediatrics.* 2015; 135(3). Available at: www.pediatrics.org/cgi/content/full/135/3/e756
6. Committee on Adolescence; Council on Clinical and Information Technology, Blythe MJ, Del Beccaro MA. Standards for health information technology to ensure adolescent privacy. *Pediatrics.* 2012;130(5):987–990
7. HealthIT.gov. Meaningful use. Available at: https://www.healthit.gov/topic/meaningful-use-and-macra/meaningful-use. Accessed April 18, 2018
8. Anoshiravani A, Gaskin GL, Groshek MR, Kuelbs C, Longhurst CA. Special requirements for electronic medical records in adolescent medicine. *J Adolesc Health.* 2012;51(5):409–414
9. Society for Adolescent Health and Medicine, Gray SH, Pasternak RH, Gooding HC, et al. Recommendations for electronic health record use for delivery of adolescent health care. *J Adolesc Health.* 2014;54(4):487–490
10. Center for Connected Health Policy. About telehealth. Available at: https://www.cchpca.org/about/about-telehealth. Accessed April 18, 2018
11. Burke BL Jr, Hall RW; Section on Telehealth Care. Telemedicine: pediatric applications. *Pediatrics.* 2015;136(1). Available at: www.pediatrics.org/cgi/content/full/136/1/e293
12. Committee on Pediatric Workforce, Marcin JP, Rimsza ME, Moskowitz WB. The use of telemedicine to address access and physician workforce shortages. *Pediatrics.* 2015;136(1): 202–209
13. American Health Information Management Association. Fundamentals of the legal health record and designated record set. Available at: http://library.ahima.org/doc?oid=104008#.WLSV_G8rLX4. Accessed April 18, 2018
14. Weithorn LA, Campbell SB. The competency of children and adolescents to make informed treatment decisions. *Child Dev.* 1982; 53(6):1589–1598
15. Cohen GJ, Weitzman CC; Committee on Psychosocial Aspects of Child and Family Health; Section on Developmental and Behavioral Pediatrics. Helping children and families deal with divorce and separation. *Pediatrics.* 2016;138(6): e20163020
16. Bourgeois FC, Nigrin DJ, Harper MB. Preserving patient privacy and confidentiality in the era of personal health records. *Pediatrics.* 2015;135(5). Available at: www.pediatrics.org/cgi/content/full/135/5/e1125
17. Temple MW, Sisk B, Krams LA, Schneider JH, Kirkendall ES, Lehmann CU. Trends in use of electronic health records in pediatric office settings. *J Pediatr.* 2019; 206:134-171.e2
18. Sharko M, Wilcox L, Hong MK, Ancker JS. Variability in adolescent portal privacy features: how the unique privacy needs of the adolescent patient create a complex decision-making process. *J Am Med Inform Assoc.* 2018;25(8): 1008–1017
19. Guttmacher Institute. An overview of consent to reproductive health services by young people. Available at: https://www.guttmacher.org/state-policy/explore/overview-minors-consent-law. Accessed April 18, 2018
20. US Department of Health & Human Services. Health Insurance Portability and Accountability Act Enforcement Rule, 45 CFR §160(c–e) (2013)
21. *Byrne v Avery Center for Obstetrics and Gynecology,* No. 18904, 2014 WL 5507439 (Conn 2014)
22. *R.K. v St. Mary's Medical Center,* 735 S.E.2d 715 (WVa 2012)
23. Guttmacher Institute. Protecting confidentiality for individuals insured as dependents. Available at: https://www.guttmacher.org/print/state-policy/explore/protecting-confidentiality-individuals-insured-dependents. Accessed April 18, 2018

Emergency Contraception

- *Policy Statement*

POLICY STATEMENT Organizational Principles to Guide and Define the Child Health Care System and/or Improve the Health of all Children

American Academy of Pediatrics

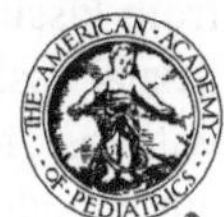

DEDICATED TO THE HEALTH OF ALL CHILDREN™

Emergency Contraception

Krishna K. Upadhya, MD, MPH, FAAP, COMMITTEE ON ADOLESCENCE

abstract

Despite significant declines over the past 2 decades, the United States continues to experience birth rates among teenagers that are significantly higher than other high-income nations. Use of emergency contraception (EC) within 120 hours after unprotected or underprotected intercourse can reduce the risk of pregnancy. Emergency contraceptive methods include oral medications labeled and dedicated for use as EC by the US Food and Drug Administration (ulipristal and levonorgestrel), the "off-label" use of combined oral contraceptives, and insertion of a copper intrauterine device. Indications for the use of EC include intercourse without use of contraception; condom breakage or slippage; missed or late doses of contraceptives, including the oral contraceptive pill, contraceptive patch, contraceptive ring, and injectable contraception; vomiting after use of oral contraceptives; and sexual assault. Our aim in this updated policy statement is to (1) educate pediatricians and other physicians on available emergency contraceptive methods; (2) provide current data on the safety, efficacy, and use of EC in teenagers; and (3) encourage routine counseling and advance EC prescription as 1 public health strategy to reduce teenaged pregnancy.

Children's National Health System, Washington, District of Columbia

Policy statements from the American Academy of Pediatrics benefit from expertise and resources of liaisons and internal (AAP) and external reviewers. However, policy statements from the American Academy of Pediatrics may not reflect the views of the liaisons or the organizations or government agencies that they represent.

Dr Upadhya was responsible for all aspects of revising and writing the policy statement with input from reviewers and the Board of Directors; she approves the final manuscript as submitted.

The guidance in this statement does not indicate an exclusive course of treatment or serve as a standard of medical care. Variations, taking into account individual circumstances, may be appropriate.

All policy statements from the American Academy of Pediatrics automatically expire 5 years after publication unless reaffirmed, revised, or retired at or before that time.

This document is copyrighted and is property of the American Academy of Pediatrics and its Board of Directors. All authors have filed conflict of interest statements with the American Academy of Pediatrics. Any conflicts have been resolved through a process approved by the Board of Directors. The American Academy of Pediatrics has neither solicited nor accepted any commercial involvement in the development of the content of this publication.

DOI: https://doi.org/10.1542/peds.2019-3149

Address correspondence to Krishna K. Upadhya, MD, MPH, FAAP. E-mail: kupadhya@childrensnational.org

PEDIATRICS (ISSN Numbers: Print, 0031-4005; Online, 1098-4275).

Copyright © 2019 by the American Academy of Pediatrics

FINANCIAL DISCLOSURE: The author has indicated she has no financial relationships relevant to this article to disclose.

FUNDING: No external funding.

POTENTIAL CONFLICT OF INTEREST: The author has indicated she has no potential conflicts of interest to disclose.

To cite: Upadhya KK, AAP COMMITTEE ON ADOLESCENCE. Emergency Contraception. *Pediatrics.* 2019;144(6): e20193149

BACKGROUND INFORMATION

Emergency contraception (EC) refers to methods of contraception that are used after sexual intercourse to reduce the risk of pregnancy. Methods currently available in the United States are (1) ulipristal acetate (UPA), an oral progesterone receptor agonist-antagonist; (2) levonorgestrel (LNG), an oral progestin; (3) the copper intrauterine device (Cu-IUD); and (4) off-label use of combined oral contraceptives (Yuzpe method). EC can reduce the risk of pregnancy if used up to 120 hours after unprotected intercourse, and hormonal emergency contraceptive pills (ECPs) are more likely to be effective the sooner they are used.[1] Use of EC after unprotected or underprotected intercourse remains an important strategy to reduce unintended pregnancies among adolescents and women.

By the age of 19 years, approximately two-thirds of youth will have initiated sexual intercourse.[2] Most teenagers report first intercourse with a steady partner and consensual sex.[3] Approximately 11% of US high school students report experiencing a forced sexual experience ranging from kissing to forced intercourse.[4] Sexual assault is 1 factor associated with risk for unintended pregnancy among adolescents.[5] Youth with developmental and other disabilities may be at even higher risk of experiencing sexual abuse or assault than their peers are.[6,7] Improved use of contraception, not declines in sexual activity, has been the most significant contributor to the decline in pregnancy risk among US teenagers over the past decade.[8] Pediatricians have an important role to play in enabling adolescent access to all available contraceptive methods to address the Healthy People 2020 objective of continuing to reduce adolescent pregnancy in the United States.[9]

The most commonly used methods of contraception reported by teenagers who have had intercourse in the United States are the condom, followed by withdrawal, the oral contraceptive pill, and ECPs.[2] Condoms are important for protection against sexually transmitted infections (STIs) as well as pregnancy, and the oral contraceptive pill can be an effective method for pregnancy prevention; however, both methods require strict adherence by the user to be maximally effective. Withdrawal is not recommended because of its relatively low effectiveness for pregnancy prevention and because it provides no protection against STIs. Although the American Academy of Pediatrics (AAP) and other medical organizations recommend the use of intrauterine devices (IUDs) and implants as the most effective methods for adolescents,[10,11] rates of use of these methods remain low. The most recent analysis from the Centers for Disease Control and Prevention (CDC) indicates that only 3% of 15- to 19-year-olds who have ever had sex have used an IUD, and 3% report ever having used an implant.[12]

EC is the only contraceptive method designed to prevent pregnancy after intercourse. Indications for the use of EC include intercourse without use of contraception; condom breakage or slippage; missed or late doses of contraceptives, including the oral contraceptive pill, contraceptive patch, contraceptive ring, and injectable contraception; vomiting after use of oral contraceptive pills, and sexual assault. ECPs include products labeled and approved by the US Food and Drug Administration (FDA) for use as EC (levonorgestrel and UPA) and the off-label use of combination oral contraceptives (the Yuzpe method) that have been described in the literature since 1974.[13] Insertion of a Cu-IUD within 5 days of unprotected intercourse is an additional method of EC available in the United States. Insertion of a Cu-IUD is the most effective method of EC and has the extra benefit of providing ongoing contraception when left in place.[1]

Studies have shown that adolescents are more likely to use ECPs when they have been supplied or prescribed in advance of need.[14] As of August 2013, levonorgestrel EC is approved for over-the-counter sale throughout the United States to people of all ages[15]; however, barriers to access include cost and availability in pharmacies.[16] Surveys suggest that most practicing pediatricians and pediatric residents do not routinely counsel patients about EC and do not prescribe it.[17–21] This policy statement provides updated guidance on all methods of EC available to US adolescents (Table 1) and ongoing policy and access issues.

EC METHODS

EC Pills

UPA Progesterone Agonist-Antagonist

In August 2010, the FDA approved a progesterone agonist-antagonist, UPA, for use as an EC.[22] UPA binds to the human progesterone receptor, thereby preventing the binding of progesterone, and inhibits ovulation. Ulipristal, sold under the brand name ella (Watson, Morristown, NJ), is a single pill containing 30 mg of UPA and is indicated for use up to 120 hours after unprotected intercourse. It is important for patients to be counseled that onset of menses after UPA use may be later than expected and a pregnancy test is indicated if the patient does not have a period within 3 weeks. UPA is currently available by prescription only, regardless of age, and many pharmacies do not have it in stock.

Progestin-Only Pills

Levonorgestrel EC was approved by the FDA in 1999 under the brand name Plan B and is currently marketed under several names, including Plan B One Step (Teva Women's Health, Woodcliff Lake, NJ), Take Action (Teva Women's Health), Next Choice One Dose (Actavis Pharma, Inc, Parsippany, NJ), and My Way (Gavis Pharmaceuticals, Somerset, NJ). Although levonorgestrel EC originally consisted of 2 pills, current regimens are packaged as a single pill with 1.5 mg of levonorgestrel. Package labeling indicates that levonorgestrel EC should be taken within 72 hours of unprotected intercourse; however, data support that use up to 120 hours after intercourse may prevent pregnancy.[23,24] Adolescents should be instructed to take 1.5 mg of levonorgestrel as soon as possible and up to 120 hours after unprotected intercourse. Adolescents should be aware that the medicine is less likely to be effective when taken at 120 hours when compared with immediate use. No physical examination or pregnancy testing is required before use. Adolescents are advised to test for pregnancy (at home or in a clinic) if they do not have a period within 3 weeks of EC use. It is important for patients to know that levonorgestrel use may cause the next period to come sooner

TABLE 1 Selected Regimens for EC Available in the United States

Brand	First Dose	Second Dose, 12 h Later	Ethinyl Estradiol per Dose, µg	Levonorgestrel per Dose, mg
Progestin-only pills				
Next Choice or Plan B	2 pills	None	0	1.5
Plan B One Step	1 pill	None	0	1.5
Ovrette	20 pills	20 pills	0	0.75
Other ECP: ella	30 mg of UPA	—	—	—
IUD: Paragard	Insert within 120 h of unprotected intercourse	Insert within 120 h of unprotected intercourse	NA	NA
Combined estrogen and progestin pills				
Ovral	2 white pills	2 white pills	100	0.5
Levora	4 white pills	4 white pills	120	0.6
Nordette	4 light-orange pills	4 light-orange pills	120	0.6
Seasonale	4 pink pills	4 pink pills	120	0.6
Triphasil	4 yellow pills	4 yellow pills	120	0.5
Alesse	5 pink pills	5 pink pills	120	0.5

Additional combinations are available at https://ec.princeton.edu/questions/dose.html#dose. NA, not applicable.

than expected.[1] Because use of ECPs may result in a delay in ovulation, it is imperative to counsel patients to abstain from intercourse or use condoms for pregnancy prevention until the next menses.

Combined Hormonal Regimens (Yuzpe Method)

The use of combination oral contraceptives for EC is commonly referred to as the Yuzpe method.[13] Used since 1974, its acceptability and efficacy were limited by adverse effects of nausea and vomiting. The Yuzpe method involves taking 2 doses of pills 12 hours apart, each containing a minimum of 100 µg of ethinyl estradiol and a minimum of 500 µg of levonorgestrel. Other pill formulations used for EC are included in Table 1. Similar information is available from the Office of Population Research at Princeton University, which maintains a comprehensive source of information on EC (http://ec.princeton.edu/). The availability of many combination oral contraceptives with norgestrel or levonorgestrel makes this alternative particularly helpful when there is no or limited access to an EC product. Although combination oral contraceptives have not been labeled specifically for EC, the CDC "Selected Practice Recommendations for Contraceptive Use" and professional organizations such as the American College of Obstetricians and Gynecologists acknowledge the use of combination oral contraceptives as safe and effective for EC.[25,26]

IUD

Studies have established that the insertion of a Cu-IUD within 5 days of unprotected or underprotected intercourse is the most effective method of EC.[27–29] It must be inserted by a trained provider. In comparison with ECPs, the effectiveness of the Cu-IUD for EC results from the copper component and is not believed to vary by time of insertion within 120 hours of unprotected or underprotected sex.

The mechanisms of action of hormonal IUDs differ from those of the Cu-IUD, and hormonal IUDs have not been approved for use as EC. One published study found that women presenting for EC who desired an IUD for contraception could be offered levonorgestrel ECPs and also have a hormonal IUD placed at the same visit for ongoing contraception.[30]

COMPARATIVE EFFECTIVENESS OF ECPS

The effectiveness of oral EC depends on inhibiting ovulation and is affected by the timing of use within the menstrual cycle. A recently published meta-analysis of ECP trial data compared the effectiveness of EC methods. Pooled data from trials suggest that UPA resulted in fewer pregnancies than levonorgestrel did (relative risk, 0.59; 95% confidence interval, 0.35–0.99; 2 randomized controlled trials, n = 3448; I^2 = 0%; high-quality evidence).[1] Levonorgestrel also resulted in fewer pregnancies than the Yuzpe method did (relative risk, 0.57; 95% confidence interval, 0.39–0.84; 6 randomized controlled trials, n = 4750; I^2 = 23%; high-quality evidence).[1] It should be noted, however, that current CDC guidance does not indicate a preference for UPA over levonorgestrel regimens.

Two secondary analyses of ECP trial data identified that repeat unprotected intercourse in the same cycle was associated with EC failure.[31,32] The delay of ovulation from ECPs highlights the need for abstinence or contraception after ECP use.

EFFECT OF BMI ON EFFECTIVENESS OF ALL METHODS

Efficacy of the Cu-IUD is not affected by body weight. CDC recommendations indicate that young women in need of EC who do not wish to use a Cu-IUD or who do not have access to IUD insertion should be offered ECPs regardless of their weight.

Although no clinical trials have specifically evaluated the impact of BMI on the effectiveness of oral EC, meta-analyses have suggested that both levonorgestrel and UPA may be less effective in adolescents and women who are overweight.[31–33] In response to these data and labeling changes to EC products in Europe, the FDA conducted its own review of the evidence and issued a statement in 2016 indicating that the data regarding BMI and the effectiveness of levonorgestrel EC are conflicting and made no labeling changes. The FDA stated that there are no safety concerns with the use of levonorgestrel EC in women with BMI greater than 25 or with body weight greater than 165 pounds and that the most important factor affecting the medication's effectiveness is how quickly it is taken after unprotected or underprotected intercourse.[34]

ADVERSE EFFECTS AND CONTRAINDICATIONS

The only contraindication for use of EC is known pregnancy. According to the CDC Medical Eligibility Criteria for Contraceptive Use, pregnancy is an absolute contraindication for insertion of a Cu-IUD (category 4).[35] ECPs are not indicated for use in patients with documented or suspected pregnancy; however, according to CDC Medical Eligibility Criteria, no harms to the woman, pregnancy, or fetus of inadvertent ECP use during pregnancy are known to exist.[35] Use of ECPs will not disrupt a pregnancy that is implanted in the uterus, and ECPs are not abortifacients. Years of use of hormonal contraceptives indicate that there is no risk of teratogenicity from use of levonorgestrel EC or the Yuzpe method. There have also been no reports of fetal malformations after the use of UPA. Finally, repeat use of ECPs should prompt discussion of more effective, ongoing contraception, but there is no specific limit on repeated use, including within the same cycle. As noted below, however, the use of hormonal contraceptives within 5 days of UPA may reduce the effectiveness of UPA.

Ulipristal

The most common adverse effects reported by users of UPA include headache (18%), nausea (12%), and abdominal pain (12%).[36] It is recommended to redose UPA if vomiting occurs within 3 hours of the initial dose. For clinicians who are providing this medication in a setting where the patient is discharged before 3 hours after the dose and without an ongoing relationship with the patient (ie, emergency departments or urgent care), it may be important to discuss provisions for repeat dosing with patients if indicated.

Levonorgestrel-Only Methods

The most common adverse effect reported after use of levonorgestrel EC is heavier menstrual bleeding; spotting may also be reported.[37] The rate of nausea and vomiting with levonorgestrel EC is approximately half that with the Yuzpe method, and the routine use of antiemetics is not indicated. If vomiting does occur within 3 hours of use, the dose should be taken again. Repeated use of levonorgestrel EC is associated with the same adverse effects as 1-time use. A Cochrane Review of the subject found no serious adverse effects in trials of repeated use.[38]

Yuzpe and Estrogen-Containing Methods

The most common adverse effects that occur during the first 24 to 48 hours of using estrogen-containing EC methods are nausea (~50%) and vomiting (~20%), which seem to be unaffected by food intake.[39–41] The severity and incidence of nausea and vomiting can be decreased significantly by using an antiemetic 1 hour before an estrogen-containing regimen. Antiemetics are ineffective if taken after nausea is already present.[41] If vomiting occurs within 3 hours of a dose, the dose should be repeated. As with daily use of oral contraceptives, other adverse effects might include fatigue, breast tenderness, headache, abdominal pain, and dizziness. It should be noted that CDC Medical Eligibility Criteria indicate that benefits of estrogen-containing pills for EC generally outweigh the risks of use even in adolescents or women with health conditions, such as thromboembolic disease (ie, category 2).[35]

Cu-IUD

The Cu-IUD can be inserted within 5 days of the first act of unprotected sexual intercourse as EC. Otherwise, eligibility criteria and initiation procedures for the Cu-IUD are the same for emergency or nonemergency Cu-IUD insertion. Pain with insertion is possible with use of the Cu-IUD for EC, and some patients may be fearful of pain and/or the required pelvic examination. Events associated with ongoing use of the Cu-IUD include expulsion (~6% in first year) and heavy menstrual bleeding and/or painful periods (~12%). Contraindications for Cu-IUD use include anatomic features that prevent insertion, Wilson disease, and signs of active cervical and/or pelvic infection.[35] Of note, negative STI test results are not required before the insertion of an IUD. However, if an adolescent has not been screened for gonorrhea and *Chlamydia* according to screening guidelines,[42] screening can be performed at the time of IUD insertion, and IUD insertion should not be delayed. The American College of Obstetricians and Gynecologists Long-Acting Reversible Contraception Program provides links to resources for clinicians who are interested in obtaining training on IUD insertion (www.acog.org/About-ACOG/ACOG-Departments/Long-Acting-Reversible-Contraception).

OTHER CLINICAL CONSIDERATIONS

Initiating Contraception After Use of ECPs

Although there is no specific contraindication for repeated use of EC, it should be emphasized to patients that ECPs are intended for emergency use and routine use of ECPs to prevent pregnancy is not as effective as the regular use of other forms of contraception. Ongoing hormonal contraceptives may be initiated or resumed immediately after use of levonorgestrel ECPs or the Yuzpe method; however, condoms or abstinence should be used in addition for 7 days for back-up protection.[25] Initiation of ongoing hormonal contraceptives after the use of UPA should be delayed for 5 days to minimize the risk of interference with UPA activity.[25] Prescriptions or a supply of hormonal contraceptives can be given at the time of UPA provision; however, patients should be instructed not to initiate them until 5 days after the dose of UPA. In addition, as with levonorgestrel or the Yuzpe method, patients should be counseled to abstain from intercourse or use condoms for 7 days after the initiation of ongoing contraception or until the start of their next period, whichever occurs first.[25]

Assessing for STI Risk

The discussion of EC methods with patients must include the fact that none of these methods protect from STIs. Because of the cooccurring risk of STIs, offering STI testing at the visit for EC or encouraging patients to schedule follow-up visits for STI testing or treatment are advisable. In addition, follow-up visits are an important time to discuss options for ongoing contraception, abstinence, and consensual intercourse. Although EC is exclusively for use by individuals at risk of pregnancy, it is important for young men to be counseled on this method as well as on condom use and the regular use of other contraceptive methods so that they can communicate with their at-risk partners about optimal contraceptive use.

ADOLESCENTS AND EC: AWARENESS AND ACCESS

Data from the CDC indicate that the use of EC by female teenagers who had sexual intercourse at least once has increased over the past decade from 8% in 2002 to 22% in 2011 to 2013.[2] This increase is likely related to regulatory changes that increased nonprescription access to levonorgestrel EC during this time. Despite the FDA approval of levonorgestrel for over-the-counter access without an age restriction, additional access barriers remain. In its most recent survey, the American Society for Emergency Contraception found that only 64% of pharmacies have ECPs in stock on their shelves, and among those that do, nearly half use a lock of some kind requiring employee assistance to obtain it from the shelf.[16] Additionally, despite multiple brand-name and generic products on the market, the cost of levonorgestrel ECPs remains at $40 to $50, on average. This cost may be prohibitive, so pediatricians are encouraged to be aware of other resources for patients to obtain affordable ECPs, which may include college health services, school-based clinics, or Title X clinics. Insurance coverage may help with the cost barrier; however, coverage may vary by plan. In addition to the cost barrier, some stores also continue to enforce an unjustified age restriction on purchase.[16]

Access to UPA is also often limited. One study in Hawaii reported data from a secret-shopper study of pharmacies throughout the state that found that less than 3% had UPA in stock at the time of the request.[43] The average cost of UPA in studied pharmacies was approximately $50. Another study of pharmacy availability of UPA was conducted in Massachusetts and reported that 7% of pharmacies surveyed had UPA in stock.[44]

Although EC methods are indicated for use only in patients at risk of pregnancy, previous AAP policy statements advised that educating adolescent male patients is important.[45] Evidence suggests that most male teenagers are not knowledgeable about EC.[45–47] One study conducted among an older adolescent and young adult population (ages 18–25 years) recruited from a Job Corps site and a free clinic in Los Angeles surveyed male and female participants and found that 18% of male participants reported having a partner who had previously used EC.[48] Significantly fewer male than female participants in that study reported having received information about EC from a health care provider. Another study of a younger convenience sample of sexually experienced adolescent male participants (ages 13–24 years) in Denver reported that only 42% had heard of EC.[49] One study explored how willing young men are to accept an advanced supply of EC in a clinic setting and found that a majority who were offered EC accepted it.[46]

It is important that information about EC be included in all contraceptive and STI counseling for adolescents wherever these visits occur: the primary care office, the emergency department, specialty clinics, or inpatient units. Discussions should include indications for use and how patients can access EC in a timely fashion. Yet, provider communication about EC remains low and differs by patient characteristics. Findings from a nationally representative sample of sexually active 15- to 24-year-old women in the 2011–2015 National Survey of Family Growth found that provider communication about EC during a visit for a pelvic examination or Papanicolaou test was infrequent (19%) compared with communication about birth control (67%) and differed by patient characteristics, including race and/or ethnicity and insurance status.[50] For example, a higher proportion of non-Hispanic black (25%) and Hispanic (27%) women reported receiving provider counseling about EC than did non-Hispanic white (14%) women. Reasons for differences in the reporting of counseling by race and/or ethnicity have not been identified by research to date. Adolescents with disabilities (both physical and cognitive) and their families should be counseled on EC as part of routine anticipatory guidance,[51] especially because data suggest that children with disabilities have 2 times the risk of being sexual assaulted compared with children without disabilities.[52] Offering advance prescription of ECPs is encouraged.

Laws allowing minors to consent to birth control services, including EC, without parents and rights to confidentiality vary by state. The Guttmacher Institute regularly updates information on the general categories of reproductive health services to which minors can consent by state.[53] Minors in special circumstances, such as those in the foster care or juvenile justice systems, may face unique barriers to access and confidentiality.[54] State laws regarding reporting age of consent for sexual activity and mandated reporting of sexual activity involving minors also vary by state.[55]

PERSONAL BELIEFS FOR PHYSICIANS AND PHARMACISTS

Despite the fact that hormonal EC will not disrupt an established pregnancy and studies showing that access to EC does not make it more likely that adolescents will engage in more sex or less likely that they will use condoms or other contraceptives,[56–58] public and medical discourse indicates that personal values of physicians and pharmacists continue to affect access to EC, particularly for adolescents.[59–63] Some physicians decline to provide EC to teenagers, regardless of the circumstance,[20] and others may provide EC only if sexual assault has occurred.[20,64] These decisions by physicians and pharmacists have important adverse consequences for adolescents in their ability to access EC.

A physician's decision to provide EC at a time of need but not in advance of need may be related to the physician's beliefs about whether it is acceptable for teenagers to have sex.[20] Often, physicians hold conflicting values when approaching reproductive health issues with teenagers. Physicians may object to unprotected intercourse or intercourse outside of marriage, but they may also feel the need to prevent unwanted pregnancy among teenagers. It is important that pediatricians are aware of the ways in which the underlying beliefs they bring to their clinical practice affect the care that they provide.

The AAP has issued a policy statement on refusal to provide information or treatment on the basis of conscience, stating that pediatricians have a duty to inform their patients about relevant, legally available treatment options to which they object and have a moral obligation to refer patients to other physicians who will provide and educate about those services.[65]

Pediatricians may also encounter situations in which adolescents and their parents differ in their acceptance of sexual intercourse and contraception. Recognizing the importance of parents and families to adolescent health and helping adolescents make decisions with which they are comfortable can be challenging. In these cases, it is important for pediatricians to be knowledgeable about the rights of the adolescent with regard to consent for contraception in their state and ensure that adolescents are aware of these rights. Pediatricians can also be an important source of information for parents to help them communicate with their adolescents and to educate them about the importance of contraception and other prevention strategies to reduce risks associated with sexual activity if their adolescents make the decision to have sex.

SUMMARY AND RECOMMENDATIONS

We recommend the following.

1. Pediatricians should be aware that sexual behavior is prevalent among teenagers and that many sexually active teenagers may be the victims of sexual assault. Despite the availability of hormonal and long-acting contraceptives, the pregnancy prevention methods most commonly used by US teenagers are condoms and withdrawal. EC is an important back-up method to which all teenagers should have access.
2. Indications for use of EC include unprotected or underprotected intercourse, such as failure to use any form of contraception; sexual assault; and imperfect contraceptive use (eg, condom breakage or slippage and missed or late doses of oral contraceptive pills, contraceptive patch, contraceptive ring, or injectable contraception).
3. Pediatricians should provide ECPs (levonorgestrel or UPA) or Cu-IUD insertion to adolescents and young adults who are in immediate need of EC. In addition, the AAP recommends that pediatricians provide prescriptions and/or a supply of ECPs (with refills and condoms) so adolescents have them on hand in case of future need (ie, advanced provision).

When a visit is not possible, ECPs can safely be prescribed over the phone without requiring a pregnancy test.

4. ECPs are most effective in decreasing risk of pregnancy when used as soon as possible, but may be used up to 120 hours after unprotected or underprotected intercourse. Adolescents should be instructed to use EC as soon as possible after unprotected intercourse and to then schedule a follow-up appointment with their primary provider to address the need for STI testing and ongoing contraception.
5. Advanced provision of ECPs increases the likelihood that teenagers will use EC when needed, reduces the time to use, and does not decrease condom or other contraceptive use. Levonorgestrel ECPs are available to male and female patients regardless of age without a prescription but may be expensive when purchased over the counter and are often covered by insurance with a prescription. UPA is available by prescription only. Pediatricians should be aware that the stock of available ECPs, especially UPA, may vary by pharmacy and that local patterns of availability, cost, insurance coverage, and sources of low-cost EC in their practice area may affect the ability of their patients to obtain recommended services.
6. When a dedicated ECP product or Cu-IUD are not options, the use of combined oral contraceptive pills for EC (Yuzpe method) may be recommended. Adverse effects may include nausea, vomiting, and abdominal pain, and coadministration of an antiemetic may be considered with this method.
7. Meta-analyses have suggested that both levonorgestrel and UPA may be less effective in individuals who are overweight. Efficacy of the Cu-IUD is not affected by weight. Patients who do not wish to use a Cu-IUD or do not have access to IUD insertion should be offered EC pills regardless of their weight.
8. Repeat episodes of unprotected sex during the same cycle after the use of ECPs increase the risk of pregnancy because they work by delaying ovulation. Adolescents who use ECPs should be counseled to abstain or use another method to prevent pregnancy until their next period. Ongoing hormonal contraceptives may be initiated immediately after the use of levonorgestrel ECPs or the Yuzpe method. Ongoing hormonal contraceptives should not be initiated sooner than 5 days after the use of UPA to minimize the risk of interference with UPA activity. Nonhormonal methods (eg, condoms) may be initiated immediately after ECP use.
9. The AAP recommends that all adolescents receive counseling about EC as part of routine anticipatory guidance in the context of a discussion on sexual health and family planning regardless of current intentions for sexual behavior. In addition, it is important that information about EC be included in all contraceptive and STI counseling for adolescents wherever these visits occur, including emergency departments, clinics, and hospitals. Information provided should include indications for use and options for access, including over-the-counter availability and advance prescription or supply if available in the clinic. It is important that pediatricians also provide this counseling to adolescents with physical and cognitive disabilities and their parents. At the policy level, pediatricians should advocate for low-cost or free, nonprescription access to ECPs for teenagers regardless of age and insurance coverage of EC without cost sharing to further reduce cost barriers.

LEAD AUTHORS

Krishna K. Upadhya, MD, MPH, FAAP

COMMITTEE ON ADOLESCENCE, 2016–2017

Cora C. Breuner, MD, MPH, FAAP, Chairperson
Elizabeth M. Alderman, MD, FAAP, FSAHM
Laura K. Grubb, MD, FAAP
Laurie L. Hornberger, MD, MPH, FAAP
Makia E. Powers, MD, MPH, FAAP
Krishna K. Upadhya, MD, FAAP
Stephenie B. Wallace, MD, FAAP

LIAISONS

Liwei L. Hua, MD, PhD – *American Academy of Child and Adolescent Psychiatry*
Margo Lane, MD – *Canadian Pediatric Society*
Meredith Loveless, MD – *American College of Obstetricians and Gynecologists*
Seema Menon, MD – *North American Society of Pediatric and Adolescent Gynecology*
Lauren B. Zapata, PhD, MSPH – *Centers for Disease Control and Prevention*

STAFF

Karen Smith
James Baumberger, MPP

ABBREVIATIONS

AAP: American Academy of Pediatrics
CDC: Centers for Disease Control and Prevention
Cu-IUD: copper intrauterine device
EC: emergency contraception
ECP: emergency contraceptive pill
FDA: US Food and Drug Administration
IUD: intrauterine device
STI: sexually transmitted infection
UPA: ulipristal acetate

REFERENCES

1. Shen J, Che Y, Showell E, Chen K, Cheng L. Interventions for emergency contraception. *Cochrane Database Syst Rev*. 2017;8(8):CD001324

2. Martinez GM, Abma JC. Sexual activity, contraceptive use, and childbearing of teenagers aged 15–19 in the United States. *NCHS Data Brief.* 2015;(209):1–8

3. Martinez G, Copen CE, Abma JC. Teenagers in the United States: sexual activity, contraceptive use, and childbearing, 2006–2010 national survey of family growth. *Vital Health Stat 23.* 2011;(31):1–35

4. Kann L, McManus T, Harris WA, et al. Youth risk behavior surveillance - United States, 2015. *MMWR Surveill Summ.* 2016;65(6):1–174

5. Trent M, Clum G, Roche KM. Sexual victimization and reproductive health outcomes in urban youth. *Ambul Pediatr.* 2007;7(4):313–316

6. Helton JJ, Gochez-Kerr T, Gruber E. Sexual abuse of children with learning disabilities. *Child Maltreat.* 2018;23(2): 157–165

7. Casteel C, Martin SL, Smith JB, Gurka KK, Kupper LL. National study of physical and sexual assault among women with disabilities. *Inj Prev.* 2008; 14(2):87–90

8. Lindberg L, Santelli J, Desai S. Understanding the decline in adolescent fertility in the United States, 2007–2012. *J Adolesc Health.* 2016; 59(5):577–583

9. US Department of Health and Human Services. Healthy People 2020 objectives: family planning. Available at: https://www.healthypeople.gov/2020/topics-objectives/topic/family-planning/objectives. Accessed September 30, 2018

10. Ott MA, Sucato GS; Committee on Adolescence. Contraception for adolescents. *Pediatrics.* 2014;134(4). Available at: www.pediatrics.org/cgi/content/full/134/4/e1257

11. American College of Obstetricians and Gynecologists. ACOG Committee Opinion No. 735: adolescents and long-acting reversible contraception: implants and intrauterine devices. *Obstet Gynecol.* 2018;131(5):e130–e139

12. Abma JC, Martinez GM. Sexual activity and contraceptive use among teenagers in the United States, 2011–2015. *Natl Health Stat Rep.* 2017; (104):1–23

13. Yuzpe AA, Thurlow HJ, Ramzy I, Leyshon JI. Post coital contraception–A pilot study. *J Reprod Med.* 1974;13(2):53–58

14. Meyer JL, Gold MA, Haggerty CL. Advance provision of emergency contraception among adolescent and young adult women: a systematic review of literature. *J Pediatr Adolesc Gynecol.* 2011;24(1):2–9

15. Rowan A. Obama administration yields to the courts and the evidence, allows emergency contraception to be sold without restrictions. Available at: https://www.guttmacher.org/gpr/2013/06/obama-administration-yields-courts-and-evidence-allows-emergency-contraception-be-sold. Accessed January 7, 2019

16. American Society for Emergency Contraception. Inching towards progress: ASEC's 2015 pharmacy access study. Available at: http://americansocietyforec.org/uploads/3/4/5/6/34568220/asec_2015_ec_access_report_1.pdf. Accessed February 13, 2017

17. Sills MR, Chamberlain JM, Teach SJ. The associations among pediatricians' knowledge, attitudes, and practices regarding emergency contraception. *Pediatrics.* 2000;105(4, pt 2):954–956

18. Golden NH, Seigel WM, Fisher M, et al. Emergency contraception: pediatricians' knowledge, attitudes, and opinions. *Pediatrics.* 2001;107(2): 287–292

19. Lim SW, Iheagwara KN, Legano L, Coupey SM. Emergency contraception: are pediatric residents counseling and prescribing to teens? *J Pediatr Adolesc Gynecol.* 2008;21(3):129–134

20. Upadhya KK, Trent ME, Ellen JM. Impact of individual values on adherence to emergency contraception practice guidelines among pediatric residents: implications for training. *Arch Pediatr Adolesc Med.* 2009;163(10):944–948

21. Batur P, Cleland K, McNamara M, Wu J, Pickle S; EC Survey Group. Emergency contraception: a multispecialty survey of clinician knowledge and practices. *Contraception.* 2016;93(2):145–152

22. Pharma HRA. FDA advisory committee unanimously recommends approval of HRA pharma's ulipristal acetate for emergency contraception. 2010. Available at: https://ec.princeton.edu/news/HRA_Ella_PR.pdf. Accessed January 7, 2019

23. von Hertzen H, Piaggio G, Ding J, et al; WHO Research Group on Post-ovulatory Methods of Fertility Regulation. Low dose mifepristone and two regimens of levonorgestrel for emergency contraception: a WHO multicentre randomised trial. *Lancet.* 2002; 360(9348):1803–1810

24. Rodrigues I, Grou F, Joly J. Effectiveness of emergency contraceptive pills between 72 and 120 hours after unprotected sexual intercourse. *Am J Obstet Gynecol.* 2001;184(4):531–537

25. Curtis KM, Jatlaoui TC, Tepper NK, et al. U.S. selected practice recommendations for contraceptive use, 2016. *MMWR Recomm Rep.* 2016; 65(4):1–66

26. American College of Obstetricians and Gynecologists. Practice Bulletin No. 152: emergency contraception. *Obstet Gynecol.* 2015;126(3):e1–e11

27. Cleland K, Zhu H, Goldstuck N, Cheng L, Trussell J. The efficacy of intrauterine devices for emergency contraception: a systematic review of 35 years of experience. *Hum Reprod.* 2012;27(7): 1994–2000

28. Wu S, Godfrey EM, Wojdyla D, et al. Copper T380A intrauterine device for emergency contraception: a prospective, multicentre, cohort clinical trial. *BJOG.* 2010;117(10): 1205–1210

29. Turok DK, Godfrey EM, Wojdyla D, et al. Copper T380 intrauterine device for emergency contraception: highly effective at any time in the menstrual cycle. *Hum Reprod.* 2013;28(10): 2672–2676

30. Turok DK, Sanders JN, Thompson IS, et al. Preference for and efficacy of oral levonorgestrel for emergency contraception with concomitant placement of a levonorgestrel IUD: a prospective cohort study. *Contraception.* 2016;93(6):526–532

31. Moreau C, Trussell J. Results from pooled Phase III studies of ulipristal acetate for emergency contraception. *Contraception.* 2012;86(6):673–680

32. Glasier A, Cameron ST, Blithe D, et al. Can we identify women at risk of

pregnancy despite using emergency contraception? Data from randomized trials of ulipristal acetate and levonorgestrel. *Contraception.* 2011; 84(4):363–367

33. Kapp N, Abitbol JL, Mathé H, et al. Effect of body weight and BMI on the efficacy of levonorgestrel emergency contraception. *Contraception.* 2015; 91(2):97–104

34. US Food and Drug Administration. FDA communication on levonorgestrel emergency contraceptive effectiveness and weight. Available at: https://www.fda.gov/Drugs/DrugSafety/PostmarketDrugSafetyInformationforPatientsandProviders/ucm109775.htm. Accessed January 3, 2019

35. Curtis KM, Tepper NK, Jatlaoui TC, et al. US medical eligibility criteria for contraceptive use, 2016. *MMWR Recomm Rep.* 2016;65(3):1–103

36. US Food and Drug Administration. Highlights of prescribing information: ella (ulipristal acetate) tablet. Revised March 2015. Available at: www.accessdata.fda.gov/drugsatfda_docs/label/2015/022474s007lbl.pdf. Accessed January 3, 2019

37. US Food and Drug Administration. Highlights of prescribing information: Plan B One-Step tablet (levonorgestrel) 1.5mg for oral use. Revised July 2009. Available at: www.accessdata.fda.gov/drugsatfda_docs/label/2009/021998lbl.pdf. Accessed January 3, 2019

38. Halpern V, Raymond EG, Lopez LM. Repeated use of pre- and postcoital hormonal contraception for prevention of pregnancy. *Cochrane Database Syst Rev.* 2010;(1):CD007595

39. Ellertson C, Webb A, Blanchard K, et al. Modifying the Yuzpe regimen of emergency contraception: a multicenter randomized controlled trial. *Obstet Gynecol.* 2003;101(6): 1160–1167

40. Percival-Smith RK, Abercrombie B. Postcoital contraception with dl-norgestrel/ethinyl estradiol combination: six years experience in a student medical clinic. *Contraception.* 1987;36(3):287–293

41. Raymond EG, Creinin MD, Barnhart KT, et al. Meclizine for prevention of nausea associated with use of emergency contraceptive pills: a randomized trial. *Obstet Gynecol.* 2000;95(2):271–277

42. Workowski KA, Bolan GA; Centers for Disease Control and Prevention. Sexually transmitted diseases treatment guidelines, 2015. *MMWR Recomm Rep.* 2015;64(RR-03):1–137

43. Bullock H, Steele S, Kurata N, et al. Pharmacy access to ulipristal acetate in Hawaii: is a prescription enough? *Contraception.* 2016;93(5):452–454

44. Brant A, White K, St Marie P. Pharmacy availability of ulipristal acetate emergency contraception: an audit study. *Contraception.* 2014;90(3): 338–339

45. Committee on Adolescence. Emergency contraception. *Pediatrics.* 2012;130(6): 1174–1182

46. Garbers S, Bell DL, Ogaye K, Marcell AV, Westhoff CL, Rosenthal SL. Advance provision of emergency contraception to young men: an exploratory study in a clinic setting [published online ahead of print April 17, 2018]. *Contraception.* doi:10.1016/j.contraception.2018.04.005

47. Marcell AV, Waks AB, Rutkow L, et al. What do we know about males and emergency contraception? A synthesis of the literature. *Perspect Sex Reprod Health.* 2012;44(3):184–193

48. Schrager SM, Olson J, Beharry M, et al. Young men and the morning after: a missed opportunity for emergency contraception provision? *J Fam Plann Reprod Health Care.* 2015;41(1):33–37

49. Richards MJ, Peters M, Sheeder J, Kaul P. Contraception and adolescent males: an opportunity for providers. *J Adolesc Health.* 2016;58(3):366–368

50. Liddon N, Steiner RJ, Martinez GM. Provider communication with adolescent and young females during sexual and reproductive health visits: findings from the 2011–2015 National Survey of Family Growth. *Contraception.* 2018;97(1):22–28

51. Murphy NA, Elias ER. Sexuality of children and adolescents with developmental disabilities. *Pediatrics.* 2006;118(1):398–403

52. Hibbard RA, Desch LW; American Academy of Pediatrics Committee on Child Abuse and Neglect; American Academy of Pediatrics Council on Children With Disabilities. Maltreatment of children with disabilities. *Pediatrics.* 2007;119(5):1018–1025

53. Guttmacher Institute. Minors' access to contraceptive services. 2018. Available at: https://www.guttmacher.org/state-policy/explore/minors-access-contraceptive-services. Accessed April 5, 2018

54. Dudley TI. Bearing injustice: foster care, pregnancy prevention, and the law. *Law Justice.* 2013;28(1):77–115

55. US Department of Health and Human Services. Statutory rape: a guide to state laws and reporting requirements. 2004. Available at: https://aspe.hhs.gov/report/statutory-rape-guide-state-laws-and-reporting-requirements. Accessed April 12, 2018

56. Stewart HE, Gold MA, Parker AM. The impact of using emergency contraception on reproductive health outcomes: a retrospective review in an urban adolescent clinic. *J Pediatr Adolesc Gynecol.* 2003;16(5):313–318

57. Gold MA, Wolford JE, Smith KA, Parker AM. The effects of advance provision of emergency contraception on adolescent women's sexual and contraceptive behaviors. *J Pediatr Adolesc Gynecol.* 2004;17(2): 87–96

58. Raine TR, Harper CC, Rocca CH, et al. Direct access to emergency contraception through pharmacies and effect on unintended pregnancy and STIs: a randomized controlled trial. *JAMA.* 2005;293(1):54–62

59. Conard LA, Fortenberry JD, Blythe MJ, Orr DP. Pharmacists' attitudes toward and practices with adolescents. *Arch Pediatr Adolesc Med.* 2003;157(4): 361–365

60. Grimes DA. Emergency contraception: politics trumps science at the U.S. Food and Drug Administration. *Obstet Gynecol.* 2004;104(2): 220–221

61. Pruitt SL, Mullen PD. Contraception or abortion? Inaccurate descriptions of emergency contraception in newspaper articles, 1992-2002. *Contraception.* 2005;71(1):14–21

62. Karasz A, Kirchen NT, Gold M. The visit before the morning after: barriers to preprescribing emergency

contraception. *Ann Fam Med.* 2004;2(4): 345–350

63. Fairhurst K, Wyke S, Ziebland S, Seaman P, Glasier A. "Not that sort of practice": the views and behaviour of primary care practitioners in a study of advance provision of emergency contraception. *Fam Pract.* 2005;22(3): 280–286

64. Miller MK, Mollen CJ, O'Malley D, et al. Providing adolescent sexual health care in the pediatric emergency department: views of health care providers. *Pediatr Emerg Care.* 2014;30(2): 84–90

65. Committee on Bioethics. Policy statement–Physician refusal to provide information or treatment on the basis of claims of conscience. *Pediatrics.* 2009;124(6):1689–1693

Executive Summary: Criteria for Critical Care of Infants and Children: PICU Admission, Discharge, and Triage Practice Statement and Levels of Care Guidance

- *Policy Statement*

POLICY STATEMENT Organizational Principles to Guide and Define the Child Health Care System and/or Improve the Health of all Children

American Academy of Pediatrics

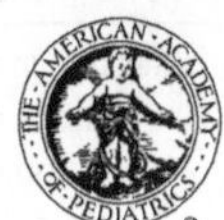

DEDICATED TO THE HEALTH OF ALL CHILDREN™

Executive Summary: Criteria for Critical Care of Infants and Children: PICU Admission, Discharge, and Triage Practice Statement and Levels of Care Guidance

Benson S. Hsu, MD, MBA, FAAP,[a] Vanessa Hill, MD, FAAP,[b] Lorry R. Frankel, MD, FCCM,[c] Timothy S. Yeh, MD, MCCM,[d] Shari Simone, CRNP, DNP, FCCM, FAANP, FAAN,[e] Marjorie J. Arca, MD, FACS, FAAP,[f] Jorge A. Coss-Bu, MD,[g] Mary E. Fallat, MD, FACS, FAAP,[h] Jason Foland, MD,[i] Samir Gadepalli, MD, MBA,[j] Michael O. Gayle, BS, MD, FCCM,[k] Lori A. Harmon, RRT, MBA, CPHQ,[l] Christa A. Joseph, RN, MSN,[m] Aaron D. Kessel, BS, MD,[n] Niranjan Kissoon, MD, MCCM,[o] Michele Moss, MD, FCCM,[p] Mohan R. Mysore, MD, FAAP, FCCM,[q] Michele E. Papo, MD, MPH, FCCM,[r] Kari L. Rajzer-Wakeham, CCRN, MSN, PCCNP, RN,[s] Tom B. Rice, MD,[t] David L. Rosenberg, MD, FAAP, FCCM,[u] Martin K. Wakeham, MD,[v,t] Edward E. Conway, Jr, MD, FCCM, MS,[w] Michael S.D. Agus, MD, FAAP, FCCM[x]

abstract

This is an executive summary of the 2019 update of the 2004 guidelines and levels of care for PICU. Since previous guidelines, there has been a tremendous transformation of Pediatric Critical Care Medicine with advancements in pediatric cardiovascular medicine, transplant, neurology, trauma, and oncology as well as improvements of care in general PICUs. This has led to the evolution of resources and training in the provision of care through the PICU. Outcome and quality research related to admission, transfer, and discharge criteria as well as literature regarding PICU levels of care to include volume, staffing, and structure were reviewed and included in this statement as appropriate. Consequently, the purposes of this significant update are to address the transformation of the field and codify a revised set of guidelines that will enable hospitals, institutions, and individuals in developing the appropriate PICU for their community needs. The target audiences of the practice statement and guidance are broad and include critical care professionals; pediatricians; pediatric subspecialists; pediatric surgeons; pediatric surgical subspecialists; pediatric imaging physicians; and other members of the patient care team such as nurses, therapists, dieticians, pharmacists, social workers, care coordinators, and hospital administrators who make daily administrative and clinical decisions in all PICU levels of care.

[a]Pediatric Critical Care, Sanford School of Medicine, University of South Dakota, Vermillion, South Dakota; [b]Hospital Medicine, Baylor College of Medicine and Children's Hospital of San Antonio, San Antonio, Texas; [c]Department of Pediatrics and Critical Care Services, California Pacific Medical Center, San Francisco, California; [d]Department of Pediatrics, Saint Barnabas Medical Center, Livingston, New Jersey; [e]PICU, Medical Center, University of Maryland, Baltimore, Maryland; [f]Divisions of Pediatric Surgery and [t]Pediatric Critical Care Medicine, [v]Medical College of Wisconsin and Children's Hospital of Wisconsin, Milwaukee, Wisconsin; [g]Pediatrics and Critical Care Medicine, Baylor College of Medicine and Texas Children's Hospital, Houston, Texas; [h]Division of Pediatric Surgery, University of Louisville and Norton Children's Hospital, Louisville, Kentucky; [i]Pediatric Intensive Care, Studer Family Children's Hospital, Ascension Sacred Heart, Pensacola, Florida; [j]Division of Pediatric Surgery, University of Michigan, Ann Arbor, Michigan; [k]Pediatric Intensive Care, Wolfson Children's Hospital, Jacksonville, Florida; [l]Department of Quality, Society of Critical Care Medicine, Mount Prospect, Illinois; [m]Pediatric Intensive Care, Children's Hospital Oakland, Oakland, California; [n]Pediatric Critical Care Medicine, Cohen Children's Medical Center, New Hyde Park, New York; [o]Medical Affairs, British Columbia Children's Hospital, Vancouver, Canada; [p]Pediatric Critical Care Medicine, Arkansas Children's Hospital, Little Rock, Arkansas;

To cite: Hsu BS, Hill V, Frankel LR, et al. Executive Summary: Criteria for Critical Care of Infants and Children: PICU Admission, Discharge, and Triage Practice Statement and Levels of Care Guidance. *Pediatrics*. 2019; 144(4):e20192433

BACKGROUND INFORMATION

Pediatric critical care medicine has evolved over the last 3 decades into a highly respected, board-certified specialty that has become an

TABLE 1 Recommendations Summary

Recommendations
Recommended PICU level of care admission criteria
Patients who are appropriately triaged according to level of illness and services provided in community, tertiary, or quaternary PICU facilities will have comparable outcomes and quality of care. The specifics of each PICU level of care described above serve as a reference for minimum standards of quality care to guide appropriate PICU admissions and promote optimal patient outcomes.
Individual hospitals and their PICU leadership team should develop admission criteria to assist in the placement of critically ill children that are aligned with their PICU level of care.
Pediatric patients requiring specialized service interventions such as cardiac, neurologic, or trauma-related surgery have improved outcomes when cared for in a quaternary or tertiary ICU, and early interfacility transfer to the appropriate regional facility should be the standard of care.
Congenital heart surgery should only be performed in a hospital that has a PICU with a dedicated pediatric cardiac intensive care team, including but not restricted to pediatric intensivists and nurses with expertise in cardiac intensive care, cardiovascular surgeon with pediatric expertise, pediatric perfusionists, pediatric cardiologists, and pediatric cardiac anesthesiologists.
Recommended ICU structure and provider staffing model
Expertise in the care of the critically ill child is required in all PICU levels of care.
All critically ill children admitted to any PICU should be cared for by a pediatric intensivist who is board eligible, board certified, or undergoing maintenance of certification as primary provider while in the ICU setting.
Trauma patients should be cared for by both the trauma service (including trainees) and the PICU service in a collaborative manner. The ACS requires that surgeons be the primary provider on all patients admitted with traumatic injuries. Programs in which the attending surgeon has training and certification in surgical critical care may (institution specific) allow for the primary attending to be a surgeon with such expertise working with the PICU attending.
Burn patients should be comanaged by the burn surgeon of record (discipline may be pediatric surgery, general surgery, or plastic surgery) and the PICU service.
In a PICU that supports an ACS-verified children's surgical center, an ICU team that demonstrates direct surgeon involvement in the day-to-day management of the surgical needs of the patient is essential. Both PICU and surgery services must be promptly available 24 h per d.
Any level of PICU that supports advanced ACGME training programs such as pediatric residency, general surgery residency, pediatric critical care medicine fellowships, pediatric surgery fellowships, and pediatric surgical critical care fellowships (among others) will promote the participation of trainees in interprofessional care of patients providing appropriate communication and collaboration. Clear delineation of responsibilities will be sought on each patient. This requirement reflects the common program requirements outlined by the ACGME.
A qualified medical provider (in quaternary facility PICUs, the qualified medical provider should be a critical care specialist) who is able to respond within 5 min to all emergent patient issues (eg, airway management or cardiopulmonary resuscitation) is necessary for optimal patient outcomes in all levels of PICU. Specialized or quaternary facility PICUs have a minimum of an in-house critical care fellow.
A qualified surgical provider who is able to respond readily to emergency surgical issues in critically ill patients should be available. The designation of qualified is defined by the surgical problem, and availability should be commensurate with the level of care of the PICU and level of ACS Children's Surgery Verification of the institution.
Night coverage response requirement for pediatric intensivists who are not in house, primarily in community and tertiary PICUs, includes being readily available by telephone and present in the PICU within 30 min of request.
Recommended ICU personnel and resources
The ICU structure and care delivery model components that are essential in all PICU levels of care include nursing staff and respiratory therapists with PICU expertise as well as multidisciplinary rounds. In tertiary and quaternary facility PICUs, 24/7 in-house coverage, a dedicated clinical pharmacist, a social worker, a child life specialist, and palliative care services are necessary.
All PICUs should have access to an on-site pediatric pharmacist who is available for daily rounds, pharmacy support, and ongoing educational activities.
All providers, including pediatric hospitalists, nurse practitioners, and physician assistants who provide first-line night coverage in PICUs, must be skilled in advanced airway, intravenous and intraosseous line placement, and ventilator management.
All PICUs must have access to a transfer and transport program that can ensure the safe and timely movement of a critically ill or injured child from a community hospital to an institution with a higher PICU level of care.

indispensable service for inpatient programs of most children's hospitals as well as a highly valued resource supporting most community-based programs. The earlier published guidelines for pediatric critical care medicine were used to help establish the basic needs for a state-of-the-art PICU. These guidelines were used by both physician leadership and policy makers to advocate for personnel, supplies, and space that were unique to PICUs. However, there has been a tremendous transformation of pediatric critical care medicine over the past 10 years, with explosive growth in specialized PICUs in pediatric cardiovascular medicine, transplant, neurology, trauma, and oncology as well as improvements of care in general PICUs. This has led to the evolution in both human and material resources and training in more highly specialized areas such as cardiovascular medicine, neurosurgical ICUs, and trauma care.[1,2]

STATEMENT OF PROBLEM

To provide a 2019 update of the American Academy of Pediatrics and Society of Critical Care Medicine's 2004 *Guidelines and levels of care for PICUs.*[3]

EVIDENCE BASIS

Methodology

A group of nationally and internationally recognized clinical experts in pediatric critical care medicine made up the pediatric critical care admission guidelines task force. The task force reviewed the work of the previous guidelines and made decisions regarding topic selection inclusion. The topic selection for the guidelines addressed PICU characteristics and interventions by the PICU level of care, including quaternary or specialized, tertiary, and community. Interventions addressed included PICU admission, team structure, transport and transfer mechanisms, outreach programs, and quality metrics.

TABLE 1 Continued

Recommendations
Quaternary facilities or specialized PICUs have access to a critical care transport program with a dedicated trained pediatric team and specialized equipment.
When PICUs require outsourcing of critical care transport activities, the transport service team members must all have training in pediatric emergency and critical care.
Recommended performance improvement and patient safety
Quaternary facilities and tertiary levels of PICUs should participate in academic pursuits.
All quaternary facilities and tertiary levels of PICUs should be involved in providing peer community outreach education such as educational conferences, technical skill competencies, stabilization, and resuscitation (eg, PALS education).
Community and tertiary PICUs should be involved in providing community outreach through educational events that focus on technical skills needed for stabilization, resuscitation, and communication for the triage and transport of critically ill and injured children. These activities might include case conferences.
All levels of PICU should provide feedback to referral centers after transfer of a patient to a PICU, which is essential for both quality improvement and education.
Recommended equipment and technology
Some emergency resuscitative therapies such as invasive and noninvasive respiratory support and central line access can be safely performed in community PICUs.
Renal replacement therapies (peritoneal dialysis, continuous hemofiltration and hemodialysis, and intermittent hemodialysis) may be offered in a community-based PICU when appropriately trained support personnel, which must include a nephrologist, are present.
All PICU levels must have access to helium-oxygen. In selected PICUs, epoprostenol sodium, nitric oxide, and anesthetic agents may be used if appropriate personnel and equipment are available for the safe delivery and monitoring of these agents.
The following are appropriate indications for PICU transfer from a community to a tertiary or quaternary level of care: intracranial pressure monitoring, acute hepatic failure leading to coma, congenital heart disease with unstable cardiorespiratory status, need for temporary cardiac pacing, head injury with initial GCS ≤8, multiple traumatic injuries, or heart failure requiring an interventional cardiologist. For complicated burns >10% TBSA, access to a specialized burn unit or burn center is recommended.
Recommended PICU discharge and transfer criteria
Each PICU should have clearly defined criteria for escalation and de-escalation of resources and, therefore, level of PICU required on the basis of the physiologic status of the patient.
All levels of PICU should have policies and protocols in place that specify when the patient's physiologic status requires escalation of care, with transfer to a more appropriate level of care as expeditiously as needed.
When a patient's physiologic status improves, discharge from the PICU can occur in many ways:
Transfer to an appropriate acute care bed within that facility
Return transfer to the referring facility
Transfer to a skilled nursing or rehabilitation facility
Discharge from the PICU to home
After discharge from the PICU, the following should take place:
Appropriate communication with the accepting facility, including oral handoff, a clear and concise written summary, and exchange of necessary health information
Discharge planning and communication with the family or caregivers if going home
Communication with the primary care physician who will assume care of the child once the patient is returned to the community
Communication with subspecialists caring for the child and appropriate follow-up arranged as necessary
As needed, careful care coordination with outpatient services such as but not limited to:
Delivery and instruction in the use of durable medical equipment
Home pharmacy and nutrition support
Ongoing rehabilitation needs such as occupational or physical therapy
Ancillary support as required

ACGME, Accreditation Council for Graduate Medical Education; ACS, American College of Surgeons; GCS, Glasgow Coma Scale; PALS, Pediatric Advanced Life Support; TBSA, total body surface area.

A comprehensive literature search on the topics and agreed-on questions determined by the task force was performed by a dedicated Society of Critical Care Medicine librarian in selected biomedical databases. The 2004 guidelines and levels of care for PICUs served as the starting point for searches in Medline (Ovid), Embase (Ovid), and PubMed on articles published from 2004 to 2016. Members of the task force received the set of citations and abstracts relevant to the section of the guidelines; references not directly related to the content area were excluded from the review. The full-text articles were retrieved and reviewed to determine appropriate inclusion for appraisal.

The admission to the PICU literature search identified 832 articles. The review of article titles resulted in 299 relevant articles, of which all abstracts were reviewed. The full text of 75 articles and 12 additional articles obtained by hand searching reference lists were reviewed. Twenty-one relevant pediatric studies in which outcomes related to pediatric level of care, specialized PICU, patient volume, or personnel were evaluated were found. The discharge and unplanned readmission literature search yielded 68 articles. The full text of 24 articles and 6 additional articles obtained by hand searching reference lists were reviewed. No articles were found in which PICU discharge criteria were evaluated, and only 14 relevant studies were found in which outcomes related to unplanned PICU readmissions were evaluated. Since publication of the 2004 revised guidelines, evidence on evaluating the impact of the level of PICU care on patient outcomes remains limited. After deliberation, the task force determined that the strength and quality of the current pediatric evidence for the selected topics was insufficient to use the Grading of Recommendations, Assessment, Development, and Evaluation system in supporting evidence-based recommendations. The sparse literature and the nature of the questions under review did not lend itself to the use of the population, intervention, comparison, and outcome format. Therefore,

TABLE 2 PICU Resources by Level of Care

Resources by Organ System	Quaternary or Specialized Facility	Tertiary	Community
Cardiovascular			
Hemodynamic monitoring			
Noninvasive	Essential	Essential	Essential
Invasive	Essential	Essential	Essential
Inotropic support	Essential	Essential	Essential
Echocardiogram (24-h availability)	Essential	Essential	Essential
ECMO or ECLS	Essential	Optional	NE
VADs	Essential	Optional	NE
Transplant: heart	Desirable	Optional	NE
Gastrointestinal			
Upper and lower endoscopy	Essential	Essential	Desirable
Transplant: liver	Desirable	Optional	NE
Hematologic			
Plasmapheresis or leukapheresis	Essential	Essential	Desirable
Transplant: bone marrow	Essential	Optional	NE
Neurologic			
Intracranial pressure monitoring	Essential	Essential	Desirable
External ventricular drain	Essential	Essential	Desirable
Lumbar drain	Essential	Essential	Desirable
Continuous EEG	Essential	Essential	Optional
Video EEG	Essential	Essential	Optional
Respiratory			
Noninvasive ventilation (HFNC, CPAP, BIPAP, NPV)	Essential	Essential	Essential
Conventional mechanical ventilation	Essential	Essential	Essential
Advanced mechanical ventilation (HIFV, HFOV)	Essential	Essential	Desirable
Conventional inhalation therapies (heliox or continuous albuterol)	Essential	Essential	Essential
Nitric oxide	Essential	Essential	Desirable
Advanced inhalation gases (flolan or anesthetic agents)	Essential	Desirable	Optional
Bronchoscopy	Essential	Essential	Desirable
Transplant: lungs	Desirable	Optional	NE
Renal			
Continuous renal replacement therapy	Essential	Essential	Optional
Hemodialysis	Essential	Essential	Optional
Peritoneal dialysis	Essential	Essential	Optional
Charcoal hemofiltration	Essential	Essential	Desirable
Transplant: kidney	Essential	Optional	NE
Radiology			
Diagnostic imaging, including CT (24-h availability)	Essential	Essential	Essential
Advanced Diagnostic Imaging, including MRI (with sedation)	Essential	Essential	Desirable
Interventional neuroradiology	Essential	Desirable	Optional
Interventional cardiology	Essential	Desirable	Optional
Cardiac MRI	Essential	Desirable	Optional

BIPAP, biphasic positive airway pressure; CPAP, continuous positive airway pressure; CT, computed tomography; ECLS, extracorporeal life support; ECMO, extracorporeal membrane oxygenation; HFNC, high-flow nasal cannula; HFOV, high-frequency oscillatory ventilation; HIFV, high-inspiratory flow ventilation; NE, not expected; NPV, negative pressure ventilation; VAD, ventricular assist device.

a modified Delphi process was undertaken, seeking expert opinion to develop consensus-based recommendations where gaps in the evidence exist.

Modified Delphi Methodology

Members were selected to be on the panel on the basis of their experience as PICU directors, administrators, or other leadership roles and were chosen to represent a variety of hospital settings, from academic centers to community hospitals. The American Academy of Pediatrics also appointed a hospitalist and critical care physician liaison to serve on the panel and to assist in the development of the guideline. An American College of Critical Care Board of Regents member served as a liaison to the committee to support its work.

The guidelines panel consisted of 2 groups: a voting group consisting of 30 members and a writing group of 20 members. The voting panel used an iterative collaborative approach to formulate 30 statements on the basis of the literature review and common practice. Five of the 30 statements were multicomponent statements specific to PICU level of care, including team structure, technology, education and training, academic pursuits, and indications for transfer to a tertiary or quaternary PICU.

TABLE 3 PICU Level of Care Matched to Personnel

Staff	Qualifications	Roles	Quaternary or Specialized	Tertiary	Community
Leadership					
Medical director	• Board certified for pediatric critical care medicine after completion of an ACGME-accredited pediatric critical care medicine fellowship • Participates in training to meet ongoing education and certification requirements	• Primary attending physician • Provides consultation for PICU patients • Participates in development, review, and implementation of policies • Supervises quality control and assessment activities • Supervises and coordinates all medical staff education and competencies • Participates in program development, including budgetary preparation and policy implementation • Available to the PICU 24 h per d, 7 d per wk for both clinical and administrative issues (or similar qualified physician)	Essential	Essential	Essential
Nurse manager or director	• Training and expertise in pediatric critical care • Master's degree in pediatric nursing or nursing administration • Participates in education and training to meet ongoing education and certification requirements	• Ensures appropriate nurse to patient ratios • Participates in development, review, and implementation of unit and nursing policies and procedures • Assurance of nursing orientation and competency, performance reviews • Participates in program development, including budgetary preparation and policy implementation • Participates in development of quality improvement projects • Available to PICU for clinical and administrative issues 24 h per d (or qualified designee)	Essential; nurse to patient ratios: 1:1, 1:2, 2:1	Essential; nurse to patient ratios: 1:1, 1:2	Essential; nurse to patient ratios: 1:1, 1:2
Surgical director or leader	• Board certified for pediatric surgery after completion of an ACGME-accredited pediatric surgery fellowship. Additional certification in surgical critical care is desirable but not required.	• A children's surgeon who serves within the medical leadership structure of the PICU (who may be designated as the surgical director) and is responsible for setting policies and defining administrative needs related to PICU patients with general or subspecialty pediatric surgical needs	Essential	Essential	Desirable (a general surgeon with pediatric interest would be an alternative)
Trauma director	• Board certified for pediatric surgery after completion of an ACGME-accredited pediatric surgery fellowship	• A children's surgeon who serves within the medical leadership structure of the PICU (who may be designated as the trauma director) and is responsible for setting policies and defining administrative needs related to PICU patients with traumatic injuries (the surgical director or leader may serve in this capacity for nontrauma centers)	Essential	Essential	Desirable (a general surgeon with pediatric interest would be an alternative)

TABLE 3 Continued

Staff	Qualifications	Roles	Quaternary or Specialized	Tertiary	Community
Primary medical and surgical providers					
Pediatric intensivist or equivalent	• Board eligible or board certified in pediatric critical care medicine after training in an ACGME-accredited program • Participates in training to meet ongoing education and certification requirements for pediatric critical care	• Physician in-house 24 h per d • Available in ≤30 min (24 h per d) • Provides medical care and oversight for care provided by physicians in training, NPs, and PAs for all PICU patients • Participates in development of quality improvement projects	Essential	Essential (desirable: physician in-house 24 h per d)	Essential (optional: physician in-house 24 h per d)
Pediatric surgeon	• Board certified for pediatric surgery after completion of an ACGME-accredited pediatric surgery fellowship. Additional certification in surgical critical care is desirable but not required • Participates in training to meet ongoing education and certification requirements for pediatric surgery	• Available in ≤1 h to the PICU • Provides surgical care and oversight for care provided by physicians in training, NPs, and PAs • Participates in development of quality improvement projects	Essential	Essential	Desirable (a general surgeon with pediatric interest would be an alternative)
Other physicians: hospitalists, pediatric trainees, surgical trainees	• Postgraduate year 2 level or higher assigned to PICU • ACGME-accredited pediatric or surgery critical care with focus on pediatric critical care residency program Participate in training to meet ongoing education and certification requirements	• In house PICU coverage 24 h/d within ACGME restrictions • Participates in monitoring of quality improvement projects	Essential (may include combination of hospitalists and NPs)	Essential (may include combination of hospitalists and NPs)	Desirable (may include combination of hospitalists and NPs)
APPs or NPs	• Training and expertise in pediatric critical care • Pediatric NP certification; preferred acute care • Master of science in nursing or doctorate in nursing practice • Participates in training to meet ongoing education and certification requirements	• Provide collaborative, comprehensive management of PICU patients • Performance of advanced therapeutic procedures • Participate in development of quality improvement projects	Desirable (may include combination of hospitalists and NPs)	Desirable (may include combination of hospitalists and NPs)	Desirable (may include combination of hospitalists and NPs)
PA	• Training and expertise in pediatric critical care • Graduate of PA program • Participates in training to meet ongoing education and certification requirements	• Direct patient management with physician supervision • Performance of advanced therapeutic procedures • Participates in monitoring of quality improvement	Desirable (may include combination of hospitalists and PAs)	Desirable (may include combination of hospitalists and PAs)	Desirable (may include combination of hospitalists and PAs)

TABLE 3 Continued

Staff	Qualifications	Roles	Quaternary or Specialized	Tertiary	Community
Additional medical and surgical providers					
Pediatric medical subspecialists	• Cardiologist • Pulmonologist • Neonatologist	• Available 24 h per d	Essential	Essential	Essential
	• Nephrologist • Hematologist and/or oncologist • Endocrinologist • Gastroenterologist • Neurologist • Infectious disease specialist	• Available 24 h per d	Essential	Essential	Desirable
	Interventional cardiologist • Allergist • Geneticist • Rheumatologist • Child advocacy • Cardiovascular surgeon	• Available 24 h per d	Essential	Desirable	Optional
Pediatric surgical subspecialists	• Neurosurgeon • Otolaryngologist • Orthopedic surgeon • Ophthalmologist • Plastic surgeon • Urologist	• Available in ≤1 h to the PICU	Essential	Desirable (essential: nonpediatric)	Optional (desirable: nonpediatric)
Pediatric anesthesia	• Anesthesiologist	• Available in ≤1 h to the PICU	Essential	Essential	Desirable (essential: nonpediatric)
Pediatric radiologists	• Radiologist	• Available 24 h per d	Essential	Essential	Desirable (essential: nonpediatric)
	• Interventional radiologist	• Available 24 h per d	Essential	Essential	Desirable (essential: nonpediatric)
	• Neuroendovascular	• Available 24 h per d	Essential	Desirable	Optional
Psychiatrist or psychologist		• Available for consultation	Essential	Essential	Essential
Nursing staff					
RNs	• Bachelor of science in nursing degree preferred • Hospitals with magnet designation require <10% non-BSN RNs • Completion of PICU orientation • Continuing education requirements for licensure renewal • BLS and PALS • Pediatric CCRN certification • Maintenance of designated PICU competencies	• Provision of continuous care based on the needs and characteristics of the patient • Provision of physiologic assessments, implementation, and evaluation of responses to treatment plan • Skilled in advanced technology monitoring • Appropriate No. nurses trained in highly specialized therapies such as CRRT and roles, including: Charge nurse Arrest team nurse	Essential	Essential (desirable: pediatric CCRN certification)	Essential (desirable: pediatric CCRN certification)

TABLE 3 Continued

Staff	Qualifications	Roles	Quaternary or Specialized	Tertiary	Community
		Transport team nurse Trauma team nurse • Preceptor for novice nurses • Participates in development and monitoring of quality improvement projects			
Nurse educator or clinical nurse specialist	• Training and expertise in pediatric critical care • Master of science in nursing or education or doctorate or DNP prepared • Pediatric nursing expertise • Pediatric CCRN certification • BLS and PALS	• Participates in and coordinates nursing staff education • Clinical resource for nursing staff • Participates in development of quality improvement projects • Participates in clinical research efforts	Essential	Essential	Desirable
Nursing assistants or unlicensed personnel		• Assists RNs in patient care tasks • Supervised by nursing staff	Desirable	Desirable	Optional
Respiratory therapy staff					
Supervisor	• Registered respiratory therapist with training and expertise in pediatric critical care	• Responsible for training therapists • Clinical resource for therapists	Essential	Essential	Essential
Respiratory therapists	• Registered respiratory therapist • BLS and PALS • Demonstrate competence with pediatric mechanical ventilation • Adjunctive respiratory therapies including gases	• Therapist assigned to PICU 24 h per d • Skill in management of pediatric patients with respiratory disease • Maintenance of equipment and quality control and review	Essential	Essential	Essential
Other team members					
Pediatric pharmacist	• Pediatric clinical doctor of pharmacy	• Available 24 h per d	Essential	Essential	Desirable (essential: nonpediatric)
Rehabilitation services	• Physical therapist, occupational therapist, and speech therapist	• Available for consultation	Essential	Essential	Essential
Nutritionist or clinical dietitian		• Available for consultation	Essential	Essential	Essential
Social worker		• Available for consultation	Essential	Essential	Essential
Clergy		• Available for consultation	Essential	Essential	Essential
Child life specialist		• Available for consultation	Essential	Essential	Desirable
Pain team		• Available for consultation	Essential	Essential	Desirable
Palliative care		• Available for consultation	Essential	Desirable	Desirable
Rapid response team		• Available 24 h per d	Essential	Essential	Essential
Transport team		• Available 24 h per d	Essential	Essential	Desirable
Ethics committee		• Available for consultation	Essential	Essential	Essential
Quality and safety		• Available for consultation	Essential	Essential	Essential
Legal or risk management		• Available for consultation	Essential	Essential	Essential
Biomedical technician		• In-hospital or available within 1 h, 24 h per d	Essential	Essential	Essential
Radiology services		• Available in ≤1 h	Essential	Essential	Essential
Laboratory services		• Available 24 h per d	Essential	Essential	Essential

TABLE 3 Continued

Staff	Qualifications	Roles	Quaternary or Specialized	Tertiary	Community
		• Provide basic hematologic, chemistry, blood gas, and toxicology analysis			
Blood bank services		• Available 24 h per d	Essential	Essential	Essential
Neurodiagnostic services		• EEG available on call for emergencies	Essential	Essential	Desirable
Unit clerk		• Staffed 24 h per d	Essential	Essential	Desirable

ACGME, Accreditation Council for Graduate Medical Education; APP, advanced practice provider; BLS, basic life support; BSN, bachelor of science in nursing; CCRN, critical care registered nurse; CRRT, continuous renal replacement therapy; DNP, doctor of nursing practice; NP, nurse practitioner; PA, physician assistant; PALS, Pediatric Advanced Life Support; RN, registered nurse.

These statements were then presented via an online anonymous voting tool to a voting group by using a 3-cycle interactive forecasting Delphi method. With each cycle of voting, statements were refined on the basis of votes received and comments. Consensus was deemed achieved once 80% or higher scores from the voting group were recorded on any given statement or when there was consensus after review of comments provided by voters. Of the 25 final statements, 17 met the consensus cutoff score. The writing panel evaluated the survey data and together with literature findings formulated admission recommendations.

RECOMMENDATIONS

Critically ill or injured pediatric patients should be cared for in a child- and family-centered environment by a multidisciplinary pediatric critical care team. Three levels of care are described in these recommendations on the basis of the results of the Delphi survey and expert panel consensus: community-based PICU, tertiary PICU, and quaternary or specialized PICU.

Community medical center PICUs play an important role in health care systems that provide care to infants and children. In the previously published guidelines, these centers were categorized as level II PICUs. These units provide a broad range of services and resources that may differ on the basis of institution, hospital size, and referral base. The majority of these will be located in general medical-surgical institutions with the capability of treating pediatric patients. Tertiary PICUs provide advanced care for many medical and surgical illnesses in infants and children. In the previously published guidelines, these units were categorized as level I PICUs, as distinguished from level II PICUs. Tertiary PICUs should provide advanced ventilatory support such as high-frequency oscillatory ventilation and inotropic management but would not be expected to provide extracorporeal membrane oxygenation support. There would be ready access to most pediatric medical subspecialties but there may not be in-house coverage. A quaternary or specialized PICU facility provides regional care and serves large populations or has a large catchment area. The center should provide comprehensive care to all complex patients. Uniquely, a specialized PICU provides diagnosis-specific care for select patient populations. This highest level of PICU facility should have readily available resources to support an American College of Surgeons (ACS) verified Level I or Level II Children's Surgical Center or Level I or Level II Pediatric Trauma Center. Of note, premature newborns are not addressed in these guidelines unless they require complex cardiovascular surgical interventions.

Specific recommendations are detailed in Table 1 regarding the PICU level of care admission criteria, the structure and provider staffing model, the personnel and resources, the quality metrics and education, the equipment and technology, and the discharge and transfer criteria. Table 2 reveals the necessary resources needed for each level of care. Table 3 reveals the personnel needed, including the qualifications, competencies, roles, and responsibilities based on each level of PICU.

This practice statement and guidance address important specifications for each PICU level of care, including the team structure and resources, technology and equipment, education and training, quality metrics, admission and discharge criteria, and indications for transfer to a higher level of care. The sparse high-quality evidence led the panel to use a modified Delphi process to seek expert opinion to develop consensus-based recommendations where gaps in the evidence exist. Despite this limitation, the members of the task force believe these recommendations provide guidance to practitioners in making informed decisions regarding pediatric admission or transfer to the appropriate level of care to achieve best outcomes. Additional well-designed clinical investigations are needed to determine and address the confounding factors that impact admission, discharge, and transfer of children in all levels of PICUs.

ACKNOWLEDGMENTS

We thank the members of the previous PICU admission and levels of care guidelines task forces for their preliminary contributions. The members of the ADT task force acknowledge the limitations of this practice statement and guidance. As a result of the vast medical and health care management information to consider, constraints to evaluate rapidly available new evidence, human fallibility, and other considerations, readers should use their judgment on how best to apply our suggestions and recommendations.

ABBREVIATION

ACS: American College of Surgeons

[q]Pediatrics, Critical Care Medicine, College of Medicine, Medical Center, University of Nebraska, Omaha, Nebraska; [r]PICU, Medical City Children's Hospital, Dallas, Texas; [s]Pediatric Critical Care Medicine, Children's Hospital of Wisconsin, Wauwatosa, Wisconsin; [u]Pediatrics and Pediatric Intensive Care, Grand Strand Medical Center, Myrtle Beach, South Carolina; [w]Pediatrics and Pediatric Critical Care Medicine, Jacobi Medical Center, the Bronx, New York; and [x]Division of Medical Critical Care, Boston Children's Hospital and Harvard Medical School, Harvard University, Boston, Massachusetts

Policy statements from the American Academy of Pediatrics benefit from expertise and resources of liaisons and internal (AAP) and external reviewers. However, policy statements from the American Academy of Pediatrics may not reflect the views of the liaisons or the organizations or government agencies that they represent.

The guidance in this statement does not indicate an exclusive course of treatment or serve as a standard of medical care. Variations, taking into account individual circumstances, may be appropriate.

All policy statements from the American Academy of Pediatrics automatically expire 5 years after publication unless reaffirmed, revised, or retired at or before that time.

This document is copyrighted and is property of the American Academy of Pediatrics and its Board of Directors. All authors have filed conflict of interest statements with the American Academy of Pediatrics. Any conflicts have been resolved through a process approved by the Board of Directors. The American Academy of Pediatrics has neither solicited nor accepted any commercial involvement in the development of the content of this publication.

DOI: https://doi.org/10.1542/peds.2019-2433

Address correspondence to Benson S. Hsu, MD, MBA, FAAP. E-mail: benson.hsu@usd.edu

PEDIATRICS (ISSN Numbers: Print, 0031-4005; Online, 1098-4275).

Copyright © 2019 by the American Academy of Pediatrics

FINANCIAL DISCLOSURE: The authors have indicated they have no financial relationships relevant to this article to disclose.

FUNDING: No external funding.

POTENTIAL CONFLICT OF INTEREST: The authors have indicated they have no potential conflicts of interest to disclose.

REFERENCES

1. Committee on Hospital Care of the American Academy of Pediatrics; Pediatric Section of the Society of Critical Care Medicine. Guidelines and levels of care for pediatric intensive care units. Committee on Hospital Care of the American Academy of Pediatrics and Pediatric Section of the Society of Critical Care Medicine. *Pediatrics*. 1993; 92(1):166–175
2. Rosenberg DI, Moss MM; American College of Critical Care Medicine of the Society of Critical Care Medicine. Guidelines and levels of care for pediatric intensive care units. *Crit Care Med*. 2004;32(10):2117–2127
3. American Academy of Pediatrics, Society of Critical Care Medicine. Criteria for critical care of infants and children: PICU admission, discharge, and triage practice statement and levels of care guidance. *Crit Care Med*. 2019; in press

Fish, Shellfish, and Children's Health: An Assessment of Benefits, Risks, and Sustainability

• *Technical Report*

TECHNICAL REPORT

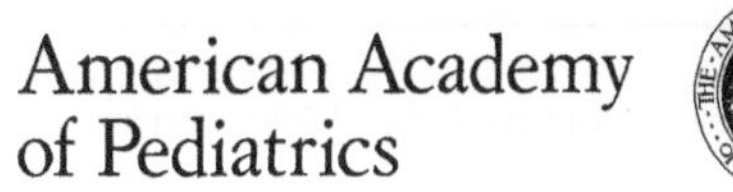
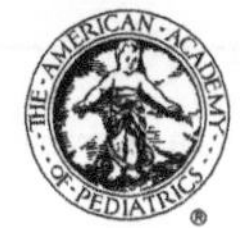

DEDICATED TO THE HEALTH OF ALL CHILDREN™

Fish, Shellfish, and Children's Health: An Assessment of Benefits, Risks, and Sustainability

Aaron S. Bernstein, MD, MPH, FAAP,[a] Emily Oken, MD, MPH,[b] Sarah de Ferranti, MD, MPH, FAAP,[c] COUNCIL ON ENVIRONMENTAL HEALTH, COMMITTEE ON NUTRITION

abstract

American children eat relatively little fish and shellfish in comparison with other sources of animal protein, despite the health benefits that eating fish and shellfish may confer. At the same time, fish and shellfish may be sources of toxicants. This report serves to inform pediatricians about available research that elucidates health risks and benefits associated with fish and shellfish consumption in childhood as well as the sustainability of fish and shellfish harvests.

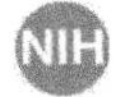

Departments of [a]Pediatrics and [c]Cardiology, Boston Children's Hospital and Harvard Medical School, Harvard University, Boston, Massachusetts; and [b]Department of Population Medicine, Harvard Pilgrim Health Care, Boston, Massachusetts

This document is copyrighted and is property of the American Academy of Pediatrics and its Board of Directors. All authors have filed conflict of interest statements with the American Academy of Pediatrics. Any conflicts have been resolved through a process approved by the Board of Directors. The American Academy of Pediatrics has neither solicited nor accepted any commercial involvement in the development of the content of this publication.

Technical reports from the American Academy of Pediatrics benefit from expertise and resources of liaisons and internal (AAP) and external reviewers. However, technical reports from the American Academy of Pediatrics may not reflect the views of the liaisons or the organizations or government agencies that they represent.

The guidance in this report does not indicate an exclusive course of treatment or serve as a standard of medical care. Variations, taking into account individual circumstances, may be appropriate.

All technical reports from the American Academy of Pediatrics automatically expire 5 years after publication unless reaffirmed, revised, or retired at or before that time.

DOI: https://doi.org/10.1542/peds.2019-0999

Address correspondence to Aaron S. Bernstein, MD, MPH, FAAP. Email: aaron.bernstein@childrens.harvard.edu

PEDIATRICS (ISSN Numbers: Print, 0031-4005; Online, 1098-4275).

Copyright © 2019 by the American Academy of Pediatrics

To cite: Bernstein AS, Oken E, de Ferranti S, AAP COUNCIL ON ENVIRONMENTAL HEALTH, AAP COMMITTEE ON NUTRITION. Fish, Shellfish, and Children's Health: An Assessment of Benefits, Risks, and Sustainability. *Pediatrics*. 2019;143(6): e20190999

Fish and shellfish are, in general, good sources of low-fat protein rich in several essential vitamins and minerals as well as, in certain instances, the essential nutrients omega-3 long-chain polyunsaturated fatty acids (n-3 LCPUFAs). Some guidance is available and accessible to pediatric health care providers or families to assist them with navigating fish and shellfish choices, but most sources focus on consumption by adults or pregnant women[1] and do not directly address childhood consumption. This report provides an overview of the potential risks and benefits associated with childhood consumption of fish and shellfish. Whenever possible, it draws on research performed with children. However, in instances when such evidence is not available, it will examine prenatal and adult evidence.

This report also addresses the sustainability of fish and shellfish choices. Approximately 90% of fisheries worldwide are exploited at or above maximum sustainable yield. As a result, any guidance on fish consumption must consider sustainability to protect the viability of fisheries.

An overview of the report can be found in Table 1.

NUTRIENT VALUE OF FISH CONSUMPTION

All fish are protein dense and have little or no sugar or saturated fat. Many species contain high levels of vitamin D and calcium. Some shellfish

TABLE 1 Technical Report Summary

In this report, we cover 4 areas related to seafood: nutrition, potential health benefits, toxicants, and sustainability. An overview of evidence in each of these areas is provided here with the sections of the report providing detail on specific studies.	
Nutrition	• Compared with other animal protein, such as beef, pork, or chicken, fish have a favorable nutrient profile (see Table 2) and are a good source of lean protein, calcium, vitamin D, and n-3 LCPUFAs.
Potential Health Benefits	Childhood fish consumption has been associated with the following: • prevention of allergic disorders. Fish oil supplement intake in childhood has been associated with the following: • reduced hospitalization and number of pain crises in sickle cell disease, based on limited data. Studies that have evaluated the effects of either childhood fish consumption and/or n-3 LCPUFA intake and had mixed (ie, positive and/or negative) or null results for the following: • treatment of ADHD symptoms; • treatment of depressive symptoms; • treatment of allergic diseases; • prevention or treatment of inflammatory bowel disease flares; • cognitive development, including memory, processing speed, and IQ; • hyperlipidemia; and • prevention or treatment of hypertension. For some diseases, evidence suggests that fish oil supplementation may benefit children who have below average n-3 LCPUFA levels. Studies that have revealed benefits from fish oil supplementation often rely on daily administration of high-dose formulations, which may be difficult for children to comply with. Fish oil supplements sold in the United States are not FDA approved, and as such, their contents may not be as advertised on the product label.
Toxicants	• Some fish species can be a source of MeHg, which can damage the developing nervous system in utero. • Many accessible resources provide guidance on which species of which to limit intake or avoid (see Resources). • POPs, such as PCBs, can be found in fish, especially in fish caught in freshwater; other animal protein sources may contain as much PCBs and other POPs as many fish and shellfish. • Fish and shellfish captured in freshwater bodies in the United States may have high concentrations of pollutants and populations that regularly consume freshwater fish, and shellfish may be at higher risk of harms from these toxicants.
Sustainability	• Approximately 30% of global fish stocks are overexploited; a further 60% are harvested at or near their maximum sustainable yield. Medical and governmental organizations have encouraged greater seafood consumption for Americans, which may add pressure to declining wild fisheries and promote unsustainable aquaculture practice. • Shrimp is the most commonly consumed seafood in the United States; much of the shrimp comes from highly unsustainable overseas fisheries, which exact heavy environmental and human tolls. • US fisheries, wild or farmed, are some of the best managed in the world, even if not all are sustainably harvested. • In comparison with conventional red meat production in the United States, most wild catch fisheries and best practice aquaculture have favorable water, greenhouse gas, and pollution footprints.

species have high iron content. Other trace nutrients, such as selenium and iodine, are present in many fish and shellfish species as well. The health benefits of consumption of these nutrients have been documented extensively elsewhere[2–7] and will not be reviewed here, but a summary table describing which fish and shellfish species provide various nutrients is provided in Table 2.

Some fish are a rich source of the n-3 LCPUFAs, eicosapentaenoic acid (EPA), and docosahexaenoic acid (DHA). n-3 LCPUFAs are essential nutrients and, as such, must be consumed in the diet. Humans also can elongate and desaturate short-chain "parent" polyunsaturated fatty acids such as linoleic acid, present in nuts and seeds, into LCPUFAs, but this process is inefficient and unlikely to result in sufficient levels for optimal health among most individuals.[8] Fish are the primary natural dietary source for DHA and EPA. These fatty acids can also be concentrated from algal sources and in this form have been added to infant formula and foods such as milk, yogurt, and pasta and increasingly are taken as supplements. n-3 LCPUFAs are structural components of neurons in the brain and eye and have anti-inflammatory and immunomodulatory properties, and many researchers have investigated the potential benefits of fish or n-3 LCPUFA consumption in early life for neurodevelopmental and atopic outcomes, which are summarized in later sections of this report.

STUDIES OF FISH CONSUMPTION

Prevention of Allergic Disease

The majority of observational studies conducted to date have shown that maternal fish consumption likely

TABLE 2 Nutritional and Toxicant Contents for Various Animal Based Foods (Per 100 g Raw, Unless Otherwise Specified)

	Kcal	Protein (g)	Total fat (g) (rounded to nearest whole No.)	Sat fat (g) (rounded to nearest whole No.)	Cholesterol (mg)	DHA + EPA omega-3 (mg)	Calcium (mg)	Vitamin D (IU)	Iron (mg)	Mercury mean[a] (CV) mg/kg (ppm)[b]
Fish										
Catfish	95	16	3	1	58	364	14	500	0.3	0.118 (4.97)
Atlantic cod	82	18	1	0	43	184	16	36	0.4	0.070 (3.70)
Flounder	70	12	2	0	45	245	21	113	0.2	0.119 (3.42)
Haddock	74	16	1	0	54	131	11	18	0.2	0.164 (4.59)
Halibut (Pacific)	91	19	1	0	49	194	7	190	0.8	0.261 (4.32)
Pangasius, swai, or basa[c]	74	15	2	0	36	0	10	54	0.1	[d]
Pollock, Alaskan[e]	70	17	0	0	61	62	15	73	0.22	0.58 (5.93)
Rainbow trout (wild)	119	20	3	1	59	587	67	265[f]	0.7	0.344 (3.00)
Salmon (farmed Atlantic)	208	20	13	3	55	1866	9	441	0.3	0.026 (2.91)
Salmon (wild Alaskan Chinook or King)	187	20	12	2	61	1150	42	425[g]	0.8	0.067 (1.59)
Sardine, Atlantic canned in oil, with bone	208	25	11	2	142	1480	382	193	2.9	0.079 (2.56)
Swordfish	144	20	7	2	66	754	5	558	0.4	0.893 (2.30)
Tilapia	96	20	2	1	50	91	10	124	0.6	0.019 (4.99)
Tuna (albacore, canned in water)	128	24	3	1	42	862	14	80[h]	1.0	0.328 (2.92)
Tuna (light or skipjack, canned in water)	116	26	1	0	30	281	11	47	1.5	0.118 (2.55)
Tuna (yellowfin)	109	24	1	0	39	100	4	69	0.8	0.143 (4.80)
Shellfish										
Blue crab	87	18	1	0	78	549	89	0	0.7	0.110 (5.40)
Clams[i]	86	15	1	0	30	107	39	1	1.6	0.028
Lobster	77	17	1	0	127	176	84	0	0.3	0.153 (2.06)
Scallops	69	12	3	0	24	106	6	1	0.4	0.40 (3.65)
Shrimp	85	20	1	0	161	61	64	0	1.62	0.053 (4.03)
Other animal protein										
Bologna (beef)	299	11	26	10	57	4	21	28	1.3	ND
Chicken breast with skin	172	21	9	3	64	30	11	16	0.7	0[j]
Chicken leg with skin	214	16	16	4	79	14	8	2	0.7	0[f]
Eggs	143	6	5	3	186	58	56	82	1.8	0[f]
Milk, whole (with vitamin D supplemented)	61	3	3	2	10	0	113	51	0	0[f] (NA)
Pork chops, meat and fat	170	20	9	3	69	0	19	21	0.63	ND
Sirloin steak, trimmed to 1/8" fat	201	20	13	5	75	0	24	7[k]	1.61	ND

Nutritional data from US Department of Agriculture Food Composition Database unless otherwise noted (https://ndb.nal.usda.gov/ndb/foods). Typical seafood serving size (84 g/3 oz). Recommended daily allowances: Vitamin D: 600 IU, ages 1–18 years, male or female. Calcium: 0–6 months, 200 mg; 7–12 months, 260 mg; 1–3 years, 700 mg; 4–8 years, 1 g; 9–18 years, 1.3 g. Iron: 0–6 months, 0.27 mg; 7–12 months, 11 g; 1–3 years, 7 mg; 4–8 years, 10 mg; 9–13 years, 8 mg; 14–18 years, 11–15 mg (male or female); pregnant women, 27 mg; lactating women, 10 mg. CV, coefficient of variation; NA, not applicable; ND, no data.

[a] Mercury data from Karimi R, Fitzgerald TP, Fisher NS. A quantitative synthesis of mercury in commercial seafood and implications for exposure in the United States. *Environ Health Perspect.* 2012;120(11):1512–1519. The FDA has set an action level of 1 ppm per edible portion. Fish that exceed this level may be pulled from the marketplace by the FDA.

[b] More detailed information on mercury content of seafood can be found in Table 3.

[c] Data from UK Department of Health Analysis of Fish and Fish Products, 2013. Available at: https://www.gov.uk/government/uploads/system/uploads/attachment_data/file/167923/Nutrient_analysis_of_fish_and_fish_products_-_Analytical_Report.pdf.

[d] No reliable data available. Available at: http://www.seafoodhealthfacts.org/description-top-commercial-seafood-items/pangasius for more information on Pangasius.

[e] Omega 3, calcium, vitamin D, and iron data from Canada's nutrient profile database, as values were unavailable from US Department of Agriculture. Available at: https://food-nutrition.canada.ca/cnf-fce/index-eng.jsp.

[f] Vitamin D data from Canada's nutrient profile database, as values were unavailable from US Department of Agriculture. Available at: https://food-nutrition.canada.ca/cnf-fce/index-eng.jsp.

[g] Vitamin D content for wild Chinook salmon obtained from Nutrition Canada's nutrient profile database, as values were unavailable from US Department of Agriculture. Available at: https://food-nutrition.canada.ca/cnf-fce/index-eng.jsp.

[h] Vitamin D data from Canada's nutrient profile database, as values were unavailable from US Department of Agriculture. Available at https://food-nutrition.canada.ca/cnf-fce/index-eng.jsp.

[i] US Department of Agriculture nutrition information based on "mixed" species. Mercury data for clams includes softshell, Pacific littleneck, cockle, geoduck, and hard.

[j] Data from FDA Market Basket studies 1996–2011. Available at: http://www.fda.gov/downloads/Food/FoodScienceResearch/TotalDietStudy/UCM184301.pdf.

[k] Vitamin D data from Canada's nutrient profile database as values unavailable from US Department of Agriculture. Available at https://food-nutrition.canada.ca/cnf-fce/index-eng.jsp.

TABLE 3 MeHg Content of Selected Fish (Adapted from Karimi et al)

Seafood Item	Grand			
	Mean Hg (ppm) a	Samples (Total) b	SDw	SEw
Anchovies (all)	0.103	455	0.197	0.041
Bass (Chilean)	0.357	100	0.185	0.041
Bass (freshwater, all)	0.170	149	0.361	0.059
Bass (saltwater, black, white, striped)	0.288	1660	1.004	0.150
Bass, striped (all)	0.285	1367	1.155	0.140
Bass, striped (farmed)	0.028	15	NA	NA
Bass, striped (wild)	0.295	1311	1.147	0.134
Bluefish	0.351	1019	0.965	0.145
Butterfish	0.054	109	0.112	0.021
Carp (all)	0.156	477	0.521	0.095
Catfish (all)	0.118	1757	0.586	0.087
Catfish (wild, all species)	0.144	1396	0.513	0.078
Catfish, channel (wild)	0.120	521	0.253	0.038
Catfish (farmed, all species)	0.012	320	0.073	0.008
Clams (all)	0.028	1027	0.177	0.032
Clams, hard	0.047	181	0.130	0.026
Clams, geoduck	0.030	11	0.049	0.021
Clams, cockle	0.054	122	0.404	0.073
Clams, Pacific littleneck	0.022	18	0.022	0.009
Clams, softshell	0.016	471	0.249	0.020
Cod (all)	0.087	2115	0.358	0.038
Cod, Atlantic (farmed)	0.034	24	NA	NA
Cod, Atlantic (wild)	0.070	1452	0.261	0.017
Cod, Pacific	0.144	431	0.260	0.038
Crab (all)	0.098	1564	0.453	0.086
Crab (blue, king, and snow)	0.095	1087	0.526	0.098
Crab, blue	0.110	864	0.594	0.103
Crab, Dungeness	0.120	264	0.225	0.037
Crab, king	0.027	203	0.154	0.032
Crab, snow	0.110	20	0.187	0.073
Crawfish (all)	0.034	206	0.104	0.019
Croaker (all)	0.092	856	0.308	0.058
Croaker, Atlantic	0.069	572	0.135	0.025
Croaker, white	0.169	193	0.344	0.066
Cuttlefish	0.134	156	0.275	0.085
Eel (all)	0.186	986	0.608	0.111
Eel (wild)	0.216	659	0.551	0.110
Eel (farmed)	0.066	220	0.163	0.027
Flatfish (flounder, plaice, sole)	0.110	3070	0.417	0.079
Flounder (all)	0.119	1687	0.406	0.075
Flounder, summer	0.121	427	0.216	0.042
Flounder, windowpane	0.152	84	0.152	0.037
Flounder, winter	0.070	302	0.228	0.039
Freshwater perch (all)	0.141	1295	0.745	0.110
Grouper (all)	0.417	643	0.804	0.196
Haddock (all)	0.164	226	0.752	0.166
Hake (all)	0.146	739	0.489	0.090
Halibut (all)	0.254	3532	0.703	0.060
Halibut, Pacific	0.261	3111	1.127	0.053
Halibut, Greenland	0.183	138	0.630	0.120
Herring (all)	0.043	1277	0.174	0.026
Herring, Atlantic	0.037	973	0.119	0.015
Herring, Pacific	0.060	194	0.300	0.048
Lingcod	0.363	333	0.952	0.128
Lobster (all)	0.153	344	0.315	0.070
Lobster, American	0.200	142	0.367	0.075
Lobster, spiny	0.100	62	0.137	0.035
Mackerel (all)	0.586	2481	3.237	0.450
Mackerel, Atlantic	0.045	191	0.192	0.037

influences risk of atopy in offspring.[9] Available research also suggests that eating fish early in life can prevent certain allergic diseases, including asthma, eczema, and allergic rhinitis.

In more than a dozen observational studies, the associations of fish consumption in infancy and childhood with atopy risk have been evaluated. In a prospective observational study of more than 4000 Swedish infants who did not have eczema or recurrent wheeze in the first year of life, Kull et al[10] found a dose-dependent association of greater fish consumption with lower risks for asthma, eczema, allergic rhinitis, and sensitization, even when controlling for smoking, maternal age, existence of parental allergies, and breastfeeding. They also found an inverse association between age at introduction of fish and atopy risk: children who consumed fish between 3 and 8 months of age had lower risks for asthma (adjusted odds ratio [OR], 0.73; 95% confidence interval [CI]: 0.55 to 0.97), eczema (adjusted OR, 0.77; 95% CI: 0.64 to 0.92), allergic rhinitis (adjusted OR, 0.77; 95% CI: 0.60 to 0.97), and allergic sensitization (adjusted OR, 0.78; 95% CI: 0.64 to 0.95) compared with children introduced to fish at 9 months or older. A subsequent study of this cohort found that the benefits of consuming 2 or more fish meals per month by age 1 extended to 12 years of age.[11]

Further research corroborates the potential for early fish consumption having durable protective effects. Goksör et al[12] found that introduction of fish before 9 months of age independently reduced the risk (adjusted OR, 0.6; 95% CI: 0.4 to 0.96) of current atopic asthma (defined by respiratory symptoms plus positive skin prick test result) at school age. A 2013 meta-analysis of 3 studies found that fish consumption in infancy was inversely related to childhood asthma incidence, with children who ate the most fish having

TABLE 3 Continued

Seafood Item	Grand			
	Mean Hg (ppm) a	Samples (Total) b	SDw	SEw
Mackerel, chub	0.099	129	0.166	0.033
Mackerel, king	1.101	821	3.470	0.383
Mackerel, Spanish	0.440	1168	1.105	0.097
Marlin (all)	1.517	821	7.495	1.654
Marlin, blue	2.465	364	9.532	2.120
Marlin, striped	0.861	179	2.356	0.528
Marlin, white	0.695	56	0.518	0.120
Monkfish	0.174	92	0.117	0.024
Mullet	0.050	638	0.152	0.027
Mussels (all)	0.028	755	0.106	0.016
Ocean perch	0.117	262	0.421	0.082
Orange roughy	0.513	152	0.569	0.103
Oysters (all)	0.020	5310	0.178	0.013
Oysters, Eastern	0.018	4573	0.161	0.009
Oysters, Pacific	0.039	290	0.171	0.025
Pike	0.404	1374	1.328	0.101
Plaice	0.148	282	0.576	0.137
Pollock (all)	0.058	540	0.342	0.059
Pollock, Atlantic	0.160	79	0.330	0.053
Pollock, Pacific/Alaska	0.050	235	0.145	0.027
Porgy	0.065	169	0.143	0.027
Sablefish	0.243	477	0.620	0.080
Salmon (all)	0.048	2818	0.143	0.023
Salmon, Atlantic (farmed)	0.026	145	0.077	0.020
Salmon, Atlantic (wild)	0.058	95	0.083	0.015
Salmon, Chinook, farmed	0.017	4	0.024	0.017
Salmon, Chinook, wild	0.067	580	0.106	0.013
Salmon, chum	0.046	456	0.139	0.018
Salmon, coho	0.044	567	0.065	0.007
Salmon, pink	0.037	222	0.064	0.009
Salmon, sockeye	0.039	396	0.026	0.004
Salmon (canned)	0.035	61	0.042	0.012
Sardine (all)	0.079	1007	0.201	0.036
Scallops (all)	0.040	336	0.148	0.033
Seabass, black	0.120	139	0.118	0.032
Shad (all)	0.077	93	0.099	0.031
Shad, American	0.067	76	0.095	0.019
Shark (all)	0.882	3722	2.504	0.462
Shark, blacktip	0.882	250	1.249	0.274
Shark, blue	0.664	50	1.516	0.480
Shark, mako	1.259	166	1.995	0.464
Shark, sandbar	0.869	115	1.141	0.301
Shark, thresher	0.622	119	1.874	0.421
Shrimp (all)	0.053	935	0.212	0.038
Shrimp, brown	0.077	72	0.083	0.053
Shrimp, pink	0.083	49	0.079	0.024
Shrimp, white	0.057	113	0.136	0.016
Skate (all)	0.138	70	0.093	0.036
Smelt	0.025	175	0.086	0.019
Snapper (all)	0.230	1244	0.514	0.104
Snapper, gray	0.233	699	0.595	0.068
Snapper, red	0.243	279	0.725	0.168
Sole	0.086	1101	0.310	0.056
Squid	0.044	728	0.130	0.024
Swordfish	0.893	1726	2.052	0.296
Tilapia	0.019	129	0.097	0.027
Tilefish (all)	0.883	109	2.962	0.695
Tilefish, Atlantic	0.171	47	0.195	0.049
Tilefish, Gulf of Mexico	1.445	61	0.324	0.059

a 25% lower risk of developing asthma than those who ate the least.[13]

Another prospective cohort of Swedish infants found that introduction of fish between 6 and 8 months of age substantially reduced rates of infantile eczema (OR, 0.6; 95% CI: 0.5 to 0.7; $P < .001$), and children who did not consume fish were 2.7 times more likely to have eczema than those who ate fish 3 or more times a week (95% CI: 1.80 to 4.13; $P < .001$).[14] Oien et al[15] found that infants who ate fish once a week or more were 38% less likely to have eczema at 2 years. In this study, the mean age of introducing fish was 9 months. In contrast, in a trial among 123 pregnant women who were randomly assigned to consume 2 weekly servings of salmon or their usual diet low in fish, there was no difference in rates of infantile eczema at 6 months.[16]

Results from other studies (eg, Hesselmar et al[17]) support the potential for early introduction of fish to prevent other allergic disease, such as allergic rhinitis. Alm et al[14] found that children who were given fish before 9 months were half as likely to develop allergic rhinitis by 4.5 years of age in a prospective cohort of Swedish children.

Of note, some evidence suggests that prenatal shellfish consumption (as opposed to finfish) may increase risk of food allergy. In their analysis of early childhood diet, Pelé et al[18] found that maternal prenatal shellfish intake at least once a month was associated with a higher risk of any food allergy before age 2 (adjusted OR, 1.62; 95% CI: 1.11 to 2.37) compared with intake less than once per month while controlling for fish intake. Leermakers et al[19] similarly found that 1 to 13 g of shellfish consumption per week, on average, during the first trimester of pregnancy marginally increased risk of childhood wheezing and eczema

TABLE 3 Continued

Seafood Item	Grand			
	Mean Hg (ppm) a	Samples (Total) b	SDw	SEw
Trout (freshwater, wild and unknown status)	0.344	2804	1.030	0.087
Trout, lake	0.349	2748	1.268	0.080
Trout (freshwater, farmed)	0.029	178	0.066	0.015
Tuna (fresh/frozen, all)	0.450	3780	1.619	0.340
Tuna, albacore	0.317	296	0.475	0.103
Tuna, Atlantic bonito	0.499	263	2.200	0.359
Tuna, bigeye	0.582	376	1.113	0.222
Tuna, blackfin	0.856	159	0.972	0.231
Tuna, bluefin (farmed)	0.455	108	0.540	0.156
Tuna, bluefin (wild)	0.796	514	2.408	0.542
Tuna, skipjack	0.198	341	0.320	0.083
Tuna, yellowfin	0.270	1183	0.797	0.125
Tuna, albacore (canned)	0.328	1362	0.955	0.113
Tuna, light (canned or packed)	0.118	972	0.300	0.038
Tuna, yellowfin (canned)	0.143	298	0.688	0.098
Weakfish/seatrout (all)	0.361	2105	1.348	0.193
Whitefish (all)	0.106	2721	0.707	0.051
Whiting	0.040	27	0.056	0.015

Adapted from Karimi R, Fitzgerald TP, Fisher NS. A quantitative synthesis of mercury in commercial seafood and implications for exposure in the United States. Environ Health Perspect. 2012;120(11):1512–1519. NA, not applicable; SEw, weighted SE; SDw, weighted SD.

(OR, 1.20; 95% CI: 1.04 to 1.40; OR, 1.18; 95% CI: 1.01 to 1.37, respectively) after controlling for fish intake.

Regarding the timing of introduction of fish and the risks related to atopic disease, a 2008 American Academy of Pediatrics clinical report revised previous guidance, which had recommended delaying consumption until 3 years for infants and children with a strong family history of allergic disease.[20] The 2008 guidance states that the evidence is not adequate to delay introduction of foods beyond 4 to 6 months.[21] More research is needed to clarify the effects of earlier introduction of fish and shellfish, particularly to at-risk infants.

STUDIES OF N-3 LCPUFA SUPPLEMENTATION

Prevention of Allergic Disease

Results of observational studies, such as those cited previously, have suggested that fish consumption in early childhood may protect against allergic disease, but they are subject to unmeasured confounding.

Randomized trials in which children are assigned to fish consumption or placebo are implausible, but such trials can be completed with n-3 LCPUFAs delivered via fish oil supplements. Such studies can help determine if n-3 LCPUFAs may account for allergy prevention as well as other health outcomes that may be associated with fish consumption.

The results of all fish oil trials carry caveats. First, although the studies cited here used fish oil supplements in which the contents were standardized (although substantially different doses of EPA and DHA were used across studies), no assurance exists that over-the-counter supplements sold in the United States contain fatty acids in the amounts and types specified on the labels. Second, studies tend to use high doses of n-3 LCPUFAs, which may not be well tolerated by children. A recent review of 75 fish oil supplement studies in children found dropout rates of 17% and adherence rates of 85%, although most studies lacked adequate data on measures of compliance.[22] Last, adverse events are not routinely reported. Although generally thought to be benign, fish oil supplements may carry certain risks, such as elevated low-density lipoprotein (LDL) cholesterol.[23] Among possible side effects, weight gain has most often not been a consequence of fish oil supplementation, although some longitudinal studies, especially of children born prematurely, have documented greater weight in those receiving supplements (for example, Kennedy et al[24]).

A Cochrane systematic review analyzed data from 8 randomized controlled trials of pre- and postnatal fish oil supplementation for effects on childhood allergy. These studies evaluated food allergy, eczema, allergic rhinitis, and/or asthma (or wheeze). The metanalysis conducted found that among children born to women who consumed fish oil supplements, immunoglobulin E (IgE)-mediated food allergy was less likely in children younger than 1 year (relative risk [RR] 0.13; 95% CI: 0.02 to 0.95), and any IgE-mediated allergy was less likely in children 12 to 36 months of age (RR 0.66; 95% CI: 0.44 to 0.98). No benefit was observed for eczema, allergic rhinitis, or asthma between birth and 3 years of age. Findings did not differ based on maternal history of asthma or prenatal or postnatal supplementation of the mother.[25]

Since that review, 2 randomized trials have been published. The first is a follow-up to one of the trials included in the Cochrane review. The original study began in 1990[26] and randomly assigned 533 women to consume a fish oil supplement, olive oil, or no oil capsules after 30 weeks' gestation. At 24 years' follow-up, adults born to mothers who received supplementation were less likely to need medications for asthma as compared with individuals born to mothers who received olive oil supplements (hazard ratio, 0.54; 95% CI: 0.32 to 0.90).[27] A second randomized trial of n-3 LCPUFA supplementation among more than 700 women in the third trimester of pregnancy found that supplementation reduced symptoms of asthma at 3 years of age (hazard ratio, 0.69; 95% CI: 0.49 to 0.97) and especially among children born to women who had the lowest serum n-3 LCPUFA levels at study entry.[28]

If a protective effect against asthma and allergy of n-3 LCPUFAs or of fish consumption exists, an outstanding question is when the optimal time of introduction may be. Studies suggest that introduction before 9 months of age may be preferable to postponing until 1 year.[12,14,29]

Treatment of Allergic Disease

The potential of fish and fish oil to prevent allergic disease raises the question as to whether they may be effective treatments for allergic disease. Few studies have investigated these questions. Hodge et al[30] found that among a group of 39 children 8 to 12 years of age, supplementation with n-3 LCPUFA did not affect lung function, day or night symptoms, peak flow rates, or medication use at 3 or 6 months after the start of the intervention. Similarly, no effect on allergic outcomes including sensitization, eczema, asthma, or food allergy was found in a randomized study of 420 infants born to Australian women with history of atopy.[31] In this study, infants received daily supplements from birth to 6 months and dropout rates were substantially higher in the fish oil supplement arm as compared with the placebo arm of the study (28.4% vs 16.8%).

In a study of 29 Japanese children with prolonged hospitalization for severe asthma, fish oil supplementation over 10 months reduced sensitivity to acetylcholine and induced bronchospasm as well as asthmatic symptoms based on a standardized asthma severity scale. Despite the small size of this study, it had several unique strengths. The children in this study largely received the same diet, air to breathe, and other potential exposures because they shared the same environment. They were also monitored by nurses and physicians in the hospital who assessed them with standardized outcome measures.[32]

Inflammatory Bowel Disease

The anti-inflammatory properties of n-3 LCPUFAs have prompted research on whether they may ameliorate or prevent inflammatory diseases, including Crohn disease and ulcerative colitis. A recent Cochrane review evaluated 6 studies on the use of fish oil supplements to maintain remission in Crohn disease. When all studies were considered, a benefit was observed of n-3 LCPUFA therapy for maintenance of remission at 12 months (RR, 0.77; 95% CI: 0.61 to 0.98). However, these 6 studies had heterogenous results ($I^2 = 0.58$), leading the reviewers to perform an analysis of the 2 most robust studies that had less potential bias. With just these 2 studies, the point estimate of the RR remained below 1, but the 95% CI crossed the null.[33] Of note, in the studies reviewed, only 1 was conducted with children. In this study, 38 children were randomly assigned to receive acetylsalicylic acid along with n-3 LCPUFAs or acetylsalicylic acid with an olive oil supplement every day for a year. Children receiving n-3 LCPUFAs had lower relapse rates at 1 year (61 vs 95%).[34]

Costea et al[35] recently published an observational analysis of 182 children with Crohn disease in which they assessed whether dietary intake of n-3 and omega-6 (n-6) fatty acids may interact with variants of genes that regulate fatty acid metabolism to affect susceptibility to Crohn disease. They found that children who consumed a higher dietary ratio of n-6/n-3 fatty acids were more susceptible to Crohn disease if they were also carriers of specific variants of CYP4F3 and FADS2 genes, which are both involved in the metabolism of polyunsaturated fatty acids.[35]

Metanalyses have not found clinical benefit of fish oil supplementation for ulcerative colitis, either for induction therapy or maintenance of remission,[36–38] although the data in these analyses come exclusively from adult studies.

Neurologic and Cognitive Development

LCPUFAs, especially DHA, are essential structural components of the brain and eye. Animal studies have shown that severe deprivation can result in blindness and impaired cognitive development.[39] Only 1 study has directly assessed the value of childhood consumption of fish or shellfish consumption in childhood for neurodevelopment. In that study, 232 Norwegian kindergarteners were randomly assigned to consume fatty fish (herring or mackerel) or meat (chicken, lamb, and/or beef) 3 times a week for 16 weeks. When controlling for the amount of fish or meat the children otherwise ate, children randomly assigned to consume fish scored higher on the Wechsler Preschool and Primary Scale of Intelligence, third edition (WPPSI-III) (fish 20.4; 95% CI: 17.5 to 23.3, vs meat 15.2; 95% CI: 12.4 to 18.0; $P = .0060$).[40] A separate randomized study evaluated the effect of fish consumption on attention and processing speed among adolescents but the study had poor compliance.[41] No trials have evaluated longer-term effects of childhood fish intake.

Some observational studies suggest that maternal prenatal consumption of fish may benefit neurodevelopment. Hibbeln et al,[42] for example, investigated a cohort of 11 875 women who had seafood consumption assessed at 32 weeks' gestation. After controlling for confounders, including prenatal smoking and psychosocial stressors via a family adversity index,* these investigators found that seafood intake during pregnancy of less than 340 g per week was associated with higher risk of children being in the lowest quartile for verbal IQ (no seafood consumption compared with mothers who consumed more than 340 g per week: OR, 1.48; 95% CI: 1.16 to 1.90; 1–340 g seafood consumption per week compared with no seafood consumption: OR, 1.09; 95% CI: 0.92 to 1.29, a nonsignificant result, but for the overall trend in consumption, $P = .004$). Low maternal seafood intake was also associated with increased risk of worse outcomes for prosocial behavior, fine motor, communication, and social development scores.[42]

In addition, Oken et al[43] found among a cohort of 25 446 Danish children that higher maternal prenatal fish intake and greater duration of breastfeeding were each independently associated with improved development in multiple domains at 18 months after controlling for socioeconomic status, smoking, maternal depression, and other relevant covariates.

In the US-based Project Viva cohort, Oken et al[44,45] have found that maternal prenatal fish consumption above 2 weekly servings was associated with better cognition during infancy and early childhood. The best cognitive test scores were seen among children of mothers who ate more fish but had lower mercury levels. More recently, they followed the same cohort to midchildhood (6–10 years) and saw no evidence of either benefit from prenatal fish intake or harm from prenatal mercury exposure, suggesting perhaps that intervening factors during childhood might attenuate the influence of these prenatal exposures.[46]

Several other studies have investigated the effects of n-3 LCPUFA supplementation on neurodevelopment and cognitive skills and whether they may be of use to improve academic performance.[47–53] Results of such research are mixed and have been summarized by Joffre et al.[54]

A study of 154 Arctic Quebecois Inuit children 10 to 13 years of age found that those with higher cord blood n-3 LCPUFA concentrations had shorter FN400 latency and larger late positive component amplitude,† findings that suggest these children had more robust memory responses to stimuli.[55]

A randomized controlled crossover trial of 409 Aboriginal Australian children aged 6 to 12 years found that fish oil supplement administered over 40 weeks resulted in more advanced drawings in the Draw-A-Person test (a global measure of cognitive maturity and intellectual ability) compared with administration of a placebo containing palm oil and a trace of fish oil to provide odor and taste consistent with the experimental treatment.[56]

Another study evaluated 183 second-grade children from Northern Cape Province of South Africa randomly assigned to consume fish flour-based spread or placebo made from pulverized rusk (twice-baked bread) over 6 months. Dropout rates were similar (about 10%) in both groups. In an intention-to-treat analysis, those children who consumed the fish flour spread containing DHA and EPA had better recognition and discrimination of words as assessed by the *Hopkins Verbal Learning Test* (estimated effect size, 0.80; 95% CI: 0.15 to 1.45; and estimated effect size, 1.10; 95% CI: 0.30 to 1.91, respectively). They also performed better on the spelling portion of the *Hopkins Verbal Learning Test* (estimated effect size, 2.81 points; 95% CI: 0.59 to 5.02).[57] This study contrasts with findings from a randomized trial of 183 children from Jakarta, Indonesia, and Adelaide, South Australia, which found no effect of DHA and EPA supplementation on similar outcomes.[58] Such opposing results may reflect the baseline levels of DHA and EPA in the population studied, with greater benefit to those with lower levels at baseline.

Richardson et al[59] have found in a randomized trial that supplementation with n-3 LCPUFA (derived from algae) improved reading skills in a cohort of 74 healthy children 7 to 9 years of age from the United Kingdom through supplementation with n-3 LCPUFA (derived from algae) whose baseline reading performance was in the lowest quintile.

In a notable study that did not show a benefit of supplementation, Makrides et al[60] conducted a double-blind, multicenter, randomized controlled trial of 2399 Australian women to determine if increasing DHA during the last half of pregnancy affects maternal depression or the neurodevelopment of their children. Mothers received fish oil capsules providing 800 mg/day of DHA or matched vegetable oil placebo without DHA from study entry to birth. Children were assessed at 18 months by using the Bayley Scales of Infant and Toddler Development. Maternal supplementation neither improved depressive symptoms nor early childhood language or cognitive development.[60] Follow-up of this cohort at 7 years of age likewise found no effect of supplementation in infancy.[61,62]

* The index is a 38-point battery of questions that cover a broad array of psychosocial variables including housing security, exposure to crime and violence, substance abuse, maternal mental health, and income.

† The FN400 latency refers to a finding on EEG associated with the brain's response to an external stimulus. A shorter latency implies faster processing of stimuli input. The late positive component on EEG assesses explicit recognition memory with larger amplitude associated with better memory retrieval.

Behavioral and Mental Health

Ample evidence from animal studies makes clear that extreme deficiencies in n-3 LCPUFA during gestation or early life can profoundly and adversely affect the developing brain, and several observational studies in children have identified low levels of n-3 PUFAs to be associated with cognitive and/or behavioral problems.[63–65] Despite these findings, studies of whether n-3 LCPUFA may be of value in the management or treatment of a variety of conditions, including attention-deficit/hyperactivity disorder (ADHD), Tourette disorder,[66] or depression, have found supplementation to be, at best, of limited value.

ADHD

In 2011, Bloch and Qawasmi[67] conducted a meta-analysis to estimate the potential effect of n-3 LCPUFA supplementation on ADHD symptoms. They included 10 trials involving 699 children and identified a small effect of n-3 LCPUFA supplementation for ADHD (standardized mean difference [SMD], 0.31; 95% CI: 0.16 to 0.47), with higher doses of EPA yielding greater improvement in ADHD symptoms (β = .36; 95% CI: 0.01 to 0.72; t = 2.30; P = .04, R^2 = 0.37). These benefits were modest in comparison with those observed with standard pharmacotherapy. However, a 2012 Cochrane review that evaluated 13 trials with more than 1000 participants found no benefit of n-3 LCPUFA supplementation on ADHD symptoms in children.[68] Bloch and Qawasmi's[67] meta-analysis and the Cochrane review evaluated much of the same evidence.

In a 2014 double-blind randomized controlled trial of 95 children with ADHD diagnoses based on *Diagnostic and Statistical Manual of Mental Disorders, Fourth Edition* criteria, participants were assigned to n-3 LCPUFA supplementation or placebo over 16 weeks. Supplementation resulted in an improvement in working memory (pretrial, 97.51 ± 10.04; posttrial, 101.78 ± 11.47; F = 5.54; P = .019) and digit span (pretrial, 12.46 ± 2.42; posttrial, 14.11 ± 2.78; F = 9.73; P = .003) compared with placebo, as assessed by the HAWIK-IV scale.[69]

Several other more recent studies, including randomized trials, have produced conflicting results, making firm conclusions about the efficacy of supplementation for management of ADHD difficult.[70–72]

Depression

n-3 LCPUFAs have been studied in the prevention and treatment of depression in both adults and children. The rationale behind n-3 LCPUFAs use is that their anti-inflammatory effects, their importance to neuroplasticity and neurogenesis, and their ability to affect serotonin and dopamine signaling in the brain, which might influence mood.[73] A recent meta-analysis by Grosso et al[74] of 11 randomized controlled trials enrolling mostly adult patients with major depression or depressive symptoms showed that DHA and EPA supplementation resulted in a pooled (DHA and EPA) SMD of 0.38 (95% CI: 0.18 to 0.59), which suggests a beneficial effect of n-3 fatty acids on depressed mood compared with placebo. Other meta-analyses have not found a beneficial effect and suggest that positive results are attributable to publication bias and methodologic shortcomings.[75] Grosso et al[74] suggest that such findings may relate to heterogeneity in symptoms and/or diagnoses in research subjects and formulations of fatty acid supplements, which they assert were better addressed in their study.

Cross-sectional pediatric studies have demonstrated lower erythrocyte DHA levels in patients with major depression.[76,77] Trials that have explored whether fish consumption was associated with depressive symptoms have had mixed results,[78,79] as have trials in which n-3 LCPUFAs were used in treatment of depression in children.[77,80]

Sickle Cell Disease

LCPUFAs have been shown to improve the membrane flexibility of red blood cells in animals and humans,[81,82] prompting interest in whether they may be of benefit to patients with sickle cell disease. Two studies have examined the potential of n-3 LCPUFAs to ameliorate symptoms of sickle cell disease. Tomer et al[83] conducted a randomized controlled trial in 2001, showing that supplementation reduced the number of pain crises from 7.8 to 3.1 per year in a small sample of sickle cell patients. A larger study of 128 Sudanese children and adults ranging from 2 to 24 years found that n-3 LCPUFA supplementation more than halved pain episodes (4.6 to 2.7 per year, $P < .01$) and decreased hospitalization for pain crisis from a median of 1 to 0 per year ($P < .0001$). Severe anemia was reduced from 16.4% to 3.2% per year and transfusion from 16.4% to 4.5% per year.[84]

Lipids

A substantial body of research in adults has evaluated the potential of n-3 LCPUFA supplementation to affect lipid profiles and has generally found modest effects of n-3 LCPUFA consumption on lipid profiles, especially on triglycerides. A 2006 meta-analysis by Balk et al[85] including 21 randomized controlled trials of fish oil found that triglycerides decreased 27 mg/dL (95% CI: 20 to 33), high-density lipoprotein increased 1.6 mg/dL (95% CI: 0.8 to 2.3), and LDL increased 6 mg/dL (95% CI: 3 to 8) in those who received fish oil versus controls.

Research on children has been much more limited. A study involving 201 fifth- and sixth-graders with obesity from Campeche, Mexico, assigned participants to metformin or n-3 LCPUFA supplement (360 mg of EPA and 240 mg of DHA) 3 times a day for 12 weeks. Those receiving the fish oil supplement had increases in high-density lipoprotein (2.12 mg/dL; 95% CI: 0.61 to 3.63) and decreases in triglycerides (−26.35 mg/dL; 95% CI: −40.78 to −11.91). No change in LDL or total cholesterol was observed.[86] Another randomized placebo controlled trial of 4 g of n-3 LCPUFA daily in 29 adolescents with hypertriglyceridemia, although underpowered, showed decreases in triglyceride levels that were not significantly different from placebo (experimental group, −54 ± 27 mg/dL; placebo, −34 ± 26 mg/dL).[87] A recent randomized, double-blind, crossover trial comparing 4 g of fish oil daily for 8 weeks with placebo by Gidding et al[88] similarly found that in a group of 42 adolescents with elevated LDL and triglycerides, those who received supplementation had lower triglycerides than those who received placebo, but the difference was not significant (−52 ± 16 vs −16 ± 16 mg/dL). No difference was found in LDL levels.[88] Given these results, changes in lipids are likely to be at best modest and may require large (eg, 1000 mg or more) doses of n-3 LCPUFAs.

Effects of n-3 LCPUFAs for children with nonalcoholic fatty liver disease have also been studied. In a randomized trial of 40 children with biopsy-proven nonalcoholic liver disease, children who received the supplement had improvements in liver steatosis, improved insulin sensitivity, and, consistent with some of the studies presented above, lower triglycerides.[89]

Blood Pressure

Dozens of randomized controlled trials have evaluated fish oil supplementation effects on blood pressure in middle-aged adults and found that high-dose (eg, ≥3 g/day) n-3 LCPUFA supplementation results in modest decreases in systolic and diastolic blood pressure. A 2014 meta-analysis of 70 randomized controlled trials found that when compared with placebo, EPA and DHA supplementation reduced systolic blood pressure (−1.52 mm Hg; 95% CI: −2.25 to −0.79) and diastolic blood pressure (−0.99 mm Hg; 95% CI: −1.54 to −0.44).[90] This is consistent with another previous meta-analysis of 36 double-blinded randomized trials of fish oil and blood pressure in which high levels of fish oil consumption (3.7 g/day) lowered systolic blood pressure by 1.7 mm Hg (95% CI: 0.3–3.1) and diastolic blood pressure by 1.5 mm Hg (95% CI: 0.6–2.3).[91] Given the size of blood pressure change, these effects are unlikely to be clinically relevant.

Effects of n-3 LCPUFA in childhood on blood pressure have been less well studied and results have not been consistent, although several have suggested that supplementation may elevate blood pressure, especially for boys. This evidence comes from observational studies[92] as well as randomized trials[93] of fish oil supplementation to infants. The studies have revealed elevations in blood pressure. Asserhøj et al[94] recruited 122 Danish mothers and randomly assigned their offspring to receive fish oil or olive oil during the first 4 months of lactation. In a follow-up of 98 children at 7 years, boys who received fish oil had unexpectedly higher diastolic and mean arterial blood pressure (6 mm Hg) than those who received olive oil. No difference was found among girls.[94] Higher diastolic blood pressure (~3 mm Hg) was observed at 10 years of age in girls, but not boys, from a group of children born at less than 35 weeks' gestation and with birth weight <2000 g who were randomly assigned to receive a formula supplemented with n-3 LCPUFA (from tuna oil) and γ linoleic acid or a formula without fatty acid supplement through 9 months postterm.[24] The difference between boys and girls became insignificant, however, after controlling for current weight, which suggests that the observed blood pressure difference may be mediated through weight. Of note, in the Asserhøj et al[94] study, children receiving fish oil supplements had higher BMI at 2.5 years, but the higher BMI did not persist at 7 years.

A multicenter European study, in which 147 children born between 37 and 42 weeks' gestation with birth weight between 2500 and 4000 g were randomly assigned to receive formula supplemented with n-3 and n-6 LCPUFAs (DHA, EPA, and α-linoleic acid, all sourced from egg yolks) or placebo through age 4 months yielded contrary results. At age 6 years, supplemented infants had lower mean blood pressure (mean difference, −3.0 mm Hg; 95% CI: −5.4 to −0.5 mm Hg) and diastolic blood pressure (mean difference, −3.6 mm Hg; 95% CI: −6.5 to −0.6 mm Hg) than the control group.[95] These results, and those from the Asserhøj et al[94] study, which compared n-3 with n-6 LCPUFA supplementation, raise the question as to whether n-6 LCPUFAs may be responsible for a greater effect than n-3 LCPUFAs on blood pressure in children. Although this specific question has not been addressed by other well-designed studies, Rytter et al[96] followed 180 children born to mothers randomly assigned to receive fish oil or olive oil supplements in the last trimester of pregnancy at 19 years of age and found no effect on blood pressure from prenatal supplementation.

POTENTIAL HARMS OF EATING FISH AND SHELLFISH

Methylmercury (MeHg) pollution is a primary reason for parents to avoid feeding their children some fish and for expectant mothers to avoid consumption of some fish during pregnancy. Available evidence indicates that prenatal and, to a lesser extent in most cases, postnatal mercury exposure has been associated with decrements in memory, attention, language, IQ, and visual-motor skills in childhood.[97–99] Mercury exposure during pregnancy may promote preterm delivery as well.[100] Several reviews present the consequences of mercury exposure in utero.[97]

Mercury bioaccumulates in marine and freshwater food chains. Most of the mercury found in humans comes from contaminated fish. Elemental mercury enters the environment primarily through coal combustion and artisanal and small-scale gold mining as well as natural emissions, for example, from volcanoes. Bacteria convert elemental to organic (methyl) mercury, a form that is readily absorbed after ingestion. Given the increased use of coal for energy in recent decades, especially in Asia, mercury levels in the world's oceans have increased and are expected to increase substantially, with a possible doubling by 2050 from 1995 levels.[101]

The US Food and Drug Administration (FDA) and Environmental Protection Agency have provided fish consumption guidance in the United States aimed at preventing harmful exposure to mercury that is intended for the average American consumer and not necessarily for populations that may have higher consumption of freshwater fish.[102] These recommendations are based on cohort studies in the Faroe Islands, Seychelles Islands, and New Zealand in which health consequences from prenatal mercury exposure have been examined, although the diets of these populations do not represent the typical American diet. The Faroese, for instance, consume large amounts of whale blubber, and the Seychellois eat 12 meals with fish per week. In addition, the primary analysis in the Seychelles and New Zealand studies did not control for fish consumption, so any benefit of n-3 LCPUFAs on neurodevelopment may have masked harmful mercury effects.[103] This was demonstrated in the Faroe Islands cohort, which had neurodevelopmental outcomes assessed while controlling for maternal fish consumption and found that beneficial effects of fish consumption concealed the deleterious effects of MeHg.[103] These analyses of the Faroe Island data also confirmed the beneficial association of fish consumption with child neurocognitive outcomes.

Largely based on findings from the Faroe Islands study, the US Environmental Protection Agency's reference dose (RfD) for MeHg is 0.1 µg/kg of body weight per day.[104] The RfD for mercury is an estimated daily intake likely to be without appreciable risk of harm over a lifetime, even for the most sensitive populations, and employs an uncertainty factor of 10 based on variability in concentrations of cord blood and maternal blood and for differences in how MeHg may be metabolized in different people. The MeHg RfD was calculated with the intent of preventing fetal neurologic harm from maternal consumption. The RfD assumes that the fetal brain is the organ most sensitive to the effects of MeHg, and thus the RfD should protect everyone, including children, from harm. As a result, no governmental guidance for MeHg in other populations, including children and nonpregnant adults, has been given.

On the basis of representative data from the NHANES, the number of women in the United States with MeHg blood levels reflecting intake above the RfD has decreased considerably since 1990, and, as a result, the number of potentially adversely affected children has decreased as well.[105] An analysis by Mahaffey et al[106] based on NHANES data from 1990 to 2000 found that each year more than 300 000 children are born in the United States with in utero exposure to MeHg at levels that may cause neurologic harm. The same analysis using data from the 2000–2010 NHANES found that only 75 000 children might have been exposed in utero to mercury at levels above the RfD.[105] Of note, neither of these analyses accounted for observed trends in maternal blood mercury with increasing age, with older women having higher blood mercury concentrations.[107] In subsequent NHANES research, researchers have also identified that women living on the Atlantic and Pacific coasts, and to a lesser extent Gulf coast, are likely to have higher blood mercury concentrations (see Fig 1).[108]

Beyond this, little research is available to inform specific recommendations for fish consumption in young children to prevent harms from mercury exposure.

Persistent Organic Pollutants

Aside from mercury, several other pollutants commonly found in fish and shellfish have raised concern for their detrimental health effects. These include a large group of chemicals known as persistent organic pollutants (POPs). POPs are organic compounds that resist breakdown and are lipid soluble. These properties make it possible for long-range transport of POPs after they are released into the environment and also enable them to bioaccumulate within animals and humans and biomagnify within food chains. As a result, some of the animals with the highest POP burdens live in the Arctic circle (for example, polar bears, which are at the apex of the marine food chain).

Polychlorinated Biphenyls

Polychlorinated biphenyls (PCBs) are POPs that comprise a group of

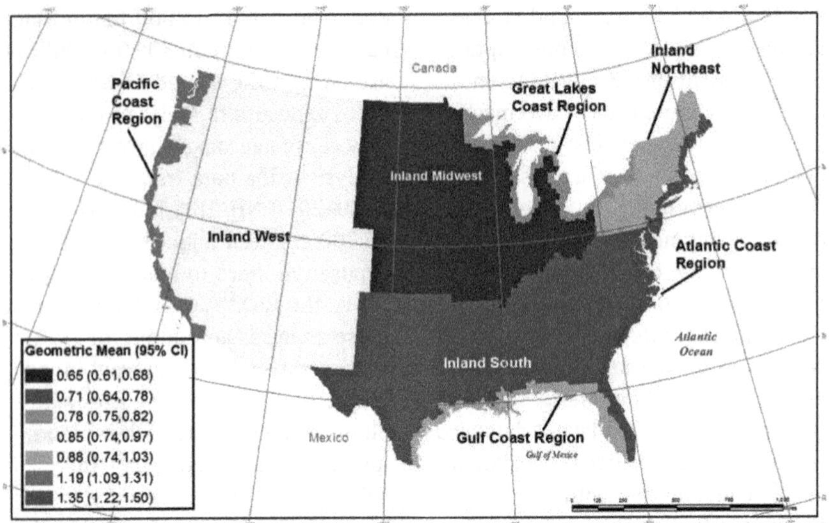

FIGURE 1
Map of whole blood mercury concentration (geometric mean and 95% CI [μg/L]) in women of childbearing ages by coastal or inland regions for NHANES 1999–2010. (Reprinted with permission from Cusack L, Smit E, Kile ML, Harding AK. Regional and temporal trends in blood mercury concentrations and fish consumption in women of child bearing age in the United States using NHANES data from 1999 to 2010. *Environ Health*. 2017;16(1):10.)

chemicals that have a biphenyl structure with between 1 and 10 chlorine atoms. Roughly 130 different PCB molecules, known as congeners, have been used commercially, and most commercial preparations contained mixtures of these congeners. They most often can be found near industrial sites where they were produced or disposed of and can contaminate fish in the surrounding rivers and harbors. Studies over several decades have found that PCBs can adversely affect the developing fetus and young children. In utero PCB exposure has been associated with lower birth weight,[109–113] acute lymphoblastic leukemia and non-Hodgkin's lymphoma,[114–116] obesity,[117,118] immune system dysfunction and impairment,[119–121] asthma,[122] motor and cognitive developmental deficits as assessed on the Bayley Scale and other instruments,[123–127] and lowered IQ.[128,129] Research on postnatal exposure is limited. Exposure through breastfeeding may both increase and decrease IgE-mediated allergy.[119] Children with higher blood levels of PCBs may have impairments in gonadal and pubertal development.[130,131] Studies on the effects of PCB blood levels on growth have yielded conflicting results.[110,132,133]

Because of health concerns, PCBs were banned in the United States in 1977. However, they have persisted in the environment, contaminating water, soil, and air and have made their way into fish and, as a result, humans, albeit at declining levels with the passage of time.[134]

Fish concentrations of PCBs vary widely. They tend to be highest in freshwater fish at the top of their local ecosystem's food chain. The Environmental Protection Agency maintains a Web site that provides information on local fish advisories across the United States that can identify local water bodies and species with potentially high levels of PCBs (http://fishadvisoryonline.epa.gov/General.aspx).

Although fish can be a significant source of dietary PCBs, most exposure for Americans is from red meat and dairy consumption.[135] On a per-weight basis, butter and processed meats may have as much PCBs as fish, if not more.[136]

Of note, several studies have investigated concentrations of PCBs in fish oil supplements, and 1 recent study examined pediatric supplements in particular. Ashley et al[137] analyzed PCBs in 13 over-the-counter children's fish oil supplements. Every supplement analyzed contained PCBs, with a mean concentration of 9 ± 8 ng PCBs/g, resulting in a mean daily exposure of 2.5 to 50.3 ng PCBs/day depending on suggested serving size. The trophic level of the fish species or purification method used to produce the supplement did not predict the amount of PCB it contained, although the sample sizes were limited.[137] The Environmental Protection Agency has established RfDs for several PCB mixtures, including Aroclor 1016 at 0.00007 mg/kg of body weight per day. Based on the supplements in the Ashley et al[137] study, several of them, if taken as directed, would result in exposures that exceed this RfD. Also, given the wide range of PCB and n-3 LCPUFA content in the samples, they might provide more or less PCB/g n-3 LCPUFA than wild-caught salmon, a fish that usually has high n-3 LCPUFA and low PCB content.[137]

Dioxins

A dioxin is a member of a class of organochlorine chemicals that originate from, among other sources, waste incineration, paper bleaching, pesticide production, metal smelting, and production of polyvinyl chloride plastics. Dioxins are highly toxic POPs known to cause reproductive and developmental problems, damage to the immune system, and cancer.[138] Dioxin levels in the US population have declined substantially in recent years because of regulations and are expected to continue to fall. Compared with other pollutants, dioxins are rarely a cause for freshwater fish advisories from the

Environmental Protection Agency.[139] In 2010, for example, only 2 of 533 fish consumption advisories were made on the basis of dioxins (not including dioxin-like PCBs) in the United States. These advisories were for the Hudson River of New York and Trinity River of Texas.[139] Dioxins are present in fish and can be at high concentrations in freshwater fish; however, the levels are often lower than in beef, butter, and cheese.[136]

Toxicant Avoidance

In general, PCBs and other POPs, because they are fat soluble, are found at higher concentrations in fatty fish and are concentrated in fatty tissue. Removing the fatty skin and broiling or baking rather than frying fish may decrease exposure.[140,141] MeHg, in contrast, tends to be stored in protein rather than in fat and is distributed throughout the flesh of the fish. Thus, removing the skin or fatty tissue does not reduce mercury exposure. For both POPs and mercury, the trophic level of the species on the food web is a major determinant of pollution burdens aside from where the fish or shellfish was raised or lived.

Mercury levels in fish are proportional to their age, size, and trophic level, as well as the amount of mercury contamination in the water where the fish lived and ate. Although certain species have generally been considered to have higher mercury concentrations in their flesh than others, variability in mercury levels even within the same species can be marked.[142] For example, the median concentration of mercury in canned light tuna is 0.128 ppm (μg/g), with a range from 0 to 0.889 ppm; the concentration in canned albacore tuna is 0.338 ppm, ranging from 0 to 0.853 ppm. A 25-kg child consuming 4 oz (113 g) of canned light tuna (a whole can is 5 oz) would, on average, consume 0.08 μg of mercury/kg of body weight (approximately 80% of the RfD) but could get none or as much as 0.57 μg/kg (>5 times RfD) depending on the size, source, and trophic level of the particular fish included in the can.[143]

Increasingly, guidance is available that provides information on nutrients, toxicants, and sustainability by fish species. See Resources for examples.

Fish and Shellfish Poisoning

Fish and shellfish, and in particular bivalve shellfish, such as oysters, clams, scallops, and mussels, can become contaminated with toxins produced by algae. If these toxins are ingested by humans, they can cause several syndromes, some of which may be life-threatening, including amnesic shellfish poisoning, diarrheal shellfish poisoning, neurotoxic shellfish poisoning, paralytic shellfish poisoning, and ciguatera fish poisoning. Because all of these toxins are heat stable, cooking does not prevent intoxication. In recent decades, coastal harmful algal blooms that contained the toxins that cause these syndromes occurred nationwide more than 60 times annually. Although shellfish poisoning syndromes were only rarely reported to the Centers for Disease Control and Prevention between 1990 and 2008,[144] estimates of the true incidence are likely 15 000 cases per year or more in the United States for ciguatera alone.[145] Most ciguatera cases from fish harvested in US waters originate from fisheries in the eastern Gulf of Mexico and around the southern coast of Florida as well as Hawaii. Caribbean fisheries also may be affected. Recent research has suggested that climate change may increase the risk of ciguatera fish poisoning.[146]

Freshwater Fish and Vulnerable Populations

Consuming freshwater fish captured from US waters carries unique risks compared with seafood, given the high concentrations of pollutants that can be found in certain water bodies, particularly POPs and MeHg. The Environmental Protection Agency maintains a database of local fish advisories (see Resources) that provide guidance on when toxicants may be present in lakes and rivers around the nation. Most states have similar databases available on the Internet as well.

For some children, freshwater fish may be a large part of their diets; therefore, fish consumption may carry heightened risk. Some American Indian children, for instance, have been found to have high exposure to PCBs, other POPs, and mercury through eating freshwater fish.[147,148]

SUSHI

Sushi has become an increasingly popular part of the American diet, including for children. Raw fish and shellfish in sushi carry increased risk for transmitting foodborne illnesses. On the basis of data reported to the Centers for Disease Control and Prevention, sushi accounted for 0.3% of all foodborne illnesses in the United States between 1998 and 2015 (see https://wwwn.cdc.gov/foodborneoutbreaks/). No evidence supports guidance on the right age to introduce raw fish and shellfish. In places where sushi consumption is more common than in the United States, parents may introduce sushi containing raw fish as early as children can eat solid foods or delay until children enter elementary school.

A NUTRITIONAL COMPARISON

Although some potential toxicants may be more likely to come from consumption of certain forms of fish, most fish, with some notable exceptions, have favorable nutritional and overall health qualities compared with other forms of animal protein. In the United States, red meat and chicken represent the majority of childhood animal protein consumption. On average, less than 10% of children's animal protein intake comes from fish.[149] PCBs and dioxins may be found in beef and other animal products in much higher concentrations than in most fish, with the possible exception of farmed salmon or certain freshwater fish.[136]

SUSTAINABILITY

Just under 60% of fisheries worldwide are harvested at their maximum sustainable yield, and 30% are overexploited.[150] Several recent and notable instances of complete collapses of fisheries include the Northwest Atlantic cod fishery off the coast of New England and Canada. The depletion of fish stocks has had major consequences for the nutrition of coastal populations, especially in resource-limited nations, where the void left by declining fish stocks has resulted in increased consumption of other animal proteins that may have less healthful profiles, including bushmeat.[151]

Fishery practices also have implications for those who work in them. In the United States, fishers and those working at sea to catch fish have the second-highest on-the-job mortality rate.[152] Research has also shown that children may be trafficked into labor in the fisheries workforce, with dire consequences. One study found that 19% of boys trafficked in the Mekong region of southeast Asia were forced to labor in fisheries. Many of these children were found to have witnessed or experienced violence and exposure to violence, and this was associated with increased risk for depression, anxiety, and posttraumatic stress disorder as well as suicidality.[153] Shrimp, the most consumed seafood in the United States,[154] comes predominantly from this region.[155]

Because of potential health benefits related to consuming fish and n-3 LCPUFAs, medical and government organizations have encouraged greater fish consumption among Americans. Such guidance, if realized, may put further pressure on fish stocks and promote unsustainable aquaculture, although specific data to describe the relationship are lacking.[156]

AQUACULTURE

A rapid increase in fish and shellfish farming, or aquaculture, in industrialized and resource-limited nations, and especially in China, has occurred over the past 2 decades. Aquaculture now provides for at least half of the fish and shellfish consumed worldwide (see Fig 2).[157]

The Sustainability of Aquaculture

Aquaculture technology and practice has advanced considerably in recent decades to make aquaculture a much more sustainable enterprise. However, among the aquaculture products in need of improvement are 2 that have particular importance to the American diet. Shrimp are the most consumed seafood in the United States, with the average American consuming approximately 4 lb per year; 94% of shrimp are imported, and almost all are farm raised.[158,159] Shrimp farms in Southeast Asia and Central and South America have resulted in the loss of millions of hectares of mangrove forest, and shrimp farms account for roughly one-third of mangrove forest loss worldwide.[160] Mangrove forests serve many functions to coastal ecosystems, including providing breeding grounds for wild fish and shellfish. Mangrove forests also are vital contributors to the health of coral reefs and seagrass beds, both among the greatest repositories of marine biodiversity.[161] Shrimp farms have also been the sources of severe nutrient and chemical pollution as crowded pens generate tremendous amounts of waste and require chemical inputs, such as antibiotics and disinfectants, that can harm people exposed to these pollutants.[162] In contrast to shrimp farming, much of the other farm-raised shellfish, such as mussels and oysters, are some of the most sustainably raised seafood available.

Farmed Salmon

Salmon is the most widely consumed noncanned fish in the United States,

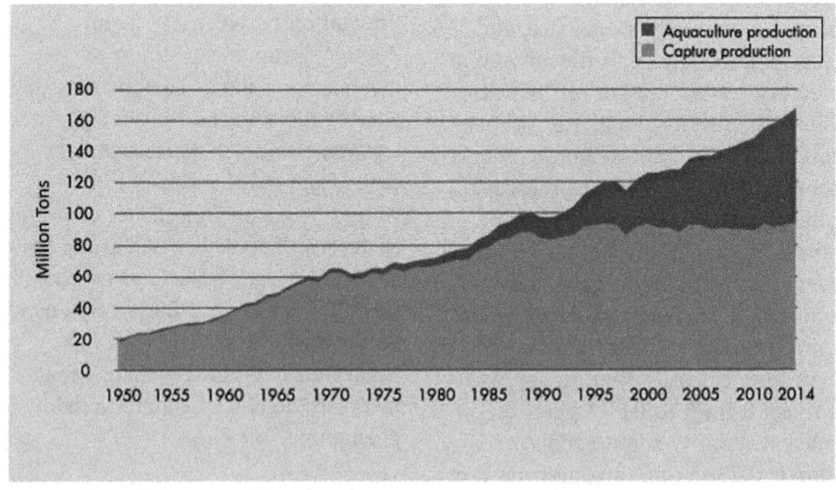

FIGURE 2
Food and Agricultural Organization of the United Nations' data on global wild and aquaculture fish production. (Reprinted with permission from Food and Agricultural Organization of the United Nations. The State of World Fisheries and Aquaculture 2016. Contributing to Food Security and Nutrition for All. Rome, Italy; Food and Agricultural Organization of the United Nations; 2016:3.)

and over the past 35 years, the majority of salmon eaten has shifted from wild to farm raised. An influential 2004 study in *Science* reported that farmed salmon had levels of PCBs, dioxins, and other POPs severalfold higher than wild-caught salmon.[163] However, critics have argued that the potential health harms of consuming the PCBs in farm-raised salmon are more than offset by the health benefits of salmon's nutritional profile.[164] In addition, among other concerns, farmed salmon has been a source of local pollution from chemical additives (eg, antibiotics) and nutrient overload as well as disease spread, given high animal density and escapes of nonnative salmon species into local ecosystems. Salmon, as carnivores, have also historically been fed fishmeal when farmed, requiring 1.5 to 3 lb of feed for every pound of salmon.

Progress has been made in recent years to address problems associated with salmon farming. Some operations now approximate 1:1 fish-in to fish-out ratios (ie, 1 lb of wild fish in salmon feed produces 1 lb of farmed salmon), scarcely use chemicals, and have greatly reduced disease spread and escapes through better monitoring and lower-density farming.[165] Experiments with vegetarian feeds and other fishmeal and oil substitutes have shown promise at further reducing reliance on wild fish stocks for long-chain omega-3 fatty acids. Experiments with vegetarian feeds and substituting a yeast for anchovies as a source of omega-3 fatty acids have shown promise in further reducing reliance on wild fish stocks.[118] (Note that the original source of all n-3 LCPUFAs in the oceans are phytoplankton).

Most salmon farms do not yet meet cutting-edge standards for production that limit undesirable environmental and health impacts. Guidance on identifying those operations engaged in best practices can be found from a variety of sources (see Resources). Many major retail outlets have embraced selling seafood that is recommended by major ocean conservation groups.[166]

The Sustainability of Aquaculture Compared With Beef, Poultry, and Pork

Comparing the resource intensity of aquaculture to other animal protein sources, most farmed fish and seafood has a comparable, if not favorable, profile. On a per-calorie basis, beef is by far the most resource-intensive animal protein: it takes about 10 times more irrigated water and 4 times more nitrogen fertilizer and produces about 10 times more greenhouse gas emissions when compared with pork or poultry.[167] Many species of farmed seafood have a carbon footprint roughly equivalent to or less than pork and poultry, although it can vary greatly, especially with long-distance transit.[168,169] Shrimp eaten in America mostly comes from Southeast Asian nations (Indonesia, India, and Thailand, in particular) and has a disproportionately large carbon footprint, in part because of transport but largely because of mangrove forest loss. Shrimp sourced from these regions can have a carbon footprint an order of magnitude greater than beef.[170,171]

Fifty percent or more of salmon is farm raised. Farmed salmon comes mostly from Canada, Chile, or Norway.[172] Studies of farmed salmon from these countries have found farmed salmon to have a carbon footprint of approximately 2 kg carbon dioxide equivalent/1000 kcal salmon, which is similar to pork or poultry.[168,173]

Sustainably Raised and Caught Fish and Shellfish

The United States has some of the best-managed fisheries (wild or farmed) in the world, and although all are not sustainably harvested, all are managed toward that direction even if they have not achieved sustainable harvests to date. The Magnusson Stevens Act (Pub Law No. 109–479 [2006]) serves as the foundation of the US regulation of fisheries and has established a framework to promote the application of the best available science to fisheries management. As a result, identifying the products of American fisheries may be the best first pass assessment of sustainability. Thorough sustainability assessments of fish and shellfish have been conducted by several nongovernmental organizations for many years. These initiatives are summarized in the Resources section of this report.

CONCLUSIONS

Despite the favorable nutritional and, in many cases, sustainability profile of fish and shellfish, children in the United States eat relatively little of them as compared with other animal protein sources, and seafood consumption by children has declined every year since 2007 to levels not seen since the early 1980s.[149,174] Some evidence suggests that federal mercury advisories on fish consumption may have pushed people away from eating fish in general and canned tuna in particular.[175] Evidence-based expert guidance has largely advised that seafood should have a larger place in the American diet. The recent Scientific Report of the 2015 Dietary Guidelines Advisory Committee, for instance, stated, "The Committee concurs with the Joint WHO/FAO Consultancy that, for the majority of commercial wild and farmed species, neither the risks of mercury nor organic pollutants outweigh the health benefits of seafood consumption, such as decreased cardiovascular disease risk and improved infant neurodevelopment. However, any assessment evaluates evidence within a time frame and contaminant composition can change rapidly based on the contamination conditions at the location of wild catch and altered production practices for farmed seafood."[176]

Even if fish and shellfish have a favorable nutritional profile compared with other forms of animal protein, available research to substantiate specific health benefits from fish and shellfish consumption in children remains limited. Further research is needed to clarify the value of fish and shellfish consumption in childhood to health.

RESOURCES

An Interactive Map of Freshwater Fish Advisories in the United States

https://fishadvisoryonline.epa.gov/General.aspx (Note that results can be limited to active advisories. In some instances, the last update may be >10 years ago. If this is the case, there is often a link to a state database to look for newer information.)

Environmental Protection Agency Fish and Shellfish Advisories and Safe Eating Guidelines

https://www.epa.gov/choose-fish-and-shellfish-wisely/fish-and-shellfish-advisories-and-safe-eating-guidelines

Monterrey Bay Aquarium Seafood Watch

Seafoodwatch.org

Mercury in Seafood: A Guide for Health Care Professionals

http://safinacenter.org/documents/2015/05/mercury-seafood-guide-health-care.pdf (sustainability, mercury)

LEAD AUTHORS

Aaron S. Bernstein, MD, MPH, FAAP
Emily Oken, MD, MPH
Sarah de Ferranti, MD, MPH, FAAP

COUNCIL ON ENVIRONMENTAL HEALTH, 2017–2018

Jennifer Ann Lowry, MD, FAAP, Chairperson
Samantha Ahdoot, MD, FAAP
Carl R. Baum, MD, FACMT, FAAP
Aaron S. Bernstein, MD, FAAP
Aparna Bole, MD, FAAP
Lori G. Byron, MD, FAAP
Philip J. Landrigan, MD, MSc, FAAP
Steven M. Marcus, MD, FAAP
Susan E. Pacheco, MD, FAAP
Adam J. Spanier, MD, PhD, MPH, FAAP
Alan D. Woolf, MD, MPH, FAAP

LIAISONS

John M. Balbus, MD, MPH – *National Institute of Environmental Health Sciences*
Nathaniel G. DeNicola, MD, MSc – *American Congress of Obstetricians and Gynecologists*
Ruth A. Etzel, MD, PhD, FAAP – *US Environmental Protection Agency*
Diane E. Hindman, MD, FAAP – *Section on Pediatric Trainees*
Mary Ellen Mortensen, MD, MS – *Centers for Disease Control and Prevention/National Center for Environmental Health*
Mary H. Ward, PhD – *National Cancer Institute*

STAFF

Paul Spire

COMMITTEE ON NUTRITION

Steven A. Abrams, MD, FAAP
George J. Fuchs, III, MD, FAAP
Jae Hong Kim, MD, PhD, FAAP
C. Wesley Lindsey, MD, FAAP
Sheela Natesh Magge, MD, MSCE, FAAP
Ellen S. Rome, MD, MPH, FAAP
Sarah J. Schwarzenberg, MD, FAAP

LIAISONS

Jeff Critch, MD – *Canadian Paediatric Society*
Janet M. de Jesus, MS, RD – *National Institutes of Health*
Andrea Lotze, MD, FAAP – *Food and Drug Administration*
Cria G. Perrine, PhD – *Centers for Disease Control and Prevention*
Valery Soto, MS, RD, LD – *US Department of Agriculture*

STAFF

Debra L. Burrowes, MHA

ACKNOWLEDGMENT

The authors thank Barton Seaver for his review of the sustainability sections of this report.

ABBREVIATIONS

ADHD: attention-deficit/hyperactivity disorder
CI: confidence interval
DHA: docosahexaenoic acid
EPA: eicosapentaenoic acid
FDA: US Food and Drug Administration
IgE: immunoglobulin E
LCPUFA: long-chain polyunsaturated amino acid
LDL: low-density lipoprotein
MeHg: methylmercury
n-3: omega-3
n-6: omega-6
OR: odds ratio
PCB: polychlorinated biphenyl
POP: persistent organic pollutant
RfD: reference dose
RR: relative risk

FINANCIAL DISCLOSURE: Dr Bernstein has received no funding for this project. Dr de Ferranti has received royalties for UpToDate articles on cholesterol and cardiovascular risk factors in childhood, the New England Congenital Cardiology Foundation, and the National Heart, Lung, and Blood Institute Pediatric Heart Network. Dr Oken has received funding from the National Institutes of Health (P30 ES00002, P30 DK040561, R01 ES016314, K24 HD069408 P30 DK092924, R01AI102960) and royalties for an UpToDate article on Fish Consumption During Pregnancy. Funded by the National Institutes of Health (NIH).

FUNDING: No external funding.

POTENTIAL CONFLICT OF INTEREST: The authors have indicated they have no potential conflicts of interest to disclose.

REFERENCES

1. Oken E, Choi AL, Karagas MR, et al. Which fish should I eat? Perspectives influencing fish consumption choices. *Environ Health Perspect.* 2012;120(6): 790–798
2. Saggese G, Vierucci F, Boot AM, et al. Vitamin D in childhood and adolescence: an expert position statement. *Eur J Pediatr.* 2015;174(5): 565–576
3. Greer FR, Krebs NF; American Academy of Pediatrics Committee on Nutrition. Optimizing bone health and calcium intakes of infants, children, and adolescents. *Pediatrics.* 2006;117(2): 578–585
4. Oski FA. Iron deficiency in infancy and childhood. *N Engl J Med.* 1993;329(3): 190–193
5. Rayman MP. Selenium and human health. *Lancet.* 2012;379(9822): 1256–1268
6. Bougma K, Aboud FE, Harding KB, Marquis GS. Iodine and mental development of children 5 years old and under: a systematic review and meta-analysis. *Nutrients.* 2013;5(4): 1384–1416
7. Zimmermann MB. The adverse effects of mild-to-moderate iodine deficiency during pregnancy and childhood: a review. *Thyroid.* 2007;17(9):829–835
8. Arterburn LM, Hall EB, Oken H. Distribution, interconversion, and dose response of n-3 fatty acids in humans. *Am J Clin Nutr.* 2006;83(suppl 6):S1467S–S1476S
9. Kremmyda L-S, Vlachava M, Noakes PS, Diaper ND, Miles EA, Calder PC. Atopy risk in infants and children in relation to early exposure to fish, oily fish, or long-chain omega-3 fatty acids: a systematic review. *Clin Rev Allergy Immunol.* 2011;41(1):36–66
10. Kull I, Bergström A, Lilja G, Pershagen G, Wickman M. Fish consumption during the first year of life and development of allergic diseases during childhood. *Allergy.* 2006;61(8):1009–1015
11. Magnusson J, Kull I, Rosenlund H, et al. Fish consumption in infancy and development of allergic disease up to age 12 y. *Am J Clin Nutr.* 2013;97(6): 1324–1330
12. Goksör E, Alm B, Pettersson R, et al. Early fish introduction and neonatal antibiotics affect the risk of asthma into school age. *Pediatr Allergy Immunol.* 2013;24(4):339–344
13. Yang H, Xun P, He K. Fish and fish oil intake in relation to risk of asthma: a systematic review and meta-analysis. *PLoS One.* 2013;8(11):e80048
14. Alm B, Aberg N, Erdes L, et al. Early introduction of fish decreases the risk of eczema in infants. *Arch Dis Child.* 2009;94(1):11–15
15. Oien T, Storrø O, Johnsen R. Do early intake of fish and fish oil protect against eczema and doctor-diagnosed asthma at 2 years of age? A cohort study. *J Epidemiol Community Health.* 2010;64(2):124–129
16. Noakes PS, Vlachava M, Kremmyda L-S, et al. Increased intake of oily fish in pregnancy: effects on neonatal immune responses and on clinical outcomes in infants at 6 mo. *Am J Clin Nutr.* 2012; 95(2):395–404
17. Hesselmar B, Saalman R, Rudin A, Adlerberth I, Wold A. Early fish introduction is associated with less eczema, but not sensitization, in infants. *Acta Paediatr.* 2010;99(12):1861–1867
18. Pelé F, Bajeux E, Gendron H, et al. Maternal fish and shellfish consumption and wheeze, eczema and food allergy at age two: a prospective cohort study in Brittany, France. *Environ Health.* 2013;12:102
19. Leermakers ETM, Sonnenschein-van der Voort AMM, Heppe DHM, et al. Maternal fish consumption during pregnancy and risks of wheezing and eczema in childhood: the Generation R Study. *Eur J Clin Nutr.* 2013;67(4):353–359
20. American Academy of Pediatrics. Committee on Nutrition. Hypoallergenic infant formulas. *Pediatrics.* 2000;106(2 pt 1):346–349
21. Greer FR, Sicherer SH, Burks AW; American Academy of Pediatrics Committee on Nutrition; American Academy of Pediatrics Section on Allergy and Immunology. Effects of early nutritional interventions on the development of atopic disease in infants and children: the role of maternal dietary restriction, breastfeeding, timing of introduction of complementary foods, and hydrolyzed formulas. *Pediatrics.* 2008;121(1): 183–191
22. van der Wurff ISM, Meyer BJ, de Groot RHM. A review of recruitment, adherence and drop-out rates in omega-3 polyunsaturated fatty acid supplementation trials in children and adolescents. *Nutrients.* 2017;9(5):474
23. Farmer A, Montori V, Dinneen S, Clar C. Fish oil in people with type 2 diabetes mellitus. *Cochrane Database Syst Rev.* 2001;(3):CD003205
24. Kennedy K, Ross S, Isaacs EB, et al. The 10-year follow-up of a randomised trial of long-chain polyunsaturated fatty acid supplementation in preterm infants: effects on growth and blood pressure. *Arch Dis Child.* 2010;95(8):588–595
25. Gunaratne AW, Makrides M, Collins CT. Maternal prenatal and/or postnatal n-3 long chain polyunsaturated fatty acids (LCPUFA) supplementation for preventing allergies in early childhood. *Cochrane Database Syst Rev.* 2015;(7): CD010085
26. Olsen SF, Østerdal ML, Salvig JD, et al. Fish oil intake compared with olive oil intake in late pregnancy and asthma in the offspring: 16 y of registry-based follow-up from a randomized controlled trial. *Am J Clin Nutr.* 2008;88(1):167–175
27. Hansen S, Strøm M, Maslova E, et al. Fish oil supplementation during pregnancy and allergic respiratory disease in the adult offspring. *J Allergy Clin Immunol.* 2017;139(1):104–111.e4
28. Bisgaard H, Stokholm J, Chawes BL, et al. Fish oil-derived fatty acids in pregnancy and wheeze and asthma in offspring. *N Engl J Med.* 2016;375(26): 2530–2539
29. Alm B, Goksör E, Thengilsdottir H, et al. Early protective and risk factors for allergic rhinitis at age 4½ yr. *Pediatr Allergy Immunol.* 2011;22(4):398–404
30. Hodge L, Salome CM, Hughes JM, et al. Effect of dietary intake of omega-3 and omega-6 fatty acids on severity of asthma in children. *Eur Respir J.* 1998; 11(2):361–365
31. D'Vaz N, Meldrum SJ, Dunstan JA, et al. Postnatal fish oil supplementation in

high-risk infants to prevent allergy: randomized controlled trial. *Pediatrics.* 2012;130(4):674–682

32. Nagakura T, Matsuda S, Shichijyo K, Sugimoto H, Hata K. Dietary supplementation with fish oil rich in omega-3 polyunsaturated fatty acids in children with bronchial asthma. *Eur Respir J.* 2000;16(5):861–865

33. Lev-Tzion R, Griffiths AM, Leder O, Turner D. Omega 3 fatty acids (fish oil) for maintenance of remission in Crohn's disease. *Cochrane Database Syst Rev.* 2014;(2):CD006320

34. Romano C, Cucchiara S, Barabino A, Annese V, Sferlazzas C. Usefulness of omega-3 fatty acid supplementation in addition to mesalazine in maintaining remission in pediatric Crohn's disease: a double-blind, randomized, placebo-controlled study. *World J Gastroenterol.* 2005;11(45):7118–7121

35. Costea I, Mack DR, Lemaitre RN, et al. Interactions between the dietary polyunsaturated fatty acid ratio and genetic factors determine susceptibility to pediatric Crohn's disease. *Gastroenterology.* 2014;146(4):929–931

36. Turner D, Steinhart AH, Griffiths AM. Omega 3 fatty acids (fish oil) for maintenance of remission in ulcerative colitis. *Cochrane Database Syst Rev.* 2007;(3):CD006443

37. De Ley M, de Vos R, Hommes DW, Stokkers P. Fish oil for induction of remission in ulcerative colitis. *Cochrane Database Syst Rev.* 2007;(4):CD005986

38. Turner D, Shah PS, Steinhart AH, Zlotkin S, Griffiths AM. Maintenance of remission in inflammatory bowel disease using omega-3 fatty acids (fish oil): a systematic review and meta-analyses. *Inflamm Bowel Dis.* 2011;17(1):336–345

39. Neuringer M, Connor WE, Lin DS, Barstad L, Luck S. Biochemical and functional effects of prenatal and postnatal omega 3 fatty acid deficiency on retina and brain in rhesus monkeys. *Proc Natl Acad Sci USA.* 1986;83(11):4021–4025

40. Øyen J, Kvestad I, Midtbø LK, et al. Fatty fish intake and cognitive function: FINS-KIDS, a randomized controlled trial in preschool children. *BMC Med.* 2018;16(1):41

41. Handeland K, Øyen J, Skotheim S, et al. Fatty fish intake and attention performance in 14-15 year old adolescents: FINS-TEENS - a randomized controlled trial. *Nutr J.* 2017;16(1):64

42. Hibbeln JR, Davis JM, Steer C, et al. Maternal seafood consumption in pregnancy and neurodevelopmental outcomes in childhood (ALSPAC study): an observational cohort study. *Lancet.* 2007;369(9561):578–585

43. Oken E, Østerdal ML, Gillman MW, et al. Associations of maternal fish intake during pregnancy and breastfeeding duration with attainment of developmental milestones in early childhood: a study from the Danish National Birth Cohort. *Am J Clin Nutr.* 2008;88(3):789–796

44. Oken E, Wright RO, Kleinman KP, et al. Maternal fish consumption, hair mercury, and infant cognition in a U.S. Cohort. *Environ Health Perspect.* 2005;113(10):1376–1380

45. Oken E, Radesky JS, Wright RO, et al. Maternal fish intake during pregnancy, blood mercury levels, and child cognition at age 3 years in a US cohort. *Am J Epidemiol.* 2008;167(10):1171–1181

46. Oken E, Rifas-Shiman SL, Amarasiriwardena C, et al. Maternal prenatal fish consumption and cognition in mid childhood: mercury, fatty acids, and selenium. *Neurotoxicol Teratol.* 2016;57:71–78

47. Gould JF, Smithers LG, Makrides M. The effect of maternal omega-3 (n-3) LCPUFA supplementation during pregnancy on early childhood cognitive and visual development: a systematic review and meta-analysis of randomized controlled trials. *Am J Clin Nutr.* 2013;97(3):531–544

48. Makrides M, Gould JF, Gawlik NR, et al. Four-year follow-up of children born to women in a randomized trial of prenatal DHA supplementation. *JAMA.* 2014;311(17):1802–1804

49. Willatts P, Forsyth S, Agostoni C, Casaer P, Riva E, Boehm G. Effects of long-chain PUFA supplementation in infant formula on cognitive function in later childhood. *Am J Clin Nutr.* 2013;98(2):S536–S542

50. Campoy C, Escolano-Margarit MV, Anjos T, Szajewska H, Uauy R. Omega 3 fatty acids on child growth, visual acuity and neurodevelopment. *Br J Nutr.* 2012;107(suppl 2):S85–S106

51. Isaacs EB, Ross S, Kennedy K, Weaver LT, Lucas A, Fewtrell MS. 10-year cognition in preterms after random assignment to fatty acid supplementation in infancy. *Pediatrics.* 2011;128(4). Available at: www.pediatrics.org/cgi/content/full/128/4/e890

52. Brew BK, Toelle BG, Webb KL, Almqvist C, Marks GB; CAPS Investigators. Omega-3 supplementation during the first 5 years of life and later academic performance: a randomised controlled trial. *Eur J Clin Nutr.* 2015;69(4):419–424

53. Helland IB, Smith L, Saarem K, Saugstad OD, Drevon CA. Maternal supplementation with very-long-chain n-3 fatty acids during pregnancy and lactation augments children's IQ at 4 years of age. *Pediatrics.* 2003;111(1). Available at: www.pediatrics.org/cgi/content/full/111/1/e39

54. Joffre C, Nadjar A, Lebbadi M, Calon F, Laye S. n-3 LCPUFA improves cognition: the young, the old and the sick. *Prostaglandins Leukot Essent Fatty Acids.* 2014;91(1–2):1–20

55. Boucher O, Burden MJ, Muckle G, et al. Neurophysiologic and neurobehavioral evidence of beneficial effects of prenatal omega-3 fatty acid intake on memory function at school age. *Am J Clin Nutr.* 2011;93(5):1025–1037

56. Parletta N, Cooper P, Gent DN, Petkov J, O'Dea K. Effects of fish oil supplementation on learning and behaviour of children from Australian Indigenous remote community schools: a randomised controlled trial. *Prostaglandins Leukot Essent Fatty Acids.* 2013;89(2–3):71–79

57. Dalton A, Wolmarans P, Witthuhn RC, van Stuijvenberg ME, Swanevelder SA, Smuts CM. A randomised control trial in schoolchildren showed improvement in cognitive function after consuming a bread spread, containing fish flour from a marine source. *Prostaglandins Leukot Essent Fatty Acids.* 2009;80(2–3):143–149

58. Osendarp SJ, Baghurst KI, Bryan J, et al; NEMO Study Group. Effect of a 12-mo micronutrient intervention on learning

and memory in well-nourished and marginally nourished school-aged children: 2 parallel, randomized, placebo-controlled studies in Australia and Indonesia. *Am J Clin Nutr.* 2007; 86(4):1082–1093

59. Richardson AJ, Burton JR, Sewell RP, Spreckelsen TF, Montgomery P. Docosahexaenoic acid for reading, cognition and behavior in children aged 7-9 years: a randomized, controlled trial (the DOLAB Study). *PLoS One.* 2012;7(9): e43909

60. Makrides M, Gibson RA, McPhee AJ, Yelland L, Quinlivan J, Ryan P; DOMInO Investigative Team. Effect of DHA supplementation during pregnancy on maternal depression and neurodevelopment of young children: a randomized controlled trial. *JAMA.* 2010;304(15):1675–1683

61. Collins CT, Gibson RA, Anderson PJ, et al. Neurodevelopmental outcomes at 7 years' corrected age in preterm infants who were fed high-dose docosahexaenoic acid to term equivalent: a follow-up of a randomised controlled trial. *BMJ Open.* 2015;5(3): e007314

62. Gould JF, Treyvaud K, Yelland LN, et al. Seven-year follow-up of children born to women in a randomized trial of prenatal DHA supplementation. *JAMA.* 2017;317(11):1173–1175

63. Gow RV, Hibbeln JR. Omega-3 fatty acid and nutrient deficits in adverse neurodevelopment and childhood behaviors. *Child Adolesc Psychiatr Clin N Am.* 2014;23(3):555–590

64. Montgomery P, Burton JR, Sewell RP, Spreckelsen TF, Richardson AJ. Low blood long chain omega-3 fatty acids in UK children are associated with poor cognitive performance and behavior: a cross-sectional analysis from the DOLAB study. *PLoS One.* 2013;8(6): e66697

65. Kohlboeck G, Glaser C, Tiesler C, et al; LISAplus Study Group. Effect of fatty acid status in cord blood serum on children's behavioral difficulties at 10 y of age: results from the LISAplus Study. *Am J Clin Nutr.* 2011;94(6):1592–1599

66. Gabbay V, Babb JS, Klein RG, et al. A double-blind, placebo-controlled trial of ω-3 fatty acids in Tourette's disorder. *Pediatrics.* 2012;129(6). Available at: www.pediatrics.org/cgi/content/full/129/6/e1493

67. Bloch MH, Qawasmi A. Omega-3 fatty acid supplementation for the treatment of children with attention-deficit/hyperactivity disorder symptomatology: systematic review and meta-analysis. *J Am Acad Child Adolesc Psychiatry.* 2011;50(10):991–1000

68. Gillies D, Sinn JK, Lad SS, Leach MJ, Ross MJ. Polyunsaturated fatty acids (PUFA) for attention deficit hyperactivity disorder (ADHD) in children and adolescents. *Cochrane Database Syst Rev.* 2012;(7):CD007986

69. Widenhorn-Müller K, Schwanda S, Scholz E, Spitzer M, Bode H. Effect of supplementation with long-chain ω-3 polyunsaturated fatty acids on behavior and cognition in children with attention deficit/hyperactivity disorder (ADHD): a randomized placebo-controlled intervention trial. *Prostaglandins Leukot Essent Fatty Acids.* 2014;91(1–2): 49–60

70. Stevenson J, Buitelaar J, Cortese S, et al. Research review: the role of diet in the treatment of attention-deficit/hyperactivity disorder–an appraisal of the evidence on efficacy and recommendations on the design of future studies. *J Child Psychol Psychiatry.* 2014;55(5):416–427

71. Sonuga-Barke EJS, Brandeis D, Cortese S, et al; European ADHD Guidelines Group. Nonpharmacological interventions for ADHD: systematic review and meta-analyses of randomized controlled trials of dietary and psychological treatments. *Am J Psychiatry.* 2013;170(3):275–289

72. Dean AJ, Bor W, Adam K, Bowling FG, Bellgrove MAA. A randomized, controlled, crossover trial of fish oil treatment for impulsive aggression in children and adolescents with disruptive behavior disorders. *J Child Adolesc Psychopharmacol.* 2014;24(3): 140–148

73. Crupi R, Marino A, Cuzzocrea S. n-3 fatty acids: role in neurogenesis and neuroplasticity. *Curr Med Chem.* 2013; 20(24):2953–2963

74. Grosso G, Pajak A, Marventano S, et al. Role of omega-3 fatty acids in the treatment of depressive disorders: a comprehensive meta-analysis of randomized clinical trials. *PLoS One.* 2014;9(5):e96905

75. Bloch MH, Hannestad J. Omega-3 fatty acids for the treatment of depression: systematic review and meta-analysis. *Mol Psychiatry.* 2012;17(12):1272–1282

76. Pottala JV, Talley JA, Churchill SW, Lynch DA, von Schacky C, Harris WS. Red blood cell fatty acids are associated with depression in a case-control study of adolescents. *Prostaglandins Leukot Essent Fatty Acids.* 2012;86(4–5): 161–165

77. McNamara RK, Strimpfel J, Jandacek R, et al. Detection and treatment of long-chain omega-3 fatty acid deficiency in adolescents with SSRI-resistant major depressive disorder. *PharmaNutrition.* 2014;2(2):38–46

78. Murakami K, Miyake Y, Sasaki S, Tanaka K, Arakawa M. Fish and n-3 polyunsaturated fatty acid intake and depressive symptoms: Ryukyus Child Health Study. *Pediatrics.* 2010;126(3). Available at: www.pediatrics.org/cgi/content/full/126/3/e623

79. Oddy WH, Hickling S, Smith MA, et al. Dietary intake of omega-3 fatty acids and risk of depressive symptoms in adolescents. *Depress Anxiety.* 2011; 28(7):582–588

80. Nemets H, Nemets B, Apter A, Bracha Z, Belmaker RH. Omega-3 treatment of childhood depression: a controlled, double-blind pilot study.*Am J Psychiatry.* 2006;163(6):1098–1100

81. Wandersee NJ, Maciaszek JL, Giger KM, et al. Dietary supplementation with docosahexanoic acid (DHA) increases red blood cell membrane flexibility in mice with sickle cell disease. *Blood Cells Mol Dis.* 2015;54(2):183–188

82. Cartwright IJ, Pockley AG, Galloway JH, Greaves M, Preston FE. The effects of dietary omega-3 polyunsaturated fatty acids on erythrocyte membrane phospholipids, erythrocyte deformability and blood viscosity in healthy volunteers. *Atherosclerosis.* 1985;55(3):267–281

83. Tomer A, Kasey S, Connor WE, Clark S, Harker LA, Eckman JR. Reduction of pain episodes and prothrombotic activity in sickle cell disease by dietary n-3 fatty acids. *Thromb Haemost.* 2001; 85(6):966–974

84. Daak AA, Ghebremeskel K, Hassan Z, et al. Effect of omega-3 (n-3) fatty acid supplementation in patients with sickle cell anemia: randomized, double-blind, placebo-controlled trial. *Am J Clin Nutr.* 2013;97(1):37–44

85. Balk EM, Lichtenstein AH, Chung M, Kupelnick B, Chew P, Lau J. Effects of omega-3 fatty acids on serum markers of cardiovascular disease risk: a systematic review. *Atherosclerosis.* 2006;189(1):19–30

86. Juárez-López C, Klünder-Klünder M, Madrigal-Azcárate A, Flores-Huerta S. Omega-3 polyunsaturated fatty acids reduce insulin resistance and triglycerides in obese children and adolescents. *Pediatr Diabetes.* 2013; 14(5):377–383

87. de Ferranti SD, Milliren CE, Denhoff ER, et al. Using high-dose omega-3 fatty acid supplements to lower triglyceride levels in 10- to 19-year-olds. *Clin Pediatr (Phila).* 2014;53(5):428–438

88. Gidding SS, Prospero C, Hossain J, et al. A double-blind randomized trial of fish oil to lower triglycerides and improve cardiometabolic risk in adolescents. *J Pediatr.* 2014;165(3):497–503.e2

89. Nobili V, Bedogni G, Alisi A, et al. Docosahexaenoic acid supplementation decreases liver fat content in children with non-alcoholic fatty liver disease: double-blind randomised controlled clinical trial. *Arch Dis Child.* 2011;96(4): 350–353

90. Miller PE, Van Elswyk M, Alexander DD. Long-chain omega-3 fatty acids eicosapentaenoic acid and docosahexaenoic acid and blood pressure: a meta-analysis of randomized controlled trials. *Am J Hypertens.* 2014;27(7):885–896

91. Geleijnse JM, Giltay EJ, Grobbee DE, Donders ART, Kok FJ. Blood pressure response to fish oil supplementation: metaregression analysis of randomized trials. *J Hypertens.* 2002;20(8): 1493–1499

92. Damsgaard CT, Stark KD, Hjorth MF, et al. n-3 PUFA status in school children is associated with beneficial lipid profile, reduced physical activity and increased blood pressure in boys. *Br J Nutr.* 2013;110(7):1304–1312

93. Lauritzen L, Eriksen SE, Hjorth MF, et al. Maternal fish oil supplementation during lactation is associated with reduced height at 13 years of age and higher blood pressure in boys only. *Br J Nutr.* 2016;116(12):2082–2090

94. Asserhøj M, Nehammer S, Matthiessen J, Michaelsen KF, Lauritzen L. Maternal fish oil supplementation during lactation may adversely affect long-term blood pressure, energy intake, and physical activity of 7-year-old boys. *J Nutr.* 2009;139(2):298–304

95. Forsyth JS, Willatts P, Agostoni C, Bissenden J, Casaer P, Boehm G. Long chain polyunsaturated fatty acid supplementation in infant formula and blood pressure in later childhood: follow up of a randomised controlled trial. *BMJ.* 2003;326(7396):953

96. Rytter D, Christensen JH, Bech BH, Schmidt EB, Henriksen TB, Olsen SF. The effect of maternal fish oil supplementation during the last trimester of pregnancy on blood pressure, heart rate and heart rate variability in the 19-year-old offspring. *Br J Nutr.* 2012;108(8):1475–1483

97. Karagas MR, Choi AL, Oken E, et al. Evidence on the human health effects of low-level methylmercury exposure. *Environ Health Perspect.* 2012;120(6): 799–806

98. Axelrad DA, Bellinger DC, Ryan LM, Woodruff TJ. Dose-response relationship of prenatal mercury exposure and IQ: an integrative analysis of epidemiologic data. *Environ Health Perspect.* 2007;115(4):609–615

99. Cohen JT, Bellinger DC, Shaywitz BA. A quantitative analysis of prenatal methyl mercury exposure and cognitive development. *Am J Prev Med.* 2005; 29(4):353–365

100. Xue F, Holzman C, Rahbar MH, Trosko K, Fischer L. Maternal fish consumption, mercury levels, and risk of preterm delivery. *Environ Health Perspect.* 2007; 115(1):42–47

101. Sunderland EM, Krabbenhoft DP, Moreau JW, Strode SA, Landing WM. Mercury sources, distribution, and bioavailability in the North Pacific Ocean: insights from data and models. *Global Biogeochem Cycles.* 2009;23(2): 1–14

102. US Food and Drug Administration. Advice about eating fish, from the Environmental Protection Agency and Food and Drug Administration. 2017. Available at: https://www.federalregister.gov/documents/2017/01/19/2017-01073/advice-about-eating-fish-from-the-environmental-protection-agency-and-food-and-drug-administration. Accessed April 22, 2019

103. Budtz-Jørgensen E, Grandjean P, Weihe P. Separation of risks and benefits of seafood intake. *Environ Health Perspect.* 2007;115(3):323–327

104. Rice DC, Schoeny R, Mahaffey K. Methods and rationale for derivation of a reference dose for methylmercury by the U.S. EPA. *Risk Anal.* 2003;23(1): 107–115

105. US Environmental Protection Agency. Trends in blood mercury concentrations and fish consumption among U.S. Women of childbearing age. NHANES, 1999–2010. 2013. Available at: https://www.epa.gov/sites/production/files/2018-11/documents/trends-blood-mercury-concentrations-report.pdf. Accessed October 16, 2014

106. Mahaffey KR, Clickner RP, Bodurow CC. Blood organic mercury and dietary mercury intake: National Health and Nutrition Examination Survey, 1999 and 2000. *Environ Health Perspect.* 2004; 112(5):562–570

107. Mortensen ME, Caudill SP, Caldwell KL, Ward CD, Jones RL. Total and methyl mercury in whole blood measured for the first time in the U.S. population: NHANES 2011-2012. *Environ Res.* 2014; 134:257–264

108. Cusack LK, Smit E, Kile ML, Harding AK. Regional and temporal trends in blood mercury concentrations and fish consumption in women of child bearing Age in the united states using NHANES data from 1999-2010. *Environ Health.* 2017;16(1):10

109. Govarts E, Nieuwenhuijsen M, Schoeters G, et al; OBELIX; ENRIECO. Birth weight and prenatal exposure to polychlorinated biphenyls (PCBs) and dichlorodiphenyldichloroethylene (DDE): a meta-analysis within 12 European Birth Cohorts. *Environ Health Perspect.* 2012;120(2):162–170

110. Karmaus W, Zhu X. Maternal concentration of polychlorinated

biphenyls and dichlorodiphenyl dichlorethylene and birth weight in Michigan fish eaters: a cohort study. *Environ Health.* 2004;3(1):1

111. Murphy LE, Gollenberg AL, Buck Louis GM, Kostyniak PJ, Sundaram R. Maternal serum preconception polychlorinated biphenyl concentrations and infant birth weight. *Environ Health Perspect.* 2010;118(2): 297–302

112. Casas M, Nieuwenhuijsen M, Martínez D, et al. Prenatal exposure to PCB-153, p,p'-DDE and birth outcomes in 9000 mother-child pairs: exposure-response relationship and effect modifiers. *Environ Int.* 2015;74:23–31

113. Papadopoulou E, Caspersen IH, Kvalem HE, et al. Maternal dietary intake of dioxins and polychlorinated biphenyls and birth size in the Norwegian Mother and Child Cohort Study (MoBa). *Environ Int.* 2013;60:209–216

114. Ward MH, Colt JS, Metayer C, et al. Residential exposure to polychlorinated biphenyls and organochlorine pesticides and risk of childhood leukemia. *Environ Health Perspect.* 2009;117(6):1007–1013

115. Zani C, Toninelli G, Filisetti B, Donato F. Polychlorinated biphenyls and cancer: an epidemiological assessment. *J Environ Sci Health C Environ Carcinog Ecotoxicol Rev.* 2013;31(2):99–144

116. Freeman MD, Kohles SS. Plasma levels of polychlorinated biphenyls, non-Hodgkin lymphoma, and causation. *J Environ Public Health.* 2012;2012: 258981

117. Tang-Péronard JL, Heitmann BL, Andersen HR, et al. Association between prenatal polychlorinated biphenyl exposure and obesity development at ages 5 and 7 y: a prospective cohort study of 656 children from the Faroe Islands. *Am J Clin Nutr.* 2014;99(1):5–13

118. Valvi D, Mendez MA, Martinez D, et al. Prenatal concentrations of polychlorinated biphenyls, DDE, and DDT and overweight in children: a prospective birth cohort study. *Environ Health Perspect.* 2012;120(3): 451–457

119. Grandjean P, Poulsen LK, Heilmann C, Steuerwald U, Weihe P. Allergy and sensitization during childhood associated with prenatal and lactational exposure to marine pollutants. *Environ Health Perspect.* 2010;118(10):1429–1433

120. Leijs MM, Koppe JG, Olie K, van Aalderen WMC, de Voogt P, ten Tusscher GW. Effects of dioxins, PCBs, and PBDEs on immunology and hematology in adolescents. *Environ Sci Technol.* 2009; 43(20):7946–7951

121. Weisglas-Kuperus N, Patandin S, Berbers GA, et al. Immunologic effects of background exposure to polychlorinated biphenyls and dioxins in Dutch preschool children. *Environ Health Perspect.* 2000;108(12): 1203–1207

122. Hansen S, Strøm M, Olsen SF, et al. Maternal concentrations of persistent organochlorine pollutants and the risk of asthma in offspring: results from a prospective cohort with 20 years of follow-up. *Environ Health Perspect.* 2014;122(1):93–99

123. Gladen BC, Rogan WJ, Hardy P, Thullen J, Tingelstad J, Tully M. Development after exposure to polychlorinated biphenyls and dichlorodiphenyl dichloroethene transplacentally and through human milk. *J Pediatr.* 1988;113(6):991–995

124. Koopman-Esseboom C, Weisglas-Kuperus N, de Ridder MA, Van der Paauw CG, Tuinstra LG, Sauer PJ. Effects of polychlorinated biphenyl/dioxin exposure and feeding type on infants' mental and psychomotor development. *Pediatrics.* 1996;97(5):700–706

125. Park H-Y, Hertz-Picciotto I, Sovcikova E, Kocan A, Drobna B, Trnovec T. Neurodevelopmental toxicity of prenatal polychlorinated biphenyls (PCBs) by chemical structure and activity: a birth cohort study. *Environ Health.* 2010;9:51

126. Park H-Y, Park J-S, Sovcikova E, et al. Exposure to hydroxylated polychlorinated biphenyls (OH-PCBs) in the prenatal period and subsequent neurodevelopment in eastern Slovakia. *Environ Health Perspect.* 2009;117(10): 1600–1606

127. Boucher O, Muckle G, Jacobson JL, et al. Domain-specific effects of prenatal exposure to PCBs, mercury, and lead on infant cognition: results from the Environmental Contaminants and Child Development Study in Nunavik. *Environ Health Perspect.* 2014;122(3):310–316

128. Jacobson JL, Jacobson SW. Intellectual impairment in children exposed to polychlorinated biphenyls in utero. *N Engl J Med.* 1996;335(11):783–789

129. Stewart PW, Lonky E, Reihman J, Pagano J, Gump BB, Darvill T. The relationship between prenatal PCB exposure and intelligence (IQ) in 9-year-old children. *Environ Health Perspect.* 2008;116(10): 1416–1422

130. Korrick SA, Lee MM, Williams PL, et al. Dioxin exposure and age of pubertal onset among Russian boys. *Environ Health Perspect.* 2011;119(9):1339–1344

131. Rennert A, Wittsiepe J, Kasper-Sonnenberg M, et al. Prenatal and early life exposure to polychlorinated dibenzo-p-dioxins, dibenzofurans and biphenyls may influence dehydroepiandrosterone sulfate levels at prepubertal age: results from the Duisburg birth cohort study. *J Toxicol Environ Health A.* 2012;75(19–20): 1232–1240

132. Jackson LW, Lynch CD, Kostyniak PJ, McGuinness BM, Louis GMB. Prenatal and postnatal exposure to polychlorinated biphenyls and child size at 24 months of age. *Reprod Toxicol.* 2010;29(1):25–31

133. Burns JS, Williams PL, Sergeyev O, et al. Serum dioxins and polychlorinated biphenyls are associated with growth among Russian boys. *Pediatrics.* 2011; 127(1). Available at: www.pediatrics.org/cgi/content/full/127/1/e59

134. Xue J, Liu SV, Zartarian VG, Geller AM, Schultz BD. Analysis of NHANES measured blood PCBs in the general US population and application of SHEDS model to identify key exposure factors. *J Expo Sci Environ Epidemiol.* 2014; 24(6):615–621

135. Schecter A, Colacino J, Haffner D, et al. Perfluorinated compounds, polychlorinated biphenyls, and organochlorine pesticide contamination in composite food samples from Dallas, Texas, USA. *Environ Health Perspect.* 2010;118(6): 796–802

136. Schecter A, Cramer P, Boggess K, et al. Intake of dioxins and related compounds from food in the U.S. population. *J Toxicol Environ Health A.* 2001;63(1):1–18

137. Ashley JTF, Ward JS, Anderson CS, et al. Children's daily exposure to polychlorinated biphenyls from dietary supplements containing fish oils. *Food Addit Contam Part A Chem Anal Control Expo Risk Assess*. 2013;30(3):506–514

138. National Institute of Environmental Health Sciences. Dioxins. 2012. Available at: www.niehs.nih.gov/health/materials/dioxins_new_508.pdf

139. US Environmental Protection Agency. National listing of fish advisories: technical fact sheet. 2010. Available at: http://water.epa.gov/scitech/swguidance/fishshellfish/fishadvisories/technical_factsheet_2010.cfm#figure4. Accessed October 18, 2014

140. Rawn DFK, Breakell K, Verigin V, et al. Impacts of cooking technique on polychlorinated biphenyl and polychlorinated dioxins/furan concentrations in fish and fish products with intake estimates. *J Agric Food Chem*. 2013;61(4):989–997

141. Bayen S, Barlow P, Lee HK, Obbard JP. Effect of cooking on the loss of persistent organic pollutants from salmon. *J Toxicol Environ Health A*. 2005;68(4):253–265

142. Karimi R, Fitzgerald TP, Fisher NS. A quantitative synthesis of mercury in commercial seafood and implications for exposure in the United States. *Environ Health Perspect*. 2012;120(11):1512–1519

143. Oken E. Seafood consumption in pregnancy. UptoDate. Available at: https://www.uptodate.com/contents/fish-consumption-and-marine-n-3-long-chain-polyunsaturated-fatty-acid-supplementation-in-pregnancy. Accessed April 22, 2019

144. Gould LH, Walsh KA, Vieira AR, et al; Centers for Disease Control and Prevention. Surveillance for foodborne disease outbreaks - United States, 1998-2008. *MMWR Surveill Summ*. 2013;62(2):1–34

145. Pennotti R, Scallan E, Backer L, Thomas J, Angulo FJ. Ciguatera and scombroid fish poisoning in the United States. *Foodborne Pathog Dis*. 2013;10(12):1059–1066

146. Kibler SR, Tester PA, Kunkel KE, Moore SK, Litaker RW. Effects of ocean warming on growth and distribution of dinoflagellates associated with ciguatera fish poisoning in the Caribbean. *Ecol Modell*. 2015;316:194–210

147. Gochfeld M, Burger J. Disproportionate exposures in environmental justice and other populations: the importance of outliers. *Am J Public Health*. 2011;101(suppl 1):S53–S63

148. Kuhnlein HV, Chan HM. Environment and contaminants in traditional food systems of northern indigenous peoples. *Annu Rev Nutr*. 2000;20(1):595–626

149. Daniel CR, Cross AJ, Koebnick C, Sinha R. Trends in meat consumption in the USA. *Public Health Nutr*. 2011;14(4):575–583

150. Gerber LR, Karimi R, Fitzgerald TP. Sustaining seafood for public health. *Front Ecol Environ*. 2012;10(9):487–493

151. Brashares JS, Arcese P, Sam MK, Coppolillo PB, Sinclair ARE, Balmford A. Bushmeat hunting, wildlife declines, and fish supply in West Africa. *Science*. 2004;306(5699):1180–1183

152. US Bureau of Labor Statistics. National census of fatal occupational injuries. Available at: https://www.bls.gov/news.release/pdf/cfoi.pdf. Accessed April 22, 2019

153. Kiss L, Yun K, Pocock N, Zimmerman C. Exploitation, violence, and suicide risk among child and adolescent survivors of human trafficking in the greater Mekong subregion. *JAMA Pediatr*. 2015;169(9):e152278

154. Bentley J, Kantor L; US Department of Agriculture, Economic Research Service. Food availability (per capita) data system. Available at: https://www.ers.usda.gov/data-products/food-availability-per-capita-data-system/. Accessed September 10, 2018

155. NOAA Office of Science and Technology. Annual trade data by product, country/association. Available at: https://www.st.nmfs.noaa.gov/commercial-fisheries/foreign-trade/applications/annual-product-by-countryassociation. Accessed September 10, 2018

156. Greene J, Ashburn SM, Razzouk L, Smith DA. Fish oils, coronary heart disease, and the environment. *Am J Public Health*. 2013;103(9):1568–1576

157. Food and Agricultural Organization of the United Nations. *The State of World Fisheries and Aquaculture 2016*. Rome, Italy: Food Security and Nutrition Organization; 2016

158. National Oceanic and Atmospheric Administration. FishWatch: the surprising sources of your favorite seafoods. 2015. Available at: www.fishwatch.gov/features/top10seafoods_and_sources_10_10_12.html. Accessed July 21, 2015

159. Consumer Reports. How safe is your shrimp? 2015. Available at: www.consumerreports.org/cro/magazine/2015/06/shrimp-safety/index.htm

160. Van Lavieren H, Spalding M, Alongi D, Kainuma M, Clüsener-Godt M, Adeel Z. Securing the future of mangroves, a policy brief. 2012 Available at https://en.unesco.org/news/policy-brief-securing-future-mangroves. Accessed April 26, 2019

161. Barbier EB. Natural barriers to natural disasters: replanting mangroves after the tsunami. *Front Ecol Environ*. 2006;4(3):124–131

162. Coscorbi A. Farmed shrimp: worldwide overview. 2004. Available at: http://www.seafoodwatch.org/-/m/sfw/pdf/reports/s/mba_seafoodwatch_farmedshrimpreport.pdf. Accessed April 22, 2019

163. Hites RA, Foran JA, Carpenter DO, Hamilton MC, Knuth BA, Schwager SJ. Global assessment of organic contaminants in farmed salmon. *Science*. 2004;303(5655):226–229

164. Mozaffarian D, Rimm EB. Fish intake, contaminants, and human health: evaluating the risks and the benefits. *JAMA*. 2006;296(15):1885–1899

165. Howard BC. Salmon farming gets leaner and greener. *National Geographic*. March 19. 2014. Available at: http://news.nationalgeographic.com/news/2014/03/140319-salmon-farming-sustainable-aquaculture/. Accessed July 21, 2015

166. Potts J, Wilkings A, Lynch M, McFatridge S. *State of Sustainability Initiatives Review: Standards and the Blue Economy*. Winnipeg, Canada: International Institute for Sustainable Development; 2016

167. Eshel G, Shepon A, Makov T, Milo R. Land, irrigation water, greenhouse gas, and reactive nitrogen burdens of meat, eggs, and dairy production in the

United States. *Proc Natl Acad Sci USA.* 2014;111(33):11996–12001

168. Ziegler F, Winther U, Hognes ES, Emanuelsson A, Sund V, Ellingsen H. The carbon footprint of Norwegian seafood products on the global seafood market. *J Ind Ecol.* 2013;17(1):103–116

169. Nijdam D, Rood T, Westhoek H. The price of protein: review of land use and carbon footprints from life cycle assessments of animal food products and their substitutes. *Food Policy.* 2012; 37(6):760–770

170. Stokstad E. The carbon footprint of a shrimp cocktail. *Science News.* February 17, 2012. Available at: http://news.sciencemag.org/earth/2012/02/carbon-footprint-shrimp-cocktail. Accessed July 31, 2015

171. Kauffman JB, Heider C, Norfolk J, Payton F. Carbon stocks of intact mangroves and carbon emissions arising from their conversion in the Dominican Republic. *Ecol Appl.* 2014;24(3):518–527

172. National Oceanic and Atmospheric Administration. NOAA - FishWatch: farmed Atlantic Salmon. FishWatch U.S. seafood facts. 2015. Available at: www.fishwatch.gov/seafood_profiles/species/salmon/species_pages/atlantic_salmon_farmed.htm. Accessed July 31, 2015

173. US Department of Agriculture. USDA's National Agricultural Statistics Service: aquaculture. 2015. Available at: https://www.nass.usda.gov/Statistics_by_State/Florida/Publications/Aquaculture/

174. Lowther A, Liddel M. *Fisheries of the United States.* Silver Spring, MD: National Marine Fisheries Service Office of Science and Technology; 2014

175. Oken E, Kleinman KP, Berland WE, Simon SR, Rich-Edwards JW, Gillman MW. Decline in fish consumption among pregnant women after a national mercury advisory. *Obstet Gynecol.* 2003; 102(2):346–351

176. Dietary Guidelines Advisory Committee to the US Department of Health and Human Services and the US Department of Agriculture. Scientific Report of the 2015 Dietary Guidelines Advisory Committee. Appendix E-2.38: evidence portfolio part D. Chapter 5: food sustainability and safety. 2015. Available at: http://health.gov/dietaryguidelines/2015-scientific-report/14-appendix-e2/e2-38.asp

Guidelines for Monitoring and Management of Pediatric Patients Before, During, and After Sedation for Diagnostic and Therapeutic Procedures

- *Clinical Report*

American Academy of Pediatrics

DEDICATED TO THE HEALTH OF ALL CHILDREN™

Guidelines for Monitoring and Management of Pediatric Patients Before, During, and After Sedation for Diagnostic and Therapeutic Procedures

Charles J. Coté, MD, FAAP, Stephen Wilson, DMD, MA, PhD, AMERICAN ACADEMY OF PEDIATRICS, AMERICAN ACADEMY OF PEDIATRIC DENTISTRY

abstract

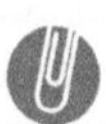

The safe sedation of children for procedures requires a systematic approach that includes the following: no administration of sedating medication without the safety net of medical/dental supervision, careful presedation evaluation for underlying medical or surgical conditions that would place the child at increased risk from sedating medications, appropriate fasting for elective procedures and a balance between the depth of sedation and risk for those who are unable to fast because of the urgent nature of the procedure, a focused airway examination for large (kissing) tonsils or anatomic airway abnormalities that might increase the potential for airway obstruction, a clear understanding of the medication's pharmacokinetic and pharmacodynamic effects and drug interactions, appropriate training and skills in airway management to allow rescue of the patient, age- and size-appropriate equipment for airway management and venous access, appropriate medications and reversal agents, sufficient numbers of appropriately trained staff to both carry out the procedure and monitor the patient, appropriate physiologic monitoring during and after the procedure, a properly equipped and staffed recovery area, recovery to the presedation level of consciousness before discharge from medical/dental supervision, and appropriate discharge instructions. This report was developed through a collaborative effort of the American Academy of Pediatrics and the American Academy of Pediatric Dentistry to offer pediatric providers updated information and guidance in delivering safe sedation to children.

This document is copyrighted and is property of the American Academy of Pediatrics and its Board of Directors. All authors have filed conflict of interest statements with the American Academy of Pediatrics. Any conflicts have been resolved through a process approved by the Board of Directors. The American Academy of Pediatrics has neither solicited nor accepted any commercial involvement in the development of the content of this publication.

Clinical reports from the American Academy of Pediatrics benefit from expertise and resources of liaisons and internal (AAP) and external reviewers. However, clinical reports from the American Academy of Pediatrics may not reflect the views of the liaisons or the organizations or government agencies that they represent.

The guidance in this report does not indicate an exclusive course of treatment or serve as a standard of medical/dental care. Variations, taking into account individual circumstances, may be appropriate.

All clinical reports from the American Academy of Pediatrics automatically expire 5 years after publication unless reaffirmed, revised, or retired at or before that time.

DOI: https://doi.org/10.1542/peds.2019-1000

PEDIATRICS (ISSN Numbers: Print, 0031-4005; Online, 1098-4275).

Copyright © 2019 by the American Academy of Pediatric Dentistry and American Academy of Pediatrics. This report is also being published in Pediatr Dent 2019;41(4): in press. The articles are identical. Either citation can be used when citing this report.

FINANCIAL DISCLOSURE: The authors have indicated they do not have a financial relationship relevant to this article to disclose.

FUNDING: No external funding.

To cite: Coté CJ, Wilson S. AMERICAN ACADEMY OF PEDIATRICS, AMERICAN ACADEMY OF PEDIATRIC DENTISTRY. Guidelines for Monitoring and Management of Pediatric Patients Before, During, and After Sedation for Diagnostic and Therapeutic Procedures. *Pediatrics.* 2019;143(6):e20191000

INTRODUCTION

The number of diagnostic and minor surgical procedures performed on pediatric patients outside of the traditional operating room setting has increased in the past several decades. As a consequence of this change and the increased awareness of the importance of providing analgesia and anxiolysis, the need for sedation for procedures in physicians' offices, dental offices, subspecialty procedure suites, imaging facilities, emergency departments, other inpatient hospital settings, and ambulatory surgery centers also has increased markedly.[1–52] In recognition of this need for both elective and emergency use of sedation in nontraditional settings, the American Academy of Pediatrics (AAP) and the American Academy of Pediatric Dentistry (AAPD) have published a series of guidelines for the monitoring and management of pediatric patients during and after sedation for a procedure.[53–58] The purpose of this updated report is to unify the guidelines for sedation used by medical and dental practitioners; to add clarifications regarding monitoring modalities, particularly regarding continuous expired carbon dioxide measurement; to provide updated information from the medical and dental literature; and to suggest methods for further improvement in safety and outcomes. This document uses the same language to define sedation categories and expected physiologic responses as The Joint Commission, the American Society of Anesthesiologists (ASA), and the AAPD.[56,57,59–61]

This revised statement reflects the current understanding of appropriate monitoring needs of pediatric patients both during and after sedation for a procedure.* The monitoring and care outlined may be exceeded at any time on the basis of the judgment of the responsible practitioner. Although intended to encourage high-quality patient care, adherence to the recommendations in this document cannot guarantee a specific patient outcome. However, structured sedation protocols designed to incorporate these safety principles have been widely implemented and shown to reduce morbidity.† These practice recommendations are proffered with the awareness that, regardless of the intended level of sedation or route of drug administration, the sedation of a pediatric patient represents a continuum and may result in respiratory depression, laryngospasm, impaired airway patency, apnea, loss of the patient's protective airway reflexes, and cardiovascular instability.‡

Procedural sedation of pediatric patients has serious associated risks.§ These adverse responses during and after sedation for a diagnostic or therapeutic procedure may be minimized, but not completely eliminated, by a careful preprocedure review of the patient's underlying medical conditions and consideration of how the sedation process might affect or be affected by these conditions: for example, children with developmental disabilities have been shown to have a threefold increased incidence of desaturation compared with children without developmental disabilities.[74,78,103] Appropriate drug selection for the intended procedure, a clear understanding of the sedating medication's pharmacokinetics and pharmacodynamics and drug interactions, as well as the presence of an individual with the skills needed to rescue a patient from an adverse response are critical.# Appropriate physiologic monitoring and continuous observation by personnel not directly involved with the procedure allow for the accurate and rapid diagnosis of complications and initiation of appropriate rescue interventions.** The work of the Pediatric Sedation Research Consortium has improved the sedation knowledge base, demonstrating the marked safety of sedation by highly motivated and skilled practitioners from a variety of specialties practicing the above modalities and skills that focus on a culture of sedation safety.[45,83,95,128–138] However, these groundbreaking studies also show a low but persistent rate of potential sedation-induced life-threatening events, such as apnea, airway obstruction, laryngospasm, pulmonary aspiration, desaturation, and others, even when the sedation is provided under the direction of a motivated team of specialists.[129] These studies have helped define the skills needed to rescue children experiencing adverse sedation events.

The sedation of children is different from the sedation of adults. Sedation in children is often administered to relieve pain and anxiety as well as to modify behavior (eg, immobility) so as to allow the safe completion of a procedure. A child's ability to control his or her own behavior to cooperate for a procedure depends both on his or her chronologic age and cognitive/emotional development. Many brief procedures, such as suture of a minor laceration, may be accomplished with distraction and guided imagery techniques, along with the use of topical/local anesthetics and minimal sedation, if needed.[175–181] However, longer procedures that require immobility involving children younger than 6 years or those with developmental delay often require an increased depth of sedation to gain control of their behavior.[86,87,103] Children younger than 6 years (particularly those younger than 6 months) may be at greatest risk of an adverse event.[129] Children in this age group are particularly vulnerable to the sedating medication's effects on

* Refs 3, 4, 11, 18, 20, 21, 23, 24, 33, 39, 41, 44, 47, 51, and 62–73

† Refs 11, 23, 24, 27, 30–33, 35, 39, 41, 44, 47, 51, and 74–84

‡ Refs 38, 43, 45, 47, 48, 59, 62, 63, and 85–112

§ Refs 2, 5, 38, 43, 45, 47, 48, 62, 63, 71, 83, 85, 88–105, and 107–138

Refs 42, 48, 62, 63, 92, 97, 99, 125–127, 132, 133, and 139–158

** Refs 44, 63, 64, 67, 68, 74, 90, 96, 110, and 159–174

respiratory drive, airway patency, and protective airway reflexes.[62,63] Other modalities, such as careful preparation, parental presence, hypnosis, distraction, topical local anesthetics, electronic devices with age-appropriate games or videos, guided imagery, and the techniques advised by child life specialists, may reduce the need for or the needed depth of pharmacologic sedation.[29,46,49,182–211]

Studies have shown that it is common for children to pass from the intended level of sedation to a deeper, unintended level of sedation,[85,88,212,213] making the concept of rescue essential to safe sedation. Practitioners of sedation must have the skills to rescue the patient from a deeper level than that intended for the procedure. For example, if the intended level of sedation is "minimal," practitioners must be able to rescue from "moderate sedation"; if the intended level of sedation is "moderate," practitioners must have the skills to rescue from "deep sedation"; if the intended level of sedation is "deep," practitioners must have the skills to rescue from a state of "general anesthesia." The ability to rescue means that practitioners must be able to recognize the various levels of sedation and have the skills and age- and size-appropriate equipment necessary to provide appropriate cardiopulmonary support if needed.

These guidelines are intended for all venues in which sedation for a procedure might be performed (hospital, surgical center, freestanding imaging facility, dental facility, or private office). Sedation and anesthesia in a nonhospital environment (eg, private physician's or dental office, freestanding imaging facility) historically have been associated with an increased incidence of "failure to rescue" from adverse events, because these settings may lack immediately available backup. Immediate activation of emergency medical services (EMS) may be required in such settings, but the practitioner is responsible for life-support measures while awaiting EMS arrival.[63,214] Rescue techniques require specific training and skills.[63,74,215,216] The maintenance of the skills needed to rescue a child with apnea, laryngospasm, and/or airway obstruction include the ability to open the airway, suction secretions, provide continuous positive airway pressure (CPAP), perform successful bag-valve-mask ventilation, insert an oral airway, a nasopharyngeal airway, or a laryngeal mask airway (LMA), and, rarely, perform tracheal intubation. These skills are likely best maintained with frequent simulation and team training for the management of rare events.[128,130,217–220] Competency with emergency airway management procedure algorithms is fundamental for safe sedation practice and successful patient rescue (see Figs 1, 2, and 3).[215,216,221–223]

Practitioners should have an in-depth knowledge of the agents they intend to use and their potential complications. A number of reviews and handbooks for sedating pediatric patients are available.[††] There are specific situations that are beyond the scope of this document. Specifically, guidelines for the delivery of general anesthesia and monitored anesthesia care (sedation or analgesia), outside or within the operating room by anesthesiologists or other practitioners functioning within a department of anesthesiology, are addressed by policies developed by the ASA and by individual departments of anesthesiology.[234] In addition, guidelines for the sedation of patients undergoing mechanical ventilation in a critical care environment or for providing analgesia for patients postoperatively, patients with chronic painful conditions, and patients in hospice care are beyond the scope of this document.

Suggested Management of Airway Obstructions

Reposition the airway → successful
↓ unsuccessful
Perform a jaw thrust → successful
↓ unsuccessful
Insert oral airway → successful
↓ unsuccessful
Call for help
↓
Insert nasal trumpet → successful
↓ unsuccessful
Insert supraglottic device (LMA or other) → successful
↓ unsuccessful
Tracheal intubation → successful
↓ unsuccessful
Surgical airway

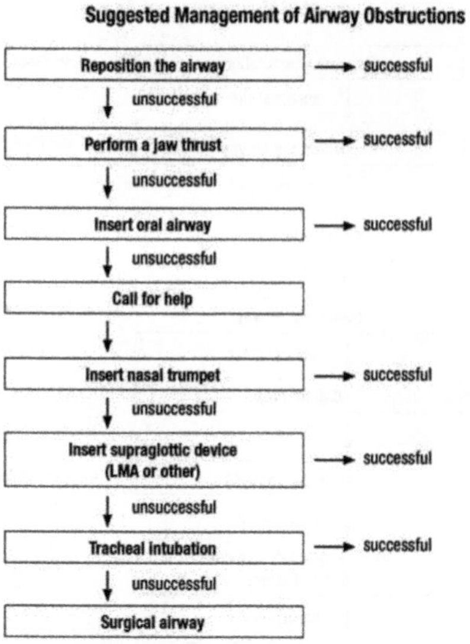

FIGURE 1
Suggested management of airway obstruction.

GOALS OF SEDATION

The goals of sedation in the pediatric patient for diagnostic and therapeutic procedures are as follows: (1) to guard the patient's safety and welfare; (2) to minimize physical discomfort and pain; (3) to control anxiety, minimize psychological trauma, and maximize the potential for amnesia; (4) to

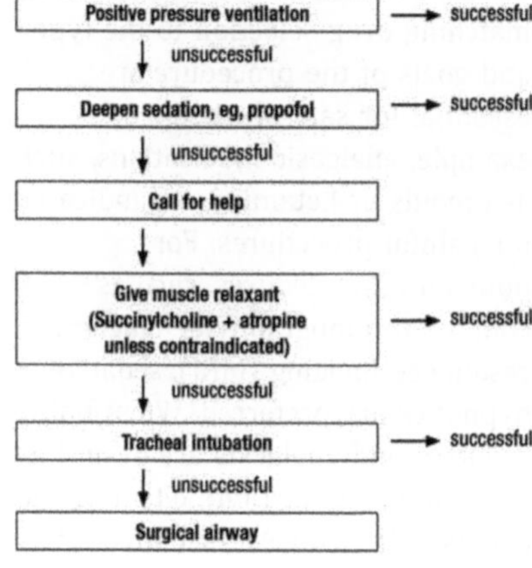

FIGURE 2
Suggested management of laryngospasm.

†† Refs 30, 39, 65, 75, 171, 172, 201, 224–233

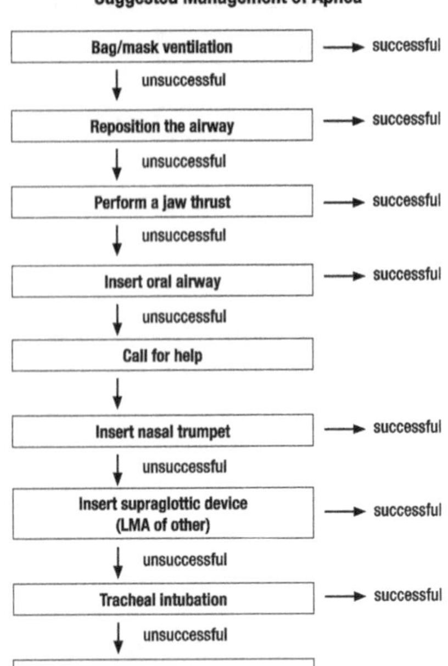

FIGURE 3
Suggested management of apnea.

modify behavior and/or movement so as to allow the safe completion of the procedure; and (5) to return the patient to a state in which discharge from medical/dental supervision is safe, as determined by recognized criteria (Supplemental Appendix 1).

These goals can best be achieved by selecting the lowest dose of drug with the highest therapeutic index for the procedure. It is beyond the scope of this document to specify which drugs are appropriate for which procedures; however, the selection of the fewest number of drugs and matching drug selection to the type and goals of the procedure are essential for safe practice. For example, analgesic medications, such as opioids or ketamine, are indicated for painful procedures. For nonpainful procedures, such as computed tomography or magnetic resonance imaging (MRI), sedatives/hypnotics are preferred. When both sedation and analgesia are desirable (eg, fracture reduction), either single agents with analgesic/sedative properties or combination regimens are commonly used. Anxiolysis and amnesia are additional goals that should be considered in the selection of agents for particular patients. However, the potential for an adverse outcome may be increased when 2 or more sedating medications are administered.[62,127,136,173,235] Recently, there has been renewed interest in noninvasive routes of medication administration, including intranasal and inhaled routes (eg, nitrous oxide; see below).[236]

Knowledge of each drug's time of onset, peak response, and duration of action is important (eg, the peak electroencephalogram (EEG) effect of intravenous midazolam occurs at ~4.8 minutes, compared with that of diazepam at ~1.6 minutes[237–239]). Titration of drug to effect is an important concept; one must know whether the previous dose has taken full effect before administering additional drugs.[237] Drugs that have a long duration of action (eg, intramuscular pentobarbital, phenothiazines) have fallen out of favor because of unpredictable responses and prolonged recovery. The use of these drugs requires a longer period of observation even after the child achieves currently used recovery and discharge criteria.[62,238–241] This concept is particularly important for infants and toddlers transported in car safety seats; re-sedation after discharge attributable to residual prolonged drug effects may lead to airway obstruction.[62,63,242] In particular, promethazine (Phenergan; Wyeth Pharmaceuticals, Philadelphia, PA) has a "black box warning" regarding fatal respiratory depression in children younger than 2 years.[243] Although the liquid formulation of chloral hydrate is no longer commercially available, some hospital pharmacies now are compounding their own formulations. Low-dose chloral hydrate (10–25 mg/kg), in combination with other sedating medications, is used commonly in pediatric dental practice.

GENERAL GUIDELINES

Candidates

Patients who are in ASA classes I and II are frequently considered appropriate candidates for minimal, moderate, or deep sedation (Supplemental Appendix 2). Children in ASA classes III and IV, children with special needs, and those with anatomic airway abnormalities or moderate to severe tonsillar hypertrophy present issues that require additional and individual consideration, particularly for moderate and deep sedation.[68,244–249] Practitioners are encouraged to consult with appropriate subspecialists and/or an anesthesiologist for patients at increased risk of experiencing adverse sedation events because of their underlying medical/surgical conditions.

Responsible Person

The pediatric patient shall be accompanied to and from the treatment facility by a parent, legal guardian, or other responsible person. It is preferable to have 2 adults accompany children who are still in car safety seats if transportation to and from a treatment facility is provided by 1 of the adults.[250]

Facilities

The practitioner who uses sedation must have immediately available facilities, personnel, and equipment to manage emergency and rescue situations. The most common serious complications of sedation involve compromise of the airway or depressed respirations resulting in airway obstruction, hypoventilation, laryngospasm, hypoxemia, and apnea. Hypotension and cardiopulmonary arrest may occur, usually from the inadequate recognition and treatment of respiratory compromise.‡‡ Other rare complications also may include

‡‡ Refs 42, 48, 92, 97, 99, 125, 132, and 139–155

seizures, vomiting, and allergic reactions. Facilities providing pediatric sedation should monitor for, and be prepared to treat, such complications.

Back-up Emergency Services

A protocol for immediate access to back-up emergency services shall be clearly outlined. For nonhospital facilities, a protocol for the immediate activation of the EMS system for life-threatening complications must be established and maintained.[44] It should be understood that the availability of EMS does not replace the practitioner's responsibility to provide initial rescue for life-threatening complications.

On-site Monitoring, Rescue Drugs, and Equipment

An emergency cart or kit must be immediately accessible. This cart or kit must contain the necessary age- and size-appropriate equipment (oral and nasal airways, bag-valve-mask device, LMAs or other supraglottic devices, laryngoscope blades, tracheal tubes, face masks, blood pressure cuffs, intravenous catheters, etc) to resuscitate a nonbreathing and unconscious child. The contents of the kit must allow for the provision of continuous life support while the patient is being transported to a medical/dental facility or to another area within the facility. All equipment and drugs must be checked and maintained on a scheduled basis (see Supplemental Appendices 3 and 4 for suggested drugs and emergency life support equipment to consider before the need for rescue occurs). Monitoring devices, such as electrocardiography (ECG) machines, pulse oximeters with size-appropriate probes, end-tidal carbon dioxide monitors, and defibrillators with size-appropriate patches/paddles, must have a safety and function check on a regular basis as required by local or state regulation. The use of emergency checklists is recommended, and these should be immediately available at all sedation locations; they can be obtained from http://www.pedsanesthesia.org/.

Documentation

Documentation prior to sedation shall include, but not be limited to, the following recommendations:

1. Informed consent: The patient record shall document that appropriate informed consent was obtained according to local, state, and institutional requirements.[251,252]
2. Instructions and information provided to the responsible person: The practitioner shall provide verbal and/or written instructions to the responsible person. Information shall include objectives of the sedation and anticipated changes in behavior during and after sedation.[163,253–255] Special instructions shall be given to the adult responsible for infants and toddlers who will be transported home in a car safety seat regarding the need to carefully observe the child's head position to avoid airway obstruction. Transportation in a car safety seat poses a particular risk for infants who have received medications known to have a long half-life, such as chloral hydrate, intramuscular pentobarbital, or phenothiazine because deaths after procedural sedation have been reported.[62,63,238,242,256,257] Consideration for a longer period of observation shall be given if the responsible person's ability to observe the child is limited (eg, only 1 adult who also has to drive). Another indication for prolonged observation would be a child with an anatomic airway problem, an underlying medical condition such as significant obstructive sleep apnea (OSA), or a former preterm infant younger than 60 weeks' postconceptional age. A 24-hour telephone number for the practitioner or his or her associates shall be provided to all patients and their families. Instructions shall include limitations of activities and appropriate dietary precautions.

Dietary Precautions

Agents used for sedation have the potential to impair protective airway reflexes, particularly during deep sedation. Although a rare occurrence, pulmonary aspiration may occur if the child regurgitates and cannot protect his or her airway.[95,127,258] Therefore, the practitioner should evaluate preceding food and fluid intake before administering sedation. It is likely that the risk of aspiration during procedural sedation differs from that during general anesthesia involving tracheal intubation or other airway manipulations.[259,260] However, the absolute risk of aspiration during elective procedural sedation is not yet known; the reported incidence varies from ~1 in 825 to ~1 in 30 037.[95,127,129,173,244,261] Therefore, standard practice for fasting before elective sedation generally follows the same guidelines as for elective general anesthesia; this requirement is particularly important for solids, because aspiration of clear gastric contents causes less pulmonary injury than aspiration of particulate gastric contents.[262,263]

For emergency procedures in children undergoing general anesthesia, the reported incidence of pulmonary aspiration of gastric contents from 1 institution is ~1 in 373 compared with ~1 in 4544 for elective anesthetics.[262] Because there are few published studies with adequate statistical power to provide guidance to the practitioner regarding the safety or risk of pulmonary aspiration of gastric contents during procedural sedation,[§§] it is unknown whether the risk of aspiration is

---

§§ Refs 95, 127, 129, 173, 244, 259–261, and 264–268

reduced when airway manipulation is not performed/anticipated (eg, moderate sedation). However, if a deeply sedated child requires intervention for airway obstruction, apnea, or laryngospasm, there is concern that these rescue maneuvers could increase the risk of pulmonary aspiration of gastric contents. For children requiring urgent/emergent sedation who do not meet elective fasting guidelines, the risks of sedation and possible aspiration are as-yet unknown and must be balanced against the benefits of performing the procedure promptly. For example, a prudent practitioner would be unlikely to administer deep sedation to a child with a minor condition who just ate a large meal; conversely, it is not justifiable to withhold sedation/analgesia from the child in significant pain from a displaced fracture who had a small snack a few hours earlier. Several emergency department studies have reported a low to zero incidence of pulmonary aspiration despite variable fasting periods[260,264,268]; however, each of these reports has, for the most part, clearly balanced the urgency of the procedure with the need for and depth of sedation.[268,269] Although emergency medicine studies and practice guidelines generally support a less restrictive approach to fasting for brief urgent/emergent procedures, such as care of wounds, joint dislocation, chest tube placement, etc, in healthy children, further research in many thousands of patients would be desirable to better define the relationships between various fasting intervals and sedation complications.[262–270]

Before Elective Sedation

Children undergoing sedation for elective procedures generally should follow the same fasting guidelines as those for general anesthesia (Table 1).[271] It is permissible for routine necessary medications (eg, antiseizure medications) to be taken with a sip of clear liquid or water on the day of the procedure.

TABLE 1 Appropriate Intake of Food and Liquids Before Elective Sedation

Ingested Material	Minimum Fasting Period, h
Clear liquids: water, fruit juices without pulp, carbonated beverages, clear tea, black coffee	2
Human milk	4
Infant formula	6
Nonhuman milk: because nonhuman milk is similar to solids in gastric emptying time, the amount ingested must be considered when determining an appropriate fasting period.	6
Light meal: a light meal typically consists of toast and clear liquids. Meals that include fried or fatty foods or meat may prolong gastric emptying time. Both the amount and type of foods ingested must be considered when determining an appropriate fasting period.	6

Source: American Society of Anesthesiologists. Practice guidelines for preoperative fasting and the use of pharmacologic agents to reduce the risk of pulmonary aspiration: application to healthy patients undergoing elective procedures. An updated report by the American Society of Anesthesiologists Committee on Standards and Practice Parameters. Available at: https://www.asahq.org/For-Members/Practice-Management/Practice-Parameters.aspx. For emergent sedation, the practitioner must balance the depth of sedation versus the risk of possible aspiration; see also Mace et al[272] and Green et al.[273]

For the Emergency Patient

The practitioner must always balance the possible risks of sedating nonfasted patients with the benefits of and necessity for completing the procedure. In particular, patients with a history of recent oral intake or with other known risk factors, such as trauma, decreased level of consciousness, extreme obesity (BMI ≥95% for age and sex), pregnancy, or bowel motility dysfunction, require careful evaluation before the administration of sedatives. When proper fasting has not been ensured, the increased risks of sedation must be carefully weighed against its benefits, and the lightest effective sedation should be used. In this circumstance, additional techniques for achieving analgesia and patient cooperation, such as distraction, guided imagery, video games, topical and local anesthetics, hematoma block or nerve blocks, and other techniques advised by child life specialists, are particularly helpful and should be considered.[29,49,182–201,274,275]

The use of agents with less risk of depressing protective airway reflexes, such as ketamine, or moderate sedation, which would also maintain protective reflexes, may be preferred.[276] Some emergency patients requiring deep sedation (eg, a trauma patient who just ate a full meal or a child with a bowel obstruction) may need to be intubated to protect their airway before they can be sedated.

Use of Immobilization Devices (Protective Stabilization)

Immobilization devices, such as papoose boards, must be applied in such a way as to avoid airway obstruction or chest restriction.[277–281] The child's head position and respiratory excursions should be checked frequently to ensure airway patency. If an immobilization device is used, a hand or foot should be kept exposed, and the child should never be left unattended. If sedating medications are administered in conjunction with an immobilization device, monitoring must be used at a level consistent with the level of sedation achieved.

Documentation at the Time of Sedation

1. Health evaluation: Before sedation, a health evaluation shall be performed by an appropriately

licensed practitioner and reviewed by the sedation team at the time of treatment for possible interval changes.[282] The purpose of this evaluation is not only to document baseline status but also to determine whether the patient has specific risk factors that may warrant additional consultation before sedation. This evaluation also facilitates the identification of patients who will require more advanced airway or cardiovascular management skills or alterations in the doses or types of medications used for procedural sedation.

An important concern for the practitioner is the widespread use of medications that may interfere with drug absorption or metabolism and therefore enhance or shorten the effect time of sedating medications. Herbal medicines (eg, St John's wort, ginkgo, ginger, ginseng, garlic) may alter drug pharmacokinetics through inhibition of the cytochrome P450 system, resulting in prolonged drug effect and altered (increased or decreased) blood drug concentrations (midazolam, cyclosporine, tacrolimus).[283–292] Kava may increase the effects of sedatives by potentiating γ-aminobutyric acid inhibitory neurotransmission and may increase acetaminophen-induced liver toxicity.[293–295] Valerian may itself produce sedation that apparently is mediated through the modulation of γ-aminobutyric acid neurotransmission and receptor function.[291,296–299] Drugs such as erythromycin, cimetidine, and others may also inhibit the cytochrome P450 system, resulting in prolonged sedation with midazolam as well as other medications competing for the same enzyme systems.[300–304] Medications used to treat HIV infection, some anticonvulsants, immunosuppressive drugs, and some psychotropic medications (often used to treat children with autism spectrum disorder) may also produce clinically important drug-drug interactions.[305–314] Therefore, a careful drug history is a vital part of the safe sedation of children. The practitioner should consult various sources (a pharmacist, textbooks, online services, or handheld databases) for specific information on drug interactions.[315–319] The US Food and Drug Administration issued a warning in February 2013 regarding the use of codeine for postoperative pain management in children undergoing tonsillectomy, particularly those with OSA. The safety issue is that some children have duplicated cytochromes that allow greater than expected conversion of the prodrug codeine to morphine, thus resulting in potential overdose; codeine should be avoided for postprocedure analgesia.[320–324]

The health evaluation should include the following:

- age and weight (in kg) and gestational age at birth (preterm infants may have associated sequelae such as apnea of prematurity); and
- health history, including (1) food and medication allergies and previous allergic or adverse drug reactions; (2) medication/drug history, including dosage, time, route, and site of administration for prescription, over-the-counter, herbal, or illicit drugs; (3) relevant diseases, physical abnormalities (including genetic syndromes), neurologic impairments that might increase the potential for airway obstruction, obesity, a history of snoring or OSA,[325–328] or cervical spine instability in Down syndrome, Marfan syndrome, skeletal dysplasia, and other conditions; (4) pregnancy status (as many as 1% of menarchal females presenting for general anesthesia at children's hospitals are pregnant)[329–331] because of concerns for the potential adverse effects of most sedating and anesthetic drugs on the fetus[329,332–338]; (5) history of prematurity (may be associated with subglottic stenosis or propensity to apnea after sedation); (6) history of any seizure disorder; (7) summary of previous relevant hospitalizations; (8) history of sedation or general anesthesia and any complications or unexpected responses; and (9) relevant family history, particularly related to anesthesia (eg, muscular dystrophy, malignant hyperthermia, pseudocholinesterase deficiency).

The review of systems should focus on abnormalities of cardiac, pulmonary, renal, or hepatic function that might alter the child's expected responses to sedating/analgesic medications. A specific query regarding signs and symptoms of sleep-disordered breathing and OSA may be helpful. Children with severe OSA who have experienced repeated episodes of desaturation will likely have altered mu receptors and be analgesic at opioid levels one-third to one-half those of a child without OSA[325–328,339,340]; lower titrated doses of opioids should be used in this population. Such a detailed history will help to determine which patients may benefit from a higher level of care by an appropriately skilled health care provider, such as an anesthesiologist. The health evaluation should also include:

- vital signs, including heart rate, blood pressure, respiratory rate, room air oxygen saturation, and temperature (for some children who are very upset or noncooperative, this may not be possible and a note should be written to document this circumstance);
- physical examination, including a focused evaluation of the airway (tonsillar hypertrophy, abnormal anatomy [eg, mandibular hypoplasia], high Mallampati score [ie, ability to visualize only the hard palate or tip of the uvula]) to determine whether there is an increased risk of airway obstruction[74,341–344];

- physical status evaluation (ASA classification [see Appendix 2]); and
- name, address, and telephone number of the child's home or parent's, or caregiver's cell phone; additional information such as the patient's personal care provider or medical home is also encouraged.

For hospitalized patients, the current hospital record may suffice for adequate documentation of presedation health; however, a note shall be written documenting that the chart was reviewed, positive findings were noted, and a management plan was formulated. If the clinical or emergency condition of the patient precludes acquiring complete information before sedation, this health evaluation should be obtained as soon as feasible.

2. Prescriptions. When prescriptions are used for sedation, a copy of the prescription or a note describing the content of the prescription should be in the patient's chart along with a description of the instructions that were given to the responsible person. **Prescription medications intended to accomplish procedural sedation must not be administered without the safety net of direct supervision by trained medical/dental personnel.** The administration of sedating medications at home poses an unacceptable risk, particularly for infants and preschool-aged children traveling in car safety seats because deaths as a result of this practice have been reported.[63,257]

Documentation During Treatment

The patient's chart shall contain a time-based record that includes the name, route, site, time, dosage/kilogram, and patient effect of administered drugs. Before sedation, a "time out" should be performed to confirm the patient's name, procedure to be performed, and laterality and site of the procedure.[59] During administration, the inspired concentrations of oxygen and inhalation sedation agents and the duration of their administration shall be documented. Before drug administration, special attention must be paid to the calculation of dosage (ie, mg/kg); for obese patients, most drug doses should likely be adjusted lower to ideal body weight rather than actual weight.[345] When a programmable pump is used for the infusion of sedating medications, the dose/kilogram per minute or hour and the child's weight in kilograms should be double-checked and confirmed by a separate individual. The patient's chart shall contain documentation at the time of treatment that the patient's level of consciousness and responsiveness, heart rate, blood pressure, respiratory rate, expired carbon dioxide values, and oxygen saturation were monitored. Standard vital signs should be further documented at appropriate intervals during recovery until the patient attains predetermined discharge criteria (Appendix 1). A variety of sedation scoring systems are available that may aid this process.[212,238,346–348] Adverse events and their treatment shall be documented.

Documentation After Treatment

A dedicated and properly equipped recovery area is recommended (see Appendices 3 and 4). The time and condition of the child at discharge from the treatment area or facility shall be documented, which should include documentation that the child's level of consciousness and oxygen saturation in room air have returned to a state that is safe for discharge by recognized criteria (see Appendix 1). Patients receiving supplemental oxygen before the procedure should have a similar oxygen need after the procedure. Because some sedation medications are known to have a long half-life and may delay a patient's complete return to baseline or pose the risk of re-sedation[62,104,256,349,350] and because some patients will have complex multiorgan medical conditions, a longer period of observation in a less intense observation area (eg, a step-down observation area) before discharge from medical/dental supervision may be indicated.[239] Several scales to evaluate recovery have been devised and validated.[212,346–348,351,352] A simple evaluation tool may be the ability of the infant or child to remain awake for at least 20 minutes when placed in a quiet environment.[238]

CONTINUOUS QUALITY IMPROVEMENT

The essence of medical error reduction is a careful examination of index events and root-cause analysis of how the event could be avoided in the future.[353–359] Therefore, each facility should maintain records that track all adverse events and significant interventions, such as desaturation; apnea; laryngospasm; need for airway interventions, including the need for placement of supraglottic devices such as an oral airway, nasal trumpet, or LMA; positive-pressure ventilation; prolonged sedation; unanticipated use of reversal agents; unplanned or prolonged hospital admission; sedation failures; inability to complete the procedure; and unsatisfactory sedation, analgesia, or anxiolysis.[360] Such events can then be examined for the assessment of risk reduction and improvement in patient/family satisfaction.

PREPARATION FOR SEDATION PROCEDURES

Part of the safety net of sedation is using a systematic approach so as to not overlook having an important drug, piece of equipment, or monitor immediately available at the time of a developing emergency. To avoid this problem, it is helpful to use an acronym that allows the same setup and checklist for every procedure. A commonly used acronym useful in planning and preparation for a procedure is **SOAPME**, which represents the following:

S = Size-appropriate suction catheters and a functioning suction apparatus (eg, Yankauer-type suction)

O = an adequate Oxygen supply and functioning flow meters or other devices to allow its delivery

A = size-appropriate Airway equipment (eg, bag-valve-mask or equivalent device [functioning]), nasopharyngeal and oropharyngeal airways, LMA, laryngoscope blades (checked and functioning), endotracheal tubes, stylets, face mask

P = Pharmacy: all the basic drugs needed to support life during an emergency, including antagonists as indicated

M = Monitors: functioning pulse oximeter with size-appropriate oximeter probes,[361,362] end-tidal carbon dioxide monitor, and other monitors as appropriate for the procedure (eg, noninvasive blood pressure, ECG, stethoscope)

E = special Equipment or drugs for a particular case (eg, defibrillator)

SPECIFIC GUIDELINES FOR INTENDED LEVEL OF SEDATION

Minimal Sedation

Minimal sedation (old terminology, "anxiolysis") is a drug-induced state during which patients respond normally to verbal commands. Although cognitive function and coordination may be impaired, ventilatory and cardiovascular functions are unaffected. Children who have received minimal sedation generally will not require more than observation and intermittent assessment of their level of sedation. Some children will become moderately sedated despite the intended level of minimal sedation; should this occur, then the guidelines for moderate sedation apply.[85,363]

Moderate Sedation

Moderate sedation (old terminology, "conscious sedation" or "sedation/analgesia") is a drug-induced depression of consciousness during which patients respond purposefully to verbal commands or after light tactile stimulation. No interventions are required to maintain a patent airway, and spontaneous ventilation is adequate. Cardiovascular function is usually maintained. The caveat that loss of consciousness should be unlikely is a particularly important aspect of the definition of moderate sedation; drugs and techniques used should carry a margin of safety wide enough to render unintended loss of consciousness unlikely. Because the patient who receives moderate sedation may progress into a state of deep sedation and obtundation, the practitioner should be prepared to increase the level of vigilance corresponding to what is necessary for deep sedation.[85]

Personnel

The Practitioner

The practitioner responsible for the treatment of the patient and/or the administration of drugs for sedation must be competent to use such techniques, to provide the level of monitoring described in these guidelines, and to manage complications of these techniques (ie, to be able to rescue the patient). Because the level of intended sedation may be exceeded, the practitioner must be sufficiently skilled to rescue a child with apnea, laryngospasm, and/or airway obstruction, including the ability to open the airway, suction secretions, provide CPAP, and perform successful bag-valve-mask ventilation should the child progress to a level of deep sedation. Training in, and maintenance of, advanced pediatric airway skills is required (eg, pediatric advanced life support [PALS]); regular skills reinforcement with simulation is strongly encouraged.[79,80,128,130,217–220,364]

Support Personnel

The use of moderate sedation shall include the provision of a person, in addition to the practitioner, whose responsibility is to monitor appropriate physiologic parameters and to assist in any supportive or resuscitation measures, if required. This individual may also be responsible for assisting with interruptible patient-related tasks of short duration, such as holding an instrument or troubleshooting equipment.[60] This individual should be trained in and capable of providing advanced airway skills (eg, PALS). The support person shall have specific assignments in the event of an emergency and current knowledge of the emergency cart inventory. The practitioner and all ancillary personnel should participate in periodic reviews, simulation of rare emergencies, and practice drills of the facility's emergency protocol to ensure proper function of the equipment and coordination of staff roles in such emergencies.[133,365–367] It is recommended that at least 1 practitioner be skilled in obtaining vascular access in children.

Monitoring and Documentation

Baseline

Before the administration of sedative medications, a baseline determination of vital signs shall be documented. For some children who are very upset or uncooperative, this may not be possible, and a note should be written to document this circumstance.

During the Procedure

The physician/dentist or his or her designee shall document the name, route, site, time of administration, and dosage of all drugs administered. If sedation is being directed by a physician who is not personally administering the medications, then recommended practice is for the qualified health care provider administering the medication to confirm the dose verbally before administration. There shall be continuous monitoring of oxygen saturation and heart rate; when bidirectional verbal communication between the provider and patient is appropriate and possible (ie, patient is developmentally able and purposefully communicates), monitoring of ventilation by (1) capnography (preferred) or (2) amplified, audible pretracheal stethoscope (eg, Bluetooth technology)[368–371] or precordial stethoscope is strongly recommended. If bidirectional verbal communication is not appropriate or not possible, monitoring of ventilation by capnography (preferred), amplified, audible pretracheal stethoscope, or precordial stethoscope is required. Heart rate, respiratory rate, blood pressure, oxygen saturation, and expired carbon dioxide values should be recorded, at minimum, every 10 minutes in a time-based record. Note that the exact value of expired carbon dioxide is less important than simple assessment of continuous respiratory gas exchange. In some situations in which there is excessive patient agitation or lack of cooperation or during certain procedures such as bronchoscopy, dentistry, or repair of facial lacerations capnography may not be feasible, and this situation should be documented. For uncooperative children, it is often helpful to defer the initiation of capnography until the child becomes sedated. Similarly, the stimulation of blood pressure cuff inflation may cause arousal or agitation; in such cases, blood pressure monitoring may be counterproductive and may be documented at less frequent intervals (eg, 10–15 minutes, assuming the patient remains stable, well oxygenated, and well perfused). Immobilization devices (protective stabilization) should be checked to prevent airway obstruction or chest restriction. If a restraint device is used, a hand or foot should be kept exposed. The child's head position should be continuously assessed to ensure airway patency.

After the Procedure

The child who has received moderate sedation must be observed in a suitably equipped recovery area, which must have a functioning suction apparatus as well as the capacity to deliver >90% oxygen and positive-pressure ventilation (bag-valve mask) with an adequate oxygen capacity as well as age- and size-appropriate rescue equipment and devices. The patient's vital signs should be recorded at specific intervals (eg, every 10–15 minutes). If the patient is not fully alert, oxygen saturation and heart rate monitoring shall be used continuously until appropriate discharge criteria are met (see Appendix 1). Because sedation medications with a long half-life may delay the patient's complete return to baseline or pose the risk of re-sedation, some patients might benefit from a longer period of less intense observation (eg, a step-down observation area where multiple patients can be observed simultaneously) before discharge from medical/dental supervision (see section entitled "Documentation Before Sedation" above).[62,256,349,350] A simple evaluation tool may be the ability of the infant or child to remain awake for at least 20 minutes when placed in a quiet environment.[238] Patients who have received reversal agents, such as flumazenil or naloxone, will require a longer period of observation, because the duration of the drugs administered may exceed the duration of the antagonist, resulting in re-sedation.

Deep Sedation/General Anesthesia

"Deep sedation" ("deep sedation/analgesia") is a drug-induced depression of consciousness during which patients cannot be easily aroused but respond purposefully after repeated verbal or painful stimulation (eg, purposefully pushing away the noxious stimuli). Reflex withdrawal from a painful stimulus is not considered a purposeful response and is more consistent with a state of general anesthesia. The ability to independently maintain ventilatory function may be impaired. Patients may require assistance in maintaining a patent airway, and spontaneous ventilation may be inadequate. Cardiovascular function is usually maintained. A state of deep sedation may be accompanied by partial or complete loss of protective airway reflexes. Patients may pass from a state of deep sedation to the state of general anesthesia. In some situations, such as during MRI, one is not usually able to assess responses to stimulation, because this would defeat the purpose of sedation, and one should assume that such patients are deeply sedated.

"General anesthesia" is a drug-induced loss of consciousness during which patients are not arousable, even by painful stimulation. The ability to independently maintain ventilatory function is often impaired. Patients often require assistance in maintaining a patent airway, and positive-pressure ventilation may be required because of depressed spontaneous ventilation or drug-induced depression of neuromuscular function. Cardiovascular function may be impaired.

Personnel

During deep sedation and/or general anesthesia of a pediatric patient in a dental facility, there must be at least 2 individuals present with the patient throughout the procedure. These 2 individuals must have appropriate training and up-to-date certification in patient rescue, as delineated below, including drug administration and PALS or Advanced Pediatric Life Support (APLS). One of these 2 must be an independent observer who is independent of performing or assisting with the dental procedure. This individual's sole responsibility is to administer drugs and constantly observe the patient's vital signs, depth of sedation, airway patency, and adequacy of ventilation. The independent observer must, at a minimum, be trained in PALS (or APLS) and capable of managing any airway, ventilatory, or cardiovascular emergency event resulting from the deep sedation and/or general anesthesia. The independent observer must be trained and skilled to establish intravenous access and draw up and administer rescue medications. The independent observer must have the training and skills to rescue a nonbreathing child; a child with airway obstruction; or a child with hypotension, anaphylaxis, or cardiorespiratory arrest, including the ability to open the airway, suction secretions, provide CPAP, insert supraglottic devices (oral airway, nasal trumpet, or laryngeal mask airway), and perform successful bag-valve-mask ventilation, tracheal intubation, and cardiopulmonary resuscitation. The independent observer in the dental facility, as permitted by state regulation, must be 1 of the following: a physician anesthesiologist, a certified registered nurse anesthetist, a second oral surgeon, or a dentist anesthesiologist. The second individual, who is the practitioner in the dental facility performing the procedure, must be trained in PALS (or APLS) and capable of providing skilled assistance to the independent observer with the rescue of a child experiencing any of the adverse events described above.

During deep sedation and/or general anesthesia of a pediatric patient in a hospital or surgicenter setting, at least 2 individuals must be present with the patient throughout the procedure with skills in patient rescue and up-to-date PALS (or APLS) certification, as delineated above. One of these individuals may either administer drugs or direct their administration by the skilled independent observer. The skills of the individual directing or administering sedation and/or anesthesia medications must include those described in the previous paragraph. Providers who may fulfill the role of the skilled independent observer in a hospital or surgicenter, as permitted by state regulation, must be a physician with sedation training and advanced airway skills, such as, but not limited to, a physician anesthesiologist, an oral surgeon, a dentist anesthesiologist, or other medical specialists with the requisite licensure, training, and competencies; a certified registered nurse anesthetist or certified anesthesiology assistant; or a nurse with advanced emergency management skills, such as several years of experience in the emergency department, pediatric recovery room, or intensive care setting (ie, nurses who are experienced with assisting the individual administering or directing sedation with patient rescue during life-threatening emergencies).

Equipment

In addition to the equipment needed for moderate sedation, an ECG monitor and a defibrillator for use in pediatric patients should be readily available.

Vascular Access

Patients receiving deep sedation should have an intravenous line placed at the start of the procedure or have a person skilled in establishing vascular access in pediatric patients immediately available.

Monitoring

A competent individual shall observe the patient continuously. Monitoring shall include all parameters described for moderate sedation. Vital signs, including heart rate, respiratory rate, blood pressure, oxygen saturation, and expired carbon dioxide, must be documented at least every 5 minutes in a time-based record. Capnography should be used for almost all deeply sedated children because of the increased risk of airway/ventilation compromise. Capnography may not be feasible if the patient is agitated or uncooperative during the initial phases of sedation or during certain procedures, such as bronchoscopy or repair of facial lacerations, and this circumstance should be documented. For uncooperative children, the capnography monitor may be placed once the child becomes sedated. Note that if supplemental oxygen is administered, the capnograph may underestimate the true expired carbon dioxide value; of more importance than the numeric reading of exhaled carbon dioxide is the assurance of continuous respiratory gas exchange (ie, continuous waveform). Capnography is particularly useful for patients who are difficult to observe (eg, during MRI or in a darkened room).[##]

The physician/dentist or his or her designee shall document the name, route, site, time of administration, and dosage of all drugs administered. If sedation is being directed by a physician who is not personally administering the medications, then recommended practice is for the nurse administering the medication to confirm the dose verbally before administration. The inspired concentrations of inhalation sedation agents and oxygen and the duration of administration shall be documented.

Postsedation Care

The facility and procedures followed for postsedation care shall conform

[##] Refs 64, 67, 72, 90, 96, 110, 159–162, 164–170, and 372–375

TABLE 2 Comparison of Moderate and Deep Sedation Equipment and Personnel Requirements

	Moderate Sedation	Deep Sedation
Personnel	An observer who will monitor the patient but who may also assist with interruptible tasks; should be trained in PALS	An independent observer whose only responsibility is to continuously monitor the patient; trained in PALS
Responsible practitioner	Skilled to rescue a child with apnea, laryngospasm, and/or airway obstruction including the ability to open the airway, suction secretions, provide CPAP, and perform successful bag-valve-mask ventilation; recommended that at least 1 practitioner should be skilled in obtaining vascular access in children; trained in PALS	Skilled to rescue a child with apnea, laryngospasm, and/or airway obstruction, including the ability to open the airway, suction secretions, provide CPAP, perform successful bag-valve-mask ventilation, tracheal intubation, and cardiopulmonary resuscitation; training in PALS is required; at least 1 practitioner skilled in obtaining vascular access in children immediately available
Monitoring	Pulse oximetry ECG recommended Heart rate Blood pressure Respiration Capnography recommended	Pulse oximetry ECG required Heart rate Blood pressure Respiration Capnography required
Other equipment	Suction equipment, adequate oxygen source/supply	Suction equipment, adequate oxygen source/supply, defibrillator required
Documentation	Name, route, site, time of administration, and dosage of all drugs administered Continuous oxygen saturation, heart rate, and ventilation (capnography recommended); parameters recorded every 10 minutes	Name, route, site, time of administration, and dosage of all drugs administered; continuous oxygen saturation, heart rate, and ventilation (capnography required); parameters recorded at least every 5 minutes
Emergency checklists	Recommended	Recommended
Rescue cart properly stocked with rescue drugs and age- and size-appropriate equipment (see Appendices 3 and 4)	Required	Required
Dedicated recovery area with rescue cart properly stocked with rescue drugs and age- and size-appropriate equipment (see Appendices 3 and 4) and dedicated recovery personnel; adequate oxygen supply	Recommended; initial recording of vital signs may be needed at least every 10 minutes until the child begins to awaken, then recording intervals may be increased	Recommended; initial recording of vital signs may be needed for at least 5-minute intervals until the child begins to awaken, then recording intervals may be increased to 10–15 minutes
Discharge criteria	See Appendix 1	See Appendix 1

to those described under "moderate sedation." The initial recording of vital signs should be documented at least every 5 minutes. Once the child begins to awaken, the recording intervals may be increased to 10 to 15 minutes. Table 2 summarizes the equipment, personnel, and monitoring requirements for moderate and deep sedation.

Special Considerations

Neonates and Former Preterm Infants

Neonates and former preterm infants require specific management, because immaturity of hepatic and renal function may alter the ability to metabolize and excrete sedating medications,[376] resulting in prolonged sedation and the need for extended postsedation monitoring. Former preterm infants have an increased risk of postanesthesia apnea,[377] but it is unclear whether a similar risk is associated with sedation, because this possibility has not been systematically investigated.[378]

Other concerns regarding the effects of anesthetic drugs and sedating medications on the developing brain are beyond the scope of this document. At this point, the research in this area is preliminary and inconclusive at best, but it would seem prudent to avoid unnecessary exposure to sedation if the procedure is unlikely to change medical/dental management (eg, a sedated MRI purely for screening purposes in preterm infants).[379–382]

Local Anesthetic Agents

All local anesthetic agents are cardiac depressants and may cause central nervous system excitation or depression. Particular weight-based attention should be paid to cumulative dosage in all children.[118,120,125,383–386] To ensure that the patient will not receive an excessive dose, the maximum allowable safe dosage (eg, mg/kg) should be calculated before administration. There may be enhanced sedative effects when the highest recommended doses of local anesthetic drugs are used in combination with other sedatives or opioids (see Tables 3 and 4 for limits and conversion tables of commonly used local anesthetics).[118,125,387–400] In general, when administering local anesthetic drugs, the practitioner should aspirate frequently to minimize the likelihood that the needle is in a blood vessel; lower doses should be used when injecting into vascular tissues.[401] If high doses or injection of amide local anesthetics

TABLE 3 Commonly Used Local Anesthetic Agents for Nerve Block or Infiltration: Doses, Duration, and Calculations

Local Anesthetic	Maximum Dose With Epinephrine,[a] mg/kg		Maximum Dose Without Epinephrine, mg/kg		Duration of Action,[b] min
	Medical	Dental	Medical	Dental	
Esters					
Procaine	10.0	6	7	6	60–90
Chloroprocaine	20.0	12	15	12	30–60
Tetracaine	1.5	1	1	1	180–600
Amides					
Lidocaine	7.0	4.4	4	4.4	90–200
Mepivacaine	7.0	4.4	5	4.4	120–240
Bupivacaine	3.0	1.3	2.5	1.3	180–600
Levobupivacaine[c]	3.0	2	2	2	180–600
Ropivacaine	3.0	2	2	2	180–600
Articaine[d]	—	7	—	7	60–230

Maximum recommended doses and durations of action are shown. Note that lower doses should be used in very vascular areas.

[a] These are maximum doses of local anesthetics combined with epinephrine; lower doses are recommended when used without epinephrine. Doses of amides should be decreased by 30% in infants younger than 6 mo. When lidocaine is being administered intravascularly (eg, during intravenous regional anesthesia), the dose should be decreased to 3 to 5 mg/kg; long-acting local anesthetic agents should not be used for intravenous regional anesthesia.

[b] Duration of action is dependent on concentration, total dose, and site of administration; use of epinephrine; and the patient's age.

[c] Levobupivacaine is not available in the United States.

[d] Use in pediatric patients under 4 years of age is not recommended.

(bupivacaine and ropivacaine) into vascular tissues is anticipated, then the immediate availability of a 20% lipid emulsion for the treatment of local anesthetic toxicity is recommended (Tables 3 and 5).[402–409] Topical local anesthetics are commonly used and encouraged, but the practitioner should avoid applying excessive doses to mucosal surfaces where systemic uptake and possible toxicity (seizures, methemoglobinemia) could result and to remain within the manufacturer's recommendations regarding allowable surface area application.[410–415]

Pulse Oximetry

Newer pulse oximeters are less susceptible to motion artifacts and may be more useful than older oximeters that do not contain updated software.[416–420] Oximeters that change tone with changes in hemoglobin saturation provide immediate aural warning to everyone within hearing distance. The oximeter probe must be properly positioned; clip-on devices are easy to displace, which may produce artifactual data (under- or overestimation of oxygen saturation).[361,362]

TABLE 4 Local Anesthetic Conversion Chart

Concentration, %	mg/mL
4.0	40
3.0	30
2.5	25
2.0	20
1.0	10
0.5	5
0.25	2.5
0.125	1.25

Capnography

Expired carbon dioxide monitoring is valuable to diagnose the simple presence or absence of respirations, airway obstruction, or respiratory depression, particularly in patients sedated in less-accessible locations, such as in MRI machines or darkened rooms.*** In patients receiving supplemental oxygen, capnography facilitates the recognition of apnea or airway obstruction several minutes before the situation would be detected just by pulse oximetry. In this situation, desaturation would be delayed due to increased oxygen reserves; capnography would enable earlier intervention.[161] One study in children sedated in the emergency department found that the use of capnography reduced the incidence of hypoventilation and desaturation (7% to 1%).[174] The use of expired carbon dioxide monitoring devices is now required for almost all deeply sedated children (with rare exceptions), particularly in situations in which other means of assessing the adequacy of ventilation are limited. Several manufacturers have produced nasal cannulae that allow simultaneous delivery of oxygen and measurement of expired carbon dioxide values.[421,422,427] Although these devices can have a high degree of false-positive alarms, they are also very accurate for the detection of complete airway obstruction or apnea.[164,168,169] Taping the sampling line under the nares under an oxygen face mask or nasal hood will provide similar information. The exact measured value is less important than the simple answer to the question: Is the child exchanging air with each breath?

*** Refs 64, 66, 67, 72, 90, 96, 110, 159–162, 164–170, 372–375, and 421–427

Processed EEG (Bispectral Index)

Although not new to the anesthesia community, the processed EEG (bispectral index [BIS]) monitor is slowly finding its way into the sedation literature.[428] Several studies

TABLE 5 Treatment of Local Anesthetic Toxicity

1. Get help. Ventilate with 100% oxygen. Alert nearest facility with cardiopulmonary bypass capability.
2. Resuscitation: airway/ventilatory support, chest compressions, etc. Avoid vasopressin, calcium channel blockers, β-blockers, or additional local anesthetic. Reduce epinephrine dosages. Prolonged effort may be required.
3. Seizure management: benzodiazepines preferred (eg, intravenous midazolam 0.1–0.2 mg/kg); avoid propofol if cardiovascular instability.
4. Administer 1.5 mL/kg 20% lipid emulsion over ~1 minute to trap unbound amide local anesthetics. Repeat bolus once or twice for persistent cardiovascular collapse.
5. Initiate 20% lipid infusion (0.25 mL/kg per minute) until circulation is restored; double the infusion rate if blood pressure remains low. Continue infusion for at least 10 minutes after attaining circulatory stability. Recommended upper limit of ~10 mL/kg.
6. A fluid bolus of 10–20 mL/kg balanced salt solution and an infusion of phenylephrine (0.1 μg/kg per minute to start) may be needed to correct peripheral vasodilation.

Source: https://www.asra.com/advisory-guidelines/article/3/checklist-for-treatment-of-local-anesthetic-systemic-toxicity.

have attempted to use BIS monitoring as a means of noninvasively assessing the depth of sedation. This technology was designed to examine EEG signals and, through a variety of algorithms, correlate a number with depth of unconsciousness: that is, the lower the number, the deeper the sedation. Unfortunately, these algorithms are based on adult patients and have not been validated in children of varying ages and varying brain development. Although the readings correspond quite well with the depth of propofol sedation, the numbers may paradoxically go up rather than down with sevoflurane and ketamine because of central excitation despite a state of general anesthesia or deep sedation.[429,430] Opioids and benzodiazepines have minimal and variable effects on the BIS. Dexmedetomidine has minimal effect with EEG patterns, consistent with stage 2 sleep.[431] Several sedation studies have examined the utility of this device and degree of correlation with standard sedation scales.[347,363,432–435] It appears that there is some correlation with BIS values in moderate sedation, but there is not a reliable ability to distinguish between deep sedation and moderate sedation or deep sedation from general anesthesia.[432] Presently, it would appear that BIS monitoring might provide useful information only when used for sedation with propofol[363]; in general, it is still considered a research tool and not recommended for routine use.

Adjuncts to Airway Management and Resuscitation

The vast majority of sedation complications can be managed with simple maneuvers, such as supplemental oxygen, opening the airway, suctioning, placement of an oral or nasopharyngeal airway, and bag-mask-valve ventilation. Rarely, tracheal intubation is required for more prolonged ventilatory support. In addition to standard tracheal intubation techniques, a number of supraglottic devices are available for the management of patients with abnormal airway anatomy or airway obstruction. Examples include the LMA, the cuffed oropharyngeal airway, and a variety of kits to perform an emergency cricothyrotomy.[436,437]

The largest clinical experience in pediatrics is with the LMA, which is available in multiple sizes, including those for late preterm and term neonates. The use of the LMA is now an essential addition to advanced airway training courses, and familiarity with insertion techniques can be life-saving.[438–442] The LMA can also serve as a bridge to secure airway management in children with anatomic airway abnormalities.[443,444] Practitioners are encouraged to gain experience with these techniques as they become incorporated into PALS courses.

Another valuable emergency technique is intraosseous needle placement for vascular access. Intraosseous needles are available in several sizes; insertion can be life-saving when rapid intravenous access is difficult. A relatively new intraosseous device (EZ-IO Vidacare, now part of Teleflex, Research Triangle Park, NC) is similar to a hand-held battery-powered drill. It allows rapid placement with minimal chance of misplacement; it also has a low-profile intravenous adapter.[445–450] Familiarity with the use of these emergency techniques can be gained by keeping current with resuscitation courses, such as PALS and advanced pediatric life support.

Patient Simulators

High-fidelity patient simulators are now available that allow physicians, dentists, and other health care providers to practice managing a variety of programmed adverse events, such as apnea, bronchospasm, and laryngospasm.[133,220,450–452] The use of such devices is encouraged to better train medical professionals and teams to respond more effectively to rare events.[128,131,451,453–455] One study that simulated the quality of cardiopulmonary resuscitation compared standard management of ventricular fibrillation versus rescue with the EZ-IO for the rapid establishment of intravenous access and placement of an LMA for establishing a patent airway in adults; the use of these devices resulted in more rapid establishment of vascular access and securing of the airway.[456]

Monitoring During MRI

The powerful magnetic field and the generation of radiofrequency emissions necessitate the use of special equipment to provide continuous patient monitoring throughout the MRI scanning procedure.[457–459] MRI-compatible pulse oximeters and capnographs capable of continuous function during scanning should be used in any sedated or restrained pediatric patient. Thermal injuries can result if appropriate precautions are not taken; the practitioner is cautioned to avoid coiling of all wires (oximeter, ECG) and to place the oximeter probe as far from the magnetic coil as possible to diminish the possibility of injury. ECG monitoring during MRI has been associated with thermal injury; special MRI-compatible ECG pads are essential to allow safe monitoring.[460–463] If sedation is achieved by using an infusion pump, then either an MRI-compatible pump is required or the pump must be situated outside of the room with long infusion tubing so as to maintain infusion accuracy. All equipment must be MRI compatible, including laryngoscope blades and handles, oxygen tanks, and any ancillary equipment. All individuals, including parents, must be screened for ferromagnetic materials, phones, pagers, pens, credit cards, watches, surgical implants, pacemakers, etc, before entry into the MRI suite.

Nitrous Oxide

Inhalation sedation/analgesia equipment that delivers nitrous oxide must have the capacity of delivering 100% and never less than 25% oxygen concentration at a flow rate appropriate to the size of the patient. Equipment that delivers variable ratios of nitrous oxide >50% to oxygen that covers the mouth and nose must be used in conjunction with a calibrated and functional oxygen analyzer. All nitrous oxide-to-oxygen inhalation devices should be calibrated in accordance with appropriate state and local requirements. Consideration should be given to the National Institute of Occupational Safety and Health Standards for the scavenging of waste gases.[464] Newly constructed or reconstructed treatment facilities, especially those with piped-in nitrous oxide and oxygen, must have appropriate state or local inspections to certify proper function of inhalation sedation/analgesia systems before any delivery of patient care.

Nitrous oxide in oxygen, with varying concentrations, has been successfully used for many years to provide analgesia for a variety of painful procedures in children.[14,36,49,98,465–493] The use of nitrous oxide for minimal sedation is defined as the administration of nitrous oxide of ≤50% with the balance as oxygen, without any other sedative, opioid, or other depressant drug before or concurrent with the nitrous oxide to an otherwise healthy patient in ASA class I or II. The patient is able to maintain verbal communication throughout the procedure. It should be noted that although local anesthetics have sedative properties, for purposes of this guideline they are not considered sedatives in this circumstance. If nitrous oxide in oxygen is combined with other sedating medications, such as chloral hydrate, midazolam, or an opioid, or if nitrous oxide is used in concentrations >50%, the likelihood for moderate or deep sedation increases.[107,197,492,494,495] In this situation, the practitioner is advised to institute the guidelines for moderate or deep sedation, as indicated by the patient's response.[496]

LEAD AUTHORS

Charles J. Coté, MD, FAAP
Stephen Wilson, DMD, MA, PhD

AMERICAN ACADEMY OF PEDIATRICS

AMERICAN ACADEMY OF PEDIATRIC DENTISTRY

STAFF

Jennifer Riefe, MEd
Raymond J. Koteras, MHA

ABBREVIATIONS

AAP: American Academy of Pediatrics
AAPD: American Academy of Pediatric Dentistry
ASA: American Society of Anesthesiologists
BIS: bispectral index
CPAP: continuous positive airway pressure
ECG: electrocardiography
EEG: electroencephalogram/electroencephalography
EMS: emergency medical services
LMA: laryngeal mask airway
MRI: magnetic resonance imaging
OSA: obstructive sleep apnea
PALS: pediatric advanced life support

POTENTIAL CONFLICT OF INTEREST: The authors have indicated they have no potential conflicts of interest to disclose.

REFERENCES

1. Milnes AR. Intravenous procedural sedation: an alternative to general anesthesia in the treatment of early childhood caries. *J Can Dent Assoc.* 2003;69:298–302

2. Law AK, Ng DK, Chan KK. Use of intramuscular ketamine for endoscopy sedation in children. *Pediatr Int.* 2003;45(2):180–185

3. Flood RG, Krauss B. Procedural sedation and analgesia for children in the emergency department. *Emerg Med Clin North Am.* 2003;21(1):121–139

4. Jaggar SI, Haxby E. Sedation, anaesthesia and monitoring for bronchoscopy. *Paediatr Respir Rev.* 2002;3(4):321–327

5. de Blic J, Marchac V, Scheinmann P. Complications of flexible bronchoscopy in children: prospective study of 1,328 procedures. *Eur Respir J.* 2002;20(5):1271–1276

6. Mason KP, Michna E, DiNardo JA, et al. Evolution of a protocol for ketamine-induced sedation as an alternative to general anesthesia for interventional radiologic procedures in pediatric patients. *Radiology.* 2002;225(2):457–465

7. Houpt M. Project USAP 2000—use of sedative agents by pediatric dentists: a 15-year follow-up survey. *Pediatr Dent.* 2002;24(4):289–294

8. Vinson DR, Bradbury DR. Etomidate for procedural sedation in emergency medicine. *Ann Emerg Med.* 2002;39(6):592–598

9. Everitt IJ, Barnett P. Comparison of two benzodiazepines used for sedation of children undergoing suturing of a laceration in an emergency department. *Pediatr Emerg Care.* 2002;18(2):72–74

10. Karian VE, Burrows PE, Zurakowski D, Connor L, Poznauskis L, Mason KP. The development of a pediatric radiology sedation program. *Pediatr Radiol.* 2002;32(5):348–353

11. Kaplan RF, Yang CI. Sedation and analgesia in pediatric patients for procedures outside the operating room. *Anesthesiol Clin North America.* 2002;20(1):181–194, vii

12. Wheeler DS, Jensen RA, Poss WB. A randomized, blinded comparison of chloral hydrate and midazolam sedation in children undergoing echocardiography. *Clin Pediatr (Phila).* 2001;40(7):381–387

13. Hain RD, Campbell C. Invasive procedures carried out in conscious children: contrast between North American and European paediatric oncology centres. *Arch Dis Child.* 2001;85(1):12–15

14. Kennedy RM, Luhmann JD. Pharmacological management of pain and anxiety during emergency procedures in children. *Paediatr Drugs.* 2001;3(5):337–354

15. Kanagasundaram SA, Lane LJ, Cavalletto BP, Keneally JP, Cooper MG. Efficacy and safety of nitrous oxide in alleviating pain and anxiety during painful procedures. *Arch Dis Child.* 2001;84(6):492–495

16. Younge PA, Kendall JM. Sedation for children requiring wound repair: a randomised controlled double blind comparison of oral midazolam and oral ketamine. *Emerg Med J.* 2001;18(1):30–33

17. Ljungman G, Gordh T, Sörensen S, Kreuger A. Lumbar puncture in pediatric oncology: conscious sedation vs. general anesthesia. *Med Pediatr Oncol.* 2001;36(3):372–379

18. Poe SS, Nolan MT, Dang D, et al. Ensuring safety of patients receiving sedation for procedures: evaluation of clinical practice guidelines. *Jt Comm J Qual Improv.* 2001;27(1):28–41

19. D'Agostino J, Terndrup TE. Chloral hydrate versus midazolam for sedation of children for neuroimaging: a randomized clinical trial. *Pediatr Emerg Care.* 2000;16(1):1–4

20. Green SM, Kuppermann N, Rothrock SG, Hummel CB, Ho M. Predictors of adverse events with intramuscular ketamine sedation in children. *Ann Emerg Med.* 2000;35(1):35–42

21. Hopkins KL, Davis PC, Sanders CL, Churchill LH. Sedation for pediatric imaging studies. *Neuroimaging Clin N Am.* 1999;9(1):1–10

22. Bauman LA, Kish I, Baumann RC, Politis GD. Pediatric sedation with analgesia. *Am J Emerg Med.* 1999;17(1):1–3

23. Bhatt-Mehta V, Rosen DA. Sedation in children: current concepts. *Pharmacotherapy.* 1998;18(4):790–807

24. Morton NS, Oomen GJ. Development of a selection and monitoring protocol for safe sedation of children. *Paediatr Anaesth.* 1998;8(1):65–68

25. Murphy MS. Sedation for invasive procedures in paediatrics. *Arch Dis Child.* 1997;77(4):281–284

26. Webb MD, Moore PA. Sedation for pediatric dental patients. *Dent Clin North Am.* 2002;46(4):803–814, xi

27. Malviya S, Voepel-Lewis T, Tait AR, Merkel S. Sedation/analgesia for diagnostic and therapeutic procedures in children. *J Perianesth Nurs.* 2000;15(6):415–422

28. Zempsky WT, Schechter NL. Office-based pain managemen: the 15-minute consultation. *Pediatr Clin North Am.* 2000;47(3):601–615

29. Kennedy RM, Luhmann JD. The "ouchless emergency department": getting closer: advances in decreasing distress during painful procedures in the emergency department. *Pediatr Clin North Am.* 1999;46(6):1215–1247, vii–viii

30. Rodriguez E, Jordan R. Contemporary trends in pediatric sedation and analgesia. *Emerg Med Clin North Am.* 2002;20(1):199–222

31. Ruess L, O'Connor SC, Mikita CP, Creamer KM. Sedation for pediatric diagnostic imaging: use of pediatric and nursing resources as an alternative to a radiology department sedation team. *Pediatr Radiol.* 2002;32(7):505–510

32. Weiss S. Sedation of pediatric patients for nuclear medicine procedures. *Semin Nucl Med.* 1993;23(3):190–198

33. Wilson S. Pharmacologic behavior management for pediatric dental treatment. *Pediatr Clin North Am.* 2000;47(5):1159–1175

34. McCarty EC, Mencio GA, Green NE. Anesthesia and analgesia for the ambulatory management of fractures in children. *J Am Acad Orthop Surg.* 1999;7(2):81–91

35. Egelhoff JC, Ball WS Jr, Koch BL, Parks TD. Safety and efficacy of sedation in children using a structured sedation program. *AJR Am J Roentgenol.* 1997;168(5):1259–1262

36. Heinrich M, Menzel C, Hoffmann F, Berger M, Schweinitz DV. Self-administered procedural analgesia

using nitrous oxide/oxygen (50:50) in the pediatric surgery emergency room: effectiveness and limitations. *Eur J Pediatr Surg*. 2015;25(3):250–256

37. Hoyle JD Jr, Callahan JM, Badawy M, et al; Traumatic Brain Injury Study Group for the Pediatric Emergency Care Applied Research Network (PECARN). Pharmacological sedation for cranial computed tomography in children after minor blunt head trauma. *Pediatr Emerg Care*. 2014;30(1):1–7
38. Chiaretti A, Benini F, Pierri F, et al. Safety and efficacy of propofol administered by paediatricians during procedural sedation in children. *Acta Paediatr*. 2014;103(2):182–187
39. Pacheco GS, Ferayorni A. Pediatric procedural sedation and analgesia. *Emerg Med Clin North Am*. 2013;31(3): 831–852
40. Griffiths MA, Kamat PP, McCracken CE, Simon HK. Is procedural sedation with propofol acceptable for complex imaging? A comparison of short vs. prolonged sedations in children. *Pediatr Radiol*. 2013;43(10):1273–1278
41. Doctor K, Roback MG, Teach SJ. An update on pediatric hospital-based sedation. *Curr Opin Pediatr*. 2013;25(3): 310–316
42. Alletag MJ, Auerbach MA, Baum CR. Ketamine, propofol, and ketofol use for pediatric sedation. *Pediatr Emerg Care*. 2012;28(12):1391–1395; quiz: 1396–1398
43. Jain R, Petrillo-Albarano T, Parks WJ, Linzer JF Sr, Stockwell JA. Efficacy and safety of deep sedation by non-anesthesiologists for cardiac MRI in children. *Pediatr Radiol*. 2013;43(5): 605–611
44. Nelson T, Nelson G. The role of sedation in contemporary pediatric dentistry. *Dent Clin North Am*. 2013;57(1):145–161
45. Monroe KK, Beach M, Reindel R, et al. Analysis of procedural sedation provided by pediatricians. *Pediatr Int*. 2013;55(1):17–23
46. Alexander M. Managing patient stress in pediatric radiology. *Radiol Technol*. 2012;83(6):549–560
47. Macias CG, Chumpitazi CE. Sedation and anesthesia for CT: emerging issues for providing high-quality care. *Pediatr Radiol*. 2011;41(suppl 2):517–522
48. Andolfatto G, Willman E. A prospective case series of pediatric procedural sedation and analgesia in the emergency department using single-syringe ketamine-propofol combination (ketofol). *Acad Emerg Med*. 2010;17(2): 194–201
49. Brown SC, Hart G, Chastain DP, Schneeweiss S, McGrath PA. Reducing distress for children during invasive procedures: randomized clinical trial of effectiveness of the PediSedate. *Paediatr Anaesth*. 2009;19(8):725–731
50. Yamamoto LG. Initiating a hospital-wide pediatric sedation service provided by emergency physicians. *Clin Pediatr (Phila)*. 2008;47(1):37–48
51. Doyle L, Colletti JE. Pediatric procedural sedation and analgesia. *Pediatr Clin North Am*. 2006;53(2):279–292
52. Todd DW. Pediatric sedation and anesthesia for the oral surgeon. *Oral Maxillofac Surg Clin North Am*. 2013; 25(3):467–478, vi–vii
53. Committee on Drugs, Section on Anesthesiology, American Academy of Pediatrics. Guidelines for the elective use of conscious sedation, deep sedation, and general anesthesia in pediatric patients. *Pediatrics*. 1985; 76(2):317–321
54. American Academy of Pediatric Dentistry. Guidelines for the elective use of conscious sedation, deep sedation, and general anesthesia in pediatric patients. *ASDC J Dent Child*. 1986;53(1):21–22
55. Committee on Drugs, American Academy of Pediatrics. Guidelines for monitoring and management of pediatric patients during and after sedation for diagnostic and therapeutic procedures. *Pediatrics*. 1992;89(6 pt 1): 1110–1115
56. Committee on Drugs, American Academy of Pediatrics. Guidelines for monitoring and management of pediatric patients during and after sedation for diagnostic and therapeutic procedures: addendum. *Pediatrics*. 2002;110(4):836–838
57. American Academy of Pediatrics, American Academy of Pediatric Dentistry. Guidelines on the elective use of minimal, moderate, and deep sedation and general anesthesia for pediatric dental patients. 2011. Available at: http://www.aapd.org/media/policies_guidelines/g_sedation.pdf. Accessed May 27, 2016
58. Coté CJ, Wilson S; American Academy of Pediatrics; American Academy of Pediatric Dentistry; Work Group on Sedation. Guidelines for monitoring and management of pediatric patients during and after sedation for diagnostic and therapeutic procedures: an update. *Pediatrics*. 2006;118(6): 2587–2602
59. The Joint Commission. Comprehensive Accreditation Manual for Hospitals (CAMH): the official handbook. Oakbrook Terrace, IL: The Joint Commission; 2014
60. American Society of Anesthesiologists Task Force on Sedation and Analgesia by Non-Anesthesiologists. Practice guidelines for sedation and analgesia by non-anesthesiologists. *Anesthesiology*. 2002;96(4):1004–1017
61. Committee of Origin: Ad Hoc on Non-Anesthesiologist Privileging. Statement on granting privileges for deep sedation to non-anesthesiologist sedation practitioners. 2010. Available at: http://www.asahq.org/~/media/sites/asahq/files/public/resources/standards-guidelines/advisory-on-granting-privileges-for-deep-sedation-to-non-anesthesiologist.pdf. Accessed May 27, 2016
62. Coté CJ, Karl HW, Notterman DA, Weinberg JA, McCloskey C. Adverse sedation events in pediatrics: analysis of medications used for sedation. *Pediatrics*. 2000;106(4):633–644
63. Coté CJ, Notterman DA, Karl HW, Weinberg JA, McCloskey C. Adverse sedation events in pediatrics: a critical incident analysis of contributing factors. *Pediatrics*. 2000;105(4 pt 1): 805–814
64. Kim G, Green SM, Denmark TK, Krauss B. Ventilatory response during dissociative sedation in children-a pilot study. *Acad Emerg Med*. 2003;10(2): 140–145
65. Coté CJ. Sedation for the pediatric patient: a review. *Pediatr Clin North Am*. 1994;41(1):31–58
66. Mason KP, Burrows PE, Dorsey MM, Zurakowski D, Krauss B. Accuracy of

capnography with a 30 foot nasal cannula for monitoring respiratory rate and end-tidal CO2 in children. *J Clin Monit Comput.* 2000;16(4):259–262

67. McQuillen KK, Steele DW. Capnography during sedation/analgesia in the pediatric emergency department. *Pediatr Emerg Care.* 2000;16(6):401–404

68. Malviya S, Voepel-Lewis T, Tait AR. Adverse events and risk factors associated with the sedation of children by nonanesthesiologists. *Anesth Analg.* 1997;85(6):1207–1213

69. Coté CJ, Rolf N, Liu LM, et al. A single-blind study of combined pulse oximetry and capnography in children. *Anesthesiology.* 1991;74(6):980–987

70. Guideline SIGN; Scottish Intercollegiate Guidelines Network. SIGN Guideline 58: safe sedation of children undergoing diagnostic and therapeutic procedures. *Paediatr Anaesth.* 2008;18(1):11–12

71. Peña BM, Krauss B. Adverse events of procedural sedation and analgesia in a pediatric emergency department. *Ann Emerg Med.* 1999;34(4 pt 1):483–491

72. Smally AJ, Nowicki TA. Sedation in the emergency department. *Curr Opin Anaesthesiol.* 2007;20(4):379–383

73. Ratnapalan S, Schneeweiss S. Guidelines to practice: the process of planning and implementing a pediatric sedation program. *Pediatr Emerg Care.* 2007;23(4):262–266

74. Hoffman GM, Nowakowski R, Troshynski TJ, Berens RJ, Weisman SJ. Risk reduction in pediatric procedural sedation by application of an American Academy of Pediatrics/American Society of Anesthesiologists process model. *Pediatrics.* 2002;109(2):236–243

75. Krauss B. Management of acute pain and anxiety in children undergoing procedures in the emergency department. *Pediatr Emerg Care.* 2001; 17(2):115–122; quiz: 123–125

76. Slovis TL. Sedation and anesthesia issues in pediatric imaging. *Pediatr Radiol.* 2011;41(suppl 2):514–516

77. Babl FE, Krieser D, Belousoff J, Theophilos T. Evaluation of a paediatric procedural sedation training and credentialing programme: sustainability of change. *Emerg Med J.* 2010;27(8):577–581

78. Meredith JR, O'Keefe KP, Galwankar S. Pediatric procedural sedation and analgesia. *J Emerg Trauma Shock.* 2008;1(2):88–96

79. Priestley S, Babl FE, Krieser D, et al. Evaluation of the impact of a paediatric procedural sedation credentialing programme on quality of care. *Emerg Med Australas.* 2006;18(5–6):498–504

80. Babl F, Priestley S, Krieser D, et al. Development and implementation of an education and credentialing programme to provide safe paediatric procedural sedation in emergency departments. *Emerg Med Australas.* 2006;18(5–6):489–497

81. Cravero JP, Blike GT. Pediatric sedation. *Curr Opin Anaesthesiol.* 2004;17(3): 247–251

82. Shavit I, Keidan I, Augarten A. The practice of pediatric procedural sedation and analgesia in the emergency department. *Eur J Emerg Med.* 2006;13(5):270–275

83. Langhan ML, Mallory M, Hertzog J, Lowrie L, Cravero J; Pediatric Sedation Research Consortium. Physiologic monitoring practices during pediatric procedural sedation: a report from the Pediatric Sedation Research Consortium. *Arch Pediatr Adolesc Med.* 2012;166(11):990–998

84. Primosch RE. Lidocaine toxicity in children—prevention and intervention. *Todays FDA.* 1992;4:4C–5C

85. Dial S, Silver P, Bock K, Sagy M. Pediatric sedation for procedures titrated to a desired degree of immobility results in unpredictable depth of sedation. *Pediatr Emerg Care.* 2001;17(6):414–420

86. Maxwell LG, Yaster M. The myth of conscious sedation. *Arch Pediatr Adolesc Med.* 1996;150(7):665–667

87. Coté CJ. "Conscious sedation": time for this oxymoron to go away! *J Pediatr.* 2001;139(1):15–17; discussion: 18–19

88. Motas D, McDermott NB, VanSickle T, Friesen RH. Depth of consciousness and deep sedation attained in children as administered by nonanaesthesiologists in a children's hospital. *Paediatr Anaesth.* 2004;14(3):256–260

89. Cudny ME, Wang NE, Bardas SL, Nguyen CN. Adverse events associated with procedural sedation in pediatric patients in the emergency department. *Hosp Pharm.* 2013;48(2):134–142

90. Mora Capín A, Míguez Navarro C, López López R, Marañón Pardillo R. Usefulness of capnography for monitoring sedoanalgesia: influence of oxygen on the parameters monitored [in Spanish]. *An Pediatr (Barc).* 2014;80(1):41–46

91. Frieling T, Heise J, Kreysel C, Kuhlen R, Schepke M. Sedation-associated complications in endoscopy—prospective multicentre survey of 191142 patients. *Z Gastroenterol.* 2013; 51(6):568–572

92. Khutia SK, Mandal MC, Das S, Basu SR. Intravenous infusion of ketamine-propofol can be an alternative to intravenous infusion of fentanyl-propofol for deep sedation and analgesia in paediatric patients undergoing emergency short surgical procedures. *Indian J Anaesth.* 2012; 56(2):145–150

93. Kannikeswaran N, Chen X, Sethuraman U. Utility of endtidal carbon dioxide monitoring in detection of hypoxia during sedation for brain magnetic resonance imaging in children with developmental disabilities. *Paediatr Anaesth.* 2011;21(12):1241–1246

94. McGrane O, Hopkins G, Nielson A, Kang C. Procedural sedation with propofol: a retrospective review of the experiences of an emergency medicine residency program 2005 to 2010. *Am J Emerg Med.* 2012;30(5):706–711

95. Mallory MD, Baxter AL, Yanosky DJ, Cravero JP; Pediatric Sedation Research Consortium. Emergency physician-administered propofol sedation: a report on 25,433 sedations from the Pediatric Sedation Research Consortium. *Ann Emerg Med.* 2011; 57(5):462–468.e1

96. Langhan ML, Chen L, Marshall C, Santucci KA. Detection of hypoventilation by capnography and its association with hypoxia in children undergoing sedation with ketamine. *Pediatr Emerg Care.* 2011;27(5):394–397

97. David H, Shipp J. A randomized controlled trial of ketamine/propofol versus propofol alone for emergency department procedural sedation. *Ann Emerg Med.* 2011;57(5):435–441

98. Babl FE, Belousoff J, Deasy C, Hopper S, Theophilos T. Paediatric procedural sedation based on nitrous oxide and ketamine: sedation registry data from Australia. *Emerg Med J.* 2010;27(8): 607–612

99. Lee-Jayaram JJ, Green A, Siembieda J, et al. Ketamine/midazolam versus etomidate/fentanyl: procedural sedation for pediatric orthopedic reductions. *Pediatr Emerg Care.* 2010; 26(6):408–412

100. Melendez E, Bachur R. Serious adverse events during procedural sedation with ketamine. *Pediatr Emerg Care.* 2009; 25(5):325–328

101. Misra S, Mahajan PV, Chen X, Kannikeswaran N. Safety of procedural sedation and analgesia in children less than 2 years of age in a pediatric emergency department. *Int J Emerg Med.* 2008;1(3):173–177

102. Green SM, Roback MG, Krauss B, et al; Emergency Department Ketamine Meta-Analysis Study Group. Predictors of airway and respiratory adverse events with ketamine sedation in the emergency department: an individual-patient data meta-analysis of 8,282 children. *Ann Emerg Med.* 2009;54(2): 158–168.e1–e4

103. Kannikeswaran N, Mahajan PV, Sethuraman U, Groebe A, Chen X. Sedation medication received and adverse events related to sedation for brain MRI in children with and without developmental disabilities. *Paediatr Anaesth.* 2009;19(3):250–256

104. Ramaswamy P, Babl FE, Deasy C, Sharwood LN. Pediatric procedural sedation with ketamine: time to discharge after intramuscular versus intravenous administration. *Acad Emerg Med.* 2009;16(2):101–107

105. Vardy JM, Dignon N, Mukherjee N, Sami DM, Balachandran G, Taylor S. Audit of the safety and effectiveness of ketamine for procedural sedation in the emergency department. *Emerg Med J.* 2008;25(9):579–582

106. Capapé S, Mora E, Mintegui S, García S, Santiago M, Benito J. Prolonged sedation and airway complications after administration of an inadvertent ketamine overdose in emergency department. *Eur J Emerg Med.* 2008; 15(2):92–94

107. Babl FE, Oakley E, Seaman C, Barnett P, Sharwood LN. High-concentration nitrous oxide for procedural sedation in children: adverse events and depth of sedation. *Pediatrics.* 2008;121(3). Available at: www.pediatrics.org/cgi/content/full/121/3/e528

108. Mahar PJ, Rana JA, Kennedy CS, Christopher NC. A randomized clinical trial of oral transmucosal fentanyl citrate versus intravenous morphine sulfate for initial control of pain in children with extremity injuries. *Pediatr Emerg Care.* 2007;23(8):544–548

109. Sacchetti A, Stander E, Ferguson N, Maniar G, Valko P. Pediatric Procedural Sedation in the Community Emergency Department: results from the ProSCED registry. *Pediatr Emerg Care.* 2007; 23(4):218–222

110. Anderson JL, Junkins E, Pribble C, Guenther E. Capnography and depth of sedation during propofol sedation in children. *Ann Emerg Med.* 2007;49(1): 9–13

111. Luhmann JD, Schootman M, Luhmann SJ, Kennedy RM. A randomized comparison of nitrous oxide plus hematoma block versus ketamine plus midazolam for emergency department forearm fracture reduction in children. *Pediatrics.* 2006;118(4). Available at: www.pediatrics.org/cgi/content/full/118/4/e1078

112. Waterman GD Jr, Leder MS, Cohen DM. Adverse events in pediatric ketamine sedations with or without morphine pretreatment. *Pediatr Emerg Care.* 2006;22(6):408–411

113. Moore PA, Goodson JM. Risk appraisal of narcotic sedation for children. *Anesth Prog.* 1985;32(4):129–139

114. Nahata MC, Clotz MA, Krogg EA. Adverse effects of meperidine, promethazine, and chlorpromazine for sedation in pediatric patients. *Clin Pediatr (Phila).* 1985;24(10):558–560

115. Brown ET, Corbett SW, Green SM. Iatrogenic cardiopulmonary arrest during pediatric sedation with meperidine, promethazine, and chlorpromazine. *Pediatr Emerg Care.* 2001;17(5):351–353

116. Benusis KP, Kapaun D, Furnam LJ. Respiratory depression in a child following meperidine, promethazine, and chlorpromazine premedication: report of case. *ASDC J Dent Child.* 1979; 46(1):50–53

117. Garriott JC, Di Maio VJ. Death in the dental chair: three drug fatalities in dental patients. *J Toxicol Clin Toxicol.* 1982;19(9):987–995

118. Goodson JM, Moore PA. Life-threatening reactions after pedodontic sedation: an assessment of narcotic, local anesthetic, and antiemetic drug interaction. *J Am Dent Assoc.* 1983; 107(2):239–245

119. Jastak JT, Pallasch T. Death after chloral hydrate sedation: report of case. *J Am Dent Assoc.* 1988;116(3):345–348

120. Jastak JT, Peskin RM. Major morbidity or mortality from office anesthetic procedures: a closed-claim analysis of 13 cases. *Anesth Prog.* 1991;38(2):39–44

121. Kaufman E, Jastak JT. Sedation for outpatient dental procedures. *Compend Contin Educ Dent.* 1995;16(5):462–466; quiz: 480

122. Wilson S. Pharmacological management of the pediatric dental patient. *Pediatr Dent.* 2004;26(2): 131–136

123. Sams DR, Thornton JB, Wright JT. The assessment of two oral sedation drug regimens in pediatric dental patients. *ASDC J Dent Child.* 1992;59(4):306–312

124. Geelhoed GC, Landau LI, Le Souëf PN. Evaluation of SaO2 as a predictor of outcome in 280 children presenting with acute asthma. *Ann Emerg Med.* 1994;23(6):1236–1241

125. Chicka MC, Dembo JB, Mathu-Muju KR, Nash DA, Bush HM. Adverse events during pediatric dental anesthesia and sedation: a review of closed malpractice insurance claims. *Pediatr Dent.* 2012;34(3):231–238

126. Lee HH, Milgrom P, Starks H, Burke W. Trends in death associated with pediatric dental sedation and general anesthesia. *Paediatr Anaesth.* 2013; 23(8):741–746

127. Sanborn PA, Michna E, Zurakowski D, et al. Adverse cardiovascular and respiratory events during sedation of pediatric patients for imaging examinations. *Radiology.* 2005;237(1): 288–294

128. Shavit I, Keidan I, Hoffmann Y, et al. Enhancing patient safety during pediatric sedation: the impact of simulation-based training of nonanesthesiologists. *Arch Pediatr Adolesc Med.* 2007;161(8):740–743

129. Cravero JP, Beach ML, Blike GT, Gallagher SM, Hertzog JH; Pediatric Sedation Research Consortium. The incidence and nature of adverse events during pediatric sedation/anesthesia with propofol for procedures outside the operating room: a report from the Pediatric Sedation Research Consortium. *Anesth Analg.* 2009;108(3): 795–804

130. Blike GT, Christoffersen K, Cravero JP, Andeweg SK, Jensen J. A method for measuring system safety and latent errors associated with pediatric procedural sedation. *Anesth Analg.* 2005;101(1):48–58

131. Cravero JP, Havidich JE. Pediatric sedation—evolution and revolution. *Paediatr Anaesth.* 2011;21(7):800–809

132. Havidich JE, Cravero JP. The current status of procedural sedation for pediatric patients in out-of-operating room locations. *Curr Opin Anaesthesiol.* 2012;25(4):453–460

133. Hollman GA, Banks DM, Berkenbosch JW, et al. Development, implementation, and initial participant feedback of a pediatric sedation provider course. *Teach Learn Med.* 2013;25(3):249–257

134. Scherrer PD, Mallory MD, Cravero JP, Lowrie L, Hertzog JH, Berkenbosch JW; Pediatric Sedation Research Consortium. The impact of obesity on pediatric procedural sedation-related outcomes: results from the Pediatric Sedation Research Consortium. *Paediatr Anaesth.* 2015;25(7):689–697

135. Emrath ET, Stockwell JA, McCracken CE, Simon HK, Kamat PP. Provision of deep procedural sedation by a pediatric sedation team at a freestanding imaging center. *Pediatr Radiol.* 2014; 44(8):1020–1025

136. Kamat PP, McCracken CE, Gillespie SE, et al. Pediatric critical care physician-administered procedural sedation using propofol: a report from the Pediatric Sedation Research Consortium Database. *Pediatr Crit Care Med.* 2015;16(1):11–20

137. Couloures KG, Beach M, Cravero JP, Monroe KK, Hertzog JH. Impact of provider specialty on pediatric procedural sedation complication rates. *Pediatrics.* 2011;127(5). Available at: www.pediatrics.org/cgi/content/full/127/5/e1154

138. Metzner J, Domino KB. Risks of anesthesia or sedation outside the operating room: the role of the anesthesia care provider. *Curr Opin Anaesthesiol.* 2010;23(4):523–531

139. Patel KN, Simon HK, Stockwell CA, et al. Pediatric procedural sedation by a dedicated nonanesthesiology pediatric sedation service using propofol. *Pediatr Emerg Care.* 2009; 25(3):133–138

140. Koo SH, Lee DG, Shin H. Optimal initial dose of chloral hydrate in management of pediatric facial laceration. *Arch Plast Surg.* 2014;41(1):40–44

141. Ivaturi V, Kriel R, Brundage R, Loewen G, Mansbach H, Cloyd J. Bioavailability of intranasal vs. rectal diazepam. *Epilepsy Res.* 2013;103(2–3):254–261

142. Mandt MJ, Roback MG, Bajaj L, Galinkin JL, Gao D, Wathen JE. Etomidate for short pediatric procedures in the emergency department. *Pediatr Emerg Care.* 2012;28(9):898–904

143. Tsze DS, Steele DW, Machan JT, Akhlaghi F, Linakis JG. Intranasal ketamine for procedural sedation in pediatric laceration repair: a preliminary report. *Pediatr Emerg Care.* 2012;28(8):767–770

144. Jasiak KD, Phan H, Christich AC, Edwards CJ, Skrepnek GH, Patanwala AE. Induction dose of propofol for pediatric patients undergoing procedural sedation in the emergency department. *Pediatr Emerg Care.* 2012; 28(5):440–442

145. McMorrow SP, Abramo TJ. Dexmedetomidine sedation: uses in pediatric procedural sedation outside the operating room. *Pediatr Emerg Care.* 2012;28(3):292–296

146. Sahyoun C, Krauss B. Clinical implications of pharmacokinetics and pharmacodynamics of procedural sedation agents in children. *Curr Opin Pediatr.* 2012;24(2):225–232

147. Sacchetti A, Jachowski J, Heisler J, Cortese T. Remifentanil use in emergency department patients: initial experience. *Emerg Med J.* 2012;29(11): 928–929

148. Shah A, Mosdossy G, McLeod S, Lehnhardt K, Peddle M, Rieder M. A blinded, randomized controlled trial to evaluate ketamine/propofol versus ketamine alone for procedural sedation in children. *Ann Emerg Med.* 2011;57(5): 425–433.e2

149. Herd DW, Anderson BJ, Keene NA, Holford NH. Investigating the pharmacodynamics of ketamine in children. *Paediatr Anaesth.* 2008;18(1): 36–42

150. Sharieff GQ, Trocinski DR, Kanegaye JT, Fisher B, Harley JR. Ketamine-propofol combination sedation for fracture reduction in the pediatric emergency department. *Pediatr Emerg Care.* 2007; 23(12):881–884

151. Herd DW, Anderson BJ, Holford NH. Modeling the norketamine metabolite in children and the implications for analgesia. *Paediatr Anaesth.* 2007;17(9): 831–840

152. Herd D, Anderson BJ. Ketamine disposition in children presenting for procedural sedation and analgesia in a children's emergency department. *Paediatr Anaesth.* 2007;17(7):622–629

153. Heard CM, Joshi P, Johnson K. Dexmedetomidine for pediatric MRI sedation: a review of a series of cases. *Paediatr Anaesth.* 2007;17(9):888–892

154. Heard C, Burrows F, Johnson K, Joshi P, Houck J, Lerman J. A comparison of dexmedetomidine-midazolam with propofol for maintenance of anesthesia in children undergoing magnetic resonance imaging. *Anesth Analg.* 2008; 107(6):1832–1839

155. Hertzog JH, Havidich JE. Non-anesthesiologist-provided pediatric procedural sedation: an update. *Curr Opin Anaesthesiol.* 2007;20(4):365–372

156. Petroz GC, Sikich N, James M, et al. A phase I, two-center study of the pharmacokinetics and pharmacodynamics of dexmedetomidine in children. *Anesthesiology.* 2006;105(6):1098–1110

157. Potts AL, Anderson BJ, Warman GR, Lerman J, Diaz SM, Vilo S. Dexmedetomidine pharmacokinetics in pediatric intensive care—a pooled

analysis. *Paediatr Anaesth.* 2009;19(11): 1119–1129

158. Mason KP, Lerman J. Dexmedetomidine in children: current knowledge and future applications [review]. *Anesth Analg.* 2011;113(5):1129–1142

159. Sammartino M, Volpe B, Sbaraglia F, Garra R, D'Addessi A. Capnography and the bispectral index—their role in pediatric sedation: a brief review. *Int J Pediatr.* 2010;2010:828347

160. Yarchi D, Cohen A, Umansky T, Sukhotnik I, Shaoul R. Assessment of end-tidal carbon dioxide during pediatric and adult sedation for endoscopic procedures. *Gastrointest Endosc.* 2009;69(4):877–882

161. Lightdale JR, Goldmann DA, Feldman HA, Newburg AR, DiNardo JA, Fox VL. Microstream capnography improves patient monitoring during moderate sedation: a randomized, controlled trial. *Pediatrics.* 2006;117(6). Available at: www.pediatrics.org/cgi/content/full/117/6/e1170

162. Yldzdaş D, Yapcoglu H, Ylmaz HL. The value of capnography during sedation or sedation/analgesia in pediatric minor procedures. *Pediatr Emerg Care.* 2004;20(3):162–165

163. Connor L, Burrows PE, Zurakowski D, Bucci K, Gagnon DA, Mason KP. Effects of IV pentobarbital with and without fentanyl on end-tidal carbon dioxide levels during deep sedation of pediatric patients undergoing MRI. *AJR Am J Roentgenol.* 2003;181(6):1691–1694

164. Primosch RE, Buzzi IM, Jerrell G. Monitoring pediatric dental patients with nasal mask capnography. *Pediatr Dent.* 2000;22(2):120–124

165. Tobias JD. End-tidal carbon dioxide monitoring during sedation with a combination of midazolam and ketamine for children undergoing painful, invasive procedures. *Pediatr Emerg Care.* 1999;15(3):173–175

166. Hart LS, Berns SD, Houck CS, Boenning DA. The value of end-tidal CO2 monitoring when comparing three methods of conscious sedation for children undergoing painful procedures in the emergency department. *Pediatr Emerg Care.* 1997; 13(3):189–193

167. Marx CM, Stein J, Tyler MK, Nieder ML, Shurin SB, Blumer JL. Ketamine-midazolam versus meperidine-midazolam for painful procedures in pediatric oncology patients. *J Clin Oncol.* 1997;15(1):94–102

168. Croswell RJ, Dilley DC, Lucas WJ, Vann WF Jr. A comparison of conventional versus electronic monitoring of sedated pediatric dental patients. *Pediatr Dent.* 1995;17(5):332–339

169. Iwasaki J, Vann WF Jr, Dilley DC, Anderson JA. An investigation of capnography and pulse oximetry as monitors of pediatric patients sedated for dental treatment. *Pediatr Dent.* 1989;11(2):111–117

170. Anderson JA, Vann WF Jr. Respiratory monitoring during pediatric sedation: pulse oximetry and capnography. *Pediatr Dent.* 1988;10(2):94–101

171. Rothman DL. Sedation of the pediatric patient. *J Calif Dent Assoc.* 2013;41(8): 603–611

172. Scherrer PD. Safe and sound: pediatric procedural sedation and analgesia. *Minn Med.* 2011;94(3):43–47

173. Srinivasan M, Turmelle M, Depalma LM, Mao J, Carlson DW. Procedural sedation for diagnostic imaging in children by pediatric hospitalists using propofol: analysis of the nature, frequency, and predictors of adverse events and interventions. *J Pediatr.* 2012;160(5): 801–806.e1

174. Langhan ML, Shabanova V, Li FY, Bernstein SL, Shapiro ED. A randomized controlled trial of capnography during sedation in a pediatric emergency setting. *Am J Emerg Med.* 2015;33(1): 25–30

175. Vetri Buratti C, Angelino F, Sansoni J, Fabriani L, Mauro L, Latina R. Distraction as a technique to control pain in pediatric patients during venipuncture: a narrative review of literature. *Prof Inferm.* 2015;68(1):52–62

176. Robinson PS, Green J. Ambient versus traditional environment in pediatric emergency department. *HERD.* 2015; 8(2):71–80

177. Singh D, Samadi F, Jaiswal J, Tripathi AM. Stress reduction through audio distraction in anxious pediatric dental patients: an adjunctive clinical study. *Int J Clin Pediatr Dent.* 2014;7(3):149–152

178. Attar RH, Baghdadi ZD. Comparative efficacy of active and passive distraction during restorative treatment in children using an iPad versus audiovisual eyeglasses: a randomised controlled trial. *Eur Arch Paediatr Dent.* 2015;16(1):1–8

179. McCarthy AM, Kleiber C, Hanrahan K, et al. Matching doses of distraction with child risk for distress during a medical procedure: a randomized clinical trial. *Nurs Res.* 2014;63(6): 397–407

180. Guinot Jimeno F, Mercadé Bellido M, Cuadros Fernández C, Lorente Rodríguez AI, Llopis Pérez J, Boj Quesada JR. Effect of audiovisual distraction on children's behaviour, anxiety and pain in the dental setting. *Eur J Paediatr Dent.* 2014;15(3):297–302

181. Gupta HV, Gupta VV, Kaur A, et al. Comparison between the analgesic effect of two techniques on the level of pain perception during venipuncture in children up to 7 years of age: a quasi-experimental study. *J Clin Diagn Res.* 2014;8(8):PC01–PC04

182. Newton JT, Shah S, Patel H, Sturmey P. Non-pharmacological approaches to behaviour management in children. *Dent Update.* 2003;30(4):194–199

183. Peretz B, Bimstein E. The use of imagery suggestions during administration of local anesthetic in pediatric dental patients. *ASDC J Dent Child.* 2000;67(4): 263–267, 231

184. Iserson KV. Hypnosis for pediatric fracture reduction. *J Emerg Med.* 1999; 17(1):53–56

185. Rusy LM, Weisman SJ. Complementary therapies for acute pediatric pain management. *Pediatr Clin North Am.* 2000;47(3):589–599

186. Langley P. Guided imagery: a review of effectiveness in the care of children. *Paediatr Nurs.* 1999;11(3):18–21

187. Ott MJ. Imagine the possibilities! Guided imagery with toddlers and pre-schoolers. *Pediatr Nurs.* 1996;22(1): 34–38

188. Singer AJ, Stark MJ. LET versus EMLA for pretreating lacerations: a randomized trial. *Acad Emerg Med.* 2001;8(3):223–230

189. Taddio A, Gurguis MG, Koren G. Lidocaine-prilocaine cream versus tetracaine gel for procedural pain in children. *Ann Pharmacother.* 2002; 36(4):687–692

190. Eichenfield LF, Funk A, Fallon-Friedlander S, Cunningham BB. A clinical study to evaluate the efficacy of ELA-Max (4% liposomal lidocaine) as compared with eutectic mixture of local anesthetics cream for pain reduction of venipuncture in children. *Pediatrics.* 2002;109(6):1093–1099

191. Shaw AJ, Welbury RR. The use of hypnosis in a sedation clinic for dental extractions in children: report of 20 cases. *ASDC J Dent Child.* 1996;63(6): 418–420

192. Stock A, Hill A, Babl FE. Practical communication guide for paediatric procedures. *Emerg Med Australas.* 2012;24(6):641–646

193. Barnea-Goraly N, Weinzimer SA, Ruedy KJ, et al; Diabetes Research in Children Network (DirecNet). High success rates of sedation-free brain MRI scanning in young children using simple subject preparation protocols with and without a commercial mock scanner—the Diabetes Research in Children Network (DirecNet) experience. *Pediatr Radiol.* 2014;44(2):181–186

194. Ram D, Shapira J, Holan G, Magora F, Cohen S, Davidovich E. Audiovisual video eyeglass distraction during dental treatment in children. *Quintessence Int.* 2010;41(8):673–679

195. Lemaire C, Moran GR, Swan H. Impact of audio/visual systems on pediatric sedation in magnetic resonance imaging. *J Magn Reson Imaging.* 2009; 30(3):649–655

196. Nordahl CW, Simon TJ, Zierhut C, Solomon M, Rogers SJ, Amaral DG. Brief report: methods for acquiring structural MRI data in very young children with autism without the use of sedation. *J Autism Dev Disord.* 2008; 38(8):1581–1590

197. Denman WT, Tuason PM, Ahmed MI, Brennen LM, Cepeda MS, Carr DB. The PediSedate device, a novel approach to pediatric sedation that provides distraction and inhaled nitrous oxide: clinical evaluation in a large case series. *Paediatr Anaesth.* 2007;17(2): 162–166

198. Harned RK II, Strain JD. MRI-compatible audio/visual system: impact on pediatric sedation. *Pediatr Radiol.* 2001; 31(4):247–250

199. Slifer KJ. A video system to help children cooperate with motion control for radiation treatment without sedation. *J Pediatr Oncol Nurs.* 1996; 13(2):91–97

200. Krauss BS, Krauss BA, Green SM. Videos in clinical medicine: procedural sedation and analgesia in children. *N Engl J Med.* 2014;370(15):e23

201. Wilson S. Management of child patient behavior: quality of care, fear and anxiety, and the child patient. *Pediatr Dent.* 2013;35(2):170–174

202. Kamath PS. A novel distraction technique for pain management during local anesthesia administration in pediatric patients. *J Clin Pediatr Dent.* 2013;38(1):45–47

203. Asl Aminabadi N, Erfanparast L, Sohrabi A, Ghertasi Oskouei S, Naghili A. The impact of virtual reality distraction on pain and anxiety during dental treatment in 4-6 year-old children: a randomized controlled clinical trial. *J Dent Res Dent Clin Dent Prospect.* 2012;6(4):117–124

204. El-Sharkawi HF, El-Housseiny AA, Aly AM. Effectiveness of new distraction technique on pain associated with injection of local anesthesia for children. *Pediatr Dent.* 2012;34(2): e35–e38

205. Adinolfi B, Gava N. Controlled outcome studies of child clinical hypnosis. *Acta Biomed.* 2013;84(2):94–97

206. Peretz B, Bercovich R, Blumer S. Using elements of hypnosis prior to or during pediatric dental treatment. *Pediatr Dent.* 2013;35(1):33–36

207. Huet A, Lucas-Polomeni MM, Robert JC, Sixou JL, Wodey E. Hypnosis and dental anesthesia in children: a prospective controlled study. *Int J Clin Exp Hypn.* 2011;59(4):424–440

208. Al-Harasi S, Ashley PF, Moles DR, Parekh S, Walters V. Hypnosis for children undergoing dental treatment. *Cochrane Database Syst Rev.* 2010;8:CD007154

209. McQueen A, Cress C, Tothy A. Using a tablet computer during pediatric procedures: a case series and review of the "apps". *Pediatr Emerg Care.* 2012; 28(7):712–714

210. Heilbrunn BR, Wittern RE, Lee JB, Pham PK, Hamilton AH, Nager AL. Reducing anxiety in the pediatric emergency department: a comparative trial. *J Emerg Med.* 2014;47(6):623–631

211. Tyson ME, Bohl DD, Blickman JG. A randomized controlled trial: child life services in pediatric imaging. *Pediatr Radiol.* 2014;44(11):1426–1432

212. Malviya S, Voepel-Lewis T, Tait AR, Merkel S, Tremper K, Naughton N. Depth of sedation in children undergoing computed tomography: validity and reliability of the University of Michigan Sedation Scale (UMSS). *Br J Anaesth.* 2002;88(2):241–245

213. Gamble C, Gamble J, Seal R, Wright RB, Ali S. Bispectral analysis during procedural sedation in the pediatric emergency department. *Pediatr Emerg Care.* 2012;28(10):1003–1008

214. Domino KB. Office-based anesthesia: lessons learned from the closed claims project. *ASA Newsl.* 2001;65:9–15

215. American Heart Association. *Pediatric Advance Life Support Provider Manual.* Dallas, TX: American Heart Association; 2011

216. American Academy of Pediatrics, American College of Emergency Physicians. *Advanced Pediatric Life Support,* 5th ed.. Boston, MA: Jones and Bartlett Publishers; 2012

217. Cheng A, Brown LL, Duff JP, et al; International Network for Simulation-Based Pediatric Innovation, Research, and Education (INSPIRE) CPR Investigators. Improving cardiopulmonary resuscitation with a CPR feedback device and refresher simulations (CPR CARES Study): a randomized clinical trial. *JAMA Pediatr.* 2015;169(2):137–144

218. Nishisaki A, Nguyen J, Colborn S, et al. Evaluation of multidisciplinary simulation training on clinical performance and team behavior during tracheal intubation procedures in a pediatric intensive care unit. *Pediatr Crit Care Med.* 2011;12(4):406–414

219. Howard-Quijano KJ, Stiegler MA, Huang YM, Canales C, Steadman RH. Anesthesiology residents' performance of pediatric resuscitation during

a simulated hyperkalemic cardiac arrest. *Anesthesiology.* 2010;112(4): 993–997

220. Chen MI, Edler A, Wald S, DuBois J, Huang YM. Scenario and checklist for airway rescue during pediatric sedation. *Simul Healthc.* 2007;2(3): 194–198

221. Wheeler M. Management strategies for the difficult pediatric airway. In: Riazi J, ed. *The Difficult Pediatric Airway.* 16th ed. Philadelphia, PA: W.B. Saunders Company; 1998:743–761

222. Sullivan KJ, Kissoon N. Securing the child's airway in the emergency department. *Pediatr Emerg Care.* 2002; 18(2):108–121; quiz: 122–124

223. Levy RJ, Helfaer MA. Pediatric airway issues. *Crit Care Clin.* 2000;16(3): 489–504

224. Krauss B, Green SM. Procedural sedation and analgesia in children. *Lancet.* 2006;367(9512):766–780

225. Krauss B, Green SM. Sedation and analgesia for procedures in children. *N Engl J Med.* 2000;342(13):938–945

226. Ferrari L, ed. *Anesthesia and Pain Management for the Pediatrician,* 1st ed. Baltimore, MD: John Hopkins University Press; 1999

227. Malvyia S. *Sedation Analgesia for Diagnostic and Therapeutic Procedures,* 1st ed. Totowa, NJ: Humana Press; 2001

228. Yaster M, Krane EJ, Kaplan RF, Coté CJ, Lappe DG. *Pediatric Pain Management and Sedation Handbook.* 1st ed. St. Louis, MO: Mosby-Year Book, Inc.; 1997

229. Cravero JP, Blike GT. Review of pediatric sedation. *Anesth Analg.* 2004;99(5): 1355–1364

230. Deshpande JK, Tobias JD. *The Pediatric Pain Handbook.* 1st ed. St. Louis, MO: Mosby; 1996

231. Mace SE, Barata IA, Cravero JP, et al; American College of Emergency Physicians. Clinical policy: evidence-based approach to pharmacologic agents used in pediatric sedation and analgesia in the emergency department. *Ann Emerg Med.* 2004; 44(4):342–377

232. Alcaino EA. Conscious sedation in paediatric dentistry: current philosophies and techniques. *Ann R Australas Coll Dent Surg.* 2000;15: 206–210

233. Tobias JD, Cravero JP. *Procedural Sedation for Infants, Children, and Adolescents.* Elk Grove Village, IL: American Academy of Pediatrics; 2015

234. Committee on Standards and Practice Parameters. *Standards for Basic Anesthetic Monitoring.* Chicago, IL: American Society of Anesthesiologists; 2011

235. Mitchell AA, Louik C, Lacouture P, Slone D, Goldman P, Shapiro S. Risks to children from computed tomographic scan premedication. *JAMA.* 1982; 247(17):2385–2388

236. Wolfe TR, Braude DA. Intranasal medication delivery for children: a brief review and update. *Pediatrics.* 2010; 126(3):532–537

237. Bührer M, Maitre PO, Crevoisier C, Stanski DR. Electroencephalographic effects of benzodiazepines. II. Pharmacodynamic modeling of the electroencephalographic effects of midazolam and diazepam. *Clin Pharmacol Ther.* 1990;48(5):555–567

238. Malviya S, Voepel-Lewis T, Ludomirsky A, Marshall J, Tait AR. Can we improve the assessment of discharge readiness? A comparative study of observational and objective measures of depth of sedation in children. *Anesthesiology.* 2004;100(2): 218–224

239. Coté CJ. Discharge criteria for children sedated by nonanesthesiologists: is "safe" really safe enough? *Anesthesiology.* 2004;100(2):207–209

240. Pershad J, Palmisano P, Nichols M. Chloral hydrate: the good and the bad. *Pediatr Emerg Care.* 1999;15(6):432–435

241. McCormack L, Chen JW, Trapp L, Job A. A comparison of sedation-related events for two multiagent oral sedation regimens in pediatric dental patients. *Pediatr Dent.* 2014;36(4):302–308

242. Kinane TB, Murphy J, Bass JL, Corwin MJ. Comparison of respiratory physiologic features when infants are placed in car safety seats or car beds. *Pediatrics.* 2006;118(2):522–527

243. Wyeth Pharmaceuticals. *Wyeth Phenergan (Promethazine HCL) Tablets and Suppositories* [package insert]. Philadelphia, PA: Wyeth Pharmaceuticals; 2012

244. Caperell K, Pitetti R. Is higher ASA class associated with an increased incidence of adverse events during procedural sedation in a pediatric emergency department? *Pediatr Emerg Care.* 2009; 25(10):661–664

245. Dar AQ, Shah ZA. Anesthesia and sedation in pediatric gastrointestinal endoscopic procedures: a review. *World J Gastrointest Endosc.* 2010;2(7): 257–262

246. Kiringoda R, Thurm AE, Hirschtritt ME, et al. Risks of propofol sedation/anesthesia for imaging studies in pediatric research: eight years of experience in a clinical research center. *Arch Pediatr Adolesc Med.* 2010;164(6): 554–560

247. Thakkar K, El-Serag HB, Mattek N, Gilger MA. Complications of pediatric EGD: a 4-year experience in PEDS-CORI. *Gastrointest Endosc.* 2007;65(2): 213–221

248. Jackson DL, Johnson BS. Conscious sedation for dentistry: risk management and patient selection. *Dent Clin North Am.* 2002;46(4):767–780

249. Malviya S, Voepel-Lewis T, Eldevik OP, Rockwell DT, Wong JH, Tait AR. Sedation and general anaesthesia in children undergoing MRI and CT: adverse events and outcomes. *Br J Anaesth.* 2000;84(6): 743–748

250. O'Neil J, Yonkman J, Talty J, Bull MJ. Transporting children with special health care needs: comparing recommendations and practice. *Pediatrics.* 2009;124(2):596–603

251. Committee on Bioethics, American Academy of Pediatrics. Informed consent, parental permission, and assent in pediatric practice *Pediatrics.* 1995;95(2):314–317

252. Committee on Pediatric Emergency Medicine; Committee on Bioethics. Consent for emergency medical services for children and adolescents. *Pediatrics.* 2011;128(2):427–433

253. Martinez D, Wilson S. Children sedated for dental care: a pilot study of the 24-hour postsedation period. *Pediatr Dent.* 2006;28(3):260–264

254. Kaila R, Chen X, Kannikeswaran N. Postdischarge adverse events related to sedation for diagnostic imaging in children. *Pediatr Emerg Care.* 2012; 28(8):796–801

255. Treston G, Bell A, Cardwell R, Fincher G, Chand D, Cashion G. What is the nature of the emergence phenomenon when using intravenous or intramuscular ketamine for paediatric procedural sedation? *Emerg Med Australas.* 2009; 21(4):315–322

256. Malviya S, Voepel-Lewis T, Prochaska G, Tait AR. Prolonged recovery and delayed side effects of sedation for diagnostic imaging studies in children. *Pediatrics.* 2000;105(3):E42

257. Nordt SP, Rangan C, Hardmaslani M, Clark RF, Wendler C, Valente M. Pediatric chloral hydrate poisonings and death following outpatient procedural sedation. *J Med Toxicol.* 2014;10(2):219–222

258. Walker RW. Pulmonary aspiration in pediatric anesthetic practice in the UK: a prospective survey of specialist pediatric centers over a one-year period. *Paediatr Anaesth.* 2013;23(8): 702–711

259. Babl FE, Puspitadewi A, Barnett P, Oakley E, Spicer M. Preprocedural fasting state and adverse events in children receiving nitrous oxide for procedural sedation and analgesia. *Pediatr Emerg Care.* 2005;21(11): 736–743

260. Roback MG, Bajaj L, Wathen JE, Bothner J. Preprocedural fasting and adverse events in procedural sedation and analgesia in a pediatric emergency department: are they related? *Ann Emerg Med.* 2004;44(5):454–459

261. Vespasiano M, Finkelstein M, Kurachek S. Propofol sedation: intensivists' experience with 7304 cases in a children's hospital. *Pediatrics.* 2007; 120(6). Available at: www.pediatrics.org/cgi/content/full/120/6/e1411

262. Warner MA, Warner ME, Warner DO, Warner LO, Warner EJ. Perioperative pulmonary aspiration in infants and children. *Anesthesiology.* 1999;90(1): 66–71

263. Borland LM, Sereika SM, Woelfel SK, et al. Pulmonary aspiration in pediatric patients during general anesthesia: incidence and outcome. *J Clin Anesth.* 1998;10(2):95–102

264. Agrawal D, Manzi SF, Gupta R, Krauss B. Preprocedural fasting state and adverse events in children undergoing procedural sedation and analgesia in a pediatric emergency department. *Ann Emerg Med.* 2003;42(5):636–646

265. Green SM. Fasting is a consideration—not a necessity—for emergency department procedural sedation and analgesia. *Ann Emerg Med.* 2003;42(5): 647–650

266. Green SM, Krauss B. Pulmonary aspiration risk during emergency department procedural sedation—an examination of the role of fasting and sedation depth. *Acad Emerg Med.* 2002; 9(1):35–42

267. Treston G. Prolonged pre-procedure fasting time is unnecessary when using titrated intravenous ketamine for paediatric procedural sedation. *Emerg Med Australas.* 2004;16(2):145–150

268. Pitetti RD, Singh S, Pierce MC. Safe and efficacious use of procedural sedation and analgesia by nonanesthesiologists in a pediatric emergency department. *Arch Pediatr Adolesc Med.* 2003;157(11): 1090–1096

269. Thorpe RJ, Benger J. Pre-procedural fasting in emergency sedation. *Emerg Med J.* 2010;27(4):254–261

270. Paris PM, Yealy DM. A procedural sedation and analgesia fasting consensus advisory: one small step for emergency medicine, one giant challenge remaining. *Ann Emerg Med.* 2007;49(4):465–467

271. American Society of Anesthesiologists Committee. Practice guidelines for preoperative fasting and the use of pharmacologic agents to reduce the risk of pulmonary aspiration: application to healthy patients undergoing elective procedures: an updated report by the American Society of Anesthesiologists Committee on Standards and Practice Parameters. *Anesthesiology.* 2011;114(3):495–511

272. Mace SE, Brown LA, Francis L, et al Clinical policy: Critical issues in the sedation of pediatric patients in the emergency department. *Ann Emerg Med.* 2008;51:378–399

273. Green SM, Roback MG, Miner JR, Burton JH, Krauss B. Fasting and emergency department procedural sedation and analgesia: a consensus-based clinical practice advisory. *Ann Emerg Med.* 2007;49(4):454–461

274. Duchicela S, Lim A. Pediatric nerve blocks: an evidence-based approach. *Pediatr Emerg Med Pract.* 2013;10(10): 1–19; quiz: 19–20

275. Beach ML, Cohen DM, Gallagher SM, Cravero JP. Major adverse events and relationship to nil per os status in pediatric sedation/anesthesia outside the operating room: a report of the Pediatric Sedation Research Consortium. *Anesthesiology.* 2016; 124(1):80–88

276. Green SM, Krauss B. Ketamine is a safe, effective, and appropriate technique for emergency department paediatric procedural sedation. *Emerg Med J.* 2004;21(3):271–272

277. American Academy of Pediatrics Committee on Pediatric Emergency Medicine. The use of physical restraint interventions for children and adolescents in the acute care setting. *Pediatrics.* 1997;99(3):497–498

278. American Academy of Pediatrics Committee on Child Abuse and Neglect. Behavior management of pediatric dental patients. *Pediatrics.* 1992;90(4): 651–652

279. American Academy of Pediatric Dentistry. Guideline on protective stabilization for pediatric dental patients. *Pediatr Dent.* 2013;35(5): E169–E173

280. Loo CY, Graham RM, Hughes CV. Behaviour guidance in dental treatment of patients with autism spectrum disorder. *Int J Paediatr Dent.* 2009; 19(6):390–398

281. McWhorter AG, Townsend JA; American Academy of Pediatric Dentistry. Behavior symposium workshop A report—current guidelines/revision. *Pediatr Dent.* 2014;36(2):152–153

282. American Society of Anesthesiologists CoSaPP. Practice advisory for preanesthesia evaluation an updated report by the American Society of Anesthesiologists Task Force on Preanesthesia Evaluation. *Anesthesiology.* 2012;116:1–17

283. Gorski JC, Huang SM, Pinto A, et al. The effect of echinacea (Echinacea purpurea root) on cytochrome P450 activity in vivo. *Clin Pharmacol Ther.* 2004;75(1):89–100

284. Hall SD, Wang Z, Huang SM, et al. The interaction between St John's wort and an oral contraceptive. *Clin Pharmacol Ther.* 2003;74(6):525–535

285. Markowitz JS, Donovan JL, DeVane CL, et al. Effect of St John's wort on drug metabolism by induction of cytochrome P450 3A4 enzyme. *JAMA.* 2003;290(11):1500–1504

286. Spinella M. Herbal medicines and epilepsy: the potential for benefit and adverse effects. *Epilepsy Behav.* 2001;2(6):524–532

287. Wang Z, Gorski JC, Hamman MA, Huang SM, Lesko LJ, Hall SD. The effects of St John's wort (Hypericum perforatum) on human cytochrome P450 activity. *Clin Pharmacol Ther.* 2001;70(4):317–326

288. Xie HG, Kim RB. St John's wort-associated drug interactions: short-term inhibition and long-term induction? *Clin Pharmacol Ther.* 2005;78(1):19–24

289. Chen XW, Sneed KB, Pan SY, et al. Herb-drug interactions and mechanistic and clinical considerations. *Curr Drug Metab.* 2012;13(5):640–651

290. Chen XW, Serag ES, Sneed KB, et al. Clinical herbal interactions with conventional drugs: from molecules to maladies. *Curr Med Chem.* 2011;18(31):4836–4850

291. Shi S, Klotz U. Drug interactions with herbal medicines. *Clin Pharmacokinet.* 2012;51(2):77–104

292. Saxena A, Tripathi KP, Roy S, Khan F, Sharma A. Pharmacovigilance: effects of herbal components on human drugs interactions involving cytochrome P450. *Bioinformation.* 2008;3(5):198–204

293. Yang X, Salminen WF. Kava extract, an herbal alternative for anxiety relief, potentiates acetaminophen-induced cytotoxicity in rat hepatic cells. *Phytomedicine.* 2011;18(7):592–600

294. Teschke R. Kava hepatotoxicity: pathogenetic aspects and prospective considerations. *Liver Int.* 2010;30(9):1270–1279

295. Izzo AA, Ernst E. Interactions between herbal medicines and prescribed drugs: an updated systematic review. *Drugs.* 2009;69(13):1777–1798

296. Ang-Lee MK, Moss J, Yuan CS. Herbal medicines and perioperative care. *JAMA.* 2001;286(2):208–216

297. Abebe W. Herbal medication: potential for adverse interactions with analgesic drugs. *J Clin Pharm Ther.* 2002;27(6):391–401

298. Mooiman KD, Maas-Bakker RF, Hendrikx JJ, et al. The effect of complementary and alternative medicines on CYP3A4-mediated metabolism of three different substrates: 7-benzyloxy-4-trifluoromethyl-coumarin, midazolam and docetaxel. *J Pharm Pharmacol.* 2014;66(6):865–874

299. Carrasco MC, Vallejo JR, Pardo-de-Santayana M, Peral D, Martín MA, Altimiras J. Interactions of Valeriana officinalis L. and Passiflora incarnata L. in a patient treated with lorazepam. *Phytother Res.* 2009;23(12):1795–1796

300. von Rosensteil NA, Adam D. Macrolide antibacterials: drug interactions of clinical significance. *Drug Saf.* 1995;13(2):105–122

301. Hiller A, Olkkola KT, Isohanni P, Saarnivaara L. Unconsciousness associated with midazolam and erythromycin. *Br J Anaesth.* 1990;65(6):826–828

302. Mattila MJ, Idänpään-Heikkilä JJ, Törnwall M, Vanakoski J. Oral single doses of erythromycin and roxithromycin may increase the effects of midazolam on human performance. *Pharmacol Toxicol.* 1993;73(3):180–185

303. Olkkola KT, Aranko K, Luurila H, et al. A potentially hazardous interaction between erythromycin and midazolam. *Clin Pharmacol Ther.* 1993;53(3):298–305

304. Senthilkumaran S, Subramanian PT. Prolonged sedation related to erythromycin and midazolam interaction: a word of caution. *Indian Pediatr.* 2011;48(11):909

305. Flockhart DA, Oesterheld JR. Cytochrome P450-mediated drug interactions. *Child Adolesc Psychiatr Clin N Am.* 2000;9(1):43–76

306. Yuan R, Flockhart DA, Balian JD. Pharmacokinetic and pharmacodynamic consequences of metabolism-based drug interactions with alprazolam, midazolam, and triazolam. *J Clin Pharmacol.* 1999;39(11):1109–1125

307. Young B. Review: mixing new cocktails: drug interactions in antiretroviral regimens. *AIDS Patient Care STDS.* 2005;19(5):286–297

308. Gonçalves LS, Gonçalves BM, de Andrade MA, Alves FR, Junior AS. Drug interactions during periodontal therapy in HIV-infected subjects. *Mini Rev Med Chem.* 2010;10(8):766–772

309. Brown KC, Paul S, Kashuba AD. Drug interactions with new and investigational antiretrovirals. *Clin Pharmacokinet.* 2009;48(4):211–241

310. Pau AK. Clinical management of drug interaction with antiretroviral agents. *Curr Opin HIV AIDS.* 2008;3(3):319–324

311. Moyal WN, Lord C, Walkup JT. Quality of life in children and adolescents with autism spectrum disorders: what is known about the effects of pharmacotherapy? *Paediatr Drugs.* 2014;16(2):123–128

312. van den Anker JN. Developmental pharmacology. *Dev Disabil Res Rev.* 2010;16(3):233–238

313. Pichini S, Papaseit E, Joya X, et al. Pharmacokinetics and therapeutic drug monitoring of psychotropic drugs in pediatrics. *Ther Drug Monit.* 2009;31(3):283–318

314. Tibussek D, Distelmaier F, Schönberger S, Göbel U, Mayatepek E. Antiepileptic treatment in paediatric oncology—an interdisciplinary challenge. *Klin Padiatr.* 2006;218(6):340–349

315. Wilkinson GR. Drug metabolism and variability among patients in drug response. *N Engl J Med.* 2005;352(21):2211–2221

316. Salem F, Rostami-Hodjegan A, Johnson TN. Do children have the same vulnerability to metabolic drug–drug interactions as adults? A critical analysis of the literature. *J Clin Pharmacol.* 2013;53(5):559–566

317. Funk RS, Brown JT, Abdel-Rahman SM. Pediatric pharmacokinetics: human development and drug disposition.

Pediatr Clin North Am. 2012;59(5): 1001–1016

318. Anderson BJ. My child is unique: the pharmacokinetics are universal. *Paediatr Anaesth.* 2012;22(6):530–538

319. Elie V, de Beaumais T, Fakhoury M, Jacqz-Aigrain E. Pharmacogenetics and individualized therapy in children: immunosuppressants, antidepressants, anticancer and anti-inflammatory drugs. *Pharmacogenomics.* 2011;12(6): 827–843

320. Chen ZR, Somogyi AA, Reynolds G, Bochner F. Disposition and metabolism of codeine after single and chronic doses in one poor and seven extensive metabolisers. *Br J Clin Pharmacol.* 1991;31(4):381–390

321. Gasche Y, Daali Y, Fathi M, et al. Codeine intoxication associated with ultrarapid CYP2D6 metabolism. *N Engl J Med.* 2004; 351(27):2827–2831

322. Kirchheiner J, Schmidt H, Tzvetkov M, et al. Pharmacokinetics of codeine and its metabolite morphine in ultra-rapid metabolizers due to CYP2D6 duplication. *Pharmacogenomics J.* 2007;7(4):257–265

323. Voronov P, Przybylo HJ, Jagannathan N. Apnea in a child after oral codeine: a genetic variant—an ultra-rapid metabolizer. *Paediatr Anaesth.* 2007; 17(7):684–687

324. Kelly LE, Rieder M, van den Anker J, et al. More codeine fatalities after tonsillectomy in North American children. *Pediatrics.* 2012;129(5). Available at: www.pediatrics.org/cgi/content/full/129/5/e1343

325. Farber JM. Clinical practice guideline: diagnosis and management of childhood obstructive sleep apnea syndrome. *Pediatrics.* 2002;110(6): 1255–1257; author reply: 1255–1257

326. Schechter MS; Section on Pediatric Pulmonology, Subcommittee on Obstructive Sleep Apnea Syndrome. Technical report: diagnosis and management of childhood obstructive sleep apnea syndrome. *Pediatrics.* 2002;109(4). Available at: www.pediatrics.org/cgi/content/full/109/4/e69

327. Marcus CL, Brooks LJ, Draper KA, et al; American Academy of Pediatrics. Diagnosis and management of childhood obstructive sleep apnea syndrome. *Pediatrics.* 2012;130(3): 576–584

328. Coté CJ, Posner KL, Domino KB. Death or neurologic injury after tonsillectomy in children with a focus on obstructive sleep apnea: Houston, we have a problem! *Anesth Analg.* 2014;118(6): 1276–1283

329. Wheeler M, Coté CJ. Preoperative pregnancy testing in a tertiary care children's hospital: a medico-legal conundrum. *J Clin Anesth.* 1999;11(1): 56–63

330. Neuman G, Koren G. Safety of procedural sedation in pregnancy. *J Obstet Gynaecol Can.* 2013;35(2): 168–173

331. Larcher V. Developing guidance for checking pregnancy status in adolescent girls before surgical, radiological or other procedures. *Arch Dis Child.* 2012;97(10):857–860

332. August DA, Everett LL. Pediatric ambulatory anesthesia. *Anesthesiol Clin.* 2014;32(2):411–429

333. Maxwell LG. Age-associated issues in preoperative evaluation, testing, and planning: pediatrics. *Anesthesiol Clin North America.* 2004;22(1):27–43

334. Davidson AJ. Anesthesia and neurotoxicity to the developing brain: the clinical relevance. *Paediatr Anaesth.* 2011;21(7):716–721

335. Reddy SV. Effect of general anesthetics on the developing brain. *J Anaesthesiol Clin Pharmacol.* 2012;28(1):6–10

336. Nemergut ME, Aganga D, Flick RP. Anesthetic neurotoxicity: what to tell the parents? *Paediatr Anaesth.* 2014; 24(1):120–126

337. Olsen EA, Brambrink AM. Anesthesia for the young child undergoing ambulatory procedures: current concerns regarding harm to the developing brain. *Curr Opin Anaesthesiol.* 2013; 26(6):677–684

338. Green SM, Coté CJ. Ketamine and neurotoxicity: clinical perspectives and implications for emergency medicine. *Ann Emerg Med.* 2009;54(2):181–190

339. Brown KA, Laferrière A, Moss IR. Recurrent hypoxemia in young children with obstructive sleep apnea is associated with reduced opioid requirement for analgesia. *Anesthesiology.* 2004;100(4):806–810; discussion: 5A

340. Moss IR, Brown KA, Laferrière A. Recurrent hypoxia in rats during development increases subsequent respiratory sensitivity to fentanyl. *Anesthesiology.* 2006;105(4):715–718

341. Litman RS, Kottra JA, Berkowitz RJ, Ward DS. Upper airway obstruction during midazolam/nitrous oxide sedation in children with enlarged tonsils. *Pediatr Dent.* 1998;20(5): 318–320

342. Fishbaugh DF, Wilson S, Preisch JW, Weaver JM II. Relationship of tonsil size on an airway blockage maneuver in children during sedation. *Pediatr Dent.* 1997;19(4):277–281

343. Heinrich S, Birkholz T, Ihmsen H, Irouschek A, Ackermann A, Schmidt J. Incidence and predictors of difficult laryngoscopy in 11,219 pediatric anesthesia procedures. *Paediatr Anaesth.* 2012;22(8):729–736

344. Kumar HV, Schroeder JW, Gang Z, Sheldon SH. Mallampati score and pediatric obstructive sleep apnea. *J Clin Sleep Med.* 2014;10(9):985–990

345. Anderson BJ, Meakin GH. Scaling for size: some implications for paediatric anaesthesia dosing. *Paediatr Anaesth.* 2002;12(3):205–219

346. Ramsay MA, Savege TM, Simpson BR, Goodwin R. Controlled sedation with alphaxalone-alphadolone. *BMJ.* 1974; 2(5920):656–659

347. Agrawal D, Feldman HA, Krauss B, Waltzman ML. Bispectral index monitoring quantifies depth of sedation during emergency department procedural sedation and analgesia in children. *Ann Emerg Med.* 2004;43(2): 247–255

348. Cravero JP, Blike GT, Surgenor SD, Jensen J. Development and validation of the Dartmouth Operative Conditions Scale. *Anesth Analg.* 2005;100(6): 1614–1621

349. Mayers DJ, Hindmarsh KW, Sankaran K, Gorecki DK, Kasian GF. Chloral hydrate disposition following single-dose administration to critically ill neonates and children. *Dev Pharmacol Ther.* 1991;16(2):71–77

350. Terndrup TE, Dire DJ, Madden CM, Davis H, Cantor RM, Gavula DP. A prospective analysis of intramuscular meperidine, promethazine, and chlorpromazine in pediatric emergency department patients. *Ann Emerg Med.* 1991;20(1):31–35

351. Macnab AJ, Levine M, Glick N, Susak L, Baker-Brown G. A research tool for measurement of recovery from sedation: the Vancouver Sedative Recovery Scale. *J Pediatr Surg.* 1991;26(11):1263–1267

352. Chernik DA, Gillings D, Laine H, et al. Validity and reliability of the Observer's Assessment of Alertness/Sedation Scale: study with intravenous midazolam. *J Clin Psychopharmacol.* 1990;10(4):244–251

353. Bagian JP, Lee C, Gosbee J, et al. Developing and deploying a patient safety program in a large health care delivery system: you can't fix what you don't know about. *Jt Comm J Qual Improv.* 2001;27(10):522–532

354. May T, Aulisio MP. Medical malpractice, mistake prevention, and compensation. *Kennedy Inst Ethics J.* 2001;11(2):135–146

355. Kazandjian VA. When you hear hoofs, think horses, not zebras: an evidence-based model of health care accountability. *J Eval Clin Pract.* 2002;8(2):205–213

356. Connor M, Ponte PR, Conway J. Multidisciplinary approaches to reducing error and risk in a patient care setting. *Crit Care Nurs Clin North Am.* 2002;14(4):359–367, viii

357. Gosbee J. Human factors engineering and patient safety. *Qual Saf Health Care.* 2002;11(4):352–354

358. Tuong B, Shnitzer Z, Pehora C, et al. The experience of conducting Mortality and Morbidity reviews in a pediatric interventional radiology service: a retrospective study. *J Vasc Interv Radiol.* 2009;20(1):77–86

359. Tjia I, Rampersad S, Varughese A, et al. Wake Up Safe and root cause analysis: quality improvement in pediatric anesthesia. *Anesth Analg.* 2014;119(1):122–136

360. Bhatt M, Kennedy RM, Osmond MH, et al; Consensus Panel on Sedation Research of Pediatric Emergency Research Canada (PERC);Pediatric Emergency Care Applied Research Network (PECARN). Consensus-based recommendations for standardizing terminology and reporting adverse events for emergency department procedural sedation and analgesia in children. *Ann Emerg Med.* 2009;53(4):426–435.e4

361. Barker SJ, Hyatt J, Shah NK, Kao YJ. The effect of sensor malpositioning on pulse oximeter accuracy during hypoxemia. *Anesthesiology.* 1993;79(2):248–254

362. Kelleher JF, Ruff RH. The penumbra effect: vasomotion-dependent pulse oximeter artifact due to probe malposition. *Anesthesiology.* 1989;71(5):787–791

363. Reeves ST, Havidich JE, Tobin DP. Conscious sedation of children with propofol is anything but conscious. *Pediatrics.* 2004;114(1). Available at: www.pediatrics.org/cgi/content/full/114/1/e74

364. Maher EN, Hansen SF, Heine M, Meers H, Yaster M, Hunt EA. Knowledge of procedural sedation and analgesia of emergency medicine physicians. *Pediatr Emerg Care.* 2007;23(12):869–876

365. Fehr JJ, Boulet JR, Waldrop WB, Snider R, Brockel M, Murray DJ. Simulation-based assessment of pediatric anesthesia skills. *Anesthesiology.* 2011;115(6):1308–1315

366. McBride ME, Waldrop WB, Fehr JJ, Boulet JR, Murray DJ. Simulation in pediatrics: the reliability and validity of a multiscenario assessment. *Pediatrics.* 2011;128(2):335–343

367. Fehr JJ, Honkanen A, Murray DJ. Simulation in pediatric anesthesiology. *Paediatr Anaesth.* 2012;22(10):988–994

368. Martinez MJ, Siegelman L. The new era of pretracheal/precordial stethoscopes. *Pediatr Dent.* 1999;21(7):455–457

369. Biro P. Electrically amplified precordial stethoscope. *J Clin Monit.* 1994;10(6):410–412

370. Philip JH, Raemer DB. An electronic stethoscope is judged better than conventional stethoscopes for anesthesia monitoring. *J Clin Monit.* 1986;2(3):151–154

371. Hochberg MG, Mahoney WK. Monitoring of respiration using an amplified pretracheal stethoscope. *J Oral Maxillofac Surg.* 1999;57(7):875–876

372. Fredette ME, Lightdale JR. Endoscopic sedation in pediatric practice. *Gastrointest Endosc Clin N Am.* 2008;18(4):739–751, ix

373. Deitch K, Chudnofsky CR, Dominici P. The utility of supplemental oxygen during emergency department procedural sedation and analgesia with midazolam and fentanyl: a randomized, controlled trial. *Ann Emerg Med.* 2007;49(1):1–8

374. Burton JH, Harrah JD, Germann CA, Dillon DC. Does end-tidal carbon dioxide monitoring detect respiratory events prior to current sedation monitoring practices? *Acad Emerg Med.* 2006;13(5):500–504

375. Wilson S, Farrell K, Griffen A, Coury D. Conscious sedation experiences in graduate pediatric dentistry programs. *Pediatr Dent.* 2001;23(4):307–314

376. Allegaert K, van den Anker JN. Clinical pharmacology in neonates: small size, huge variability. *Neonatology.* 2014;105(4):344–349

377. Coté CJ, Zaslavsky A, Downes JJ, et al. Postoperative apnea in former preterm infants after inguinal herniorrhaphy: a combined analysis. *Anesthesiology.* 1995;82(4):809–822

378. Havidich JE, Beach M, Dierdorf SF, Onega T, Suresh G, Cravero JP. Preterm versus term children: analysis of sedation/anesthesia adverse events and longitudinal risk. *Pediatrics.* 2016;137(3):1–9

379. Nasr VG, Davis JM. Anesthetic use in newborn infants: the urgent need for rigorous evaluation. *Pediatr Res.* 2015;78(1):2–6

380. Sinner B, Becke K, Engelhard K. General anaesthetics and the developing brain: an overview. *Anaesthesia.* 2014;69(9):1009–1022

381. Yu CK, Yuen VM, Wong GT, Irwin MG. The effects of anaesthesia on the developing brain: a summary of the clinical evidence. *F1000 Res.* 2013;2:166

382. Davidson A, Flick RP. Neurodevelopmental implications of the use of sedation and analgesia in

neonates. *Clin Perinatol.* 2013;40(3): 559–573

383. Lönnqvist PA. Toxicity of local anesthetic drugs: a pediatric perspective. *Paediatr Anaesth.* 2012;22(1):39–43

384. Wahl MJ, Brown RS. Dentistry's wonder drugs: local anesthetics and vasoconstrictors. *Gen Dent.* 2010;58(2): 114–123; quiz: 124–125

385. Bernards CM, Hadzic A, Suresh S, Neal JM. Regional anesthesia in anesthetized or heavily sedated patients. *Reg Anesth Pain Med.* 2008;33(5):449–460

386. Ecoffey C. Pediatric regional anesthesia —update. *Curr Opin Anaesthesiol.* 2007; 20(3):232–235

387. Aubuchon RW. Sedation liabilities in pedodontics. *Pediatr Dent.* 1982;4: 171–180

388. Fitzmaurice LS, Wasserman GS, Knapp JF, Roberts DK, Waeckerle JF, Fox M. TAC use and absorption of cocaine in a pediatric emergency department. *Ann Emerg Med.* 1990;19(5):515–518

389. Tipton GA, DeWitt GW, Eisenstein SJ. Topical TAC (tetracaine, adrenaline, cocaine) solution for local anesthesia in children: prescribing inconsistency and acute toxicity. *South Med J.* 1989; 82(11):1344–1346

390. Gunter JB. Benefit and risks of local anesthetics in infants and children. *Paediatr Drugs.* 2002;4(10):649–672

391. Resar LM, Helfaer MA. Recurrent seizures in a neonate after lidocaine administration. *J Perinatol.* 1998;18(3): 193–195

392. Yagiela JA. Local anesthetics. In: Yagiela JA, Dowd FJ, Johnson BS, Mariotti AJ, Neidle EA, eds. *Pharmacology and Therapeutics for Dentistry.* 6th ed. St. Louis, MO: Mosby, Elsevier; 2011: 246–265

393. Haas DA. An update on local anesthetics in dentistry. *J Can Dent Assoc.* 2002; 68(9):546–551

394. Malamed SF. Anesthetic considerations in dental specialties. In: Malamed SF, ed. *Handbook of Local Anesthesia.* 6th ed. St. Louis, MO: Elsevier; 2013:277–291

395. Malamed SF. The needle. In: Malamed SF, ed. *Handbook of Local Anesthetics.* 6th ed. St Louis, MO: Elsevier; 2013: 92–100

396. Malamed SF. Pharmacology of local anesthetics. In: Malamed SF, ed. *Handbook of Local Anesthesia.* 6th ed. St. Louis, MO: Elsevier; 2013:25–38

397. Ram D, Amir E. Comparison of articaine 4% and lidocaine 2% in paediatric dental patients. *Int J Paediatr Dent.* 2006;16(4):252–256

398. Jakobs W, Ladwig B, Cichon P, Ortel R, Kirch W. Serum levels of articaine 2% and 4% in children. *Anesth Prog.* 1995; 42(3–4):113–115

399. Wright GZ, Weinberger SJ, Friedman CS, Plotzke OB. Use of articaine local anesthesia in children under 4 years of age—a retrospective report. *Anesth Prog.* 1989;36(6):268–271

400. Malamed SF, Gagnon S, Leblanc D. A comparison between articaine HCl and lidocaine HCl in pediatric dental patients. *Pediatr Dent.* 2000;22(4): 307–311

401. American Academy of Pediatric Dentistry, Council on Clinical Affairs. Guidelines on use of local anesthesia for pediatric dental patients. Chicago, IL: American Academy of Pediatric Dentistry; 2015. Available at: http://www.aapd.org/media/policies_guidelines/g_localanesthesia.pdf. Accessed May 27, 2016

402. Ludot H, Tharin JY, Belouadah M, Mazoit JX, Malinovsky JM. Successful resuscitation after ropivacaine and lidocaine-induced ventricular arrhythmia following posterior lumbar plexus block in a child. *Anesth Analg.* 2008;106(5):1572–1574

403. Eren CS, Tasyurek T, Guneysel O. Intralipid emulsion treatment as an antidote in lipophilic drug intoxications: a case series. *Am J Emerg Med.* 2014; 32(9):1103–1108

404. Evans JA, Wallis SC, Dulhunty JM, Pang G. Binding of local anaesthetics to the lipid emulsion Clinoleic™ 20%. *Anaesth Intensive Care.* 2013;41(5):618–622

405. Presley JD, Chyka PA. Intravenous lipid emulsion to reverse acute drug toxicity in pediatric patients. *Ann Pharmacother.* 2013;47(5):735–743

406. Li Z, Xia Y, Dong X, et al. Lipid resuscitation of bupivacaine toxicity: long-chain triglyceride emulsion provides benefits over long- and medium-chain triglyceride emulsion. *Anesthesiology.* 2011;115(6):1219–1228

407. Maher AJ, Metcalfe SA, Parr S. Local anaesthetic toxicity. *Foot.* 2008;18(4): 192–197

408. Corman SL, Skledar SJ. Use of lipid emulsion to reverse local anesthetic-induced toxicity. *Ann Pharmacother.* 2007;41(11):1873–1877

409. Litz RJ, Popp M, Stehr SN, Koch T. Successful resuscitation of a patient with ropivacaine-induced asystole after axillary plexus block using lipid infusion. *Anaesthesia.* 2006;61(8): 800–801

410. Raso SM, Fernandez JB, Beobide EA, Landaluce AF. Methemoglobinemia and CNS toxicity after topical application of EMLA to a 4-year-old girl with molluscum contagiosum. *Pediatr Dermatol.* 2006;23(6):592–593

411. Larson A, Stidham T, Banerji S, Kaufman J. Seizures and methemoglobinemia in an infant after excessive EMLA application. *Pediatr Emerg Care.* 2013; 29(3):377–379

412. Tran AN, Koo JY. Risk of systemic toxicity with topical lidocaine/prilocaine: a review. *J Drugs Dermatol.* 2014;13(9): 1118–1122

413. Young KD. Topical anaesthetics: what's new? *Arch Dis Child Educ Pract Ed.* 2015;100(2):105–110

414. Gaufberg SV, Walta MJ, Workman TP. Expanding the use of topical anesthesia in wound management: sequential layered application of topical lidocaine with epinephrine. *Am J Emerg Med.* 2007;25(4):379–384

415. Eidelman A, Weiss JM, Baldwin CL, Enu IK, McNicol ED, Carr DB. Topical anaesthetics for repair of dermal laceration. *Cochrane Database Syst Rev.* 2011;6:CD005364

416. Next-generation pulse oximetry. *Health Devices.* 2003;32(2):49–103

417. Barker SJ. "Motion-resistant" pulse oximetry: a comparison of new and old models. *Anesth Analg.* 2002;95(4): 967–972

418. Malviya S, Reynolds PI, Voepel-Lewis T, et al. False alarms and sensitivity of conventional pulse oximetry versus the Masimo SET technology in the pediatric

postanesthesia care unit. *Anesth Analg.* 2000;90(6):1336–1340

419. Barker SJ, Shah NK. Effects of motion on the performance of pulse oximeters in volunteers. *Anesthesiology.* 1996; 85(4):774–781

420. Barker SJ, Shah NK. The effects of motion on the performance of pulse oximeters in volunteers (revised publication). *Anesthesiology.* 1997;86(1): 101–108

421. Colman Y, Krauss B. Microstream capnogrpay technology: a new approach to an old problem. *J Clin Monit Comput.* 1999;15(6):403–409

422. Wright SW. Conscious sedation in the emergency department: the value of capnography and pulse oximetry. *Ann Emerg Med.* 1992;21(5):551–555

423. Roelofse J. Conscious sedation: making our treatment options safe and sound. *SADJ.* 2000;55(5):273–276

424. Wilson S, Creedon RL, George M, Troutman K. A history of sedation guidelines: where we are headed in the future. *Pediatr Dent.* 1996;18(3):194–199

425. Miner JR, Heegaard W, Plummer D. End-tidal carbon dioxide monitoring during procedural sedation. *Acad Emerg Med.* 2002;9(4):275–280

426. Vascello LA, Bowe EA. A case for capnographic monitoring as a standard of care. *J Oral Maxillofac Surg.* 1999; 57(11):1342–1347

427. Coté CJ, Wax DF, Jennings MA, Gorski CL, Kurczak-Klippstein K. Endtidal carbon dioxide monitoring in children with congenital heart disease during sedation for cardiac catheterization by nonanesthesiologists. *Paediatr Anaesth.* 2007;17(7):661–666

428. Bowdle TA. Depth of anesthesia monitoring. *Anesthesiol Clin.* 2006;24(4): 793–822

429. Rodriguez RA, Hall LE, Duggan S, Splinter WM. The bispectral index does not correlate with clinical signs of inhalational anesthesia during sevoflurane induction and arousal in children. *Can J Anaesth.* 2004;51(5): 472–480

430. Overly FL, Wright RO, Connor FA Jr, Fontaine B, Jay G, Linakis JG. Bispectral analysis during pediatric procedural sedation. *Pediatr Emerg Care.* 2005; 21(1):6–11

431. Mason KP, O'Mahony E, Zurakowski D, Libenson MH. Effects of dexmedetomidine sedation on the EEG in children. *Paediatr Anaesth.* 2009; 19(12):1175–1183

432. Malviya S, Voepel-Lewis T, Tait AR, Watcha MF, Sadhasivam S, Friesen RH. Effect of age and sedative agent on the accuracy of bispectral index in detecting depth of sedation in children. *Pediatrics.* 2007;120(3). Available at: www.pediatrics.org/cgi/content/full/120/3/e461

433. Sadhasivam S, Ganesh A, Robison A, Kaye R, Watcha MF. Validation of the bispectral index monitor for measuring the depth of sedation in children. *Anesth Analg.* 2006;102(2):383–388

434. Messieha ZS, Ananda RC, Hoffman WE, Punwani IC, Koenig HM. Bispectral Index System (BIS) monitoring reduces time to discharge in children requiring intramuscular sedation and general anesthesia for outpatient dental rehabilitation. *Pediatr Dent.* 2004;26(3): 256–260

435. McDermott NB, VanSickle T, Motas D, Friesen RH. Validation of the bispectral index monitor during conscious and deep sedation in children. *Anesth Analg.* 2003;97(1):39–43

436. Schmidt AR, Weiss M, Engelhardt T. The paediatric airway: basic principles and current developments. *Eur J Anaesthesiol.* 2014;31(6):293–299

437. Nagler J, Bachur RG. Advanced airway management. *Curr Opin Pediatr.* 2009; 21(3):299–305

438. Berry AM, Brimacombe JR, Verghese C. The laryngeal mask airway in emergency medicine, neonatal resuscitation, and intensive care medicine. *Int Anesthesiol Clin.* 1998; 36(2):91–109

439. Patterson MD. Resuscitation update for the pediatrician. *Pediatr Clin North Am.* 1999;46(6):1285–1303

440. Diggs LA, Yusuf JE, De Leo G. An update on out-of-hospital airway management practices in the United States. *Resuscitation.* 2014;85(7):885–892

441. Wang HE, Mann NC, Mears G, Jacobson K, Yealy DM. Out-of-hospital airway management in the United States. *Resuscitation.* 2011;82(4):378–385

442. Ritter SC, Guyette FX. Prehospital pediatric King LT-D use: a pilot study. *Prehosp Emerg Care.* 2011;15(3): 401–404

443. Selim M, Mowafi H, Al-Ghamdi A, Adu-Gyamfi Y. Intubation via LMA in pediatric patients with difficult airways. *Can J Anaesth.* 1999;46(9):891–893

444. Munro HM, Butler PJ, Washington EJ. Freeman-Sheldon (whistling face) syndrome: anaesthetic and airway management. *Paediatr Anaesth.* 1997; 7(4):345–348

445. Horton MA, Beamer C. Powered intraosseous insertion provides safe and effective vascular access for pediatric emergency patients. *Pediatr Emerg Care.* 2008;24(6):347–350

446. Gazin N, Auger H, Jabre P, et al. Efficacy and safety of the EZ-IO™ intraosseous device: out-of-hospital implementation of a management algorithm for difficult vascular access. *Resuscitation.* 2011; 82(1):126–129

447. Frascone RJ, Jensen J, Wewerka SS, Salzman JG. Use of the pediatric EZ-IO needle by emergency medical services providers. *Pediatr Emerg Care.* 2009; 25(5):329–332

448. Neuhaus D. Intraosseous infusion in elective and emergency pediatric anesthesia: when should we use it? *Curr Opin Anaesthesiol.* 2014;27(3): 282–287

449. Oksan D, Ayfer K. Powered intraosseous device (EZ-IO) for critically ill patients. *Indian Pediatr.* 2013;50(7):689–691

450. Santos D, Carron PN, Yersin B, Pasquier M. EZ-IO(®) intraosseous device implementation in a pre-hospital emergency service: a prospective study and review of the literature. *Resuscitation.* 2013;84(4):440–445

451. Tan GM. A medical crisis management simulation activity for pediatric dental residents and assistants. *J Dent Educ.* 2011;75(6):782–790

452. Schinasi DA, Nadel FM, Hales R, Boswinkel JP, Donoghue AJ. Assessing pediatric residents' clinical performance in procedural sedation: a simulation-based needs assessment. *Pediatr Emerg Care.* 2013;29(4):447–452

453. Rowe R, Cohen RA. An evaluation of a virtual reality airway simulator. *Anesth Analg.* 2002;95(1):62–66

454. Medina LS, Racadio JM, Schwid HA. Computers in radiology—the sedation, analgesia, and contrast media computerized simulator: a new approach to train and evaluate radiologists' responses to critical incidents. *Pediatr Radiol.* 2000;30(5): 299–305

455. Blike G, Cravero J, Nelson E. Same patients, same critical events—different systems of care, different outcomes: description of a human factors approach aimed at improving the efficacy and safety of sedation/analgesia care. *Qual Manag Health Care.* 2001;10(1):17–36

456. Reiter DA, Strother CG, Weingart SD. The quality of cardiopulmonary resuscitation using supraglottic airways and intraosseous devices: a simulation trial. *Resuscitation.* 2013; 84(1):93–97

457. Schulte-Uentrop L, Goepfert MS. Anaesthesia or sedation for MRI in children. *Curr Opin Anaesthesiol.* 2010; 23(4):513–517

458. Schmidt MH, Downie J. Safety first: recognizing and managing the risks to child participants in magnetic resonance imaging research. *Account Res.* 2009;16(3):153–173

459. Chavhan GB, Babyn PS, Singh M, Vidarsson L, Shroff M. MR imaging at 3.0 T in children: technical differences, safety issues, and initial experience. *Radiographics.* 2009;29(5):1451–1466

460. Kanal E, Shellock FG, Talagala L. Safety considerations in MR imaging. *Radiology.* 1990;176(3):593–606

461. Shellock FG, Kanal E. Burns associated with the use of monitoring equipment during MR procedures. *J Magn Reson Imaging.* 1996;6(1):271–272

462. Shellock FG. Magnetic resonance safety update 2002: implants and devices. *J Magn Reson Imaging.* 2002;16(5): 485–496

463. Dempsey MF, Condon B, Hadley DM. MRI safety review. *Semin Ultrasound CT MR.* 2002;23(5):392–401

464. Department of Health and Human Services, Centers for Disease Control and PreventionCriteria for a Recommended Standard: Waste Anesthetic Gases: Occupational Hazards in Hospitals. 2007. Publication 2007-151. Available at: http://www.cdc.gov/niosh/docs/2007-151/pdfs/2007-151.pdf. Accessed May 27, 2016

465. O'Sullivan I, Benger J. Nitrous oxide in emergency medicine. *Emerg Med J.* 2003;20(3):214–217

466. Kennedy RM, Luhmann JD, Luhmann SJ. Emergency department management of pain and anxiety related to orthopedic fracture care: a guide to analgesic techniques and procedural sedation in children. *Paediatr Drugs.* 2004;6(1): 11–31

467. Frampton A, Browne GJ, Lam LT, Cooper MG, Lane LG. Nurse administered relative analgesia using high concentration nitrous oxide to facilitate minor procedures in children in an emergency department. *Emerg Med J.* 2003;20(5):410–413

468. Everitt I, Younge P, Barnett P. Paediatric sedation in emergency department: what is our practice? *Emerg Med (Fremantle).* 2002;14(1):62–66

469. Krauss B. Continuous-flow nitrous oxide: searching for the ideal procedural anxiolytic for toddlers. *Ann Emerg Med.* 2001;37(1):61–62

470. Otley CC, Nguyen TH. Conscious sedation of pediatric patients with combination oral benzodiazepines and inhaled nitrous oxide. *Dermatol Surg.* 2000; 26(11):1041–1044

471. Luhmann JD, Kennedy RM, Jaffe DM, McAllister JD. Continuous-flow delivery of nitrous oxide and oxygen: a safe and cost-effective technique for inhalation analgesia and sedation of pediatric patients. *Pediatr Emerg Care.* 1999; 15(6):388–392

472. Burton JH, Auble TE, Fuchs SM. Effectiveness of 50% nitrous oxide/50% oxygen during laceration repair in children. *Acad Emerg Med.* 1998;5(2): 112–117

473. Gregory PR, Sullivan JA. Nitrous oxide compared with intravenous regional anesthesia in pediatric forearm fracture manipulation. *J Pediatr Orthop.* 1996;16(2):187–191

474. Hennrikus WL, Shin AY, Klingelberger CE. Self-administered nitrous oxide and a hematoma block for analgesia in the outpatient reduction of fractures in children. *J Bone Joint Surg Am.* 1995; 77(3):335–339

475. Hennrikus WL, Simpson RB, Klingelberger CE, Reis MT. Self-administered nitrous oxide analgesia for pediatric fracture reductions. *J Pediatr Orthop.* 1994;14(4):538–542

476. Wattenmaker I, Kasser JR, McGravey A. Self-administered nitrous oxide for fracture reduction in children in an emergency room setting. *J Orthop Trauma.* 1990;4(1):35–38

477. Gamis AS, Knapp JF, Glenski JA. Nitrous oxide analgesia in a pediatric emergency department. *Ann Emerg Med.* 1989;18(2):177–181

478. Kalach N, Barbier C, el Kohen R, et al. Tolerance of nitrous oxide-oxygen sedation for painful procedures in emergency pediatrics: report of 600 cases [in French]. *Arch Pediatr.* 2002; 9(11):1213–1215

479. Michaud L, Gottrand F, Ganga-Zandzou PS, et al. Nitrous oxide sedation in pediatric patients undergoing gastrointestinal endoscopy. *J Pediatr Gastroenterol Nutr.* 1999;28(3):310–314

480. Baskett PJ. Analgesia for the dressing of burns in children: a method using neuroleptanalgesia and Entonox. *Postgrad Med J.* 1972;48(557):138–142

481. Veerkamp JS, van Amerongen WE, Hoogstraten J, Groen HJ. Dental treatment of fearful children, using nitrous oxide. Part I: treatment times. *ASDC J Dent Child.* 1991;58(6):453–457

482. Veerkamp JS, Gruythuysen RJ, van Amerongen WE, Hoogstraten J. Dental treatment of fearful children using nitrous oxide. Part 2: the parent's point of view. *ASDC J Dent Child.* 1992;59(2): 115–119

483. Veerkamp JS, Gruythuysen RJ, van Amerongen WE, Hoogstraten J. Dental treatment of fearful children using nitrous oxide. Part 3: anxiety during sequential visits. *ASDC J Dent Child.* 1993;60(3):175–182

484. Veerkamp JS, Gruythuysen RJ, Hoogstraten J, van Amerongen WE. Dental treatment of fearful children using nitrous oxide. Part 4: anxiety after two years. *ASDC J Dent Child.* 1993; 60(4):372–376

485. Houpt MI, Limb R, Livingston RL. Clinical effects of nitrous oxide conscious sedation in children. *Pediatr Dent.* 2004; 26(1):29–36

486. Shapira J, Holan G, Guelmann M, Cahan S. Evaluation of the effect of nitrous oxide and hydroxyzine in controlling the behavior of the pediatric dental patient. *Pediatr Dent.* 1992;14(3):167–170

487. Primosch RE, Buzzi IM, Jerrell G. Effect of nitrous oxide-oxygen inhalation with scavenging on behavioral and physiological parameters during routine pediatric dental treatment. *Pediatr Dent.* 1999;21(7):417–420

488. McCann W, Wilson S, Larsen P, Stehle B. The effects of nitrous oxide on behavior and physiological parameters during conscious sedation with a moderate dose of chloral hydrate and hydroxyzine. *Pediatr Dent.* 1996;18(1): 35–41

489. Wilson S, Matusak A, Casamassimo PS, Larsen P. The effects of nitrous oxide on pediatric dental patients sedated with chloral hydrate and hydroxyzine. *Pediatr Dent.* 1998;20(4):253–258

490. Pedersen RS, Bayat A, Steen NP, Jacobsson ML. Nitrous oxide provides safe and effective analgesia for minor paediatric procedures—a systematic review [abstract]. *Dan Med J.* 2013; 60(6):A4627

491. Lee JH, Kim K, Kim TY, et al. A randomized comparison of nitrous oxide versus intravenous ketamine for laceration repair in children. *Pediatr Emerg Care.* 2012;28(12):1297–1301

492. Seith RW, Theophilos T, Babl FE. Intranasal fentanyl and high-concentration inhaled nitrous oxide for procedural sedation: a prospective observational pilot study of adverse events and depth of sedation. *Acad Emerg Med.* 2012;19(1):31–36

493. Klein U, Robinson TJ, Allshouse A. End-expired nitrous oxide concentrations compared to flowmeter settings during operative dental treatment in children. *Pediatr Dent.* 2011;33(1):56–62

494. Litman RS, Kottra JA, Berkowitz RJ, Ward DS. Breathing patterns and levels of consciousness in children during administration of nitrous oxide after oral midazolam premedication. *J Oral Maxillofac Surg.* 1997;55(12):1372–1377; discussion: 1378–1379

495. Litman RS, Kottra JA, Verga KA, Berkowitz RJ, Ward DS. Chloral hydrate sedation: the additive sedative and respiratory depressant effects of nitrous oxide. *Anesth Analg.* 1998;86(4): 724–728

496. American Academy of Pediatric Dentistry, Council on Clinical Affairs. Guideline on use of nitrous oxide for pediatric dental patients. Chicago, IL: American Academy of Pediatric Dentistry; 2013. Available at: http://www.aapd.org/media/policies_guidelines/g_nitrous.pdf. Accessed May 27, 2016

Health and Mental Health Needs of Children in US Military Families

• *Clinical Report*

CLINICAL REPORT Guidance for the Clinician in Rendering Pediatric Care

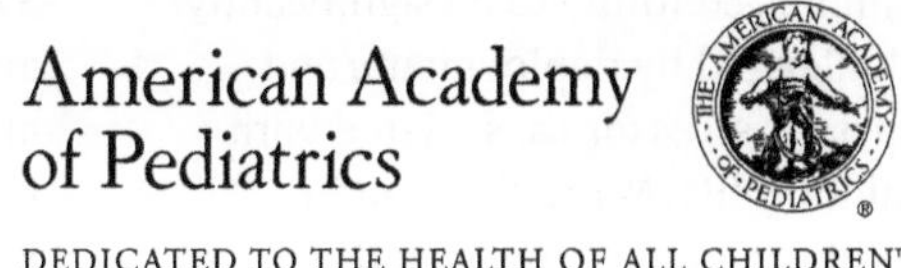

Health and Mental Health Needs of Children in US Military Families

CDR Chadley R. Huebner, MD, MPH, FAAP, SECTION ON UNIFORMED SERVICES, COMMITTEE ON PSYCHOSOCIAL ASPECTS OF CHILD AND FAMILY HEALTH

abstract

Children in US military families share common experiences and unique challenges, including parental deployment and frequent relocation. Although some of the stressors of military life have been associated with higher rates of mental health disorders and increased health care use among family members, there are various factors and interventions that have been found to promote resilience. Military children often live on or near military installations, where they may attend Department of Defense–sponsored child care programs and schools and receive medical care through military treatment facilities. However, many families live in remote communities without access to these services. Because of this wide geographic distribution, military children are cared for in both military and civilian medical practices. This clinical report provides a background to military culture and offers practical guidance to assist civilian and military pediatricians caring for military children.

Department of Pediatrics, Naval Medical Center, San Diego, California

Dr Huebner was responsible for revising and writing this clinical report with consideration of the input of all reviewers and the board of directors and approved the final manuscript as submitted.

The views expressed herein are those of the author and do not necessarily reflect the official policy or position of the Department of the Navy, Department of Defense, or the US Government.

This document is copyrighted and is property of the American Academy of Pediatrics and its Board of Directors. All authors have filed conflict of interest statements with the American Academy of Pediatrics. Any conflicts have been resolved through a process approved by the Board of Directors. The American Academy of Pediatrics has neither solicited nor accepted any commercial involvement in the development of the content of this publication.

Clinical reports from the American Academy of Pediatrics benefit from expertise and resources of liaisons and internal (AAP) and external reviewers. However, clinical reports from the American Academy of Pediatrics may not reflect the views of the liaisons or the organizations or government agencies that they represent.

The guidance in this report does not indicate an exclusive course of treatment or serve as a standard of medical care. Variations, taking into account individual circumstances, may be appropriate.

All clinical reports from the American Academy of Pediatrics automatically expire 5 years after publication unless reaffirmed, revised, or retired at or before that time.

DOI: https://doi.org/10.1542/peds.2018-3258

Address correspondence to Chadley R. Huebner, MD, MPH, FAAP. E-mail: chadley74@yahoo.com

PEDIATRICS (ISSN Numbers: Print, 0031-4005; Online, 1098-4275).

Copyright © 2019 by the American Academy of Pediatrics

FINANCIAL DISCLOSURE: The author has indicated he has no financial relationships relevant to this article to disclose.

To cite: Huebner CR, AAP SECTION ON UNIFORMED SERVICES, AAP COMMITTEE ON PSYCHOSOCIAL ASPECTS OF CHILD AND FAMILY HEALTH. Health and Mental Health Needs of Children in US Military Families. *Pediatrics.* 2019;143(1):e20183258

INTRODUCTION

Children who are military connected have unique needs and experiences compared with peers of the same age. These experiences often include frequent moves, prolonged separations, and deployments of family members. Although these challenges may be familiar to military and civilian health care providers working at military treatment facilities, up to 50% of children who are military connected receive care in the civilian sector.[1–3] The American Academy of Pediatrics (AAP) clinical report "Health and Mental Health Needs of Children in US Military Families" was published in 2013 to assist pediatric health care providers who care for military children who have been affected by deployment.[4] In that report, the cycle of deployment was described as well as the common reactions to deployment and the effects of wartime deployment on children at different developmental stages. Age-based recommendations were provided to assist family members, and additional resources were provided to assist pediatricians.

Since the publication of the last AAP clinical report, military families continue to be significantly challenged by deployments and various stressors associated with military life. Many children in military families live in settings remote from a military community, and civilian health care providers are faced with caring for military children in their practices. This updated clinical report is intended to provide a background of the military culture, to serve as a tool to help navigate the military health care system, and to provide resources that may assist families and the broader health care community, especially during periods of transition and relocation.

DEMOGRAPHICS

The Department of Defense (DOD) remains the nation's largest government agency and employer; 1.3 million men and women serve on active duty, 818 000 in the National Guard and Reserve and more than 2 million military retirees.[5,6] Active duty personnel are members of the US Armed Forces who serve in a full-time duty status. Approximately 88% of active duty forces are stationed in the continental United States and US territories, whereas the remainder are stationed at installations throughout the world but primarily in East Asia (5%) and Europe (5.1%).[5] According to the DOD, military personnel are composed of 17.7% officers with an average age of 34.6 years and 82.3% enlisted personnel with an average age of 27.1 years.[5,7] Most enlisted personnel have a high school diploma, and 8% have a bachelor's degree or higher; the majority of officers (85%) have a bachelor's degree or higher.[5]

Approximately 58% of the 2.2 million members serving on active duty and the National Guard and Reserve have families, and 40% have at least 2 children.[1,3] There are an estimated 1.7 million children of active duty and reserve military personnel, of whom 37.8% are 0 to 5 years of age, 31.6% are 6 to 11 years of age, and 23.8% are 12 to 18 years of age.[5] When including active duty personnel, reserve personnel, and veterans, it is estimated that there are 4 million children who are military connected, with the largest group age ≤5 years.[7]

MILITARY CULTURE

The military is a well-defined institution with a distinct hierarchy and organizational structure. Service members come from ethnically and geographically diverse backgrounds and join the military for a variety of reasons, including the propensity to serve, educational benefits, and financial motivations.[8] Redmond et al[9] described the military workplace culture as a unique environment with unifying characteristics, including discipline, self-sacrifice, cohesiveness, and emphasis on core values. Military service is associated with numerous traditions and common experiences that engender a sense of camaraderie among members who have proudly served.

Military personnel are a relatively young workforce, are more likely to marry young, and have a high proportion of children that are of preschool age.[10] Military personnel are generally paid favorably in comparison with their civilian equivalents; however, additional stressors of the military lifestyle, such as relocation, results in spousal underemployment and unemployment.[11] Military life is often defined by prolonged separation and frequent moves, with many simultaneous stressors in a short time.[10]

Children growing up in military families often share common experiences with each other, such as living on base or post, attending DOD schools, frequent moves, and prolonged separations from a parent. These experiences create a common bond and camaraderie among peers. This sense of identity may be influential in later career choices because children of veterans are more likely than their civilian peers to enlist.[12]

Conversely, military children may feel heightened pressure to conform, behave, and wear their parent's military rank.[1] Davis et al[2] reported that early research portrayed the military family as authoritarian with children who were behaviorally challenged; however, subsequent research has revealed no psychosocial differences from nonmilitary families. Padden and Agazio[13] described 4 major stressors for military children: relocation, family separation, adaptation to danger, and a unique military culture. Socioeconomic challenges include financial stressors among junior enlisted personnel[14] and rates of food insecurity similar to the national average.[15]

RELOCATION

One of the most common aspects of military life is frequent relocation. Active duty personnel receive orders to their respective duty stations for a tour of duty, which is generally 2 to 3 years in length. These orders may be designated as accompanied or unaccompanied, in which the former authorizes dependents' travel and sponsorship at the new duty station and the latter does not. Unaccompanied orders are generally 1 to 2 years in length and are often a result of the nature of the assignment or a dependent family member having medical needs that exceed the capabilities of the local military medical treatment facility.

Military families are geographically mobile, moving at a rate 2.4 times more frequent than that of their civilian counterparts.[7,10,16] Military children may experience a move every 2 to 4 years and can transition between schools up to 9 times by the age of 18 years.[1,17] Because of the frequent mobility, there is often a lack of continuity of health care[1] and limited employment opportunities for nonmilitary spouses.[10]

In a large population study of military youth, there were increased mental health encounters if a geographic move occurred in the past year.[18] This study also revealed that adolescents who were affected had increased psychiatric hospitalizations and emergency department visits. Because families often move away from extended family support, they often refer to the military community as a surrogate family that provides a support network.

Although children of reservists are typically geographically more stable than their active duty counterparts, they often live in nonmilitary communities without resources or knowledge specific to the military.[1] They may feel isolated from the community,[10] and services may not be as readily available.[2] Veteran families may also feel isolated and have challenges when transitioning to civilian communities,[10] where familiar military programs may not exist and there may no longer be access to many of the benefits that were associated with active duty service.[12]

Although moves may be stressful, Clever and Segal[10] asserted that some research has demonstrated increased resilience in military children, including decreased school problems and enhanced development of positive attitudes about moves.[19] Protective factors may include effective support systems, such as living in a military community and military programs designed to address relocation challenges, which may include family newcomer orientations, command sponsorship programs, and programs intended to assist children in connecting with peers at the prospective duty station before the move.

DEPLOYMENT

One of the characteristics of military life that is well known to the public is deployment. Research has found that more than 2 million children of military families have had a parent deployed since 2001.[1] Service members may be deployed to areas throughout the world in support of combat operations or peacekeeping missions for periods ranging from several weeks to more than a year. During this time, family members often remain at home to adapt to life without the military service member or temporarily move to areas where they may have support from extended family members.

The deployment cycle, as described by Pincus et al,[20] consists of 5 stages (predeployment, deployment, sustainment, redeployment, and postdeployment) that each present various emotional challenges to family members. Recommendations to assist family members during each of these stages have been offered by various authors[4,13,20] and serve as a valuable framework for pediatricians caring for children affected by deployment.

Impact of Deployment

Multiple studies have explored the effects of deployment on families and children who are military connected. The stressors associated with deployment, including prolonged family separation, potential injury or death of a service member, and traumatic experiences, can have a cumulative negative effect on the entire family unit. Aranda et al[21] found that 1 in 4 military children have an emotional-behavioral challenge associated with deployment. One study revealed an 11% increase in mental and behavioral health outpatient visits in children 3 to 8 years of age during parental deployment.[22] An additional study evaluating the effect of deployment on children 5 to 12 years of age showed increased child psychosocial morbidity with parental stress and decreased morbidity with military supports.[3]

A 2014 systematic review explored literature examining the impact of parental deployment–related mental health problems on children's outcomes.[23] Of the 42 studies reviewed, the authors found that outcomes were negatively affected by caregiver stress and mental health, and there was evidence of increased child maltreatment and substance abuse. The authors found that family communication was a protective factor, and interventions should be aimed at addressing these challenges. Another 2015 systematic review revealed that a child's age and development, parental mental health and coping abilities, available resources, and resilience factors influenced coping abilities in children affected by military deployment.[24]

Mustillo et al[25] evaluated the timing and duration of deployment on children ages 10 years and younger and whether deployment was associated with any particular type of emotional-behavioral disorder. The authors identified increased anxiety in children ages 3 to 5 years if there was a recent long deployment. For older children ages 6 to 10 years, there was evidence of a long-term impact of parental deployment at the time of their birth, including more peer problems and behavioral problems. This study and others suggested differential effects on the basis of developmental age.[4,26] In a telephone survey involving children 11 to 17 years of age and their home caregivers, increased length of deployment and poor mental health of the caregiver who was not deployed was associated with more challenges for children in dealing with the deployment.[27] Another study of 6- to 12-year-old children and their civilian parent who was not deployed demonstrated increased depression and externalizing symptoms associated with parental distress and cumulative length of parental combat deployment as well as increased anxiety symptoms.[28] The aforementioned research was focused on the immediate effects of wartime deployment, and more longitudinal studies are needed to assess the long-term effects.[29]

Deployment Interventions

Given the challenges associated with deployment, numerous programs have been established to assist service members and their families. Nelson et al[7] described several family-based intervention programs that have been established to increase resilience, combat stress, and improve family functioning: Families OverComing Under Stress,[30] After Deployment: Adaptive Parenting Tools,[31] and the STRoNG Intervention for families with young children.[32] Additional programs that may assist families with younger children in preparing for the stress of the deployment cycle include Sesame Workshop's Talk, Listen, Connect initiative[33] and child-parent psychotherapy–based interventions.[34]

Health Care Use

Research has revealed various challenges associated with deployment, including a decline in academics, increased behavioral problems during deployment, increased emergency and specialist visits, and somatic symptoms.[1,35] A systematic review of 26 studies found an association between increased deployment-related stress and mental health problems in parents and young children as well as increased use of mental health resources.[36] One of these studies demonstrated an increase in outpatient and well-child visits during deployment for children of married parents, which may be attributed to the effect of deployment-related stress on the spouse who was not deployed.[37] Conversely, the authors found decreased visits for children of single parents, which may be attributed to a decreased effect of deployment on a nonparent caregiver or lack of familiarity navigating the health care system. Another study showed an increase in specialist visits and antidepressant and/or anxiolytic medication use among children during deployment. Additionally, a shift from military treatment facilities to civilian facilities during deployment was observed, which may be indicative of a temporary family relocation while the active duty service member was deployed.[38] Finally, research has shown a 7% increase in outpatient visits for children younger than 2 years during the deployment of a parent[37] as well as an increased effect of deployment on children if it occurred during the developmental or attachment period.[39]

Abuse and/or Neglect

Deployment and relocation stressors are concerning for an increased risk of child maltreatment.[40] Cozza et al[41] demonstrated an increased risk of neglect among deployed families compared with families that were never deployed, and a systematic review found an increased risk of child maltreatment, including neglect and physical abuse.[36] Furthermore, there is an increased risk at the time of redeployment,[1] making it important to continue to provide resources once a service member who was deployed returns.

Various programs are available to assist families with abuse prevention, and there are also resources available if abuse has occurred, including the Family Advocacy Program (FAP).[42] FAP professionals interact with families in a variety of ways, including parent workshops and support programs, and conduct investigations when allegations of abuse are made. Because civilian providers may not be aware of the FAP, they may report concerns about child maltreatment to local child protective services without also notifying the local FAP office. Wood et al[40] found that only 42% of cases of medically diagnosed maltreatment were reported to the FAP, compared with 90% reported to child protective services, meaning that many families do not receive timely and appropriate military-specific services.

The DOD has various programs to support families with young children. The New Parent Support Program is an FAP that uses licensed clinicians, nurses, and home-visiting specialists to serve families with young children. A variety of services are available through this program, including home visits, parenting classes, and linkages to community and DOD resources. More information on this valuable program may be found at http://www.militaryonesource.mil/-/the-new-parent-support-program.[43]

RESILIENCE

Despite many of the inherent challenges of military life, multiple studies indicate increased resilience among children who are military connected. Easterbrooks et al[44] noted that most research on military children is focused on deficits rather than the strengths and supports that promote resilience. The authors cite several studies that describe positive outcomes, including enhanced family bonding during deployment, resilience through shared experiences, and enhanced social connections. Aranda et al[21] found that although school-aged children had increased psychosocial morbidity during parental wartime deployment, they had lower baseline psychosocial symptoms than those of civilian peers. Resilience is key in all phases of deployment, and effective support networks may improve coping skills.[2] There is usually not a difference in psychological symptoms in military children during nondeployed seasons, although there may be a "dose effect" with repeated deployments.[21]

Research has examined factors that promote resilience. Parental mental health and parental adjustment to deployment may impact a child's resilience[11]; therefore, it is important to consider the family dynamic when caring for military children. A longitudinal study across the deployment cycle found that socialization with other military children during a deployment was a protective factor that led to better functioning.[45] An ecological model[46] that includes various systems of influence on an individual, such as family and community, has been suggested as a framework to identify the effects of military deployment and separations on children,[26,47] and effective interventions to promote resilience should be designed and tailored at each level.

CHILD CARE AND EDUCATION

Child Care System

The DOD runs the nation's largest employee-sponsored child care system, which consists of 900 child development centers, 300 school-age care program sites, 4500 family child care homes, and subsidized civilian child care.[48] Child development centers are located on most military installations throughout the world and provide child care to children from ages 6 weeks to 5 years. School-age care programs are available for children ages 5 to 12 years and are typically located at schools or youth centers. Additional child care services may be provided in other settings, including on- or off-base child care homes, providing more flexible hours and servicing a wider age range. Services at DOD-sponsored child care sites are income based, and some families may receive subsidies for civilian child care if space is unavailable through military care centers and if they meet specific income qualifications.[48]

Despite the immensity of the child care system, a 2008 study by the RAND Corporation revealed that only a small fraction of the military population was reached by these programs.[49] In this study, only 7% of military members were served by child development centers, and fewer than half of families with children younger than 6 years of age were using DOD-sponsored child care. Child development centers were found to be costlier and less flexible than other options, such as family child care homes. An increased awareness of the various child care options can assist families who are seeking child care arrangements, and additional information may be found at http://www.militaryonesource.mil/-/military-child-care-programs.[50]

Education System

Approximately 13% of children with an active duty parent attend a Department of Defense Education Activity (DODEA) school.[7] DODEA operates 166 schools for 72 000 children enrolled in kindergarten through 12th grade; is located in 7 states, 11 countries, and 2 territories; and also provides support for 1.2 million students who are military connected in public schools in the United States.[51,52] DODEA schools are accredited by the Commission on Accreditation and School Improvement and use a comprehensive curriculum and standardized assessments, including the National Assessment of Educational Progress.[52]

Although continuity of education through DODEA provides many advantages for transient military children, the vast majority of military children attend civilian schools. Astor et al[53] referenced research that revealed that the average military student attends 9 schools between kindergarten and 12th grade.[54] The authors remarked that civilian schools may be less familiar with the needs of military children. Because of increased risks of academic challenges and social problems,[55] it is recommended that military children are provided a supportive environment, which can serve as a protective factor. To facilitate the challenges civilian schools may encounter with military issues, there is a partnership grant with DODEA and public schools to assist civilian schools[11] with children who are military connected. School liaison officers serve as a valuable resource and are available near military installations worldwide (http://www.dodea.edu/Partnership/schoolLiaisonOfficers.cfm).[56]

MILITARY HEALTH SYSTEM

The Military Health System is a global health care delivery system dedicated to supporting the nation's military mission.[57] It is a single-payer umbrella system[2] that serves 9.4 million beneficiaries at an annual cost of approximately $50 billion.[57,58] The Assistant Secretary of Defense for Health Affairs oversees the Defense Health Agency, which manages regional Tricare contracts and the centralized Military Health System while integrating direct and purchased health care systems.[59] Each service branch is responsible for ensuring medical readiness of its operational forces and provides direct health care to beneficiaries at 54 inpatient hospitals and 377 ambulatory clinics throughout the world.[57]

There are multiple Tricare plans available. Eligibility is dependent on service status and enrollment in the Defense Enrollment Eligibility Reporting System. All health care plans are in compliance with the coverage requirements for the Affordable Care Act.[60] The most recent changes to Tricare occurred on January 1, 2018, with several changes to health plans, coverage limits, and regional contractors.[61] Most dependents of active duty members are enrolled in the Tricare Prime program if they live in Prime Service Areas, usually near a military treatment facility.[62] This is a managed care option in which beneficiaries receive direct care at military facilities or from network providers and generally do not pay out of pocket.[58] Tricare Select (Formerly Tricare Standard and Extra) is a fee-for-service plan with deductibles and cost sharing that is available to beneficiaries who do not meet eligibility for Prime or choose not to enroll in Prime and generally receive purchased care through network providers outside of military treatment facilities.[58,63]

There are different Tricare regions throughout the United States administered by a managed care support contractor.[64] Tricare-authorized providers can work directly with the managed care support contractor for claims processing and any management assistance. Additional information for providers can be found at www.tricare.mil/Providers.[64]

MILITARY CHILDREN WITH SPECIAL HEALTH CARE NEEDS

Approximately 220 000 active duty and reserve military personnel have a family member with special needs,[65] including 20% of children who are military connected.[66] In fiscal year 2015, 1.79 million children ages 6 months to 21 years were enrolled in the Military Health System, 17.3% of whom had noncomplex chronic needs and 5.6% of whom had complex chronic needs.[57]

Although subspecialty care may be available at military treatment facilities, children with special health care needs often receive services through civilian network providers, who may be unfamiliar with the military system. In a survey of military family support providers, the most common challenges included navigating systems, child behavioral problems, parental stress and child care, relocation, and the therapy and/or insurance referral process.[65,67] To assist parents of children with special needs, the Office of Community Support for Military Families with Special Needs published the DOD *Special Needs Tool Kit: Birth to 18*.[68] This resource provides valuable information for families navigating early intervention programs and special education services, relocating, accessing Tricare benefits, and connecting to support services.

In addition, the Office of Special Needs provides an early intervention and special education directory to assist families with transitions during relocation to different communities, which is available through the Military OneSource Web site (www.militaryonesource.mil).[69] For military children located overseas who qualify for early intervention services, Educational and Developmental Intervention Services provides comprehensive developmental services, including early childhood special education, speech therapy, occupational therapy, physical therapy, social work, and child psychology. For children ages 3 to 21 years who qualify for special education services, DODEA schools provide special education services while collaborating with Educational and Developmental Intervention Services for medically related services in the school setting.

Exceptional Family Member Program

The Exceptional Family Member Program (EFMP) is a DOD program that provides services for families with special health care or educational needs. There are currently more than 128 000 military family members enrolled in the EFMP,[47,70] with approximately two-thirds of these being children and youth.[65] Any active duty family member with a chronic medical condition or special education need should be enrolled in the EFMP. In a survey of EFMP family support providers across all branches, the largest proportion of disabilities cited included autism spectrum disorders and attention-deficit/hyperactivity disorder.[23,65]

For children of an active duty service member with a chronic medical condition, a DD Form 2792 documenting medical diagnoses and therapeutic needs is required from their pediatrician and should be taken by the family to their respective EFMP service coordinator to complete the enrollment process. The educational form (DD Form 2792-1) should be completed by an early intervention program or school special education program provider if the child is receiving Individuals with Disabilities Education Act Part C or Part B services, respectively. An EFMP quick reference guide is available on the Military OneSource Web site (www.militaryonesource.mil) and may be used to guide families and providers when enrolling in the EFMP. Enrollment in the EFMP is mandatory for dependents of active duty members and ensures that medical and educational needs can be met when service members are considered for various duty stations.

Overseas Screening

Overseas suitability screening (OSS) is a process that active duty service members and their family members undergo once they are identified for an overseas assignment. Because of limited medical service capabilities in overseas environments, OSS reviewers take these factors into consideration when making a determination. Families undergoing this process should bring required OSS and EFMP paperwork to their provider for completion and return these to their screening coordinator.

If a determination is made by the receiving overseas medical facility that the patient's medical needs exceed local capability and capacity or if the environment may exacerbate a medical condition, then the service member may receive unaccompanied orders to the overseas location or may be reconsidered for an alternative duty assignment in an area with the required services to preserve family cohesiveness and avoid unnecessary costs for early returns because of lack of available services.

EXTENDED CARE HEALTH OPTION

The Tricare Extended Care Health Option (ECHO) program is a supplemental benefit for active duty family members with a qualifying condition, such as autism spectrum disorders, intellectual disability, serious physical disabilities, and neuromuscular developmental conditions.[71] It is a monthly cost share based on the sponsor's rank that ranges from $25 to $250 per month, with an annual coverage limit of $36 000.[71] Services covered by ECHO may include durable medical equipment, in-home medical services, rehabilitative services, respite care, and transportation.[71] ECHO eligibility is contingent on enrollment in the EFMP.

AUTISM CARE DEMONSTRATION

Military children with autism spectrum disorders are eligible for applied behavioral analysis (ABA) therapy through the Tricare Autism Care Demonstration (ACD).[72] Eligibility for dependents of active duty members and some activated reservists is contingent on EFMP and ECHO enrollment, whereas dependents of retirees are eligible for ACD services without EFMP and ECHO enrollment. Once a diagnosis of autism is received, a referral for ABA therapy is placed to the regional Tricare contractor, who will then authorize an initial 6 months of ABA therapy.[67] The ACD provides services totaling $195 million in yearly expenditures,[57] with cost shares and copayments dependent on the family's Tricare health plan.[72]

Military families with children with autism spectrum disorders face challenges, including delays in reestablishing therapeutic services and lack of provider continuity because of relocation.[57,73] Given the unique burdens of military families, recommendations are to identify autism spectrum disorders in children early, have a tiered menu of services available, and consider telehealth options for parent training.[74,75] In addition, early identification and improving access to early intervention may be cost-effective measures to ensure sustainability of the military autism benefit.[76]

SUGGESTIONS FOR PEDIATRICIANS CARING FOR MILITARY CHILDREN

Cultural Competency

Most US medical students will care for a patient who is military connected in their career. Prospective military physicians who receive medical training through the F. Edward Hébert School of Medicine at the Uniformed Services University of the Health Sciences or civilian medical schools through the Health Professions Scholarship Program are exposed early in their careers to military medicine through clerkships and research opportunities. Furthermore, military residency programs have served a vital role in training military physicians to serve our nation in operational settings and military treatment facilities throughout the world.

Although military physicians are familiar with military culture and the military medical system, their civilian colleagues may not have received similar training opportunities. Gleeson and Hemmer[77] have recommended competency training in medical schools, including military history taking, providing opportunities for clinical rotations through military treatment facilities, and encouraging medical students who are military connected to share their experiences in medical schools. Graduate medical education as well as printed and online information may serve as effective routes for increased cultural competency.[74]

Research indicates that 56% of providers outside of military treatment facilities do not ask for the military status of families,[78] and recommendations have been made for community capacity building through increased cultural awareness, asking families about military status, and implementation of clinical practice measures aimed at improving coordination of care between health care systems.[79] To assist providers, the Department of Veterans Affairs has created the Veterans Affairs Community Provider Toolkit,[80] which provides additional information on military culture.

Screening

Given the increased stressors associated with the military lifestyle and the associated behavioral risks, incorporating a behavioral screening tool can assist the pediatrician in the office setting. The Pediatric Symptom Checklist was used in 1 study during parental deployment and revealed increased internalizing behaviors, externalizing behaviors, and school problems.[21] The AAP, in a recent clinical report, recommends behavioral and emotional screening as a routine component in pediatric practice, and references multiple resources available on its Web site (http://www2.aap.org/commpeds/dochs/mentalhealth/KeyResources.html).[81]

Although broad-scale behavioral screening tools are effective, a mechanism to identify military children in practice would be a helpful adjunct. Chandra and London[29] recommend routinely identifying children who are military connected in practices as well as taking a military history at intake.[23] A school identifier has been proposed to assist in school-district resourcing for military students,[11] and schools may serve as a primary resource for pediatricians to identify issues that may influence the academic, social, and behavioral health of children in military families. The Have You Ever Served in the Military? campaign by the American Academy of Nursing designed a pocket card to assist clinicians caring for veterans.[82] An expanded American Academy of Nursing initiative, I Serve 2, has been launched to identify military children in practice by asking the question, "Do you have a parent who has or is serving in the military?" and to provide a modified pocket guide to assist clinicians caring for military children.[1] Furthermore, Hisle-Gorman et al[39] have also suggested not only asking families about their military status but also directly asking about deployment schedules and parental health as well as gaining familiarization with local support systems for military families.

Advocacy

Efforts to advocate for military children can occur at many levels. Lester and Flake[47] note that military children are influenced by many factors, and understanding these systems from an ecological framework may influence outcomes. In addition to the individual- and family-based interactions discussed in this report, advocacy efforts can occur at the community and national level. There have been several large-scale legislative actions and national campaigns in support of military children and their families, including the Military Family Act of 1985 and Joining Forces.[2] April has been designated as the Month of the Military Child, during which time awareness is brought to the forefront. The *Eunice Kennedy Shriver* National Institute of Child Health and Human Development and the HSC Foundation sponsored a conference in April 2014 to raise awareness for children with special health care needs who are military connected and provided an excellent summary of the latest challenges and research surrounding the military child.[66] (conference summary can be found at: https://www.nichd.nih.gov/news/resources/spotlight/120214-military-families). Aronson et al[65] have stressed that health care professionals, schools, and communities should proactively reach out to military families.

Psychosocial support resources are also available to assist families that may be affected by disasters or grief and bereavement. Two AAP clinical reports are available to assist pediatricians: "Providing Psychosocial Support to Children and Families in the Aftermath of Disasters and Crises"[83] and "Supporting the Grieving Child and Family."[84]

Navigating the Military Health System

This clinical report provides a review of the current literature and identifies some of the programs available for children with connections to the military. One of the key ways providers can assist military families is through effectively navigating the military health care system and coordinating with community agencies and local support networks. The following list provides general recommendations that may provide additional assistance to providers caring for children who are military connected.

RECOMMENDATIONS

Screening

1. Establish a clinical process to identify children who are military connected and document it in the electronic medical record.
2. Take a thorough military history, including parental deployment history, relocation, and parental mental health.
3. Integrate an evidence-based behavioral and emotional rating scale in your practice to identify children who are at risk.

Deployment

1. Gain familiarization with the deployment cycle and common reactions to deployment.
2. Provide a linkage to community-based resources for families of service members who are deployed, including mental health services and evidence-based intervention programs that promote resilience:
   a. Families OverComing Under Stress (http://focusproject.org),
   b. After Deployment: Adaptive Parenting Tools (ADAPT): http://www.cehd.umn.edu/fsos/research/adapt/default.asp,[31]
   c. STRoNG Intervention for families with young children,[32] and
   d. Sesame Workshop's Talk, Listen, Connect initiative: http://www.sesameworkshop.org/what-we-do/our-initiatives/military-families/.[33]

Relocation

1. Help new families in the local community connect with local military resources and community agencies.
2. Prepare families for an upcoming move through online resources for spouses at Military

OneSource[85] (militaryonesource.mil/for-spouses) and for children at Military Kids Connect (militarykidsconnect.dcoe.mil/).

3. Work with local schools to implement a program identifying military children and provide resources to assist with transitions.

Special Needs

1. For children with special health care needs, complete EFMP paperwork and ask the family member to turn in the completed copy to their local EFMP office. The EFMP Quick Reference Guide, which includes the DD Form 2792 to be completed by the medical provider, may be found on the Military OneSource Web site at: http://download.militaryonesource.mil/12038/MOS/ResourceGuides/EFMP-QuickReferenceGuide.pdf.[86]
2. Provide families with contact information for the ECHO program to assist with any additional coverage that may not be afforded by the Tricare benefit.
3. Additional resources that are valuable in assisting families with children with special needs include:
   a. the EFMP special needs tool kit,[68] (http://download.militaryonesource.mil/12038/EFMP/PTK_SCORs/ParentToolkit_Apr2014.pdf), and
   b. Specialized Training of Military Parents (http://stompproject.blogspot.com).

Tricare

1. For providers interested in becoming a Tricare-approved provider, refer to the Tricare Web site for additional information at https://tricare.mil/Providers.[64]
2. For assistance with navigating Tricare, contact information for regional contractors can be found at https://tricare.mil/Providers.[64]
3. Generally, prior authorization or referrals are not required of Tricare beneficiaries for initial outpatient mental health care with providers who are Tricare authorized.[87] Pediatricians can assist families connecting with an authorized Tricare provider by referring them to www.tricare.mil/findaprovider.[88]
4. Please refer to the following for additional Tricare information:
   a. Tricare Prime (https://tricare.mil/Plans/HealthPlans/Prime),[62]
   b. Tricare Select (https://tricare.mil/Plans/HealthPlans/TS),[63] and
   c. Tricare Mental Health Care (https://tricare.mil/mentalhealth).[89]

Overseas Screening

1. Pediatricians can work with overseas screening coordinators by completing any requested forms and providing an up-to-date assessment of a patient's medical needs.
2. Overseas hospitals frequently publish possible disqualifying conditions on their Web sites, which can help families be prepared and manage expectations.
3. In the case of an overseas screening denial, pediatricians can clarify any concerns with the overseas screening office and provide any additional documentation as needed to facilitate a thorough review of the case.

Additional Resources

1. Comprehensive resources for pediatricians and families:
   a. Military OneSource (www.militaryonesource.mil) and
   b. The National Military Family Association (www.militaryfamily.org).
2. New parent support:
   a. The New Parent Support Program (http://www.militaryonesource.mil/-/the-new-parent-support-program)[43] and
   b. Zero to Three (https://www.zerotothree.org/resources/series/honoring-our-babies-and-toddlers#the-resources).
3. Education:
   a. the Military Child Education Coalition (www.militarychild.org) and
   b. DODEA (www.dodea.edu).
4. Child care: Military Child Care (www.militarychildcare.com);
5. Autism:
   a. Operation Autism (www.operationautismonline.org) and
   b. Autism Care Demonstration: https://tricare.mil/Plans/SpecialPrograms/ACD/GettingCare.[90]
6. Advocacy:
   a. AAP Section on Uniformed Services (https://www.aap.org/en-us/about-the-aap/Committees-Councils-Sections/Section-on-Uniformed-Services/Pages/default.aspx) and
   b. Clearinghouse for Military Family Readiness (www.militaryfamilies.psu.edu).

ACKNOWLEDGMENT

The author would like to thank Lisa Serow for reviewing the report from a parent's perspective.

LEAD AUTHOR

CDR Chadley R. Huebner, MD, MPH, FAAP

SECTION ON UNIFORMED SERVICES EXECUTIVE COMMITTEE, 2018–2019

COL Catherine A. Kimball-Eayrs, MD, IBCLC, FAAP, Chairperson
LCDR Bridget K. Cunningham, MD, FAAP
Lt Col Brian M. Faux, MD, FAAP
LCDR Christopher W. Foster, MD, FAAP
Lt Col Courtney Anne Judd, MD, MPH, FAAP
COL Keith M. Lemmon, MD, FAAP
CDR Lisa M. Mondzelewski, MD, MPH, FAAP
COL Martin E. Weisse, MD, FAAP
Lt Col Lauren J. Wolf, MD, FAAP
CAPT David Wong, MD, FAAP

LIAISONS

COL Patrick Wilson Hickey, MD, FAAP – *Uniformed Services University of the Health Sciences*
CPT Elizabeth Marx Perkins, MD, FAAP – *Section on Pediatric Trainees*

STAFF

Jackie P. Burke

COMMITTEE ON PSYCHOSOCIAL ASPECTS OF CHILD AND FAMILY HEALTH, 2018–2019

Arthur Lavin, MD, FAAP, Chairperson
George Askew, MD, FAAP
Rebecca Baum, MD, FAAP
Evelyn Berger-Jenkins MD, MPH, FAAP
Thresia B. Gambon, MD, MBA, MPH, FAAP
Arthur Lavin, MD, FAAP
Gerri Mattson, MD, FAAP
Raul Montiel-Esparza, MD, FAAP
Arwa Nasir, MBBS, MSc, MPH, FAAP
Lawrence Sagin Wissow, MD, MPH, FAAP

LIAISONS

Sharon Berry, PhD, ABPP– *Society of Pediatric Psychology*
Edward R. Christophersen, PhD, FAAP (hon) – *Society of Pediatric Psychology*
Norah Johnson, PhD, RN, CPNP – *National Association of Pediatric Nurse Practitioners*
Abigail Schlesinger, MD – *American Academy of Child and Adolescent Psychiatry*
Amy Starin, PhD, LCSW – *National Association of Social Workers*

STAFF

Karen S. Smith

ABBREVIATIONS

AAP: American Academy of Pediatrics
ABA: applied behavioral analysis
ACD: Autism Care Demonstration
DOD: Department of Defense
DODEA: Department of Defense Education Activity
ECHO: Extended Care Health Option
EFMP: Exceptional Family Member Program
FAP: Family Advocacy Program
OSS: overseas suitability screening

FUNDING: No external funding.

POTENTIAL CONFLICT OF INTEREST: The author has indicated he has no potential conflicts of interest to disclose.

REFERENCES

1. Rossiter AG, Dumas MA, Wilmoth MC, Patrician PA. "I Serve 2": meeting the needs of military children in civilian practice. *Nurs Outlook*. 2016;64(5):485–490
2. Davis BE, Blaschke GS, Stafford EM. Military children, families, and communities: supporting those who serve. *Pediatrics*. 2012;129(suppl 1):S3–S10
3. Flake EM, Davis BE, Johnson PL, Middleton LS. The psychosocial effects of deployment on military children. *J Dev Behav Pediatr*. 2009;30(4):271–278
4. Siegel BS, Davis BE; Committee on Psychosocial Aspects of Child and Family Health; Section on Uniformed Services. Health and mental health needs of children in US military families. *Pediatrics*. 2013;131(6). Available at: www.pediatrics.org/cgi/content/full/131/6/e2002
5. Department of Defense. 2016 demographics. Profile of the military community. Available at: http://download.militaryonesource.mil/12038/MOS/Reports/2016-Demographics-Report.pdf. Accessed June 7, 2018
6. Department of Defense. Our story. Available at: https://www.defense.gov/About/. Accessed July 17, 2017
7. Nelson SC, Baker MJ, Weston CG. Impact of military deployment on the development and behavior of children. *Pediatr Clin North Am*. 2016;63(5):795–811
8. Woodruff T, Kelty R, Segal DR. Propensity to serve and motivation to enlist among American combat soldiers. *Armed Forces Soc*. 2016;32(3):353–366
9. Redmond SA, Wilcox SL, Campbell S, et al. A brief introduction to the military workplace culture. *Work*. 2015;50(1):9–20
10. Clever M, Segal DR. The demographics of military children and families. *Future Child*. 2013;23(2):13–39
11. Cozza SJ, Lerner RM, Haskins R. Social policy report. Military and veteran families and children: policies and programs for health maintenance and positive development. 2014. Available at: https://www.srcd.org/sites/default/files/documents/spr283_final.pdf. Accessed September 23, 2017
12. Sherman MD. Children of military veterans: an overlooked population. Available at: https://www.srcd.org/sites/default/files/documents/spr283_final.pdf. Accessed September 6, 2017
13. Padden D, Agazio J. Caring for military families across the deployment cycle. *J Emerg Nurs*. 2013;39(6):562–569
14. Hosek J, Wadsworth SM. Economic conditions of military families. *Future Child*. 2013;23(2):41–59
15. Wax SG, Stankorb SM. Prevalence of food insecurity among military households with children 5 years of age and younger. *Public Health Nutr*. 2016;19(13):2458–2466
16. Cooney R, De Angelis K, Segal MW. Moving with the military: race, class, and gender differences in the employment consequences of tied migration. *Race, Gender & Class*. 2011;18(1/2):360–384

17. National Military Family Association. Education revolution: Their right. Our fight. Available at: https://www.militaryfamily.org/info-resources/education/education-revolution/. Accessed July 19, 2017

18. Millegan J, McLay R, Engel C. The effect of geographic moves on mental healthcare utilization in children. *J Adolesc Health.* 2014;55(2):276–280

19. Weber EG, Weber DK. Geographic relocation frequency, resilience, and military adolescent behavior. *Mil Med.* 2005;170(7):638–642

20. Pincus SH, House R, Christenson J, Adler LE. The emotional cycle of deployment: a military family perspective. *US Army Med Dep J.* 2001;2(5):15–23

21. Aranda MC, Middleton LS, Flake E, Davis BE. Psychosocial screening in children with wartime-deployed parents. *Mil Med.* 2011;176(4):402–407

22. Gorman GH, Eide M, Hisle-Gorman E. Wartime military deployment and increased pediatric mental and behavioral health complaints. *Pediatrics.* 2010;126(6):1058–1066

23. Creech SK, Hadley W, Borsari B. The impact of military deployment and reintegration on children and parenting: a systematic review. *Prof Psychol Res Pr.* 2014;45(6):452–464

24. Bello-Utu CF, DeSocio JE. Military deployment and reintegration: a systematic review of child coping. *J Child Adolesc Psychiatr Nurs.* 2015;28(1):23–34

25. Mustillo S, Wadsworth SM, Lester P. Parental deployment and well-being in children: results from a new study of military families. *J Emot Behav Disord.* 2015;24(2):82–91

26. Masten AS. Competence, risk, and resilience in military families: conceptual commentary. *Clin Child Fam Psychol Rev.* 2013;16(3):278–281

27. Chandra A, Lara-Cinisomo S, Jaycox LH, et al. Children on the homefront: the experience of children from military families. *Pediatrics.* 2010;125(1):16–25

28. Lester P, Peterson K, Reeves J, et al. The long war and parental combat deployment: effects on military children and at-home spouses. *J Am Acad Child Adolesc Psychiatry.* 2010;49(4):310–320

29. Chandra A, London AS. Unlocking insights about military children and families. *Future Child.* 2013;23(2):187–198

30. FOCUS Project. FOCUS: Resilience training for military families. Available at: http://focusproject.org/. Accessed August 29, 2017

31. University of Minnesota. ADAPT - after deployment: adaptive parenting tools. Available at: www.cehd.umn.edu/fsos/research/adapt/default.asp. Accessed September 3, 2017

32. Rosenblum KL, Muzik M. STRoNG intervention for military families with young children. *Psychiatr Serv.* 2014;65(3):399

33. Sesame Workshop. Talk, listen, connect: arming military families with love, laughter, and practical tools for deployment. Available at: www.sesameworkshop.org/what-we-do/our-initiatives/military-families/. Accessed September 3, 2017

34. Osofsky JD, Chartrand MM. Military children from birth to five years. *Future Child.* 2013;23(2):61–77

35. Johnson HL, Ling CG. Caring for military children in the 21st century. *J Am Assoc Nurse Pract.* 2013;25(4):195–202

36. Trautmann J, Alhusen J, Gross D. Impact of deployment on military families with young children: a systematic review. *Nurs Outlook.* 2015;63(6):656–679

37. Eide M, Gorman G, Hisle-Gorman E. Effects of parental military deployment on pediatric outpatient and well-child visit rates. *Pediatrics.* 2010;126(1):22–27

38. Larson MJ, Mohr BA, Adams RS, et al. Association of military deployment of a parent or spouse and changes in dependent use of health care services. *Med Care.* 2012;50(9):821–828

39. Hisle-Gorman E, Harrington D, Nylund CM, Tercyak KP, Anthony BJ, Gorman GH. Impact of parents' wartime military deployment and injury on young children's safety and mental health. *J Am Acad Child Adolesc Psychiatry.* 2015;54(4):294–301

40. Wood JN, Griffis HM, Taylor CM, et al. Under-ascertainment from healthcare settings of child abuse events among children of soldiers by the U.S. Army Family Advocacy Program. *Child Abuse Negl.* 2017;63:202–210

41. Cozza SJ, Whaley GL, Fisher JE, et al. Deployment status and child neglect types in the U.S. Army. *Child Maltreat.* 2018;23(1):25–33

42. Military OneSource. The Family Advocacy Program. Available at: www.militaryonesource.mil/-/the-family-advocacy-program. Accessed September 3, 2017

43. Military OneSource. The new parent support program. Available at: http://www.militaryonesource.mil/-/the-new-parent-support-program. Accessed November 18, 2018

44. Easterbrooks MA, Ginsburg K, Lerner RM. Resilience among military youth. *Future Child.* 2013;23(2):99–120

45. Meadows SO, Tanielian T, Karney B, et al. The Deployment Life Study: longitudinal analysis of military families across the deployment cycle. *Rand Health Q.* 2017;6(2):7

46. Bronfenbrenner U, Morris PA. The bioecological model of human development. In: Damon W, Lerner RM, eds. *Handbook of Child Psychology.* Vol. 1. 6th ed. Hoboken, NJ: John Wiley & Sons, Inc; 2007

47. Lester P, Flake E. How wartime military service affects children and families. *Future Child.* 2013;23(2):121–141

48. Floyd L, Phillips DA. Child care and other support programs. *Future Child.* 2013;23(2):79–97

49. Zellman GL, Gates SM, Cho M, Shaw R. Options for improving the military child care system. 2008. Available at: https://www.rand.org/content/dam/rand/pubs/occasional_papers/2008/RAND_OP217.sum.pdf. Accessed July 28, 2017

50. Military OneSource. Military child care programs. Available at: http://www.militaryonesource.mil/-/military-child-care-programs. Accessed November 18, 2018

51. Department of Defense Education Activity. Community strategic plan volume 1: school years 2013/14–2017/18. 2013. Available at: www.

dodea.edu/CSP/upload/CSP_130703.pdf. Accessed July 28, 2017

52. Department of Defense Education Activity. About DoDEA - DoDEA schools worldwide. Available at: www.dodea.edu/aboutDoDEA/today.cfm. Accessed June 8, 2018

53. Astor RA, De Pedro KT, Gilreath TD, Esqueda MC, Benbenishty R. The promotional role of school and community contexts for military students. *Clin Child Fam Psychol Rev.* 2013;16(3):233–244

54. Kitmitto S, Huberman M, Blankenship C, Hannan S, Norris D, Christenson B. Educational options and performance of military-connected school districts research study – final report. 2011. Available at: www.dodea.edu/Partnership/upload/AIR-Research-Study-2011.pdf. Accessed September 3, 2017

55. Chandra A, Martin LT, Hawkins SA, Richardson A. The impact of parental deployment on child social and emotional functioning: perspectives of school staff. *J Adolesc Health.* 2010;46(3):218–223

56. US Department of Defense Education Activity. School liaison officers. Available at: http://www.dodea.edu/Partnership/schoolLiaisonOfficers.cfm. Accessed November 18, 2018

57. Defense Health Agency. Evaluation of the TRICARE program: Fiscal year 2017 report to Congress. Available at: https://health.mil/Reference-Center/Reports/2017/06/08/Evaluation-of-the-TRICARE-Program. Accessed June 25, 2017

58. Task Force on Defense Personnel. *Health, Health Care, and a High-Performance Force.* Washington, DC: Bipartisan Policy Center; 2017

59. Military Health System. Defense Health Agency. Available at: http://health.mil/dha. Accessed August 17, 2017

60. Tricare. Plan finder. Available at: https://www.tricare.mil/Home/Plans/PlanFinder. Accessed August 17, 2017

61. Tricare. About us - changes. Available at: https://tricare.mil/changes. Accessed February 4, 2018

62. Tricare. TRICARE Prime. Available at: https://tricare.mil/Plans/HealthPlans/Prime. Accessed February 4, 2018

63. Tricare. TRICARE Select. Available at: https://tricare.mil/Plans/HealthPlans/TS. Accessed February 4, 2018

64. Military Health System. Information for TRICARE providers. Available at: https://tricare.mil/Providers. Accessed August 17, 2017

65. Aronson KR, Kyler SJ, Moeller JD, Perkins DF. Understanding military families who have dependents with special health care and/or educational needs. *Disabil Health J.* 2016;9(3):423–430

66. Eunice Kennedy Shriver National Institute of Child Health and Human Development. Military-connected children with special health care needs and their families. 2014. Available at: https://www.nichd.nih.gov/news/resources/spotlight/120214-military-families. Accessed November 18, 2018

67. Tricare. Getting care. Available at: https://www.tricare.mil/Plans/SpecialPrograms/ACD/GettingCare. Accessed July 31, 2017

68. Department of Defense. Special needs parent tool kit: birth to 18. 2014. Available at: http://download.militaryonesource.mil/12038/EFMP/PTK_SCORs/ParentToolkit_Apr2014.pdf. Accessed September 23, 2017

69. Military OneSource. Education directory for children with special needs. Available at: http://apps.militaryonesource.mil/MOS/f?p=EFMP_DIRECTORY:HOME:0. Accessed September 3, 2017

70. Department of Defense. *Annual Report to the Congressional Defense Committees on Support for Military Families with Special Needs.* Washington, DC: Department of Defense; 2015

71. Tricare. Extended care health option. 2016. Available at: https://tricare.mil/-/media/Files/TRICARE/Publications/FactSheets/ECHO_FS.ashx. Accessed July 31, 2017

72. Tricare. Autism care demonstration. 2016. Available at: https://www.tricare.mil/Plans/SpecialPrograms/ACD. Accessed July 31, 2017

73. Davis JM, Finke EH. The experience of military families with children with autism spectrum disorders during relocation and separation. *J Autism Dev Disord.* 2015;45(7):2019–2034

74. Meyer E. Case report: military subcultural competency. *Mil Med.* 2013;178(7):e848–e850

75. Davis JM, Finke E, Hickerson B. Service delivery experiences and intervention needs of military families with children with ASD. *J Autism Dev Disord.* 2016;46(5):1748–1761

76. Klin A, Wetherby AM, Woods J, et al. Toward innovative, cost-effective, and systemic solutions to improve outcomes and well-being of military families affected by autism spectrum disorder. *Yale J Biol Med.* 2015;88(1):73–79

77. Gleeson TD, Hemmer PA. Providing care to military personnel and their families: how we can all contribute. *Acad Med.* 2014;89(9):1201–1203

78. Kilpatrick DG, Best CL, Smith DW, Kudler H, Cornelison-Grant V. *Serving Those Who Have Served: Educational Needs of Health Care Providers Working With Military Members, Veterans, and Their Families.* Charleston, SC: Medical University of South Carolina Department of Psychiatry, National Crime Victims Research and Treatment Center; 2011

79. Kudler H, Porter RI. Building communities of care for military children and families. *Future Child.* 2013;23(2):163–185

80. Community Provider Toolkit. Welcome to the community provider toolkit. Available at: https://www.mentalhealth.va.gov/communityproviders/index.asp. Accessed August 29, 2017

81. Weitzman C, Wegner L; Section on Developmental and Behavioral Pediatrics; Committee on Psychosocial Aspects of Child and Family Health; Council on Early Childhood; Society for Developmental and Behavioral Pediatrics; American Academy of Pediatrics. Promoting optimal development: screening for behavioral and emotional problems [published correction appears in *Pediatrics.* 2015;135(2):946]. *Pediatrics.* 2015;135(5):384–395

82. Have You Ever Served in the Military? Pocket card & posters. Available at: www.haveyoueverserved.com/

pocket-card--posters.html. Accessed August 22, 2017

83. Schonfeld DJ, Demaria T; Disaster Preparedness Advisory Council; Committee on Psychosocial Aspects of Child and Family Health. Providing psychosocial support to children and families in the aftermath of disasters and crises. *Pediatrics.* 2015;136(4). Available at: www.pediatrics.org/cgi/content/full/136/4/e1120

84. Schonfeld DJ, Demaria T; Committee on Psychosocial Aspects of Child and Family Health; Disaster Preparedness Advisory Council. Supporting the grieving child and family. *Pediatrics.* 2016;138(3):e20162147

85. Military OneSource. For spouses. Available at: www.militaryonesource.mil/for-spouses. Accessed November 18, 2018

86. Military OneSource. Quick reference guide. Available at: http://download.militaryonesource.mil/12038/MOS/ResourceGuides/EFMP-QuickReferenceGuide.pdf. Accessed November 18, 2018

87. Tricare. Mental health care and substance use disorder services. 2017. Available at: https://tricare.mil/-/media/Files/TRICARE/Publications/FactSheets/Mental_Health_FS.ashx. Accessed September 4, 2017

88. Tricare. Find a doctor. Available at: www.tricare.mil/findaprovider. Accessed November 18, 2018

89. Tricare. Mental health care. Available at: https://tricare.mil/mentalhealth. Accessed November 18, 2018

90. Tricare. Getting care. Available at: https://tricare.mil/Plans/SpecialPrograms/ACD/GettingCare. Accessed November 18, 2018

Health Supervision for Children With Neurofibromatosis Type 1

• *Clinical Report*

CLINICAL REPORT Guidance for the Clinician in Rendering Pediatric Care

American Academy of Pediatrics

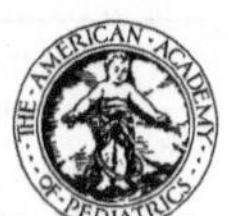

DEDICATED TO THE HEALTH OF ALL CHILDREN™

Health Supervision for Children With Neurofibromatosis Type 1

David T. Miller, MD, PhD, FAAP,[a] Debra Freedenberg, MD, PhD, FAAP,[b] Elizabeth Schorry, MD,[c] Nicole J. Ullrich, MD, PhD,[d] David Viskochil, MD, PhD,[e] Bruce R. Korf, MD, PhD, FAAP,[f] COUNCIL ON GENETICS, AMERICAN COLLEGE OF MEDICAL GENETICS AND GENOMICS

abstract

Neurofibromatosis type 1 (NF1) is a multisystem disorder that primarily involves the skin and peripheral nervous system. Its population prevalence is approximately 1 in 3000. The condition is usually recognized in early childhood, when pigmentary manifestations emerge. Although NF1 is associated with marked clinical variability, most children affected follow patterns of growth and development within the normal range. Some features of NF1 can be present at birth, but most manifestations emerge with age, necessitating periodic monitoring to address ongoing health and developmental needs and minimize the risk of serious medical complications. In this report, we provide a review of the clinical criteria needed to establish a diagnosis, the inheritance pattern of NF1, its major clinical and developmental manifestations, and guidelines for monitoring and providing intervention to maximize the health and quality of life of a child affected.

[a]Division of Genetics and Genomics and [d]Department of Neurology, Harvard Medical School, Harvard University and Boston Children's Hospital, Boston, Massachusetts; [b]Texas Department of State Health Services, Austin, Texas; [c]Division of Human Genetics, Cincinnati Children's Hospital Medical Center, Cincinnati, Ohio; [e]Division of Medical Genetics, Department of Pediatrics, University of Utah, Salt Lake City, Utah; and [f]Department of Genetics, University of Alabama at Birmingham, Birmingham, Alabama

Dr Miller led the working group, served as liaison between the working group and the American College of Medical Genetics, reviewed and updated literature references, and drafted several sections; Dr Freedenberg served as liaison between the working group and the American Academy of Pediatrics; Drs Schorry, Ullrich, and Viskochil reviewed and updated literature references and drafted several sections; Dr Korf cochaired the working group, reviewed and updated literature references, and drafted several sections; and all authors approved the final manuscript as submitted and agree to be accountable for all aspects of the work. *This document is copyrighted and is property of the American Academy of Pediatrics and its Board of Directors. All authors have filed conflict of interest statements with the American Academy of Pediatrics. Any conflicts have been resolved through a process approved by the Board of Directors. The American Academy of Pediatrics has neither solicited nor accepted any commercial involvement in the development of the content of this publication.*

Clinical reports from the American Academy of Pediatrics benefit from expertise and resources of liaisons and internal (AAP) and external reviewers. However, clinical reports from the American Academy of Pediatrics may not reflect the views of the liaisons or the organizations or government agencies that they represent.

The guidance in this report does not indicate an exclusive course of treatment or serve as a standard of medical care. Variations, taking into account individual circumstances, may be appropriate.

To cite: Miller DT, Freedenberg D, Schorry E, et al. AAP COUNCIL ON GENETICS, AAP AMERICAN COLLEGE OF MEDICAL GENETICS AND GENOMICS. Health Supervision for Children With Neurofibromatosis Type 1. *Pediatrics.* 2019;143(5):e20190660

INTRODUCTION

Neurofibromatosis type 1 (NF1) is 1 of the most common inherited genetic conditions, affecting approximately 1 in 3000 individuals.[1] NF1 is a multisystem disorder in which some features may be present at birth but most are age-related manifestations. Since the publication of the article "Health Supervision for Children With Neurofibromatosis," the health supervision and treatment rationale has evolved, necessitating this update.[2] In this report, we only address issues concerning the diagnosis and management of NF1, which should not be confused with neurofibromatosis type 2, a separate and distinct disorder that typically presents in childhood and adolescence with cutaneous and vestibular schwannomas and has an incidence of 1 in 33 000 and a prevalence of less than 1 in 50 000.[1] Most pediatricians and pediatric medical subspecialists follow multiple children with NF1 in their practices, and NF1 has a wide spectrum of health implications. This document seeks to educate and provide guidance for the clinician on the current understanding of the

TABLE 1 NIH Consensus Development Conference Criteria

Clinical Criteria	Clinical Pearls
1. Six or more CALMs equal to or greater than 5 mm in longest diameter in prepubertal patients and 15 mm in longest diameter in postpubertal patients	• 2–3 or fewer CALMs are normal in the population
	• Typically, CALMs are present since infancy in people with NF1
	• Typically have smooth edges
2. Two or more neurofibromas of any type or 1 plexiform neurofibroma	• Dermal and subcutaneous neurofibromas not typically detectable until later in childhood
	• Plexiform neurofibroma typically changes the color and/or texture of overlying skin
3. Freckling in the axillary or inguinal regions (Crowe sign)	• Not typically detectable until age 5 or later
	• Freckling in areas not exposed to the sun is unexpected in people without NF1
4. Optic glioma (OPG)	• Not detectable without direct ophthalmoscopy
	• May be present in infancy
	• Early detection critical for preserving vision
5. Two or more iris hamartomas (Lisch nodules) (Fig 1)	• Occurrence is age related (rarely present in infants and toddlers; present in about half of children by school age; present in most teenagers)
	• Not detectable (without slit-lamp examination)
	• Does not affect vision
6. A distinctive osseous lesion, such as sphenoid wing dysplasia or long-bone dysplasia (with associated cortical thickening and medullary canal narrowing), with or without pseudoarthrosis	• Tibial dysplasia is the most common type of bone dysplasia
	• Infants and toddlers with anterior-lateral tibial bowing on examination should have tibial radiographs and referral to orthopedics
7. A first-degree relative (parent, sibling, or child) with NF1 according to the aforementioned criteria	• Parent who is affected should have some symptoms even if mildly affected (100% penetrance)
	• NF1 does not skip a generation

Two or more criteria are required to establish the diagnosis of NF1. Adapted from Neurofibromatosis. Conference statement. National Institutes of Health Consensus Development Conference. *Arch Neurol.* 1988;45(5):575–578; National Institutes of Health Consensus Development Conference Statement: neurofibromatosis. Bethesda, Md., USA, July 13-15, 1987. *Neurofibromatosis.* 1988;1(3):172–178; and DeBella K, Szudek J, Friedman JM. Use of the national institutes of health criteria for diagnosis of neurofibromatosis 1 in children. *Pediatrics.* 2000;105(3, pt 1):608–614.

pathophysiology of NF1, health supervision for children with NF1, and the role of the medical home in caring for children with NF1.

DIAGNOSIS AND DIFFERENTIAL DIAGNOSIS

In a National Institutes of Health (NIH) consensus development conference regarding NF1, 7 criteria were demarcated, of which 2 or more are required to establish the diagnosis of NF1 (see Table 1).[3–6] The diagnosis of NF1 in nonfamilial pediatric cases may be difficult because certain clinical manifestations are age dependent. The variability of clinical expressivity in NF1 also makes it difficult to predict future manifestations of NF1 in a child who is affected.

The diagnosis of NF1 in a child is usually first suspected on the basis of café-au-lait macules (CALMs) (Fig 2). The differential diagnosis (Table 2) includes other conditions that present with CALMs or other pigmentary manifestations. In general, CALMs in NF1 have uniform and regular borders ("coast of California"). Atypical CALMs that are irregularly shaped ("coast of Maine") or have heavy pigment compared with adjacent skin may be seen in NF1, but if typical CALMs are not also present, other conditions should be considered. Other signs and symptoms delineate these conditions, and referral to a specialist experienced in diagnosing NF1 and related conditions (usually a medical geneticist, dermatologist, or neurologist) may be helpful to establish a diagnosis. Finally, there are individuals who have fair complexion with up to 6 lightly pigmented, irregularly marginated CALMs who may have a pigmentary dysplasia unrelated to an underlying medical condition.[7]

There are families in which individuals have typical multiple CALMs inherited as an autosomal dominant trait with no other manifestations of NF1. Some of these

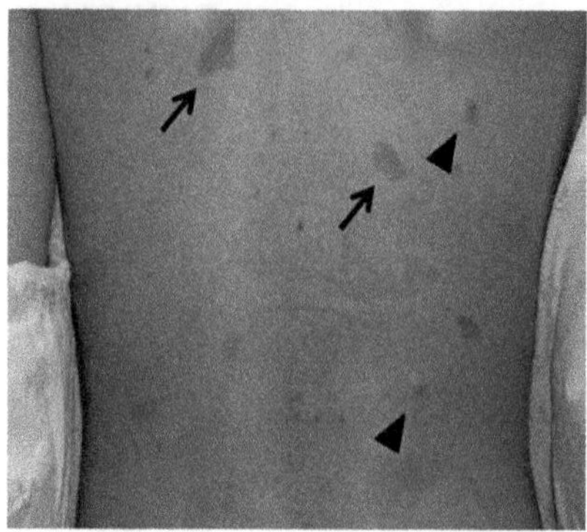

FIGURE 1
Multiple CALMs over the back and cutaneous neurofibromas below the right scapula and right side of the lower back.

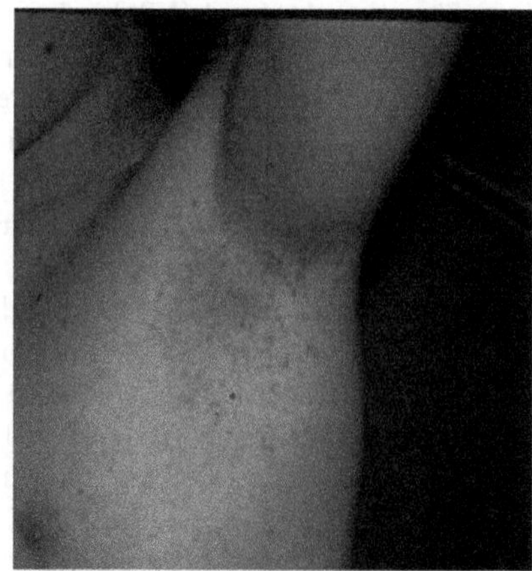

FIGURE 2
Axillary freckling.

TABLE 2 Differential Diagnosis of Patients With CALMs

Diagnosis	Clinical Features
Legius syndrome	• Typical NF1-like CALMs; mild freckling • No neurofibromas or OPGs • Similar cognitive impairment
McCune-Albright syndrome	• Jagged (coast of Maine) CALMs • Polyostotic fibrous dysplasia with fracture • Precocious puberty or other tumors • No neurofibromas
Noonan syndrome	• Typical CALMs but fewer • Lentigines rather than Crowe sign freckling • Pulmonic valve stenosis with neck webbing • Short stature, cryptorchidism, pectus excavatum, curly hair, distinctive facial gestalt
Silver-Russell syndrome	• Typical CALMs but fewer; no freckling • Intrauterine growth retardation with postnatal growth retardation, normocephaly • Fifth digit clinodactyly, hypospadias, body asymmetry
Chromosomal or DNA instability syndromes: FS, BS, MMRCS	• Atypical CALMs; no freckles • Postnatal growth retardation with microcephaly • UV sensitivity (BS), brain and blood cancers (MMRCS), congenital malformations (FS)
PTEN hamartoma tumor syndrome	• Typical CALMs but fewer; no freckles • CALMs of the glans and/or penile shaft in males • Macrocephaly (≥3 SD from mean) • Hypotonia, family history of thyroid and breast cancer
Chromosomal mosaicism and ring chromosomes	• Atypical CALMs; pigmentary dysplasia • Intellectual disability • Growth retardation with microcephaly • Body asymmetry
Sotos syndrome, Nevoid basal cell carcinoma syndrome, neurofibromatosis type 2, epidermal nevus syndrome, Carney syndrome	• Atypical CALMs; no freckling • Physical manifestations distinct from NF1

BS, Bloom syndrome; FS, Fanconi syndrome; MMRCS, mismatch repair cancer syndrome; PTEN, Phosphatase and tensin homolog.

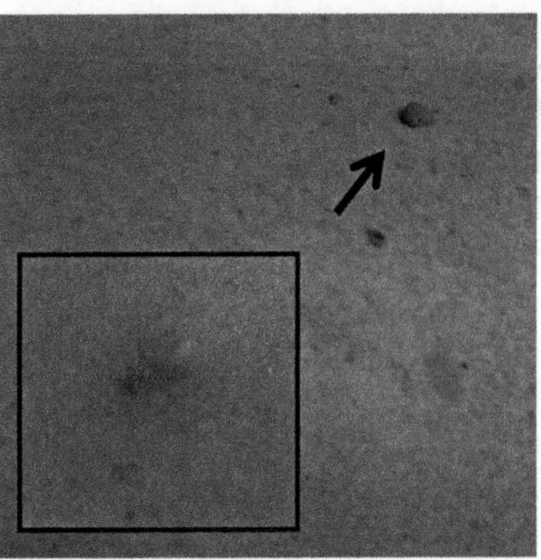

FIGURE 3
Close-up of a 9 mm sessile cutaneous neurofibroma (cNF; inset) and 12mm globular cNF from the same individual. The globular cNF protrudes further from the surrounding skin surface, but both are benign lesions.

families are genetically linked to the *NF1* locus and carry an *NF1* pathogenic variant. There are also other, less common, conditions associated with CALMs. The condition that could appear most similar to NF1 is Legius syndrome, which is caused by pathogenic variants in *SPRED1*, which encodes a protein that also functions within the Ras signaling pathway. People with Legius syndrome have multiple CALMs, intertriginous freckling (Fig 3), learning disabilities, and relative macrocephaly that is indistinguishable from findings in mild cases of NF1.[8] Other manifestations of NF1, such as neurofibromas or other tumors, ophthalmologic findings, and skeletal manifestations, are not present in families with Legius syndrome.[9] The absence of neurofibromas in adults with multiple CALMs in an extended pedigree is helpful to establish a diagnosis of Legius syndrome versus NF1, and molecular testing for *SPRED1* versus *NF1* should be considered in these cases.[9]

GENETICS

NF1 is inherited in an autosomal dominant fashion, although approximately half of individuals affected have sporadic cases caused by a new (or de novo) *NF1* gene mutation, hereafter called a pathogenic sequence variant (PSV). There is complete penetrance (ie, everyone with a pathogenic change in the *NF1* gene will show some features of NF1), although expression is extremely variable, even within members of the same family. An individual with NF1 (whether familial or de novo) has a 50% chance of having a child with NF1 with each pregnancy. In contrast, unaffected parents of a child with a new PSV have a low risk of recurrence in siblings of the child who is affected. The *NF1* gene encodes a protein called neurofibromin, which functions to regulate the Ras signaling pathway that controls cell proliferation. Cells in tumors associated with NF1, such as Schwann cells in neurofibromas, have a PSV of both *NF1* alleles: the germ-line PSV and a somatically acquired PSV of the other allele. *NF1*, therefore, functions as a tumor-suppressor gene.

Role of Genetic Testing in Diagnosis

Molecular diagnosis of NF1 is available on the basis of analysis of DNA for a pathogenic variant in the *NF1* gene. Testing can be performed on any source of DNA, usually a blood specimen. Thousands of distinct PSVs have been identified in different patients; most lead to loss of function of the gene product, as expected for a tumor-suppressor gene.[10,11]

Thus far, only 4 genotype-phenotype correlations have been established:

1. A deletion of the entire *NF1* gene and more than 10 surrounding genes, comprising 1.4 to 1.5 Mb of DNA, leads to a severe phenotype with intellectual disability, a large burden of neurofibromas, and increased risk of malignant peripheral nerve sheath tumors (MPNSTs) and cardiovascular malformations.[12]
2. A specific 3-base deletion in exon 22 (National Center for Biotechnology Information nomenclature) of the *NF1* gene (c.2970-2972 delAAT) leads to a mild phenotype characterized by CALMs and skinfold freckles with no neurofibromas.[13]
3. Amino acid substitution at codon 1809 (which encodes arginine) is associated with pigmentary features but not neurofibromas, although these patients may also have a Noonan syndrome–like phenotype, including pulmonic stenosis and short stature.[14]
4. Some missense or splicing variants are associated with "spinal NF1," in which there are often few pigmentary findings, few or no dermal neurofibromas, and normal cognitive ability but large numbers of internal tumors involving spinal nerve roots and deep peripheral nerves.[15]

NF1 genetic testing may be performed for purposes of diagnosis or to assist in genetic counseling and family planning. If a child fulfills diagnostic criteria for NF1, molecular genetic confirmation is usually unnecessary. For a young child who presents only with CALMs, *NF1* genetic testing can confirm a suspected diagnosis before a second feature, such as skinfold freckling, appears. Some families may wish to establish a definitive diagnosis as soon as possible and not wait for this second feature, and genetic testing can usually resolve the issue. With a sensitivity rate of 95%, genetic testing is considered highly reliable, although a negative test does not completely rule out the condition.

In rare instances, CALMs may be associated with either of the 2 specific *NF1* PSVs noted above, in which case neurofibromas are unlikely to occur. Also, Legius syndrome, associated with the *SPRED1* gene, can present with multiple CALMs, sometimes with skinfold freckling, but without other features of NF1.[8,9] Some laboratories will initially perform *NF1* testing on a child with multiple CALMs and then test for *SPRED1* if *NF1* testing is negative. It is also possible to test only for *SPRED1* and then to assume that *NF1* is most likely if *SPRED1* testing is negative,[16] although many parents whose child is undergoing genetic testing might prefer to have a definitive diagnosis. Genetic testing for the *NF1* gene can also be helpful in children who present with atypical features such as isolated plexiform neurofibromas, optic glioma, or tibial dysplasia. Blood testing in such instances is usually negative because the genetic changes may have occurred only in the affected tissue. In such cases, testing of tissue obtained from a lesion might be positive and indicative of somatic mosaicism. Children who present with "segmental NF1" (who usually have a limited distribution of CALMs and/or skinfold freckles or, sometimes, of neurofibromas) can also be diagnosed with somatic mosaicism after a biopsy of affected tissue and molecular testing of either melanocytes from CALMs or Schwann cells from neurofibromas.[17] This protocol usually does not guide clinical management, so it is rarely followed, although it can be helpful for adults who are concerned about the possibility of genetic transmission by way of gonadal *NF1* mutation mosaicism and wish to identify the specific PSV for future prenatal testing.

Knowledge of the *NF1* PSV can enable testing of other family members and prenatal diagnostic testing. Because the penetrance of NF1 is essentially 100% by adolescence, a careful physical examination usually suffices to establish the diagnosis in a relative at risk for having inherited the mutant allele. People with NF1 have a 50% risk for each of their offspring to be affected and can be offered prenatal testing or preimplantation genetic diagnosis. Prenatal testing requires previous knowledge of the specific PSV in the affected individual. The unaffected parents of a child who is sporadically affected have a low probability of having another child who is affected, barring the occurrence of germ-line mosaicism or a new de novo PSV in a subsequent pregnancy. The latter scenario has been reported but is expected to occur less often than germ-line mosaicism.[18] Prenatal testing could be performed if the PSV of the child who is sporadically affected is known. Typically, families are counseled that the recurrence risk is 1% or less for parents who are clinically unaffected.

Summary and Recommendations About Genetic Testing

The following can be summarized about genetic testing:

- can confirm a suspected diagnosis before a clinical diagnosis is possible;
- can differentiate NF1 from Legius syndrome;
- may be helpful in children who present with atypical features;
- usually does not predict future complications; and
- may not detect all cases of NF1; a negative genetic test rules out

a diagnosis of NF1 with 95% (but not 100%) sensitivity.

SKIN

Cutaneous pigmentary manifestations are the most common and most well-recognized features of NF1 in children. The morphology and significance of CALMs have already been noted. Axillary and inguinal freckles (Fig 3), commonly referred to as Crowe sign, are small (1–2 mm) pigmented macules that appear in skinfold regions (eg, axillae, inguinal regions, and the neck), typically beginning at about 3 to 5 years of age. In some cases, there may be similar diffuse freckling all over the body. The only importance of skinfold freckling is as 1 of the diagnostic criteria for NF1. Additional skin manifestations include juvenile xanthogranulomas (JXGs) and nevus anemicus.[19] JXGs are small, waxy, yellowish nodules that appear on the skin in a small percentage of young children with NF1. They typically resolve spontaneously. It has been suggested that JXGs might be associated with leukemia in children with NF1,[20] but studies reveal that either they are not a risk factor for leukemia or the risk is too low to warrant surveillance for leukemia.[19,21] Nevus anemicus is a flat skin macule that is paler than surrounding skin; unlike surrounding skin, it will not turn red when rubbed. Nevus anemicus may occur in up to half of individuals with NF1.[22] Pruritus is a common symptom in individuals with NF1, and topical lotions and antihistamines are minimally effective. In older children, gabapentin can be helpful.

NEUROFIBROMAS

Nonmalignant Cutaneous and Subcutaneous Neurofibromas

Various types of neurofibromas are common manifestations of NF1. Cutaneous neurofibromas typically emerge in the teenage years and increase in numbers with increasing age (Fig 4). Sometimes they may be seen in younger children, often visible with side lighting as subtle skin bumps. Neurofibromas are present in almost all adults with NF1 (although the numbers vary greatly), and they usually first appear on the trunk and then extend to the extremities, neck, and face. Some people may have relatively low numbers of small cutaneous neurofibromas, and others may be carpeted with hundreds or even thousands. They often have a mild purplish coloration and may either be raised above the skin or pucker subcutaneously. Cutaneous neurofibromas are benign tumors; however, by virtue of sheer numbers and ready visualization, these tumors can significantly affect quality of life. Removal of neurofibromas by a plastic surgeon or dermatologist can be recommended if they rub on clothing or cause discomfort. Laser surgery and electrodessication have been used by some providers, although long-term outcome data are not available.

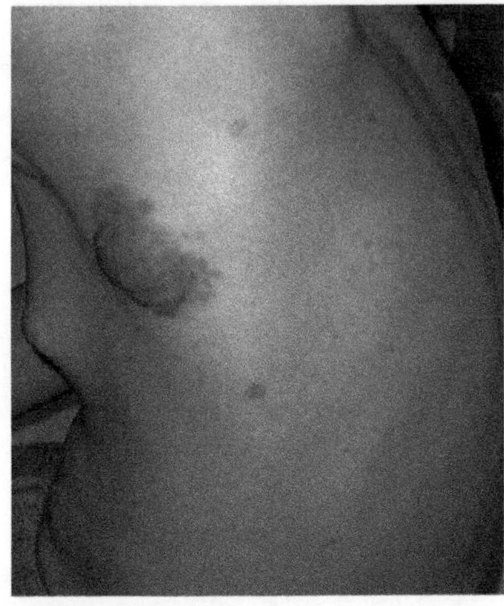

FIGURE 4
Plexiform neurofibroma adjacent to the left axilla.

Summary and Recommendations About Skin and Cutaneous Neurofibromas

The following can be summarized about skin and cutaneous neurofibromas:

- cutaneous manifestations are the usual presenting symptoms of NF1;
- pruritus is common among patients with NF1;
- the number of CALMs does not predict severity of NF1;
- cutaneous neurofibromas (other than cutaneous plexiform neurofibromas) are not at risk for malignant transformation but may have significant impact on quality of life; and
- in a child with NF1, it is not possible to predict future neurofibroma burden.

Plexiform Neurofibromas

Plexiform neurofibromas are a distinct type of neurofibroma that arise from 1 or multiple nerve trunks or branches (Fig 5). Unlike cutaneous neurofibromas, plexiform neurofibromas often come to attention early in childhood and are believed to be congenital lesions. Plexiform neurofibromas are found in approximately 50% of individuals with NF1 by whole-body MRI in adults, but less than 20% of individuals will require any intervention during childhood.[23–25] Plexiform neurofibromas may have overlying skin manifestations (such as thickened orange-peel overlying skin with a purplish brown coloration), may also have an

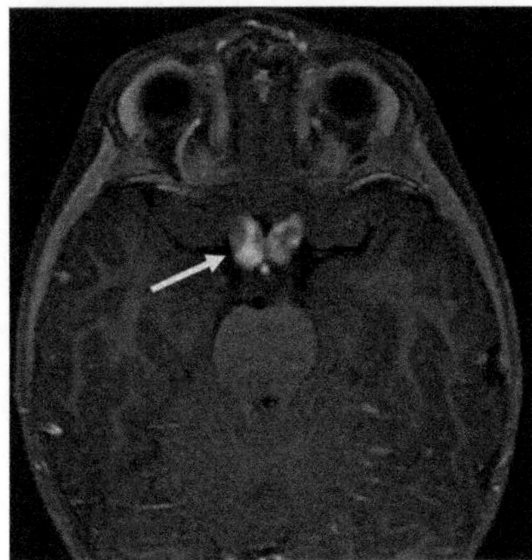

FIGURE 5
OPG affecting the right (greater than left) optic pathway (arrow).

associated hairy patch or region of hyperpigmentation, and may tend to have a heterogeneous texture or nodularity on palpation. Plexiform neurofibromas can occur in any area of the body, including the head and neck, orbit, extremities, thorax, paraspinal nerve roots, abdomen, and pelvis. These tumors may be asymptomatic or can cause pain and morbidity by compression of adjacent structures. Plexiform neurofibromas are usually difficult to remove in their entirety because of interdigitation into normal tissues and peripheral nerves. Persistent pain at the site of a plexiform neurofibroma may indicate transformation to an MPNST (see Malignancies Related to NF1). Nodular neurofibromas are a subtype of plexiform neurofibromas that have a relatively homogenous appearance on MRI and are more likely to have an atypical histology on biopsy; these tumors may be a precursor to MPNSTs.

Summary and Recommendations About Plexiform Neurofibromas

The following can be summarized about plexiform neurofibromas:

- believed to be congenital lesions;
- are present in approximately 50% of people with NF1, but less than 20% will require any intervention during childhood; and
- are benign tumors that may transform into MPNSTs (usually accompanied by symptoms such as pain, rapid growth, or neurologic dysfunction).

GLIOMAS OF THE CENTRAL NERVOUS SYSTEM

Optic Pathway Gliomas

Optic pathway gliomas (OPGs) (Fig 6) are the most common central nervous system (CNS)–associated tumor seen in children with NF1 and can be detected in approximately 15% to 20% of pediatric patients with NF1.[26,27] Symptomatic OPGs are most commonly detected in children

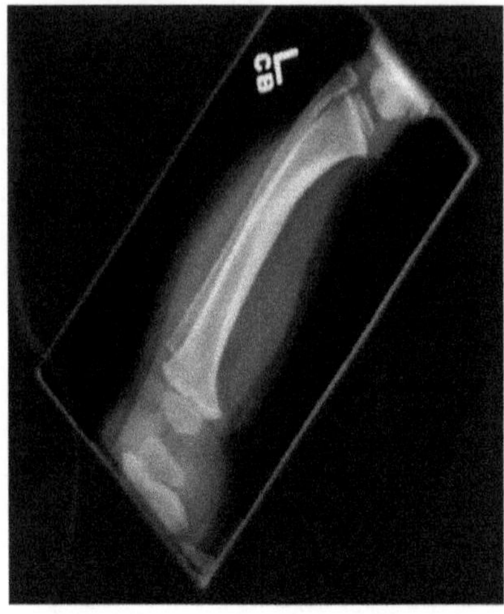

FIGURE 6
Anterior bowing of the left tibia. Note cortical thickening with medullary narrowing proximal to the segment of anterior bowing. The fibula is also bowed.

younger than 6 years during ophthalmologic surveillance (before any vision complaint). The majority of OPGs are classified as pilocytic astrocytomas (World Health Organization grade 1). The large majority of these lesions remain indolent without effect on vision; however, a small percentage can lead to vision loss and other morbidity such as precocious puberty. There is no way to reliably predict which tumors will result in a decrease in visual acuity or visual function. Lesions located in the optic chiasm and posterior optic tracts appear more likely to require treatment than those in the prechiasmatic optic nerve. Lesions located close to or involving the hypothalamus are more likely to result in precocious puberty.[27] Data also have revealed that female patients with OPGs are more likely to progress and require treatment, but both male and female patients should have the same surveillance.[28–30]

Children with known or suspected NF1 should undergo screening and surveillance ophthalmologic examinations at least annually from the time of diagnosis of NF1 or suspected NF1 by an ophthalmologist familiar with management of NF1, and this examination should be performed more frequently or repeated if there is concern. OPGs most often develop before 6 years of age, when it may be difficult to obtain a reliable ophthalmologic evaluation and when children are less likely to complain of visual symptoms. For these reasons, there has been some suggestion to screen more frequently, such as every 6 months, before 6 years of age, but this has not yet become standard practice.[31] The use of screening and surveillance neuroimaging in the setting of NF1 also is controversial; the Optic Pathway Task Force has recommended against the use of screening MRI,[26] but others have suggested that outcomes may be improved by early detection in young children.[32,33] Because of the potential for glioma to have contiguous involvement of the hypothalamus, regular monitoring for early pubertal development and monitoring for acceleration in linear growth is recommended for all patients. There is consensus that ophthalmologic examination should be performed at least annually, and decisions about more frequent surveillance or the use of diagnostic imaging in the child who is asymptomatic are best made by the ophthalmologist and clinicians caring for each patient.

OPGs in people with NF1 have a better prognosis than sporadic OPGs in people without NF1. Treatment is considered when there is decrease of visual function such as decrease in visual acuity, constriction of visual fields, change in color vision, or afferent pupillary defect. After treatment, two-thirds of people have stabilization or improvement of vision. Traditional chemotherapy (vincristine and carboplatin) is often used initially, although there are newer targeted, NF1-specific treatments in the pipeline that may be used in cases of progression or recurrence. Radiotherapy and surgery

TABLE 3 Indications for Neuroimaging Studies in Children With NF1

Indications for Consideration of Neuroimaging Studies
• Focal sensory or motor symptoms
• New onset of seizures
• Headaches that are increasing in frequency or severity
• Signs of increased intracranial pressure (headaches, visual disturbance, increased lethargy)
• Transient ischemic attack or stroke-like symptoms
• Decline in visual acuity or visual fields
• Precocious puberty or accelerated growth
• Head and neck plexiform neurofibromas increasing in size or with new development of pain
• Encephalopathy or cognitive deterioration
• Extremity asymmetry (ie, leg-length discrepancy)

are usually contraindicated except in rare situations.

Summary and Recommendations About OPGs

The following can be summarized about OPGs:

- highest morbidity is in children younger than 6 years, but young children are not likely to report symptoms;
- less than half of patients with OPGs develop vision loss or other symptoms;
- changes in linear growth rate may reveal the presence of OPGs affecting the hypothalamic-pituitary axis, but this can be treated by an endocrinologist (if needed) and is not an indication for chemotherapy;
- treatment with modified chemotherapy is often effective in halting further vision loss and/or improving vision, so early treatment is crucial;
- surveillance by a pediatric ophthalmologist familiar with NF1 (at least annually); and
- neuroimaging is an option as a baseline study and is mandatory for signs and symptoms outlined in Table 3.

Characteristic MRI Findings, Low-Grade Gliomas, and Brainstem Expansions

One of the most frequent findings in patients with NF1 is the occurrence of hyperintense lesions on T2-weighted MRI of the brain. These are located predominantly in the basal ganglia, brainstem, and cerebellum. They have been called "unidentified bright objects," "focal areas of signal intensity [FASI]," "NF [neurofibromatosis] spots," or "spongiform changes" because the true nature and significance of these lesions is still undetermined. The most proper designation at this time is "T2 hyperintensities." These lesions become evident between 2 and 10 years of age, and then regress by the second decade.

If an MRI-based T2-weighted hyperintensity reveals contrast enhancement or mass effect, a low-grade glioma should be suspected. Low-grade gliomas in people with NF1 can occur anywhere in the brain.[34] The brainstem is a common region to have both T2-weighted hyperintensities and low-grade gliomas; the latter are often accompanied by expansion of the brainstem with or without enhancement. Similar to OPGs, a biopsy is rarely performed on brainstem gliomas to avoid iatrogenic symptoms. Brainstem gliomas are typically benign and progress clinically in only one-third or fewer of cases.[35] Children with NF1 and a known brainstem-expansive lesion are monitored for development of clinical symptoms referable to the location such as headache, hydrocephalus, or cranial nerve dysfunction. Similar to OPGs, NF1-associated brainstem gliomas are more indolent than those not associated with NF1 and most often do not require clinical intervention or treatment, suggesting that conservative management is optimal.

Malignancies Related to NF1

The most frequent neoplasms associated with NF1 in children are MPNSTs, gliomas, pheochromocytomas, and leukemia. Malignant tumors are the most worrisome complications of NF1. Malignancy, mainly MPNSTs, and cardiovascular complications are the major causes of reduced life expectancy in NF1, but this is reflective mostly of adults. Life expectancy is decreased by 8 to 15 years.[36,37]

MPNSTs usually arise by malignant transformation of an existing plexiform or nodular neurofibroma. For individuals with NF1, there is a lifetime risk of 8% to 13% to develop an MPNST, which typically develops during or after young adulthood.[38] Treatment involves surgical resection, radiotherapy, and chemotherapy; however, 5-year survival remains at less than 20%. The primary care provider should be alert to the possibility of malignant transformation in a patient who has a known plexiform neurofibroma with the development of pain (especially persistent pain or pain that wakes the patient from sleep), rapid growth, or change in consistency (eg, from soft and pliable to firm and hard). Patients and families should also be educated in reporting such symptoms for potential referral to a sarcoma specialist. Patients who are symptomatic should undergo MRI of the affected area and consideration of a positron emission tomography with radiographic computed tomography (PET-CT) scan, which, in some larger studies, has been shown to help in distinguishing benign neurofibromas from MPNSTs.[39,40] These tumors are staged and treated as malignant soft-tissue sarcomas, preferably at a dedicated sarcoma center. Targeted medical therapies for MPNSTs are under exploration but have not been as effective as wide surgical resection and are only used as adjuvant therapy for surgery.

Other pediatric malignancies occur less frequently in NF1, including low- to high-grade astrocytomas, rhabdomyosarcoma, pheochromocytoma, and juvenile myelomonocytic leukemia.[41] High-grade astrocytomas tend to occur in older people, and low-grade astrocystomas and/or gliomas of the posterior fossa can be symptomatic. Pheochromocytomas can lead to increased catecholamine concentrations and consequent hypertension but are rare in children with NF1. Most experts recommend screening for pheochromocytoma if there is an acute and dramatic increase in heart rate and/or blood pressure. Pheochromocytoma is often diagnosed incidentally in patients with NF1 because of a higher frequency of imaging for other neoplasms.[42] Breast cancer occurs more frequently in young adults with NF1 than in the general population.[43,44]

Summary and Recommendations About Malignancies Related to NF1

The following can be summarized about malignancies related to NF1:

- MPNSTs most often develop within a plexiform neurofibroma;
- diagnostic imaging is an option to assess the extent of a plexiform neurofibroma at the time of diagnosis and is clinically indicated for signs and symptoms outlined this section above and/or in Table 3; a fludeoxyglucose PET-CT scan may be useful in detecting malignant transformation of a plexiform neurofibroma;
- hypertension may be indicative of pheochromocytoma, but most hypertension is detected incidentally;
- there is an increased risk of breast cancer in young adults with NF1; and
- other types of malignancy may occur in NF1.

NEUROLOGIC MANIFESTATIONS

Individuals with NF1 are more susceptible to developing headaches, particularly common migraine headaches.[45] Brain MRI may be indicated depending on the acuity of symptoms but is not necessary if the headaches are easily controlled and if neurologic examination is normal. Brain MRI would be indicated for signs or symptoms suggestive of a new intracranial mass such as symptoms of increased intracranial pressure, a new neurologic deficit with apparent or possible CNS origin, or new onset of seizures (Table 3). Once an acute process is ruled out, headaches in NF1 can be managed as they would be for similar-type headaches in the general population. A referral to a headache specialist may be indicated for headaches that are frequent and/or difficult to control with nonprescription medication. Typical lifestyle modifications for sufferers of common migraines should be offered to the person with NF1 and headaches once more-acute pathology has been ruled out.

Individuals with NF1 are more susceptible to developing seizures compared with the general population. This higher risk of seizures may be attributable, at least in part, to structural or vascular changes in the individual with NF1.[46] Seizures can occur at any age, are usually focal, and warrant concern about a focal CNS lesion; neuroimaging with brain MRI is recommended at presentation with new onset of seizure.

SUMMARY AND RECOMMENDATIONS ABOUT HEADACHES AND SEIZURES

The following can be summarized about headaches and seizures:

- headaches (often migraine) are more common among individuals with NF1;
- imaging is often not needed for a headache that can be controlled with nonprescription medication if neurologic examination is normal, and the approach to treatment is usually the same as for similar-type headaches in a patient without NF1;
- seizures are more common among patients with NF1, and an initial seizure should prompt consideration for neuroimaging; and
- other indications for neuroimaging are summarized in Table 3.

IMAGING CONSIDERATIONS

As described in preceding sections, diagnostic imaging is often used in the care of patients with NF1 for applications such as tumor surveillance (assessment of burden of tumor and progression). It has been standard practice to use clinical assessment to determine if, when, and where to image. MRI is the most common modality for imaging of plexiform neurofibromas and brain lesions such as OPGs and low-grade gliomas. In addition to MRI, PET-CT may be indicated in the assessment of possible malignant transformation of a neurofibroma. The value of imaging to assess the extent of a plexiform neurofibroma in the absence of evidence of progression is debatable because treatment decisions are typically based on clinical, and not radiographic, progression. Therefore, decisions about whether, when, and where to image are judgments best left to providers experienced in caring for children with NF1.

NEURODEVELOPMENTAL

Infants and toddlers with NF1 may have mild motor developmental delays, such as muscular hypotonia, which typically improves slowly through childhood. The NF1 population has an increased incidence of speech and language issues (particularly oromotor deficits, including speech dyspraxia, which can improve with appropriate speech therapy), velopharyngeal insufficiency, misarticulation, and disfluency.[47,48] Problems with hearing are not typical for patients with NF1, and any suspicion about hearing problems should be approached as they would be for any other pediatric patient.

Approximately 50% of individuals with NF1 have some type of learning problem.[49,50] Intellectual disability occurs in a minority of patients at a rate slightly higher than that in the general population. Intellectual disability should increase suspicion for chromosome 17 microdeletion involving the *NF1* locus, and the microdeletion has other implications such as increased tumor burden and risk of malignancy (including MPNSTs). Typical learning difficulties include problems with executive function and nonverbal learning disabilities such as reduced processing speed. Attention-deficit/hyperactivity disorder also occurs in at least 50% of individuals with NF1, and approaches to treatment are akin to those used in the general population.[49] Having a diagnosis of NF1 does not result in a predictable pattern of learning disability, so each person with NF1 should be carefully monitored and offered psychoeducational and/or neuropsychological and academic testing at the first sign of any academic or social concerns. The goal of such testing is to determine specific areas of strength and weakness and to provide appropriate interventions such as a 504 plan or an individualized education program. A diagnosis of NF1 may help underscore the need for speech, occupational, and/or physical therapy.

Some studies have suggested that NF1 increases susceptibility to autism spectrum disorder, especially in the realm of communication skills.[51–53] Many individuals with NF1, particularly teenagers, demonstrate difficulty with social pragmatics, and this can adversely affect social adjustment, even without a formal diagnosis of autism spectrum disorder. Individuals with NF1 typically have a personality profile with delayed social maturity compared with peers. For this, and perhaps other reasons, they often experience anxiety. Efforts to help in learning coping skills for social anxiety are often indicated.

SUMMARY AND RECOMMENDATIONS ABOUT DEVELOPMENTAL ISSUES

The following can be summarized about developmental issues:

- learning difficulties are common among patients with NF1 and typically are more severe among patients with an *NF1* microdeletion or complete gene deletion;
- speech articulation difficulties are common, and many patients with NF1 require speech therapy;
- executive function and attention are often affected, and neuropsychological testing is desirable to identify the particular challenges faced by each individual;
- a 504 accommodation plan and/or an individualized education program can be considered for school;
- social difficulties are common, but the rate of autism is unknown; consider referral to psychotherapy for social anxiety or coping difficulties;
- the evaluating therapists and educators must communicate back to the primary care provider regarding developmental and educational progress and additional recommendations; and
- support adherence with "2017 Recommendations for Preventive Pediatric Health Care" from the American Academy of Pediatrics.[54]

SKELETAL GROWTH

NF1-related skeletal abnormalities include macrocephaly, short stature, and osteopenia as well as localized bone dysplasias. Macrocephaly and relative macrocephaly (ie, head size disproportionately larger than height) typically require no special follow-up. Congenital hydrocephalus is not more common in NF1, but acquired hydrocephalus attributable to aqueductal stenosis can occur. Postnatal growth delay is seen in approximately one-third of children, and the pubertal growth spurt is slightly reduced. Height growth velocity is typically normal for both sexes during childhood, and growth charts made specifically for children with NF1 are available.[55]

The etiologies of relative macrocephaly and short stature are not understood. Some children have responded to growth-hormone therapy to treat short stature. Although short-term tumor induction has not been observed in those treated with growth hormone, the presence of insulin-like growth factor receptors in Schwann cells is concerning for long-term induction of tumors if treated with growth-hormone therapy. Growth-hormone therapy in NF1 is implemented cautiously and is generally reserved for people who have poor growth velocity and documented test results of low growth-hormone stimulation (ie, $<$5 ng/mL). Children with NF1 who have accelerated growth velocity or tall stature in childhood with or without precocious puberty should be evaluated for associated gliomas (OPGs) involving the chiasm and/or hypothalamic-pituitary axis. Disproportionate growth of the extremities, including leg-length discrepancy, is generally associated with plexiform neurofibromas causing local bone growth acceleration and soft-tissue hypertrophy.

Childhood osteopenia is frequent in NF1, but there is only a slightly increased risk for fractures.[56] The etiology of osteopenia is unknown, although it may be related to decreased musculoskeletal strength and poor neuromuscular coordination, leading to decreased bone remodeling. Children with NF1 have a higher prevalence of insufficient concentrations of serum (25-hydroxycholecalciferol) vitamin D, which modulates calcium and phosphorus bone metabolism (important in bone deposition). Periodic assessment of vitamin D concentrations, especially in higher latitudes, cultures without vitamin D fortification of food, and children who have less sun exposure, are helpful in determining the need for and dosing of vitamin D supplementation.

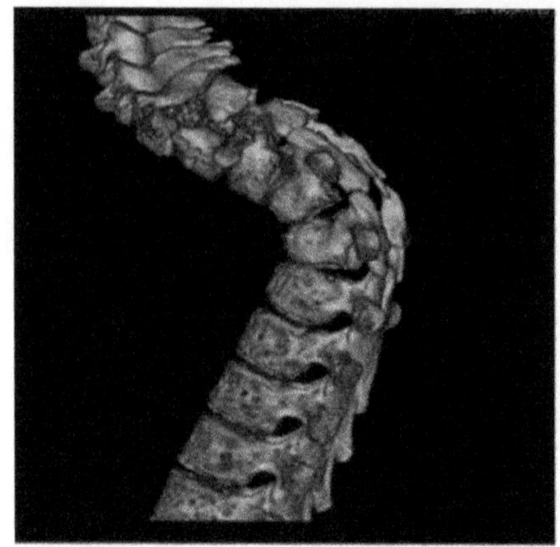

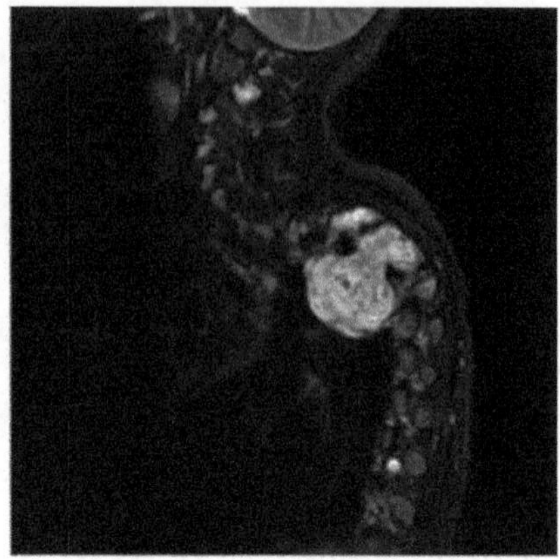

FIGURE 7
Dystrophic scoliosis in a patient with NF1. The image on the left shows a computed tomography reconstruction of the vertebral column revealing acute angle kyphoscoliosis. The image on the right, from the same patient, reveals a relatively large paraspinal plexiform neurofibroma in the area of spinal deformity.

A few distinctive skeletal manifestations are part of the NF1 diagnostic criteria (sphenoid wing dysplasia, dystrophic scoliosis, and long-bone dysplasia[57,58]). Although each of these is relatively uncommon, individually occurring in fewer than 10% of individuals with NF1, each can cause significant morbidity, underscoring the need for careful surveillance. These skeletal anomalies arise as focal manifestations, usually unilateral or involving a short segment of the spine. Sphenoid wing dysplasia is typically congenital, and at least half of cases develop ipsilateral periorbital plexiform neurofibromas. Long-bone dysplasia (especially of the tibia), defined on radiographs as a thickened cortex with a narrowed medullary cavity with or without cysts, usually emerges in late infancy or in toddlers with both anterior and lateral bowing (Fig 7). This dysplasia can progress to fracture with poor bone healing, resulting in pseudarthrosis; therefore, tibial radiography is recommended in children with anterior tibial bowing before they begin to walk. More than two-thirds of infants presenting with congenital pseudarthrosis of the tibia have NF1.

In addition to typical scoliosis that usually arises in early adolescence, children with NF1 also can have dystrophic scoliosis (Fig 8), which is a short-segment, sharply angulated curve associated with underlying vertebral-body and rib abnormalities and sometimes with adjacent plexiform neurofibromas. Specific features of dystrophic scoliosis include vertebral scalloping, penciling of ribs, spindling of transverse processes, and wedging of one or more vertebral bodies. This condition generally presents in early childhood and progresses rapidly over a few years, requiring surgical intervention with spine appliances through the growth years until definitive spinal fusion can be performed. Other distinctive focal skeletal manifestations include nonossifying fibromas of the distal femur or proximal tibia, cranial bone defects, giant-cell tumor of the jaw, and ossifying subperiosteal hematomas.

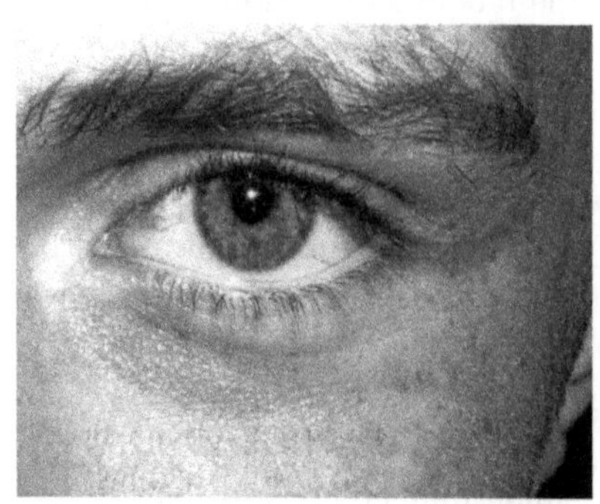

FIGURE 8
Multiple Lisch nodules with peripheral clustering between 3:30 and 8:30.

Chest-wall deformities, such as pectus excavatum or carinatum, occur in approximately one-third of individuals with NF1; this manifestation overlaps with other RASopathy conditions, primarily Noonan syndrome. Localized bone erosions and/or bone dysplasia (sphenoid wing dysplasia) can occur with adjacent growth of plexiform neurofibromas, especially scalp neurofibromas. Dental abnormalities and increased caries may also occur.[59]

Summary and Recommendations of Skeletal Features

General Skeletal Features

The following can be summarized about general skeletal features:

- macrocephaly is typically benign;
- short stature may necessitate an endocrinology referral;
- accelerated growth and/or early puberty indicates referral to endocrinology and brain MRI for a hypothalamic tumor; and
- osteopenia and vitamin D insufficiency is frequent in NF1 in children.

Specific Skeletal Features

The following can be summarized about specific skeletal features:

- sphenoid wing dysplasia is often associated with unilateral periorbital plexiform neurofibromas;
- dystrophic scoliosis and long-bone dysplasia require clinical surveillance and early orthopedic referral; and
- nonossifying fibromas, pectus anomalies, and cranial bone defects do not usually require intervention.

Other Medical Complications

Approximately one-third of patients with NF1 develop serious medical complications; however, with the variability of clinical manifestations and the progressive nature of NF1, it is not possible to determine the prognosis after establishing a diagnosis, especially at a young age. The reported incidence of complications in NF1 varies from study to study, mostly because of biased patient selection by age and specialty referral but also because of inconsistent use of diagnostic criteria and variable use of imaging. The rate of complications is often overestimated because most studies involve patients in hospitals or referral clinics.

VASCULAR

A wide range of congenital cardiac anomalies, vascular stenoses and aneurysms, and cerebrovascular lesions are associated with NF1. NF1 vasculopathy can involve different-sized vessels, ranging from small arterioles to the aorta, and, in many cases, remains asymptomatic.[60] Renal artery stenosis, with and without internal renal arteriopathy, is the most frequent site of symptomatic vasculopathy and can be an important cause of hypertension in children with NF1.[60] The prevalence of hypertension in children and teenagers with NF1 is higher than that in the general population and is often related to vascular lesions (renal artery stenosis, aortic stenosis, and coarctation).[61] The true prevalence may be lower than reported in studies that are based on patients at specialty clinics but still necessitates regular assessment of blood pressure in patients with NF1.

Essential hypertension is also a frequent occurrence in teenage patients with NF1. Workup of hypertension in the pediatric age group should include Doppler ultrasonography of the aorta and renal arteries, renal arteriography, or magnetic resonance angiography.

Congenital heart disease occurs more commonly in patients with NF1 than in the general population, with a frequency of 2% reported in a large international NF1 database. Pulmonic stenosis is by far the most common congenital heart defect seen in NF1.[60,62] Other cardiac malformations include atrial septal defect, ventricular septal defect, aortic coarctation, tetralogy of Fallot, mitral valve prolapse, and hypertrophic cardiomyopathy.[62,63] Congenital cardiac malformations and hypertrophic cardiomyopathy may be more common in patients with large *NF1* deletions.[64] Children with NF1 and a cardiac murmur or those with microdeletion of the *NF1* locus should be evaluated with a cardiology examination and echocardiography. It remains unclear whether screening of all patients with NF1 with echocardiography is indicated; however, those with a large deletion should be evaluated.[64]

Cerebrovascular abnormalities are seen in 2.5% to 6% of children with NF1 screened by MRI or magnetic resonance angiography of the brain.[65] Stenotic lesions, particularly of the internal carotid, middle cerebral, or anterior cerebral arteries, are most common, although aneurysms can also be seen. Lesions may remain stable and asymptomatic but can also develop progressive narrowing over time, leading to an increased risk for stroke and focal neurologic signs. Moyamoya syndrome, a progressive stenosis of internal carotid arteries with concomitant formation of tortuous arterial collaterals, occurs in a subset of patients, particularly those with a history of cranial radiotherapy.[66] Outcomes of NF1 cerebrovascular disease may be improved by treatment with antiplatelet agents such as aspirin and revascularization surgery for those with progressive lesions.[66] Radiotherapy to the brain should be avoided when at all possible for children with NF1 because of the risk of moyamoya syndrome.

SUMMARY AND RECOMMENDATIONS FOR VASCULAR COMPLICATIONS

The following can be summarized about vascular complications:

- Examination of the newborn should include attention to the increased risk of congenital heart malformations such as pulmonic stenosis. Referral to cardiology and/or consideration for an echocardiogram should be based on the clinical examination.
- Blood pressure should be monitored at least annually.
- Persistent hypertension requires assessment of large vessels, including renal arteries.
- Moyamoya syndrome responds well to revascularization surgery, but patients should continue receiving prophylactic-aspirin therapy under the direction of a neurosurgeon even after successful surgery.
- Neuroimaging is an option as a baseline study and is mandatory for signs and symptoms outlined in Table 3.

GASTROINTESTINAL

Constipation and midgastric abdominal pain are common in children with NF1. A recent study revealed that 30% of a small group of children with NF1 met diagnostic criteria for constipation, including an enlarged rectal diameter.[67] Management with diet modification and gentle stool softeners, such as polyethylene glycol, is often helpful. Abdominal migraine has been reported

TABLE 4 Health Supervision Guidelines for Children With NF1

	Infancy, 1 mo to 1 y	Early Childhood, 1–5 y	Late Childhood 5 y to Puberty	Adolescence and Young Adulthood (Postpubertal)
Genetic counseling				
Genetic etiology	X[a]	—	—	X[b]
Genetic testing	As needed[c]	As needed[c]	As needed[c]	As needed[c]
Future reproductive planning	X[a]	—	X[b]	X[d]
Medical evaluation and treatment[e]				
Monitor growth rate	X	Annual	Annual[f]	Annual
Measure head circumference	X	X	X	—
Blood pressure	—	Annual	Annual[fg]	Annual[f]
Attention to cardiac examination	X	—	—	—
Skin examination	X	Annual	Annual	Annual
Bone examination or scoliosis examination	X[b]	Annual	Annual[f]	Annual[f]
Neurologic examination	X	Annual	Annual[f]	Annual[f]
Ophthalmologic examination	Annual	Annual	Annual	As needed
Monitor precocious puberty	—	Annual[f]	Annual[f]	—
Diagnostic imaging examinations[e]	As needed[e]	As needed[e]	As needed[e]	As needed[e]
Developmental and psychosocial evaluation[g]	X	X	X	X
Anticipatory guidance; phenotype review[h]	X[a]	X[b]	X[b]	X[b]
Family support	X	X	X	X
Support groups	X	X	X[b]	X[b]
Long-term planning	X	X	X[b]	X[b]
Sexual and reproductive issues	—	—	X[b]	X

X indicates to be performed; —, not applicable.
a Or at the time of diagnosis.
b At least once in this time period.
c See discussion.
d Before transition to adult care.
e As needed for significant abnormalities and/or new signs.
f Advise for more frequent visits as indicated.
g Ensure compliance with "2017 Recommendations for Preventive Pediatric Health Care" from the American Academy of Pediatrics.[54] "Developmental and psychosocial evaluation" in this table should follow the standard recommendations for pediatric preventive care.
h Anticipatory guidance; phenotype review: review age-related medical and developmental issues of NF1 with the patient and family, including the following: issues related to motor and language development and potential need for early intervention (eg, speech therapy); learning and behavioral problems (eg, attention-deficit/hyperactivity disorder), school performance, and potential need for neuropsychological testing; and anticipatory guidance about concerning signs and symptoms related to plexiform neurofibromas.

as a cause of episodic abdominal pain in children with NF1 and may be more common than anatomic causes of abdominal pain.[68] Treatment with migraine medications, such as propranolol and cyproheptadine, can be helpful. Plexiform neurofibromas involving the mesentery or retroperitoneum are only rarely a source of abdominal pain, vomiting, and abdominal mass. Intestinal polyps occasionally occur, with pathology consistent with neurofibromas or schwannomas. Gastrointestinal stromal tumors (GISTs) are benign tumors of the small intestine that can cause gastrointestinal bleeding and abdominal pain in patients with NF1.[69] GISTs are rare in childhood and do not respond to tyrosine kinase inhibitors, unlike some GISTs that occur in the general population and can be treated by these medications.

SUMMARY AND RECOMMENDATIONS FOR GASTROINTESTINAL COMPLICATIONS

The following can be summarized about gastrointestinal complications:

- Constipation is common in children with NF1, but treatment does not differ from other children.
- Midgastric abdominal pain is more common in children with NF1, and abdominal migraine should be considered as a possible cause; abdominal tumors are a less common cause of abdominal pain.

MEDICAL HOME AND TRANSITION

The primary care medical home is valuable for children with NF1. In addition to the broad principles of the medical home, surveillance plans for medical, developmental, and behavioral issues are important in NF1, especially during childhood. Determination of appropriate referrals to pediatric medical subspecialists are also important to optimize care.[70,71] Health supervision guidance is outlined in several sections in this document and in Table 4. Referral to and coordination with community-based services, especially educational and behavioral services, are frequently necessary. Collaboration with pediatric medical subspecialists and programs, particularly genetics, neurology, ophthalmology, orthopedics, oncology, and dermatology, at regional referral centers on an ongoing basis can be helpful for primary care clinicians and families.

NF1 is a lifelong condition, and some of the complications are more likely to occur among adults with the disorder. These include many of the tumor-related complications, ranging from quality-of-life concerns to potentially life-threatening complications. Adults with NF1 also may continue to face social and vocational challenges because of the cognitive profile associated with the disorder. Medical and psychosocial supports should be continued for young adults. The American Academy of Pediatrics offers detailed guidance on how to plan and execute better health care transitions for all patients,[72] including a step-by-step algorithm. Patients with NF1 benefit from avoiding a gap in care during the transition from pediatric to adult providers.[73]

INTO THE FUTURE: PROSPECTS FOR MEDICAL TREATMENT OF NF1

The mechanisms that underlie various complications of NF1 are gradually coming to light, and this is leading to the development of new approaches to therapy. Examples are drugs that target the Ras signaling mechanism that is regulated by the *NF1* gene product or molecules that mediate communication between cells that are important in tumor formation. Preclinical studies and human clinical trials are underway, for the most part, by using drugs that were originally developed for treatment of other disorders that involve aberrant cell signaling such as cancer.[74] Medical therapy for various features of NF1 are likely to become increasingly available; clinical trials can be identified through ClinicalTrials.gov, and sources such as the Children's Tumor Foundation (www.ctf.org) provide up-to-date information on current treatment. This is a time of great hope for individuals with NF1 and their families, with the prospect of new treatments that will significantly improve quality of life and health in the years to come.

Pediatricians can play a critical role in improving outcomes by identifying signs that can lead to a diagnosis and by conducting appropriate surveillance. There are also potential new therapies, primarily for tumor-related aspects of NF1, that are currently in clinical trials and not yet part of standard clinical practice. A few key areas that will benefit from future efforts toward a systematic review to facilitate evidence-based practice guidelines include the following: optimal ophthalmologic, orthopedic, and neuropsychological assessments for timely interventions. Likewise, more data are needed to determine if and when to perform surveillance imaging by whole-body or regional MRI for routine tumor surveillance.[23,24,75]

SUPPORT GROUPS AND RESOURCES

The following are support groups and resources:

Children's Tumor Foundation (includes information about NF1 clinic locations): 120 Wall Street, New York, New York 10005-3904 (phone: 800-323-7938 [toll free] or 212-344-6633; fax: 212-747-0004; e-mail: info@ctf.org; Web site: www.ctf.org);

Neurofibromatosis Network: 213 South Wheaton Avenue, Wheaton, Illinois 60187 (phone: 800-942-6825; fax: 630-510-8508; e-mail: admin@nfnetwork.org; Web site: www.nfnetwork.org); and

ClinicalTrials.gov: a service of the US NIH, ClinicalTrials.gov is a registry and results database of publicly and privately supported clinical studies of human participants conducted around the world (Web site: https://clinicaltrials.gov/).

LEAD AUTHORS

David T. Miller, MD, PhD, FAAP
Debra Freedenberg, MD, PhD, FAAP
Elizabeth Schorry, MD
Nicole J. Ullrich, MD, PhD
David Viskochil, MD, PhD
Bruce R. Korf, MD, PhD, FAAP

COUNCIL ON GENETICS EXECUTIVE COMMITTEE, 2018–2019

Emily Chen, MD, PhD, FAAP, Co-Chairperson
Tracy L. Trotter, MD, FAAP, Co-Chairperson
Susan A. Berry, MD, FAAP
Leah W. Burke, MD, FAAP
Timothy A. Geleske, MD, FAAP
Rizwan Hamid, MD, FAAP
Robert J. Hopkin, MD, FAAP
Wendy J. Introne, MD, FAAP
Michael J. Lyons, MD, FAAP
Angela E. Scheuerle, MD, FAAP
Joan M. Stoler, MD, FAAP

FORMER COUNCIL ON GENETICS EXECUTIVE COMMITTEE MEMBERS

Debra Freedenberg, MD, PhD, FAAP
Marilyn C. Jones, MD, FAAP

LIAISONS

Katrina M. Dipple, MD, PhD – *American College of Medical Genetics*
Melissa A. Parisi, MD, PhD – *Eunice Kennedy Shriver National Institute of Child Health and Human Development*
Britton D. Rink, MD – *American College of Obstetricians and Gynecologists*
Joan A. Scott, MS, CGC – *Health Resources and Services Administration, Maternal and Child Health Bureau*
Stuart K. Shapira, MD, PhD – *Centers for Disease Control and Prevention*

STAFF

Paul Spire

ABBREVIATIONS

CALM: café-au-lait macule
CNS: central nervous system
GIST: gastrointestinal stromal tumor
JXG: juvenile xanthogranuloma
MPNST: malignant peripheral nerve sheath tumor
NF1: neurofibromatosis type 1
NIH: National Institutes of Health
OPG: optic pathway glioma
PET-CT: positron emission tomography with radiographic computed tomography
PSV: pathogenic sequence variant

All clinical reports from the American Academy of Pediatrics automatically expire 5 years after publication unless reaffirmed, revised, or retired at or before that time.

DOI: https://doi.org/10.1542/peds.2019-0660

Address correspondence to David T. Miller, MD, PhD, FAAP. Email: David.Miller2@childrens.harvard.edu

PEDIATRICS (ISSN Numbers: Print, 0031-4005; Online, 1098-4275).

Copyright © 2019 by the American Academy of Pediatrics

FINANCIAL DISCLOSURE: Dr Korf has consulting or advisory committee relationships with Accolade, AstraZeneca, Envision Genomics, Genome Medical, Neurofibromatosis Initiative, the Neurofibromatosis Therapeutic Acceleration Project, and Novartis and serves as an editor with the American Society of Human Genetics; Dr Miller had a part-time clinical consulting relationship with Claritas Genomics, which concluded in August 2017; Dr Viskochil has a consulting relationship with Genzyme-Sanofi and research relationships with Armagen, Shire, and Ultragenyx; and Drs Freedenberg, Schorry, and Ullrich have indicated they have no financial relationships relevant to this article to disclose.

FUNDING: No external funding.

POTENTIAL CONFLICT OF INTEREST: The authors have indicated they have no potential conflicts of interest to disclose.

REFERENCES

1. Evans DG, Howard E, Giblin C, et al. Birth incidence and prevalence of tumor-prone syndromes: estimates from a UK family genetic register service. *Am J Med Genet A*. 2010; 152A(2):327–332
2. Hersh JH; American Academy of Pediatrics Committee on Genetics. Health supervision for children with neurofibromatosis. *Pediatrics*. 2008; 121(3):633–642
3. Neurofibromatosis. Conference statement. National Institutes of Health Consensus Development Conference. *Arch Neurol*. 1988;45(5):575–578
4. National Institutes of Health Consensus Development Conference Statement: neurofibromatosis. Bethesda, Md., USA, July 13-15, 1987. *Neurofibromatosis*. 1988;1(3):172–178
5. DeBella K, Szudek J, Friedman JM. Use of the national institutes of health criteria for diagnosis of neurofibromatosis 1 in children. *Pediatrics*. 2000;105(3, pt 1):608–614
6. Gutmann DH, Aylsworth A, Carey JC, et al. The diagnostic evaluation and multidisciplinary management of neurofibromatosis 1 and neurofibromatosis 2. *JAMA*. 1997;278(1): 51–57
7. St John J, Summe H, Csikesz C, Wiss K, Hay B, Belazarian L. Multiple café au lait spots in a group of fair-skinned children without signs or symptoms of neurofibromatosis type 1. *Pediatr Dermatol*. 2016;33(5):526–529
8. Brems H, Chmara M, Sahbatou M, et al. Germline loss-of-function mutations in SPRED1 cause a neurofibromatosis 1-like phenotype. *Nat Genet*. 2007;39(9): 1120–1126
9. Messiaen L, Yao S, Brems H, et al. Clinical and mutational spectrum of neurofibromatosis type 1-like syndrome [published correction appears in *JAMA*. 2010;303(24):2477]. *JAMA*. 2009;302(19): 2111–2118
10. Messiaen LM, Callens T, Mortier G, et al. Exhaustive mutation analysis of the NF1 gene allows identification of 95% of mutations and reveals a high frequency of unusual splicing defects. *Hum Mutat*. 2000;15(6):541–555
11. Wimmer K, Yao S, Claes K, et al. Spectrum of single- and multiexon NF1 copy number changes in a cohort of 1,100 unselected NF1 patients. *Genes Chromosomes Cancer*. 2006;45(3): 265–276
12. Pasmant E, Sabbagh A, Spurlock G, et al; members of the NF France Network. NF1 microdeletions in neurofibromatosis type 1: from genotype to phenotype. *Hum Mutat*. 2010;31(6):E1506–E1518
13. Upadhyaya M, Huson SM, Davies M, et al. An absence of cutaneous neurofibromas associated with a 3-bp inframe deletion in exon 17 of the NF1 gene (c.2970-2972 delAAT): evidence of a clinically significant NF1 genotype-phenotype correlation. *Am J Hum Genet*. 2007;80(1):140–151
14. Rojnueangnit K, Xie J, Gomes A, et al. High incidence of Noonan syndrome features including short stature and pulmonic stenosis in patients carrying NF1 missense mutations affecting p. Arg1809: genotype-phenotype correlation. *Hum Mutat*. 2015;36(11): 1052–1063
15. Ruggieri M, Polizzi A, Spalice A, et al. The natural history of spinal neurofibromatosis: a critical review of clinical and genetic features. *Clin Genet*. 2015;87(5):401–410
16. Muram TM, Stevenson DA, Watts-Justice S, et al. A cost savings approach to SPRED1 mutational analysis in individuals at risk for neurofibromatosis type 1. *Am J Med Genet A*. 2013;161A(3):467–472
17. Maertens O, Brems H, Vandesompele J, et al. Comprehensive NF1 screening on cultured Schwann cells from neurofibromas. *Hum Mutat*. 2006; 27(10):1030–1040
18. Upadhyaya M, Majounie E, Thompson P, et al. Three different pathological lesions in the NF1 gene originating de novo in a family with neurofibromatosis type 1. *Hum Genet*. 2003;112(1):12–17
19. Ferrari F, Masurel A, Olivier-Faivre L, Vabres P. Juvenile xanthogranuloma and nevus anemicus in the diagnosis of neurofibromatosis type 1. *JAMA Dermatol*. 2014;150(1):42–46
20. Zvulunov A, Barak Y, Metzker A. Juvenile xanthogranuloma, neurofibromatosis, and juvenile chronic myelogenous

leukemia. World statistical analysis. *Arch Dermatol.* 1995;131(8):904–908

21. Cambiaghi S, Restano L, Caputo R. Juvenile xanthogranuloma associated with neurofibromatosis 1: 14 patients without evidence of hematologic malignancies. *Pediatr Dermatol.* 2004; 21(2):97–101
22. Marque M, Roubertie A, Jaussent A, et al. Nevus anemicus in neurofibromatosis type 1: a potential new diagnostic criterion. *J Am Acad Dermatol.* 2013;69(5):768–775
23. Mautner VF, Asuagbor FA, Dombi E, et al. Assessment of benign tumor burden by whole-body MRI in patients with neurofibromatosis 1. *Neuro Oncol.* 2008; 10(4):593–598
24. Plotkin SR, Bredella MA, Cai W, et al. Quantitative assessment of whole-body tumor burden in adult patients with neurofibromatosis. *PLoS One.* 2012;7(4): e35711
25. Prada CE, Rangwala FA, Martin LJ, et al. Pediatric plexiform neurofibromas: impact on morbidity and mortality in neurofibromatosis type 1. *J Pediatr.* 2012;160(3):461–467
26. Listernick R, Louis DN, Packer RJ, Gutmann DH. Optic pathway gliomas in children with neurofibromatosis 1: consensus statement from the NF1 Optic Pathway Glioma Task Force. *Ann Neurol.* 1997;41(2):143–149
27. Listernick R, Charrow J, Gutmann DH. Intracranial gliomas in neurofibromatosis type 1. *Am J Med Genet.* 1999;89(1):38–44
28. Fisher MJ, Loguidice M, Gutmann DH, et al. Visual outcomes in children with neurofibromatosis type 1-associated optic pathway glioma following chemotherapy: a multicenter retrospective analysis. *Neuro Oncol.* 2012;14(6):790–797
29. Fisher MJ, Loguidice M, Gutmann DH, et al. Gender as a disease modifier in neurofibromatosis type 1 optic pathway glioma. *Ann Neurol.* 2014;75(5):799–800
30. Diggs-Andrews KA, Brown JA, Gianino SM, Rubin JB, Wozniak DF, Gutmann DH. Sex is a major determinant of neuronal dysfunction in neurofibromatosis type 1. *Ann Neurol.* 2014;75(2):309–316
31. Caen S, Cassiman C, Legius E, Casteels I. Comparative study of the ophthalmological examinations in neurofibromatosis type 1. Proposal for a new screening algorithm. *Eur J Paediatr Neurol.* 2015;19(4):415–422
32. Blazo MA, Lewis RA, Chintagumpala MM, Frazier M, McCluggage C, Plon SE. Outcomes of systematic screening for optic pathway tumors in children with neurofibromatosis type 1. *Am J Med Genet A.* 2004;127A(3):224–229
33. Prada CE, Hufnagel RB, Hummel TR, et al. The use of magnetic resonance imaging screening for optic pathway gliomas in children with neurofibromatosis type 1. *J Pediatr.* 2015;167(4):851–856.e1
34. Gutmann DH, Rasmussen SA, Wolkenstein P, et al. Gliomas presenting after age 10 in individuals with neurofibromatosis type 1 (NF1). *Neurology.* 2002;59(5):759–761
35. Ullrich NJ, Raja AI, Irons MB, Kieran MW, Goumnerova L. Brainstem lesions in neurofibromatosis type 1. *Neurosurgery.* 2007;61(4):762–766; discussion 766–767
36. Evans DG, O'Hara C, Wilding A, et al. Mortality in neurofibromatosis 1: in North West England: an assessment of actuarial survival in a region of the UK since 1989 [published correction appears in *Eur J Hum Genet.* 2013;21(9): 1031]. *Eur J Hum Genet.* 2011;19(11): 1187–1191
37. Uusitalo E, Leppävirta J, Koffert A, et al. Incidence and mortality of neurofibromatosis: a total population study in Finland. *J Invest Dermatol.* 2015;135(3):904–906
38. Evans DG, Huson SM, Birch JM. Malignant peripheral nerve sheath tumours in inherited disease. *Clin Sarcoma Res.* 2012;2(1):17
39. Tsai LL, Drubach L, Fahey F, Irons M, Voss S, Ullrich NJ. [^{18}F]-fluorodeoxyglucose positron emission tomography in children with neurofibromatosis type 1 and plexiform neurofibromas: correlation with malignant transformation. *J Neurooncol.* 2012;108(3):469–475
40. Meany H, Dombi E, Reynolds J, et al. 18-fluorodeoxyglucose-positron emission tomography (FDG-PET) evaluation of nodular lesions in patients with neurofibromatosis type 1 and plexiform neurofibromas (PN) or malignant peripheral nerve sheath tumors (MPNST). *Pediatr Blood Cancer.* 2013; 60(1):59–64
41. Seminog OO, Goldacre MJ. Risk of benign tumours of nervous system, and of malignant neoplasms, in people with neurofibromatosis: population-based record-linkage study. *Br J Cancer.* 2013; 108(1):193–198
42. Shinall MC, Solórzano CC. Pheochromocytoma in neurofibromatosis type 1: when should it be suspected? *Endocr Pract.* 2014; 20(8):792–796
43. Seminog OO, Goldacre MJ. Age-specific risk of breast cancer in women with neurofibromatosis type 1. *Br J Cancer.* 2015;112(9):1546–1548
44. Uusitalo E, Rantanen M, Kallionpää RA, et al. Distinctive cancer associations in patients with neurofibromatosis type 1. *J Clin Oncol.* 2016;34(17):1978–1986
45. Pinho RS, Fusão EF, Paschoal JKSF, et al. Migraine is frequent in children and adolescents with neurofibromatosis type 1. *Pediatr Int.* 2014;56(6):865–867
46. Ostendorf AP, Gutmann DH, Weisenberg JL. Epilepsy in individuals with neurofibromatosis type 1. *Epilepsia.* 2013;54(10):1810–1814
47. Thompson HL, Viskochil DH, Stevenson DA, Chapman KL. Speech-language characteristics of children with neurofibromatosis type 1. *Am J Med Genet A.* 2010;152A(2):284–290
48. Alivuotila L, Hakokari J, Visnapuu V, et al. Speech characteristics in neurofibromatosis type 1. *Am J Med Genet A.* 2010;152A(1):42–51
49. Lehtonen A, Howie E, Trump D, Huson SM. Behaviour in children with neurofibromatosis type 1: cognition, executive function, attention, emotion, and social competence. *Dev Med Child Neurol.* 2013;55(2):111–125
50. Coutinho V, Kemlin I, Dorison N, Billette de Villemeur T, Rodriguez D, Dellatolas G. Neuropsychological evaluation and parental assessment of behavioral and motor difficulties in children with neurofibromatosis type 1. *Res Dev Disabil.* 2016;48:220–230

51. Garg S, Green J, Leadbitter K, et al. Neurofibromatosis type 1 and autism spectrum disorder. *Pediatrics*. 2013; 132(6). Available at: www.pediatrics.org/cgi/content/full/132/6/e1642
52. Garg S, Lehtonen A, Huson SM, et al. Autism and other psychiatric comorbidity in neurofibromatosis type 1: evidence from a population-based study. *Dev Med Child Neurol*. 2013;55(2): 139–145
53. Walsh KS, Vélez JI, Kardel PG, et al. Symptomatology of autism spectrum disorder in a population with neurofibromatosis type 1. *Dev Med Child Neurol*. 2013;55(2):131–138
54. Committee on Practice and Ambulatory Medicine; Bright Futures Periodicity Schedule Workgroup. 2017 recommendations for preventive pediatric health care. *Pediatrics*. 2017; 139(4):e20170254
55. Clementi M, Milani S, Mammi I, Boni S, Monciotti C, Tenconi R. Neurofibromatosis type 1 growth charts. *Am J Med Genet*. 1999;87(4): 317–323
56. George-Abraham JK, Martin LJ, Kalkwarf HJ, et al. Fractures in children with neurofibromatosis type 1 from two NF clinics. *Am J Med Genet A*. 2013; 161A(5):921–926
57. Elefteriou F, Kolanczyk M, Schindeler A, et al. Skeletal abnormalities in neurofibromatosis type 1: approaches to therapeutic options. *Am J Med Genet A*. 2009;149A(10):2327–2338
58. Crawford AH, Schorry EK. Neurofibromatosis in children: the role of the orthopaedist. *J Am Acad Orthop Surg*. 1999;7(4):217–230
59. Javed F, Ramalingam S, Ahmed HB, et al. Oral manifestations in patients with neurofibromatosis type-1: a comprehensive literature review. *Crit Rev Oncol Hematol*. 2014;91(2):123–129
60. Friedman JM, Arbiser J, Epstein JA, et al. Cardiovascular disease in neurofibromatosis 1: report of the NF1 Cardiovascular Task Force. *Genet Med*. 2002;4(3):105–111
61. Dubov T, Toledano-Alhadef H, Chernin G, Constantini S, Cleper R, Ben-Shachar S. High prevalence of elevated blood pressure among children with neurofibromatosis type 1. *Pediatr Nephrol*. 2016;31(1):131–136
62. Lin AE, Birch PH, Korf BR, et al. Cardiovascular malformations and other cardiovascular abnormalities in neurofibromatosis 1. *Am J Med Genet*. 2000;95(2):108–117
63. Tedesco MA, Di Salvo G, Natale F, et al. The heart in neurofibromatosis type 1: an echocardiographic study. *Am Heart J*. 2002;143(5):883–888
64. Nguyen R, Mir TS, Kluwe L, et al. Cardiac characterization of 16 patients with large NF1 gene deletions. *Clin Genet*. 2013;84(4):344–349
65. Rea D, Brandsema JF, Armstrong D, et al. Cerebral arteriopathy in children with neurofibromatosis type 1. *Pediatrics*. 2009;124(3). Available at: www.pediatrics.org/cgi/content/full/124/3/e476
66. Koss M, Scott RM, Irons MB, Smith ER, Ullrich NJ. Moyamoya syndrome associated with neurofibromatosis type 1: perioperative and long-term outcome after surgical revascularization. *J Neurosurg Pediatr*. 2013;11(4): 417–425
67. Pedersen CE, Krogh K, Siggaard C, Joensson IM, Haagerup A. Constipation in children with neurofibromatosis type 1. *J Pediatr Gastroenterol Nutr*. 2013; 56(2):229–232
68. Heuschkel R, Kim S, Korf B, Schneider G, Bousvaros A. Abdominal migraine in children with neurofibromatosis type 1: a case series and review of gastrointestinal involvement in NF1. *J Pediatr Gastroenterol Nutr*. 2001; 33(2):149–154
69. Yamamoto H, Tobo T, Nakamori M, et al. Neurofibromatosis type 1-related gastrointestinal stromal tumors: a special reference to loss of heterozygosity at 14q and 22q. *J Cancer Res Clin Oncol*. 2009;135(6):791–798
70. Medical Home Initiatives for Children With Special Needs Project Advisory Committee; American Academy of Pediatrics. The medical home. *Pediatrics*. 2002;110(1, pt 1):184–186
71. Stille C, Turchi RM, Antonelli R, et al; Academic Pediatric Association Task Force on Family-Centered Medical Home. The family-centered medical home: specific considerations for child health research and policy. *Acad Pediatr*. 2010;10(4):211–217
72. Cooley WC, Sagerman PJ; American Academy of Pediatrics; American Academy of Family Physicians; American College of Physicians; Transitions Clinical Report Authoring Group. Supporting the health care transition from adolescence to adulthood in the medical home. *Pediatrics*. 2011;128(1):182–200
73. Van Lierde A, Menni F, Bedeschi MF, et al. Healthcare transition in patients with rare genetic disorders with and without developmental disability: neurofibromatosis 1 and Williams-Beuren syndrome. *Am J Med Genet A*. 2013;161A(7):1666–1674
74. Dombi E, Baldwin A, Marcus LJ, et al. Activity of selumetinib in neurofibromatosis type 1-related plexiform neurofibromas. *N Engl J Med*. 2016;375(26):2550–2560
75. Evans DGR, Salvador H, Chang VY, et al. Cancer and central nervous system tumor surveillance in pediatric neurofibromatosis 1. *Clin Cancer Res*. 2017;23(12):e46–e53

Identifying Child Abuse Fatalities During Infancy

- *Clinical Report*

CLINICAL REPORT Guidance for the Clinician in Rendering Pediatric Care

American Academy of Pediatrics

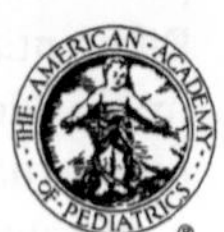

DEDICATED TO THE HEALTH OF ALL CHILDREN™

Identifying Child Abuse Fatalities During Infancy

Vincent J. Palusci, MD, MS, FAAP,[a] Council on Child Abuse and Neglect, Amanda J. Kay, MD, MPH, FAAP,[b] Erich Batra, MD, FAAP,[c] Section on Child Death Review and Prevention, Rachel Y. Moon, MD, FAAP,[d] Task Force on Sudden Infant Death Syndrome, NATIONAL ASSOCIATION OF MEDICAL EXAMINERS, Tracey S. Corey, MD,[e] Thomas Andrew, MD,[f] Michael Graham, MD[g]

abstract

When a healthy infant dies suddenly and unexpectedly, it is critical to correctly determine if the death was caused by child abuse or neglect. Sudden unexpected infant deaths should be comprehensively investigated, ancillary tests and forensic procedures should be used to more-accurately identify the cause of death, and parents deserve to be approached in a nonaccusatory manner during the investigation. Missing a child abuse death can place other children at risk, and inappropriately approaching a sleep-related death as maltreatment can result in inappropriate criminal and protective services investigations. Communities can learn from these deaths by using multidisciplinary child death reviews. Pediatricians can support families during investigation, advocate for and support state policies that require autopsies and scene investigation, and advocate for establishing comprehensive and fully funded child death investigation and reviews at the local and state levels. Additional funding is also needed for research to advance our ability to prevent these deaths.

[a]School of Medicine, New York University, New York, New York; [b]Department of Pediatrics, Christiana Care Health Systems, Wilmington, Delaware; [c]Departments of Pediatrics and Family and Community Medicine, College of Medicine, Pennsylvania State University, Hershey, Pennsylvania; [d]Department of Pediatrics, School of Medicine, University of Virginia, Charlottesville, Virginia; [e]Associate Medical Examiner, Florida Districts 5 & 24 Medical Examiner's Office, Leesburg, Florida; [f]Consultant, White Mountain Forensic Consulting Services, Concord, New Hampshire; and [g]Department of Pathology, School of Medicine, St Louis University, St Louis, Missouri

Drs Palusci, Kay, Moon, Corey, Andrew, and Graham conceptualized this clinical report and each wrote sections of the draft; and all authors reviewed and revised subsequent drafts and approved the final manuscript as submitted.

This document is copyrighted and is property of the American Academy of Pediatrics and its Board of Directors. All authors have filed conflict of interest statements with the American Academy of Pediatrics. Any conflicts have been resolved through a process approved by the Board of Directors. The American Academy of Pediatrics has neither solicited nor accepted any commercial involvement in the development of the content of this publication.

Clinical reports from the American Academy of Pediatrics benefit from expertise and resources of liaisons and internal (AAP) and external reviewers. However, clinical reports from the American Academy of Pediatrics may not reflect the views of the liaisons or the organizations or government agencies that they represent.

The guidance in this report does not indicate an exclusive course of treatment or serve as a standard of medical care. Variations, taking into account individual circumstances, may be appropriate.

To cite: Palusci VJ, AAP Council on Child Abuse and Neglect, Kay AJ, AAP Council on Child Abuse and Neglect, AAP Section on Child Death Review and Prevention, AAP Task Force on Sudden Infant Death Syndrome, NATIONAL ASSOCIATION OF MEDICAL EXAMINERS. Identifying Child Abuse Fatalities During Infancy. *Pediatrics.* 2019;144(3): e20192076

INTRODUCTION

More than 60 years ago, the medical community began a search to understand and prevent the sudden unexpected deaths of apparently healthy infants. Sudden refers to the fact that death comes without warning, and unexpected means that there is no preexisting condition known that could have reasonably predicted it. In an effort to further study and categorize these deaths, the term sudden infant death syndrome (SIDS) was coined.[1,2] Almost simultaneously, medical professionals recognized the realities of child abuse.[3–6] Since then, public and professional awareness of sudden unexpected infant death and fatal child abuse have increased, and well-validated reports of homicide and child abuse have appeared in the medical literature and in the lay press.[7–9] The US Commission on the Elimination of Child Abuse and Neglect Fatalities has noted significant undercounting of child abuse fatalities and has called for improved identification and prevention of these deaths.[10] Differentiating deaths from abuse from sudden infant deaths that are unintentional, however, can be a difficult diagnostic decision.[11–13] Clinicians and pathologists need an appropriately high index of suspicion of abuse, and additional funding for improved identification and research into the causes and prevention of these fatalities is needed. This report updates a previous statement[14] on the basis of new publications from the American Academy of Pediatrics (AAP) and other updated research to assist in the identification and prevention of child maltreatment fatality.

SUDDEN UNEXPLAINED INFANT DEATH

The term SIDS was introduced in the 1960s as the medical community attempted to better identify and define the sudden, unexpected, and unexplained deaths of infants and young children.[15,16] Throughout the ensuing decades, there was an increase in the depth and breadth of autopsy procedures and ancillary testing and sophistication and detail of death investigation, including scene investigation and caregiver interviews. Knowledge has increased about less-obvious causes of death, such as inborn errors of metabolism, primary cardiac dysrhythmias, and occult seizures.[17,18] Coinciding with improved investigative techniques, there has been a diagnostic shift away from using SIDS as a cause of death, and in its place, many medical examiners and coroners classify infant deaths occurring in an unsafe sleep environment as having an "undetermined cause" or "accidental asphyxiation in an unsafe sleep environment" because they cannot attribute these deaths with certainty specifically to the sleep environment. Because of this diagnostic shift, sleep-related infant deaths are now often grouped as "sudden unexpected infant deaths."[19–21]

In the United States over a number of years through 2015, sudden unexpected infant death is the primary category of death in vital statistics for children between 1 and 12 months of age, with a peak incidence between 1 and 4 months of age, and with 90% of these before the age of 6 months.[21–23] Rates in 2013 were 2 to 3 times higher among non-Hispanic African American and American Indian or Alaskan Native children when compared with non-Hispanic white children (172.4 and 177.6 vs 84.5 deaths per 100 000 live births, respectively).[22] Increased risk for SIDS has been found in epidemiological studies with prone and side sleep positions, prenatal and postnatal tobacco and opioid exposure, sleeping on a soft surface, sharing a sleep surface with others, overheating, late or no prenatal care, young maternal age, preterm birth, low birth weight, and male sex.[24–30] Breastfeeding, pacifier use, immunizations, and room sharing without bed-sharing have been identified as protective factors. There is no evidence that recurrent episodes of cyanosis, apnea, or apparent life-threatening events (sometimes called "near-miss SIDS" and now called brief resolved unexplained events [BRUEs][11]) increase the risk.

Despite extensive research, our understanding of the causes of sudden unexpected infant death remains incomplete.[15] There have been varying guidelines published to facilitate research and administrative purposes with a growing consensus that these deaths can be described as unexplained only when:

1. A complete autopsy has been performed, including examination of the cranium and the cranial contents, and the gross and microscopic findings fail to demonstrate an anatomic cause of death;
2. There is no evidence of acute or remote inflicted trauma, significant natural disease, or significant and contributory unintentional trauma as judged by radiologic imaging, postmortem examination, and reliable clinical history;
3. Other causes and/or mechanisms of death, including meningitis, sepsis, aspiration, pneumonia, myocarditis, trauma, dehydration, fluid and electrolyte imbalance, significant congenital defects, inborn metabolic disorders, asphyxia, drowning, burns, and poisoning, have been sufficiently excluded as a cause of death;
4. Comprehensive testing has revealed no evidence of toxic exposure to alcohol, drugs, or other substances that may have contributed to death; and
5. Thorough review of the clinical history and death- and incident-scene investigation have revealed no cause of death.

CHILD MALTREATMENT FATALITY

Child abuse causes and contributes to infant death in a number of ways. In data from the US National Child Abuse and Neglect Data System, it was noted in 2016 that of the estimated 1750 child maltreatment deaths, almost half involved infants younger than 1 year, a rate of 20.63 per 100 000 children in the population younger than 1 year.[31] Most maltreatment fatalities are attributed to neglect, with or without additional physical abuse. Factors identified in families with increased risk for child maltreatment fatality include poverty, previous or current involvement with child protective services, unrelated male caregivers, and previous unexplained death or nonaccidental trauma of other infants.[32–37] In recent literature, it is suggested that natural or accidental deaths are more commonly reported than child abuse fatalities, with approximately 3700 sudden unexpected infant deaths in 2015 in the United States.[16] However, deaths reported as child maltreatment fatalities are believed to be underestimates, with more than triple the number officially reported being estimated to occur.[10,31]

Closed head injury is considered the leading cause of fatal abuse, with a peak incidence at 1 to 2 months of age, a time period that overlaps with sudden unexpected infant deaths.[38] Several findings, such as subdural hematoma, retinal hemorrhages, optic nerve sheath hemorrhages, rib fractures, and classic metaphyseal lesions, have most frequently been identified.[39] Characteristics may include the absence of a history of trauma as well as the absence of external evidence of impact to the head, skull fractures, subdural hemorrhage, or hypoxic-ischemic changes. Some additional causes of child abuse fatalities have been found to be intentional asphyxia; abdominal, thoracic, and other trauma; and poisoning.[30]

It may be difficult to differentiate among a natural infant death, an unintentional or accidental infant death, and an intentional or neglectful infant death when findings of maltreatment are absent. Parents have been observed trying to suffocate and harm their infants,[7,40–42] and estimates of the incidence of infanticide among cases designated as sudden infant death have ranged from 1% to 10%.[43] Certain circumstances in the medical history can indicate increased risk for intentional suffocation,[44] including:

- recurrent cyanosis, apnea, or BRUEs occurring only while in the care of the same person;
- age at death older than 6 months;
- previous unexpected or unexplained deaths of 1 or more siblings;
- simultaneous or nearly simultaneous death of twins; and
- previous death of an infant under the care of the same unrelated person.

INITIAL MANAGEMENT OF SUDDEN UNEXPECTED INFANT DEATH

It is critical to identify whether child abuse or neglect has contributed to an infant's death. Missing a child abuse death can place other children at risk, and inappropriately labeling a sleep-related death as a homicide can result in an inappropriate criminal investigation and possible prosecution. Comprehensive medical evaluation, scene investigation, and autopsy are critical to improving identification and reporting of the cause of an infant's death.[45]

Most sudden unexpected infant deaths occur at home. Parents are shocked, bewildered, and distressed. Parents who are innocent of blame in their infant's death often feel responsible, nonetheless, and imagine ways in which they might have contributed to or prevented the tragedy, and they often feel remorse, guilt, and fear of consequences.[45] Grief and long-term effects of such stress are significant, especially for remaining children in the home.[46–50] The appropriate ethical medical professional response to every child death must be compassionate, empathic, supportive, and nonaccusatory.[51] Inadvertent comments and accusatory questioning by medical personnel and investigators are likely to cause additional stress. It is important for those in contact with parents during this time to remain nonaccusatory and to allow them to begin the process of grieving while a thorough death investigation is conducted. Concerns about unsafe sleep and bed-sharing as possible contributors to a child's death should be shared with parents as appropriate at some time during the investigation. The National Institute of Justice and National Institute of Standards and Technology have identified key principles and resources to assist medical examiners and families during investigation.[51]

The likelihood of a repetition of sudden unexpected infant death within a sibship in the medical literature is unclear.[52–54] Although repetitive sudden unexpected infant deaths occurring within the same family should compel investigators to consider the possibility of serial homicide,[8] it is important to remember that infant deaths within a sibship can also be explained by a heritable disorder that is undefined and/or unrecognized at the time of investigation, 2 separate and unrelated natural disease processes, or an unrecognized environmental hazard. When an infant's sudden unexpected death has been thoroughly evaluated and alternate genetic, environmental, accidental, or inflicted causes have been carefully excluded, parents can be informed that the risk in subsequent children is not likely increased. Parents can be given a clearly stated, honest, and forthright conclusion, even if that conclusion lacks the solidity of a specific diagnosis, such as pneumonia or congenital heart disease.[55] Good communication with parents should include an adequate explanation that "undetermined" simply means "unable to be determined" or "we do not know." The term undetermined does not necessarily imply that a death is suspicious and should not diminish parental access to appropriate grief counseling. It can be explained to parents that the investigation might enable them and their physician to understand why their infant died and how other children in the family, including children born later, might be affected.

Depending on local protocols and statutes, and if permitted by the medical examiner, the family may be given a supervised opportunity to see and hold the infant and collect materials once death has been pronounced.[56] It is suggested that an unrelated professional remain with the family throughout this period to serve as a witness should issues regarding postmortem artifacts arise. Professionals need to have the many immediate issues that require attention addressed, including baptism, grief counseling, funeral arrangements, religious support, resolution of breastfeeding, and the reactions of surviving siblings. All parents can be provided with information about sudden unexpected infant death and how to contact the medical examiner's or coroner's office and local support groups.[57–59]

INVESTIGATION

It continues to be difficult to distinguish fatal child abuse by autopsy alone.[60,61] In the absence of a complete investigation of the circumstances of death and case review, child maltreatment is missed, familial and genetic diseases go unrecognized, public health threats are overlooked, inadequate medical care goes undetected, product safety issues remain unidentified, and progress in understanding the causes and mechanisms of unexpected infant death is delayed.[10,18,51,52,61,62] A thorough investigation can remove the shroud of suspicion while maintaining good communication with families.

A comprehensive scene investigation is one essential leg of a complete and thorough infant death investigation.[61] Personnel on first-response teams should have specific training to make observations at the scene, including position of the infant; marks on the body; pattern and distribution of livor mortis; rigor mortis; location of the infant when found, including type of bed, crib, or other sleep environment and any defects in it; amount and position of clothing and bedding; room temperature; type of ventilation and heating; and reaction of the caregivers. Medics and emergency department personnel should be trained to distinguish normal findings from trauma attributable to abuse. Death investigators should be trained and skilled in the recognition of potentially important environmental features, such as cigarette or other smoke, the presence of drugs or alcohol, sources of carbon monoxide in the sleep room of the deceased infant, or a wet bathtub or infant bathing area. Appropriate consultations by medical examiners and coroners with available medical specialists (eg, general pediatrician, child abuse pediatrician, pediatric pathologist, pediatric radiologist, and/or pediatric neuropathologist) can also be invaluable. Doll reenactment has become an increasingly valuable investigative tool, as well.[61]

If standard and case-appropriate toxicology tests are not performed, infant deaths attributable to accidental or deliberate poisoning will be missed.[63] In 1 review of autopsies in the early 1990s, it was found that 17 (40%) of 43 infants who died before 2 days of age without an obvious cause of death at autopsy had toxicological evidence of cocaine exposure.[64] In a separate review of 600 infant deaths, evidence of cocaine exposure in 16 infants (2.7%) younger than 8 months who died suddenly and unexpectedly was revealed.[65] Lethal concentrations of opioids, cocaine, and many other drugs are not well established in infancy, and blood and liver concentrations must always be interpreted in the context of the complete investigation.

POSTMORTEM IMAGING

Radiographic skeletal surveys and computed tomography (CT) imaging performed before autopsy may reveal evidence of traumatic skeletal injury or skeletal abnormalities indicative of a naturally occurring illness. The presence of both old and new traumatic injuries as well as fractures specific for abuse may suggest inflicted injuries and may lend focus to the postmortem examination, investigation of the circumstances of death, and police investigation. Ideally, such imaging should only be performed at the direction of the medical examiner or coroner, and it is helpful for medical examiners and coroners to create protocols for this to occur. The skeletal survey and/or CT scans should be performed according to American College of Radiology guidelines as recommended for living infants in whom abuse is suspected and reviewed by a radiologist experienced in identifying the sometimes subtle radiologic changes seen with abuse as well as findings that may be confused with inflicted injuries.[66] It is also important to review medical history for any previous medical encounters that included imaging that could show evidence of previous injuries or normal variants. Thorough documentation of all sites of suspected skeletal injury may require additional procedures, including, but not limited to, specimen resection, high-detail specimen radiography, CT, and histologic analysis to assess aging.

PATHOLOGY

For infants who die suddenly and unexpectedly, the AAP and the National Association of Medical Examiners have endorsed universal performance of autopsies by forensic pathologists experienced in the evaluation of infant death and qualified in forensic pathology by the American Board of Pathology. The forensic pathologist performing the autopsy should have access to specialists and reference laboratories for consultation and ancillary testing. Medical specialist consultants may include but are not limited to neuropathologists, ophthalmologic pathologists, pediatric neurologists, cardiac specialists, geneticists, pediatric pathologists, pediatric radiologists, and child abuse pediatricians. Reference laboratories may include but are not limited to postmortem toxicology laboratories, clinical pathology laboratories, and laboratories screening for inborn errors of metabolism. Historically, postmortem findings in cases of fatal child abuse have included evidence of intracranial injuries, retinal hemorrhages, abdominal trauma (eg, liver laceration, hollow viscous perforation, or intramural hematoma), fractures, bruises, burns, or drowning.[67–69]

Testing for inborn errors of metabolism is considered by many to be a routine ancillary test in the evaluation of an unexplained infant death. When these deaths have occurred more than once within a sibship, a thorough evaluation to exclude or confirm an inborn error of metabolism is essential.[70] Analysis of blood and bile may facilitate diagnosis of a fatal inborn error of metabolism. Blood tests for evaluation of many metabolic disorders are now available at low cost, and many states include testing for a number of metabolic diseases on their newborn metabolic screening panel. However, a negative newborn screen result does not eliminate an inborn error of metabolism as the cause of death, so additional postmortem testing may be considered. If an inborn error of metabolism is suspected by autopsy findings (eg, hepatic steatosis) or history (eg, previous unexpected deaths in childhood in the family), the forensic pathologist may elect to retain additional tissues such as brain, liver, kidney, heart, muscle, adrenal gland, and/or pancreas for further analysis. In any case in which the medical examiner is unable to demonstrate an adequate reason for death, a blood sample can be retained for potential future analysis.

More recently, it has been suggested that genetic mutations associated with cardiac rhythm disturbances, such as prolonged QT syndrome, catecholaminergic ventricular paroxysmal tachycardia, and others, are responsible for up to 10% of cases of sudden unexpected infant death.[71,72] In addition, associations with sleep suggest that sleep is a significant risk factor for sudden unexpected death in epilepsy and that the prone position might be an important contributory factor.[73,74] Identification of a possible index case thus warrants referral of the family for comprehensive genetic counseling and additional testing. However, the cost of routine genetic testing may be beyond the capacity of some medical examiner's or coroner's offices, but it may be possible to obtain payment for genetic testing via the family's health insurance carrier.

MULTIDISCIPLINARY CASE REVIEW

Multidisciplinary case reviews of child fatalities have been recommended.[75] In all states, child death review teams have been established to review child fatalities, and improved case identification and evidence for prevention strategies in many jurisdictions are offered in such reviews.[76–78] The focus of such teams varies, ranging from infant or child deaths with accidental or homicidal manner to all childhood deaths from all causes. Many child fatality review teams routinely review sudden unexpected infant deaths. Ideally, a multidisciplinary child death review team should include child welfare or child protective services, law enforcement, public health, the medical examiner or coroner, a pediatrician with expertise in child maltreatment, a forensic pathologist, a representative of the emergency medical services system, a pediatric pathologist, public health and school officials, a local prosecutor, and other agencies pertinent to the case.[79] The proceedings of these committees should be confidential and protected by appropriate state or local laws. Sharing data among agencies should be allowed to ensure that information in community systems can be used to identify areas of prevention and to correctly attribute the cause of death. In addition, surviving and subsequent siblings may need to be protected, and services need to be provided for family members to address the immediate and long-term effects of the death. A growing number of pediatricians and medical examiners and coroners in several jurisdictions are currently receiving support from the Centers for Disease Control and Prevention for a sudden unexpected infant death case reporting system to review cases using standard data collection forms and procedures.[80,81]

RECOMMENDATIONS

The following recommendations are made to improve the identification of child abuse fatalities during infancy:

- A thorough assessment of each unexpected infant fatality should be completed. Such evaluation could include, but would not be limited to, careful history-taking by emergency responders and medical personnel at the time of death with transmission of this information to the medical examiner or coroner; prompt investigation with doll reenactment of the scene at which the infant was found lifeless or unresponsive; careful interviews of household members by knowledgeable, culturally sensitive professionals, such as police, death investigators, prosecutors, and child protective services professionals who have the legal authority and mandate to conduct such investigations; complete autopsy performed by a forensic pathologist within 24 hours of death, including examination of all major body cavities, including cranial contents and microscopic examination of major organs; photographs; radiographic examination, including skeletal survey; toxicological and metabolic screening; collection of medical history through interviews of caregivers and key medical providers; and review of previous medical charts.
- There should be consultations as needed with available local or in-state medical specialists (eg, pediatrician, child abuse pediatrician, pediatric pathologist, pediatric radiologist, pediatric neurologist) by medical examiners and coroners and consideration of intentional asphyxia, especially in cases of unexpected infant death in siblings and with a history of recurrent cyanosis, apnea, or BRUEs witnessed only by a single caregiver.
- Pediatricians, other health care professionals, and investigators should maintain an unbiased, nonaccusatory approach to parents during investigation and provide services or referral to address grief and stresses for surviving family members.
- Because an investigation may require an extended period of time,

pediatricians can advocate for proper death certification and prompt communication to parents and the use of consistent diagnostic categories on death certificates as soon as possible after review; work with families to obtain information from the medical examiner and offer to meet with families to review findings; reinforce Safe to Sleep guidelines for other children; and refer families to social services agencies as needed and for further assessment if potential inheritable conditions are identified.

- There should be review of collected data and prevention strategies by child death review teams with participation of the medical examiner or coroner. Child death review teams at both the state and local levels should include pediatricians who serve as expert members in reviewing case files of the medical examiner and other agencies, particularly for deaths of children who were their patients; information should be shared with providers caring for the family to the extent allowable by law.
- Pediatricians should continue to support the Safe to Sleep campaign and the adoption of safe sleep practices, child death review, and other strategies focusing on ways to reduce the risk of infant sleep-related and maltreatment deaths.
- Pediatricians can work with their state AAP chapters to advocate for and support state policies that require autopsies for sudden unexpected infant deaths and that establish comprehensive and fully funded child death investigation and review systems at the local and state levels. Pediatricians can also advocate for additional funding for research into the causes, identification, and prevention of sudden unexpected infant fatality.

LEAD AUTHORS

Vincent J. Palusci, MD, MS, FAAP
Amanda J. Kay, MD, MPH, FAAP
Erich Batra, MD, FAAP
Rachel Y. Moon, MD, FAAP
Tracey S. Corey, MD
Thomas Andrew, MD
Michael Graham, MD

COUNCIL ON CHILD ABUSE AND NEGLECT EXECUTIVE COMMITTEE, 2018–2020

Andrew P. Sirotnak, MD, FAAP, Chairperson
Emalee G. Flaherty, MD, FAAP, Immediate Past Chairperson
CAPT Amy R. Gavril, MD, MSCI, FAAP
Amanda Bird Hoffert Gilmartin, MD, FAAP
Suzanne B. Haney, MD, FAAP, Chairperson-Elect
Sheila M. Idzerda, MD, FAAP
Antoinette "Toni" Laskey, MD, MPH, MBA, FAAP
Lori A. Legano, MD, FAAP
Stephen A. Messner, MD, FAAP
Bethany Anne Mohr, MD, FAAP
Rebecca L. Moles, MD, FAAP
Shalon Marie Nienow, MD, FAAP
Vincent J. Palusci, MD, MS, FAAP

LIAISONS

Beverly Fortson, PhD – *Centers for Disease Control and Prevention*
Brooks Keeshin, MD, FAAP – *American Academy of Child and Adolescent Psychiatry*
Elaine Stedt, MSW, ACSW – *Administration for Children, Youth and Families, Office on Child Abuse and Neglect*
Anish Raj, MD – *Section on Pediatric Trainees*

STAFF

Tammy Piazza Hurley

SECTION ON CHILD DEATH REVIEW AND PREVENTION, 2018–2020

Erich Batra, MD, FAAP, Chairperson
Carol Berkowitz, MD, FAAP
Amanda Kay, MD, MPH, FAAP
Howard Needelman, MD, FAAP
Timothy Corden, MD, MPH, FAAP

STAFF

Florence Rivera, MPH

TASK FORCE ON SUDDEN INFANT DEATH SYNDROME, 2016–2018

Rachel Y. Moon, MD, FAAP, Chairperson
Robert Darnall, MD, FAAP
Lori Feldman-Winter, MD, MPH, FAAP
Michael Goodstein, MD, FAAP
Fern R. Hauck, MD, MS, FAAP

CONSULTANTS

Carrie Shapiro-Mendoza, PhD – *Centers for Disease Control and Prevention*
Marion Koso-Thomas, MD – *Eunice Kennedy Shriver National Institute of Child Health and Human Development*

STAFF

James Couto, MA

NATIONAL ASSOCIATION OF MEDICAL EXAMINERS

Tracey S. Corey, MD
Thomas Andrew, MD
Michael Graham, MD

ABBREVIATIONS

AAP: American Academy of Pediatrics
BRUE: brief resolved unexplained event
CT: computed tomography
SIDS: sudden infant death syndrome

All clinical reports from the American Academy of Pediatrics automatically expire 5 years after publication unless reaffirmed, revised, or retired at or before that time.

DOI: https://doi.org/10.1542/peds.2019-2076

Address correspondence to Vincent J. Palusci, MD, MS, FAAP. E-mail: vincent.palusci@nyulangone.org

PEDIATRICS (ISSN Numbers: Print, 0031-4005; Online, 1098-4275).

Copyright © 2019 by the American Academy of Pediatrics

FINANCIAL DISCLOSURE: The authors have indicated they have no financial relationships relevant to this article to disclose.

FUNDING: No external funding.

POTENTIAL CONFLICT OF INTEREST: The authors have indicated they have no potential conflicts of interest to disclose.

REFERENCES

1. Werne J, Garrow I. Sudden apparently unexplained death during infancy. I. Pathologic findings in infants found dead. *Am J Pathol.* 1953;29(4):633–675
2. Adelson L, Kinney ER. Sudden and unexpected death in infancy and childhood. *Pediatrics.* 1956;17(5): 663–699
3. Caffey J. Multiple fractures in the long bones of infants suffering from chronic subdural hematoma. *Am J Roentgenol Radium Ther.* 1946;56(2):163–173
4. Silverman FN. The roentgen manifestations of unrecognized skeletal trauma in infants. *Am J Roentgenol Radium Ther Nucl Med.* 1953;69(3): 413–427
5. Adelson L. Slaughter of the innocents. A study of forty-six homicides in which the victims were children. *N Engl J Med.* 1961;264:1345–1349
6. Kempe CH, Silverman FN, Steele BF, Droegemueller W, Silver HK. The battered-child syndrome. *JAMA.* 1962; 181:17–24
7. Southall DP, Plunkett MC, Banks MW, Falkov AF, Samuels MP. Covert video recordings of life-threatening child abuse: lessons for child protection. *Pediatrics.* 1997;100(5):735–760
8. Firstman R, Talan J. *The Death of Innocents: A True Story of Murder, Medicine, and High-Stakes Science.* New York, NY: Bantam Books; 1997
9. Heisler T. As overdose deaths pile up, a medical examiner quits the morgue. New York Times. October 7, 2017. Available at: www.nytimes.com/2017/10/07/us/drug-overdose-medical-examiner.html. Accessed October 7, 2017
10. US Commission to Eliminate Child Abuse and Neglect Fatalities. *Within Our Reach: A National Strategy to Eliminate Child Abuse and Neglect Fatalities.* Washington, DC: Government Printing Office; 2016
11. Tieder JS, Bonkowsky JL, Etzel RA, et al; Subcommittee on Apparent Life Threatening Events. Brief resolved unexplained events (formerly apparent life-threatening events) and evaluation of lower-risk infants [published correction appears in Pediatrics. 2016; 138(2):e20161487]. *Pediatrics.* 2016; 137(5):e20160590
12. Reece RM. Fatal child abuse and sudden infant death syndrome: a critical diagnostic decision. *Pediatrics.* 1993; 91(2):423–429
13. Byard R, Krous H. Suffocation, shaking or sudden infant death syndrome: can we tell the difference? *J Paediatr Child Health.* 1999;35(5):432–433
14. Hymel KP; American Academy of Pediatrics; Committee on Child Abuse and Neglect; National Association of Medical Examiners. Distinguishing sudden infant death syndrome from child abuse fatalities. *Pediatrics.* 2006; 118(1):421–427
15. Moon RY; Task Force on Sudden Infant Death Syndrome. SIDS and other sleep-related infant deaths: evidence base for 2016 updated recommendations for a safe infant sleeping environment. *Pediatrics.* 2016;138(5):e20162940
16. Task Force on Sudden Infant Death Syndrome. SIDS and other sleep-related infant deaths: updated 2016 recommendations for a safe infant sleeping environment. *Pediatrics.* 2016; 138(5):e20162938
17. Corey TS, Hanzlick R, Howard J, Nelson C, Krous H; NAME Ad Hoc Committee on Sudden Unexplained Infant Death. A functional approach to sudden unexplained infant deaths. *Am J Forensic Med Pathol.* 2007;28(3): 271–277
18. Loughrey CM, Preece MA, Green A. Sudden unexpected death in infancy (SUDI). *J Clin Pathol.* 2005;58(1):20–21
19. Malloy MH, MacDorman M. Changes in the classification of sudden unexpected infant deaths: United States, 1992-2001. *Pediatrics.* 2005; 115(5):1247–1253
20. Shapiro-Mendoza CK, Tomashek KM, Anderson RN, Wingo J. Recent national trends in sudden, unexpected infant deaths: more evidence supporting a change in classification or reporting. *Am J Epidemiol.* 2006;163(8):762–769
21. Matthews TJ, MacDorman MF, Thoma ME. Infant mortality statistics from the 2013 period linked birth/infant death data set. *Natl Vital Stat Rep.* 2015;64(9): 1–30
22. Parks SE, Erck Lambert AB, Shapiro-Mendoza CK. Racial and ethnic trends in sudden unexpected infant deaths: United States, 1995-2013. *Pediatrics.* 2017;139(6):e20163844
23. Erck Lambert AB, Parks SE, Shapiro-Mendoza CK. National and state trends in sudden unexpected infant death: 1990-2015. *Pediatrics.* 2018;141(3): e20173519
24. Hoffman HJ, Hillman LS. Epidemiology of the sudden infant death syndrome: maternal, neonatal, and postneonatal risk factors. *Clin Perinatol.* 1992;19(4): 717–737
25. Ponsonby AL, Dwyer T, Gibbons LE, Cochrane JA, Wang YG. Factors potentiating the risk of sudden infant death syndrome associated with the prone position. *N Engl J Med.* 1993; 329(6):377–382
26. Kemp JS, Nelson VE, Thach BT. Physical properties of bedding that may increase risk of sudden infant death syndrome in prone-sleeping infants. *Pediatr Res.* 1994;36(1, pt 1):7–11
27. Jeffery HE, Megevand A, Page H. Why the prone position is a risk factor for sudden infant death syndrome. *Pediatrics.* 1999;104(2, pt 1):263–269
28. MacDorman MF, Cnattingius S, Hoffman HJ, Kramer MS, Haglund B. Sudden infant death syndrome and smoking in the United States and Sweden. *Am J Epidemiol.* 1997;146(3):249–257
29. Fleming PJ, Blair PS, Bacon C, et al; Confidential Enquiry into Stillbirths and Deaths Regional Coordinators and

Researchers. Environment of infants during sleep and risk of the sudden infant death syndrome: results of 1993-5 case-control study for confidential inquiry into stillbirths and deaths in infancy. *BMJ.* 1996;313(7051):191–195

30. Palusci VJ, Covington TM. Child maltreatment deaths in the U.S. National Child Death Review Case Reporting System. *Child Abuse Negl.* 2014;38(1):25–36
31. US Department of Health and Human Services, Administration for Children and Families, Administration on Children, Youth and Families, Children's Bureau. Child maltreatment. Available at: www.acf.hhs.gov/programs/cb/research-data-technology/statistics-research/child-maltreatment. Accessed December 16, 2018
32. Schnitzer PG, Ewigman BG. Child deaths resulting from inflicted injuries: household risk factors and perpetrator characteristics. *Pediatrics.* 2005;116(5). Available at: www.pediatrics.org/cgi/content/full/116/5/e687
33. Schnitzer PG, Covington TM, Kruse RL. Assessment of caregiver responsibility in unintentional child injury deaths: challenges for injury prevention. *Inj Prev.* 2011;17(suppl 1):i45–i54
34. Deans KJ, Thackeray J, Askegard-Giesmann JR, et al. Mortality increases with recurrent episodes of nonaccidental trauma in children. *J Trauma Acute Care Surg.* 2013;75(1):161–165
35. Farrell CA, Fleegler EW, Monuteaux MC, et al. Community poverty and child abuse fatalities in the United States. *Pediatrics.* 2017;139(5):e20161616
36. Putnam-Hornstein E, Schneiderman JU, Cleves MA, Magruder J, Krous HF. A prospective study of sudden unexpected infant death after reported maltreatment. *J Pediatr.* 2014;164(1):142–148
37. Putnam-Hornstein E, Cleves MA, Licht R, Needell B. Risk of fatal injury in young children following abuse allegations: evidence from a prospective, population-based study. *Am J Public Health.* 2013;103(10):e39–e44
38. Christian CW, Block R; Committee on Child Abuse and Neglect; American Academy of Pediatrics. Abusive head trauma in infants and children. *Pediatrics.* 2009;123(5):1409–1411
39. Choudhary AK, Servaes S, Slovis TL, et al. Consensus statement on abusive head trauma in infants and young children. *Pediatr Radiol.* 2018;48(8):1048–1065
40. Chadwick DL, Kirschner RH, Reece RM, et al. Shaken baby syndrome–a forensic pediatric response. *Pediatrics.* 1998;101(2):321–323
41. Meadow R. Suffocation, recurrent apnea, and sudden infant death. *J Pediatr.* 1990;117(3):351–357
42. Bass C, Glaser D. Early recognition and management of fabricated or induced illness in children. *Lancet.* 2014;383(9926):1412–1421
43. Milroy CM, Kepron C. Ten percent of SIDS cases are murder—or are they? *Acad Forensic Pathol.* 2017;7(2):163–170
44. Rosen CL, Frost JD Jr, Bricker T, et al. Two siblings with recurrent cardiorespiratory arrest: Munchausen syndrome by proxy or child abuse? *Pediatrics.* 1983;71(5):715–720
45. American Academy of Pediatrics Committee on Pediatric Emergency Medicine; American College of Emergency Physicians Pediatric Emergency Medicine Committee; Emergency Nurses Association Pediatric Committee. Death of a child in the emergency department. *Pediatrics.* 2014;134(1):198–201
46. Garner AS, Shonkoff JP; Committee on Psychosocial Aspects of Child and Family Health; Committee on Early Childhood, Adoption, and Dependent Care; Section on Developmental and Behavioral Pediatrics. Early childhood adversity, toxic stress, and the role of the pediatrician: translating developmental science into lifelong health. *Pediatrics.* 2012;129(1). Available at: www.pediatrics.org/cgi/content/full/129/1/e224
47. Yu Y, Liew Z, Cnattingius S, et al. Association of mortality with the death of a sibling in childhood. *JAMA Pediatr.* 2017;171(6):538–545
48. Levetown M; American Academy of Pediatrics Committee on Bioethics. Communicating with children and families: from everyday interactions to skill in conveying distressing information. *Pediatrics.* 2008;121(5). Available at: www.pediatrics.org/cgi/content/full/121/5/e1441
49. Wender E; Committee on Psychosocial Aspects of Child and Family Health. Supporting the family after the death of a child. *Pediatrics.* 2012;130(6):1164–1169
50. American Academy of Pediatrics. Committee on Psychosocial Aspects of Child and Family Health. The pediatrician and childhood bereavement. *Pediatrics.* 2000;105(2):445–447
51. Scientific Working Group for Medicolegal Death Investigation. *Principles for Communicating with Next of Kin During Medicolegal Death Investigations.* Washington, DC: National Institute of Justice; 2012. Available at: http://swgmdi.org/images/nokguidelinesforcommunicationwithnok6.14.12%202.pdf. Accessed January 23, 2018
52. Oyen N, Skjaerven R, Irgens LM. Population-based recurrence risk of sudden infant death syndrome compared with other infant and fetal deaths. *Am J Epidemiol.* 1996;144(3):300–305
53. Irgens LM, Skjaerven R, Peterson DR. Prospective assessment of recurrence risk in sudden infant death syndrome siblings. *J Pediatr.* 1984;104(3):349–351
54. Irgens LM, Oyen N, Skjaerven R. Recurrence of sudden infant death syndrome among siblings. *Acta Paediatr Suppl.* 1993;82(suppl 389):23–25
55. Crandall LG, Reno L, Himes B, Robinson D. The diagnostic shift of SIDS to undetermined: are there unintended consequences? *Acad Forensic Pathol.* 2017;7(2):212–220
56. Rudd RA, Marain LC, Crandall L. To hold or not to hold: medicolegal death investigation practices during unexpected child death investigations and the experiences of next of kin. *Am J Forensic Med Pathol.* 2014;35(2):132–139
57. National Sudden Infant Death Syndrome/Infant Death Resource Center. Responding to a sudden, unexpected infant death: the professional's role. Available at: https://

www.ncemch.org/suid-sids/documents/SIDRC/ProfessionalRole.pdf. Accessed October 13, 2017

58. First Candle. First candle. Available at: www.firstcandle.org. Accessed October 13, 2017

59. Association of SIDS and Infant Mortality Programs. Bereavement counseling for sudden infant death syndrome (SIDS) and infant mortality: core competencies for the health care professional. Available at: https://www.nwsids.org/documents/BereavementCounselingforInfantMortality.pdf. Accessed January 7, 2019

60. Case ME. Distinguishing accidental from inflicted head trauma at autopsy. *Pediatr Radiol.* 2014;44(suppl 4):S632–S640

61. Centers for Disease Control and Prevention, Maternal and Infant Health Branch, Division of Reproductive Health. *Sudden, Unexplained Infant Death Investigation: Guidelines for the Scene Investigator.* Atlanta, GA: Centers for Disease Control and Prevention; 2007. Available at: https://www.cdc.gov/sids/pdf/508suidiguidelinessingles_tag508.pdf. Accessed January 6, 2018

62. Diebold-Hargrave KL. Best practices: infant death scene recreation and investigation. *Acad Forensic Pathol.* 2011;1(4):356–361

63. Perrot LJ, Nawojczyk S. Nonnatural death masquerading as SIDS (sudden infant death syndrome). *Am J Forensic Med Pathol.* 1988;9(2):105–111

64. Rogers C, Hall J, Muto J. Findings in newborns of cocaine-abusing mothers. *J Forensic Sci.* 1991;36(4):1074–1078

65. Mirchandani HG, Mirchandani IH, Hellman F, et al. Passive inhalation of free-base cocaine ('crack') smoke by infants. *Arch Pathol Lab Med.* 1991;115(5):494–498

66. Section on Radiology; American Academy of Pediatrics. Diagnostic imaging of child abuse. *Pediatrics.* 2009;123(5):1430–1435

67. Brown RH. The battered child syndrome. *J Forensic Sci.* 1976;21(1):65–70

68. Lauer B, ten Broeck E, Grossman M. Battered child syndrome: review of 130 patients with controls. *Pediatrics.* 1974;54(1):67–70

69. Scott PD. Fatal battered baby cases. *Med Sci Law.* 1973;13(3):197–206

70. Harpey JP, Charpentier C, Paturneau-Jouas M. Sudden infant death syndrome and inherited disorders of fatty acid beta-oxidation. *Biol Neonate.* 1990;58(suppl 1):70–80

71. Ackerman MJ. State of postmortem genetic testing known as the cardiac channel molecular autopsy in the forensic evaluation of unexplained sudden cardiac death in the young. *Pacing Clin Electrophysiol.* 2009;32(suppl 2):S86–S89

72. Cunningham KS, Pollanen M. Evolution of a molecular autopsy program from within a death investigation system. *Acad Forensic Pathol.* 2015;5(2):211–220

73. Milroy C, Parai J. Sudden unexpected death in epilepsy (SUDEP) and certification. *Acad Forensic Pathol.* 2015;5(1):59–66

74. Ali A, Wu S, Issa NP, et al. Association of sleep with sudden unexpected death in epilepsy. *Epilepsy Behav.* 2017;76:1–6

75. Committee on Child Abuse and Neglect; Committee on Injury, Violence, and Poison Prevention; Council on Community Pediatrics. American Academy of Pediatrics. Policy statement–child fatality review. *Pediatrics.* 2010;126(3):592–596

76. Palusci VJ, Haney ML. Strategies to prevent child maltreatment and integration into practice. *APSAC Adv.* 2010;22(1):8–17

77. Schnitzer PG, Covington TM, Wirtz SJ, Verhoek-Oftedahl W, Palusci VJ. Public health surveillance of fatal child maltreatment: analysis of 3 state programs. *Am J Public Health.* 2008;98(2):296–303

78. Palusci VJ, Yager S, Covington TM. Effects of a citizens review panel in preventing child maltreatment fatalities. *Child Abuse Negl.* 2010;34(5):324–331

79. Centers for Disease Control and Prevention, National Center for Injury Prevention and Control. *National Action Plan for Child Injury Prevention.* Atlanta, GA: Centers for Disease Control and Prevention, National Center for Injury Prevention and Control; 2012

80. Burns KM, Bienemann L, Camperlengo L, et al; Sudden Death in the Young Case Registry Steering Committee. The sudden death in the young case registry: collaborating to understand and reduce mortality. *Pediatrics.* 2017;139(3):e20162757

81. Shapiro-Mendoza CK, Camperlengo LT, Kim SY, Covington T. The sudden unexpected infant death case registry: a method to improve surveillance. *Pediatrics.* 2012;129(2). Available at: www.pediatrics.org/cgi/content/full/129/2/e486

The Impact of Racism on Child and Adolescent Health

- *Policy Statement*

POLICY STATEMENT Organizational Principles to Guide and Define the Child Health Care System and/or Improve the Health of all Children

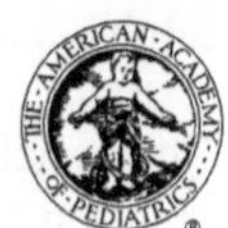

American Academy of Pediatrics

DEDICATED TO THE HEALTH OF ALL CHILDREN™

The Impact of Racism on Child and Adolescent Health

Maria Trent, MD, MPH, FAAP, FSAHM,[a] Danielle G. Dooley, MD, MPhil, FAAP,[b] Jacqueline Dougé, MD, MPH, FAAP,[c] SECTION ON ADOLESCENT HEALTH, COUNCIL ON COMMUNITY PEDIATRICS, COMMITTEE ON ADOLESCENCE

abstract

The American Academy of Pediatrics is committed to addressing the factors that affect child and adolescent health with a focus on issues that may leave some children more vulnerable than others. Racism is a social determinant of health that has a profound impact on the health status of children, adolescents, emerging adults, and their families. Although progress has been made toward racial equality and equity, the evidence to support the continued negative impact of racism on health and well-being through implicit and explicit biases, institutional structures, and interpersonal relationships is clear. The objective of this policy statement is to provide an evidence-based document focused on the role of racism in child and adolescent development and health outcomes. By acknowledging the role of racism in child and adolescent health, pediatricians and other pediatric health professionals will be able to proactively engage in strategies to optimize clinical care, workforce development, professional education, systems engagement, and research in a manner designed to reduce the health effects of structural, personally mediated, and internalized racism and improve the health and well-being of all children, adolescents, emerging adults, and their families.

[a]Division of Adolescent and Young Adult Medicine, Department of Pediatrics, School of Medicine, Johns Hopkins University, Baltimore, Maryland; [b]Division of General Pediatrics and Community Health and Child Health Advocacy Institute, Children's National Health System, Washington, District of Columbia; and [c]Medical Director, Howard County Health Department, Columbia, Maryland

Drs Trent, Dooley, and Dougé worked together as a writing team to develop the manuscript outline, conduct the literature search, develop the stated policies, incorporate perspectives and feedback from American Academy of Pediatrics leadership, and draft the final version of the manuscript; and all authors approved the final manuscript as submitted.

This document is copyrighted and is property of the American Academy of Pediatrics and its Board of Directors. All authors have filed conflict of interest statements with the American Academy of Pediatrics. Any conflicts have been resolved through a process approved by the Board of Directors. The American Academy of Pediatrics has neither solicited nor accepted any commercial involvement in the development of the content of this publication.

Policy statements from the American Academy of Pediatrics benefit from expertise and resources of liaisons and internal (AAP) and external reviewers. However, policy statements from the American Academy of Pediatrics may not reflect the views of the liaisons or the organizations or government agencies that they represent.

The guidance in this statement does not indicate an exclusive course of treatment or serve as a standard of medical care. Variations, taking into account individual circumstances, may be appropriate.

All policy statements from the American Academy of Pediatrics automatically expire 5 years after publication unless reaffirmed, revised, or retired at or before that time.

DOI: https://doi.org/10.1542/peds.2019-1765

Address correspondence to Maria Trent, MD. E-mail: mtrent2@jhmi.edu

To cite: Trent M, Dooley DG, Dougé J, AAP SECTION ON ADOLESCENT HEALTH, AAP COUNCIL ON COMMUNITY PEDIATRICS, AAP COMMITTEE ON ADOLESCENCE. The Impact of Racism on Child and Adolescent Health. *Pediatrics.* 2019;144(2):e20191765

STATEMENT OF THE PROBLEM

Racism is a "system of structuring opportunity and assigning value based on the social interpretation of how one looks (which is what we call 'race') that unfairly disadvantages some individuals and communities, unfairly advantages other individuals and communities, and saps the strength of the whole society through the waste of human resources."[1] Racism is a social determinant of health[2] that has a profound impact on the health status of children, adolescents, emerging adults, and their families.[3–8] Although progress has been made toward racial equality and equity,[9] the evidence to support the continued negative impact of racism on health and well-being through implicit and explicit biases, institutional structures, and interpersonal relationships is clear.[10] Failure to address racism will continue to undermine health equity for all children, adolescents, emerging adults, and their families.

The social environment in which children are raised shapes child and adolescent development, and pediatricians are poised to prevent and respond to environmental circumstances that undermine child health. Pediatrics as a field has yet to systematically address the influence of racism on child health outcomes and to prepare pediatricians to identify, manage, mitigate, or prevent risks and harms. Recognizing that racism has significant adverse effects on the individual who receives, commits, and observes racism,[11,12] substantial investments in dismantling structural racism are required to facilitate the societal shifts necessary for optimal development of children in the United States. The American Academy of Pediatrics (AAP) is committed to reducing the ongoing costs and burden of racism to children, the health care system, and society.[13,14]

Today's children, adolescents, and emerging adults are increasingly diverse. Strategies to address health and developmental issues across the pediatric life span that incorporate ethnicity, culture, and circumstance are critical to achieving a reduction in health disparities. Accordingly, pediatrics should be at the forefront of addressing racism as a core social determinant. The inclusion of racism is in alignment with the health equity pillar of the AAP strategic plan.[15] In a series of workshops in 2016 during national meetings of pediatricians, 3 strategic actions were identified: (1) development of a task force within the AAP to address racism and other forms of discrimination that impact the health status and outcomes of minority youth, (2) development of a policy statement on racism, and (3) integration of evidence-based anticipatory guidance about racism into *Bright Futures*.[16]

The objective of this policy statement is to provide an evidence-based document focused on the role of racism in child and adolescent development and health outcomes. This policy statement will allow pediatricians to implement recommendations in practice that will better address the factors that make some children more vulnerable than others.[13] The statement also builds on existing AAP policy recommendations associated with other social determinants of health, such as poverty, housing insecurity, child health equity, immigration status, and early childhood adversity.[9,17–19]

RACISM AS A CORE DETERMINANT OF CHILD HEALTH

Racism is a core social determinant of health that is a driver of health inequities.[20–22] The World Health Organization defines social determinants of health as "the conditions in which people are born, grow, live, work, and age." These determinants are influenced by economic, political, and social factors linked to health inequities (avoidable inequalities in health between groups of people within populations and between countries). These health inequities are not the result of individual behavior choices or genetic predisposition but are caused by economic, political, and social conditions, including racism.[23]

The impact of racism has been linked to birth disparities and mental health problems in children and adolescents.[6,24–30] The biological mechanism that emerges from chronic stress leads to increased and prolonged levels of exposure to stress hormones and oxidative stress at the cellular level. Prolonged exposure to stress hormones, such as cortisol, leads to inflammatory reactions that predispose individuals to chronic disease.[31] As an example, racial disparities in the infant mortality rate remain,[32] and the complications of low birth weight have been associated with perceived racial discrimination and maternal stress.[25,33,34]

Investments in policies to address social determinants of health, such as poverty, have yielded improvements in the health of children. The Food Stamp Program, a War on Poverty initiative first developed in the 1930s during the Great Depression and later revived in the 1960s, is linked to improvements in birth outcomes.[35] Efforts in education, housing, and child health insurance have also led to improved health outcomes for issues such as lead poisoning, injuries, asthma, cancer, neurotoxicity, cardiovascular disease, and mental health problems.[20,36,37] Expansion of child health insurance has improved health care access for children, with significant gains for African American and Hispanic children in terms of access to well-child, doctor, and dental visits.[38] Despite these improvements, it is important to recognize that children raised in African American, Hispanic, and American Indian populations continue to face higher risks of parental unemployment and to reside in families with significantly lower household net wealth relative to white children in the United States, posing barriers to equal opportunities and services that optimize health and vocational outcomes.[39–45]

Juvenile justice involvement is also a critical social determinant of health. Because racial inequity continues to shape the juvenile justice system, this area is a modern example of race being an important determinant of short- and long-term outcomes. The AAP published a statement in 2011[46] focusing on key health issues of justice-involved youth, which was recently revised to include an in-depth discussion on racial and ethnic inequalities for this population.[47] Although the overall rates of youth incarceration have decreased, African American, Hispanic, and American

Indian youth continue to be disproportionately represented.[48] While incarcerated, youth experience additional adverse experiences, such as solitary confinement and abuse, that have the potential to undermine socioemotional development and general developmental outcomes.[49–51] Differential treatment of youth offenders on the basis of race shapes an individual's participation and ultimate function in society. This type of modern racism must be recognized and addressed if the United States seeks to attain health equity.[52]

THE DEVELOPMENT OF RACE AS A CONSTRUCT

Race as a social construct is rooted in history and remains a mechanism through which social class has been controlled over time. Flawed science was used to solidify the permanence of race, reinforce the notions of racial superiority, and justify differential treatment on the basis of phenotypic differences as people from different parts of the world came in contact with each other.[53] Race emerged as a social classification used to assign dominance of some social classes over others.[53] Scientific, anthropologic, and historical inquiry further solidified race as a social construct.[54] Modern science, however, has demonstrated that there is only 1 biological race and that the clines (phenotypic differences in skin and eye color, hair texture, and bone structure) at the core of early anthropologic research were insufficient to establish different races among human beings. Dr Francis Collins, former director of the National Human Genome Project and presently the director of the National Institutes of Health, has affirmed that humans are 99.9% the same at the level of their genome.[55] Despite this, efforts to collect, organize, and categorize individuals on the basis of the plausibility of the 0.01% human variation remain a force of scientific discovery, innovation, and medical-pharmaceutical collaborations.[56] Rather than focusing on preventing the social conditions that have led to racial disparities, science and society continue to focus on the disparate outcomes that have resulted from them, often reinforcing the posited biological underpinnings of flawed racial categories.[57] Although race used in these ways has been institutionalized, linked to health status, and impeded our ability to improve health and eliminate health disparities,[58,59] it remains a powerful measure that must be better measured, carefully used, and potentially replaced to mark progress in pediatric health disparities research.[60,61]

As such, it is important to examine the historical underpinnings of race used as a tool for subjugation. American racism was transported through European colonization. It began with the subjugation, displacement, and genocide of American Indian populations and was subsequently bolstered by the importation of African slaves to frame the economy of the United States. Although institutions such as slavery were abolished more than a century ago, discriminatory policies, such as Jim Crow laws, were developed to legalize subjugation. As the United States expanded west in North America and into Alaska and the Pacific Islands, the diversity of populations encompassing the United States also expanded. Native Hawaiian and Pacific Islander, Alaskan native, Asian American, and Latino American populations have experienced oppression and similar exclusions from society.[62–65] Although some racial and/or ethnic groups have received reparations[66] and fared better than others over time, remnants of these policies remain in place today and continue to oppress the advancement of people from historically aggrieved groups.[67–72]

Through these underpinnings, racism became a socially transmitted disease passed down through generations, leading to the inequities observed in our population today. Although the endemic nature of racism has powerful impacts on perceived and actual health outcomes, it is also important to note that other forms of discrimination (eg, sex, religion, sexual orientation, immigrant status, and disability status) are actively at play and have created a syndemic with the potential to undermine child and family health further. It is important to address racism's impact on the health and well-being of children, adolescents, and emerging adults to avoid perpetuating a health system that does not meet the needs of all patients.[52] Pediatricians are uniquely positioned to both prevent and mitigate the consequences of racism as a key and trusted source of support for pediatric patients and their families.

CHILDHOOD EXPERIENCES OF RACISM

Children can distinguish the phenotypic differences associated with race during infancy[73–75]; therefore, effective management of difference as normative is important in a diverse society. To identify, address, and manage the impacts of racism on child health, it is critical that pediatricians understand 3 key levels through which racism operates: (1) institutional, (2) personally mediated, and (3) internalized. The experience of race is also impacted by other identities that people have related to ethnicity, sex, religious affiliation, immigrant status, family composition, sexuality, disability, and others that must be navigated alongside race. Much of the discussion to date related to the historical underpinnings of race deals with institutionalized (or structural) racism, expressed through patterns of social institutions (eg, governmental organizations, schools, banks, and courts of law) that implicitly or explicitly discriminate against individuals from historically marginalized groups.[22,52,76,77] Children experience the outputs of structural racism through place (where they live), education (where they learn), economic means (what they have), and legal means (how their rights are executed). Research has identified the role of implicit and explicit personally mediated racism (racism characterized by assumptions about the abilities, motives, or intents of others on the basis of race)[78] as a factor affecting health care delivery and general health outcomes.[79–86] The impacts of structural and personally mediated racism may result in internalized racism (internalizing racial stereotypes about one's racial group). A positive racial identity mediates experiences of discrimination and generates optimal youth development outcomes.[12,87,88] The importance of a prosocial identity is critical during adolescence, when young people must navigate the impacts of social status and awareness of personally mediated discrimination based on race.[89–91]

Although children and adolescents who are the targets of racism experience the most significant impact, bystanders are also adversely affected by racism. As an example, young adults who were bystanders to racism and other forms of victimization as youth experience profound physiologic and psychological effects when asked to recall the memory of a past anchoring event as a victim or bystander that are comparable to those experienced by first responders after a major disaster. Three core features that characterized the abusive event(s) were as follows: (1) an individual gets hurt psychologically or physically, (2) a power differential exists (eg, age, size and/or stature, or status) versus the target individual resulting in domination and erosion of the target's self-esteem, and (3) the abuse is repetitive, causing stress levels to increase because of anticipation of future events.[11] Internalized negative stereotypes related to race can unconsciously erode self-perception and capacity and may later play out in the form of stereotype threat or the fear of confirming a negative stereotype of one's race.[91] Stereotype threats can undermine academic and vocational attainment, key developmental milestones for the victim. Underachievement then reinforces the stereotype held by both the perpetrator and victim, further enhancing the vulnerability of the victim and the bystander to repeated acts of overt or covert victimization. These observations suggest that universal interventions to eliminate racism (experienced as a victim or bystander) from the lives of children and to engage in active societal antiracism bystander behavioral intervention may optimize well-being for all children and the adults who care for them. For individual intervention to occur, however, bystanders must identify critical situations, view them as an emergency, develop a sense of personal responsibility, have self-efficacy to succeed with the intervention, perceive the costs of nonintervention as high, and consciously decide to help.[11,92] Research has demonstrated that racism has an effect on health across racial groups in communities reporting high levels of racism[93] but that racially diverse environments, such as schools, can benefit all youth by improving cognitive skills such as critical thinking and problem-solving.[94]

RACISM AT THE INTERSECTION OF EDUCATION AND CHILD AND ADOLESCENT HEALTH

Educational and vocational attainment are key developmental outcomes that pediatricians monitor to assess for successful growth and development. After accounting for sleep and time spent at home, children spend a significant portion of their time in educational settings.[95–97] Educational achievement is an important predictor of long-term health and economic outcomes for children. Adults with a college degree live longer and have lower rates of chronic disease than those who did not graduate from college.[98] It is critical for pediatricians to recognize the institutional, personally mediated, and internalized levels of racism that occur in the educational setting because education is a critical social determinant of health for children.[99]

Disparities in educational access and attainment, along with racism experienced in the educational setting, affect the trajectory of academic achievement for children and adolescents and ultimately impact health. Chronic absenteeism, defined as missing ≥10% of school days in an academic year, is a strong predictor of educational achievement. Chronic absenteeism disproportionately affects children of color, children living in poverty, children with disabilities, and children with chronic diseases.[100] In high school, 21.2% of Hispanic, 23.4% of African American, and 27.5% of American Indian children were chronically absent in 2013–2014 compared with 17.3% of white children.[101] Immigration enforcement and the fear of apprehension by authorities can negatively affect school attendance for Hispanic and black immigrants, thereby perpetuating inequalities in attendance.[102] According to the National Center for Education Statistics, the graduation rate for white students nationally in 2015–2016 was 88% compared with 76% for African American students, 72% for American Indian students, and 79% for Hispanic students.[103] Disparities in chronic absenteeism and high school graduation rates prevent children from realizing the full benefits of educational attainment and can increase the development of chronic disease and reduce overall life expectancy.[104]

Although the landmark US Supreme Court case *Brown v Board of Education* banned government-sponsored segregation and laid a foundation for equal access to a quality public education, the US Department of Education continues to report institutional or structural inequality in educational access and outcomes,[105] even in the most diverse and well-resourced communities in the United States. Students from historically aggrieved groups have less access to experienced teachers, advanced coursework, and resources and are also more harshly punished for minor behavioral infractions occurring in the school setting.[105] They are less likely to be identified for and receive special education services,[106] and in some states, school districts with more nonwhite children receive lower funding at any given poverty level than districts with more white children.[107]

Children may also experience personally mediated racism early in their schooling, which may be internalized and ultimately affect their interactions with others.[108] Early teacher-child interactions are important for long-term academic outcomes. The relationship of teacher to student across ages and grade levels influences school adjustment, literacy, math skills, grade point average, and scholastic aptitude test scores.[109–111] Given the critical nature of the student-teacher relationship, it is important to explore how racism and implicit bias affect this dynamic. Student-teacher racial mismatch can impact academic performance, with studies showing that African American children are more likely to receive a worse assessment of their behavior when they have a non-Hispanic white teacher than when they have an African American teacher.[112] This finding may result from racial bias in teachers' expectations of their students, with data demonstrating that white and other non–African American teachers are more likely than African American teachers to predict that African American students would not finish high school.[113] Similarly, data indicate that teachers may underestimate the ability of African American and Latino students, which can lead to lower grade point averages and fewer years of schooling.[114] African American students who have 1 African American teacher in elementary school are more likely to graduate from high school and enroll in college than their peers who do not have an African American teacher; the proposed mechanism for this improved long-term educational outcome is the exposure to a role model early in the educational experience.[115] These findings indicate the importance of ensuring a diverse teacher workforce, particularly as the population of students in US schools continues to diversify.[116] School racial climate, which refers to norms, curricula, and interactions around race and diversity within the school setting, also impacts educational outcomes for students.[117] Students who had a positive perception of school racial climate had higher academic achievement and fewer disciplinary issues.[118] Racial inequities in school discipline begin early, and school discipline has long-term consequences for children. Although federal civil rights laws prohibit discrimination in the administration of discipline in public schools, the US Government Accountability Office found that African American and American Indian students are overrepresented among students experiencing suspension.[119] Data from the US Department of Education confirm that a disproportionate number of African American children receive more than 1 out-of-school suspension in preschool and overall in kindergarten through grade 12 are suspended 3 times more and expelled 1.9 times more than white students.[120] To mediate the effects of institutional and personally mediated racism in the educational setting and prevent internalized racism, studies show that a positive, strong racial or ethnic identity and parental engagement in families is protective against the negative effects of racial discrimination on academic outcomes.[121–123]

HOW PEDIATRICIANS CAN ADDRESS AND AMELIORATE THE EFFECTS OF RACISM ON CHILDREN AND ADOLESCENTS

Pediatricians and other child health professionals must be prepared to discuss and counsel families of all races on the effects of exposure to racism as victims, bystanders, and perpetrators.[124–126] Pediatricians can implement systems in their practices that ensure that all patients and families know that they are welcome, that they will be treated with mutual respect, and that high-quality care will be delivered regardless of background using the tenets of family- and patient-centered care.[127] To do this, it is critical for pediatricians to examine their own biases.[128] Pediatricians can advocate for community initiatives and collaborate with government and community-based organizations to help redress biases and inequities in the health, justice, and educational systems. These strategies may optimize developmental outcomes and reduce exposure to adverse events that dramatically alter the lived experiences, health, and perceived self-value of youth.[48,129,130]

Optimizing Clinical Practice

In practice, pediatricians and other child health care providers encounter children every day who have experienced racism. There are interventions available for use in the medical home that can identify and potentially ameliorate inequities.

- Create a culturally safe medical home[131] where the providers acknowledge and are sensitive to the racism that children and families experience by integrating patient- and family-centered communication strategies and evidence-based screening tools that incorporate valid measures of perceived and experienced racism into clinical practice.[132–136]
- Use strategies such as the Raising Resisters approach during anticipatory guidance to provide support for youth and families to (1) recognize racism in all forms, from subversive to blatant displays of racism; (2) differentiate racism from other forms of unfair treatment and/or routine developmental stressors; (3) safely oppose the negative messages and/or behaviors of others; and (4) counter or replace those messages and experiences with something positive.[137,138]
- Train clinical and office staff in culturally competent care according to national standards for culturally and linguistically appropriate services.[139,140]
- Assess patients for stressors (eg, bullying and/or cyberbullying on the basis of race)[141] and social determinants of health often associated with racism (eg, neighborhood safety, poverty, housing inequity, and academic access) to connect families to resources.[9,142,143]
- Assess patients who report experiencing racism for mental health conditions, including signs of posttraumatic stress, anxiety, grief, and depressive symptoms, using validated screening tools and a trauma-informed approach to make referrals to mental health services as needed.[144]
- Integrate positive youth development approaches,[145] including racial socialization,[123,146] to identify strengths and assess youth and families for protective factors,[9] such as a supportive extended family network, that can help mitigate exposure to racist behaviors.[138]
- Infuse cultural diversity into AAP-recommended early literacy–promotion programs[147] to ensure that there is a representation of authors, images, and stories that reflect the cultural diversity of children served in pediatric practice.
- Encourage pediatric practices and local chapters to embrace the challenge of testing best practices using Community Access to Child Health grants and participation in national quality-improvement projects to examine the effectiveness of office-based interventions designed to address the impact of racism on patient outcomes.
- Encourage practices and chapters to develop resources for families with civil rights concerns, including medicolegal partnerships and referrals to agencies responsible for enforcing civil rights laws.
- Encourage pediatric-serving organizations within local communities, including pediatric practices, hospitals, and health maintenance organizations, to conduct internal quality-assurance assessments that include analyses of quality of care and patient satisfaction by race and to initiate improvement protocols as needed to improve health outcomes and community trust.

Optimizing Workforce Development and Professional Education

- Advocate for pediatric training programs that are girded by competencies and subcompetencies related to effective patient and family communication across differences in pediatric populations.[148,149]
- Encourage policies to foster interactive learning communities that promote cultural humility (eg, self-awareness, lifelong commitment to self-evaluation, and commitment to managing power imbalances)[150,151] and provide simulation opportunities to ensure new pediatricians are competent to deliver culturally appropriate and patient- and family-centered care.[152–155]
- Integrate active learning strategies, such as simulation[156] and language immersion,[157] to adequately prepare pediatric residents to serve the most diverse pediatric population to date to exist in the United States[158] and lead diverse and interdisciplinary pediatric care teams.[159]
- Advocate for policies and programs that diversify the pediatric workforce and provide ongoing professional education for pediatricians in practice as a strategy to reduce implicit biases and improve safety and quality in the health care delivery system.[160–162]

Optimizing Systems Through Community Engagement, Advocacy, and Public Policy

- Acknowledge that health equity is unachievable unless racism is addressed through interdisciplinary partnerships with other organizations that have developed campaigns against racism.[163,164]
- Engage community leaders to create safe playgrounds and healthy food markets to reduce disparities in obesity and undernutrition in neighborhoods affected by poverty.
- Advocate for improvements in the quality of education in segregated urban, suburban, and rural communities designed to better optimize vocational attainment and educational milestones for all students.

- Support local educational systems by connecting with and supporting school staff. The AAP Council on School Health provides resources to help physicians engage and interact with their school system and provides guidelines around the role of school physicians and school health personnel.[165,166]
- Advocate for federal and local policies that support implicit-bias training in schools and robust training of educators in culturally competent classroom management to improve disparities in academic outcomes and disproportionate rates of suspension and expulsion among students of color, reflecting a systemic bias in the educational system.[167]
- Advocate for increased access to support for mental health services in schools designed to help teachers better manage students with disruptive classroom behaviors and to reduce racial disparities in school expulsion.[144,168,169]
- Advocate for curricula that are multicultural, multilingual, and reflective of the communities in which children in their practices attend school.[170]
- Advocate for policies and programs that diversify the teacher workforce to mitigate the effects of the current demographic mismatch of teachers and students that affects academic attitudes and attainment for all students.[115,171]
- Advocate for evidence-based programs that combat racism in the education setting at a population level.[172–174]
- Encourage community-level advocacy with members of those communities disproportionately affected by racism to develop policies that advance social justice.[19,175]
- Advocate for alternative strategies to incarceration for management of nonviolent youth behavior.[50,176,177]
- Collaborate with first responders and community police to enhance positive youth engagement by sharing expertise on child and adolescent development and mental health, considering potential differences in culture, sex, and background.[178]
- Advocate for fair housing practices, including access to housing loans and rentals that prohibit the persistence of historic "redlining."[179]

Optimizing Research

- Advocate for funding and dissemination of rigorous research that examine the following:
  1. the impact of perceived and observed experiences of discrimination on child and family health outcomes[180];
  2. the role of self-identification versus perceived race on child health access, status, and outcomes[52];
  3. the impact of workforce development activities on patient satisfaction, trust, care use, and pediatric health outcomes[161];
  4. the impact of policy changes and community-level interventions on reducing the health effects of racism and other forms of discrimination on youth development; and
  5. integration of the human genome as a way to identify critical biomarkers that can be used to improve human health rather than continue to classify people on the basis of their minor genetic differences and countries of origin.[55]

CONCLUSIONS

Achieving decisive public policies, optimized clinical service delivery, and community change with an activated, engaged, and diverse pediatric workforce is critically important to begin untangling the thread of racism sewn through the fabric of society and affecting the health of pediatric populations. Pediatricians must examine and acknowledge their own biases and embrace and advocate for innovative policies and cross-sector partnerships designed to improve medical, economic, environmental, housing, judicial, and educational equity for optimal child, adolescent, and emerging adult developmental outcomes.

SECTION ON ADOLESCENT HEALTH EXECUTIVE COMMITTEE, 2018–2019

Maria E. Trent, MD, MPH, FAAP, Chairperson
Robert M. Cavanaugh Jr, MD, FAAP
Amy E. Lacroix, MD, FAAP
Jonathon Fanburg, MD, MPH, FAAP
Maria H. Rahmandar, MD, FAAP
Laurie L. Hornberger, MD, MPH, FAAP
Marcie B. Schneider, MD, FAAP
Sophia Yen, MD, MPH, FAAP

STAFF

Karen S. Smith

COUNCIL ON COMMUNITY PEDIATRICS EXECUTIVE COMMITTEE, 2018–2019

Lance Alix Chilton, MD, FAAP, Chairperson
Andrea E. Green, MD, FAAP
Kimberley Jo Dilley, MD, MPH, FAAP
Juan Raul Gutierrez, MD, FAAP
James H. Duffee, MD, MPH, FAAP
Virginia A. Keane, MD, FAAP
Scott Daniel Krugman, MD, MS, FAAP
Carla Dawn McKelvey, MD, MPH, FAAP
Julie Michelle Linton, MD, FAAP
Jacqueline Lee Nelson, MD, FAAP
Gerri Mattson, MD, FAAP

LIAISON

Donene Feist

STAFF

Dana Bennett-Tejes, MA, MNM

COMMITTEE ON ADOLESCENCE, 2018–2019

Cora C. Breuner, MD, MPH, FAAP, Chairperson
Elizabeth M. Alderman, MD, FSAHM, FAAP
Laura K. Grubb, MD, MPH, FAAP
Janet Lee, MD, FAAP

Makia E. Powers, MD, MPH, FAAP
Maria H. Rahmandar, MD, FAAP
Krishna K. Upadhya, MD, FAAP
Stephenie B. Wallace, MD, FAAP

LIAISONS

Liwei L. Hua, MD, PhD – *American Academy of Child and Adolescent Psychiatry*
Geri D. Hewitt, MD – *American College of Obstetricians and Gynecologists*
Seema Menon, MD – *North American Society of Pediatric and Adolescent Gynecology*
Ellie E. Vyver, MD, FRCPC, FAAP – *Canadian Pediatric Society*
Lauren B. Zapata, PhD, MSPH – *Centers for Disease Control and Prevention*

STAFF

Karen S. Smith

ACKNOWLEDGMENTS

We are grateful for internal review and critical feedback by Drs Benard Dreyer, Olanrewaju Falusi, Renee Jenkins, Judith Palfrey, Krishna Upadhya, Joseph Wright, Jonathan Klein, Janie Ward, Michael Lindsey, Lance Chilton, James Duffee, Andrea Green, Julie Linton, Virginia Keane, Jackie Nelson, Raul Gutierrez, Lase Ajayi, Lee Beers, Nathaniel Beers, Heidi Schumacher, and Tonya Vidal Kinlow.

ABBREVIATION

AAP: American Academy of Pediatrics

PEDIATRICS (ISSN Numbers: Print, 0031-4005; Online, 1098-4275).

Copyright © 2019 by the American Academy of Pediatrics

FINANCIAL DISCLOSURE: The authors have indicated they have no financial relationships relevant to this article to disclose.

FUNDING: No external funding.

POTENTIAL CONFLICT OF INTEREST: The authors have indicated they have no potential conflicts of interest to disclose.

REFERENCES

1. Jones CP, Truman BI, Elam-Evans LD, et al. Using "socially assigned race" to probe white advantages in health status. *Ethn Dis*. 2008;18(4):496–504
2. Paradies Y, Ben J, Denson N, et al. Racism as a determinant of health: a systematic review and meta-analysis. *PLoS One*. 2015;10(9):e0138511
3. Berman G, Paradies Y. Racism, disadvantage and multiculturalism: towards effective anti-racist praxis. *Ethn Racial Stud*. 2010;33(2):214–232
4. Elias A, Paradies Y. Estimating the mental health costs of racial discrimination. *BMC Public Health*. 2016;16(1):1205
5. Heard-Garris NJ, Cale M, Camaj L, Hamati MC, Dominguez TP. Transmitting Trauma: a systematic review of vicarious racism and child health. *Soc Sci Med*. 2018;199:230–240
6. Pachter LM, Coll CG. Racism and child health: a review of the literature and future directions. *J Dev Behav Pediatr*. 2009;30(3):255–263
7. Paradies Y. Defining, conceptualizing and characterizing racism in health research. *Crit Public Health*. 2006;16(2):144–157
8. Pachter LM, Bernstein BA, Szalacha LA, García Coll C. Perceived racism and discrimination in children and youths: an exploratory study. *Health Soc Work*. 2010;35(1):61–69
9. Council on Community Pediatrics. Poverty and child health in the United States. *Pediatrics*. 2016;137(4):e20160339
10. Institute of Medicine, Committee on Improving the Health, Safety, and Well-Being of Young Adults. B: diversity and the effects of bias and discrimination on young adults' health and well-being. In: Bonnie RJ, Stroud C, Breiner H, eds. *Investing in the Health and Well-Being of Young Adults*. Washington, DC: National Academies Press; 2015. Available at: https://www.nap.edu/download/18869. Accessed August 22, 2017
11. Janson GR, Hazler RJ. Trauma reactions of bystanders and victims to repetitive abuse experiences. *Violence Vict*. 2004;19(2):239–255
12. Clark K, Clark M. The development of consciousness of self and the emergence of racial identification in Negro preschool children. *J Soc Psychol*. 1939;10:98
13. American Academy of Pediatrics. Blueprint for children. Available at: https://www.aap.org/en-us/Documents/BluePrintForChildren.pdf. Accessed August 22, 2017
14. Szilagyi PG, Dreyer BP, Fuentes-Afflick E, Coyne-Beasley T, First L. The road to tolerance and understanding. *Pediatrics*. 2017;139(6):e20170741
15. American Academy of Pediatrics. American Academy Pediatrics five-year strategic plan. Available at: https://www.aap.org/en-us/about-the-aap/aap-facts/Pages/Strategic-Plan.aspx. Accessed September 13, 2018
16. Hagan JF, Shaw JS, Duncan PM, eds. *Bright Futures: Guidelines for Health Supervision of Infants, Children, and Adolescents*. 4th ed. Elk Grove Village, IL: American Academy of Pediatrics; 2017
17. Council on Community Pediatrics. Providing care for immigrant, migrant, and border children. *Pediatrics*. 2013;131(6). Available at: www.pediatrics.org/cgi/content/full/131/6/e2028
18. Council on Community Pediatrics. Providing care for children and adolescents facing homelessness and housing insecurity. *Pediatrics*. 2013;131(6):1206–1210

19. American Academy of Pediatrics, Council on Community Pediatrics and Committee on Native American Child Health. Policy statement: health equity and children's rights. *Pediatrics*. 2010; 125(4):838–849. Reaffirmed October 2013

20. Gee GC, Walsemann KM, Brondolo E. A life course perspective on how racism may be related to health inequities. *Am J Public Health*. 2012;102(5):967–974

21. Gee GC. Leveraging the social determinants to build a culture of health. 2016. Available at: https://healthequity.globalpolicysolutions.org/wp-content/uploads/2016/12/RWJF_SDOH_Final_Report-002.pdf. Accessed March 19, 2019

22. Gee GC, Ford CL. Structural racism and health inequities: old issues, new directions. *Du Bois Rev*. 2011;8(1): 115–132

23. The World Health Organization. Social determinants of health. Available at: www.who.int/social_determinants/thecommission/finalreport/key_concepts/en/. Accessed August 24, 2017

24. Nyborg VM, Curry JF. The impact of perceived racism: psychological symptoms among African American boys. *J Clin Child Adolesc Psychol*. 2003; 32(2):258–266

25. Dominguez TP, Dunkel-Schetter C, Glynn LM, Hobel C, Sandman CA. Racial differences in birth outcomes: the role of general, pregnancy, and racism stress. *Health Psychol*. 2008;27(2): 194–203

26. Viner RM, Ozer EM, Denny S, et al. Adolescence and the social determinants of health. *Lancet*. 2012; 379(9826):1641–1652

27. Hogben M, Leichliter JS. Social determinants and sexually transmitted disease disparities. *Sex Transm Dis*. 2008;35(suppl 12):S13–S18

28. Crosby RA, Holtgrave DR. The protective value of social capital against teen pregnancy: a state-level analysis. *J Adolesc Health*. 2006;38(5):556–559

29. Upchurch DM, Mason WM, Kusunoki Y, Kriechbaum MJ. Social and behavioral determinants of self-reported STD among adolescents. *Perspect Sex Reprod Health*. 2004;36(6):276–287

30. Slopen N, Williams DR. Discrimination, other psychosocial stressors, and self-reported sleep duration and difficulties. *Sleep (Basel)*. 2014;37(1):147–156

31. Cohen S, Janicki-Deverts D, Doyle WJ, et al. Chronic stress, glucocorticoid receptor resistance, inflammation, and disease risk. *Proc Natl Acad Sci USA*. 2012;109(16):5995–5999

32. Riddell CA, Harper S, Kaufman JS. Trends in differences in US mortality rates between black and white infants. *JAMA Pediatr*. 2017;171(9):911–913

33. Lu MC, Kotelchuck M, Hogan V, Jones L, Wright K, Halfon N. Closing the Black-White gap in birth outcomes: a life-course approach. *Ethn Dis*. 2010; 20(1,suppl 2):S2–S62–S76

34. Gadson A, Akpovi E, Mehta PK. Exploring the social determinants of racial/ethnic disparities in prenatal care utilization and maternal outcome. *Semin Perinatol*. 2017;41(5):308–317

35. Almond D, Hoynes HW, Whitmore Schanzenbach D. Inside the War on Poverty: impact of food stamps on birth outcomes. Available at: https://www.irp.wisc.edu/publications/dps/pdfs/dp135908.pdf. Accessed March 19, 2019

36. Robert Wood Johnson Foundation; Pew Charitable Trusts. Health Impact Assessment and Housing: opportunities for the Housing Sector. Available at: www.pewtrusts.org/~/media/assets/2016/03/opportunities_for_the_housing_sector.pdf. Accessed August 29, 2017

37. US Office of the Surgeon General. *The Surgeon General's Call to Action to Promote Healthy Homes*. Rockville, MD: Office of the Surgeon General; 2009

38. Larson K, Cull WL, Racine AD, Olson LM. Trends in access to health care services for US children: 2000-2014. *Pediatrics*. 2016;138(6):e20162176

39. Matthew DB, Rodrigue E, Reeves RV; Brookings Institute. Time for justice: tackling race inequalities in health and housing. 2016. Available at: https://www.brookings.edu/research/time-for-justice-tackling-race-inequalities-in-health-and-housing/. Accessed September 13, 2018

40. Jones J; Economic Policy Institute. Unemployment of black and Hispanic workers remains high relative to white workers. 2018. Available at: https://www.epi.org/publication/unemployment-of-black-and-hispanic-workers-remains-high-relative-to-white-workers-in-16-states-and-the-district-of-columbia-the-african-american-unemployment-rate-is-at-least-twice-the-rate-of-white/. Accessed March 12, 2019

41. US Department of Labor, Bureau of Labor Statistics. Labor force statistics from Current Population Survey. 2019. Available at: https://www.bls.gov/web/empsit/cpsee_e16.htm. Accessed March 12, 2019

42. US Department of Labor, Bureau of Labor Statistics. Labor market trends for American Indians and Alaskan natives 2000-2017. Available at: https://www.bls.gov/opub/ted/2018/labor-market-trends-for-american-indians-and-alaska-natives-2000-17.htm. Accessed March 12, 2019

43. History D. The Native American Power movement. 2016. Available at: www.digitalhistory.uh.edu/disp_textbook.cfm?smtID=2&psid=3348. Accessed March 12, 2019

44. Dettling LJ, Hsu JW, Jacobs L, et al. Recent trends in wealth-holding by race and ethnicity: evidence from the survey of consumer finances. 2017. Available at: https://www.federalreserve.gov/econres/notes/feds-notes/recent-trends-in-wealth-holding-by-race-and-ethnicity-evidence-from-the-survey-of-consumer-finances-20170927.htm. Accessed March 12, 2019

45. Henderson T; Pew Charitable Trusts. The (very) few places with no black-white income gap. Stateline. 2016. Available at: www.pewtrusts.org/en/research-and-analysis/blogs/stateline/2016/11/10/the-very-few-places-with-no-black-white-income-gap. Accessed March 12, 2019

46. Committee on Adolescence. Health care for youth in the juvenile justice system. *Pediatrics*. 2011;128(6):1219–1235

47. American Academy of Pediatrics, Committee on Adolescence. Health care for youth in the juvenile justice system. *Pediatrics*. 2011;128(6):1219–1235. Reaffirmed May 2015

48. Kruger DJ, De Loney EH. The association of incarceration with community health and racial health disparities. *Prog*

Community Health Partnersh. 2009;3(2): 113–121

49. Lambie I, Randell I. The impact of incarceration on juvenile offenders. *Clin Psychol Rev.* 2013;33(3):448–459

50. Development Services Group I. Alternatives to detention and confinement. 2014. Available at: https://www.ojjdp.gov/mpg/litreviews/AlternativesToDetentionand Confinement.pdf. Accessed August 29, 2017

51. Whitley K, Rozel JS. Mental health care of detained youth and solitary confinement and restraint within juvenile detention facilities. *Child Adolesc Psychiatr Clin N Am.* 2016;25(1): 71–80

52. Jones CP, Jones CY, Perry GS, Barclay G, Jones CA. Addressing the social determinants of children's health: a cliff analogy. *J Health Care Poor Underserved.* 2009;20(suppl 4):1–12

53. Sussman RW. *The Myth of Race: The Troubling Persistence of an Unscientific Idea.* Cambridge, MA: Harvard University Press; 2014

54. United Nations Educational, Scientific and Cultural Organization. *Four Statements on the Race Question.* Paris, France: Oberthur-Rennes; 1969. Available at: http://unesdoc.unesco.org/images/0012/001229/122962eo.pdf. Accessed August 22, 2017

55. Collins FS. What we do and don't know about 'race', 'ethnicity', genetics and health at the dawn of the genome era. *Nat Genet.* 2004;36(suppl 11):S13–S15

56. Fullwiley D. Race and genetics: attempts to define the relationship. *Biosocieties.* 2007;2:221–237

57. National Research Council. *Measuring Racial Discrimination.* Washington, DC: National Academies Press; 2004. Available at: https://www.nap.edu/catalog/10887/measuring-racial-discrimination. Accessed June 16, 2019

58. Bhopal R, Donaldson L. White, European, Western, Caucasian, or what? Inappropriate labeling in research on race, ethnicity, and health. *Am J Public Health.* 1998;88(9):1303–1307

59. Fullilove MT. Comment: abandoning "race" as a variable in public health research–an idea whose time has come. *Am J Public Health.* 1998;88(9): 1297–1298

60. Bamshad M. Genetic influences on health: does race matter? *JAMA.* 2005; 294(8):937–946

61. Cheng TL, Goodman E; Committee on Pediatric Research. Race, ethnicity, and socioeconomic status in research on child health. *Pediatrics.* 2015;135(1). Available at: www.pediatrics.org/cgi/content/full/135/1/e225

62. National Public Radio. Hawaii is diverse, but far from paradise. 2009. Available at: https://www.npr.org/templates/story/story.php?storyId=120431126. Accessed April 5, 2019

63. Iggiagruk Hensley WL. There are two versions of the story of how the U.S. purchased Alaska from Russia. *Smithsonian Magazine.* March 29, 2017. Available at: https://www.smithsonianmag.com/history/why-russia-gave-alaska-americas-gateway-arctic-180962714/. Accessed April 6, 2019

64. US Department of State, Office of the Historian. Chinese immigration and the Chinese Exclusion Acts. Available at: https://history.state.gov/milestones/1866-1898/chinese-immigration. Accessed April 6, 2019

65. Japanese Americans Citizens League. Asian American history. Available at: https://jacl.org/asian-american-history/. Accessed April 5, 2019

66. Qureshi B; National Public Radio. From wrong to right: a U.S apology for Japanese internment. 2013. Available at: https://www.npr.org/sections/codeswitch/2013/08/09/210138278/japanese-internment-redress. Accessed April 5, 2019

67. Robert Wood Johnson Foundation. Discrimination: experiences and views on effects of discrimination across major population groups in the United States. Available at: https://www.rwjf.org/en/library/research/2017/10/discrimination-in-america–experiences-and-views.html. Accessed April 5, 2019

68. US Department of State, Office of the Historian. Indian treaties and the Native American Removal Act of 1830. Available at: https://history.state.gov/milestones/1830-1860/indian-treaties. Accessed August 24, 2017

69. US Department of State, Office of the Historian. 1830-1860 diplomacy and westward expansion. Available at: https://history.state.gov/milestones/1830-1860/foreword. Accessed August 24, 2017

70. Franklin JH. *From Slavery to Freedom.* 9th ed. New York, NY: McGraw-Hill; 2010

71. Rothstein R. *The Color of Law.* New York, NY: W.W. Norton & Co; 2017

72. Alexander M. *The New Jim Crow.* New York, NY: New Press; 2012

73. Xiao NG, Quinn PC, Liu S, Ge L, Pascalis O, Lee K. Older but not younger infants associate own-race faces with happy music and other-race faces with sad music. *Dev Sci.* 2018;21(2):e12537

74. Vogel M, Monesson A, Scott LS. Building biases in infancy: the influence of race on face and voice emotion matching. *Dev Sci.* 2012;15(3):359–372

75. Sangrigoli S, De Schonen S. Recognition of own-race and other-race faces by three-month-old infants. *J Child Psychol Psychiatry.* 2004;45(7):1219–1227

76. Jones CP. Levels of racism: a theoretic framework and a gardener's tale. *Am J Public Health.* 2000;90(8):1212–1215

77. Carmichael S, Hamilton CV. *Black Power: The Politics of Liberation in America.* New York, NY: Vintage Books; 1967

78. Jones CP. Invited commentary: "race," racism, and the practice of epidemiology. *Am J Epidemiol.* 2001; 154(4):299–304; discussion 305–306

79. Riera A, Walker DM. The impact of race and ethnicity on care in the pediatric emergency department. *Curr Opin Pediatr.* 2010;22(3):284–289

80. Laster M, Soohoo M, Hall C, et al. Racial-ethnic disparities in mortality and kidney transplant outcomes among pediatric dialysis patients. *Pediatr Nephrol.* 2017;32(4):685–695

81. Goyal MK, Kuppermann N, Cleary SD, Teach SJ, Chamberlain JM. Racial disparities in pain management of children with appendicitis in emergency departments. *JAMA Pediatr.* 2015;169(11):996–1002

82. Johnson TJ, Weaver MD, Borrero S, et al. Association of race and ethnicity with management of abdominal pain in the emergency department. *Pediatrics.*

2013;132(4). Available at: www.pediatrics.org/cgi/content/full/132/4/e851

83. Wickrama KA, Bae D, O'Neal CW. Black-white disparity in young adults' disease risk: an investigation of variation in the vulnerability of black young adults to early and later adversity. *J Adolesc Health*. 2016;59(2):209–214

84. Mulia N, Zemore SE. Social adversity, stress, and alcohol problems: are racial/ethnic minorities and the poor more vulnerable? *J Stud Alcohol Drugs*. 2012;73(4):570–580

85. Call KT, McAlpine DD, Johnson PJ, Beebe TJ, McRae JA, Song Y. Barriers to care among American Indians in public health care programs. *Med Care*. 2006;44(6):595–600

86. Puumala SE, Burgess KM, Kharbanda AB, et al. The role of bias by emergency department providers in care for American Indian children. *Med Care*. 2016;54(6):562–569

87. Rivas-Drake D, Seaton EK, Markstrom C, et al; Ethnic and Racial Identity in the 21st Century Study Group. Ethnic and racial identity in adolescence: implications for psychosocial, academic, and health outcomes. *Child Dev*. 2014;85(1):40–57

88. Brody GH, Yu T, Miller GE, Chen E. Discrimination, racial identity, and cytokine levels among African-American adolescents. *J Adolesc Health*. 2015;56(5):496–501

89. Cheng ER, Cohen A, Goodman E. The role of perceived discrimination during childhood and adolescence in understanding racial and socioeconomic influences on depression in young adulthood. *J Pediatr*. 2015;166(2):370–7.e1

90. Muuss R. *Theories of Adolescence*. 6th ed. New York, NY: McGraw Hill; 1996

91. Steele CM. *Whistling Vivaldi: How Stereotypes Affect Us and What We Can Do (Issues of Our Time)*. New York, NY: W.W. Norton & Co; 2011

92. Fischer P, Krueger JI, Greitemeyer T, et al. The bystander-effect: a meta-analytic review on bystander intervention in dangerous and non-dangerous emergencies. *Psychol Bull*. 2011;137(4):517–537

93. Leitner JB, Hehman E, Ayduk O, Mendoza-Denton R. Blacks' death rate due to circulatory diseases is positively related to whites' explicit racial bias. *Psychol Sci*. 2016;27(10):1299–1311

94. Wells AS, Fox L, Cordova D. How racially diverse schools and classrooms can benefit all students. 2016. Available at: https://tcf.org/content/report/how-racially-diverse-schools-and-classrooms-can-benefit-all-students/?agreed=1. Accessed September 14, 2018

95. National Center for Education Statistics. Schools and Staffing Survey (SASS). Available at: https://nces.ed.gov/surveys/sass/tables/sass0708_035_s1s.asp. Accessed August 25, 2017

96. Hofferth SL, Sandberg JF. How American children spend their time. *J Marriage Fam*. 2001;63:295–308

97. US Department of Health and Human Services, Office on Adolescent Health. A day in the life. Available at: https://www.hhs.gov/ash/oah/facts-and-stats/day-in-the-life/index.html. Accessed September 13, 2018

98. Robert Wood Johnson Foundation. The relationship between school attendance and health. 2016. Available at: https://www.rwjf.org/en/library/research/2016/09/the-relationship-between-school-attendance-and-health.html. Accessed September 13, 2018

99. McGill N; American Public Health Association. Education attainment linked to health throughout lifespan: exploring social determinants of health. *Nations Health*. 2016;46(6):1–19

100. Allison MA, Attisha E; Council on School Health. The link between school attendance and good health. *Pediatrics*. 2019;143(2):e20183648

101. US Department of Education. Chronic absenteeism in the nation's schools. Available at: https://www2.ed.gov/datastory/chronicabsenteeism.html#intro. Accessed August 25, 2017

102. Aranda E, Vaquera E. Racism, the immigration enforcement regime, and the implications for racial inequality in the lives of undocumented young adults. *Sociol Race Ethn (Thousand Oaks)*. 2015;1:104

103. National Center for Education Statistics. Public high school graduation rates. 2018. Available at: https://nces.ed.gov/programs/coe/indicator_coi.asp. Accessed September 13, 2018

104. Virginia Commonwealth University, Center on Health and Society. Education: it matters to health more than ever before. Available at: https://societyhealth.vcu.edu/work/the-projects/education-it-matters-more-to-health-than-ever-before.html. Accessed August 25, 2017

105. US Department of Education. Equity of opportunity. Available at: https://www.ed.gov/equity. Accessed August 25, 2017

106. Morgan PL, Farkas G, Hilliemeier MM, Maczuga S. Replicated evidence of racial and ethnic disparities in disability identification in U.S. schools. *Educ Res*. 2017;46(6):305–322

107. White GB. The data are damning: how race influences school funding. *The* Atlantic. September 30, 2015. Available at: https://www.theatlantic.com/business/archive/2015/09/public-school-funding-and-the-role-of-race/408085/. Accessed September 14, 2018

108. Derman-Sparks L, Ramsey G. *What If All the Kids Are White? Multicultural/Anti-Bias Education With White Children*. 2nd ed. New York, NY: Teachers' College Press; 2011

109. Birch SH, Ladd GW. The teacher-child relationship and children's early school adjustment. *J Sch Psychol*. 1997;35(1):61–79

110. Lowenstein AE, Friedman-Krauss AH, Raver CC, Jones SM, Pess RA. School climate, teacher-child closeness, and low-income children's academic skills in kindergarten. *J Educ Develop Psychol*. 2015;5(2):89–108

111. Alvidrez J, Weinstein RS. Early teacher perceptions and later student academic achievement. *J Educ Psychol*. 1999;91(4):731–746

112. Bates LA, Glick JE. Does it matter if teachers and schools match the student? Racial and ethnic disparities in problem behaviors. *Soc Sci Res*. 2013;42(5):1180–1190

113. Gershenson S, Holt S, Papageorge NW. Who believes in me? The effect of student–teacher demographic match on teacher expectations. *Econ Educ Rev*. 2016;52:209–224

114. Cherng H. If they think I can: teacher bias and youth of color expectations and achievement. *Soc Sci Res*. 2017;66: 170–186

115. Gershenson S, Hart CMD, Lindsay CA, Papageorge NW. IZA DP No. 10630: the long run impacts of same-race teachers. Available at: http://ftp.iza.org/dp10630.pdf. Accessed June 16, 2019

116. National Center for Education Statistics. Fast facts: back to school statistics. 2018. Available at: https://nces.ed.gov/fastfacts/display.asp?id=372. Accessed March 12, 2019

117. Byrd CM. *Student Perceptions of Racial Climate in Secondary Education: Effects of Climate's Multiple Dimensions on Academic Achievement and Motivation*. Ann Arbor, MI: University of Michigan, Horace H. Rackham School of Graduate Studies; 2012

118. Mattison E, Aber MS. Closing the achievement gap: the association of racial climate with achievement and behavioral outcomes. *Am J Community Psychol*. 2007;40(1–2):1–12

119. US Government Accountability Office (GAO). K-12 education: discipline disparities for black students, boys, and students with disabilities (GAO-18-258). 2018. Available at: https://www.gao.gov/products/GAO-18-258. Accessed March 12, 2019

120. US Department of Education, Office on Civil Rights. 2013-2014 civil rights data: a first look. 2016. Available at: https://www2.ed.gov/about/offices/list/ocr/docs/2013-14-first-look.pdf. Accessed March 12, 2019

121. Wong CA, Eccles JS, Sameroff A. The influence of ethnic discrimination and ethnic identification on African American adolescents' school and socioemotional adjustment. *J Pers*. 2003;71(6):1197–1232

122. Caughy MO, O'Campo PJ, Randolph SM, Nickerson K. The influence of racial socialization practices on the cognitive and behavioral competence of African American preschoolers. *Child Dev*. 2002; 73(5):1611–1625

123. Anderson AT, Jackson A, Jones L, Kennedy DP, Wells K, Chung PJ. Minority parents' perspectives on racial socialization and school readiness in the early childhood period. *Acad Pediatr*. 2015;15(4):405–411

124. Waseem M, Paul A, Schwartz G, et al. Role of pediatric emergency physicians in identifying bullying. *J Emerg Med*. 2017;52(2):246–252

125. Juvonen J, Graham S, Schuster MA. Bullying among young adolescents: the strong, the weak, and the troubled. *Pediatrics*. 2003;112(6, pt 1):1231–1237

126. Committee on Injury, Violence, and Poison Prevention. Policy statement–Role of the pediatrician in youth violence prevention. *Pediatrics*. 2009;124(1):393–402

127. Committee on Hospital Care and Institute For Patient- and Family-Centered Care. Patient- and family-centered care and the pediatrician's role. *Pediatrics*. 2012;129(2):394–404

128. Lang KR, Dupree CY, Kon AA, Dudzinski DM. Calling out implicit racial bias as a harm in pediatric care. *Camb Q Healthc Ethics*. 2016;25(3):540–552

129. Society for Adolescent Health and Medicine. International youth justice systems: promoting youth development and alternative approaches: a position paper of the society for adolescent health and medicine. *J Adolesc Health*. 2016;59(4):482–486

130. Barnert ES, Dudovitz R, Nelson BB, et al. How does incarcerating young people affect their adult health outcomes? *Pediatrics*. 2017;139(2):e20162624

131. Richardson S, Williams T. Why is cultural safety essential in health care? *Med Law*. 2007;26(4):699–707

132. Gibbons FX, Roberts ME, Gerrard M, et al. The impact of stress on the life history strategies of African American adolescents: cognitions, genetic moderation, and the role of discrimination. *Dev Psychol*. 2012;48(3): 722–739

133. Landrine H, Klonoff EA. The schedule of racist events: a measure of racial discrimination and a study of its negative physical and mental health consequences. *J Black Psychol*. 1996; 22(2):144–168

134. Pachter LM, Szalacha LA, Bernstein BA, Coll CG. Perceptions of Racism in Children and Youth (PRaCY): properties of a self-report instrument for research on children's health and development. *Ethn Health*. 2010;15(1):33–46

135. American Academy of Pediatrics. Engaging patients and families: providing culturally effective care toolkit. Available at: https://www.aap.org/en-us/professional-resources/practice-transformation/managing-patients/Pages/effective-care.aspx. Accessed March 12, 2019

136. National Resource Center for Patient/Family-Centered Medical Home. What is medical home? Available at: https://medicalhomeinfo.aap.org/overview/Pages/Whatisthemedicalhome.aspx. Accessed March 12, 2019

137. Ward JV. Raising resisters: the role of truth telling in the psycho-logical development of African American girls. In: Weis L, Fine M, eds. *Construction Sites: Excavating Race, Class and Gender Among Urban Youth*. New York, NY: Teachers College Press; 2000:64

138. Ward JV. *The Skin We're in: Teaching Our Teens to be Emotional Strong, Socially Smart, and Spiritually Connected*. New York, NY: Free Press; 2002

139. Barksdale CL, Rodick WH III, Hopson R, Kenyon J, Green K, Jacobs CG. Literature review of the national CLAS standards: policy and practical implications in reducing health disparities. *J Racial Ethn Health Disparities*. 2017;4(4): 632–647

140. US Department of Health and Human Services. National CLAS standards. Available at: https://www.thinkculturalhealth.hhs.gov/clas. Accessed August 29, 2017

141. Brown P, Tierney C. Media role in violence and the dynamics of bullying. *Pediatr Rev*. 2011;32(10):453–454

142. Slopen N, Shonkoff JP, Albert MA, et al. Racial disparities in child adversity in the U.S.: interactions with family immigration history and income. *Am J Prev Med*. 2016;50(1):47–56

143. Sampson RJ, Wilson WJ. Toward a theory of race, crime, and urban inequality. In: Hagan J, Peterson RD, eds. *Crime and Inequality*. Stanford, CA: Stanford University Press; 1995:56

144. Marsac ML, Kassam-Adams N, Hildenbrand AK, et al. Implementing a trauma-informed approach in

pediatric health care networks. *JAMA Pediatr.* 2016;170(1):70–77

145. Ginsburg KR, Kinsman SB. *Reaching Teens: Strength-Based Communication Strategies to Build Resilience and Support Healthy Adolescent Development.* Elk Grove, IL: American Academy of Pediatrics; 2014

146. Gaskin A; American Psychological Association. Racial socialization: ways parents can teach their children about race. 2015. Available at: www.apa.org/pi/families/resources/newsletter/2015/08/racial-socialization.aspx. Accessed March 12, 2019

147. High PC, Klass P; Council on Early Childhood. Literacy promotion: an essential component of primary care pediatric practice. *Pediatrics.* 2014;134(2):404–409

148. Sectish TC, Zalneraitis EL, Carraccio C, Behrman RE. The state of pediatrics residency training: a period of transformation of graduate medical education. *Pediatrics.* 2004;114(3):832–841

149. Carraccio C, Burke AE. Beyond competencies and milestones: adding meaning through context. *J Grad Med Educ.* 2010;2(3):419–422

150. Cross T, Bazron B, Dennis K, Isaacs M, eds. *Towards a Culturally Competent System of Care.* Washington, DC: CASSP Technical Assistance Center, Center for Child Health and Mental Health Policy, Georgetown University Child Development Center; 1989

151. Tervalon M, Murray-García J. Cultural humility versus cultural competence: a critical distinction in defining physician training outcomes in multicultural education. *J Health Care Poor Underserved.* 1998;9(2):117–125

152. Saha S, Beach MC, Cooper LA. Patient centeredness, cultural competence and healthcare quality. *J Natl Med Assoc.* 2008;100(11):1275–1285

153. Saha S, Korthuis PT, Cohn JA, Sharp VL, Moore RD, Beach MC. Primary care provider cultural competence and racial disparities in HIV care and outcomes. *J Gen Intern Med.* 2013;28(5):622–629

154. Ho MJ, Yao G, Lee KL, Hwang TJ, Beach MC. Long-term effectiveness of patient-centered training in cultural competence: what is retained? What is lost? *Acad Med.* 2010;85(4):660–664

155. Paez KA, Allen JK, Beach MC, Carson KA, Cooper LA. Physician cultural competence and patient ratings of the patient-physician relationship. *J Gen Intern Med.* 2009;24(4):495–498

156. Maguire MS, Kottenhahn R, Consiglio-Ward L, Smalls A, Dressler R. Using a poverty simulation in graduate medical education as a mechanism to introduce social determinants of health and cultural competency. *J Grad Med Educ.* 2017;9(3):386–387

157. Barkin S, Balkrishnan R, Manuel J, Hall MA. Effect of language immersion on communication with Latino patients. *N C Med J.* 2003;64(6):258–262

158. Federal Interagency Forum on Child and Family Statistics. America's children in brief: key national indicators of well-being, 2018. Available at: https://www.childstats.gov/americaschildren/demo.asp. Accessed August 25, 2017

159. Katkin JP, Kressly SJ, Edwards AR, et al; Task Force on Pediatric Practice Change. Guiding principles for team-based pediatric care. *Pediatrics.* 2017;140(2):e20171489

160. Hall WJ, Chapman MV, Lee KM, et al. Implicit racial/ethnic bias among health care professionals and its influence on health care outcomes: a systematic review. *Am J Public Health.* 2015;105(12):e60–e76

161. Committee on Pediatric Workforce. Enhancing pediatric workforce diversity and providing culturally effective pediatric care: implications for practice, education, and policy making. *Pediatrics.* 2013;132(4). Reaffirmed October 2015. Available at: www.pediatrics.org/cgi/content/full/132/4/e1105

162. The Joint Commission. Implicit bias in healthcare. 2016. Available at: https://www.jointcommission.org/assets/1/23/Quick_Safety_Issue_23_Apr_2016.pdf. Accessed March 12, 2019

163. Jee-Lyn Garcia J, Sharif MZ. Black lives matter: a commentary on racism and public health. *Am J Public Health.* 2015;105(8):e27–e30

164. American Public Health Association. Racism and health. Available at: https://www.apha.org/topics-and-issues/health-equity/racism-and-health. Accessed December 19, 2017

165. Devore CD, Wheeler LS; Council on School Health; American Academy of Pediatrics. Role of the school physician. *Pediatrics.* 2013;131(1):178–182

166. Council on School Health. The role of the school nurse in providing school health services. *J Sch Nurs.* 2008;24(5):269–274

167. van den Bergh L, Denessen E, Hornstra L, Voeten M, Holland RW. The implicit prejudiced attitudes of teachers: relations to teacher expectations and the ethnic achievement gap. *Am Educ Res J.* 2010;47(2):527

168. Mendelson T, Tandon SD, O'Brennan L, Leaf PJ, Ialongo NS. Brief report: moving prevention into schools: the impact of a trauma-informed school-based intervention. *J Adolesc.* 2015;43:142–147

169. Gilliam WS, Maupin AN, Reyes CR. Early childhood mental health consultation: results of a statewide random-controlled evaluation. *J Am Acad Child Adolesc Psychiatry.* 2016;55(9):754–761

170. Southern Poverty Law Center. Perspectives for a diverse America. Available at: www.tolerance.org/sites/default/files/general/Perspectives%20for%20a%20Diverse%20America%20User%20Experience.pdf. Accessed August 26, 2017

171. Gershenson S, Dee TS; Brookings Institute. The insidiousness of unconscious bias. 2017. Available at: https://www.brookings.edu/blog/brown-center-chalkboard/2017/03/20/the-insidiousness-of-unconscious-bias-in-schools/. Accessed March 12, 2019

172. Kirwan Institute, Ohio State University. Interventions to address racialized discipline disparities and school "push out." Available at: http://kirwaninstitute.osu.edu/wp-content/uploads/2014/05/ki-interventions.pdf. Accessed November 24, 2017

173. Southern Poverty Law Center. Teaching tolerance. Available at: https://www.splcenter.org/teaching-tolerance. Accessed August 26, 2017

174. National Child Traumatic Stress Network. Addressing race and trauma in the classroom: a resource for educators. 2017. Available at: https://

www.nctsn.org/resources/addressing-race-and-trauma-classroom-resource-educators. Accessed March 12, 2019

175. Boyd RW, Ellison AM, Horn IB. Police, equity, and child health. *Pediatrics*. 2016;137(3):e20152711

176. The Pew Charitable Trusts/Research & Analysis. Re-examining juvenile incarceration: high cost, poor outcomes spark shift to alternatives. 2015. Available at: https://www.pewtrusts.org/en/research-and-analysis/issue-briefs/2015/04/reexamining-juvenile-incarceration. Accessed March 12, 2019

177. Chamberlain P, Reid JB. Comparison of two community alternatives to incarceration for chronic juvenile offenders. *J Consult Clin Psychol*. 1998; 66(4):624–633

178. Bostic JQ, Thurau L, Potter M, Drury SS. Policing the teen brain. *J Am Acad Child Adolesc Psychiatry*. 2014;53(2): 127–129

179. Mitchell B, Franco J. *HOLC "Redlining" Maps: The Persistent Structure of Segregation and Economic Inequality*. Washington, DC: National Community Reinvestment Coalition; 2018. Available at: https://ncrc.org/holc/. Accessed April 5, 2019

180. Heard-Garris N, Williams DR, Davis M. Structuring research to address discrimination as a factor in child and adolescent health. *JAMA Pediatr*. 2018; 172(10):910–912

Improving Health and Safety at Camp

- *Policy Statement*

POLICY STATEMENT Organizational Principles to Guide and Define the Child Health Care System and/or Improve the Health of all Children

American Academy of Pediatrics

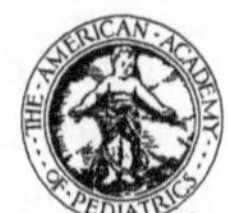

DEDICATED TO THE HEALTH OF ALL CHILDREN™

Improving Health and Safety at Camp

Michael J. Ambrose, MD, FAAP,[a] Edward A. Walton, MD, FAAP,[b] COUNCIL ON SCHOOL HEALTH

abstract

The American Academy of Pediatrics has created recommendations for health appraisal and preparation of young people before participation in day, resident, or family camps and to guide health and safety practices at camp. These recommendations are intended for parents and families, primary health care providers, and camp administration and health center staff. Although camps have diverse environments, there are general guidelines that apply to all situations and specific recommendations that are appropriate under special conditions. This policy statement has been reviewed and is supported by the American Camp Association and Association of Camp Nursing.

BENEFITS OF THE CAMP EXPERIENCE

For more than 150 years, children have been attending camp.[1] Today, more than 14 000 day and resident camps exist in the United States, and approximately 14 million children attend day or resident camp supported by 1.5 million staff members.[2] When there is a successful match between a camp's philosophy, practices, and methods and a child's developmental, experiential, and temperamental readiness, abilities, and nature, the camp experience has been proven to have a lasting effect on psychosocial development, with positive effects on self-esteem, peer relationships, independence, leadership, values, and willingness to try new things.[3] Camps can also offer an opportunity to overcome a lack of connection with the natural environment, which has been associated with depression, attention disorders, and obesity.[4] In addition, research has shown that camps are safe.[5]

Camp health care providers can expect to care for campers with any of the physical and emotional conditions seen daily by primary care providers. Because of these issues, the precamp health evaluation is extremely important. Parents, camp administrators, and camp health care providers should openly share consented information to help ensure that a camper is appropriately prepared for his or her new camp environment. In addition, parents and families should prepare their child for camp. Camp administration must create appropriate policies and procedures and work in cooperation with local health care providers and facilities to ensure off-site support is in place (eg, hospitals, police department, and fire department).

[a]St Joseph Mercy Hospital, Ann Arbor, Michigan; and [b]Ascension St John Hospital, Detroit, Michigan

Dr Ambrose conceptualized and designed the initial manuscript and revised the final manuscript; Dr Walton conceptualized and designed the initial manuscript; and both authors approved the final manuscript as submitted and agree to be accountable for all aspects of the work.

This document is copyrighted and is property of the American Academy of Pediatrics and its Board of Directors. All authors have filed conflict of interest statements with the American Academy of Pediatrics. Any conflicts have been resolved through a process approved by the Board of Directors. The American Academy of Pediatrics has neither solicited nor accepted any commercial involvement in the development of the content of this publication.

Policy statements from the American Academy of Pediatrics benefit from expertise and resources of liaisons and internal (AAP) and external reviewers. However, policy statements from the American Academy of Pediatrics may not reflect the views of the liaisons or the organizations or government agencies that they represent.

The guidance in this statement does not indicate an exclusive course of treatment or serve as a standard of medical care. Variations, taking into account individual circumstances, may be appropriate.

All policy statements from the American Academy of Pediatrics automatically expire 5 years after publication unless reaffirmed, revised, or retired at or before that time.

DOI: https://doi.org/10.1542/peds.2019-1355

Address correspondence to Michael J. Ambrose, MD, FAAP. E-mail: ambrosem@gmail.com

PEDIATRICS (ISSN Numbers: Print, 0031-4005; Online, 1098-4275).

Copyright © 2019 by the American Academy of Pediatrics

FINANCIAL DISCLOSURE: Dr Ambrose has indicated he is CEO and Founder of DocNetwork, Inc, an electronic health record system for camps, child care, and schools. Dr Walton has idicated he has no financial disclosures related to this article to disclose.

FUNDING: No external funding.

To cite: Ambrose MJ, Walton EA, AAP COUNCIL ON SCHOOL HEALTH. Improving Health and Safety at Camp. *Pediatrics.* 2019;144(1):e20191355

ROLE OF PARENTS AND GUARDIANS AND PRIMARY CARE PROVIDERS

Roles of parents and guardians and primary care providers include the following:

1. Before choosing a camp, parents or guardians should be encouraged to assess their child's interests, skills, and overall physical, mental, and emotional well-being and evaluate his or her ability to effectively participate in a particular camp setting. Camp Web sites, mission statements, and promotional handouts can help guide parents when choosing an appropriate camping environment for their child. Although many camps are inclusive and able to care for campers with chronic illnesses or specific psychosocial needs, camping programs for children with special needs are available (eg, camps for children with cancer, diabetes, asthma, attention-deficit/hyperactivity disorder [ADHD], autism spectrum disorder, and learning disabilities). Camps for special populations exist, including camps for lesbian, gay, bisexual, transgender, or questioning youth; grief and bereavement camps; and camps for gifted and talented children. The locations of camp programs may vary as well, with some camp programs being run on college and university campuses and others being run by municipalities (eg, parks and recreation). Before enrolling their child, parents should be aware of preadmission medical requirements for campers and the scope of health services available at camp. Parents are encouraged to discuss all camper health needs, including any special physical, emotional, or dietary needs, with camp health staff and camp directors before enrolling their child and before the start of the program.[6]
2. Some day and overnight camps offer programs that require an increased level of physical fitness because of strenuous activities and/or geographic factors, such as altitude or remote location. These camps may require a more extensive health evaluation relevant to the nature, conditions, and activities of the camp. Exact health requirements for participation will depend on the program. All campers, including day campers, resident campers, and family campers, should provide the camp with a complete health record before the first day of camp. The health record should be completed by the child's parents and/or guardians with input from the camper's primary care provider. This health record includes an annual review of the camper's health by a licensed health care provider and an annual physical examination as required by the program. It is recommended that the annual review and physical examination be completed by the child's primary care provider who is well known to him or her. This recommendation is consistent with those of *Bright Futures: Guidelines for Health Supervision of Infants, Children, and Adolescents, Fourth Edition.*[7] The appropriateness of the camp's program for the individual camper should be addressed during that review. The health care provider should be provided with pertinent information about the camp before the visit. For children with ongoing health care needs, it is important that the health record be updated before their arrival at camp.

The annual review should include a comprehensive health history, which addresses significant illnesses, surgeries, injuries, allergies, medications, and the present state of physical health of the child. The annual review should also include a history of the child's mental, emotional, and social health, including any family stressors and history of emotional trauma. Campers with clinically significant medical or psychosocial histories or those with conditions requiring long-term management should undergo further review by the medical provider before participation (eg, asthma, diabetes, anaphylactic allergies, mood or anxiety disorders, and ADHD). An action plan appropriate to the camper's condition and to the camp program should be created by the camper's medical provider and provided to the camp as needed (eg, asthma action plan, seizure action plan, and allergy action plan).[8] If provided, this plan should also address all medications, both prescription and over the counter, to be used by the individual while at camp.[9] The medical provider should perform the annual review on the basis of current practice guidelines, physician examination, history, and any appropriate testing, and if no obvious reasons for exclusion from camp have been identified, parents must also consider the child's individual risks and benefits of participation and understand that clearance is not a guarantee against adverse outcomes or future medical problems.

Written orders from a licensed health care provider should be obtained for prescription medications, medically indicated diets, physical activity limitations, or special medical devices.

3. Once the health record has been submitted to the camp, parents and guardians are responsible for providing the program with any changes in the camper's health status, allergies, medications, or recent travel before the camper arrives. Elective interruption in medications (ie, drug holidays) should be avoided in campers on long-term psychotropic therapy or those on maintenance therapy required for a chronic medical condition. If elective interruption

is in the best interest of the child, this should be disclosed to the camp before the camper arrives.[10–12]

4. Before starting camp, all campers and staff should be in compliance with the recommended childhood immunization schedule published annually by the American Academy of Pediatrics (AAP), the Advisory Committee on Immunization Practices of the Centers for Disease Control and Prevention (CDC), and the American Academy of Family Physicians.[13] Camp administrators should be aware that individual states might require other immunizations in addition to those recommended by these organizations. Immunization requirements for participation at camp provide a safe environment for those participating. Nonmedical exemptions to required immunizations are inappropriate, and these exemptions should be eliminated by camps. Participation by campers and staff who are incompletely immunized or unimmunized because of nonmedical exemptions is inappropriate for individual, public health, and ethical reasons. Camps should support medical exemptions to specific immunizations as determined for each individual (eg, those with congenital conditions, with compromised immune systems, or taking specific medications).[14] Individuals traveling internationally as part of a camp program should consult the CDC "Travelers' Health" Web site[15] or visit a traveler's clinic for information regarding particular immunization requirements or health concerns that may be associated with their destination.
5. Some inexperienced campers may experience acute psychological distress associated with separation from home and loved ones, commonly known as homesickness. Primary care providers may recommend the following interventions to provide help for prospective campers and their parents because they have been found to significantly reduce the incidence and severity of homesickness[11]:
   - involve the child in the process of choosing and preparing for camp;
   - discuss homesickness openly, be positive about the upcoming camp experience, and avoid expressing personal doubts or concerns;
   - arrange practice time away from home with friends or relatives before camp; and
   - frame the time to be spent at camp in comparison with previous enjoyable experiences the child may have had of similar duration.

Although homesickness is traditionally believed to affect resident campers, younger children attending day camp may suffer from homesickness as well. Parents should avoid making "pick-up" arrangements in the event of homesickness because these arrangements may undermine the child's confidence in his or her own independence.[11] Health care providers should discuss these interventions as part of the anticipatory guidance associated with the health evaluation before camp.

ROLE OF THE CAMP

Roles of the camp include the following:

1. Camp administrative officials should have a clear understanding of the essential functions of a camper insofar as their specific camp program is concerned.[16] It is the responsibility of the camp to provide parents, children, and primary health care providers with expectations for successful participation in the camp program. Certain camp activities may increase the risk of complications from specific medical conditions (eg, horseback riding, which may trigger an asthma exacerbation). It should be a combined effort of parents, health care providers, and camp personnel to identify children who might be at risk and specify the extent of accommodations necessary for safe participation for those children.
2. All camps should have written health policies and protocols that have been reviewed and approved by a physician with specialized training in children's health, preferably a pediatrician or family physician. These policies and protocols should be tailored to the training and scope of practice of the on-site camp health care providers and should be developed with the input of those individuals.[17,18] Camp administrators should inquire as to the previous training and camp experiences of camp health care providers and provide additional training or support if necessary. It is strongly recommended that camp health care providers have specialized training in children's health, including all physicians, nurses, nurse practitioners, and physician assistants who will provide care to children while they are at camp. If pediatric health care providers practice a subspecialty, their knowledge and practice of general pediatrics should be assessed before arrival to camp.[19]

Camp health policies and protocols should address both major and minor illnesses and injuries and include information on the camp's relationship and coordination with local emergency services.[20] Local emergency medical service providers should be contacted by camp directors before camp begins to ensure a prompt and coordinated response in the event of an emergency.[21,22] Camps should also establish relationships with local dentists and/or orthodontists who are willing to treat dental emergencies if the need arises as well as with local mental health professionals. The AAP encourages its members to cooperate with local camps in reviewing such policies and protocols and by providing medical support if practical.

3. The 2009–2010 H1N1 influenza pandemic, the emergence of methicillin-resistant *Staphylococcus aureus*, and the Zika and West Nile virus epidemics have highlighted the need for increased screening and surveillance at camps. There is increased importance for camps to teach good hygiene practices, including good hand-washing and coughing and/or sneeze behaviors and to ensure the appropriate use of insect repellent.[5] Camps should have management plans for infectious disease outbreaks in place.[23] These plans should include guidance for caring for ill campers or staff and for isolating ill people from the healthy population. Camp health care providers should also be aware of health hazards that are particular to their area (eg, Lyme disease and Rocky Mountain spotted fever).[24] A camp emergency plan should also be created because children are particularly vulnerable and limited in their ability to escape or protect themselves from harm in the event that a natural or manmade disaster occurs.[25]

For resident camps, all campers and staff should undergo a screening supervised by camp health providers on arrival. This screening should assess the potential for communicable diseases, establish a health status baseline, and identify health problems, such as febrile illness or lice. Children with febrile illness (temperature higher than 38°C) should be isolated from the general camp population until they have been fever free for 24 hours. Camps should abandon "no-nit" policies, and children with active lice infestations should be allowed to return to camp activities after treatment.[26] Updated medication orders and health history should also be made available to camp health staff on initial arrival at camp.

4. Whenever possible, camper medications should be sent to camp before the camper arrives so that camp health care providers have adequate time to review and sort all medications and address any concerns. Camp health care providers with appropriate knowledge and training should be responsible for the safe storage, transport, and administration of medications. Relying on handwritten instructions when administering medications can lead to medication errors.[27] The use of an electronic medication administration record is encouraged to minimize the potential for human error and ensure the right camper, right drug, right dose, right route, right time, and right documentation when administering medications. Prepackaged medication services should be considered to reduce preventable medication errors and eliminate the risk of missed medications or incorrect dosing. A protocol should be established for safe transport of medications during out-of-camp trips, and a determination should be made by the on-site health care provider as to the skill of camp personnel to administer medications and the safety of sending a particular child on the trip.[9]

5. Camps that maintain over-the-counter and emergency medication, oxygen, or other emergency equipment should routinely check supplies and expiration dates and ensure that necessary training has been completed. Recent guidelines support the use of automated external defibrillators (AEDs) in children 1 year or older.[28] All camps should have an AED on-site. Camps with an AED should comply with local regulations regarding required protocols and training in their use. Campers should be instructed in the use of personal emergency medications or medical devices, such as inhalers or epinephrine autoinjectors, before arrival at camp. Many states have legislation allowing camps to stock unassigned epinephrine autoinjectors, and some states have laws requiring that camps stock unassigned epinephrine devices. Camps should review local regulations and requirements for stocking unassigned epinephrine and other emergency medications for seizures, diabetes mellitus, or opioid overdose. Parents should also make clear to the camp staff primarily responsible for their campers the situations that may require use of these medications and whether the children are competent to carry or administer the medication themselves. Specific protocols and training for administration of these medications or use of specialized equipment by the camper, counselors, or other unlicensed providers should be created. These devices should be kept in locations that are easily accessible to individuals who may need them.[9,29]

6. Use of an electronic health record to capture camper and staff medical information that is compliant with federal guidelines is encouraged to ensure easy

access to medical records and emergency contact information at all times.[30,31] The parent or guardian with legal custody should be clearly indicated. Protocols for parental notification should be established. In addition, if a chronic condition exists, the child's primary care physician and any subspecialty physicians should be identified by name, telephone number, and e-mail, and the date of the last health care visit should be noted.[32] Written or electronic authorization to obtain treatment, to transport children in camp vehicles for nonemergency care, and to share medical information should be provided by the parent or guardian.[33] Camps should make their requirements for health insurance coverage clear, and parents or guardians should ensure that their insurance policy is in force at the camp's location. Supplemental travel and emergency medical insurance may be recommended for travel camps or camps where higher-risk activities occur. Confidentiality of health information should be maintained.[34]

7. All illnesses and injuries should be documented for campers and staff. This documentation should be consistent with state or local licensing requirements and allow for surveillance of the camp illness and injury profile.[5] Documentation in the "SOAP" note format (subjective, objective, assessment, and plan), a widely adopted documentation format for interdisciplinary health care providers, to capture a camper's or staff's initial visit and monitor progress during follow-up care is encouraged.[35]
8. It is important for all camps to have personnel who can administer on-site first aid irrespective of their distance from definitive medical care (eg, cardiopulmonary resuscitation, epinephrine for anaphylaxis, glucagon for hypoglycemia, and rescue treatments for seizures). A health care provider or staff member with the appropriate training must be on duty at all times, both at camp and on off-site trips. This statement does not address specific camp staff training issues; however, those who are involved in waterfront activities, including lifeguards, should be certified in cardiopulmonary resuscitation.
9. Pediatric campers with food allergies are at greater risk for exposure and anaphylaxis when outside their usual environment. Children with food allergies represent about 8% of the pediatric population, with nearly 40% of those children having a history of severe reaction requiring immediate intervention.[36] Those who are directly responsible for care of the camper's with food allergies should receive hands-on training to recognize anaphylaxis and administer epinephrine. Camps should create and provide their food allergy policies to families before the start of camp and discuss those policies with food vendors. Cross-contamination prevention policies should be established, including washing tables before and after meals, hand-washing practices, serving peanut butter in packets with separate utensils, and not allowing food in camper cabins.
10. Head injuries can cause long-term symptoms and complications, and appropriate management is essential for reducing physical and cognitive deficits.[37] Camp activities should be designed to limit the risk of head injuries, and camps should provide the proper equipment and supervision to decrease the incidence and severity of head injuries. Camp staff should have a clear understanding of the definition, signs, and symptoms of concussion and should follow CDC and state-specific return-to-play guidelines before an individual with a head injury participates in competitive or recreational activities to avoid reinjury or prolonged recovery. If a qualified health care provider is not available on-site to evaluate children with suspected head injuries, children should be taken to the nearest medical facility for urgent evaluation.[38]
11. Camp staff should be trained to effectively respond to camper mental, emotional, and social health needs. Many children who attend camp will have had a diagnosis of ADHD, autism spectrum disorder, or eating disorders, among other diagnoses. Camps should educate their staff about mental health problems, teach staff to support campers who need extra help, and help facilitate communication with parents. Camps should consider using a camp social worker who can assist with psychosocial concerns. A full-time administrator who oversees health care at the camp should also be considered for continuity of care during camp because many camp physicians and nurses rotate and may only be present for short periods of time.[39]
12. Obesity and related cardiovascular risk factors are important health priorities, and camp communities should adhere to principles of healthy living.[40] Food that is served and sold in camps should, at least, follow federal guidelines for school nutrition. Camp staff should model healthy food choices for their campers. Food

should not be used as a reward, nor should withholding food be used as a punishment. At least 30 minutes of daily physical activity should be included as a component of any camp program. Plain water should be available throughout the day, and sweetened beverages, including sports drinks, should be strictly limited or simply not used.[41]

13. The principles promoted in this statement apply to all camps. It should be noted, however, that inclusion of children with disabilities and other special health care needs may require the establishment of additional assessments and services, and it is strongly recommended that all camps adhere to the Americans with Disabilities Act and make the necessary accommodations to maintain an atmosphere of inclusion for all. Appropriate pairing of the camper with camp facilities and camp resources should take place at the application stage of camp enrollment.[42] Camps should address accessibility and have equipment available so that all campers and staff can participate in camp activities (eg, adaptive bath chairs and pool lifts). Camp staff should be trained to assist campers who require help with routine activities of daily living, such as dressing, bathing, and toileting.[32] In addition, camp personnel should be familiar with the health and safety guidelines for child care centers developed by the AAP, American Public Health Association, and Maternal and Child Health Bureau and should adhere to those appropriate to their programs and facilities.[43]

Parents and guardians should feel confident that their children are ready for camp and that their chosen camp is well prepared to care for their children. To this end, the AAP offers the aforementioned recommendations for creating a healthy and safe camp experience.

ADDITIONAL RESOURCES

American Academy of Pediatrics. Coding at the AAP. Available at: https://www.aap.org/en-us/professional-resources/practice-transformation/getting-paid/Coding-at-the-AAP/Pages/default.aspx.

American Camp Association. American Camp Association's accreditation process guide. Available at: https://www.acacamps.org/staff-professionals/accreditation-standards/accreditation.

American Camp Association. Health forms and records. Available at: www.acacamps.org/resource-library/forms/health-forms-records.

Donoghue EA, Kraft CA. Managing Chronic Health Needs Children in Child Care and School. Elk Grove Village, IL: American Academy of Pediatrics; 2009.

Erceg LE, Pravda M. The Basics of Camp Nursing, 2nd ed. Monterey, CA: Healthy Learning; 2009.

Harris SS, Anderson SJ, eds. Care of the Young Athlete. 2nd ed. Elk Grove Village, IL: American Academy of Pediatrics; 2010.

Louv R. Last Child in the Woods. Chapel Hill, NC: Algonquin Books; 2008.

Thuber CA, Malinowski JC. The Summer Camp Handbook. Los Angeles, CA: Perspective Publishing; 2000.

Thurber CA. The Secret Ingredients of Summer Camp Success: How to Have the Most Fun with the Least Homesickness [DVD/CD]. Martinsville, IN: American Camp Association; 2006.

LEAD AUTHORS

Michael J. Ambrose, MD, FAAP
Edward A. Walton, MD, FAAP

CONSULTANTS

Tracey Gaslin, PhD, CPNP, FNP-BC, CRNI, Association of Camp Nursing
Linda Ebner Erceg, RN, MS, PHN, Association of Camp Nursing

COUNCIL ON SCHOOL HEALTH, 2018–2019

Marc Lerner, MD, FAAP, Chairperson
Cheryl De Pinto, MD, MPH, FAAP, Chairperson-Elect
Marti Baum, MD, FAAP
Nathaniel Savio Beers, MD, MPA, FAAP
Sara Bode, MD, FAAP
Erica J. Gibson, MD, FAAP
Peter Gorski, MD, MPA, FAAP
Chris Kjolhede, MD, MPH, FAAP
Sonja C. O'Leary, MD, FAAP
Heidi Schumacher, MD, FAAP
Adrienne Weiss-Harrison, MD, FAAP

FORMER EXECUTIVE COMMITTEE MEMBERS

Mandy Allison, MD, MSPH, FAAP
Richard Ancona, MD, FAAP
Elliott Attisha, DO, FAAP
Breena Welch Holmes, MD, FAAP, Immediate Past Chairperson
Jeffrey Okamoto MD, FAAP, Past Chairperson
Thomas Young, MD, FAAP

LIAISONS

Susan Hocevar Adkins, MD, FAAP
Laurie Combe, MN, RN, NCSN
Delaney Gracy, MD, FAAP
Shashank Joshi, MD, FAAP

FORMER LIAISONS

Nina Fekaris, MS, BSN, RN, NCSN
Linda Grant, MD, MPH
Veda Charmaine Johnson, MD, FAAP
Sheryl Kataoka, MD, MSHS
Sandra Leonard, DNP, RN, FNP

STAFF

Stephanie Domain, MS

ABBREVIATIONS

AAP: American Academy of Pediatrics
ADHD: attention-deficit/hyperactivity disorder
AED: automated external defibrillator
CDC: Centers for Disease Control and Prevention

POTENTIAL CONFLICT OF INTEREST: Dr Ambrose has indicated he is CEO and Founder of DocNetwork, Inc, an electronic health record system for camps, child care, and schools. Dr Walton has indicated he has no potential conflicts of interest to disclose.

REFERENCES

1. American Camp Association. 100 year anniversary of the American Camp Association. Available at: www.acacamp.org/anniversary/. Accessed November 25, 2018
2. American Camp Association. ACA facts and trends. Available at: www.acacamps.org/press-room/aca-facts-trends. Accessed November 25, 2018
3. American Camp Association. Directions: youth outcomes of the camp experience. Available at: https://www.acacamps.org/sites/default/files/resource_library/report-directions-youth-development-outcomes.pdf. Accessed November 25, 2018
4. Louv R. *Last Child in the Woods*. Chapel Hill, NC: Algonquin Books; 2005
5. American Camp Association. Healthy camp study impact report 2006–2010. Available at: https://www.acacamps.org/sites/default/files/downloads/Healthy-Camp-Study-Impact-Report.pdf. Accessed November 25, 2018
6. American Camp Association. Healthy Camp Toolbox. Available at: www.acacamps.org/resource-library/research/healthy-camp-toolbox. Accessed November 25, 2018
7. Hagan J, Shaw J, Duncan P, eds. *Bright Futures: Guidelines for Health Supervision of Infants, Children and Adolescents*, 4th ed. Itasca, IL: American Academy of Pediatrics; 2017
8. American Academy of Pediatrics Council on School Health. Medical emergencies occurring at school. *Pediatrics*. 2008;122(4):887–894. Reaffirmed September 2011
9. American Academy of Pediatrics Council on School Health. Policy statement–guidance for the administration of medication in school. *Pediatrics*. 2009;124(4):1244–1251. Reaffirmed February 2013
10. Reiff MI, ed. *ADHD: A Complete and Authoritative Guide*. Itasca, IL: American Academy of Pediatrics; 2004
11. Thurber CA, Walton E; American Academy of Pediatrics Council on School Health. Preventing and treating homesickness. *Pediatrics*. 2007;119(1):192–201
12. Pelham WE, Gnagy EM, Greiner AR, et al. Behavioral versus behavioral and pharmacological treatment in ADHD children attending a summer treatment program. *J Abnorm Child Psychol*. 2000;28(6):507–525
13. Committee on Infectious Diseases. Recommended childhood and adolescent immunization schedules: United States, 2018. *Pediatrics*. 2018;141(3):e20180083
14. Committee on Practice and Ambulatory Medicine; Committee on Infectious Diseases; Committee on State Government Affairs; Council on School Health; Section on Administration and Practice Management. Medical versus nonmedical immunization exemptions for child care and school attendance. *Pediatrics*. 2016;138(3):e20162145
15. Centers for Disease Control and Prevention. Traveler's health. 2018. Available at: http://wwwnc.cdc.gov/travel. Accessed November 25, 2018
16. Erceg LE, Pravda M. *The Basics of Camp Nursing*. 2nd ed. Monterey, CA: Healthy Learning; 2009
17. American Academy of Pediatrics Committee on Pediatric Workforce. Scope of practice issues in the delivery of pediatric health care. *Pediatrics*. 2013;131(6):1211–1216. Reaffirmed October 2015
18. Association of Camp Nursing. *The Scope and Standards of Camp Nursing Practice*. 3rd ed. Bemidji, MN: Association of Camp Nurses; 2017
19. American Camp Association. Health care providers: who's best for my camp? Available at: https://www.acacamps.org/resource-library/camping-magazine/health-care-providers-whos-best-my-camp. Accessed November 25, 2018
20. American Camp Association. Communicable diseases and infestations. Available at: https://www.acacamps.org/staff-professionals/core-competencies/health-wellness/communicable-diseases-infestations. Accessed November 25, 2018
21. American Academy of Pediatrics; Committee on Pediatric Emergency Medicine; American College of Emergency Physicians; Pediatric Committee; Emergency Nurses Association Pediatric Committee. Joint policy statement–guidelines for care of children in the emergency department. *Pediatrics*. 2009;124(4):1233–1243
22. Walton EA, Maio RF, Hill EM. Camp health services in the state of Michigan. *Wilderness Environ Med*. 2004;15(4):274–283
23. Centers for Disease Control and Prevention. CDC guidance for day and residential camp responses to influenza during the 2010 summer camp season. 2010. Available at: www.cdc.gov/h1n1flu/camp.htm. Accessed November 25, 2018
24. American Academy of Pediatrics Committee on Infectious Diseases. American Academy of Pediatrics. Committee on Infectious Diseases. Prevention of Lyme disease. *Pediatrics*. 2000;105(1, pt 1):142–147
25. Chang M, Sielaff A, Bradin S, Walker K, Ambrose M, Hashikawa A. Assessing disaster preparedness among select children's summer camps in the United States and Canada. *South Med J*. 2017;110(8):502–508
26. Devore CD, Schutze GE; Council on School Health and Committee on Infectious Diseases, American Academy of Pediatrics. Head lice [published correction appears in *Pediatrics*. 2015;135(5):e1355–e1365]. *Pediatrics*. 2015;135(5). Available at: www.pediatrics.org/cgi/content/full/135/5/e1355
27. The Joint Commission. Preventing pediatric medication errors. *Sentinel Event Alert*. 2008;(39):1–4

28. American Heart Association. *Pediatric Advanced Life Support (PALS) Provider Manual.* 16th ed. Dallas, TX: American Heart Association; 2016

29. Schellpfeffer NR, Leo HL, Ambrose M, Hashikawa AN. Food allergy trends and epinephrine autoinjector presence in summer camps. *J Allergy Clin Immunol Pract.* 2017;5(2):358–362

30. National Coordinator for Health Information Technology. About ONC. Available at: https://www.healthit.gov/topic/about-onc. Accessed November 25, 2018

31. Spooner SA; Council on Clinical Information Technology, American Academy of Pediatrics. Special requirements of electronic health record systems in pediatrics. *Pediatrics.* 2007;119(3):631–637

32. American Academy of Pediatrics Committee on Pediatric Emergency Medicine and Council on Clinical Information Technology; American College of Emergency Physicians Pediatric Emergency Medicine Committee. Policy statement–emergency information forms and emergency preparedness for children with special health care needs. *Pediatrics.* 2010;125(4):829–837. Reaffirmed October 2014

33. Fanaroff JM; Committee on Medical Liability and Risk Management. Consent by proxy for nonurgent pediatric care. *Pediatrics.* 2017;139(2):e20163911

34. United States Department of Health and Human Services. Health information privacy. Available at: www.hhs.gov/ocr/privacy. Accessed November 25, 2018

35. American Camp Association. Health and wellness standards resources. Available at: www.acacamps.org/resource-library/accreditation-standards/health-wellness-standards-resources. Accessed November 25, 2018

36. Gupta RS, Springston EE, Warrier MR, et al. The prevalence, severity, and distribution of childhood food allergy in the United States. *Pediatrics.* 2011; 128(1). Available at: www.pediatrics.org/cgi/content/full/128/1/e9

37. Halstead ME, Walter KD, Moffatt K; Council on Sports Medicine and Fitness. Sport-related concussion in children and Adolescents. *Pediatrics.* 2018; 142(6):e20183074

38. Centers for Disease Control and Prevention. Heads Up. Available at: https://www.cdc.gov/headsup. Accessed November 25, 2018

39. American Camp Association. Mental health. 2017. Available at: www.acacamps.org/staff-professionals/core-competencies/health-wellness/mental-health. Accessed November 25, 2018

40. Koplan JP, Liverman CT, Kraak VI; Committee on Prevention of Obesity in Children and Youth. Preventing childhood obesity: health in the balance: executive summary. *J Am Diet Assoc.* 2005;105(1):131–138

41. American Academy of Pediatrics Council on School Health. Soft drinks in school. *Pediatrics.* 2004;113(1, pt 1): 152–154

42. American Camp Association. Americans with Disabilities Act (ADA) - applicability to camps. 2018. Available at: https://www.acacamps.org/about/who-we-are/public-policy/americans-disabilities-act-ada-applicability-camps. Accessed November 25, 2018

43. American Academy of Pediatrics; American Public Health Association; National Resource Center for Health and Safety in Child Care and Early Education. *Caring for Our Children: National Health and Safety Performance Standards: Guidelines for Early Care and Early Education Programs.* 3rd ed. Elk Grove Village, IL: American Academy of Pediatrics; 2011

Incorporating Recognition and Management of Perinatal Depression Into Pediatric Practice

- *Policy Statement*

POLICY STATEMENT Organizational Principles to Guide and Define the Child Health Care System and/or Improve the Health of all Children

American Academy of Pediatrics

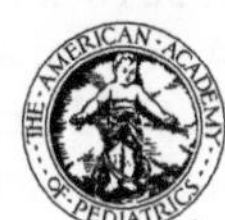

DEDICATED TO THE HEALTH OF ALL CHILDREN™

Incorporating Recognition and Management of Perinatal Depression Into Pediatric Practice

Marian F. Earls, MD, MTS, FAAP,[a,b] Michael W. Yogman, MD, FAAP,[c] Gerri Mattson, MD, MSPH, FAAP,[d,e] Jason Rafferty, MD, MPH, EdM, FAAP,[f,g,h] COMMITTEE ON PSYCHOSOCIAL ASPECTS OF CHILD AND FAMILY HEALTH

abstract

Perinatal depression (PND) is the most common obstetric complication in the United States. Even when screening results are positive, mothers often do not receive further evaluation, and even when PND is diagnosed, mothers do not receive evidence-based treatments. Studies reveal that postpartum depression (PPD), a subset of PND, leads to increased costs of medical care, inappropriate medical treatment of the infant, discontinuation of breastfeeding, family dysfunction, and an increased risk of abuse and neglect. PPD, specifically, adversely affects this critical early period of infant brain development. PND is an example of an adverse childhood experience that has potential long-term adverse health complications for the mother, her partner, the infant, and the mother-infant dyad. However, PND can be treated effectively, and the stress on the infant can be buffered. Pediatric medical homes should coordinate care more effectively with prenatal providers for women with prenatally diagnosed maternal depression; establish a system to implement PPD screening at the 1-, 2-, 4-, and 6-month well-child visits; use community resources for the treatment and referral of the mother with depression; and provide support for the maternal-child (dyad) relationship, including breastfeeding support. State chapters of the American Academy of Pediatrics, working with state departments of public health, public and private payers, and maternal and child health programs, should advocate for payment and for increased training for PND screening and treatment. American Academy of Pediatrics recommends advocacy for workforce development for mental health professionals who care for young children and mother-infant dyads, and for promotion of evidence-based interventions focused on healthy attachment and parent-child relationships.

[a]Community Care of North Carolina, Raleigh, North Carolina; [b]Department of Pediatrics at the School of Medicine, University of North Carolina, Chapel Hill, North Carolina; [c]Department of Pediatrics, Harvard Medical School, Boston, Massachusetts; [d]Department of Maternal and Child Health at the Gillings School of Global Public Health, Chapel Hill, North Carolina; [e]Wake County Health and Human Services, Raleigh, North Carolina; [f]Department of Pediatrics, Thundermist Health Centers, Woonsocket, Rhode Island; [g]Department of Child Psychiatry, Emma Pendleton Bradley Hospital, East Providence, Rhode Island; and [h]Department of Psychiatry and Human Behavior, Warren Alpert Medical School of Brown University, Providence, Rhode Island

Drs Earls, Yogman, Mattson, and Rafferty conceptualized the statement, drafted the initial manuscript, reviewed and revised the manuscript, approved the final manuscript as submitted, and agree to be accountable for all aspects of the work.

This document is copyrighted and is property of the American Academy of Pediatrics and its Board of Directors. All authors have filed conflict of interest statements with the American Academy of Pediatrics. Any conflicts have been resolved through a process approved by the Board of Directors. The American Academy of Pediatrics has neither solicited nor accepted any commercial involvement in the development of the content of this publication.

Policy statements from the American Academy of Pediatrics benefit from expertise and resources of liaisons and internal (AAP) and external reviewers. However, policy statements from the American Academy of Pediatrics may not reflect the views of the liaisons or the organizations or government agencies that they represent.

The guidance in this statement does not indicate an exclusive course of treatment or serve as a standard of medical care. Variations, taking into account individual circumstances, may be appropriate.

To cite: Earls MF, Yogman MW, Mattson G, et al; AAP Committee on Psychosocial Aspects of Child and Family Health. Incorporating Recognition and Management of Perinatal Depression Into Pediatric Practice. *Pediatrics.* 2019;143(1):e20183259

BACKGROUND INFORMATION

A 2010 clinical report from the American Academy of Pediatrics (AAP) described the rationale and need for screening for postpartum depression (PPD) in pediatric primary care.[1] Although primary care clinicians (PCCs) have improved the rates of integrating screening in practice since then, according to the 2013 periodic survey of AAP members, less than half of pediatricians screened mothers for depression. The expanding understanding of the effects of adverse childhood experiences, the recognition of screening as an evidence-based recommendation by the US Preventive Services Task Force (USPSTF),[2,3] and the statement of the Centers for Medicare and Medicaid Services (CMS)[4,5] for support of the coverage of PPD screening under Early and Periodic Screening, Diagnostic and Treatment services have emphasized that it is time to close the gap in rates of screening.

Maternal depression affects the whole family.[6] This policy statement focuses specifically on the effects of maternal depression on the young infant and the role of the pediatric PCC (physician, nurse practitioner, or physician assistant) in identifying PPD and referring the mother-infant dyad for treatment. Perinatal depression (PND) is a major or minor depressive disorder, with an episode occurring during pregnancy or within the first year after the birth of a child. A family history of depression, substance use, marital discord, family violence, isolation, poverty, difficult infant temperament, young maternal age, chronic illness, and a personal history of depression increase the risk of PND.[7] In addition, the risk is also higher with multiple births, preterm birth, and congenital or acquired physical or neurodevelopmental deficits in the infant. Stressful transitions, such as returning to work, may also be a risk factor. Minority, immigrant, and refugee populations are especially at risk because they face the added stress of adjusting to and learning to function in a new environment without as much local family support and with added financial concerns or cultural barriers (language or not asking for help because of cultural norms or lack of awareness of resources).[8,9]

Pediatric PCCs are in a good position to recognize the signs of PPD because they are in frequent contact with parents of infants. PND peaks in women 18 to 44 years of age. In general, as many as 12% of all women who are pregnant or in the postpartum period experience depression in a given year, and 11% to 18% of women report postpartum depressive symptoms. The prevalence in women with low income is estimated to be double at 25%. Moreover, adolescent mothers with low income report depressive symptoms at a rate of 40% to 60%.[1] Minor depression peaks at 2 to 3 months postpartum, and the peak for major depression is at 6 weeks postpartum. There is another peak for depression at 6 months postpartum. Depression in a parent is known to have a profound effect on infants and other children in the family. A growing understanding of early brain development reveals the ecobiodevelopmental factors that determine lifelong physical and mental health. In fact, according to a study by the Centers for Disease Control and Prevention, PPD is 1 of the most common adverse childhood experiences that are associated with the costliest adverse adult health outcomes.[10]

Studies have documented that maternal health care costs associated with PPD are 90% higher than those for comparison groups of women who are postpartum and do not have PPD; the difference is attributable to increased use of mental health services and emergency department visits by both mothers and children. Overall, costs to employers for US workers with PPD, including worker absence and lost productivity, are $44 billion per year and $12.4 billion in health care costs.[11,12]

PPD has a spectrum ranging from milder symptoms of "postpartum blues" to PPD and postpartum psychosis (PPP). It is estimated that 50% to 80% of all mothers experience postpartum blues after childbirth. These symptoms are transient (beginning a few days after childbirth and lasting up to 2 weeks), but they do not impair function. Symptoms include crying, depressed mood, irritability, anxiety, and confusion.

PPD meets the criteria of the *Diagnostic and Statistical Manual of Mental Disorders, Fifth Edition* as a major depressive disorder. Anxiety is a common component of PPD.[13] If a woman experiences PPD, she is likely to experience it with subsequent pregnancies. However, PPD can also affect mothers with subsequent pregnancies even without a previous history with earlier births.

PPP is a relatively rare event. Only 1 to 2 per 1000 women experience PPP after childbirth. Occurring in the first 4 weeks after childbirth, impairment is serious and may include paranoia, mood shifts, hallucinations and/or delusions, and suicidal and/or homicidal thoughts. PPP requires immediate medical attention.

Fathers also suffer from PPD, with a prevalence rate that varies from 2% to as high as 25%, with an increase to 50% when the mother experiences PPD.[14–19] Although the rate of paternal depression is higher when the mother has PPD (which compounds the effect on children), a father who is not depressed is 1 protective factor for children of mothers with depression. Fathers are less likely to seek help. They are more likely to present with symptoms of substance use, domestic violence, and undermining breastfeeding instead of sadness.[20]

IMPACT ON THE INFANT, DYAD, AND FAMILY

Research on early brain development, toxic stress, epigenetics, and adverse childhood experiences has revealed the physiologic effect of the infant's environment on health, development, and learning in the short- and long-term.[21] An infant in the environment of significant maternal depression is at risk for toxic stress and its consequences. Toxic stress is an unhealthy prolonged activation of the stress response unbuffered by a caregiver. Physiologic responses to stress in the infant's environment affect the infant's social-emotional development. The infant, therefore, is at risk for impaired social interaction and delays in language, cognitive, and social-emotional development.

Sequelae of untreated maternal PPD include failure to implement the injury-prevention components from anticipatory guidance (eg, car safety seats and electrical plug covers),[22] failure to implement preventive health practices for the child (eg, Back to Sleep campaign),[22–25] and difficulty managing chronic health conditions (such as asthma or disabilities) in the young child.[23,26] Families with a parent who is depressed (ie, any parental depression) overuse health care and emergency facilities, often presenting with somatic complaints.[26]

Untreated PPD can lead to impaired parent-child interaction, discontinuation of breastfeeding, child abuse and neglect, and family dysfunction.[27] In extreme situations, it can result in suicide or infanticide. With PPD, there is potential immediate impairment of parenting. PPD can:

- hinder bonding, reciprocal interaction, and healthy attachment;
- distort perception of the infant's behavior;
- cause the mother to be less sensitive and attuned, indifferent, or more controlling; and
- impair the mother's attention to, and judgment for, health and safety.

Because maternal depression compromises bonding, the mother-child relationship may create an environment in which the infant withdraws from daily activities and may avoid interaction. In this situation, the infant is at risk for failure to thrive and attachment disorders of infancy (reactive attachment disorder or other trauma, stress and deprivation disorder, or relationship-specific disorder of infancy and early childhood, as defined in the *Diagnostic Classification of Mental Health and Developmental Disorders of Infancy and Early Childhood*).[28]

Early response to PPD is urgent. If the mother continues to experience depression and there is no intervention for the mother-infant relationship, the child's developmental issues are likely to persist and be less responsive to intervention over time. Long-term effects extend to preschoolers and older children. Maternal depression in infancy also is predictive of cortisol levels in preschoolers, and these changes in levels are linked with anxiety, social wariness, and withdrawal.[29–32] As they age, children of mothers who are untreated for PPD often have poor self-control, poor peer relationships, school problems, and aggression. These children may need special education services, can experience grade retention, and may exit school early.[33] Attachment disorders, behavior problems, and depression and other mood disorders can occur into childhood and adolescence.[34]

THE ROLE OF THE MEDICAL HOME

PCCs caring for infants have crucial opportunities to promote healthy social-emotional development, to prevent (beginning at prenatal visits) and/or ameliorate the effects of toxic stress,[35] and to provide routine screening for PPD in early infancy. Pediatric PCCs also have the opportunity to perform depression screening in pregnant mothers at sibling visits. Pediatric medical homes can establish a system to implement screening and to identify and use community resources for the further assessment and treatment of the mother with depression as well as for the support of the mother-child dyad. Identification and coordinating access to treatment of PPD are evidence-based examples of the successful buffering of toxic stress or an adverse childhood experience by pediatricians. Despite previous recommendations, less than half of pediatricians screened mothers for maternal depression in the 2013 periodic survey of AAP members, and it is now time to close the gap.[36,37]

There is much support for primary care incorporating these approaches. The AAP policy statement "The Future of Pediatrics: Mental Health Competencies for Pediatric Primary Care" recognizes the unique advantage the PCC has for surveillance, screening, and working with families to improve mental health outcomes.[38] The AAP Task Force on Mental Health promotes the use of a common-factors approach to engage families and build an alliance for addressing mental health issues. *Bright Futures: Guidelines for Health Supervision of Infants, Children, and Adolescents, fourth Edition*[39] places particular emphasis on engaging families in identifying parental strengths and discussing social determinants of health. Screening for PPD in the medical home is consistent with this 2-generation emphasis.

IMPLEMENTATION

The infant and the mother-infant dyad relationship are the primary concerns of the pediatric PCC. Treatment, when focused solely on the adult, is often less effective than treatment that is focused on the mother-infant dyad. Apart from the adolescent mother who is a patient of the pediatric practice, the mother is generally not the pediatric PCC's patient, but concern extends to the mother herself as well as to her partner. Using a validated tool to screen for depression is 1 of the ways PCCs engage families about psychosocial risks. PCCs (often using a formal surveillance tool or standardized questions) also ask about homelessness, food insecurity, domestic violence, tobacco use, substance use, guns in the home, etc, so they can link the family with community resources, if needed, to reduce the risk for the child. The pediatric PCC also manages the child closely to monitor the possible effects of these risk factors. Referral and follow-up for the infant and mother-infant dyad are the major areas of focus for the pediatric PCC, but knowledge of community resources to which to refer the parent, including knowing how to access community mental health crisis services, is essential to implementing an office process for screening. Implementation often requires a quality improvement approach to office process.

Concerns may be raised regarding liability for the pediatric PCC because the mother is not the patient of that visit. Screening for PPD is performed for the benefit of the infant because the well-being of the infant is inextricably linked to the mother-infant dyad. The pediatric PCC's focus is the dyad, and the PCC is facilitating referral for the mother, not providing treatment.

Surveillance and Screening

Over the course of routine well-child care, the pediatric PCC and the family are developing a longitudinal relationship. A crucial part of this relationship is eliciting parent, family, and child strengths and risks. Psychosocial screening and surveillance for risk and protective factors is an integral part of routine care. Pediatric PCCs need to be aware of and promote protective factors, such as parental knowledge and skills about child development and caregiving, good parental or caregiver physical and mental health, positive father or partner involvement, strong emotional bonding or attachment between infant or child and parent or caregiver, and social supports (ie, friends, neighbors, relatives, faith-based groups, and other agencies). According to resilience theory, an individual's resilience is determined by balancing risk and protective factors in the face of adversity.[40] Promotion of family protective factors promotes resiliency. For example, a father who is not depressed is one protective factor for infants of mothers with depression.

The prenatal visit to the pediatric office is an excellent opportunity for the pediatric PCC and expectant parent(s) to discuss strengths and stressors during pregnancy, including depression.[35] The pediatric PCC may be able to provide anticipatory guidance and to initiate supportive strategies for the mother for the benefit of the infant, even before the infant's birth. Obstetricians and other obstetric providers who identify depression during pregnancy can be especially encouraged to refer prospective parents to pediatricians prenatally so that postpartum management of PND is coordinated. Communication between the obstetrician and pediatric PCC is desirable for this reason. The American College of Obstetricians and Gynecologists specifically recommends this collaboration between obstetricians and their pediatric colleagues.[41] In turn, pediatric PCCs would encourage communication on behalf of the infant.

On the basis of knowledge regarding peak occurrence times for PPD, routine screening in which a validated screening tool is used should occur at well-infant visits at 1, 2, 4, and 6 months. Repeated screening at these visits allows for a mother who may not be comfortable disclosing initially to do so at a later visit, and it maximizes the opportunity to engage a dyad that may miss 1 or more of the recommended well-infant visits. Components of documentation in the infant's chart include the type of screening tool used, results, discussion with the mother or parents (whether positive or negative), and a follow-up and referral plan if indicated. There is no reason to open a chart on the mother because she is not receiving treatment. Although not the focus of this statement, it should also be noted that there are recommendations that PPD screening should be performed for the parents of infants who are hospitalized and the parents of infants up to 1 year of age seen in the emergency department.[42,43]

Pediatricians should be encouraged to consider screening the partner as well at the 6-month visit with the Edinburgh Postpartum Depression Scale (EPDS), either in person if the partner is present or by having the partner fill out the screen at home and mail it back. If the partner is male, this process is more feasible if the pediatrician has identified referral resources when he screens positive for depression.

Screening tools for PPD include the EPDS (note that the EPDS is now included within the Survey of Well-being of Young Children [SWYC]) or the Patient Health Questionnaire. The EPDS is completed by the mother, and a score of 10 or greater indicates possible depression. The EPDS also contains 2 questions regarding anxiety. Screening for PPD by using the EPDS has now been validated for men as well as women.[20]

It should be noted that screening is not diagnostic. A positive screen result indicates a risk that depression is present, and the purpose of referral is to clarify the diagnosis and offer the indicated treatment.

As with other screening implementations, it is essential for the practice to understand and prepare for referral and linkages with appropriate resources for children and/or families who are identified as at risk.

Follow-up, Referral, Treatment

When screening reveals a concern, next steps include communication and demystification, support, identification of community and family resources, and referrals as indicated.

Immediate action is necessary if question 10 on the EPDS is positive (indicating possible suicidality), if question 9 on the Patient Health Questionnaire 9 is positive (indicating possible suicidality), if the mother expresses concern about her or her infant's safety, or if the PCC suspects that the mother is suicidal, homicidal, severely depressed, manic, or psychotic. As with any mental health crisis in which suicidality is a concern, referral to emergency mental health services (most communities have mental health crisis teams or services) is needed, and the mother should only leave with her support person or under the care of community resources, such as mental health crisis services or emergency medical services.

When a depression screen result is positive, management will vary according to the degree of concern and need. Because the mother is not the patient of the pediatrician, a detailed discussion of treatment of the mother is outside the scope of this article, but a Cochrane review of a few studies of mothers with PPD revealed that there is no difference between the effectiveness of antidepressants and psychological and/or psychosocial treatments.[44] At the very least, management will require support and demystification. Management of PPD includes:

- demystification (reducing guilt and shame by emphasizing how common these feelings are);
- support resources (family and community); and
- referrals for the mother (to a mental health professional or the mother's PCC or obstetrician), for the mother-infant dyad, for the child (for targeted promotion of social-emotional development and early intervention [EI]), and for the mother who is breastfeeding (for lactation support from an experienced provider).

Regardless of the referral arrangement, a key component is a follow-up with the mother to be certain that she is receiving treatment and that depressive symptoms are decreased. Such follow-up could be conducted by a designated referral person on the practice staff.

Demystification removes the mystery about maternal depression, acknowledging that PPD happens to many women, that the mother is not at fault or a "bad" mother, that depression is treatable, and that the PCC is a resource. A brief intervention at the visit would involve:

- promoting the strength of the mother-infant relationship;
- encouraging the mother and reassuring her regarding any concerns about breastfeeding;
- encouraging understanding and responding to the infant's cues;
- encouraging reading and talking to the infant;
- encouraging routines for predictability and security, sleep, diet, exercise, and stress relief;
- promoting realistic expectations and prioritizing important things; and
- encouraging social connections.

To follow-up on the impact on the infant and dyad, use of a screening tool for infant social-emotional development is appropriate. One such tool, the Baby Pediatric Symptom Checklist, is brief and in the public domain as part of the SWYC. It screens for irritability, inflexibility, and difficulty with routines. The Ages & Stages Questionnaires: Social-Emotional, Second Edition is another infant social-emotional screening tool (not in the public domain). It is completed by the parent, has a single cutoff score, and screens affect, self-regulation, adaptive functioning, autonomy, compliance, and communication.[45–47]

If there are concerns about attachment and bonding, the dyad needs referral to a mental health professional with expertise in the treatment of young children. Evidence-based interventions for the dyad (child's age 0–5 years) include child-parent psychotherapy, Circle of Security (www.circleofsecurityinternational.com), and Attachment and Biobehavioral Catch-up.[46,47] These interventions are used to address the dyadic relationship in high-risk families and are often used in situations of abuse and neglect or interpersonal violence, and with Circle of Security, in the setting of PND. A key component of follow-up is comanagement (and standardized communication) with the mental health professional serving the dyad.

If the practice has an integrated mental health professional, such as a licensed clinical social worker or counselor, that team member can provide immediate triage for a positive screen, administer secondary screens, offer support and follow-up, facilitate referrals, and coordinate follow-up with the PCC.

Referral to EI services for children from birth to 3 years of age through Part C of the Individuals with Disabilities Education Act is also important to address the dyad relationship.[48–50] EI in the home can provide modeling for interaction and play to prevent toxic stress and promote healthy development. However, in many states, it is difficult to access EI services because of eligibility processes. This difficulty is attributable in part to funding limitations, leading to more restrictive eligibility, but the crucial issue is that the domain of social-emotional development may not be included in eligibility criteria. Given the inextricable connection of social-emotional development to cognitive and language development, such eligibility policies can be detrimental to children and families.

Community resources include Early Head Start, Healthy Start, home visiting programs, and other community organizations. Other community resources for the family include public health nurses, lactation specialists, parent educators, parent support groups, parent-child groups, and postpartum support groups.

Coding and Billing

The AAP, along with the USPSTF[2,3] and the CMS,[4,5] recognizes that PPD screens are a measure of risk in the infant's environment, and therefore, billing is appropriate at the infant's visit, with the infant as the patient. *Current Procedural Terminology* code 96161 (effective as of January 2017) allows reporting of the administration of a caregiver-focused health risk assessment (eg, parent depression screen) for the benefit of the patient. However, because billing codes may vary by payer and by state, PCCs are advised to consult AAP state chapter pediatric councils and payers for updated coding guidance. When a screen result is positive, the PCC should be familiar with coding on the basis of counseling time and complexity when indicated.

CONCLUSIONS

The 2010 AAP clinical report[1] acknowledged that PPD leads to adverse effects on infant brain development, family dysfunction, cessation of breastfeeding, inappropriate medical treatment of the infant, and increased costs of medical care. Since that time, PCCs in several states have successfully implemented screening and have built referral relationships for evidence-based interventions, for community resources for the treatment and referral of the mother with depression, and for resources to support the mother-child (dyad) relationship.

National recognition of toxic stress, adverse childhood experiences, and the importance of trauma-informed care has led to recommendations for recognition and intervention from professional and policy organizations, including the USPSTF and CMS as well as the AAP. Recognizing and building resilience against toxic stress, education, and advocacy has been a focus of the national advocacy campaign of the AAP Section on Pediatric Trainees (https://www.aap.org/en-us/advocacy-and-policy/aap-health-initiatives/resilience/Pages/default.aspx).[51]

The pediatric PCC has a unique opportunity to identify PPD and help prevent untoward developmental and mental health outcomes for the infant and family. Screening has proven successful in several initiatives and locations and can be implemented in office workflow by PCCs caring for infants and their families. Intervention and referral are optimized by collaborative relationships with community resources and/or by collocated and/or integrated mental health in primary care.

RECOMMENDATIONS

Routine screening for PPD should be integrated into well-child visits at 1, 2, 4, and 6 months of age. This screening schedule is recommended in *Bright Futures: Guidelines for Health Supervision of Infants, Children, and Adolescents, Fourth Edition*.[39] PPD screening has also been recognized as evidence based according to the USPSTF (Grade B recommendation; see accompanying technical report[52]). Training and continuing medical education programs should be available for all pediatric providers on the subject of PPD screening and referral.[4]

OPPORTUNITIES FOR ADVOCACY

1. AAP chapters, other stakeholders, and state public health agencies and officials can increase awareness of the need for PND screening as outlined in the obstetric and pediatric periodicity of care schedules. Advocacy should be conducted with commercial payers to ensure payment for PND screening and related services.

2. In keeping with current CMS recommendations, state Medicaid programs may pay for PPD screening under Early and Periodic Screening, Diagnostic and Treatment using a validated screening instrument, such as the EPDS, Patient Health Questionnaire, or the SWYC.

3. The AAP can collaborate with the American College of

Obstetricians and Gynecologists to encourage prenatal referral of all mothers to the PCC of the infant so that care is coordinated and integrated for families at a high risk for PPD.[53]

4. Screening of mothers for PPD by pediatricians at least once during the first 6 months after birth should be part of quality metrics used for payment.
5. Establishment of consultation and referral resources to improve access to treatment of mothers identified with PPD should be advocated.
6. Workforce development should be promoted for mental health providers who care for young children and the parent-infant dyad.
7. Evidence-based interventions focused on healthy attachment and parent-child relationships should be promoted.
8. Federal funding should be advocated for states to establish, improve, or maintain programs for screening, assessment, and treatment services for women who are pregnant or who have given birth within the preceding 12 months, as required under the 21st Century Cures Act of 2016 (Public Law 114–255).
9. Inclusion of social-emotional development as a domain for eligibility in Part C programs should be supported.
10. Creation of postpartum support networks in local communities should be encouraged by partnering with local businesses and nonprofits.
11. Media campaigns and messaging to counteract stigma associated with PND should be encouraged.

LEAD AUTHORS

Marian Earls, MD, FAAP
Michael Yogman, MD, FAAP
Gerri Mattson, MD, MSPH, FAAP
Jason Rafferty, MD, MPH, EdM

COMMITTEE ON PSYCHOSOCIAL ASPECTS OF CHILD AND FAMILY HEALTH, 2016–2017

Michael Yogman, MD, FAAP Chairperson
Rebecca Baum, MD, FAAP
Thresia Gambon, MD, FAAP
Arthur Lavin, MD, FAAP
Gerri Mattson, MD, MSPH, FAAP
Jason Rafferty, MD, MPH, EdM
Lawrence Wissow, MD, MPH, FAAP

LIAISONS

Sharon Berry, PhD – *Society of Pediatric Psychology*
Terry Carmichael, MSW – *National Association of Social Workers*
Edward R. Christopherson, PhD, FAAP (hon) – *Society of Pediatric Psychology*
Norah Johnson, PhD, RN, CPNP-PC – *National Association of Pediatric Nurse Practitioners*
L. Read Sulik, MD, FAAP – *American Academy of Child and Adolescent Psychiatry*

STAFF

Stephanie Domain, MS

ABBREVIATIONS

AAP: American Academy of Pediatrics
CMS: Centers for Medicare and Medicaid Services
EI: early intervention
EPDS: Edinburgh Postpartum Depression Scale
PCC: primary care clinician
PND: perinatal depression
PPD: postpartum depression
PPP: postpartum psychosis
SWYC: Survey of Well-being of Young Children
USPSTF: US Preventive Services Task Force

All policy statements from the American Academy of Pediatrics automatically expire 5 years after publication unless reaffirmed, revised, or retired at or before that time.

DOI: https://doi.org/10.1542/peds.2018-3259

Address Correspondence to Marian Earls, MD, MTS, FAAP. Email: mearls@communitycarenc.org

PEDIATRICS (ISSN Numbers: Print, 0031-4005; Online, 1098-4275).

Copyright © 2019 by the American Academy of Pediatrics

FINANCIAL DISCLOSURE: The authors have indicated they have no financial relationships relevant to this article to disclose.

FUNDING: No external funding.

POTENTIAL CONFLICT OF INTEREST: The authors have indicated they have no potential conflicts of interest to disclose.

REFERENCES

1. Earls MF; Committee on Psychosocial Aspects of Child and Family Health; American Academy of Pediatrics. Incorporating recognition and management of perinatal and postpartum depression into pediatric practice. *Pediatrics*. 2010;126(5):1032–1039
2. US Preventive Services Task Force. Final recommendation statement. Depression in adults: screening. 2016. Available at: https://www.uspreventiveservicestaskforce.org/Page/Document/RecommendationStatementFinal/depression-in-adults-screening1. Accessed February 2, 2018
3. Siu AL, Bibbins-Domingo K, Grossman DC, et al; US Preventive Services Task Force (USPSTF). Screening for depression in adults: US Preventive Services Task Force recommendation statement. *JAMA*. 2016;315(4):380–387
4. Centers for Medicare and Medicaid Services. CMCS Informational Bulletin,

May 11, 2016. Maternal depression screening and treatment: a critical role for Medicaid in the care of mothers and children. Available at: https://www.medicaid.gov/federal-policy-guidance/downloads/cib051116.pdf. Accessed July 22, 2018

5. Olin SS, McCord M, Stein REK, et al. Beyond Screening: A Stepped Care Pathway for Managing Postpartum Depression in Pediatric Settings. *J Womens Health (Larchmt).* 2017;26(9):966–975
6. Isaacs M. *Community Care Networks for Depression in Low-Income Communities and Communities of Color: A Review of the Literature.* Washington, DC: Howard University School of Social Work and National Alliance of Multiethnic Behavioral Health Associations; 2004
7. Kahn RS, Wise PH, Wilson K. Maternal smoking, drinking and depression: a generational link between socioeconomic status and child behavior problems [abstract]. *Pediatr Res.* 2002;51(pt 2):191A
8. Doe S, LoBue S, Hamaoui A, Rezai S, Henderson CE, Mercado R. Prevalence and predictors of positive screening for postpartum depression in minority parturients in the South Bronx. *Arch Womens Ment Health.* 2017;20(2):291–295
9. Cebollos M, Wallace G, Goodwin G. Postpartum depression among African-American and Latina mothers living in small cities, towns, and rural communities. *J Racial Ethn Health Disparities.* 2017;4(5):916–927
10. Felitti VJ, Anda RF, Nordenberg D, et al. Relationship of childhood abuse and household dysfunction to many of the leading causes of death in adults. The Adverse Childhood Experiences (ACE) study. *Am J Prev Med.* 1998;14(4):245–258
11. Witters D, Liu D, Agrawal S. Depression costs U.S. workplaces $23 billion in absenteeism. 2013. Available at: http://news.gallup.com/poll/163619/depression-costs-workplaces-billion-absenteeism.aspx. Accessed February 2, 2018
12. Dagher RK, McGovern PM, Dowd BE, Gjerdingen DK. Postpartum depression and health services expenditures among employed women. *J Occup Environ Med.* 2012;54(2):210–215
13. Ross LE, McLean LM. Anxiety disorders during pregnancy and the postpartum period: a systematic review. *J Clin Psychiatry.* 2006;67(8):1285–1298
14. Davis RN, Davis MM, Freed GL, Clark SJ. Fathers' depression related to positive and negative parenting behaviors with 1-year-old children. *Pediatrics.* 2011;127(4):612–618
15. Chang JJ, Halpern CT, Kaufman JS. Maternal depressive symptoms, father's involvement, and the trajectories of child problem behaviors in a US national sample. *Arch Pediatr Adolesc Med.* 2007;161(7):697–703
16. Goodman JH. Paternal postpartum depression, its relationship to maternal postpartum depression, and implications for family health. *J Adv Nurs.* 2004;45(1):26–35
17. Edmondson OJ, Psychogiou L, Vlachos H, Netsi E, Ramchandani PG. Depression in fathers in the postnatal period: assessment of the Edinburgh Postnatal Depression Scale as a screening measure. *J Affect Disord.* 2010;125(1–3):365–368
18. Ramchandani PG, Psychogiou L, Vlachos H, et al. Paternal depression: an examination of its links with father, child and family functioning in the postnatal period. *Depress Anxiety.* 2011;28(6):471–477
19. Paulson JF, Bazemore SD. Prenatal and postpartum depression in fathers and its association with maternal depression: a meta-analysis. *JAMA.* 2010;303(19):1961–1969
20. Rochlen AB. Men in (and out of) therapy: central concepts, emerging directions, and remaining challenges. *J Clin Psychol.* 2005;61(6):627–631
21. Garner AS, Shonkoff JP; Committee on Psychosocial Aspects of Child and Family Health; Committee on Early Childhood, Adoption, and Dependent Care; Section on Developmental and Behavioral Pediatrics. Early childhood adversity, toxic stress, and the role of the pediatrician: translating developmental science into lifelong health. *Pediatrics.* 2012;129(1). Available at: www.pediatrics.org/cgi/content/full/129/1/e224
22. McLennan JD, Kotelchuck M. Parental prevention practices for young children in the context of maternal depression. *Pediatrics.* 2000;105(5):1090–1095
23. Chung EK, McCollum KF, Elo IT, Lee HJ, Culhane JF. Maternal depressive symptoms and infant health practices among low-income women. *Pediatrics.* 2004;113(6). Available at: www.pediatrics.org/cgi/content/full/113/6/e523
24. Kavanaugh M, Halterman JS, Montes G, Epstein M, Hightower AD, Weitzman M. Maternal depressive symptoms are adversely associated with prevention practices and parenting behaviors for preschool children. *Ambul Pediatr.* 2006;6(1):32–37
25. Paulson JF, Dauber S, Leiferman JA. Individual and combined effects of postpartum depression in mothers and fathers on parenting behavior. *Pediatrics.* 2006;118(2):659–668
26. Sills MR, Shetterly S, Xu S, Magid D, Kempe A. Association between parental depression and children's health care use. *Pediatrics.* 2007;119(4). Available at: www.pediatrics.org/cgi/content/full/119/4/e829
27. Ip S, Chung M, Raman G, et al. *Breastfeeding and Maternal and Infant Health Outcomes in Developed Countries.* Rockville, MD: Agency for Health Research and Quality; 2007:130–131
28. Zero to Three. *DC:0-5: Diagnostic Classification of Mental Health and Developmental Disorders of Infancy and Early Childhood.* Washington, DC: Zero to Three; 2016
29. Beardslee WR, Versage EM, Gladstone TR. Children of affectively ill parents: a review of the past 10 years. *J Am Acad Child Adolesc Psychiatry.* 1998;37(11):1134–1141
30. Smider NA, Essex MJ, Kalin NH, et al. Salivary cortisol as a predictor of socioemotional adjustment during kindergarten: a prospective study. *Child Dev.* 2002;73(1):75–92
31. Essex MJ, Klein MH, Cho E, Kalin NH. Maternal stress beginning in infancy may sensitize children to later stress exposure: effects on cortisol and behavior. *Biol Psychiatry.* 2002;52(8):776–784

32. Essex MJ, Klein MH, Miech R, Smider NA. Timing of initial exposure to maternal major depression and children's mental health symptoms in kindergarten. *Br J Psychiatry.* 2001;179:151–156

33. Lahti M, Savolainen K, Tuovinen S, et al. Maternal depressive symptoms during and after pregnancy and psychiatric problems in children. *J Am Acad Child Adolesc Psychiatry.* 2017;56(1):30–39.e7

34. Netsi E, Pearson RM, Murray L, Cooper P, Craske MG, Stein A. Association of persistent and severe postnatal depression with child outcomes. *JAMA Psychiatry.* 2018;75(3):247–253

35. Yogman M, Lavin A, Cohen G; Committee on Psychosocial Aspects of Child and Family Health. The prenatal visit. *Pediatrics.* 2018;142(1):e20181218

36. Kerker BD, Storfer-Isser A, Stein RE, et al. Identifying maternal depression in pediatric primary care: changes over a decade. *J Dev Behav Pediatr.* 2016;37(2):113–120

37. Yogman MW. Postpartum depression screening by pediatricians: time to close the gap. *J Dev Behav Pediatr.* 2016;37(2):157

38. Committee on Psychosocial Aspects of Child and Family Health; Task Force on Mental Health. Policy statement–the future of pediatrics: mental health competencies for pediatric primary care. *Pediatrics.* 2009;124(1):410–421

39. Hagan J, Shaw JS, Duncan PM, eds. *Bright Futures: Guidelines for Health Supervision of Infants, Children, and Adolescents.* 4th ed. Elk Grove Village, IL: American Academy of Pediatrics; 2017

40. Luthar SS, Cicchetti D, Becker B. The construct of resilience: a critical evaluation and guidelines for future work. *Child Dev.* 2000;71(3):543–562

41. Committee on Obstetric Practice. The American College of Obstetricians and Gynecologists Committee opinion no. 630. Screening for perinatal depression. *Obstet Gynecol.* 2015;125(5):1268–1271

42. Trost MJ, Molas-Torreblanca K, Man C, Casillas E, Sapir H, Schrager SM. Screening for maternal postpartum depression during infant hospitalizations. *J Hosp Med.* 2016;11(12):840–846

43. Emerson BL, Bradley ER, Riera A, Mayes L, Bechtel K. Postpartum depression screening in the pediatric emergency department. *Pediatr Emerg Care.* 2014;30(11):788–792

44. Molyneaux E, Howard LM, McGeown HR, Karia AM, Trevillion K. Antidepressant treatment for postnatal depression. *Cochrane Database Syst Rev.* 2014;(9):CD002018

45. Weitzman C, Wegner L; Section on Developmental and Behavioral Pediatrics; Committee on Psychosocial Aspects of Child and Family Health; Council on Early Childhood; Society for Developmental and Behavioral Pediatrics; American Academy of Pediatrics. Promoting optimal development: screening for behavioral and emotional problems [published correction appears in *Pediatrics.* 2015;135(5):946]. *Pediatrics.* 2015;135(2):384–395

46. Gleason MM, Goldson E, Yogman MW; Council on Early Childhood; Committee on Psychosocial Aspects of Child and Family Health; Section on Developmental and Behavioral Pediatrics. Addressing early childhood emotional and behavioral problems. *Pediatrics.* 2016;138(6):e20163025

47. Council on Early Childhood; Committee on Psychosocial Aspects of Child and Family Health; Section on Developmental and Behavioral Pediatrics. Addressing early childhood emotional and behavioral problems. *Pediatrics.* 2016;138(6):e20163023

48. Pilowsky DJ, Wickramaratne P, Talati A, et al. Children of depressed mothers 1 year after the initiation of maternal treatment: findings from the STAR*D-Child Study. *Am J Psychiatry.* 2008;165(9):1136–1147

49. Foster CE, Webster MC, Weissman MM, et al. Remission of maternal depression: relations to family functioning and youth internalizing and externalizing symptoms. *J Clin Child Adolesc Psychol.* 2008;37(4):714–724

50. Cicchetti D, Rogosch FA, Toth SL. The efficacy of toddler-parent psychotherapy for fostering cognitive development in offspring of depressed mothers. *J Abnorm Child Psychol.* 2000;28(2):135–148

51. American Academy of Pediatrics. Resilience project. Available at: https://www.aap.org/en-us/advocacy-and-policy/aap-health-initiatives/resilience/Pages/default.aspx. Accessed July 22, 2018

52. Rafferty J, Mattson G, Earls M, Yogman M; Committee on Psychosocial Aspects of Child and Family Health. Incorporating recognition and management of perinatal depression into pediatric practice. *Pediatrics.* 2018;143(1):e20183260

53. American College of Obstetricians and Gynecologists' Committee on Obstetric Practice; Association of Women's Health, Obstetric and Neonatal Nurses. Committee opinion no. 666: optimizing postpartum care. *Obstet Gynecol.* 2016;127(6):e187–e192

Incorporating Recognition and Management of Perinatal Depression Into Pediatric Practice

- *Technical Report*

TECHNICAL REPORT

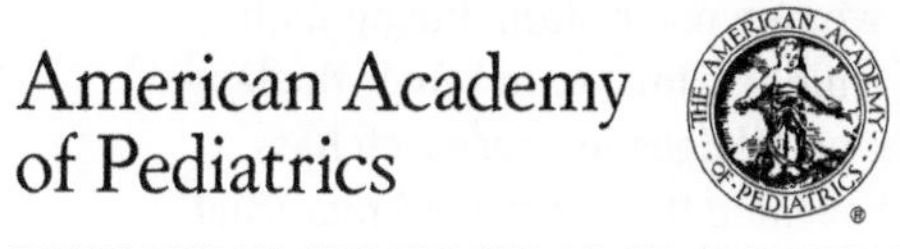

Incorporating Recognition and Management of Perinatal Depression Into Pediatric Practice

Jason Rafferty, MD, MPH, EdM, FAAP,[a,b,c] Gerri Mattson, MD, MSPH, FAAP,[d,e] Marian F. Earls, MD, MTS, FAAP,[f,g] Michael W. Yogman, MD, FAAP,[h] COMMITTEE ON PSYCHOSOCIAL ASPECTS OF CHILD AND FAMILY HEALTH

abstract

Perinatal depression is the most common obstetric complication in the United States, with prevalence rates of 15% to 20% among new mothers. Untreated, it can adversely affect the well-being of children and families throught increasing the risk for costly complications during birth and lead to deterioration of core supports, including partner relationships and social networks. Perinatal depression contributes to long-lasting, and even permanent, consequences for the physical and mental health of parents and children, including poor family functioning, increased risk of child abuse and neglect, delayed infant development, perinatal obstetric complications, challenges with breastfeeding, and costly increases in health care use. Perinatal depression can interfere with early parent-infant interaction and attachment, leading to potentially long-term disturbances in the child's physical, emotional, cognitive, and social development. Fortunately, perinatal depression is identifiable and treatable. The US Preventive Services Task Force, Centers for Medicare and Medicaid Services, and many professional organizations recommend routine universal screening for perinatal depression in women to facilitate early evidence-based treatment and referrals, if necessary. Despite significant gains in screening rates from 2004 to 2013, a minority of pediatricians routinely screen for postpartum depression, and many mothers are still not identified or treated. Pediatric primary care clinicians, with a core mission of promoting child and family health, are in an ideal position to implement routine postpartum depression screens at several well-child visits throughout infancy and to provide mental health support through referrals and/or the interdisciplinary services of a pediatric patient-centered medical home model.

[a]Department of Pediatrics, Thundermist Health Centers, Providence, Rhode Island; [b]Department of Child Psychiatry, Emma Pendeltom Bradley Hospital, East Providence, Rhode Island; [c]Department of Psychiatry and Human Behavior, Warren Alpert Medical School of Brown University, Providence, Rhode Island; [d]Wake County Health and Human Services, Raleigh, North Carolina; [e]Department of Maternal and Child Health, Gillings School of Global Public Health, and [f]Department of Pediatrics, School of Medicine, University of North Carolina, Chapel Hill, North Carolina; [g]Community Care of North Carolina, Raleigh, North Carolina; and [h]Department of Pediatrics, Harvard Medical School, Boston, Massachusetts

Drs Rafferty, Mattson, Earls, and Yogman conceptualized the statement and drafted, reviewed, and revised the initial manuscript; and all authors approved the final manuscript as submitted and agree to be accountable for all aspects of the work.

This document is copyrighted and is property of the American Academy of Pediatrics and its Board of Directors. All authors have filed conflict of interest statements with the American Academy of Pediatrics. Any conflicts have been resolved through a process approved by the Board of Directors. The American Academy of Pediatrics has neither solicited nor accepted any commercial involvement in the development of the content of this publication.

Technical reports from the American Academy of Pediatrics benefit from expertise and resources of liaisons and internal (AAP) and external reviewers. However, technical reports from the American Academy of Pediatrics may not reflect the views of the liaisons or the organizations or government agencies that they represent.

The guidance in this report does not indicate an exclusive course of treatment or serve as a standard of medical care. Variations, taking into account individual circumstances, may be appropriate.

To cite: Rafferty J, Mattson G, Earls MF, et al. Incorporating Recognition and Management of Perinatal Depression Into Pediatric Practice. *Pediatrics.* 2019;143(1):e20183260

BACKGROUND

Depression is experienced by women most often during their childbearing years.[1] Over the last several decades, research has revealed that untreated maternal depression during pregnancy or the first year after childbirth can have significant adverse effects on the well-being of women, infants, and their families. Maternal depression experienced around the time of childbirth can increase the risk for costly complications during birth and can contribute to long-lasting and even permanent effects on the child's development.[2] Only in the last decade has universal screening for maternal depressive symptoms during the perinatal period been recommended by professional health care associations, including the American College of Obstetricians and Gynecologists (ACOG),[3] American Academy of Family Physicians (AAFP),[4] and American Academy of Pediatrics (AAP).[1] However, screening remains far from universal. In 1 study, nearly 6 out of 10 women screening positive on the Edinburgh Postnatal Depression Scale (EPDS) had not spoken to a health care professional about their symptoms or concerns.[5] It is estimated that 50% of women who are depressed during and after pregnancy have their depression go undiagnosed and untreated, which makes it the most underdiagnosed and undertreated obstetric complication.[6] However, most mothers (80%) report being comfortable with the idea of being screened for depression.[7] Among pediatricians, 90% in 1 study reported assuming responsibility for identifying maternal depression, but most (71%) rarely or never assessed for it, and almost all (93%) reported having never or rarely provided mental health referrals.[8] From 2004 to 2013, screening rates by pediatricians for maternal depression increased from 13% to only 44% in periodic surveys by a number of organizations, including the AAP.[9] Inadequate perinatal depression screening rates and limited access to evidence-based treatment are attributable to the stigma associated with mental health, patient apprehension about openly admitting to emotional struggles, limits in provider education and skill sets, and systemic limitations around delivery of and payment for screening.[7,10,11]

There has been increased attention given to perinatal depression, including the release of the US Surgeon General's Report on Mental Health in 2000 in which postpartum depression and psychosis was mentioned,[12] the 2000 report of the US Surgeon General's Conference on Children's Mental Health,[13] and a recent review article in the *New England Journal of Medicine*.[14] Congress designated increased funding to address screening and treatment of perinatal depression through the Health Resources and Services Administration's Maternal and Child Health Bureau in 2004.[2] In 2018, Congress designated $5 million for programs used to address maternal perinatal depression in the 2018 Omnibus Funding Bill (public law 114–255). This funding will be used to support state grants primarily aimed at establishing, improving, and maintaining programs to train professionals to screen and treat for maternal perinatal depression.

The most recent update of the AAP's *Bright Futures: Guidelines for Health Supervision of Infants, Children, and Adolescents, Fourth Edition* includes a recommendation for pediatric providers to screen for postpartum depression at 4 well-child visits in the first 6 months of life and refer to appropriate evaluation and treatment services for the mother and infant when indicated.[15] In 2009, the AAP released a policy statement, "The Future of Pediatrics: Mental Health Competencies for Pediatric Primary Care," emphasizing the unique role pediatric providers have in screening for mental health concerns in children and families, including parental depressive symptoms, and working with families to improve mental health outcomes.[16] The National Academy of Sciences published its report on parental depression in 2009, emphasizing the role of the AAP Medical Home Initiative in reducing perinatal depression occurrence.[17,18] It was followed by a clinical report from the AAP that was focused on recognition and management of perinatal and postpartum depression in 2010[1] and the US Healthy People 2020 objectives to reduce the proportion of mothers experiencing perinatal depression (maternal, infant, and child health objective 34) and to improve overall maternal and child perinatal health.[19] It is within this context that the National Institute for Health Care Management released a report concluding:

> *The consequences of allowing maternal depression to go underdiagnosed and untreated are detrimental to the health of all mothers and their children. Knowing a woman's risk of developing depression peaks during her childbearing years, it is vital for all health care providers to recognize the symptoms of depression and understand the risk factors associated with maternal depression to identify and treat depression as soon as possible.*[2]

In 2016, the US Preventive Services Task Force (USPSTF) reviewed available research and asserted that direct and indirect evidence shows a "moderate net benefit" to screening for perinatal depression because it contributes to a significant reduction in overall prevalence of depression and associated morbidities.[20,21] In addition, in 2016, the Centers for Medicare and Medicaid Services (CMS) sent a directive to all state Medicaid directors clarifying that maternal postpartum depression screening can be billed under well-infant visits as a "screening of the caregiver."[22] Both the USPSTF and CMS encourage universal maternal postpartum depression screening by pediatric providers, with appropriate payment by insurers. The USPSTF specifically states that "screening should be implemented with adequate systems in place to ensure accurate diagnosis, effective treatment, and appropriate follow up."[21] This requires close partnerships between pediatricians, family physicians, adult primary care physicians, and obstetricians, mental health providers, and other community agencies.

Recent research also has begun to examine the influence of a father's affective state on a child's early development and well-being.[23,24] Available evidence indicates that fathers independently experience higher rates of depression after the birth of a child, which adversely influences parenting and positive interactions.[25] Paternal depression may present differently with substance use (alcohol and drug-related comorbidity), domestic violence, and compulsive behavior, which impairs parenting and can undermine breastfeeding.[26,27] There are virtually no empirical studies on the rates or effects of depression among same-sex partners or nonbiological parents.

This technical report aims to review the definitions of perinatal depression, along with its epidemiology, to discuss the serious consequences for child development and to highlight efforts across the country that have demonstrated effectiveness in increasing early screening and treatment. The technical report reviews the evidence and rationale underlying recommendations in an accompanying policy statement[28] concerning the role of the pediatric provider as a clinician and advocate in ensuring timely identification of perinatal depression and referral to evidence-based treatment programs. With this report, we provide an update to the 2010 clinical report from the AAP on this subject.[1]

DEFINITIONS

Perinatal depression is characterized by an episode of major depression, including 2 weeks of depressed mood and neurovegetative symptoms (alterations in sleep, appetite, concentration, energy level, etc), as described in the *Diagnostic and Statistical Manual of Mental Disorders, Fifth Edition (DSM-5)*, occurring during pregnancy or after delivery. Although the diagnostic criteria for major depressive disorder (MDD) did not undergo significant change between the fourth edition and the *DSM-5*, the specifier "with perinatal onset" replaced the traditional distinction between antenatal and postpartum onset.[29] The reason for this change is that 50% of MDD identified during the postpartum period actually begins before delivery.[30] With this change, there is emphasis on the utility of early screening, detection, and management throughout pregnancy, not just after delivery. In fact, in 2015, the ACOG released a committee opinion recommending mothers be screened for depression at least once during the perinatal period[3] expanding the window for recommended screening into the antenatal period. Despite changes in nomenclature and disease conceptualization, much of the literature and current guidelines continue to reference only depression after delivery using the term, "postpartum depression."

There is controversy around the time course of perinatal depression, with the *DSM-5* referencing symptom onset occurring any time during pregnancy or within 4 weeks of delivery. However, many professional organizations, including the ACOG, expand the criteria to include onset of symptoms up to 12 months after delivery. Although most of the biological factors influencing mood may be less relevant at the later stage, there are significant ongoing psychosocial stressors that increase risk, especially with the added responsibilities of caring for an infant.[3]

Perinatal depression is 1 of a few recognized mood disorders that may occur around pregnancy and delivery (Table 1). "Postpartum blues" is a transient state of increased emotional reactivity occurring in approximately 50% to 80% of mothers after labor and delivery. They may cry more easily, be irritable, or demonstrate emotional lability. Peak onset is 3 to 5 days after delivery, often when women begin lactating, and duration is days to weeks. Psychiatric history, environmental stress, cultural context, and breastfeeding do not seem to be related.[2,31] Mothers with postpartum blues do not meet *DSM-5* criteria for a mood disorder, and treatment is generally supportive, because symptoms generally lessen and resolve with time.

"Postpartum psychosis" is a rare event with an estimated incidence of 2 in every 1000 deliveries. Often, the onset is within the first 1 to 4 weeks of delivery, with agitation, irritability, mood lability, delusions, and disorganized behavior. Often, it is conceptualized as on a spectrum with perinatal depression, but the preponderance of data suggests that postpartum psychosis is an overt presentation of bipolar disorder.[33] In the *DSM-5*, such a patient may meet criteria for major depression or bipolar disorder (type I or II) with psychotic features or a brief psychotic episode. Again, the "with peripartum onset" specifier is added if onset is within 4 weeks of delivery.[30] Risk factors include personal and family history of bipolar depression and schizoaffective disorder. Hormonal shifts, sleep deprivation, environmental stress, and stopping mood-stabilizing medications are believed to be

TABLE 1 Characteristics of Postpartum Blues, Perinatal Depression, and Postpartum Psychosis

Type	Course	Prevalence	Symptoms
Postpartum blues	Onset in first few wk after labor, peaks at 3–5 d postpartum (with lactation), and usually resolves in <2 wk.	50%–80% of mothers	Crying, weeping Sadness Irritability Exaggerated sense of empathy Anxiety Mood lability ("ups and downs") Feeling overwhelmed Insomnia Fatigue and/or exhaustion Frustration
Perinatal depression		15%–20% of mothers from conception to 1 y postpartum	Persistent sadness, emptiness, hopelessness, frequent crying, irritability Loss of interest in caring for self and/or child, enjoyable activities, and/or poor bonding with infant (attachment) Changes in appetite or wt
Prenatal depression	Onset during pregnancy, peaks in first trimester, then declines. Symptoms last at least 2 wk.	Up to 13% of mothers (incidence: 2%–7%)	Insomnia or hypersomnia Fatigue and/or exhaustion, decreased motivation Poor concentration or indecisiveness; difficulty remembering
Postpartum depression	After delivery, rates increase and peak at 3 mo postpartum. Symptoms present any time in the first y after delivery and last at least 2 wk.	Up to 10% mothers (incidence: about 7%). Up to 4% of fathers (incidence 4%–25%)[32]	Feelings of worthlessness, guilt, inadequacy Suicidal thoughts Possibly anxiety, including bizarre thoughts, obsessions, and/or fears
Postpartum psychosis	Onset 1–4 wk postpartum.	1–2 cases in every 1000 new mothers	Auditory hallucinations and delusions (including commands and/or beliefs that need to harm the infant) Visual hallucinations Agitation, irritability, anger Insomnia Mood lability or highly elevated mood Disorganized thoughts and behaviors High levels of anxiety Paranoia; distrusting of others Confusion Thoughts of harming or killing self, others, or the infant

Adapted from Santoro K, Peabody H. *Identifying and Treating Maternal Depression: Strategies and Considerations for Health Plans. NIHCM Foundation Issue Brief.* Washington DC: National Institutes of Health Care Management; 2010:3.

contributing factors. Postpartum psychosis is an emergency, because there is risk of infanticide and up to a 70-fold increased risk of suicide.[33]

EPIDEMIOLOGY

Various sources estimate up to 15% to 20% of women experience perinatal depression in the United States, with worldwide prevalence almost double in low-income countries.[3,9,34–36] The Centers for Disease Control and Prevention surveyed 29 reporting areas across the United States in the 2009 Pregnancy Risk Assessment Monitoring System (PRAMS) (most recent published data) and found a prevalence of self-reported depressive symptoms ranging from 7.7% in Illinois to 19.9% in Arkansas.[37] The Agency for Healthcare Research and Quality conducted a systematic review as part of its Evidence-Based Practice Program in 2015, reviewing 30 epidemiological studies of perinatal depression (as confirmed by clinical assessment or structured interview). They estimated that at any given time, 12.7% of women meet criteria for an episode of MDD during pregnancy, with an additional 7.1% meeting criteria in the first 3 months postpartum. The rate of newly diagnosed cases or incidence of MDD during pregnancy was 7.5% during pregnancy and 6.5% in the first 3 months postpartum.[35] Authors of a more recent large epidemiological study found comparable results, with period prevalence rates of 12.4% during pregnancy and 9.6% in the postpartum period; incidence rates were 2.2% and 6.8%, respectively.[38] Studies have suggested that even higher rates of postpartum depression may be seen in low-income or ethnically diverse populations, teenagers, individuals with a previous history of perinatal depression, and those with a personal

TABLE 2 Risk Factors for Perinatal Depression

Risk Factors	Additional Risk Factors Specific for Depression After Delivery
History of depression	Depression before or during pregnancy
History of anxiety	Anxiety before or during pregnancy
Preexisting stressor or relationship issues	Experiencing stressful life events during pregnancy or the early postpartum period
Lack of social support	Traumatic birth experience
Unintended, unwanted pregnancy	Preterm birth and/or infant admission to neonatal intensive care
Medicaid insurance or uninsured	Breastfeeding problems
Domestic and/or family violence	
Lower income or socioeconomic status	
Lower education	
Smoking and substance use	
Single status	
Young parents (<30 y of age)	
Having previous children	

As reviewed in Lancaster et al,[49] Robertson et al,[50] and Underwood et al.[42]

or family history of postpartum depression or major depression.[7,36,39]

The prevalence of depression during pregnancy is highest during the second 2 trimesters.[40] Controlling for antenatal medical complications and past maternal psychiatric history, including depression, in late pregnancy has been shown to be associated with obstetric and pediatric complications, including increased need for epidural analgesia, operative deliveries, preterm birth, and neonatal intensive care admissions.[41] In the postpartum period, peak prevalence is at 3 months after delivery (12.9%) and then remains steady through 7 months at 9.9% to 10.6%.[35] A recent study in New Zealand revealed that even at 9 months postpartum, more than 5% of women endorsed significant depressive symptoms.[42] These figures provide further empirical support for the expanded definition of perinatal depression with a time course of up to 1 year postpartum and the expanded time frame of monitoring for symptoms.

The incidence of paternal postpartum depression ranges from 4% to 25% in community samples,[32] and maternal postpartum depression was identified as the strongest predictor, with 24% to 50% incidence in families in which there was also maternal postpartum depression.[23] New fathers are 1.38 times more likely to be depressed than age-matched males.[43] In at least 2 prevalence studies, 4% of fathers experienced clinical depression in the first year of the child's life.[44,45] In an 18-city study, 18% of fathers of children enrolled in Early Head Start had symptoms of depression, and fathers with depression had higher rates of substance use.[23] In general, men are more likely to avoid emotional expression, deny vulnerability, and not seek help, which may help explain discrepancies in prevalence rates.[46,47]

RISK FACTORS AND COMORBIDITIES

Multiple conditions are believed to increase the risk for perinatal depression (Table 2), although it is often difficult to clearly distinguish confounding factors and comorbidities. It was identified in PRAMS data from 2004 to 2005 that younger, non-Hispanic African American mothers were most likely to report postpartum depression symptoms.[48] The PRAMS data also revealed that women who had lower educational attainment and who received Medicaid benefits for their deliveries were more likely to report depressive symptoms. In all or nearly all of the 17 states participating in PRAMS, depressive symptoms were significantly associated with 5 possible co-occurring issues or comorbidities: use of tobacco during the last 3 months of pregnancy, physical abuse before or during pregnancy, partner-related stress, traumatic stress, and financial stress during pregnancy.[48] In 14 states, maternal depressive symptoms were significantly correlated with delivery of an infant with low birth weight and experiencing emotional stress during pregnancy. NICU admission was associated with maternal depressive symptoms in 9 states.[48]

It is documented that maternal stress, whether attributable to complications of the pregnancy or the mother's psychosocial situation, may contribute to and result from perinatal depression. Perinatal depression is strongly associated with previous miscarriage, past pregnancy complications, chronic medical disease, and shorter gestation and labor.[51] Psychosocial risk factors for perinatal depression include low socioeconomic status, being a single mother, being a teenager, having low self-esteem, prenatal anxiety, substance use, poverty, history of mood disorder, family history or past medical history of depression, having poor social support, and experiencing general life stress.[49,50,52,53] Having an infant with a difficult temperament is also a risk factor for perinatal depression, but a mother's perception of her inability to soothe her infant has a stronger association with postpartum depression than the actual duration of infant crying or fussing.[54]

Unwanted and unplanned pregnancies and relationship stress, including domestic violence and lack of social support, also have strong associations with perinatal depression.[49,55] Perinatal depression may be comorbid with marital discord, divorce, family violence (verbal and/or physical), and substance use and abuse.[56] The directionality of effect and potential reinforcement between these issues and perinatal depression is complex and warrants more study.

The etiology of perinatal depression is likely multifactorial, but there is evidence for a significant genetic basis. Familial trends in MDD are well established: first-degree relatives of someone with MDD have nearly 3 times the risk of developing it than those without such a family history.[57] Among women with a family history of postpartum depression, 42% experienced depression after their first delivery compared with only 15% of women with no such family history.[58]

Depression and anxiety are common comorbidities in the general population, with almost 60% of individuals with a diagnosis of MDD meeting criteria for an anxiety disorder at some point during their lifetime.[59,60] Depression and anxiety are also comorbidities in the perinatal period; in 1 review, anxiety had the strongest correlation with antepartum depression.[49] Biologically, studies have revealed that women with perinatal depression have abnormal stress hormone levels, particularly increased cortisol secretion, which is believed to be an underlying factor in anxiety symptoms.[61] Maternal anxiety is independently related to obstetric and pediatric complications, which compound the risk for perinatal depression. Anxiety symptoms in pregnancy are associated with preterm birth, low birth weight infants,[62] increased rate of cesarean delivery, reduced duration of breastfeeding, and increased maternal health care use within 2 weeks of delivery.[63] Maternal anxiety has also been connected to altered infant immune system function,[64] altered patterns of infant gastrointestinal microorganism growth,[65] and some limited research suggests that neural structures are modified that may predispose the child for anxiety disorders.[66] In terms of fathers, a correlation has also been documented between fathers who have preterm infants and higher levels of self-reported depression and anxiety symptoms.[67]

EFFECTS AND CONSEQUENCES

Effect on the Parent-Child Dyadic Relationship

In a classic experiment from the 1970s, researchers manipulated interactions between mothers and infants, illustrating that infants not only attempt to spontaneously initiate social exchanges but also modulate affect and attention around the presence and absence of reciprocal response. In the experiment, mothers first engaged in face-to-face reciprocal interactions (eg, when the child smiled, the mother smiled back, etc) in a laboratory with their 2- to 6-month-old infants. Mothers were then instructed to leave the room and reenter sitting opposite the infant with a "still face" (ie, an unresponsive "poker face"). In response, the infants reacted with fussiness, averting their gazes, slumping in their infant seats, and then reattempting to elicit interaction with a smile before finally giving up.[68] In later replications, exposure to the still face produced physiologic changes in the infants, such as increase in heart rate and decreased vagal tone.[69] When the mother reentered and again responded reciprocally, the infant's behavior and physiologic changes recover. This paradigm has been repeated with fathers and their infants demonstrating identical results,[70] and limited additional research further support the important role of paternal attachment.[71,72] This study ultimately reveals that the emotional life of an infant is heavily influenced by social interactions, particularly with parents, and the loss of parental engagement and reciprocity can be emotionally, behaviorally, and physiologically distressing, even if just temporarily.

"Attachment" describes the emotional connection between a child and parent that is characterized by a desire for closeness to maintain a sense of security, especially during times of stress and separation.[73–75] From a psychoanalytic perspective, the primary dyadic relationship serves as a prototype for all future social interactions.[74] Furthermore, the model is transactional, so rejection from a parent may cause the child to interpret the parent as rejecting as well as the self as unlovable.[76] From an organizational perspective, children progress through a hierarchy of relevant developmental tasks, each building on each other. Early effects of being raised by a parent who is emotionally absent and depressed, if sustained, can carry forward and adversely influence future adaptation.[77] Research suggests that parent-child relationships or attachment likely influences a child's ability to integrate positive representations of parents and of the self.[78] Therefore, high-quality parent-child dyadic interaction facilitates a secure attachment, which is 1 important factor in promoting early life resiliency, emotional regulation, and cognitive development.[79] Adaptations to the still-face experiment described provide some support for this claim, because infants at 6 months of age who were assessed as "securely attached" with their parents recovered faster with more "positive expression" immediately after the still-face exposure.[80]

Supportive behaviors by mothers that have been identified as especially important for cognitive and socioemotional development include following the child's interests and attention, responding contingently, and stimulating the child's engagement with his or her environment through verbal and practical encouragement. Parents who are depressed speak less, are less responsive (eg, smiling), present with flat affect, and express more negative emotions.[81–83] Mothers and fathers who are depressed are less likely to engage in enrichment activities with their child, including reading, singing, and storytelling.[25] Mothers with perinatal depression also demonstrate less reciprocal interaction; distorted perceptions of the infant's behavior, particularly rejection; less positive attribution, leading the child to irritability; less sensitivity and attunement; apathy; and lower rates of breastfeeding.[84,85]

Ultimately, insecure mother-child attachment is associated with social withdrawal from daily activities and less interaction. As early as 2 months of age, infants look at mothers who are depressed less, and infants of mothers with a history of poorly or untreated perinatal depression tend to demonstrate poor behavioral regulation, less explorative play, and lower activity levels. The infants have poor orientation skills and tracking, lower activity level, and irritable temperament. There is an increased risk of feeding and sleeping problems as well as failure to thrive.[81,86,87] Infants of mothers with untreated perinatal depression cry a lot because of difficulty with both self-comforting and being soothed by others. They may be apathetic, avoidant, clingy, or indifferent, and they tend not to exhibit any maternal preference or anxiety around strangers. Long-term impact of insecure attachment extends to preschool and older children with anxiety, behavior problems, poor peer relationships, school problems, and depression.[88] Such behaviors may even serve to worsen a parent's sense of worthlessness, rejection, and depression.[89]

Effect on the Child

In the prenatal period, maternal stress and depression negatively affect fetal growth and development.[90] Stress hormones, such as cortisol, are chronically elevated in states of generalized anxiety and depression, and they readily pass through the placenta. Animal and human studies reveal that increased maternal cortisol levels have been associated with decreased placental size, increased rates of fetal growth restriction, and premature delivery.[91–93] Norepinephrine, another stress hormone, does not cross the placenta, but it may influence the placental environment through peripheral effects, including increasing uterine arterial resistance and decreasing blood flow and oxygenation, resulting in fetal growth deprivation. Norepinephrine has also been associated with increased risk of preeclampsia.[94] Consequently, in 1 study, it was found that antenatal maternal depression led to a 34% increase in the odds of a developmental delay using the Denver II Developmental Screen in children at 18 months of age. This effect was statistically significant and independent of any postnatal depression.[95]

In the postpartum period, the still-face experiment revealed that social development starts early. In the experiment, infants demonstrated basic abilities to connect facial expression to emotional states, to have social and emotional awareness of others in their environment, and to adjust affect and attention in response to their parent. It also revealed that the absence of reciprocal interactions can have emotional consequences, including distress and withdrawal. This basic understanding of early emotional states combined with attachment research has given rise to transactional or social relational models of development. These models suggest that a child's emotional regulation, as well as possibly the child's physical, cognitive, and social well-being, depends heavily on close, intimate parent-infant relationships that begin early in life. Through mutually reinforcing and reciprocal interaction patterns, infants develop building blocks for social exchanges and future relationships, including the skill of turn taking, which is the basis for the pragmatics of language development. The theory suggests that as the child grows, his or her network of relationships becomes complex, which may promote more advanced levels of interactions, such as language and coordinated behaviors.[96–98] It would follow that physical, social, and cognitive development are likely inextricably linked, and disruption of early reciprocal relationships may have long-term adverse effects on overall development and health.

This reasoning has been supported by the body of research investigating adverse childhood experiences (ACEs), such as abuse, neglect, and family dysfunction. In a retrospective 1998 study of a large adult population, it was found that ACEs were common, which may point to high levels of resiliency present in childhood.[99] Those with high levels of risk behaviors and disease as adults (eg, obesity, smoking, depression, suicidality) reported being exposed to multiple ACEs as children. Childhood exposure to household mental illness, such as perinatal depression, was 1 of the more common ACEs reported, and it was often associated with other ACEs, such as exposure to parental substance use or domestic violence. The conclusion has been that accumulation of ACEs throughout childhood as well as their presence during particularly sensitive periods, such as early childhood, may have long-lasting effects on development and overall health into adulthood and may even contribute to an intergenerational cycle of recurring ACEs.[99,100]

Since the original ACEs study was conducted in 1998, there has been growing evidence, including prospective studies, directly associating perinatal depression with increased risk for problematic psychological and socioemotional development in children over time.[101–105] The longer a mother continues to experience depression, the more likely the child's developmental issues are to persist with less response to intervention.[106–108] In 1 study of children with internalizing symptoms (anxiety, depression), a history of maternal depression during the child's first 2 years of life was the best predictor of elevation in baseline cortisol levels at 7 years of age.[109] Prolonged cortisol elevation in preschool children predisposes them to anxiety disorders and social withdrawal.[110–112] Children of mothers with perinatal depression have been documented to have lower standardized scores of mental and motor development, poorer self-control, and social adjustment difficulties up to 5 years of age. Children of mothers with depression also had lower IQ with more attentional problems and difficulty with mathematical reasoning up to 11 years of age.[88,112,113]

In addition to primary associations with poor long-term outcomes for the child, untreated perinatal depression is also strongly tied with other unfavorable states and events that may add to the adverse effect on a child's overall health and development, including the following:

- child abuse and neglect;
- failure to implement the injury-prevention components from anticipatory guidance (eg, car safety seat and electrical plug covers)[114,115];
- failure to implement preventive health practices for the child (eg, Back to Sleep)[114,116–119]; and
- difficulty managing chronic health conditions such as asthma or disabilities in the young child.[117,120]

Families with a parent with depression have been reported to overuse health care and emergency facilities because of somatic complaints[120] and often fall behind on well-child visits and immunizations.[121] Perinatal depression also reduces a mother's chances of continued breastfeeding because of decreased satisfaction, more reported complications, and lower self-efficacy.[84]

The adverse effect of accumulating ACEs on child development may be mediated through the development of toxic stress, or the state of excessive, persistent, repetitive, and/or uncontrollable adversity without the buffering of a safe, stable, nurturing, and responsive parent to promote adaptive coping. Over time, toxic stress has consequences on brain architecture and disrupts multiple organ systems through chronic activation of stress hormone responses, cytokines, and immune modulators. The association between toxic stress states in early childhood and impaired language, cognitive and socioemotional development, and even lifelong disease has been independently validated.[122–124]

There is growing evidence that perinatal depression in parents contributes to elevated stress hormone levels in infants, suggesting that it is likely a contributing factor to toxic stress states. In 1 study, children exposed to mothers with postpartum depression had elevated levels of salivary cortisol levels during infancy[125] and at 3 years of age compared with children in a control group.[126] This effect was also revealed with adolescents at 13 years of age after controlling for current maternal or adolescent depression, experience of undesirable life events by the adolescent, maternal partner conflict, and duration of maternal depression.[127] Therefore, not only is the parent with depression impaired in his or her ability to function as a supportive buffer of adversity, but also, there may be a direct long-term activation of the child's stress responses. Persistent elevation of cortisol can disrupt the developing brain's architecture in the areas of the amygdala, hippocampus, and prefrontal cortex, affecting learning, memory, and behavioral and emotional adaptation.[122–124]

Animal studies with rats reveal compelling evidence for a causal relationship between maternal behaviors and stress reactivity in offspring through individual differences in neuronal gene expression transmitted from mother to pup through parenting behaviors in the first week of life. There is natural variation in maternal rat licking and/or grooming and nursing behaviors, so litters were split between mothers varying in levels of such behaviors. Pups exposed to less maternal care not only went on to provide less care to their own future young but also demonstrated increased gene expression in brain regions regulating behavioral and endocrine responses to stress.[128]

The influence of paternal depression on children and families has only recently been explored.[27,72] A large study from the United Kingdom revealed that paternal postpartum depression, when maternal postpartum depression was controlled for, was associated with adverse emotional and behavioral outcomes in children at 3 to 5 years of age, particularly conduct disorder in sons.[44] Fathers with depression negatively interact not only with their partners but also with their child, including being less likely to play with the child outside.[25] Furthermore, it is well documented that a father's affective state mirrors that of the mother, so there may be a compounded adverse effect on the child's social and emotional development.[23,71]

Fortunately, perinatal depression is identifiable and treatable. Early identification via screening increases access to timely care and significantly reduces the potential negative consequences for the child and family. Even brief psychosocial interventions within primary care settings have shown to be efficacious.[129] Recent studies have revealed that supports to increase maternal engagement and responsiveness can reverse gene expression patterns related to stress via epigenetic pathways and, thereby, buffer initial adverse effects of perinatal depression (DNA methylation and neuroendocrine functioning).[130]

PREVENTION

Antenatal Depression

Prevention of perinatal depression is challenging, given the complex biopsychosocial factors that influence the entire perinatal period. Historically, much of the focus has been exclusively on reducing risk factors, comorbidities, and adverse outcomes related to depression in the postpartum period, particularly on childhood development. There is growing evidence that untreated antenatal depression is 1 of the highest risk factors for meeting criteria for postpartum depression.[51,94,131,132] Early identification and management of depressive symptoms antenatally are needed to optimize the postpartum environment and prevent such symptoms from persisting.[50,131,133] Recommendations by several professional organizations, such as the Centers for Disease Control and Prevention,[48] the National Center for Children in Poverty,[134] the Center on the Developing Child,[123] the AAFP,[4] and the ACOG[3] have included screening women for depression routinely by antenatal providers, such as obstetricians, family physicians, nurse midwives, behavioral health providers, and other primary care clinicians.

Ideally, pediatric providers can collaborate with obstetric antenatal care providers so that maternal risk factors for perinatal depression are accurately communicated through all transitions of care.[133] Establishing this line of communication can be facilitated through a prenatal visit with the pediatric provider.[135] A prenatal visit with the pediatric provider is the first visit recommended in *Bright Futures: Guidelines for Health Supervision of Infants, Children, and Adolescents, Fourth Edition.*[15] An AAP clinical report defines the prenatal visit as important in building a relationship with the mother and father, coordinating services, and providing key anticipatory guidance and prevention education in the context of the upcoming birth.[135] If there are identified risk factors for perinatal depression, this visit allows the pediatric patient-centered medical home (PPCMH) to coordinate resources for the anticipated primary care and mental health needs of the mother and the mother-child dyad. More research is needed to understand and promote dyadic mother-child and parent-child mental health across the entire perinatal continuum.[131] Advocacy is needed to ensure payment to pediatric providers for prenatal visits and services.[135]

Postpartum Depression

A variety of interventions have revealed some success in preventing postpartum depression. Delivery room companions who provide early support with child-mother interaction combined with home visitation programs with nursing interventions, including cognitive behavioral therapy (CBT), have been shown to be successful, particularly for women at risk for depression, minorities, and underserved populations.[136–138] In another study, midwives were trained to provide individualized emotional support to mothers throughout their pregnancy, which led to improved continuity of care between antenatal and postpartum providers and reductions in symptoms of postpartum maternal depression.[139] In addition, prenatal childbirth classes or weekly parenting classes offered postpartum are potentially effective educational environments in which mothers and fathers can be engaged with messages around postpartum parental depression recognition and prevention.[139]

Finally, Practical Resources for Effective Postpartum Parenting (PREPP)[140] is 1 promising brief mother-infant dyadic intervention. PREPP is aimed at promoting the infant's sleep while reducing fussing and/or crying. This is achieved through integrating evidence-based caregiving techniques, traditional psychotherapy approaches, psychoeducation, and mindfulness meditation through a training program for at-risk women. As a result, mothers reported an increased sense of accomplishment, rest, and effectiveness while the incidence and severity of postpartum depression symptoms declined. PREPP revealed strong effects on reducing depression symptoms at 6 weeks, but the effect was not sustained beyond that period.[140] This suggests a role for pediatric providers in providing ongoing parenting education along with evidence-based strategies for coping with stress.

SCREENING

National and State Integrated Screening Systems

Despite the growing empirical evidence and support for screening for perinatal depression that leads to early identification and referrals for effective treatment, implementation of screening by pediatricians has been slowly increasing from 13% in 2001 to 47% in 2013 in periodic surveys.[9,21] In January 2016, the USPSTF completed its most recent review of the evidence for perinatal depression screening, providing a "grade B recommendation" for implementation. The task force found that there is a moderate net benefit to screening for perinatal depression, particularly when treatment such as psychotherapy or counseling can be made readily available.[20,141,142] Moderate net benefit refers to a situation in which the evidence supporting a prevention practice indicates a determined effect on health outcomes, but assessing the magnitude of effect may be limited by issues with the number, size, quality, consistency, and generalizability of available studies. The report specifically stated that there is "… convincing evidence that screening of pregnant and postpartum women in primary care improves the accurate identification of depression" and "… adequate evidence that programs combining depression screening with adequate support systems in place improve clinical outcomes for pregnant and postpartum women."[143]

In May 2016, CMS sent an informational bulletin (https://www.medicaid.gov/federal-policy-guidance/downloads/cib051116.pdf) to all state Medicaid directors stating, "since maternal depression screening is for the direct benefit of the child, state Medicaid agencies may allow such screening to be claimed as a service for the child as part of the Early and Periodic Screening, Diagnostic, and Treatment benefit." State programs can train providers to screen and refer mothers with positive screens if necessary, and states are eligible for Medicaid administrative matching funds to help with the cost of training.

The Well-Women Task Force is a collaborative initiative hosted by the ACOG. Existing guidelines were reviewed to develop consensus recommendations on the care of adolescent and adult women. This task force asserted that, in addition to providers offering annual screening for depression in adolescent and adult women using a validated tool, additional screening for depression is specifically recommended in the postpartum period.[144] The 2017 *Bright Futures: Guidelines for Health Supervision of Infants, Children, and Adolescents, Fourth Edition* recommendations from the AAP also now include screening for maternal depression by the 1-, 2-, 4-, and 6-month well-child visits.[15]

On the state level, health care providers, academic centers, Medicaid programs, legislatures, and local professional bodies, including AAP chapters, have been working for decades to incorporate maternal perinatal depression screening with standardized tools into prenatal, postpartum, and periodic well-child visits. Ideally, screening would be conducted within a system of care that also provides access to additional mental health evaluation and treatment when concerns are identified. Although such interdisciplinary integration is not always available or feasible, progress has been made. New Jersey and Illinois (2008) were the first to pass legislative requirements for perinatal depression screening, which resulted in increased awareness, conducted assessments, and referrals for treatment. In 2010, Massachusetts policymakers led the way by creating a statewide Postpartum Depression Commission to advocate for screening and treatment and to monitor implementation. Several other states have since made efforts to provide training and support even without a formal legislative mandate. In addition, a growing number of state Medicaid programs are now paying for perinatal depression screening. For more information on related state laws and policies, contact AAP State Advocacy at stgov@aap.org. Many states have developed quality improvement programs, community support groups, media campaigns, and other resources to improve both provider and public awareness of the need for early identification and treatment of perinatal depression.[145] Ultimately, such state-level efforts have fostered early identification and treatment of affected parents and have increased public awareness of screening protocols and procedures and appropriate referrals for additional family assessment, support, and treatment. The recent AAP recommendations are for universal screening of infant behavior and development[146] and partnering with mental health care providers to implement evidence-based treatments during early childhood.[147] These recommendations are increasingly being adopted by pediatric providers in all states.[15] An important aspect of screening is to also assess for common perinatal depression comorbidities that adversely affect child development, behavior, and the family environment, including substance use, domestic violence, and food insecurity. Standardized screening tools are now, more than ever, being used to assess for such comorbidities.[148]

State perinatal depression screening efforts were also aided when the National Quality Forum developed a quality measure (National Quality Forum Measure 1401) that assesses whether a maternal perinatal depression screen was administered to a patient's mother at 1 face-to-face visit with her provider during the first 6 months of the child's life.[149] This measure was endorsed by the CMS for the Electronic Health Record Incentive Program in March 2013.[150] The quality measure was anticipated to help with the adoption of perinatal depression screening by providers participating in Meaningful Use Incentive programs, although these programs have since been modified.

Role of the Primary Pediatric Clinician and the PPCMH

Perinatal depression is a pertinent issue for the primary care clinician because of the significant risks to the health and well-being of the infant and the family.[2] Pediatric primary care practices, particularly those identifying as PPCMHs, can build a system to implement postpartum depression screening, to connect affected families to supportive community resources, and to refer parents for additional treatment when indicated.[1]

Early identification and appropriate treatment of perinatal depression can result in more favorable outcomes for the expectant and postpartum mother,[143] her infant, and the entire family.[1] As mentioned, prevention and screening for risk factors and comorbidities of perinatal depression start well before birth in the preconception and antenatal periods where obstetric providers, midwives, and family and adult primary care practitioners are optimally positioned. The ACOG has specific recommendations for antenatal screening as well as collaboration between obstetric providers and their pediatric colleagues to facilitate ongoing assessment, treatment, and support for women with perinatal depression and their families.[3] Ideally, this occurs through handoffs that include important information on antenatal screening, risk factors, and comorbidities of perinatal depression, particularly the existence of any intimate partner violence, substance use, or obstetric complications. The prenatal visit, recommended by the 2017 *Bright Futures: Guidelines for Health Supervision of Infants, Children, and Adolescents, Fourth Edition* recommendations from the AAP, is an opportunity for obtaining such information, assessing existing supports, and providing direct education to potential parents about expectations during the first few days of a child's life and the symptoms of perinatal depression.[15,135,151]

In the postpartum period, the USPSTF and CMS recommend screening of parents by pediatric providers caring for infants with a validated tool at the 1-, 2-, 4-, and 6-month well-child visits. This recommendation is supported by the current understanding of when postpartum depression peaks in prevalence. Repeated screenings are important, because mothers who may not be comfortable disclosing initially may do so at later visits as trust and familiarity builds with the pediatric provider. Perinatal depression is also associated with missed appointments, so having multiple screening times also increases the probability that such families are screened and maximizes opportunities for identification of concerns and engagement in ongoing supports and pediatric health surveillance. Pediatric providers can also screen for and promote healthy social-emotional development in the infant using general developmental and specific social-emotional screening tools when risks factors for or maternal symptoms of postpartum depression are present. In the postpartum period, the parents' primary care and mental health providers are important partners that can communicate with and work with pediatric providers to prevent, buffer, and ameliorate the adverse effects of postpartum depression on the family.[81–83,142]

The PPCMH setting provides an interdisciplinary infrastructure to both implement postpartum depression screening and respond to specific concerns. PPCMHs may have embedded services or expertise from multiple disciplines, including care managers, lactation consultants, social workers, and pediatric mental health providers. Collocating or integrating mental health and pediatric primary care services has been shown to help with access to and compliance with mental health services for infants, children, and their parents. Having these services collocated or integrated also facilitates communication across services, particularly using a shared medical record.[152,153]

Over the well-child visit schedule, the pediatric provider, ideally as a part of a PPCMH, develops a longitudinal relationship with the infant and his or her parents starting at an early age. As trust is built in the provider-patient relationship, it provides opportunities to emphasize the importance of both infant and parental mental health.[16] Well-child visits have an important role in assessing social determinants of health and promoting healthy social-emotional development in young children.[15,16,154] In addition, well visits offer opportunities for screening for psychosocial stressors and concerns, including parental depression, as mentioned previously, as well as intimate partner violence, substance use, poverty, food insecurity, and homelessness.[154] These psychosocial issues can have a compounding effect with perinatal depression and can promote an environment of toxic stress.[155] Recognized in the AAP policy statement, "The Future of Pediatrics:

Mental Health Competencies for Pediatric Primary Care,"[16] is the unique advantage of the primary care clinician, particularly in a PPCMH context, for surveillance, screening, and addressing child and parental mental health outcomes through:

- longitudinal, trusting relationship with the family, including the creation of a safe space for discussion of psychosocial issues;
- family centeredness, including attention to the parents' emotional needs;
- unique opportunities for prevention and anticipatory guidance, including communication and discussion with families in a way that fosters early detection and intervention of emerging social-emotional and mental health concerns and problems;
- understanding of common social-emotional and learning issues in the context of development;
- experience in coordinating with and referring to a broad range of relevant specialists and community-based agencies, particularly those that are focused on the care of children with special health care needs and their families; and
- familiarity with chronic care principles and practice improvement.[156]

Several validated and effective screening instruments for perinatal depression have been developed and are readily available (reviewed in detail below).[1,3] However, despite having access to these screening tools, many physicians do not screen for perinatal depression.[8,21] Many barriers to screening for perinatal depression are reported by providers, including the lack of time to screen and competing demands, inadequate knowledge about the validated tools available and how to appropriately document findings, lack of or insufficient reimbursement to screen and discuss results, and fears associated with legal implications of screening.[7,10] Studies reveal that providers who rely solely on observational cues and do not use validated tools to screen tend to underdiagnose parental depression.[157,158] As a result, many women may erroneously attribute their changes in mood, fatigue, sleep, eating, body weight, and other symptoms of postpartum depression to their pregnancy and do not seek necessary support.[3]

There is some evidence that screening for perinatal depression can also be conducted effectively in emergency department and pediatric inpatient settings for the mother of an infant in the first year of life.[159,160]

Perinatal Depression Screening Tools

Multiple screening tools exist that can efficiently identify patients at risk for perinatal depression, and most are available free online (Table 3). If there is an interest in reproducing any of these tools, it is important to check with the authors and/or developers of the tools to honor any of the copyright requirements and/or requests for permission for use. Before using any screening tool, it is also important to have detailed policies and protocols about how to address identified depressive symptoms, including follow-up or referral to a licensed mental health provider, if necessary. Knowledge of appropriate emergency mental health resources is important. Immediate action is required at any time during the administration of a screening tool if a parent expresses any concern about the infant's safety or if the parent reports being (or pediatric provider suspects the parent is) suicidal, homicidal, severely depressed, manic, or psychotic.[161] Appropriate documentation of perinatal depression screenings includes the screen used, results, discussion with the parent including anticipatory guidance, and the plan for follow-up and/or referrals.[6]

The EPDS[163] is a free, widely-used 10-question instrument that is used specifically to screen for perinatal depression. The EPDS was originally developed for screening postpartum women in outpatient, home-visiting settings or at the 6- to 8-week postpartum examination. The tool has been validated with numerous populations and is available in Spanish[164] and for fathers.[165–167] Of note, it includes reverse-scored items that can be used to assess reliability of responses. The most recent 2016 recommendations of the USPSTF clearly conclude that there is sufficient evidence to support the use of the EPDS as an effective screening tool for depression in pregnant and postpartum women.[20] The Survey of Well-being of Young Children (SWYC) (www.theSWYC.org) is a validated developmental and psychosocial screening tool that now includes the EPDS in the 2-, 4-, and 6-month questionnaires (available in English, Spanish, Burmese, Nepali, and Portuguese).[168] The EPDS has some benefit in identifying anxiety disorders as well but is not focused on somatic symptoms or parent-infant relationships.

A total score of 10 or more on the EPDS is a positive screen indicating a concern for depression, which necessitates further discussion in which providers can clarify the findings, determine acuity of concerns, and, if necessary, make appropriate referrals for further assessment and treatment of the parent (as described below).[129,163] It is important to note that similar to all screening tools, the EPDS is not a diagnostic instrument. In situations in which there is any indication of suicidal ideation (on the EPDS question 10 or in discussion), if the parent expresses concern about his or her ability to maintain the infant's safety, or if the pediatric provider suspects that the parent is suicidal or

TABLE 3 Valid Screening Tools for Perinatal Depression

Screening Tool	No. Items	Sensitivity and Specificity[a,b]	Available for Free
EPDS	10	Mothers (score >9–12) Sensitivity 80%–90% Specificity 80%–90% Fathers (score >10) Sensitivity 90% Specificity 78%	Yes[c]
PDSS	35	Sensitivity 80%–90% Specificity 80%–90%	No http://www.wpspublish.com/store/p/2902/postpartum-depression-screening- scale-pdss
PHQ-2	2	Sensitivity 100% Specificity 44.3%–65.7%	Yes[c]
PHQ-9	9	Sensitivity 75%–89% Specificity 83%–91%	Yes[c]
Beck Depression Inventory–II	21	Sensitivity 75%–90% Specificity 80%–90%	No http://www.pearsonclinical.com/psychology/products/100000159/beck-depression-inventoryii-bdi-ii.html

All of the above screening tools take <10 min to complete, on average, and are available in Spanish.

[a] Validity specifically for postpartum depression as reviewed in Myers et al.[162]

[b] For EDPS only; as reviewed in Siu et al.[21]

[c] Indicated free screening tools are available on the AAP Web site: https://www.aap.org/en-us/advocacy-and-policy/aap-health-initiatives/Screening/Pages/Screening-Tools.aspx; https://brightfutures.aap.org/materials-and-tools/tool-and-resource-kit/Pages/Developmental-Behavioral-Psychosocial-Screening-and-Assessment-Forms.aspx.

homicidal, it is considered a positive screen that warrants an immediate evaluation for safety of the parent and/or infant, often in an emergency psychiatric setting. Immediate action with a referral to an emergency psychiatric setting has also been recommended with scores greater than 20 or if there is clinical concern that the parent may be severely depressed, manic, or psychotic.[163]

The accuracy of the EPDS as a screening tool in pregnant and postpartum women has been established by a recent USPSTF review of 23 studies (n = 5298) comparing the accuracy of the EPDS with a diagnostic interview. Sensitivity of the EPDS using a cutoff of 13 ranged from 0.67 (95% confidence interval [CI], 0.18–0.96) to 0.8 (95% CI, 0.81–1.00) for the detection of MDD. Specificity for detecting MDD was consistently 0.87 or higher.[20,141,143] Two studies in this review were conducted in the United States (1 specifically among African American women) demonstrating an average sensitivity of approximately 0.80. The positive predictive value for detecting MDD would be 47% to 64% in a population with a 10% prevalence of MDD.[143,169,170] The Agency for Healthcare Research and Quality also reviewed validity statistics for various screening tools among postpartum women specifically and found that the EPDS had a sensitivity of 80% to 90% and specificity of 80% to 90%.[162] Higher cutoff scores for EPDS have been proposed (up to a threshold of 13) to limit false-positive results.[171] Recently, shorter versions of the EPDS have been validated, including a 2-question screen for adolescent mothers.[172]

The EPDS has demonstrated cross-cultural sensitivity,[163] including the Spanish version, which showed acceptable performance characteristics.[143] The EPDS is also available in French, Dutch, Swedish, Spanish, Chinese, Thai, Turkish, and Arabic. Cutoff scores may vary in different populations.[173]

One screen that has been used over the last decade in some primary care settings is the Patient Health Questionnaire-2 (PHQ-2).[174,175] The PHQ-2 is a simple, free general depression screening tool (ie, not limited to use in the postpartum period or with women) with 2 questions about depressed mood and anhedonia that are derived from the longer 9-question Patient Health Questionnaire-9 (PHQ-9) (discussed in the following paragraph). The PHQ-2 does not include a question about suicidality. The PHQ-2 has been studied in both primary care and obstetric populations.[176] The 2 questions in the PHQ-2 are:

1. Over the past 2 weeks, have you ever felt down, depressed, or hopeless?
2. Over the past 2 weeks, have you felt little interest or pleasure in doing things?

A person is asked to choose 1 of 4 possible choices for each question that comes closest to how he or she has been feeling: not at all (0), several days (1), more than half the days (2), or nearly every day (3). A score of 3 out of a maximum of 6 is the accepted cutoff for a positive screen, with a sensitivity of 83% and a specificity of 92% for MDD.[176] Studies in postpartum populations, specifically, reveal that the sensitivity of the PHQ-2 is 100% and the specificity is 44.3% to 65.7%.[162]

The most recent USPSTF review[143] concluded that no studies of screening in pregnant or postpartum women conducted with the PHQ-2 met methodologic inclusion criteria. As a result, the USPSTF currently has determined that there is not sufficient evidence to support the use of the PHQ-2 at this time as a primary screening tool in pregnant and postpartum women.[20] Yet many practices continue to use it as an initial screen. If a parent screens positive with the PHQ-2, then the recommendation is that it be followed up with a more comprehensive screening tool (eg, PHQ-9, discussed in the following paragraph, or the EPDS).[174,175]

The longer 9-question PHQ-9 has been used as a primary screening instrument for perinatal depression and to monitor for worsening or improvement of perinatal depression symptoms over time.[177] The PHQ-9 has also been widely used to screen nonpregnant adults[178] and adolescents for depression.[179] The diagnostic validity of the PHQ-9 has been established in both primary care and obstetrical clinics,[179,180] although the USPSTF concluded that the data were insufficient for specific use in postpartum depression screening. In addition to the questions from the PHQ-2, the PHQ-9 also asks how often over the past 2 weeks the person has been bothered by different problems related to sleep, lack of energy, feeling bad or letting someone down (feeling like a failure), appetite, concentration, speaking slowly, or being restless. Similar to the PHQ-2, the respondent is asked to choose 1 of 4 responses for symptoms corresponding to how often they are experienced, ranging from not at all to nearly every day. The PHQ-9 specifically asks about suicidal thoughts and how any of the identified symptoms affect the respondent's ability to function at work, at home, or in interacting with other people. Scores of 5, 10, 15, and 20 on the PHQ-9 represent mild, moderate, moderately severe, and severe depression, respectively. PHQ-9 scores ≥10 had a sensitivity of 88% and specificity of 88% for MDD[180] and among postpartum women had a specificity of 75% to 89% and specificity of 83% to 91%.[162] However, the most recent USPSTF review[143] concluded that no studies of screening in pregnant or postpartum women conducted using the PHQ-9 met methodologic inclusion criteria. Although the USPSTF currently has determined that there is not sufficient evidence to support the use of the PHQ-9 specifically in pregnant and postpartum women,[20] it still continues to be used widely.

Other screens are available with a cost and may be used by adult and mental health providers during the pregnancy or postpartum period and much less often by pediatric primary care clinicians. However, some adult and pediatric providers may choose to use these in partnership with mental health providers who are collocated, integrated, or linked with an obstetric, family medicine, or pediatric practice. The Beck Depression Inventory (BDI-II)[181] is a 21-question scale that is a self-report tool used to provide more feedback on severity of depressive symptoms. This tool is currently endorsed by the USPSTF[141] as an effective screening tool for postpartum depression and also continues to be endorsed by the USPSTF for use in screening all adolescents between 12 and 18 years of age for depression.[182] Two additional tools are the Hamilton Depression Rating Scale (HAM-D)[183] and the Postpartum Depression Screening Scale (PDSS). The Hamilton Depression Rating Scale uses an interview format and is mostly used in research settings. The PDSS is a 35-question screen that identifies patients at high risk for depression but is less commonly used.[184] Among postpartum women, the PDSS has a sensitivity and specificity of 80% to 90%.[162] It should be noted that these screening tools include constitutional symptoms such as insomnia, changes in appetite, low energy, etc, which may be normative in pregnancy, so their specificity is lower for perinatal depression.[3]

A drawback to these currently less commonly used questionnaires is that they tend to yield higher estimates than clinician-administered interviews, so clinical assessment is recommended but often not conducted. Also, studies differ in their methods in terms of cutoff scores, reporting of cutoff scores, and use of scores as continuous measures in analysis.[61] Just as with the EPDS, these other questionnaires are only screening tools, and they do not diagnose MDD or perinatal depression. Diagnosis requires a face-to-face clinical assessment and, in some circumstances, referral for clinical correlation by an appropriately licensed health care professional.[129]

Infant Assessment

Routine well-child visits allow for pediatric providers to assess and promote healthy early child development, including assessing overall family strengths and supports and the child's social-emotional adjustment.[15,142,146] Identified developmental concerns and delays in an infant may be the only indication of perinatal depression, difficulty with early adjustment as a new family, as well as many other factors. When developmental delays are present in the child, they often increase the stress and decrease the perceived efficacy experienced by the mother.[185] Therefore, several screening tools (some are free online) can be used to assess the child's social-emotional development, family supports, and early family adjustments. These tools can be used whenever there are developmental concerns or delays, particularly if the mother presents with other risk factors identified or has been previously diagnosed with perinatal depression. These tools include the

Ages and Stages Questionnaire Social Emotional-2,[186] the Early Childhood Screening Assessment,[187] the SWYC,[148,168] and the Baby Pediatric Symptom Checklist, which is included in the SWYC,[188,189] among others. Guidance on these and other similar screening tools is available in a policy statement and technical report about early childhood emotional and behavioral problems.[147]

DIAGNOSIS AND TREATMENT

As discussed, screening tools alone are inadequate for diagnosing perinatal depression, but when they indicate concerns, the pediatric provider's role is to discuss results and facilitate referral for appropriate supports and treatment. Some PPCMHs may have mental health, social work, lactation support, and other such services collocated or even integrated directly into a visit, which decreases stigma and improves access.[153,190] In the context of discussing screening results, an opportunity exists to validate parents' experiences and inquire about existing supports available to them and their family in times of transient acute stress. These supports may include extended family, friends, and even therapists or counselors who are providing mental health treatment. It is also a time when careful attention can be given to assessing for any risk of suicide or harm to the infant as well as the presence of other psychosocial stressors or comorbidities in addition to depression.

As was previously discussed, rates of intimate partner violence and substance use are elevated in families in which a parent has perinatal depression symptoms. If there is specific concern for domestic or intimate partner violence or substance use, especially in the perinatal period, then state agencies may require notification. Many national and community agencies are available to support families as well. Information about local organizations available to support victims of intimate partner violence can be accessed through the National Domestic Violence Hotline at http://www.thehotline.org or 1-800-799-SAFE.

A positive screen leads to a discussion with the parent about the specific mental health concerns and symptoms identified in the screening tool and/or during a patient encounter.[142] There is literature showing that, in addition to pediatric providers, such a discussion can be conducted by the parent's primary care provider, obstetric provider, or a licensed mental health provider with perinatal expertise.[129] There may be times when the screening is positive, without suicidal ideation or risk of harm to the infant, and the mother is not interested in a referral for further evaluation and diagnosis. It is important for the pediatric provider and/or other members of the PPCMH to inquire about existing supports and clarify the psychosocial concerns and comorbidities, such as domestic violence and substance use, that may affect the welfare of the infant and to follow-up to monitor the abatement of risk.

When a screen is positive in "low-risk" situations, without suicidal ideation or risk of harm to the infant, a pediatric provider may consider recommending the mother to follow-up with her obstetric or primary care provider for additional discussion and also closely monitoring the infant and mother with a visit or telephone call before the next scheduled well-child visit. The pediatric provider may also recommend adjustments in schedule to provide adequate sleep, additional supports from community agencies such as quality child care, home visiting, mother's morning out programs, or other programs. There are additional office-based interventions that a pediatric provider can implement that will be discussed below.[1] In discussion with the parent and family, it may be determined that referrals to mental health and specialty providers are necessary for diagnostic evaluation, psychotherapy, or even consideration of psychiatric medication management.[142]

In "high-risk" situations in which there are concerns for suicidal ideation, risk of harm to the infant, or severe mental illness, there may be urgent or emergent need for referral to an emergency psychiatric setting for evaluation and treatment.

Regardless of the level of risk or modality of treatment, it is important to explain to parents the assessed need for follow-up or referral, specifically if further evaluation and treatment is necessary by a parent's primary care provider or a mental health specialist. If perinatal depression is ultimately diagnosed, then reassurance can be offered that pediatric providers can work with such adult providers and community organizations to support the parent and his or her ability to best care for the child. Consideration of risk factors, parent's previous psychiatric history, and former treatments, if known by the pediatric provider at the time of referral, is important to communicate through the transition in care to develop an accurate risk profile.[3,191]

Access to Treatment

Although progress is being made in identifying and effectively treating perinatal depression, the cumulative shortfalls in mothers receiving effective treatment are still large. In a recent study, only 49% of women with antenatal depression and 30.8% of women with postpartum depression were screened and identified in practice. In addition, 13.6% of women with antenatal depression and 15.8% of women with postpartum depression received any treatment, and only

8.6% of women with antenatal depression and 6.3% of women with postpartum depression received adequate treatment. Ultimately, 4.8% of women with antenatal depression and 3.2% of women with postpartum depression achieved remission.[192]

Despite the consequences of untreated perinatal depression and the presence of a range of options for effective, evidence-based treatment, most mothers with perinatal depression do not seek therapy and treatment for themselves and their infants.[11,193] Mothers may not seek therapy because of concern about perceptions of others (ie, stigma), cost and a lack of insurance coverage, need for child care during the mental health visit, lack of access to a trained provider and lack of knowledge about perinatal depression, unrealistic beliefs about coping with being a mother, feelings of failure, and fears about using mental health services.[11] These challenges are compounded by the symptoms of depression, especially low energy and motivation, which adversely affect a mother's ability to access help.

Fortunately, data suggest that when providers speak to patients about their depression, they are more likely to become engaged and seek treatment. Use of provider notification systems and motivational interviewing techniques can assist providers in engaging their patients in discussions about their depression.[194] A study from the University of Michigan found that a single motivational interviewing session can increase rates of treatment adherence, particularly through the process of identifying and challenging practical and psychological barriers to care.[195]

In many pediatric clinics and PPCMHs, care coordinators have a significant role in developing and maintaining a referral network of community resources and specialty providers for perinatal depression. They can often follow through to ensure patients are able to access necessary specialty providers in a timely manner.[16,196] An integrated frontline mental health provider, such as a licensed clinical social worker or counselor, can provide immediate triage for a positive screen, conduct additional assessments, offer support, and coordinate follow-up and referrals for the infant, mother, and family. Regardless of whether a clinic has a care coordinator or integrated mental health provider, many sources emphasize the importance of close working relationships and communication between pediatric providers and mental health providers, adult primary care providers, and other agencies in the community with expertise in the evaluation, treatment, and/or support of the mother with perinatal depression and the mother-infant dyad.[1,3]

Emergency and/or Urgent Situations

Many screening tools have critical thresholds above which they recommend that the pediatric provider take immediate action, which usually means referring the parent to an emergency psychiatric setting to ensure safety with timely evaluation and treatment. If question 10 inquiring about suicidality on the EPDS is positive,[161,163] if question 9 inquiring about suicidality on the PHQ-9 is positive, if the parent expresses concern about maintaining the infant's safety during any screening, or if the pediatric provider is concerned at any time with screening that the parent is suicidal, homicidal, severely depressed, manic, or psychotic, immediate evaluation is warranted in an emergency psychiatric setting (ie, calling 911) or by a crisis team that can respond directly to the provider (if available in the community).[161] Although the ultimate goal is to support the mother so she can best care for her child, in a situation in which the mother requires immediate evaluation, it is important that someone is available to specifically maintain care for the infant. An ideal process is that the mother is not left alone at any time, and if sent to an emergency psychiatric setting, the mother is accompanied by a trusted adult or staff member.

If the provider's level of concern is elevated but an emergency intervention is deemed not necessary, precautions are taken to promote safety, including having the mother leave with a support person (not alone), ensuring adequate supervision of the mother and infant at home, composing a specific safety plan (including phone numbers and steps for accessing help urgently), and scheduling close follow-up. Pediatric providers can be prepared by having a current list of contacts for pediatric and adult emergency mental health providers on hand. Fortunately, most positive perinatal depression screens do not necessitate urgent or emergency action by the pediatric provider.[197] Intervention for the mother ranges from support, to therapy, to therapy plus medication, to emergency mental health services and hospitalization.[198,199]

Infant and/or Dyadic Interventions

In promoting evidence-based mental health treatments for infants and their mothers with perinatal depression, most approaches caution against implying any blame or carrying an exclusive focus on challenges faced by the mother. Strengths-based approaches that are focused on the infant-mother dyad are promoted on the basis of some evidence of efficacy in generally addressing attachment issues and developmental concerns in other settings.[147,200,201] Most of these dyadic interventions are focused on infant-mother attachment, but limited evidence is now suggesting the importance of supporting attachment with fathers and nontraditional families.[202] For example, there are specific evidence-based dyadic interventions that have been used with high-risk families, often in the setting of interpersonal violence or abuse, such as Child Parent Dyadic Psychotherapy[203] and Attachment and Biobehavioral Catch-up.[204] Circle of Security[205] has been specifically validated for use specifically with mothers with perinatal depression and their infants.[147,201] Videotaped interactions of mothers and their infants with feedback and coaching has shown efficacy.[94]

Dyadic psychotherapy is an evolving field. These interventions may not be readily available in all areas and require mental health providers to obtain specialized training. Pediatric providers can play an important role in advocating for increased availability of such services, specialized training, and availability of a specialized workforce with experience working with young children, parents, and families.

Office-Based Supportive Management by Pediatric Providers

Pediatric providers can have an important role in partnering with parents, families, and various other involved providers to manage and support parents with perinatal depression. However, considering the demands placed on pediatric providers in most settings, it is essential to evaluate what is feasible and effective for any given practice and in the context of each individual family. It is important that the pediatric provider consider collaborating closely with the mother's adult providers, mental health care providers, and various local agencies to provide optimal support for the mother-child dyad within the entire family structure.

When time and resources allow, pediatric providers can offer parents in low-risk situations office-based interventions. Components of most office-based interventions include:

- explanation and open dialogue with the mother and family to help reduce stigma, normalize the stress faced by new families, and ultimately, foster early identification of those who may need additional resources ("demystification");
- communication about the potential impact on the infant and need for infant screenings and surveillance;
- initial and ongoing support, which includes providing validation and empathy for the mother's experiences and identifying community resources to promote family wellness; and
- reinforcement, when necessary, through referrals to evidence-based treatment programs. Referrals may take the form of a mental health provider for the parent or lactation support for the mother, as will be discussed later.

Demystification is directed at removing the mystery about maternal and paternal depression—that postpartum depression can affect any parent, that it is not the parents' fault, and that it does not imply "bad" parenting. Depression is treatable, and the support facilitated by the pediatric provider for appropriate intervention is an essential ingredient.[1] Having an infant and expanding the family is a transition that can be difficult when there are other stressors involved. However, many parents also experience resiliency factors, such as stable housing, adequate family and/or friend supports, and access to care, which may help attenuate the risk of perinatal depression.

The AAP Task Force on Mental Health promoted the use of a common factors approach to routine mental health assessment[206] to engage families and build an alliance.[16] *Bright Futures: Guidelines for Health Supervision of Infants, Children, and Adolescents, Fourth Edition* provides health promotion themes, including family support, child development, and mental health. Specifically, it includes surveillance for parental socioemotional well-being and for social determinants of health.[15] The common factors theory asserts that therapies can be designed for broad classes of people rather than specific individuals who are deemed "at-risk" or fit a specific diagnostic category.[206] The common factors theory emphasizes that providers can influence behavioral change in patients and families through specific evidence-based interaction approaches, such as motivational interviewing, integrated into routine visits. A mnemonic for a group of common factors that can be routinely assessed and monitored throughout the scheduled well-child visits is "HELLPPP," which stands for hope, empathy, language, loyalty, permission, partnership, and plan.[206] In the absence of an urgent psychiatric crisis, pediatric providers can build alliance and common understanding over time that will foster greater disclosure and recognition of mental health needs and social-emotional concerns. For example, pediatric providers may recognize the need for anticipatory guidance and education on parenting and lifestyle issues (eg, sleep, exercise, diet, rest) that ultimately could mitigate the risk of depression and promote the mental health of parents and children. More details are available on the AAP Mental Health Initiatives site, with a resource in the AAP Mental Health Toolkit at https://www.aap.org/en-us/advocacy-and-policy/aap-health-initiatives/Mental-Health/Pages/Primary-Care-Tools.aspx.

Following is an example of how a brief intervention can be designed by using the common factors approach within the context of a PPCMH to provide support to a parent when there are concerns for perinatal depression:

- Hope: increase the parent's hopefulness by describing realistic expectations and reinforcing the value and strengths of the mother-infant relationship and understanding and responding to the infant's cues;
- Empathy: communicate empathy by listening attentively;
- Language: use the parent's language to reflect your understanding of the concerns for perinatal depression;
- Loyalty: communicate loyalty to the parent by expressing your support and commitment to help;
- Permission: ask for permission to share information;
- Partnership: partner to work together to address common concerns; and
- Plan:
    - encourage infant and parent routines for predictability and security;
    - encourage focus on wellness: sleep, diet, exercise, stress relief;
    - Ask about concerns regarding breastfeeding, and support and/or encourage if the mother is able to breastfeed. It is important to address specific worries and try to reassure the mother when she is doing well with the breastfeeding and her infant is adequately gaining weight;
    - encourage social connections and supports;
    - depending on the degree of concern from the perinatal depression screening, refer the parent and infant dyad to mental health providers who use evidence-based treatments, and follow-up closely; and
    - make referrals to a variety of agencies and efforts in your local community as available and described below.[206]

Other brief interventions that could take place when there are concerns for postpartum depression could include:

- encourage understanding and response to the infant's cues; emphasize the importance of observing nonverbal behavior;
- encourage routines for predictability and security;
- encourage focus on wellness (sleep, diet, exercise, stress relief);
- acknowledge personal experiences;
- promote realistic expectations and prioritizing important things; and
- encourage social involvement and bolster social networks and supports.

Partnering With Community Agencies

Mental health providers are an important resource, but many community agencies can also provide essential support, such as home-based services or partial hospitalization programs that specialize in addressing stressors of the postpartum period. Part C of the Individuals with Disabilities in Education Act (IDEA) governs how states and community organizations and programs provide services to infants and children from birth to 3 years of age with disabilities or developmental delays, with or without an established condition. This legislation supports early intervention programs that provide family-centered services to help children from birth to age 3 develop skills necessary to promote health and positive development in early life. Early intervention programs can provide education and assessment targeting the infant-parent dyad, often by modeling positive interactions and play.[1,207] However, in many areas, early intervention referrals can be difficult to facilitate because of limitations in state-specific eligibility requirements (emphasizing cognitive, motor, and language delays but not social-emotional delays) and insufficient funding. Inadequate funding may also limit the ability of such services to provide adequate and uniform interventions addressing social-emotional developmental delays for infants and the mother-infant dyad across sites.[207] These challenges to accessing early intervention are concerning given the inextricable connection of social-emotional development to physical health, language acquisition, and cognitive development.

Early Head Start, Head Start, home-visiting programs, and postpartum support groups are additional examples of community resources that are available in many areas. There are opportunities in various regions for public health nurses, lactation specialists, parent educators, and facilitators of family support groups (see http://www.motherwoman.org or www.postpartum.net) to form partnerships with pediatric providers aimed at reducing perinatal depression.

In Massachusetts, the legislature has funded an adjunct to the Massachusetts Child Psychiatry Access Project (MCPAP) called MCPAP for Moms. This statewide project improves access through providing immediate consultation and referral services to pediatric providers and other providers when a positive perinatal depression screen is identified in the community. Furthermore, MCPAP for Moms has created a toolkit for pediatric providers that is available free of charge (www.mcpapformoms.org). The Substance Abuse and Mental Health Services Administration also has a similar toolkit that describes how community service agencies can approach perinatal depression, specifically through forming effective partnerships with pediatric providers.[208]

Psychotherapy and Psychological Interventions

Several validated individual psychological treatments are offered by mental health professionals to help mothers with perinatal depression.[199] Psychotherapy is often preferred by women over medication during the perinatal period because of perceived adverse effects of medication on pregnancy and with breastfeeding.[209] Many women identified with mild to moderate postpartum depression are optimally treated with psychotherapy and do not require medication.[198]

The USPSTF[143] evaluated the efficacy of psychological treatment with trials in postpartum women, revealing a 28% to 59% reduction in symptoms of depression at follow-up compared with usual care. All 10 trials of a CBT intervention showed an increased likelihood of remission from depressive symptoms with short-term treatment (7–8 months). At the 1-year follow-up, there was a 35% increase in remission rates with CBT compared with usual care (pooled relative risk, 1.34; 95% CI, 1.19–1.50).[20] There is little risk of adverse effects from psychotherapy. In women with antenatal depression, CBT-based interventions have also been shown to be effective in preventing depression recurrence during the perinatal period.[136] The USPSTF has recommended that clinicians consider CBT or other evidence-based counseling, such as interpersonal psychotherapy, when managing depression in pregnant or breastfeeding women.[141,199]

Different methods of delivering interpersonal psychotherapy and CBT are being developed and preliminarily show reduction in depression prevalence. These methods include postpartum telephone-based and telecare sessions using CBT, relaxation techniques, and problem-solving strategies,[210] Internet-based CBT,[211,212] and home-based CBT.[213] A recent Cochrane review evaluated computer or Internet-based interventions to address perinatal depressive symptoms and suggested promising trends, but such interventions are largely still in development.[212] Small studies of additional alternative treatment options, including yoga, massage, light therapy, acupuncture, and omega-3 fatty acids in fish oil, show some limited efficacy, but more research is needed.[4,214] There are no formal recommendations for these treatments at this time.

Psychotropic Medications*

Pharmacologic treatment of depression is often indicated during pregnancy and/or lactation. Review and discussion of the risk of untreated versus treated depression is advised. Consideration of each patient's previous disease and treatment history, along with the risk profile for individual pharmacologic agents, is important when selecting pharmacologic therapy with the greatest likelihood of treatment success. Psychotropic medications, particularly antidepressants such as selective serotonin reuptake inhibitors (SSRIs), may have a role in the management of postpartum depression depending on the presenting symptoms and needs of individual parents. Most often, psychotropic medications are managed through referrals to adult primary care, psychiatric, or other qualified mental health professionals. However, pediatric providers can still play a role in dispelling myths, providing education, and responding to specific concerns about medications that a parent may have, particularly as they relate to the health and welfare of the infant. A detailed discussion comparing psychotherapy and psychopharmacology is outside the scope of this article, but a Cochrane review of a few studies consisting of mothers with postpartum depression showed that there is no difference between the effectiveness of antidepressants and psychological or psychosocial treatments.[215]

Despite the availability of effective medications, many mothers prefer not to use psychotropic medications in the perinatal period because of the fear of adverse effects.[216] Discussions about the risks and benefits of using or withholding medications are important for parents to have with their own adult health care providers so they can make informed decisions regarding the role of antidepressant medications used antenatally or in the postpartum period, especially while breastfeeding. Studies about the long-term effects on the infant of maternal antidepressant medication use, such as SSRIs, during pregnancy are mixed, because it is difficult to control for many other cooccurring factors that may influence birth outcomes, including maternal illness or problematic health behaviors.[216] In 1 study, mothers made a list of potential risks and benefits of treatment with medication in the context of their therapeutic goals for a healthy pregnancy and postpartum period. An exercise like this should be conducted in partnership with appropriate providers, including the parent's prescriber, who can provide accurate information.[4,198] The pediatric provider can also play an important role in reinforcing and

* This section on pharmacological management of perinatal depression is being included to provide context to the pediatric provider; it is not to imply that pediatric providers would or should be instituting psychiatric care for adult parents. It is acknowledged that even when referred to appropriate mental health specialists, parents will often still return to pediatric providers caring for their children with questions or concerns. This section is not meant to be an exhaustive resource, but rather it is used to provide a basic overview of core understandings around perinatal psychopharmacology that may be relevant.

sharing accurate information about various treatment options.

Untreated and severe perinatal depression poses significant risk for morbidity and occasionally mortality for the mother and fetus during pregnancy. Studies have demonstrated that the risks associated with untreated depression are far more detrimental (including suicide) than the unclearly associated risks of growth effects, neurobehavioral outcomes, preterm birth, low birth weight, structural malformations, and respiratory distress, which vary among studies.[198,217–219] Yet, many mothers choose to stop taking psychotropic medications during pregnancy, although they report significant symptoms of depression, placing them at high risk for the sequela of perinatal depression.[209] In mothers who are suicidal, homicidal, manic, or psychotic, there is often an urgent need for medication in the context of an emergency or inpatient psychiatric setting.[198]

The AAFP,[4] ACOG,[3] Academy of Breastfeeding Medicine (ABM),[191] and American Psychiatric Association[198] endorse the appropriate use of antidepressant medications during the perinatal period. The ABM recommends consideration of each patient's previous disease and treatment history, along with the risk profiles for individual treatments when choosing the treatment with the greatest likelihood of treatment effect.[191] The ABM states that in the "setting of moderate to severe depression, the benefits of [psychotropic medication] treatment likely outweigh the risks of the medication to the mother or infant."[191] Therefore, antidepressant medications can be an important option to consider for parents with perinatal depression symptoms, particularly if their symptoms are not responsive to therapy or they have previous positive response to medications.

Detailed guidance in regard to specific medications is outside the scope of this article, but SSRIs have become the mainstay of treatment of moderate to severe major perinatal depression because of their favorable profiles of adverse reactions.

Parents often express concerns to and have questions for pediatric providers regarding the use of antidepressant medication while breastfeeding. There is increasing evidence to support the safe use of these medications during lactation. The ABM has developed a clinical protocol on the use of antidepressants in breastfeeding mothers but stipulates, "[There is] no widely accepted algorithm for antidepressant medication treatment of depression in lactating women."[191] In the context of breastfeeding, it has again been asserted that the benefit of effectively treating perinatal depression far outweighs the risks to the infant through breastfeeding.[220,221] Clinical studies in breastfeeding patients who are using sertraline, fluvoxamine, and paroxetine suggest that the transfer of these medications into human milk is low and that there is even lower uptake by the infant. No or minimal adverse effects on infants have been reported after the use of these 3 medications in lactating mothers themselves.[216,220,221] Sertraline was preferred over the other 2 drugs, because many studies have shown that human milk and infant plasma have low to undetectable concentrations of this drug.[216]

Many parents may experience combined or sequential treatment with psychotherapy, such as CBT, and antidepressant medication management. This may implicate multiple providers, which emphasizes the importance of collateral communication. Evidence suggests that combined treatment may lead to even further benefit[198] and may be preferred for some women with high risk of relapse and co-occurring conditions, such as anxiety disorders.[199] More studies are needed to evaluate the relative efficacy of different psychotherapeutic approaches as well as other psychological and psychosocial treatments, with and without medication.[199]

CODING AND BILLING

Given the 2016 recommendations by the USPSTF and CMS, providers are encouraged to bill for perinatal depression screening at 1-, 2-, 4- and 6-month well-child visits. However, coding may vary by state or payer. The AAP Web site, state AAP chapters, and specific payers can be consulted with any questions. A new *Current Procedural Terminology* code, 96161, for the administration of a mother-focused health risk assessment for the benefit of the patient was approved by the American Medical Association in 2016. Providers can consider the opportunity to bill for time-based counseling and coordination of care with a separate evaluation and management code with a 25 modifier when there are significant concerns for maternal depression.

CONCLUSIONS

There is strong evidence that parental, particularly maternal, depression during pregnancy and the first year after childbirth (perinatal depression) has profound negative consequences on the well-being of women and infants, including family dysfunction, disruption of critical infant brain development, cessation of breastfeeding, and increased health care use, and may place the child at increased risk for future anxiety and depression. A growing body of research shows that fathers are also at increased risk of perinatal depression, which can magnify the adverse effects on an infant's social-emotional development.[23,45,167] Perinatal depression is the most prevalent ACE and can lead to toxic stress and present challenges to essential early attachments between children and their parents.[100]

With a core responsibility to promote the well-being of children and the benefit of longitudinal relationships with families, pediatric providers have a critical role in screening and supporting parents and their infants with concerns for perinatal depression. This responsibility includes supporting parents at risk for or with a diagnosis of perinatal depression and communicating and working with adult obstetric, primary care, and/or mental health providers. If indicated, referrals to community agencies or specialty providers may be necessary for support, diagnostic evaluation, or treatment.

Over the past decade, multiple professional health care and regulatory bodies have recommended routine perinatal depression screening. Most recently, both the USPSTF and CMS have reviewed the evidence and have recommended screening consistent with those asserted by the AAP's *Bright Futures: Guidelines for Health Supervision of Infants, Children, and Adolescents, Fourth Edition*. These recommendations have encouraged, even mandated, many commercial insurers to pay for screening. Medicaid programs are now encouraged to cover and pay for screening for perinatal depression. The recommendation for maternal depression screening is once during pregnancy and then during the infant's well visits at 1, 2, 4, and 6 months of age.[15,20] However, despite the efforts of many state and local AAP and AAFP chapters and other advocacy groups, perinatal depression screening remains far from universal in clinical practice or payment.[140] As more providers are screening and identifying psychosocial risk factors in diverse clinical settings, more emphasis needs to be put on improving collaboration and transitions of care throughout the perinatal period. Finally, there are many models around the country of creative and effective interventions to promote early identification and treatment of perinatal depression. Best practices and evidence-based treatments for parents and the parent-infant dyad need to be identified, advocated for, and brought to scale to allow access to care to promote the best outcomes for women and their infants.

LEAD AUTHORS

Jason Rafferty, MD, MPH, EdM, FAAP
Gerri Mattson, MD, MPH, FAAP
Marian Earls, MD, FAAP
Michael W. Yogman, MD, FAAP

COMMITTEE ON PSYCHOSOCIAL ASPECTS OF CHILD AND FAMILY HEALTH, 2016–2017

Michael W. Yogman, MD, FAAP, Chairperson
Thresia B. Gambon, MD, FAAP
Arthur Lavin, MD, FAAP
Gerri Mattson, MD, FAAP
Jason Richard Rafferty, MD, MPH, EdM
Lawrence Sagin Wissow, MD, MPH, FAAP

LIAISONS

Sharon Berry, PhD, LP – *Society of Pediatric Psychology*
Terry Carmichael, MSW – *National Association of Social Workers*
Edward R. Christophersen, PhD, FAAP – *Society of Pediatric Psychology*
Norah L. Johnson, PhD, RN, CPNP-BC – *National Association of Pediatric Nurse Practitioners*
Leonard Read Sulik, MD, FAAP – *American Academy of Child and Adolescent Psychiatry*

STAFF

Stephanie Domain, MS

ABBREVIATIONS

AAFP: American Academy of Family Physicians
AAP: American Academy of Pediatrics
ABM: Academy of Breastfeeding Medicine
ACE: adverse childhood experience
ACOG: American College of Obstetricians and Gynecologists
CBT: cognitive behavioral therapy
CI: confidence interval
CMS: Centers for Medicare and Medicaid Services
DSM-5: *Diagnostic and Statistical Manual of Mental Disorders, Fifth Edition*
EPDS: Edinburgh Postnatal Depression Scale
MCPAP: Massachusetts Child Psychiatry Access Project
MDD: major depressive disorder
PDSS: Postpartum Depression Screening Scale
PHQ-2: Patient Health Questionnaire-2
PHQ-9: Patient Health Questionnaire-9
PPCMH: pediatric patient-centered medical home
PRAMS: Pregnancy Risk Assessment Monitoring System
PREPP: Practical Resources for Effective Postpartum Parenting
SSRI: selective serotonin reuptake inhibitor
SWYC: Survey of Well-being of Young Children
USPSTF: US Preventive Services Task Force

All technical reports from the American Academy of Pediatrics automatically expire 5 years after publication unless reaffirmed, revised, or retired at or before that time.

DOI: https://doi.org/10.1542/peds.2018-3260

Address correspondence to Jason Rafferty, MD, MPH, EdM, FAAP. Email: Jason_Rafferty@mail.harvard.edu

PEDIATRICS (ISSN Numbers: Print, 0031-4005; Online, 1098-4275).

Copyright © 2019 by the American Academy of Pediatrics

FINANCIAL DISCLOSURE: The authors have indicated they have no financial relationships relevant to this article to disclose.

FUNDING: No external funding.

POTENTIAL CONFLICT OF INTEREST: The authors have indicated they have no potential conflicts of interest to disclose.

REFERENCES

1. Earls MF; Committee on Psychosocial Aspects of Child and Family Health American Academy of Pediatrics. Incorporating recognition and management of perinatal and postpartum depression into pediatric practice. *Pediatrics*. 2010;126(5):1032–1039
2. Santoro K, Peabody H. *Identifying and Treating Maternal Depression: Strategies & Considerations for Health Plans. NIHCM Foundation Issue Brief.* Washington, DC: National Institutes of Health Care Management; 2010
3. Committee on Obstetric Practice. The American College of Obstetricians and Gynecologists Committee opinion no. 630. Screening for perinatal depression. *Obstet Gynecol*. 2015;125(5):1268–1271
4. Hirst KP, Moutier CY. Postpartum major depression. *Am Fam Physician*. 2010;82(8):926–933
5. Declerq ER, Sakala C, Corry MP, Applebaum S, Risher P. *Listening to Mothers: Report of the First National U.S. Survey of Women's Childbearing Experiences*. New York, NY: Maternity Center Association; 2002
6. Chaudron LH, Szilagyi PG, Tang W, et al. Accuracy of depression screening tools for identifying postpartum depression among urban mothers. *Pediatrics*. 2010;125(3). Available at: www.pediatrics.org/cgi/content/full/125/3/e609
7. Gjerdingen DK, Yawn BP. Postpartum depression screening: importance, methods, barriers, and recommendations for practice. *J Am Board Fam Med*. 2007;20(3):280–288
8. Leiferman JA, Dauber SE, Heisler K, Paulson JF. Primary care physicians' beliefs and practices toward maternal depression. *J Womens Health (Larchmt)*. 2008;17(7):1143–1150
9. Kerker BD, Storfer-Isser A, Stein RE, et al. Identifying maternal depression in pediatric primary care: changes over a decade. *J Dev Behav Pediatr*. 2016;37(2):113–120
10. Nutting PA, Rost K, Dickinson M, et al. Barriers to initiating depression treatment in primary care practice. *J Gen Intern Med*. 2002;17(2):103–111
11. Bilszta J, Ericksen J, Buist A, Milgrom J. Women's experiences of postnatal depression – beliefs and attitudes as barriers to care. *Aust J Adv Nurs*. 2010;27(3):44–54
12. US Department of Health and Human Services. *Mental Health: A Report of the Surgeon General*. Washington, DC: US Public Health Service; 1999
13. US Public Health Service. *Report of the Surgeon General's Conference on Children's Mental Health: A National Action Agenda*. Washington, DC: US Department of Health and Human Services; 2000
14. Stewart DE, Vigod S. Postpartum depression. *N Engl J Med*. 2016;375(22):2177–2186
15. Hagan JF, Shaw JS, Duncan PM, eds. *Bright Futures: Guidelines for Health Supervision of Infants, Children, and Adolescents*. 4th ed. Elk Grove Village, IL: American Academy of Pediatrics; 2017
16. Committee on Psychosocial Aspects of Child and Family Health and Task Force on Mental Health. Policy statement–the future of pediatrics: mental health competencies for pediatric primary care. *Pediatrics*. 2009;124(1):410–421
17. Institute of Medicine. *Depression in Parents, Parenting, and Children. Opportunities to Improve Identification, Treatment, and Prevention.* Washington, DC: National Academies Press; 2009
18. Medical Home Initiatives for Children With Special Needs Project Advisory Committee; American Academy of Pediatrics. The medical home. *Pediatrics*. 2002;110(1 pt 1):184–186
19. Office of Disease Prevention and Health Promotion. *Healthy People 2020. ODPHP Publication No. B0132*. Washington, DC: US Department of Health and Human Services, Office of Disease Prevention and Health Promotion; 2010
20. O'Connor E, Rossom RC, Henninger M, Groom HC, Burda BU. Primary care screening for and treatment of depression in pregnant and postpartum women: evidence report and systematic review for the US Preventive Services Task Force. *JAMA*. 2016;315(4):388–406
21. Siu AL, Bibbins-Domingo K, Grossman DC, et al; US Preventive Services Task Force (USPSTF). Screening for depression in adults: US Preventive Services Task Force recommendation statement. *JAMA*. 2016;315(4):380–387
22. Wachino V; Center for Medicaid and CHIP Services. *Maternal Depression Screening: A Critical Role for Medicaid in the Care of Mothers and Children*. Baltimore, MD: Department of Health and Human Services; 2016. Available at: https://www.medicaid.gov/federal-policy-guidance/downloads/cib051116.pdf. Accessed February 5, 2018
23. Goodman JH. Paternal postpartum depression, its relationship to maternal postpartum depression, and

implications for family health. *J Adv Nurs.* 2004;45(1):26–35

24. Yogman M, Garfield CF; Committee on Psychosocial Aspects of Child and Family Health. Fathers' roles in the care and development of their children: the role of pediatricians. *Pediatrics.* 2016;138(1):e20161128
25. Paulson JF, Dauber S, Leiferman JA. Individual and combined effects of postpartum depression in mothers and fathers on parenting behavior. *Pediatrics.* 2006;118(2):659–668
26. Cochran SV. Assessing and treating depression in men. In: Brooks GR, Good GE, eds. *The New Handbook of Psychotherapy and Counseling With Men.* Vol 1. San Francisco, CA: Jossey-Bass; 2001:3–21
27. Edward KL, Castle D, Mills C, Davis L, Casey J. An integrative review of paternal depression. *Am J Men Health.* 2015;9(1):26–34
28. Earls M, Yogman M, Mattson G, Rafferty J; American Academy of Pediatrics, Committee on Psychosocial Aspects of Child and Family Health. Incorporating recognition and management of perinatal and postpartum depression into pediatric practice. *Pediatrics.* 2018;143(1):e20183259
29. Uher R, Payne JL, Pavlova B, Perlis RH. Major depressive disorder in DSM-5: implications for clinical practice and research of changes from DSM-IV. *Depress Anxiety.* 2014;31(6):459–471
30. American Psychiatric Association. *Diagnostic and Statistical Manual of Mental Disorders (DSM-5).* 5th ed. Washington, DC: American Psychiatric Publishing; 2013
31. Miller LJ. Postpartum depression. *JAMA.* 2002;287(6):762–765
32. Stadtlander L. Paternal postpartum depression. *Int J Childbirth Educ.* 2015;30(2):11–13
33. Sit D, Rothschild AJ, Wisner KL. A review of postpartum psychosis. *J Womens Health (Larchmt).* 2006;15(4):352–368
34. O'Hara MW. Postpartum depression: what we know. *J Clin Psychol.* 2009;65(12):1258–1269
35. Gavin NI, Gaynes BN, Lohr KN, Meltzer-Brody S, Gartlehner G, Swinson T. Perinatal depression: a systematic review of prevalence and incidence. *Obstet Gynecol.* 2005;106(5 pt 1):1071–1083
36. Hearn G, Iliff A, Jones I, et al. Postnatal depression in the community. *Br J Gen Pract.* 1998;48(428):1064–1066
37. Robbins CL, Zapata LB, Farr SL, et al; Centers for Disease Control and Prevention (CDC). Core state preconception health indicators - pregnancy risk assessment monitoring system and behavioral risk factor surveillance system, 2009. *MMWR Surveill Summ.* 2014;63(3):1–62
38. Banti S, Mauri M, Oppo A, et al. From the third month of pregnancy to 1 year postpartum. Prevalence, incidence, recurrence, and new onset of depression. Results from the perinatal depression-research & screening unit study. *Compr Psychiatry.* 2011;52(4):343–351
39. Evins GG, Theofrastous JP, Galvin SL. Postpartum depression: a comparison of screening and routine clinical evaluation. *Am J Obstet Gynecol.* 2000;182(5):1080–1082
40. Bennett HA, Einarson A, Taddio A, Koren G, Einarson TR. Prevalence of depression during pregnancy: systematic review. *Obstet Gynecol.* 2004;103(4):698–709
41. Chung TK, Lau TK, Yip AS, Chiu HF, Lee DT. Antepartum depressive symptomatology is associated with adverse obstetric and neonatal outcomes. *Psychosom Med.* 2001;63(5):830–834
42. Underwood L, Waldie K, D'Souza S, Peterson ER, Morton S. A review of longitudinal studies on antenatal and postnatal depression. *Arch Women Ment Health.* 2016;19(5): 711–720
43. Giallo R, D'Esposito F, Christensen D, et al. Father mental health during the early parenting period: results of an Australian population based longitudinal study. *Soc Psychiatry Psychiatr Epidemiol.* 2012;47(12):1907–1966
44. Ramchandani P, Stein A, Evans J, O'Connor TG; ALSPAC Study Team. Paternal depression in the postnatal period and child development: a prospective population study. *Lancet.* 2005;365(9478):2201–2205
45. Escribà-Agüir V, Artazcoz L. Gender differences in postpartum depression: a longitudinal cohort study. *J Epidemiol Community Health.* 2011;65(4):320–326
46. Mansfield AK, Addis ME, Mahalik JR. "Why won't he go to the doctor?": the psychology of men's help seeking. *Int J Mens Health.* 2003;2(2):93–109
47. Rochlen AB. Men in (and out of) therapy: central concepts, emerging directions, and remaining challenges. *J Clin Psychol.* 2005;61(6):627–631
48. Centers for Disease Control and Prevention (CDC). Prevalence of self-reported postpartum depressive symptoms–17 states, 2004-2005. *MMWR Morb Mortal Wkly Rep.* 2008;57(14):361–366
49. Lancaster CA, Gold KJ, Flynn HA, Yoo H, Marcus SM, Davis MM. Risk factors for depressive symptoms during pregnancy: a systematic review. *Am J Obstet Gynecol.* 2010;202(1):5–14
50. Robertson E, Grace S, Wallington T, Stewart DE. Antenatal risk factors for postpartum depression: a synthesis of recent literature. *Gen Hosp Psychiatry.* 2004;26(4):289–295
51. Larsson C, Sydsjö G, Josefsson A. Health, sociodemographic data, and pregnancy outcome in women with antepartum depressive symptoms. *Obstet Gynecol.* 2004;104(3):459–466
52. Woods SM, Melville JL, Guo Y, Fan MY, Gavin A. Psychosocial stress during pregnancy. *Am J Obstet Gynecol.* 2010;202(1):61.e1–61.e7
53. Underwood L, Waldie KE, D'Souza S, Peterson ER, Morton SM. A longitudinal study of pre-pregnancy and pregnancy risk factors associated with antenatal and postnatal symptoms of depression: evidence from growing up in New Zealand. *Matern Child Health J.* 2017;21(4):915–931
54. Radesky JS, Zuckerman B, Silverstein M, et al. Inconsolable infant crying and maternal postpartum depressive symptoms. *Pediatrics.* 2013;131(6). Available at: www.pediatrics.org/cgi/content/full/131/6/e1857
55. Lee AM, Lam SK, Sze Mun Lau SM, Chong CS, Chui HW, Fong DY.

Prevalence, course, and risk factors for antenatal anxiety and depression. *Obstet Gynecol.* 2007;110(5):1102–1112

56. Kahn RS, Wise PH, Wilson K. Maternal smoking, drinking and depression: a generational link between socioeconomic status and child behavior problems [abstract]. *Pediatr Res.* 2002;51(pt 2):191A
57. Sullivan PF, Neale MC, Kendler KS. Genetic epidemiology of major depression: review and meta-analysis. *Am J Psychiatry.* 2000;157(10):1552–1562
58. Forty L, Jones L, Macgregor S, et al. Familiality of postpartum depression in unipolar disorder: results of a family study. *Am J Psychiatry.* 2006;163(9):1549–1553
59. Kessler RC, Berglund P, Demler O, et al; National Comorbidity Survey Replication. The epidemiology of major depressive disorder: results from the National Comorbidity Survey Replication (NCS-R). *JAMA.* 2003;289(23):3095–3105
60. Ross LE, McLean LM. Anxiety disorders during pregnancy and the postpartum period: a systematic review. *J Clin Psychiatry.* 2006;67(8):1285–1298
61. Brummelte S, Galea LA. Depression during pregnancy and postpartum: contribution of stress and ovarian hormones. *Prog Neuropsychopharmacol Biol Psychiatry.* 2010;34(5):766–776
62. Ding XX, Wu YL, Xu SJ, et al. Maternal anxiety during pregnancy and adverse birth outcomes: a systematic review and meta-analysis of prospective cohort studies. *J Affect Disord.* 2014;159:103–110
63. Paul IM, Downs DS, Schaefer EW, Beiler JS, Weisman CS. Postpartum anxiety and maternal-infant health outcomes. *Pediatrics.* 2013;131(4). Available at: www.pediatrics.org/cgi/content/full/131/4/e1218
64. O'Connor TG, Winter MA, Hunn J, et al. Prenatal maternal anxiety predicts reduced adaptive immunity in infants. *Brain Behav Immun.* 2013;32:21–28
65. Zijlmans MA, Korpela K, Riksen-Walraven JM, de Vos WM, de Weerth C. Maternal prenatal stress is associated with the infant intestinal microbiota. *Psychoneuroendocrinology.* 2015;53:233–245
66. Rifkin-Graboi A, Meaney MJ, Chen H, et al. Antenatal maternal anxiety predicts variations in neural structures implicated in anxiety disorders in newborns. *J Am Acad Child Adolesc Psychiatry.* 2015;54(4):313–321.e2
67. Pace CC, Spittle AJ, Molesworth CM, et al. Evolution of depression and anxiety symptoms in parents of very preterm infants during the newborn period. *JAMA Pediatr.* 2016;170(9):863–870
68. Tronick E, Als H, Adamson L, Wise S, Brazelton TB. The infant's response to entrapment between contradictory messages in face-to-face interaction. *J Am Acad Child Psychiatry.* 1978;17(1):1–13
69. Tronick EZ. Emotions and emotional communication in infants. *Am Psychol.* 1989;44(2):112–119
70. Braungart-Rieker J, Garwood MM, Powers BP, Notaro PC. Infant affect and affect regulation during the still-face paradigm with mothers and fathers: the role of infant characteristics and parental sensitivity. *Dev Psychol.* 1998;34(6):1428–1437
71. Fuertes M, Faria A, Beeghly M, Lopes-dos-Santos P. The effects of parental sensitivity and involvement in caregiving on mother-infant and father-infant attachment in a Portuguese sample. *J Fam Psychol.* 2016;30(1):147–156
72. Lucassen N, Tharner A, Prinzie P, et al. Paternal history of depression or anxiety disorder and infant-father attachment. *Infant Child Dev.* 2017;27(2):e2070
73. Bowlby J. Attachment and loss. In: *Attachment.* Vol 1. 2nd ed. New York, NY: Basic Books; 1969/1982
74. Ainsworth MS, Bowlby J. An ethological approach to personality development. *Am Psychol.* 1991;46(4):333–341
75. Bretherton I. The origins of attachment theory: John Bowlby and Mary Ainsworth. *Dev Psychol.* 1992;28(5):759–775
76. Bretherton I. Open communication and internal working models: their role in the development of attachment relationships.*Nebr Symp Motiv.* 1988;36:57–113
77. Toth SL, Rogosch FA, Sturge-Apple M, Cicchetti D. Maternal depression, children's attachment security, and representational development: an organizational perspective. *Child Dev.* 2009;80(1):192–208
78. Steele M, Steele H, Johansson M. Maternal predictors of children's social cognition: an attachment perspective. *J Child Psychol Psychiatry.* 2002;43(7):861–872
79. Letourneau NM. Fostering resiliency in infants and young children through parent-infant interaction. *Infants Young Child.* 1997;9(3):36–45
80. Cohn JF, Campbell SB, Ross S. Infant response in the still-face paradigm at 6 months predicts avoidant and secure attachments at 12 months. *Dev Psychopathol.* 1991;3(4): 367–376
81. Righetti-Veltema M, Conne-Perréard E, Bousquet A, Manzano J. Postpartum depression and mother-infant relationship at 3 months old. *J Affect Disord.* 2002;70(3):291–306
82. Korja R, Savonlahti E, Ahlqvist-Björkroth S, et al; PIPARI Study Group. Maternal depression is associated with mother-infant interaction in preterm infants. *Acta Paediatr.* 2008;97(6):724–730
83. Flykt M, Kanninen K, Sinkkonen J, Punamaki RL. Maternal depression and dyadic interaction: the role of maternal attachment style. *Infant Child Dev.* 2010;19:530–550
84. Dennis CL, McQueen K. Does maternal postpartum depressive symptomatology influence infant feeding outcomes? *Acta Paediatr.* 2007;96(4):590–594
85. Agency for Healthcare Research and Quality. *Breastfeeding and Maternal and Infant Health Outcomes in Developed Countries. Evidence Report 153.* Rockville, MD: Agency for Healthcare Research and Quality; 2007:130–131
86. Zero to Three. *Diagnostic Classification of Mental Health and Developmental Disorders of Infancy and Early Childhood (DC: 0-3R).* Washington, DC: Zero to Three; 2005
87. Murray L, Cooper PJ. The impact of postpartum depression on child

development. *Int Rev Psychiatry.* 1996;8(1):55–63

88. Beardslee WR, Versage EM, Gladstone TR. Children of affectively ill parents: a review of the past 10 years. *J Am Acad Child Adolesc Psychiatry.* 1998;37(11):1134–1141

89. Weinberg MK, Tronick EZ. Infant affective reactions to the resumption of maternal interaction after the still-face. *Child Dev.* 1996;67(3):905–914

90. Londono Tobon A, Diaz Stransky A, Ross DA, Stevens HE. Effects of maternal prenatal stress: mechanisms, implications, and novel therapeutic interventions. *Biol Psychiatry.* 2016;80(11):e85–e87

91. Rondó PH, Ferreira RF, Nogueira F, Ribeiro MC, Lobert H, Artes R. Maternal psychological stress and distress as predictors of low birth weight, prematurity and intrauterine growth retardation. *Eur J Clin Nutr.* 2003;57(2):266–272

92. French NP, Hagan R, Evans SF, Godfrey M, Newnham JP. Repeated antenatal corticosteroids: size at birth and subsequent development. *Am J Obstet Gynecol.* 1999;180(1 pt 1):114–121

93. Reinisch JM, Simon NG, Karow WG, Gandelman R. Prenatal exposure to prednisone in humans and animals retards intrauterine growth. *Science.* 1978;202(4366):436–438

94. Field T, Diego M, Hernandez-Reif M. Prenatal depression effects on the fetus and newborn: a review. *Infant Behav Dev.* 2006;29(3):445–455

95. Deave T, Heron J, Evans J, Emond A. The impact of maternal depression in pregnancy on early child development. *BJOG.* 2008;115(8):1043–1051

96. Evangelou M. *Early Years Learning and Development: Literature Review.* Washington, DC: Department for Children, Schools and Families; 2009

97. Sameroff AJ, MacKenzie MJ. A quarter-century of the transactional model: how have things changed? *Zero to Three.* 2003;24(1):14–22

98. Sameroff AJ. Transactional models in early social relations. *Hum Dev.* 1975;18(1–2):65–79

99. Felitti VJ, Anda RF, Nordenberg D, et al. Relationship of childhood abuse and household dysfunction to many of the leading causes of death in adults. The Adverse Childhood Experiences (ACE) study. *Am J Prev Med.* 1998;14(4):245–258

100. McDonnell CG, Valentino K. Intergenerational effects of childhood trauma: evaluating pathways among maternal ACEs, perinatal depressive symptoms, and infant outcomes. *Child Maltreat.* 2016;21(4):317–326

101. Verbeek T, Bockting CL, van Pampus MG, et al. Postpartum depression predicts offspring mental health problems in adolescence independently of parental lifetime psychopathology. *J Affect Disord.* 2012;136(3):948–954

102. Avan B, Richter LM, Ramchandani PG, Norris SA, Stein A. Maternal postnatal depression and children's growth and behaviour during the early years of life: exploring the interaction between physical and mental health. *Arch Dis Child.* 2010;95(9): 690–695

103. Murray L, Halligan SL, Cooper PJ. Effects of postnatal depression on mother-infant interactions, and child development. In: Bremner G, Wachs T, eds. *The Wiley-Blackwell Handbook of Infant Development.* London, United Kingdom: John Wiley; 2010:192–220

104. Essex MJ, Klein MH, Miech R, Smider NA. Timing of initial exposure to maternal major depression and children's mental health symptoms in kindergarten. *Br J Psychiatry.* 2001;179:151–156

105. Lahti M, Savolainen K, Tuovinen S, et al. Maternal depressive symptoms during and after pregnancy and psychiatric problems in children. *J Am Acad Child Adolesc Psychiatry.* 2017;56(1):30–39.e7

106. Brennan PA, Hammen C, Andersen MJ, Bor W, Najman JM, Williams GM. Chronicity, severity, and timing of maternal depressive symptoms: relationships with child outcomes at age 5. *Dev Psychol.* 2000;36(6): 759–766

107. Campbell SB, Cohn JF, Meyers T. Depression in first-time mothers: mother-infant interaction and depression chronicity. *Dev Psychol.* 1995;31(3):349–357

108. Teti DM, Gelfand DM, Messinger DS, Isabella R. Maternal depression and the quality of early attachment: an examination of infants, preschoolers, and their mothers. *Dev Psychol.* 1995;31(3):364–376

109. Ashman SB, Dawson G, Panagiotides H, Yamada E, Wilkinson CW. Stress hormone levels of children of depressed mothers. *Dev Psychopathol.* 2002;14(2):333–349

110. Smider NA, Essex MJ, Kalin NH, et al. Salivary cortisol as a predictor of socioemotional adjustment during kindergarten: a prospective study. *Child Dev.* 2002;73(1):75–92

111. Essex MJ, Klein MH, Cho E, Kalin NH. Maternal stress beginning in infancy may sensitize children to later stress exposure: effects on cortisol and behavior. *Biol Psychiatry.* 2002;52(8):776–784

112. Kersten-Alvarez LE, Hosman CM, Riksen-Walraven JM, van Doesum KT, Smeekens S, Hoefnagels C. Early school outcomes for children of postpartum depressed mothers: comparison with a community sample. *Child Psychiatry Hum Dev.* 2012;43(2):201–218

113. Milgrom J, Westley DT, Gemmill AW. The mediating role of maternal responsiveness in some longer term effects of postnatal depression on infant development. *Infant Behav Dev.* 2004;27(4):443–454

114. McLennan JD, Kotelchuck M. Parental prevention practices for young children in the context of maternal depression. *Pediatrics.* 2000;105(5):1090–1095

115. Moore T, Kotelchuck M. Predictors of urban fathers' involvement in their child's health care. *Pediatrics.* 2004;113(3 pt 1):574–580

116. Santona A, Tagini A, Sarracino D, et al. Maternal depression and attachment: the evaluation of mother-child interactions during feeding practice. *Front Psychol.* 2015;6:1235

117. Chung EK, McCollum KF, Elo IT, Lee HJ, Culhane JF. Maternal depressive symptoms and infant health practices among low-income women. *Pediatrics.* 2004;113(6). Available at: www.pediatrics.org/cgi/content/full/113/6/e523

118. Kavanaugh M, Halterman JS, Montes G, Epstein M, Hightower AD, Weitzman M. Maternal depressive symptoms are adversely associated with prevention practices and parenting behaviors for preschool children. *Ambul Pediatr.* 2006;6(1):32–37

119. Paulson JF, Bazemore SD. Prenatal and postpartum depression in fathers and its association with maternal depression: a meta-analysis. *JAMA.* 2010;303(19):1961–1969

120. Sills MR, Shetterly S, Xu S, Magid D, Kempe A. Association between parental depression and children's health care use. *Pediatrics.* 2007;119(4). Available at: www.pediatrics.org/cgi/content/full/119/4/e829

121. Field T. Postpartum depression effects on early interactions, parenting, and safety practices: a review. *Infant Behav Dev.* 2010;33(1):1–6

122. Shonkoff JP, Boyce WT, Cameron J, et al. *Excessive Stress Disrupts the Architecture of the Developing Brain. Working Paper No. 3.* Cambridge, MA: Centre on the Developing Child, Harvard University; 2009. Available at: http://developingchild.harvard.edu. Accessed February 5, 2018

123. Shonkoff JP, Duncan GJ, Yoshikawa H, Guyer B, Magnuson K, Philips D. *Maternal Depression Can Undermine the Development of Young Children. Working Paper No. 8.* Cambridge, MA: Centre on the Developing Child, Harvard University; 2009. Available at: http://developingchild.harvard.edu. Accessed February 5, 2018

124. Garner AS, Shonkoff JP; Committee on Psychosocial Aspects of Child and Family Health; Committee on Early Childhood, Adoption, and Dependent Care; Section on Developmental and Behavioral Pediatrics. Early childhood adversity, toxic stress, and the role of the pediatrician: translating developmental science into lifelong health. *Pediatrics.* 2012;129(1). Available at: www.pediatrics.org/cgi/content/full/129/1/e224

125. Brennan PA, Pargas R, Walker EF, Green P, Newport DJ, Stowe Z. Maternal depression and infant cortisol: influences of timing, comorbidity and treatment. *J Child Psychol Psychiatry.* 2008;49(10):1099–1107

126. Hessl D, Dawson G, Frey K, et al. A longitudinal study of children of depressed mothers: psychobiological findings related to stress. In: Hann DM, Huffman LC, Lederhendler KK, Minecke D, eds. *Advancing Research on Developmental Plasticity: Integrating the Behavioral Sciences and the Neurosciences of Mental Health.* Bethesda, MD: National Institutes of Mental Health; 1998:256

127. Halligan SL, Herbert J, Goodyer IM, Murray L. Exposure to postnatal depression predicts elevated cortisol in adolescent offspring. *Biol Psychiatry.* 2004;55(4):376–381

128. Francis D, Diorio J, Liu D, Meaney MJ. Nongenomic transmission across generations of maternal behavior and stress responses in the rat. *Science.* 1999;286(5442):1155–1158

129. Olin SC, Kerker B, Stein RE, et al. Can postpartum depression be managed in pediatric primary care? *J Womens Health (Larchmt).* 2016;25(4):381–390

130. Conradt E, Hawes K, Guerin D, et al. The contributions of maternal sensitivity and maternal depressive symptoms to epigenetic processes and neuroendocrine functioning. *Child Dev.* 2016;87(1):73–85

131. Bonari L, Pinto N, Ahn E, Einarson A, Steiner M, Koren G. Perinatal risks of untreated depression during pregnancy. *Can J Psychiatry.* 2004;49(11):726–735

132. Waters CS, Hay DF, Simmonds JR, van Goozen SH. Antenatal depression and children's developmental outcomes: potential mechanisms and treatment options. *Eur Child Adolesc Psychiatry.* 2014;23(10):957–971

133. Stowe ZN, Hostetter AL, Newport DJ. The onset of postpartum depression: implications for clinical screening in obstetrical and primary care. *Am J Obstet Gynecol.* 2005;192(2):522–526

134. Knitzer J, Theberge S, Johnson K. *Reducing maternal depression and its impact on young children: toward a responsive early childhood policy framework. Project Thrive Issue Brief, 2.* New York, NY: National Center for Children in Poverty; 2008

135. Yogman M, Lavin A, Cohen G; Committee on Psychosocial Aspects of Child and Family Health. The prenatal visit. *Pediatrics.* 2018;142(1):e20181218

136. Ogrodniczuk JS, Piper WE. Preventing postnatal depression: a review of research findings. *Harv Rev Psychiatry.* 2003;11(6):291–307

137. Stuart-Parrigon K, Stuart S. Perinatal depression: an update and overview. *Curr Psychiatry Rep.* 2014;16(9):468

138. Sockol LE. A systematic review of the efficacy of cognitive behavioral therapy for treating and preventing perinatal depression. *J Affect Disord.* 2015;177:7–21

139. Zauderer C. Postpartum depression: how childbirth educators can help break the silence. *J Perinat Educ.* 2009;18(2):23–31

140. Werner EA, Gustafsson HC, Lee S, et al. PREPP: postpartum depression prevention through the mother-infant dyad. *Arch Women Ment Health.* 2016;19(2):229–242

141. O'Connor E, Rossom RC, Henninger M. *Screening for Depression in Adults: An Updated Systematic Evidence Review for the US Preventive Services Task Force: Evidence Synthesis No. 128. AHRQ Publication No. 14-05208-EF-1.* Rockville, MD: Agency for Healthcare Research and Quality; 2016

142. Olin SS, McCord M, Stein REK, et al. Beyond screening: a stepped care pathway for managing postpartum depression in pediatric settings. *J Womens Health (Larchmt).* 2017;26(9):966–975

143. Yogman MW. Postpartum depression screening by pediatricians: time to close the gap. *J Dev Behav Pediatr.* 2016;37(2):157–157

144. Conry JA, Brown H. Well-woman task force: components of the well-woman visit.*Obset Gynecol.* 2015;126(4):697–701

145. Rhodes AM, Segre LS. Perinatal depression: a review of US legislation and law. *Arch Women Ment Health.* 2013;16(4):259–270

146. Weitzman C, Wegner L; Section on Developmental and Behavioral Pediatrics; Committee on Psychosocial Aspects of Child and Family Health; Council on Early Childhood; Society for Developmental and Behavioral Pediatrics; American Academy

of Pediatrics. Promoting optimal development: screening for behavioral and emotional problems [published correction appears in *Pediatrics.* 2015;135(5):946]. *Pediatrics.* 2015;135(2):384–395

147. Gleason MM, Goldson E, Yogman MW; Council on Early Childhood; Committee on Psychosocial Aspects of Child and Family Health; Section on Developmental and Behavioral Pediatrics. Addressing early childhood emotional and behavioral problems. *Pediatrics.* 2016;138(6): e20163025

148. Sheldrick RC, Perrin EC. Evidence-based milestones for surveillance of cognitive, language, and motor development. *Acad Pediatr.* 2013;13(6):577–586

149. National Quality Forum. *Perinatal and Reproductive Health Endorsement Maintenance: Technical Report.* Washington, DC: National Quality Forum; 2012:1–92. Available at: www.qualityforum.org/Publications/2012/06/Perinatal_and_Reproductive_Health_Endorsement_Maintenance.aspx. Accessed February 5, 2018

150. Centers for Medicare and Medicaid Services. *An Introduction to EHR Incentive Programs for Eligible Professionals: 2014 Clinical Quality Measure (CQM) Electronic Reporting Guide.* Washington, DC: Department of Health and Human Services; 2015. Available at: www.cms.gov/Regulations-and-Guidance/Legislation/EHRIncentivePrograms/Downloads/CQM2014_GuideEP.pdf. Accessed February 5, 2018

151. Scharf RJ, Scharf GJ, Stroustrup A. Developmental milestones [published correction appears in *Pediatr Rev.* 2016;37(6):266]. *Pediatrics.* 2016;37(1):25–37; quiz 38, 47

152. Kinman CR, Gilchrist EC, Payne-Murphy JC, Miller BF. *Provider- and Practice-Level Competencies for Integrated Behavioral Health in Primary Care: A Literature Review. Contract No. HHSA 290-2009-00023I.* Rockville, MD: Agency for Healthcare Research and Quality; 2015

153. Williams J, Shore SE, Foy JM. Co-location of mental health professionals in primary care settings: three North Carolina models. *Clin Pediatr (Phila).* 2006;45(6): 537–543

154. Council on Community Pediatrics. Poverty and child health in the United States. *Pediatrics.* 2016;137(4):e20160339

155. Garg A, Dworkin PH. Applying surveillance and screening to family psychosocial issues: implications for the medical home. *J Dev Behav Pediatr.* 2011;32(5):418–426

156. Wagner EH. Chronic disease management: what will it take to improve care for chronic illness? *Eff Clin Pract.* 1998;1(1):2–4

157. Heneghan AM, Morton S, DeLeone NL. Paediatricians' attitudes about discussing maternal depression during a paediatric primary care visit. *Child Care Health Dev.* 2007;33(3):333–339

158. Heneghan AM, Silver EJ, Bauman LJ, Stein RE. Do pediatricians recognize mothers with depressive symptoms? *Pediatrics.* 2000;106(6):1367–1373

159. Emerson BL, Bradley ER, Riera A, Mayes L, Bechtel K. Postpartum depression screening in the pediatric emergency department. *Pediatr Emerg Care.* 2014;30(11):788–792

160. Trost MJ, Molas-Torreblanca K, Man C, Casillas E, Sapir H, Schrager SM. Screening for maternal postpartum depression during infant hospitalizations. *J Hosp Med.* 2016;11(12):840–846

161. Seehusen DA, Baldwin LM, Runkle GP, Clark G. Are family physicians appropriately screening for postpartum depression? *J Am Board Fam Pract.* 2005;18(2):104–112

162. Myers ER, Aubuchon-Endsley N, Bastian LA, et al. *Efficacy and Safety of Screening for Postpartum Depression: Comparative Effectiveness Review, 106. AHRQ Publication No. 13-EHC064-EF.* Rockville, MD: Agency for Healthcare Research and Quality; 2013. Available at: https://effectivehealthcare.ahrq.gov/topics/depression-postpartum-screening/research. Accessed February 5, 2018

163. Cox JL, Holden JM, Sagovsky R. Detection of postnatal depression. Development of the 10-item Edinburgh Postnatal Depression Scale. *Br J Psychiatry.* 1987;150:782–786

164. Alvarado R, Jadresic E, Guajardo V, Rojas G. First validation of a Spanish-translated version of the Edinburgh postnatal depression scale (EPDS) for use in pregnant women. A Chilean study. *Arch Women Ment Health.* 2015;18(4):607–612

165. Massoudi P, Hwang CP, Wickberg B. How well does the Edinburgh Postnatal Depression Scale identify depression and anxiety in fathers? A validation study in a population based Swedish sample. *J Affect Disord.* 2013;149(1–3):67–74

166. Matthey S, Barnett B, Kavanagh DJ, Howie P. Validation of the Edinburgh Postnatal Depression Scale for men, and comparison of item endorsement with their partners. *J Affect Disord.* 2001;64(2–3):175–184

167. Ramchandani PG, Stein A, O'Connor TG, Heron J, Murray L, Evans J. Depression in men in the postnatal period and later child psychopathology: a population cohort study. *J Am Acad Child Adolesc Psychiatry.* 2008;47(4):390–398

168. Perrin E. *The Survey of Wellbeing of Young Children.* Boston, MA: Tufts Medical Center; 2012. Available at: https://www.floatinghospital.org/The-Survey-of-Wellbeing-of-Young-Children/Age-Specific-Forms. Accessed November 27, 2018

169. Beck CT, Gable RK. Comparative analysis of the performance of the Postpartum Depression Screening Scale with two other depression instruments. *Nurs Res.* 2001;50(4):242–250

170. Tandon SD, Cluxton-Keller F, Leis J, Le HN, Perry DF. A comparison of three screening tools to identify perinatal depression among low-income African American women. *J Affect Disord.* 2012;136(1–2):155–162

171. Buist AE, Barnett BE, Milgrom J, et al. To screen or not to screen–that is the question in perinatal depression. *Med J Aust.* 2002;177(suppl):S101–S105

172. Venkatesh KK, Zlotnick C, Triche EW, Ware C, Phipps MG. Accuracy of brief screening tools for identifying postpartum depression among

adolescent mothers. *Pediatrics.* 2014;133(1). Available at: www.pediatrics.org/cgi/content/full/133/1/e45

173. Montazeri A, Torkan B, Omidvari S. The Edinburgh Postnatal Depression Scale (EPDS): translation and validation study of the Iranian version. *BMC Psychiatry.* 2007;7:11

174. Olson AL, Dietrich AJ, Prazar G, Hurley J. Brief maternal depression screening at well-child visits. *Pediatrics.* 2006;118(1):207–216

175. Olson AL, Dietrich AJ, Prazar G, et al. Two approaches to maternal depression screening during well child visits. *J Dev Behav Pediatr.* 2005;26(3):169–176

176. Kroenke K, Spitzer RL, Williams JB. The Patient Health Questionnaire-2: validity of a two-item depression screener. *Med Care.* 2003;41(11):1284–1292

177. Löwe B, Unützer J, Callahan CM, Perkins AJ, Kroenke K. Monitoring depression treatment outcomes with the patient health questionnaire-9. *Med Care.* 2004;42(12):1194–1201

178. Wittkampf KA, Naeije L, Schene AH, Huyser J, van Weert HC. Diagnostic accuracy of the mood module of the Patient Health Questionnaire: a systematic review. *Gen Hosp Psychiatry.* 2007;29(5):388–395

179. Richardson LP, McCauley E, Grossman DC, et al. Evaluation of the Patient Health Questionnaire-9 Item for detecting major depression among adolescents. *Pediatrics.* 2010;126(6):1117–1123

180. Kroenke K, Spitzer RL, Williams JB. The PHQ-9: validity of a brief depression severity measure. *J Gen Intern Med.* 2001;16(9):606–613

181. Beck AT, Steer RA, Ball R, Ranieri W. Comparison of Beck Depression Inventories -IA and -II in psychiatric outpatients. *J Pers Assess.* 1996;67(3):588–597

182. Forman-Hoffman V, McClure E, McKeeman J, et al. Screening for major depressive disorder in children and adolescents: a systematic review for the U.S. Preventive Services Task Force. *Ann Intern Med.* 2016;164(5):342–349

183. Ji S, Long Q, Newport DJ, et al. Validity of depression rating scales during pregnancy and the postpartum period: impact of trimester and parity. *J Psychiatr Res.* 2011;45(2):213–219

184. Beck CT. A checklist to identify women at risk for developing postpartum depression. *J Obstet Gynecol Neonatal Nurs.* 1998;27(1):39–46

185. Baker BL, McIntyre LL, Blacher J, Crnic K, Edelbrock C, Low C. Pre-school children with and without developmental delay: behaviour problems and parenting stress over time. *J Intellect Disabil Res.* 2003;47(pt 4–5):217–230

186. Squires J, Bricker D, Twombly E. *Ages & Stages Questionnaires: A Parent-Completed Child Monitoring System for Social-Emotional Behaviors.* 2nd ed. Baltimore, MD: Paul Brooks Publishing Co; 2015. Available at: https://agesandstages.com. Accessed February 5, 2018

187. Gleason MM, Zeanah CH, Dickstein S. Recognizing young children in need of mental health assessment: development and preliminary validity of the early childhood screening assessment. *Infant Ment Health J.* 2010;31(3):335–357

188. Sheldrick RC, Henson BS, Merchant S, Neger EN, Murphy JM, Perrin EC. The Preschool Pediatric Symptom Checklist (PPSC): development and initial validation of a new social/emotional screening instrument. *Acad Pediatr.* 2012;12(5):456–467

189. Sheldrick RC, Henson BS, Neger EN, Merchant S, Murphy JM, Perrin EC. The baby pediatric symptom checklist: development and initial validation of a new social/emotional screening instrument for very young children. *Acad Pediatr.* 2013;13(1):72–80

190. Ader J, Stille CJ, Keller D, Miller BF, Barr MS, Perrin JM. The medical home and integrated behavioral health: advancing the policy agenda. *Pediatrics.* 2015;135(5):909–917

191. Sriraman NK, Melvin K, Meltzer-Brody S; Academy of Breastfeeding Medicine Protocol Committee. ABM clinical protocol #18: use of antidepressants in breastfeeding mothers. *Breastfeed Med.* 2015;10(6):290–299

192. Cox EQ, Sowa NA, Meltzer-Brody SE, Gaynes BN. The perinatal depression treatment cascade: baby steps toward improving outcomes. *J Clin Psychiatry.* 2016;77(9):1189–1200

193. Brealey SD, Hewitt C, Green JM, Morrell J, Gilbody S. Screening for postnatal depression: is it acceptable to women and healthcare professionals? A systematic review and meta-synthesis. *J Reprod Infant Psychol.* 2010;28(4):328–344

194. Marcus SM. Depression during pregnancy: rates, risks and consequences–Motherisk Update 2008. *Can J Clin Pharmacol.* 2009;16(1):e15–e22

195. Marcus SM, Barry KL, Flynn HA, Blow FC. *Improving Detection, Prevention and Treatment of Depression and Substance Abuse in Childbearing Women: Critical Variables in Pregnancy and Pre-Pregnancy Planning.* Ann Arbor, MI: University of Michigan Clinical Ventures, Faculty Group Practice; 1998

196. Thota AB, Sipe TA, Byard GJ, et al; Community Preventive Services Task Force. Collaborative care to improve the management of depressive disorders: a community guide systematic review and meta-analysis. *Am J Prev Med.* 2012;42(5):525–538

197. Howard LM, Flach C, Mehay A, Sharp D, Tylee A. The prevalence of suicidal ideation identified by the Edinburgh Postnatal Depression Scale in postpartum women in primary care: findings from the RESPOND trial. *BMC Pregnancy Childbirth.* 2011;11(1):57

198. Yonkers KA, Wisner KL, Stewart DE, et al. The management of depression during pregnancy: a report from the American Psychiatric Association and the American College of Obstetricians and Gynecologists. *Gen Hosp Psychiatry.* 2009;31(5):403–413

199. Stuart S, Koleva H. Psychological treatments for perinatal depression. *Best Pract Res Clin Obstet Gynaecol.* 2014;28(1):61–70

200. Forman DR, O'Hara MW, Stuart S, Gorman LL, Larsen KE, Coy KC. Effective treatment for postpartum depression is not sufficient to improve the developing mother-child relationship. *Dev Psychopathol.* 2007;19(2):585–602

201. Council on Early Childhood; Committee on Psychosocial Aspects of Child and Family Health; Section on Developmental and Behavioral Pediatrics. Addressing early childhood emotional and behavioral problems. *Pediatrics*. 2016;138(6):e20163023

202. Gaskin-Butler VT, McKay K, Gallardo G, Salman-Engin S, Little T, McHale JP. Thinking 3 rather than 2+1: how a coparenting framework can transform infant mental health efforts with unmarried African American parents. *Zero to Three*. 2015;35(5):49–58

203. Willheim E. Dyadic psychotherapy with infants and young children: child-parent psychotherapy. *Child Adolesc Psychiatric Clin N Am*. 2013;22(2):215–239

204. Cassidy J, Woodhouse SS, Sherman LJ, Stupica B, Lejuez CW. Enhancing infant attachment security: an examination of treatment efficacy and differential susceptibility. *J Dev Psychopathol*. 2011;23(1):131–148

205. Marvin R, Cooper G, Hoffman K, Powell B. The Circle of Security project: attachment-based intervention with caregiver-pre-school child dyads. *Attach Hum Dev*. 2002;4(1):107–124

206. Wissow L, Anthony B, Brown J, et al. A common factors approach to improving the mental health capacity of pediatric primary care. *Adm Policy Ment Health*. 2008;35(4):305–318

207. Feinberg E, Donahue S, Bliss R, Silverstein M. Maternal depressive symptoms and participation in early intervention services for young children. *Matern Child Health J*. 2012;16(2):336–345

208. Substance Abuse and Mental Health Services Administration. *Depression in Mothers: More Than the Blues—A Toolkit for Family Service Providers. HHS Publication No. (SMA) 14-4878*. Rockville, MD: Substance Abuse and Mental Health Services Administration; 2014

209. van Schaik DJ, Klijn AF, van Hout HP, et al. Patients' preferences in the treatment of depressive disorder in primary care. *Gen Hosp Psychiatry*. 2004;26(3):184–189

210. Ugarriza DN, Schmidt L. Telecare for women with postpartum depression. *J Psychosoc Nurs Ment Health Serv*. 2006;44(1):37–45

211. Sheeber LB, Seeley JR, Feil EG, et al. Development and pilot evaluation of an Internet-facilitated cognitive-behavioral intervention for maternal depression. *J Consult Clin Psychol*. 2012;80(5):739–749

212. Ashford MT, Olander EK, Ayers S. Computer- or web-based interventions for perinatal mental health: a systematic review. *J Affect Disord*. 2016;197:134–146

213. Ammerman RT, Putnam FW, Altaye M, Stevens J, Teeters AR, Van Ginkel JB. A clinical trial of in-home CBT for depressed mothers in home visitation. *Behav Ther*. 2013;44(3):359–372

214. Freeman MP, Hibbeln JR, Wisner KL, Brumbach BH, Watchman M, Gelenberg AJ. Randomized dose-ranging pilot trial of omega-3 fatty acids for postpartum depression. *Acta Psychiatr Scand*. 2006;113(1):31–35

215. Molyneaux E, Howard LM, McGeown HR, Karia AM, Trevillion K. Antidepressant treatment for postnatal depression. *Cochrane Database Syst Rev*. 2014;(9):CD002018

216. McDonagh MS, Matthews A, Phillipi C, et al. Depression drug treatment outcomes in pregnancy and the postpartum period: a systematic review and meta-analysis. *Obstet Gynecol*. 2014;124(3):526–534

217. Grigoriadis S. The effects of antidepressant medications on mothers and babies. *J Popul Ther Clin Pharmacol*. 2014;21(3):e533–e541

218. Andersen JT, Andersen NL, Horwitz H, Poulsen HE, Jimenez-Solem E. Exposure to selective serotonin reuptake inhibitors in early pregnancy and the risk of miscarriage. *Obstet Gynecol*. 2014;124(4):655–661

219. Meltzer-Brody S. Treating perinatal depression: risks and stigma. *Obstet Gynecol*. 2014;124(4):653–654

220. Rowe H, Baker T, Hale TW. Maternal medication, drug use, and breastfeeding. *Child Adolesc Psychiatr Clin N Am*. 2015;24(1):1–20

221. Hale TW. *Medication and Mother's Milk 2012: A Manual of Lactational Pharmacology*. 15th ed. Amarillo, TX: Hale Publishing LP; 2012

Institutional Ethics Committees

- *Policy Statement*

POLICY STATEMENT Organizational Principles to Guide and Define the Child Health Care System and/or Improve the Health of all Children

American Academy of Pediatrics

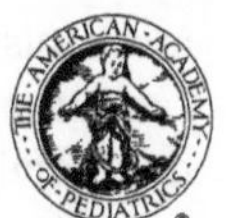

DEDICATED TO THE HEALTH OF ALL CHILDREN™

Institutional Ethics Committees

Margaret Moon, MD, MPH, FAAP, COMMITTEE ON BIOETHICS

abstract

In hospitals throughout the United States, institutional ethics committees (IECs) have become a standard vehicle for the education of health professionals about biomedical ethics, for the drafting and review of hospital policy, and for clinical ethics case consultation. In addition, there is increasing interest in a role for the IEC in organizational ethics. Recommendations are made about the membership and structure of an IEC, and guidance is provided for those serving on an IEC.

School of Medicine, Johns Hopkins University, Baltimore, Maryland

Dr Moon was responsible for all aspects of revising and writing this statement and approved the final manuscript as submitted.

This document is copyrighted and is property of the American Academy of Pediatrics and its Board of Directors. All authors have filed conflict of interest statements with the American Academy of Pediatrics. Any conflicts have been resolved through a process approved by the Board of Directors. The American Academy of Pediatrics has neither solicited nor accepted any commercial involvement in the development of the content of this publication.

Policy statements from the American Academy of Pediatrics benefit from expertise and resources of liaisons and internal (AAP) and external reviewers. However, policy statements from the American Academy of Pediatrics may not reflect the views of the liaisons or the organizations or government agencies that they represent.

The guidance in this statement does not indicate an exclusive course of treatment or serve as a standard of medical care. Variations, taking into account individual circumstances, may be appropriate.

All policy statements from the American Academy of Pediatrics automatically expire 5 years after publication unless reaffirmed, revised, or retired at or before that time.

DOI: https://doi.org/10.1542/peds.2019-0659

Address correspondence to Margaret Moon, MD, MPH, FAAP. E-mail: mmoon4@jhmi.edu

PEDIATRICS (ISSN Numbers: Print, 0031-4005; Online, 1098-4275).

Copyright © 2019 by the American Academy of Pediatrics

FINANCIAL DISCLOSURE: The author has indicated she has no financial relationships relevant to this article to disclose.

FUNDING: No external funding.

POTENTIAL CONFLICT OF INTEREST: The author has indicated she has no potential conflicts of interest to disclose.

To cite: Moon M, AAP COMMITTEE ON BIOETHICS. Institutional Ethics Committees. *Pediatrics.* 2019; 143(5):e20190659

INTRODUCTION

Institutional ethics committees (IECs) have evolved considerably since the 1983 President's Commission report on foregoing life-sustaining treatment[1] suggested that hospitals establish ethics committees to assist with decisions regarding the use of life-sustaining interventions and since the American Academy of Pediatrics (AAP) published its 1984 statement concerning infant bioethics committees.[2] At that time, ethics committees were the exception, with only 1% of hospitals having standing ethics committees.[1] A decade later, the Joint Commission on Accreditation of Healthcare Organizations (now The Joint Commission) included standards requiring hospitals to establish a "mechanism to consider ethical issues in patient care," and in 1999, Medicare began requiring participating hospitals to inform patients about resources for ethics consultation.[3,4] Currently, IECs are the norm, present in more than 95% of hospitals.[5]

Although IECs arose as mechanisms for implementing federal regulations about treatment of infants and children who were disabled,[3] modern IECs primarily serve to promote ethical practice through activities such as (1) case consultation, (2) provision of ethics education to health care communities, (3) review and development of policies related to ethical issues in patient care, and (4) provision of a forum for discussion of pressing ethical issues or concerns within the hospital community. An additional function of IECs in some institutions includes participation, with institutional leadership, in organizational ethics. For the purposes of this statement, the IEC function is separate from the research review committees present in most academic institutions.

The AAP supports the availability and use of an IEC as an important mechanism for the discussion and resolution of ethical issues raised in the individual and institutional provision of patient care. Additionally, the AAP recognizes the value of IEC integration in a more comprehensive ethics program, including policy development and organizational ethics. The AAP recognizes that although the structure and function of IECs will vary depending on institutions, there are elements common to all ethics committees.

In this statement, we discuss the 3 most common roles for an IEC: (1) clinical case consultation; (2) education of health care professionals, patients, and other health care employees; and (3) development and review of institutional policy concerning ethical issues in patient care. Additionally, we will review the emerging role for IECs in organizational leadership and quality improvement. Finally, we will describe the structure and membership of an IEC and current commentary on competencies and standards for IEC members providing case consultation.

ROLES OF AN IEC IN CLINICAL ETHICS CASE CONSULTATION

For the majority of physician-patient-family encounters in pediatrics, conflicts about the scope, value, and desirability of medical interventions are rare. Problems occur when there are conflicts or uncertainty about the goals of care, the value of a specific intervention as it relates to those goals, and the moral implications of medical choices and when communication about these conflicts breaks down. When conflicts or uncertainties occur and communication is difficult, an IEC may be asked for assistance in resolving the ethical issues implicit in the conflict. It is important to note that some requests for ethics committee consultation may involve concerns that are not strictly ethical in nature. Ethics committees may appropriately serve to support staff affected by moral distress related to difficult clinical situations, to lead or coordinate family meetings, or to advise medical staff leadership on medical staff professionalism concerns. These roles may be accepted at the discretion of the committee leadership, in cooperation with the institutional leadership.

The American Society for Bioethics and Humanities (ASBH) has been developing guidance on ethics case consultation. The ASBH identifies 2 core tasks of clinical ethics case consultation: (1) identify and analyze the nature of the value uncertainty and (2) facilitate the building of a "principled ethical resolution."[6,7] The AAP recognizes that there are a range of approaches to providing clinical ethics consultation service. The defining characteristics of the case consultation activity are that (1) it is initiated by a request for assistance; (2) it involves a specific patient, family, or both; and (3) it is documented in an appropriate manner. An IEC that is engaged in providing ethics consultations should have a policy and procedure statement that includes the following:

- who can request a consultation;
- how the IEC is contacted;
- who responds to the request;
- how the consultation is conducted;
- who is to be included in the consultation;
- proper notification of affected persons;
- protection of patient confidentiality;
- how the consultation is documented;
- whether, in some circumstances, an ethics consultation is required; and
- the advisory nature of the consultant's recommendations.

Access to ethics consultation should be open to patients, families, surrogates, staff, and members of the medical team. Information about the availability and process of ethics consultation should be widely distributed to patients, parents, family members, physicians, nurses, and other individuals who may have reason to call on the consultative services of the IEC. Although ethics consultation is most common within the inpatient setting, the need for consultation in the outpatient setting should be recognized and supported by institutions. Research has revealed disparities in access to ethics consultation between inpatient and outpatient settings and between large and small communities.[8,9] Some IECs, especially those in large institutions, may be able to offer support to nonaffiliated community physicians as requested.

The consultation process may involve a team from the IEC, a solo consultant representing the IEC, or, in some cases, an outside consultant. The process of consultation will include review of the clinical situation and will generally include interactions with the patient and family as well as the clinical team.

The following guidance should apply to providing ethics consultation to promote fairness and accountability:

1. Any patient, parent or guardian, or family member should be able to initiate an ethics consultation.
2. The patient and parent or guardian should be able to refuse to participate in an ethics consultation without concern for negative repercussions.
3. The refusal of a patient or parent or guardian to participate in an ethics consultation should not obstruct the ability of an ethics committee to provide consultation services to physicians, nurses, and other concerned staff.
4. Any physician, nurse, or other health care provider who is

involved in the care of the patient should be able to request an ethics consultation without fear of reprisal.

5. The process of consultation should be open to all persons involved in the patient's care yet conducted in a manner that respects patient and family confidentiality and privacy.
6. Anonymous requests for consultation are not recommended. In situations in which fear of reprisal limits open discussion of the issues, the identity of the person(s) requesting consultation may be kept confidential.
7. The primary care pediatrician should be invited to participate in the consultation to support existing physician-family relationships.

Three models of case consultation and deliberation generally have been used: (1) an individual consultant who reports on a periodic basis to the entire committee, (2) a small team of committee members, or (3) a meeting of the entire committee. Each model has advantages and disadvantages. In some circumstances, consultation provided by a single person from the IEC may suffice. In others, a variation of these models may be the best way to accommodate institutional needs. Although an individual consultant may respond in a timely and flexible manner, such an approach risks losing the diversity and range of perspectives offered by a group. In most situations, small consultation teams made up of individuals of varying personal and professional backgrounds are recommended to balance a timely and flexible response with the value of diverse points of view.

IECs and their members should attend to the following concerns in developing a reasonable process for ethics consultation:

- IECs must concern themselves with questions of procedural fairness and confidentiality. They must have a mechanism for involving or advising patients and others who are the subjects of consultation, and they must respect the privacy and confidentiality of all persons affected by all aspects of IEC consultation.
- IECs must have means of keeping current with relevant bioethics literature and health law, including information relevant to infants, children, and adolescents. They should also know which circumstances usually warrant further consultation or review (from authorities in ethics, medicine, or law) and when hospital counsel or judicial involvement should be sought.
- IECs should work to define appropriate competencies for those who participate in ethics consultation and develop a program to create and maintain those competencies.
- IECs should adopt a code of ethics and professionalism for ethics consultants that emphasizes competence, integrity, management of conflicts of interest, and justice.[10]

Failure to develop and then follow reasonable policies and procedures for ethics consultation violates standards of The Joint Commission and general standards of professionalism. Information about the institution's policies and procedures related to ethical issues in patient care should be included in routine training for staff who interact with patients. Furthermore, guidance on how to raise ethics concerns should be easily accessible for patients, parents or guardians, and hospital personnel.

The quality of an ethics consultation rests first on the IEC's ability to identify and explicate the ethical issues driving the perceived conflict or uncertainty and then provide a forum for open discussion of the medical, moral, and legal issues surrounding the difficult situation. The authority, whether institutional, moral, or legal, of an ethics consultant and an IEC is limited.[11,12] The AAP supports the view that the recommendations from an ethics consultation are advisory only. Although case law, statutory law, and state regulations may be discussed within an ethics consultation, the mere fact that an IEC was involved in a case is of uncertain value in providing legal protection to the participants.[13,14] Improved communication, clarification of differences and available options, and careful documentation of the decisional process may reduce the potential for future legal action.[15] All ethics consultations should be documented in the committee records, and, in most cases, a summary of the consultation should be included in the patient's medical record. The form and extent of chart documentation of ethics consultations may vary depending on local hospital regulations and requirements.[16,17]

In critiques of the role of IECs in case consultation, lack of regulation and professional standards, inadequate focus on potential conflicts of interest,[18] and inadequate reviews of quality and efficacy have been cited.[19] Although The Joint Commission has established standards regarding access to discussion of ethical concerns, there has been no specific guidance about requirements for ethics consultants. Surveys of ethics consultants and hospital IECs revealed wide variation in the type and extent of training in ethics, and ethics consultation varied widely among ethics consultants and hospitals.[5,20] The ASBH has identified core skills for ethics consultants, including assessment skills, process skills, and interpersonal skills. The skills and knowledge necessary to participate as a member or leader of such a consultation team varies with one's role in the process. This is reflected in the ASBH's recommended set of knowledge competencies for ethics consultants, including basic and advanced skills.[21] Beyond establishing and maintaining competencies for consultation, IECs should develop mechanisms to evaluate the quality and outcomes of their work.[22]

Ethics Education

An IEC should have a major role in educating all health care professionals, employees, and administrative staff in the ethical foundations of patient care and institutional relationships. Although it is evident that ethical issues occur frequently in routine patient care,[8,23] requests for IEC consultation are relatively rare.[5] IECs should take the lead in educating clinicians to enhance their capacities to identify and manage ethics concerns independently while encouraging appropriate use of ethics consultation. Such education can occur as traditional didactic presentations, as ad hoc discussions about common clinical situations, or as 1 aspect of clinical case consultation. It is particularly valuable to develop interprofessional ethics education programs to enhance communication within teams about ethics concerns.[24] Whenever possible, students and house officers should be included in these educational opportunities. Additionally, an IEC may serve the larger community by including community education and community engagement in its mission. Most importantly, an IEC should, itself, engage in continuing education and ongoing training for all its members to ensure the highest quality clinical ethics consultations and to keep members abreast of the changing dynamic of clinical care.

Policy Review and Development and Quality Improvement

In addition to involvement in case consultation and in educating patients, families, and staff members about ethical issues, the functions of an IEC generally include the drafting and review of institutional policy and procedures specifically related to ethical issues in clinical care. Policies for the limitation or withdrawal of various treatments (such as cardiopulmonary resuscitation, medically provided fluid and nutrition, medical or physician orders for life-sustaining–treatment rules, and organ donation) often have been drafted with IEC involvement. The IEC also may be involved in drafting other policies with ethical importance, such as the ability of hospital employees to object to participating in certain aspects of patient care, the resolution of conflict, and certain aspects of relevant business practices.

The IEC role may include both response to administrative requests for policy review and development and proactive identification of issues with ethical ramifications that warrant an institutional policy and procedure. IECs, especially through the process of ethics consultation, are well positioned to identify structural or organizational factors that may be at the root of recurrent ethical problems. IECs may consider an expanded approach to consultation that allows a focus on proactive identification and prevention of ethical problems, especially systems-level factors that are likely to create ethics problems or hinder their resolutions. Specifically, IECs should work to include critical reflection on institutional factors that contribute to ethical conflicts.[25]

THE ROLE OF AN IEC IN ORGANIZATIONAL ETHICS

Health care institutions must identify a process for addressing organization-level ethical issues. A model to integrate the IEC more completely in organizational structure has been proposed by various authors.[26–28] The integrated ethics model for an IEC includes the traditional case consultation function with an expanded role in proactive policy development and leadership on organizational ethics. It is based in a focus on ethics as integral to quality of care.[29] The AAP supports integration of the IEC into an institution's process for establishing and promoting organizational ethics but notes that including organizational ethics in the purview of the IEC raises specific questions about its structure, function, and member qualifications.[30] An IEC whose function includes organizational ethics and policy development should establish standards of membership, process, and self-improvement specific to organizational ethics issues and to the organizational structure of its home institution.

MEMBERSHIP AND STRUCTURE OF AN IEC

The membership of an IEC should be multidisciplinary with sufficient knowledge and experience to address the range of ethical issues brought to the committee. The varied tasks of an IEC (consultation, education, and policy review and development) reveal the need for a broad variety of skills, knowledge, and experience. In light of the increasing complexity of medical and information technologies and the persistent effect of resource allocation and business practices on ethical issues, an IEC may need to seek and incorporate the advice of consultants to address specific issues of concern. In some institutions, an IEC large enough to include a sufficient diversity of personal, community, and professional views as well as the requisite knowledge base and skill sets may suffer limited efficiency. It may be appropriate for the larger IEC to delegate certain tasks to smaller subgroups (such as providing ethics consultation or drafting specific policies) while retaining the authority for coordination, oversight, and approval of activities of the subcommittees.

Two important issues concerning IEC structure are (1) the participation of the hospital attorney, risk manager, or hospital administrator in the IEC and (2) the presence of >1 IEC in an institution. The hospital attorney or risk manager may experience a conflict of interest between a duty to protect the institution and a duty to protect the patient's interest. Such conflicts should be recognized prospectively, and, in some circumstances, the consultation team may choose to restrict the hospital attorney, risk manager, or other administrators to function as ex officio advisors on specific legal or administrative matters.[20] Many IECs have found that the inclusion of nonhospital attorneys familiar with ethical issues is beneficial. In addressing organizational ethics issues, nonhospital attorney membership may be essential.

A single multidisciplinary IEC should have authority over all IEC subcommittees addressing consultative, educational, nursing, pediatric, or administrative concerns. The existence of special interest ethics committees, such as an infant care review committee or a nursing ethics committee, can undermine the diverse multidisciplinary context that is the strength of an IEC and may weaken the IEC's capacity to assist with development of organizational policies that support ethical practice throughout the institution. The presence of multiple IECs may create a sense that the process and deliberations of 1 IEC are not inclusive and may lead to unwarranted inconsistency in implementation of ethically critical policies and procedures. Institutions that find a need to maintain special interest ethics committees should include specific mechanisms to monitor and mediate these risks. An IEC may fulfill its functions whether it reports to the medical staff, hospital administration, or board of directors; however, because some ethical issues may involve conflicts between the clinical, administrative, and financial commitments of an institution, the reporting structure should be able to protect the IEC from manipulation.[8]

At institutions with academic affiliations, the IEC may coexist with an academic bioethics program engaged in teaching, research, and ethics consultation. Nevertheless, the IEC should retain oversight within an institution for ethics consultation, policy review, and education when these functions have been delegated to such programs.

SERVING ON AN IEC

IEC membership requires a commitment to acquire and then maintain the knowledge sufficient to address the complex issues faced by an IEC. Each IEC should establish a continuing education program designed to assist IEC members in fulfilling the stated mission of the IEC, especially as new issues emerge. A prospective IEC member should be comfortable with the committee's general mission statement, policies, and operation and the required responsibilities with respect to these functions. Anyone asked to be a member of an IEC should assess his or her commitment to acquiring and then maintaining a sufficient level of knowledge in bioethics appropriate to the tasks of the IEC. Expertise specific to ethical issues that arise in the care of pediatric patients is necessary for any IEC that will participate in pediatric case consultation. Core knowledge components specific to ethical issues involving minors are included in the ASBH guide on competencies in clinical ethics consultation.[22]

There is ongoing discussion of the role of quality attestation or certification of IEC members, specifically those who participate in ethics case consultation.[31] As noted previously, the ASBH has proposed a set of knowledge and skills-based competencies for ethics consultants. Certification programs for ethics consultants have emerged, although there remains no regulatory requirement for certification, and the impact of such professionalization of the field of ethics consultation has raised significant debate.[32,33] Institutional capacity to offer specific training for IEC members involved in consultation may vary. It is incumbent on the institution and the IEC to recognize the stakes involved in ethics consultation and to ensure that the process includes high-quality, well-informed, well-educated, and competent consultants. It is important, particularly, to note that although clinical experience is often necessary to untangle the details of an ethics case, it is generally not sufficient to engage competently in clinical ethics consultation. Even when an experienced clinician possesses considerable skill in talking with patients and families about the difficult practical and moral problems faced in complex and uncertain situations, clinical experience must be supplemented with a basic knowledge of ethical theory, health policy, law, and clinical ethics literature.[7] Many successful ethics consultants are nonclinicians supported by access to clinical expertise.

An IEC might permit different levels of member involvement, ranging from simply attending general committee meetings, discussing and drafting institutional policy, or participating in ethics consultation to leading an ethics consultation team, depending on the skills and experience of each member.

If engaged in clinical ethics consultation, it is reasonable to ask what one's legal liability might be in offering this service. An IEC should clarify the extent to which IEC proceedings are discoverable and whether its members are covered by liability insurance. The question of legal liability is difficult to answer except in general terms. Responsibility increases with authority, so it is generally riskier for IECs to direct than to simply advise.[32] States vary in legal protections afforded IEC members.[33] However, the likelihood that IEC members will be held legally liable for the actions arising from a consultation is both historically rare and practically remote.[33,34] Nevertheless, IECs and their members have an important opportunity to help set the standards for their own work by careful attention to continuing education, preparation, policy, procedure, and documentation.[14,35,36] IEC policies and procedures should be part of the institutional policy structure, and institutions should protect individual IEC members from liability that might arise in the course of official duties.

RECOMMENDATIONS

1. An IEC should have responsibility within an institution for oversight of clinical ethics consultation, review of policies relevant to ethical issues in patient care, and education of professional, administrative, and support staff about ethical issues, regardless of whether these functions are delegated to other subcommittees or programs.
2. Institutional policies and procedures for review of ethics concerns should be included in staff training; information on how to raise ethics concerns should be available to patients, families, and staff.
3. An IEC may play an important role, along with institutional administration, in organizational ethics and quality improvement.
4. Membership on an IEC should be diverse and reflect different perspectives within the hospital and general community.
5. An IEC that is engaged in clinical ethics consultations should have clearly articulated policies and procedures that conform to ethical principles of fairness and confidentiality.
6. An IEC should establish continuing education and training programs that ensure that IEC members attain and maintain the competencies required to perform their specific duties within the IEC.
7. Independent ethics committees within a single institution should be dissolved or restructured to report to the larger IEC.
8. IECs within a general hospital setting should ensure an adequate degree of multidisciplinary expertise for addressing ethical issues specific to pediatrics.

LEAD AUTHOR

Margaret Moon, MD, MPH, FAAP

COMMITTEE ON BIOETHICS, 2017–2018

Robert C. Macauley, MD, MDiv, FAAP, Chairperson
Gina Marie Geis, MD, FAAP
Naomi Tricot Laventhal, MD, FAAP
Douglas J. Opel, MD, MPH, FAAP
William R. Sexson, MD, MAB, FAAP
Mindy B. Statter, MD, FAAP

LIAISONS

Mary Lynn Dell, MD, DMin – *American Academy of Child and Adolescent Psychiatry*
Douglas S. Diekema, MD, MPH, FAAP – *American Board of Pediatrics*
Ginny Ryan, MD – *American College of Obstetricians and Gynecologists*
Nanette Elster, JD, MPH – *Legal Consultant*

STAFF

Florence Rivera, MPH

ABBREVIATIONS

AAP: American Academy of Pediatrics
ASBH: American Society for Bioethics and Humanities
IEC: institutional ethics committee

REFERENCES

1. President's Commission for the Study of Ethical Problems in Medicine and Biomedical and Behavioral Research. *Deciding to Forego Life-Sustaining Treatment: A Report on the Ethical, Medical, and Legal Issues in Treatment Decisions.* Washington, DC: US Government Printing Office; 1983
2. American Academy of Pediatrics Infant Bioethics Task Force and Consultants: guidelines for infant bioethics committees. *Pediatrics.* 1984;74(2): 306–310
3. The Joint Commission. *Hospital Accreditation Standards.* Oakbrook Terrace, IL: The Joint Commission; 2012
4. Health Care Financing Administration; Department of Health and Human Services. Medicare and Medicaid programs; hospital conditions of participation: patients' rights. *Fed Regist.* 1999;64(127):36070–36089
5. Fox E, Myers S, Pearlman RA. Ethics consultation in United States hospitals: a national survey. *Am J Bioeth.* 2007; 7(2):13–25
6. Dubler NN, Liebman CB. *Bioethics Mediation: A Guide to Shaping Shared Solutions, Revised and Expanded Edition.* Nashville, TN: Vanderbilt University Press; 2011
7. American Society for Bioethics and Humanities. *Core Competencies for Health Care Ethics Consultation.* Glenview, IL: American Society for Bioethics and Humanities; 2010
8. DuVal G, Clarridge B, Gensler G, Danis M. A national survey of U.S. internists' experiences with ethical dilemmas and ethics consultation. *J Gen Intern Med.* 2004;19(3):251–258
9. Barina R, Trancik EK. Moving ethics into ambulatory care: the future of Catholic health care ethics in shifting delivery trends. *Health Care Ethics USA.* 2013; 21(2):1–5
10. American Society for Bioethics and Humanities. *Code of Ethics and Professional Responsibilities for Healthcare Ethics Consultants.* Glenview, IL: American Society for Bioethics and Humanities; 2014. Available at: http://asbh.org/uploads/publications/ASBH%20Code%20of%

20Ethics.pdf. Accessed November 3, 2017

11. Adams DM. Ethics expertise and moral authority: is there a difference? *Am J Bioeth.* 2013;13(2):27–28
12. Agich GJ. Authority in ethics consultation. *J Law Med Ethics.* 1995; 23(3):273–283
13. Murphy CA. Searching for proper judicial recognition of hospital ethics committees in decisions to forego medical treatment. *Gold Gate Law Rev.* 1990;20(2):319–344
14. Sontag DN. Are clinical ethics consultants in danger? An analysis of the potential legal liability of individual clinical ethicists. *Univ PA Law Rev.* 2002; 151(2):667–705
15. Levinson W, Roter DL, Mullooly JP, Dull VT, Frankel RM. Physician-patient communication. The relationship with malpractice claims among primary care physicians and surgeons. *JAMA.* 1997;277(7):553–559
16. Bruce CR, Smith ML, Tawose OM, Sharp RR. Practical guidance for charting ethics consultations. *HEC Forum.* 2014; 26(1):79–93
17. Dubler NN. The art of the chart note in clinical ethics consultation and bioethics mediation: conveying information that can be understood and evaluated. *J Clin Ethics.* 2013;24(2): 148–155
18. Spielman B. Has faith in health care ethics consultants gone too far? Risks of an unregulated practice and a model act to contain them. *Marquette Law Rev.* 2001;85(1):161–221
19. Magill G. Quality in ethics consultations. *Med Health Care Philos.* 2013;16(4): 761–774
20. Kesselheim JC, Johnson J, Joffe S. Ethics consultation in children's hospitals: results from a survey of pediatric clinical ethicists. *Pediatrics.* 2010;125(4):742–746
21. Tarzian AJ; ASBH Core Competencies Update Task Force 1. Health care ethics consultation: an update on core competencies and emerging standards from the American Society for Bioethics and Humanities' core competencies update task force. *Am J Bioeth.* 2013; 13(2):3–13
22. American Society for Bioethics and Humanities Clinical Ethics Task Force. *Improving Competencies in Clinical Ethics Consultation: An Education Guide.* 2nd ed. Glenview, IL: American Society for Bioethics and Humanities; 2009
23. Carrese JA, Antommaria AH, Berkowitz KA, et al; American Society for Bioethics and Humanities Clinical Ethics Consultation Affairs Standing Committee. HCEC pearls and pitfalls: suggested do's and don't's for healthcare ethics consultants. *J Clin Ethics.* 2012;23(3):234–240
24. Moon M, Taylor HA, McDonald EL, Hughes MT, Carrese JA. Everyday ethics issues in the outpatient clinical practice of pediatric residents. *Arch Pediatr Adolesc Med.* 2009;163(9):838–843
25. Interprofessional Education Collaborative Expert Panel. *Core Competencies for Interprofessional Collaborative Practice: Report of an Expert Panel.* Washington, DC: Interprofessional Education Collaborative; 2011
26. Opel DJ, Wilfond BS, Brownstein D, Diekema DS, Pearlman RA. Characterisation of organisational issues in paediatric clinical ethics consultation: a qualitative study. *J Med Ethics.* 2009;35(8):477–482
27. Foglia MB, Pearlman RA. Integrating clinical and organizational ethics. A systems perspective can provide an antidote to the "silo" problem in clinical ethics consultations. *Health Prog.* 2006; 87(2):31–35
28. Spencer EM. A new role for institutional ethics committees: organizational ethics. *J Clin Ethics.* 1997;8(4):372–376
29. Fox E, Bottrell MM, Berkowitz KA, Chanko BL, Foglia MB, Pearlman RA. IntegratedEthics: an innovative program to improve ethics quality in health care. *Innov J.* 2010;15(2):1–36
30. Foglia MB, Fox E, Chanko B, Bottrell MM. Preventive ethics: addressing ethics quality gaps on a systems level. *Jt Comm J Qual Patient Saf.* 2012;38(3): 103–111
31. Ells C. Healthcare ethics committees' contribution to review of institutional policy. *HEC Forum.* 2006;18(3):265–275
32. Kodish E, Fins JJ, Braddock C III, et al. Quality attestation for clinical ethics consultants: a two-step model from the American Society for Bioethics and Humanities. *Hastings Cent Rep.* 2013; 43(5):26–36
33. Burda M. Certifying clinical ethics consultants: who pays? *J Clin Ethics.* 2011;22(2):194–199
34. Fox E. Strategies to improve health care ethics consultation: bridging the knowledge gap. *AMA J Ethics.* 2016; 18(5):528–533
35. Pope TM. Legal briefing: healthcare ethics committees. *J Clin Ethics.* 2011; 22(1):74–93
36. Annas G, Grodin M. Hospital ethics committees, consultants, and courts. *AMA J Ethics.* 2016;18(5):554–559

The Link Between School Attendance and Good Health

- *Policy Statement*

POLICY STATEMENT Organizational Principles to Guide and Define the Child Health Care System and/or Improve the Health of all Children

American Academy of Pediatrics

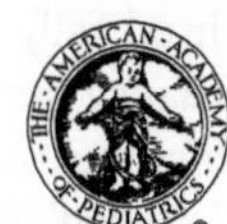

DEDICATED TO THE HEALTH OF ALL CHILDREN™

The Link Between School Attendance and Good Health

Mandy A. Allison, MD, MSPH, FAAP,[a] Elliott Attisha, DO, FAAP,[b] COUNCIL ON SCHOOL HEALTH

abstract

More than 6.5 million children in the United States, approximately 13% of all students, miss 15 or more days of school each year. The rates of chronic absenteeism vary between states, communities, and schools, with significant disparities based on income, race, and ethnicity. Chronic school absenteeism, starting as early as preschool and kindergarten, puts students at risk for poor school performance and school dropout, which in turn, put them at risk for unhealthy behaviors as adolescents and young adults as well as poor long-term health outcomes. Pediatricians and their colleagues caring for children in the medical setting have opportunities at the individual patient and/or family, practice, and population levels to promote school attendance and reduce chronic absenteeism and resulting health disparities. Although this policy statement is primarily focused on absenteeism related to students' physical and mental health, pediatricians may play a role in addressing absenteeism attributable to a wide range of factors through individual interactions with patients and their parents and through community-, state-, and federal-level advocacy.

[a]Department of Pediatrics, University of Colorado Anschutz Medical Campus, Adult and Child Consortium for Health Outcomes Research and Delivery Science, School of Medicine, University of Colorado, and Children's Hospital Colorado, Aurora, Colorado; and [b]Detroit Public Schools Community District, Detroit, Michigan

This document is copyrighted and is property of the American Academy of Pediatrics and its Board of Directors. All authors have filed conflict of interest statements with the American Academy of Pediatrics. Any conflicts have been resolved through a process approved by the Board of Directors. The American Academy of Pediatrics has neither solicited nor accepted any commercial involvement in the development of the content of this publication.

Policy statements from the American Academy of Pediatrics benefit from expertise and resources of liaisons and internal (AAP) and external reviewers. However, policy statements from the American Academy of Pediatrics may not reflect the views of the liaisons or the organizations or government agencies that they represent.

The guidance in this statement does not indicate an exclusive course of treatment or serve as a standard of medical care. Variations, taking into account individual circumstances, may be appropriate.

All policy statements from the American Academy of Pediatrics automatically expire 5 years after publication unless reaffirmed, revised, or retired at or before that time.

DOI: https://doi.org/10.1542/peds.2018-3648

Address correspondence to Mandy A. Allison. E-mail: Mandy.Allison@ucdenver.edu

PEDIATRICS (ISSN Numbers: Print, 0031-4005; Online, 1098-4275).

Copyright © 2019 by the American Academy of Pediatrics

FINANCIAL DISCLOSURE: The authors have indicated they have no financial relationships relevant to this article to disclose.

FUNDING: No external funding.

POTENTIAL CONFLICT OF INTEREST: The authors have indicated they have no potential conflicts of interest to disclose.

To cite: Allison MA, Attisha E, AAP COUNCIL ON SCHOOL HEALTH. The Link Between School Attendance and Good Health. *Pediatrics.* 2019;143(2):e20183648

STATEMENT OF THE PROBLEM

What Is Chronic Absenteeism?

Chronic absenteeism broadly refers to missing too much school for any reason, including excused and unexcused absences as well as suspensions. The US Department of Education's Office of Civil Rights has used a definition of missing 15 or more days over the course of a school year.[1] Most researchers and a growing number of states have defined chronic absenteeism as missing 10% (or around 18 days) of the entire school year. Some organizations suggest using 10%, because it promotes earlier identification of poor attendance throughout the school year. For example, identifying students who have missed just 2 days in the first month of school predicts chronic absence throughout the year.[2]

Chronic absence is different than truancy. The definition of truancy also varies but usually refers to when a student willfully misses school, and the absence is "unexcused."[3] Although students who are truant may be chronically absent, focusing solely on truancy may miss those students who miss excessive amounts of school for "excused" reasons. Regardless of whether absences are unexcused or excused, chronic absenteeism typically results in poor academic outcomes and is linked to poor health outcomes.

Factors such as poverty, unstable housing conditions, poor parental health, and racial or ethnic minority status are associated with poor child health outcomes and are known in the medical and public health communities as social determinants of health.[4–6] Students living in poverty are more likely than students from higher-income families to be chronically absent from school.[7,8] Factors associated with chronic absenteeism include poorer overall health,[9,10] unstable housing conditions,[11] transportation difficulties, and exposure to violence.[12] Students who change schools within the school year are also more likely to experience absenteeism.[13] In addition, youth may be called on to care for sick family members or stay home with younger siblings when a parent or primary caregiver is sick or cannot take time off work, and this is more likely to occur among low-income families.[14] Finally, authors of some studies have found that students from racial and ethnic minority groups and those who are English language learners are more likely to be chronically absent than students who are not in these groups.[1]

Children with a history of maltreatment or exposure to major trauma, such as witnessing domestic violence or experiencing a natural disaster, are more likely than those without these exposures to experience absenteeism, truancy, school suspension, and school dropout.[15–17] These children are also more likely to experience other risk factors for chronic absenteeism, including poor mental and behavioral health, poverty, homelessness, and frequent school changes.[15,16,18] Children who are living in foster care are more likely to transfer schools within a year compared with the general school population; however, this effect is mitigated among children with more stable (3 months or longer) foster care placements.[16] Although reliable data are lacking regarding the effect of immigrant or refugee status on school attendance, immigrant and refugee children are likely to have 1 or more risk factors for poor school outcomes, including poverty, racial or ethnic minority status, and exposure to major trauma.[17,19]

Why Does Chronic Absenteeism Matter?

Chronic absenteeism can occur as early as preschool and kindergarten and has been shown to be related to future chronic absenteeism, grade retention, and poor academic achievement, particularly for social skills and reading.[3,8,20,21] Among elementary school students, absenteeism is highest in kindergarten and first grade, then decreases until middle school. At least 10% of kindergarten and first-grade students miss a month or more of the school year.[21] Absenteeism tends to increase again in middle school and high school, with an estimated 19% of all high school students being chronically absent.[1] A national map of chronic absenteeism based on the US Department of Education's 2013–2014 Civil Rights Data Collection reveals wide geographic variation in chronic absenteeism and describes variations on the basis of race and ethnicity, with African American, Hispanic, American Indian, and Pacific Islander students experiencing higher rates of chronic absenteeism than their white and Asian American peers.[22]

Students with poor attendance score lower than their peers who attend school regularly on national skills assessments, regardless of race or ethnicity.[3] Chronic absenteeism can be a better predictor of school failure than test scores. In 1 study, students with high test scores who missed at least 2 weeks of school during the semester were more likely to have failing grades than students with low test scores who regularly attended school.[23] Chronic absenteeism as early as sixth grade is predictive of dropping out of school.[3]

The literature reveals that poor school performance is associated with poor adult health outcomes. Compared with adults with higher educational attainment, those with low educational attainment are more likely to be unemployed or work at a part-time or lower-paying job.[24] Those with lower educational attainment are less likely to report having a fulfilling job, feeling that they have control over their lives, and feeling that they have high levels of social support.[24,25] This lack of control and social support is thought to be associated with poor health attributable to difficulty adhering to healthy behaviors, psychological processes such as depression, and biological processes such as increased inflammation and reduced immune system function.[26] Adults with lower educational attainment are also more likely to smoke and less likely to exercise, which are directly linked to poor health outcomes.[24,25] Not earning a high school diploma is associated with increased mortality risk or lower life expectancy.[27] Conversely, obtaining advanced degrees and additional years of education are associated with a reduced mortality risk.[27] Over the past 20 years, disparities in mortality rates based on educational attainment are worsening for preventable causes of death.[28]

Chronic absenteeism is associated with engaging in health risk behaviors, including smoking cigarettes or marijuana, alcohol and other drug use, and risky sexual behavior, such as having 4 or more sexual partners.[29] For every year a student delays alcohol or drug use, his or her odds of regular school attendance in subsequent quarters increase.[30] Students' experiences of teenage pregnancy, violence, unintentional injury, and suicide attempts are associated with chronic absenteeism.[31–33] Roughly 30% to 40% of female teenage dropouts are mothers, with teenage pregnancy being the number 1 cause of high school dropout for adolescent female students.[34] Poor school attendance is also associated with juvenile delinquency; in 1 study of youth in Mississippi from 2003 to 2013, authors found that those with chronic absenteeism had 3.5-times higher odds of being arrested or referred to the juvenile justice system.[35]

Causes of School Absenteeism

Students may be frequently absent from school for a wide variety of reasons. In the publication, "The Importance of Being in School: A Report on Absenteeism in the Nation's Public Schools," Balfanz and Byrnes[36] describe 3 broad categories of causes: "(1) students who cannot attend school due to illness, family responsibilities, housing instability, the need to work or involvement with the juvenile justice system; (2) students who will not attend school to avoid bullying, unsafe conditions, harassment and embarrassment; and (3) students who do not attend school because they, or their parents, do not see the value in attending school, they have something else they would rather do, or nothing stops them from skipping school."[36] An additional category (ie, "myths") is also thought to cause problem absenteeism. Myths include when students and their families do not realize that missing just 2 days a month can be a problem, think that it is a problem only if absences are unexcused, or do not think absences are a problem for younger children in preschool through grade school.[14] Finally, school suspension and expulsion, as early as preschool, have increasingly been identified as causes of chronic absenteeism that disproportionately affect African American students and students with emotional and behavioral disorders and attention-deficit/hyperactivity disorder.[37–42]

Most studies of health-related causes of school absence have been conducted by authors focusing on a specific health condition and determining whether that condition is associated with missing school. Common health conditions that have been associated with school absenteeism include influenza infection,[43,44] group A streptococcal pharyngitis,[45] gastroenteritis,[46] fractures,[47–49] poorly controlled asthma,[50–54] type 1 diabetes mellitus,[55] chronic fatigue,[56,57] chronic pain[58–62] (including headaches and abdominal pain), seizures,[63] poor oral health,[64–67] dental pain,[68,69] and obesity.[70–73] Experienced clinicians know that mental health conditions may present with physical health complaints, including some of those listed above that have been associated with frequent absences. Few studies have been conducted to identify groups of children with higher absenteeism and lower absenteeism and determine which health conditions are most prevalent among those with higher absenteeism.[74] Therefore, it is a challenge to clearly define which health conditions cause more absenteeism than others. In addition, although more data are needed, the data that exist and the authors' clinical knowledge suggest that the most common health-related causes of school absenteeism likely vary among communities.

Although occasional absences attributable to health conditions can be expected, absences can quickly add up and lead to chronic absenteeism if a child experiences multiple health conditions, unrecognized or undertreated conditions, or lack of access to care. Absenteeism attributable to physical health conditions can be compounded by the presence of mental or behavioral health conditions and socioeconomic factors.

Children with disabilities are more likely to be chronically absent than children without disabilities.[1] Similarly, children and youth with special health care needs tend to have more school absences than children without.[75–77] School performance, including absenteeism, of children and youth with special health care needs has been shown to be affected by risk and protective factors at the child, family, and system levels (eg, socioeconomic factors, the presence or absence of care coordination, and school climate and accommodations).[75,76,78–80] Children with moderate-to-severe autism spectrum disorder may be at particular risk for disruptive behaviors that affect their own and other students' learning. Students with autism spectrum disorder who display disruptive behaviors at school may be more likely to be excluded or absent from school.[81,82]

School absenteeism has been associated with mental health conditions and substance use disorders.[83–86] Longitudinal cohort studies have revealed that conduct disorder and depressive symptoms can lead to frequent absenteeism and, conversely, that frequent absenteeism can lead to conduct disturbances and depressive symptoms.[87] Youth who are truant, defined as willfully refusing to attend school, are more likely than youth who attend school regularly to be diagnosed with oppositional defiant disorder, conduct disorder, depression, and tobacco, alcohol, and marijuana abuse.

Studies have been used to examine school absenteeism by using a socioecologic model considering individual-, family-, and school-level factors. Authors of these studies have found that individual factors (such as hyperactivity, conduct problems, and poor perceived health), family factors (such as low maternal education and high levels of unemployment), and school factors (such as not feeling safe or not feeling treated with respect at school) all contributed to students' poor attendance.[88] Issues that are likely to be brought up during a visit to a health care provider include bullying, gender identity and sexuality, and adverse childhood experiences (ACEs). In-person and electronic bullying have been shown to be associated with school absenteeism.[89] Lesbian, gay, bisexual, transgender, queer, and questioning youth have been shown to be at risk for poor school connectedness, and poor school connectedness is a risk for poor attendance.[90] Finally, students with higher numbers of ACEs are more likely to have chronic absenteeism than students with fewer ACEs.[91]

EVIDENCE FOR PHYSICAL AND MENTAL HEALTH INTERVENTIONS TO IMPROVE SCHOOL ATTENDANCE

Many organizations are making multidisciplinary efforts to promote school attendance at community, state, and national levels. Although the body of evidence about effective interventions to improve school attendance is growing, high-quality evaluation has been limited by the lack of routine measurement of chronic absenteeism and differences in how schools and local educational agencies measure and define absenteeism and attendance.[36] Several national organizations and collaborations are working to promote school attendance by bringing together stakeholders from diverse sectors, including education, law enforcement, juvenile justice, public health, and health care. Summaries of additional evidence and information about strategies to promote school attendance and address chronic absenteeism are available from these organizations and are listed in the Additional Resources section below.

Infection Prevention

Interventions used to improve hand hygiene practices in schools include increased frequency of hand-washing and use of hand sanitizers. It is suggested in a 2016 review of 18 randomized controlled trials that hand hygiene interventions can be used to promote good hand hygiene practices among children and school staff and can be used to reduce the incidence of respiratory tract illness symptoms, symptoms attributable to influenza, and school absenteeism.[92] Evidence was mixed for hand hygiene interventions to reduce absenteeism attributable to gastrointestinal tract illness.[92] The effects of school-based infection prevention measures have been best studied for influenza. In addition to studies of hand hygiene interventions,[93] school-located influenza vaccination programs have been shown to reduce school absenteeism during influenza season.[94] Finally, school immunization requirements have been shown to increase immunization coverage in the community, and high levels of coverage are necessary for the prevention of outbreaks of vaccine-preventable diseases that could lead to school absenteeism.[95]

School Nurses

School nurses play a significant role in student success and attendance. The American Academy of Pediatrics (AAP) and the National Association of School Nurses recommend a minimum of 1 full-time professional school nurse in every school, recognizing that the ideal nurse-to-student ratio varies depending on the needs of the student population.[96,97] Healthy People 2020 includes goals to have a school nurse-to-student ratio of 1:750 in elementary and secondary schools.[98] School nurses have the expertise to identify and intervene on health issues that may affect the learning environment and are critical team members for ensuring that students' individualized education programs, 504 plans, or health care plans are appropriately designed and implemented.[96,97,99] Given the complexity of studying nursing services in the school setting and the paucity of research funding and researchers studying school nursing services, data regarding the effect of school nurses on school attendance are limited. One study revealed that 95% of students seen by a school nurse for illness or injury are able to return to class compared with 82% of students seen by an unlicensed school employee.[100] Studies have also revealed that the addition of full-time school nurses reduces illness-related absenteeism among children with asthma compared with children with asthma in schools with part-time school nurses.[101,102] One literature review revealed that school nurses can improve attendance among students with chronic absenteeism and that lower nurse-to-student ratios were associated with improved school-level attendance rates.[103] Many schools have nurse coverage only part-time, and some schools do not have nurse coverage at all[104]; therefore, a health aide or other school personnel may provide some school health services. The services provided by health aides or other school personnel are essential when a nurse is not available, but these other providers typically do not have nursing training.

School-Based Health Centers

School-based health centers (SBHCs) have been shown to improve education outcomes, including grade point average and high school graduation,[105] and have been recommended by the Community Preventive Services Task Force to improve both education and health outcomes in low-income communities.[106] SBHCs provide health services to students who otherwise may have been sent home or missed school because of illnesses and injuries or attending medical appointments for management of chronic health problems. School-based health services can include preventive services, dental services, and mental or behavioral health services.[107] Research has shown SBHCs can reduce absenteeism. Authors of a study of SBHC users in Seattle found that those who used the clinic for medical purposes had a significant increase in attendance over nonusers.[108,109] African American male SBHC users were 3 times more likely to stay in school than their peers who did not use the SBHC. Authors of 2 studies in New York found that students enrolled in SBHCs had more time in class, better attendance, and fewer hospitalizations attributable to asthma.[110,111] Authors of another study found a 50% decrease in absenteeism and 25% decrease in tardiness for high school students who received school-based mental health services.[112] Overall, SBHCs have been shown to improve school attendance for students who use SBHCs for physical and mental health care, with greater improvement for those using SBHCs for physical health.[108,110,113]

Mental Health Care

Authors of a recent review of children's mental health services provided in schools or in other community-based or clinic settings found that educational outcomes, including school attendance, are infrequently measured.[114] The authors of this review did suggest that mental health treatment was associated with improved overall educational outcomes for children. Investigators found that providing cognitive behavioral therapy for students identified with "school refusing" can improve attendance as well as anxiety and depressive symptoms.[115,116] "Trauma-informed schools" are schools in which the adults in the school community are prepared to recognize and respond to those who have been affected by trauma.[117] These schools are focused on the life experiences of a student and how the experiences may affect the student's behavior and performance at school. In addition, these schools provide individual mental health interventions for students and/or link students and families to services in the community. Although research in this area is new and ongoing, a trauma-informed approach at schools appears to reduce school suspensions and expulsions and improve attendance and school performance.[117] Overall, more evidence is needed, specifically regarding the effectiveness of school-based mental health services and trauma-informed approaches for improving school attendance.[118,119]

School Policies and Programs

Policies that promote a positive school climate can promote attendance.[120] As defined by the National School Climate Center, "School climate refers to the quality and character of school life. School climate is based on patterns of students', parents' and school personnel's experience of school life and reflects norms, goals, values, interpersonal relationships, teaching and learning practices, and organizational structures."[121] The concepts of school climate and school connectedness are closely related, and research reveals that students who feel a connection with their school are more likely to attend and less likely to engage in risky behaviors.[32] The Centers for Disease Control and Prevention (CDC) has identified specific strategies to improve school connectedness.[122] The CDC also provides technical guidance regarding prevention of youth violence, including bullying, for schools and communities. This guidance suggests strategies including universal school-based programs for strengthening youth skills, connecting youth to caring adults and activities through mentoring and after-school programs, and creating protective community environments including a positive school climate. It is suggested in evidence that these strategies can be used to reduce youth violence and, in turn, improve school connectedness, attendance, and academic success.[123] Although many of these strategies are directed toward education professionals in the schools, they include engaging with community partners such as health care professionals. Some researchers suggest rewarding students for good attendance with parties, gift certificates, or other types of special recognition results in higher attendance rates.[124]

Parent Interventions

Schools that communicate effectively with all parents, regardless of language or culture, provide parents with a specific school contact person who can address their questions and concerns, and provide workshops about school attendance for parents have higher attendance rates.[124,125] Strong parental monitoring and parental involvement (eg, when a parent knows whether his or her child is attending school) are related to lower levels of delinquency, which is associated to better school attendance.[126] In 1 study conducted in 2014–2015 among students in kindergarten through 11th grade in Philadelphia, authors indicated that simply informing parents of their children's absences from school can help reduce subsequent absenteeism; this may be partly because parents have misbeliefs about how much their child has been absent.[14,127] Schools that build strong partnerships with families and the community have shown improved student attendance.[125] In addition to school nurses and other members of the school health team, school counselors can play a key role in developing these partnerships.[128,129]

Coordinated School Health

The CDC's Whole School, Whole Community, Whole Child model provides a framework for health and educational professionals to promote students' health and academic achievement.[130,131] The components of this model are health education; physical education and physical activity; nutrition environment and services; health services; counseling, psychological, and social services; social and emotional climate; physical environment; employee wellness; family engagement; and community involvement. Although not all of these components have been studied in relation to school attendance, authors of a recent comprehensive summary of the literature indicate that each component plays a role in improving children's academic performance.[132] Aspects of nutrition services (breakfast at school); health services (nursing services); counseling, psychological, and social services (school-based mental health care); social and emotional school climate (school connectedness); physical environment (full-spectrum lighting, reduction of physical threats, indoor air quality); family engagement; and community involvement have all been associated with improved school attendance.[132]

RECOMMENDATIONS

Pediatricians could address school attendance in their office-based practices and communities and/or states or nationally as advocates using a tiered approach. The office-based approaches could include members of the health care team, such as front office staff, medical assistants, nurses, or care coordinators, to reduce the burden on the pediatrician.

Tier 1

These office-based and advocacy approaches promote school attendance for all youth.

Office-Based

- Routinely ask at preventive care visits and sick visits about the number of absences a student has experienced. Consider adding questions about the number of missed school days in the previous month and the name of the school each patient is currently attending in templates in the paper or electronic medical record;
- Encourage parents to bring copies of their child's report card or share data available from their child's online school information system during preventive visits. These data sources usually include information about school absences and tardiness;
- Praise patients and caregivers when patients are regularly attending school, meaning they miss no more than a day per month on average;
- Talk about the effects of school absences on school performance and future wellness. Talk about how absences can add up. Stress the value of developing strong attendance habits as early as preschool;
- Support parents in addressing barriers to attendance;
- Ask families of children with chronic health issues, such as asthma, allergies, and seizures, if they have an action plan at school. Help complete school action plans so that families feel secure sending their children to school. When needed, work with the school nurse to adjust the action plan when there is a change in a patient's condition. Some states and national organizations or foundations have developed standardized forms for asthma,[133] allergy,[134] and seizure action plans[135];
- Encourage families to share their concerns about their children's health with their school nurse;
- Assist families in documenting and interpreting their children's medical needs or disability for an individualized education program or 504 plan to help them establish services to optimize learning opportunities[99,136];
- Promote school attendance by using handouts, posters, or videos in your waiting area (see links to resources below), working with community partners (eg, during September Attendance Awareness Month campaigns: http://awareness.attendanceworks.org/), and communicating via your practice Web site or social media;
- Educate yourself and your office staff about the appropriate and inappropriate reasons to exclude a child from school. Additional information about appropriate school inclusion and exclusion criteria can be found in the following publications from the AAP: *Managing Infectious Disease in Child Care and Schools: A Quick Reference Guide*[137] and the chapter on school health in the *Red Book: 2015 Report of the Committee on Infectious Diseases*[138];
- Provide firm guidance on when a child should stay home if sick and how to avoid absences from minor illness or anxiety (links to resource below);
- Learn about resources in the community and connect families with resources that can improve the well-being of the entire family (eg, family counseling, food pantries, housing assistance) as described in more detail in the "Poverty and Child Health in the United States" policy statement[139]; and
- Routinely ask about whether your patients have experienced out-of-school suspension or expulsion and assist patients and families affected by suspension and expulsion (more

detail in the "Out-of-School Suspension and Expulsion" policy statement).[42]

Population-Based

Pediatricians are encouraged to be advocates and supporters of children's health. Available opportunities may include the following:

- Work with AAP chapter leaders to advocate at the school, school district, state school board, and state legislative levels for policies and interventions known to promote school attendance. These interventions can include policies and approaches that promote a positive school climate and avoid suspension and expulsion.[42,121] Advocate for funding to ensure adequate numbers of school support personnel, including school nurses and school counselors, and for school-based medical, oral, and behavioral health services[96,140];
- Encourage and collaborate with community leaders (faith leaders, public officials, businesses) to develop and deliver consistent and coordinated community-specific and culturally salient messages that inform the public about the importance of regular school attendance at all ages, starting in early childhood;
- Educate and collaborate with school professionals about appropriate and inappropriate reasons for exclusion (eg, some schools continue to exclude children with head lice from school despite a strong, evidence-based recommendation to avoid exclusion from school for head lice).[141] AAP chapter leaders and the Council on School Health can provide assistance in these efforts;
- Support school districts' efforts to improve children's and families' access to health insurance and medical services;
- Serve as a school physician or on a school board, school or school district health services advisory committee, or wellness committee to develop policies and practices that promote school attendance[142];
- Work with your state school board, department of education, or school districts (local educational agencies) to encourage schools to consistently collect and share data with public health and health care providers on chronic absence by grade, school, and neighborhood, because chronic absence is often an indicator that children and families are struggling with health-related issues. Develop and promote strategies that encourage data sharing and are compliant with existing privacy laws;
- Work with schools to identify physical and mental health conditions that are significantly contributing to school absenteeism among their students and help identify interventions to address these conditions; and
- Encourage public health departments to compare chronic absence data and available health metrics to identify where collaborative action would be helpful.

Tier 2

In addition to the approaches described in tier 1, pediatricians can use the following office-based interventions for patients who are missing 2 or 3 days of school per month (~10% of total school time):

- Prevent, identify, and treat physical and mental health conditions that are contributing to school absences. Collaboration with school and mental health professionals is essential in the treatment of youth with psychosomatic symptoms that result in poor school attendance;
- When possible, identify psychosocial risk factors and health factors among a patient's caregivers that may be contributing to the patient's school absenteeism and refer the caregiver to appropriate resources in the community;
- Avoid writing excuses for school absences when the absence was not appropriate and avoid backdating to justify absences;
- Strongly encourage patients who are well enough to attend school to return to school immediately after their medical appointments, so they do not miss the entire day;
- Avoid contributing to school absences. In concordance with the medical home concepts of providing accessible, continuous, and family-centered care, consider offering extended office hours and encourage families to make preventive care appointments and follow-up appointments for times outside of regular school hours[143];
- Communicate and collaborate with school professionals and community partners to manage the health conditions of your patients with chronic absenteeism. The school nurse is usually the best first contact.[96] The AAP publication *Managing Chronic Health Needs in Child Care and Schools*[136] is a reference that may be particularly useful in the child care or preschool settings, where a school nurse or child care health consultant may not be readily available; and
- Encourage parents of students with excessive absences to seek a formal school team meeting (often termed a school study team) to discuss how the school and family can cooperate to address the issue. Specifically, parents can request that their student be considered for participation in their school's behavioral intervention system.[144]

Tier 3

In addition to the approaches described in tiers 1 and 2, pediatricians can use the following office-based interventions for patients who have severe chronic absenteeism and are missing 4 or more days of school per month (~15% of total school time):

- Encourage the school or school district to provide services such as intensive case management and mentorship, communicate and collaborate with professionals providing support services in school, and serve as your patient's advocate and medical expert; and
- Children are eligible for home or hospital educational services from the public schools if they have a legitimate medical reason for absences. The use of these services should be clearly justified on the basis of the patient's medical presentation. The goal should be for these services to be time limited. Communicate and collaborate with school professionals to decide whether out-of-school instruction is appropriate, develop a time line for out-of-school instruction, develop a reentry plan, and identify whether an alternative to out-of-school instruction is appropriate.

ADDITIONAL RESOURCES

Organizations Addressing School Attendance

- America's Promise Alliance, Grad Nation (http://www.americaspromise.org/program/gradnation);
- Attendance Works (http://www.attendanceworks.org/);
- Everyone Graduates Center (http://www.every1graduates.org/);
- Healthy Schools Campaign (https://healthyschoolscampaign.org/);
- National Center for Education Statistics, Every School Day Counts (https://nces.ed.gov/); and
- National Center for School Engagement (http://schoolengagement.org/).

Links to Resources to Share With Patients and Parents

- Handouts to give to parents (http://www.attendanceworks.org/resources/handouts-for-families/);
- Video to show in waiting room (http://www.attendanceworks.org/tools/for-parents/bringing-attendance-home-video/); and
- Mobile-friendly Web site geared to preteenagers, teenagers, and their parents (https://getschooled.com/dashboard).

LEAD AUTHORS

Mandy Allison, MD, MSPH, FAAP
Elliott Attisha, DO, FAAP

COUNCIL ON SCHOOL HEALTH EXECUTIVE COMMITTEE, 2017–2018

Marc Lerner, MD, FAAP, Chairperson
Cheryl Duncan De Pinto, MD, MPH, FAAP, Chairperson Elect
Elliott Attisha, DO, FAAP
Nathaniel Savio Beers, MD, MPA, FAAP
Erica J. Gibson, MD, FAAP
Peter Gorski, MD, MPA, FAAP
Chris Kjolhede, MD, MPH, FAAP
Sonja C. O'Leary, MD, FAAP
Heidi Schumacher, MD, FAAP
Adrienne Weiss-Harrison, MD, FAAP

FORMER EXECUTIVE COMMITTEE MEMBERS

Mandy Allison, MD, MSPH, FAAP
Richard Ancona, MD, FAAP
Breena Welch Holmes, MD, FAAP, Immediate Past Chairperson
Jeffrey Okamoto, MD, FAAP, FAAP, Past Chairperson
Thomas Young, MD, FAAP

CONSULTANTS

Hedy Chang – *Attendance Works*
Ken Seeley – *National Center for School Engagement*

LIAISONS

Susan Hocevar Adkins, MD, FAAP
Laurie Combe, MN, RN, NCSN
Veda Charmaine Johnson, MD, FAAP
Shashank Joshi, MD, FAAP

FORMER LIAISONS

Nina Fekaris, MS, BSN, RN, NCSN
Linda Grant, MD, MPH
Sheryl Kataoka, MD, MSHS
Sandra Leonard, DNP, RN, FNP

STAFF

Madra Guinn-Jones, MPH
Stephanie Domain, MS

ABBREVIATIONS

AAP: American Academy of Pediatrics
ACE: adverse childhood experience
CDC: Centers for Disease Control and Prevention
SBHC: school-based health center

REFERENCES

1. US Department of Education Office for Civil Rights. 2013-2014 civil rights data collection, a first look. 2016. Available at: http://www2.ed.gov/about/offices/list/ocr/docs/2013-14-first-look.pdf. Accessed November 16, 2016
2. Baltimore Education Research Consortium. Why September matters: improving student attendance. 2014. Available at: http://baltimore-berc.org/wp-content/uploads/2014/08/SeptemberAttendanceBriefJuly2014.pdf. Accessed November 16, 2016
3. Ginsburg A, Jordan P, Chang H. Absences add up: how school attendance influences student success. 2014. Available at: https://www.attendanceworks.org/wp-content/uploads/2017/05/Absenses-Add-Up_September-3rd-2014.pdf. Accessed December 21, 2018
4. Larson K, Russ SA, Crall JJ, Halfon N. Influence of multiple social risks on children's health. *Pediatrics*. 2008; 121(2):337–344
5. Cutts DB, Meyers AF, Black MM, et al. US housing insecurity and the health of very young children. *Am J Public Health*. 2011;101(8):1508–1514
6. Schickedanz A, Dreyer BP, Halfon N. Childhood poverty: understanding and

preventing the adverse impacts of a most-prevalent risk to pediatric health and well-being. *Pediatr Clin North Am.* 2015;62(5):1111–1135

7. Carlson JA, Mignano AM, Norman GJ, et al. Socioeconomic disparities in elementary school practices and children's physical activity during school. *Am J Health Promot.* 2014;28 (suppl 3):S47–S53
8. Chang HN, Romero M. *Present, Engaged, and Accounted for: The Critical Importance of Addressing Chronic Absence in the Early Grades.* New York, NY: National Center for Children in Poverty; 2008
9. Hughes DC, Ng S. Reducing health disparities among children. *Future Child.* 2003;13(1):153–167
10. Bloom B, Dey AN. Summary health statistics for U.S. children: National Health Interview Survey, 2004. *Vital Health Stat 10.* 2006;(227):1–85
11. Rafferty Y. The legal rights and educational problems of homeless children and youth. *Educ Eval Policy Anal.* 1995;17(1):39–61
12. Ramirez M, Wu Y, Kataoka S, et al. Youth violence across multiple dimensions: a study of violence, absenteeism, and suspensions among middle school children. *J Pediatr.* 2012;161(3): 542–546.e2
13. The University of Utah Utah Education Policy Center. Research brief: chronic absenteeism. 2012. Available at: www.attendanceworks.org/wordpress/wp-content/uploads/2014/04/UTAH-Chronic-AbsenteeismResearch-Brief-July-2012.pdf. Accessed November 16, 2016
14. Ad Council. California attendance parent survey results. 2015. Available at: https://oag.ca.gov/sites/all/files/agweb/pdfs/tr/toolkit/QuantitativeResearchReport.pdf. Accessed December 21, 2018
15. Downer JT, Booren LM, Lima OK, Luckner AE, Pianta RC. The Individualized Classroom Assessment Scoring System (inCLASS): preliminary reliability and validity of a system for observing preschoolers' competence in classroom interactions. *Early Child Res Q.* 2010;25(1):1–16
16. Romano E, Babchishin L, Marquis R, Fréchette S. Childhood maltreatment and educational outcomes. *Trauma Violence Abuse.* 2015;16(4):418–437
17. Porche MV, Fortuna LR, Lin J, Alegria M. Childhood trauma and psychiatric disorders as correlates of school dropout in a national sample of young adults. *Child Dev.* 2011;82(3):982–998
18. Fantuzzo JW, Perlman SM, Dobbins EK. Types and timing of child maltreatment and early school success: a population-based investigation. *Child Youth Serv Rev.* 2011;33(8):1404–1411
19. Block K, Cross S, Riggs E, Gibbs L. Supporting schools to create an inclusive environment for refugee students. *Int J Inclusive Educ.* 2014; 18(12):1337–1355
20. Connolly F, Olson LS. Early elementary performance and attendance in Baltimore city schools' pre-kindergarten and kindergarten. 2012. Available at: https://files.eric.ed.gov/fulltext/ED535768.pdf. Accessed December 21, 2018
21. Bruner C, Discher A, Chang H. Chronic elementary absenteeism: a problem hidden in plain sight. November 2011. Available at: https://www.edweek.org/media/chronicabsence-15chang.pdf. Accessed December 21, 2018
22. US Department of Education. Chronic absenteeism in the nation's schools: the geography of chronic absenteeism. 2016. Available at: https://www2.ed.gov/datastory/chronicabsenteeism.html#three. Accessed January 30, 2018
23. Allensworth EM, Easton JQ. What matters for staying on-track and graduating in Chicago public high schools. 2007. Available at: https://consortium.uchicago.edu/sites/default/files/publications/07 What Matters Final.pdf. Accessed December 21, 2018
24. Ross CE, Wu C-l. The links between education and health. *Am Sociol Rev.* 1995;60(5):719–745
25. Rogers RG, Hummer RA, Everett BG. Educational differentials in US adult mortality: an examination of mediating factors. *Soc Sci Res.* 2013;42(2):465–481
26. Uchino BN. Social support and health: a review of physiological processes potentially underlying links to disease outcomes. *J Behav Med.* 2006;29(4): 377–387
27. Lawrence EM, Rogers RG, Zajacova A. Educational attainment and mortality in the United States: effects of degrees, years of schooling, and certification. *Popul Res Policy Rev.* 2016;35(4): 501–525
28. Miech R, Pampel F, Kim J, Rogers RG. The enduring association between education and mortality: the role of widening and narrowing disparities. *Am Sociol Rev.* 2011;76(6):913–934
29. Eaton DK, Brener N, Kann LK. Associations of health risk behaviors with school absenteeism. Does having permission for the absence make a difference? *J Sch Health.* 2008;78(4): 223–229
30. Engberg J, Morral AR. Reducing substance use improves adolescents' school attendance. *Addiction.* 2006; 101(12):1741–1751
31. Gottfried MA. Chronic absenteeism and its effects on students' academic and socioemotional outcomes. *J Educ Stud Placed Risk.* 2014;19(2):53–75
32. Hawkrigg S, Payne DN. Prolonged school non-attendance in adolescence: a practical approach. *Arch Dis Child.* 2014;99(10):954–957
33. Barnet B, Arroyo C, Devoe M, Duggan AK. Reduced school dropout rates among adolescent mothers receiving school-based prenatal care. *Arch Pediatr Adolesc Med.* 2004;158(3):262–268
34. Freudenberg N, Ruglis J. Reframing school dropout as a public health issue. *Prev Chronic Dis.* 2007;4(4):A107
35. Robertson AA, Walker CS. Predictors of justice system involvement: maltreatment and education. *Child Abuse Negl.* 2018;76:408–415
36. Balfanz R, Byrnes V. *The Importance of Being in School: A Report on Absenteeism in the Nation's Public Schools.* Baltimore, MD: Johns Hopkins University Center for Social Organization of Schools; 2012:4–9
37. Council of State Governments Justice Center; Public Policy Research Institute at Texas A&M University. Breaking schools' rules: a statewide study of how school discipline relates to students' success and juvenile justice involvement. 2011. Available at: https://csgjusticecenter.org/wp-content/uploads/2012/08/Breaking_Schools_Rules_

Report_Final.pdf. Accessed August 29, 2017

38. Michail S. Understanding school responses to students' challenging behaviour: a review of literature. *Improv Sch.* 2011;14(2):156–171

39. Skiba RJ, Horner RH, Chung C-G, Rausch MK, May SL, Tobin T. Race is not neutral: a national investigation of African American and Latino disproportionality in school discipline. *Sch Psychol Rev.* 2011;40(1):85–107

40. U.S. Department of Education. School climate and discipline: know the data. 2016. Available at: https://www2.ed.gov/policy/gen/guid/school-discipline/data.html. Accessed August 29, 2017

41. Achilles GM, McLaughlin MJ, Croninger RG. Sociocultural correlates of disciplinary exclusion among students with emotional, behavioral, and learning disabilities in the SEELS national dataset. *J Emotional Behav Disord.* 2007;15(1):33–45

42. Council on School Health. Out-of-school suspension and expulsion. *Pediatrics.* 2013;131(3). Available at: www.pediatrics.org/cgi/content/full/131/3/e1000

43. Graitcer SB, Dube NL, Basurto-Davila R, et al. Effects of immunizing school children with 2009 influenza A (H1N1) monovalent vaccine on absenteeism among students and teachers in Maine. *Vaccine.* 2012;30(32):4835–4841

44. King JC Jr, Beckett D, Snyder J, Cummings GE, King BS, Magder LS. Direct and indirect impact of influenza vaccination of young children on school absenteeism. *Vaccine.* 2012;30(2):289–293

45. Pfoh E, Wessels MR, Goldmann D, Lee GM. Burden and economic cost of group A streptococcal pharyngitis. *Pediatrics.* 2008;121(2):229–234

46. Prazuck T, Compte-Nguyen G, Pelat C, Sunder S, Blanchon T. Reducing gastroenteritis occurrences and their consequences in elementary schools with alcohol-based hand sanitizers. *Pediatr Infect Dis J.* 2010;29(11):994–998

47. Hyman JE, Gaffney JT, Epps HR, Matsumoto H. Impact of fractures on school attendance. *J Pediatr Orthop.* 2011;31(2):113–116

48. Sesko AM, Choe JC, Vitale MA, Ugwonali O, Hyman JE. Pediatric orthopaedic injuries: the effect of treatment on school attendance. *J Pediatr Orthop.* 2005;25(5):661–665

49. Hyman JE, Jewetz ST, Matsumoto H, Choe JC, Vitale MG. Risk factors for school absence after acute orthopaedic injury in New York city. *J Pediatr Orthop.* 2007;27(4):415–420

50. Meng YY, Babey SH, Wolstein J. Asthma-related school absenteeism and school concentration of low-income students in California. *Prev Chronic Dis.* 2012;9:E98

51. Mizan SS, Shendell DG, Rhoads GG. Absence, extended absence, and repeat tardiness related to asthma status among elementary school children. *J Asthma.* 2011;48(3):228–234

52. Basch CE. Asthma and the achievement gap among urban minority youth. *J Sch Health.* 2011;81(10):606–613

53. Shendell DG, Alexander MS, Sanders DL, Jewett A, Yang J. Assessing the potential influence of asthma on student attendance/absence in public elementary schools. *J Asthma.* 2010;47(4):465–472

54. Dean BB, Calimlim BM, Kindermann SL, Khandker RK, Tinkelman D. The impact of uncontrolled asthma on absenteeism and health-related quality of life. *J Asthma.* 2009;46(9):861–866

55. Parent KB, Wodrich DL, Hasan KS. Type 1 diabetes mellitus and school: a comparison of patients and healthy siblings. *Pediatr Diabetes.* 2009;10(8):554–562

56. Bakker RJ, van de Putte EM, Kuis W, Sinnema G. Risk factors for persistent fatigue with significant school absence in children and adolescents. *Pediatrics.* 2009;124(1). Available at: www.pediatrics.org/cgi/content/full/124/1/e89

57. Crawley E, Sterne JA. Association between school absence and physical function in paediatric chronic fatigue syndrome/myalgic encephalopathy. *Arch Dis Child.* 2009;94(10):752–756

58. Logan DE, Simons LE, Carpino EA. Too sick for school? Parent influences on school functioning among children with chronic pain. *Pain.* 2012;153(2):437–443

59. Gorodzinsky AY, Hainsworth KR, Weisman SJ. School functioning and chronic pain: a review of methods and measures. *J Pediatr Psychol.* 2011;36(9):991–1002

60. Logan DE, Simons LE, Kaczynski KJ. School functioning in adolescents with chronic pain: the role of depressive symptoms in school impairment. *J Pediatr Psychol.* 2009;34(8):882–892

61. Saps M, Seshadri R, Sztainberg M, Schaffer G, Marshall BM, Di Lorenzo C. A prospective school-based study of abdominal pain and other common somatic complaints in children. *J Pediatr.* 2009;154(3):322–326

62. Logan DE, Simons LE, Stein MJ, Chastain L. School impairment in adolescents with chronic pain. *J Pain.* 2008;9(5):407–416

63. Aguiar BV, Guerreiro MM, McBrian D, Montenegro MA. Seizure impact on the school attendance in children with epilepsy. *Seizure.* 2007;16(8):698–702

64. Seirawan H, Faust S, Mulligan R. The impact of oral health on the academic performance of disadvantaged children. *Am J Public Health.* 2012;102(9):1729–1734

65. Piovesan C, Antunes JL, Mendes FM, Guedes RS, Ardenghi TM. Influence of children's oral health-related quality of life on school performance and school absenteeism. *J Public Health Dent.* 2012;72(2):156–163

66. Jackson SL, Vann WF Jr, Kotch JB, Pahel BT, Lee JY. Impact of poor oral health on children's school attendance and performance. *Am J Public Health.* 2011;101(10):1900–1906

67. Blumenshine SL, Vann WF Jr, Gizlice Z, Lee JY. Children's school performance: impact of general and oral health. *J Public Health Dent.* 2008;68(2):82–87

68. Thikkurissy S, Glazer K, Amini H, Casamassimo PS, Rashid R. The comparative morbidities of acute dental pain and acute asthma on quality of life in children. *Pediatr Dent.* 2012;34(4):e77–e80

69. Guarnizo-Herreño CC, Wehby GL. Children's dental health, school performance, and psychosocial well-being. *J Pediatr.* 2012;161(6):1153–1159

70. Li Y, Raychowdhury S, Tedders SH, Lyn R, Lòpez-De Fede A, Zhang J. Association between increased BMI and severe school absenteeism among US children and adolescents: findings from a national survey, 2005-2008. *Int J Obes.* 2012;36(4):517–523
71. Baxter SD, Royer JA, Hardin JW, Guinn CH, Devlin CM. The relationship of school absenteeism with body mass index, academic achievement, and socioeconomic status among fourth-grade children. *J Sch Health.* 2011; 81(7):417–423
72. Rappaport EB, Daskalakis C, Andrel J. Obesity and other predictors of absenteeism in Philadelphia school children. *J Sch Health.* 2011;81(6): 341–344
73. Shore SM, Sachs ML, Lidicker JR, Brett SN, Wright AR, Libonati JR. Decreased scholastic achievement in overweight middle school students. *Obesity (Silver Spring).* 2008;16(7):1535–1538
74. Jones R, Hoare P, Elton R, Dunhill Z, Sharpe M. Frequent medical absences in secondary school students: survey and case-control study. *Arch Dis Child.* 2009;94(10):763–767
75. Forrest CB, Bevans KB, Riley AW, Crespo R, Louis TA. School outcomes of children with special health care needs. *Pediatrics.* 2011;128(2):303–312
76. Bethell C, Forrest CB, Stumbo S, Gombojav N, Carle A, Irwin CE. Factors promoting or potentially impeding school success: disparities and state variations for children with special health care needs. *Matern Child Health J.* 2012;16(suppl 1):S35–S43
77. Reuben CA, Pastor PN. The effect of special health care needs and health status on school functioning. *Disabil Health J.* 2013;6(4):325–332
78. O'Connor M, Howell-Meurs S, Kvalsvig A, Goldfeld S. Understanding the impact of special health care needs on early school functioning: a conceptual model. *Child Care Health Dev.* 2015;41(1):15–22
79. Willits KA, Troutman-Jordan ML, Nies MA, Racine EF, Platonova E, Harris HL. Presence of medical home and school attendance: an analysis of the 2005-2006 national survey of children with special healthcare needs. *J Sch Health.* 2013;83(2):93–98
80. Turchi RM, Berhane Z, Bethell C, Pomponio A, Antonelli R, Minkovitz CS. Care coordination for CSHCN: associations with family-provider relations and family/child outcomes. *Pediatrics.* 2009;124(suppl 4): S428–S434
81. Fitzpatrick SE, Srivorakiat L, Wink LK, Pedapati EV, Erickson CA. Aggression in autism spectrum disorder: presentation and treatment options. *Neuropsychiatr Dis Treat.* 2016;12: 1525–1538
82. Pas ET, Johnson SR, Larson KE, Brandenburg L, Church R, Bradshaw CP. Reducing behavior problems among students with autism spectrum disorder: coaching teachers in a mixed-reality setting. *J Autism Dev Disord.* 2016;46(12):3640–3652
83. Egger HL, Costello EJ, Angold A. School refusal and psychiatric disorders: a community study. *J Am Acad Child Adolesc Psychiatry.* 2003;42(7): 797–807
84. Bernstein GA, Garfinkel BD. School phobia: the overlap of affective and anxiety disorders. *J Am Acad Child Psychiatry.* 1986;25(2):235–241
85. Gase LN, Kuo T, Coller K, Guerrero LR, Wong MD. Assessing the connection between health and education: identifying potential leverage points for public health to improve school attendance. *Am J Public Health.* 2014; 104(9):e47–e54
86. Hallfors D, Vevea JL, Iritani B, Cho H, Khatapoush S, Saxe L. Truancy, grade point average, and sexual activity: a meta-analysis of risk indicators for youth substance use. *J Sch Health.* 2002;72(5):205–211
87. Wood JJ, Lynne-Landsman SD, Langer DA, et al. School attendance problems and youth psychopathology: structural cross-lagged regression models in three longitudinal data sets. *Child Dev.* 2012;83(1):351–366
88. Ingul JM, Klöckner CA, Silverman WK, Nordahl HM. Adolescent school absenteeism: modelling social and individual risk factors. *Child Adolesc Ment Health* 2012;17(2):93–100
89. Steiner RJ, Rasberry CN. Brief report: associations between in-person and electronic bullying victimization and missing school because of safety concerns among U.S. high school students. *J Adolesc.* 2015;43:1–4
90. Seelman KL, Forge N, Walls NE, Bridges N. School engagement among LGBTQ high school students: the roles of safe adults and gay–straight alliance characteristics. *Child Youth Serv Rev.* 2015;57:19–29
91. Stempel H, Cox-Martin M, Bronsert M, Dickinson LM, Allison MA. Chronic school absenteeism and the role of adverse childhood experiences. *Acad Pediatr.* 2017;17(8):837–843
92. Willmott M, Nicholson A, Busse H, MacArthur GJ, Brookes S, Campbell R. Effectiveness of hand hygiene interventions in reducing illness absence among children in educational settings: a systematic review and meta-analysis. *Arch Dis Child.* 2016;101(1): 42–50
93. Stebbins S, Cummings DA, Stark JH, et al. Reduction in the incidence of influenza A but not influenza B associated with use of hand sanitizer and cough hygiene in schools: a randomized controlled trial. *Pediatr Infect Dis J.* 2011;30(11):921–926
94. Hull HF, Ambrose CS. The impact of school-located influenza vaccination programs on student absenteeism: a review of the U.S. literature. *J Sch Nurs.* 2011;27(1):34–42
95. Committee on Practice and Ambulatory Medicine; Committee on Infectious Diseases; Committee on State Government Affairs; Council on School Health; Section on Administration and Practice Management. Medical versus nonmedical immunization exemptions for child care and school attendance. *Pediatrics.* 2016;138(3):e20162145
96. Council on School Health. Role of the school nurse in providing school health services. *Pediatrics.* 2016;137(6): e20160852
97. National Association of School Nurses. School nurse workload: staffing for safe care (position statement). 2015. Available at: https://www.nasn.org/advocacy/professional-practice-documents/position-statements/ps-workload. Accessed December 21, 2018
98. Office of Disease Prevention and Health Promotion. Healthy people 2020. ECBP-5.

2016. Available at: https://www.healthypeople.gov/2020/topics-objectives/topic/educational-and-community-based-programs/objectives. December 21, 2018

99. Lipkin PH, Okamoto J; Council on Children with Disabilities; Council on School Health. The individuals with disabilities education act (IDEA) for children with special educational needs. *Pediatrics*. 2015;136(6). Available at: www.pediatrics.org/cgi/content/full/136/6/e1650

100. Pennington N, Delaney E. The number of students sent home by school nurses compared to unlicensed personnel. *J Sch Nurs*. 2008;24(5):290–297

101. Telljohann SK, Dake JA, Price JH. Effect of full-time versus part-time school nurses on attendance of elementary students with asthma. *J Sch Nurs*. 2004;20(6):331–334

102. Rodriguez E, Rivera DA, Perlroth D, Becker E, Wang NE, Landau M. School nurses' role in asthma management, school absenteeism, and cost savings: a demonstration project. *J Sch Health*. 2013;83(12):842–850

103. Maughan E. The impact of school nursing on school performance: a research synthesis. *J Sch Nurs*. 2003;19(3):163–171

104. Willgerodt MA, Brock DM, Maughan ED. Public school nursing practice in the United States. *J Sch Nurs*. 2018;34(3):232–244

105. Knopf JA, Finnie RK, Peng Y, et al; Community Preventive Services Task Force. School-based health centers to advance health equity: a community guide systematic review. *Am J Prev Med*. 2016;51(1):114–126

106. Community Preventive Services Task Force. School-based health centers to promote health equity: recommendation of the Community Preventive Services Task Force. *Am J Prev Med*. 2016;51(1):127–128

107. The School-Based Health Alliance. 2013-2014 census report of school-based health centers. 2015. Available at: www.sbh4all.org/school-health-care/national-census-of-school-based-health-centers/. Accessed September 5, 2017

108. Walker SC, Kerns SE, Lyon AR, Bruns EJ, Cosgrove TJ. Impact of school-based health center use on academic outcomes. *J Adolesc Health*. 2010;46(3):251–257

109. McCord MT, Klein JD, Foy JM, Fothergill K. School-based clinic use and school performance. *J Adolesc Health*. 1993;14(2):91–98

110. Van Cura M. The relationship between school-based health centers, rates of early dismissal from school, and loss of seat time. *J Sch Health*. 2010;80(8):371–377

111. Webber MP, Carpiniello KE, Oruwariye T, Lo Y, Burton WB, Appel DK. Burden of asthma in inner-city elementary schoolchildren: do school-based health centers make a difference? *Arch Pediatr Adolesc Med*. 2003;157(2):125–129

112. Gall G, Pagano ME, Desmond MS, Perrin JM, Murphy JM. Utility of psychosocial screening at a school-based health center. *J Sch Health*. 2000;70(7):292–298

113. Geierstanger SP, Amaral G, Mansour M, Walters SR. School-based health centers and academic performance: research, challenges, and recommendations. *J Sch Health*. 2004;74(9):347–352

114. Becker KD, Brandt NE, Stephan SH, Chorpita BF. A review of educational outcomes in the children's mental health treatment literature. *Adv Sch Ment Health Promot*. 2014;7(1):5–23

115. King NJ, Tonge BJ, Heyne D, et al. Cognitive-behavioral treatment of school-refusing children: a controlled evaluation. *J Am Acad Child Adolesc Psychiatry*. 1998;37(4):395–403

116. Pina AA, Zerr AA, Gonzales NA, Ortiz CD. Psychosocial interventions for school refusal behavior in children and adolescents. *Child Dev Perspect*. 2009;3(1):11–20

117. McInerney M, McKlindon A; Education Law Center. Unlocking the door to learning: trauma-informed classrooms & transformational schools. 2014. Available at: https://www.elc-pa.org/resource/unlocking-the-door-to-learning-trauma-informed-classrooms-and-transformational-schools/. Accessed December 21, 2018

118. Daly BP, Sander MA, Nicholls EG, Medhanie A, Vanden Berk E, Johnson J. Three-year longitudinal study of school behavior and academic outcomes: results from a comprehensive expanded school mental health program. *Adv Sch Ment Health Promot*. 2014;7(1):24–41

119. Kang-Yi CD, Mandell DS, Hadley T. School-based mental health program evaluation: children's school outcomes and acute mental health service use. *J Sch Health*. 2013;83(7):463–472

120. Thapa A, Cohen J, Guffey S, Higgins-D'Alessandro A. A review of school climate research. *Rev Educ Res*. 2013;83(3):357–385

121. National School Climate Center. What is School Climate? 2016. Available at: https://www.schoolclimate.org/about/our-approach/what-is-school-climate. Accessed December 21, 2018

122. Centers for Disease Control and Prevention. School Connectedness: Strategies for Increasing Protective Factors Among Youth. Atlanta, GA: US Department of Health and Human Services; 2009. Available at: www.cdc.gov/healthyyouth/protective/pdf/connectedness.pdf. Accessed December 21, 2018

123. David-Ferdon C, Vivolo-Kantor AM, Dahlberg LL, Marshall KJ, Rainford N, Hall JE. *A Comprehensive Technical Package for the Prevention of Youth Violence and Associated Risk Behaviors*. Atlanta, GA: National Center for Injury Prevention and Control, Centers for Disease Control and Prevention; 2016

124. Epstein JL, Sheldon SB. Present and accounted for: improving student attendance through family and community involvement. *J Educ Res*. 2002;95(5):308–318

125. Sheldon SB. Improving student attendance with school, family, and community partnerships. *J Educ Res*. 2007;100(5):267–275

126. Monahan KC, VanDerhei S, Bechtold J, Cauffman E. From the school yard to the squad car: school discipline, truancy, and arrest. *J Youth Adolesc*. 2014;43(7):1110–1122

127. Rogers T, Feller A. Reducing student absences at scale by targeting parents' misbeliefs. 2018. Nature Human

Behaviour. doi: 10.1038/s41562-018-0328-1

128. Epstein JL, Van Voorhis FL. School counselors' roles in developing partnerships with families and communities for student success. *Prof Sch Couns.* 2010;14(1):1–14

129. American School Counselor Association. The school counselor and school-family-community partnerships. 2010. Available at: https://www.schoolcounselor.org/asca/media/asca/PositionStatements/PS_Partnerships.pdf. Accessed August 29, 2017

130. Centers for Disease Control and Prevention. Whole School, Whole Community, Whole Child (WSCC) Model. 2018. Available at: https://www.cdc.gov/healthyyouth/wscc/model.htm. Accessed December 21, 2018

131. Lewallen TC, Hunt H, Potts-Datema W, Zaza S, Giles W. The Whole School, Whole Community, Whole Child model: a new approach for improving educational attainment and healthy development for students. *J Sch Health.* 2015;85(11): 729–739

132. Michael SL, Merlo CL, Basch CE, Wentzel KR, Wechsler H. Critical connections: health and academics. *J Sch Health.* 2015;85(11):740–758

133. National Association of School Nurses. Asthma. 2017. Available at: https://www.nasn.org/nasn/nasn-resources/practice-topics/asthma. Accessed August 29, 2017

134. National Association of School Nurses. Food allergies and anaphylaxis. 2017. Available at: https://www.nasn.org/nasn/nasn-resources/practice-topics/food-allergies. Accessed August 29, 2017

135. Epilepsy Foundation. Seizure action plan. 2008. Available at: https://www.epilepsy.com/sites/core/files/atoms/files/seizure-action-plan-pdf_0.pdf. Accessed August 29, 2017

136. Donoghue EA, Kraft CA. *Managing Chronic Health Needs in Child Care and Schools: A Quick Reference Guide*, 2nd ed. American Academy of Pediatrics; 2018

137. Shope TR, Aronson SS, eds. *Managing Infectious Diseases in Child Care and Schools: A Quick Reference Guide.* 3rd ed. Elk Grove Village, IL: American Academy of Pediatrics; 2013

138. Committee on Infectious Diseases American Academy of Pediatrics. *Red Book: 2015 Report of the Committee on Infectious Diseases.* 30th ed. Elk Grove Village, IL: American Academy of Pediatrics; 2015

139. American Academy of Pediatrics; Council on Community Pediatrics. Policy statement: Poverty and Child Health in the United States. *Pediatrics.* 2016; 137(4):e20160339

140. American School Counselor Association. *ASCA National Model: A Framework for School Counseling Programs.* 3rd ed.Alexandria, VA: American School Counselor Association; 2012. Available at: https://schoolcounselor.org/Ascanationalmodel/media/ANM-templates/ANMExecSumm.pdf. Accessed August 29, 2017

141. Devore CD, Schutze GE; Council on School Health and Committee on Infectious Diseases, American Academy of Pediatrics. Head lice [published correction appears in *Pediatrics.* 2015;136(4):781–782]. *Pediatrics.* 2015;135(5). Available at: www.pediatrics.org/cgi/content/full/135/5/e1355

142. Devore CD, Wheeler LS; Council on School Health; American Academy of Pediatrics. Role of the school physician. *Pediatrics.* 2013;131(1):178–182

143. Medical Home Initiatives for Children With Special Needs Project Advisory Committee; American Academy of Pediatrics. The medical home. *Pediatrics.* 2002;110(1 pt 1): 184–186

144. Positive Behavioral Interventions & Supports. Positive Behavioral Interventions & Supports. 2016. Available at: https://www.pbis.org. Accessed December 21, 2018

Management of Infants at Risk for Group B Streptococcal Disease

- *Clinical Report*

CLINICAL REPORT Guidance for the Clinician in Rendering Pediatric Care

American Academy of Pediatrics 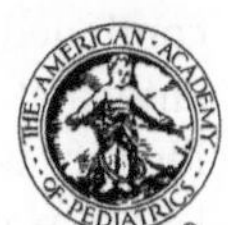

DEDICATED TO THE HEALTH OF ALL CHILDREN™

Management of Infants at Risk for Group B Streptococcal Disease

Karen M. Puopolo, MD, PhD, FAAP,[a,b] Ruth Lynfield, MD, FAAP,[c] James J. Cummings, MD, MS, FAAP,[d] COMMITTEE ON FETUS AND NEWBORN, COMMITTEE ON INFECTIOUS DISEASES

abstract

Group B streptococcal (GBS) infection remains the most common cause of neonatal early-onset sepsis and a significant cause of late-onset sepsis among young infants. Administration of intrapartum antibiotic prophylaxis is the only currently available effective strategy for the prevention of perinatal GBS early-onset disease, and there is no effective approach for the prevention of late-onset disease. The American Academy of Pediatrics joins with the American College of Obstetricians and Gynecologists to reaffirm the use of universal antenatal microbiologic-based testing for the detection of maternal GBS colonization to facilitate appropriate administration of intrapartum antibiotic prophylaxis. The purpose of this clinical report is to provide neonatal clinicians with updated information regarding the epidemiology of GBS disease as well current recommendations for the evaluation of newborn infants at risk for GBS disease and for treatment of those with confirmed GBS infection. This clinical report is endorsed by the American College of Obstetricians and Gynecologists (ACOG), July 2019, and should be construed as ACOG clinical guidance.

[a]Department of Pediatrics, Perelman School of Medicine, University of Pennsylvania, Philadelphia, Pennsylvania; [b]Children's Hospital of Philadelphia, Philadelphia, Pennsylvania; [c]Minnesota Department of Health, St Paul, Minnesota; and [d]Departments of Pediatrics and Bioethics, Alden March Bioethics Institute, Albany Medical College, Albany, New York

This document is copyrighted and is property of the American Academy of Pediatrics and its Board of Directors. All authors have filed conflict of interest statements with the American Academy of Pediatrics. Any conflicts have been resolved through a process approved by the Board of Directors. The American Academy of Pediatrics has neither solicited nor accepted any commercial involvement in the development of the content of this publication.

Clinical reports from the American Academy of Pediatrics benefit from expertise and resources of liaisons and internal (AAP) and external reviewers. However, clinical reports from the American Academy of Pediatrics may not reflect the views of the liaisons or the organizations or government agencies that they represent.

The guidance in this report does not indicate an exclusive course of treatment or serve as a standard of medical care. Variations, taking into account individual circumstances, may be appropriate.

All clinical reports from the American Academy of Pediatrics automatically expire 5 years after publication unless reaffirmed, revised, or retired at or before that time.

DOI: https://doi.org/10.1542/peds.2019-1881

Address correspondence to Karen M. Puopolo, MD, PhD. E-mail: puopolok@email.chop.edu

PEDIATRICS (ISSN Numbers: Print, 0031-4005; Online, 1098-4275).

Copyright © 2019 by the American Academy of Pediatrics

To cite: Puopolo KM, Lynfield R, Cummings JJ, AAP COMMITTEE ON FETUS AND NEWBORN, AAP COMMITTEE ON INFECTIOUS DISEASES. Management of Infants at Risk for Group B Streptococcal Disease. *Pediatrics.* 2019;144(2): e20191881

The Centers for Disease Control and Prevention (CDC) first published consensus guidelines on the prevention of perinatal group B streptococcal (GBS) disease in 1996. These guidelines were developed in collaboration with the American Academy of Pediatrics (AAP), the American College of Obstetricians and Gynecologists (ACOG), the American College of Nurse-Midwives, the American Academy of Family Physicians, and other stakeholder organizations[1] on the basis of available evidence as well as expert opinion. The 1996 consensus guidelines recommended either an antenatal culture–based or risk factor–based approach for the administration of intrapartum antibiotic prophylaxis (IAP) to prevent invasive neonatal GBS early-onset disease (EOD).[1] The guidelines were updated in 2002 primarily on the basis of new data from a CDC multistate retrospective cohort study in which authors found universal screening for group B streptococci (*Streptococcus agalactiae*) was >50% more effective at preventing the disease compared to a risk-based approach.[2,3] In 2010, the CDC once again revised the GBS perinatal prevention guidelines and continued to endorse the universal antenatal culture–based approach to identify women who would receive IAP to prevent GBS EOD.[4] Notable changes in the 2010 revision addressed the use of IAP for women in preterm labor and those with preterm prelabor rupture of membranes (PROM), the choice of specific antibiotics for IAP, and the use of nucleic acid amplification tests (NAATs) to identify maternal GBS colonization. The 2010 revision included a neonatal management algorithm for secondary prevention of GBS EOD that was widely adopted by neonatal physicians as a means of managing risk of all bacterial causes of early-onset sepsis (EOS).[5] With implementation of universal maternal antenatal screening and IAP, the national incidence of GBS EOD has declined from 1.8 cases per 1000 live births in 1990 to 0.23 cases per 1000 live births in 2015.[6]

Evolving epidemiology, newly published data, and changing practice standards inform periodic review of practice guidelines. In 2017, representatives from the CDC, AAP, ACOG, and other stakeholder organizations agreed to review and revise the 2010 GBS guidelines. A consensus was reached that the AAP would revise neonatal care recommendations and ACOG would revise obstetric care guidelines. These separate but aligned publications replace the CDC 2010 GBS perinatal guidance.

This clinical report addresses the epidemiology, microbiology, disease pathogenesis, and management strategies for neonatal early- and late-onset GBS infection. Maternal management is addressed in ACOG Committee Opinion No. 782, "Prevention of Group B Streptococcal Early-Onset Disease in Newborns."[7] This clinical report is endorsed by the American College of Obstetricians and Gynecologists (ACOG), July 2019, and should be construed as ACOG clinical guidance.

CURRENT EPIDEMIOLOGY OF NEONATAL GBS INFECTION

Early-Onset GBS Infection

GBS EOD is defined as isolation of group B *Streptococcus* organisms from blood, cerebrospinal fluid (CSF), or another normally sterile site from birth through 6 days of age.[8] Active Bacterial Core surveillance (ABCs), performed in collaboration with the CDC in 10 states from 2006 to 2015, found that the overall incidence of GBS EOD declined from 0.37 cases per 1000 live births in 2006 to 0.23 cases per 1000 live births in 2015.[6] Meningitis was diagnosed in 9.5% of infants with GBS EOD. CSF culture-positive GBS EOD occurred in the absence of bacteremia in 9.1% of early-onset meningitis cases (incidence: approximately 2.5 cases per 1 million live births).[6] Infants born at <37 weeks' gestation account for 28% of all GBS cases; approximately 15% of cases occur among preterm infants with very low birth weight (<1500 g).[6,9] Overall, GBS infection accounts for approximately 45% of all cases of culture-confirmed EOS among term infants and approximately 25% of all EOS cases that occur among infants with very low birth weight.[9,10] Death attributable to GBS EOD occurs primarily among preterm infants: the current case fatality ratio is 2.1% among term infants and 19.2% among those born at <37 weeks' gestation.[6]

GBS EOD primarily presents clinically at or shortly after birth. The majority of infants become symptomatic by 12 to 24 hours of age[11–13]; during the 2006–2015 period of ABCs, 94.7% of GBS EOD cases were diagnosed ≤48 hours after birth.[6] The incidence of newborn infants discharged from a birth hospital and readmitted to a hospital with GBS EOD within 6 days of age was approximately 0.3 cases per 100 000 live births in the ABCs. Although potentially an underestimate, this finding was consistent with data from the Northern California Kaiser Permanente health care system, which found the incidence of newborn infants readmitted to the hospital within the first week after hospital discharge with culture-confirmed infection attributable to any bacteria to be approximately 5 cases per 100 000 live births.[14] Globally, outside the United States, an estimated 200 000 cases of GBS EOD occurred in 2015. Stillbirth, GBS EOD, and late-onset GBS cases combined contribute to an estimated 150 000 fetal and neonatal deaths throughout the world, with the largest concentration of GBS perinatal deaths occurring in Africa.[15]

Late-Onset GBS Disease

GBS late-onset disease (LOD) is defined as isolation of GBS from a normally sterile site from 7 to 89 days of age.[8] Rarely, very–late-onset GBS disease may occur after 3 months of age, primarily among infants born very preterm or infants with immunodeficiency syndromes.[16,17] GBS LOD rates have not changed with widespread use of IAP. GBS LOD incidence was stable over the 2006–2015 ABCs study period, with an average incidence of 0.31 cases per 1000 live births.[6] The median age at presentation with GBS LOD was 34 days (interquartile range: 20–49 days). Bacteremia was identified in approximately 93% of GBS LOD, and bacteremia without focus was the most common form of disease. Group B streptococci were isolated from CSF in 20.7% of cases, and meningitis was diagnosed in 31.4% of cases. Cultures of bone and joint and peritoneal fluid yielded group B streptococci in 1.8% of cases. CSF culture-positive GBS LOD occurred in the absence of bacteremia in approximately 20% of late-onset meningitis cases (incidence: 1.9 cases per 100 000 live births). Infants born at <37 weeks' gestation account for approximately 42% of all GBS LOD cases, and death attributable to GBS LOD occurs in preterm infants at roughly twice the rate of term infants (7.8% vs 3.4%, respectively).[6] GBS LOD complicated by meningitis has a higher patient fatality rate than those with other syndromes.

PATHOGENESIS OF AND RISK FACTORS FOR GBS INFECTION

EOD

Group B *Streptococcus* emerged as the primary bacterial cause of EOS in the 1970s, and subsequent studies identified maternal GBS colonization as the primary risk factor for GBS-specific EOS.[18–20] The most common pathogenesis of GBS EOD is that of ascending colonization of the uterine compartment with group B streptococci that are present in the maternal gastrointestinal and genitourinary flora. Infection occurs with subsequent colonization and invasive infection of the fetus and/or fetal aspiration of infected amniotic fluid. This pathogenesis primarily occurs during labor for term infants, but the timing is less certain among preterm infants for whom intraamniotic infection may be the cause of PROM and/or preterm labor.[21] Rarely, GBS EOD may develop at or near term before the onset of labor, potentially because of group B streptococci traversing exposed but intact membranes. GBS EOD also is associated with stillbirth.[22,23]

Maternal colonization is a prerequisite for GBS EOD. Authors of a recent meta-analysis estimated that globally, GBS colonization was detected at vaginal and/or rectal sites in 18% of pregnant women, with regional variation of 11% to 35%.[24] Authors of most clinical studies in the United States have found colonization rates of 20% to 30% among pregnant women,[14,25–28] with variation by maternal age and race. Colonization can be ongoing or intermittent among pregnant and nonpregnant women.[28,29] Transmission of group B streptococci from mother to infant usually occurs shortly before or during delivery. In the absence of IAP, approximately 50% of newborn infants born to mothers positive for GBS become colonized with group B streptococci, and of those, 1% to 2% will develop GBS EOD.[30–33]

Multiple clinical characteristics associated with greater risk of maternal GBS colonization and with the pathogenesis of GBS EOD are predictive of neonatal disease.[20,21,34–43] Lower gestational age is associated with less effective opsonic, neutrophil-mediated defenses in the infant as well as lower levels of protective maternally derived antibody.[44–46] Increased duration of rupture of membranes (ROM) promotes the process of ascending colonization and infection of the uterine compartment and fetus. Maternal intrapartum fever may reflect the maternal inflammatory response to evolving intraamniotic bacterial infection and is an important predictor of neonatal early-onset infection. African American race and, less consistently, a maternal age <20 years have been associated with a higher risk of GBS EOD.[10,34,37,39] The independent contribution of these factors remains unclear because maternal age and race are also associated with higher rates of GBS colonization, preterm birth, and socioeconomic disadvantage, and African American race has been associated with a greater likelihood of missed antenatal screening.[37,41] The delivery of a previous infant with GBS EOD is associated with increased risk in a subsequent delivery,[3] a factor that may be related to poor maternal antibody responses to colonizing strains or other immune- or strain-specific factors.[42] GBS bacteriuria is associated with a high level of maternal colonization and increased risk of neonatal colonization and disease.[41,47] Finally, obstetric practices that may promote ascending bacterial infection, such as the frequency of intrapartum vaginal examinations, invasive fetal monitoring, and membrane sweeping, have been associated with GBS EOD in some observational studies.[39,44] Such studies are difficult to interpret because of confounding; available data are not sufficient to determine if these procedures are associated with an increased risk for GBS EOD. Current ACOG guidance addresses the appropriate use of these procedures among GBS-colonized women.[7] Administration of IAP in women with GBS colonization minimizes the impact of intrapartum obstetric procedures on the risk of neonatal GBS EOD.

LOD

A positive GBS screen result in the mother at the time of birth and at the time of LOD diagnosis is significantly associated with LOD.[48,49] Maternal colonization is not universally present in LOD cases, however, suggesting that horizontal acquisition of group B streptococci from nonmaternal caregivers may also be part of the pathogenesis of GBS LOD. GBS LOD is strongly associated with preterm birth.[6,48–53] In studies from Washington in 1992 to 2011 and Houston in 1995 to 2000, it was found that the risk for LOD increased for each week of decreasing gestation and 40% to 50% of all LOD occurs among infants born <37 weeks' gestation.[48,50] Maternal age <20 years and African American race are variably associated with neonatal GBS LOD in United States studies.[10,48,50,51] Other clinical intrapartum factors predictive of GBS EOD (maternal intrapartum fever, duration of ROM) are not predictive of LOD. Authors of a population-based study in Italy found that group B streptococci could be cultured from a mother's milk in approximately 25% of cases that occurred in breastfed infants,[49] and authors of case reports associate colonized human milk with GBS LOD.[54] However, human milk–associated GBS antibody is protective against GBS LOD,[55] and it remains unclear whether human milk is simply a marker of heavy maternal and infant colonization or a source of infection.

GBS Virulence

Bacterial factors promote invasive GBS infection. Group B streptococci are characterized by immunologically distinct surface polysaccharide capsules that define 10 serotypes (types I, Ia, and II–IX). Worldwide, serotypes I–V account for 98% of carriage and 97% of infant invasive strains; serotype III accounts for approximately 25% of colonizing strains and approximately 62% of invasive infant strains, with regional variation.[24,56] Surveillance data in the United States for invasive strains from 2006 to 2015 revealed that 93.1% of GBS EOD cases were attributable to serotypes Ia (27.3%), III (27.3%), II (15.6%), V (14.2%), and Ib (8.8%); the proportion attributable to the emerging serotype IV ranged from 3.4% to 11.3% over the study period.[6] Serotype III accounted for approximately 56.2% of 1387 GBS LOD cases during 2006–2015, with serotypes Ia (20%), V (8.3%), IV (6.2%), and Ib (6.1%) making up most of the remaining serotypes. The capsular polysaccharide of all GBS serotypes resists complement deposition and inhibits opsonophagocytosis. Maternally derived, serotype-specific antibody to maternal colonizing GBS isolates is protective against newborn infection.[44,45] Group B streptococci express multiple additional virulence factors, including surface proteins such as the α and β C-proteins that promote adherence and immune evasion, pore-forming toxins such as β-hemolysin and CAMP factor, and secreted proteases such as the C5a peptidase that cleaves complement.[57] Strains vary in their expression of virulence factors, many of which are highly regulated by 2-component regulatory systems.[58–62] The hypervirulent serotype III multilocus sequence type 17 (ST17), for example, is commonly found in cases of GBS meningitis.[6,23]

IAP FOR THE PREVENTION OF EARLY-ONSET GBS INFECTION

Prevention of Perinatal GBS Infection

Multiple observational studies and 1 randomized controlled trial have revealed that the administration of intrapartum antibiotics before delivery interrupts vertical transmission of group B streptococci and decreases the incidence of invasive GBS EOD.[30–32,63] IAP is hypothesized to prevent neonatal GBS disease in 3 ways: (1) by temporarily decreasing maternal vaginal GBS colonization burden; (2) by preventing surface and mucus membrane colonization of the fetus or newborn; and (3) by reaching levels in newborn bloodstream above the minimum inhibitory concentration (MIC) of the antibiotic for killing group B streptococci.[30,31] Current clinical practices are focused on the identification of women at highest risk of GBS colonization and/or of transmission of group B streptococci to the newborn infant to facilitate targeted administration of IAP.

The ACOG currently recommends universal antenatal testing of pregnant women for GBS colonization by using vaginal-rectal cultures obtained at 36 0/7 to 37 6/7 weeks' gestation.[7] GBS testing is also recommended for pregnant women who present in preterm labor and/or with PROM before 37 0/7 weeks' gestation. If maternal GBS colonization is identified by antenatal urine culture, it does not need to be reconfirmed by vaginal-rectal culture. GBS vaginal-rectal culture is optimally performed by using a broth enrichment step, followed by GBS identification by using traditional microbiologic methods or by NAAT-based methods. At some centers, NAATs may be used to perform real-time, point-of-care screening of women who present in labor with unknown GBS status. Point-of care NAAT-based screening is not the primary recommended approach to determine maternal colonization status, both because of variable reported sensitivity of the point-of-care NAAT as compared to traditional culture and because most NAAT-based testing cannot be used to determine the antibiotic susceptibility of colonizing GBS isolates among women with a penicillin allergy.

Updated ACOG recommendations address the indications for IAP.[7] IAP at the time of presentation for delivery is indicated for all women with GBS colonization identified by antenatal vaginal-rectal culture, for women with GBS bacteriuria identified at any point during pregnancy, for women with a history of a previous infant with GBS disease, and for women who present in preterm labor and/or with PROM at <37 0/7 weeks' gestation. Women who present in labor at ≥37 0/7 weeks' gestation with unknown GBS status should receive IAP if risk factors develop during labor (maternal intrapartum temperature ≥100.4°F [38°C] or duration of ROM ≥18 hours) or if the result of an available point-of-care NAAT is positive for group B streptococci. If a woman with unknown status has a negative point-of-care NAAT test result but develops intrapartum risk factors, IAP should be administered because the sensitivity of the NAAT may be decreased without an enrichment incubation step. Women with GBS colonization in one pregnancy have an estimated 50% risk of colonization in a subsequent pregnancy.[64] Therefore, current ACOG recommendations state that if a woman with unknown GBS status presents in labor and is known to have had GBS colonization in a previous pregnancy, IAP may be considered.

Recommended Antibiotics for GBS IAP to Prevent Neonatal GBS EOD

Group B streptococci remain susceptible to β-lactam antibiotics, and penicillin G and ampicillin are the antibiotics best studied for prevention of neonatal infection.

Penicillin G administered to the mother readily crosses the placenta, reaching peak cord blood concentrations by 1 hour and rapidly declining by 4 hours, reflecting elimination of the antibiotic by the fetal kidney into amniotic fluid.[65] Ampicillin has been detected in cord blood within 30 minutes and in amniotic fluid within 45 minutes of administration to the mother.[30] Ampicillin concentrations measured in 115 newborn infants at 4 hours of age were found to be greater than the GBS MIC if maternal IAP dosing occurred at least 15 minutes before delivery.[66] Ampicillin IAP decreases maternal vaginal colonization and prevents neonatal surface colonization in 97% of cases if IAP is administered at least 2 hours before delivery.[30,32] Penicillin G has a narrower antimicrobial spectrum compared to ampicillin and therefore remains the preferred agent, but ampicillin is acceptable.

Alternative Antibiotics for GBS IAP

Cefazolin is recommended for GBS IAP for women with a penicillin allergy who are at low risk for anaphylaxis[7] and has similar pharmacokinetics and mechanisms of action as ampicillin. Cefazolin rapidly crosses the placenta and is detected in cord blood and amniotic fluid at levels above the GBS MIC within 20 minutes after maternal administration.[67–70]

Clindamycin is recommended for GBS IAP for women with a penicillin allergy who are at high risk for anaphylaxis and who are colonized with GBS known to be susceptible to clindamycin.[7] Group B streptococci are increasingly resistant to clindamycin as well as to macrolide antibiotics such as erythromycin. In reports from the ABCs from 2016, authors found that 42% of GBS isolates were resistant to clindamycin and 54% were resistant to erythromycin.[71] Because of both poor placental kinetics and high levels of resistance, erythromycin is no longer recommended for GBS IAP.[7] Antibiotic susceptibility data for the maternal colonizing GBS isolate should be available to support the use of clindamycin for IAP in women who report a penicillin allergy. Several studies inform the potential efficacy of clindamycin prophylaxis.[72–75] Authors of 1 study of 21 women colonized with clindamycin-susceptible GBS isolates found vaginal GBS colony counts declined with administration of clindamycin IAP.[72] Clindamycin administered intravenously to 23 women for high-risk penicillin allergy resulted in cord blood concentrations that were 37% to 160% of maternal concentrations and within therapeutic ranges in 22 of the 23.[75] However, clindamycin undergoes hepatic metabolism and is poorly excreted in fetal urine and, therefore, does not reach significant concentrations in amniotic fluid until multiple doses are administered.[73,74] The clinical effectiveness of clindamycin as IAP administered a median of 6 hours before delivery was only 22% compared to no IAP in an ABCs study that included women treated with clindamycin during the time periods of 1998–1999 and 2003–2004.[76]

Vancomycin is recommended for use as GBS IAP for women with a penicillin allergy who are at high risk for anaphylaxis if colonized with clindamycin-resistant GBS isolates. Although authors of older studies using ex vivo perfusion models with placental lobules suggested that vancomycin crosses the placental poorly, authors of a subsequent study of 13 women undergoing elective cesarean delivery found cord blood concentrations of vancomycin greater than the GBS MIC within 30 minutes of maternal drug administration.[77,78] Authors of recent studies compared cord blood vancomycin concentrations after vancomycin was administered to pregnant women using standard dosing and maternal weight-based dosing.[79,80] Therapeutic maternal and cord blood vancomycin concentrations were achieved in most cases with weight-based dosing. The ACOG currently recommends weight-based dosing for vancomycin when this agent is indicated for IAP.

Current data support the use of clindamycin and vancomycin as alternative medications for GBS IAP when maternal allergy precludes the use of β-lactam antibiotics. These medications are likely to provide some protection against GBS infection for both mother and newborn infant when antimicrobial susceptibility testing supports the use of these second-line agents. In addition, new ACOG recommendations encouraging the use of penicillin allergy testing in pregnant women with uncertain or undocumented histories of penicillin reactions are intended to increase the number of pregnant women who can safely receive β-lactam–based regimens for GBS IAP.[7]

IAP and GBS EOD

The pharmacokinetics and pharmacodynamics of ampicillin, penicillin, and cefazolin suggest that effective GBS EOD prophylaxis may be achieved within 2 to 4 hours of maternal administration. The clinical effectiveness of different durations of GBS IAP was evaluated by using a data set including 7691 births collected as part of the ABCs system from 2003 to 2004. In this study, the administration of different durations of penicillin or ampicillin (≥4; 2–<4; or <2 hours before delivery) were compared to no administration to evaluate the effectiveness of each in preventing GBS EOD. Although all regimens were effective compared to no IAP, administration of IAP at ≥4 hours before delivery was most effective in preventing GBS EOD.[76] This study was limited by the fact that 85% of the cases occurred among infants born to women who screened negative for GBS or whose GBS status was unknown, meaning that in most cases, GBS IAP was administered in response to risk factors and not as prophylaxis for known maternal GBS colonization. Despite this limitation, this study, combined with the time-dependent bactericidal mechanism of action of β-lactam antibiotics, supports the effectiveness of ampicillin and penicillin administered at least 4 hours before delivery. No data specifically inform the clinical effectiveness of cefazolin IAP, but the pharmacokinetics and mechanism of bacterial killing action for cefazolin are similar enough to those of penicillin and ampicillin that the administration of cefazolin can be considered to provide adequate prophylaxis against GBS EOD. Although data regarding the pharmacokinetics of clindamycin and vancomycin have been published, evidence regarding their clinical efficacy is more limited. Therefore, for the purpose of newborn GBS EOD risk assessment, when non–β-lactam antibiotics of any duration are administered for GBS IAP, such treatment should be considered as not fully adequate in neonatal risk calculation.

IAP and GBS LOD

There is no epidemiological evidence to suggest a protective effect of GBS IAP for the prevention of GBS LOD. This observation is likely attributable to the dynamic nature of GBS colonization. Early studies of IAP demonstrated initial maternal vaginal and/or rectal GBS clearance with IAP, followed by recolonization with group B streptococci within 24 to 48 hours after birth.[30] Authors of a study in Italy found that approximately 25% of infants born to mothers with GBS colonization who received GBS IAP were colonized by 1 month of age. Molecular analysis revealed the infant colonization was attributable to the same strain colonizing the mother antepartum.[81] Similarly, authors of a longitudinal cohort study conducted in Japan from 2014 to 2015 observed that among neonates born to mothers with GBS colonization who received IAP, approximately 20% were colonized with group B streptococci at 1 week and/or 1 month of age.[82] The authors also observed that 6.5% of infants born to mothers who screened negative for GBS were colonized at 1 week and/or 1 month of age, likely as a result of horizontal transmission from newly colonized mothers as well as from other contacts.

RISK ASSESSMENT FOR EARLY-ONSET GBS INFECTION

Because the pathogenesis of GBS EOD begins with vertical transmission of group B streptococci from mother to fetus and newborn infant, the strongest predictor of GBS EOD is maternal GBS colonization. Other factors that are important to the pathogenesis of GBS EOD, such as the virulence of the maternal colonizing isolate and the presence of maternal serotype-specific protective antibody, cannot be known to the physician at the time of neonatal risk assessment. The remaining clinical risk factors for GBS EOD are the same as those for EOS caused by other common bacterial causes of EOS, including gestational age at birth, intraamniotic infection, and duration of ROM. The administration of GBS IAP and the administration of intrapartum antibiotics in response to obstetric concern for intraamniotic infection both decrease this risk. The newborn infant's condition at birth and evolving condition over the first 12 to 24 hours after birth are strong predictors of early-onset infection attributable to any pathogen.[12,13]

Previous guidance on GBS EOD risk assessment presented challenges to physicians because of practical difficulties in establishing the obstetric diagnosis of maternal chorioamnionitis or intraamniotic infection, absence of guidance on what defines abnormal laboratory test results in the newborn infant, and a lack of clear definitions for newborn clinical illness. Each of these concerns are addressed in detail in the current AAP clinical reports on management of neonates with suspected or proven early-onset bacterial sepsis.[83,84] In summary, at this time, evidence supports the following:

- The ACOG provides guidance regarding intraamniotic infection[85]; neonatal risk assessment can be informed by this guidance. The definitive diagnosis of intraamniotic infection is that made by amniotic fluid Gram-stain and/or culture or by placental histopathologic testing. Such clear diagnostic information will rarely be available at the time of delivery for infants born at or near term. Suspected intraamniotic infection is defined as a single maternal intrapartum temperature ≥39.0°C or maternal temperature of 38.0°C to 38.9°C in combination with 1 or more of maternal leukocytosis, purulent cervical drainage, or fetal tachycardia. Recognizing the uncertainties surrounding the diagnosis of intraamniotic infection, the ACOG recommends that intrapartum antibiotic therapy be administered whenever intra-amniotic infection is diagnosed or suspected and should be considered when otherwise unexplained isolated maternal temperature 38.0°C to 38.9°C is present.[85]
- The routine measurement of complete blood cell counts or inflammatory markers such as C-reactive protein alone in newborn infants to determine risk of GBS EOD is not justified given the poor test performance of these in predicting what is currently a low-incidence disease.[86–89]
- Newborn clinical illness consisting of abnormal vital signs (eg, tachycardia, tachypnea, and/or temperature instability), supplemental oxygen requirement and/or need for continuous positive airway pressure, mechanical ventilation, or blood pressure support can be used to predict early-onset infection.[13] There is no evidence that hypoglycemia occurring in isolation

in otherwise well-appearing infants is a risk factor for GBS EOD or EOS. A newborn's clinical condition often evolves in the hours after birth, and physicians must exercise judgment to distinguish transitional instability from signs of clinical illness.

Clinicians should recognize that GBS EOD can occur among term infants born to mothers who have screened negative for GBS. Authors of 1 single-center study with policies mandating universal screening-based GBS IAP found that over an 8-year period, 17 GBS EOD cases occurred among term infants and 14 of 17 (82.4%) of the mothers had screened negative for GBS.[90] Multistate ABCs data in 2003–2004 identified 189 cases of GBS EOD among term infants and determined that 116 of 189 (61.4%) occurred among infants born to women who screened negative for GBS.[37] GBS EOD may occur in infants of mothers who screened negative for GBS because of changes in maternal colonization status during the interval from screening to presentation for delivery or because of an incorrect technique in obtaining vaginal and rectal screening cultures or in laboratory processing. Studies comparing antepartum culture to intrapartum culture or intrapartum molecular identification techniques reveal that approximately 7% to 8% of women who screen negative for GBS will be identified as positive for GBS at the time of delivery.[27,91] In some proportion of these cases, additional risk factors for EOS were present, but GBS EOD can develop in newborn infants without additional risk, and these will only be identified when they develop signs of illness.

Nonetheless, most infants who develop GBS EOD will do so in the setting of specific risk factors. In the current era of widespread use of GBS IAP, the clinical approach to risk of GBS EOD should be the same as that for all bacterial causes of early-onset infection. As addressed in the AAP clinical reports on management of neonates with suspected or proven early-onset bacterial sepsis,[83,84] risk of early-onset infection should be considered separately for infants born at or near term (≥35 weeks' gestation) and those preterm (≤34 6/7 weeks' gestation). A summary of the management strategies provided in the previous AAP reports are provided here.

There Are 3 Current Approaches to Risk Assessment Among Infants Born at ≥35 Weeks' Gestation

- Categorical risk assessment: Categorical risk factor assessment uses risk factor threshold values to identify infants at increased risk for

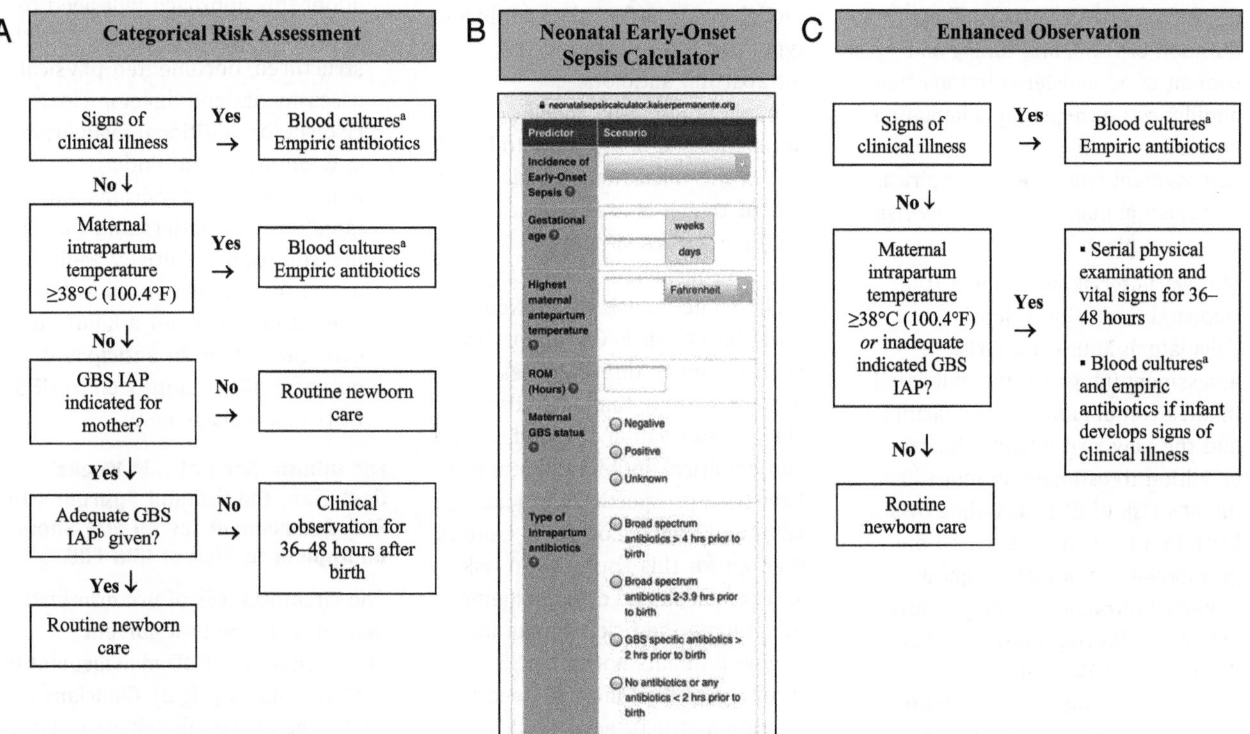

FIGURE 1

Options for EOS risk assessment among infants born ≥35 weeks' gestation. A, Categorical risk assessment. B, Neonatal Early-Onset Sepsis Calculator. The screenshot of the Neonatal Early-Onset Sepsis Calculator (https://neonatalsepsiscalculator.kaiserpermanente.org/) was used with permission from Kaiser-Permanente Division of Research. C, Enhanced observation. [a] Consider lumbar puncture and CSF culture before initiation of empiric antibiotics for infants who are at the highest risk of infection, especially those with critical illness. Lumbar puncture should not be performed if the infant's clinical condition would be compromised, and antibiotics should be administered promptly and not deferred because of procedure delays. [b] Adequate GBS IAP is defined as the administration of penicillin G, ampicillin, or cefazolin ≥4 hours before delivery.

GBS EOD (Fig 1A). Different versions of this approach have been published since 1996 and are based on infection epidemiology and expert opinion. For the purpose of categorical risk assessment, maternal intrapartum temperature ≥38.0°C is used as a surrogate for intraamniotic infection. The administration of penicillin G, ampicillin, or cefazolin ≥4 hours before delivery is considered adequate GBS IAP; other antibiotics or other durations of treatment <4 hours are considered inadequate when using this approach. Substantial data have been reported on the impact of using categorical risk factors to manage the risk of GBS EOD.[3,14,36,40] However, the risk is highly variable among the newborn infants recommended to receive empirical treatment in this approach, ranging from slightly lower than the baseline population risk to significantly higher, depending on the gestational age, duration of ROM, and timing and content of administered intrapartum antibiotics. Consequently, a limitation of this approach is that categorical management will result in empirical treatment of many relatively low-risk newborn infants.

- Multivariate risk assessment (the Neonatal Early-Onset Sepsis Calculator): Multivariate risk assessment integrates the individual infant's combination of risk factors and the newborn infant's clinical condition to estimate an individual infant's risk of EOS, including GBS EOD. Predictive models based on gestational age at birth, highest maternal intrapartum temperature, maternal GBS colonization status, duration of ROM, and type and duration of intrapartum antibiotic therapies have been developed and validated.[13,38] These models are available as a Web-based Neonatal Early-Onset Sepsis Calculator (Fig 1B) (https://neonatalsepsiscalculator.kaiserpermanente.org) that includes recommended clinical actions to be taken at specific levels of predicted risk. The models begin with the previous probability of infection, and because they predict all bacterial causes of EOS and not only GBS EOD, physicians in the United States should enter a previous probability of 0.5/1000, unless local incidence of EOS is known to differ from the national incidence of EOS among term infants. The models do account for the content and timing of GBS-specific IAP. When using these models, only penicillin, ampicillin, or cefazolin should be considered as "GBS-specific antibiotics." The administration of clindamycin or vancomycin alone for IAP for any duration is currently recommended to be entered as "no antibiotics." Because the models were developed to predict risk of all bacterial causes of EOS (and not just GBS EOD), and because these models account for other antibiotic types and indications for intrapartum antibiotic administration, "GBS specific antibiotics >2 hours prior to birth" is 1 of the calculator variables. The 2-hour timing is used because multiple factors in addition to GBS IAP are considered when using the multivariate models in the Neonatal Early-Onset Sepsis Calculator. Used in this manner, threshold risk estimates prompting enhanced clinical observation or blood culture and empirical antibiotic therapy have been prospectively validated in large newborn cohorts.[14,92] Centers that opt for this approach to risk assessment should develop methods to calculate the risk estimate for all newborn infants born at ≥35 weeks' gestation and will need to develop a structured approach to close clinical observation of infants at specific levels of estimated risk.
- Risk assessment based on newborn clinical condition: A final approach to GBS EOD risk assessment is to rely on clinical signs of illness to identify infants who may be at increased risk of infection. Among term infants, good clinical condition at birth is associated with an approximately 60% to 70% reduction in risk for early-onset infection.[13] Under this approach, infants who appear ill at birth and those who develop signs of illness over the first 48 hours after birth are treated empirically with antibiotics.[93–95] One center reported the use of clinical observation for initially well-appearing infants born at ≥34 to 35 weeks' gestation to mothers with the obstetric diagnosis of chorioamnionitis. Whether observed in a setting with continuous monitoring or with serial examinations during maternal-infant couplet care, this center ultimately administered empirical antibiotics to 5% to 12% of such infants.[94,95] Centers that adopt this approach will need to establish processes to ensure serial, structured, documented physical assessments and develop clear criteria for additional evaluation and empirical antibiotic administration. Physicians and families must understand that the identification of initially well-appearing infants who develop clinical illness is not a failure of care, but rather an anticipated outcome of this approach to GBS EOD risk management.

For Infants Born at ≤34 Weeks' Gestation, the Optimal Approach to Risk Assessment for All EOS Should Be Applied to Risk of GBS EOD

The circumstances of preterm birth may provide the best current approach to GBS EOD management for preterm infants (Fig 2). Clinicians may adopt one of the following strategies to develop institutional approaches best suited to their local resources and structure of care (Fig 1).

- Preterm infants at highest risk for EOS: Infants born preterm because of cervical insufficiency, preterm labor, PROM, intraamniotic infection, and/or acute and otherwise unexplained onset of nonreassuring fetal status are at the highest risk of EOS and GBS EOD. The administration of GBS IAP may decrease the risk of infection among these infants, but the most reasonable approach to these infants is to obtain a blood culture and start empirical antibiotic treatment. A lumbar puncture for culture and analysis of CSF should be considered in clinically ill infants when there is a high suspicion for GBS EOD, unless the procedure will compromise the neonate's clinical condition.

- Preterm infants at lower risk for EOS: Preterm infants at lowest risk for all EOS and for GBS EOD are those born under circumstances that include all of these criteria[96,97]: (1) maternal and/or fetal indications for preterm birth (such as maternal preeclampsia or other noninfectious medical illness, placental insufficiency, or fetal growth restriction), (2) birth by cesarean delivery, and (3) absence of labor, attempts to induce labor, or any ROM before delivery. Acceptable initial approaches to these infants include (1) no laboratory evaluation and no empirical antibiotic therapy or (2) blood culture and clinical monitoring. For infants who do not improve after initial stabilization and/or those who have severe systemic instability, the administration of empirical antibiotics may be reasonable but is not mandatory.
- Infants delivered for maternal and/or fetal indications but who are ultimately born by vaginal or cesarean delivery after efforts to induce labor and/or with ROM before delivery are subject to factors associated with the pathogenesis of GBS EOD. If the mother has an indication for GBS IAP and adequate IAP (penicillin, ampicillin, or cefazolin ≥4 hours before delivery) is not given or if any other concern for infection arises during the process of delivery, the infant should be managed as recommended above for preterm infants at higher risk for GBS EOD. Otherwise, an acceptable approach to these infants is close observation for those infants who are well appearing at birth and to obtain a blood culture and to initiate antibiotic therapy for infants with respiratory and/or cardiovascular instability after birth.

CLINICAL PRESENTATION AND TREATMENT OF GBS INFECTION

Newborn infants with GBS EOD may present with signs of illness ranging from tachycardia, tachypnea, or lethargy to severe cardiorespiratory failure, persistent pulmonary hypertension of the newborn, and perinatal encephalopathy. GBS LOD most commonly occurs as bacteremia without a focus and is often characterized by fever (≥38°C) as well as lethargy, poor feeding,

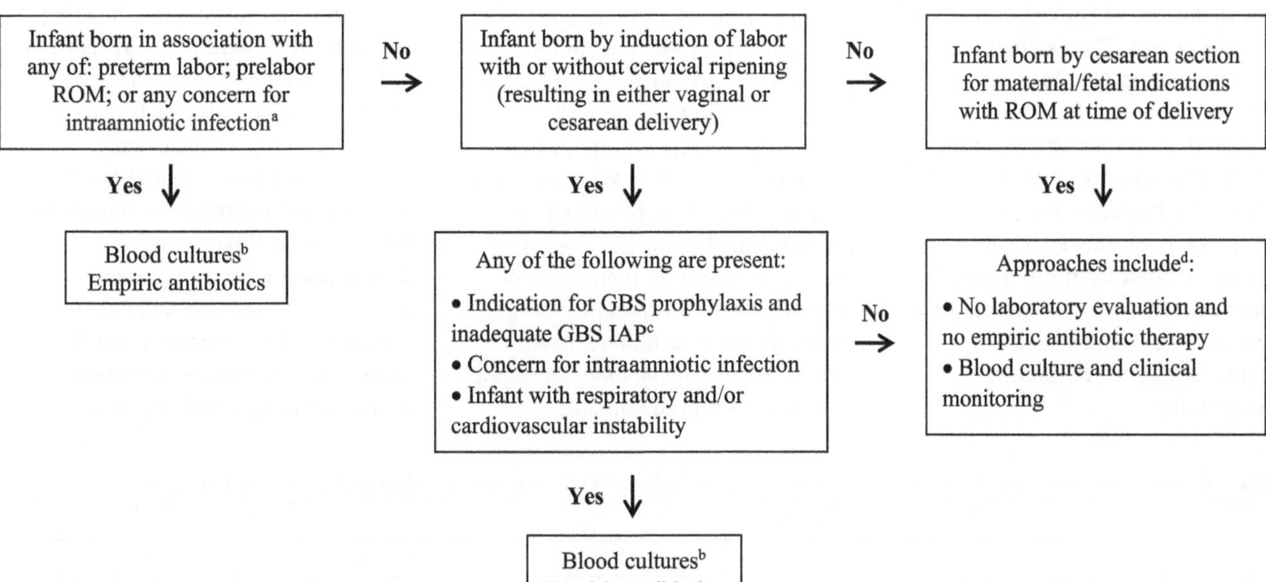

FIGURE 2

EOS risk assessment among infants born ≤34 weeks' gestation. [a] Intraamniotic infection should be considered when a pregnant woman presents with unexplained decreased fetal movement and/or there is sudden and unexplained poor fetal testing. [b] Lumbar puncture and CSF culture should be performed before initiation of empiric antibiotics for infants who are at the highest risk of infection unless the procedure would compromise the infant's clinical condition. Antibiotics should be administered promptly and not deferred because of procedural delays. [c] Adequate GBS IAP is defined as the administration of penicillin G, ampicillin, or cefazolin ≥4 hours before delivery. [d] For infants who do not improve after initial stabilization and/or those who have severe systemic instability, the administration of empiric antibiotics may be reasonable but is not mandatory.

irritability, tachypnea, grunting, or apnea. Infants with LOD meningitis can also have nonspecific signs such as irritability, poor feeding, vomiting, and temperature instability as well as signs suggestive of central nervous systems involvement such as bulging fontanelle or seizures. Focal syndromes such as pneumonia, bone or joint infection, cellulitis, or adenitis often have findings that point to the site of infection. Osteomyelitis frequently is insidious and may not be associated with fever. Complications are common for meningitis and can include neurodevelopment impairment, hearing loss, persistent seizure disorders, or cerebrovascular disease.[98]

Evaluation for GBS disease is the same as that for all forms of sepsis in the newborn and young infant.[83,84] Blood culture, lumbar puncture for culture and analysis of CSF, and markers of inflammation are discussed in detail in the AAP clinical reports on management of neonates with suspected or proven early-onset bacterial sepsis. The evaluation for GBS LOD should also include urine culture. If bone or joint infection is suspected, additional studies can include radiographs, MRI, and bone or joint fluid culture. When meningitis is diagnosed, cranial imaging is often useful to assess for complications such as ventriculitis or brain abscess. Cultures should include testing for antibiotic susceptibility.

Empirical and Definitive Treatment

Antibiotics initiated because of concern for GBS EOD are the same as those for all bacterial causes of EOS until the results of cultures are available. GBS neonatal disease isolates remain susceptible to β-lactam antibiotics, although ABCs has identified rare isolates of group B streptococci with mutations in penicillin-binding proteins leading to elevated MICs (nonsusceptibility) to β-lactam antibiotics.[99] Ampicillin, together with an aminoglycoside, is the primary recommended therapy for infants up to 7 days of age. The empirical addition of broader-spectrum therapy should be considered if there is strong clinical concern for ampicillin-resistant infection in a critically ill newborn, particularly among neonates with very low birth weight.[100–102] Among previously healthy infants in the community, if the infant is not critically ill and there is no evidence of meningitis, ampicillin and ceftazidime together are recommended as empirical therapy for those 8 to 28 days of age; ceftriaxone therapy is recommended under these circumstances for infants 29 to 90 days of age. For all previously healthy infants in the community from 8 to 90 days of age, vancomycin should be added to recommended empirical therapy if there is evidence of meningitis or critical illness to expand coverage, including for β-lactam–resistant *Streptococcus pneumoniae*. The choice of empirical therapy among continuously hospitalized preterm infants beyond 72 hours of age is guided by multiple factors, including the presence of central venous catheters and local hospital microbiology. The empirical choice for such infants should include an antibiotic to which group B streptococci are susceptible, such as a β-lactam, cephalosporin, or vancomycin. When group B streptococci are identified in culture, penicillin G is the drug of choice, with ampicillin as an acceptable alternative therapy.

See Table 1 for dose and interval guidance. The length of antibiotic treatment is generally 10 days for bacteremia without focus and 14 days for uncomplicated meningitis; antibiotics should be given intravenously for the entire course. Longer therapy is used when there is a prolonged or complicated course. Some experts recommend a second lumbar puncture for CSF culture 24 to 48 hours after the start of antibiotics. Additional lumbar punctures and intracranial imaging are advised if there is not resolution of CSF infection, if neurologic abnormalities persist, or if focal deficits develop. Osteoarticular infection should be treated for 3 to 4 weeks and ventriculitis should be treated for at least 4 weeks. Consultation with a pediatric infectious disease specialist should be considered for meningitis and for cases with site-specific infection. Audiology testing and ongoing

TABLE 1 Recommended Intravenous Antibiotic Treatment Regimens for Confirmed Early- and Late-Onset GBS Bacteremia and Meningitis

	GA ≤34 wk		GA >34 wk	
	PNA ≤7 d	PNA >7 d	PNA ≤7 d	PNA >7 d
Bacteremia				
Ampicillin	50 mg/kg every 12 h	75 mg/kg every 12 h	50 mg/kg every 8 h	50 mg/kg every 8 h
Penicillin G	50 000 U/kg every 12 h	50 000 U/kg every 8 h	50 000 U/kg every 12 h	50 000 U/kg every 8 h
Meningitis				
Ampicillin	100 mg/kg every 8 h	75 mg/kg every 6 h	100 mg/kg every 8 h	75 mg/kg q 6 h
Penicillin G	150 000 U/kg every 8 h	125 000 U/kg every 6 h	150 000 U/kg every 8 h	125 000 U/kg every 6 h

Adapted from Table 4.2. Antibacterial Drugs for Neonates (<28 Postnatal Days of Age). In: Kimberlin DW, Brady MT, Jackson MA, Long SS, eds. *Red Book: 2018 Report of the Committee on Infectious Diseases*. 31st ed. Itasca, IL: American Academy of Pediatrics; 2018:915-919. GA, gestational age; PNA, postnatal age.

audiologic monitoring, if indicated, should be arranged before discharge.

Multiple Births

When invasive GBS infection occurs in an infant who is 1 of multiple births, the birth siblings should be observed carefully for signs of infection and treated empirically if signs of illness occur. There is no evidence to support full antibiotic treatment courses in the absence of confirmed GBS disease.

Recurrent GBS Disease

Recurrent neonatal and young infant GBS disease can occur after completed appropriate treatment of the primary infection.[103,104] Authors of a population-based study conducted in Japan[53] during 2011 to 2015 found that recurrence occurred in 2.8% of cases of neonatal GBS infection. Recurrent cases were identified 3 to 54 days after completion of the therapy for the first occurrence. Recurrent cases are generally caused by the same GBS serotype that caused the primary infection, and persistent mucosal colonization and poor neonatal antibody responses to the first infection likely contribute to the pathogenesis of recurrent infection. Recurrent disease is not preventable by extension of recommended antibiotic courses nor by the addition of rifampin to eradicate mucosal colonization.[105] Parents should be counseled about the possibility of recurrent GBS disease after treatment of both GBS EOD and LOD.

FUTURE DIRECTIONS

Intrapartum Antibiotics, the Microbiome, and Childhood Health

GBS IAP and the administration of intrapartum antibiotics because of concern for maternal intraamniotic infection combined result in approximately 30% of pregnant women receiving antibiotics around the time of delivery. The composition of the gut microbiota develops and diversifies from birth through early childhood, and disruption of the microbiota during this critical period may have enduring health consequences. Perinatal antibiotic administration is associated with abnormal host development in animal models.[106–108] Human epidemiological studies have associated early infant antibiotic exposures with increased risks of atopic and allergic disorders as well as increases in early childhood weight gain.[109–112] Several human studies report differences in the composition of the maternal vaginal[113] and infant gut microbiome associated with the use of IAP, with effects on both the diversity and richness of identified species.[114–119] The differences observed vary with the mode of delivery and duration of breastfeeding; differences were detected as long as 12 months after birth in 1 study.[115] Changes in the initial constitution of neonatal gut microbiota in response to IAP are not unexpected; GBS IAP is administered with the intent of altering the content of the newborn infant's initial microflora exposure at delivery to decrease colonization with a significant neonatal pathogen. Whether the secondary effects of IAP on the microbiome influence short- and long-term childhood health outcomes is unknown and an area of active investigation.

GBS Vaccine Development

Multiple gaps remain in GBS disease prevention. Neonatal EOD continues to occur in the United States, primarily among preterm infants, term infants born to women with cultures negative for antenatal GBS, and infants born to mothers with reported β-lactam allergy that precludes maximally effective IAP. The incidence of GBS LOD has not been affected by IAP. In addition, group B *Streptococcus* is a cause of stillbirth and of invasive infection among pregnant and postpartum women as well as among the elderly and those whose health is compromised by diabetes or malignancy.[15,120] Furthermore, GBS disease is a worldwide problem, particularly among resource-limited countries where IAP is not a readily available preventive strategy. Effective, multivalent vaccines administered to pregnant women and at-risk nonpregnant adults could potentially prevent many of these issues. Preclinical and human phase I and II studies have been completed revealing the safety and immunogenicity of glycoconjugate GBS vaccines.[121–123] Current ABCs reveals that 99% of infections are caused by 6 GBS serotypes, suggesting that a hexavalent vaccine could be widely effective.[6]

SUMMARY OF RECOMMENDATIONS

1. The AAP supports the maternal policies and procedures for the prevention of perinatal GBS disease as recommended by the ACOG.
2. For the purpose of neonatal management, the administration of intrapartum penicillin G, ampicillin, or cefazolin can provide adequate IAP against neonatal early-onset GBS disease. For women at high risk of anaphylaxis to β-lactam antibiotics, clindamycin and vancomycin should be administered as recommended by the ACOG and will likely provide some protection against GBS EOD in exposed newborn infants. However, there is currently insufficient clinical efficacy evidence to consider the administration of these antibiotics equivalent to β-lactam antibiotics for the purpose of neonatal risk assessment.
3. Risk assessment for early-onset GBS disease should follow the general principles established in the AAP clinical reports on management of neonates with suspected or proven early-onset bacterial sepsis.[83,84] These principles include the following:
   - separate consideration of infants born at ≥35 0/7 weeks'

gestation and those born at ≤34 6/7 weeks' gestation;
  - infants born at ≥35 0/7 weeks' gestation may be assessed for risk of early-onset GBS infection with a categorical algorithm by using multivariate models such as the Neonatal Early-Onset Sepsis Calculator or with enhanced clinical observation; and
  - infants born at ≤34 6/7 weeks' gestation are at highest risk for early-onset infection from all causes, including group B streptococci, and may be best approached by using the circumstances of preterm birth to determine management.
4. Early-onset GBS infection is diagnosed by blood or CSF culture. Common laboratory tests such as the complete blood cell count and C-reactive protein do not perform well in predicting early-onset infection, particularly among well-appearing infants at lowest baseline risk of infection.
5. Evaluation for late-onset GBS disease should be based on clinical signs of illness in the infant. Diagnosis is based on the isolation of group B streptococci from blood, CSF, or other normally sterile sites. Late-onset GBS disease occurs among infants born to mothers who had positive GBS screen results as well as those who had negative screen results during pregnancy. Adequate IAP does not protect infants from late-onset GBS disease.
6. Empirical antibiotic therapy for early-onset and late-onset GBS disease differs by postnatal age at the time of evaluation. Penicillin G is the preferred antibiotic for definitive treatment of GBS disease in infants; ampicillin is an acceptable alternative.

COMMITTEE ON FETUS AND NEWBORN, 2018–2019

James Cummings, MD, MS, FAAP, Chairperson
Ivan Hand, MD, FAAP
Ira Adams-Chapman, MD, FAAP
Brenda Poindexter, MD, FAAP
Dan L. Stewart, MD, FAAP
Susan W. Aucott, MD, FAAP
Karen M. Puopolo, MD, PhD, FAAP
Jay P. Goldsmith, MD, FAAP
Meredith Mowitz, MD, FAAP
Kristi Watterberg, MD, FAAP, Immediate Past Chairperson

LIAISONS

Timothy Jancelewicz, MD – *American Academy of Pediatrics Section on Surgery*
Michael Narvey, MD – *Canadian Pediatric Society*
Russell Miller, MD – *American College of Obstetricians and Gynecologists*
RADM Wanda Barfield, MD, MPH – *Centers for Disease Control and Prevention*
Erin Keels, DNP, APRN, NNP-BC – *National Association of Neonatal Nurses*

STAFF

Jim Couto, MA

COMMITTEE ON INFECTIOUS DISEASES, 2018–2019

Yvonne A. Maldonado, MD, FAAP, Chairperson
Theoklis E. Zaoutis, MD, MSCE, FAAP, Vice Chairperson
Ritu Banerjee, MD, PhD, FAAP
Elizabeth D. Barnett MD, FAAP
James D. Campbell, MD, MS, FAAP
Jeffrey S. Gerber, MD, PhD, FAAP
Athena P. Kourtis, MD, PhD, MPH, FAAP
Ruth Lynfield, MD, FAAP
Flor M. Munoz, MD, MSc, FAAP
Dawn Nolt, MD, MPH, FAAP
Ann-Christine Nyquist, MD, MSPH, FAAP
Sean T. O'Leary, MD, MPH, FAAP
Mark H. Sawyer, MD, FAAP
William J. Steinbach, MD, FAAP
Ken Zangwill, MD, FAAP

EX OFFICIO

David W. Kimberlin, MD, FAAP – *Red Book Editor*
Henry H. Bernstein, DO, MHCM, FAAP – *Red Book Online Associate Editor*
H. Cody Meissner, MD, FAAP – *Visual Red Book Associate Editor*

LIAISONS

Amanda C. Cohn, MD, FAAP – *Centers for Disease Control and Prevention*
Jamie Deseda-Tous, MD – *Sociedad Latinoamericana de Infectología Pediátrica*
Karen M. Farizo, MD – *US Food and Drug Administration*
Marc Fischer, MD, FAAP – *Centers for Disease Control and Prevention*
Natasha B. Halasa, MD, MPH, FAAP – *Pediatric Infectious Diseases Society*
Nicole Le Saux, MD, FRCP(C) – *Canadian Paediatric Society*
Scot B. Moore, MD, FAAP – *Committee on Practice Ambulatory Medicine*
Neil S. Silverman, MD – *American College of Obstetricians and Gynecologists*
Jeffrey R. Starke, MD – FAAP, *American Thoracic Society*
James J. Stevermer, MD, MSPH, FAAFP – *American Academy of Family Physicians*
Kay M. Tomashek, MD, MPH, DTM – *National Institutes of Health*

STAFF

Jennifer M. Frantz, MPH

ACKNOWLEDGMENTS

The American Academy of Pediatrics thanks Stephanie Schrag, DPhil, Epidemiology Team Lead, Respiratory Diseases Branch, Centers for Disease Control and Prevention, and Carol Baker, MD, McGovern Medical School, University of Texas-Houston, for their partnership and contributions to the development of this clinical report.

ABBREVIATIONS

AAP: American Academy of Pediatrics
ABCs: Active Bacterial Core surveillance
ACOG: American College of Obstetricians and Gynecologists
CDC: Centers for Disease Control and Prevention
CSF: cerebrospinal fluid
EOD: early-onset disease
EOS: early-onset sepsis
GBS: group B streptococcal
IAP: intrapartum antibiotic prophylaxis
LOD: late-onset disease
MIC: minimum inhibitory concentration
NAAT: nucleic acid amplification test
PROM: prelabor rupture of membranes
ROM: rupture of membranes

FINANCIAL DISCLOSURE: The authors have indicated they have no financial relationships relevant to this article to disclose.

FUNDING: No external funding.

POTENTIAL CONFLICT OF INTEREST: The authors have indicated they have no potential conflicts of interest to disclose.

REFERENCES

1. Centers for Disease Control and Prevention. Prevention of perinatal group B streptococcal disease: a public health perspective [published correction appears in *MMWR Morb Mortal Wkly Rep.* 1996;45(31):679]. *MMWR Recomm Rep.* 1996;45(RR-7): 1–24
2. Schrag S, Gorwitz R, Fultz-Butts K, Schuchat A. Prevention of perinatal group B streptococcal disease. Revised guidelines from CDC. *MMWR Recomm Rep.* 2002;51(RR-11):1–22
3. Schrag SJ, Zell ER, Lynfield R, et al; Active Bacterial Core Surveillance Team. A population-based comparison of strategies to prevent early-onset group B streptococcal disease in neonates. *N Engl J Med.* 2002;347(4): 233–239
4. Verani JR, McGee L, Schrag SJ; Division of Bacterial Diseases, National Center for Immunization and Respiratory Diseases, Centers for Disease Control and Prevention (CDC). Prevention of perinatal group B streptococcal disease--revised guidelines from CDC, 2010. *MMWR Recomm Rep.* 2010;59(RR-10):1–36
5. Mukhopadhyay S, Taylor JA, Von Kohorn I, et al. Variation in sepsis evaluation across a national network of nurseries. *Pediatrics.* 2017;139(3): e0162845
6. Nanduri SA, Petit S, Smelser C, et al. Epidemiology of invasive early-onset and late-onset group B streptococcal disease in the United States, 2006 to 2015: multistate laboratory and population-based surveillance. *JAMA Pediatr.* 2019;173(3):224–233
7. American College of Obstetricians and Gynecologists. Prevention of group B streptococcal early-onset disease in newborns: ACOG Committee Opinion, Number 782. *Obstet Gynecol.* 2019; 134(1):e19–e40
8. American Academy of Pediatrics. Group B streptococcal infections. In: Kimberlin DW, Brady MT, Jackson MA, Long SS, eds. *Red Book: 2018 Report of the Committee on Infectious Diseases.* 31st ed. Itasca, IL: American Academy of Pediatrics; 2018:762–768
9. Schrag SJ, Farley MM, Petit S, et al. Epidemiology of invasive early-onset neonatal sepsis, 2005 to 2014. *Pediatrics.* 2016;138(6):e20162013
10. Weston EJ, Pondo T, Lewis MM, et al. The burden of invasive early-onset neonatal sepsis in the United States, 2005-2008. *Pediatr Infect Dis J.* 2011;30(11): 937–941
11. Baker CJ. Early onset group B streptococcal disease. *J Pediatr.* 1978; 93(1):124–125
12. Escobar GJ, Li DK, Armstrong MA, et al. Neonatal sepsis workups in infants >/=2000 grams at birth: a population-based study. *Pediatrics.* 2000;106(2 pt 1):256–263
13. Escobar GJ, Puopolo KM, Wi S, et al. Stratification of risk of early-onset sepsis in newborns ≥ 34 weeks' gestation. *Pediatrics.* 2014;133(1):30–36
14. Kuzniewicz MW, Puopolo KM, Fischer A, et al. A quantitative, risk-based approach to the management of neonatal early-onset sepsis. *JAMA Pediatr.* 2017;171(4):365–371
15. Seale AC, Bianchi-Jassir F, Russell NJ, et al. Estimates of the burden of group B streptococcal disease worldwide for pregnant women, stillbirths, and children. *Clin Infect Dis.* 2017;65(suppl_2):S200–S219
16. Hussain SM, Luedtke GS, Baker CJ, Schlievert PM, Leggiadro RJ. Invasive group B streptococcal disease in children beyond early infancy. *Pediatr Infect Dis J.* 1995;14(4):278–281
17. Guilbert J, Levy C, Cohen R, Delacourt C, Renolleau S, Flamant C; Bacterial meningitis group. Late and ultra late onset *Streptococcus* B meningitis: clinical and bacteriological data over 6 years in France. *Acta Paediatr.* 2010; 99(1):47–51
18. Boyer KM, Gadzala CA, Burd LI, Fisher DE, Paton JB, Gotoff SP. Selective intrapartum chemoprophylaxis of neonatal group B streptococcal early-onset disease. I. Epidemiologic rationale. *J Infect Dis.* 1983;148(5): 795–801
19. Baker CJ, Barrett FF. Transmission of group B streptococci among parturient women and their neonates. *J Pediatr.* 1973;83(6):919–925
20. Benitz WE, Gould JB, Druzin ML. Risk factors for early-onset group B streptococcal sepsis: estimation of odds ratios by critical literature review. *Pediatrics.* 1999;103(6). Available at: www.pediatrics.org/cgi/content/full/103/6/e77
21. Goldenberg RL, Hauth JC, Andrews WW. Intrauterine infection and preterm delivery. *N Engl J Med.* 2000;342(20): 1500–1507
22. Gibbs RS, Roberts DJ. Case records of the Massachusetts General Hospital. Case 27-2007. A 30-year-old pregnant woman with intrauterine fetal death. *N Engl J Med.* 2007;357(9): 918–925
23. Nan C, Dangor Z, Cutland CL, Edwards MS, Madhi SA, Cunnington MC. Maternal group B *Streptococcus*-related stillbirth: a systematic review. *BJOG.* 2015;122(11):1437–1445
24. Russell NJ, Seale AC, O'Driscoll M, et al; GBS Maternal Colonization Investigator Group. Maternal colonization with group B *Streptococcus* and serotype distribution worldwide: systematic review and meta-analyses. *Clin Infect Dis.* 2017;65(suppl_2):S100–S111
25. Campbell JR, Hillier SL, Krohn MA, Ferrieri P, Zaleznik DF, Baker CJ. Group B streptococcal colonization and serotype-specific immunity in pregnant women at delivery. *Obstet Gynecol.* 2000;96(4):498–503

26. Buchan BW, Faron ML, Fuller D, Davis TE, Mayne D, Ledeboer NA. Multicenter clinical evaluation of the Xpert GBS LB assay for detection of group B *Streptococcus* in prenatal screening specimens. *J Clin Microbiol.* 2015;53(2): 443–448

27. Young BC, Dodge LE, Gupta M, Rhee JS, Hacker MR. Evaluation of a rapid, real-time intrapartum group B streptococcus assay. *Am J Obstet Gynecol.* 2011;205(4):372.e1–372.e6

28. Hansen SM, Uldbjerg N, Kilian M, Sørensen UB. Dynamics of *Streptococcus agalactiae* colonization in women during and after pregnancy and in their infants. *J Clin Microbiol.* 2004;42(1):83–89

29. Meyn LA, Moore DM, Hillier SL, Krohn MA. Association of sexual activity with colonization and vaginal acquisition of group B *Streptococcus* in nonpregnant women. *Am J Epidemiol.* 2002;155(10): 949–957

30. Yow MD, Mason EO, Leeds LJ, Thompson PK, Clark DJ, Gardner SE. Ampicillin prevents intrapartum transmission of group B streptococcus. *JAMA.* 1979; 241(12):1245–1247

31. Boyer KM, Gadzala CA, Kelly PD, Gotoff SP. Selective intrapartum chemoprophylaxis of neonatal group B streptococcal early-onset disease. III. Interruption of mother-to-infant transmission. *J Infect Dis.* 1983;148(5):810–816

32. de Cueto M, Sanchez MJ, Sampedro A, Miranda JA, Herruzo AJ, Rosa-Fraile M. Timing of intrapartum ampicillin and prevention of vertical transmission of group B streptococcus. *Obstet Gynecol.* 1998;91(1):112–114

33. Russell NJ, Seale AC, O'Sullivan C, et al. Risk of early-onset neonatal group B streptococcal disease with maternal colonization worldwide: systematic review and meta-analyses. *Clin Infect Dis.* 2017;65(suppl_2):S152–S159

34. Schuchat A, Oxtoby M, Cochi S, et al. Population-based risk factors for neonatal group B streptococcal disease: results of a cohort study in metropolitan Atlanta. *J Infect Dis.* 1990; 162(3):672–677

35. Schuchat A, Deaver-Robinson K, Plikaytis BD, Zangwill KM, Mohle-Boetani J, Wenger JD; The Active Surveillance Study Group. Multistate case-control study of maternal risk factors for neonatal group B streptococcal disease. *Pediatr Infect Dis J.* 1994;13(7): 623–629

36. Schuchat A, Zywicki SS, Dinsmoor MJ, et al. Risk factors and opportunities for prevention of early-onset neonatal sepsis: a multicenter case-control study. *Pediatrics.* 2000;105(1 pt 1):21–26

37. Van Dyke MK, Phares CR, Lynfield R, et al. Evaluation of universal antenatal screening for group B streptococcus. *N Engl J Med.* 2009;360(25):2626–2636

38. Puopolo KM, Draper D, Wi S, et al. Estimating the probability of neonatal early-onset infection on the basis of maternal risk factors. *Pediatrics.* 2011; 128(5). Available at: www.pediatrics.org/cgi/content/full/128/5/e1155

39. Zaleznik DF, Rench MA, Hillier S, et al. Invasive disease due to group B Streptococcus in pregnant women and neonates from diverse population groups. *Clin Infect Dis.* 2000;30(2): 276–281

40. Mukhopadhyay S, Dukhovny D, Mao W, Eichenwald EC, Puopolo KM. 2010 perinatal GBS prevention guideline and resource utilization. *Pediatrics.* 2014; 133(2):196–203

41. Heath PT, Balfour GF, Tighe H, Verlander NQ, Lamagni TL, Efstratiou A; HPA GBS Working Group. Group B streptococcal disease in infants: a case control study. *Arch Dis Child.* 2009;94(9):674–680

42. Carstensen H, Christensen KK, Grennert L, Persson K, Polberger S. Early-onset neonatal group B streptococcal septicaemia in siblings. *J Infect.* 1988; 17(3):201–204

43. Persson K, Bjerre B, Elfström L, Polberger S, Forsgren A. Group B streptococci at delivery: high count in urine increases risk for neonatal colonization. *Scand J Infect Dis.* 1986; 18(6):525–531

44. Baker CJ, Kasper DL. Correlation of maternal antibody deficiency with susceptibility to neonatal group B streptococcal infection. *N Engl J Med.* 1976;294(14):753–756

45. Baker CJ, Carey VJ, Rench MA, et al. Maternal antibody at delivery protects neonates from early onset group B streptococcal disease. *J Infect Dis.* 2014;209(5):781–788

46. Collins A, Weitkamp JH, Wynn JL. Why are preterm newborns at increased risk of infection? *Arch Dis Child Fetal Neonatal Ed.* 2018;103(4):F391–F394

47. Adair CE, Kowalsky L, Quon H, et al. Risk factors for early-onset group B streptococcal disease in neonates: a population-based case-control study. *CMAJ.* 2003;169(3):198–203

48. Pintye J, Saltzman B, Wolf E, Crowell CS. Risk factors for late-onset group B streptococcal disease before and after implementation of universal screening and intrapartum antibiotic prophylaxis. *J Pediatric Infect Dis Soc.* 2016;5(4): 431–438

49. Berardi A, Rossi C, Lugli L, et al; GBS Prevention Working Group, Emilia-Romagna. Group B streptococcus late-onset disease: 2003-2010. *Pediatrics.* 2013;131(2). Available at: www.pediatrics.org/cgi/content/full/131/2/e361

50. Lin FY, Weisman LE, Troendle J, Adams K. Prematurity is the major risk factor for late-onset group B streptococcus disease. *J Infect Dis.* 2003;188(2): 267–271

51. Jordan HT, Farley MM, Craig A, et al; Active Bacterial Core Surveillance (ABCs)/Emerging Infections Program Network, CDC. Revisiting the need for vaccine prevention of late-onset neonatal group B streptococcal disease: a multistate, population-based analysis. *Pediatr Infect Dis J.* 2008; 27(12):1057–1064

52. Bartlett AW, Smith B, George CR, et al. Epidemiology of late and very late onset group B streptococcal disease: fifteen-year experience from two Australian tertiary pediatric facilities. *Pediatr Infect Dis J.* 2017;36(1):20–24

53. Matsubara K, Hoshina K, Kondo M, et al. Group B streptococcal disease in infants in the first year of life: a nationwide surveillance study in Japan, 2011-2015. *Infection.* 2017;45(4): 449–458

54. Zimmermann P, Gwee A, Curtis N. The controversial role of breast milk in GBS late-onset disease. *J Infect.* 2017; 74(suppl 1):S34–S40

55. Le Doare K, Kampmann B. Breast milk and Group B streptococcal infection: vector of transmission or vehicle for protection? *Vaccine*. 2014;32(26): 3128–3132

56. Madrid L, Seale AC, Kohli-Lynch M, et al; Infant GBS Disease Investigator Group. Infant group B streptococcal disease incidence and serotypes worldwide: systematic review and meta-analyses. *Clin Infect Dis*. 2017;65(suppl_2): S160–S172

57. Patras KA, Nizet V. Group B streptococcal maternal colonization and neonatal disease: molecular mechanisms and preventative approaches. *Front Pediatr*. 2018;6:27

58. Jiang SM, Cieslewicz MJ, Kasper DL, Wessels MR. Regulation of virulence by a two-component system in group B streptococcus. *J Bacteriol*. 2005;187(3): 1105–1113

59. Tazi A, Bellais S, Tardieux I, Dramsi S, Trieu-Cuot P, Poyart C. Group B Streptococcus surface proteins as major determinants for meningeal tropism. *Curr Opin Microbiol*. 2012; 15(1):44–49

60. Klinzing DC, Ishmael N, Dunning Hotopp JC, et al. The two-component response regulator LiaR regulates cell wall stress responses, pili expression and virulence in group B *Streptococcus*. *Microbiology*. 2013;159(pt 7):1521–1534

61. Mu R, Cutting AS, Del Rosario Y, et al. Identification of CiaR regulated genes that promote group B streptococcal virulence and interaction with brain endothelial cells. *PLoS One*. 2016;11(4): e0153891

62. Périchon B, Szili N, du Merle L, et al. Regulation of PI-2b pilus expression in hypervirulent *Streptococcus agalactiae* ST-17 BM110. *PLoS One*. 2017;12(1): e0169840

63. Boyer KM, Gotoff SP. Prevention of early-onset neonatal group B streptococcal disease with selective intrapartum chemoprophylaxis. *N Engl J Med*. 1986; 314(26):1665–1669

64. Turrentine MA, Colicchia LC, Hirsch E, et al. Efficiency of screening for the recurrence of antenatal group B *Streptococcus* colonization in a subsequent pregnancy: a systematic review and meta-analysis with independent patient data. *Am J Perinatol*. 2016;33(5):510–517

65. Barber EL, Zhao G, Buhimschi IA, Illuzzi JL. Duration of intrapartum prophylaxis and concentration of penicillin G in fetal serum at delivery. *Obstet Gynecol*. 2008; 112(2 pt 1):265–270

66. Berardi A, Pietrangiolillo Z, Bacchi Reggiani ML, et al. Are postnatal ampicillin levels actually related to the duration of intrapartum antibiotic prophylaxis prior to delivery? A pharmacokinetic study in 120 neonates. *Arch Dis Child Fetal Neonatal Ed*. 2018; 103(2):F152–F156

67. Brown CEL, Christmas JT, Bawdon RE. Placental transfer of cefazolin and piperacillin in pregnancies remote from term complicated by Rh isoimmunization. *Am J Obstet Gynecol*. 1990;163(3):938–943

68. Groff SM, Fallatah W, Yang S, et al. Effect of maternal obesity on maternal-fetal transfer of preoperative cefazolin at cesarean section. *J Pediatr Pharmacol Ther*. 2017;22(3):227–232

69. Fiore Mitchell T, Pearlman MD, Chapman RL, Bhatt-Mehta V, Faix RG. Maternal and transplacental pharmacokinetics of cefazolin. *Obstet Gynecol*. 2001;98(6):1075–1079

70. Allegaert K, van Mieghem T, Verbesselt R, et al. Cefazolin pharmacokinetics in maternal plasma and amniotic fluid during pregnancy. *Am J Obstet Gynecol*. 2009;200(2):170.e1–170.e7

71. Centers for Disease Control and Prevention. Active bacterial core surveillance (ABCs): bact facts interactive. Available at: https://wwwn.cdc.gov/BactFacts/index.html. Accessed February 20, 2019

72. Knight KM, Thornburg LL, McNanley AR, Hardy DJ, Vicino D, Glantz JC. The effect of intrapartum clindamycin on vaginal group B streptococcus colony counts. *J Matern Fetal Neonatal Med*. 2012; 25(6):747–749

73. Weinstein AJ, Gibbs RS, Gallagher M. Placental transfer of clindamycin and gentamicin in term pregnancy. *Am J Obstet Gynecol*. 1976;124(7):688–691

74. Philipson A, Sabath LD, Charles D. Transplacental passage of erythromycin and clindamycin. *N Engl J Med*. 1973;288(23):1219–1221

75. Wear CD, Towers CV, Brown MS, Weitz B, Porter S, Wolfe L. Transplacental passage of clindamycin from mother to neonate. *J Perinatol*. 2016;36(11): 960–961

76. Fairlie T, Zell ER, Schrag S. Effectiveness of intrapartum antibiotic prophylaxis for prevention of early-onset group B streptococcal disease. *Obstet Gynecol*. 2013;121(3):570–577

77. Nanovskaya T, Patrikeeva S, Zhan Y, Fokina V, Hankins GD, Ahmed MS. Transplacental transfer of vancomycin and telavancin. *Am J Obstet Gynecol*. 2012;207(4):331.e1–331.e6

78. Laiprasert J, Klein K, Mueller BA, Pearlman MD. Transplacental passage of vancomycin in noninfected term pregnant women. *Obstet Gynecol*. 2007; 109(5):1105–1110

79. Towers CV, Weitz B. Transplacental passage of vancomycin. *J Matern Fetal Neonatal Med*. 2018;31(8):1021–1024

80. Onwuchuruba CN, Towers CV, Howard BC, Hennessy MD, Wolfe L, Brown MS. Transplacental passage of vancomycin from mother to neonate. *Am J Obstet Gynecol*. 2014;210(4):352.e1–352.e4

81. Berardi A, Rossi C, Creti R, et al. Group B streptococcal colonization in 160 mother-baby pairs: a prospective cohort study. *J Pediatr*. 2013;163(4):1099–104.e1

82. Toyofuku M, Morozumi M, Hida M, et al. Effects of intrapartum antibiotic prophylaxis on neonatal acquisition of group B streptococci. *J Pediatr*. 2017; 190:169–173.e1

83. Puopolo KM, Benitz WE, Zaoutis TE; Committee on Fetus and Newborn; Committee on Infectious Diseases. Management of neonates born at ≥35 0/7 weeks' gestation with suspected or proven early-onset bacterial sepsis. *Pediatrics*. 2018;142(6):e20182894

84. Puopolo KM, Benitz WE, Zaoutis TE; Committee on Fetus and Newborn; Committee on Infectious Diseases. Management of neonates born at ≤34 6/7 weeks' gestation with suspected or proven early-onset bacterial sepsis. *Pediatrics*. 2018;142(6):e20182896

85. Committee on Obstetric Practice. Committee opinion no. 712: intrapartum management of intraamniotic infection. *Obstet Gynecol*. 2017;130(2):e95–e101

86. Newman TB, Puopolo KM, Wi S, Draper D, Escobar GJ. Interpreting complete blood counts soon after birth in newborns at risk for sepsis. *Pediatrics.* 2010;126(5):903–909

87. Hornik CP, Benjamin DK, Becker KC, et al. Use of the complete blood cell count in early-onset neonatal sepsis. *Pediatr Infect Dis J.* 2012;31(8):799–802

88. Newman TB, Draper D, Puopolo KM, Wi S, Escobar GJ. Combining immature and total neutrophil counts to predict early onset sepsis in term and late preterm newborns: use of the I/T^2. *Pediatr Infect Dis J.* 2014;33(8):798–802

89. Benitz WE. Adjunct laboratory tests in the diagnosis of early-onset neonatal sepsis. *Clin Perinatol.* 2010;37(2):421–438

90. Puopolo KM, Madoff LC, Eichenwald EC. Early-onset group B streptococcal disease in the era of maternal screening. *Pediatrics.* 2005;115(5):1240–1246

91. El Helali N, Nguyen JC, Ly A, Giovangrandi Y, Trinquart L. Diagnostic accuracy of a rapid real-time polymerase chain reaction assay for universal intrapartum group B streptococcus screening. *Clin Infect Dis.* 2009;49(3):417–423

92. Dhudasia MB, Mukhopadhyay S, Puopolo KM. Implementation of the sepsis risk calculator at an academic birth hospital. *Hosp Pediatr.* 2018;8(5):243–250

93. Berardi A, Fornaciari S, Rossi C, et al. Safety of physical examination alone for managing well-appearing neonates ≥ 35 weeks' gestation at risk for early-onset sepsis. *J Matern Fetal Neonatal Med.* 2015;28(10):1123–1127

94. Joshi NS, Gupta A, Allan JM, et al. Clinical monitoring of well-appearing infants born to mothers with chorioamnionitis. *Pediatrics.* 2018;141(4):e20172056

95. Joshi NS, Gupta A, Allan JM, et al. Management of chorioamnionitis-exposed infants in the newborn nursery using a clinical examination-based approach. *Hosp Pediatr.* 2019;9(4):227–233

96. Mukhopadhyay S, Puopolo KM. Clinical and microbiologic characteristics of early-onset sepsis among very low birth weight infants: opportunities for antibiotic stewardship. *Pediatr Infect Dis J.* 2017;36(5):477–481

97. Puopolo KM, Mukhopadhyay S, Hansen NI, et al; NICHD Neonatal Research Network. Identification of extremely premature infants at low risk for early-onset sepsis. *Pediatrics.* 2017;140(5):e20170925

98. Tibussek D, Sinclair A, Yau I, et al. Late-onset group B streptococcal meningitis has cerebrovascular complications. *J Pediatr.* 2015;166(5):1187–1192.e1

99. Metcalf BJ, Chochua S, Gertz RE Jr, et al; Active Bacterial Core surveillance team. Short-read whole genome sequencing for determination of antimicrobial resistance mechanisms and capsular serotypes of current invasive Streptococcus agalactiae recovered in the USA. *Clin Microbiol Infect.* 2017;23(8):574.e7–574.e14

100. Schrag SJ, Hadler JL, Arnold KE, Martell-Cleary P, Reingold A, Schuchat A. Risk factors for invasive, early-onset *Escherichia coli* infections in the era of widespread intrapartum antibiotic use. *Pediatrics.* 2006;118(2):570–576

101. Puopolo KM, Eichenwald EC. No change in the incidence of ampicillin-resistant, neonatal, early-onset sepsis over 18 years. *Pediatrics.* 2010;125(5). Available at: www.pediatrics.org/cgi/content/full/125/5/e1031

102. Moore MR, Schrag SJ, Schuchat A. Effects of intrapartum antimicrobial prophylaxis for prevention of group-B-streptococcal disease on the incidence and ecology of early-onset neonatal sepsis. *Lancet Infect Dis.* 2003;3(4):201–213

103. Green PA, Singh KV, Murray BE, Baker CJ. Recurrent group B streptococcal infections in infants: clinical and microbiologic aspects. *J Pediatr.* 1994;125(6 pt 1):931–938

104. Moylett EH, Fernandez M, Rench MA, Hickman ME, Baker CJ. A 5-year review of recurrent group B streptococcal disease: lessons from twin infants. *Clin Infect Dis.* 2000;30(2):282–287

105. Fernandez M, Rench MA, Albanyan EA, Edwards MS, Baker CJ. Failure of rifampin to eradicate group B streptococcal colonization in infants. *Pediatr Infect Dis J.* 2001;20(4):371–376

106. Cox LM, Yamanishi S, Sohn J, et al. Altering the intestinal microbiota during a critical developmental window has lasting metabolic consequences. *Cell.* 2014;158(4):705–721

107. Cho I, Yamanishi S, Cox L, et al. Antibiotics in early life alter the murine colonic microbiome and adiposity. *Nature.* 2012;488(7413):621–626

108. Leclercq S, Mian FM, Stanisz AM, et al. Low-dose penicillin in early life induces long-term changes in murine gut microbiota, brain cytokines and behavior. *Nat Commun.* 2017;8:15062

109. Kummeling I, Stelma FF, Dagnelie PC, et al. Early life exposure to antibiotics and the subsequent development of eczema, wheeze, and allergic sensitization in the first 2 years of life: the KOALA Birth Cohort Study. *Pediatrics.* 2007;119(1). Available at: www.pediatrics.org/cgi/content/full/119/1/e225

110. Risnes KR, Belanger K, Murk W, Bracken MB. Antibiotic exposure by 6 months and asthma and allergy at 6 years: findings in a cohort of 1,401 US children. *Am J Epidemiol.* 2011;173(3):310–318

111. Metsälä J, Lundqvist A, Virta LJ, Kaila M, Gissler M, Virtanen SM. Mother's and offspring's use of antibiotics and infant allergy to cow's milk. *Epidemiology.* 2013;24(2):303–309

112. Saari A, Virta LJ, Sankilampi U, Dunkel L, Saxen H. Antibiotic exposure in infancy and risk of being overweight in the first 24 months of life. *Pediatrics.* 2015;135(4):617–626

113. Roesch LF, Silveira RC, Corso AL, et al. Diversity and composition of vaginal microbiota of pregnant women at risk for transmitting Group B *Streptococcus* treated with intrapartum penicillin. *PLoS One.* 2017;12(2):e0169916

114. Aloisio I, Mazzola G, Corvaglia LT, et al. Influence of intrapartum antibiotic prophylaxis against group B *Streptococcus* on the early newborn gut composition and evaluation of the anti-*Streptococcus* activity of *Bifidobacterium* strains. *Appl Microbiol Biotechnol.* 2014;98(13):6051–6060

115. Azad MB, Konya T, Persaud RR, et al; CHILD Study Investigators. Impact of maternal intrapartum antibiotics,

method of birth and breastfeeding on gut microbiota during the first year of life: a prospective cohort study. *BJOG.* 2016;123(6):983–993

116. Corvaglia L, Tonti G, Martini S, et al. Influence of intrapartum antibiotic prophylaxis for group B streptococcus on gut microbiota in the first month of life. *J Pediatr Gastroenterol Nutr.* 2016; 62(2):304–308

117. Stearns JC, Simioni J, Gunn E, et al. Intrapartum antibiotics for GBS prophylaxis alter colonization patterns in the early infant gut microbiome of low risk infants. *Sci Rep.* 2017;7(1):16527

118. Nogacka A, Salazar N, Suárez M, et al. Impact of intrapartum antimicrobial prophylaxis upon the intestinal microbiota and the prevalence of antibiotic resistance genes in vaginally delivered full-term neonates. *Microbiome.* 2017;5(1):93

119. Pärnänen K, Karkman A, Hultman J, et al. Maternal gut and breast milk microbiota affect infant gut antibiotic resistome and mobile genetic elements. *Nat Commun.* 2018;9(1):3891

120. Edwards MS, Baker CJ. Group B streptococcal infections in elderly adults. *Clin Infect Dis.* 2005;41(6): 839–847

121. Madhi SA, Cutland CL, Jose L, et al. Safety and immunogenicity of an investigational maternal trivalent group B streptococcus vaccine in healthy women and their infants: a randomised phase 1b/2 trial. *Lancet Infect Dis.* 2016; 16(8):923–934

122. Hillier SL, Ferrieri P, Edwards MS, et al. A phase 2, randomized, control trial of group B streptococcus (GBS) type III capsular polysaccharide-tetanus toxoid (GBS III-TT) vaccine to prevent vaginal colonization with GBS III. *Clin Infect Dis.* 2019;68(12):2079–2086

123. Dzanibe S, Madhi SA. Systematic review of the clinical development of group B streptococcus serotype-specific capsular polysaccharide-based vaccines. *Expert Rev Vaccines.* 2018; 17(7):635–651

Mental Health Competencies for Pediatric Practice

- *Policy Statement*

POLICY STATEMENT Organizational Principles to Guide and Define the Child Health Care System and/or Improve the Health of all Children

American Academy of Pediatrics

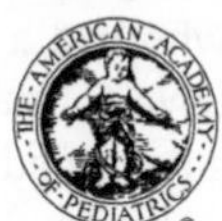

DEDICATED TO THE HEALTH OF ALL CHILDREN™

Mental Health Competencies for Pediatric Practice

Jane Meschan Foy, MD, FAAP,[a] Cori M. Green, MD, MS, FAAP,[b] Marian F. Earls, MD, MTS, FAAP,[c] COMMITTEE ON PSYCHOSOCIAL ASPECTS OF CHILD AND FAMILY HEALTH, MENTAL HEALTH LEADERSHIP WORK GROUP

abstract

Pediatricians have unique opportunities and an increasing sense of responsibility to promote healthy social-emotional development of children and to prevent and address their mental health and substance use conditions. In this report, the American Academy of Pediatrics updates its 2009 policy statement, which proposed competencies for providing mental health care to children in primary care settings and recommended steps toward achieving them. This 2019 policy statement affirms the 2009 statement and expands competencies in response to science and policy that have emerged since: the impact of adverse childhood experiences and social determinants on mental health, trauma-informed practice, and team-based care. Importantly, it also recognizes ways in which the competencies are pertinent to pediatric subspecialty practice. Proposed mental health competencies include foundational communication skills, capacity to incorporate mental health content and tools into health promotion and primary and secondary preventive care, skills in the psychosocial assessment and care of children with mental health conditions, knowledge and skills of evidence-based psychosocial therapy and psychopharmacologic therapy, skills to function as a team member and comanager with mental health specialists, and commitment to embrace mental health practice as integral to pediatric care. Achievement of these competencies will necessarily be incremental, requiring partnership with fellow advocates, system changes, new payment mechanisms, practice enhancements, and decision support for pediatricians in their expanded scope of practice.

[a]*Department of Pediatrics, School of Medicine, Wake Forest University, Winston-Salem, North Carolina;* [b]*Department of Pediatrics, Weill Cornell Medicine, Cornell University, New York, New York; and* [c]*Community Care of North Carolina, School of Medicine, University of North Carolina at Chapel Hill, Chapel Hill, North Carolina*

Policy statements from the American Academy of Pediatrics benefit from expertise and resources of liaisons and internal (AAP) and external reviewers. However, policy statements from the American Academy of Pediatrics may not reflect the views of the liaisons or the organizations or government agencies that they represent.

Drs Foy, Green, and Earls contributed to the drafting and revising of this manuscript; and all authors approved the final manuscript as submitted.

The guidance in this statement does not indicate an exclusive course of treatment or serve as a standard of medical care. Variations, taking into account individual circumstances, may be appropriate.

All policy statements from the American Academy of Pediatrics automatically expire 5 years after publication unless reaffirmed, revised, or retired at or before that time.

To cite: Foy JM, Green CM, Earls MF , AAP COMMITTEE ON PSYCHOSOCIAL ASPECTS OF CHILD AND FAMILY HEALTH, MENTAL HEALTH LEADERSHIP WORK GROUP. Mental Health Competencies for Pediatric Practice. *Pediatrics.* 2019; 144(5):e20192757

INTRODUCTION

A total of 13% to 20% of US children and adolescents experience a mental* disorder in a given year.[1] According to the seminal Great Smoky Mountain Study, which has followed a cohort of rural US youth since 1992, 19% of youth manifested impaired mental functioning without meeting the criteria for diagnosis as a mental disorder (ie, subthreshold symptoms).[2] The authors of this study have since shown that adults who had a childhood mental disorder have 6 times the odds of at least 1 adverse adult outcome in the domain of health, legal, financial, or social functioning compared with adults without childhood disorders, even after controlling for childhood psychosocial hardships. Adults who had impaired functioning and subthreshold psychiatric symptoms during childhood—termed "problems" in this statement—have 3 times the odds of adverse outcomes as adults.[3] These findings underscore the importance to adult health of both mental health disorders and mental health problems during childhood.

The prevalence of mental health disorders and problems (collectively termed "conditions" in this statement) in children and adolescents is increasing and, alarmingly, suicide rates are now the second leading cause of death in young people from 10 to 24 years of age.[4–6] Furthermore, nearly 6 million children were considered disabled in 2010–2011, an increase of more than 15% from a decade earlier; among these children, reported disability related to physical illnesses decreased by 11.8%, whereas disability related to neurodevelopmental and mental health conditions increased by 20.9%.[5] Although the highest rates of reported neurodevelopmental and mental health disabilities were seen in children living in poverty, the greatest increase in prevalence of reported neurodevelopmental and mental health disabilities occurred, unexpectedly, among children living in socially advantaged households (income ≥400% of the federal poverty level).[5]

Comorbid mental health conditions often complicate chronic physical conditions, decreasing the quality of life for affected children and increasing the cost of their care.[7–12] Because of stigma, shortages of mental health specialists, administrative barriers in health insurance plans, cost, and other barriers to mental health specialty care, an estimated 75% of children with mental health disorders go untreated.[13–16] Primary care physicians are the sole physician managers of care for an estimated 4 in 10 US children with attention-deficit/hyperactivity disorder (ADHD) and one-third with mental disorders overall.[17]

In 2009, the American Academy of Pediatrics (AAP) issued a policy statement, "The Future of Pediatrics: Mental Health Competencies for Pediatric Primary Care," proposing competencies—skills, knowledge, and attitudes—requisite to providing mental health care of children in primary care settings and recommending steps toward achieving them.[18] In the policy, the AAP documented the many forces driving the need for enhancements in pediatric mental health practice.

Updates to the Previous Statement

In the years since publication of the original policy statement on mental health competencies, increases in childhood mental health morbidity and mortality and a number of other developments have added to the urgency of enhancing pediatric mental health practice. A federal parity law has required that insurers cover mental health and physical health conditions equivalently.[19,20] Researchers have shown that early positive and adverse environmental influences—caregivers' protective and nurturing relationships with the child, social determinants of health, traumatic experiences (ecology), and genetic influences (biology)—interact to affect learning capacities, adaptive behaviors, lifelong physical and mental health, and adult productivity, and pediatricians have a role to play in addressing chronic stress and adverse early childhood experiences.[21–24] Transformative changes in the health care delivery system—payment for value, system- and practice-level integration of mental health and medical services, crossdiscipline accountability for outcomes, and the increasing importance of the family- and patient-centered medical home—all have the potential to influence mental health care delivery.[25–27] Furthermore, improving training and competence in mental health care for future pediatricians—pediatric subspecialists as well as primary care pediatricians—has become a national priority of the American Board of Pediatrics[28,29] and the Association of Pediatric Program Directors.[30]

In this statement, we (1) discuss the unique aspects of the pediatrician's role in mental health care; (2) articulate competencies needed by the pediatrician to promote healthy social-emotional development, identify risks and emerging symptoms, prevent or mitigate impairment from mental health symptoms, and address the mental health and substance use conditions prevalent among children and adolescents in the United States; and (3) recommend achievable next steps toward enhancing mental health practice to support pediatricians in providing mental health care. The accompanying technical report, "Achieving the Pediatric Mental Health Competencies," is focused on strategies to train future pediatricians and prepare practices for achieving the competencies.[31]

Uniqueness of the Pediatrician's Role in Mental Health Care

Traditional concepts of mental health care as well as mental health payment systems build on the assumption that treatment must follow the diagnosis of a disorder. However, this diagnostic approach does not take into account the many opportunities afforded pediatricians, both in general and subspecialty practice, to promote mental health and to offer primary and secondary prevention. Nor do these traditional concepts address the issue that many children have impaired functioning although they do not meet the diagnostic criteria for a specific mental disorder. Consequently, pediatric mental health competencies differ in some important respects from competencies of mental health professionals. The unique role of pediatricians in mental health care stems from the "primary care advantage," which is a developmental mind-set, and their role at the front lines of children's health care.[32] Primary care pediatricians typically see their patients longitudinally, giving them the opportunity to develop a trusting and empowering therapeutic relationship with patients and their families; to promote social-emotional health with every contact, whether for routine health supervision, acute care, or care of a child's chronic medical or developmental condition; to prevent mental health problems through education and anticipatory guidance; and to intervene in a timely way if and when risks, concerns, or symptoms emerge. Recognizing the longitudinal and close relationships that many pediatric subspecialists have with patients and families, the authors of this statement have expanded the concept of primary care advantage to the "pediatric advantage."

Pediatric subspecialists, like pediatric primary care clinicians, need basic mental health competencies. Children and adolescents with somatic manifestations of mental health problems often present to pediatric medical subspecialists or surgical specialists for evaluation of their symptoms; awareness of mental health etiologies has the potential to prevent costly and traumatic workups and expedite referral for necessary mental health services.[33] Children and adolescents with chronic medical conditions have a higher prevalence of mental health problems than do their peers without those conditions; and unrecognized mental health problems, particularly anxiety and depression, often drive excessive use of medical services in children with a chronic illness and impede adherence to their medical treatment.[34] Furthermore, children and adolescents with serious and life-threatening medical and surgical conditions often experience trauma, such as painful medical procedures, disfigurement, separation from loved ones during hospitalizations, and their own and their loved ones' fears about prognosis.[35] For these reasons, mental health competencies involving clinical assessment, screening, early intervention, referral, and comanagement are relevant to pediatric subspecialists who care for children with chronic conditions. Subspecialists have the additional responsibility of coordinating any mental health services they provide with patients' primary care clinicians to prevent duplication of effort, connect children and families to accessible local resources, and reach agreement on respective roles in monitoring patients' mental health care.

Integration of Mental Health Care Into Pediatric Workflow

The AAP Task Force on Mental Health (2004–2010) spoke to the importance of enhancing pediatricians' mental health practice while recognizing that incorporating mental health care into a busy pediatric practice can be a daunting prospect. The task force offered an algorithm, the "Primary Care Approach to Mental Health Care," depicting a process by which mental health services can be woven into practice flow, and tied each step in the algorithm to *Current Procedural Terminology* coding guidance that can potentially support those mental health–related activities in a fee-for-service environment.[32] The AAP Mental Health Leadership Work Group (2011–present) recently updated this to the "Algorithm: A Process for Integrating Mental Health Care Into Pediatric Practice" (see Fig 1). The AAP has a number of resources to assist with coding for mental health care.

The pediatric process for identifying and managing mental health problems is similar to the iterative process of caring for a child with fever and no focal findings: the clinician's initial assessment of the febrile child's severity of illness determines if there is a serious problem that urgently requires further diagnostic evaluation and treatment; if not, the clinician advises the family on symptomatic care and watchful waiting and advises the family to return for further assessment if symptoms persist or worsen. Similarly, a mental health concern of the patient, family, or child care and/or school personnel (or scheduling of a routine health supervision visit [algorithm step 1]) triggers a preliminary psychosocial assessment (algorithm step 2). This initial assessment can be expedited by use of previsit collection of data and screening tools (electronic or paper and pencil), which the clinician can review in advance of the visit, followed by a brief interview and observations to explore findings (both positive and negative) and the opportunity to highlight the child's and family's strengths, an important element of supportive, family-centered care. Finding a problem that is not simply a normal behavioral variation (algorithm step 3) necessitates triage for a psychiatric and/or social emergency and, if indicated, immediate care in the subspecialty or social service system (algorithm steps 9 and 10). In making these determinations, it is important to understand the family context, namely, the added risks conferred by adverse social determinants of health, which may exacerbate the problem and precipitate an emergency.

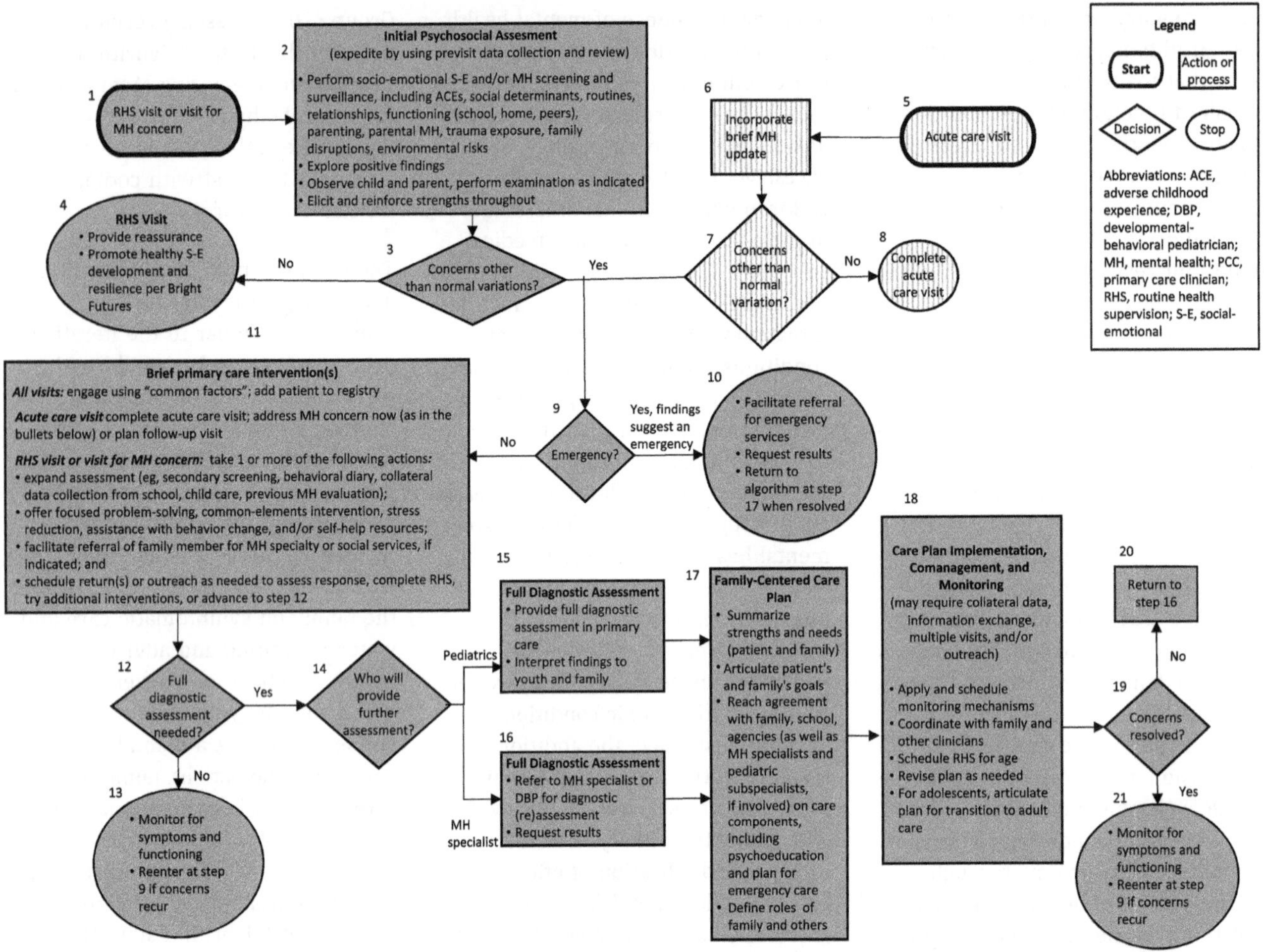

FIGURE 1
Mental health (MH) care in pediatric practice. ACE, adverse childhood experience; RHS, routine health supervision; S-E, social-emotional.

Intervention will need to include supports to address social determinants.

If an identified problem is not an emergency, the clinician can undertake 1 or more brief interventions, as time allows, during the current visit or at follow-up visit(s) (algorithm step 11). These interventions may include iteratively expanding the assessment, for example, by using secondary screening tools, gathering information from school personnel or child care providers, or having the family create a diary of problem behaviors and their triggers. Brief interventions may also include referral of a family member for assistance in addressing his or her own social or mental health problems that may be contributing to the child's difficulties. In addition, brief interventions may include evidence-informed techniques to address the child's symptoms, as described in the section immediately below.

When indicated by findings of the assessment and/or by failure to respond to brief therapeutic interventions, a full diagnostic assessment can be performed, either by the pediatrician (algorithm step 15) at a follow-up visit or through referral to a specialist (algorithm step 16), followed by the steps of care planning and implementation, comanagement, and monitoring the child's progress (algorithm steps 17 and 18).

Brief Interventions: Addressing Mental Health Symptoms in the Context of a Busy Pediatric Practice

Although disorder-specific, standardized psychosocial treatments have been a valuable advance in the mental health field generally, their real-world application to the care of children and adolescents has been limited by the fact that many young people are "diagnostically heterogeneous"; that is, they manifest symptoms of multiple disorders or problems, and their manifestations are variably triggered by events and by their social environment. These limitations led researchers in the field of psychotherapy to develop and successfully apply "transdiagnostic" approaches to the care of children and adolescents, addressing multiple disorders and problems by using a single protocol and allowing for more flexibility in selecting and sequencing interventions.[36]

A number of transdiagnostic approaches are proving to be adaptable for use as brief interventions in pediatric settings. The goals of brief therapeutic interventions for children and adolescents with emerging symptoms of mild to moderate severity are to improve the patient's functioning, reduce distress in the patient and parents, and potentially prevent a later disorder. For children and adolescents identified as needing mental health and/or developmental-behavioral specialty involvement, goals of brief interventions are to help overcome barriers to their accessing care, to ameliorate symptoms and distress while awaiting completion of the referral, and to monitor the patient's functioning and well-being while awaiting higher levels of care. Brevity of these interventions, ideally no more than 10 to 15 minutes per session, mitigates disruption to practice flow. Although formal evaluation of these adaptations is in its early stages, authors of studies suggest that they can be readily learned by pediatric clinicians and are beneficial to the child and family.[37] Table 1 is used to excerpt several of these adaptations from a summary by Wissow et al.[37]

All of these approaches feature prominently in the pediatric mental health competencies; 2 require further explanation.

"Common-factors" communication skills, so named because they are components of effective interventions common to diverse therapies across multiple diagnoses, are foundational among the proposed pediatric mental health competencies. These communication techniques include clinician interpersonal skills that help to build a therapeutic alliance—the felt bond between the clinician and patient and/or family, a powerful factor in facilitating emotional and psychological healing—which, in turn, increases the patient and/or family's optimism, feelings of well-being, and willingness to work toward improved health. Other common-factors techniques target feelings of anger, ambivalence, and hopelessness, family conflicts, and barriers to behavior change and help seeking. Still other techniques keep the discussion focused, practical, and organized. These techniques come from family therapy, cognitive therapy, motivational interviewing, family engagement, family-focused pediatrics, and solution-focused therapy.[38] They have been proven useful and effective in addressing mental health symptoms in pediatrics across the age spectrum and can be readily acquired by experienced clinicians.[39] Importantly, when time is short, the clinician can also use them to bring a visit to a supportive close while committing his or her loyalty and further assistance to the patient and family—that is, reinforcing the therapeutic alliance, even as he or she accommodates to the rapid pace of the practice.

See Table 2 for the HELP mnemonic, developed by the AAP Task Force on Mental Health to summarize components of the common-factors approach.

"Common-elements" approaches can also be used as brief interventions. They differ from common factors in that instead of applying to a range of diagnoses that are not causally related, common elements are semispecific components of psychosocial therapies that apply to a group of related conditions.[40–43] In this approach, the clinician caring for a patient who manifests a cluster of causally related symptoms—for example, fearfulness and avoidant behaviors—draws interventions from evidence-based psychosocial therapies for a related set of disorders—in this example, anxiety disorders. Thus, as a first-line intervention to help an anxious child, the pediatrician coaches the parent to provide gradual exposure to feared activities or objects and to model brave behavior—common elements in a number of effective psychosocial treatments for anxiety disorders. Such interventions can be definitive or a means to reduce distress and ameliorate symptoms while a child is awaiting mental health specialty assessment and/or care. Table 3 is used to summarize promising common-elements approaches applicable to common pediatric primary care problems.

Certain evidence-based complementary and integrative medicine approaches may also lend themselves to brief interventions: for example, relaxation and other self-regulation therapies reveal promise

TABLE 1 Promising Adaptations of Mental Health Treatment for Primary Care

Pediatric Settings	Parallels in Mental Health Services
Emphasis on patient-centered care and joint decision-making building trust and activation	Common-factors psychotherapeutic processes promoting engagement, optimism, alliance
Initial treatment often presumptive or relatively nonspecific	Stepped-care models with increasing specificity of diagnosis and intensity of treatment
Treatment based on brief counseling focused on patient-identified problems	"Common elements"
Links with community services, advice addressing family and social determinants	Peer and/or family navigators

Adapted from Wissow LS, van Ginneken N, Chandna J, Rahman A. Integrating children's mental health into primary care. *Pediatr Clin North Am.* 2016; 63(1):101.

TABLE 2 Common-Factors Approach: HELP Build a Therapeutic Alliance

H = Hope

Hope facilitates coping. Increase the family's hopefulness by describing your realistic expectations for improvement and reinforcing the strengths and assets you see in the child and family. Encourage concrete steps toward whatever is achievable.

E = Empathy

Communicate empathy by listening attentively, acknowledging struggles and distress, and sharing happiness experienced by the child and family.

L^2 = Language, Loyalty

Use the child or family's own language (not a clinical label) to reflect your understanding of the problem as they see it and to give the child and family an opportunity to correct any misperceptions.

Communicate loyalty to the family by expressing your support and your commitment to help now and in the future.

P^3 = Permission, Partnership, Plan

Ask the family's permission for you to ask more in-depth and potentially sensitive questions or make suggestions for further evaluation or management.

Partner with the child and family to identify any barriers or resistance to addressing the problem, find strategies to bypass or overcome barriers, and find agreement on achievable steps (or simply an achievable first step) aligned with the family's motivation. The more difficult the problem, the more important is the promise of partnership.

On the basis of the child's and family's preferences and sense of urgency, establish a plan (or incremental first step) through which the child and family will take some action(s), work toward greater readiness to take action, or monitor the problem and follow-up with you. (The plan might include, eg, keeping a diary of symptoms and triggers, gathering information from other sources such as the child's school, making lifestyle changes, applying parenting strategies or self-management techniques, reviewing educational resources about the problem or condition, initiating specific treatment, seeking referral for further assessment or treatment, or returning for further family discussion.)

Adapted from Foy JM; American Academy of Pediatrics, Task Force on Mental Health. Enhancing pediatric mental health care: algorithms for primary care. *Pediatrics*. 2010;125(suppl 3): S110.

in assisting children to manage stress and build their resilience to trauma and social adversities.[43] Other brief interventions include coaching parents in managing a particular behavior (eg, "time-out" for disruptive behavior[44]) or, more broadly, strategies to reduce stress in the household and to foster a sense of closeness and emotional security, for example, reading together,[45] sharing outdoor time,[46] or parent-child "special time"—a regularly scheduled period as brief as 5 to 10 minutes set aside for a one-on-one, interactive activity of the child's choice.[47] Self-help resources may also be useful (eg, online depression management).[48] Encouragement of healthy habits, such as sufficient sleep (critically important to children's mental health and resilience as well as their parents'), family meals, active play, time and content limits on media exposure, and prosocial activities with peers can be used as "universal" brief interventions across an array of presenting problems as well as a means to promote mental wellness and resilience.[49]

For a more detailed summary of psychosocial interventions and the evidence supporting them, see PracticeWise Evidence-Based Child and Adolescent Psychosocial Interventions at www.aap.org/mentalhealth. Psychosocial interventions that have been studied in primary care are listed in Common Elements of Evidence-Based Practice Amenable to Primary Care: Indications and Sources at www.aap.org/mentalhealth. With training, pediatricians can achieve competence in applying brief interventions such as these in primary care or, potentially, subspecialty settings.[37,50–52]

MENTAL HEALTH COMPETENCIES

The Accreditation Council for Graduate Medical Education has organized competencies into 6 domains: patient care, medical knowledge, interpersonal and communication skills, practice-based learning and improvement, professionalism, and systems-based practice.[53] We have used this framework to develop a detailed outline of pediatric mental health competencies for use by pediatric educators; this outline is available at www.aap.org/mentalhealth. Competencies most salient to this statement are listed in Tables 4 and 5.

Clinical Skills

All pediatricians need skills to promote mental health, efficiently perform psychosocial assessments, and provide primary and secondary preventive services (eg, anticipatory guidance, screening). They need to be able to triage for psychiatric emergencies (eg, suicidal or homicidal intent, psychotic thoughts) and social emergencies (eg, child abuse or neglect, domestic violence, other imminent threats to safety).

TABLE 3 Most Frequently Appearing Common Elements in Evidence-Based Practices, Grouped by Common Presenting Problems in Pediatric Primary Care

Presenting Problem Area	Most Common Elements of Related Evidence-Based Practices
Anxiety	Graded exposure, modeling
ADHD and oppositional problems	Tangible rewards, praise for child and parent, help with monitoring, time-out, effective commands and limit setting, response cost
Low mood	Cognitive and/or coping methods, problem-solving strategies, activity scheduling, behavioral rehearsal, social skills building

Adapted from Wissow LS, van Ginneken N, Chandna J, Rahman A. Integrating children's mental health into primary care. *Pediatr Clin North Am*. 2016; 63(1):103.

TABLE 4 Core Pediatric Mental Health Competencies: Clinical Skills

Pediatricians providing care to children and adolescents can maximize the patient's and family's health, agency, sense of safety, respect, and partnership by developing competence in performing the following activities:
Promotion and primary prevention
Promote healthy emotional development by providing anticipatory guidance on healthy lifestyles and stress management
Routinely gather an age-appropriate psychosocial history, applying appropriate tools to assist with data gathering
Secondary prevention
Identify and evaluate risk factors to healthy emotional development and emerging symptoms that could cause impairment or suggest future mental health problems, applying appropriate tools to assist with screening and refer to community resources when appropriate (ie, parenting programs)
Assessment
Recognize mental health emergencies such as suicide risk, severe functional impairment, and complex mental health symptoms that require urgent mental health specialty care
Analyze and interpret results from mental health screening, history, physical examination, and observations to determine what brief interventions may be useful and whether a full diagnostic assessment is needed
Diagnose school-aged children and adolescents with the following disorders: ADHD, common anxiety disorders (separation anxiety disorder, social phobia, generalized anxiety disorder), depression, and substance use
Treatment
Apply fundamental (common factors, motivational interviewing) communications skills to engage youth and families and overcome barriers to their help seeking for identified social and mental health problems
Apply common-factors skills and common elements of evidence-based psychosocial treatments to initiate the care of the following:
Children and youth with medical and developmental conditions who manifest comorbid mental health symptoms
Depressed mothers and their children
Infants and young children manifesting difficulties with communication and/or attachment or other signs and symptoms of emotional distress (eg, problematic sleep, eating behaviors)
Children and adolescents presenting with the following:
Anxious or avoidant behaviors
Exposure to trauma or loss
Impulsivity and inattention, with or without hyperactivity
Low mood or withdrawn behaviors
Disruptive or aggressive behaviors
Substance use
Learning difficulties
When a higher level of care is needed for symptoms listed above, integrate patient and/or family strengths, needs, and preferences, the clinician's own skills, and available resources into development of a care plan for children and adolescents with mental health problem(s), alone, with the practice care team, or in collaboration with mental health specialists
Demonstrate proficiency in selecting, prescribing, and monitoring (for response and adverse effects) ADHD medications and selective serotonin reuptake inhibitors that have a safety and efficacy profile appropriate to use in pediatric care
Develop a contingency or crisis plan for a child or adolescent
Develop a safety plan with patients and parents for children and adolescents who are suicidal and/or depressed
Apply strategies to actively monitor adverse and positive effects of nonpharmacologic and pharmacologic therapy
Facilitate a family's and patient's engagement with and transfer of trust (ie, "warm handoff") to a mental health professional
Demonstrate an accurate understanding of privacy regulations
Refer, collaborate, comanage, and participate as a team member in coordinating mental health care with specialists and in transitioning adolescents with mental health needs to adult primary care and mental health specialty providers

Pediatricians need to be able to establish a therapeutic alliance with the patient and family and take initial action on any identified mental health and social concerns, as described above. All pediatricians also need to know how to organize the care of patients who require mental health specialty referral or consultation, facilitate transfer of trust to mental health specialists, and coordinate their patients' mental health care with other clinicians, reaching previous agreement on respective roles, such as who will prescribe and monitor medications and how communication will take place. The care team might include any of the individuals listed in Table 6, on- or off-site. For a discussion of collaborative care models that integrate services of mental health and pediatric professionals, see the accompanying technical report.[31]

The clinical role of the pediatrician will depend on the patient's condition and level of impairment, interventions and supports needed, patient and family priorities and preferences, pediatrician's self-perception of efficacy and capacity, and accessibility of community services.

Disorders such as maladaptive aggression[54,55] and bipolar disorder[56] may require medications for which pediatricians will need specialized training or consultation from physician mental health specialists to prescribe (eg, antipsychotics, lithium). Comanagement—formally defined as "collaborative and coordinated care that is conceptualized, planned, delivered, and evaluated by 2 or more health care providers"[57]—is a successful

TABLE 5 Core Pediatric Mental Health Competencies: Practice Enhancements

Pediatricians providing care to children and adolescents can improve the quality of their practice's (and network's) mental health services by developing competence in performing the following activities
Establish collaborative and consultative relationships—within the practice, virtually, or off-site—and define respective roles in assessment, treatment, coordination of care, exchange of information, and family support
Build a practice team culture around a shared commitment to embrace mental health care as integral to pediatric practice and an understanding of the impact of trauma on child well-being
Establish systems within the practice (and network) to support mental health services; elements may include the following:
Preparation of office staff and professionals to create an environment of respect, agency, confidentiality, safety, and trauma-informed care;
Preparation of office staff and professionals to identify and manage patients with suicide risk and other mental health emergencies;
Electronic health record prompts and culturally and/or linguistically appropriate educational materials to facilitate offering anticipatory guidance and to educate youth and families on mental health and substance use topics and resources;
Routines for gathering the patient's and family's psychosocial history, conducting psychosocial and/or behavioral assessment;
Registries, evidence-based protocols, and monitoring and/or tracking mechanisms for patients with positive psychosocial screen results, adverse childhood experiences and social determinants of health, behavioral risks, and mental health problems;
Directory of mental health and substance use disorder referral sources, school-based resources, and parenting and family support resources in the region;
Mechanisms for coordinating the care provided by all collaborating providers through standardized communication; and
Tools for facilitating coding and billing specific to mental health.
Systematically analyze the practice by using quality improvement methods with the goal of mental health practice improvement

approach for complex mental conditions in children and adolescents. Both general pediatricians and pediatric subspecialists will benefit from these collaborative skills. These skills also enable pediatricians to help adolescents with mental health conditions and their families transition the adolescent's care to adult primary and mental health specialty care at the appropriate time, as pediatricians do other patients with special health care needs.

Misperceptions about privacy regulations (eg, the Health Insurance Portability and Accountability Act of 1996,[58] federal statutes and regulations regarding substance abuse treatment [42 US Code § 290dd–2; 42 Code of Federal Regulations 2.11],[59] and state-specific regulations) often impede collaboration by limiting communication among clinicians who are providing services. In most instances, pediatricians are, in fact, allowed to exchange information with other clinicians involved in a patient's care, even without the patient or guardian's consent. Pediatricians need an accurate understanding of privacy regulations to ensure that all clinicians involved in the mutual care of a patient share information in an appropriate and timely way (see https://www.aap.org/en-us/advocacy-and-policy/aap-health-initiatives/Mental-Health/Pages/HIPAA-Privacy-Rule-and-Provider-to-Provider-Communication.aspx).

TABLE 6 Potential Mental Health Care Team Members

Patient and family
One or more PCC
Any other pediatric team member who has forged a bond of trust with the family (eg, nurse, front desk staff, medical assistant)
Mental health medical consultant (eg, child psychiatrist, developmental-behavioral pediatrician, adolescent specialist, pediatric neurologist), directly involved or consulting with PCC by phone or telemedicine link
Psychologist, social worker, advanced practice nurse, substance use counselor, early intervention specialist, or other licensed specialist(s) trained in the relevant evidence-based psychosocial therapy
School-based professionals (eg, guidance counselor, social worker, school nurse, school psychologist)
Representative of involved social service agency
Medical subspecialist(s) or surgical specialist
Parent educator
Peer navigator
Care manager

PCC, primary care clinician.

Other necessary clinical skills are specific to the age, presenting problem of the patient, and type of therapy required, as described in the following sections.

Infants and Preschool-aged Children

For infants and preschool-aged children, the signs and symptoms of emotional distress may be varied and nonspecific and may manifest themselves in the child, in the parent, or in their relationship. When consistently outside the range of normal development, these young children and families typically require specialized diagnostic assessment (based on the *Diagnostic Classification of Mental Health and Developmental Disorders of Infancy and Early Childhood*[60]), intensive parenting interventions, and treatment by developmental-behavioral specialists or mental health specialists with expertise in early childhood. Consequently, pediatric mental health competencies for the care of this age group involve overcoming any barriers to referral, guiding the family in nurturing and stimulating the child, counseling on parenting and behavioral management techniques, referring for diagnostic assessment and dyadic (attachment-focused) therapy as indicated, and comanaging care. When social risk factors are identified (eg, maternal depression, poverty, food insecurity), the pediatrician's role is to connect the family to needed resources.

School-aged Children and Adolescents

The AAP Task Force on Mental Health identified common manifestations of mental health problems in school-aged children and adolescents as depression (low mood), anxious and avoidant behaviors, impulsivity and inattention (with or without hyperactivity), disruptive behavior and aggression, substance use, and learning difficulty and developed guidance to assist pediatric clinicians in addressing these problems.[61] Recognizing that 75% of children who need mental health services do not receive them, the AAP went on to publish a number of additional educational resources on these topics, specifically for pediatricians.[62–64] Additional tools are available online at www.aap.org/mentalhealth. Children and adolescents who have experienced trauma may manifest any combination of these symptoms.[65,66] Children and adolescents with an underlying mental condition may present with somatic symptoms (eg, headache, abdominal pain, chest pain, limb pain, fatigue) or eating abnormalities.[67,68] Furthermore, children and adolescents may experience impaired functioning at home, at school, or with peers, even in the absence of symptoms that reach the threshold for a diagnosis.[2,69,70]

Once a pediatrician has identified a child or adolescent with 1 or more of these manifestations of a possible mental health condition (collectively termed "mental health concerns" in this statement, indicating that they are undifferentiated as to disorder, problem, or normal variation), the pediatrician needs skills to differentiate normal variations from problems from disorders and to diagnose, at a minimum, conditions for which evidence-based primary care assessment and treatment guidance exists—currently ADHD,[71] depression,[72,73] and substance use.[74] Pediatricians also need knowledge and skills to diagnose anxiety disorders, which are among the most common disorders of childhood, often accompany and adversely affect the care of chronic medical conditions, and when associated with no more than mild to moderate impairment, are often amenable to pediatric treatment.[66] A number of disorder-specific rating scales and functional assessment tools are applicable to use in pediatrics, both to assist in diagnosis and to monitor the response to interventions; these have been described and referenced in the document "Mental Health Tools for Pediatrics" at www.aap.org/mentalhealth.

Although the diagnostic assessment of children presenting with aggressive behaviors often requires mental health specialty involvement, pediatricians can use a stepwise approach to begin the assessment and offer guidance in selecting psychosocial interventions in the community for further diagnosis and treatment, as outlined in the guideline, "Treatment of Maladaptive Aggression in Youth (T-MAY)," available at www.ahrq.gov/sites/default/files/wysiwyg/chain/practice-tools/tmay-final.pdf.

Pharmacologic and Psychosocial Therapies

Many pharmacologic and psychosocial therapies have been proven effective in treating children with mental health disorders. Pharmacologic therapies may be more familiar to pediatricians than psychosocial therapies; however, psychosocial therapies, either alone or in combination with pharmacologic therapies, may be more effective in some circumstances. For example, American Academy of Child and Adolescent Psychiatry guidelines recommend at least 2 trials of psychosocial treatment before starting medication in young children up to 5 years of age.[75] Studies involving children and adolescents in several specific age groups have revealed the advantage of combined psychosocial and medication treatment over either type of therapy alone for ADHD in 7- to 9-year-old children,[76] common anxiety disorders in 7- to 9-year-old children,[77] and depression in 12- to 17-year-old children,[78] and benefits of combined therapy likely go well beyond these age groups. Furthermore, many children with mild or subthreshold anxiety or depression are likely to benefit from psychosocial therapy, mind-body approaches, and self-help resources without medication.[48,66,79] Although pediatricians may feel pressured to prescribe only medication in these and other situations because it is generally more accessible and/or expedient,[80] knowledge of these other approaches is necessary to offer children these choices. If needed community services are not available, pediatricians can use common-elements approaches in the pediatric office and advocate for evidence-based therapies to be offered by the mental health community.

Certain disorders (ADHD, common anxiety disorders, depression), if associated with no more than moderate impairment, are amenable to primary care medication management because there are indicated medications with a well-established safety profile (eg, a variety of ADHD medications and certain selective serotonin reuptake inhibitors).[81] Ideally, pediatric subspecialists would also be knowledgeable about these medications, their adverse effects, and their interactions with medications prescribed in their subspecialty practice. Necessary clinical skills are summarized in Table 4.

Practice Enhancements

Effective mental health care requires the support of office and network systems. Competencies requisite to establishing and sustaining these systems are outlined in Table 5.

PROGRESS TO DATE

Despite many efforts to enhance the competence of pediatric residents and practicing pediatricians (see accompanying technical report "Achieving the Pediatric Mental Health Competencies"[31]), change in mental health practice during the last decade has been modest, as measured by the AAP's periodic surveys of members. National data reveal that in 2013, only 57% of pediatricians were consistently treating ADHD and less than a quarter were treating any other disorder.[82] Although fewer barriers were reported in 2013 than in 2004, most pediatricians surveyed in 2013 reported that they had inadequate training in treating child mental health problems, a lack of confidence to counsel children, and limited time for these problems.[83]

In the accompanying technical report, we address the barriers of training and confidence.[31] The barrier of limited time for mental health care may one day become an artifact of volume-based care and the payment systems that have incentivized it. Value-based payment, expanded clinical care teams, and integration of mental health care into pediatric settings may provide new incentives and opportunities for mental health practice, improve quality of care, and result in improved outcomes for both physical and mental health conditions. In the interim, the AAP recognizes that although the proposed competencies are necessary to meet the needs of children, pediatricians will necessarily achieve them through incremental steps that rely on improved third-party payment for their mental health services and access to expertise in mental health coding and billing to support the time required for mental health practice.

RECOMMENDATIONS

The recommendations that follow build on the 2009 policy statement[18] and assumptions drawn from review of available literature; the recognized, well-documented, and growing mental health needs of the pediatric population; expert opinion of the authoring bodies; and review and feedback by additional relevant AAP entities. There are striking geographic variations in access to pediatric mental health services from state to state and within states, from urban to rural areas.[84] By engaging in the kind of partnerships described in the first point below, pediatricians can prioritize their action steps and implement them, incrementally, in accordance with their community's needs. With the pediatric advantage in mind, the AAP recommends that pediatricians engage in the following:

partner with families, youth, and other child advocates; mental health, adolescent, and developmental specialists; teachers; early childhood educators; health and human service agency leaders; local and state chapters of mental health specialty organizations; and/or AAP chapter and national leaders with the goal of improving the organizational and financial base of mental health care, depending on the needs of a particular community or practice; this might include such strategies as:

advocating with insurers and payers for appropriate payment to pediatricians and mental health specialists for their mental health services (see the Chapter Action Kit in Resources);

using appropriate coding and billing practices to support mental health services in a fee-for-service payment environment (see Chapter Action Kit in Resources);

participating in development of models of value-based and bundled payment for integrated mental health care (see the AAP Practice Transformation Web site in Resources); and/or

identifying gaps in key mental health services in their communities and advocating to address deficiencies (see Chapter Action Kit in Resources);

pursue quality improvement and maintenance of certification activities that enhance their mental health practice, prioritizing suicide prevention (see Quality Improvement and/or Maintenance of Certification in Resources);

explore collaborative care models of practice, such as integration of a mental health specialist as a member of the medical home team, consultation with a child psychiatrist or developmental-behavioral pediatrician, or telemedicine technologies that both enhance patients' access to mental health specialty care and grow the competence and confidence of involved pediatricians (see AAP Mental Health Web site in Resources);

build relationships with mental health specialists (including school-based providers) with whom they can collaborate in enhancing their mental health knowledge and skills, in identifying and providing emergency care to children and adolescents at risk for suicide, and in comanaging children with primary mental health conditions and physical conditions with mental health comorbidities (see Chapter Action Kit in Resources);

pursue educational strategies (eg, participation in a child psychiatry consultation network, collaborative office rounds, learning collaborative, miniature fellowship, AAP chapter, or health system network initiative) suited to their own learning style and skill level for incrementally achieving the mental health competencies outlined in Tables 4 and 5 (see accompanying technical report for in-depth discussion of educational strategies);

advocate for innovations in medical school education, residency and fellowship training, and continuing medical education activities to increase the knowledge base and skill level of future pediatricians in accordance with the mental health competencies outlined in Tables 4 and 5; and

promote and participate in research on the delivery of mental health services in pediatric primary care and subspecialty settings.

In the accompanying technical report,[31] we highlight successful educational initiatives and suggest promising strategies for achieving the mental health competencies through innovations in the training of medical students, pediatric residents, fellows, preceptors, and practicing pediatricians and through support in making practice enhancements.

CONCLUSIONS

The AAP recognizes pediatricians' unique opportunities to promote children's healthy socioemotional development, strengthen children's resilience to the many stressors that face them and their families, and recognize and address the mental health needs that emerge during childhood and adolescence. These opportunities flow from the pediatric advantage, which includes longitudinal, trusting, and empowering relationships with patients and their families and the nonstigmatizing, family friendliness of pediatric practices. Fully realizing this advantage will depend on pediatricians developing or honing their mental health knowledge and skills and enhancing their mental health practice. To that end, this statement outlines mental health competencies for pediatricians, incorporating evidence-based clinical approaches that are feasible within pediatrics, supported by collaborative relationships with mental health specialists, developmental-behavioral pediatricians, and others at both the community and practice levels.

Enhancements in pediatric mental health practice will also depend on system changes, new methods of financing, access to reliable sources of information about existing evidence and new science, decision support, and innovative educational methods (discussed in the accompanying technical report[31]). For this reason, attainment of the competencies proposed in this statement will, for most pediatricians, be achieved incrementally over time. Gains are likely to be substantial, including the improved well-being of children, adolescents, and families and enhanced satisfaction of pediatricians who care for them.

RESOURCES

AAP Clinical Tools and/or Tool Kits

AAP clinical tools and/or tool kits include the following:

Addressing Mental Health Concerns in Primary Care: A Clinician's Toolkit;

Health Insurance Portability and Accountability Act of 1996 Privacy Rule and Provider to Provider Communication;

Mental Health Initiatives Chapter Action Kit; and

AAP Coding Fact Sheets (AAP log-on required).

AAP Policies

AAP policies include the following:

ADHD: Clinical Practice Guideline for the Diagnosis, Evaluation, and Treatment of Attention-Deficit/Hyperactivity Disorder in Children and Adolescents (November 2011);

Guidelines for Adolescent Depression in Primary Care (GLAD-PC): Part I. Practice Preparation, Identification, Assessment, and Initial Management (endorsed by the AAP March 2018);

Guidelines for Adolescent Depression in Primary Care (GLAD-PC): Part II. Treatment and Ongoing Management (endorsed by the AAP March 2018);

Policy Statement: Incorporating Recognition and Management of Perinatal and Postpartum Depression Into Pediatric Practice (January 2019);

Technical Report: Incorporating Recognition and Management of Perinatal and Postpartum Depression Into Pediatric Practice (January 2019);

Policy Statement: Early Childhood Adversity, Toxic Stress, and the Role of the Pediatrician: Translating Developmental Science Into Lifelong Health (January 2012; reaffirmed July 2016);

Technical Report: The Lifelong Effects of Early Childhood Adversity and Toxic Stress (January 2012; reaffirmed July 2016);

Clinical Report: Mind-Body Therapies in Children and Youth (September 2016);

The Prenatal Visit (July 2018);

Clinical Report: Promoting Optimal Development: Screening for Behavioral and Emotional Problems (February 2015);

Policy Statement: Substance Use Screening, Brief Intervention, and Referral to Treatment (July 2016); and

Clinical Report: Substance Use Screening, Brief Intervention, and Referral to Treatment (July 2016).

Quality Improvement and/or Maintenance of Certification

Quality improvement and/or Maintenance of Certification resources include the following:

Education in Quality Improvement for Pediatric Practice: Bright Futures - Middle Childhood and Adolescence;

Education in Quality Improvement for Pediatric Practice: Substance Use - Screening, Brief Intervention, Referral to Treatment; and

American Board of Pediatrics Quality Improvement Web site.

AAP Publications

AAP publications include the following:

AAP Developmental Behavioral Pediatrics, Second Edition;

Mental Health Care of Children and Adolescents: A Guide for Primary Care Clinicians;

Promoting Mental Health in Children and Adolescents: Primary Care Practice and Advocacy;

Pediatric Psychopharmacology for Primary Care;

Quick Reference Guide to Coding Pediatric Mental Health Services 2019; and

Thinking Developmentally.

AAP Reports

AAP reports include the following:

Improving Mental Health Services in Primary Care: A Call to Action for the Payer Community (AAP log-on required); and

Reducing Administrative and Financial Barriers.

Web Sites

Web site resources include the following:

AAP Mental Health Web site;

AAP Practice Transformation Web site;

National Center for Medical Home Implementation;

The Resilience Project; and

Screening Technical Assistance and Resource Center.

Lead Authors

Jane Meschan Foy, MD, FAAP

Cori M. Green, MD, MS, FAAP

Marian F. Earls, MD, MTS, FAAP

Committee on Psychosocial Aspects of Child and Family Health, 2018–2019

Arthur Lavin, MD, FAAP, Chairperson

George LaMonte Askew, MD, FAAP

Rebecca Baum, MD, FAAP

Evelyn Berger-Jenkins, MD, FAAP

Thresia B. Gambon, MD, FAAP

Arwa Abdulhaq Nasir, MBBS, MSc, MPH, FAAP

Lawrence Sagin Wissow, MD, MPH, FAAP

Former Committee on Psychosocial Aspects of Child and Family Health Members

Michael Yogman, MD, FAAP, Former Chairperson

Gerri Mattson, MD, FAAP

Jason Richard Rafferty, MD, MPH, EdM, FAAP

Liaisons

Sharon Berry, PhD, ABPP, LP – *Society of Pediatric Psychology*

Edward R. Christophersen, PhD, FAAP – *Society of Pediatric Psychology*

Norah L. Johnson, PhD, RN, CPNP-BC – *National Association of Pediatric Nurse Practitioners*

Abigail Boden Schlesinger, MD – *American Academy of Child and Adolescent Psychiatry*

Rachel Shana Segal, MD – *Section on Pediatric Trainees*

Amy Starin, PhD – *National Association of Social Workers*

Mental Health Leadership Work Group, 2017–2018

Marian F. Earls, MD, MTS, FAAP, Chairperson

Cori M. Green, MD, MS, FAAP

Alain Joffe, MD, MPH, FAAP

Staff

Linda Paul, MPH

ABBREVIATIONS

AAP: American Academy of Pediatrics
ADHD: attention-deficit/hyperactivity disorder

*The term "mental" throughout this statement is intended to encompass "behavioral," "psychiatric," "psychological," "emotional," and "substance use" as well as family context and community-related concerns. Accordingly, factors affecting mental health include precipitants such as child abuse and neglect, separation or divorce of parents, domestic violence, parental or family mental health issues, natural disasters, school crises, military deployment of children's loved ones, incarceration of a loved one, and the grief and loss accompanying any of these issues or the illness or death of family members. Mental also is intended to encompass somatic manifestations of psychosocial issues, such as eating disorders and gastrointestinal symptoms. This use of the term is not to suggest that the full range or severity of all mental health conditions and concerns falls within the scope of pediatric practice but, rather, that children and adolescents may suffer from the full range and severity of mental health conditions and psychosocial stressors. As such, children with mental health needs, similar to children with special physical and developmental needs, are children for whom pediatricians provide care in the medical home and in subspecialty practice.

This document is copyrighted and is property of the American Academy of Pediatrics and its Board of Directors. All authors have filed conflict of interest statements with the American Academy of Pediatrics. Any conflicts have been resolved through a process approved by the Board of Directors. The American Academy of Pediatrics has neither solicited nor accepted any commercial involvement in the development of the content of this publication.

DOI: https://doi.org/10.1542/peds.2019-2757

Address correspondence to Jane Meschan Foy, MD, FAAP. E-mail: foy.jane@gmail.com

PEDIATRICS (ISSN Numbers: Print, 0031-4005; Online, 1098-4275).

Copyright © 2019 by the American Academy of Pediatrics

FINANCIAL DISCLOSURE: The authors have indicated they have no financial relationships relevant to this article to disclose.

FUNDING: No external funding.

POTENTIAL CONFLICT OF INTEREST: The authors have indicated they have no potential conflicts of interest to disclose.

REFERENCES

1. Perou R, Bitsko RH, Blumberg SJ, et al; Centers for Disease Control and Prevention (CDC). Mental health surveillance among children–United States, 2005-2011. *MMWR Suppl.* 2013; 62(2):1–35
2. Burns BJ, Costello EJ, Angold A, et al. Children's mental health service use across service sectors. *Health Aff (Millwood).* 1995;14(3):147–159
3. Copeland WE, Wolke D, Shanahan L, Costello EJ. Adult functional outcomes of common childhood psychiatric problems: a prospective, longitudinal study. *JAMA Psychiatry.* 2015;72(9): 892–899
4. Slomski A. Chronic mental health issues in children now loom larger than physical problems. *JAMA.* 2012;308(3): 223–225
5. Houtrow AJ, Larson K, Olson LM, Newacheck PW, Halfon N. Changing trends of childhood disability, 2001-2011. *Pediatrics.* 2014;134(3):530–538
6. Heron M. Deaths: Leading causes for 2016. National Vital Statistics Reports; Vol 67. *No 6.* Hyattsville, MD: National Center for Health Statistics. 2018. Available at: https://www.cdc.gov/nchs/data/nvsr/nvsr67/nvsr67_06.pdf. Accessed September 22, 2019
7. Suryavanshi MS, Yang Y. Clinical and economic burden of mental disorders among children with chronic physical conditions, United States, 2008-2013. *Prev Chronic Dis.* 2016;13:E71
8. Barlow JH, Ellard DR. The psychosocial well-being of children with chronic disease, their parents and siblings: an overview of the research evidence base. *Child Care Health Dev.* 2006;32(1):19–31
9. Perrin JM, Gnanasekaran S, Delahaye J. Psychological aspects of chronic health conditions. *Pediatr Rev.* 2012;33(3): 99–109
10. Hood KK, Beavers DP, Yi-Frazier J, et al. Psychosocial burden and glycemic control during the first 6 years of diabetes: results from the SEARCH for Diabetes in Youth study. *J Adolesc Health.* 2014;55(4):498–504
11. Shomaker LB, Tanofsky-Kraff M, Stern EA, et al. Longitudinal study of depressive symptoms and progression of insulin resistance in youth at risk for adult obesity. *Diabetes Care.* 2011; 34(11):2458–2463
12. Roy-Byrne PP, Davidson KW, Kessler RC, et al. Anxiety disorders and comorbid medical illness. *Gen Hosp Psychiatry.* 2008;30(3):208–225
13. American Academy of Child and Adolescent Psychiatry, Committee on Health Care Access and Economics Task Force on Mental Health. Improving mental health services in primary care: reducing administrative and financial barriers to access and collaboration. *Pediatrics.* 2009;123(4):1248–1251
14. Merikangas KR, He JP, Brody D, et al. Prevalence and treatment of mental disorders among US children in the 2001-2004 NHANES. *Pediatrics.* 2010; 125(1):75–81
15. Merikangas KR, He JP, Burstein M, et al. Service utilization for lifetime mental disorders in U.S. adolescents: results of the National Comorbidity Survey-Adolescent Supplement (NCS-A). *J Am Acad Child Adolesc Psychiatry.* 2011; 50(1):32–45
16. Whitney DG, Peterson MD. US national and state-level prevalence of mental health disorders and disparities of mental health care use in children. *JAMA Pediatr.* 2019;173(4):389–391
17. Anderson LE, Chen ML, Perrin JM, Van Cleave J. Outpatient visits and medication prescribing for US children with mental health conditions. *Pediatrics.* 2015;136(5). Available at: www.pediatrics.org/cgi/content/full/136/5/e1178
18. Committee on Psychosocial Aspects of Child and Family Health and Task Force on Mental Health. Policy statement--The future of pediatrics: mental health competencies for pediatric primary care. *Pediatrics.* 2009;124(1):410–421
19. Centers for Medicare & Medicaid Services (CMS), HHS. Medicaid and Children's Health Insurance Programs; Mental Health Parity and Addiction Equity Act of 2008; the application of mental health parity requirements to coverage offered by Medicaid managed care organizations, the Children's Health Insurance Program (CHIP), and alternative benefit plans. Final rule. *Fed Regist.* 2016;81(61):18389–18445
20. Cauchi R, Hanson K; National Conference of State Legislators. Mental health benefits: state laws mandating or regulating. 2015. Available at: www.ncsl.org/research/health/mental-health-benefits-state-mandates.aspx. Accessed September 8, 2017
21. Garner AS, Shonkoff JP; Committee on Psychosocial Aspects of Child and Family Health; Committee on Early Childhood, Adoption, and Dependent Care; Section on Developmental and Behavioral Pediatrics. Early childhood adversity, toxic stress, and the role of the pediatrician: translating developmental science into lifelong health. *Pediatrics.* 2012;129(1). Available at: www.pediatrics.org/cgi/content/full/129/1/e224
22. Shonkoff JP, Garner AS; Committee on Psychosocial Aspects of Child and

Family Health; Committee on Early Childhood, Adoption, and Dependent Care; Section on Developmental and Behavioral Pediatrics. The lifelong effects of early childhood adversity and toxic stress. *Pediatrics*. 2012;129(1). Available at: www.pediatrics.org/cgi/content/full/129/1/e232

23. McLaughlin KA, Greif Green J, Gruber MJ, et al. Childhood adversities and first onset of psychiatric disorders in a national sample of US adolescents. *Arch Gen Psychiatry*. 2012;69(11): 1151–1160

24. Levine ME, Cole SW, Weir DR, Crimmins EM. Childhood and later life stressors and increased inflammatory gene expression at older ages. *Soc Sci Med*. 2015;130:16–22

25. Council on Children with Disabilities and Medical Home Implementation Project Advisory Committee. Patient- and family-centered care coordination: a framework for integrating care for children and youth across multiple systems. *Pediatrics*. 2014;133(5). Available at: www.pediatrics.org/cgi/content/full/133/5/e1451

26. Croghan TW, Brown JD. *Integrating Mental Health Treatment Into the Patient Centered Medical Home*. Rockville, MD: Agency for Healthcare Research and Quality; 2010

27. Internal Revenue Service, Department of the Treasury; Employee Benefits Security Administration, Department of Labor; Centers for Medicare & Medicaid Services, Department of Health and Human Services. Final rules under the Paul Wellstone and Pete Domenici Mental Health Parity and Addiction Equity Act of 2008; technical amendment to external review for multi-state plan program. Final rules. *Fed Regist*. 2013;78(219):68239–68296

28. Leslie L; American Board of Pediatrics. Finding allies to address children's mental and behavioral needs. 2016. Available at: https://blog.abp.org/blog/finding-allies-address-childrens-mental-and-behavioral-needs. Accessed September 12, 2017

29. McMillan JA, Land M Jr, Leslie LK. Pediatric residency education and the behavioral and mental health crisis: a call to action. *Pediatrics*. 2017;139(1): e20162141

30. McMillan JA, Land ML Jr, Rodday AM, et al. Report of a joint Association of Pediatric Program Directors-American Board of Pediatrics workshop: Preparing Future Pediatricians for the Mental Health Crisis. *J Pediatr*. 2018; 201:285–291

31. Green CM, Foy JM, Earls MF; American Academy of Pediatrics, Committee on Psychosocial Aspects of Child and Family Health; Mental Health Leadership Work Group. Technical report: achieving the pediatric mental health competencies. *Pediatrics*. 2019;144(5): e20192758

32. Foy JM; American Academy of Pediatrics, Task Force on Mental Health. Enhancing pediatric mental health care: report from the American Academy of Pediatrics Task Force on Mental Health. Introduction. *Pediatrics*. 2010;125(suppl 3):S69–S74

33. Samsel C, Ribeiro M, Ibeziako P, DeMaso DR. Integrated behavioral health care in pediatric subspecialty clinics. *Child Adolesc Psychiatr Clin N Am*. 2017;26(4): 785–794

34. Bernal P. Hidden morbidity in pediatric primary care. *Pediatr Ann*. 2003;32(6): 413–418–422

35. Janssen JS. Medical trauma. Available at: https://www.socialworktoday.com/news/enews_0416_1.shtml. Accessed November 3, 2018

36. Marchette LK, Weisz JR. Practitioner Review: empirical evolution of youth psychotherapy toward transdiagnostic approaches. *J Child Psychol Psychiatry*. 2017;58(9):970–984

37. Wissow LS, van Ginneken N, Chandna J, Rahman A. Integrating children's mental health into primary care. *Pediatr Clin North Am*. 2016;63(1):97–113

38. Wissow L, Anthony B, Brown J, et al. A common factors approach to improving the mental health capacity of pediatric primary care. *Adm Policy Ment Health*. 2008;35(4):305–318

39. Wissow LS, Gadomski A, Roter D, et al. Improving child and parent mental health in primary care: a cluster-randomized trial of communication skills training. *Pediatrics*. 2008;121(2): 266–275

40. Chorpita BF, Daleiden EL, Weisz JR. Identifying and selecting the common elements of evidence based interventions: a distillation and matching model. *Ment Health Serv Res*. 2005;7(1):5–20

41. Chorpita BF, Daleiden EL, Park AL, et al. Child STEPs in California: a cluster randomized effectiveness trial comparing modular treatment with community implemented treatment for youth with anxiety, depression, conduct problems, or traumatic stress. *J Consult Clin Psychol*. 2017;85(1):13–25

42. Tynan WD, Baum R. *Adapting Psychosocial Interventions to Primary Care. Mental Health Care of Children and Adolescents: A Guide for Primary Care Clinicians*. Itasca, IL: American Academy of Pediatrics; 2018

43. Kemper KJ, Vora S, Walls R; Task Force on Complementary and Alternative Medicine; Provisional Section on Complementary, Holistic, and Integrative Medicine. American Academy of Pediatrics. The use of complementary and alternative medicine in pediatrics. *Pediatrics*. 2008; 122(6):1374–1386. Reaffirmed January 2013

44. Sanders MR, Bor W, Morawska A. Maintenance of treatment gains: a comparison of enhanced, standard, and self-directed Triple P-Positive Parenting Program. *J Abnorm Child Psychol*. 2007;35(6):983–998

45. High PC, Klass P; Council on Early Childhood. Literacy promotion: an essential component of primary care pediatric practice. *Pediatrics*. 2014; 134(2):404–409

46. Yogman M, Garner A, Hutchinson J, Hirsh-Pasek K, Golinkoff RM; Committee on Psychosocial Aspects of Child and Family Health; Council on Communications and Media. The power of play: a pediatric role in enhancing development in young children. *Pediatrics*. 2018;142(3):e20182058

47. Howard BJ. Guidelines for Special Time. In: Jellinek M, Patel BP, Froehle MC, eds. *Bright Futures in Practice: Mental Health—Volume II. Tool Kit*. Arlington, VA: National Center for Education in Maternal and Child Health; 2002

48. van Straten A, Cuijpers P, Smits N. Effectiveness of a Web-based self-help intervention for symptoms of depression, anxiety, and stress:

randomized controlled trial. *J Med Internet Res*. 2008;10(1):e7

49. Foy JM, ed. *Promoting Mental Health in Children and Adolescents: Primary Care Practice and Advocacy*. Itasca, IL: American Academy of Pediatrics; 2018

50. Weersing VR, Brent DA, Rozenman MS, et al. Brief behavioral therapy for pediatric anxiety and depression in primary care: a randomized clinical trial. *JAMA Psychiatry*. 2017;74(6): 571–578

51. Walkup JT, Mathews T, Green CM. Transdiagnostic behavioral therapies in pediatric primary care: looking ahead. *JAMA Psychiatry*. 2017;74(6):557–558

52. Leslie LK, Mehus CJ, Hawkins JD, et al. Primary health care: potential home for family-focused preventive interventions. *Am J Prev Med*. 2016;51(4 suppl 2): S106–S118

53. Accreditation Council on Graduate Medical Education. ACGME core competencies. Available at: https://www.ecfmg.org/echo/acgme-core-competencies.html. Accessed March 9, 2018

54. Knapp P, Chait A, Pappadopulos E, Crystal S, Jensen PS; T-MAY Steering Group. Treatment of maladaptive aggression in youth: CERT guidelines I. Engagement, assessment, and management. *Pediatrics*. 2012;129(6). Available at: www.pediatrics.org/cgi/content/full/129/6/e1562

55. Scotto Rosato N, Correll CU, Pappadopulos E, Chait A, Crystal S, Jensen PS; Treatment of Maladaptive Aggressive in Youth Steering Committee. Treatment of maladaptive aggression in youth: CERT guidelines II. Treatments and ongoing management. *Pediatrics*. 2012;129(6). Available at: www.pediatrics.org/cgi/content/full/129/6/e1577

56. Shain BN; Committee on Adolescence. Collaborative role of the pediatrician in the diagnosis and management of bipolar disorder in adolescents. *Pediatrics*. 2012;130(6). Available at: www.pediatrics.org/cgi/content/full/130/6/e1725

57. Stille CJ. Communication, comanagement, and collaborative care for children and youth with special healthcare needs. *Pediatr Ann*. 2009; 38(9):498–504

58. American Academy of Pediatrics. Mental health initiatives: HIPAA privacy rule and provider to provider communication. Available at: https://www.aap.org/en-us/advocacy-and-policy/aap-health-initiatives/Mental-Health/Pages/HIPAA-Privacy-Rule-and-Provider-to-Provider-Communication.aspx. Accessed March 9, 2018

59. Office of the Federal Register. Confidentiality of substance use disorder patient records. Available at: https://www.federalregister.gov/documents/2017/01/18/2017-00719/confidentiality-of-substance-use-disorder-patient-records. Accessed March 9, 2018

60. Zero to Three. *DC:0-5 Diagnostic Classification of Mental Health and Developmental Disorders of Infancy and Early Childhood*. Washington, DC: Zero to Three; 1994. Available at: https://www.zerotothree.org/our-work/dc-0-5. Accessed November 1, 2017

61. American Academy of Pediatrics. *Addressing Mental Health Concerns in Primary Care: A Clinician's Toolkit*. Elk Grove Village, IL: American Academy of Pediatrics; 2010

62. Adam H, Foy J. *Signs and Symptoms in Pediatrics*. Elk Grove Village, IL: American Academy of Pediatrics; 2015

63. McInerny TK, Adam HM, Campbell DE, eds, et al. *Textbook of Pediatric Care*, 2nd ed. Elk Grove Village, IL: American Academy of Pediatrics; 2016

64. American Academy of Pediatrics. Pediatric care online. Available at: https://pediatriccare.solutions.aap.org/Pediatric-Care.aspx. Accessed November 3, 2018

65. Knapp P. The Iterative Mental Health Assessment. In: Foy JM, ed. *Mental Health Care of Children and Adolescents: A Guide for Primary Care Clinicians*, vol. Vol 1. Itasca, IL: American Academy of Pediatrics; 2018:pp 173–226

66. Wissow LS. Anxiety and Trauma-Related Distress. In: Foy JM, ed. *Mental Health Care of Children and Adolescents: A Guide for Primary Care Clinicians*, vol. Vol 1. Itasca, IL: American Academy of Pediatrics; 2018:pp 433–456

67. Baum R, Campo J. Medically Unexplained Symptoms. In: Foy JM, ed. *Mental Health Care of Children and Adolescents: A Guide for Primary Care Clinicians*, vol. Vol 1. Itasca, IL: American Academy of Pediatrics; 2018:pp 649–659

68. Schneider M, Fisher M. Eating Abnormalities. In: Foy JM, ed. *Mental Health Care of Children and Adolescents: A Guide for Primary Care Clinicians*, vol. Vol 1. Itasca, IL: American Academy of Pediatrics; 2018:pp 477–506

69. Angold A, Costello EJ, Farmer EM, Burns BJ, Erkanli A. Impaired but undiagnosed. *J Am Acad Child Adolesc Psychiatry*. 1999;38(2):129–137

70. Lewinsohn PM, Shankman SA, Gau JM, Klein DN. The prevalence and co-morbidity of subthreshold psychiatric conditions. *Psychol Med*. 2004;34(4): 613–622

71. Wolraich M, Brown L, Brown RT, et al; Subcommittee on Attention-Deficit/Hyperactivity Disorder; Steering Committee on Quality Improvement and Management. ADHD: clinical practice guideline for the diagnosis, evaluation, and treatment of attention-deficit/hyperactivity disorder in children and adolescents. *Pediatrics*. 2011;128(5): 1007–1022

72. Zuckerbrot RA, Cheung A, Jensen PS, Stein REK, Laraque D; GLAD-PC Steering Group. Guidelines for Adolescent Depression in Primary Care (GLAD-PC): part I. practice preparation, identification, assessment, and initial management. *Pediatrics*. 2018;141(3): e20174081

73. Cheung AH, Zuckerbrot RA, Jensen PS, Laraque D, Stein REK; GLAD-PC STEERING GROUP. Guidelines for Adolescent Depression in Primary Care (GLAD-PC): part II. Treatment and ongoing management. *Pediatrics*. 2018;141(3): e20174082

74. Levy SJ, Williams JF; Committee on Substance Use and Prevention. Substance use screening, brief intervention, and referral to treatment. *Pediatrics*. 2016;138(1):e20161211

75. Gleason MM, Egger HL, Emslie GJ, et al. Psychopharmacological treatment for very young children: contexts and guidelines. *J Am Acad Child Adolesc Psychiatry*. 2007;46(12):1532–1572

76. The MTA Cooperative Group. Multimodal Treatment Study of Children with ADHD. A 14-month randomized clinical trial of treatment strategies for attention-deficit/hyperactivity disorder. *Arch Gen Psychiatry.* 1999;56(12):1073–1086

77. Walkup JT, Albano AM, Piacentini J, et al. Cognitive behavioral therapy, sertraline, or a combination in childhood anxiety. *N Engl J Med.* 2008;359(26):2753–2766

78. March J, Silva S, Petrycki S, et al; Treatment for Adolescents With Depression Study (TADS) Team. Fluoxetine, cognitive-behavioral therapy, and their combination for adolescents with depression: Treatment for Adolescents With Depression Study (TADS) randomized controlled trial. *JAMA.* 2004;292(7):807–820

79. Wissow LS. Low Mood. In: Foy JM, ed. *Mental Health Care of Children and Adolescents: A Guide for Primary Care Clinicians*, vol. Vol 1. Itasca, IL: American Academy of Pediatrics; 2018: pp 617–636

80. Smith BL. Inappropriate prescribing. *Monit Psychol.* 2012;43(6):36

81. Riddle MA, ed. *Pediatric Psychopharmacology for Primary Care.* Elk Grove Village, IL: American Academy of Pediatrics; 2015

82. Stein RE, Storfer-Isser A, Kerker BD, et al. Beyond ADHD: how well are we doing? *Acad Pediatr.* 2016;16(2):115–121

83. Horwitz SM, Storfer-Isser A, Kerker BD, et al. Barriers to the identification and management of psychosocial problems: changes from 2004 to 2013. *Acad Pediatr.* 2015;15(6):613–620

84. Hudson CG. Disparities in the geography of mental health: implications for social work. *Soc Work.* 2012;57(2):107–119

Metabolic and Bariatric Surgery for Pediatric Patients With Severe Obesity

• *Technical Report*

TECHNICAL REPORT

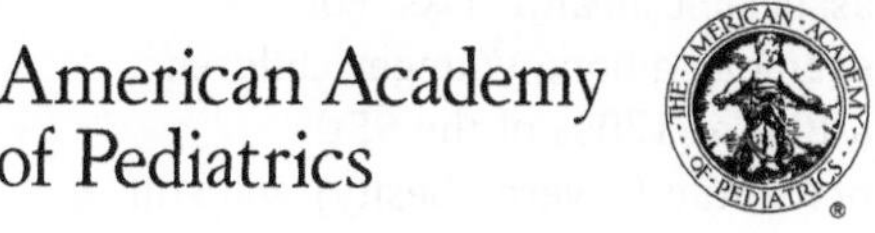

Metabolic and Bariatric Surgery for Pediatric Patients With Severe Obesity

Christopher F. Bolling, MD, FAAP,[a] Sarah C. Armstrong, MD, FAAP,[b] Kirk W. Reichard, MD, MBA, FAAP,[c] Marc P. Michalsky, MD, FACS, FAAP, FASMBS,[d] SECTION ON OBESITY, SECTION ON SURGERY

abstract

Severe obesity affects the health and well-being of millions of children and adolescents in the United States and is widely considered to be an "epidemic within an epidemic" that poses a major public health crisis. Currently, few effective treatments for severe obesity exist. Metabolic and bariatric surgery are existing but underuse treatment options for pediatric patients with severe obesity. Roux-en-Y gastric bypass and vertical sleeve gastrectomy are the most commonly performed metabolic and bariatric procedures in the United States and have been shown to result in sustained short-, mid-, and long-term weight loss, with associated resolution of multiple obesity-related comorbid diseases. Substantial evidence supports the safety and effectiveness of surgical weight loss for children and adolescents, and robust best practice guidelines for these procedures exist.

[a]Department of Pediatrics, College of Medicine, University of Cincinnati and Cincinnati Children's Hospital Medical Center, Cincinnati, Ohio; [b]Departments of Pediatrics and Population Health Sciences, Duke Center for Childhood Obesity Research, and Duke Clinical Research Institute, Duke University, Durham, North Carolina; [c]Division of Pediatric Surgery, Nemours/Alfred I. duPont Hospital for Children, Wilmington, Delaware; and [d]Department of Pediatric Surgery, College of Medicine, The Ohio State University and Nationwide Children's Hospital, Columbus, Ohio

Technical reports from the American Academy of Pediatrics benefit from expertise and resources of liaisons and internal (AAP) and external reviewers. However, technical reports from the American Academy of Pediatrics may not reflect the views of the liaisons or the organizations or government agencies that they represent.

Dr Armstrong conceptualized and contributed to the content for the initial manuscript, contributed the clinical perspective of the recommendations, and contributed to revisions and critical edits of the entire manuscript; Dr Bolling conceptualized and contributed to the content for the initial manuscript, was responsible for the initial drafting of the manuscript, contributed the clinical perspective of the recommendations, and contributed to revisions and critical edits of the entire manuscript; Drs Michalsky and Reichard conceptualized and contributed to the content for the initial manuscript, contributed the surgical perspective and the enrollment criteria table, and contributed to revisions and critical edits of the entire manuscript; and all authors approved the final manuscript as submitted and agree to be accountable for all aspects of the work.

The guidance in this report does not indicate an exclusive course of treatment or serve as a standard of medical care. Variations, taking into account individual circumstances, may be appropriate.

All technical reports from the American Academy of Pediatrics automatically expire 5 years after publication unless reaffirmed, revised, or retired at or before that time.

To cite: Bolling CF, Armstrong SC, Reichard KW, et al. AAP SECTION ON OBESITY, SECTION ON SURGERY. Metabolic and Bariatric Surgery for Pediatric Patients With Severe Obesity. *Pediatrics.* 2019;144(6):e20193224

DEFINITION OF SEVERE OBESITY AND EPIDEMIOLOGY

This technical report uses the term "pediatric" in reference to a person under 18 years of age. Although the term "adolescent" may be defined differently in various studies and clinical settings, this technical report uses "adolescent" to refer to a person aged 13 to 18 years. Although BMI percentile for age and sex is widely used to define weight status in the pediatric population regarding underweight, normal weight, overweight, and obesity, the BMI percentile, BMI *z* score, and several other established methods of measurement have significant limitations when applied to populations at the highest and lowest ends of the obesity spectrum. In addition, these measures often do not change greatly even when significant weight loss occurs. For these reasons, the preferred method of reporting weight status in severe obesity is as a percentage over the 95th BMI percentile for age and sex.[1]

Although adults with class 2 obesity have an absolute BMI of 35 or higher, direct correlation within the pediatric population requires some additional consideration. Specifically, because BMI values increase over time from age 2 to 18 years, the use of absolute BMI is generally not considered an accurate surrogate for adiposity and may either over- or underestimate associated health risks. For example, among younger children, a BMI at 120% of the 95th percentile (severe obesity) will still be well below an absolute BMI of 35. In addition, adolescents, who are often near adult heights, can have a BMI of 35, thereby meeting the adult definition of class 2 obesity, but this BMI may be below 120% of the 95th percentile. As a result, severe obesity in children and adolescents is defined as having a BMI ≥35 or a BMI that is ≥120% of the 95th percentile for age and sex, whichever is lower. This definition of "severe obesity," per the American Heart Association, is an appropriate point of reference for use in children and adolescents 2 years and older.[1,2] Cut points to define severe obesity are meant to identify patients at greatest risk for developing chronic and progressive disease states (ie, hypertension, impaired glucose metabolism, dyslipidemia, etc) because of their weight status.[1] The World Health Organization's classification of obesity in adults, which is helpful in discussing the likelihood of comorbidities, has prompted the use of obesity classifications in youth. Class 2 obesity is defined as having a BMI ≥120% of the 95th percentile or BMI ≥35, and class 3 obesity is defined as having a BMI ≥140% of the 95th percentile or BMI ≥40. As with many illnesses, patient populations of racial or ethnic minorities or with limited resources experience the majority of disease burden. African American and Hispanic populations have been shown to have 1.5 to 2 times the prevalence of severe obesity when compared with age-matched white counterparts.[1] American Indian youth are also at increased risk for severe obesity and especially weight-related type 2 diabetes mellitus.[3] In addition, when controlling for race and ethnicity, lower socioeconomic status is associated with higher prevalence of severe obesity; this effect is most pronounced in girls and is present across all age groups.[4]

Prevalence of obesity remains well above historic norms and continues to increase in low-income populations and in certain racial and ethnic populations.[5] In addition, the prevalence of severe obesity is increasing at a greater rate among all groups and most significantly among adolescents.[2] Data from 2014 reveal that nearly 10% of adolescents were identified as having class 2 obesity (BMI ≥120% of the 95th percentile or BMI ≥35) and that 5% were identified as having class 3 obesity (BMI ≥140% of the 95th percentile or BMI ≥40). These results represent a dramatic increase from the estimated rate of class 2 obesity or higher in 1999 as 1.3%.[6] When combined with the high probability of corresponding obesity in adulthood[7] and the anticipated cumulative impact of related comorbid diseases, the prevalence of severe obesity has been appropriately described as an "epidemic within an epidemic."

The increase of severe obesity and its associated illnesses has resulted in a treatment crisis. Although behavioral and lifestyle interventions will be successful for certain individuals, the overall outcomes of behavioral and lifestyle interventions are discouraging when viewed as a solution for a larger number of patients with severe obesity.[8–12] Youth with severe obesity require effective intervention to prevent a lifetime of illness and poor quality of life.

CONSIDERATIONS FOR PURSUING METABOLIC AND BARIATRIC SURGERY

Patient age as well as multiple variables related to developmental maturity factor into the decision and optimal timing for metabolic and bariatric surgery. Recent data from the Teen-Longitudinal Assessment of Bariatric Surgery (Teen-LABS) study reveal that patients undergoing a weight loss procedure (ages 12–28 years, with a mean age of 17 years) demonstrate a direct correlation between increasing preoperative BMI and a higher probability of presenting with multiple comorbid conditions and/or associated cardiovascular risk factors.[13,14] Furthermore, evidence suggests that individuals who present with the highest BMI levels at the time of surgical intervention (ie, BMI >50) are less likely to achieve a nonobesity state (ie, BMI <30) after a successful operation.[15,16] Correspondingly, recent data from the Teen-LABS consortium have revealed that increased weight loss after bariatric surgery, female sex, and younger age at the time of surgical intervention serve to independently predict an increased likelihood of improvement in a number of cardiovascular risk factors (ie, elevated blood pressure, dyslipidemia, and abnormally elevated levels of high-sensitivity C-reactive protein).[14] Additionally, resolution of comorbid disease occurs before a normal weight is achieved. Collectively, such results suggest that optimal timing of metabolic and bariatric surgery for children and adolescents, designed to maximize long-term health benefits, warrants further research, clinical consideration, and potential refinements.

Barriers to insurance coverage occur for more than half of adolescents seeking treatment, which delay care.[17] These barriers are especially acute for patients from racial and ethnic minorities.[18,19] These barriers seem most related to economic disadvantage.[20] For a patient who meets criteria and whose family wishes to pursue surgical treatment, the process would ideally begin as soon as possible. Clinicians can balance the child's psychological and developmental understanding of the procedure and the likelihood of successful weight loss through behavioral modifications with potential benefits for health and quality of life with surgical intervention.

Preparing a patient for metabolic and bariatric surgery starts with a realistic discussion of the available treatment options (ie, choosing a specific weight loss procedure) and likely expected outcomes with the patient and family. At present time, payers often require documentation of previous weight loss attempts and frequently require documentation of other related medical and behavioral evaluations. Although success rates are low, some youth with severe obesity will respond to behavioral interventions. Documentation of these interventions, even when unsuccessful, can assist in preparing a patient for surgical intervention. Understanding various payer-specific mandates for approval of insurance coverage of surgical weight loss can be both confusing and time consuming for health care providers and patients and their families. An equally important part of the initial conversation with a patient and family is the identification of a local or regional tertiary care facility that is equipped to provide ongoing bariatric surgical care to the pediatric population.

Ideally, early communication with a local or regional center may serve to streamline the process by establishing the need for various mandatory components of the preoperative evaluation. Although most centers rely on comprehensive multidisciplinary resources to conduct the necessary preoperative evaluation, the development of a focused collaboration between a pediatric weight loss center and a pediatric or other primary care practice can serve to expedite the process. Whether conducted entirely by the referring practice, by the weight loss treatment center, or as an established collaborative effort, the preoperative evaluation may include evidence of regular visits with the multidisciplinary weight loss team and evidence that comorbid conditions have been screened for and appropriately managed. Additionally, a multidisciplinary weight loss team can screen for and treat genetic disorders (eg, Bardet-Biedl syndrome and Prader-Willi syndrome) and selective hormonal abnormalities (eg, proopiomelanocortin mutations and leptin deficiency) that can be medically managed. A comprehensive evaluation by a behavioral health clinician is essential early in the process to document the child's psychological well-being or to document an effective treatment plan, if indicated, for behavioral health concerns. In addition, a pediatric mental health clinician who has experience with obesity is able to document that the child has the necessary social and emotional support to follow through with required postoperative lifestyle modifications.

The patient's primary care pediatrician plays an important role in the perioperative period by monitoring progress and recognizing and reporting symptoms to the surgical program. Long-term follow-up requires monitoring the patient's progress, including weight regain and nutritional status. Adolescent girls undergoing metabolic and bariatric surgery have a higher risk for pregnancy than peers,[21] and pediatricians can discuss this risk and develop a family-planning approach before surgery. Specific discussions related to reproductive health and various options for appropriate contraception can be a shared decision between the provider and patient as well as the family, as desired by the patient.

Studies reveal a small risk for anemia and bone mineral density loss among adolescents after metabolic and bariatric surgery.[22] Evidence on specific pre- and postoperative laboratory studies is lacking. Pediatricians or surgeons may obtain routine laboratory test results as indicated by the procedure and patient. Particular attention should be focused on the need to monitor and address potential long-term micronutrient deficiencies in the postoperative period. Although psychosocial functioning and health-related quality of life usually improve after metabolic and bariatric surgery,[10] pediatric patients with preexisting emotional concerns may require additional and ongoing evaluation postoperatively. In addition, adolescents may develop risk-taking behaviors, including increased use of alcohol, increased sexual activity, and suicide ideation, after surgery.[21,23–25]

COMMON WEIGHT LOSS PROCEDURES AND THEIR OUTCOMES

Roux-en-Y Gastric Bypass

Roux-en-Y gastric bypass (RYGB) has been considered the gold standard for the surgical management of severe obesity in adults[26–28] and adolescents.[29–31] Like all contemporary weight loss operations, RYGB is performed by using minimally invasive surgical techniques (ie, laparoscopic surgery) and results in significant and sustained weight loss from alterations in appetite, satiety, and regulation of energy balance.[32] RYGB requires the creation a small proximal gastric pouch in combination with an accompanying roux limb of jejunum, which effectively excludes the remaining stomach (ie, gastric remnant), and proximal small bowel from the stream of ingested enteral content. The resulting anatomy creates a direct conduit between the newly established gastric pouch and jejunum, resulting in a "downstream" exposure of enteral content to the important biliopancreatic enzymes.

Vertical Sleeve Gastrectomy

Vertical sleeve gastrectomy (VSG) emerged as an alternative weight loss procedure in both adults and youth in the mid-2000s and is currently the most common bariatric operation performed in the United States.[27,33] Current evidence suggests that altered gastric emptying and neurohormonal mechanisms may also be involved in achieving weight loss.[34] The VSG involves removal of ~80% of the stomach (consisting of the entire greater curve), resulting in a gastric sleeve (60–100 mL capacity). Creation of a uniformly fashioned sleeve is typically accomplished by using surgical dilators as a guide that range in size from 36F to 44F catheter diameter. Because the pylorus and distal antrum are anatomically preserved, gastric filling and emptying remain largely intact, resulting in enhanced postprandial satiety while avoiding the intestinal "dumping syndrome" that can occur after RYGB. Because VSG does not include creation of a gastrojejunostomy (ie, intestinal bypass), malabsorption and the complications stemming from more complex surgical anatomy are less frequent.[35] As is the case in adults,[26] major complications in adolescents after VSG are less common than after RYGB and include staple-line leak, stricture formation, and bleeding.[36] Nutritional complications are also less common with VSG than with RYGB and include iron deficiency and vitamin B_{12} deficiency, presumably related to decreased production of intrinsic factor resulting from the loss of the gastric fundus.[36]

Laparoscopic Adjustable Gastric Band

The laparoscopic adjustable gastric band (LAGB) is an implantable device consisting of a silastic belt lined by a soft, low-pressure, adjustable balloon that is placed around the proximal portion of the stomach in a circumferential fashion (ie, immediately beneath the gastroesophageal junction). The creation of a "pseudo-pouch" at the proximal end of the stomach limits food intake and promotes early satiety because of its restrictive properties. The balloon is connected to a small subcutaneous fluid reservoir positioned on the abdominal wall. In an outpatient setting, the volume of the balloon lining the band may be adjusted by percutaneous infusion or aspiration of sterile water from the subcutaneous port. The ability to modulate the narrowness of the band limits food intake but does not affect physiologic pathways regulating energy balance, appetite, or satiety. as in RYGB or VSG. Although initially believed to be a desirable option for the adolescent population on the basis of several short-term safety and efficacy reports,[27] a relative paucity of longitudinal outcomes in combination with reports of weight regain and high device-explant rates in both adult[37] and adolescent[38] populations have dampened enthusiasm for this procedure. Complications associated with LAGB include port and catheter disruption, proximal gastric pouch dilatation, gastric erosion, and esophageal dysfunction. Explant rates may exceed 20%, and those procedures are associated with increased morbidity.[39] To date, use of the adjustable gastric band has been restricted to individuals 18 years and older by the US Food and Drug Administration.

Complications and Outcomes

Surgical complications after bariatric surgery in adolescents are infrequent, with the majority being defined as minor (15%) and occurring in the early postoperative period (eg, postoperative nausea and dehydration).[35,36,40] Major perioperative complications (30 days) occurred in 8% of Teen-LABS participants. In addition, reoperation before hospital discharge was required in 2.7%, which is similar to recent outcomes reported in a large adult series.[41] Micronutrient deficiencies are common after both RYGB (iron, 66%; vitamin B_{12}, 8%; folate, 6%) and VSG (iron, 32%; folate, 10%).[36] Vitamin D deficiency is common preoperatively among teenagers with obesity and does not change significantly after surgery.[36] Folate deficiency is a concern for female patients of childbearing age.[36] However, most longitudinal studies of adolescent metabolic and bariatric surgery do not assess nutrient deficiency or follow a patient through subsequent pregnancy to assess for related complications.[40] In addition, although data related to psychosocial complications after weight loss surgery in adolescents are relatively sparse, recent data citing an increased risk of poor mental health in the postoperative time period among individuals with higher levels of anxiety, depression, and poor mental health highlights the need for long-term follow-up.[25] Although no perioperative deaths were reported in the Teen-LABS, Adolescent Morbid Obesity Surgery (AMOS), or Follow-up of Adolescent Bariatric Surgery at 5 Plus Years (FABS-5+) cohorts, 3 deaths (0.3%) occurred postoperatively at 9 months (related to infectious colitis),[16] 3.3 years (related to hypoglycemic complications in a patient with type 1 diabetes),[36] and 6 years (unrelated), respectively, collectively representing a recently reported 0.3% mortality rate.[40]

Several recent prospective multi-institutional studies have helped to define weight loss and comorbidity outcomes for bariatric surgical procedures in adolescents. The Teen-LABS study consortium has published 3-year outcomes from the first large (242 subjects), prospective, observational study in patients younger than 19 years undergoing RYGB and VSG, with an overall follow-up rate of 89%.[36] Although the study was not specifically designed to detect between-group differences, total weight loss at 3 years was 27% in all patients and was similar for both procedures. Comorbidity resolution rates, including type 2 diabetes mellitus (95%), hypertension (80%), and dyslipidemia (66%), exceeded those reported in similar adult cohorts.[25] In a more recent analysis, researchers examined changes in overall prevalence of baseline cardiovascular disease risk factors in the same cohort as well as predictors of such change. There was an 85% reduction in the overall multiplicity of associated risk factors, whereby one-third (33%) of study participants had ≥3 risk factors at baseline (preoperatively), with only 5% demonstrating a similar degree by 3 years.[14] Improvements in certain variables (ie, dyslipidemia, elevated blood pressure, impaired glucose metabolism, and systemic inflammation) in association with increasing weight loss were not unexpected. Investigators also observed in postanalysis studies that after surgery, younger participants were more likely to experience improvements in dyslipidemia and elevated high-sensitivity C-reactive protein levels compared with older patients and that female patients were more likely than male patients to experience significant improvements in blood pressure. These results are novel and offer new insights into long-term outcomes and support ongoing refinement in the evolving selection criteria and optimal timing of bariatric surgery in this age group.[14]

In the AMOS study, a prospective, controlled, and nonrandomized interventional study, researchers compared 80 adolescents undergoing RYGB with a matched cohort of adults of a parallel study after metabolic and bariatric surgery as well as a matched control group of adolescents undergoing conventional medical treatment of obesity in Sweden.[42] Recently reported outcomes from this comparative analysis revealed a significant reduction in both weight and BMI at 5 years among adolescents that was strikingly similar to results observed among the parallel adult subjects. In addition, the study authors reported substantial improvements in several comorbidities and cardiovascular risk factors. These results compared favorably with those of the adolescent nonsurgical control group. Furthermore, the AMOS study revealed a 92% resolution in elevated liver transaminase levels in patients after surgery versus an 18% resolution rate in control patients.[39] To date, the FABS-5+ study is the longest prospective longitudinal analysis of subjects undergoing adolescent metabolic and bariatric surgery, consisting of 58 adolescent patients undergoing RYGB (mean age, 17.1 years), with a mean follow-up of 8.0 years (range, 5.4–12.5 years). The FABS-5+ study revealed a 29% long-term reduction in preoperative BMI as well as a significant reduction in elevated blood pressure, type 2 diabetes mellitus, and dyslipidemia.[16] The effect on type 2 diabetes mellitus is especially striking. Surgical intervention results in better outcomes than medical management in youth with severe obesity and type 2 diabetes mellitus.[43,44]

In no prospective studies is the efficacy of the various weight loss surgery procedures in pediatric patients directly compared, but a recent meta-analysis revealed that 1-year outcomes favored laparoscopic RYGB over LAGB, with intermediate results achieved in a small group of patients who underwent laparoscopic VSG.[45] In 1 single institutional retrospective comparison, adolescents undergoing laparoscopic VSG lost twice as much weight as those undergoing LAGB at 24 months.[46] Two smaller retrospective studies suggest similar weight loss in adults and adolescents after laparoscopic VSG (1 and 2 years) and LAGB (1 year).[27] Finally, in a single-institution longitudinal-outcome study of adolescents undergoing laparoscopic RYGB, the total weight loss percentage (37%) was independent of the baseline BMI, and patients with lower baseline BMIs were more likely to achieve normal weight at 1 year.[15] The results of this analysis raise the possibility of a therapeutic "ceiling effect" and may, if confirmed, support the need for changes in current referral patterns so that potential candidates may benefit from surgical consultation before reaching extremely high BMI levels (ie, ≥50).

Clear evidence pointing to "the best" or most appropriate weight loss procedure for pediatric patients with severe obesity remains elusive. RYGB was, by far, the most common weight loss surgical procedure used among adolescents in the early 2000s,[47] with LAGB gaining popularity later in the decade,[48] only to be followed quickly by the emergence of the VSG as a primary operation. Although an analysis of weight loss surgical procedural prevalence in the United States from the early 2010s reveals an equal proportion of VSGs and RYGBs, more recent data have suggested that VSG has become the most commonly performed weight loss operation among adolescents, reflecting a pattern similar to the one observed in the adult population.[33] As in the adult population, the use of the LAGB in adolescents has dramatically declined in frequency.[33,35] Despite the presence of comparative results between RYGB and VSG that suggest similar surgical outcomes, there is still a need for prospective studies, controlling for confounding variables and potential selection bias.

THE CURRENT CLIMATE FOR PEDIATRIC METABOLIC AND BARIATRIC SURGERY

Access to Care

No unified reporting system tracks the overall procedural prevalence of pediatric metabolic and bariatric surgery in the United States. This paucity of data prevents the establishment of an accurate assessment of current access to bariatric surgical care. According to recent cross-sectional data, approximately 4 million adolescents have severe obesity.[6] In a recent analysis of discharge data obtained from the Healthcare Cost and Utilization Project Kids' Inpatient Database, Kelleher et al[49] showed an increase in procedural prevalence from 0.8 per 100 000 adolescents in 2000 to 2.3 per 100 000 in 2003, resulting in approximately 1000 cases per year. However, the investigators reported no subsequent change in the annual rate of adolescent weight loss procedures between 2003 and 2009.[49] In an additional report, Zwintscher et al[48] identified as many as 1600 adolescent patients from the same database, suggesting that procedural prevalence has likely continued to increase, albeit representing a fraction of the overall procedural prevalence when compared with the adult population. Low rates of metabolic and bariatric surgery in the adolescent population are likely to be multifactorial. Availability of surgical options, physician attitudes regarding surgery, and individual assessment of likely patient outcome from surgery all appear to influence whether patients are referred for surgical evaluation.[50,51]

For example, recent reports from both the United States and the United Kingdom highlight the potential impact of differing attitudes toward the use of metabolic and bariatric surgery in the pediatric population (including the potential differences in associated referral patterns) among medical versus surgical health care providers.[50,52] In addition, recent data used to examine insurance coverage for adolescent metabolic and bariatric surgery in the United States reveal reduced approvals in comparison with those for adults seeking similar coverage.[17] In this multi-institutional review, Inge et al[17] showed that payers initially approved metabolic and bariatric surgery for less than half of adolescents who met the requirements. In contrast, payers initially approved 80% to 85% of adults who met similar criteria. Ultimately, 80% of adolescents received insurance approval, but it required patients, physicians, families, and support staff to engage in complex and time-consuming appeals processes. Adolescents seeking metabolic and bariatric surgery were required to appeal unfavorable coverage decisions as many as 5 times before obtaining the required authorization. The implications of such disparity in access to specialized health care compared with adults with severe obesity undergoing bariatric surgery, commonly during the fifth or sixth generation of life, becomes even more compelling considering the cumulative impact of numerous obesity-related disorders potentially leading to reduced quality of life and early mortality in younger patients. Limited studies indicate that the improvement in comorbidities may enhance the cost-effectiveness of adolescent metabolic and bariatric surgery.[53,54]

Best Practice Guidelines and National Accreditation Standards

Metabolic and bariatric surgery in the treatment of severe obesity was first described in the late 1950s and early 1960s in the adult population and led to the establishment of formalized clinical guidelines in the 1990s with the release of the National Institutes of Health consensus guidelines statement.[55] A corresponding framework for clinical eligibility in the pediatric population, however, has only emerged within the past 2 decades. Initial consensus-driven recommendations were predicated on the previously established adult clinical guidelines, including an overall assessment of related comorbid diseases in combination with the use of anthropomorphic criteria (ie, minimal BMI).[56] In contrast to the adult model, these initial recommendations called for a more conservative approach regarding minimal eligibility criteria (ie, BMI ≥40 in the presence of severe obesity-related comorbidities or BMI ≥50 with or without severe comorbid disease). The most recently updated guidelines from the American Society of Metabolic and Bariatric Surgery (ASMBS) follow evidence from several ongoing studies revealing favorable results.[57–59] In these updated guidelines, absolute age limits are eliminated, the World Health Organization weight classification is adopted, and the weight and comorbidity guidelines are brought into alignment with adult recommendations. Unlike clinical situations in which competing guidelines confuse care, the recommendations for weight loss surgery in children and adolescents are aligned and evidence based, yet they are not uniformly applied, creating barriers to accessing recommended care.

Consensus recommendations related to clinical criteria will likely continue to evolve in the decades to come. Best practice guidelines published by the ASMBS and pediatric-specific metabolic and bariatric surgery accreditation standards established by the joint ASMBS and American College of Surgeons Metabolic and Bariatric Surgery Quality Improvement Program establish a robust framework for the safe delivery of surgical weight management in the context of a multidisciplinary care model.[60] Clinical programs seeking pediatric accreditation within the Metabolic and Bariatric Surgery Quality Improvement Program are required to demonstrate access to child- and adolescent-specific clinical care resources designed to deliver optimal age-appropriate care. Such resources include incorporation of pediatric health care providers with expertise in general pediatric medicine, nutrition, anesthesia, and behavioral disciplines (www.mbsaqip.org).

Multidisciplinary Care Model

With recent interest in metabolic and bariatric surgery as safe and effective treatments of severe pediatric obesity, several important age-specific considerations have led to the development of child- and adolescent-specific clinical standards for perioperative evaluation, corresponding surgical care, and long-term follow-up. In expert recommendations established during the 2011 Children's Hospital Association multidisciplinary collaborative panel, FOCUS on a Fitter Future, which was commissioned to establish and disseminate expert recommendations pertaining to all aspects of childhood obesity prevention and treatment strategies, Michalsky et al[61] presented a consensus-driven road map for institutional development of age-appropriate weight loss surgical care. As a primary goal of the expert panel report, the authors highlighted the importance of multidisciplinary care, which maximizes child- and adolescent-specific health care resources to deliver optimal care. The report emphasized the need for an institutional commitment to a culture of clinical excellence and safety during the delivery of age-appropriate weight loss surgical care. The report also offered a point-by-point set of recommendations, including establishment of a "medical home" (ie, including the need to establish routine communication among members of the multidisciplinary weight loss team and the patient's primary care provider). Key components of the medical home for pediatric patients with severe obesity include the establishment of a "medical leader," a qualified pediatric medical provider with experience in the screening and treatment of common obesity-related comorbid conditions. The team of medical home providers may also include an adolescent-specific behavioral health specialist, a dedicated registered dietitian familiar with the management of individuals undergoing metabolic and bariatric surgery, a licensed social worker, and medical subspecialists required on a case-by-case basis (ie, cardiology, nephrology, gastroenterology and hepatology, endocrinology, etc).

The ASMBS has published best practice guidelines that include contemporary and consensus-driven clinical inclusion criteria.[57] A joint ASMBS–American College of Surgeons national accreditation standard recommendation details specific requirements for the delivery of weight loss surgical care for individuals younger than 18 years. All groups strongly support the thoughtful delivery of complex care for an emerging and vulnerable population. The Teen-LABS consortium has also published contemporary examples for implementation of this general framework for institutions considering the establishment of pediatric surgical weight management programs.[62] These works, along with the accompanying policy statement, "Pediatric Metabolic and Bariatric Surgery: Evidence, Barriers, and Best Practices,"[63] provide a coordinated and reinforcing view of the role of metabolic and bariatric surgery for youth with severe obesity.

CONCLUSIONS

Severe obesity in children and adolescents is a worsening health crisis in the United States. Unfortunately, severe obesity has few effective treatments. The application of metabolic and bariatric surgery in the pediatric population provides evidence-based effective treatment of severe obesity and related comorbid diseases.[14,16,36,42] Improved access to metabolic and bariatric surgery for pediatric patients with severe obesity is urgently needed. American Academy of Pediatrics policy recommendations regarding metabolic and bariatric surgery in pediatric patients can be found in the accompanying policy statement, "Pediatric Metabolic and Bariatric Surgery: Evidence, Barriers, and Best Practices."[63]

LEAD AUTHORS

Christopher F. Bolling, MD, FAAP
Sarah C. Armstrong, MD, FAAP
Kirk W. Reichard, MD, MBA, FAAP
Marc P. Michalsky, MD, FACS, FAAP, FASMBS

SECTION ON OBESITY EXECUTIVE COMMITTEE, 2017–2018

Christopher F. Bolling, MD, FAAP, Chairperson
Sarah C. Armstrong, MD, FAAP
Matthew Allen Haemer, MD, MPH, FAAP
Natalie Digate Muth, MD, MPH, RD, FAAP
John Conrad Rausch, MD, MPH, FAAP
Victoria Weeks Rogers, MD, FAAP

LIAISON

Marc P. Michalsky, MD, FACS, FAAP, FASMBS

CONSULTANT

Stephanie Walsh, MD, FAAP

STAFF

Mala Thapar, MPH

SECTION ON SURGERY EXECUTIVE COMMITTEE, 2017–2018

Kurt F. Heiss, MD, FAAP, Chairperson
Gail Ellen Besner, MD, FAAP
Cynthia D. Downard, MD, FAAP
Mary Elizabeth Fallat, MD, FAAP
Kenneth William Gow, MD FACS, FAAP

STAFF

Vivian Baldassari Thorne

ABBREVIATIONS

AMOS: Adolescent Morbid Obesity Surgery
ASMBS: American Society of Metabolic and Bariatric Surgery
FABS-5+: Follow-up of Adolescent Bariatric Surgery at 5 Plus Years
LAGB: laparoscopic adjustable gastricband
RYGB: Roux-en-Y gastric bypass
Teen-LABS: Teen-Longitudinal Assessment of Bariatric Surgery
VSG: vertical sleeve gastrectomy

This document is copyrighted and is property of the American Academy of Pediatrics and its Board of Directors. All authors have filed conflict of interest statements with the American Academy of Pediatrics. Any conflicts have been resolved through a process approved by the Board of Directors. The American Academy of Pediatrics has neither solicited nor accepted any commercial involvement in the development of the content of this publication.

DOI: https://doi.org/10.1542/peds.2019-3224

Address correspondence to Christopher F. Bolling, MD, FAAP. E-mail: bolling.cf@gmail.com

PEDIATRICS (ISSN Numbers: Print, 0031-4005; Online, 1098-4275).

Copyright © 2019 by the American Academy of Pediatrics

FINANCIAL DISCLOSURE: Dr Armstrong disclosed that she has a research relationship with AstraZeneca. Drs Bolling, Michalsky, and Reichard have indicated they have no financial relationships relevant to this article to disclose.

FUNDING: No external funding.

POTENTIAL CONFLICT OF INTEREST: The authors have indicated they have no potential conflicts of interest to disclose.

REFERENCES

1. Kelly AS, Barlow SE, Rao G, et al; American Heart Association Atherosclerosis, Hypertension, and Obesity in the Young Committee of the Council on Cardiovascular Disease in the Young, Council on Nutrition, Physical Activity and Metabolism, and Council on Clinical Cardiology. Severe obesity in children and adolescents: identification, associated health risks, and treatment approaches: a scientific statement from the American Heart Association. *Circulation*. 2013;128(15):1689–1712
2. Flegal KM, Wei R, Ogden CL, et al. Characterizing extreme values of body mass index-for-age by using the 2000 Centers for Disease Control and Prevention growth charts. *Am J Clin Nutr*. 2009;90(5):1314–1320
3. Wheelock KM, Sinha M, Knowler WC, et al. Metabolic risk factors and type 2 diabetes incidence in American Indian children. *J Clin Endocrinol Metab*. 2016;101(4):1437–1444
4. Skelton JA, Cook SR, Auinger P, Klein JD, Barlow SE. Prevalence and trends of severe obesity among US children and adolescents. *Acad Pediatr*. 2009;9(5):322–329
5. Ogden CL, Carroll MD, Curtin LR, Lamb MM, Flegal KM. Prevalence of high body mass index in US children and adolescents, 2007-2008. *JAMA*. 2010;303(3):242–249
6. Skinner AC, Skelton JA. Prevalence and trends in obesity and severe obesity among children in the United States, 1999-2012. *JAMA Pediatr*. 2014;168(6):561–566
7. Freedman DS, Mei Z, Srinivasan SR, Berenson GS, Dietz WH. Cardiovascular risk factors and excess adiposity among overweight children and adolescents: the Bogalusa Heart Study. *J Pediatr*. 2007;150(1):12–17.e2
8. Danielsson P, Kowalski J, Ekblom Ö, Marcus C. Response of severely obese children and adolescents to behavioral treatment. *Arch Pediatr Adolesc Med*. 2012;166(12):1103–1108
9. Johnston CA, Tyler C, Palcic JL, et al. Smaller weight changes in standardized body mass index in response to treatment as weight classification increases. *J Pediatr*. 2011;158(4):624–627
10. Kalarchian MA, Levine MD, Arslanian SA, et al. Family-based treatment of severe

pediatric obesity: randomized, controlled trial. *Pediatrics*. 2009;124(4): 1060–1068

11. Knop C, Singer V, Uysal Y, et al. Extremely obese children respond better than extremely obese adolescents to lifestyle interventions. *Pediatr Obes*. 2015;10(1):7–14

12. Levine MD, Ringham RM, Kalarchian MA, Wisniewski L, Marcus MD. Is family-based behavioral weight control appropriate for severe pediatric obesity? *Int J Eat Disord*. 2001;30(3): 318–328

13. Michalsky MP, Inge TH, Simmons M, et al; Teen-LABS Consortium. Cardiovascular risk factors in severely obese adolescents: the Teen Longitudinal Assessment of Bariatric Surgery (Teen-LABS) study. *JAMA Pediatr*. 2015;169(5):438–444

14. Michalsky MP, Inge TH, Jenkins TM, et al; Teen-LABS Consortium. Cardiovascular risk factors after adolescent bariatric surgery. *Pediatrics*. 2018;141(2): e20172485

15. Inge TH, Jenkins TM, Zeller M, et al. Baseline BMI is a strong predictor of nadir BMI after adolescent gastric bypass. *J Pediatr*. 2010;156(1): 103–108.e1

16. Inge TH, Jenkins TM, Xanthakos SA, et al. Long-term outcomes of bariatric surgery in adolescents with severe obesity (FABS-5+): a prospective follow-up analysis. *Lancet Diabetes Endocrinol*. 2017;5(3):165–173

17. Inge TH, Boyce TW, Lee M, et al. Access to care for adolescents seeking weight loss surgery. *Obesity (Silver Spring)*. 2014;22(12):2593–2597

18. Wee CC, Huskey KW, Bolcic-Jankovic D, et al. Sex, race, and consideration of bariatric surgery among primary care patients with moderate to severe obesity. *J Gen Intern Med*. 2014;29(1): 68–75

19. Stanford FC, Jones DB, Schneider BE, et al. Patient race and the likelihood of undergoing bariatric surgery among patients seeking surgery. *Surg Endosc*. 2015;29(9):2794–2799

20. Wallace AE, Young-Xu Y, Hartley D, Weeks WB. Racial, socioeconomic, and rural-urban disparities in obesity-related bariatric surgery. *Obes Surg*. 2010; 20(10):1354–1360

21. Roehrig HR, Xanthakos SA, Sweeney J, Zeller MH, Inge TH. Pregnancy after gastric bypass surgery in adolescents. *Obes Surg*. 2007;17(7):873–877

22. Kaulfers AM, Bean JA, Inge TH, Dolan LM, Kalkwarf HJ. Bone loss in adolescents after bariatric surgery. *Pediatrics*. 2011;127(4). Available at: www.pediatrics.org/cgi/content/full/127/4/e956

23. Ratcliff MB, Reiter-Purtill J, Inge TH, Zeller MH. Changes in depressive symptoms among adolescent bariatric candidates from preoperative psychological evaluation to immediately before surgery. *Surg Obes Relat Dis*. 2011;7(1):50–54

24. Zeller MH, Washington GA, Mitchell JE, et al; Teen-LABS Consortium; TeenView Study Group. Alcohol use risk in adolescents 2 years after bariatric surgery. *Surg Obes Relat Dis*. 2017; 13(1):85–94

25. Järvholm K, Karlsson J, Olbers T, et al. Characteristics of adolescents with poor mental health after bariatric surgery. *Surg Obes Relat Dis*. 2016; 12(4):882–890

26. Zhang Y, Wang J, Sun X, et al. Laparoscopic sleeve gastrectomy versus laparoscopic Roux-en-Y gastric bypass for morbid obesity and related comorbidities: a meta-analysis of 21 studies [published correction appears in *Obes Surg*. 2015;25(1):27]. *Obes Surg*. 2015;25(1):19–26

27. Zitsman JL, Inge TH, Reichard KW, et al. Pediatric and adolescent obesity: management, options for surgery, and outcomes. *J Pediatr Surg*. 2014;49(3): 491–494

28. Courcoulas AP, Christian NJ, Belle SH, et al; Longitudinal Assessment of Bariatric Surgery (LABS) Consortium. Weight change and health outcomes at 3 years after bariatric surgery among individuals with severe obesity. *JAMA*. 2013;310(22):2416–2425

29. Soper RT, Mason EE, Printen KJ, Zellweger H. Gastric bypass for morbid obesity in children and adolescents. *J Pediatr Surg*. 1975;10(1):51–58

30. Anderson AE, Soper RT, Scott DH. Gastric bypass for morbid obesity in children and adolescents. *J Pediatr Surg*. 1980;15(6):876–881

31. Wittgrove AC, Buchwald H, Sugerman H, Pories W; American Society for Bariatric Surgery. Surgery for severely obese adolescents: further insight from the American Society for Bariatric Surgery. *Pediatrics*. 2004;114(1): 253–254

32. Eickhoff H. Central modulation of energy homeostasis and cognitive performance after bariatric surgery. *Adv Neurobiol*. 2017;19:213–236

33. Reames BN, Finks JF, Bacal D, Carlin AM, Dimick JB. Changes in bariatric surgery procedure use in Michigan, 2006-2013. *JAMA*. 2014;312(9):959–961

34. Benaiges D, Más-Lorenzo A, Goday A, et al. Laparoscopic sleeve gastrectomy: more than a restrictive bariatric surgery procedure? *World J Gastroenterol*. 2015;21(41): 11804–11814

35. Inge TH, Zeller MH, Jenkins TM, et al; Teen-LABS Consortium. Perioperative outcomes of adolescents undergoing bariatric surgery: the Teen-Longitudinal Assessment of Bariatric Surgery (Teen-LABS) study. *JAMA Pediatr*. 2014;168(1): 47–53

36. Inge TH, Courcoulas AP, Jenkins TM, et al; Teen-LABS Consortium. Weight loss and health status 3 years after bariatric surgery in adolescents. *N Engl J Med*. 2016;374(2):113–123

37. Himpens J, Cadière GB, Bazi M, et al. Long-term outcomes of laparoscopic adjustable gastric banding. *Arch Surg*. 2011;146(7):802–807

38. Zitsman JL, DiGiorgi MF, Fennoy I, et al. Adolescent laparoscopic adjustable gastric banding (LAGB): prospective results in 137 patients followed for 3 years. *Surg Obes Relat Dis*. 2015; 11(1):101–109

39. Altieri MS, Yang J, Telem DA, et al. Lap band outcomes from 19,221 patients across centers and over a decade within the state of New York. *Surg Endosc*. 2016;30(5):1725–1732

40. Shoar S, Mahmoudzadeh H, Naderan M, et al. Long-term outcome of bariatric surgery in morbidly obese adolescents: a systematic review and meta-analysis of 950 patients with a minimum of

3 years follow-up. *Obes Surg.* 2017; 27(12):3110–3117

41. Flum DR, Belle SH, King WC, et al; Longitudinal Assessment of Bariatric Surgery (LABS) Consortium. Perioperative safety in the longitudinal assessment of bariatric surgery. *N Engl J Med.* 2009;361(5):445–454
42. Olbers T, Beamish AJ, Gronowitz E, et al. Laparoscopic Roux-en-Y gastric bypass in adolescents with severe obesity (AMOS): a prospective, 5-year, Swedish nationwide study. *Lancet Diabetes Endocrinol.* 2017;5(3):174–183
43. Zeitler P, Hirst K, Pyle L, et al; TODAY Study Group. A clinical trial to maintain glycemic control in youth with type 2 diabetes. *N Engl J Med.* 2012;366(24): 2247–2256
44. Inge TH, Laffel LM, Jenkins TM, et al; Teen–Longitudinal Assessment of Bariatric Surgery (Teen-LABS) and Treatment Options of Type 2 Diabetes in Adolescents and Youth (TODAY) Consortia. Comparison of surgical and medical therapy for type 2 diabetes in severely obese adolescents. *JAMA Pediatr.* 2018;172(5):452–460
45. Black JA, White B, Viner RM, Simmons RK. Bariatric surgery for obese children and adolescents: a systematic review and meta-analysis. *Obes Rev.* 2013; 14(8):634–644
46. Pedroso FE, Gander J, Oh PS, Zitsman JL. Laparoscopic vertical sleeve gastrectomy significantly improves short term weight loss as compared to laparoscopic adjustable gastric band placement in morbidly obese adolescent patients. *J Pediatr Surg.* 2015;50(1):115–122
47. Schilling PL, Davis MM, Albanese CT, Dutta S, Morton J. National trends in adolescent bariatric surgical procedures and implications for surgical centers of excellence [published correction appears in *J Am Coll Surg.* 2008;207(3):458]. *J Am Coll Surg.* 2008;206(1):1–12
48. Zwintscher NP, Azarow KS, Horton JD, Newton CR, Martin MJ. The increasing incidence of adolescent bariatric surgery. *J Pediatr Surg.* 2013;48(12): 2401–2407
49. Kelleher DC, Merrill CT, Cottrell LT, Nadler EP, Burd RS. Recent national trends in the use of adolescent inpatient bariatric surgery: 2000 through 2009. *JAMA Pediatr.* 2013; 167(2):126–132
50. Woolford SJ, Clark SJ, Gebremariam A, Davis MM, Freed GL. To cut or not to cut: physicians' perspectives on referring adolescents for bariatric surgery. *Obes Surg.* 2010;20(7):937–942
51. Michalsky MP. Adolescent bariatric surgery in the United Kingdom; a call for continued study and open dialogue. *Arch Dis Child.* 2014;99(10):885–886
52. Penna M, Markar S, Hewes J, et al. Adolescent bariatric surgery–thoughts and perspectives from the UK. *Int J Environ Res Public Health.* 2013;11(1): 573–582
53. Bairdain S, Samnaliev M. Cost-effectiveness of adolescent bariatric surgery. *Cureus.* 2015;7(2):e248
54. Klebanoff MJ, Chhatwal J, Nudel JD, et al. Cost-effectiveness of bariatric surgery in adolescents with obesity. *JAMA Surg.* 2017;152(2):136–141
55. Gastrointestinal surgery for severe obesity. Proceedings of a National Institutes of Health Consensus Development Conference. March 25-27, 1991, Bethesda, MD. *Am J Clin Nutr.* 1992;55(suppl 2):487S–619S
56. Inge TH, Garcia V, Daniels S, et al. A multidisciplinary approach to the adolescent bariatric surgical patient. *J Pediatr Surg.* 2004;39(3):442–447; discussion 446–447
57. Michalsky M, Reichard K, Inge T, Pratt J, Lenders C; American Society for Metabolic and Bariatric Surgery. ASMBS pediatric committee best practice guidelines. *Surg Obes Relat Dis.* 2012;8(1):1–7
58. Pratt JS, Lenders CM, Dionne EA, et al. Best practice updates for pediatric/adolescent weight loss surgery. *Obesity (Silver Spring).* 2009;17(5):901–910
59. Pratt JSA, Browne A, Browne NT, et al. ASMBS pediatric metabolic and bariatric surgery guidelines, 2018. *Surg Obes Relat Dis.* 2018;14(7):882–901
60. Blackstone R, Dimick JB, Nguyen NT. Accreditation in metabolic and bariatric surgery: pro versus con. *Surg Obes Relat Dis.* 2014;10(2):198–202
61. Michalsky M, Kramer RE, Fullmer MA, et al. Developing criteria for pediatric/adolescent bariatric surgery programs. *Pediatrics.* 2011;128(suppl 2):S65–S70
62. Michalsky MP, Inge TH, Teich S, et al; Teen-LABS Consortium. Adolescent bariatric surgery program characteristics: the Teen Longitudinal Assessment of Bariatric Surgery (Teen-LABS) study experience. *Semin Pediatr Surg.* 2014;23(1):5–10
63. Armstrong SC, Bolling CF, Michalsky MP, Reichard KW; American Academy of Pediatrics, Section on Obesity and Section on Surgery. Pediatric metabolic and bariatric surgery: evidence, barriers, and best practices. *Pediatrics.* 2019;144(6):e20193223

Neonatal Provider Workforce

- *Technical Report*

TECHNICAL REPORT

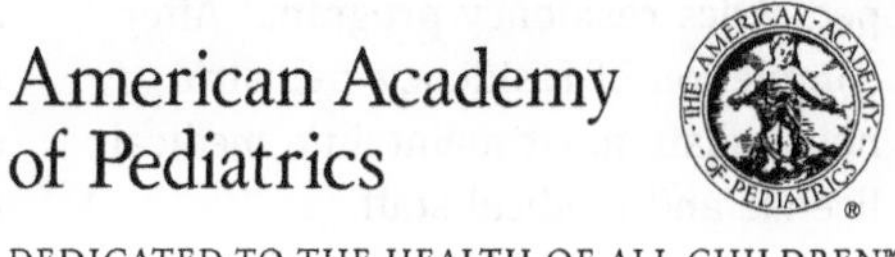

Neonatal Provider Workforce

Erin L. Keels, DNP, APRN-CNP, NNP-BC,[a,b] Jay P. Goldsmith, MD, FAAP,[c] COMMITTEE ON FETUS AND NEWBORN

abstract

This technical report reviews education, training, competency requirements, and scopes of practice of the different neonatal care providers who work to meet the special needs of neonatal patients and their families in the NICU. Additionally, this report examines the current workforce issues of NICU providers, offers suggestions for establishing and monitoring quality and safety of care, and suggests potential solutions to the NICU provider workforce shortages now and in the future.

[a]National Association of Neonatal Nurses, Chicago, Illinois; [b]Nationwide Children's Hospital, Columbus, Ohio; and [c]Department of Pediatrics, Tulane University, New Orleans, Louisiana

Technical reports from the American Academy of Pediatrics benefit from expertise and resources of liaisons and internal (AAP) and external reviewers. However, technical reports from the American Academy of Pediatrics may not reflect the views of the liaisons or the organizations or government agencies that they represent.

On behalf of the Committee on Fetus and Newborn, Drs Keels and Goldsmith conducted a thorough literature review, synthesized currently available information, authored and edited the manuscript, and approved the final manuscript as submitted.

The guidance in this report does not indicate an exclusive course of treatment or serve as a standard of medical care. Variations, taking into account individual circumstances, may be appropriate.

All technical reports from the American Academy of Pediatrics automatically expire 5 years after publication unless reaffirmed, revised, or retired at or before that time.

This document is copyrighted and is property of the American Academy of Pediatrics and its Board of Directors. All authors have filed conflict of interest statements with the American Academy of Pediatrics. Any conflicts have been resolved through a process approved by the Board of Directors. The American Academy of Pediatrics has neither solicited nor accepted any commercial involvement in the development of the content of this publication.

DOI: https://doi.org/10.1542/peds.2019-3147

Address correspondence to Erin L. Keels, DNP, APRN-CNP, NNP-BC. E-mail: Erin.keels@nationwidechildrens.org

PEDIATRICS (ISSN Numbers: Print, 0031-4005; Online, 1098-4275).

Copyright © 2019 by the American Academy of Pediatrics

FINANCIAL DISCLOSURE: The authors have indicated they have no financial relationships relevant to this article to disclose.

FUNDING: No external funding.

POTENTIAL CONFLICT OF INTEREST: The authors have indicated they have no potential conflicts of interest to disclose.

To cite: Keels EL, Goldsmith JP, AAP COMMITTEE ON FETUS AND NEWBORN. Neonatal Provider Workforce. *Pediatrics.* 2019;144(6):e20193147

To meet the critical and complex health needs of preterm neonates and neonates who are ill in the NICU, collaborative teams of health care providers work to render timely, safe, effective, efficient, and evidence-based care.[1] Many NICU provider teams include neonatologists, advanced practice registered nurses (APRNs), physician assistants (PAs), pediatric hospitalists, neonatal fellows, and pediatric residents.[1] In collaboration, these providers work together to consistently provide high-quality care throughout the neonatal hospitalization.

Training and licensure are different for the various NICU provider groups. Most APRNs and PAs working in NICUs have completed master's or doctoral degree programs that require the acquisition of certain cognitive abilities and technical skills aimed at producing safe and effective patient care.[2,3] Neonatal nurse practitioners (NNPs) and pediatric nurse practitioners (PNPs) are registered nurses with advanced education and training to enable them to care for neonatal, infant, and pediatric patients, respectively, as APRNs.[4] PAs are educated as medical generalists in programs that include pediatric and adult medicine.[5] After graduating from a master's- or doctoral-level academic program and achieving national certification and state licensure, APRNs and PAs typically complete medical staff credentialing and a period of orientation to the provider role in the NICU on the basis of demonstrated skill sets and competencies. Pediatric hospitalists are physicians who have completed a graduate medical school program as well as a pediatric residency program that requires proficiency and skills in all areas of pediatrics, including neonatal medicine.[6] A minimum number of months in the newborn nursery and NICU settings are required as part of any

Accreditation Council for Graduate Medical Education (ACGME)–certified pediatrics residency program.[7] After completion of residency, pediatric hospitalists must maintain a medical license and medical staff credentialing for their specific scope of practice. Neonatal fellows are physicians who have also completed graduate medical school as well as a pediatric residency program and are currently completing advanced subspecialty training in neonatology.[8] Pediatric residents are physician trainees who have completed graduate medical school but have not yet completed their pediatric residency program.[7] These physician trainees may have received different amounts of training, experience, and technical instruction in neonatal intensive care.[9]

The continued revision of pediatric resident duty hours prescribed by the ACGME has resulted in less availability of the pediatric resident workforce to care for patients in the NICU.[10,11] This trend has further reduced training time and skill acquisition of these trainees and has shifted much of the work of providing care in many NICUs onto other providers, such as pediatric hospitalists, NNPs, and PAs.[11] Concurrently, there appears to be a growing national workforce shortage of NNPs and insufficient numbers of PAs and pediatric hospitalists practicing in neonatal intensive care to fill the gap, challenging many neonatal programs' abilities to adequately staff their NICUs with providers.[2,11,12] This challenge has caused some programs to consider using various providers in different roles across NICU settings.[11] Further guidance from national professional organizations and other groups may be useful regarding the use of these various provider types.

This technical report reviews education, training, competency requirements, and scopes of practice of the different neonatal care providers who work to meet the specialized needs of neonatal patients and their families in the NICU. Additionally, this report examines the current workforce issues of the NICU providers, offers suggestions for establishing and monitoring quality and safety of care, and suggests potential solutions to the NICU provider workforce shortages now and in the future.

TEAM-BASED COLLABORATIVE CARE

In 2010, the Best Practices Innovation Collaborative of the Institute of Medicine (IOM) Roundtable on Value and Science-Driven Health Care defined team-based, collaborative care as the delivery of health services to individuals, families, and/or communities by at least 2 health providers who work collaboratively with patients to accomplish shared goals and achieve coordinated, high-quality care.[13] Collaboration, from the Latin term meaning "working" or laboring together, requires effective leadership, skillful communication, and sharing of information in an environment in which help can be sought and obtained freely and easily.[14] This often requires skills and practice in crew resource management, performance review, communication, and simulation.

NICU provider team composition varies widely across the United States and, in addition to the neonatologist, may include pediatric hospitalists, NNPs, PNPs, PAs, neonatal fellows, and medical, APRN, and PA trainees.[1] The knowledge base, scope of practice, and skill sets for each type of provider will vary on the basis of formal education, certification and/or licensure, clinical experience, medical staff privileging, state practice laws, and job descriptions. However, a certain basic set of behavioral competencies, cognitive abilities, and technical skills is necessary for all neonatal providers to practice in the specialized and high-risk setting of the NICU. The ACGME provides direction on the development of competencies, skills, and abilities for pediatric residents and neonatal fellows,[7,8] which is largely beyond the scope of this article. However, it may be helpful to understand the educational preparation, competencies, scope of practice, and workforce issues of the pediatric hospitalists, APRNs, and PAs who work in the NICU to develop shared basic competencies for all neonatal providers.

Pediatric Physician Hospitalists

Pediatric hospitalists are physicians whose primary professional focus is the general medical care of pediatric patients who are hospitalized. Pediatric hospitalist activities include patient care, teaching, quality improvement, research, and leadership related to hospital care.[15,16] Clinical responsibilities and practice sites of pediatric hospitalists vary significantly and may include general inpatient pediatric care, emergency department care, perioperative surgical and medical subspecialty care, delivery room services, newborn nursery care, and NICU coverage.[15,16] Some pediatricians pursue long-term careers in hospital medicine in the hospitalist role and have gained valuable experience and clinical expertise in the field. Others may be hired to work as a hospitalist for a discreet amount of time, during which they can gain additional clinical experience before entering a general practice or a subspecialty fellowship.

The Section on Hospital Medicine was established within the American Academy of Pediatrics (AAP) in 1998.[6] Within the Section on Hospital Medicine is the Neonatal Hospitalists Subcommittee, which focuses on the care of newborn infants who are hospitalized. Formal pediatric hospitalist fellowship training programs are offered in growing numbers of academic centers across the United States.[17] The field of pediatric hospital medicine (PHM) will be an American Board of Pediatrics (ABP)–certified subspecialty starting in 2019.[18]

Some pediatric hospitalists working in the NICU environment may be graduates of PHM fellowship programs and may have additional training in the care of children who are hospitalized. Other pediatricians working in the hospitalist role are pediatric residency graduates and will have varying levels of NICU experience, depending on their training program and subsequent years of clinical experience. The 6 ACGME core competencies for residents include patient care, medical knowledge, professionalism, interpersonal and communication skills, practice-based learning and improvement, and systems-based learning.[19] The competencies are aimed at trainees in a particular specialty (ie, pediatrics). After graduation from a pediatric residency program, successful board certification by the ABP validates foundational knowledge in pediatric care.[20] Individual state licensure grants authority to practice as a physician, and behavioral and procedural competencies for the neonatal and pediatric populations are confirmed through organizational credentialing and periodic review.[21]

In 2010, core competencies for pediatric hospitalist programs were developed in an effort to standardize and improve inpatient training programs.[22] These core competencies include common clinical diagnoses and conditions, core skills, specialized clinical services (including newborn care and delivery room management), and health care systems to support and advance child health.[22] These core competencies are continually being updated and revised. In addition, the Neonatal Hospitalist Subcommittee of the AAP Section on Hospital Medicine is helping to develop and review goals and objectives related to delivery room management and common neonatal conditions for PHM fellowship curriculum as well as for the PHM subspecialty board certification examination.[18]

As PHM programs, fellowships, and subspecialty board certification become more formally established and grow in popularity, there will likely be an increasing workforce of pediatric hospitalists in the future. Many pediatric hospitalists possess the expertise necessary to care for newborn infants who are hospitalized and may become more commonly used in the nursery and NICU settings.

APRNs

APRNs are registered nurses who have gained additional education, training, certification, and licensure to practice as providers.[23] The 4 APRN roles are certified nurse practitioners (NPs), clinical nurse specialists, certified nurse midwives, and certified registered nurse anesthetists.[23] National certification examinations are required for each of these categories of advanced practice nursing within 1 of 6 population foci: adult-gerontology, family and/or across the life span, pediatrics, psychiatric-mental health, neonatology, or women's health. In addition, the populations of adult-gerontology and pediatrics includes separate certifications in either acute care or primary care.[23] State-specific nurse practice acts regulate APRN licensure, certification, and education requirements.[23] To decrease variability among states, the Consensus Model for APRN Regulation was introduced in 2008 to help define and standardize these requirements.[23] Although progress has been noted, variation among states continues to exist, most notably related to physician oversight of practice. Some states require formal agreements between the APRN and physician(s) related to supervised or collaborative practice, and other states have independent APRN practices.[23,24]

Commonly, APRNs in neonatal care include the neonatal clinical nurse specialist to direct care, education, and continuous improvement in outcomes for a population of patients and the NNP to provide care to individuals or populations of patients.[25] In some settings, the primary care–certified pediatric nurse practitioner (PC PNP) and/or the acute care–certified pediatric nurse practitioner (AC PNP) may provide care for various populations within the neonatal service line or NICU within their respective scopes of practice, such as a neonatal follow-up clinic visit for PNPs certified in primary care or inpatient NICU care of older infants with chronic conditions, such as bronchopulmonary dysplasia or congenital heart lesions, for PNPs certified in acute care.[26]

Per the Consensus Model for APRN Regulation, the APRN scope of practice is defined as the culmination of the formal graduate- or doctoral-level education and board certification in one or more of the population foci previously mentioned and is then further delineated by variable state practice rules and organizational bylaws and policies.[23] General competencies for all NPs are developed by the National Organization of Nurse Practitioner Faculties (NONPF) and include scientific foundations, leadership, quality, practice inquiry, technology and informatics literacy, policy, health care delivery systems, ethics, and independent practice.[4,27] APRN professional organizations, such as the National Association of Neonatal Nurses (NANN), use the NONPF recommendations to develop competencies for the specific NP practice populations to guide education standards and clinical practice.[28,29]

NNPs

NNPs are APRNs educated at the graduate or doctoral level and are nationally board certified to care for high-risk neonates across the care continuum, from preterm and term birth to the age of 2 years.[25,28,29] NNP academic graduate training programs follow the *Education Standards and Curriculum Guidelines for Neonatal Nurse Practitioner Programs.*[29] In addition to didactic instruction, NNP graduate students acquire supervised clinical preceptorship hours in delivery rooms; in level II, level III, and level IV NICUs; and in follow-up and well-infant programs.[29] The clinical preceptorship experiences include a wide variety of neonatal populations and disease processes as well as opportunities to build expertise in communication, collaboration, transitions of care, and family-centered care strategies.[29]

After graduation, successful national board certification by the National Certification Corporation validates foundational knowledge competency in neonatal care.[23,30] Individual state licensure grants authority to practice as an APRN, and behavioral and procedural competencies are confirmed through organizational credentialing and periodic review.[1] The NANN has developed a process for initial and ongoing neonatal competency maintenance and recommends that each NNP become and remain technically competent in endotracheal intubation, umbilical line insertion, needle-chest thoracentesis, and arterial puncture at a minimum.[31] NNPs maintain their certification in 3-year cycles with a core-competency knowledge assessment and targeted continuing education based on their assessments.[25]

Care to high-risk infants by NNPs has been found to be safe, of high quality, and cost-effective.[32–36] Accordingly, the role of the NNP in the care of high-risk neonatal patients has been endorsed by the AAP[37] and in the *Guidelines for Perinatal Care.*[1] To monitor the quality of individuals and teams of NNPs, the NANN has developed a policy with recommendations on NNP-related quality metrics associated with neonatal care.[38]

Currently, the demand for NNPs outpaces the supply, and a national NNP workforce shortage exists for a variety of reasons.[39] In a 2016 workforce survey, there were 5433 certified NNPs in the United States.[40] Of the 1100 survey respondents, the average age was 49 years, 72% worked at least 35 hours per week, and more than half reported that they regularly worked more than their scheduled hours because of staffing vacancies.[40] The shortage of NNPs is felt at the bedside, where NNPs may have higher-than-recommended workloads, creating frustration and burnout, which may further challenge recruitment and retention endeavors.[39,41] In a 2014 workforce survey, 5% of respondents planned to retire by the year 2020.[39] At last count, 35 academic programs across the United States reported graduating 240 NNP students each year,[42] although that number has increased to more than 300 recently (S. Bellini, DNP, APRN, NNP-BC, CNE, personal communication, 2017), which is approximately 1.6% of all newly graduated NPs entering the workforce in the United States.[43] Strategic modeling of the current NNP workforce predicts that the shortage may last for up to 10 years unless innovative recruitment and retention strategies are used to deal with this issue.[41]

PNPs

PNPs provide care to children from late preterm and term birth through adulthood.[43,44] Through formal graduate or doctoral training, PNPs become nationally certified in acute care, primary care, or both.[43] AC PNP training programs are focused on the care of the child with acutely changing and/or unstable physiology and include advanced physiology and pharmacology of the infant, child, or adolescent and neonatal content on topics such as congenital heart lesions, chronic lung disease, and sepsis.[4] PC PNP training programs are focused on comprehensive, chronic, and continuous care; transitions in care; wellness; and prevention.[4] Typical PC PNP neonatal curriculum includes immunizations, breastfeeding, and common childhood diseases.[4] Invasive neonatal procedures are not part of the scope of practice for PC PNPs. Moreover, none of the AC PNP or PC PNP competencies, recommended curricula from the NONPF, or national PNP certification examination guidelines include content related to fetal or preterm infant physiology, pathophysiology, or management of high-risk preterm infants.[4] However, AC PNP national certification examination content does include competencies related to ventilator management, noninvasive positive-pressure ventilation, enteral and parenteral nutrition, diagnostic imaging, and laboratory test interpretation.[4] The management of high-risk deliveries and preterm infants who are critically ill and/or have low birth weight is not included in the national competencies for PNPs by the NONPF.[4] However, because the Consensus Model for APRN Regulation has not been fully adopted and/or implemented in every state, inconsistent state nursing regulations and variable practices in individual organizations exist.[24]

Currently, there are approximately 18 000 certified PNPs in the United States, which represents 0.6% of all NPs.[43] A PNP workforce shortage exists for reasons similar to the NNP workforce shortage, including a limited number of academic programs, faculty shortages, low enrollment, and difficulties with securing clinical sites and preceptors.[45,46] Strategic modeling predicts that the shortage could continue for 13 years unless innovative strategies for recruitment and retention are implemented.[47]

PAs

PAs are nationally certified, state-licensed medical professionals who practice medicine on health care teams.[48,49] Medical education at the graduate level prepares PAs to take medical histories, perform physical examinations, order and interpret results of laboratory tests, diagnose illnesses, develop and manage treatment plans, prescribe medications, and assist in surgery. PA programs include didactic content across the life span and clinical hours in a variety of settings, leading to a foundation in general medical knowledge.[49,50] Programs average 27 months in length and include 2000 hours of clinical rotations.[50]

Before beginning to practice, PA-program graduates must pass a national certification examination administered by the National Commission on Certification of Physician Assistants (NCCPA) and obtain a state license.[50] PAs must recertify every 10 years and complete at least 100 hours of continuing medical education (CME) every 2 years.[50] Neither recertification nor CME requirements are specific to neonatal care.

PAs prepare to practice in neonatology either by receiving further specialized education in the clinical workplace or through hospital-based postgraduate programs,[51] allowing each hospital-based program to develop its own curricula and competencies to meet the needs of the organization. Other centers may not have formal PA postgraduate training programs; instead, newly hired PAs who do not have neonatal experience receive additional training in the clinical setting of unspecified scope and length of time.

The PA scope of practice is determined by education and experience, variable state laws that include degree of physician oversight, policies of employers and facilities, and the needs of patients.[50,52] PAs practice in every setting and specialty. Of 123 000 practicing PAs, approximately 4% (approximately 2400) practice in pediatrics.[53] An estimated 500 PAs work in neonatal-perinatal or pediatric critical care medicine, and the rest work in various pediatric subspecialties.[53]

Studies have revealed that PAs provide safe, high-quality, cost-effective care to infants. These studies demonstrate that PAs provide care that is equal in quality to that of other neonatal and pediatric providers and complement the work of attending and resident physicians.[32,54–56] PAs are important members of the NICU provider team, as described the *Guidelines for Perinatal Care*.[1]

The PA workforce has experienced robust growth over recent years. Overall employment of PAs is projected to grow 37% from 2016 to 2026, much faster than the average for all occupations, creating potential for PAs to help fill the need for neonatal providers.[57–59] The National Center for Health Workforce Analysis predicts that PAs in pediatric subspecialties will experience growth of 185% between 2010 and 2025.[60] Growth in the overall number of PAs and strategies to recruit PAs to neonatology may help increase overall numbers of neonatal providers.

COMPETENCY, SAFETY, AND PATIENT OUTCOMES

Typically, health care providers acquire competence through education and training that begins during preclinical care settings and continues over a continuum of time, leading to the emergence of expertise from novice to expert.[61,62] In the IOM publication *Health Professions Education: A Bridge to Quality*, essential skills for all health care professionals' education and preparation are identified to provide the foundation on which other specialty or population-based competencies are further delineated to meet the goals of safe, effective, efficient, patient-centered, timely, and equitable health care.[63,64]

In addition to the IOM competencies, the ABP (adopted by the ACGME), national PA organizations (the NCCPA, the Accreditation Review Commission on Education for the Physician Assistant, the American Academy of Physician Assistants [AAPA], and the Physician Assistant Education Association), and the NONPF have each developed some neonatal competencies to guide the provision of safe and effective care.[4,19,22,27,50,63,65] Simplistically, these core competencies can be organized into 3 broad categories: knowledge-based, procedural, and behavioral competencies. The organizations and their core competencies are summarized in Table 1.

Knowledge-Based Competency

Neonatal-perinatal medicine and NNP board certification examinations validate knowledge-based competencies specifically focused on the care of the preterm and high-risk neonate.[30,67] Other providers working in the NICU have variable amounts of neonatal knowledge gained during their academic programs, clinical experiences, and past professional practices. It is important for all NICU providers to have a basic knowledge base and understanding of fetal and neonatal physiology, typical neonatal conditions and diseases, skills in

TABLE 1 Core Competencies by Organization

Professional Organization	Core Competencies
AAP Section on Hospital Medicine[22]	Common clinical diagnoses and conditions Core skills Specialized clinical services Health care systems: supporting and advancing child health
ABP and ACGME[19,66]	Patient care Medical knowledge Professionalism Interpersonal and communication skills Practice-based learning and improvement Systems-based learning
IOM (now the National Academy of Medicine)[63]	Provision of patient-centered care Interdisciplinary teamwork Employment of evidence-based practice Application of quality improvement strategies Use of informatics
NONPF[4,27]	Scientific foundations Leadership Quality Practice inquiry Technology and informatics literacy Policy Health care delivery systems Ethics Independent practice
NCCPA, Accreditation Review Commission on Education for the Physician Assistant, AAPA, Physician Assistant Education Association[50,65]	Medical knowledge Interpersonal and communication skills Patient care Professionalism Practice-based learning and improvement Systems-based practice

physical examination and health assessment, and pharmacology. This knowledge can be obtained during a formal academic program, during an employment orientation period, and throughout the provider's career through clinical experience and CME. These knowledge-based competencies enable providers to effectively perform comprehensive physical examinations and take medical histories, develop plans for initial care and stabilization, and order laboratory tests, radiologic studies, medications, and treatments for infants with acute and chronic illnesses.[30,67] Skills in discharge planning (which include medication reconciliation and management), in assessment of ongoing needs for nutrition and durable medical equipment, in making appropriate referrals, and in educating and preparing parents for their infant's discharge, including health promotion and disease-prevention activities, are also important attributes for all NICU providers.[1,68]

Procedural Competency

The ACGME Neonatal Fellowship Program requirements provide general guidance on procedural competencies for trainees, which includes general principles of critical care and neonatal resuscitation, venous and arterial access, evacuation of air leaks, endotracheal intubation, preparation for transport, ventilator support, continuous monitoring, and temperature control.[8] Use of didactic instruction, simulation, and supervised performance is recommended to establish basic competencies.[8]

Likewise, the National Association of Neonatal Nurse Practitioners (NANNP), a subsidiary of the NANN that is focused on issues specific to neonatal APRNs, has delineated the necessary procedural competency for both practicing and student NNPs.[28,29] Neonatal procedures are taught in classrooms and/or simulation laboratories and are performed in the clinical setting under the supervision and mentorship of a competent preceptor.[29] Documentation of initial competency is required.[29] National certification for AC PNPs requires competency in pediatric critical care, including mechanical ventilation, continuous monitoring, and invasive procedures.[4] In some programs, PA students may be exposed to neonatal procedures during their formal academic program and clinical rotations. Other avenues for PAs to become proficient in neonatology include hospital-based postgraduate neonatal training programs and courses[69] and additional training in the clinical setting as an employed PA. The definition of procedural competency is elusive and is not satisfied by the completion of an arbitrary number of procedures alone but includes ongoing instruction and/or feedback, simulation, and practice.[70] The recommendation for NNPs from the NANNP is no less than 3 performances of each procedure to be documented annually.[28] If the NNP does not meet these requirements, other provisions can be made to ensure competency.[28] National recommendations for procedural review for NNPs include logged procedures as well as practice laboratories, proctored simulation, and review of policy and procedural guidelines. Documentation of procedures are kept by each NNP, including what procedures were performed, success rates, and complications. Data obtained from the logs are a necessary component for quality improvement purposes.[28,38]

In consideration of the basic knowledge and procedural experience of NICU provider roles, we present in Table 2 procedures that are required and those that are recommended for hospitalists, NNPs, AC PNPs, and PAs in the NICU. Use of a quality improvement approach may be helpful to establish initial competence and confidence.[71] Formal instruction and simulation can be completed, along with direct supervision by a credentialed and competent provider for initial procedural attempts, on patients in the NICU. Initial and ongoing competency can be documented through the use of procedure logs, observation, and/or proctored simulations and policy and procedure reviews.[72–74]

TABLE 2 Essential Neonatal Procedures

Required neonatal procedures for all neonatal providers
Neonatal resuscitation, according to the American Heart Association and AAP Neonatal Resuscitation Program
Management of airway: positive-pressure ventilation with bag or mask, nasal continuous positive airway pressure, and endotracheal intubation
Umbilical line insertion
Needle-chest thoracentesis
Other procedures that may be recommended depending on the practice site (NICU-designated level) and patient population
Chest tube placement
Arterial blood gas sampling
Peripheral arterial line insertion
Lumbar puncture
Peripherally inserted central catheters
Suprapubic bladder taps
Exchange transfusion
Ventricular reservoir taps
Intraosseous cannulation and infusion
Abdominal paracentesis
Pericardiocentesis or pericardial tap

Behavioral Competency

The ABP, ACGME, various national PA organizations, and the NONPF provide guidance on behavioral competency in areas such as practiced-based learning and quality improvement, self-assessment, interpersonal and communication skills, professionalism, and systems-based practice.[3–5,7,8,16,19,20,67] These emphasize independent and interprofessional practice; analytic skills for evaluating and providing evidence-based, patient-centered care; and advanced knowledge of health care delivery systems and are in accordance with the IOM recommendations for health professions education.[63,64] At a minimum, NICU providers must be able to make complex decisions through analytical thinking and practice inquiry, communicate and collaborate with neonatologists and other health care providers, use and analyze information technology, develop effective teamwork and quality improvement skills, use patient- and family-centered care practices, and incorporate evidence-based practice, safety, and knowledge of hospital and unit policy to promote the delivery of high-quality, safe, and cost-effective care to neonates.[4,8] Behavioral competencies are developed through structured education, mentorship, experience, and feedback, which may include individual coaching, team debriefings, simulations, and root-cause analysis exercises, and can be part of all providers' developmental process in training and throughout their careers.[8,29] Periodic assessment of behavioral competencies can be conducted and included in initial and ongoing performance evaluations.[63]

Initial and Ongoing Neonatal Competency Acquisition and Maintenance

The *Guidelines for Perinatal Care, Eighth Edition* recommends that procedures are established for the initial granting and subsequent maintenance of privileges, ensuring that the proper professional credentials are in place for each NICU provider.[1] Each institution is responsible to ensure that the neonatal provider, whether physician, APRN, or PA, has the formal education, experience, and board certification to function within the requested scope of clinical and professional privileges. The credentialing process is best developed through a collaborative effort between nursing administration and the medical staff governing body by using guidance from national bodies regarding the core competencies.[1] Hospitals accredited by The Joint Commission require physician and nonphysician health care providers, including APRNs and PAs, to obtain privileges to practice through a process of medical staff credentialing.[75] Diagnostic and therapeutic services allowed by state and federal law may be further restricted by the hospital and/or medical staff.[21,75] Procedural privileges may be limited by professional degree, experience, or lack of ability to demonstrate appropriate training or competence to a credentialing body.[21,75]

Once an individual is credentialed, plans for initial and periodic reviews of safety and quality care can be developed, for individuals to maintain requested privileges, through a practice such as the focused professional practice evaluation and ongoing professional practice evaluation processes for those organizations accredited by The Joint Commission.[76,77]

POTENTIAL STRATEGIES TO ADDRESS WORKFORCE SHORTAGE OF NEONATAL PROVIDERS

Strategies to address provider workforce shortages in the NICU can include attempting to reduce the workload (ie, reduce the number of patients admitted to the NICU and/or shorten the length of stay) and/or increase the number of providers. In addition to declining birth rates in the United States,[78] new care strategies may potentially change the acuity and locations where newborn infants receive their care and, over time, may lead to a redistribution and change the workloads of the NICU provider workforce. These emerging care strategies include limiting elective cesarean deliveries to 39 weeks' gestation or greater[79,80]; treating infants with neonatal abstinence syndrome outside of the NICU[81]; reducing the need for antibiotic administration and, therefore, length of hospital stay for mothers with intraamniotic inflammation or infection[82]; reducing NICU admissions for treatment of hypoglycemia with intravenous glucose administration by using dextrose or glucose gel[83]; and reducing length of NICU stay through quality improvement strategies, such as decreasing the incidence of central line–associated bloodstream infections.[84]

Strategies to increase the NICU provider workforce have mostly been concentrated on increasing the use of pediatric hospitalists, NNPs, and PAs.[11,15,39–41,45–47] Workforce surveys conducted by the NANNP have delineated the existing and future NNP workforce needs.[39,40] The authors noted that education, recruitment, and retention of NNPs were key areas of focus to increase supply.[39,40]

Education for NNPs has evolved over 5 decades from certificate programs, to bachelor's and master's degrees in nursing, to the doctorate of nursing practice degree, which could slow the NNP pipeline further.[85,86] Barriers to obtaining this education are lack of higher degree (ie, doctorate of nursing) programs, funding of faculty, access to preceptors, and federal and state regulations.[87] Regulations posed by the US Department of Education related to long-distance learning have had an effect on NNP education and have contributed to a drop in enrollment in states with significantly restrictive requirements.[87] Collaboration among educational institutions may be a strategy to overcome restrictive regulations and minimize costs and faculty needs.[39] Locally, neonatal programs and hospitals can increase efforts to recruit more neonatal nurses within the workplace to pursue higher education as an NNP and offer tuition reimbursement or scholarships to assist with the financial burden.[88] This strategy capitalizes on the professional expertise of neonatal nurses, facilitating success and easing the transition into the APRN role. A shortage of university nursing faculty is another limitation of enrollment in academic programs. The NANNP has led a strategy to support NNP programs to prepare expert NNP clinicians to become educators in clinical faculties. It is hoped that this effort to increase faculty will enable an increase in the student cohort size and consequently increase the numbers of newly graduated NNPs in the workforce.[39]

Recruitment of NNPs is vital to the NICU provider workforce. Practicing NNPs should contribute to recruitment efforts by serving as clinical preceptors for NNP students.[25] Mentoring programs for novice NNPs have been shown to be valuable recruitment tools for NNP practices and hospitals. Offering longer orientation or residency programs is attractive to new graduates as well.

Retention of NNPs in the workforce is another important aspect of maintaining the NNP supply. With an aging workforce, any additional reduction in manpower from burnout and early retirement will compound the workforce deficit and increase demand. The scope of responsibility for NNPs includes the NICU provider role along with other roles, such as transport NNP, educator, delivery room resuscitation, cross-coverage for physician housestaff, and well-infant consultations, etc.[25] Adequate staffing ratios are required to balance the needs of the unit with safe and effective care to neonates.[39] Consideration of patient load and acuity will help reduce burnout and increase job satisfaction.[39] In hospitals that maintain 24-hour work shifts, ensuring downtime for NNPs is critical to safe and competent care.[39] Other strategies may include creating shorter shift lengths and devising creative scheduling techniques to offer better work-life balance in an attempt to increase longevity of the NNP role.[39,40]

AC PNPs, acting within their scope of practice, can be used as NICU providers for term and older infants, such as those with surgical conditions and chronic medical conditions. PC PNPs, working within their scope of practice, could be used to perform well-newborn and other types of consultations, discharge education, care coordination, and neurodevelopmental follow-up. This team-based collaborative model capitalizes on the unique skill sets of each provider. However, the PNP workforce pipeline suffers from many of the same or similar issues as the NNP pipeline, and it is likely that applying some of the above recruitment and retention strategies may help.[45–47] Additionally, some PNPs may consider achieving additional certification as an NNP through a post–master's certification academic program.

Efforts to increase the PA workforce in the NICU have included the addition of postgraduate training programs,[69] and more hospitals are hiring PAs and providing onboarding for those without specific NICU experience. As the total population of PAs continues to increase, offering optional rotations through the NICU during student coursework and clinical rotations, creating more postgraduate training opportunities in neonatology for PAs, and formalizing neonatal PA orientation programs may increase the numbers of these providers in neonatology. Reynolds and Bricker[51] note that PAs "represent a historically underutilized resource to resolve neonatology's workforce issues."

Pediatric hospitalists have completed a formal pediatrics residency program and are licensed physicians who can be used as NICU providers within their scope of practice. Hospitalists can currently achieve board certification through the ABP in the field of general pediatrics[20] and, if eligible, may also soon be able to obtain board certification in PHM.[18] The AAP Section on Hospital Medicine and its Neonatal Hospitalists Subcommittee are developing and reviewing content on delivery room care and common neonatal conditions for PHM fellowship programs and for the PHM board certification process.[18] Recruitment and retention of pediatric hospitalists who are focused on newborn care and work as providers in the NICU may be helpful to the overall NICU provider workforce. The scope of responsibility for pediatric and neonatal hospitalists may include clinical responsibilities for delivery room resuscitation, transport, cross-coverage for housestaff, well-newborn consultation and care, and the care of selected newborn infants in the intermediate and intensive care nurseries.[6,15] In addition, many pediatric hospitalists also serve as educators, researchers, and leaders of committees and quality improvement activities.[6,15] Adequate staffing ratios are important to the practice environment and are required to balance the needs of the unit with safe and effective care to neonates. Consideration of patient load, acuity, and need for academic and professional development will help reduce burnout and increase longevity and job satisfaction of pediatric and neonatal hospitalists.

In addition to the pipeline, recruitment, and retention strategies mentioned previously, efforts should also be focused on effective use and quality-outcomes metrics of all neonatal providers to improve effectiveness and efficiency issues and to improve the quality of care delivered to the neonate who is hospitalized.

SUMMARY AND CONCLUSIONS

- The NICU provider workforce consists of a variety of professionals in varied stages of their careers with a wide range of degrees, training, experience, skills, and competencies.
- Increasing collaboration of neonatologists with other NICU providers (pediatric hospitalists, APRNs, and PAs) and physician trainees will be necessary to meet the needs of the NICU population going forward.
- The skill level, experience, and competency of neonatology physician trainees (residents and fellows) and NICU providers (PAs, pediatric hospitalists, and PNPs) can be variable, although the training model for NNPs is well developed and may serve as a model for other NICU providers.
- All neonatal providers should possess a basic set of knowledge, procedural, and behavioral-based competencies to provide safe and effective care.
- It is the responsibility of the medical and nursing leadership of the NICU, with the assistance of the hospital credentialing committee, to develop and periodically review competency criteria for all NICU providers.
- Competency criteria, such as those developed by the AAP, ACGME, AAPA, and NONPF, can help guide the development and evaluation of NICU providers to provide high-quality, safe, and cost-effective

care to the high-risk NICU population.

- Strategies to increase the overall NICU provider workforce should be evaluated and thoughtfully employed at the national and state levels to remove barriers to education, training, and practice.
- Ultimately, the attending neonatologist is responsible for the care given by NICU providers under his or her supervision and/or collaboration. He or she should be involved in the development and periodic review of competency criteria and should ensure that malpractice liability protection, of the institution or obtained personally, covers adverse events that may involve members of the neonatal care team.

LEAD AUTHORS

Erin L. Keels, DNP, APRN-CNP, NNP-BC
Jay P. Goldsmith, MD, FAAP

COMMITTEE ON FETUS AND NEWBORN, 2018–2019

James J. Cummings, MD, FAAP, Chairperson
Ira S. Adams-Chapman, MD, FAAP
Susan Wright Aucott, MD, FAAP
Jay P. Goldsmith, MD, FAAP
Ivan L. Hand, MD, FAAP
Sandra E. Juul, MD, PhD, FAAP
Brenda Bradley Poindexter, MD, MS, FAAP
Karen Marie Puopolo, MD, PhD, FAAP
Dan L. Stewart, MD, FAAP
Wanda D. Barfield, MD, MPH, FAAP, RADM, USPHS

LIAISONS

Yasser El-Sayed, MD – *American College of Obstetricians and Gynecologists*
Erin L. Keels, DNP, APRN, NNP-BC – *National Association of Neonatal Nurses*
Meredith Mowitz, MD, MS, FAAP – *AAP Section on Neonatal-Perinatal Medicine*
Michael Ryan Narvey, MD, FAAP – *Canadian Pediatric Society*
Tonse N.K. Raju, MD, DCH, FAAP – *National Institutes of Health*
Kasper S. Wang, MD, FACS, FAAP – *Section on Surgery*

STAFF

Jim Couto, MA

ABBREVIATIONS

AAP: American Academy of Pediatrics
AAPA: American Academy of Physician Assistants
ABP: American Board of Pediatrics
ACGME: Accreditation Council for Graduate Medical Education
AC PNP: acute care–certified pediatric nurse practitioner
APRN: advanced practice registered nurse
CME: continuing medical education
IOM: Institute of Medicine
NANN: National Association of Neonatal Nurses
NANNP: National Association of Neonatal Nurse Practitioners
NCCPA: National Commission on Certification of Physician Assistants
NNP: neonatal nurse practitioner
NONPF: National Organization of Nurse Practitioner Faculties
NP: nurse practitioner
PA: physician assistant
PC PNP: primary care–certified pediatric nurse practitioner
PHM: pediatric hospital medicine
PNP: pediatric nurse practitioner

REFERENCES

1. American Academy of Pediatrics Committee on Fetus and Newborn; American Academy of Pediatrics Committee on Fetus and Newborn. In: Kilpatrick SJ, Papile LA, Macones GA, eds. *Guidelines for Perinatal Care*, 8th ed. Elk Grove Village, IL: American Academy of Pediatrics Publishing; 2017
2. National Association of Neonatal Nurses. *Neonatal Nurse Practitioner Workforce. Position Statement #3058.* Chicago, IL: National Association of Neonatal Nurses; 2013
3. Accreditation Review Commission on Education for the Physician Assistant. *Accreditation Standards for Physician Assistant Education.* 4th ed. Johns Creek, GA: Accreditation Review Commission on Education for the Physician Assistant; 2018. Available at: www.arc-pa.org/wp-content/uploads/2018/06/Standards-4th-Ed-March-2018.pdf. Accessed October 30, 2018
4. National Organization of Nurse Practitioner Faculties. Population focused nurse practitioner competencies. 2013. Available at: https://cdn.ymaws.com/www.nonpf.org/resource/resmgr/Competencies/CompilationPopFocusComps2013.pdf. Accessed October 25, 2019
5. American Academy of Physician Assistants. PA education—preparation for excellence. 2016. Available at: https://www.aapa.org/wp-content/uploads/2016/12/Issue_Brief_PA_Education.pdf. Accessed October 31, 2018
6. American Academy of Pediatrics; Section on Hospital Medicine. Guiding principles for pediatric hospital medicine programs. *Pediatrics*. 2013; 132(4):782–786
7. Accreditation Council for Graduate Medical Education. ACGME program requirements for graduate medical education in neonatal-perinatal medicine. Available at: www.acgme.org/portals/0/pfassets/2013-pr-faq-pif/329_neonatal_perinatal_peds_07012013.pdf. Accessed December 1, 2018
8. Accreditation Council for Graduate Medical Education. ACGME program requirements for graduate medical education in neonatal-perinatal medicine. 2007. Available at: http://www.acgme.org/Portals/0/PFAssets/2013-PR-FAQ-PIF/329_neonatal_perinatal_peds_07012013.pdf. Accessed October 25, 2019
9. Sawyer T, Foglia E, Hatch LD, et al. Improving neonatal intubation safety: a journey of a thousand miles. *J Neonatal Perinatal Med*. 2017;10(2): 125–131
10. Accreditation Council for Graduate Medical Education. Summary of changes to ACGME common program requirements Section VI. Available at: https://www.acgme.org/What-We-Do/Accreditation/Common-Program-Requirements/Summary-of-Proposed-

Changes-to-ACGME-Common-Program-Requirements-Section-VI. Accessed December 1, 2018

11. Freed GL, Dunham KM, Moran LM, Spera L; Research Advisory Committee of the American Board of Pediatrics. Resident work hour changes in children's hospitals: impact on staffing patterns and workforce needs. *Pediatrics*. 2012; 130(4):700–704

12. Typpo KV, Tcharmtchi MH, Thomas EJ, et al. Impact of resident duty hour limits on safety in the intensive care unit: a national survey of pediatric and neonatal intensivists. *Pediatr Crit Care Med*. 2012;13(5):578–582

13. Institute of Medicine (US) Roundtable on Value and Science-Driven Health Care. In: Yong PL, Olsen LA, McGinnis JM, eds. *Value in Health Care: Accounting for Cost, Quality, Safety, Outcomes, and Innovation*. Washington, DC: National Academies Press (US); 2010

14. Merriam-Webster. Collaborate. Available at: https://www.merriam-webster.com/dictionary/collaborate. Accessed May 13, 2018

15. Freed GL, Brzoznowski K, Neighbors K, Lakhani I; American Board of Pediatrics, Research Advisory Committee. Characteristics of the pediatric hospitalist workforce: its roles and work environment. *Pediatrics*. 2007; 120(1):33–39

16. Section on Hospital Medicine. Guiding principles for pediatric hospital medicine programs. *Pediatrics*. 2013; 132(4):782–786

17. Gosdin C, Simmons J, Yau C, et al. Survey of academic pediatric hospitalist programs in the US: organizational, administrative, and financial factors. *J Hosp Med*. 2013;8(6): 285–291

18. American Board of Pediatrics. Pediatric hospital medicine certification. 2018. Available at: https://www.abp.org/content/pediatric-hospital-medicine-certification. Accessed March 7, 2018

19. Holmboe ES, Edgar L, Hamstra S. *The Milestones Guidebook*. Chicago, IL: Accreditation Council for Graduate Medical Education; 2016. Available at: https://www.acgme.org/Portals/0/MilestonesGuidebook.pdf. Accessed March 7, 2018

20. American Board of Pediatrics. Board certification. Available at: https://www.abp.org/content/board-certification. Accessed December 1, 2018

21. Rauch DA; Committee on Hospital Care; Section on Hospital Medicine. Medical staff appointment and delineation of pediatric privileges in hospitals. *Pediatrics*. 2012;129(4):784–787

22. Stucky ER, Ottolini MC, Maniscalco J. Pediatric hospital medicine core competencies: development and methodology. *J Hosp Med*. 2010;5(6): 339–343

23. National Council of State Boards of Nursing. APRN consensus model. Available at: https://www.ncsbn.org/aprn-consensus.htm. Accessed May 13, 2018

24. National Council of State Boards of Nursing. APRN consensus implementation status. Available at: https://www.ncsbn.org/5397.htm. Accessed December 1, 2018

25. National Association of Neonatal Nurses. *Advanced Practice Registered Nurse: Role, Preparation, and Scope of Practice. Position Statement #3059*. Chicago, IL: National Association of Neonatal Nurses; 2014

26. Staebler SL, Alianiello L, Kosch B, Keels E. The long road home: neonatal long-term care. *AACN Adv Crit Care*. 2014; 25(4):330–333

27. NP Core Competencies Content Work Group, National Organization of Nurse Practitioner Faculties. Nurse practitioner core competencies content. 2017. Available at: https://cdn.ymaws.com/www.nonpf.org/resource/resmgr/competencies/2017_NPCoreComps_with_Curric.pdf. Accessed February 23, 2018

28. National Association of Neonatal Nurses. *Standard for Maintaining the Competence of Neonatal Nurse Practitioners. Position Statement #3062*. Chicago, IL: National Association of Neonatal Nurses; 2015

29. National Association of Neonatal Nurses. *Education Standards and Curriculum Guidelines for Neonatal Nurse Practitioner Programs*. Chicago, IL: National Association of Neonatal Nurses; 2014

30. National Certification Corporation. 2018 candidate guide: neonatal nurse practitioner. Available at: https://www.nccwebsite.org/content/documents/cms/nnp-candidate_guide.pdf. Accessed February 3, 2018

31. National Association of Neonatal Nurse Practitioners. *Competencies and Orientation Toolkit for Neonatal Nurse Practitioners*, 2nd ed. Chicago, IL: National Association of Neonatal Nurses; 2014

32. Carzoli RP, Martinez-Cruz M, Cuevas LL, Murphy S, Chiu T. Comparison of neonatal nurse practitioners, physician assistants, and residents in the neonatal intensive care unit. *Arch Pediatr Adolesc Med*. 1994;148(12): 1271–1276

33. Mitchell-DiCenso A, Guyatt G, Marrin M, et al. A controlled trial of nurse practitioners in neonatal intensive care. *Pediatrics*. 1996;98(6, pt 1):1143–1148

34. Karlowicz MG, McMurray JL. Comparison of neonatal nurse practitioners' and pediatric residents' care of extremely low-birth-weight infants. *Arch Pediatr Adolesc Med*. 2000; 154(11):1123–1126

35. Bosque E. Collaboration, not competition: cost analysis of neonatal nurse practitioner plus neonatologist versus neonatologist-only care models. *Adv Neonatal Care*. 2015;15(2):112–118

36. Sheldon RE, Corff K, McCann D, Kenner C. Nursing perspectives: acute care nurse practitioners in the neonatal intensive care unit: why this is a successful collaboration. *NeoReviews*. 2015;16(3):e138–e143

37. Wallman C; Committee on Fetus and Newborn. Advanced practice in neonatal nursing. *Pediatrics*. 2009; 123(6):1606–1607

38. National Association of Neonatal Nurses. *Quality Metrics. Position Statement #3068*. Chicago, IL: National Association of Neonatal Nurses; 2016

39. Kaminski MM, Meier S, Staebler S. National Association of Neonatal Nurse Practitioners (NANNP) workforce survey. *Adv Neonatal Care*. 2015;15(3): 182–190

40. Staebler S, Bissinger R. 2016 neonatal nurse practitioner workforce survey:

report of findings. *Adv Neonatal Care.* 2017;17(5):331–336

41. Schell GJ, Lavieri MS, Jankovic F, et al. Strategic modeling of the neonatal nurse practitioner workforce. *Nurs Outlook.* 2016;64(4):385–394
42. Bellini S. State of the state: NNP program update 2013. *Adv Neonatal Care.* 2013;13(5):346–348
43. American Association of Nurse Practitioners. NP fact sheet. Available at: https://www.aanp.org/all-about-nps/np-fact-sheet. Accessed April 28, 2018
44. National Association of Pediatric Nurse Practitioners; Professional Issues Committee. NAPNAP position statement on age parameters for pediatric nurse practitioner practice. *J Pediatr Health Care.* 2019;33(2):A9–A11
45. Freed GL, Moran LM, Dunham KM, Hawkins-Walsh E, Martyn KK; Research Advisory Committee of the American Board of Pediatrics. Capacity of, and demand for, pediatric nurse practitioner educational programs: a missing piece of the workforce puzzle. *J Prof Nurs.* 2015;31(4):311–317
46. Freed GL, Dunham KM, Martyn K, et al; Research Advisory Committee of the American Board of Pediatrics. Pediatric nurse practitioners: influences on career choice. *J Pediatr Health Care.* 2014;28(2):114–120
47. Schell GJ, Lavieri MS, Li X, et al. Strategic modeling of the pediatric nurse practitioner workforce. *Pediatrics.* 2015;135(2):298–306
48. American Academy of Physician Assistants. What is a PA? Available at: https://www.aapa.org/what-is-a-pa/. Accessed January 31, 2018
49. American Academy of Physician Assistants. Physician assistants at a glance. 2016. Available at https://www.aapa.org/wp-content/uploads/2019/08/What_Is_A_PA_Infographic_LetterSize_July2019.pdf. Accessed January 31, 2018
50. American Academy of Physician Assistants. PA scope of practice. 2017. Available at: https://www.aapa.org/wp-content/uploads/2017/01/Issue-brief_Scope-of-Practice_0117-1.pdf. Accessed October 31, 2018
51. Reynolds EW, Bricker JT. Nonphysician clinicians in the neonatal intensive care unit: meeting the needs of our smallest patients. *Pediatrics.* 2007;119(2):361–369
52. National Conference of State Legislatures; Association of State and Territorial Health Officials. Physician assistants overview. Available at: http://scopeofpracticepolicy.org/practitioners/physician-assistants/. Accessed December 1, 2018
53. National Commission on Certification of Physician Assistants. *2017 Specialty Report.* Duluth, GA: National Commission on Certification of Physician Assistants; 2018. Available at: http://prodcmsstoragesa.blob.core.windows.net/uploads/files/2017StatisticalProfilebySpecialty.pdf. Accessed November 8, 2018
54. Schulman M, Lucchese KR, Sullivan AC. Transition from housestaff to nonphysicians as neonatal intensive care providers: cost, impact on revenue, and quality of care. *Am J Perinatol.* 1995;12(6):442–446
55. Mathur M, Rampersad A, Howard K, Goldman GM. Physician assistants as physician extenders in the pediatric intensive care unit setting-A 5-year experience. *Pediatr Crit Care Med.* 2005;6(1):14–19
56. Hascall RL, Perkins RS, Kmiecik L, et al. PAs reduce rounding interruptions in the pediatric intensive care unit. *JAAPA.* 2018;31(6):41–45
57. Freed GL, Dunham KM, Moote MJ, Lamarand KE; American Board of Pediatrics Research Advisory Committee. Pediatric physician assistants: distribution and scope of practice. *Pediatrics.* 2010;126(5):851–855
58. Bureau of Labor Statistics, US Department of Labor. Occupational outlook handbook, physician assistants. Available at: https://www.bls.gov/ooh/healthcare/physician-assistants.htm. Accessed January 31, 2018
59. American Academy of Physician Assistants. 2013 AAPA annual survey report. Available at: https://www.aapa.org/wp-content/uploads/2016/12/Annual_Server_Data_Tables-S.pdf. Accessed January 31, 2018
60. National Center for Health Workforce Analysis. Projecting the supply of non-primary care specialty and subspecialty clinicians: 2010-2025. 2017. Available at: https://bhw.hrsa.gov/sites/default/files/bhw/nchwa/projections/clinicalspecialties.pdf. Accessed November 7, 2018
61. Merriam-Webster. Competency. Available at: https://www.merriam-webster.com/dictionary/competency. Accessed May 13, 2018
62. Kak N, Burkhalter B, Cooper M. *Measuring the Competence of Healthcare Providers.* Bethesda, MD: Quality Assurance Project; 2001. Available at: https://usaidassist.org/sites/assist/files/measuring_the_competence_of_hc_providers_qap_2001.pdf. Accessed November 8, 2018
63. Institute of Medicine (US) Committee on the Health Professions Education Summit. In: Greiner AC, Knebel E, eds. *Health Professions Education: A Bridge to Quality.* Washington, DC: National Academies Press; 2003
64. Institute of Medicine (US) Committee on Quality of Health Care in America. *Crossing the Quality Chasm: A New Health System for the 21st Century.* Washington, DC: National Academies Press (US); 2001
65. National Commission on Certification of Physician Assistants; Accreditation Review Commission on Education for the Physician Assistant; American Academy of Physician Assistants; Physician Assistant Education Association. Competencies for the physician assistant profession. 2012. Available at: https://www.aapa.org/wp-content/uploads/2017/02/PA-Competencies-updated.pdf. Accessed February 3, 2018
66. American Board of Pediatrics. ACGME core competencies. Available at: https://www.abp.org/content/acgme-core-competencies. Accessed February 3, 2018
67. American Board of Pediatrics. Neonatal-perinatal medicine certification. Available at: https://www.abp.org/content/neonatal-perinatal-medicine-certification. Accessed February 3, 2018
68. American Academy of Pediatrics Committee on Fetus and Newborn. Hospital discharge of the high-risk

neonate. *Pediatrics.* 2008;122(5): 1119–1126

69. The Association of Post Graduate PA Programs. Postgraduate PA/NP program membership roster by specialty. Available at: https://appap.org/wp-content/uploads/2019/10/APPAP-Postgraduate-PANP-Program-Membership-Roster-by-Specialty-as-of-Oct-2019.pdf. Accessed October 25, 2019
70. Sawyer T, French H, Ades A, Johnston L. Neonatal-perinatal medicine fellow procedural experience and competency determination: results of a national survey. *J Perinatol.* 2016;36(7):570–574
71. Starr M, Sawyer T, Jones M, Batra M, McPhillips H. A simulation-based quality improvement approach to improve pediatric resident competency with required procedures. *Cureus.* 2017;9(6): e1307
72. Sawyer T, Gray MM. Procedural training and assessment of competency utilizing simulation. *Semin Perinatol.* 2016;40(7): 438–446
73. Butler-O'Hara M, Marasco M, Dadiz R. Simulation to standardize patient care and maintain procedural competency. *Neonatal Netw.* 2015;34(1):18–30
74. Halamek LP. Simulation as a methodology for assessing the performance of healthcare professionals working in the delivery room. *Semin Fetal Neonatal Med.* 2013; 18(6):369–372
75. Joint Commission Resource. *Medical Staff Essentials: Your Go-To Guide*, 1st ed. Oakbrook, IL: Joint Commission Resource; 2017
76. The Joint Commission. Standards interpretation. Available at: https://www.jointcommission.org/standards_information/jcfaqdetails.aspx?StandardsFaqId=1890&ProgramId=46. Accessed February 11, 2018
77. The Joint Commission. Standards FAQ details. Available at: https://www.jointcommission.org/standards_information/jcfaqdetails.aspx?StandardsFaqId=1605&ProgramId=46 Accessed February 11, 2018
78. Martin JA, Hamilton BE, Osterman MJK, Driscoll AK, Drake P. Births: final data for 2017. *Natl Vital Stat Rep.* 2018;67(8): 1–50
79. Tita AT, Landon MB, Spong CY, et al; Eunice Kennedy Shriver NICHD Maternal-Fetal Medicine Units Network. Timing of elective repeat cesarean delivery at term and neonatal outcomes. *N Engl J Med.* 2009;360(2): 111–120
80. Chiossi G, Lai Y, Landon MB, et al; Eunice Kennedy Shriver National Institute of Child Health and Human Development (NICHD) Maternal-Fetal Medicine Units (MFMU) Network. Timing of delivery and adverse outcomes in term singleton repeat cesarean deliveries. *Obstet Gynecol.* 2013;121(3):561–569
81. Holmes AV, Atwood EC, Whalen B, et al. Rooming-in to treat neonatal abstinence syndrome: improved family-centered care at lower cost. *Pediatrics.* 2016;137(6):e20152929
82. Kuzniewicz MW, Puopolo KM, Fischer A, et al. A quantitative, risk-based approach to the management of neonatal early-onset sepsis. *JAMA Pediatr.* 2017;171(4):365–371
83. Weston PJ, Harris DL, Battin M, et al. Oral dextrose gel for the treatment of hypoglycaemia in newborn infants. *Cochrane Database Syst Rev.* 2016;(5): CD011027
84. Payne V, Hall M, Prieto J, Johnson M. Care bundles to reduce central line-associated bloodstream infections in the neonatal unit: a systematic review and meta-analysis. *Arch Dis Child Fetal Neonatal Ed.* 2018;103(5):F422–F429
85. Bellflower B, Carter MA. Primer on the practice doctorate for neonatal nurse practitioners. *Adv Neonatal Care.* 2006; 6(6):323–332
86. Pressler JL, Kenner CA. The NNP/DNP shortage: transforming neonatal nurse practitioners into DNPs. *J Perinat Neonatal Nurs.* 2009;23(3):272–278
87. Staebler S, Meier SR, Bagwell G, Conway-Orgel M. The future of neonatal advanced practice registered nurse practice: white paper. *Adv Neonatal Care.* 2016;16(1):8–14
88. Freed GL, Dunham KM, Martyn K, et al. Neonatal nurse practitioners: influences on career choice. *J Nurse Pract.* 2013;9(2):82–86

Ongoing Pediatric Health Care for the Child Who Has Been Maltreated

- *Clinical Report*

CLINICAL REPORT Guidance for the Clinician in Rendering Pediatric Care

American Academy of Pediatrics

DEDICATED TO THE HEALTH OF ALL CHILDREN™

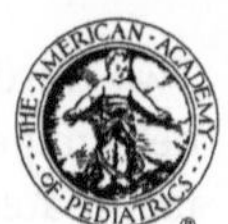

Ongoing Pediatric Health Care for the Child Who Has Been Maltreated

Emalee Flaherty, MD, FAAP,[a] Lori Legano, MD, FAAP,[b] Sheila Idzerda, MD, FAAP,[c] COUNCIL ON CHILD ABUSE AND NEGLECT

abstract

Pediatricians provide continuous medical care and anticipatory guidance for children who have been reported to state child protection agencies, including tribal child protection agencies, because of suspected child maltreatment. Because families may continue their relationships with their pediatricians after these reports, these primary care providers are in a unique position to recognize and manage the physical, developmental, academic, and emotional consequences of maltreatment and exposure to childhood adversity. Substantial information is available to optimize follow-up medical care of maltreated children. This new clinical report will provide guidance to pediatricians about how they can best oversee and foster the optimal physical health, growth, and development of children who have been maltreated and remain in the care of their biological family or are returned to their care by Child Protective Services agencies. The report describes the pediatrician's role in helping to strengthen families' and caregivers' capabilities and competencies and in promoting and maximizing high-quality services for their families in their community. Pediatricians should refer to other reports and policies from the American Academy of Pediatrics for more information about the emotional and behavioral consequences of child maltreatment and the treatment of these consequences.

[a]Department of Pediatrics, Northwestern University, Chicago, Illinois; [b]Department of Pediatrics, School of Medicine, New York University, New York, New York; and [c]Billings Clinic Bozeman Acorn Pediatrics, Bozeman, Montana

Drs Flaherty, Legano, and Idzerda conceptualized this clinical report, wrote sections of the draft, reviewed and revised subsequent drafts, and approved the final manuscript as submitted.

This document is copyrighted and is property of the American Academy of Pediatrics and its Board of Directors. All authors have filed conflict of interest statements with the American Academy of Pediatrics. Any conflicts have been resolved through a process approved by the Board of Directors. The American Academy of Pediatrics has neither solicited nor accepted any commercial involvement in the development of the content of this publication.

Clinical reports from the American Academy of Pediatrics benefit from expertise and resources of liaisons and internal (AAP) and external reviewers. However, clinical reports from the American Academy of Pediatrics may not reflect the views of the liaisons or the organizations or government agencies that they represent.

The guidance in this report does not indicate an exclusive course of treatment or serve as a standard of medical care. Variations, taking into account individual circumstances, may be appropriate.

All clinical reports from the American Academy of Pediatrics automatically expire 5 years after publication unless reaffirmed, revised, or retired at or before that time.

DOI: https://doi.org/10.1542/peds.2019-0284

Address correspondence to Emalee Flaherty, MD, FAAP. Email: e-flaherty@northwestern.edu.

PEDIATRICS (ISSN Numbers: Print, 0031-4005; Online, 1098-4275).

Copyright © 2019 by the American Academy of Pediatrics

FINANCIAL DISCLOSURE: The authors have indicated they have no financial relationships relevant to this article to disclose.

To cite: Flaherty E, Legano L, Idzerda S, AAP COUNCIL ON CHILD ABUSE AND NEGLECT. Ongoing Pediatric Health Care for the Child Who Has Been Maltreated. *Pediatrics.* 2019; 143(4):e20190284

Pediatricians provide medical care and anticipatory guidance for children who have been maltreated. Because as many as 25% of the child population has experienced some form of maltreatment, medical encounters in a pediatric practice with maltreated children are not uncommon.[1–3] Although only a small proportion of children who have been maltreated are investigated by Child Protective Services (CPS), each year, state CPS agencies determine that approximately 700 000 children have been victims of child maltreatment.[4] Approximately 75% of these children are neglected, and about 17% are physically abused; many children suffer multiple forms of maltreatment. In the United States, an estimated 1700 children die each year as a result of abuse and neglect. Child maltreatment has many long-term health, developmental, and emotional consequences for the children who survive.

Two-thirds of children who have been determined by CPS to have been maltreated will remain in the care of their families while receiving supportive and therapeutic services.[4] Even when children are placed in out-of-home care, approximately half will be returned to their families within days to months. The median length of stay in foster care for children who are later reunified with their family of origin is 8 months.[5]

Because families may continue their relationships with pediatricians despite the other disruptions and challenges they have experienced, pediatricians are ideally positioned to recognize and manage the physical, developmental, and emotional consequences of the maltreatment and to provide support and direction to the families of the children.[6] In this report, we will provide guidance to pediatricians and other primary care clinicians about the service and care for these children's physical, developmental, and cognitive needs. Pediatricians should refer to the reports from the American Academy of Pediatrics (AAP), "Clinical Considerations Related to the Behavioral Manifestations of Child Maltreatment"[7] and the forthcoming "Children Exposed to Maltreatment: Assessment and the Role of Psychotropic Medication,"[8] for information about the emotional and behavioral consequences of maltreatment and the treatment of these consequences. Previous reports have described the care of children entering foster care.[9,10] Providing care for the child remaining with the family and/or after his or her return to the family is the focus of this report. Besides the clinical care of the child, the pediatrician has a role in monitoring and supporting the family, working with the community, and advocating for appropriate interventions and services to help ensure that children grow up in safe, stable, nurturing environments.

FOLLOW-UP CARE OF THE CHILD

Children who have been maltreated need to be evaluated more frequently by the primary care clinician than other children of the same age. Certain ages and developmental stages will merit more thorough evaluations and more frequent follow-up. The clinician can follow the recommendations for youth entering foster care: 3 visits in 3 months after CPS involvement or leaving foster care and every 6 months after that.[9,11] Although much of the medical care for these children will follow along standard paths (eg, *Bright Futures: Guidelines for Health Supervision of Infants, Children, and Adolescents*[12]) certain areas deserve a more-thorough evaluation in children who have been maltreated. Typically, the child may be seen within the first week after return to his or her family, at 1 month, and again at 3 months after the transition.

The initial history should include the reason for CPS intervention, the outcome of the investigation, and any services recommended, if this information is available. Pediatricians may be aware that a patient has been reported to CPS. In some cases, the pediatrician will have been the initial reporter, and other times, a parent will have told the pediatrician about the report or subsequent investigation, possibly asking for the pediatrician's support or assistance. CPS investigators may have contacted the pediatrician during their investigation into an allegation of possible child maltreatment. When speaking to CPS, it is helpful for the pediatrician to document the name and contact information of the CPS investigator.

Pediatricians, however, report that they are not always informed of the outcome of the investigation.[13] Although in some states CPS may notify the initial reporter about the outcome of the investigation (whether it has been substantiated or unfounded), the pediatrician may not be informed of the outcome of the investigation or told about any services or interventions provided to the family. Sharing information between medical and child protection professionals can be challenging but is vital because the pediatrician can play an important role in supporting the family, ensuring that the family continues to participate in indicated services, monitoring the family for recurrent maltreatment, and preventing further maltreatment. If the CPS investigator refuses to provide information, the pediatrician can obtain parental consent and ask CPS for a multidisciplinary team meeting to discuss how he or she can best assist the family. Another strategy is to ask to speak to the investigator's supervisor or the director and explain how knowledge of the investigation and recommended services may help protect the child and assist the family with parenting. Some jurisdictions have medical directors who may be able to assist. Pennsylvania passed legislation in 2014 (Act 176) that enabled 2-way communication between CPS and the primary care physician.[14]

The pediatrician may want to ask the family if the child was placed in a cultural environment different from the family. For example, the family may speak a different language than that spoken by the family with whom the child was placed. In addition, because of the relative lack of approved American Indian foster homes, American Indian children may have been placed in non–American Indian foster homes, despite passage of the Indian Child Welfare Act (Pub L No. 95–608 [1978]).[15,16] Cultural displacement can occur when any child is placed out of his or her distinctive ethnic, linguistic, spiritual, or cultural community with any foster family who the child may view as "other."[17] American Indian children placed in white foster homes report feeling that they do not belong in either an American Indian community or in white society.[18]

If the child was placed outside the home, the pediatrician may ask about any medical problems, hospitalizations, immunizations, and other health care, including mental health care, that the child received during this placement. The parent can also be asked about referrals to subspecialists and whether their child was seen for those appointments. Although it may be challenging to obtain the medical records, the pediatrician will find it helpful to have access to the records of any medical care and mental health care provided. The parents may assist in obtaining these records if they understand the importance for both the parent and pediatrician to have this information.

The pediatrician can ask the parent about any behavioral changes or adjustment difficulties. The AAP report "Clinical Considerations Related to the Behavioral Manifestations of Child Maltreatment" discusses possible behavioral and emotional responses of a child who has been previously maltreated.[6] The pediatrician may be able to interview, separately from the parents, those children who are verbal and ask about their adjustment to the changes in their life and their return home. If the family has information about the placement home, the pediatrician can assess for possible exposures, such as lead in preschool children, secondhand tobacco smoke, and other hazards.

During adolescence, a psychosocial interview focusing on home environment, education and employment, eating, peer-related activities, drugs, sexuality, suicide or depression, and safety from injury and violence (HEEADSSS) can be conducted.[19] Using the HEEADSSS method of interviewing will help to assess the adolescent's adaptation and elicit risky health behaviors. Adolescents who have been maltreated may engage in risky behaviors, such as smoking, drug use, regular alcohol consumption, and binge drinking, which are behaviors with short- and long-term health consequences for the adolescent.[1,20,21] A history of sexual abuse during childhood is associated with risky sexual behaviors and early pregnancy.[22,23] Consider the administration of the human papillomavirus (HPV) vaccination, which can be administered as early as 9 years of age, in this high-risk population.[24]

Assessing Development, Cognition, and Academic Performance

Child maltreatment and other childhood adversities may affect brain development. Severe ongoing stress or "toxic stress" affects brain anatomy and function.[25,26] Early adverse experiences may affect the structure, organization, and activity of the brain because of the brain's plasticity.[27] Maltreatment may alter the hypothalamic-pituitary-adrenal (HPA) axis and autonomic nervous system function.[28] Exposure to adversity and early life stress, if not mitigated, may result in epigenetic changes.[29–31] Therefore, pediatricians may want to monitor developmental and social-emotional milestones, cognition, and the academic performance of the child.

Although pediatricians generally check developmental milestones in all children, children who have been neglected or have suffered abusive head trauma (AHT) will particularly benefit from having their milestones closely monitored. The etiology of both atypical developmental and behavioral delays is multifactorial.[32,33] Because drug and alcohol abuse are risk factors for child maltreatment, the risk of prenatal drug and alcohol exposure effects is increased in children who have been maltreated.[34] Therefore, the clinician may find signs of fetal alcohol spectrum disorders or behavioral issues related to other drug exposures.[35,36]

Early intervention services are often indicated to help speed up the child's acquisition of new skills. Repeated and regular surveillance and screening to assess and identify children who may be at risk for developmental delay is recommended. The AAP does not recommend or endorse 1 particular standardized screening tool. Guidance is available in the AAP policy,[37] and training and resources are available on the AAP Screening in Practices Web site, at www.aap.org/screening.

Child maltreatment is associated with an increased chance of impaired cognition and academic functioning; maltreated children are more likely to have lower grades and lower standardized test scores and IQ scores.[38–40] Academic difficulty associated with maltreatment may manifest as early as kindergarten.[41] Early maltreatment causes problems for adolescents because they may miss more days of school and complete fewer years of school compared with adolescents who were not maltreated.[38,40] Adolescents are at risk for impairment in cognitive flexibility, the ability to switch between thinking about 2 different concepts.[42–44] Cognitive flexibility is a measure of executive function. In addition to untoward changes in academic performance or school attendance, affected children may have difficulties interacting with peers. Extreme shyness, aggressive behavior, social isolation from peer groups, unstable moods, eccentric choice of clothing, or frequent use of school health services may suggest acute or unresolved victimization.[38,45] Some of these factors are also linked to the increased risk of more severe psychiatric illness.

Special attention should be given to the child's academic achievement because low school achievement is associated with low reading skills and overall educational outcome.[40] Lower academic achievement in parents may confer a higher risk of learning struggles in these children, and higher rates of family dysfunction contribute to delayed acquisition of preacademic and self-regulation skills.[46] Pediatricians can ask about school attendance because regular attendance appears to serve as a protective factor.[47]

Review of Systems

In addition to a general review of all systems, the family should be asked about the circumstances of any injuries occurring before and since the child was initially reported to CPS. Careful documentation of the circumstances of such injuries is essential.

Physical Examination

The physical examination should be guided by any current concerns or complaints, the type of maltreatment that occurred previously, and the age of the child. At each visit, the examination should include a complete head-to-toe inspection.

Growth parameters should be measured and compared with previous patterns of growth. Child maltreatment may be associated with nutritional disorders, including both growth failure and obesity.[48,49] Nutritional neglect may manifest as malnutrition.[50] The severity of the growth delay can have a long-term or permanent effect on the growth and cognitive development of the child. A child with marked malnutrition needs careful monitoring of his or her head circumference until 2 or 3 years of age as well as developmental status because severely malnourished children may never reach their full cognitive potential. All growth parameters should be followed until the pediatrician is confident that the child is on a healthy growth trajectory. Most children who have been malnourished will need to be followed more frequently than the standard health supervision schedule.[12]

Maltreatment can also be associated with obesity and eating disorders.[1,48] Childhood obesity is a concern for all children, but children subjected to maltreatment have higher rates of obesity.[48,49,51] The prevalence of obesity can persist and increase into adulthood. The British Birth Cohort, one of the largest studies to follow the effects of child maltreatment on BMI into adulthood, followed 15 000 subjects.[51] Children were not found to have increased BMI initially, but through adolescence and adulthood, BMI increased compared with those who were not maltreated. Physical abuse was associated with an odds ratio 1.67 (95% confidence interval: 1.25–2.24) gain in BMI by age 50 years. Sexual abuse and neglect are also associated with obesity.[51,52] The pediatrician may carefully follow the weight of children who were maltreated because early counseling and treatment may help to alter this trajectory.

Children who have been maltreated are also at risk for other eating disorders, such as anorexia nervosa and bulimia nervosa.[53] In particular, children who experienced physical neglect or sexual abuse are at risk for eating disorders in adolescence.[53] Maladaptive paternal behavior, described as low paternal communication with the child and low paternal time spent with the child, is also associated with eating disorders.[53]

An unclothed physical examination may reveal evidence of malnutrition or other signs of neglect and identify skin findings or other injuries suspicious for abuse. Bruises and other soft tissue injuries are the most common injury caused by child abuse.[54,55] If an infant who is not yet cruising has a bruise, the pediatrician may consider that the child may have been abused.[56] Patterned bruises and bruises on the face, ears, neck, trunk, and upper arm may also raise suspicion of abuse.[57,58] Bruises and scars resulting from previous injuries, including physical abuse, should be documented. The pediatrician should also document any new injuries. Attempts should be made to ensure that these lesions have been recognized and investigated by CPS.

An oral examination should be performed on children who have experienced maltreatment because children who have been neglected are more likely to have unmet oral health needs, and about half of children evaluated before entering foster care needed dental care.[59,60] A dental evaluation should be performed by a trained oral pediatric health care provider on all children 12 months or older.[11] It is likely that children who are reported to CPS and remain in their home have similar dental needs. Because frenulum tears in infants can be caused by child abuse, the pediatrician should also check the frenulum when performing the oral examination.[60,61]

The child's stage of sexual development is generally assessed and documented at each visit. Physicians should be sensitive to any previous trauma, particularly sexual trauma, when performing this assessment and examination. The onset of puberty in girls may be affected by abuse. Because the HPA axis is affected by child maltreatment and other adverse childhood experiences, alterations in onset of puberty can be found in children after maltreatment.[62–65] The type of abuse affects the timing of onset of puberty; a history of child sexual abuse may be associated with precocious puberty and earlier onset of puberty, and a history of severe child physical abuse is associated with both early puberty and delayed onset of puberty.[65–68]

Children and adolescents who have been sexually abused or assaulted will likely need follow-up testing for sexually transmitted infections.[69] The HPV vaccine is recommended at 9 years of age in children who have been sexually abused because these children are at high risk for HPV.[24,70] Children who are victims of sexual trauma have a greater risk of early initiation of sexual activity and pregnancy and should be counseled and tested accordingly.[70]

AHT

AHT is discussed separately in this report because it has specific physical and developmental consequences for the children who have been subjected to this form of abuse. Outcomes of AHT are related to the severity and location of the head injury or injuries. Children who are unresponsive when they first present for medical attention, those who suffer hypoxic ischemic injury, and those who present with a low Glasgow Coma Scale score tend to have the worst outcomes.[71–73] Approximately 20% of children who have suffered AHT will die as a result of their head trauma, and 60% to 80% will suffer some neurologic impairment ranging from mild to severe.[72,74–76] Children with AHT are slower to recover from their brain injury than children with similar injuries that are not the result of abuse.[77]

Children who suffered from AHT are at risk for microcephaly (from cerebral atrophy) or macrocephaly (from hydrocephalus).[78] Cerebral injury can result in a number of consequences. Cerebral palsy may evolve, often beginning with central hypotonia and a delay in motor milestones, followed by other signs, such as spasticity. Hemiparesis may lead to poor growth of 1 side of the body, causing an asymmetric body structure.[72] Cranial nerve abnormalities may also occur. Seizure disorders are a common sequela.[32,72,79] About 25% to 40% of children suffering AHT will experience visual impairment related to cortical or retinal injury.[72] Many children will also have speech and language delays. Attention-deficit disorders, self-injurious behavior, and developmental delays have all been described in children who suffered brain injury.[72,80] Global cognitive deficits, including problems in motor control, visual processing, and receptive and expressive language, have also been described.[73] Some of the cognitive, neuromotor, and behavioral sequelae may not be apparent for months or years after the injury, when a child is expected to perform higher-level cognitive activities.[81,82] Parents report particular difficulty in managing the behavior of children who suffered frontal lobe injuries caused by AHT.[72]

Autism spectrum disorder has been described in children who have suffered AHT.[72] Autism screening should follow the recommendation for pediatric well-child visits.[37,83]

Endocrine Consequences of AHT

Traumatic brain injury (TBI), including AHT, has been associated with endocrine consequences.[79,84,85] More data are available about adults who have suffered TBI, but in emerging data in children, endocrine dysregulation is reported in 5% to 90% of children after TBI.[79,85] Endocrine dysfunction is not a static situation and can evolve over time. Thus, it is important to continue to monitor a child's endocrinologic status after AHT.

Initially, TBI disrupts the HPA axis, resulting in antidiuretic hormone production and release.[85] Central diabetes insipidus is also observed at a higher rate in the short-term after an injury and is also associated with higher mortality rates. Central diabetes insipidus can occur in up to 30% of patients.[79] Both diabetes insipidus and cortical metabolism defects typically improve over the first year after injury; however, even 5 years later, approximately 30% of children who suffered mild to severe TBI will suffer from altered pituitary hormone secretion.

Growth hormone deficiency and disturbances in puberty are the most common endocrine problems that occur after TBI.[85] It is important to monitor growth over time in children who have experienced TBI by measuring height, weight, growth velocity, and pubertal staging.[79,86–88] Also, because other endocrine abnormalities can change over time, survivors of AHT should have careful growth and pubertal examinations every 6 to 12 months after the injury and then yearly, once stable. A pediatric endocrinologist will be able to recognize subtle hormone deficiencies and help guide the appropriate workup and follow-up.[85]

Adolescents Transitioning to Adult Health Care

For adolescents who may be transitioning to adult health care, it is important to connect them with providers for both their physical and mental health needs. Approximately 30% to 40% of the adolescents who have experienced child maltreatment are coping with mental health problems, and about one-third have a chronic illness or disability.[89–91] The clinician can teach adolescents the skills they will need to navigate the adult health care system.[92] Preparation for transitioning should start early: depending on their cognitive abilities, children 14 years or younger can be prepared and taught to manage their own care. Youth with special health care needs may require a longer transition process because issues such as guardianship and transfer of specialty care must be addressed.[89,92] Pediatricians can identify physicians in their community who are interested in working with adults with health care and mental health challenges.[92] In some communities, however, it may challenging to identify such physicians.

Resiliency

Children who have experienced childhood adversities, including child maltreatment, do not demonstrate a uniform response to these "childhood traumas."[93] Certain protective factors appear to buffer the child's response to these childhood adversities, including the child's temperament, personality, cognitive ability, and coping strategies and demographic variables, such as male sex, older age, and greater amount of education.[94]

The pediatrician can help build the child's resiliency. Children who have a caring and supportive adult in their life are more resilient.[95] This adult can be a parent, friend, relative, or teacher. The pediatrician can encourage the child to form relationships with supportive adults. A pediatrician who is a caring and constant individual in the child's life may help to promote the child's resiliency.[96]

Resiliency is also bolstered by a supportive family environment.[97,98] Pediatricians can help parents and caregivers be supportive and therapeutic by helping them understand the behaviors of children exposed to maltreatment.

A positive school experience may improve the child's sense of self-worth.[99] Extracurricular activities may also help to improve a child's self-esteem. In 1 study of children who had experienced violence in childhood, higher resilience was associated with greater spirituality, emotional intelligence, and support from friends.[96]

PEDIATRICIAN'S ROLE WITH PARENTS, FAMILY, AND OTHER CAREGIVERS

The pediatrician may use health care visits to determine how the child, parent(s), and other siblings are coping after a report and investigation by CPS. If the child or children were placed outside the home, the clinician may ask the parent how they are managing after the child's or children's return home. Parents are more satisfied with the child's primary care provider when stress is discussed during the visit.[100] Observing the parent-child interaction can also provide information about how they are coping. Parents generally respond positively to pediatricians when they are asked about the services or interventions they are receiving because of CPS intervention, especially if the pediatrician is open and nonjudgmental and expresses a desire to help the caregiver successfully parent their children.[101,102]

Families may perceive the CPS investigation as hostile or adversarial, and therefore they may not cooperate with CPS recommendations for services. In one study, no significant change in social support, family function, poverty, maternal education, or child behavior problems was found in households after CPS had investigated suspected maltreatment because either referrals were not made or families did not participate in the CPS-recommended services.[103] Because families may have a trusting relationship with their pediatricians, the family may respond to recommendations made by the pediatrician.

Pediatricians can better help families not only if they understand the reason for the initial report and the risk factors that may exist but also if they understand the family's response to the investigation and any services provided. Although some caregivers report that they are no better off as a result of an investigation, many caregivers report positive changes occurred as a result of CPS intervention and describe how they recognize their own role in the maltreatment reported.[102] Some parents change or reform high-risk parenting behaviors as a result of the report. Parents have demonstrated that they can learn to use the parenting techniques they learned in parenting classes.[102] Some parents identify new strengths in themselves or develop more confidence in their parenting abilities as a result of CPS intervention.[102]

If the child was placed outside the home during the CPS intervention, the pediatrician should ask the family if the child has developed new or concerning behaviors since living in other home(s). Children who return home after placement in foster care may bring with them new problem behaviors, which can add to the stress of a household.[104]

Poverty places additional stress on a family and may lead to food insecurity; therefore, the pediatrician should assess for this and other measures of poverty.[105,106] Food insecurity is not uncommon, and food insecurity is associated with both malnutrition and obesity. To assess for food insecurity, the AAP recommends the pediatrician ask the family to reply to 2 statements: (1) "Within the past 12 months, we worried whether our food would run out before we got money to buy more" (yes, no) and (2) "Within the past 12 months, the food we bought just didn't last and we didn't have money to get more" (yes, no).[105] This screen has been found to have high sensitivity and good specificity.[106] Pediatricians can learn about the resources available in their community, such as the Supplemental Nutrition Assistance Program; the Special Supplemental Nutrition Program for Women, Infants, and Children; summer food programs; and child and adult food programs, and make referrals when food insecurity is identified. Pediatricians can also advocate for adequate funding of community programs.

Recidivism: Identification and Prevention

Pediatricians should be aware that although CPS intervention may have interrupted the maltreatment, families continue to live in the same environment and may face the same challenges, such as poverty, food insecurity, interpersonal violence, substance abuse, and mental illness, as before the report to CPS. The family may have also experienced new and additional stressors, such as loss of financial support, loss of transportation, and other hurdles because of the CPS report. In addition, because CPS is still involved with the family, the CPS intervention may be an additional source of stress. The pediatrician can help the family by identifying and addressing these old and new stresses and by making referrals for appropriate services in the community, if indicated.

Most importantly, child maltreatment may recur.[107] Many factors are associated with higher rates of recurrence. Neglect is not only the most common type of child maltreatment, but it is also linked to higher rates of recurrence.[108,109] In addition, children who have suffered more than 1 type of maltreatment (eg, both physical abuse and neglect) are more likely to be maltreated again.[110] Many of the factors known to place a child at risk for maltreatment, such as poverty; poor parent-child relationships; younger children in the family; a greater number of children in the family; children with disabilities; families with low levels of family or social support; a single-parent household; caregiver mental health problems, particularly depression; and caregiver substance abuse, also are associated with higher rates of recurrence.[108,111–113] Caregivers of children with behavior problems and caregivers who were themselves abused as children are more likely to reabuse a child when the child remains in the home after a CPS report.[114]

Rates of recurrence range from approximately 1% to 2% for families considered at low risk for recurrence to greater than 65% for families at high risk.[115,116] In 1 large study of children who remained at home after child maltreatment, more than 60% were rereported within 5 years.[117] Families are at greatest risk to be rereported to CPS during the first 6 months after a case disposition.[111] Clinicians should encourage families to participate in and complete all services recommended by CPS because families who have accepted and actively engaged in services are more likely to be successful at preventing any recurrence.[118]

The pediatrician should remain alert to signs of recurrence and also understand that children who have suffered 1 type of maltreatment may suffer other types of maltreatment in the future.[110] At each visit, the pediatrician should inquire about the factors that initially placed the child at risk for maltreatment, the child's and family's adjustment, and any new stresses in the family. The family's failure to attend medical appointments may be another sign of abuse or neglect.

Families should be asked about the child's behavior and how they discipline or respond to negative behavior. The family should be counseled about appropriate discipline, and any use of corporal punishment should be discouraged. The pediatrician should discuss alternative forms of discipline appropriate to the age and development of the child. The parent should be encouraged to recognize and respond to positive behaviors in the child as a means of reinforcing these behaviors. For more guidance, refer to the AAP policy statement "Effective Discipline to Raise Healthy Resilient Children."[119]

Maternal depression is common in families involved with CPS.[120–122] Maternal depression is associated with harsh parenting, physical abuse, and increased psychological aggression.[120] Depression in fathers in the postnatal period is also associated with psychiatric disorders in their children and with family dysfunction.[123,124] Therefore, it is important to assess for depression and other signs of mental illness and to make appropriate referrals for treatment.[125,126] The Edinburgh Postnatal Depression Scale is a standardized tool to assess for maternal depression in the postpartum period, but other tools may be more appropriate to assess and identify depression in mothers and fathers of older children.[127] Pediatricians who suspect a recurrence of child maltreatment must report these suspicions to CPS, as mandated by state laws.[128] Some pediatricians are reluctant to report because they believe that they can help the family better than CPS can or because they are not certain that the child has been maltreated.[129] Some physicians fear that they will lose the family as patients if they report, but most families return for care after primary care physicians have reported them to CPS, according to 1 national study.[130] The CPS case worker, a child abuse pediatrician, or the local hospital child abuse team can serve as a resource for pediatricians when they are uncertain about their decision to report or the next steps they should take. Rather than viewing reporting as a punitive action, the pediatrician should recognize that a report to CPS may help to keep the child safe and may help the family obtain important services. In most cases, it is best for the pediatrician to tell the family that he or she plans to make a report to CPS and why the report is being made. Continuing an open and honest rapport with the family may help to maintain the family's trust.

Supporting Families

The pediatrician can ask caregivers and the children if they have friends or family members who provide emotional support. To help determine whether support is available, the pediatrician may ask whom the parents or caregivers would ask for help with the child or children if they suddenly became ill or had to be hospitalized. Likewise, the pediatrician can ask children to whom they would talk if they had problems they did not wish to discuss with their parent or caregiver. The primary care clinician can also provide emotional support by asking the caregiver and verbal children in the family about how they are feeling and coping. Caregivers found it helpful when others offered support that made them feel more secure or self-sufficient, rather than offering prescriptive interventions.[102] Supporting the family will increase the caregivers' abilities to buffer the stress for their child or children.[131]

ADVOCACY AND COLLABORATION WITH THE COMMUNITY

Communities often have resources that will help to support and strengthen families. Pediatricians should familiarize themselves with the resources available in their communities and advocate for the additional resources that are needed.

Community programs have proved to be successful in promoting parent-child interaction and helping the child's cognitive development and ultimate success. Children who have been neglected, particularly, may benefit from these programs. Reach Out and Read is a program already adopted by many pediatric practices in the country, which encourages parents to read aloud to their children from a young age.[132] Pediatricians give age-appropriate books to parents at each visit from 6 months to 5 years of age, encouraging the parents to read to their children. Reading aloud has been shown to increase the child's vocabulary and contributes to the child's subsequent reading ability. Pediatricians can help parents to understand the importance of talking to their children and reading aloud to their children beginning in infancy and how this interaction helps their child's development.

Significant disparities exist in children's early language environments, including differences in the quantity and the complexity of sentences that they hear.[133] These disparities are linked to the child's cognitive development and ultimate success in school.[134] The pediatrician can encourage and model for parents how, even from birth, they can talk to their child throughout the day.

Other resources that have been shown to be effective are home visiting programs and early childhood education programs. In home visiting programs, trained professionals visit parents and children in their home and provide support, education, and information that can help to improve parent caregiving abilities. Home visiting programs vary in form and quality.[135] The US Department of Health and Human services provides a current review of different home visiting program models and the evidence for their effectiveness.[129]

The Nurse-Family Partnership has been demonstrated to be effective in reducing risk factors for child maltreatment, but the program is only for first-time pregnancies.[136] The program begins in pregnancy and continues until the child is 2 years old. A number of randomized controlled studies have demonstrated that the program produced significant effects on women's timing and likelihood of subsequent pregnancies and number of subsequent births. In addition, these programs have increased the stability of the mothers' relationships with their partners; improved the mother-child responsive interaction; and improved the emotional development, language, mental development, and academic achievement of children born to mothers with low psychological resources.[137–139] There is also evidence that home visiting reduces the risk of child abuse and unintentional injury.[116]

Early Head Start programs have been shown to improve the child's cognitive abilities, language, attention, and health as well as decrease behavior problems.[140] Early childhood education programs can promote school readiness.[141] In addition, mothers also demonstrated improved parenting, better mental health, and more employment when their children participated in early childhood programs.[142] For school-aged children, some schools offer skilled and comprehensive support services, including assessment, counseling, mentoring, and tutoring. Primary care pediatricians should consider coordinating information, resources, and intervention with school personnel to support at-risk children and families. Other resources for the pediatrician are listed in Table 1. Pediatricians can learn more about the resources in their communities from their local CPS agencies and from social workers, child abuse teams, and child abuse pediatricians in their communities.

Parents need access to quality child care and education systems. Neighborhoods with more child care spaces relative to child care needs have demonstrated lower rates of child maltreatment.[143]

Parent training programs are designed to improve parents' child-rearing skills, increase the parents' knowledge of child development, and encourage positive child management skills. Pediatricians should determine which parent training programs are available in their communities. Rather than focusing on the children, Shonkoff, from the Center for the Developing Child, and Fisher[144] advocate focusing more resources on the adults who care for young children by strengthening their capabilities and improving the health and well-being of the parents and

TABLE 1 Resources for the Pediatrician

Resources
AAP
Bright Futures: Guidelines for Health Supervision of Infants, Children, and Adolescents provides pediatricians with guidelines for each health supervision visit. The tool and resource kit contains assessments and tools that the pediatrician can use to identify psychosocial issues, including suggestions for open-ended questions that can assess for family stress. Available at: https://brightfutures.aap.org
Connected Kids addresses violence prevention for children of different ages. Available at: https://www.aap.org/en-us/advocacy-and-policy/aap-health-initiatives/Pages/Connected-Kids.aspx
The Resilience Project provides education and resources to more effectively identify and care for children and adolescents who have been exposed to violence. Available at: https://www.aap.org/en-us/advocacy-and-policy/aap-health-initiatives/resilience/Pages/About-the-Project.aspx
Screening in Practices initiative provides training and resources to improve early childhood screening, referral, and follow-up for developmental milestones, maternal depression, and social determinants of health. Available at: www.aap.org/screening
Helping Foster and Adoptive Parents Cope with Trauma provides materials for pediatricians on how to support adoptive and foster families. Available at: http://www.aap.org/traumaguide
Council on Child Abuse and Neglect. Available at: www.aap.org/council/childabuse
AAP Policy Statement. "Abusive Head Trauma in Infants and Children." Available at: http://pediatrics.aappublications.org/content/123/5/1409
AAP Clinical Report. "The Evaluation of Children in the Primary Care Setting When Sexual Abuse is Suspected." Available at: http://pediatrics.aappublications.org/content/132/2/e558
AAP Policy Statement. "The Pediatrician's Role in Family Support and Family Support Programs." Available at: http://pediatrics.aappublications.org/content/128/6/e1680
AAP Clinical Report. "The Pediatrician's Role in Child Maltreatment Prevention." Available at: http://pediatrics.aappublications.org/content/126/4/833
AAP Clinical Report. "Evaluation for Bleeding Disorders in Suspected Child Abuse." Available at: http://pediatrics.aappublications.org/content/131/4/e1314
AAP Clinical Report. "Caregiver-Fabricated Illness in a Child: A Manifestation of Child Maltreatment." Available at: http://pediatrics.aappublications.org/content/132/3/590
AAP Clinical Report. "Evaluating Children With Fractures for Child Physical Abuse." Available at: http://pediatrics.aappublications.org/content/133/2/e477
AAP Clinical Report. "The Evaluation of Suspected Child Physical Abuse." Available at: http://pediatrics.aappublications.org/content/135/5/e1337
Center for the Study of Social Policy. Available at: https://www.cssp.org/
Centers for Disease Control and Prevention
Essentials for Childhood Framework. Available at: http://www.cdc.gov/violenceprevention/childmaltreatment/essentials.html
Preventing Multiple Forms of Violence: A Strategic Vision for Connecting the Dots. Available at: http://www.cdc.gov/violenceprevention/pdf/strategic_vision.pdf
Stop SV: A Technical Package to Prevent Sexual Violence. Available at: https://www.cdc.gov/violenceprevention/pdf/sv-prevention-technical-package.pdf
Preventing Child Abuse and Neglect: A Technical Package for Policy, Norm, and Programmatic Activities. Available at: https://www.cdc.gov/violenceprevention/pdf/can-prevention-technical-package.pdf
Pinterest board for Positive Parenting. Available at: https://www.pinterest.com/cdcgov/cdc-positive-parenting/
Connecting the Dots: An Overview of the Links Among Multiple Forms of Violence. Available at: https://www.cdc.gov/violenceprevention/pub/connecting_dots.html
Violence Education Tools Online (VetoViolence). Available at: http://vetoviolence.cdc.gov
Harvard University Center on the Developing Child. The Science of Early Childhood Series. Available at: https://developingchild.harvard.edu/resources/inbrief-science-of-ecd/
National Survey of Children's Exposure to Violence Bulletins. Available at: http://www.ojjdp.gov/publications/PubResults.asp?sei=94&PreviousPage=PubResults&strSortby=date&p=
Talk, Read, and Sing Together Every Day. Available at: https://www.ed.gov/early-learning/talk-read-sing
Too Small to Fail. Available at: http://toosmall.org/
Resilience: The Biology of Stress and the Science of Hope. Available at: http://kpjrfilms.co/resilience/

other caregivers to support the child's optimal development. They also advocate for the development of a better linkage between the services provided to the child and to the adult, what they call "two-generational programs."[144]

The Triple P (Positive Parenting Program) is a public health population-based intervention program designed to provide parenting and family support.[145–147] The program includes different intervention levels of increasing intensity. The program has shown positive effects on maltreatment and associated outcomes.[148]

Behavioral parent training programs, such as Parent-Child Interaction Therapy, The Incredible Years, and SafeCare, have been found to increase positive parenting behaviors, decrease problem behaviors in children, reduce abuse and neglect risk factors, and reduce recidivism in families involved in the child welfare system.[149] Attachment and Behavioral Catch-up therapy (10 sessions with child and mother) has been found to be effective in treating disorganized attachment, frightening parental behavior, and other atypical behavior associated with disorganized attachment.[150] More information is available in "Clinical Considerations Related to the Behavioral Manifestations of Child Maltreatment."[7]

GUIDANCE FOR PEDIATRICIANS

In summary, pediatricians can play an important role in helping children who have suffered previous maltreatment to grow and develop optimally. They can work with families to identify their strengths and stresses and develop priorities and goals that will assist families to provide a safe, nurturing environment. Pediatricians can advocate for community-based services that facilitate optimal growth and development of children.

Child

- Identify children in the practice who have been reported to CPS because of maltreatment. Using appropriate *International Statistical Classification of Diseases and Related Health Problems, 10th Revision* codes will help to track these at-risk children.
- Obtain records of any medical or mental health care provided.
- In the history, during the initial visit, include the reason for the CPS intervention, the outcome of the investigation, and any services recommended.
- Ask about any injuries occurring before and since the report to CPS.
- Assess whether cultural displacement occurred: ask if the child was placed in a cultural environment different from the family.
- Screen for possible hazardous environmental exposures, such as lead, drugs of abuse, and secondhand smoke.
- Monitor the child's growth and assess for growth failure, obesity, and eating disorders.
- Monitor the child or adolescent's development, academic progress, and emotional health.
- Monitor the child's adjustment in the home and at school.
- Be alert to signs of recurrence. The greatest risk for recurrence is during the first 6 months after a case disposition.
- Physical examination: Monitor growth parameters, look for signs of malnutrition, examine the skin for signs of previous injury or physical abuse, perform a dental evaluation on all children 12 months and older, and document the stage of sexual development at each visit.
- Help build resiliency by encouraging the child to form relationships with supportive adults.
- Children will need more frequent visits: 3 visits in 3 months and every 6 months after the maltreatment occurred and after returning home from foster care.
- AHT: If a child has suffered head trauma, follow the head circumference closely until 2 or 3 years of age, in addition to other growth parameters. Monitor development and academic performance and make appropriate referrals for intervention. Be aware that survivors of AHT may suffer from altered pituitary hormone secretion, which may persist. Carefully monitor growth and pubertal examination 6 and 12 months after the injury and annually once stable. Consider a consultation with a pediatric endocrinologist who can help guide the workup and follow-up.
- Adolescents: Assess for concerns with returning home and for risky behaviors. The HEEADSSS assessment may be used. Consider administering the HPV vaccine, which can be given as early as 9 years of age. Prepare adolescents for transition to adult providers by teaching them skills they need to navigate the adult health system.
- Children and adolescents who have been sexually abused or assaulted and who are examined soon after the assault will need follow-up testing for sexually transmitted infections.

Parent and Caregiver

- Encourage and enable family to follow through with recommendations and services provided by CPS. Focus on improving the capabilities and competencies of the child's caregivers. Identify other services that may be needed and make appropriate referrals for treatment programs for modifiable stresses, such as alcohol and drug abuse and parental depression.
- Assess how the parent(s) and other siblings are adjusting after a report to and investigation by CPS.
- Understand the family and child stresses, triggers, and dysfunction that led to the maltreatment. Provide families with the knowledge, skills, and support to raise their children. Help parents and caregivers to understand the behaviors of children associated with toxic stress. As needed, refer families to programs and resources that will help to improve their knowledge and skills and provide them with the support they need to raise their children.
- Encourage parents to talk to their children and read aloud to their children. Educate families about resources that may assist them in caring for their child, such as parental coaching programs. Recommend that preschool-aged children enroll in Head Start or other early childhood programs.
- Coordinate with school personnel to support at-risk children and families.
- Assess for food insecurity. Be aware of services such as the Supplemental Nutrition Assistance Program; the Special Supplemental Nutrition Program for Women, Infants, and Children; summer food programs; and adult and child food programs.
- Assess caregivers for depression and refer them for treatment if depression is identified.
- Assess families for their method of discipline. Any use of corporal punishment should be discouraged.
- Assess whether the parent(s) and child have friends and/or family

who provide them with emotional support.

- Work with the family to build resiliency. Fostering a positive, caring relationship between child and parent is a way to enhance resiliency.

Community and Advocacy

- To demonstrate the need for more community services, educate the community about the effects of toxic stress and adverse childhood experiences.
- Educate the community about child factors, family factors, and community factors that are protective and help to build resiliency.
- Collaborate with the community to identify vulnerabilities and effective services. Be knowledgeable about community resources for at-risk children and families. Advocate for high-quality, evidence-based services and programs, including early childhood and K-12 programs, that reduce toxic stress and mitigate the negative effects of toxic stress on the health and development of children to ensure that the services are equipped to properly address children with a history of trauma in a manner that is not punitive. Advocate for the funding of home visiting programs.
- Promote healthy community environments. Advocate for physically safe and hazard-free out-of-home placements for maltreated children. Advocate for foster placements in culturally similar environments.
- Join with the AAP chapter to work for better CPS-pediatrician communication. Join with the AAP chapter to advocate for better funding for CPS and to provide input into local and state services for children who are maltreated.
- Support policies and programs that strengthen economic supports to families and improve quality of child care and education.
- Advocate for more research to determine which strategies best help to reduce all forms of violence and how these strategies can be enhanced and translated into action in all communities.
- Consider serving on the local child protection team or other child abuse prevention programs in your local area as a consultant or advisor.

COUNCIL ON CHILD ABUSE AND NEGLECT EXECUTIVE COMMITTEE, 2017–2018

Emalee G. Flaherty, MD, FAAP, Co-Chairperson
Andrew P. Sirotnak, MD, FAAP, Co-Chairperson
Ann E. Budzak, MD, FAAP
Amy R. Gavril, MD, FAAP
Suzanne B. Haney, MD, FAAP
Sheila M. Idzerda, MD, FAAP
Antoinette "Toni" Laskey, MD, FAAP
Lori A. Legano, MD, FAAP
Stephen A. Messner, MD, FAAP
Rebecca L. Moles, MD, FAAP
Vincent J. Palsuci, MD, FAAP

LIAISONS

Sara L. Harmon, MD - *AAP Section on Pediatric Trainees*
Beverly Fortson, PhD - *Centers for Disease Control and Prevention*
Harriet MacMillan, MD - *American Academy of Child and Adolescent Psychiatry*
Elaine Stedt, MSW - *Office on Child Abuse and Neglect, Administration for Children, Youth and Families*

STAFF

Tammy Piazza Hurley

ABBREVIATIONS

AAP: American Academy of Pediatrics
AHT: abusive head trauma
CPS: Child Protective Services
HEEADSSS: home environment, education and employment, eating, peer-related activities, drugs, sexuality, suicide or depression, and safety from injury and violence
HPA: hypothalamic-pituitary-adrenal
HPV: human papillomavirus
TBI: traumatic brain injury

FUNDING: No external funding.

POTENTIAL CONFLICT OF INTEREST: The authors have indicated they have no potential conflicts of interest to disclose.

REFERENCES

1. Gilbert R, Widom CS, Browne K, Fergusson D, Webb E, Janson S. Burden and consequences of child maltreatment in high-income countries. *Lancet*. 2009;373(9657): 68–81
2. Felitti VJ, Anda RF, Nordenberg D, et al. Relationship of childhood abuse and household dysfunction to many of the leading causes of death in adults. The Adverse Childhood Experiences (ACE) study. *Am J Prev Med*. 1998;14(4): 245–258
3. Finkelhor D, Turner HA, Shattuck A, Hamby SL. Prevalence of childhood exposure to violence, crime, and abuse: results from the National Survey of Children's Exposure to Violence. *JAMA Pediatr*. 2015;169(8): 746–754
4. United States Department of Health and Human Services, Administration for Children and Families. Child maltreatment 2016. Washington, DC: Government Printing Office; 2017. Available at: https://www.acf.hhs.gov/cb/resource/child-maltreatment-

2016. Accessed September 9, 2017

5. United States Department of Health and Human Services, Administration on Children, Youth, and Famlies. *Child Welfare Outcomes 2009-2012 Report to Congress: Safety, Permanency, Well Being*. Washington, DC: Government Printing Office; 2014. Available at: https://www.acf.hhs.gov/cb/resource/cwo-09-12. Accessed September 9, 2017

6. Sege R, Flaherty E, Jones R, et al; Child Abuse Recognition and Experience Study (CARES) Study Team. To report or not to report: examination of the initial primary care management of suspicious childhood injuries. *Acad Pediatr*. 2011;11(6):460–466

7. Sege RD, Amaya-Jackson L; American Academy of Pediatrics Committee on Child Abuse and Neglect, Council on Foster Care, Adoption, and Kinship Care; American Academy of Child and Adolescent Psychiatry Committee on Child Maltreatment and Violence; National Center for Child Traumatic Stress. Clinical considerations related to the behavioral manifestations of child maltreatment. *Pediatrics*. 2017; 139(4):e20170100

8. Keeshin B, Forkey H, Fouras G, et al. Children exposed to maltreatment: assessment and the role of psychotropic medication. *Pediatrics*. 2019, In press

9. Council on Foster Care; Adoption, and Kinship Care; Committee on Adolescence, and Council on Early Childhood. Health care issues for children and adolescents in foster care and kinship care. *Pediatrics*. 2015; 136(4). Available at: www.pediatrics.org/cgi/content/full/136/4/e1131

10. Szilagyi MA, Rosen DS, Rubin D, Zlotnik S; Council on Foster Care, Adoption, and Kinship Care; Committee on Adolescence; Council on Early Childhood. Health care issues for children and adolescents in foster care and kinship care. *Pediatrics*. 2015;136(4). Available at: www.pediatrics.org/cgi/content/full/136/4/e1142

11. American Academy of Pediatrics; District II, New York State; Task Force on Health Care for Children in Foster Care. *Fostering Health: Health Care for Children and Adolescents in Foster Care*. 2nd ed. Elk Grove Village, IL: American Academy of Pediatrics; 2005

12. Hagan JF, Shaw JS, Duncan P, eds. *Bright Futures: Guidelines for Health Supervision of Infants, Children, and Adolescents*. 4th ed. Elk Grove Village, IL: American Academy of Pediatrics; 2017

13. Flaherty EG, Jones R, Sege R; Child Abuse Recognition Experience Study Research Group. Telling their stories: primary care practitioners' experience evaluating and reporting injuries caused by child abuse. *Child Abuse Negl*. 2004;28(9):939–945

14. Pennsylvania General Assembly. Domestic relations code (23 PA.C.S.), exchange of information, Pub L No. 2876: Cl 23

15. Sarche MC, Whitesell NR. Child development research in North American Native communities-looking back and moving forward: introduction. *Child Dev Perspect*. 2012;6(1):42–48

16. Leake R, Potter C, Lucero N, Gardner J, Deserly K. Findings from a national needs assessment of American Indian/Alaska native child welfare programs. *Child Welfare*. 2012;91(3):47–63

17. Phoenix A; Thomas Coram Research Unit. Diversity, difference and belonging in childhood: Issues for foster care and identities.*Social Work and Society International Online Journal*. 2016;14(2). Available at: www.socwork.net/sws/article/view/480/975. Accessed September 9, 2017

18. Westermeyer J. Cross-racial foster home placement among native American psychiatric patients. *J Natl Med Assoc*. 1977;69(4):231–236

19. Knight KM, Parr M, Walker D, Shalhoub J. Web-based training package for HEEADSSS assessment and motivational interviewing techniques: a multi-professional evaluation survey. *Med Teach*. 2010;32(9):790

20. Diaz A, Simantov E, Rickert VI. Effect of abuse on health: results of a national survey. *Arch Pediatr Adolesc Med*. 2002; 156(8):811–817

21. Hussey JM, Chang JJ, Kotch JB. Child maltreatment in the United States: prevalence, risk factors, and adolescent health consequences. *Pediatrics*. 2006; 118(3):933–942

22. Fiscella K, Kitzman HJ, Cole RE, Sidora KJ, Olds D. Does child abuse predict adolescent pregnancy? *Pediatrics*. 1998; 101(4, pt 1):620–624

23. Hillis SD, Anda RF, Dube SR, Felitti VJ, Marchbanks PA, Marks JS. The association between adverse childhood experiences and adolescent pregnancy, long-term psychosocial consequences, and fetal death. *Pediatrics*. 2004;113(2): 320–327

24. Robinson CL, Romero JR, Kempe A, Pellegrini C; Advisory Committee on Immunization Practices (ACIP) Child/Adolescent Immunization Work Group. Advisory Committee on Immunization Practices recommended immunization schedule for children and adolescents aged 18 years or younger - United States, 2017. *MMWR Morb Mortal Wkly Rep*. 2017;66(5):134–135

25. Garner AS, Shonkoff JP; Committee on Psychosocial Aspects of Child and Family Health; Committee on Early Childhood, Adoption, and Dependent Care; Section on Developmental and Behavioral Pediatrics. Early childhood adversity, toxic stress, and the role of the pediatrician: translating developmental science into lifelong health. *Pediatrics*. 2012;129(1). Available at: www.pediatrics.org/cgi/content/full/129/1/e224

26. Shonkoff JP, Garner AS; Committee on Psychosocial Aspects of Child and Family Health; Committee on Early Childhood, Adoption, and Dependent Care; Section on Developmental and Behavioral Pediatrics. The lifelong effects of early childhood adversity and toxic stress. *Pediatrics*. 2012;129(1). Available at: www.pediatrics.org/cgi/content/full/129/1/e232

27. Weiss MJ, Wagner SH. What explains the negative consequences of adverse childhood experiences on adult health? Insights from cognitive and neuroscience research. *Am J Prev Med*. 1998;14(4):356–360

28. Jaffee SR, Price TS, Reyes TM. Behavior genetics: past, present, future. *Dev Psychopathol*. 2013;25(4, pt 2):1225–1242

29. Roth TL, Lubin FD, Funk AJ, Sweatt JD. Lasting epigenetic influence of early-life adversity on the BDNF gene. *Biol Psychiatry*. 2009;65(9):760–769

30. O'Donovan A, Epel E, Lin J, et al. Childhood trauma associated with short leukocyte telomere length in posttraumatic stress disorder. *Biol Psychiatry.* 2011;70(5):465–471

31. Murgatroyd C, Patchev AV, Wu Y, et al. Dynamic DNA methylation programs persistent adverse effects of early-life stress. *Nat Neurosci.* 2009;12(12): 1559–1566

32. Nuño M, Pelissier L, Varshneya K, Adamo MA, Drazin D. Outcomes and factors associated with infant abusive head trauma in the US. *J Neurosurg Pediatr.* 2015;16(5):515–522

33. Dubowitz H. Child neglect. *Pediatr Ann.* 2014;43(11):444–445

34. Kelleher K, Chaffin M, Hollenberg J, Fischer E. Alcohol and drug disorders among physically abusive and neglectful parents in a community-based sample. *Am J Public Health.* 1994;84(10): 1586–1590

35. Hoyme HE, Kalberg WO, Elliott AJ, et al. Updated clinical guidelines for diagnosing fetal alcohol spectrum disorders. *Pediatrics.* 2016;138(2): e20154256

36. Goh PK, Doyle LR, Glass L, et al. A decision tree to identify children affected by prenatal alcohol exposure. *J Pediatr.* 2016;177:121–127.e1

37. Council on Children With Disabilities; Section on Developmental Behavioral Pediatrics; Bright Futures Steering Committee; Medical Home Initiatives for Children With Special Needs Project Advisory Committee. Identifying infants and young children with developmental disorders in the medical home: an algorithm for developmental surveillance and screening [published correction appears in *Pediatrics.* 2006; 118(4):1808–1809]. *Pediatrics.* 2006; 118(1):405–420

38. Lansford JE, Dodge KA, Pettit GS, Bates JE, Crozier J, Kaplow J. A 12-year prospective study of the long-term effects of early child physical maltreatment on psychological, behavioral, and academic problems in adolescence. *Arch Pediatr Adolesc Med.* 2002;156(8):824–830

39. Mills R, Alati R, O'Callaghan M, et al. Child abuse and neglect and cognitive function at 14 years of age: findings from a birth cohort. *Pediatrics.* 2011; 127(1):4–10

40. Perez CM, Widom CS. Childhood victimization and long-term intellectual and academic outcomes. *Child Abuse Negl.* 1994;18(8):617–633

41. Jimenez ME, Wade R Jr, Lin Y, Morrow LM, Reichman NE. Adverse experiences in early childhood and kindergarten outcomes. *Pediatrics.* 2016;137(2): e20151839

42. Spann MN, Mayes LC, Kalmar JH, et al. Childhood abuse and neglect and cognitive flexibility in adolescents. *Child Neuropsychol.* 2012;18(2):182–189

43. Tomoda A, Navalta CP, Polcari A, Sadato N, Teicher MH. Childhood sexual abuse is associated with reduced gray matter volume in visual cortex of young women. *Biol Psychiatry.* 2009;66(7):642–648

44. Tomoda A, Suzuki H, Rabi K, Sheu YS, Polcari A, Teicher MH. Reduced prefrontal cortical gray matter volume in young adults exposed to harsh corporal punishment. *Neuroimage.* 2009; 47(suppl 2):T66–T71

45. Wolfe DA, Scott K, Wekerle C, Pittman AL. Child maltreatment: risk of adjustment problems and dating violence in adolescence. *J Am Acad Child Adolesc Psychiatry.* 2001;40(3):282–289

46. Maclean MJ, Taylor CL, O'Donnell M. Pre-existing adversity, level of child protection involvement, and school attendance predict educational outcomes in a longitudinal study. *Child Abuse Negl.* 2016;51:120–131

47. Brayden RM, Deitrich-MacLean G, Dietrich MS, Sherrod KB, Altemeier WT. Evidence for specific effects of childhood sexual abuse on mental well-being and physical self-esteem. *Child Abuse Negl.* 1995;19(10):1255–1262

48. Widom CS, Czaja SJ, Bentley T, Johnson MS. A prospective investigation of physical health outcomes in abused and neglected children: new findings from a 30-year follow-up. *Am J Public Health.* 2012;102(6):1135–1144

49. Whitaker RC, Phillips SM, Orzol SM, Burdette HL. The association between maltreatment and obesity among preschool children. *Child Abuse Negl.* 2007;31(11–12):1187–1199

50. Homan GJ. Failure to thrive: a practical guide. *Am Fam Physician.* 2016;94(4): 295–299

51. Clark CJ, Spencer RA, Everson-Rose SA, et al. Dating violence, childhood maltreatment, and BMI from adolescence to young adulthood. *Pediatrics.* 2014;134(4):678–685

52. Power C, Pinto Pereira SM, Li L. Childhood maltreatment and BMI trajectories to mid-adult life: follow-up to age 50 y in a British birth cohort. *PLoS One.* 2015;10(3):e0119985

53. Johnson JG, Cohen P, Kasen S, Brook JS. Childhood adversities associated with risk for eating disorders or weight problems during adolescence or early adulthood. *Am J Psychiatry.* 2002;159(3): 394–400

54. McMahon P, Grossman W, Gaffney M, Stanitski C. Soft-tissue injury as an indication of child abuse. *J Bone Joint Surg Am.* 1995;77(8):1179–1183

55. Pau-Charles I, Darwich-Soliva E, Grimalt R. Skin signs in child abuse [in Spanish]. *Actas Dermosifiliogr.* 2012;103(2):94–99

56. Sugar NF, Taylor JA, Feldman KW; Puget Sound Pediatric Research Network. Bruises in infants and toddlers: those who don't cruise rarely bruise. *Arch Pediatr Adolesc Med.* 1999;153(4): 399–403

57. Pierce MC, Kaczor K, Acker D, Carle M, Webb T, Brenzel AJ. Bruising missed as a prognostic indicator of future fatal and near fatal child abuse. In: *Pediatric Academic Society Meeting*; May, 2008; Honolulu, HI

58. Pierce MC, Kaczor K, Aldridge S, O'Flynn J, Lorenz DJ. Bruising characteristics discriminating physical child abuse from accidental trauma. *Pediatrics.* 2010;125(1):67–74

59. Chernoff R, Combs-Orme T, Risley-Curtiss C, Heisler A. Assessing the health status of children entering foster care. *Pediatrics.* 1994;93(4):594–601

60. Fisher-Owens SA, Lukefahr JL, Tate AR; American Academy of Pediatrics, Section on Oral Health; Committee on Child Abuse and Neglect; American Academy of Pediatric Dentistry, Council on Clinical Affairs, Council on Scientific Affairs; Ad Hoc Work Group on Child Abuse and Neglect. Oral and dental aspects of child

abuse and neglect. *Pediatrics*. 2017; 140(2):e20171487

61. Thackeray JD. Frena tears and abusive head injury: a cautionary tale. *Pediatr Emerg Care*. 2007;23(10):735–737
62. Mendle J, Leve LD, Van Ryzin M, Natsuaki MN. Linking childhood maltreatment with girls' internalizing symptoms: early puberty as a tipping point. *J Res Adolesc*. 2014;24(4):689–702
63. Ryan RM, Mendle J, Markowitz AJ. Early childhood maltreatment and girls' sexual behavior: the mediating role of pubertal timing. *J Adolesc Health*. 2015; 57(3):342-347
64. Negriff S, Saxbe DE, Trickett PK. Childhood maltreatment, pubertal development, HPA axis functioning, and psychosocial outcomes: an integrative biopsychosocial model. *Dev Psychobiol*. 2015;57(8):984–993
65. Li L, Denholm R, Power C. Child maltreatment and household dysfunction: associations with pubertal development in a British birth cohort. *Int J Epidemiol*. 2014;43(4):1163–1173
66. Boynton-Jarrett R, Wright RJ, Putnam FW, et al. Childhood abuse and age at menarche. *J Adolesc Health*. 2013;52(2): 241–247
67. Zabin LS, Emerson MR, Rowland DL. Childhood sexual abuse and early menarche: the direction of their relationship and its implications. *J Adolesc Health*. 2005;36(5):393–400
68. Henrichs KL, McCauley HL, Miller E, Styne DM, Saito N, Breslau J. Early menarche and childhood adversities in a nationally representative sample. *Int J Pediatr Endocrinol*. 2014;2014(1):14
69. Seña AC, Hsu KK, Kellogg N, et al. Sexual assault and sexually transmitted infections in adults, adolescents, and children. *Clin Infect Dis*. 2015;61(suppl 8):S856–S864
70. Crawford-Jakubiak JE, Alderman EM, Leventhal JM; Committee on Child Abuse and Neglect; Committee on Adolescence. Care of the adolescent after an acute sexual assault. *Pediatrics*. 2017;139(3): e20164243
71. Duhaime AC, Christian C, Moss E, Seidl T. Long-term outcome in infants with the shaking-impact syndrome. *Pediatr Neurosurg*. 1996;24(6):292–298
72. Barlow KM, Thomson E, Johnson D, Minns RA. Late neurologic and cognitive sequelae of inflicted traumatic brain injury in infancy. *Pediatrics*. 2005;116(2). Available at: www.pediatrics.org/cgi/content/full/116/2/e174
73. Keenan HT, Hooper SR, Wetherington CE, Nocera M, Runyan DK. Neurodevelopmental consequences of early traumatic brain injury in 3-year-old children. *Pediatrics*. 2007;119(3). Available at: www.pediatrics.org/cgi/content/full/119/3/e616
74. Chevignard MP, Lind K. Long-term outcome of abusive head trauma. *Pediatr Radiol*. 2014;44(suppl 4): S548–S558
75. Peterson C, Xu L, Florence C, et al. The medical cost of abusive head trauma in the United States. *Pediatrics*. 2014; 134(1):91–99
76. Miller TR, Steinbeigle R, Wicks A, Lawrence BA, Barr M, Barr RG. Disability-adjusted life-year burden of abusive head trauma at ages 0-4. *Pediatrics*. 2014;134(6). Available at: www.pediatrics.org/cgi/content/full/134/6/e1545
77. Risen SR, Suskauer SJ, Dematt EJ, Slomine BS, Salorio CF. Functional outcomes in children with abusive head trauma receiving inpatient rehabilitation compared with children with nonabusive head trauma. *J Pediatr*. 2014;164(3):613–619.e2
78. Vadivelu S, Rekate HL, Esernio-Jenssen D, Mittler MA, Schneider SJ. Hydrocephalus associated with childhood nonaccidental head trauma. *Neurosurg Focus*. 2016;41(5):E8
79. Richmond E, Rogol AD. Traumatic brain injury: endocrine consequences in children and adults. *Endocrine*. 2014; 45(1):3–8
80. Crowe LM, Catroppa C, Babl FE, Rosenfeld JV, Anderson V. Timing of traumatic brain injury in childhood and intellectual outcome. *J Pediatr Psychol*. 2012;37(7):745–754
81. Weitlauf AS, Vehorn AC, Stone WL, Fein D, Warren ZE. Using the M-CHAT-R/F to identify developmental concerns in a high-risk 18-month-old sibling sample. *J Dev Behav Pediatr*. 2015;36(7):497–502
82. McPheeters ML, Weitlauf A, Vehorn A, et al; U.S. Preventive Services Task Force Evidence Syntheses, formerly Systematic Evidence Reviews. *Screening for Autism Spectrum Disorder in Young Children: A Systematic Evidence Review for the U.S. Preventive Services Task Force*. Rockville, MD: Agency for Healthcare Research and Quality; 2016
83. Johnson CP, Myers SM; American Academy of Pediatrics Council on Children With Disabilities. Identification and evaluation of children with autism spectrum disorders. *Pediatrics*. 2007; 120(5):1183–1215
84. De Sanctis V, Soliman AT, Elsedfy H, Soliman NA, Elalaily R, El Kholy M. Precocious puberty following traumatic brain injury in early childhood: a review of the literature. *Pediatr Endocrinol Rev*. 2015;13(1):458–464
85. Reifschneider K, Auble BA, Rose SR. Update of endocrine dysfunction following pediatric traumatic brain injury. *J Clin Med*. 2015;4(8):1536–1560
86. Acerini CL, Tasker RC, Bellone S, Bona G, Thompson CJ, Savage MO. Hypopituitarism in childhood and adolescence following traumatic brain injury: the case for prospective endocrine investigation. *Eur J Endocrinol*. 2006;155(5):663–669
87. Acerini CL, Tasker RC. Endocrine sequelae of traumatic brain injury in childhood. *Horm Res*. 2007;68(suppl 5): 14–17
88. Acerini CL, Tasker RC. Traumatic brain injury induced hypothalamic-pituitary dysfunction: a paediatric perspective. *Pituitary*. 2007;10(4):373–380
89. Council on Foster Care, Adoption, and Kinship Care And Committee on Early Childhood. Health care of youth aging out of foster care. *Pediatrics*. 2012;130(6):1170–1173
90. Jonson-Reid M, Kohl PL, Drake B. Child and adult outcomes of chronic child maltreatment. *Pediatrics*. 2012;129(5): 839–845
91. Norman RE, Byambaa M, De R, Butchart A, Scott J, Vos T. The long-term health consequences of child physical abuse, emotional abuse, and neglect: a systematic review and meta-analysis. *PLoS Med*. 2012;9(11):e1001349
92. Christian CW, Schwarz DF. Child maltreatment and the transition to

adult-based medical and mental health care. *Pediatrics.* 2011;127(1):139–145

93. Klika JB, Herrenkohl TI. A review of developmental research on resilience in maltreated children. *Trauma Violence Abuse.* 2013;14(3):222–234
94. Bonanno GA, Mancini AD. The human capacity to thrive in the face of potential trauma. *Pediatrics.* 2008;121(2):369–375
95. Heller SS, Larrieu JA, D'Imperio R, Boris NW. Research on resilience to child maltreatment: empirical considerations. *Child Abuse Negl.* 1999;23(4):321–338
96. Howell KH, Miller-Graff LE. Protective factors associated with resilient functioning in young adulthood after childhood exposure to violence. *Child Abuse Negl.* 2014;38(12):1985–1994
97. Masten AS. Global perspectives on resilience in children and youth. *Child Dev.* 2014;85(1):6–20
98. Tiet QQ, Bird HR, Davies M, et al. Adverse life events and resilience. *J Am Acad Child Adolesc Psychiatry.* 1998;37(11):1191–1200
99. Mrazek PJ, Mrazek DA. Resilience in child maltreatment victims: a conceptual exploration. *Child Abuse Negl.* 1987;11(3):357–366
100. Brown JD, Wissow LS. Discussion of maternal stress during pediatric primary care visits. *Ambul Pediatr.* 2008;8(6):368–374
101. Pietrantonio AM, Wright E, Gibson KN, Alldred T, Jacobson D, Niec A. Mandatory reporting of child abuse and neglect: crafting a positive process for health professionals and caregivers. *Child Abuse Negl.* 2013;37(2–3):102–109
102. Campbell KA, Olson LM, Keenan HT, Morrow SL. What happened next: interviews with mothers after a finding of child maltreatment in the household. *Qual Health Res.* 2017;27(2):155–169
103. Campbell KA, Cook LJ, LaFleur BJ, Keenan HT. Household, family, and child risk factors after an investigation for suspected child maltreatment: a missed opportunity for prevention. *Arch Pediatr Adolesc Med.* 2010;164(10):943–949
104. Taussig HN, Clyman RB, Landsverk J. Children who return home from foster care: a 6-year prospective study of behavioral health outcomes in adolescence. *Pediatrics.* 2001;108(1). Available at: www.pediatrics.org/cgi/content/full/108/1/e10
105. Council on Community Pediatrics; Committee on Nutrition. Promoting food security for all children. *Pediatrics.* 2015;136(5). Available at: www.pediatrics.org/cgi/content/full/136/5/e1431
106. Hager ER, Quigg AM, Black MM, et al. Development and validity of a 2-item screen to identify families at risk for food insecurity. *Pediatrics.* 2010;126(1). Available at: www.pediatrics.org/cgi/content/full/126/1/e26
107. Eastman AL, Mitchell MN, Putnam-Hornstein E. Risk of re-report: a latent class analysis of infants reported for maltreatment. *Child Abuse Negl.* 2016;55:22–31
108. White OG, Hindley N, Jones DP. Risk factors for child maltreatment recurrence: an updated systematic review. *Med Sci Law.* 2015;55(4):259–277
109. Connell CM, Vanderploeg JJ, Katz KH, Caron C, Saunders L, Tebes JK. Maltreatment following reunification: predictors of subsequent Child Protective Services contact after children return home. *Child Abuse Negl.* 2009;33(4):218–228
110. Finkelhor D, Ormrod RK, Turner HA. Re-victimization patterns in a national longitudinal sample of children and youth. *Child Abuse Negl.* 2007;31(5):479–502
111. Connell CM, Bergeron N, Katz KH, Saunders L, Tebes JK. Re-referral to child protective services: the influence of child, family, and case characteristics on risk status. *Child Abuse Negl.* 2007;31(5):573–588
112. Fluke JD, Shusterman GR, Hollinshead DM, Yuan YY. Longitudinal analysis of repeated child abuse reporting and victimization: multistate analysis of associated factors. *Child Maltreat.* 2008;13(1):76–88
113. Proctor LJ, Aarons GA, Dubowitz H, et al. Trajectories of maltreatment re-reports from ages 4 to 12: evidence for persistent risk after early exposure. *Child Maltreat.* 2012;17(3):207–217
114. Dakil SR, Sakai C, Lin H, Flores G. Recidivism in the child protection system: identifying children at greatest risk of reabuse among those remaining in the home. *Arch Pediatr Adolesc Med.* 2011;165(11):1006–1012
115. DePanfilis D, Zuravin SJ. Rates, patterns, and frequency of child maltreatment recurrences among families known to CPS. *Child Maltreat.* 1998;3(1):27–42
116. MacMillan HL, Thomas BH, Jamieson E, et al. Effectiveness of home visitation by public-health nurses in prevention of the recurrence of child physical abuse and neglect: a randomised controlled trial. *Lancet.* 2005;365(9473):1786–1793
117. Putnam-Hornstein E, Simon JD, Eastman AL, Magruder J. Risk of re-reporting among infants who remain at home following alleged maltreatment. *Child Maltreat.* 2015;20(2):92–103
118. DePanfilis D, Zuravin SJ. The effect of services on the recurrence of child maltreatment. *Child Abuse Negl.* 2002;26(2):187–205
119. Sege RD, Siegel BS; Council on Child Abuse and Neglect; Committee on Psychosocial Aspects of Child and Family Health. Effective discipline to raise healthy children. *Pediatrics.* 2018;142(6):e20183112
120. Conron KJ, Beardslee W, Koenen KC, Buka SL, Gortmaker SL. A longitudinal study of maternal depression and child maltreatment in a national sample of families investigated by child protective services. *Arch Pediatr Adolesc Med.* 2009;163(10):922–930
121. Dubowitz H, Black MM, Kerr MA, et al. Type and timing of mothers' victimization: effects on mothers and children. *Pediatrics.* 2001;107(4):728–735
122. Chaffin M, Kelleher K, Hollenberg J. Onset of physical abuse and neglect: psychiatric, substance abuse, and social risk factors from prospective community data. *Child Abuse Negl.* 1996;20(3):191–203
123. Ramchandani PG, Stein A, O'Connor TG, Heron J, Murray L, Evans J. Depression in men in the postnatal period and later child psychopathology: a population cohort study. *J Am Acad Child Adolesc Psychiatry.* 2008;47(4):390–398
124. Ramchandani PG, Psychogiou L, Vlachos H, et al. Paternal depression: an examination of its links with father, child and family functioning in the postnatal

period. *Depress Anxiety.* 2011;28(6): 471–477

125. Scott D. Early identification of maternal depression as a strategy in the prevention of child abuse. *Child Abuse Negl.* 1992;16(3):345–358
126. Earls MF; Committee on Psychosocial Aspects of Child and Family Health American Academy of Pediatrics. Incorporating recognition and management of perinatal and postpartum depression into pediatric practice. *Pediatrics.* 2010;126(5): 1032–1039
127. Cox JL, Holden JM, Sagovsky R. Detection of postnatal depression. Development of the 10-item Edinburgh postnatal depression scale. *Br J Psychiatry.* 1987; 150(6):782–786
128. U.S. Department of Health and Human Services, Administration for Children and Families. Home visiting evidence of effectiveness. Available at: http://homvee.acf.hhs.gov/. Accessed June 27, 2018
129. Flaherty EG, Sege R, Price LL, Christoffel KK, Norton DP, O'Connor KG. Pediatrician characteristics associated with child abuse identification and reporting: results from a national survey of pediatricians. *Child Maltreat.* 2006;11(4):361–369
130. Jones R, Flaherty EG, Binns HJ, et al; Child Abuse Reporting Experience Study Research Group. Clinicians' description of factors influencing their reporting of suspected child abuse: report of the Child Abuse Reporting Experience Study Research Group. *Pediatrics.* 2008;122(2): 259–266
131. Shonkoff JP. Capitalizing on advances in science to reduce the health consequences of early childhood adversity. *JAMA Pediatr.* 2016;170(10): 1003–1007
132. Zuckerman B. Promoting early literacy in pediatric practice: twenty years of reach out and read. *Pediatrics.* 2009; 124(6):1660–1665
133. Hoff E. The specificity of environmental influence: socioeconomic status affects early vocabulary development via maternal speech. *Child Dev.* 2003;74(5): 1368–1378
134. Forget-Dubois N, Dionne G, Lemelin JP, Pérusse D, Tremblay RE, Boivin M. Early child language mediates the relation between home environment and school readiness. *Child Dev.* 2009;80(3):736–749
135. Duffee JH, Mendelsohn AL, Kuo AA, Legano LA, Earls MF; Council on Community Pediatrics; Council on Early Childhood; Committee on Child Abuse and Neglect. Early childhood home visiting. *Pediatrics.* 2017;140(3):e20172150
136. Olds D, Donelan-McCall N, O'Brien R, et al. Improving the nurse-family partnership in community practice. *Pediatrics.* 2013;132(suppl 2):S110–S117
137. Olds DL, Robinson J, O'Brien R, et al. Home visiting by paraprofessionals and by nurses: a randomized, controlled trial. *Pediatrics.* 2002;110(3):486–496
138. Olds DL, Robinson J, Pettitt L, et al. Effects of home visits by paraprofessionals and by nurses: age 4 follow-up results of a randomized trial. *Pediatrics.* 2004;114(6):1560–1568
139. Olds DL, Kitzman H, Hanks C, et al. Effects of nurse home visiting on maternal and child functioning: age-9 follow-up of a randomized trial. *Pediatrics.* 2007; 120(4). Available at: www.pediatrics.org/cgi/content/full/120/4/e832
140. Love JM, Kisker EE, Ross C, et al. The effectiveness of early head start for 3-year-old children and their parents: lessons for policy and programs. *Dev Psychol.* 2005;41(6):885–901
141. High PC; American Academy of Pediatrics Committee on Early Childhood, Adoption, and Dependent Care and Council on School Health. School readiness. *Pediatrics.* 2008; 121(4). Available at: www.pediatrics.org/cgi/content/full/121/4/e1008
142. Love JM, Chazan-Cohen R, Raikes H, Brooks-Gunn J. What makes a difference: early Head Start evaluation findings in a developmental context. *Monogr Soc Res Child Dev.* 2013;78(1):vii–viii
143. Klein S. The availability of neighborhood early care and education resources and the maltreatment of young children. *Child Maltreat.* 2011;16(4):300–311
144. Shonkoff JP, Fisher PA. Rethinking evidence-based practice and two-generation programs to create the future of early childhood policy. *Dev Psychopathol.* 2013;25(4, pt 2):1635–1653
145. Prinz RJ, Sanders MR, Shapiro CJ, Whitaker DJ, Lutzker JR. Population-based prevention of child maltreatment: the U.S. Triple p system population trial. *Prev Sci.* 2009;10(1):1–12
146. Sanders MR, Bor W, Morawska A. Maintenance of treatment gains: a comparison of enhanced, standard, and self-directed Triple P-Positive Parenting Program. *J Abnorm Child Psychol.* 2007;35(6):983–998
147. Sanders MR, Burke K, Prinz RJ, Morawska A. Achieving population-level change through a system-contextual approach to supporting competent parenting. *Clin Child Fam Psychol Rev.* 2017;20(1):36–44
148. Macmillan HL, Wathen CN, Barlow J, Fergusson DM, Leventhal JM, Taussig HN. Interventions to prevent child maltreatment and associated impairment. *Lancet.* 2009;373(9659): 250–266
149. Thomas R, Zimmer-Gembeck MJ. Parent-child interaction therapy: an evidence-based treatment for child maltreatment. *Child Maltreat.* 2012;17(3):253–266
150. Bernard K, Dozier M, Bick J, Lewis-Morrarty E, Lindhiem O, Carlson E. Enhancing attachment organization among maltreated children: results of a randomized clinical trial. *Child Dev.* 2012;83(2):623–636

Organized Sports for Children, Preadolescents, and Adolescents

- *Clinical Report*

CLINICAL REPORT Guidance for the Clinician in Rendering Pediatric Care

American Academy of Pediatrics

DEDICATED TO THE HEALTH OF ALL CHILDREN™

Organized Sports for Children, Preadolescents, and Adolescents

Kelsey Logan, MD, MPH, FAAP,[a] Steven Cuff, MD, FAAP,[b] COUNCIL ON SPORTS MEDICINE AND FITNESS

abstract

Interest and participation in organized sports for children, preadolescents, and adolescents continue to grow. Because of increased participation, and younger entry age, in organized sports, appropriate practice, game schedules, and content become more important, taking into account athlete developmental stage and skills. Parental support for organized sports in general, with focus on development and fun instead of winning, has emerged as a key factor in the athlete's enjoyment of sports. Schools and community sports organizations who support multiple levels of sport (eg, recreational, competitive, elite) can include more youth who want to play sports and combat sport dropout. This report reviews the benefits and risks of organized sports as well as the roles of schools, community organizations, parents, and coaches in organized sports. It is designed to complement the American Academy of Pediatrics clinical reports "Physical Activity Assessment and Counseling in Pediatric Clinical Settings" and "Sports Specialization and Intensive Training in Young Athletes" by reviewing relevant literature on healthy organized sports for youth and providing guidance on organized sport readiness and entry. The report also provides guidance for pediatricians on counseling parents and advocating for healthy organized sports participation.

[a]Division of Sports Medicine, Cincinnati Children's Hospital Medical Center, Cincinnati, Ohio; and [b]Division of Sports Medicine, Nationwide Children's Hospital, and Department of Pediatrics, The Ohio State University College of Medicine, Columbus, Ohio

Drs Logan and Cuff served as coauthors of the manuscript and provided substantial input into its content and revision; and both authors approved the final manuscript as submitted.

This document is copyrighted and is property of the American Academy of Pediatrics and its Board of Directors. All authors have filed conflict of interest statements with the American Academy of Pediatrics. Any conflicts have been resolved through a process approved by the Board of Directors. The American Academy of Pediatrics has neither solicited nor accepted any commercial involvement in the development of the content of this publication.

Clinical reports from the American Academy of Pediatrics benefit from expertise and resources of liaisons and internal (AAP) and external reviewers. However, clinical reports from the American Academy of Pediatrics may not reflect the views of the liaisons or the organizations or government agencies that they represent.

The guidance in this report does not indicate an exclusive course of treatment or serve as a standard of medical care. Variations, taking into account individual circumstances, may be appropriate.

All clinical reports from the American Academy of Pediatrics automatically expire 5 years after publication unless reaffirmed, revised, or retired at or before that time.

DOI: https://doi.org/10.1542/peds.2019-0997

Address correspondence to Kelsey Logan, MD, MPH, FAAP. E-mail: kelsey.logan@cchmc.org

PEDIATRICS (ISSN Numbers: Print, 0031-4005; Online, 1098-4275).

Copyright © 2019 by the American Academy of Pediatrics

FINANCIAL DISCLOSURE: The authors have indicated they have no financial relationships relevant to this article to disclose.

To cite: Logan K, Cuff S, AAP COUNCIL ON SPORTS MEDICINE AND FITNESS. Organized Sports for Children, Preadolescents, and Adolescents. *Pediatrics.* 2019;143(6):e20190997

DEFINITION

For this report, organized sport is defined as physical activity that is directed by adult or youth leaders and involves rules and formal practice and competition. School and club sports are included in this definition. Physical education classes at schools do not typically fall into the category of organized sport.

INTRODUCTION

Organized sports participation has become a large part of children's and adolescents' lives over recent decades and has contributed to many positive outcomes. Health benefits from physical activity and organized sports participation may include better overall mental health in young adolescents,[1] higher bone mineral density in adult women who spent more time playing sports at 12 years of age,[2] and a decrease in cardiovascular risk, overweight, and obesity in elementary schoolchildren.[3,4] Participation in organized sports in adolescence is associated with higher physical activity[5] and better subjective health in young adulthood.[6] Remarkably, the strongest predictor of physical activity and higher level of health in male World War II veterans was shown to be whether they played a varsity sport in high school.[7] As discussed in a clinical report from the American Academy of Pediatrics (AAP) that is currently under development ("Physical Activity Assessment and Counseling in Pediatric Clinical Settings"), childhood skills developed in organized sports, such as rope jumping, kicking, and throwing, are associated with better cardiovascular fitness, both in the short-term[8] and into adolescence.[9] Organized sports participation may aid in the development of physical skills, such as hand-eye coordination, functional movement skills and strength, and academic, self-regulatory, and general life skills. It also may have positive social benefits, leading to both improved social identity and social adjustment.[10]

However, children in the United States may not be realizing the positive effects of organized sport. The United States Report Card on Physical Activity for Children and Youth has reported low grades for overall physical activity and high school sports participation.[11]

There is a small amount of data on the specific effect of organized sports participation on children with special health care needs and disabilities. Adolescents with chronic health conditions were evaluated for their participation in organized sports. Young women with a chronic health condition were found to have similar rates of organized sports participation as controls; however, young men with a chronic health condition were significantly less likely to participate, with time and having an injury or physical handicap as the main barriers.[12]

For youth with developmental disabilities, organized sports participation, particularly length of time involved in the Special Olympics, has shown to improve both psychosocial function and physical fitness.[13] Children and adolescents with neurologic disabilities (cerebral palsy, spinal cord injury, and myelomeningocele) who participate in organized sports are shown to have higher levels of physical activity, social support, self-perceived physical appearance, and self-worth.[14] A study of adults with physical disabilities showed that quality of life was higher in those who participated in adaptive sports than those who did not.[15]

There are physical activity data clearly showing low levels of cardiorespiratory fitness in children with intellectual disabilities; this fitness continues to decline as the child ages.[16] Overall, physical activity rates are shown to be lower in children with developmental disabilities, compared with the general population.[17]

This clinical report replaces a previous AAP clinical report titled "Organized Sports for Children and Preadolescents"[18] and is complementary to the AAP clinical reports "Physical Activity Assessment and Counseling in Pediatric Clinical Settings" (currently under development) and "Sports Specialization and Intensive Training in Young Athletes."[19] This report reviews the benefits and risks of organized sports as well as the roles of schools, community organizations, parents, and coaches in organized sports. Guidance for pediatricians on counseling parents and advocating for healthy organized sports participation is provided.

ROLE OF FREE PLAY AND READINESS

Children learn skills needed for organized sports through active play that is fun and developmentally appropriate (Fig 1). Given the right developmental environment, many of these skills are learned through free play, such as running, leaping, and climbing.[20] Ample opportunity for free play is necessary, especially in the preschool and elementary school years, when the basic skills needed for organized sports are being developed and combined (eg, kicking while running). A program designed to incorporate skill development into free play in kindergartners and first-graders was associated with significant improvement in a variety of motor skill tests; these improvements persisted at a 4-month follow-up.[8]

Motor skill development in childhood may ultimately be important for future health. It has been associated with level of physical activity in older childhood, with those with better motor coordination engaging in more physical activity than those with lesser skills.[21] Skill development during elementary school years may also occur with organized sports. Motor coordination is significantly higher in 6- through 9-year-olds who have consistent organized sports participation compared with those who do not participate regularly or at all.[22]

Children who feel competent in skills required for their specific organized sport have more fun and are more likely to stay in the sport than those who do not.[23] Aspects of readiness to consider are motor skill acquisition, ability to combine those skills, and attention span.[23] Children who are younger than 6 years may not possess sufficient skills and attention span, even for simple organized sports.[24]

ROLE OF SCHOOLS

In the academic year, youth spend much of their waking time at school,

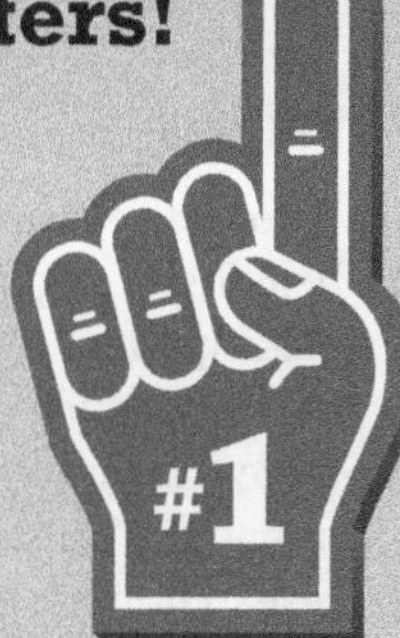

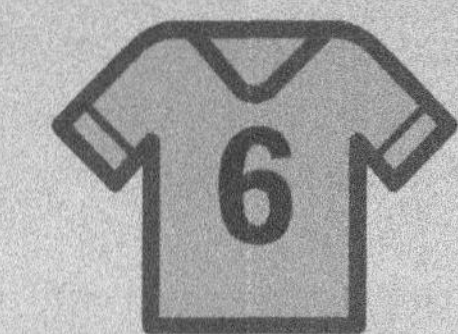

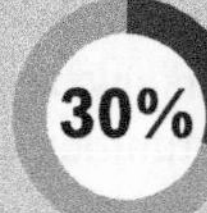

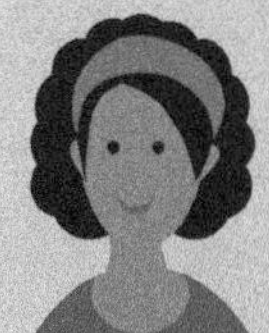

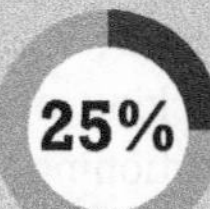

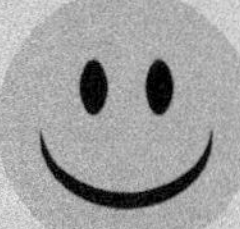

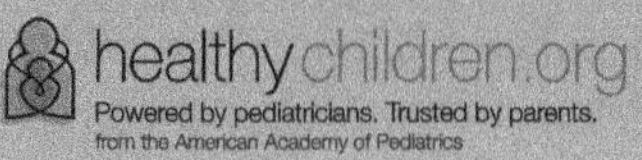

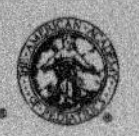

FIGURE 1
Kids and sports: let the fun win!

in a relatively controlled environment. Physical activity improves cognitive performance in school; participation in organized sports outside of school is also associated with higher cognitive performance.[25] Although there is little research on organized sports in schools, given this association, it may be prudent for schools to explore organized sports for students, whether in school or in school-sport organization partnerships.

A large study of urban Canadian youth of low socioeconomic status (SES) showed low levels of overall involvement in organized school sports, with increasing participation among boys over time[26]; participation of girls stayed stable. In the same study, participation in organized sports outside school declined over time. This may represent an opportunity for schools to increase their organized sports options as adolescents age, not decrease them, as is the current trend. However, if increasing physical activity through organized sports is the goal, just increasing opportunity has not been shown to definitively increase physical activity.[27] Elementary school students in "sports schools" (defined as simply adding more standard physical education time with specific development of bodily and sport-specific skills, at least 4.5 hours of physical education weekly), despite having more physical activity during school time than students in "normal schools" (90 minutes of physical education weekly), did not have more overall physical activity.[27] The students decreased their involvement in leisure-time organized sports, offsetting the increases they saw in physical activity at school.

In the School Health Policies and Programs Study, researchers identified "competence in motor skills and movement patterns" as a goal of most schools' physical education programs.[28] Less than 70% of schools described achieving that goal, and in an era of decreasing prevalence of physical education programming during the school day, school-based organized sports offers another resource to meet such goals.[28,29] As schools focus less on motor skill development and assessment, this may be a missed opportunity to expose young children to motor skill training and to identify children who are not accomplishing expected skills.[29]

There is some evidence of school-community partnerships that increase organized sports participation. A program that provides after-school soccer, creative writing, and service learning experiences (partnering with local elementary schools) slightly increased moderate to vigorous physical activity (MVPA) in overweight and obese youth.[30]

ROLE OF COMMUNITY ORGANIZATIONS

As the level of competition in organized sports leagues increase, those who do not desire to compete at a higher level may simply drop out of sports.[31] A study indicated that girls who do not become involved at a young age (<8 years) will likely not become involved as they get older, but boys may join sports in adolescence, even if they are not involved earlier.[31] Because some health benefits are seen with any organized sports participation, community offerings for girls and boys at multiple levels of competition could support greater participation. The business model of most community youth sports organizations has drifted toward supporting higher and higher playing levels (eg, "elite" levels). Expanding programming to all levels for all ages would create more opportunities for more athletes and potentially support financial health of the organizations.

From preadolescence through adolescence, a steep decline in physical activity is seen in girls, culminating in little physical activity by the end of adolescence, outside what is mandated at school.[32,33] This affects African American girls more than it does white girls, shown in the National Heart, Lung, and Blood Institute Growth and Health Study.[32,33] Community organizations that engage in organized sports management, partnering with schools, could focus on improving physical activity in girls, particularly if they start at a young age.

A known correlate of organized sports participation is SES. A study indicated that participation for both sexes increases as SES level increases, and those with higher SES engage in higher levels of physical activity in high school and young adulthood.[34] A barrier to organized sports participation is affordability[35]; organizations that provide low- or no-cost options may attract a higher number of low-SES youth for activities. Another barrier is transportation home from after-school activities, as demonstrated in a study of urban adolescents in after-school programs.[36] The Aspen Institute's Project Play advocates for the revitalization of in-town leagues to close gaps between organized sports participation in high- and low-SES areas.[37] Strategies to remove barriers to sport participation for families with low SES are making parents aware of existing funding opportunities, increasing funding opportunities or subsidies, and providing ways for parents to volunteer in exchange for lower fees.[38]

The average age of entry into organized sports is decreasing. To increase engagement and long-term participation, administrating organizations will need to tailor game and practice schedules and content to the appropriate child developmental level.[39]

In addition, the community youth development (CYD) framework has been proposed as a successful model to increase the benefit of organized sports through community organizations.[40] This framework includes youth in planning their organized sports activities and using their skills to contribute to the health of their community while building on participants' strengths and recognizing areas of potential growth. The basis of CYD includes addressing young people's sense of belonging, sense of mastery, and sense of generosity and mattering, culminating with the opportunity to make a difference in their own world.[40] One example of a program using CYD elements is Play it Smart, a National Football Foundation program that focuses on transferring sports skills to academics, relationships, and job readiness; this program showed a positive academic effect for participants.[41]

BENEFITS

Before discussing the perceived benefits of organized sports participation, it is worthwhile to note that much of the research on this topic has largely been observational in nature. Therefore, although such research may show statistically significant correlations, it cannot necessarily establish causality or direction of causality.

Skill Acquisition

Early development of motor skills is important because both preschool[42,43] and school-aged children[21,44] with better motor skill performance and coordination are more likely to be physically active. Unfortunately, many children do not naturally learn fundamental motor skills,[45] and low-income minority students may be at particular risk for starting preschool with delayed fundamental motor skills development.[45] Fundamental motor skills, such as running, leaping, throwing, catching, and kicking, are essential for everyday functioning and are important building blocks for higher-level sports skills. One way to help kids achieve motor skill proficiency is through organized sports participation.[24] Youth sports provide a framework in which kids can learn, practice, and develop gross motor skills.[24] Boys participating in organized sports have demonstrated better hand-eye coordination than nonparticipants, although the correlation is less strong in girls.[46] Children consistently engaged in sports also demonstrate superior gross motor coordination[22] via assessment of fundamental motor skills, and organized physical activity appears to have a greater effect on fundamental motor skill proficiency than nonorganized physical activity.[47] Similarly, seventh- and eighth-graders involved in outside sports demonstrate an association with stronger grip and back strength, along with greater vertical jump and vertical power, when compared with those who participate only in physical education classes.[48] When matched with controls, a group of 12- to 15-year-olds involved in soccer training showed associated gains in leg press strength and shuttle run speed,[49] and kindergarten through eighth-graders involved in T-ball, baseball, and softball demonstrated more advanced throwing development.[50]

Organized sports participation's effect on skill development is not limited to the acquisition of physical skills. There is extensive evidence to show that elite athletes tend to be high academic achievers.[51–55] Both parents and children from low-income families report that improved academic performance is associated with involvement in youth sports.[38] Specifically, sports participation has been associated with increased mathematic performance.[56] Among adolescents, practicing organized extracurricular physical activity is positively correlated with cognitive performance in verbal, numeric, and reasoning domains.[57] In fact, athletes taking part in multiple activities may score higher than those involved in only 1.[57] One explanation for this is that elite athletes report increased use of self-regulatory skills, such as planning, self-monitoring, evaluation, reflection, and effort.[53] More specifically, these athletes reflect more on past performance to learn and, therefore, may benefit more from the time they spend on learning.[58] Snyder and Spreitzer[59] postulate other reasons that school sports participation may enhance academics, including increased interest in the school, desire to maintain eligibility, heightened sense of self-worth, others (parents, coaches, and teachers) taking a personal interest in their classroom performance, and the hope of participating in college athletics. Furthermore, effective time management skills are essential to balance both sport and school commitments, and research shows that athletes may use their free time more efficiently than the typical adolescent[52,60] and spend more time on homework.[55] Athletes tend to be goal oriented and problem focused.[51,60] It stands to reason that these attributes carry over into the educational realm and contribute to the academic success and higher graduation rates reported in athletes compared with nonathletes.[61,62] Additionally, it has been shown that there is an association of athletic involvement with plans to attend college[63,64] and that a greater percentage of high school athletes go on to college, compared with their peers, even when controlling for SES.[55,59]

The development of life skills, defined as skills that are required to deal with the demands and challenges of everyday life,[65] is also associated with sports participation. Life skills are important predictors of future well-being, academic performance, and job satisfaction.[66] Coaches may recognize the importance of teaching nonathletic skills and values and prioritize the personal development of their athletes.[67–69] Parents use sport contexts to reinforce concepts like sportsmanship and personal responsibility, and both parents and coaches use sports to emphasize work ethic.[70] Athletes report learning experiences related to self-knowledge and emotional regulation, taking initiative, goal setting, applying effort, respect, teamwork, and leadership.[71–73] In 1 sample of high school students, athletes demonstrated significantly greater leadership ability than their nonathletic peers on the basis of scores from a standardized leadership ability test.[74] The sporting environment is also rich in feedback and instruction and is highly goal oriented, all of which may further the development of self-regulatory life skills.[58] In a recent systematic review of sports programs serving a socially vulnerable population, authors made the correlation that at least 1 life skill improved in participating youth in each study.[66] In low-income families, both parents and children identify emotional control, exploration, confidence, and discipline to be benefits associated with youth sports participation.[38] Not all programs appear to be created equally, however. Table 1 lists characteristics of a well-designed youth sports program.[66,75]

Social

Involvement in sports, particularly as a member of a sports team, may help youth to develop psychosocially and help form their social identity. Participation in organized sports is strongly associated with a positive social self-concept.[64] The team environment provides a setting for athletes to bond socially, identify with peers, and engage in personal growth and development.[76] It has also been correlated with enhanced perception of social acceptance.[77,78] Organized sports participation allows kids to work with others to achieve goals and provides an opportunity for peer interaction and for participants to learn social skills.[70] Athletes score higher on social functioning measures,[79] and high-level athletes, in particular, report significantly superior general self-concept and better peer and parent relations than nonathletes.[52] In a systematic review of the social benefits of organized sports in children and adolescents, researchers associated involvement in sports with better social skills.[10] There is evidence that such benefits may be long-lasting because a longitudinal study of sports participation in 10th grade was associated with less social isolation later in life.[62] Because organized sport programs take place in a social setting, they may provide opportunities to develop such skills as communication, conflict resolution,

TABLE 1 Characteristics of Well-Designed Sports Programs

- Positive youth-coach relationships
- Coaches who encourage kids to deal with challenges that occur during activity
- Both recreational and competitive environment
- Athletes participate in multiple sports instead of the requirement that they play only 1
- Kids have a sense of belonging to the program
- Life skills educational element
- Athletes develop skills valued by future employees:
  - Volunteering
  - Commitment to team building
  - Acceptance of rules
  - Tolerant attitude toward cultural diversity

and empathy.[66] Sports participation allows youth to experience community integration and positive intergroup relations while increasing social status and facilitating social mobility.[78,80–82] In fact, both boys and girls identify sports participation as one of the most common avenues to achieve social prestige and popularity in high school.[83] Additionally, organized sports experiences may foster citizenship, social success, positive peer relationships, and leadership skills.[81]

Social interaction is one of the most commonly reported advantages of organized sports[10] and brings together people from varied backgrounds who might not otherwise meet.[84] In children from low-income families, making new friends and learning teamwork and social skills are perceived benefits of youth sports participation.[38] Parents of Special Olympians report increased social competence and more friendships for their children, relative to others with developmental delay.[13] In a study of elementary school students, involvement in organized sports has been associated with a particularly positive effect on shy children, revealing that sports participation was positively associated with social adjustment and that this population reported significant decreases in social anxiety over time.[85] Similar findings have been confirmed in an evaluation of social anxiety in Swiss elementary schoolchildren.[86] Sports participation can help adolescents as well. Those with continuous involvement in sports activities have more friendships after the transition to high school, and female athletes experience less loneliness and social dissatisfaction during this time.[87]

Psychological

It has been well documented that sports involvement has an overall positive effect on mental health in kids of all ages. Relative to other activities, sports help develop emotional regulation,[72,73] and both parents and kids report that better emotional control and exploration are benefits of athletics.[38] Athletes report higher scores on mental health scales,[79] and teenagers participating in organized sports report fewer mental health problems and have lower odds of emotional distress compared with peers.[88–90] Members of sports clubs show greater stress resistance and have a lower prevalence of psychosomatic symptoms.[91] Sports have been inversely associated with depression in athletes, and fewer depressive symptoms and higher confidence and competence are some of the most commonly associated positive outcomes of participation.[10,77] More athletic adolescents appear better adjusted, feel less nervous and anxious, and are more often full of energy and happy about life. Athletes also feel sad, depressed, or desperate less often than those less involved in sports.[92] The protective effect of sports on mental health is further indicated by the fact that children who drop out of organized sports may experience greater psychological difficulties and social and emotional problems.[93] Sports participation may have a lasting effect on mental health, as well. Involvement in school sports during adolescence is an associated predictor of lower depression symptoms, lower perceived stress, and higher self-rated mental health in young adults.[94]

The beneficial effect of sports on mental health and depression applies to suicide, as well. After controlling for physical activity, team sports protect against feelings of hopelessness and suicidality, and organized sports participation is associated with a lower likelihood of suicidal behavior.[89,95] Furthermore, a longitudinal study of middle school and high school students showed lower rates of suicidal ideation during high school in athletes, compared with those who never played sports.[96] High school athletic involvement also significantly reduces the odds of contemplating suicide in both boys and girls, and athletic participation in adolescence was associated with a lower tendency to attempt suicide.[92,97–99] These findings may be attributed to the capacity of team sports participation to foster feelings of social support and integration.[95]

Another area in which organized sports participation has a positive influence on youth psychological development is self-esteem.[10,55,100,101] More specifically, sport club activities have a positive influence on the development of self-esteem, a finding that occurs earlier in girls than in boys.[91] This effect may be, at least in part, related to self-perceived athletic competence in this cohort.[78,101] Organized sports participation has been positively related to self-assessments of physical appearance and competence and physical and general self-esteem in both adolescent boys and girls, along with enhanced body image and a lower likelihood of body dissatisfaction.[77,78,92,102] In girls, team sport achievement experiences in early adolescence are positively associated with self-esteem in middle adolescence,[103] and earlier sports participation in girls correlates positively with self-esteem in college because it can foster physical competence, favorable body image, and more flexible attitudes about what it means to be female.[100] Organized sports programs can also help at-risk youth improve self-esteem, self-concept, and temperament.[104,105] Similarly, Special Olympics athletes demonstrate improved self-esteem and confidence, according to parent surveys.[13]

Emotional status seems to be related to the amount and intensity of involvement in sport. Athletes partaking in a greater number of organized sports, or with more hours or increased frequency, report lower levels of emotional problems, show lower depression scores, and have better feelings of well-being, respectively, compared with those with less participation.[10,106–108]

Physical Health and Weight Management

Given the epidemic of obesity and all of its accompanying medical conditions, it is important to find ways to keep kids physically active. Organized sports participation is 1 tactic to accomplish this. There is substantial association with organized sports involvement and higher levels of energy expenditure and physical activity, including MVPA.[109–119] Organized sports participation is also strongly correlated with better cardiovascular fitness in children and adolescents,[47,115,117,120] including endurance, speed, strength, and coordination.[121] On fitness tests, fifth-graders participating in recreational sports perform significantly better on measures of upper body strength and upper and lower body power than their peers.[122] Special Olympics athletes also have increased fitness, aerobic capacity, overall fitness, and strength, compared with others with developmental delay who are not involved in the program.[13]

Organized sports participation is also associated with young adult physical activity levels and physical fitness.[84,123,124] More specifically, becoming involved in organized sports at an early age may increase the likelihood of a physically active lifestyle in young adulthood,[125] and membership in a sports club during adolescence may predict a high level of physical activity later in life.[126]

The relationship between sports participation and obesity is less clear, with many studies showing no conclusive evidence of a positive correlation between organized sports participation and healthy weight status.[119] However, there is some indication that organized sports may have a role to play in reducing obesity. Early sports participation during kindergarten and first grade is associated with smaller increases in BMI during the adiposity rebound period of childhood,[4] and in elementary school, regular involvement in sports is associated with a lower likelihood of being overweight[120] and lower accumulation of body fat.[127,128] These findings hold true in older children and adolescents, as well. In middle school students, organized sports participation was associated with a reduction in the likelihood of being overweight and obese; participants had a 2% reduction in BMI.[129] Furthermore, parents and children from low-income families report weight management benefits from organized sports participation,[38] and decreased body fat and lower overall weight is correlated with Special Olympics involvement.[13]

Along with the obvious benefits of regular activity, there appear to be other ways in which organized sports participation contributes to overall physical health and weight management, such as healthy eating practices. A survey of fourth-graders suggested that greater sports participation is associated with a healthier overall eating profile, including lower consumption of soda,[130] and organized sports participation has been associated with improved caloric expenditure and reduced unnecessary snacking.[24] Adolescents involved in sports may eat breakfast more frequently and have better overall nutrient intake than their peers,[131,132] and athletes may also be more likely to eat fruits and vegetables and drink milk.*

Organized sports participation may lead to long-term health benefits, as well. Sustained participation in organized sports is associated with a lower risk of developing metabolic syndrome in adulthood.[133] In addition, kids who play ball sports during childhood appear to have a decreased risk of developing future stress fractures,[134] and involvement in impact-loading sports has a positive effect on bone mineral composition, density, and geometry, benefits that may be partially maintained even in those who do not continue participation into adulthood.[135]

Another positive effect of sports participation is the association with lower rates of substance use (excluding alcohol, which is addressed later in this report) and other risky behaviors. It is generally shown in studies that, compared with their peers, teenagers involved in sports are less likely to smoke cigarettes† and marijuana[97,132,136] and are less likely to use cocaine and other illicit drugs.[97,137–139] Both male and female adolescent athletes are more likely to report use of a condom during their last sexual encounter, and girls are less likely to engage in

* Refs 89,97,99,114,130,132,202.

† Refs 91,92,97,107,132,[137],138,[149],203,[204].

sexual behavior in general and report fewer pregnancies.[97,99,140] Finally, surveyed athletes of both sexes are less likely than nonathletes to carry a weapon.[97,99]

Adolescents participating in organized sports report fewer general health, eating, and dietary problems,[88] and athletes report higher scores on measures of general health and physical functioning, along with lower scores on a bodily pain scale, than nonathletes.[79] Given this and the other findings discussed earlier, it is unsurprising that young athletes tend to have higher overall health-related quality of life compared with their peers.[141,142]

RISKS

Burnout and Overscheduling

One concerning trend regarding organized sports participation in young athletes is that of early sports specialization. Sports specialization is the concept of intensely focusing on a single sport, typically year-round, while giving up other sports. Although early specialization may be beneficial in the few sports in which peak performance is often reached before physical maturation is complete (gymnastics, diving, figure skating), in most instances it can lead to more injuries and a higher risk of burnout.[19] In addition to sports specialization, other forms of overtraining; outside pressure from parents, coaches, and teammates; and internal stress placed on the athlete by his or her own self can all lead to burnout.[143–145] Burnout can be thought of as a syndrome comprising emotional and physical exhaustion, a reduced sense of accomplishment, and sport devaluation.[144] Common signs and symptoms include chronic joint or muscle pain, fatigue, elevated resting heart rate, decreased sport performance, personality changes, lack of enthusiasm regarding athletics, or difficulty completing usual routines.[145] Burnout can be difficult to measure but is thought to occur in between 1% and 9% of adolescent athletes.[144] A full discussion of sports specialization and burnout is beyond the scope of this report but is covered elsewhere, in the AAP clinical reports "Sports Specialization and Intensive Training in Young Athletes"[19] and "Overuse Injuries, Overtraining, and Burnout in Child and Adolescent Athletes."[145] It has been suggested that young athletes participating in more hours of sport each week than their age in years and those spending more than twice as much time in organized sports than in free play are at increased risk of suffering a serious overuse injury.[146] Kids who start concentrated training earlier in life, those who are involved in fewer extracurricular activities, and those with less unstructured play are more likely to drop out of sports[147] and, therefore, will not reap the many benefits of organized sports participation. Having an intense sports focus and its associated time commitment, along with the home schooling or participation in sports academies that often accompanies such training, can foster social isolation from peers and lead to limited social and problem-solving skills. Finally, parent and coach behaviors can adversely affect kids' organized sports experience, with 30% of young athletes reporting negative actions of parents and coaches as their reason for quitting sport.[23]

Risk-taking Behavior

As mentioned previously, adolescent athletes are less likely to smoke cigarettes and use illegal drugs than their peers. However, they are more likely to drink alcohol and use smokeless tobacco.‡ Youth involved in competitive sports have higher odds of reporting first getting drunk at an earlier age (elementary school or middle school) than peers.[148] They are also more likely to engage in binge drinking[149] and drunk driving in high school.[150] Despite lower illegal drug use overall, a recent survey showed that male adolescent athletes are more likely to be prescribed opiate medication and more likely to misuse such medication than boys who do not participate in organized sports.[151]

Some athletes, especially those involved in weight-class sports (wrestling, boxing, weightlifting, and crew), aesthetic sports (gymnastics, dance, and figure skating), and endurance sports, may engage in unhealthy weight-control practices.[152,153] Wrestlers, in particular, report multiple potentially harmful weight-cutting measures, such as overexercising, prolonged fasting, restricting fluid intake, and dehydration techniques.[152,153] Methods of dehydration include saunas and steam baths; spitting; vomiting; use of laxatives, diuretics, and diet pills; and wearing rubber suits while exercising.[152,153] Male athletes are more likely to vomit or use laxatives or diet pills for weight loss,[99] but girls are at unique risk of developing the "female athlete triad,"[154] a combination of low energy availability, menstrual dysfunction, and low bone mineral density. The female athlete triad can be triggered either by purposeful restriction of calories (sometimes associated with an eating disorder such as anorexia nervosa or bulimia nervosa) or simply from inadequate caloric intake to meet energy demands of the sport. These topics are discussed further in the AAP policy statement "Promotion of Healthy Weight-Control Practices in Young Athletes."[152]

Another unhealthy practice among athletes is the use of performance-enhancing substances, such as steroids, human growth hormone, and nutritional supplements. Although the name "nutritional supplement" implies a healthy product, use of such products can be

‡ Refs 62,97,99,136,[137],139,148,149,204–206.

dangerous because they lack regulatory oversight and have been frequently shown to be contaminated with steroids, stimulants, and other impurities.[155] Although consumption of performance-enhancing substances for the purpose of improved appearance is common in adolescents in general, usage appears to be greater in the athletic population[156] to gain a performance advantage. The lifetime prevalence rate of steroid use among adolescents ranges from 2% to 6% and is higher in the athletic population, particularly boys.[156–158] This conflicts with adult data showing a higher prevalence of steroid use in nonathletes.[159] For more details on steroid use and other performance-enhancing substances in children and adolescents, see the AAP clinical report "Use of Performance-Enhancing Substances."[156]

Bullying and Hazing

Bullying is a social issue that is prevalent throughout society, and the youth sports world is no exception. Bullying can be defined as a pattern of physical, verbal, or psychological behaviors between individuals that has the potential to be harmful, is based on an imbalance of power, and includes an absence of provocation.[160] Bullying in sports may be physical, social, or psychological. Physical contact such as hitting, kicking, or pushing or stealing or destroying equipment would be examples of physical bullying. Social bullying may involve isolating, excluding, or otherwise not accepting a player or teammate, and psychological forms of bullying include name calling, rumor spreading, threatening, and humiliating or ridiculing behavior.[160,161] Although there is no difference in the sexes when it comes to victims of bullying, male athletes are more likely to be perpetrators, and athletes of male coaches report higher rates of bullying, compared with athletes of female coaches.[162] Along with disability, sexual and gender orientation are factors that have been identified as risk factors for harassment in sport.[160] Victims of bullying in sports also tend to report weaker connections to peers, and those conducting the bullying report weaker relationships with coaches.[162]

Hazing differs somewhat from bullying in that although it may be humiliating, degrading, or dangerous, it is an expectation of someone joining a group conducted with the intention of increasing commitment to the team or organization.[161,163,164] Hazing may be conducted with or without the participant's willingness to participate.[163] Hazing activities may be physical, such as beating or paddling, branding, head shaving, kidnapping, sexual assault, or being forced to perform feats of physical endurance.[161,163] Other examples include forced alcohol consumption; being made to perform embarrassing acts, including sexual acts; being deprived of sleep or food; or being tied up, confined, or abandoned.[161,163] The incidence of hazing in youth sports varies from 5% to 17% in middle school up to 17% to 48% in high school,[163–165] although some experts believe hazing may be underreported by athletes either for fear of retribution or because they may not perceive certain activities as hazing.[166] Despite the potentially catastrophic outcomes that can and have occurred as a result of hazing, 86% of adolescent athletes report feeling that their experiences were worth it to be part of the team.[164] Because of this, it is up to coaches and team leaders to create an environment in which such behaviors are no longer acceptable.[166]

Parental Influence

Most parents undoubtedly want what is best for their children when it comes to sports. However, some parents do encourage young athletes to participate beyond their readiness or interest or inadvertently create unrealistic expectations for performance, which can cause kids to lose confidence and set them up for failure.[24,167] Pressure from parents who are too controlling in organized sports has been linked to performance anxiety.[168] Parental criticism and high expectations are both factors that have been associated with burnout in young athletes.[81] Additionally, some parents model poor behavior on the sidelines, screaming, fighting, and at times even attacking officials, which can embarrass kids and decrease their enjoyment of sport.[169,170] Negative spectator behavior on the part of parents has been shown to predict negative player behaviors as well.[170]

TABLE 2 Financial Costs Associated With Youth Sports

- Uniforms
- Equipment
- Shoes
- League registration fees
- Facility fees
- Private lessons from coaches
- Camps
- Tournament entry fees
- Travel expenses

Another way parents influence their children's organized sports participation is the amount of money spent to participate (see Table 2). Some families exhaust their savings or sacrifice vacations to pay for organized sports activities.[171] Many parents may view this as an investment, hoping their child will 1 day obtain a college scholarship or make millions of dollars as a professional athlete.[172] Unfortunately, the likelihood of either of these happening is exceptionally small. According to statistics from the National Collegiate Athletic Association, the overall percentage of high school athletes who go on to play Division 1 college football, basketball, or soccer ranges from 1.0% to 2.6%.[173] Furthermore, the amount of money parents spend on organized sports during the middle school and high school years most often exceeds the value of a college scholarship,[174] even for the rare athlete fortunate enough to obtain one.

Coach Influence (Potential for Coach Abuse)

Although most coaches presumably work with young athletes to help them succeed, coaches also face pressure to win. This pressure may lead coaches to be coercive or punitive, to encourage unsportsmanlike behavior, or to impede their players' social and personal development.[72] Some coaches try to motivate kids by yelling at them, insulting them, or calling them names.[169] Nearly half of children involved in organized sports report verbal misconduct by coaches.[169] Youth involved in sports report higher rates of inappropriate adult (those involved in the activity) behavior than those involved in other extracurricular activities.[72] Coaches sometimes get so caught up in winning that they set a bad example by cheating or fighting with other coaches, parents, and officials.[24] Children and adolescents who observe coaches behaving badly are likely to assume that sportsmanship is not a valued quality.[170] Coaches who primarily place emphasis on winning rather than advancing their athletes' best interests can end up exploiting athletes.[81] Of the three quarters of adolescent athletes who report at least 1 incident of emotional harm during their sports careers, nearly one third implicate their coach as the source of that harm.[175] Not surprisingly, athletes who are verbally intimidated or bullied by coaches often have difficulty focusing on the actual details of the game because they are preoccupied with gaining the coach's approval.[176] Coaches who are more controlling and autocratic and perceived as less encouraging and supportive are more likely to cause athletes to drop out of sports.[81,177] Even if they are not engaging in any malicious behavior, coaches may unintentionally cause harm. Many youth coaches lack adequate training in strength and conditioning principles, emergency management of sports injuries, or basic first aid, which can result in more frequent or severe injuries for youth sports participants.[24] Even worse, some athletes report feeling pressured to play while injured.[24] Punitive exercise (a coach forcing an athlete to perform significant physical exertion often not related to the athlete's sport because of athlete mistakes or performance issues) can be dangerous and is opposed by SHAPE America.[178]

TABLE 3 Role of Parents in Organized Sports

- Child's interest determines participation
- Be aware of the child's physical and developmental ability and what skills are needed for the organized sports
- Support fun, learning, and making progress in skill development
- Demonstrate positive support for participation, not for winning
- Support "sport sampling" to develop multiple skills, promote enjoyment, and reduce injury risk
- Be aware that organized sports participation alone may not offer enough physical activity for optimal health
- Support good nutrition and adequate sleep

Less commonly, athletes may even be sexually harassed or abused by a coach.[179] In a survey of Canadian adolescents, it was shown that 0.4% experienced sexual harassment and 0.5% were victims of sexual abuse at the hands of a coach,[180] and authors of an Australian analysis reported the prevalence of sexual abuse at a much higher 9.7%.[181] In the Canadian study, an additional 1.2% of athletes admitted to consensual sexual contact with a coach.[180] Although there are no published estimates of abuse rates in US athletes, there have been numerous media reports of coach-perpetrated sexual abuse in, among others, youth tennis, swimming, and martial arts in this country.[182–184] Sexual abuse of a child or teenager by a person in a position of trust (ie, coach) is a felony crime in every state.

ROLE OF PARENTS

Parents significantly influence whether their children participate in organized sports and in what environment they do so (Table 3).[185] A systematic review of parental correlates of physical activity in children and early adolescents found that parental support (eg, encouragement, facilitation) is significantly correlated with child physical activity level (including organized sports); studies on whether the parents' own physical activity level influences child physical activity level show mixed results.[185] The child's perception of parental support and positive expected outcomes from organized sports are significantly associated with participation, as is the parental belief of feeling it is important to participate in organized sports.[186] The same is likely true of youth with developmental disabilities. Parents of children with developmental disabilities who believed strongly in the benefit of physical activity reported more physical activity in their children.[17]

Parents' awareness of their own child's physical abilities, developmental trajectory, and interest is helpful when determining when to start organized sports.[24] The age of 6 years has been proposed as appropriate for most children to start organized sports because they would have achieved the skills necessary for basic participation in a variety of activities.[167] Working with their primary health care provider, parents can determine if their child has developed fundamental skills needed for most organized sports. Age-appropriate recommendations for increased physical activity and suggestions for supporting physical literacy are provided in the AAP clinical report "Physical Activity Assessment and Counseling in Pediatric Clinical Settings."

Positive behavior relating to organized sports participation (eg, empowering, teaching of life skills, supporting fun, and making progress instead of winning) is shown to increase enjoyment and decrease stress in organized sports.[171] The health of the parent-child relationship in general is also important, as shown in studies of junior athletes.[187] Pressure to intensify and succeed (win) in organized sports, while decreasing time with friends, family, and in academics, results in increased child stress and a negative outlook on the sport as a whole. Supporting the positive aspects of hard work, follow-through on commitments, and sportsmanship are shown to be associated with increased motivation for organized sports participation and better parent relationships.[188]

When parents support organized sports participation for their children, they may assume that this participation ensures they will get enough physical activity; however, this may not be true. In several studies on levels of physical activity achieved in organized sports, less than expected MVPA was demonstrated[189]; female soccer players have been shown to get ~20 minutes of MVPA for every hour of game play or practice time in 1 study.[113] In another study, both boys and girls playing in soccer games spent almost 50% of the match time sedentary.[190] Although both boys and girls across a variety of organized sports had more overall physical activity than those not in organized sports, 1 study showed that only the boys were achieving recommended physical activity levels.[111]

In addition, families with children in organized sports have been shown to have higher fast food consumption and fewer meals eaten at home because time in organized sports was prioritized over healthy eating.[191]

TABLE 4 Creating a Safe Environment to Prevent Abuse in Youth Sports: A Parent Checklist

- Review organization hiring procedures: background checks, interviews, applications, references
- Ensure formal abuse-prevention training is conducted
- Ask about organization codes of conduct, travel policies, and reporting requirements
- Rules of communication between coaches and athletes should be present (social media, texting, e-mail)
- Rules for coach and athlete contact during individual training should be established
- Sport facilities should be well maintained and provide areas for athlete privacy and safety

Adapted from LaBotz M. Creating a safe environment to prevent abuse in youth sports: a parent checklist. 2018. Available at: https://www.healthychildren.org/English/healthy-living/sports/Pages/Creating-a-Safe-Environment-to-Prevent-Abuse-in-Youth-Sports-A-Parent-Checklist.aspx. Accessed April 27, 2018.

Parents are inherently involved in decisions made about organized sports participation, both in the variety (or lack thereof) and intensity and scheduling of sports.[24] There has been much research around sports specialization, injury risk, and burnout from organized sports,[19] and the topic is fully covered in the AAP clinical report "Sports Specialization and Intensive Training in Young Athletes."[19] The current literature suggests that sports specialization is appropriate in late adolescence to decrease injury risk and promote success.[192] "Sport sampling," the concept of participating in multiple sports over childhood and early adolescence, promotes enjoyment while decreasing injuries, stress, and burnout.[193] Encouraging a variety of sports is likely to be beneficial to the young athlete in multiple ways. A recent report from the Women's Sports Foundation associated teenagers who participated in at least 2 different sports with healthier eating habits, more exercise, and better sleep habits, with lower risk of substance abuse.[194]

Parents are essential in creating environments in youth sports, especially in preventing abuse by anyone interacting with athletes, including coaches and medical staff. Parents can ask questions of both schools and youth sports organizations focused on rules of conduct and travel, abuse-prevention training, and reporting.[195] See Table 4 for a parent checklist to prevent abuse in youth sports.[195] A parent-coach partnership in creating a safe environment for sport participation is ideal.

ROLE OF COACHES

For youth, fun is named as the most rewarding part of organized sports participation.[39] In a study on the tenets of what comprises fun for young athletes, researchers found being a good sport, trying hard, and positive coaching to be highest rated.[39] Part of "fun" likely includes equal playing time, especially for younger athletes (12 years and younger) and can be a strategy for coaches to keep developing athletes involved.[196]

Design of developmentally appropriate scheduling and practices is important, keeping the focus on fun and engaging the athlete.[40] Recognizing the developmental level of children participating in organized sports is essential to designing skill acquisition and content and length of practices.[167] In addition, recognizing the role of overscheduling and fatigue on injury risk is helpful in designing the time of practices around games and tournaments, purposefully giving the young athlete time for adequate sleep and rest between bouts of physical activity.[197]

Awareness of physical activity content in practices is important; it was demonstrated in the Role of Parents section that assuming organized sports participation will meet physical activity recommendations for youth may be a mistake.[113,189,190] A coach education program focused on strategies to increase MVPA in basketball was successful in increasing MVPA and decreasing inactive time in practices.[198]

Finally, coaches and related professionals are mandated reporters of sexual abuse in most, if not all states, and should be vigilant about scrutinizing and reporting any such suspicious behavior.

ROLE OF PEDIATRICIANS

Child Evaluation and Guidance for Involvement in Organized Sport

Pediatricians have an important role in educating parents about developmental milestones leading to successful organized sports participation. Pediatricians can help parents connect the child's developmental state and achievement of skills to readiness for specific sports. For example, a 4-year-old child is not likely able to catch well and would not be ready for baseball. However, early motor skill development is important for long-term physical activity and organized sports participation. Appropriate skills can be achieved, for most children, through a combination of free play and purposeful skill development in the context of free play. More on free play can be found in the AAP clinical report "The Power of Play: A Pediatric Role in Enhancing Development in Young Children"[199] and in *Caring For Our Children: National Health and Safety Performance Standards*.[200]

Pediatricians can also reinforce that the interest in organized sports should come from the child, not the parent. Forcing children to participate in organized sports (or any physical activity) is likely to decrease fun in the activity and discourage future participation.[20]

Parental Counseling

There is a positive effect of parental support on organized sports participation.[185] Pediatricians discussing organized sports with their patients and families can address whether youth feel encouraged in organized sports endeavors and whether barriers to participation exist (eg, transportation, finances, parent ability to attend events). Educating parents about ways to show support for organized sports may be helpful in encouraging participation and, therefore, increased physical activity in their children.[186] Special attention should be paid to the physical activity and sport needs of disabled youth, recognizing that this patient population is influenced by the parental attitudes about physical activity. Because organized sports participation may not provide enough MVPA to meet physical activity recommendations,[113,189,190] pediatricians can educate parents about the need to promote physical activity in and out of organized sports.

Finding the right coaching environment for a child participating in organized sports is important, both for short-term skill development and for long-term enjoyment of physical activity and organized sports.[39] Empowering parents with knowledge about positive coaching is an important step for healthy organized participation.[24] In addition, athletes, especially disabled ones, might occasionally have physical, behavioral, or other presentations of abuse at the hands of coaches and may disclose that abuse to a pediatrician, who must then report the abuse.

Pediatricians can ask about and encourage organized sports participation in youth who may not otherwise participate: those with chronic health conditions or those who are developmentally or neurologically disabled. This is important for both the general and disabled youth populations; disabled youth are especially at risk for low fitness from low levels of physical activity. Research on other groups is lacking, but asking at-risk patients about barriers to participation and encouraging organized sports participation are valuable.

Advocacy and Policy

Pediatricians are an important part of their local community and offer knowledge specific to the development of children and adolescents that is complementary to scholastic and other community organizations. Relative to organized sports, the pediatrician is valuable in promoting healthy and safe participation.[201]

Advocacy in Schools

Knowledge about the local community's school guidelines for physical education is important. At the preschool and elementary school level, specific knowledge about motor skill acquisition programming and assessments will allow the pediatrician to promote early intervention in children who are not meeting milestones. Understanding the local school organized sports and physical education options for adolescents can help the pediatrician advocate for a wide variety of options (competitive level, sport, etc) to keep students involved in organized sports.

Advocacy in Community Programs

The pediatrician has needed expertise in advising community organized sports programs on age of start and how to promote fun, successful practices that keep children engaged and interested in sports. Advocating for practice and game schedules that allow for appropriate rest and recovery is also needed.

The pediatrician can work with community organizations to discuss barriers for organized sports in the community and how to resolve them. Encouraging community organized sports organizations to purposefully address these barriers (eg, affordability, transportation issues, scheduling, accessibility) is vital.

CONCLUSIONS

1. Organized sports participation can be an important part of overall childhood and adolescent physical, emotional, social, and psychological health.
2. Children need daily opportunity for free play to develop motor skills needed for organized sports participation.
3. Supervised motor skill acquisition in preschool and elementary school positively influences long-term participation in organized sports, physical activity, and cardiovascular health.
4. Participation in school-sponsored organized sports, relative to the entire student body, is low. Schools play a role in increasing organized sports participation by offering multiple levels of play at the junior high and high school levels, thereby retaining those athletes who do not desire to or cannot compete at high levels but want to remain involved in sports.
5. Community organizations can promote organized sports participation by identifying and promoting ways to support families with low SES. Pediatricians can be well versed in available opportunities and can use these as an adjunct to physical activity and organized sports discussions in their practices and with community organizations.
6. Parental support for organized sports participation in general and positive support (ie, encouragement, focus on fun and progress instead of winning) are important influencers of whether a child enjoys and continues organized sports. This is true for youth with disabilities as well as for all youth. However, forcing organized sports participation is not likely to have long-term benefits.
7. Parents are essential in creating safe environments in youth sports, especially in regard to preventing abuse. Parents can ask questions of both schools and youth sports organizations about hiring procedures, codes of conduct, and communication between coach and athlete.
8. Positive coaching is an important facet of organized sports. Coaches who approach organized sports with a respectful, development- and fun-focused approach to practices and performance are more likely to have athletes who enjoy and stay in organized sports.
9. Unhealthy attitudes or behaviors on the part of parents and coaches can decrease the young athlete's enjoyment of sports and contribute to burnout.
10. Involvement in sports, particularly as a member of a sports team, is an integral way for youth to develop psychosocially and help form their social identity.
11. Sports participation helps athletes develop self-esteem, correlates positively with overall mental health, and appears to have a protective effect against suicide.
12. Sports participation in some youth who are medically at risk is shown to improve well-being. This improvement in well-being is particularly evident for Special Olympics participation, for children with developmental disabilities, and for children with neurologic disabilities.
13. Youth of all ages involved in organized sports have higher levels of energy expenditure and physical activity than their nonathletic peers, and sports may be an important way to combat obesity.
14. Adolescent athletes appear less likely to smoke cigarettes and use most other illegal drugs but are more likely to consume alcohol and use performance-enhancing substances, such as steroids.
15. Bullying and hazing are common among young athletes, and it will likely be the responsibility of coaches and team leaders to decrease such practices.

LEAD AUTHORS

Kelsey Logan, MD, MPH, FAAP
Steven Cuff, MD, FAAP

COUNCIL ON SPORTS MEDICINE AND FITNESS EXECUTIVE COMMITTEE, 2017–2018

Cynthia R. LaBella, MD, FAAP, Chairperson
M. Alison Brooks, MD, MPH, FAAP, Chairperson-elect
Greg Canty, MD, FAAP
Alex B. Diamond, DO, MPH, FAAP
William Hennrikus, MD, FAAP
Kelsey Logan, MD, MPH, FAAP
Kody Moffatt, MD, FAAP
Blaise A. Nemeth, MD, MS, FAAP
K. Brooke Pengel, MD, FAAP
Andrew R. Peterson, MD, MSPH, FAAP
Paul R. Stricker, MD, FAAP

LIAISONS

Donald W. Bagnall, ATC, LAT – *National Athletic Trainers Association*
Jon Solomon – *Aspen Institute Sports and Society Program*
Mark E. Halstead, MD, FAAP – *American Medical Society for Sports Medicine*

CONSULTANTS

Avery D. Faigenbaum, EdD, FACSM
Andrew J.M. Gregory, MD, FAAP
Sarah B. Kinsella, MD, FAAP

STAFF

Anjie Emanuel, MPH

ABBREVIATIONS

AAP: American Academy of Pediatrics
CYD: community youth development
MVPA: moderate to vigorous physical activity
SES: socioeconomic status

FUNDING: No external funding.

POTENTIAL CONFLICT OF INTEREST: The authors have indicated they have no potential conflicts of interest to disclose.

REFERENCES

1. Vella SA, Swann C, Allen MS, Schweickle MJ, Magee CA. Bidirectional associations between sport involvement and mental health in adolescence. *Med Sci Sports Exerc.* 2017;49(4):687–694
2. Fehily AM, Coles RJ, Evans WD, Elwood PC. Factors affecting bone density in young adults. *Am J Clin Nutr.* 1992; 56(3):579–586
3. Hebert JJ, Klakk H, Møller NC, Grøntved A, Andersen LB, Wedderkopp N. The prospective association of organized sports participation with cardiovascular disease risk in children (the CHAMPS study-DK). *Mayo Clin Proc.* 2017;92(1):57–65
4. Dunton G, McConnell R, Jerrett M, et al. Organized physical activity in young school children and subsequent 4-year change in body mass index. *Arch Pediatr Adolesc Med.* 2012;166(8): 713–718
5. Mandic S, Bengoechea EG, Stevens E, de la Barra SL, Skidmore P. Getting kids active by participating in sport and doing it more often: focusing on what matters. *Int J Behav Nutr Phys Act.* 2012;9:86
6. Dodge T, Lambert SF. Positive self-beliefs as a mediator of the relationship between adolescents' sports participation and health in young adulthood. *J Youth Adolesc.* 2009;38(6):813–825
7. Dohle S, Wansink B. Fit in 50 years: participation in high school sports best predicts one's physical activity after age 70. *BMC Public Health.* 2013; 13:1100
8. Matvienko O, Ahrabi-Fard I. The effects of a 4-week after-school program on motor skills and fitness of kindergarten and first-grade students. *Am J Health Promot.* 2010;24(5): 299–303
9. Barnett LM, Van Beurden E, Morgan PJ, Brooks LO, Beard JR. Does childhood motor skill proficiency predict adolescent fitness? *Med Sci Sports Exerc.* 2008;40(12):2137–2144
10. Eime RM, Young JA, Harvey JT, Charity MJ, Payne WR. A systematic review of the psychological and social benefits of participation in sport for children and adolescents: informing development of a conceptual model of health through sport. *Int J Behav Nutr Phys Act.* 2013; 10:98
11. Dentro KN, Beals K, Crouter SE, et al. Results from the United States' 2014 report card on physical activity for children and youth. *J Phys Act Health.* 2014;11(suppl 1):S105–S112
12. Pittet I, Berchtold A, Akré C, Michaud PA, Surís JC. Sports practice among adolescents with chronic health conditions. *Arch Pediatr Adolesc Med.* 2009;163(6):565–571
13. Dykens EM, Rosner BA, Butterbaugh G. Exercise and sports in children and adolescents with developmental disabilities. Positive physical and psychosocial effects. *Child Adolesc Psychiatr Clin N Am.* 1998;7(4): 757–771, viii
14. Sahlin KB, Lexell J. Impact of organized sports on activity, participation, and quality of life in people with neurologic disabilities. *PM R.* 2015;7(10): 1081–1088
15. Yazicioglu K, Yavuz F, Goktepe AS, Tan AK. Influence of adapted sports on quality of life and life satisfaction in sport participants and non-sport participants with physical disabilities. *Disabil Health J.* 2012;5(4):249–253
16. Oppewal A, Hilgenkamp TI, van Wijck R, Evenhuis HM. Cardiorespiratory fitness in individuals with intellectual disabilities–a review. *Res Dev Disabil.* 2013;34(10):3301–3316
17. Pitchford EA, Siebert E, Hamm J, Yun J. Parental perceptions of physical activity benefits for youth with developmental disabilities. *Am J Intellect Dev Disabil.* 2016;121(1):25–32
18. Washington RL, Bernhardt DT, Gomez J, et al; Committee on Sports Medicine and Fitness and Committee on School Health. Organized sports for children and preadolescents. *Pediatrics.* 2001; 107(6):1459–1462
19. Brenner JS; Council on Sports Medicine and Fitness. Sports specialization and intensive training in young athletes. *Pediatrics.* 2016;138(3):e20162148
20. Loprinzi PD, Cardinal BJ, Loprinzi KL, Lee H. Benefits and environmental determinants of physical activity in children and adolescents. *Obes Facts.* 2012;5(4):597–610
21. Lopes VP, Rodrigues LP, Maia JA, Malina RM. Motor coordination as predictor of

physical activity in childhood. *Scand J Med Sci Sports*. 2011;21(5):663–669

22. Vandorpe B, Vandendriessche J, Vaeyens R, et al. Relationship between sports participation and the level of motor coordination in childhood: a longitudinal approach. *J Sci Med Sport*. 2012;15(3):220–225
23. Breuner CC. Avoidance of burnout in the young athlete. *Pediatr Ann*. 2012;41(8): 335–339
24. Merkel DL. Youth sport: positive and negative impact on young athletes. *Open Access J Sports Med*. 2013;4: 151–160
25. Ruiz JR, Ortega FB, Castillo R, et al; AVENA Study Group. Physical activity, fitness, weight status, and cognitive performance in adolescents. *J Pediatr*. 2010;157(6):917–922.e1–e5
26. O'Loughlin J, Paradis G, Kishchuk N, Barnett T, Renaud L. Prevalence and correlates of physical activity behaviors among elementary schoolchildren in multiethnic, low income, inner-city neighborhoods in Montreal, Canada. *Ann Epidemiol*. 1999;9(7):397–407
27. Møller NC, Tarp J, Kamelarczyk EF, Brønd JC, Klakk H, Wedderkopp N. Do extra compulsory physical education lessons mean more physically active children–findings from the childhood health, activity, and motor performance school study Denmark (The CHAMPS-study DK). *Int J Behav Nutr Phys Act*. 2014;11:121
28. Lee SM, Burgeson CR, Fulton JE, Spain CG. Physical education and physical activity: results from the School Health Policies and Programs Study 2006. *J Sch Health*. 2007;77(8):435–463
29. Centers for Disease Control and Prevention. Results from the School Health Policies and Practices Study. 2016. Available at: https://www.cdc.gov/healthyyouth/data/shpps/pdf/shpps-results_2016.pdf. Accessed November 19, 2017
30. Madsen K, Thompson H, Adkins A, Crawford Y. School-community partnerships: a cluster-randomized trial of an after-school soccer program. *JAMA Pediatr*. 2013;167(4):321–326
31. Howie EK, McVeigh JA, Smith AJ, Straker LM. Organized sport trajectories from childhood to adolescence and health associations. *Med Sci Sports Exerc*. 2016;48(7):1331–1339
32. Kimm SY, Glynn NW, Kriska AM, et al. Decline in physical activity in black girls and white girls during adolescence. *N Engl J Med*. 2002;347(10):709–715
33. Davis AM, Vinci LM, Okwuosa TM, Chase AR, Huang ES. Cardiovascular health disparities: a systematic review of health care interventions. *Med Care Res Rev*. 2007;64(suppl 5):S29–S100
34. Walters S, Barr-Anderson DJ, Wall M, Neumark-Sztainer D. Does participation in organized sports predict future physical activity for adolescents from diverse economic backgrounds? *J Adolesc Health*. 2009;44(3):268–274
35. Gordon-Larsen P, Griffiths P, Bentley ME, et al. Barriers to physical activity: qualitative data on caregiver-daughter perceptions and practices. *Am J Prev Med*. 2004;27(3):218–223
36. Pelcher A, Rajan S. After-school program implementation in urban environments: increasing engagement among adolescent youth. *J Sch Health*. 2016;86(8):585–594
37. The Aspen Institute Project Play. State of play 2016: trends and developments. Available at: https://assets.aspeninstitute.org/content/uploads/2016/06/State-of-Play-2016-FINAL.pdf?_ga=2.195726820.992902905.1556283441-1474546670.1556283441. Accessed April 26, 2019
38. Holt NL, Kingsley BC, Tink LN, Scherer J. Benefits and challenges associated with sport participation by children and parents from low-income families. *Psychol Sport Exerc*. 2011;12(5):490–499
39. Visek AJ, Achrati SM, Mannix H, McDonnell K, Harris BS, DiPietro L. The fun integration theory: toward sustaining children and adolescents sport participation. *J Phys Act Health*. 2015;12(3):424–433
40. Le Menestrel S, Perkins DF. An overview of how sports, out-of-school time, and youth well-being can and do intersect. *New Dir Youth Dev*. 2007;(115):13–25, 5
41. Petitpas AJ, Van Raalte JL, Cornelius AE, Presbrey J. A life skills development program for high school student-athletes. *J Prim Prev*. 2004;24(3): 325–334
42. Williams HG, Pfeiffer KA, O'Neill JR, et al. Motor skill performance and physical activity in preschool children. *Obesity (Silver Spring)*. 2008;16(6):1421–1426
43. Fisher A, Reilly JJ, Kelly LA, et al. Fundamental movement skills and habitual physical activity in young children. *Med Sci Sports Exerc*. 2005; 37(4):684–688
44. Wrotniak BH, Epstein LH, Dorn JM, Jones KE, Kondilis VA. The relationship between motor proficiency and physical activity in children. *Pediatrics*. 2006; 118(6). Available at: www.pediatrics.org/cgi/content/full/118/6/e1758
45. Stodden DF, Goodway JD, Langendorfer SJ, et al. A developmental perspective on the role of motor skill competence in physical activity: an emergent relationship. *Quest*. 2008;60(2):290–306
46. Telford RD, Cunningham RB, Telford RM, Olive LS, Byrne DG, Abhayaratna WP. Benefits of early development of eye-hand coordination: evidence from the LOOK longitudinal study. *Scand J Med Sci Sports*. 2013;23(5):e263–e269
47. Hardy LL, O'Hara BJ, Rogers K, St George A, Bauman A. Contribution of organized and nonorganized activity to children's motor skills and fitness. *J Sch Health*. 2014;84(11):690–696
48. Melekoglu T. The effects of sports participation in strength parameters in primary school students. *Procedia Soc Behav Sci*. 2015;186:1013–1018
49. Christou M, Smilios I, Sotiropoulos K, Volaklis K, Pilianidis T, Tokmakidis SP. Effects of resistance training on the physical capacities of adolescent soccer players. *J Strength Cond Res*. 2006;20(4):783–791
50. Butterfield SA, Loovis EM. Influence of age, sex, balance, and sport participation on development of throwing by children in grades K-8. *Percept Mot Skills*. 1993;76(2):459–464
51. Jonker L, Elferink-Gemser MT, Visscher C. Talented athletes and academic achievements: a comparison over 14 years. *High Abil Stud*. 2009;20(1): 55–64
52. Brettschneider WD. Risks and opportunities: adolescents in top-level sport ñ growing up with the pressures of school and training. *Eur Phys Educ Rev*. 1999;5(2):121–133

53. Jonker L, Elferink-Gemser MT, Toering TT, Lyons J, Visscher C. Academic performance and self-regulatory skills in elite youth soccer players. *J Sports Sci.* 2010;28(14):1605–1614

54. Umbach PD, Palmer MM, Kuh GD, Hannah SJ. Intercollegiate athletes and effective educational practices: winning combination or losing effort? *Res High Educ.* 2006;47(6):709–733

55. Marsh HW, Kleitman S. School athletic participation: mostly gain with little pain. *J Sport Exerc Psychol.* 2003;25(2): 205–228

56. Domazet SL, Tarp J, Huang T, et al. Associations of physical activity, sports participation and active commuting on mathematic performance and inhibitory control in adolescents. *PLoS One.* 2016;11(1):e0146319

57. Esteban-Cornejo I, Gómez-Martínez S, Tejero-González CM, et al. Characteristics of extracurricular physical activity and cognitive performance in adolescents. The AVENA study. *J Sports Sci.* 2014;32(17): 1596–1603

58. Jonker L, Elferink-Gemser MT, Visscher C. The role of self-regulatory skills in sport and academic performances of elite youth athletes. *Talent Dev Excell.* 2011;3(2):263–275

59. Snyder EE, Spreitzer E. High school athletic participation as related to college attendance among black, hispanic, and white males: a research note. *Youth Soc.* 1990;21(3):390–398

60. Durand-Bush N, Salmela JH. The development and maintenance of expert athletic performance: perceptions of world and olympic champions. *J Appl Sport Psychol.* 2002; 14(3):154–171

61. Watt SK, Moore JL. Who are student athletes? *New Dir Stud Serv.* 2001; 2001(93):7–18

62. Barber BL, Eccles JS, Stone MR. Whatever happened to the Jock, the Brain, and the Princess? Young adult pathways linked to adolescent activity involvement and social identity. *J Adolesc Res.* 2001;16(5):429–455

63. Rehberg RA, Schafer WE. Participation in interscholastic athletics and college expectations. *Am J Sociol.* 1968;73(6): 732–740

64. Marsh HW. The effects of participation in sport during the last two years of high school. *Sociol Sport J.* 1993;10(1): 18–43

65. Hodge K, Danish SJ. Promoting life skills for adolescent males through sport. In: Horne AM, Kiselica MS, eds. *Handbook of Counseling Boys and Adolescent Males: A Practitioner's Guide.* Thousand Oaks, CA: Sage; 1999:55–71

66. Hermens N, Super S, Verkooijen KT, Koelen MA. A systematic review of life skill development through sports programs serving socially vulnerable youth. *Res Q Exerc Sport.* 2017;88(4): 408–424

67. Gould D, Collins K, Lauer L, Chung Y. Coaching life skills through football: a study of award winning high school coaches. *J Appl Sport Psychol.* 2007; 19(1):16–37

68. Côté J, Salmela JH. The organizational tasks of high-performance gymnastic coaches. *Sport Psychol.* 1996;10(3): 247–260

69. McCallister SG, Blinde EM, Weiss WM. Teaching values and implementing philosophies: Dilemmas of the coach. *Phys Educator.* 2000;57(1):35–45

70. Holt NL, Tamminen KA, Tink LN, Black DE. An interpretive analysis of life skills associated with sport participation. *Qual Res Sport Exerc.* 2009;1(2):160–175

71. Holt NL, Tink LN, Mandigo JL, Fox KR. Do youth learn life skills through their involvement in high school sport? A case study? *Can J Educ.* 2008;31(1): 281–304

72. Hansen DM, Larson RW, Dworkin JB. What adolescents learn in organized youth activities: a survey of self-reported developmental experiences. *J Res Adolesc.* 2003;13(1):25–55

73. Larson RW, Hansen DM, Moneta G. Differing profiles of developmental experiences across types of organized youth activities. *Dev Psychol.* 2006;42(5): 849–863

74. Dobosz RP, Beaty LA. The relationship between athletic participation and high school students' leadership ability. *Adolescence.* 1999;34(133):215–220

75. DiCola G. In: DiCola G, ed. *Beyond the Scoreboard: Youth Employment Opportunities and Skills Development in the Sports Sector.* Geneva, Switzerland: International Labor Organization; 2006:173–192

76. Bruner MW, Balish SM, Forrest C, et al. Ties that bond: youth sport as a vehicle for social identity and positive youth development. *Res Q Exerc Sport.* 2017; 88(2):209–214

77. Boone EM, Leadbeater BJ. Game on: diminishing risks for depressive symptoms in early adolescence through positive involvement in team sports. *J Res Adolesc.* 2006;16(1):79–90

78. Balaguer I, Atienza FL, Duda JL. Self-perceptions, self-worth and sport participation in adolescents. *Span J Psychol.* 2012;15(2):624–630

79. Snyder AR, Martinez JC, Bay RC, Parsons JT, Sauers EL, Valovich McLeod TC. Health-related quality of life differs between adolescent athletes and adolescent nonathletes. *J Sport Rehabil.* 2010;19(3):237–248

80. Wankel LM, Berger BG. The psychological and social benefits of sport and physical activity. *J Leis Res.* 1990;22(2):167–182

81. Fraser-Thomas JL, Côté J, Deakin J. Youth sport programs: an avenue to foster positive youth development. *Phys Educ Sport Pedagogy.* 2005;10(1):19–40

82. Chase MA, Dummer GM. The role of sports as a social status determinant for children. *Res Q Exerc Sport.* 1992; 63(4):418–424

83. Suitor JJ, Carter RS. Jocks, nerds, babes and thugs: a research note on regional differences in adolescent gender norms. *Gend Issues.* 1999;17(3): 87–101

84. Bailey R, Hillman C, Arent S, Petitpas A. Physical activity: an underestimated investment in human capital? *J Phys Act Health.* 2013;10(3):289–308

85. Findlay LC, Coplan RJ. Come out and play: shyness in childhood and the benefits of organized sports participation. *Can J Behav Sci.* 2008; 40(3):153–161

86. Schumacher Dimech A, Seiler R. Extra-curricular sport participation: a potential buffer against social anxiety symptoms in primary school children. *Psychol Sport Exerc.* 2011;12(4):347–354

87. Bohnert AM, Aikins JW, Arola NT. Regrouping: organized activity involvement and social adjustment across the transition to high school. *New Dir Child Adolesc Dev.* 2013; 2013(140):57–75

88. Steiner H, McQuivey RW, Pavelski R, Pitts T, Kraemer H. Adolescents and sports: risk or benefit? *Clin Pediatr (Phila).* 2000;39(3):161–166

89. Harrison PA, Narayan G. Differences in behavior, psychological factors, and environmental factors associated with participation in school sports and other activities in adolescence. *J Sch Health.* 2003;73(3):113–120

90. Steptoe A, Butler N. Sports participation and emotional wellbeing in adolescents. *Lancet.* 1996;347(9018): 1789–1792

91. Brettschneider WD. Effects of sport club activities on adolescent development in Germany. *Eur J Sport Sci.* 2001;1(2): 1–11

92. Ferron C, Narring F, Cauderay M, Michaud PA. Sport activity in adolescence: associations with health perceptions and experimental behaviours. *Health Educ Res.* 1999; 14(2):225–233

93. Vella SA, Cliff DP, Magee CA, Okely AD. Associations between sports participation and psychological difficulties during childhood: a two-year follow up. *J Sci Med Sport.* 2015;18(3): 304–309

94. Jewett R, Sabiston CM, Brunet J, O'Loughlin EK, Scarapicchia T, O'Loughlin J. School sport participation during adolescence and mental health in early adulthood. *J Adolesc Health.* 2014;55(5):640–644

95. Taliaferro LA, Rienzo BA, Miller MD, Pigg RM Jr, Dodd VJ. High school youth and suicide risk: exploring protection afforded through physical activity and sport participation. *J Sch Health.* 2008; 78(10):545–553

96. Taliaferro LA, Eisenberg ME, Johnson KE, Nelson TF, Neumark-Sztainer D. Sport participation during adolescence and suicide ideation and attempts. *Int J Adolesc Med Health.* 2011;23(1):3–10

97. Pate RR, Trost SG, Levin S, Dowda M. Sports participation and health-related behaviors among US youth. *Arch Pediatr Adolesc Med.* 2000;154(9): 904–911

98. Sabo D, Miller KE, Melnick MJ, Farrell MP, Barnes GM. High school athletic participation and adolescent suicide: a nationwide US study. *Int Rev Sociol Sport.* 2005;40(1):5–23

99. Taliaferro LA, Rienzo BA, Donovan KA. Relationships between youth sport participation and selected health risk behaviors from 1999 to 2007. *J Sch Health.* 2010;80(8):399–410

100. Richman EL, Shaffer DR. If you let me play sports: how might sport participation influence the self-esteem of adolescent females? *Psychol Women Q.* 2000;24(2):189–199

101. Wagnsson S, Lindwall M, Gustafsson H. Participation in organized sport and self-esteem across adolescence: the mediating role of perceived sport competence. *J Sport Exerc Psychol.* 2014;36(6):584–594

102. Bowker A. The relationship between sports participation and self-esteem during early adolescence. *Can J Behav Sci.* 2006;38(3):214–229

103. Pedersen S, Siedman E. Team sports achievement and self-esteem development among urban adolescent girls. *Psychol Women Q.* 2004;28(4): 412–422

104. Palermo MT, Di Luigi M, Dal Forno G, et al. Externalizing and oppositional behaviors and karate-do: the way of crime prevention. A pilot study. *Int J Offender Ther Comp Criminol.* 2006; 50(6):654–660

105. Tester GJ, Watkins GG, Rouse I. The Sports Challenge international programme for identified 'at risk' children and adolescents: a Singapore study. *Asia Pac J Public Health.* 1999; 11(1):34–38

106. Sanders CE, Field TM, Diego M, Kaplan M. Moderate involvement in sports is related to lower depression levels among adolescents. *Adolescence.* 2000; 35(140):793–797

107. Michaud PA, Jeannin A, Suris JC. Correlates of extracurricular sport participation among Swiss adolescents. *Eur J Pediatr.* 2006;165(8):546–555

108. Donaldson SJ, Ronan KR. The effects of sports participation on young adolescents' emotional well-being. *Adolescence.* 2006;41(162):369–389

109. Wickel EE, Eisenmann JC. Contribution of youth sport to total daily physical activity among 6- to 12-yr-old boys. *Med Sci Sports Exerc.* 2007;39(9):1493–1500

110. Duncan SC, Duncan TE, Strycker LA, Chaumeton NR. Relations between youth antisocial and prosocial activities. *J Behav Med.* 2002;25(5): 425–438

111. Marques A, Ekelund U, Sardinha LB. Associations between organized sports participation and objectively measured physical activity, sedentary time and weight status in youth. *J Sci Med Sport.* 2016;19(2):154–157

112. Trilk JL, Pate RR, Pfeiffer KA, et al. A cluster analysis of physical activity and sedentary behavior patterns in middle school girls. *J Adolesc Health.* 2012; 51(3):292–298

113. Guagliano JM, Rosenkranz RR, Kolt GS. Girls' physical activity levels during organized sports in Australia. *Med Sci Sports Exerc.* 2013;45(1):116–122

114. Nelson TF, Stovitz SD, Thomas M, LaVoi NM, Bauer KW, Neumark-Sztainer D. Do youth sports prevent pediatric obesity? A systematic review and commentary. *Curr Sports Med Rep.* 2011;10(6): 360–370

115. Telford RM, Telford RD, Cochrane T, Cunningham RB, Olive LS, Davey R. The influence of sport club participation on physical activity, fitness and body fat during childhood and adolescence: the LOOK Longitudinal Study. *J Sci Med Sport.* 2016;19(5):400–406

116. Hebert JJ, Møller NC, Andersen LB, Wedderkopp N. Organized sport participation is associated with higher levels of overall health-related physical activity in children (CHAMPS study-DK). *PLoS One.* 2015;10(8):e0134621

117. Phillips JA, Young DR. Past-year sports participation, current physical activity, and fitness in urban adolescent girls. *J Phys Act Health.* 2009;6(1):105–111

118. Machado-Rodrigues AM, Coelho e Silva MJ, Mota J, Santos RM, Cumming SP, Malina RM. Physical activity and energy expenditure in adolescent male sport participants and nonparticipants aged 13 to 16 years. *J Phys Act Health.* 2012; 9(5):626–633

119. Lee JE, Pope Z, Gao Z. The role of youth sports in promoting children's physical activity and preventing pediatric obesity: a systematic review. *Behav Med.* 2018;44(1):62–76

120. Drenowatz C, Steiner RP, Brandstetter S, Klenk J, Wabitsch M, Steinacker JM. Organized sports, overweight, and physical fitness in primary school children in Germany. *J Obes.* 2013;2013: 935245

121. Zahner L, Muehlbauer T, Schmid M, Meyer U, Puder JJ, Kriemler S. Association of sports club participation with fitness and fatness in children. *Med Sci Sports Exerc.* 2009;41(2): 344–350

122. Hoffman JR, Kang J, Faigenbaum AD, Ratamess NA. Recreational sports participation is associated with enhanced physical fitness in children. *Res Sports Med.* 2005;13(2):149–161

123. Tammelin T, Näyhä S, Hills AP, Järvelin MR. Adolescent participation in sports and adult physical activity. *Am J Prev Med.* 2003;24(1):22–28

124. Perkins DF, Jacobs JE, Barber BL, Eccles JS. Childhood and adolescent sports participation as predictors of participation in sports and physical fitness activities during young adulthood. *Youth Soc.* 2016;35(4): 495–520

125. Kjønniksen L, Anderssen N, Wold B. Organized youth sport as a predictor of physical activity in adulthood. *Scand J Med Sci Sports.* 2009;19(5):646–654

126. Wichstrøm L, von Soest T, Kvalem IL. Predictors of growth and decline in leisure time physical activity from adolescence to adulthood. *Health Psychol.* 2013;32(7):775–784

127. Ara I, Vicente-Rodriguez G, Perez-Gomez J, et al. Influence of extracurricular sport activities on body composition and physical fitness in boys: a 3-year longitudinal study. *Int J Obes.* 2006; 30(7):1062–1071

128. Basterfield L, Reilly JK, Pearce MS, et al. Longitudinal associations between sports participation, body composition and physical activity from childhood to adolescence. *J Sci Med Sport.* 2015; 18(2):178–182

129. Quinto Romani A. Children's weight and participation in organized sports. *Scand J Public Health.* 2011;39(7): 687–695

130. Dortch KS, Gay J, Springer A, et al. The association between sport participation and dietary behaviors among fourth graders in the school physical activity and nutrition survey, 2009-2010. *Am J Health Promot.* 2014; 29(2):99–106

131. Croll JK, Neumark-Sztainer D, Story M, Wall M, Perry C, Harnack L. Adolescents involved in weight-related and power team sports have better eating patterns and nutrient intakes than non-sport-involved adolescents. *J Am Diet Assoc.* 2006;106(5):709–717

132. Baumert PW Jr, Henderson JM, Thompson NJ. Health risk behaviors of adolescent participants in organized sports. *J Adolesc Health.* 1998;22(6): 460–465

133. Yang X, Telama R, Hirvensalo M, Viikari JS, Raitakari OT. Sustained participation in youth sport decreases metabolic syndrome in adulthood. *Int J Obes.* 2009;33(11):1219–1226

134. Tenforde AS, Sainani KL, Carter Sayres L, Milgrom C, Fredericson M. Participation in ball sports may represent a prehabilitation strategy to prevent future stress fractures and promote bone health in young athletes. *PM R.* 2015;7(2):222–225

135. Tenforde AS, Fredericson M. Influence of sports participation on bone health in the young athlete: a review of the literature. *PM R.* 2011;3(9):861–867

136. Lisha NE, Crano WD, Delucchi KL. Participation in team sports and alcohol and marijuana use initiation trajectories. *J Drug Issues.* 2014;44(1): 83–93

137. Lisha NE, Sussman S. Relationship of high school and college sports participation with alcohol, tobacco, and illicit drug use: a review. *Addict Behav.* 2010;35(5):399–407

138. Naylor AH, Gardner D, Zaichkowsky L. Drug use patterns among high school athletes and nonathletes. *Adolescence.* 2001;36(144):627–639

139. Kwan M, Bobko S, Faulkner G, Donnelly P, Cairney J. Sport participation and alcohol and illicit drug use in adolescents and young adults: a systematic review of longitudinal studies. *Addict Behav.* 2014;39(3): 497–506

140. Sabo DF, Miller KE, Farrell MP, Melnick MJ, Barnes GM. High school athletic participation, sexual behavior and adolescent pregnancy: a regional study. *J Adolesc Health.* 1999;25(3): 207–216

141. Vella SA, Cliff DP, Magee CA, Okely AD. Sports participation and parent-reported health-related quality of life in children: longitudinal associations. *J Pediatr.* 2014;164(6):1469–1474

142. Eime RM, Harvey JT, Brown WJ, Payne WR. Does sports club participation contribute to health-related quality of life? *Med Sci Sports Exerc.* 2010;42(5): 1022–1028

143. DiFiori JP, Benjamin HJ, Brenner J, et al. Overuse injuries and burnout in youth sports: a position statement from the American Medical Society for Sports Medicine. *Clin J Sport Med.* 2014;24(1): 3–20

144. Gustafsson H, DeFreese JD, Madigan DJ. Athlete burnout: review and recommendations. *Curr Opin Psychol.* 2017;16:109–113

145. Brenner JS; American Academy of Pediatrics Council on Sports Medicine and Fitness. Overuse injuries, overtraining, and burnout in child and adolescent athletes. *Pediatrics.* 2007; 119(6):1242–1245

146. Jayanthi NA, LaBella CR, Fischer D, Pasulka J, Dugas LR. Sports-specialized intensive training and the risk of injury in young athletes: a clinical case-control study. *Am J Sports Med.* 2015; 43(4):794–801

147. Fraser-Thomas J, Côté J, Deakin J. Examining adolescent sport dropout and prolonged engagement from a developmental perspective. *J Appl Sport Psychol.* 2008;20(3):318–333

148. Veliz PT, Boyd CJ, McCabe SE. Competitive sport involvement and substance use among adolescents: a nationwide study. *Subst Use Misuse.* 2015;50(2):156–165

149. Rainey CJ, McKeown RE, Sargent RG, Valois RF. Patterns of tobacco and alcohol use among sedentary, exercising, nonathletic, and athletic youth. *J Sch Health.* 1996;66(1):27–32

150. Hartmann D, Massoglia M. Reassessing the relationship between high school sports participation and deviance: evidence of enduring, bifurcated effects. *Sociol Q.* 2007;48(3):485–505

151. Veliz P, Epstein-Ngo QM, Meier E, Ross-Durow PL, McCabe SE, Boyd CJ. Painfully obvious: a longitudinal examination of medical use and misuse of opioid medication among adolescent sports participants. *J Adolesc Health.* 2014;54(3):333–340

152. Carl RL, Johnson MD, Martin TJ; Council on Sports Medicine and Fitness. Promotion of healthy weight-control practices in young athletes. *Pediatrics.* 2017;140(3):e20171871

153. Patel DR, Luckstead EF. Sport participation, risk taking, and health risk behaviors. *Adolesc Med.* 2000;11(1):141–155

154. Weiss Kelly AK, Hecht S; Council on Sports Medicine and Fitness. The female athlete triad. *Pediatrics.* 2016;138(2):e20160922

155. Mathews NM. Prohibited contaminants in dietary supplements. *Sports Health.* 2018;10(1):19–30

156. LaBotz M, Griesemer BA; Council on Sports Medicine and Fitness. Use of performance-enhancing substances. *Pediatrics.* 2016;138(1):e20161300

157. Diehl K, Thiel A, Zipfel S, Mayer J, Litaker DG, Schneider S. How healthy is the behavior of young athletes? A systematic literature review and meta-analyses. *J Sports Sci Med.* 2012;11(2):201–220

158. Dodge TL, Jaccard JJ. The effect of high school sports participation on the use of performance-enhancing substances in young adulthood. *J Adolesc Health.* 2006;39(3):367–373

159. Kanayama G, Pope HG Jr. History and epidemiology of anabolic androgens in athletes and non-athletes. *Mol Cell Endocrinol.* 2018;464:4–13

160. Stirling AE, Bridges EJ, Cruz EL, Mountjoy ML; Canadian Academy of Sport and Exercise Medicine. Canadian Academy of Sport and Exercise Medicine position paper: abuse, harassment, and bullying in sport. *Clin J Sport Med.* 2011;21(5):385–391

161. Mountjoy M, Brackenridge C, Arrington M, et al. International Olympic Committee consensus statement: harassment and abuse (non-accidental violence) in sport. *Br J Sports Med.* 2016;50(17):1019–1029

162. Evans B, Adler A, Macdonald D, Côté J. Bullying victimization and perpetration among adolescent sport teammates. *Pediatr Exerc Sci.* 2016;28(2):296–303

163. Diamond AB, Callahan ST, Chain KF, Solomon GS. Qualitative review of hazing in collegiate and school sports: consequences from a lack of culture, knowledge and responsiveness. *Br J Sports Med.* 2016;50(3):149–153

164. Gershel JC, Katz-Sidlow RJ, Small E, Zandieh S. Hazing of suburban middle school and high school athletes. *J Adolesc Health.* 2003;32(5):333–335

165. Fields SK, Collins CL, Comstock RD. Violence in youth sports: hazing, brawling and foul play. *Br J Sports Med.* 2010;44(1):32–37

166. Waldron JJ, Kowalski CL. Crossing the line: rites of passage, team aspects, and ambiguity of hazing. *Res Q Exerc Sport.* 2009;80(2):291–302

167. Sport readiness in children and youth. *Paediatr Child Health.* 2005;10(6):343–344

168. Sebire SJ, Standage M, Vansteenkiste M. Examining intrinsic versus extrinsic exercise goals: cognitive, affective, and behavioral outcomes. *J Sport Exerc Psychol.* 2009;31(2):189–210

169. Shields DL, Bredemeier BL, LaVoi NM, Power FC. The sport behavior of youth, parents, and coaches: the good, the bad, and the ugly. *J Res Character Educ.* 2005;3(1):43–59

170. Arthur-Banning S, Wells MS, Baker BL, Hegreness R. Parents behaving badly? The relationship between the sportsmanship behaviors of adults and athletes in youth basketball games. *J Sport Behav.* 2009;32(1):3–18

171. Bean CN, Fortier M, Post C, Chima K. Understanding how organized youth sport maybe harming individual players within the family unit: a literature review. *Int J Environ Res Public Health.* 2014;11(10):10226–10268

172. Gregory S. How kids' sports became a $15 billion industry. *Time.* August 24, 2017. Available at: http://time.com/magazine/us/4913681/september-4th-2017-vol-190-no-9-u-s/. Accessed April 26, 2019

173. NCAA. Estimated probability of competing in college athletics. Available at: www.ncaa.org/about/resources/research/estimated-probability-competing-college-athletics. Accessed January 31, 2018

174. Hyman M. *The Most Expensive Game in Town: The Rising Cost of Youth Sports and the Toll on Today's Families.* Boston, MA: Beacon Press; 2012

175. Alexander K, Stafford A, Lewis R. *The Experiences of Children Participating in Organised Sport in the UK.* Edinburgh, Scotland: The University of Edinburgh/NSPCC Child Protection Research Centre; 2011

176. Wilson KM. When the high school coach is a bully. *NASN Sch Nurse.* 2017;32(1):33–35

177. Pelletier LG, Fortier MS, Vallerand RJ, Brière NM. Associations among perceived autonomy support, forms of self-regulation, and persistence: a prospective study. *Motiv Emot.* 2001;25(4):279–306

178. SHAPE America–Society of Health and Physical Educators. *Using Physical Activity as Punishment and/or Behavior Management (Position Statement).* Reston, VA: SHAPE America–Society of Health and Physical Educators; 2009

179. Pratt HD, Patel DR, Greydanus DE. Behavioral aspects of children's sports. *Pediatr Clin North Am.* 2003;50(4):879–899, ix

180. Parent S, Lavoie F, Thibodeau ME, Hébert M, Blais M; Team PAJ. Sexual violence experienced in the sport context by a representative sample of Quebec adolescents. *J Interpers Violence.* 2016;31(16):2666–2686

181. Leahy T, Pretty G, Tenenbaum G. Prevalence of sexual abuse in organised competitive sport in Australia. *J Sex Aggress.* 2002;8(2):16–36

182. Hohler B. Former tennis star, coach Bob Hewitt accused in abuse of young girls. *Boston Globe.* August 28, 2011. Available at: https://www.bostonglobe.com/sports/2011/08/28/tennis-star-trailed-abuse-allegations/

jWhJkNUrq45U5c6P33jkKO/story.html. Accessed April 26, 2019

183. Fuchs J. Fighting Back. *Sports Illustrated*; September 10, 2018. Available at: https://www.si.com/vault/2018/09/04/fighting-back. Accessed April 26, 2019
184. McLean S. Top USA Swimming officials under fire for alleged culture of abuse. *CNN*. February 24, 2018. Available at: https://www.cnn.com/2018/02/24/us/usa-swimming-abuse-allegations/index.html. Accessed September 23, 2018
185. Gustafson SL, Rhodes RE. Parental correlates of physical activity in children and early adolescents. *Sports Med*. 2006;36(1):79–97
186. Heitzler CD, Martin SL, Duke J, Huhman M. Correlates of physical activity in a national sample of children aged 9-13 years. *Prev Med*. 2006;42(4):254–260
187. Gould D, Lauer L, Rolo C, Jannes C, Pennisi N. Understanding the role parents play in tennis success: a national survey of junior tennis coaches. *Br J Sports Med*. 2006;40(7):632–636; discussion 636
188. Lauer L, Gould D, Roman N, Pierce M. How parents influence junior tennis players' development: qualitative narratives. *J Clin Sport Psychol*. 2010;4(1):69–92
189. Leek D, Carlson JA, Cain KL, et al. Physical activity during youth sports practices. *Arch Pediatr Adolesc Med*. 2011;165(4):294–299
190. Sacheck JM, Nelson T, Ficker L, Kafka T, Kuder J, Economos CD. Physical activity during soccer and its contribution to physical activity recommendations in normal weight and overweight children. *Pediatr Exerc Sci*. 2011;23(2):281–292
191. Chircop A, Shearer C, Pitter R, et al. Privileging physical activity over healthy eating: 'Time' to Choose? *Health Promot Int*. 2015;30(3):418–426
192. Jayanthi N, Pinkham C, Dugas L, Patrick B, Labella C. Sports specialization in young athletes: evidence-based recommendations. *Sports Health*. 2013;5(3):251–257
193. Mostafavifar AM, Best TM, Myer GD. Early sport specialisation, does it lead to long-term problems? *Br J Sports Med*. 2013;47(17):1060–1061
194. Zarrett N, Veliz P, Sabo D. Teen sport in America: why participation matters. 2018. Available at: https://www.womenssportsfoundation.org/research/article-and-report/recent-research/teen-sport-in-america/. Accessed April 26, 2019
195. LaBotz M. Creating a safe environment to prevent abuse in youth sports: a parent checklist. 2018. Available at: https://www.healthychildren.org/English/healthy-living/sports/Pages/Creating-a-Safe-Environment-to-Prevent-Abuse-in-Youth-Sports-A-Parent-Checklist.aspx. Accessed April 27, 2018
196. Lorentzen T. Allocation of playing time within team sports – a problem for discussion. *Open Review of Educational Research*. 2017;4(1):20–32
197. Luke A, Lazaro RM, Bergeron MF, et al. Sports-related injuries in youth athletes: is overscheduling a risk factor? *Clin J Sport Med*. 2011;21(4):307–314
198. Guagliano JM, Lonsdale C, Kolt GS, Rosenkranz RR, George ES. Increasing girls' physical activity during a short-term organized youth sport basketball program: a randomized controlled trial. *J Sci Med Sport*. 2015;18(4):412–417
199. Yogman M, Garner A, Hutchinson J, Hirsh-Pasek K, Golinkoff RM; Committee on Psychosocial Aspects of Child and Family Health; Council on Communications and Media. The power of play: a pediatric role in enhancing development in young children. *Pediatrics*. 2018;142(3):e20182058
200. American Academy of Pediatrics. *Caring for Our Children: National Health and Safety Performance Standards; Guidelines for Early Care and Education Programs*. 3rd ed. Aurora, CO: National Resource Center for Health and Safety in Child Care and Early Education; 2011
201. Moreno MA. Advice for patients. Children and organized sports. *Arch Pediatr Adolesc Med*. 2011;165(4):376
202. Vella SA, Cliff DP, Okely AD, Scully ML, Morley BC. Associations between sports participation, adiposity and obesity-related health behaviors in Australian adolescents. *Int J Behav Nutr Phys Act*. 2013;10:113
203. Escobedo LG, Marcus SE, Holtzman D, Giovino GA. Sports participation, age at smoking initiation, and the risk of smoking among US high school students. *JAMA*. 1993;269(11):1391–1395
204. Melnick MJ, Miller KE, Sabo DF, Farrell MP, Barnes GM. Tobacco use among high school athletes and nonatieletes: results of the 1997 youth risk behavior survey. *Adolescence*. 2001;36(144):727–747
205. Eccles JS, Barber BL, Stone M, Hunt J. Extracurricular activities and adolescent development. *J Soc Issues*. 2003;59(4):865–889
206. Eccles JS, Barber BL. Student council, volunteering, basketball, or marching band: what kind of extracurricular involvement matters? *J Adolesc Res*. 1999;14(1):10–43

Pediatric Application of Coding and Valuation Systems

- *Policy Statement*

POLICY STATEMENT Organizational Principles to Guide and Define the Child Health Care System and/or Improve the Health of all Children

American Academy of Pediatrics

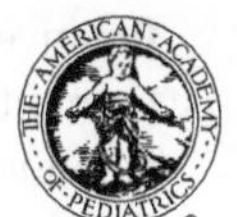

DEDICATED TO THE HEALTH OF ALL CHILDREN™

Pediatric Application of Coding and Valuation Systems

David M. Kanter, MD, MBA, FAAP,[a] Richard Lander, MD, FAAP, CIC,[b] Richard A. Molteni, MD, FAAP,[c] COMMITTEE ON CODING AND NOMENCLATURE, PRIVATE PAYER ADVOCACY ADVISORY COMMITTEE

abstract

The American Academy of Pediatrics provides this revised policy statement to address health care changes that impact procedural and visit coding and valuation as well as the incorporation of coding principles into innovative, newer payment models. This policy statement focuses solely on recommendations, and an accompanying technical report provides supplemental coding and valuation background.

[a]Mednax Services Inc, Sunrise, Florida; [b]Department of Pediatrics, University of Medicine and Dentistry of New Jersey, Newark, New Jersey; and [c]Joint Commission International and Department of Pediatrics, School of Medicine, University of Washington, Seattle, Washington

This policy statement represents a collaborative contribution of the Committee on Coding and Nomenclature (chairperson, Dr Molteni) and the Private Payer Advocacy Advisory Committee (chairperson, Dr Lander). Dr Kanter (Committee on Coding and Nomenclature) convened a workgroup of Committee on Coding and Nomenclature and Private Payer Advocacy Advisory Committee members who, over a series of meetings, established the concepts, themes, and structure of the manuscript. Incorporating guidance from Committee on Coding and Nomenclature and Private Payer Advocacy Advisory Committee members, Dr Kanter drafted the manuscript while incorporating additional recommendations from reviewers and the Board of Directors. The authors thank Linda Walsh (senior manager, health policy and coding) and Lou Terranova (senior health policy analyst) for guiding the manuscript through production.

This document is copyrighted and is property of the American Academy of Pediatrics and its Board of Directors. All authors have filed conflict of interest statements with the American Academy of Pediatrics. Any conflicts have been resolved through a process approved by the Board of Directors. The American Academy of Pediatrics has neither solicited nor accepted any commercial involvement in the development of the content of this publication.

Policy statements from the American Academy of Pediatrics benefit from expertise and resources of liaisons and internal (AAP) and external reviewers. However, policy statements from the American Academy of Pediatrics may not reflect the views of the liaisons or the organizations or government agencies that they represent.

The guidance in this statement does not indicate an exclusive course of treatment or serve as a standard of medical care. Variations, taking into account individual circumstances, may be appropriate.

To cite: Kanter DM, Lander R, Molteni RA, AAP COMMITTEE ON CODING AND NOMENCLATURE, PRIVATE PAYER ADVOCACY ADVISORY COMMITTEE. Pediatric Application of Coding and Valuation Systems. *Pediatrics.* 2019;144(4):e20192496

INTRODUCTION

The American Academy of Pediatrics (AAP) 2014 policy statement on the pediatric application of the resource-based relative value scale (RBRVS) noted that the "RBRVS system should continue to be the preferred process to establish physician payment."[1] Even in the current era of evolving models of physician payment, the RBRVS, the coding principles on which it is built, and the code sets that foster standardized communication remain the most effective systems to ensure transparency, relativity, and representative fairness in clinician service valuation. In recognition of the role these tools continue to play in the changing landscape of health care payment, the AAP Committee on Coding and Nomenclature, in collaboration with the Private Payer Advocacy Advisory Committee, provides the following recommendations that update the 2014 policy statement. These recommendations reflect the impact that these coding systems have in current payment models and clinical nomenclature, and an accompanying technical report provides instructive background information on the RBRVS, *Current Procedural Terminology* (CPT), and *International Classification of Diseases, 10th Revision, Clinical Modification* (ICD-10-CM) standardized code sets, and current payment principles.

CODING AND/OR VALUATION SYSTEM RECOMMENDATIONS

We recommend the following.

1. **Confirm the importance of the RBRVS.** The RBRVS currently remains the most effective process by which individual health care services are

valued, and the American Medical Association–Specialty Society Relative Value Scale Update Committee (RUC) is the only committee charged with developing valuation recommendations for the RBRVS. The AAP actively participates in the RUC process, which allows pediatricians to provide direct input into how pediatric services are valued and paid relative to all other medical services. Even in an era in which alternative payment models compete with fee-for-service payment, the RBRVS provides a framework to assign relative values for physician work and practice expenses. Within payment models that bundle groups of services, the elements of the RBRVS provide the basis for effectively assessing the value of the bundle. As services, especially preventive medicine visits, expand in the scope of recommended elements (such as vision, hearing, and other types of preventive screening) in response to AAP guidance, such as *Bright Futures: Recommendations for Preventive Care of Infants, Children, and Adolescents, Fourth Edition*, relative value unit (RVU) assignment allows for appropriate assessment of the overall composite service inclusive of its different components.

2. **Engage in the RUC survey process.** Effective RBRVS valuation requires clarity, relevance, and reliability in the RUC survey process. Pediatricians should understand the importance of the AAP survey in rendering RUC valuation decisions and should not allow familiar routine or repetitive experience to lead to underestimation of the work inherent in the service. Optimal nonprocedural survey tools define and quantify the unique aspects of physician work (such as facilitated care delivery and communication[2]) required to care for medically complex children, and nonprocedural services should be appropriately and competitively valued relative to procedural services. Because valuation of some types of nonprocedural work may be underrepresented relative to interventional procedures, RVUs may not be fully representative of physician productivity when comparing care dominated by nonprocedural as opposed to procedural work. In assessing physician productivity, reliance solely on RVUs could potentially underestimate nonprocedural scenarios if RVUs are not accurately reflective of the work, especially those inherent in complex pediatric care.
3. **Support Centers for Medicare and Medicaid Services (CMS) RVU publication of RUC-valued services.** Although the RUC provides valuation recommendations, the CMS maintains decision-making authority to accept or modify those recommendation for publication in its annual Medicare Physician Fee Schedule (MPFS). Currently, the CMS publishes RVUs for all Medicare-covered services; however, reliable pediatric representation requires that the CMS also publishes the RUC-recommended RVUs for those services not covered by Medicare. Most non-Medicare payers, including Medicaid and commercial insurers, rely on the published RVUs in the MPFS to construct their own independent fee schedules. Because a relatively greater number of pediatric services fall into Medicare's noncovered category, greater potential exists for nonpublication of essential pediatric services in the MPFS. The absence of noncovered services (and their RVUs) in the MPFS is especially detrimental to pediatric care and the desire of payers to reliably value the pediatric services they cover. Because many of the non-Medicare pediatric-relevant services are covered by Medicaid programs, and thus remain in the CMS domain, CMS publication of these RVUs would support Medicaid programs in establishing their own respective fee schedules. Many, if not all, of these noncovered services represent evidence- and/or consensus-based best practices advocated for by national professional societies (such as instrument-based ocular screening[3] and topical fluoride application[4]). The CMS can accommodate the publication of these noncovered RVUs through an informational approach that need not imply CMS review or acceptance but rather serves as notification of RUC-recommended values for Medicare noncovered services. Short of CMS publication of RUC-recommended values for services not covered by Medicare, the RUC should consider alternative avenues of publication to support payer access to these RVUs outside the CMS MPFS.
4. **Encourage full-spectrum acknowledgment of CPT codes and guidance.** The CPT inventory includes a broad spectrum of coded services that are relevant to pediatric care and thus should be consistently, fully, and reliably covered by payers along with payment that reflects an appropriate minimum floor (such as the current MPFS rate). Payer adherence to the full scope of CPT coding guidance should also include recognition of CPT modifiers that reflect sound coding principles and impact pediatric payment (such as modifier 22 for increased procedural services that are unusually difficult or time consuming and modifier 63 for procedures performed on infants

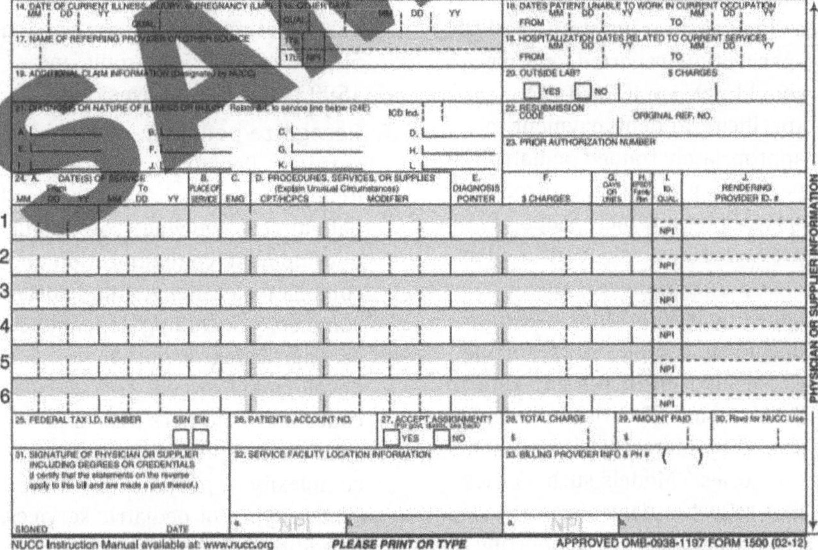
14. DATE OF CURRENT ILLNESS, INJURY, or PREGNANCY (LMP)
17. NAME OF REFERRING PROVIDER OR OTHER SOURCE
19. ADDITIONAL CLAIM INFORMATION (Designated by NUCC)
21. DIAGNOSIS OR NATURE OF ILLNESS OR INJURY
18. HOSPITALIZATION DATES RELATED TO CURRENT SERVICES
20. OUTSIDE LAB? $ CHARGES
22. RESUBMISSION CODE ORIGINAL REF. NO.
23. PRIOR AUTHORIZATION NUMBER
24. A. DATE(S) OF SERVICE B. PLACE OF SERVICE C. EMG D. PROCEDURES, SERVICES, OR SUPPLIES (Explain Unusual Circumstances) CPT/HCPCS MODIFIER E. DIAGNOSIS POINTER F. $ CHARGES G. DAYS OR UNITS H. EPSDT Family Plan I. ID. QUAL. J. RENDERING PROVIDER ID. #
1
2
3
4
5
6
25. FEDERAL TAX I.D. NUMBER SSN EIN
26. PATIENT'S ACCOUNT NO.
27. ACCEPT ASSIGNMENT? YES NO
28. TOTAL CHARGE
29. AMOUNT PAID
30. Rsvd for NUCC Use
31. SIGNATURE OF PHYSICIAN OR SUPPLIER INCLUDING DEGREES OR CREDENTIALS (I certify that the statements on the reverse apply to this bill and are made a part thereof.)
32. SERVICE FACILITY LOCATION INFORMATION
33. BILLING PROVIDER INFO & PH # ( )
SIGNED DATE
PHYSICIAN OR SUPPLIER INFORMATION
NUCC Instruction Manual available at: www.nucc.org PLEASE PRINT OR TYPE APPROVED OMB-0938-1197 FORM 1500 (02-12)

FIGURE 1

Lower half of CMS 1500 paper claim form demonstrating space limitation of only 4 ICD-10-CM codes for each line-item CPT (although 12 total ICD-10-CM codes can be entered on the claim form).

<4 kg). Comprehensive payer coverage is especially relevant to the codes and principles associated with team-based care, which is integral to the delivery of care for children with complex medical and social problems. Such team-based care is recognized by many of the recently developed transition and chronic care management services and include services that reflect efficient approaches to care delivery, such as interprofessional telephone and/or Internet consultation services. Technological evolution, site of service, or provider type should not limit payer acknowledgment of CPT coding

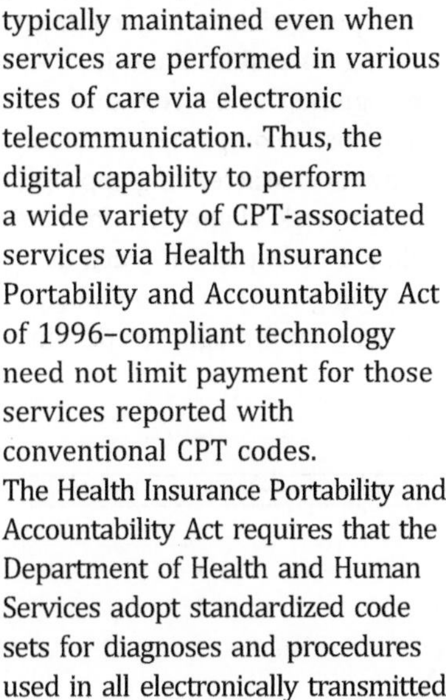
principles. Physician work is typically maintained even when services are performed in various sites of care via electronic telecommunication. Thus, the digital capability to perform a wide variety of CPT-associated services via Health Insurance Portability and Accountability Act of 1996–compliant technology need not limit payment for those services reported with conventional CPT codes. The Health Insurance Portability and Accountability Act requires that the Department of Health and Human Services adopt standardized code sets for diagnoses and procedures used in all electronically transmitted health care transactions, such as the designation of the CPT code set in representing physician services. Because children are covered by a national patchwork of payers, including Medicaid, the Children's Health Insurance Program, and other government and private payers, payer conformity in following CPT published guidance is essential in minimizing administrative burden and creating consistency in adjudicating claims. Following CPT coding guidance is especially important for immunization administration, a mainstay of pediatric physician practice and child health. Unilateral payer modification of CPT immunization administration guidance, which focuses on each vaccine component rather than each vaccine product, imposes inappropriate payment limits on immunization administration and fosters errors in claim submission. Additionally, variation in payer interpretation of CPT guidance can impede effective reporting of quality measures, such as through the Healthcare Effectiveness Data and Information Set.

5. **Develop relevant quality measures.** For newly developed alternative payment models, payers typically include quality-measure reporting to incentivize performance and the adoption of evidence-based care. Although conventional quality measures, such as those reflected by Category II CPT codes and their numerator–denominator structure, were developed for shorter-term clinical scenarios, pediatric care is unique in its focus on longer-term care of the growing and developing child within a dynamic family social fabric. The AAP recognizes the impact of social and environmental determinants of child health in pursuing its mission to attain optimal physical, intellectual, behavioral, developmental, and social health for all pediatric patients.[5] This

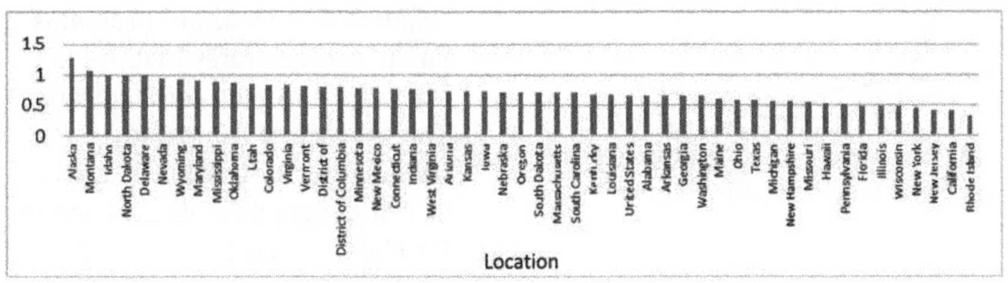

FIGURE 2

Medicaid-to-Medicare fee index for 2016 primary care services. Primary care services were defined as services subjected to the Patient Protection and Affordable Care Act's Medicaid primary care parity provision, which impacted 2013–2014 payments.[22]

unique, pediatric-focused approach to monitoring outcomes over extended periods of maturation requires creative approaches to develop meaningful quality measures. Designers of pediatric quality measures should give consideration to reporting of metrics that reflect achievement of preventive and anticipatory services rendered over extended childhood time spans and focused on longer-term outcomes.

6. **Optimize ICD-10-CM impact on payment.** Pediatricians should use the specificity of the ICD-10-CM to accurately reflect the child's conditions and complexity, yet payers must recognize that clinical specificity may be lacking when disease processes are evolving. When sufficient clinical information is not known or available about a particular health condition, the payer should recognize that the clinician can appropriately report an unspecified code without the claim being summarily denied solely on the basis of specificity.[6] Furthermore, as experts in the care of children, pediatricians should be able to provide those specialist services that fall within the scope of primary pediatric care as long as appropriate ICD-10-CM specificity is reported, and payers should not use ICD-10-CM specificity to deny payment to appropriately trained pediatricians performing those specialized services within their scope of practice. Newer payment models incorporate elaborate risk-adjustment algorithms based on diagnostic completeness, such as Department of Health and Human Services and CMS risk adjustment scored by hierarchical condition categories.[7] Models such as these that reflect patient diagnostic complexity assist in supporting resource allocation, but such risk-based models must appropriately represent the risk contributed by children with special health care needs.[8] To effectively represent the medical and social complexity that pediatricians may confront in caring for children and in recognition of the role that diagnostic comprehensiveness plays in characterizing appropriate patient risk, claim-form formatting should be expanded (such as doubling to 8) to accommodate more than 4 diagnoses per line-item service (which is the current line-item limitation for the version 5010 CMS 837P electronic and 1500 paper claim forms; Fig 1).[9]
7. **Recognize pediatric-specific services.** Pediatric care presents unique challenges because of small patient size, evolving growth and development, communication and compliance challenges, and social complexity, including dependency on adult caregivers. The development of pediatric-specific codes and modifiers assists in accurately representing the complexity of pediatric work for certain types of pediatric services. In addition to focusing on interventional procedures that merit unique pediatric specificity to support increased complexity, nonprocedural and team-based services also warrant pediatric recognition during code development to appropriately represent the pediatrician's navigation of complex social scenarios and interactive complexity.

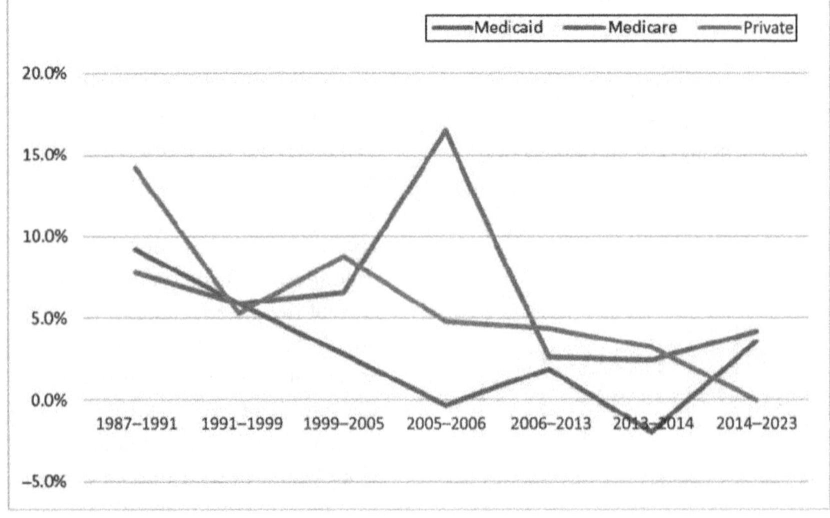

FIGURE 3
Average annual growth in Medicaid spending per enrollee compared with that of Medicare and private payers.[23]

CMS- AND/OR PAYER-FOCUSED RECOMMENDATIONS

We recommend the following.

1. **Improve comparative Medicaid payment.** Although Medicaid is jointly federally and state funded, individual state administration leads to marked variability among the nation's various Medicaid programs. Ensuring that vulnerable pediatric populations have access to appropriate care requires that Medicaid programs pay physicians rates that are at least equal to those of Medicare. The absence of comparative payment for professional services is 1 of the greatest access barriers for children and families seeking primary and specialty care. The AAP continues to voice strong support for the Medicaid program,[10] and because of its

central role in supporting health care for the family and child and because access to care is essential in maintaining pediatric health, Medicaid should fully value its services consistent with RUC recommendations and MPFS minimum thresholds. Although Medicaid has a history of physician underpayment relative to other payers,[11] the Patient Protection and Affordable Care Act's statewide 2013–2014 increase in primary care Medicaid payments to Medicare levels resulted in improved access to care.[12,13] Unfortunately, most states reverted back to historic low-payment norms when the parity program concluded. Figure 2 demonstrates 2016 Medicaid-to-Medicare fee ratios, and Fig 3 shows average annual per-enrollee growth in Medicaid compared with Medicare spending. A 2012 study revealed that the average ratio of Medicaid to Medicare primary care payments was 58%.[14] Because the burden of disease is accentuated in pediatric populations subjected to adverse socioeconomic conditions[15] and because low-income families rely on Medicaid to provide for their health care needs, Medicaid and managed Medicaid rates should at least reach parity with those of Medicare in support of access to health care. Furthermore, individual Medicaid programs should be transparent in their fee schedules, and those rates should reflect appropriate relativity among services as established by the RUC through RBRVS service valuation.

2. **Develop a national Medicaid database.** Achieving the Triple Aim of better patient and/or family care experience, better population health, and lower costs[16] will require expanded data transparency and availability to appropriately assess health care populations.[17] Effective care management requires comparative data to assist in pursuing actions and policies that support improved health.[18] The AAP encourages the development of a national database of Medicaid services capable of tracking health care use using submitted claims data based on CPT and ICD-10-CM codes and payments. By providing insight into deficiencies in care and variance in care among populations, such a database would contribute health care value to patients and families who rely on Medicaid. Although extensive claims-based administrative data are currently available for Medicare beneficiaries, the difference of that population compared with pediatric patients requires the development of Medicaid-specific data sets and publication. The AAP recognizes that the CMS is currently investing in this area through its transformation of the Medicaid Statistical Information System, an evolving national database of Medicaid program use and claims data that currently includes 42 states.[19] In an era of evolving payment models, the aggregation and analysis of administrative claims-based data provides insight into strategic allocation of resources that can guide policy while allowing for state-by-state comparison.

3. **Expedite G-code transition to CPT.** The CMS expedites code development for desired services through the introduction of temporary Healthcare Common Procedure Coding System level II G codes (a CMS-managed code set representing services, products, and supplies not otherwise addressed in CPT).[20] Although G codes represent standardized codes that may be used by any payer, G codes are primarily used by Medicare to address urgent coding requirements and are not readily incorporated into other payer systems (such as Medicaid) that are central to pediatric care. Relying primarily on G-code development, which bypasses the CPT process, has a unique impact on pediatric care because payers primarily focus on CPT coding when making coverage decisions. Pediatric care advances when services represented by new codes (such as behavioral management services) are expeditiously developed through the collaboration of CMS and CPT code developers followed by appropriate RUC valuation of the new CPT code. The AAP encourages the CMS to preferentially engage with the CPT code development process when introducing new services represented by G codes so that the development of CPT codes can occur expeditiously and potentially in parallel. In addition, while awaiting an expedited transition from G-coded services to CPT, the AAP encourages broad-scope payer recognition (especially by Medicaid) of Healthcare Common Procedure Coding System level II G codes so that pediatric patients and their physicians may benefit from newly introduced medical concepts.

4. **Align regulatory correlation with CPT codes.** Because G codes do not have widespread recognition among pediatric-relevant payers, CMS publication of regulatory guidance that focuses on G codes rather than a more universally accepted CPT code may leave a void in regulatory application. For example, in publishing its "Teaching Physician Guidance" with reference to the primary care exception that accommodates supervision of residents in a clinic setting, the CMS focuses on its annual wellness-visit G codes rather than on the parallel CPT

preventive medicine codes, which are the mainstay of pediatric preventive care.[21] Although conceptually the CPT preventive medicine visits should apply equally to the primary care exception, CMS reliance solely on the G codes fosters a lack of clarity among pediatric-relevant payers, including Medicaid as well as commercial payers. The AAP encourages the CMS and other payers to recognize the importance of inclusiveness of scope when publishing G-code guidance that also has relevance to existing parallel CPT-coded services.

LEAD AUTHORS

David M. Kanter, MD, MBA, FAAP
Richard Lander, MD, FAAP
Richard A. Molteni, MD, FAAP

COMMITTEE ON CODING AND NOMENCLATURE, 2017–2018

Richard A. Molteni, MD, FAAP, Chairperson
Margie C. Andreae, MD, FAAP
Joel F. Bradley, MD, FAAP
Eileen D. Brewer, MD, FAAP
David M. Kanter, MD, FAAP
Steven E. Krug, MD, FAAP
Edward A. Liechty, MD, FAAP
Jeffrey F. Linzer Sr, MD, FACEP, FAAP
Linda D. Parsi, MD, MBA, CPEDC, FAAP
Julia M. Pillsbury, DO, FACOP, FAAP

LIAISONS

Alexander M. Hamling, MD, FAAP – *Section on Early Career Physicians*
Kathleen K. Cain, MD, FAAP – *Section on Administration and Practice Management*
Benjamin Shain, MD, PhD – *American Academy of Child and Adolescent Psychiatry*
Samuel D. Smith, MD, FAAP – *American Pediatric Surgical Association*

STAFF

Becky Dolan, MPH, CPC, CPEDC
Teri Salus, MPA, CPC
Linda J. Walsh, MAB

PRIVATE PAYER ADVOCACY ADVISORY COMMITTEE, 2017–2018

Richard Lander, MD, FAAP, Chairperson
Mary L. Brandt, MD, FACS, FAAP
Norman "Chip" Harbaugh Jr, MD, FAAP
Mark L. Hudak, MD, FAAP
Eugene R. Hershorin, MD, FAAP
Susan J. Kressly, MD, FAAP
Elizabeth M. Peterson, MD, FAAP
Gail A. Schonfeld, MD, FAAP

STAFF

Louis A. Terranova, MHA

ABBREVIATIONS

AAP: American Academy of Pediatrics
CMS: Centers for Medicare and Medicaid Services
CPT: *Current Procedural Terminology*
ICD-10-CM: *International Classification of Diseases 10th Revision Clinical Modification*
MPFS: Medicare Physician Fee Schedule
RBRVS: resource-based relative value scale
RUC: American Medical Association–Specialty Society Relative Value Scale Update Committee
RVU: relative value unit

All policy statements from the American Academy of Pediatrics automatically expire 5 years after publication unless reaffirmed, revised, or retired at or before that time.

DOI: https://doi.org/10.1542/peds.2019-2496

Address correspondence to David M. Kanter, MD, MBA, FAAP. E-mail: david_kanter@mednax.com

PEDIATRICS (ISSN Numbers: Print, 0031-4005; Online, 1098-4275).

Copyright © 2019 by the American Academy of Pediatrics

FINANCIAL DISCLOSURE: The authors have indicated they have no financial relationships relevant to this article to disclose.

FUNDING: No external funding.

POTENTIAL CONFLICT OF INTEREST: The authors have indicated they have no potential conflicts of interest to disclose.

REFERENCES

1. Gerstle RS, Molteni RA, Andreae MC, et al; Committee on Coding and Nomenclature. Application of the resource-based relative value scale system to pediatrics. *Pediatrics*. 2014; 133(6):1158–1162
2. Foster CC, Mangione-Smith R, Simon TD. Caring for children with medical complexity: perspectives of primary care providers. *J Pediatr*. 2017;182: 275–282.e4
3. Donahue SP, Nixon CN; Section on Opthamology, American Academy of Pediatrics; Committee on Practice and Ambulatory Medicine, American Academy of Pediatrics; American Academy of Ophthalmology; American Association for Pediatric Ophthalmology and Strabismus; American Association of Certified Orthoptists. Visual system assessment in infants, children, and young adults by pediatricians. *Pediatrics*. 2016;137(1): 28–30
4. Clark MB, Slayton RL; Section on Oral Health. Fluoride use in caries

prevention in the primary care setting. *Pediatrics.* 2014;134(3):626–633

5. American Academy of Pediatrics. *Five Year Strategic Plan.* Itasca, IL: American Academy of Pediatrics; 2017. Available at: https://www.aap.org/en-us/Documents/AAP_Strategic_Plan.pdf. Accessed April 10, 2018
6. US Department of Health and Human Services, Centers for Medicare and Medicaid Services. MLN matters SE 1518: information and resources for submitting correct ICD-10 codes to Medicare. 2015. Available at: https://www.cms.gov/Outreach-and-Education/Medicare-Learning-Network-MLN/MLNMattersArticles/Downloads/SE1518.pdf. Accessed April 10, 2018
7. US Department of Health and Human Services, Centers for Medicare and Medicaid Services. Risk adjustment. Available at: https://www.cms.gov/Medicare/Health-Plans/MedicareAdvtgSpecRateStats/Risk-Adjustors.html. Accessed April 10, 2018
8. Tobias C, Comeau M, Bachman S, Honberg L. *Risk Adjustment and Other Financial Protections for Children and Youth With Special Health Care Needs in Our Evolving Health Care System.* Boston, MA: Catalyst Center; 2012. Available at: http://cahpp.org/wp-content/uploads/2015/04/risk-adjustment.pdf. Accessed April 10, 2018
9. US Department of Health and Human Services, Centers for Medicare and Medicaid Services. Medicare claims processing manual chapter 26 - completing and processing form CMS-1500 data set. Available at: https://www.cms.gov/Regulations-and-Guidance/Guidance/Manuals/downloads/clm104c26.pdf. Accessed April 10, 2018
10. Committee on Child Health Financing, American Academy of Pediatrics. Medicaid policy statement. *Pediatrics.* 2013;131(5). Available at: www.pediatrics.org/cgi/content/full/131/5/e1697
11. McManus M, Flint S, Kelly R. The adequacy of physician reimbursement for pediatric care under Medicaid. *Pediatrics.* 1991;87(6):909–920
12. Polsky D, Richards M, Basseyn S, et al. Appointment availability after increases in Medicaid payments for primary care. *N Engl J Med.* 2015;372(6):537–545
13. Tang SS, Hudak ML, Cooley DM, Shenkin BN, Racine AD. Increased Medicaid payment and participation by office-based primary care pediatricians. *Pediatrics.* 2018;141(1):e20172570
14. Rosenbaum S. Medicaid payments and access to care. *N Engl J Med.* 2014;371(25):2345–2347
15. Racine AD. Child poverty and the health care system. *Acad Pediatr.* 2016;16(3 suppl):S83–S89
16. Berwick DM, Nolan TW, Whittington J. The triple aim: care, health, and cost. *Health Aff (Millwood).* 2008;27(3):759–769
17. Freedman JD, Green L, Landon BE. All-payer claims databases - uses and expanded prospects after Gobeille. *N Engl J Med.* 2016;375(23):2215–2217
18. Fisher D, Speed C. Obstacles on the road to risk. *Health Aff.* 2017;15. Available at: http://healthaffairs.org/blog/2017/02/15/obstacles-on-the-road-to-risk/
19. Medicaid.gov. Transformed Medicaid Statistical Information System (T-MSIS). Available at: https://www.medicaid.gov/medicaid/data-and-systems/macbis/tmsis/index.html. Accessed April 10, 2018
20. Centers for Medicare and Medicaid Services. *Healthcare Common Procedure Coding System (HCPCS) Level II Coding Procedures.* Washington, DC: Centers for Medicare and Medicaid Services; 2015. Available at: https://www.cms.gov/Medicare/Coding/MedHCPCSGenInfo/Downloads/2018-11-30-HCPCS-Level2-Coding-Procedure.pdf. Accessed April 10, 2018
21. Centers for Medicare and Medicaid Services. Guidelines for teaching physicians, interns, and residents. 2018. Available at: https://www.cms.gov/Outreach-and-Education/Medicare-Learning-Network-MLN/MLNProducts/Downloads/Teaching-Physicians-Fact-Sheet-ICN006437.pdf. Accessed April 10, 2018
22. Zuckerman Z, Skopec L, Epstein M. *Medicaid Physician Fees After the ACA Primary Care Fee Bump.* Washington, DC: Urban Institute; 2017. Available at: https://www.urban.org/sites/default/files/publication/88836/2001180-medicaid-physician-fees-after-the-aca-primary-care-fee-bump_0.pdf. Accessed August 29, 2019
23. Medicaid and CHIP Payment and Access Commission. June 2016 report to Congress on Medicaid and CHIP: trends in Medicaid spending. Available at: https://www.macpac.gov/publication/june-2016-report-to-congress-on-medicaid-and-chip/. Accessed August 29, 2019

Pediatric Application of Coding and Valuation Systems

- *Technical Report*

TECHNICAL REPORT

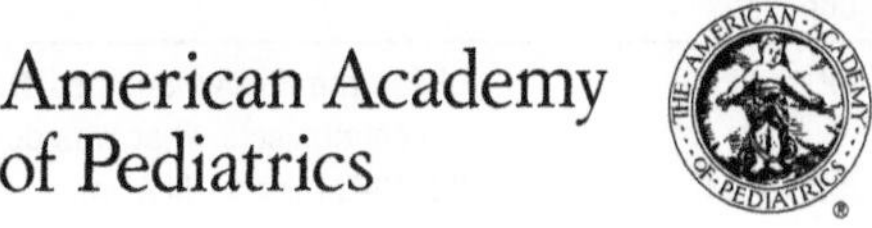

Pediatric Application of Coding and Valuation Systems

David M. Kanter, MD, MBA, FAAP,[a] Richard A. Molteni, MD, FAAP,[b] COMMITTEE ON CODING AND NOMENCLATURE

abstract

The American Academy of Pediatrics provides this technical report as supplemental background to the accompanying coding and valuation system policy statement. The rapid evolution in health care payment modeling requires that clinicians have a current appreciation of the mechanics of service representation and valuation. The accompanying policy statement provides recommendations relevant to this area, and this technical report provides a format to outline important concepts that allow for effective translation of bedside clinical events into physician payment.

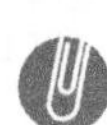

[a]Mednax Services Inc, Sunrise, Florida; and [b]Joint Commission International and Department of Pediatrics, School of Medicine, University of Washington, Seattle, Washington

This report represents a collaborative contribution from the members of the Committee on Coding and Nomenclature (COCN) (Chairperson, Dr Molteni). Through multiple meetings, COCN members established the concepts, themes, and structure of the manuscript. Incorporating guidance from COCN members, Dr Kanter (COCN) drafted the manuscript while incorporating additional recommendations from reviewers and the Board of Directors. The authors thank Linda Walsh (Senior Manager, Health Policy and Coding) for guiding the manuscript through production.

This document is copyrighted and is property of the American Academy of Pediatrics and its Board of Directors. All authors have filed conflict of interest statements with the American Academy of Pediatrics. Any conflicts have been resolved through a process approved by the Board of Directors. The American Academy of Pediatrics has neither solicited nor accepted any commercial involvement in the development of the content of this publication.

Technical reports from the American Academy of Pediatrics benefit from expertise and resources of liaisons and internal (AAP) and external reviewers. However, technical reports from the American Academy of Pediatrics may not reflect the views of the liaisons or the organizations or government agencies that they represent.

The guidance in this report does not indicate an exclusive course of treatment or serve as a standard of medical care. Variations, taking into account individual circumstances, may be appropriate.

All technical reports from the American Academy of Pediatrics automatically expire 5 years after publication unless reaffirmed, revised, or retired at or before that time.

DOI: https://doi.org/10.1542/peds.2019-2498

Address correspondence to David M. Kanter, MD, MBA, FAAP. E-mail: david_kanter@mednax.com

PEDIATRICS (ISSN Numbers: Print, 0031-4005; Online, 1098-4275).

Copyright © 2019 by the American Academy of Pediatrics

To cite: Kanter DM, Molteni RA, AAP COMMITTEE ON CODING AND NOMENCLATURE. Pediatric Application of Coding and Valuation Systems. *Pediatrics.* 2019;144(4):e20192498

STANDARDIZED CODE SETS

Under the Health Insurance Portability and Accountability Act of 1996 (HIPAA), the Secretary of the Department of Health and Human Services mandates use of standardized code sets in support of electronic health care transactions.[1] These code sets, which address diagnoses, procedures, diagnostic tests, treatments, equipment, and supplies, include *International Classification of Diseases, 10th Revision* (ICD-10); Healthcare Common Procedure Coding System (HCPCS); *Current Procedural Terminology* (CPT); National Drug Codes (NDCs); and *Current Dental Terminology* (Table 1).

The World Health Organization created the ICD-10 with adaptability for expansion and specificity for enhanced measurement, surveillance, research, and reporting across multiple domains. Clinically modified and initiated in the United States on October 1, 2015, the ICD-10 code set encompasses both the clinical modification diagnostic code set in addition to the procedure coding system used for inpatient hospital reporting of procedures. The 4 cooperating parties that oversee and manage the ICD-10 in the United States are the Centers for Medicare and Medicaid Services (CMS), the National Center for Health Statistics of the Centers for Disease Control and Prevention, the American Health Information Management Association, and the American Hospital Association.

TABLE 1 Coding Concepts

Coding or Valuation Concept	Importance
CPT	CPT is the HIPAA-mandated standardized code set by which physicians communicate what was done during the patient encounter.
ICD-10-CM	ICD-10-CM is the HIPAA-mandated standardized code set by which physicians communicate why care was rendered during the patient encounter. The reporting of an ICD code(s) linked to their respective CPT code(s) communicates a complete picture of the encounter.
HIPAA	1996 federal law designed to provide privacy standards to protect patients' medical records and other health information, including the adoption of specific code sets for diagnoses and procedures used in electronic transmission of health care data, such as in claims for payment.
CMS	A federal agency within the Department of Health and Human Services that administers the Medicare program and works in partnership with state governments to administer Medicaid and CHIP. The CMS annually publishes RVUs for its covered CPT codes in its MPFS (to which many non-Medicare payers reference with regard to payment policy and valuation).
NDC	10-digit code for reporting drug products, including vaccines (some manufacturers use an 11-digit variation).
AMA	The AMA owns and manages CPT.
CPT Editorial Panel	AMA-funded 17-member panel that develops new CPT codes as well as modifies, updates, and revises existing CPT codes as needed.
RUC	Collaboration between the AMA and CMS that allows specialty society participation in recommending values for new and revised CPT codes.
RBRVS	The Medicare mechanism by which payment for physician services are represented by assessments of resource costs (RVUs) expended to perform the service when compared with other services (relativity); based on values recommended by the RUC and forwarded to the CMS for consideration for publication in its annual MPFS.
RVUs	Measure of value for the resource costs inherent in a service relative to other services and used in calculation of the Medicare payment formula through application of a conversion factor.
NCCI edits	CMS-published Medicare and Medicaid guidance that govern reporting of combinations of CPT codes on the same date of service for the same patient. Most payers incorporate NCCI edits into their claims-processing platforms.

CHIP, Children's Health Insurance Program.

Although the *International Classification of Diseases, 10th Revision, Clinical Modification* (ICD-10-CM) remains the HIPAA-mandated code set used in communicating diagnostic selection in electronic health care transactions, additional diagnostic classification systems exist that provide physicians with greater scope and specificity in various clinical areas. For example, classification of mental health disorders is addressed through the *Diagnostic and Statistical Manual of Mental Disorders, Fifth Edition* published by the American Psychiatric Association as well as the *Diagnostic Classification of Mental and Developmental Disorders of Infancy and Early Childhood* (DC: 0–5). The DC: 0–5 classification is especially relevant to pediatrics on the basis of its expanded range and depth of mental health disorders relevant to infants and young children. (See DC: 0–5, available at https://www.zerotothree.org/our-work/dc-0-5.) Although crosswalks exist that relate DC: 0–5 to corresponding ICD-10-CM codes, the relationship between the two is not one-to-one, and DC: 0–5 is not intended to represent a claims-based diagnostic set, as is ICD-10-CM. Instead, DC: 0–5 is intended to complement ICD-10-CM through the inclusion of diagnostic directional and instructive guidance, including application of cultural variables in reaching a diagnosis, which are features not present in ICD-10-CM, a code set bound by an international framework established by the World Health Organization. Because ICD-10-CM expands each year with the inclusion of new codes, opportunities exist to pursue even greater alignment between DC: 0–5 and ICD-10-CM as ICD-10-CM continues to evolve in addressing clinical specificity.

The American Medical Association (AMA) maintains and annually publishes the CPT code set that represents procedures and services performed by physicians and qualified health care professionals. The CPT is otherwise known as level I of the HCPCS. Level II of the HCPCS represents a unique, standardized coding system used to identify products, supplies, medications, and services not otherwise represented in the CPT. HCPCS level II codes include durable medical equipment, prosthetics, orthotics, and supplies and is produced and maintained by the CMS. For example, the CMS often creates G codes as part of the level II HCPCS code set to report Medicare services not otherwise represented in the CPT. The Drug Listing Act of 1972 requires drug firms to list with the US Food and Drug Administration (FDA) drug products prepared for commercial distribution. Drug products are reported by using an NDC, a 10-digit, 3-segment number in which the first segment is assigned by the FDA and the other 2 segments are assigned by drug manufacturers. The first segment of 4 to 5 numbers identifies the labeler (such as manufacturer or distributer). The second set of 3 to 4 numbers identifies the strength and dosing form (such as capsule, liquid) and formulation of the drug by the specific manufacturer. The third 1- to 2-digit number segment identifies the package size and types (see Supplemental Information for example). Medicare, in addition to many other government and commercial payers, requires NDC code reporting when submitting claims for medications, and payers also vary in their requirement for NDC coding for vaccines. NDC codes can be found on the FDA Web site,[2] on the drug vial, or in the drug package insert.

NDC configurations may differ among manufacturers depending on when the FDA assigned the code. This lack of standardization has led to variation in the number of digits assigned to each of the 3 segments. To accommodate variation within NDC segments, an 11th digit (a leading 0) may at times be inserted into the labeler, product, or package size segment to act as a place holder to help manufacturers maintain consistency and allow better synchronization across computer systems.[3] Such variation in desired claim formatting can lead to inconsistency in reporting NDC codes to payers. In addition, payers request that administered units be appended to the NDC code on the claim form, and variation in unit measure can jeopardize claim integrity.* Proper claim formatting of NDC codes requires confirmation of approach, which may be specific to different payers.

CPT CODE DEVELOPMENT

The AMA 17-member CPT Editorial Panel (see Fig 1) meets 3 times annually to solicit input of physicians, medical device manufacturers, diagnostic test developers, and specialty society advisors in maintaining the CPT code set by adding new codes, deleting outdated codes, or modifying existing codes. The CPT Editorial Panel has created a formal code application process whereby services can be presented for consideration for publication in future CPT code sets. Through its Committee on Coding and Nomenclature, the American Academy of Pediatrics (AAP) assists its members, sections, committees, councils, and chapters in addressing clinical needs by guiding CPT code requests through the application process toward CPT Editorial Panel presentation.

When a new or modified CPT code request is approved, the CPT Editorial Panel refers the code to the American Medical Association and Specialty Society Relative Value Scale Update Committee (RUC) for valuation (see Fig 2). The multispecialty RUC represents a collaboration between the AMA and CMS and makes relative value recommendations for new, revised, and potentially misvalued codes as well as updates relative value units (RVUs) to reflect changes in medical practice.[4] Code valuation requires RUC referral to relevant specialty societies, which distribute surveys to their members to assess typical physician work expended in performing the service under consideration. Relevant specialty societies then present survey results to the RUC along with in-person specialty support for code valuation during the RUC meeting. Once code valuation is confirmed, the RUC forwards its recommendation to the CMS for consideration and publication in the Medicare Physician Fee Schedule (MPFS).

RESOURCE-BASED RELATIVE VALUE SCALE

RUC valuation of CPT services is based on resource cost allocation represented by the 3 elements of physician work, practice expense, and professional liability. RVUs are assigned to each of these elements in representing each element's contribution to resource costs relative to other types of services. Although initial physician work RVUs were based on the results of the nonsurveyed 1988 Hsiao Harvard study,[5] subsequent and current physician work RVUs are based on specialty society survey of its members with focus on the time it takes to perform the service, the

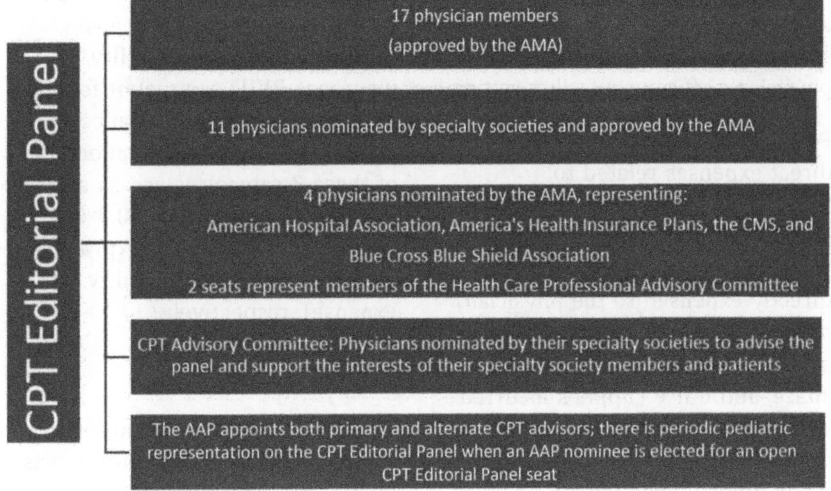

FIGURE 1
CPT Editorial Panel.

* For example, TRICARE contractors require submission of NDC codes when reporting vaccine administration, with most TRICARE contractors also requesting completion of a units field associated with the NDC number. The units field may stipulate measurement in either number of milliliters, package number for a single-dose package, or number of units for a multidose package in which 1 U equates to 1 dose within the package. If a particular contractor specifies desired units in milliliters for a 0.5-mL vaccine dose, one would specify 0.5 U on the claim rather than 1 U (see Supplemental Information and *AAP Coding Newsletter*, December 2017;13[3]).

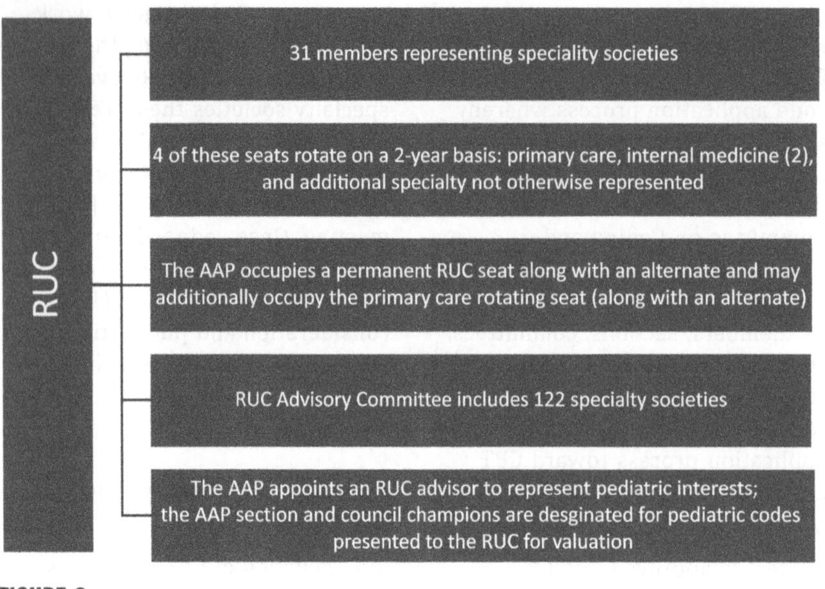

FIGURE 2
RUC.

technical skill and physical effort, the required mental effort and judgment, and stress due to the potential risk to the patient.[6] In assessing physician work RVUs, allocation of time inputs is also conceptually addressed from the perspective of intraservice time (time spent in actually performing the service) as well as pre- and postservice time (time spent preparing to perform the service and final concluding elements after performing the service). As opposed to practice expenses, physician work RVUs do not differ whether the service is performed in the physician's office or a facility setting.

Practice expense RVUs address direct expenses related to performing the service (such as clinical labor activities, medical supplies, and equipment that are directly expensed to the physician) as well as indirect expenses (such as administrative staff, building space, and office supplies incurred by the physician to manage and operate the office). Practice expense RVUs differ depending on whether the service is performed in the physician's office versus in a facility (where the costs of clinical personnel, equipment, and supplies are incurred by the facility). Because CPT codes address professional (and not facility) procedures and services, the physician incurs lower CPT practice expense RVUs for a service performed in a facility place of service as opposed to the physician's office. The RUC relies on its Practice Expense Subcommittee as well as the professional specialty societies and CMS to evaluate expense inputs for CPT services. In addition to physician work and practice expense RVUs, total service RVUs also include professional liability insurance RVUs to account for the cost of malpractice insurance premiums. Average RVU allocation of these 3 categories across all physician specialties is 50.9% (physician work), 44.8% (practice expense), and 4.3% (liability expense), respectively.[7]

THE CMS AND THE MPFS

When RVUs are designated for the target CPT service, the RUC reports its RVU recommendations to the CMS, which then has final authority to either accept, reject, or modify the RUC recommendations (with the CMS historically accepting the overwhelming majority of RUC recommendations). The CMS announces its final valuation assignments through its annually published MPFS.[8] The MPFS not only lists all CMS-accepted RVU values but also provides other useful details about the target service, including whether Medicare designates the CPT code as an active (covered) service, its procedural global package,[†] and the applicability of other types of descriptive modifiers. Although the CMS explicitly publishes its MPFS for Medicare, many other payers, including Medicaid programs and commercial plans, use information contained in the MPFS in modeling their own respective fee schedules and payment policies. Thus, specialty societies, such as the AAP, carefully focus on this CMS publication and provide comments to the CMS when necessary in support of pediatric or other specialty care. For example, in its 2018 MPFS, the CMS expressed interest in eventually modifying its evaluation and management (E/M) documentation guidelines to reduce regulatory burden and place greater emphasis on medical decision-making. In response, the AAP provided extensive comments to the CMS highlighting the uniqueness of pediatric care in documenting E/M visits and confirming the commitment of the AAP to represent pediatric interests by collaborating with the CMS through what will likely be a lengthy process of E/M modification. Along with MPFS publication of RVUs for its covered services, the CMS publishes an annual conversion factor by which the Medicare

[†] Global packages represent 0-, 10-, or 90-day postprocedural periods and specify the types of services included (bundled) in the global procedural service, such as postprocedural patient visits during the global period that are related to the procedure.

payment rate can be calculated for the respective service by using the following formula:

Medicare Payment = Annual Medicare Conversion Factor × [(Work RVU × Work Geographic Practice Cost Index (GPCI‡)) + (Practice Expense RVU × Practice Expense GPCI)]

In addition to assignment of RVUs for new services, the MPFS also addresses valuation for modified and misvalued codes. Through collaboration with the RUC, the CMS undertook sequential 5-year reviews of all code valuations from 1997 to 2012. Subsequent to that, the CMS continues to work with the RUC to reassess code valuation on the basis of request by the CMS, the public, or the RUC. For example, the RUC Relativity Assessment Workgroup selects services for valuation review on the basis of multiple factors, including newer technology impacting either work or practice expense, evolutionary shift from inpatient to outpatient site of service, high or rapid volume growth, and previously Harvard-valued with high use. Through collaboration with the CPT Editorial Panel, the CMS addresses pairings of services frequently performed together that merit bundling. In its annual MPFS, the CMS typically announces services that merit RUC revaluation (potentially misvalued codes) on the basis of any of the above factors as well as services that have experienced substantial changes in practice expense or that have experienced a substantial change in hospital length of stay or procedure time.[9]

‡ The Geographic Practice Cost Index (GPCI) is a legislatively mandated RBRVS adjustment factor that accommodates geographic variation in health care expenses. GPCIs impact work, practice expense, and malpractice expense and apply to various state- or metropolitan-based localities. The AAP provides additional detail regarding the GPCI and RBRVS calculations at https://downloads.aap.org/DOPCSP/RBRVS.pdf.

THE CMS AND THE MEDICARE ACCESS AND CHILDREN'S HEALTH INSURANCE PROGRAM REAUTHORIZATION ACT OF 2015

Through the legislative mandate of the Medicare Access and Children's Health Insurance Program Reauthorization Act (MACRA), Congress has standardized and stabilized its approach to the setting of the annual Medicare conversion factor (which establishes Medicare payment for RVU-based fee-for-service visits and procedures) while also introducing value-based elements into the fee schedule. Through MACRA legislation and subsequent Department of Health and Human Services rule writing, Medicare has instituted the following elements into the fee-for-service platform under the banner of its MACRA-legislated Quality Payment Program.[10]

- An annual 0.5% increase in the Medicare conversion factor during years 2016–2018, with a 0.25% increase in 2019;
- No annual change in the Medicare conversion factor during years 2020–2025;
- Annual conversion factor increases of either 0.25% or 0.75% beginning 2026 and thereafter (with the higher level dependent on physician threshold participation in advanced alternative payment models); and
- Clinician participation in value-based quality programs and alternative payment models that can either positively or negatively impact overall Medicare payment (with more favorable programmed increases applying to those participating in advanced alternative payment models).

The last point, referencing value-based participation, is instrumental in the CMS effort to transition Medicare from solely fee-for-service toward a payment structure in which quality and value parameters also influence payment.[11] MACRA legislation included 2 options by which Medicare physicians could pursue these value-based activities: the Merit-Based Incentive Payment System (MIPS) or the advanced alternative payment model. Under MIPS, Medicare physicians report an annual inventory of quality measures, improvement activities, promiting interoperability via electronic health record technology, and cost of care parameters, all of which can either positively or negatively impact subsequent Part B Medicare payments on the basis of a benchmarked composite score. Alternatively, Medicare physicians who participate at a given threshold volume in advanced alternative payment models (models that include not only potential upside but also downside financial risk) may bypass MIPS reporting in meeting their Quality Payment Program reporting requirements. Thus, in addition to the stabilization of the annual Medicare conversion factor, the MACRA adds a supplemental layer of Medicare Part B payment adjustment on the basis of performance in quality- and value-based clinical activities reported to the CMS via annual submission.

THE CMS AND THE NATIONAL CORRECT CODING INITIATIVE

Coding edits represent rules that address payment policy or coding guidance when reporting certain types of services together. Such edits may impact payment by either preventing the 2 services from being reported together or requiring a specific coding modifier to indicate that the 2 services sufficiently meet payer or coding guidance. Established by the CMS, the National Correct Coding Initiative (NCCI) is a widely accepted set of coding edits used by Medicare, Medicaid, and many commercial payers in addressing reporting of many combinations of code pairs. The NCCI edits are categorized by procedure-to-procedure edits (which address improper reporting of code combinations), medically unlikely edits (which address the number of units any 1 service can be reported on a given patient on the same day), and add-on edits (which require an appropriate parent code when an add-on code is also reported).[12] The CMS updates these NCCI edits quarterly, and in addition, the CMS annually publishes an NCCI Policy Manual, which provides extensive narrative background on the edits.[13] Although the CMS explicitly publishes its NCCI guidance to apply to Medicare and Medicaid claims, the widespread adoption of the NCCI by many other payers and the incorporation of NCCI edits into revenue cycle billing platforms establishes the NCCI as a de facto national coding edit policy that impacts both government and commercial claims.[14]

With Medicare accounting for 20% of national health care spending,[15] Medicare regulatory and valuation guidance significantly influences other health care systems, including Medicaid and commercial payers.[16] Not only do most Medicaid and commercial payers model their coding edits after the CMS NCCI, many payers use the Resource-Based Relative Value Scale (RBRVS)–influenced MPFS to generate their own internal fee schedules. Because of the influence that these national Medicare payment and AMA coding programs have on pediatric health care, the AAP, through its various sections, committees, councils, and chapters, engages and monitors these CMS programs in addressing the needs of pediatric physicians and their patients. Through collaboration with the CMS as well as through participation in CPT, RUC, and *International Classification of Diseases* (ICD) processes, the AAP applies its experience and knowledge of these processes by integrating the unique aspects of pediatric care into the platforms and framework that form the foundation for reporting of diagnoses, procedures, visits, and other types of patient encounters.

ROLE OF CODE SETS AND THE RBRVS IN ALTERNATIVE PAYMENT MODELS

Medicare's establishment of the Quality Payment Program under MACRA legislation represents a watershed achievement in the evolution from sole reliance on fee-for-service toward value-based alternative payment models. Alternative payment models are designed to reduce the rate of growth in health care expenditures by reducing wasteful care and encouraging efficiencies in the care of populations and episodes.[17] Although standardized code sets such as CPT and ICD have been the historical foundation for fee-for-service payment structure, such code sets will continue to play an instrumental role in the design of alternative payment models. ICD-10 especially was created to provide enhanced clinical detail, which is essential to accurately defining the populations and appropriately assigning clinical risk inherent in structuring payment bundles. Various models of hierarchical condition categories (HCCs) demonstrate the role that accurate diagnosis assignment plays in allocating risk-based payment, and diagnostic specificity has been an important long-standing feature of facility-based bundled payment diagnostic-related group models. Although the HCC models published as CMS-HCC (for Medicare Advantage) and as Health and Human Services–HCC (for non-Medicare use) provide structural detail, including stratification of infant and child, health care organizations may modify HCC models in proprietary ways that are not transparently disclosed to providers. Childhood-relevant, resource-intensive conditions often represent complex associations of chronic abnormalities (especially behavioral) exacerbated by unfavorable social health determinants, all of which may be underrepresented in proprietary risk adjustment models.[18] Many of the quality measures that represent a required reporting feature of alternative payment models include ICD-based identification of patient eligibility. The AAP monitors and participates in pediatric-relevant quality metrics through its membership with the National Quality Forum, the endorsing organization for many pediatric quality measures, including numerous Healthcare Effectiveness Data and Information Set measures.[19] Similar to the value that clinical diagnostic specificity plays in defining populations, CPT will continue to play a role in specifying the various services allocated to particular populations and episodes. Many alternative payment models represent core fee-for-service, CPT-based payment processes layered on financial risk-based performance benchmarks, which then impact subsequent, downstream payment. CPT assignment to rendering clinicians allows for identification of the physician's role in care within the model as needed for assessment of clinical contribution and patient attribution. Through leveraging of CPT valuation, understanding the relative value of services as illuminated by the RBRVS allows for strategic contracting in developing the administrative and clinical contractual framework within alternative payment models. The RBRVS and its RVU-based elements remain an effective means to track the reduction in volume and the achievement of efficiencies, which represent the goals of alternative payment models.

ADDITIONAL RESOURCES

- AMA CPT: https://www.ama-assn.org/practice-management/cpt-current-procedural-terminology;
- CMS ICD-10: https://www.cms.gov/medicare/coding/icd10/index.html;
- CMS MPFS Look-Up Tool: https://www.cms.gov/Medicare/Medicare-Fee-for-Service-Payment/PFSlookup/;
- CMS Medicare Claims Processing Manual chapter 12 (Physicians/Nonphysician Practitioners): https://www.cms.gov/Regulations-and-Guidance/Guidance/Manuals/Downloads/clm104c12.pdf;
- CMS NCCI edits: https://www.cms.gov/Medicare/Coding/NationalCorrectCodInitEd/index.html?redirect=/NationalCorrectCodinitEd/;
- CMS Quality Payment Program: https://qpp.cms.gov/;
- AAP RBRVS: What Is It and How Does It Affect Pediatrics?: https://downloads.aap.org/DOPCSP/RBRVS.pdf;
- Coding at the AAP: https://www.aap.org/en-us/professional-resources/practice-transformation/getting-paid/Coding-at-the-AAP/Pages/default.aspx;
- AAP coding hotline: https://www.aap.org/en-us/Pages/cu/Coding-Hotline-Request.aspx; and
- AMA RUC survey training video: https://www.youtube.com/watch?v=nu5unDX8VIs.

LEAD AUTHORS

David M. Kanter, MD, FAAP
Richard A. Molteni, MD, FAAP

COMMITTEE ON CODING AND NOMENCLATURE, 2017–2018

Richard A. Molteni, MD, FAAP, Chairperson
Margie C. Andreae, MD, FAAP
Joel F. Bradley, MD, FAAP
Eileen D. Brewer, MD, FAAP
David M. Kanter, MD, FAAP
Steven E. Krug, MD, FAAP
Edward A. Liechty, MD, FAAP
Jeffrey F. Linzer Sr, MD, FACEP, FAAP
Linda D. Parsi, MD, MBA, CPEDC, FAAP
Julia M. Pillsbury, DO, FACOP, FAAP

LIAISONS

Alexander M. Hamling, MD, FAAP – *Section on Early Career Physicians*
Kathleen K. Cain, MD, FAAP – *Section on Administration and Practice Management*
Benjamin Shain, MD, PhD – *American Academy of Child and Adolescent Psychiatry*
Samuel D. Smith, MD, FAAP – *American Pediatric Surgical Association*

STAFF

Becky Dolan, MPH, CPC, CPEDC
Teri Salus, MPA, CPC
Linda J. Walsh, MAB

ABBREVIATIONS

AAP: American Academy of Pediatrics
AMA: American Medical Association
CMS: Centers for Medicare and Medicaid Services
CPT: *Current Procedural Terminology*
DC: 0–5: *Diagnostic Classification of Mental and Developmental Disorders of Infancy and Early Childhood*
E/M: evaluation and management
FDA: US Food and Drug Administration
GPCI: Geographic Practice Cost Index
HCC: hierarchical condition category
HCPCS: Healthcare Common Procedure Coding System
HIPAA: Health Insurance Portability and Accountability Act of 1996
ICD: International Classification of Diseases
ICD-10: *International Classification of Diseases, 10th Revision*
ICD-10-CM: *International Classification of Diseases, 10th Revision, Clinical Modification*
MACRA: Medicare Access and Children's Health Insurance Program Reauthorization Act
MIPS: Merit-Based Incentive Payment System
MPFS: Medicare Physician Fee Schedule
NCCI: National Correct Coding Initiative
NDC: National Drug Code
RBRVS: Resource-Based Relative Value Scale
RUC: American Medical Association and Specialty Society Relative Value Scale Update Committee
RVU: relative value unit

FINANCIAL DISCLOSURE: The authors have indicated they have no financial relationships relevant to this article to disclose.

FUNDING: No external funding.

POTENTIAL CONFLICT OF INTEREST: The authors have indicated they have no potential conflicts of interest to disclose.

REFERENCES

1. Centers for Medicare and Medicaid Services. Code sets overview. Available at: https://www.cms.gov/Regulations-and-Guidance/Administrative-Simplification/Code-Sets/index.html. Accessed April 10, 2018
2. US Food and Drug Administration. National drug code directory. Available at: https://www.fda.gov/drugs/informationondrugs/ucm142438.htm. Accessed April 10, 2018
3. Optum Coding Systems. Understanding NDC and HCPCS. 2017. Available at: http://helioscomp.com/docs/default-source/White-Paper/understanding-ndc-and-hcpcs-codes.pdf. Accessed April 10, 2018
4. American Medical Association. RBRVS overview. Available at: https://www.ama-assn.org/practice-management/rbrvs-resource-based-relative-value-scale. Accessed April 10, 2018
5. Hsiao WC, Braun P, Yntema D, Becker ER. Estimating physicians' work for a resource-based relative-value scale. *N Engl J Med*. 1988;319(13):835–841
6. American Medical Association. RVS update committee (RUC). Available at: https://www.ama-assn.org/about/rvs-update-committee-ruc. Accessed April 10, 2018
7. American Medical Association. 2018 RVS update process. Available at: https://www.ama-assn.org/sites/ama-assn.org/files/corp/media-browser/public/rbrvs/ruc-update-booklet_0.pdf. Accessed April 10, 2018
8. Centers for Medicare and Medicaid Services. Physician fee schedule. Available at: https://www.cms.gov/Medicare/Medicare-Fee-for-Service-Payment/PhysicianFeeSched/. Accessed April 10, 2018
9. Centers for Medicare & Medicaid Services (CMS), HHS. Medicare program; revisions to payment policies under the physician fee schedule and other revisions to Part B for CY 2018; Medicare Shared Savings Program requirements; and Medicare Diabetes Prevention Program. Final rule. *Fed Regist*. 2017;82(219):52976–53371
10. Centers for Medicare and Medicaid Services. Quality payment program. Available at: https://qpp.cms.gov/. Accessed April 10, 2018
11. Burwell SM. Setting value-based payment goals–HHS efforts to improve U.S. health care. *N Engl J Med*. 2015; 372(10):897–899
12. Centers for Medicare and Medicaid Services. National correct coding initiative edits. Available at: https://www.cms.gov/Medicare/Coding/NationalCorrectCodInitEd/index.html. Accessed August 29, 2019
13. Centers for Medicare and Medicaid Services. NCCI policy manual archive. Available at: https://www.cms.gov/Medicare/Coding/NationalCorrectCodInitEd/NCCI-Manual-Archive.html. Accessed August 29, 2019
14. American Medical Association. *Standardization of a Code-Editing System White Paper*. Chicago, IL: American Medical Association; 2011. Available at: https://www.ncvhs.hhs.gov/wp-content/uploads/2014/05/111118p36.pdf. Accessed April 10, 2018
15. Centers for Medicare and Medicaid Services. National health expenditures 2017 Highlights. Available at: https://www.cms.gov/Research-Statistics-Data-and-Systems/Statistics-Trends-and-Reports/NationalHealthExpendData/Downloads/highlights.pdf. Accessed April 10, 2018
16. Feldman R, Dowd B, Coulam R. Medicare's role in determining prices throughout the health care system. Mercatus Working Paper. 2015. Available at: https://www.mercatus.org/system/files/Feldman-Medicare-Role-Prices-oct.pdf. Accessed April 10, 2018
17. Dafny L, Chernew M. Who will succeed with new payment models? Part I. *NEJM Catalyst*. 2017. Available at: http://catalyst.nejm.org/who-will-succeed-with-new-payment-models-part-1/. Accessed April 10, 2018
18. American Medical Association House of Delegates. Resolution 102: Effectiveness of risk assessment models in representing healthcare resources expended for infants and children, as submitted by the American Academy of Pediatrics. November 2018. Available at: https://www.ama-assn.org/system/files/2018-11/a18-resolutions.pdf. Accessed August 29, 2019
19. American Academy of Pediatrics, Division of Quality. AAP keeps children at forefront of dialogue on quality measures. *AAP News*. 2017. Available at: www.aappublications.org/news/2017/01/30/NQF013017. Accessed April 10, 2018

Pediatric Metabolic and Bariatric Surgery: Evidence, Barriers, and Best Practices

- *Policy Statement*

POLICY STATEMENT Organizational Principles to Guide and Define the Child Health Care System and/or Improve the Health of all Children

American Academy of Pediatrics

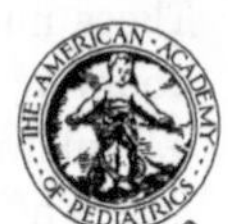

DEDICATED TO THE HEALTH OF ALL CHILDREN™

Pediatric Metabolic and Bariatric Surgery: Evidence, Barriers, and Best Practices

Sarah C. Armstrong, MD, FAAP,[a] Christopher F. Bolling, MD, FAAP,[b] Marc P. Michalsky, MD, FACS, FAAP, FASMBS,[c] Kirk W. Reichard, MD, MBA, FAAP, FACS,[d] SECTION ON OBESITY, SECTION ON SURGERY

abstract

Severe obesity among youth is an "epidemic within an epidemic" and portends a shortened life expectancy for today's children compared with those of their parents' generation. Severe obesity has outpaced less severe forms of childhood obesity in prevalence, and it disproportionately affects adolescents. Emerging evidence has linked severe obesity to the development and progression of multiple comorbid states, including increased cardiometabolic risk resulting in end-organ damage in adulthood. Lifestyle modification treatment has achieved moderate short-term success among young children and those with less severe forms of obesity, but no studies to date demonstrate significant and durable weight loss among youth with severe obesity. Metabolic and bariatric surgery has emerged as an important treatment for adults with severe obesity and, more recently, has been shown to be a safe and effective strategy for groups of youth with severe obesity. However, current data suggest that youth with severe obesity may not have adequate access to metabolic and bariatric surgery, especially among underserved populations. This report outlines the current evidence regarding adolescent bariatric surgery, provides recommendations for practitioners and policy makers, and serves as a companion to an accompanying technical report, "Metabolic and Bariatric Surgery for Pediatric Patients With Severe Obesity," which provides details and supporting evidence.

Departments of [a]Pediatrics and Population Health Sciences, Duke Center for Childhood Obesity Research, and Duke Clinical Research Institute, Duke University, Durham, North Carolina; [b]Department of Pediatrics, College of Medicine, University of Cincinnati and Cincinnati Children's Hospital Medical Center, Cincinnati, Ohio; [c]Department of Pediatric Surgery, College of Medicine, The Ohio State University and Nationwide Children's Hospital, Columbus, Ohio; and [d]Division of Pediatric Surgery, Nemours/Alfred I. duPont Hospital for Children, Wilmington, Delaware

Policy statements from the American Academy of Pediatrics benefit from expertise and resources of liaisons and internal (AAP) and external reviewers. However, policy statements from the American Academy of Pediatrics may not reflect the views of the liaisons or the organizations or government agencies that they represent.

Dr Armstrong was responsible for the initial drafting of the manuscript, conceptualized and contributed to the content of the initial manuscript, and contributed to the clinical perspective of the recommendations; Dr Bolling contributed to the clinical perspective of the recommendations and conceptualized and contributed to the content of the initial manuscript; Drs Michalsky and Reichard conceptualized and contributed to the content of the initial manuscript and contributed to the surgical perspective and the enrollment criteria table; and all authors contributed to revisions and critical edits of the entire manuscript, approved the final manuscript as submitted, and agree to be accountable for all aspects of the work.

The guidance in this statement does not indicate an exclusive course of treatment or serve as a standard of medical care. Variations, taking into account individual circumstances, may be appropriate.

All policy statements from the American Academy of Pediatrics automatically expire 5 years after publication unless reaffirmed, revised, or retired at or before that time.

To cite: Armstrong SC, Bolling CF, Michalsky MP, et al. AAP SECTION ON OBESITY, SECTION ON SURGERY. Pediatric Metabolic and Bariatric Surgery: Evidence, Barriers, and Best Practices. *Pediatrics.* 2019;144(6):e20193223

This policy statement uses the term "pediatric" in reference to a person under 18 years of age. The term "adolescent" may be defined differently in various studies and clinical settings on the basis of age or developmental stage. When making specific recommendations, this policy statement uses "adolescent" to refer to a person from age 13 years to age 18 years. "Severe" obesity (class 2 obesity or higher) is defined as having a BMI ≥35 or ≥120% of the 95th percentile for age and sex.[1] Recent data from the NHANES (2014–2016) report the prevalence of severe obesity in youth at

7.9% overall, 9.7% in 12- to 15-year-olds, and 14% in 16- to 19-year-olds. These numbers represent a near doubling since 1999 and equate to 4.5 million children in the United States affected by severe obesity.[2] These children are at high risk for developing chronic and progressive diseases, including hypertension, dyslipidemia, obstructive sleep apnea, polycystic ovarian syndrome, type 2 diabetes mellitus, fatty liver disease, bone and joint dysfunction, depression, social isolation, and poor quality of life.[3–7]

Roux-en-Y gastric bypass (RYGB) is often referred to as the gold standard for surgical management of severe obesity in adults[8,9] and adolescents[7] and is performed by using minimally invasive, laparoscopic surgical techniques. RYGB results in significant weight loss as a result of its effects on appetite, satiety, and regulation of energy balance.[9]

Vertical sleeve gastrectomy (VSG) leads to weight loss through similar effects on appetite, satiety, and regulation of energy balance and may reduce appetite through delayed gastric emptying and altered neurohormonal feedback mechanisms.[10] VSG is the most common bariatric procedure performed in adults and is becoming more common among adolescents.[11,12]

Laparoscopic adjustable gastric band (LAGB), a reversible procedure that accounted for approximately one-third of all bariatric operations in the United States a decade ago,[12] has experienced a significant decline in use among adults because of limited long-term effectiveness and higher-than-expected complication rates.[13,14] Disappointing outcomes in the context of few prospective studies in the pediatric population have resulted in a similar decline in use of LAGB among adolescents.[11] At present, LAGB is limited by the US Food and Drug Administration to people 18 years or older.

EVIDENCE

Data Quality

Evidence regarding the safety and efficacy of metabolic and bariatric surgery is outlined in detail in the accompanying technical report.[15] Data are derived from observational cohort studies, case-control series, retrospective case reports, and expert opinion. The relatively low prevalence of bariatric surgery in adolescents and the practical and ethical barriers to randomization are known limitations.

Data Sources

The Teen-Longitudinal Assessment of Bariatric Surgery (Teen-LABS) study is the largest ongoing observational cohort study of youth undergoing metabolic and bariatric surgery to date. There were 242 patients (12–28 years of age) enrolled at 5 US centers (2007–2011) undergoing RYGB (n = 161), VSG (n = 67), or LAGB (n = 14).[16] Participants had a mean age of 17 years, were mostly female (75%) and white (72%), and had a mean preoperative BMI of 53 and 4 major comorbid conditions. Although the study is still ongoing, recent publications have reported outcomes at 3 years, consisting of 99% (n = 225) of participants who have undergone RYGB or VSG.[16,17] Other data sources include the Follow-up of Adolescent Bariatric Surgery at 5 Plus Years[18] (FABS-5+) study (2001–2007), the Adolescent Morbid Obesity Surgery Study[19,20] (AMOS) (2006–2009), and the Bariatric Outcomes Longitudinal Database[21] (2004–2010). Several smaller cohort studies provide additional data.[22–24] The companion technical report further details the strengths and limitations of these studies.

Outcomes on Weight Loss and Comorbidity Resolution

Until recently, weight-loss studies have reported weight loss in different ways, making comparison between interventions challenging. In the Teen-LABS cohort, RYGB and VSG groups experienced a mean weight reduction of 27% and resolution of comorbidities at 3 years, including type 2 diabetes mellitus (95%), hypertension (74%), and dyslipidemia (66%), with an accompanying reduction overall in the prevalence of multiple concurrent cardiovascular disease risk factors (ie, 3 or more).[17] Surgical treatment is more effective than medical therapy among adolescents with severe obesity for treatment of type 2 diabetes mellitus,[25] and weight-related quality of life has also been shown to improve significantly.[16] The FABS-5+ study represents the longest-term follow-up data in adolescents to date (5–12 years; mean of 8 years) with 78% subject retention (n = 58 of 74). After RYGB, adolescents demonstrated a 29% reduction in BMI and significant improvements in elevated blood pressure, dyslipidemia, and type 2 diabetes mellitus at 8 years.[18] Results from the AMOS cohort of adolescents undergoing RYGB demonstrated a mean weight loss of 36.8 kg at 5 years. By contrast, adolescents enrolled in lifestyle modification demonstrated a mean increase in BMI of 3.3.[19,20] A 2017 meta-analysis of 24 studies reviewed outcomes for 1928 adolescent patients who received LAGB, VSG, and RYGB. In this analysis, the mean absolute BMI decrease at 6 months was 5.4% in patients who underwent LAGB, 11.5% in patients who underwent VSG, and 18% in patients who underwent RYGB. At 36 months, significant weight loss was maintained with a mean BMI reduction of 10.3% in patients who underwent LAGB, 13% in patients who underwent VSG, and 15% in patients who underwent RYGB.[26,27] More recently, an analysis of electronic health record data compared the effectiveness of bariatric procedures among pediatric patients and demonstrated a similar BMI reduction among patients who received VSG or RYGB, and a lower BMI reduction in patients who received LAGB.[28]

Complications

Surgical complications are infrequent, with the majority being defined as minor (15%) and occurring in the early postoperative period (eg, postoperative nausea and dehydration).[11,16,27] Major perioperative complications (30 days) were reported in 8% of Teen-LABS participants. In addition, 2.7% required reoperation before hospital discharge, which was similar to adults.[29] Micronutrient deficiencies are common after both RYGB (iron 66%, vitamin B_{12} 8%, and folate 6%) and VSG (iron 32% and folate 10%).[16] Vitamin D deficiency is common preoperatively among teenagers with obesity and does not change significantly after surgery.[16] Folate deficiency is a concern for females of childbearing age.[16] Long-term implications of nutrient deficiency are unknown because most longitudinal studies of pediatric metabolic and bariatric surgery do not manage patients through subsequent pregnancy to assess for related complications.[27] Among adolescents who are more severely affected by anxiety or depression at baseline, limited data suggest that they may have a higher risk for postoperative anxiety and depression.[30] Although no perioperative deaths were reported in the Teen-LABS, AMOS, or FABS-5+ cohorts, 3 deaths (0.3%) occurred—at 9 months (related to infectious colitis),[18] 3.3 years (related to hypoglycemic complications in an individual with type 1 diabetes),[16] and 6 years (unrelated), respectively, collectively representing a recently reported 0.3% mortality rate.[27]

Indications

Published adult indications for bariatric surgery,[31] longitudinal data in adolescents, and the American Society for Metabolic and Bariatric Surgery best practice recommendations[32] all contribute to 16 existing sets of recommendations for bariatric surgery in pediatric patients.[33] Key considerations include BMI, comorbid health conditions, and quality of life. As metabolic and bariatric surgery have become more widespread, outcomes have supported indications for bariatric surgery that more closely mirror adult recommendations.[24,33] Best practice guidelines (Table 1), as developed in 2018 by the American Society for Metabolic and Bariatric Surgery, recommend that bariatric surgery be considered for youth with BMI ≥35 with concurrent severe comorbid disease or for those with BMI ≥40 kg/m^2 (where comorbid disease is commonly encountered but not mandatory).[32,34] Generally accepted contraindications include a medically correctable cause of obesity, untreated or poorly controlled substance abuse, concurrent or planned pregnancy, current eating disorder, or inability to adhere to postoperative recommendations and mandatory lifestyle changes. Gaps in recommendations include a thorough discussion of patient and/or family goals and expectations; procedural preferences; detailed recommendations for perioperative care, particularly in females of childbearing age; and defined expectations and optimal timing for transition of long-term care to adult medical and/or surgical obesity care providers.[33] The presence of a disability is a relevant factor but is not an automatic contraindication, and each case warrants additional consideration.[35]

Eligibility

Determination of eligibility for bariatric surgery involves a thoughtful, shared decision-making process between the patient, parent(s) or guardian(s), and medical and surgical providers. In addition to BMI and comorbidity status, criteria include physiologic, psychological, and developmental maturity; the ability to understand risks and benefits and adhere to lifestyle modifications; decision-making capacity; and robust family and social supports leading up to and after surgery. Current longitudinal studies evaluating safety and efficacy endpoints do not apply specific age limits for the timing of surgery; thus, there is no evidence to support the application of age-based eligibility limits.[11,20]

BARRIERS

Access

Although nearly 4.5 million US adolescents have severe obesity, current estimates suggest that only a small faction undergo metabolic and bariatric surgery.[12,17,18,20,36,37] Recent estimates show a tripling of procedural prevalence in the early 2000s (0.8–2.3 per 100 000 between 2000 and 2003) with current estimates of between 1000 and 1600 cases each year.[1,38,39] Although limitations to access are

TABLE 1 Indications and Contraindications for Adolescent Metabolic and Bariatric Surgery

Wt Criteria	Comorbid Conditions
Class 2 obesity, BMI ≥35, or 120% of the 95th percentile for age and sex, whichever is lower	Clinically significant disease, including obstructive sleep apnea (AHI >5), T2DM, IIH, NASH, Blount disease, SCFE, GERD, and hypertension
Class 3 obesity, BMI ≥40, or 140% of the 95th percentile for age and sex, whichever is lower	Not required but commonly present

AHI, Apnea-Hypopnea Index; GERD, gastroesophageal reflux disease; IIH, idiopathic intracranial hypertension; NASH, nonalcoholic steatohepatitis; SCFE, slipped capital femoral epiphysis; T2DM, type 2 diabetes mellitus.

multifactorial, race and socioeconomic status have emerged as striking disparities in insurance authorization for metabolic and bariatric surgery.[40] A recent review from the Teen-LABS research consortium reports that less than half (47%) of qualifying surgical candidates received insurance coverage after an initial request for authorization. Age under 18 years was cited as the most common reason for coverage denial. In contrast, 85% of adults who met surgical criteria obtained initial insurance coverage authorization. Eleven percent of adolescents never obtained authorization despite multiple appeals.[40] Children and adolescents from racial minority groups are more likely to experience severe obesity[1,41] and related comorbid health conditions.[5] Recent data show that outcomes after adolescent bariatric surgery do not differ by race or ethnicity[21]; however, adolescents of minority groups are less likely to undergo a bariatric surgery.[42] This disparity appears most related to socioeconomic status as opposed to racial or ethnic status.[43–46] This disparity may be explained in part by inconsistent eligibility criteria for related coverage among various government-sponsored insurance programs even in the instance of medical necessity. Medical necessity is defined as "health care interventions that are evidence-based, evidence-informed, or based on consensus advisory opinion...to promote optimal growth and development in a child and to... diagnose, treat, ameliorate or palliate the effects of physical conditions."[47]

Provider Concerns

National survey data suggest that providers are reluctant to refer pediatric patients with obesity for bariatric surgery. Concerns include a lack of knowledge about the biology of obesity, surgical procedures, risks, and follow-up; a lack of awareness of surgery as an option[48]; concern for altered growth or development; and provider weight bias manifested as a belief that weight is a personal responsibility rather than a medical problem.[49,50] Existing evidence suggests that bariatric surgery does not lead to growth impairment, and among older adolescents, several studies have demonstrated that linear growth continues after surgery.[18,20,21] Recent data from a single site outside the United States routinely performing RYGB and VSG for patients with a mean age of 11.5 years have shown no adverse impact on linear growth when compared with age-matched peers receiving medical management for obesity,[51,52] although more evidence is needed to confirm this finding.

Lifestyle Counseling

Many providers prefer a "watchful waiting" approach, or long-term lifestyle management.[50] However, current evidence suggests that pediatric patients with severe obesity are unlikely to achieve a clinically significant and sustained weight reduction in lifestyle-based weight management programs[53] and that watchful waiting may lead to higher BMI and more comorbid conditions.[54–58] This concern is illustrated in a recent comparison of adolescents initially participating in a comprehensive lifestyle program before surgery (ie, delayed surgical treatment group) that showed higher starting BMI at the time of surgery when compared with adolescents who did not participate in the lifestyle program (ie, nondelayed surgical treatment group).[20] In addition, comparative data examining postoperative outcomes along the severely obese BMI spectrum (low, middle, and high) suggest that adolescents within a lower BMI range (BMI <55) at the time of bariatric surgery have a higher probability of achieving nonobese status when compared with individuals with a higher starting BMI (BMI ≥ 55).[59]

Cost-effectiveness

Bariatric surgery is more costly in the short-term than other treatment options, although this varies by the number and type of comorbidities.[60] However, long-term bariatric surgery cost-effectiveness data related to the pediatric population are limited but include several studies that suggest that surgery may become cost-effective around 5 years postoperation.[60–62] Despite economic assertions related to the use of bariatric surgery in the pediatric population, ongoing efforts to prevent obesity at the population level, including robust public health strategies, should continue to be improved and widely disseminated.[61]

BEST PRACTICES

Multidisciplinary Care

The evidence for safe and efficacious metabolic and bariatric surgery in pediatric patients is based on comprehensive care in multidisciplinary clinics involving pediatric experts on obesity, adolescent medicine, mental health, nutrition, and exercise science in addition to surgeons. The multidisciplinary care model maximizes pediatric and adolescent-specific health care resources designed to deliver optimal care.[60] These comprehensive programs follow a set of principles or best practices for pediatric metabolic and bariatric surgery. The American Society for Metabolic and Bariatric Surgery,[61] the American Heart Association,[7] and several other medical society- and institution-issued guidelines support the multidisciplinary model.[61] Although national accreditation for adolescent metabolic and bariatric surgery is recent (2014), the Metabolic and Bariatric Surgery Association Quality Improvement Program provides a resource for primary care providers to locate high-quality comprehensive adult bariatric programs with additional accreditation and pediatric-specific programs.

Adolescent-Oriented Care

Although, as described, no data exist to define an age limitation for weight-loss surgery in youth, the majority of those who undergo surgery are adolescents. The unique developmental, physiologic, and emotional needs of adolescents with respect to selection of appropriate patients for surgery, the optimal timing of surgery, and long-term follow-up are distinct from those same needs in adults. In particular, adolescent girls are more likely than adolescent boys to undergo bariatric surgery.[16,20,21,27] Some studies have noted increased pregnancy rates in adolescents after metabolic and bariatric surgery[62] and a higher risk of small-for-gestational-age births among mothers who have previously had metabolic and bariatric surgery.[63] As with other aspects of adolescent health, the provider should appropriately engage the adolescent in the decision-making process out of respect for his or her developing autonomy and ensure that the teenager has appropriate expectations for surgical outcomes. Consultation with an ethics professional may be warranted in challenging situations.

Values and Preferences

Eligibility for metabolic and bariatric surgery should be determined through a thoughtful process that considers the values of the patient and family and preference for the type of bariatric surgical procedure. These decisions may only occur after a thorough review of the effect of obesity on the adolescent's physical and emotional health and an understanding of the risks, benefits, and long-term implications of each procedure type. The relationship among the physician, patient, family, and surgical team is paramount to success. Preparing an adolescent patient for metabolic and bariatric surgery begins with a realistic discussion of these values and preferences, available treatment options, likely anticipated outcomes for weight loss, improvement in comorbid conditions, and a realistic understanding about the lifetime need for healthy lifestyle changes. Effective communication strategies, such as the teach-back method, should be used to ensure clear understanding of risks and benefits. It is important to establish the expectation for long-term psychological follow-up with patients and families early in the process.

PRACTICE-LEVEL RECOMMENDATIONS

The AAP recommends that pediatricians do the following.

1. Recognize that severe obesity (BMI ≥35 or ≥120% of the 95th percentile for age and sex, whichever is lower) places the adolescent at higher risk for liver disease, type 2 diabetes mellitus, dyslipidemias, sleep apnea, orthopedic complications, and mental health conditions even when compared with milder degrees of obesity.
2. Seek high-quality multidisciplinary centers that are experienced in assessing risks and benefits of various treatments for youth with severe obesity, including bariatric surgery, and provide referrals to where such programs are available.
3. Understand the efficacy, risks, benefits, and long-term health implications of the common metabolic and bariatric surgery procedures so that pediatricians can effectively help in family medical decision-making concerning surgical options to manage severe obesity.
4. Identify pediatric patients with severe obesity who meet criteria for surgery (Table 1), and provide timely referrals to comprehensive, multidisciplinary, pediatric-focused metabolic and bariatric surgery programs.
5. Coordinate pre- and postoperative care with the patient, family, and multidisciplinary, anesthesia, and surgical teams.
6. Monitor patients postoperatively for micronutrient deficiencies and consider providing iron, folate, and vitamin B_{12} supplementation as needed.
7. Monitor patients postoperatively for risk-taking behavior and mental health problems.

SYSTEM-LEVEL RECOMMENDATIONS

The AAP recommends that pediatricians do the following.

1. Advocate for increased access for pediatric patients of all racial, ethnic, and socioeconomic backgrounds to multidisciplinary programs that provide high-quality pediatric metabolic and bariatric surgery.

The AAP recommends that government, health, and academic medical centers do the following.

1. Use best practice guidelines outlined in this policy statement to support safe and effective multidisciplinary, pediatric-focused metabolic and bariatric surgery programs. This guidance is considered best practice because it is based on consensus expert opinion after reviewing numerous practices in various settings.
2. Consider best practice guidelines, including avoidance of unsubstantiated lower age limits, in the context of potential health care benefits and individualized patient-centered care.
3. Increase the number of and access to multidisciplinary, pediatric-focused metabolic and bariatric surgery centers, ensuring equal access to adolescents who meet criteria regardless of income, race, or ethnicity.

The AAP recommends that public and private insurers do the following.

1. Provide payment for multidisciplinary preoperative care to ensure appropriate selection of surgical candidates and for multidisciplinary postoperative care and required medications and supplements to improve surgical outcomes.
2. Provide payment for bariatric surgery from evaluation through follow-up and ongoing care for pediatric patients who meet standard criteria as set forth here.
3. Reduce barriers to pediatric metabolic and bariatric surgery (including inadequate payment, limited access, unsubstantiated exclusion criteria, and bureaucratic delays in approval requiring unnecessary and often numerous appeals) for patients who meet careful selection criteria.

CONTRAINDICATIONS

The following are contraindications:

- a medically correctable cause of obesity;
- an ongoing substance abuse problem (within the preceding 1 year);
- a medical, psychiatric, psychosocial, or cognitive condition that prevents adherence to postoperative dietary and medication regimens; and
- current or planned pregnancy within 12 to 18 months of the procedure.

LEAD AUTHORS

Sarah C. Armstrong, MD, FAAP
Christopher F. Bolling, MD, FAAP
Marc P. Michalsky, MD, FACS, FAAP, FASMBS
Kirk W. Reichard, MD, MBA, FAAP

SECTION ON OBESITY EXECUTIVE COMMITTEE, 2017–2018

Christopher F. Bolling, MD, FAAP, Chairperson
Sarah C. Armstrong, MD, FAAP
Matthew Allen Haemer, MD, MPH, FAAP
Natalie Digate Muth, MD, MPH, RD, FAAP
John Conrad Rausch, MD, MPH, FAAP
Victoria Weeks Rogers, MD, FAAP

LIAISON

Marc Michalsky, MD, FACS, FAAP

CONSULTANT

Stephanie Walsh, MD, FAAP

STAFF

Mala Thapar, MPH

SECTION ON SURGERY EXECUTIVE COMMITTEE, 2017–2018

Kurt F. Heiss, MD, FAAP, Chairperson
Gail Ellen Besner, MD, FAAP
Cynthia D. Downard, MD, FAAP
Mary Elizabeth Fallat, MD, FAAP
Kenneth William Gow, MD FACS, FAAP

STAFF

Vivian Baldassari Thorne

ABBREVIATIONS

AMOS: Adolescent Morbid Obesity Surgery Study
FABS-5+: Follow-up of Adolescent Bariatric Surgery at 5 Plus Years
LAGB: laparoscopic adjustable gastricband
RYGB: Roux-en-Y gastric bypass
Teen-LABS: Teen-Longitudinal Assessment of Bariatric Surgery
VSG: vertical sleeve gastrectomy

This document is copyrighted and is property of the American Academy of Pediatrics and its Board of Directors. All authors have filed conflict of interest statements with the American Academy of Pediatrics. Any conflicts have been resolved through a process approved by the Board of Directors. The American Academy of Pediatrics has neither solicited nor accepted any commercial involvement in the development of the content of this publication.

DOI: https://doi.org/10.1542/peds.2019-3223

Address correspondence to Sarah C. Armstrong, MD, FAAP. E-mail: sarah.c.armstrong@duke.edu

PEDIATRICS (ISSN Numbers: Print, 0031-4005; Online, 1098-4275).

Copyright © 2019 by the American Academy of Pediatrics

FINANCIAL DISCLOSURE: Dr Armstrong disclosed that she has a research relationship with AstraZeneca; Drs Bolling, Michalsky, and Reichard have indicated they have no financial relationships relevant to this article to disclose.

FUNDING: No external funding.

POTENTIAL CONFLICT OF INTEREST: The authors have indicated they have no potential conflicts of interest to disclose.

REFERENCES

1. Skinner AC, Perrin EM, Skelton JA. Prevalence of obesity and severe obesity in US children, 1999-2014. *Obesity (Silver Spring)*. 2016;24(5):1116–1123
2. Skinner AC, Ravanbakht SN, Skelton JA, Perrin EM, Armstrong SC. Prevalence of obesity and severe obesity in US children, 1999-2016. *Pediatrics*. 2018; 141(3):26
3. Li L, Pérez A, Wu LT, et al. Cardiometabolic risk factors among severely obese children and adolescents in the United States, 1999-2012. *Child Obes*. 2016;12(1):12–19
4. Jasik CB, King EC, Rhodes E, et al. Characteristics of youth presenting for weight management: retrospective national data from the POWER

study group. *Child Obes.* 2015;11(5): 630–637

5. Skinner AC, Perrin EM, Skelton JA. Cardiometabolic risks and obesity in the young. *N Engl J Med.* 2016;374(6): 592–593
6. Modi AC, Loux TJ, Bell SK, et al. Weight-specific health-related quality of life in adolescents with extreme obesity. *Obesity (Silver Spring).* 2008;16(10): 2266–2271
7. Kelly AS, Barlow SE, Rao G, et al; American Heart Association Atherosclerosis, Hypertension, and Obesity in the Young Committee of the Council on Cardiovascular Disease in the Young, Council on Nutrition, Physical Activity and Metabolism, and Council on Clinical Cardiology. Severe obesity in children and adolescents: identification, associated health risks, and treatment approaches: a scientific statement from the American Heart Association. *Circulation.* 2013;128(15): 1689–1712
8. Zhang Y, Wang J, Sun X, et al. Laparoscopic sleeve gastrectomy versus laparoscopic Roux-en-Y gastric bypass for morbid obesity and related comorbidities: a meta-analysis of 21 studies [published correction appears in *Obes Surg.* 2015;25(1):27]. *Obes Surg.* 2015;25(1):19–26
9. Courcoulas AP, Christian NJ, Belle SH, et al; Longitudinal Assessment of Bariatric Surgery (LABS) Consortium. Weight change and health outcomes at 3 years after bariatric surgery among individuals with severe obesity. *JAMA.* 2013;310(22):2416–2425
10. Benaiges D, Más-Lorenzo A, Goday A, et al. Laparoscopic sleeve gastrectomy: more than a restrictive bariatric surgery procedure? *World J Gastroenterol.* 2015; 21(41):11804–11814
11. Inge TH, Zeller MH, Jenkins TM, et al; Teen-LABS Consortium. Perioperative outcomes of adolescents undergoing bariatric surgery: the Teen-Longitudinal Assessment of Bariatric Surgery (Teen-LABS) study. *JAMA Pediatr.* 2014;168(1): 47–53
12. Reames BN, Finks JF, Bacal D, Carlin AM, Dimick JB. Changes in bariatric surgery procedure use in Michigan, 2006-2013. *JAMA.* 2014;312(9):959–961
13. Himpens J, Cadière GB, Bazi M, et al. Long-term outcomes of laparoscopic adjustable gastric banding. *Arch Surg.* 2011;146(7):802–807
14. Zitsman JL, DiGiorgi MF, Fennoy I, et al. Adolescent laparoscopic adjustable gastric banding (LAGB): prospective results in 137 patients followed for 3 years. *Surg Obes Relat Dis.* 2015; 11(1):101–109
15. Bolling CF, Armstrong SC, Reichard KW, Michalsky MP; American Academy of Pediatrics, Section on Obesity and Section on Surgery. Metabolic and bariatric surgery for adolescents with severe obesity. *Pediatrics.* 2019;144(6):e20193224
16. Inge TH, Courcoulas AP, Jenkins TM, et al; Teen-LABS Consortium. Weight loss and health status 3 years after bariatric surgery in adolescents. *N Engl J Med.* 2016;374(2):113–123
17. Michalsky MP, Inge TH, Jenkins TM, et al; Teen-LABS Consortium. Cardiovascular risk factors after adolescent bariatric surgery. *Pediatrics.* 2018;141(2):8
18. Inge TH, Jenkins TM, Xanthakos SA, et al. Long-term outcomes of bariatric surgery in adolescents with severe obesity (FABS-5+): a prospective follow-up analysis. *Lancet Diabetes Endocrinol.* 2017;5(3):165–173
19. Olbers T, Gronowitz E, Werling M, et al. Two-year outcome of laparoscopic Roux-en-Y gastric bypass in adolescents with severe obesity: results from a Swedish Nationwide Study (AMOS). *Int J Obes.* 2012;36(11):1388–1395
20. Olbers T, Beamish AJ, Gronowitz E, et al. Laparoscopic Roux-en-Y gastric bypass in adolescents with severe obesity (AMOS): a prospective, 5-year, Swedish nationwide study. *Lancet Diabetes Endocrinol.* 2017;5(3):174–183
21. Messiah SE, Lopez-Mitnik G, Winegar D, et al. Changes in weight and co-morbidities among adolescents undergoing bariatric surgery: 1-year results from the Bariatric Outcomes Longitudinal Database. *Surg Obes Relat Dis.* 2013;9(4):503–513
22. Al-Sabah SK, Almazeedi SM, Dashti SA, et al. The efficacy of laparoscopic sleeve gastrectomy in treating adolescent obesity. *Obes Surg.* 2015;25(1):50–54
23. Alqahtani AR, Antonisamy B, Alamri H, Elahmedi M, Zimmerman VA. Laparoscopic sleeve gastrectomy in 108 obese children and adolescents aged 5 to 21 years. *Ann Surg.* 2012;256(2): 266–273
24. Black JA, White B, Viner RM, Simmons RK. Bariatric surgery for obese children and adolescents: a systematic review and meta-analysis. *Obes Rev.* 2013; 14(8):634–644
25. Inge TH, Laffel LM, Jenkins TM, et al; Teen–Longitudinal Assessment of Bariatric Surgery (Teen-LABS) and Treatment Options of Type 2 Diabetes in Adolescents and Youth (TODAY) Consortia. Comparison of surgical and medical therapy for type 2 diabetes in severely obese adolescents. *JAMA Pediatr.* 2018;172(5):452–460
26. Pedroso FE, Angriman F, Endo A, et al. Weight loss after bariatric surgery in obese adolescents: a systematic review and meta-analysis. *Surg Obes Relat Dis.* 2018;14(3):413–422
27. Shoar S, Mahmoudzadeh H, Naderan M, et al. Long-term outcome of bariatric surgery in morbidly obese adolescents: a systematic review and meta-analysis of 950 patients with a minimum of 3 years follow-up. *Obes Surg.* 2017; 27(12):3110–3117
28. Inge TH, Coley RY, Bazzano LA, et al; PCORnet Bariatric Study Collaborative. Comparative effectiveness of bariatric procedures among adolescents: the PCORnet bariatric study. *Surg Obes Relat Dis.* 2018;14(9):1374–1386
29. Flum DR, Belle SH, King WC, et al; Longitudinal Assessment of Bariatric Surgery (LABS) Consortium. Perioperative safety in the longitudinal assessment of bariatric surgery. *N Engl J Med.* 2009;361(5):445–454
30. Järvholm K, Karlsson J, Olbers T, et al. Characteristics of adolescents with poor mental health after bariatric surgery. *Surg Obes Relat Dis.* 2016;12(4):882–890
31. Gastrointestinal surgery for severe obesity. Proceedings of a National Institutes of Health Consensus Development Conference. March 25-27, 1991, Bethesda, MD. *Am J Clin Nutr.* 1992;55(suppl 2):487S–619S
32. Pratt JSA, Browne A, Browne NT, et al. ASMBS pediatric metabolic and bariatric surgery guidelines, 2018. *Surg Obes Relat Dis.* 2018;14(7):882–901

33. Childerhose JE, Alsamawi A, Mehta T, et al. Adolescent bariatric surgery: a systematic review of recommendation documents. *Surg Obes Relat Dis.* 2017; 13(10):1768–1779

34. Styne DM, Arslanian SA, Connor EL, et al. Pediatric obesity-assessment, treatment, and prevention: an endocrine society clinical practice guideline. *J Clin Endocrinol Metab.* 2017;102(3):709–757

35. Hornack SE, Nadler EP, Wang J, Hansen A, Mackey ER. Sleeve gastrectomy for youth with cognitive impairment or developmental disability. *Pediatrics.* 2019;143(5):e20182908

36. Schilling PL, Davis MM, Albanese CT, Dutta S, Morton J. National trends in adolescent bariatric surgical procedures and implications for surgical centers of excellence. *J Am Coll Surg.* 2008;206(1):1–12

37. Inge TH, Courcoulas AP, Xanthakos SA. Weight loss and health status after bariatric surgery in adolescents. *N Engl J Med.* 2016;374(20):1989–1990

38. Kelleher DC, Merrill CT, Cottrell LT, Nadler EP, Burd RS. Recent national trends in the use of adolescent inpatient bariatric surgery: 2000 through 2009. *Arch Pediatr Adolesc Med.* 2013;167(2):126–132

39. Zwintscher NP, Azarow KS, Horton JD, Newton CR, Martin MJ. The increasing incidence of adolescent bariatric surgery. *J Pediatr Surg.* 2013;48(12): 2401–2407

40. Inge TH, Boyce TW, Lee M, et al. Access to care for adolescents seeking weight loss surgery. *Obesity (Silver Spring).* 2014;22(12):2593–2597

41. Ogden CL, Carroll MD, Lawman HG, et al. Trends in obesity prevalence among children and adolescents in the United States, 1988-1994 through 2013-2014. *JAMA.* 2016;315(21):2292–2299

42. Kelleher DC, Merrill CT, Cottrell LT, Nadler EP, Burd RS. Recent national trends in the use of adolescent inpatient bariatric surgery: 2000 through 2009. *JAMA Pediatr.* 2013;167(2):126–132

43. Wee CC, Huskey KW, Bolcic-Jankovic D, et al. Sex, race, and consideration of bariatric surgery among primary care patients with moderate to severe obesity. *J Gen Intern Med.* 2014;29(1):68–75

44. Stanford FC, Jones DB, Schneider BE, et al. Patient race and the likelihood of undergoing bariatric surgery among patients seeking surgery. *Surg Endosc.* 2015;29(9):2794–2799

45. Wallace AE, Young-Xu Y, Hartley D, Weeks WB. Racial, socioeconomic, and rural-urban disparities in obesity-related bariatric surgery. *Obes Surg.* 2010; 20(10):1354–1360

46. Ng J, Seip R, Stone A, et al. Ethnic variation in weight loss, but not co-morbidity remission, after laparoscopic gastric banding and Roux-en-Y gastric bypass. *Surg Obes Relat Dis.* 2015;11(1): 94–100

47. Long TF; Committee on Child Health Financing; American Academy of Pediatrics. Essential contractual language for medical necessity in children. *Pediatrics.* 2013;132(2):398–401

48. Vanguri P, Lanning D, Wickham EP, Anbazhagan A, Bean MK. Pediatric health care provider perceptions of weight loss surgery in adolescents. *Clin Pediatr (Phila).* 2014;53(1):60–65

49. Penna M, Markar S, Hewes J, et al. Adolescent bariatric surgery–thoughts and perspectives from the UK. *Int J Environ Res Public Health.* 2013;11(1): 573–582

50. Woolford SJ, Clark SJ, Gebremariam A, Davis MM, Freed GL. To cut or not to cut: physicians' perspectives on referring adolescents for bariatric surgery. *Obes Surg.* 2010;20(7):937–942

51. Alqahtani A, Elahmedi M, Qahtani AR. Laparoscopic sleeve gastrectomy in children younger than 14 years: refuting the concerns. *Ann Surg.* 2016; 263(2):312–319

52. Alqahtani AR, Elahmedi MO, Al Qahtani A. Co-morbidity resolution in morbidly obese children and adolescents undergoing sleeve gastrectomy. *Surg Obes Relat Dis.* 2014;10(5):842–850

53. Grossman DC, Bibbins-Domingo K, Curry SJ, et al; US Preventive Services Task Force. Screening for obesity in children and adolescents: US preventive services task force recommendation statement. *JAMA.* 2017;317(23):2417–2426

54. Magnussen CG, Koskinen J, Chen W, et al. Pediatric metabolic syndrome predicts adulthood metabolic syndrome, subclinical atherosclerosis, and type 2 diabetes mellitus but is no better than body mass index alone: the Bogalusa Heart Study and the Cardiovascular Risk in Young Finns Study. *Circulation.* 2010;122(16): 1604–1611

55. Li S, Chen W, Srinivasan SR, Xu J, Berenson GS. Relation of childhood obesity/cardiometabolic phenotypes to adult cardiometabolic profile: the Bogalusa Heart Study. *Am J Epidemiol.* 2012;176(suppl 7):S142–S149

56. Lai CC, Sun D, Cen R, et al. Impact of long-term burden of excessive adiposity and elevated blood pressure from childhood on adulthood left ventricular remodeling patterns: the Bogalusa Heart Study. *J Am Coll Cardiol.* 2014; 64(15):1580–1587

57. Li S, Chen W, Sun D, et al. Variability and rapid increase in body mass index during childhood are associated with adult obesity. *Int J Epidemiol.* 2015;44(6):1943–1950

58. Freedman DS, Berenson GS. Tracking of BMI *z* scores for severe obesity. *Pediatrics.* 2017;140(3):e20171072

59. Inge TH, Jenkins TM, Zeller M, et al. Baseline BMI is a strong predictor of nadir BMI after adolescent gastric bypass. *J Pediatr.* 2010;156(1): 103–108.e1

60. Michalsky M, Kramer RE, Fullmer MA, et al. Developing criteria for pediatric/ adolescent bariatric surgery programs. *Pediatrics.* 2011;128(suppl 2):S65–S70

61. Michalsky M, Reichard K, Inge T, Pratt J, Lenders C. ASMBS pediatric committee best practice guidelines. *Surg Obes Relat Dis.* 2012;8(1):1–7

62. Yau PO, Parikh M, Saunders JK, et al. Pregnancy after bariatric surgery: the effect of time-to-conception on pregnancy outcomes. *Surg Obes Relat Dis.* 2017;13(11):1899–1905

63. Johansson K, Cnattingius S, Näslund I, et al. Outcomes of pregnancy after bariatric surgery. *N Engl J Med.* 2015; 372(9):814–824

Prescribing Physical, Occupational, and Speech Therapy Services for Children With Disabilities

- *Clinical Report*

CLINICAL REPORT Guidance for the Clinician in Rendering Pediatric Care

American Academy of Pediatrics

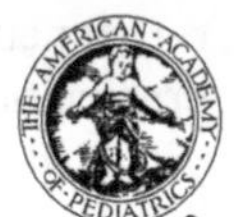

DEDICATED TO THE HEALTH OF ALL CHILDREN™

Prescribing Physical, Occupational, and Speech Therapy Services for Children With Disabilities

Amy Houtrow, MD, PhD, MPH, FAAP, FAAPMR,[a] Nancy Murphy, MD, FAAP, FAAPMR,[b] COUNCIL ON CHILDREN WITH DISABILITIES

abstract

Pediatric health care providers are frequently responsible for prescribing physical, occupational, and speech therapies and monitoring therapeutic progress for children with temporary or permanent disabilities in their practices. This clinical report will provide pediatricians and other pediatric health care providers with information about how best to manage the therapeutic needs of their patients in the medical home by reviewing the International Classification of Functioning, Disability and Health; describing the general goals of habilitative and rehabilitative therapies; delineating the types, locations, and benefits of therapy services; and detailing how to write a therapy prescription and include therapists in the medical home neighborhood.

[a]*Department of Physical Medicine and Rehabilitation and Pediatrics, University of Pittsburgh, Pittsburgh, Pennsylvania; and* [b]*Division of Pediatric Physical Medicine and Rehabilitation, Department of Pediatrics, University of Utah, Salt Lake City, Utah*

Drs Houtrow and Murphy were each responsible for all aspects of conceptualizing, writing, editing, and preparing the document for publication; and both authors approved the final manuscript as submitted.

This document is copyrighted and is property of the American Academy of Pediatrics and its Board of Directors. All authors have filed conflict of interest statements with the American Academy of Pediatrics. Any conflicts have been resolved through a process approved by the Board of Directors. The American Academy of Pediatrics has neither solicited nor accepted any commercial involvement in the development of the content of this publication.

Clinical reports from the American Academy of Pediatrics benefit from expertise and resources of liaisons and internal (AAP) and external reviewers. However, clinical reports from the American Academy of Pediatrics may not reflect the views of the liaisons or the organizations or government agencies that they represent.

The guidance in this report does not indicate an exclusive course of treatment or serve as a standard of medical care. Variations, taking into account individual circumstances, may be appropriate.

All clinical reports from the American Academy of Pediatrics automatically expire 5 years after publication unless reaffirmed, revised, or retired at or before that time.

DOI: https://doi.org/10.1542/peds.2019-0285

Address correspondence to Amy J. Houtrow, MD, PhD, MPH, FAAP, FAAPMR. E-mail: houtrow@upmc.edu

To cite: Houtrow A, Murphy N, AAP COUNCIL ON CHILDREN WITH DISABILITIES. Prescribing Physical, Occupational, and Speech Therapy Services for Children With Disabilities. *Pediatrics.* 2019;143(4):e20190285

Pediatricians and other pediatric health care providers have a vitally important role of linking children and youth with disabilities in their family-centered primary care medical homes with appropriate community-based services.[1] Pediatric providers are often asked (frequently by families) or recognize the need to prescribe habilitative and rehabilitative therapies (physical, occupational, and speech and language) for infants, children, and youth with disabilities in their clinical practices. Many general pediatric providers describe inadequate training to appropriately prescribe therapy in the various settings in which they may be available to children with disabilities.[2–5] This clinical report will review (1) the framework of the International Classification of Functioning, Disability and Health (ICF) for understanding the interaction between health conditions and personal and environmental factors that result in disability, (2) children with disabilities and the goals of habilitation and rehabilitation services, (3) the types of therapy services available with their general indications, (4) the locations in which children may receive therapy services and potential facilitators and barriers to securing therapy services, (5) the existing literature regarding the benefits of therapy and how therapy may be dosed to optimize functional outcomes, and (6) recommendations for writing therapy prescriptions. Two case examples are provided to aid the pediatric health care provider in developing expertise in addressing the therapy needs of children with disabilities in their practices.

ICF

The World Health Organization (WHO) released the ICF in 2001 as an update to the International Classification of Impairments, Disabilities, and Handicaps.[6] The WHO has developed 2 classification systems that can be used to describe an individual's health at a particular point in time. Physicians are more familiar with the WHO's International Classification of Diseases (ICD), currently in its 10th revision, which classifies diseases and other health problems. Because a diagnosis alone often does not provide a robust characterization of one's health, complementing the *International Classification of Diseases, 10th Revision*, is the ICF, a classification system with a biopsychosocial framework for describing functioning and disability associated with one's health conditions.[7]

The ICF describes the relationship between health conditions diagnosed and coded in the ICD and the personal and environmental factors that act as facilitators or barriers to functioning.[8] Houtrow and Zima[9] provided examples of the ICF and ICD together for common pediatric diagnoses in 2017. There are 3 identified levels of functioning: the body part or organ system, the person, and the person in social situations.[7] These levels correspond to body functions, activities, and participation, respectively. Disability is the umbrella term for impairments at the body part or organ system level, activity restrictions at the person level, and participation restrictions at the person-in-society level.[7] The WHO defines impairments as "problems in body function or structure such as a significant deviation or loss," activity limitations as "difficulties an individual may have in executing a task," and participation restrictions as "problems an individual may experience in involvement in life situations" (Fig 1).[7]

The ICF also includes the concepts of capacity and performance. Capacity is the individual's intrinsic ability to perform a task or an action in a standardized environment, whereas performance is how well the individual is able to actually perform the task in his or her own real-life environment.[10] These concepts are important in understanding the role of habilitative and rehabilitative therapies for children with disabilities, because achievement of skill requires extensive practice and must be integrated into the child's routine for the successful enhancement of participation in life events. In addition, the ICF framework highlights the importance of a child's environment on his or her functional outcomes.[11] The environment includes not just the physical world, such as the town where the child lives or the topography of the community, but also includes the attitudes and values of the family, community, and society at large and the technologies, services, supports, laws, and policies where the child lives.[12] Access to health and therapeutic services, the physical environment, and social supports all affect how well a child with disabilities functions in his or her daily life.[13]

CHILDHOOD DISABILITY

A child with a disability has an environmentally contextualized health-related limitation in his or her existing or emerging capacity to perform developmentally appropriate activities and participate, as desired, in society.[14] Childhood disability is on the rise, especially for children with neurodevelopmental conditions.[14–16] A childhood disability may be related to congenital or acquired health conditions and may be temporary, permanent, or progressive in nature. Common examples of health conditions associated with childhood disabilities that most pediatric health care providers encounter are autism

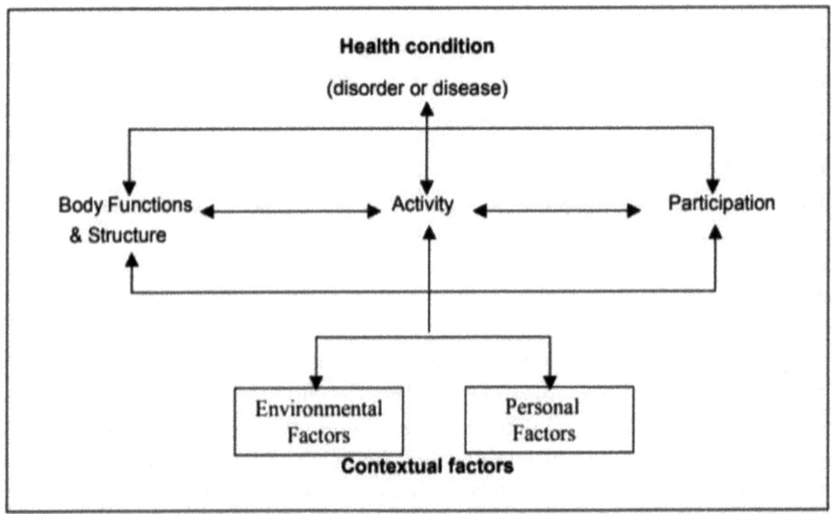

FIGURE 1
ICF. Reprinted with permission from World Health Organization. *International Classification of Functioning, Disability and Health: Toward a Common Language for Functioning, Disability and Health*. Geneva, Switzerland: World Health Organization; 2002:9.

spectrum disorder, cerebral palsy, intellectual disability, spina bifida, and acquired conditions such as traumatic brain injury or juvenile idiopathic arthritis. Temporary disability may be the result of a serious illness or injury, such as a femur fracture. Examples of progressively disabling conditions are Duchenne muscular dystrophy and cystic fibrosis. Disabilities may affect all aspects of daily life or may affect a child only in certain settings or situations, such as is sometimes the case for attention-deficit/hyperactivity disorder or when physically exerting oneself, as in the case of exercise-induced asthma and other pulmonary conditions. Some disabilities are clearly visible, and some may be less readily apparent.

THERAPEUTIC GOALS

The overarching habilitation and rehabilitation goals for children with disabilities are to help the child achieve developmentally appropriate functional skills, regardless of whether these skills existed previously for the child (rehabilitative) or are to be newly developed (habilitative); prevent maladaptive consequences; mitigate the impact of impairments of the body part or structure on the child's activities and participation; provide adaptive strategies to minimize the impacts of functional deficits; and ensure carryover into other settings through family training, support, and community integration strategies.[17] Adaptive strategies can include making environmental modifications to accommodate the child, training the child to use assistive technologies and other durable medical equipment such as walkers and wheelchairs, and helping the child develop compensatory techniques. Greater access to the physical and social worlds through adaptations provides children with disabilities greater opportunities for participation and connectedness with others and can enhance their well-being.[18]

TYPES OF THERAPY SERVICES

Although children can be supported by a range of therapies to address challenges in daily life, the 3 types of therapies detailed in this report are physical therapy, occupational therapy, and speech and language therapy. Applied behavior analysis is a therapy used frequently in autism spectrum disorder and some other conditions and is discussed in great detail in the American Academy of Pediatrics (AAP) clinical report "Management of Children With Autism Spectrum Disorders."[19] All types of therapists are valuable members of the health care team and may be involved in care delivery in multiple settings across the life course. They have important roles in direct treatment but also in family training and advocacy.[20]

Physical therapists address gross motor skills, strength building, endurance, and fitness. They also focus on prevention or reduction of impairments to achieve optimal functional mobility and participation. They help children move, often with the use of strategies to prevent the progression of impairments and through the use of adaptive equipment such as orthotics (braces) and various mobility aids such as walkers, wheelchairs, and lifts. For a child with cerebral palsy, for example, the physical therapist addresses impairments related to spasticity, weakness, poor postural control, and lack of coordination. To minimize activity limitations, the physical therapist helps the child with walking skills (among others). To address participation restrictions, the physical therapist helps the child learn to navigate a public space such as the hallways at school.[21]

Pediatric occupational therapists address upper extremity function, fine motor skills, visual-motor function, sensory processing skills, and the occupations or tasks that are expected of the child.[22] These tasks are referred to as activities of daily living (daily tasks such as feeding, eating, dressing, or toileting) and instrumental activities of daily living (complex tasks such as cooking, shopping, or using a telephone). Occupational therapists are also involved in identifying the equipment needs a child might have to perform tasks. To address impairments in the child with cerebral palsy, for example, the occupational therapist works on grasping and hand coordination; to help with an activity such as dressing, the occupational therapist works with the child to practice the skill and use an assistive device; and to aid in participation, the occupational therapist provides strategies that the child can use in and out of the classroom such as self-regulation techniques or taking notes on a keyboard versus on paper.

Speech and language pathologists, also called speech therapists, address communication and cognition.[23] They work with children with disabilities to improve their expressive language skills verbally or with alternative communication techniques. To address speech-related impairments associated with cerebral palsy, for example, the speech therapist works on oral motor skills to improve enunciation or teaches the child to use an augmentative communication device to successfully communicate with others and participate in social interactions.[24] Speech therapists also evaluate and treat swallowing problems.[23] Dysphagia is a frequently occurring impairment for children with disabilities, because many disabling conditions are associated with oropharyngeal or esophageal dysfunction. The workup for dysphagia usually includes an evaluation by a speech therapist and may also include a video fluoroscopic barium study (often referred to as a cookie swallow) or a fiber-optic endoscopic evaluation of swallow.[25] Depending on the etiology and severity of swallowing dysfunction, a multidisciplinary team that may include medical and surgical specialists such as pediatric gastroenterologists, otolaryngologists, pulmonologists, or pediatric rehabilitation medicine or complex care physicians, along with speech therapists and occupational therapists with expertise in disordered feeding, can create and execute an effective treatment plan.[25] Some tertiary care children's hospitals have dedicated feeding and swallowing clinics in which multidisciplinary assessments with recommendation can be provided. For children with complex swallowing and feeding problems, a referral to a specialized clinic may be considered.

The services provided by the 3 therapy disciplines described above often overlap with each other. Establishing coordinated goals can strengthen interdisciplinary treatment synergies.[26] For example, both physical and occupational therapists address durable medical equipment needs and help children gain skills in transitioning from 1 position to another. Speech and occupational therapists often collaborate in feeding therapy for children with poor oral motor and swallowing skills on the basis of the child's needs and the expertise of the providers involved. In addition, children who use augmentative communication or other assistive technologies often rely on the combined expertise of speech and occupational therapists to determine which devices will be most beneficial. There are numerous other examples of overlap and opportunities for synergies, but there is potential for duplication of services and payment refusal by insurance companies of which pediatric health care providers may take note. Children may also receive therapy in a group with other children with 1 or more therapy disciplines involved.[20] This approach, often called group therapy, usually targets a specific set of skills that all of the members of the group are working to achieve. Children may also receive cotreatments in which more than 1 discipline is involved in the therapeutic session, but no other children are present.

THERAPY SETTINGS

There are 4 main settings in which a child with a disability might need a therapy prescription: in the hospital, in the outpatient and/or community setting, in the child's home, and in school. In the hospital setting, the pediatric health care provider directing care might order an evaluation and treatments by a therapist. Because the pediatric medical home provider is usually not the inpatient attending physician, communications to bridge inpatient to outpatient care plans are essential. In the outpatient setting, a provider's prescription is typically needed to initiate an evaluation and treatment plan by a therapist and for those services to be covered by insurance. All states have some amount of direct access (an individual can see a therapist without a prescription), most commonly for physical therapy.[27] Regardless of the prescriber of therapies, the child's primary and subspecialty providers may all be involved in evaluating the impact of therapy on the child and participate in shared decision-making that involves collaborating to develop goals and a care plan in a mutually respectful and trusting manner with the family.[1] In the outpatient sector, there is variable access to pediatric therapists. Children with disabilities or developmental delays often have unmet needs for therapy services, especially if they have inadequate health insurance.[28–31] Some insurance plans have limited coverage for therapy services and may have high copays, have high coinsurance rates, or cap the number of visits per year. Many families report a health plan problem (inadequate coverage) as a reason for their children's unmet needs.[32–34] When access to therapy is limited, the pediatric health care provider is encouraged to help coordinate services to the extent possible and to make referrals to advocacy organizations that can help families navigate the complex web of service providers.[35] In addition, practices may find it helpful to keep a list of agencies and organizations to which to refer families handy or available on their Web site for families to access as needed. In both the inpatient and outpatient settings, therapy services are based on goals for developing new skills, regaining lost skills (such as after an illness injury or intervention), maintaining current skills at risk for decrement, making adaptations for functional loss(es), and providing accommodations.

The third location for the provision of therapy services is in the child's home. In-home therapies are less common than outpatient or school-based therapies for older children and youth but are frequently provided when the child with disabilities is young, too medically fragile to participate in outpatient therapies, or otherwise homebound. Usually, the physician documents the medical fragility for insurance companies to authorize in-home therapy. One important exception is early intervention (EI) services. For children 0 to 3 years of age, the home is the setting for EI services. Infants and young children who have disabilities, have developmental delays, or are at risk because of their diagnosed health conditions may be referred to EI for evaluation and services under the Individuals with Disabilities Education Act (IDEA) Part C.[36] Although processes and eligibility vary by state, a developmental specialist conducts a global evaluation of the child and provides play interventions to promote development. On the basis of the assessment, the infant or young child may also receive physical, occupational, speech, and/or vision therapy in the home. Providing services in the child's natural environment has been a part of IDEA Part C since its inception, with goals to enhance the development of infants and toddlers with special needs and to support families to interact and meet the needs of their children.[36] A key component of IDEA Part C EI services is an individualized family service plan.[37] Providing a medical diagnosis, documenting risk factors and findings on physical examination, and offering an informed clinical opinion, as components of the medical home, can be helpful when the child is referred or needs to be reevaluated.[36,38] The value of intervening early in a child's life is well documented[39–44]; therefore, the pediatric provider is encouraged to routinely evaluate development in line with AAP recommendations, provide support to families, collaborate with Part C programs,[45,46] and advocate on behalf of his or her patients for services. It is important to note that state-to-state variations exist because of eligibility criteria differences, including how developmental delay is defined.[36] Some infants and toddlers will also benefit from traditional outpatient therapies to supplement EI services.[36] These infants and toddlers frequently have complex medical conditions or need outpatient therapy services to achieve a specific short-term goal. Occasionally, this therapy may be provided to a child care center if a specialized arrangement is made. More information about EI services is available in the 2013 AAP clinical report "Early Intervention, IDEA Part C Services, and the Medical Home: Collaboration for Best Practice and Best Outcomes."[36]

The fourth setting for a child with a disability to receive therapies is the school. IDEA,[47] passed in 1975, legislates federal funding to states for EI (through Part C) and special education services (through Part B).[36,37] If a child needs supports or services to participate in education in the least restrictive environment, such as speech, physical, or occupational therapy, these related services are covered by IDEA Part A and can be incorporated into the child's individualized education program (IEP).[37] The specific disabilities codified in IDEA are mental retardation (now called intellectual disability), hearing impairments (including deafness), visual impairments (including blindness), speech and language impairments, orthopedic impairments, serious emotional disturbance, autism, traumatic brain injury, other health impairments, specific learning disabilities, deaf-blindness, and multiple disabilities.[48] Because IDEA uses a categorical definition of disability for children, some disabilities are, instead, covered by Section 504 of the Rehabilitation Act of 1973, which mandates the provision of accommodations so that children can receive their education in the least restrictive environment.[37] Section 504 uses a functional descriptor, that of a limitation in a major life area such as walking or speaking, instead of the IDEA categories of disabilities.[37] A therapist may evaluate the school environment and the needs for accommodations for a child's 504 plan irrespective of whether the child is placed in a regular or special education classroom.[49] It is notable that the interpretation of what constitutes school-based therapy services to promote a child's ability to participate academically can vary among service providers, districts, and states.[49] School therapies are designed to promote attainment of a student's educational goals and are often more narrowly focused than outpatient, medically based therapies. For example, an occupational therapist in the school may work on handwriting, whereas an occupational therapist in the health care system addresses many activities involving the hands, such as teeth brushing; they both address fine motor skills but with different functional tasks. Therefore, some children receiving school-based therapies also require outpatient therapy services. Nonetheless, the therapies provided in school frequently benefit the child outside of the school setting. Improved fine motor skills for handwriting can improve the child's ability to perform other fine motor tasks. Medical home providers are encouraged to help families stay abreast of school-based interventions and advocate for services when warranted. For families struggling with their school district regarding academically necessary therapy services, a referral to a medical legal partnership, their state's Disability Rights Center, or another advocacy organization may be warranted when other venues of advocacy have been exhausted.[50]

The pediatric health care provider may provide a child with a specific diagnosis, but providing a diagnosis does not necessarily mean the child will qualify for services under IDEA. For a 504 plan, the pediatric health care provider also documents the medical diagnosis and, in addition, the associated functional limitation in a major life area. Although not an actual therapy prescription, pediatric medical providers may also be asked to provide a recommendation about adaptive physical education, a protected right under IDEA.[51] For more information about IDEA and special education needs, please see the 2015 AAP clinical report "The Individuals with Disabilities Education Act (IDEA) for Children with Special Educational Needs."[37]

Regardless of the type of therapy or the setting in which it is delivered, therapists are key members of the medical home neighborhood. Strategies for communication are required to optimize service coordination and ensure that children are receiving all aspects of the medical home.[52] This effort is especially challenging for children with disabilities who often require extensive care coordination for numerous specialty services and thus are less likely to receive care in a medical home.[28]

THERAPEUTIC BENEFITS

The efficacy of therapy services to help children gain and/or maintain function and provide adaptations is well documented.[53–58] Provision of a home program with caregiver training and support is generally indicated, because carryover of skills is enhanced by frequent repetition.[59–61] To routinely perform newly achieved skills, children need practice in their own environment; having the capacity to perform a task in a structured environment can improve performance but is not enough to demonstrate achievement of a therapeutic goal.[13] Children need to demonstrate that they can routinely perform the activity in the face of challenges that exist in their environments for successful transfer of skills.[62] A home program can further enhance a child's participation in other structured activities that incorporate functional skills such as dance classes, karate, or school sports that are appropriately adapted for the child with disabilities. The time spent practicing activities with real-world carryover is part of the critical link between building capacity and performance.[13] An important role of pediatric providers in optimizing the function of children with disabilities is advocating with families for inclusion in activities that best support participation in life events. The pediatric health care provider is an ideal advocate for early involvement because of the critical early childhood period for neuroplasticity.[63,64]

Functional improvements are more likely to occur when the goals of therapy are clearly delineated and measureable,[65,66] and goal setting is a central feature of rehabilitation.[67] For sustained positive benefits from therapeutic interventions, activities can be practiced in the child's environment and reinforced by the parents or other caregivers.[2] Practice in one's natural environment is essential for success; therefore, parents and/or caregivers are encouraged to practice skill building outside of the therapeutic setting. When a therapeutic intervention is directed at 1 domain of functioning (body structures and function, activities, or participation) there can be a "ripple effect" of positive outcomes in other domains.[13,53,68] For example, strengthening the legs can lead to improved walking, which can also be associated with improved ability to navigate and participate in the classroom. Taking a holistic approach has clear value and is associated with improved therapy outcomes.[55,69–72]

Although the evidence base for the effectiveness of various therapies is increasing, not all therapeutic modalities and techniques have been shown to be efficacious, and some have harmful adverse effects and are therefore not promoted in lieu of standard or evidence-based therapies.[73–79] For example, hyperbaric oxygen for the treatment of cerebral palsy has not been shown to be efficacious and is associated with harmful adverse effects and is therefore not recommended.[78,80,81] Similarly, evidence for the benefits of patterning is lacking.[81] Treatment success that is only supported by case reports or anecdotal data and not by carefully designed research studies warrants further investigation and discussion before prescribing. Families often seek complementary or alternative treatments and may ask their pediatric health provider to advocate for these treatments on behalf of the child. In these circumstances, it is important to review the evidence and engage in a dialogue with families about the goals of treatment and how best to achieve them.[82] Other treatments and techniques are a part of a standard of care not subject to randomized controlled trials, but newer treatments and techniques require more rigorous research before conclusions can be drawn about their efficacy.[83–85] Referrals to specialists with expertise in the various therapeutic modalities and treatments may be considered by medical home providers to help determine which therapeutic interventions to prescribe. Pediatric rehabilitation medicine physicians (also known as pediatric physiatrists), neurodevelopmental pediatricians, and developmental and behavioral pediatricians are well versed in the therapeutic options that may not be standard but have evidence for efficacy.[86–95] These specialists tend to be strong medical home neighbors because of their expertise in coordinating care for children with disabilities across settings. In some cases, they may be or may become the medical home provider if the family can easily access their services and other criteria of the medical home can be met by their practices. Various forms of shared management may be explored by the primary care physician and the specialists to ensure children with disabilities are receiving optimal care.

THERAPY DOSING

Determining the appropriate dose of therapy (how much therapy, how often, and for how long) remains elusive and largely subjective.[13,22,57] Dose is determined by the minutes each therapy session is, how often it is provided, and for how long (weeks, months, years). Although much research is being conducted, there is not yet a strong evidence base to support any particular dosing strategy for specific disabilities or conditions,[22] except in unilateral hemiplegic cerebral palsy, for which high-intensity upper extremity therapy that is activity-based has been shown to improve outcomes to a greater degree than standard therapy administration (such as once a week).[96] Because of their attention spans, young children usually do well with shorter duration of therapy per session and, therefore, may need more total sessions or breaks within sessions. Children with temporary disabilities may need short-term therapy to make adaptations to their condition and recover from it. Children with new-onset disabilities, such as from traumatic injuries, frequently need intense therapy services shortly after injury often in an inpatient setting with coordinated medical and nursing care and then require ongoing therapy on a less intense schedule to optimize their outcomes.[97] Children with disabilities associated with chronic health conditions often need therapy on an ongoing basis with variable intensities on the basis of their individual functional goals.

Therapies can be dosed in an intense fashion, such as 45 to 60 minutes 2 or more times a week, especially when a short-term goal is identified and deemed quickly achievable.[21] Similarly, after a medical event or a surgery, some children with disabilities need intense therapy to regain temporarily lost function and then can return to their regular therapy schedule. A commonly delivered dose of therapy is for 30 to 60 minutes per week for an episode of care, such as during the entire school year in the case of school-based therapies.[98] This schedule is often used when a child exhibits continued progress toward goals and is at risk for a lack of progress or regression if therapy services were halted.[21] Children who are functionally stable and have attained their current functional goals may only need periodic or intermittent therapy services.[99] This is especially true of older children who may have already met most of their developmental milestones. Children with disabilities who use adaptive equipment well may only need to be checked on periodically, and when new equipment is ordered, they may need a short course of more intense therapy for training with the new device.[21] The process of therapeutic surveillance is especially important, because children with disabilities are at risk for skill regression or lack of progress because of changes in their health or changes in their environments. Reengaging therapy services quickly can help mitigate deterioration in participation and quality of life. Similarly, a child on a long-term therapeutic treatment therapy program may need to have services increased when a new problem occurs or a goal is identified on the basis of a change in functional status or developmental expectation.[21] This sudden change in therapy needs is often referred to as a burst or an episode of therapy. For example, intense gait training may be prescribed when a child is just on the cusp of developing walking skills or to incorporate efficient gait skills when gait deviations are present. Strong collaboration between the family, the treating therapists, specialists, and the pediatric medical home provider helps identify the best dosing strategies that consider the child's health, current functional status, goals, readiness for therapy, response to intervention, and cessation of services, if warranted.[21,22,100] Pediatric providers may receive requests from families for therapies that are not warranted. In these situations, family-centered, shared decision-making techniques may be used to establish goals, and then strategies to achieve these goals can be identified.[1,101] One potential strategy is to make a referral to a specialist with expertise in the evidence base for therapeutic interventions who can work with the family to develop a goal-directed plan of care that addresses concerns, such as lack of measurable progress but the need for prevention of further impairment, on which all members of the team (including family) agree.

THE THERAPY PRESCRIPTION

When a child with functional limitations needs therapy or when there is concern for developmental delay, before writing a therapy prescription, it is helpful to review past and current therapy reports (if any exist), family-identified concerns, and any findings on developmental screening or testing in addition to the goals of therapy and the expected outcomes. When prescribing initial or continuing therapy services, the provider is advised to identify the therapy discipline; the medical condition associated with the disability (or the constellation of symptoms and findings if the diagnosis is unknown), which indicates the medical necessity of the treatment; any precautions or restrictions; the goals of therapy; and the frequency and duration of treatment. Additionally, the prescription may include the specific type or modality of therapy, if 1 is desired (Fig 2). If the child recently had surgery and is in need of short-term therapy or is restricted from his or her usual therapy routine, the surgeon is often the provider who writes these prescriptions and manages restrictions such as weight-bearing precautions. After evaluation by the therapist, the provider may be asked to revise the therapy prescription on the basis of the recommendations of the therapist who participates in the development of goals and the treatment plan. See the cases in Text Boxes 1 and 2 for examples of therapy prescriptions and the elements of a therapy report.

Sample Therapy Prescription

- Patient Name:______________________ DOB:______
- Physician:_________________________ Date:______
- Diagnosis:____________________________________
- Precautions:__________________________________
- Type of Therapy:______________________________
- Frequency:_________________ Duration:__________
- Therapy Goals:________________________________
- Modalities:___________________________________
- Signature & Date: ______________________________

FIGURE 2
Sample therapy prescription. DOB, date of birth.

Providing a high level of detail in a therapy prescription may be beyond the expertise of many pediatric providers. Nonetheless, providing a clear prescription to help guide the therapy is important. Because there is a general lack of evidence for the dosing of therapy, providers are encouraged to consider the amount of functional improvement anticipated, the urgency of the need for the skill development, and how quickly the child is gaining skills. Information about the trajectory of disability associated with the condition, the evidence of the value of therapies to improve functioning, and how the individual child is expected to benefit from the interventions is also important when providing written medical justification. Providers who prefer not to write detailed therapy prescriptions can consult with pediatric rehabilitation medicine physicians, neurodevelopmental pediatricians, developmental and behavioral pediatricians, and other specialists, including physical, occupational, and speech therapists in their medical community. These types of providers can be valuable members of the medical home neighborhood and can help advance the care goals set in the child's care plan with their medical home. Pediatric providers are encouraged, nonetheless, to initiate the process for such therapies, because access to a specialist may be challenging, and the value of early engagement with therapies is well documented. Major professional organizations, existing federal guidelines, and third-party payers all emphasize the important role of physicians in determining the medical necessity for and ordering of services.[2] The choice to refer may also be affected by the severity and complexity of the child's disabilities, the family's desires, the availability of qualified specialists in the community or region, and the local or regional variations of how therapies are delivered. Pediatric medical home providers remain the locus of communication and coordination of services.[35]

Dealing With Insurance Denials

The pediatric health care provider is likely all too familiar with denials for coverage of therapy services from insurance companies. When addressing a denial, either over the phone or in writing, it behooves the provider to have some key pieces of information available to explain why the prescribed service is medically necessary: the diagnosis or diagnoses for which the service is needed, what the service is expected to accomplish (ie, how the service is reasonably likely to address the disabling condition), that there is not an equally effective less costly option, and other pertinent medical history. Pediatric health care providers may also want to familiarize themselves with the Early and Periodic Screening, Diagnosis, and Treatment (EPSDT) standards, because a majority of children with long-term disabilities are covered by Medicaid.[28,103,104] The EPSDT amendments to Medicaid direct coverage of "early and periodic" screening and diagnostic services to identify defects and chronic conditions in addition to providing coverage of health care and treatments to "correct or ameliorate" such conditions and defects.[104] This encompasses treatments that improve health outcomes as well as treatments that enable children with disabilities to achieve and maintain function.[104] Specifically, physical, occupational, and/or speech therapy are mandated pursuant to 42 US Code 1396d(a)(7) and/or 1396d(a)(11). As a result, coverage for therapy services is frequently better under Medicaid than under commercial insurance plans that limit treatments.[103] For additional reading on EPSDT, please see "EPSDT - A Guide for States: Coverage in the Medicaid Benefit for Children and Adolescents" (https://www.medicaid.gov/medicaid/benefits/downloads/epsdt_coverage_guide.pdf).

Beyond the Therapy Prescription

The primary care medical home engages in the coordination of services for children with disabilities in school, hospital, and community

BOX 1 CASE EXAMPLE OF A CHILD WITH CEREBRAL PALSY

Liam is an 11-year-old boy with spastic diplegia, a type of cerebral palsy that mainly affects the lower extremities, who has recently moved with his family from another state and is establishing care in your primary care practice. He wears braces on his lower legs and uses forearm crutches to walk, although he can walk short distances without his crutches at home. He is in the fifth grade and rides the bus with his older sister, who makes sure he gets on and off the bus safely, because he is a little impulsive and falls frequently. His mom performs his lower body dressing for him because they are often in a rush in the mornings before school. She reports that he could do all of his dressing except getting his shoes on over his braces if he had to. At school, he placed in the advanced reading group but struggles with visual perceptual tasks and has "terrible handwriting," according to his mother. The IEP meeting is next week, and prescriptions are requested by the school. The mom also wants to get him involved in therapies outside of school. Before they moved, he received physical therapy once a week and occupational therapy twice a month.

Liam has several therapeutic needs. The most pressing issue is his IEP. On the prescription for therapies at school, you document his diagnosis (spastic diplegic cerebral palsy) and the types of therapies to be provided at school (physical and occupational), the reasons he needs these therapies (mobility, safety, fine motor skills, and visual perceptual skills), the duration of therapy (entire school year), and the frequency (1–2 times per week). You also write a prescription for adaptive physical education so that the school's physical therapist can work with the gym teacher to create a safe and inclusive program for him.

To address Liam's outpatient therapy needs, you prescribe the following:

1. Physical therapy: evaluation and treatment of spastic diplegia, duration 6 months, frequency 1 to 2 times per week to address strength training, ambulation longer distances with Lofstrand crutches and gross motor skills, safety awareness (especially for getting on and off the school bus), equipment needs, stretching for spasticity management, and family training for carryover in the home environment. No restrictions.

2. Occupational therapy: evaluation and treatment of spastic diplegia, duration 6 months, frequency 1 to 2 times per week to address fine motor skills, activities of daily living (especially dressing), safety awareness, visual perceptual skills, and family training for carryover in the home environment. No restrictions.

After Liam's evaluations by the physical and occupational therapists, you receive a letter from each of them with information about the evaluations, the goals that were set, and some changes that they request. Specifically, the physical therapist thinks that Liam's balance is really impairing his progress toward ambulation without crutches. She recommends doing once-a-week hippotherapy to strengthen his core and improve his balance and would like for you to write the prescription. The occupational therapists noted that like many children with spastic diplegia, Liam has poor fine motor skills, which have really impacted his handwriting. She recommends an intense handwriting group therapy program that meets 3 afternoons a week for 2 months. She needs a special prescription for this program. After discussing the recommendations with Liam's mother, you write the prescriptions and await feedback. A few weeks later, your nurse manager reports that the hippotherapy you prescribed has been denied by Liam's insurance. The nurse shares the draft of the letter of medical justification to which you add the evidence in support of the use of hippotherapy in children with cerebral palsy and reiterate the specific goals (core strengthening and balance) along with the intended outcome of improved ambulation without an assistive device.[102] The denial is overturned. Three months later, you receive interim therapy reports from Liam's outpatient physical and occupational therapists. Each of these reports details the initial skill level Liam had when he started therapy, the specific goals they set with Liam and his mother, his achievements and his current status with a recommendation to continue the services to address existing and newly developed goals. The occupational therapist spoke to his physical therapist about shoes that would be easier for Liam to don over his orthotics because he had not been successful at achieving his lower body dressing goal with occupational therapy. The physical therapist sent a fax to your office requesting a prescription for orthotic-containing shoes. At Liam's follow-up visit, his mom indicates that she is so proud of him that he can stand without holding on to anything for nearly 1 minute and that he can get himself dressed in the morning if she makes sure he has enough time before the bus comes. She also reports that it seems easier for him to make friends because he can usually keep up with other kids if activities are modified. You agree that he seems to be making great progress, as also documented in summary reports from his therapists.

settings.[35] Regular communication between the child's care team (parents and/or caregivers, educators, therapists, subspecialists, and medical home providers) includes updates on the child's functional status, the achievement of therapy goals, identification of new goals, the planned cessation of therapy services when appropriate, and family functioning and concerns. This is especially important when children receive services in multiple settings simultaneously from multiple providers or have other vulnerabilities such as being in foster care. In addition, when the child's medical or functional status changes or when other circumstances warrant a change in treatment, the prescribing provider may need to alert the therapist(s) and delineate new precautions or goals. When a therapist notes a functional decline that is unanticipated, he or she can refer back to the pediatric health care provider who is able to evaluate the child and seek to determine the etiology for the decline and discuss findings with the family.

BOX 2 CASE EXAMPLE OF A CHILD WITH LANGUAGE DELAY

Sophia is a 2-year-old who was born at 32 weeks' gestation who has yet to say any words. At an ill visit for diarrhea, Sophia's mother shares her worries about her lack of expressive communication. You reviewed her history, which included a normal hearing screen in the NICU, no concerns on her 9-month well-child visit, and no 18-month developmental surveillance because the family had moved away and then returned to your practice. You conduct an examination that reveals that Sophia responds to her name and other noises, is happy and playful, seems to understand information and can follow commands, has normal gross motor and fine motor skills, and babbles, but mostly communicates by pointing and gesturing. After confirming normal hearing on audiology examination, you diagnose Sophia with an isolated speech delay. You refer the family to EI services and also to outpatient speech therapy. In your prescription for outpatient speech therapy, you write her diagnosis as developmental disorder of speech and language and request therapy 2 to 3 times per week, 30 minutes per session for 12 weeks to address her expressive communication skills. At reevaluation 3 months later, Sophia's expressive speech is much improved. EI services are once a week, and the outpatient speech therapist recommends decreasing the frequency of speech therapy to once a week, because most of her goals have been met. You write a new prescription for ongoing outpatient speech therapy on the basis of the recommendations of the speech therapist and your discussion with Sophia's mother.

At Sophia's 3-year well-child visit, Sophia's mother reports that EI services stopped a few months ago and that the outpatient speech therapist had tested Sophia and that her expressive language skills were in the low-normal range. Her mother reports that she speaks spontaneously with other children during play and is able to "get her point across" with adults using words. In reviewing the report from the speech therapist, you agree that services are no longer warranted, but Sophia's mother wants her to continue to get speech therapy until she tests into the midnormal range. You recognize that ongoing speech therapy services are not medically justified, so you engage in a shared decision-making process to implement a home program for continued skill development and practice, an approach to monitoring of Sophia's language skills and development closely, and a formal evaluation of her communication skills when entering school or sooner, should there be any concerns regarding her development.

Coordinating care that is organized around patient- and family-centered goals with clear communication between the health care team members is the goal to help optimize the health, function, and well-being of children with disabilities.

LEAD AUTHORS

Amy J. Houtrow, MD, PhD, MPH, FAAP
Nancy A. Murphy, MD, FAAP

COUNCIL ON CHILDREN WITH DISABILITIES EXECUTIVE COMMITTEE, 2017–2018

Dennis Z. Kuo, MD, MHS, FAAP, Chairperson
Susan Apkon, MD, FAAP
Timothy J. Brei, MD, FAAP
Lynn F. Davidson, MD, FAAP
Beth Ellen Davis, MD, MPH, FAAP
Kathryn A. Ellerbeck, MD, FAAP
Susan L. Hyman, MD, FAAP
Mary O'Connor Leppert, MD, FAAP
Garey H. Noritz, MD, FAAP
Christopher J. Stille, MD, MPH, FAAP
Larry Yin, MD, MSPH, FAAP

FORMER COUNCIL ON CHILDREN WITH DISABILITIES EXECUTIVE COMMITTEE MEMBERS

Amy J. Houtrow, MD, PhD, MPH, FAAP
Nancy Murphy, MD, FAAP
Kenneth W. Norwood, Jr, MD, FAAP, Immediate Past Chairperson

LIAISONS

Peter J. Smith, MD, MA, FAAP – *Section on Developmental and Behavioral Pediatrics*
Edwin Simpser, MD, FAAP – *Section on Home Care*
Georgina Peacock, MD, MPH, FAAP – *Centers for Disease Control and Prevention*
Marie Y. Mann, MD, MPH, FAAP – *Maternal and Child Health Bureau*
Cara Coleman, JD, MPH – *Family Voices*

STAFF

Alex Kuznetsov, RD

ABBREVIATIONS

AAP: American Academy of Pediatrics
EI: early intervention
EPSDT: Early and Periodic Screening, Diagnosis, and Treatment
ICD: International Classification of Diseases
ICF: International Classification of Functioning, Disability and Health
IDEA: Individuals with Disabilities Education Act
IEP: individualized education program
WHO: World Health Organization

PEDIATRICS (ISSN Numbers: Print, 0031-4005; Online, 1098-4275).

Copyright © 2019 by the American Academy of Pediatrics

FINANCIAL DISCLOSURE: The authors have indicated they have no financial relationships relevant to this article to disclose.

FUNDING: No external funding.

POTENTIAL CONFLICT OF INTEREST: The authors have indicated they have no potential conflicts of interest to disclose.

REFERENCES

1. Murphy NA, Carbone PS; Council on Children With Disabilities; American Academy of Pediatrics. Parent-provider-community partnerships: optimizing outcomes for children with disabilities. *Pediatrics.* 2011;128(4): 795–802

2. Sneed RC, May WL, Stencel C. Policy versus practice: comparison of prescribing therapy and durable medical equipment in medical and educational settings. *Pediatrics.* 2004; 114(5). Available at: www.pediatrics.org/cgi/content/full/114/5/e612

3. Shah RP, Kunnavakkam R, Msall ME. Pediatricians' knowledge, attitudes, and practice patterns regarding special education and individualized education programs. *Acad Pediatr.* 2013;13(5):430–435

4. Sneed RC, May WL, Stencel CS. Training of pediatricians in care of physical disabilities in children with special health needs: results of a two-state survey of practicing pediatricians and national resident training programs. *Pediatrics.* 2000;105(3, pt 1): 554–561

5. Symons AB, McGuigan D, Akl EA. A curriculum to teach medical students to care for people with disabilities: development and initial implementation. *BMC Med Educ.* 2009; 9:78

6. Dahl TH. International classification of functioning, disability and health: an introduction and discussion of its potential impact on rehabilitation services and research. *J Rehabil Med.* 2002;34(5):201–204

7. World Health Organization. *International Classification of Functioning, Disability and Health: Toward a Common Language for Functioning, Disability and Health.* Geneva, Switzerland: World Health Organization; 2002

8. Cieza A, Brockow T, Ewert T, et al. Linking health-status measurements to the international classification of functioning, disability and health. *J Rehabil Med.* 2002;34(5):205–210

9. Houtrow AJ, Zima BT. Framing childhood mental disorders within the context of disability. *Disabil Health J.* 2017;10(4):461–466

10. Almansa J, Ayuso-Mateos JL, Garin O, et al; MHADIE Consortium. The International classification of functioning, disability and health: development of capacity and performance scales. *J Clin Epidemiol.* 2011;64(12):1400–1411

11. Lollar DJ, Simeonsson RJ. Diagnosis to function: classification for children and youths. *J Dev Behav Pediatr.* 2005;26(4): 323–330

12. Schneidert M, Hurst R, Miller J, Ustün B. The role of environment in the International Classification of Functioning, Disability and Health (ICF). *Disabil Rehabil.* 2003;25(11–12):588–595

13. Gannotti ME, Christy JB, Heathcock JC, Kolobe TH. A path model for evaluating dosing parameters for children with cerebral palsy. *Phys Ther.* 2014;94(3): 411–421

14. Halfon N, Houtrow A, Larson K, Newacheck PW. The changing landscape of disability in childhood. *Future Child.* 2012;22(1):13–42

15. Houtrow AJ, Larson K, Olson LM, Newacheck PW, Halfon N. Changing trends of childhood disability, 2001-2011. *Pediatrics.* 2014;134(3):530–538

16. Boyle CA, Boulet S, Schieve LA, et al. Trends in the prevalence of developmental disabilities in US children, 1997-2008. *Pediatrics.* 2011; 127(6):1034–1042

17. Palisano RJ, Chiarello LA, King GA, Novak I, Stoner T, Fiss A. Participation-based therapy for children with physical disabilities. *Disabil Rehabil.* 2012; 34(12):1041–1052

18. Stineman MG, Streim JE. The biopsycho-ecological paradigm: a foundational theory for medicine. *PM R.* 2010;2(11): 1035–1045

19. Myers SM, Johnson CP; American Academy of Pediatrics Council on Children With Disabilities. Management of children with autism spectrum disorders. *Pediatrics.* 2007;120(5): 1162–1182

20. Hong CS, Palmer K. Occupational therapy and physiotherapy for children with disabilities. *J Fam Health Care.* 2003;13(2):38–40

21. Section on Pediatrics American Physical Therapy Association. *Dosing Considerations: Recommending School-Based Physical Therapy Interventions Under IDEA Resource Manual.* Alexandria, VA: Subcommittee on Dosing; 2014

22. Gee BM, Lloyd K, Devine N, et al. Dosage parameters in pediatric outcome studies reported in 9 peer-reviewed occupational therapy journals from 2008 to 2014: a content analysis. *Rehabil Res Pract.* 2016;2016:3580789

23. American Speech Language Hearing Association. ASHA practice policy: scope of practice in speech-language pathology. 2016. Available at: www.asha.org/policy/SP2016-00343/. Accessed September 6, 2016

24. Desch LW, Gaebler-Spira D; Council on Children With Disabilities. Prescribing assistive-technology systems: focus on children with impaired communication. *Pediatrics.* 2008;121(6):1271–1280

25. Mezoff EA. Focus on diagnosis: dysphagia. *Pediatr Rev.* 2012;33(11): 518–520

26. Palisano RJ, Begnoche DM, Chiarello LA, Bartlett DJ, McCoy SW, Chang HJ. Amount and focus of physical therapy and occupational therapy for young children with cerebral palsy. *Phys Occup Ther Pediatr.* 2012;32(4):368–382

27. American Physical Therapy Association. Levels of patient access to physical therapist services in the states. 2016. Available at: http://www.apta.org/uploadedFiles/APTAorg/Advocacy/State/Issues/Direct_Access/DirectAccessbyState.pdf. Accessed September 6, 2016

28. Houtrow AJ, Okumura MJ, Hilton JF, Rehm RS. Profiling health and health-related services for children with special health care needs with and without disabilities. *Acad Pediatr.* 2011; 11(6):508–516

29. Magnusson D, Palta M, McManus B, Benedict RE, Durkin MS. Capturing unmet therapy need among young children with developmental delay using national survey data. *Acad Pediatr.* 2016;16(2):145–153

30. McManus BM, Prosser LA, Gannotti ME. Which children are not getting their needs for therapy or mobility aids met? Data from the 2009-2010 National Survey of Children with Special Health Care Needs. *Phys Ther.* 2016;96(2): 222–231

31. Miller AR, Armstrong RW, Mâsse LC, Klassen AF, Shen J, O'Donnell ME. Waiting for child developmental and rehabilitation services: an overview of issues and needs. *Dev Med Child Neurol.* 2008;50(11):815–821

32. Kogan MD, Newacheck PW, Honberg L, Strickland B. Association between underinsurance and access to care among children with special health care needs in the United States. *Pediatrics.* 2005;116(5):1162–1169

33. Kogan MD, Newacheck PW, Blumberg SJ, et al. Underinsurance among children in the United States. *N Engl J Med.* 2010;363(9):841–851

34. Huang ZJ, Kogan MD, Yu SM, Strickland B. Delayed or forgone care among children with special health care needs: an analysis of the 2001 National Survey of Children with Special Health Care Needs. *Ambul Pediatr.* 2005;5(1):60–67

35. Council on Children with Disabilities and Medical Home Implementation Project Advisory Committee. Patient- and family-centered care coordination: a framework for integrating care for children and youth across multiple systems. *Pediatrics.* 2014;133(5). Available at: www.pediatrics.org/cgi/content/full/133/5/e1451

36. Adams RC, Tapia C; Council on Children with Disabilities. Early intervention, IDEA Part C services, and the medical home: collaboration for best practice and best outcomes. *Pediatrics.* 2013; 132(4). Available at: www.pediatrics.org/cgi/content/full/132/4/e1073

37. Lipkin PH, Okamoto J; Council on Children with Disabilities; Council on School Health. The Individuals With Disabilities Education Act (IDEA) for children with special educational needs. *Pediatrics.* 2015;136(6). Available at: www.pediatrics.org/cgi/content/full/136/6/e1650

38. Lobo MA, Paul DA, Mackley A, Maher J, Galloway JC. Instability of delay classification and determination of early intervention eligibility in the first two years of life. *Res Dev Disabil.* 2014; 35(1):117–126

39. McCormick MC, Brooks-Gunn J, Buka SL, et al. Early intervention in low birth weight premature infants: results at 18 years of age for the Infant Health and Development Program. *Pediatrics.* 2006;117(3):771–780

40. Walker SP, Chang SM, Vera-Hernández M, Grantham-McGregor S. Early childhood stimulation benefits adult competence and reduces violent behavior. *Pediatrics.* 2011;127(5): 849–857

41. Reynolds AJ, Temple JA, Robertson DL, Mann EA. Long-term effects of an early childhood intervention on educational achievement and juvenile arrest: a 15-year follow-up of low-income children in public schools. *JAMA.* 2001;285(18): 2339–2346

42. Park HY, Maitra K, Achon J, Loyola E, Rincón M. Effects of early intervention on mental or neuromusculoskeletal and movement-related functions in children born low birthweight or preterm: a meta-analysis. *Am J Occup Ther.* 2014; 68(3):268–276

43. Khetani M, Graham JE, Alvord C. Community participation patterns among preschool-aged children who have received Part C early intervention services. *Child Care Health Dev.* 2013; 39(4):490–499

44. Kingsley K, Mailloux Z. Evidence for the effectiveness of different service delivery models in early intervention services. *Am J Occup Ther.* 2013;67(4): 431–436

45. Council on Children With Disabilities; Section on Developmental Behavioral Pediatrics; Bright Futures Steering Committee; Medical Home Initiatives for Children With Special Needs Project Advisory Committee. Identifying infants and young children with developmental disorders in the medical home: an algorithm for developmental surveillance and screening [published correction appears in *Pediatrics.* 2006; 118(4):1808–1809]. *Pediatrics.* 2006; 118(1):405–420

46. Noritz GH, Murphy NA; Neuromotor Screening Expert Panel. Motor delays: early identification and evaluation [published correction appears in *Pediatrics.* 2017;140(3):e20172081]. *Pediatrics.* 2013;131(6). Available at: www.pediatrics.org/cgi/content/full/131/6/e2016

47. Individuals with Disabilities Education Act. Statute and regulations. Available at: https://sites.ed.gov/idea/statuteregulations/. Accessed January 7, 2018

48. Aron L, Loprest P. Disability and the education system. *Future Child.* 2012; 22(1):97–122

49. Cartwright JD; American Academy of Pediatrics Council on Children With Disabilities. Provision of educationally related services for children and adolescents with chronic diseases and disabling conditions. *Pediatrics.* 2007; 119(6):1218–1223

50. Zuckerman B, Sandel M, Smith L, Lawton E. Why pediatricians need lawyers to keep children healthy. *Pediatrics.* 2004;114(1):224–228

51. Murphy NA, Carbone PS; American Academy of Pediatrics Council on Children With Disabilities. Promoting the participation of children with disabilities in sports, recreation, and physical activities. *Pediatrics.* 2008; 121(5):1057–1061

52. McAllister JW, Presler E, Cooley WC. Practice-based care coordination: a medical home essential. *Pediatrics.* 2007;120(3). Available at: www.pediatrics.org/cgi/content/full/120/3/e723

53. Park EY, Kim WH. Meta-analysis of the effect of strengthening interventions in individuals with cerebral palsy. *Res Dev Disabil.* 2014;35(2):239–249

54. Dewar R, Love S, Johnston LM. Exercise interventions improve postural control in children with cerebral palsy: a systematic review. *Dev Med Child Neurol.* 2015;57(6):504–520

55. Case-Smith J, Frolek Clark GJ, Schlabach TL. Systematic review of interventions used in occupational therapy to promote motor performance for children ages birth-5 years. *Am J Occup Ther.* 2013;67(4):413–424

56. Chen YN, Liao SF, Su LF, Huang HY, Lin CC, Wei TS. The effect of long-term conventional physical therapy and independent predictive factors analysis in children with cerebral palsy. *Dev Neurorehabil.* 2013;16(5):357–362

57. Franki I, Desloovere K, De Cat J, et al. The evidence-base for basic physical therapy techniques targeting lower limb function in children with cerebral palsy: a systematic review using the International Classification of Functioning, Disability and Health as a conceptual framework. *J Rehabil Med.* 2012;44(5):385–395

58. Law MC, Darrah J, Pollock N, et al. Focus on function: a cluster, randomized controlled trial comparing child- versus context-focused intervention for young children with cerebral palsy. *Dev Med Child Neurol.* 2011;53(7):621–629

59. Novak I, Cusick A, Lannin N. Occupational therapy home programs for cerebral palsy: double-blind, randomized, controlled trial. *Pediatrics.* 2009;124(4). Available at: www.pediatrics.org/cgi/content/full/124/4/e606

60. Novak I, McIntyre S, Morgan C, et al. A systematic review of interventions for children with cerebral palsy: state of the evidence. *Dev Med Child Neurol.* 2013;55(10):885–910

61. McIntyre LL. Parent training for young children with developmental disabilities: randomized controlled trial. *Am J Ment Retard.* 2008;113(5):356–368

62. Taub E, Uswatte G. Importance for CP rehabilitation of transfer of motor improvement to everyday life. *Pediatrics.* 2014;133(1). Available at: www.pediatrics.org/cgi/content/full/133/1/e215

63. Basu AP. Early intervention after perinatal stroke: opportunities and challenges. *Dev Med Child Neurol.* 2014; 56(6):516–521

64. Yang JF, Livingstone D, Brunton K, et al. Training to enhance walking in children with cerebral palsy: are we missing the window of opportunity? *Semin Pediatr Neurol.* 2013;20(2):106–115

65. Bower E, McLellan DL, Arney J, Campbell MJ. A randomised controlled trial of different intensities of physiotherapy and different goal-setting procedures in 44 children with cerebral palsy. *Dev Med Child Neurol.* 1996;38(3):226–237

66. Thornton A, Licari M, Reid S, Armstrong J, Fallows R, Elliott C. Cognitive Orientation to (Daily) Occupational Performance intervention leads to improvements in impairments, activity and participation in children with developmental coordination disorder. *Disabil Rehabil.* 2016;38(10):979–986

67. Wade DT. Goal setting in rehabilitation: an overview of what, why and how. *Clin Rehabil.* 2009;23(4):291–295

68. Sakzewski L, Carlon S, Shields N, Ziviani J, Ware RS, Boyd RN. Impact of intensive upper limb rehabilitation on quality of life: a randomized trial in children with unilateral cerebral palsy. *Dev Med Child Neurol.* 2012;54(5):415–423

69. Kreider CM, Bendixen RM, Huang YY, Lim Y. Review of occupational therapy intervention research in the practice area of children and youth 2009-2013. *Am J Occup Ther.* 2014;68(2):e61–e73

70. Case-Smith J. Systematic review of interventions to promote social-emotional development in young children with or at risk for disability. *Am J Occup Ther.* 2013;67(4):395–404

71. Morgan C, Novak I, Badawi N. Enriched environments and motor outcomes in cerebral palsy: systematic review and meta-analysis. *Pediatrics.* 2013;132(3). Available at: www.pediatrics.org/cgi/content/full/132/3/e735

72. Gillett J. The Pediatric Acquired Brain Injury Community Outreach Program (PABICOP) - an innovative comprehensive model of care for children and youth with an acquired brain injury. *NeuroRehabilitation.* 2004; 19(3):207–218

73. Ziring PR, Brazdziunas D, Cooley WC; American Academy of Pediatrics; Committee on Children with Disabilities. The treatment of neurologically impaired children using patterning. *Pediatrics.* 1999;104(5, pt 1):1149–1151. Reaffirmed May 2018

74. Zimmer M, Desch L; Section On Complementary And Integrative Medicine; Council on Children with Disabilities; American Academy of Pediatrics. Sensory integration therapies for children with developmental and behavioral disorders. *Pediatrics.* 2012;129(6): 1186–1189

75. Bailes AF, Greve K, Burch CK, Reder R, Lin L, Huth MM. The effect of suit wear during an intensive therapy program in children with cerebral palsy. *Pediatr Phys Ther.* 2011;23(2):136–142

76. Lacey DJ, Stolfi A, Pilati LE. Effects of hyperbaric oxygen on motor function in children with cerebral palsy. *Ann Neurol.* 2012;72(5):695–703

77. Novak I, Badawi N. Last breath: effectiveness of hyperbaric oxygen treatment for cerebral palsy. *Ann Neurol.* 2012;72(5):633–634

78. Goldfarb C, Genore L, Hunt C, et al. Hyperbaric oxygen therapy for the treatment of children and youth with autism spectrum disorders: an evidence-based systematic review. *Res Autism Spectr Disord.* 2016;29–30:1–7

79. Weitlauf AS, Sathe N, McPheeters ML, Warren ZE. Interventions targeting sensory challenges in autism spectrum disorder: a systematic review. *Pediatrics.* 2017;139(6):e20170347

80. McDonagh MS, Morgan D, Carson S, Russman BS. Systematic review of hyperbaric oxygen therapy for cerebral palsy: the state of the evidence. *Dev Med Child Neurol.* 2007;49(12):942–947

81. Collet JP, Vanasse M, Marois P, et al; HBO-CP Research Group. Hyperbaric oxygen for children with cerebral palsy: a randomised multicentre trial. *Lancet.* 2001;357(9256):582–586

82. McClafferty H, Vohra S, Bailey M, et al; Section on Integrative Medicine. Pediatric integrative medicine. *Pediatrics.* 2017;140(3):e20171961

83. Meyer-Heim A, van Hedel HJ. Robot-assisted and computer-enhanced therapies for children with cerebral palsy: current state and clinical implementation. *Semin Pediatr Neurol.* 2013;20(2):139–145

84. Case-Smith J, Weaver LL, Fristad MA. A systematic review of sensory processing interventions for children with autism spectrum disorders. *Autism.* 2015;19(2):133–148

85. Fasoli SE, Ladenheim B, Mast J, Krebs HI. New horizons for robot-assisted therapy in pediatrics. *Am J Phys Med Rehabil.* 2012;91(11, suppl 3):S280–S289

86. Chen YP, Pope S, Tyler D, Warren GL. Effectiveness of constraint-induced movement therapy on upper-extremity function in children with cerebral palsy: a systematic review and meta-analysis

of randomized controlled trials. *Clin Rehabil*. 2014;28(10):939–953

87. Facchin P, Rosa-Rizzotto M, Visonà Dalla Pozza L, et al; GIPCI Study Group. Multisite trial comparing the efficacy of constraint-induced movement therapy with that of bimanual intensive training in children with hemiplegic cerebral palsy: postintervention results. *Am J Phys Med Rehabil*. 2011;90(7):539–553

88. Huang HH, Fetters L, Hale J, McBride A. Bound for success: a systematic review of constraint-induced movement therapy in children with cerebral palsy supports improved arm and hand use. *Phys Ther*. 2009;89(11):1126–1141

89. Sakzewski L, Ziviani J, Abbott DF, Macdonell RA, Jackson GD, Boyd RN. Equivalent retention of gains at 1 year after training with constraint-induced or bimanual therapy in children with unilateral cerebral palsy. *Neurorehabil Neural Repair*. 2011;25(7):664–671

90. Snider L, Korner-Bitensky N, Kammann C, Warner S, Saleh M. Horseback riding as therapy for children with cerebral palsy: is there evidence of its effectiveness? *Phys Occup Ther Pediatr*. 2007;27(2):5–23

91. Sterba JA. Does horseback riding therapy or therapist-directed hippotherapy rehabilitate children with cerebral palsy? *Dev Med Child Neurol*. 2007;49(1):68–73

92. Sterba JA, Rogers BT, France AP, Vokes DA. Horseback riding in children with cerebral palsy: effect on gross motor function. *Dev Med Child Neurol*. 2002; 44(5):301–308

93. Whalen CN, Case-Smith J. Therapeutic effects of horseback riding therapy on gross motor function in children with cerebral palsy: a systematic review. *Phys Occup Ther Pediatr*. 2012;32(3): 229–242

94. Zadnikar M, Kastrin A. Effects of hippotherapy and therapeutic horseback riding on postural control or balance in children with cerebral palsy: a meta-analysis. *Dev Med Child Neurol*. 2011;53(8):684–691

95. Lee J, Yun CK. Effects of hippotherapy on the thickness of deep abdominal muscles and activity of daily living in children with intellectual disabilities. *J Phys Ther Sci*. 2017;29(4):779–782

96. Sakzewski L, Ziviani J, Boyd RN. Efficacy of upper limb therapies for unilateral cerebral palsy: a meta-analysis. *Pediatrics*. 2014;133(1). Available at: www.pediatrics.org/cgi/content/full/133/1/e175

97. Tepas JJ III, Leaphart CL, Pieper P, et al. The effect of delay in rehabilitation on outcome of severe traumatic brain injury. *J Pediatr Surg*. 2009;44(2): 368–372

98. Majnemer A, Shikako-Thomas K, Lach L, et al; QUALA Group. Rehabilitation service utilization in children and youth with cerebral palsy. *Child Care Health Dev*. 2014;40(2):275–282

99. Bailes AF, Reder R, Burch C. Development of guidelines for determining frequency of therapy services in a pediatric medical setting. *Pediatr Phys Ther*. 2008;20(2):194–198

100. Palisano RJ, Murr S. Intensity of therapy services: what are the considerations? *Phys Occup Ther Pediatr*. 2009;29(2): 107–112

101. Adams RC, Levy SE; Council on Children With Disabilities. Shared decision-making and children with disabilities: pathways to consensus. *Pediatrics*. 2017;139(6):e20170956

102. Kwon JY, Chang HJ, Yi SH, Lee JY, Shin HY, Kim YH. Effect of hippotherapy on gross motor function in children with cerebral palsy: a randomized controlled trial. *J Altern Complement Med*. 2015; 21(1):15–21

103. Rosenbaum S, Wise PH. Crossing the Medicaid-private insurance divide: the case of EPSDT. *Health Aff (Millwood)*. 2007;26(2):382–393

104. Goldstein MM, Rosenbaum S. From EPSDT to EHBs: the future of pediatric coverage design under government financed health insurance. *Pediatrics*. 2013;131(suppl 2):S142–S148

Prevention of Drowning

- *Policy Statement*

POLICY STATEMENT Organizational Principles to Guide and Define the Child Health Care System and/or Improve the Health of all Children

American Academy of Pediatrics

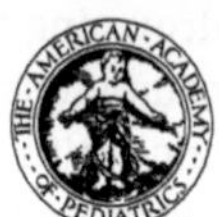

DEDICATED TO THE HEALTH OF ALL CHILDREN™

Prevention of Drowning

Sarah A. Denny, MD, FAAP,[a] Linda Quan, MD, FAAP,[b] Julie Gilchrist, MD, FAAP,[c] Tracy McCallin, MD, FAAP,[d,e] Rohit Shenoi, MD, FAAP,[e,f] Shabana Yusuf, MD, Med, FAAP,[e,f] Benjamin Hoffman, MD, FAAP,[g] Jeffrey Weiss, MD, FAAP,[h] COUNCIL ON INJURY, VIOLENCE, AND POISON PREVENTION

abstract

Drowning is a leading cause of injury-related death in children. In 2017, drowning claimed the lives of almost 1000 US children younger than 20 years. A number of strategies are available to prevent these tragedies. As educators and advocates, pediatricians can play an important role in the prevention of drowning.

[a]College of Medicine, The Ohio State University and Nationwide Children's Hospital, Columbus, Ohio; [b]School of Medicine, University of Washington and Seattle Children's Hospital, Seattle, Washington; [c]US Public Health Service, Rockville, Maryland; [d]Children's Hospital of San Antonio, San Antonio, Texas; [e]Baylor College of Medicine and [f]Texas Children's Hospital, Houston, Texas; [g]Oregon Health and Science University and Doernbecher Children's Hospital, Portland, Oregon; and [h]College of Medicine, University of Arizona and Phoenix Children's Hospital, Phoenix, Arizona

Dr Denny led the authorship group; Drs Quan, Gilchrist, McCallin, Yusuf, and Shenoi contributed sections; Dr Hoffman provided significant early review; Dr Weiss authored the previous policy statement that formed the basis of this document; and all authors approved the final manuscript as submitted.

This document is copyrighted and is property of the American Academy of Pediatrics and its Board of Directors. All authors have filed conflict of interest statements with the American Academy of Pediatrics. Any conflicts have been resolved through a process approved by the Board of Directors. The American Academy of Pediatrics has neither solicited nor accepted any commercial involvement in the development of the content of this publication.

Policy statements from the American Academy of Pediatrics benefit from expertise and resources of liaisons and internal (AAP) and external reviewers. However, policy statements from the American Academy of Pediatrics may not reflect the views of the liaisons or the organizations or government agencies that they represent.

The guidance in this statement does not indicate an exclusive course of treatment or serve as a standard of medical care. Variations, taking into account individual circumstances, may be appropriate.

All policy statements from the American Academy of Pediatrics automatically expire 5 years after publication unless reaffirmed, revised, or retired at or before that time.

DOI: https://doi.org/10.1542/peds.2019-0850

Address correspondence to Sarah A. Denny, MD, FAAP. E-mail: sarah.denny@nationwidechildrens.org

To cite: Denny SA, Quan L, Gilchrist J, et al. AAP COUNCIL ON INJURY, VIOLENCE, AND POISON PREVENTION. Prevention of Drowning. *Pediatrics.* 2019;143(5):e20190850

BACKGROUND

Drowning is the leading cause of injury death in US children 1 to 4 years of age and the third leading cause of unintentional injury death among US children and adolescents 5 to 19 years of age.[1] In 2017, drowning claimed the lives of almost 1000 US children. Fortunately, childhood unintentional drowning fatality rates have decreased steadily from 2.68 per 100 000 in 1985 to 1.11 per 100 000 in 2017. Rates of drowning death vary with age, sex, and race and/or ethnicity, with toddlers and male adolescents at highest risk. After 1 year of age, male children of all ages are at greater risk of drowning than female children. Overall, African American children have the highest drowning fatality rates, followed in order by American Indian and/or Alaskan native, white, Asian American and/or Pacific Islander, and Hispanic children. For the period 2013–2017, the highest drowning death rates were seen in white male children 0 to 4 years of age (3.44 per 100 000), American Indian and/or Alaskan native children 0 through 4 years (3.58), and African American male adolescents 15 to 19 years of age (4.06 per 100 000).[1]

Drowning is also a significant source of morbidity for children. In 2017, an estimated 8700 children younger than 20 years of age visited a hospital emergency department for a drowning event, and 25% of those children were hospitalized or transferred for further care.[1] Most victims of nonfatal drowning recover fully with no neurologic deficits, but severe long-term neurologic deficits are seen with extended submersion times (>6 minutes), prolonged resuscitation efforts, and lack of early bystander-initiated cardiopulmonary resuscitation (CPR).[2–4]

The American Academy of Pediatrics issues this revised policy statement because of new information and research regarding (1) populations at increased risk, (2) racial and sociodemographic disparities in drowning rates, (3) water competency (water-safety knowledge and attitudes, basic swim skills, and response to a swimmer in trouble),[5,6] (4) when children are in and around water (the need for close, constant, attentive, and capable adult supervision and life jacket use in children and adults), (5) when children are not expected to be around water (the importance of physical barriers to prevent drowning), and (6) the drowning chain of survival and importance of bystander CPR (Table 1).

CLASSIFICATION OF DROWNING

In 2002, the World Congress on Drowning and the World Health Organization revised the definition of drowning to "the process of experiencing respiratory impairment from submersion/immersion in liquid." Drowning outcomes are classified as "death," "no morbidity," or "morbidity" (further divided into "moderately disabled," "severely disabled," "vegetative state/coma," and "brain death"). The drowning process is a continuum that can be interrupted by rescue at any point in that process, with varying sequelae from no symptoms to death. Terms such as wet, dry, secondary, active, near, passive, and silent drowning should not be used. The 2002 revised definition and classification is more consistent with other medical conditions and injuries and should help in drowning surveillance and collection of more reliable and comprehensive epidemiological information.[7]

TABLE 1 Top Tips for Pediatricians

Assess all children for drowning risk on the basis of risk and age and prioritize evidence-based strategies:
- barriers; - supervision; - swim lessons; - life jackets; and - CPR.

POPULATIONS WITH INCREASED DROWNING RISK

Certain populations, because of behavior, skill, environment, or underlying medical condition, are at increased risk of drowning.

Toddlers

For the period 2013–2017, the highest rate of drowning occurred in the 0- to 4-year age group (2.19 per 100 000 population), with children 12 to 36 months of age being at highest risk (3.31). Most infants drown in bathtubs and buckets, whereas the majority of preschool-aged children drown in swimming pools.[8] The primary problem for this young age group is lack of barriers to prevent unanticipated, unsupervised access to water, including in swimming pools, hot tubs and spas, bathtubs, natural bodies of water, and standing water in homes (buckets, tubs, and toilets). The Consumer Product Safety Commission (CPSC) found that 69% of children younger than 5 years of age were not expected to be at or in the pool at the time of a drowning incident.[9]

Adolescents

Adolescents (15–19 years of age) have the second highest fatal drowning rate. In this age group, just less than three-quarters of all drownings occur in natural water settings, and this age group makes up half of childhood drownings in natural water.[10] In 2016, Safe Kids Worldwide reported that the natural water fatal drowning rate for adolescents 15 to 17 years old was more than 3 times higher than that for children 5 to 9 years old and twice the rate for children younger than 5 years of age.[11] The increased risk for fatal drowning in adolescents can be attributed to multiple factors, including overestimation of skills, underestimation of dangerous situations, engaging in high-risk and impulsive behaviors, and substance use.[12] Alcohol is a leading risk factor, contributing to 30% to 70% of recreational water deaths among US adolescents and adults.[13]

UNDERLYING MEDICAL CONDITIONS

Epilepsy

Drowning is the most common cause of death from unintentional injury for people with epilepsy,[14] and children with epilepsy are at greater risk of drowning, both in bathtubs and in swimming pools.[15] The relative risk of fatal and nonfatal drowning in patients with epilepsy varies greatly but is 7.5- to 10-fold higher than that in children without seizures[15,16] and varies with age, severity of illness, degree of exposure to water, and level of supervision.[15–17] Parents and caregivers of children with active epilepsy should provide direct supervision around water at all times, including swimming pools and bathtubs. Whenever possible, children with epilepsy should shower instead of bathe[17] and swim only at locations where there is a lifeguard. Children with poorly controlled epilepsy should have a discussion with their neurologist or pediatrician before any swim activity.

Autism

Children with autism spectrum disorder (ASD) are also at increased risk of drowning,[18] especially those younger than 15 years of age[18] and those with greater degrees of intellectual disability.[19] Wandering is the most commonly reported behavior leading to drowning, accounting for nearly 74% of fatal drowning incidents among children with autism.[20]

Cardiac Arrhythmias

Exertion while swimming can trigger arrhythmia among individuals with long QT syndrome.[21] Although the condition is rare and such cases represent a small percentage of drownings, long QT syndrome, as well as Brugada syndrome and catecholaminergic polymorphic ventricular tachycardia, should be considered as a possible cause for unexplained submersion injuries among proficient swimmers in low-risk settings.[22]

SOCIODEMOGRAPHIC FACTORS

There continue to be significant racial and socioeconomic disparities in drowning rates among children. For many, cultural beliefs and traditions may prevent children from swimming.[23,24] Furthermore, for some religious and ethnic groups, single-sex aquatic settings are required,[25] and clothing that protects modesty according to religious norms may not be allowed in some pools. Socioeconomically, the multiple swim lessons required to achieve basic water competency can be costly or difficult given limited access and transportation. Moreover, decreased municipal funding for swimming pools, for swimming programs, and for lifeguards has limited access to swim lessons and safe water recreational sites for many communities.

These barriers may be surmounted through community-based programs targeting high-risk groups by providing free or low-cost swim lessons, developing special programs to address cultural concerns as well as developing swim lessons for youth with developmental disabilities, changing pool policies to meet the needs of specific communities, using culturally and linguistically appropriate instructors to deliver swim lessons, and working with both health care and faith communities to refer patients and their families to swim programs.[25–27]

WATER COMPETENCY, SWIM LESSONS, AND SWIM SKILLS

Water competency is the ability to anticipate, avoid, and survive common drowning situations.[6] The components of water competency include water-safety awareness, basic swim skills, and the ability to recognize and respond to a swimmer in trouble. Swim lessons and swim skills alone cannot prevent drowning. Learning to swim needs to be seen as a component of water competency that also includes knowledge and awareness of local hazards and/or risks and of one's own limitations; how to wear a life jacket (previously referred to as "wearable personal flotation device"); and ability to recognize and respond to a swimmer in distress, call for help, and perform safe rescue and CPR.[5]

Evidence reveals that many children older than 1 year will benefit from swim lessons.[28] Swim lessons are increasingly available for a wide range of children, including those with various health conditions and disabilities such as ASD. A parent or caregiver's decision about when to initiate swim lessons must be individualized on the basis of a variety of factors, including comfort with being in water, health status, emotional maturity, and physical and cognitive limitations. Although swim lessons provide 1 layer of protection from drowning, swim lessons do not "drown proof" a child, and parents must continue to provide barriers to prevent unintended access when not in the water and closely supervise children when in and around water.

In contrast, infants younger than 1 year are developmentally unable to learn the complex movements, such as breathing, necessary to swim. They may manifest reflexive swimming movement under the water but cannot effectively raise their heads to breathe.[29] There is no evidence to suggest that infant swimming programs for those younger than 1 year are beneficial.

Basic swim skills include ability to enter the water, surface, turn around, propel oneself for at least 25 yards, float on or tread water, and exit the water.[30] Importantly, performance of these water-survival skills, usually learned in a pool, is affected by the aquatic environment (water temperature, water depth, water movement, clothing, and distance), and demonstration of skills in 1 aquatic environment may not transfer to another. There is tremendous variability among swim lessons, and not every program will be right for each child. Parents and caregivers should investigate options for swim lessons in their community before enrollment to make sure that the program meets their needs and the needs of the child. High-quality swim lessons provide more experiential training, including swimming in clothes, in life jackets, falling in, and practicing self-rescue. Achieving basic water-competency swim skills requires multiple lessons, and acquisition of water competency is a protracted process that involves learning in conjunction with developmental maturation. There is a need for a broad and coordinated research agenda to address not only the efficacy of swim lessons for children age 1 to 4 years but also the many components of water competency for the child and parent or caregiver.

DROWNING-PREVENTION STRATEGIES

The Haddon Matrix paradigm for injury prevention is used to identify interventions aimed at changing the environment, the individual at risk, and/or the agent of injury (in this case, water).[31] Experts generally recommend that multiple "layers of protection" be used to prevent drowning because it is unlikely that any single strategy will prevent drowning deaths and injuries. The Haddon Matrix (Table 2) reveals examples of interventions before the drowning event, during the drowning event, and after the drowning event at the levels of the individual, environment, and policy. Five major interventions are evidence based: 4-sided pool fencing, life jackets, swim lessons, supervision, and lifeguards (with descending levels of evidence).

Installation of 4-sided fencing (at least 4 ft tall) with self-closing and self-latching gates that completely isolates the pool from the house and yard is the most studied and effective drowning-prevention strategy for the young child, preventing more than 50% of swimming-pool drownings of young children.[32,33] Life jackets are now also well proven to prevent drowning fatalities. Some data reveal that swim lessons may lower drowning rates among children,[27] including those 1 to 4 years of age.[28] Lifeguards and CPR training also appear to be effective.[2,4,34–36] However, data regarding the value of other potential preventive strategies, such as pool covers and pool alarms, are lacking. Interventions to prevent drowning are discussed in detail in the accompanying technical report (available online soon).

Inadequate supervision is often cited as a contributing factor for childhood drowning, especially for younger children.[11,37,38] Adequate supervision, described as close, constant, and attentive supervision of young children in or around any water, is a primary and absolutely essential preventive strategy.[27] For beginning swimmers, adequate supervision is "touch supervision," in which the supervising adult is within arm's reach of the child so he or she can pull the child out of the water if the child's head becomes submerged under water. Evaluated interventions shown to increase the quality of supervision include swim lessons in which the need for continued parental supervision is emphasized,[39] and a study in Bangladesh revealed that adult supervision, in addition to the physical barrier of playpens, significantly reduced the risk of drowning in children ages 1 to 5 years.[27] Supervision should include being capable of recognizing and responding appropriately to a child in distress. Supervision is critical for safety in children with ASD and other disabilities. The National Autism Association's Big Red Safety Box[40] contains information for parents, schools, and first responders and suggests a safety plan in public places where there is a handoff of supervision so that children with ASD and other disabilities do not wander off.

Although supervision is an essential layer of protection when children are

TABLE 2 Haddon Matrix for Drowning-Prevention Strategies

	Personal	Equipment	Physical Environment	Social Environment
Before the event	**Provide close, constant, and attentive supervision of children and poor swimmers**	**Install 4-sided fencing that isolates the pool from the house and yard**	**Swim where lifeguards are present**	Mandate 4-sided residential pool fencing
	Clear handoff supervision responsibilities	Install self-closing and latching gates	Attend to warning signage	Mandate life jacket wear
	Develop water competency, including water-safety knowledge, basic swim skills, and ability to recognize and respond to a swimmer in trouble	**Wear life jackets**	Swim at designated swim sites	Adopt the Model Aquatic Health Code
	Evaluate preexisting health condition	Install compliant pool drains	Remove toys from pools when not in use to reduce temptation for children to enter the pool	Increase availability of lifeguards
	Know how to choose and fit a life jacket	Install door locks	Empty water buckets and wading pools	Increase access to affordable and culturally compatible swim lessons
	Avoid substance use	Enclosures for open bodies of water	—	Close high-risk waters during high-risk times
	Know the water's hazards, conditions	Promote life jacket–loaner programs	—	Develop designated open-water swim sites
	Swim at a designated swim site	Role model life jacket use by adults	—	Enforce boating under the influence laws
	Learn CPR	Make rescue devices available at swim sites	—	—
	Take a boater education course	Phone access to call for help	—	—
	—	Ensure functional watercraft	—	—
Event	Water-survival skills	Rescue device available	—	EMS system
After the event	**Early bystander CPR**	AED	—	Advanced medical care
	Bystander response	Rescue equipment	—	—

The Model Aquatic Health Code provides guidelines and standards for equipment, for staffing and training, and for monitoring swimming pools. Bold indicates the most evidence-based interventions. AED, automated external defibrillator.

expected to be in or around the water, barriers must be in place to prevent unintended access of children to water during nonswim times. Drowning is silent and only takes a minute. Those children with highest drowning risk are 12 to 36 months of age. Developmentally, they are curious and lack the judgement or awareness of the dangers of water, so barriers, such as 4-sided fencing and door locks, are critical in preventing access when the caregiver is distracted by other children, meal preparation, etc.

The Model Aquatic Health Code,[41] developed by the Centers for Disease Control and Prevention (CDC), is based on science and best practices to help guide policy makers and aquatic leaders on pool and spa safety. The Model Aquatic Health Code provides guidelines and standards for equipment, for staffing and training, and for monitoring swimming pools. Similar attention and effort are needed for open-water swim sites.

DROWNING CHAIN OF SURVIVAL

The drowning chain of survival (Fig 1) refers to a series of steps that, when enacted, attempt to reduce mortality associated with drowning. The steps of the chain are as follows: (1) prevent drowning, (2) recognize distress, (3) provide flotation, (4) remove from water, and (5) provide care as needed. The chain starts with prevention, the most important and effective step to reducing morbidity and mortality from drowning.[42] Rescue and resuscitation of a drowning victim must occur within minutes to save lives and reduce morbidity in nonfatal drownings and underscores the critically time-sensitive role of the parent or supervising adult.

IMPORTANCE OF BYSTANDER CPR

Immediate resuscitation at the submersion site, even before the arrival of emergency medical services (EMS) personnel, is the most effective means to improve outcomes in the event of a drowning incident.[2,3] Prompt initiation of bystander CPR, with a focus on airway and rescue breathing before compressions[43] and activation of prehospital advanced cardiac life support for the pediatric submersion victim, have the greatest impact on survival and prognosis.[4,44] Current guidelines recommend that drowning victims who require any form of resuscitation (including only rescue breaths) be transported to the emergency department for evaluation and monitoring, even if they appear alert with effective cardiopulmonary function at the scene.[43]

PREVENTION OF DROWNING RECOMMENDATIONS

Parents and Caregivers

1. Parents and caregivers should never (even for a moment) leave young children alone or in the care of another child while in or near bathtubs, pools, spas, or wading pools and when near irrigation ditches, ponds, or other open standing water.
2. Parents and caregivers must be aware of drowning risks associated with hazards in the home.
   - Infant bath seats can tip over, and children can slip out of them and drown in even a few inches of water in the bathtub. Infants should always be with an adult when sitting in a bath seat in a bathtub.[45]
   - Water should be emptied from containers, such as pails and buckets, immediately after use.
   - To prevent drowning in toilets, young children should not be left alone in the bathroom, and toilet locks may be helpful.
   - Parents and caregivers should prevent unsupervised access to the bathroom, swimming pool, or open water.
3. Whenever infants and toddlers (or noncompetent swimmers) are in or around water, a supervising adult with swim skills should be within an arm's length, providing constant touch supervision. Even with older children and better swimmers, the eyes and attention of the supervising adult should still be constantly focused on the child. This "water watcher" should not be engaged in other distracting activities that can compromise this attention, including using the telephone (eg, texting), socializing, tending chores, or drinking alcohol, and there needs to be a clear handoff of responsibility from one water watcher to the next. Supervision must be close, constant, and attentive. In case of an emergency, the supervising adult must be able to recognize a child in distress, safely perform a rescue, initiate CPR, and call for help. Parents need to recognize that lifeguards are only 1 layer of protection, and children in and near the water require constant caregiver supervision, even if a lifeguard is present.
4. To prevent unintended access, families should install a 4-ft, 4-sided isolation fence that separates the pool from the house and the rest of the yard with a self-closing, self-latching gate. Detailed guidelines for safety barriers for home pools are available online from the CPSC.[46] Families of children with ASD or other disabilities who are at risk for wandering off should identify local hazards and work with the community on pool fencing and mitigation of hazards.
5. Although data are lacking, families may consider supplemental pool alarms and weight-bearing pool covers as additional layers of protection;

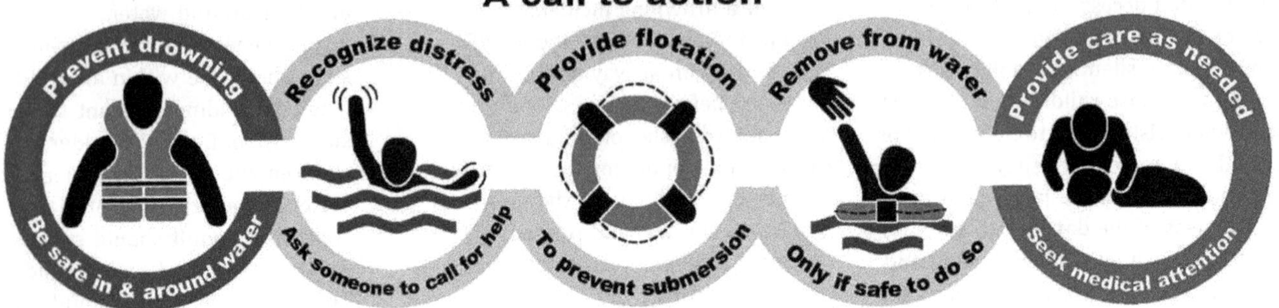

FIGURE 1
Drowning chain of survival. (Reprinted with permission from Szpilman D, Webber J, Quan L, et al. Creating a drowning chain of survival. *Resuscitation.* 2014;85[9]:1151.)

however, neither alarms nor pool covers are a substitute for adequate fencing and adult supervision. Importantly, some types of pool covers, such as thin plastic solar covers, should not be used as a means of protection because they might increase risk of drowning.

6. Parents, caregivers, and pool owners should learn CPR and keep a telephone and rescue equipment approved by the US Coast Guard (eg, life buoys, life jackets, and a reach tool such as a shepherd's crook) poolside. Older children and adolescents should learn CPR.
7. Children and parents should learn to swim and learn water-safety skills. Because children develop at different rates, not all children will be ready to learn to swim at exactly the same age. There is evidence that swim lessons may reduce the risk of drowning, including for those 1 to 4 years of age. A parent's decision about starting swim lessons or water-survival skills training at an early age must be individualized on the basis of the child's frequency of exposure to water, emotional maturity, physical and cognitive limitations, and health concerns related to swimming pools. Parents should be reminded that swim lessons will not drown proof a child of any age. It is critical that swim instructors stress this message as well as the need for constant supervision around water. Swim ability must be considered as only 1 part of water competence and a multilayered protection plan that involves effective pool barriers; close, constant, and attentive supervision; life jacket use; training in CPR and the use of an automated external defibrillator; and lifeguards. Children need to be taught never to swim alone and never to swim without adult supervision.
8. Parents should monitor their child's progress during swim lessons and continue their lessons at least until basic water competence is achieved. Basic swim skills include ability to enter the water, surface, turn around, propel oneself for at least 25 yards, float on or tread water, and exit the water.
9. Any time a young child visits a home or business where access to water exists (eg, pool, hot tub, open water), parents and/or guardians should carefully assess the premises to ensure that basic barriers are in place, such as sliding door locks and pool fences with closed gates in good working order, and ensure that supervision will be consistent with the preceding recommendations.
10. All children and adolescents should be required to wear US Coast Guard–approved life jackets whenever they are in or on watercraft, and all adults should wear life jackets when boating to model safe behavior and to facilitate their ability to help their child in case of emergency. Small children and nonswimmers should wear life jackets when they are near water and when swimming. Parents and caregivers should ensure that any life jacket is approved by the US Coast Guard because many do not meet safety requirements. Information about fitting and choosing US Coast Guard–approved life jackets is available at the US Coast Guard Web site.[47] Parents should not use air-filled swimming aids (such as inflatable arm bands, neck rings, or "floaties") in place of life jackets. These aids can deflate and are not designed to keep swimmers safe.
11. Jumping or diving into water can result in devastating spinal injury. Parents and children should know the depth of the

water and the location of underwater hazards before jumping or diving or permitting children to jump or dive. The first entry into any body of water should be feet first.

12. When selecting an open body of water in which their children will swim, parents should select sites with lifeguards and designated areas for swimming. Even for the strongest of swimmers, it is important to consider weather, tides, waves, and water currents in selecting a safe location for recreational swimming. Swimmers should know what to do in case of rip currents: swim where there is a lifeguard, and if caught in a rip current, remain calm and either swim out of the rip current parallel to the shore (do not try to swim against the current) or tread water until safely out of the current and able to return to shore or signal for help.[48]
13. Parents and children should recognize drowning risks in cold seasons. Children should refrain from walking, skating, or riding on weak or thawing ice on any body of water.

Pediatricians

1. Pediatricians should know the leading causes of drowning in their location so they can appropriately tailor their prevention guidance to caregivers. Pediatricians can provide specific targeted messages by age, sex, high risk of drowning, and geographical location.
2. Children with special health care needs should have tailored anticipatory guidance related to drowning risks. Children with epilepsy, ASD, and cardiac arrhythmias are at particular risk. When swimming or taking a bath, children of any age with epilepsy should be supervised closely by an adult at all times.[15] Children with poorly controlled seizures should discuss water safety with their physician before swim activities.
3. Counseling parents and adolescents about water safety provides an opportunity to stress the problems related to alcohol and drug use during any activity. Specifically, the discussion should include a warning about the increased drowning risk that results when alcohol or illicit drugs are used when swimming or boating. Because male adolescents have high risk of water-based injuries, they warrant extra counseling.
4. Pediatricians should help facilitate a conversation between caregivers and their children about levels of water competency to decrease the frequency of children or parents overestimating swimming skills and equipping older children with the ability to make informed decisions when not in the presence of their parent or guardian.
5. Pediatricians should support the inclusion of CPR training in high school health classes.

COMMUNITY INTERVENTIONS AND ADVOCACY OPPORTUNITIES

Pediatricians

1. Pediatricians should work with legislators and serve as a voice for children to pass policy that decreases the risk of drowning, including, but not limited to, policy on fencing, boating, life jackets, safety of aquatic environments, boating under the influence, and EMS systems. Pediatricians should partner with public health and policy leaders to address the issue of childhood drowning by implementing effective evidence-based interventions.
2. Pediatricians should use the term "nonfatal drowning" (rather than "near drowning") when speaking to families and the media to avoid confusion and misconceptions associated with the other terms previously used. There has been much misinformation circulated in recent years regarding dry drowning and secondary drowning.[49] Pediatricians should educate caregivers that dry and secondary drowning are not medically accurate terms. Pediatricians can address parental concerns by providing reassurance that nonfatal or fatal drownings do not occur at a later time in patients with no previous symptoms.
3. Pediatricians should partner with community groups to increase access to life jackets through life jacket–loaner programs at swimming and boating sites.
4. Pediatricians should work with community partners to provide access to programs that develop water-competency swim skills for all children, especially those from low-income and diverse families and those with developmental disabilities. Pediatricians can identify and support programs to increase the access to high-quality, culturally sensitive, and affordable programs.[26]

Pool Operators

1. Community pools should have certified lifeguards with current CPR certification.
2. Pool owners and operators should adopt the Model Aquatic Health Code to ensure that best practices are being used to keep the pool and spa environment safe.
3. Owners of private pools and spas and managers of public pools should be made aware of entrapment and/or entanglement risks and of the laws mandating drain covers and filter pump equipment needed to prevent these injuries that primarily involve children.[50,51]

Policy Makers

1. Policy makers should pass legislation or building codes to mandate 4-sided isolation pool fencing for new and existing residential pools at the local and state level. Local governments should inspect and strictly enforce pool fencing requirements because this has been shown to be effective in reducing drowning.[52]
2. Policy makers should work with recreation and boating agencies to support legislation mandating that life jackets be worn by adolescents and by caregivers of children when boating.[53] When adults model appropriate behavior by wearing life jackets, children and adolescents are more likely to do so as well.[53]
3. States and communities should pass legislation and adopt regulations to establish basic safety requirements for natural swimming areas and public and private recreational facilities (eg, mandating the presence of certified lifeguards in designated swimming areas).[54]
4. States and communities should enforce laws that prohibit alcohol and other drug use by all watercraft occupants, not just operators.
5. State and local EMS personnel, medical examiners, health departments, and child-death–review teams should use consistent systematic reporting of information on the circumstances of drowning events. Periodic review of these data is critical in the development of drowning-prevention strategies appropriate for the geographic area.
6. Local governmental agencies should adopt the Model Aquatic Health Code for swimming pools, with better inspection and enforcement of swimming-pool safety standards.[41]
7. Because we lack a robust evidence base, a coordinated research agenda must be established to inform future policy, and federal funding should be secured to advance this research.

APPENDIX: RESOURCES FOR PEDIATRICIANS AND FAMILIES

1. The American Academy of Pediatrics Web site (http://www.aap.org) contains educational materials for parents from the The Injury Prevention Program about home water hazards for young children, life jackets and life preservers, pool safety, and water safety for school-aged children. It also has links to water-safety information from the CPSC, the CDC, and Safe Kids Worldwide.
2. The Safe Kids Worldwide Web site[55] contains information about pools and hot tubs, drain covers and safety vacuum release systems to prevent entrapment, and safety checklists (in English and Spanish) about pools, spas, open-water swimming and boating, and home water safety. It also has links to a national research study about pool and spa safety. It has some nice materials for children, including boating-safety coloring pages. One can download a color water watcher badge from this site.
3. The CDC Web site (http://www.cdc.gov) contains a water-related injuries factsheet, CDC research and information on water safety and water-related illnesses and injuries, and a link to the Web-based Injury Statistics Query and Report System. The CDC Childhood Injury Report contains state-specific information about drowning and other injuries.[56]
4. The CPSC Web site (https://www.poolsafely.gov/) has pool-safely materials for parents, grandparents, and caregivers, including supervision, fencing and other barriers, drain covers, and CPR. It also includes information about the Virginia Graeme Baker Pool and Spa Safety Act and a list of manufacturers of approved drain covers and safety vacuum release systems. The publications section contains safety-barrier guidelines for home pools and a family education brochure about preventing childhood drowning. Specific information on fencing can be found online.[46]
5. The US Coast Guard Web site (http://www.uscgboating.org/) contains detailed information and tip sheets about life jackets, vessel safety checks, approved online boating-safety courses, and beach safety. It also has links to sites with information about safety and boating regulations as well as links to statistics, research, and surveys about boating and boating crashes and injury. Specific information on the right-fit life jacket can be found online.[47]
6. The American Heart Association Web site[57] contains information on CPR courses for the community and health professionals.
7. The National Autism Association Web site[40] contains many resources for families of children with ASD, including a Family Wandering Emergency Plan, MedicAlert tools, wireless window and door alarms, and many other helpful tools to keep children safe.
8. The Water Safety USA Web site (https://www.watersafetyusa.org/) contains information on water competency, water watchers, and water safety.

LEAD AUTHORS

Sarah A. Denny, MD, FAAP
Linda Quan, MD, FAAP
CAPT Julie Gilchrist, MD, FAAP
Tracy McCallin, MD, FAAP
Rohit Shenoi, MD, FAAP
Shabana Yusuf, MD, MEd, FAAP
Benjamin Hoffman, MD, FAAP
Jeffrey Weiss, MD, FAAP

COUNCIL ON INJURY, VIOLENCE, AND POISON PREVENTION, 2018–2019

Benjamin Hoffman, MD, FAAP, Chairperson
Phyllis F. Agran, MD, MPH, FAAP
Sarah A. Denny, MD, FAAP
Michael Hirsh, MD, FAAP
Brian Johnston, MD, MPH, FAAP
Lois K. Lee, MD, MPH, FAAP
Kathy Monroe, MD, FAAP
Judy Schaechter, MD, MBA, FAAP
Milton Tenenbein, MD, FAAP
Mark R. Zonfrillo, MD, MSCE, FAAP
Kyran Quinlan, MD, MPH, FAAP, Immediate Past Chairperson

LIAISONS

Lynne Janecek Haverkos, MD, MPH, FAAP – *National Institute of Child Health and Human Development*
Jonathan D. Midgett, PhD – *Consumer Product Safety Commission*
Bethany Miller, MSW, Med – *Health Resources and Services Administration*
Alexander W. (Sandy) Sinclair – *National Highway Traffic Safety Administration*
Richard Stanwick, MD, FAAP – *Canadian Pediatric Society*

STAFF

Bonnie Kozial

ACKNOWLEDGMENT

We write this article in memory of our friend and colleague, Ruth Brenner, MD, FAAP, and in appreciation for her significant contributions to the field of drowning prevention and policy and for her commitment to the American Academy of Pediatrics.

ABBREVIATIONS

ASD: autism spectrum disorder
CDC: Centers for Disease Control and Prevention
CPR: cardiopulmonary resuscitation
CPSC: Consumer Product Safety Commission
EMS: emergency medical services

PEDIATRICS (ISSN Numbers: Print, 0031-4005; Online, 1098-4275).

Copyright © 2019 by the American Academy of Pediatrics

FINANCIAL DISCLOSURE: The authors have indicated they have no financial relationships relevant to this article to disclose.

FUNDING: No external funding.

POTENTIAL CONFLICT OF INTEREST: Dr Quan has provided expert witness testimony in a drowning case in 2018; the other authors have indicated they have no potential conflicts of interest to disclose.

REFERENCES

1. Centers for Disease Control and Prevention. Welcome to WISQARS™. Available at: https://www.cdc.gov/injury/wisqars/index.html. Accessed March 7, 2019
2. Kyriacou DN, Arcinue EL, Peek C, Kraus JF. Effect of immediate resuscitation on children with submersion injury. *Pediatrics*. 1994;94(2, pt 1):137–142
3. Suominen P, Baillie C, Korpela R, Rautanen S, Ranta S, Olkkola KT. Impact of age, submersion time and water temperature on outcome in near-drowning. *Resuscitation*. 2002;52(3):247–254
4. Quan L, Wentz KR, Gore EJ, Copass MK. Outcome and predictors of outcome in pediatric submersion victims receiving prehospital care in King County, Washington. *Pediatrics*. 1990;86(4):586–593
5. Stallman RK, Moran Dr K, Quan L, Langendorfer S. From swimming skill to water competence: towards a more inclusive drowning prevention future. *International Journal of Aquatic Research and Education*. 2017;10(2):3. Available at: https://scholarworks.bgsu.edu/ijare/vol10/iss2/. Accessed March 7, 2019
6. Water Safety USA. Become water competent. Available at: https://www.watersafetyusa.org/water-competency.html. Accessed March 8, 2019
7. Idris AH, Berg RA, Bierens J, et al; American Heart Association. Recommended guidelines for uniform reporting of data from drowning: the "Utstein style". *Circulation*. 2003;108(20):2565–2574
8. Brenner RA, Trumble AC, Smith GS, Kessler EP, Overpeck MD. Where children drown, United States, 1995. *Pediatrics*. 2001;108(1):85–89
9. US Consumer Product Safety Commission. How to plan for the unexpected: preventing child drownings. Available at: https://cpsc.gov/safety-education/safety-guides/pools-and-spas. Accessed October 31, 2018
10. Mackay JM, Samuel E, Green A. *Hidden Hazards: An Exploration of Open Water Drowning and Risks for Children*. Washington, DC: Safe Kids Worldwide; 2018
11. Mackay JM, Steel A, Dykstra H, Wheeler T, Samuel E, Green A. *Keeping Kids Safe in and Around Water: Exploring Misconceptions that Lead to Drowning*. Washington, DC: Safe Kids Worldwide; 2016
12. Wu Y, Huang Y, Schwebel DC, Hu G. Unintentional child and adolescent drowning mortality from 2000 to 2013 in 21 countries: analysis of the WHO Mortality Database. *Int J Environ Res Public Health*. 2017;14(8):E875
13. Browne ML, Lewis-Michl EL, Stark AD. Watercraft-related drownings among New York State residents, 1988-1994. *Public Health Rep*. 2003;118(5):459–463
14. Lhatoo SD, Sander JW. Cause-specific mortality in epilepsy. *Epilepsia*. 2005;46 (suppl 11):36–39
15. Diekema DS, Quan L, Holt VL. Epilepsy as a risk factor for submersion injury in children. *Pediatrics*. 1993;91(3):612–616
16. Kemp AM, Sibert JR. Epilepsy in children and the risk of drowning. *Arch Dis Child*. 1993;68(5):684–685

17. Bell GS, Gaitatzis A, Bell CL, Johnson AL, Sander JW. Drowning in people with epilepsy: how great is the risk? *Neurology*. 2008;71(8):578–582

18. Guan J, Li G. Injury mortality in individuals with autism. *Am J Public Health*. 2017;107(5):791–793

19. Shavelle RM, Strauss DJ, Pickett J. Causes of death in autism. *J Autism Dev Disord*. 2001;31(6):569–576

20. Guan J, Li G. Characteristics of unintentional drowning deaths in children with autism spectrum disorder. *Inj Epidemiol*. 2017;4(1):32

21. Choi G, Kopplin LJ, Tester DJ, Will ML, Haglund CM, Ackerman MJ. Spectrum and frequency of cardiac channel defects in swimming-triggered arrhythmia syndromes. *Circulation*. 2004;110(15):2119–2124

22. Semple-Hess J, Campwala R. Pediatric submersion injuries: emergency care and resuscitation. *Pediatr Emerg Med Pract*. 2014;11(6):1–21; quiz 21–22

23. Irwin CC, Irwin RL, Ryan TD, Drayer J. The legacy of fear: is fear impacting fatal and non-fatal drowning of African American children? *J Black Stud*. 2011; 42(4):561–576

24. Quan L, Crispin B, Bennett E, Gomez A. Beliefs and practices to prevent drowning among Vietnamese-American adolescents and parents. *Inj Prev*. 2006; 12(6):427–429

25. Moore E, Ali M, Graham E, Quan L. Responding to a request: gender-exclusive swims in a Somali community. *Public Health Rep*. 2010;125(1):137–140

26. Stempski S, Liu L, Grow HM, et al. Everyone Swims: a community partnership and policy approach to address health disparities in drowning and obesity. *Health Educ Behav*. 2015;42 (suppl 1):106S–114S

27. Rahman F, Bose S, Linnan M, et al. Cost-effectiveness of an injury and drowning prevention program in Bangladesh. *Pediatrics*. 2012;130(6). Available at: www.pediatrics.org/cgi/content/full/130/6/e1621

28. Brenner RA, Taneja GS, Haynie DL, et al. Association between swimming lessons and drowning in childhood: a case-control study. *Arch Pediatr Adolesc Med*. 2009;163(3):203–210

29. American Red Cross. ACFASP scientific review: minimum age for swimming lessons. 2009. Available at: https://scholarworks.bgsu.edu/ijare/vol3/iss4/13/. Accessed March 24, 2019

30. Quan L, Ramos W, Harvey C, et al. Toward defining water competency: an American Red Cross definition. *International Journal of Aquatic Research and Education*. 2015;9(1): 12–23

31. Haddon W Jr. The changing approach to the epidemiology, prevention, and amelioration of trauma: the transition to approaches etiologically rather than descriptively based. *Am J Public Health Nations Health*. 1968;58(8):1431–1438

32. Cody BE, Quraishi AY, Dastur MC, Mickalide AD. *Clear Danger: A National Study of Childhood Drowning and Related Attitudes and Behaviors*. Washington, DC: National Safe Kids Campaign; 2004

33. Thompson DC, Rivara FP. Pool fencing for preventing drowning in children. *Cochrane Database Syst Rev*. 2000;(2): CD001047

34. Gilchrist J, Branche C. Lifeguard effectiveness. In: Tipton M, Wooler A, eds. *The Science of Beach Lifeguarding*. Boca Raton, FL: CRC Press; 2016:29–36

35. Cummings P, Mueller BA, Quan L. Association between wearing a personal floatation device and death by drowning among recreational boaters: a matched cohort analysis of United States Coast Guard data. *Inj Prev*. 2011;17(3):156–159

36. Stempski S, Schiff M, Bennett E, Quan L. A case-control study of boat-related injuries and fatalities in Washington State. *Inj Prev*. 2014;20(4):232–237

37. Quan L, Pilkey D, Gomez A, Bennett E. Analysis of paediatric drowning deaths in Washington State using the child death review (CDR) for surveillance: what CDR does and does not tell us about lethal drowning injury. *Inj Prev*. 2011;17(suppl 1):i28–i33

38. Petrass LA, Blitvich JD, Finch CF. Lack of caregiver supervision: a contributing factor in Australian unintentional child drowning deaths, 2000-2009. *Med J Aust*. 2011;194(5):228–231

39. Moran K, Stanley T. Toddler drowning prevention: teaching parents about water safety in conjunction with their child's in-water lessons. *Int J Inj Contr Saf Promot*. 2006;13(4):254–256

40. National Autism Association. NAA's big red safety box. Available at: http://nationalautismassociation.org/big-red-safety-box/. Accessed March 4, 2019

41. Centers for Disease Control and Prevention. The Model Aquatic Health Code (MAHC): an all-inclusive model public swimming pool and spa code. Available at: https://www.cdc.gov/mahc/index.html. Accessed January 14, 2019

42. Szpilman D, Webber J, Quan L, et al. Creating a drowning chain of survival. *Resuscitation*. 2014;85(9):1149–1152

43. Lavonas EJ, Drennan IR, Gabrielli A, et al. Part 10: special circumstances of resuscitation: 2015 American Heart Association guidelines update for cardiopulmonary resuscitation and emergency cardiovascular care [published correction appears in *Circulation*. 2016;134(9):e122]. *Circulation*. 2015;132(18, suppl 2): S501–S518

44. Tobin JM, Ramos WD, Pu Y, Wernicki PG, Quan L, Rossano JW. Bystander CPR is associated with improved neurologically favourable survival in cardiac arrest following drowning. *Resuscitation*. 2017;115:39–43

45. Rauchschwalbe R, Brenner RA, Smith GS. The role of bathtub seats and rings in infant drowning deaths. *Pediatrics*. 1997;100(4). Available at: www.pediatrics.org/cgi/content/full/100/4/e1

46. US Consumer Product Safety Commission. Safety barrier guidelines for residential pools: preventing child drownings. 2012. Available at: https://www.cpsc.gov/s3fs-public/362%20Safety%20Barrier%20Guidelines%20for%20Pools.pdf. Accessed February 19, 2019

47. US Coast Guard. How to choose the right life jacket. Available at: www.uscgboating.org/images/howtochoosetherightlifejacket_brochure.pdf. Accessed January 11, 2019

48. US Lifesaving Association. Rip currents. Available at: https://www.usla.org/page/ripcurrents. Accessed March 7, 2019

49. Szpilman D, Sempsrott J, Webber J, et al. 'Dry drowning' and other myths. *Cleve Clin J Med*. 2018;85(7):529–535

50. Quraishi AY, Morton S, Cody BE, Wilcox R. *Pool and Spa Drowning: A National Study of Drain Entrapment and Pool Safety Measures*. Washington, DC: Safe Kids Worldwide; 2006

51. US Consumer Product Safety Commission. 1999-2007 reported circulation/suction entrapments associated with pools, hot tubs, spas, and whirlpools, 2008 memorandum. 2008. Available at: https://cpsc.gov/s3fs-public/pdfs/entrap08.pdf. Accessed January 17, 2019

52. van Weerdenburg K, Mitchell R, Wallner F. Backyard swimming pool safety inspections: a comparison of management approaches and compliance levels in three local government areas in NSW. *Health Promot J Austr*. 2006;17(1):37–42

53. Chung C, Quan L, Bennett E, Kernic MA, Ebel BE. Informing policy on open water drowning prevention: an observational survey of life jacket use in Washington State. *Inj Prev*. 2014; 20(4):238–243

54. World Health Organization. *Guidelines for Safe Recreational Water Environments: Coastal and Fresh Waters*. Vol 1. Geneva, Switzerland: World Health Organization; 2003

55. Safe Kids Worldwide. Water safety at home. Available at: https://www.safekids.org/watersafety. Accessed January 14, 2019

56. Centers for Disease Control and Prevention. CDC Childhood Injury Report. Available at: http://www.cdc.gov/safechild/Child_Injury_Data.html. Accessed January 14, 2019

57. American Heart Association. CPR & first aid training classes. Available at: https://cpr.heart.org/AHAECC/CPRAndECC/FindACourse/UCM_473162_CPR-First-Aid-Training-Classes-American-Heart-Association.jsp. Accessed January 14, 2019

Principles of Pediatric Patient Safety: Reducing Harm Due to Medical Care

- *Policy Statement*

POLICY STATEMENT Organizational Principles to Guide and Define the Child Health Care System and/or Improve the Health of all Children

American Academy of Pediatrics 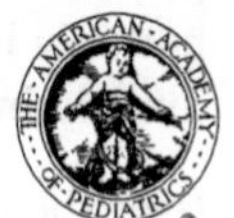

DEDICATED TO THE HEALTH OF ALL CHILDREN™

Principles of Pediatric Patient Safety: Reducing Harm Due to Medical Care

Brigitta U. Mueller, MD, MHCM, CPPS, CPHQ, FAAP,[a,b] Daniel Robert Neuspiel, MD, MPH, FAAP,[c] Erin R. Stucky Fisher, MD, FAAP,[d] COUNCIL ON QUALITY IMPROVEMENT AND PATIENT SAFETY, COMMITTEE ON HOSPITAL CARE

abstract

Pediatricians render care in an increasingly complex environment, which results in multiple opportunities to cause unintended harm. National awareness of patient safety risks has grown since the National Academy of Medicine (formerly the Institute of Medicine) published its report "To Err Is Human: Building a Safer Health System" in 1999. Patients and society as a whole continue to challenge health care providers to examine their practices and implement safety solutions. The depth and breadth of harm incurred by the practice of medicine is still being defined as reports continue to reveal a variety of avoidable errors, from those that involve specific high-risk medications to those that are more generalizable, such as patient misidentification and diagnostic error. Pediatric health care providers in all practice environments benefit from having a working knowledge of patient safety language. Pediatric providers should serve as advocates for best practices and policies with the goal of attending to risks that are unique to children, identifying and supporting a culture of safety, and leading efforts to eliminate avoidable harm in any setting in which medical care is rendered to children. In this Policy Statement, we provide an update to the 2011 Policy Statement "Principles of Pediatric Patient Safety: Reducing Harm Due to Medical Care."

[a]Johns Hopkins All Children's Hospital, St Petersburg, Florida; [b]School of Medicine, Johns Hopkins University, Baltimore, Maryland; [c]Levine Children's Hospital, Atrium Health, Charlotte, North Carolina; and [d]Department of Pediatrics, University of California San Diego and Rady Children's Hospital San Diego, San Diego, California

Drs Mueller, Neuspiel, and Fisher assisted with the conceptualization and design of this work, acquired and reviewed appropriate literature, and drafted, reviewed, and revised the manuscript; and all authors approved the final manuscript as submitted.

This document is copyrighted and is property of the American Academy of Pediatrics and its Board of Directors. All authors have filed conflict of interest statements with the American Academy of Pediatrics. Any conflicts have been resolved through a process approved by the Board of Directors. The American Academy of Pediatrics has neither solicited nor accepted any commercial involvement in the development of the content of this publication.

Policy statements from the American Academy of Pediatrics benefit from expertise and resources of liaisons and internal (AAP) and external reviewers. However, policy statements from the American Academy of Pediatrics may not reflect the views of the liaisons or the organizations or government agencies that they represent.

The guidance in this statement does not indicate an exclusive course of treatment or serve as a standard of medical care. Variations, taking into account individual circumstances, may be appropriate.

All policy statements from the American Academy of Pediatrics automatically expire 5 years after publication unless reaffirmed, revised, or retired at or before that time.

DOI: https://doi.org/10.1542/peds.2018-3649

Address correspondence to Brigitta U. Mueller, MD, MHCM, CPPS, CPHQ, FAAP. Email: bmuelle6@jhmi.edu

To cite: Mueller BU, Neuspiel DR, Fisher ERS, AAP COUNCIL ON QUALITY IMPROVEMENT AND PATIENT SAFETY, COMMITTEE ON HOSPITAL CARE. Principles of Pediatric Patient Safety: Reducing Harm Due to Medical Care. *Pediatrics.* 2019; 143(2):e20183649

BACKGROUND INFORMATION

Patient safety is defined as the prevention of harm to patients.[1] Although patient safety is only 1 of the 6 domains of quality of care defined by the National Academy of Medicine (formerly the Institute of Medicine [IOM]),[2] it is undoubtedly one of the most important. There are real and growing concerns regarding pediatric errors and harms reported related to specific populations, such as with the use of temporary names in newborn care,[3] as well as issues spanning all populations, such as diagnostic errors in ambulatory and hospital settings[4] and information technology errors in prescribing.[5] Pediatricians in all practice settings can help champion the concept that patient safety means preventing injury to children caused not only by life's accidents but also directly by the health care system.

Over the past several years, patient safety has become a key priority for health systems. Since the publication of the 1999 IOM report "To Err Is Human: Building a Safer Health System," there have been dramatic increases in research, standards, collaborative efforts, education, and measures focused on patient safety.[1,6–9] Much has been learned about pediatric patient safety. However, despite increased awareness, harm to patients is still common and has not shown a significant decline.[10] Errors still affect as many as one-third of all hospitalized children[11,12] and an unknown number of children in ambulatory settings.

In this Policy Statement, we summarize the current understanding of issues and practices to minimize pediatric medical errors and improve the quality of care. Three key issues are the focus in this Policy Statement: the significance of pediatric patient safety, the science behind the culture of safety, and strategies to ensure patient safety.

STATEMENT OF THE PROBLEM: SIGNIFICANCE OF PEDIATRIC PATIENT SAFETY

Pediatric medical errors and patient harm both differ in several ways from the errors and harms associated with adults. Children are at greater risk of medication errors than are adults because of childhood development, demographics, dependency on parents and other care providers, and the different epidemiology of medical conditions.[13] Errors in prescribing, dispensing, and administering medications represent a substantial portion of the preventable medical errors in children despite electronic prescribing.[5,14–17] Electronic health records (EHRs) are most often designed for adults and have limited effectiveness in reducing a variety of pediatric-specific errors. Moreover, these EHRs may cause increases in errors and harms until they are modified with customized decision support, such as weight-based and body surface area–based dosing.[18–20]

Reasons for the unique attributes of patient safety problems and solutions for children are multifactorial. Woods et al[21] detailed these factors as involving 3 key domains: (1) physical characteristics (eg, weight-based medication dosing), (2) developmental issues (eg, physical or mental age), and (3) issues regarding legal status as a minor (ie, lack of adult assistance in care of confidential health concerns). Layered onto these distinguishing characteristics is a general patient safety approach that involves 3 main components: (1) awareness of the epidemiology of errors and the institution of methods for error identification; (2) the integration of improvement science, including a safety culture, into daily work; and (3) the creation and implementation of core patient-safety solutions. Each of these components can be incorporated into pediatric patient safety risk assessment and solution development, with attention paid to the unique domains of pediatric patient safety risks.[21]

Pediatric errors in the inpatient setting have been reviewed by several investigators.[22–24] A study of hospitalized, pediatric, nonnewborn patients in the United States revealed a medication error rate of 1.81 to 2.96 per 100 discharges.[25] Teaching hospitals and settings where patients had more complex medical needs showed significantly higher error rates, whereas sex, payer, and zip code did not significantly affect outcomes. Among 10 778 orders in 1120 admissions reviewed by Kaushal et al[14] in 2 academic pediatric hospitals, there were 616 medication errors (5.7%), or 55 medication errors per 100 admissions. They also identified 26 adverse drug events (0.24%), of which 5 (19%) were preventable by using computerized physician order entry (CPOE) or unit-based clinical pharmacists. Serious errors occurred more often in critical-care settings, and potential adverse drug events occurred 3 times more frequently among pediatric patients than among adults. This 2001 publication predated significant EHR use, and the authors cited CPOE as a potential solution but also identified the need for ward-based clinical pharmacists. A 2016 study of 41 pediatric inpatient facilities in which a validated tool was used revealed that these pediatric CPOE systems were able to be used to identify 62% of potential medication errors in test scenarios, but this ability to detect errors varied widely across the sites, from 23% to 91%, and had no association with the EHR vendor.[26] Importantly for pediatric care, in which dose calculation errors are common, institutions did fairly well in this study when identifying dosing errors for a single inappropriate dose. An average of 81.1% (95% confidence interval 72.7%–89.5%) of these errors were identified across all 41 sites, suggesting that customized EHRs can aid in error avoidance. Other studies, including one in which a trigger tool was used, have revealed myriad nonmedication harms, with total rates as high as 40 harms per 100 patients.[27] Harms reported include accidental extubation, pressure ulcers, patient misidentification, delays in diagnosis, intravenous infiltrates, and other adverse events attributed to communication, training, and systems failures.[27] In children with chronic diseases, who by nature have a greater number of medications and medical interventions, the error rate can be higher.[28] In the Vermont Oxford Network, an analysis of medical errors in NICUs revealed that 47% of the cases involved medications, 14%

involved errors in the administration of or method of using a treatment, 11% involved patient misidentification, and 7% involved delays or errors in diagnosis.[8,29,30]

Pediatric errors in emergency department (ED) settings may be attributable to multiple factors, including incorrect patient identification, lack of experience of many ED staff with pediatric patients versus with adults, and challenges with performing technical procedures in and calculating medication doses for children.[31,32] Other sources of error include communication between prehospital and ED staff; among ED staff, particularly during change-of-shift sign off; between ED and inpatient staff; and between ED staff and family members. The use of a standardized hand-off process has been shown to decrease errors.[33,34] Other important sources of errors in the ED include diagnostic mistakes, medication errors unrelated to dose calculation, and environmental deficits, such as equipment malfunction. In a Canadian pediatric ED, 100 prescribing errors and 39 medication administration errors occurred per 1000 patients.[35]

Pediatric errors in the ambulatory setting have more limited published studies despite the fact that children have far more outpatient than hospital care interactions.[16,36,37] The Learning From Errors in Ambulatory Pediatrics study revealed 147 medical errors reported in 14 practices over 4 months (no denominator was reported).[38] The largest group of errors was attributed to medical treatment (37%). Other errors included patient identification (22%); preventive care, including immunizations (15%); diagnostic testing (13%); patient communication (8%); and less frequent causes. Among medical treatment errors, 85% were medication errors. Of these, 55% were related to prescribing errors, 30% were related to failure to order, 11% were related to administration, 2% were related to transcribing, and 2% were dispensing errors. In a prospective cohort study at 6 pediatric practices in or near Boston, Massachusetts, over a 2-month period, 3% of 1788 patients had preventable adverse drug events.[39] The preventive strategies with the most potential to reduce errors were determined to be improved communication between providers and parents and between pharmacists and parents. Among new prescriptions for 22 common medications in outpatient pediatric clinics, 15% were issued with potential dosing errors.[40] In addition, drug samples are often dispensed with inadequate documentation.[15] Children with special health care needs have been reported to be at higher risk for medication errors.[36,37,41]

In a general pediatric practice with 26 000 visits per year, Neuspiel et al[16] reported 216 medical errors over a 30-month period from 2008 to 2010. The most frequent reports in both paper and electronic systems were of misfiled or incorrectly entered patient information (32%), laboratory tests being delayed or not being performed (13%), medication prescription or dispensing errors (11%), immunization errors (10%), a requested appointment or referral not being given (7%), and delays in office care (7%); together, these errors comprised 80% of all reports. In this practice, a voluntary, nonpunitive, multidisciplinary team approach was effective in improving error reporting, investigating causes of reported errors, and implementing safety promotion strategies.

In addition to these setting-specific errors, the National Academies of Sciences, Engineering, and Medicine has turned attention to diagnostic decision-making as perhaps the most frequent source of medical error. Errors or delay in diagnosis may be caused by cognitive errors, such as premature closure (the tendency to prematurely end the decision-making process without considering other possible diagnoses), posterior probability error (the likelihood that diagnosis is overly influenced by previous events), and failures attributable to inexperience, fatigue, or lack of training.[4] The use of inappropriate or outmoded tests or therapies or failure to act on results of monitoring or testing are frequently cited as a basis for malpractice litigation. Of closed pediatric malpractice claims from 2003 to 2012 in the United States, the most frequent cause reported was error in diagnosis.[42] In balance with this is the awareness of potential harms caused by unnecessary medical care and overdiagnosis. The Choosing Wisely campaign (choosingwisely.org) was initiated to reduce overuse in certain conditions and diseases. This campaign includes statements from national societies, including the American Academy of Pediatrics (AAP),[43] regarding conditions for which best evidence supports not performing certain tests or treatments that by themselves can lead to a diagnosis or treatment based on incidental findings.[44] When applied judiciously, these recommendations can lead to a reduction in potential errors and harm events via avoidance of the event itself.

THE SCIENCE OF PATIENT SAFETY

The Safety Culture

In addition to understanding the epidemiology of medical harm to children, the awareness and attitudes of health care providers regarding patient safety are important. Specifically, a culture of safety is fundamental for avoiding patient harm and emphasizes the improvement of systems rather than blaming individual people. This culture supports responding to errors or potential errors in real time, with the expectation being to escalate or "stop the line" when safety is of concern. Society is demanding a safer health care system. State and federal agencies (eg, the Centers for Medicare and Medicaid Services), certifying organizations (eg, The Joint Commission and the American Board of Pediatrics), and professional societies (eg, the AAP) also have patient safety expectations.[45,46] These combined forces are placing greater pressure on the health care community to develop a culture of safety in which leaders and members understand and act on the basis of a systems approach.

Human-Factors Perspective

A culture of safety addresses human fallibility by concentrating on the conditions under which people work and building defenses to avert errors or mitigate their effects.[47] The culture of safety does not focus on errors of individual people because errors within organizations that deal with high-hazard processes rarely have their ultimate cause rooted in individual behavior.[48] High-reliability organizations recognize variability as a constant and are focused on minimizing that variability and its effects. The basis for this framework in health care rests on research in high-hazard industries (eg, aviation, nuclear power, and petrochemical industries) that have significantly decreased the incidence of catastrophic events.[49,50] Although the complexity of medical care may present difficulties in creating a culture of safety, the science of human factors (the focus on how people interact with each other and their environment) provides common principles that can endow health care providers with the resilience to avoid errors and adverse events.

The optimal culture of safety requires an organizational culture that supports 3 key elements: reporting, flexibility, and learning. The goal of a culture of safety is to be an informed culture with constant attentiveness and commitment to avoiding failures by endorsing a reluctance to accept simple explanations for errors that occur (by adhering to a structured investigation of events), commitment to resilience (with debriefing and support after events and integrating consistent skills training), deference to expertise (in which any member of the team can assume a leadership role for a given event on the basis of expertise and skills), and sensitivity to systems-based practices (by promoting team training, communication, and awareness of the effect of the environment on patient care).[51]

For an organization to be informed, it needs to have a "reporting culture." In a reporting culture, providers collect, analyze, and disseminate data about medical errors and adverse events. In this culture, frontline staff with direct patient care contact are willing and able to report errors and adverse events without fear of retribution. Crucial to this culture are the abilities of staff as well as patients and families to communicate easily, confidentially, or anonymously to entities that are separate from those with disciplinary functions. Those filing reports also need to be provided with timely and useful feedback.[16,52,53]

Organizations with a "just culture" encourage and reward error reporting by maintaining a nonpunitive environment. A just culture focuses on a systems approach to human fallibility while holding accountable those who intend to harm or intentionally fail to adhere to policies and procedures that are designed to keep patients safe.[54]

An optimal culture of safety has a "flexible culture" that is capable of adapting effectively to changing demands. A flexible culture depends on staff who consistently adhere to proven protocols and standards and leaders who are chosen not merely by rank but instead by expertise. For the care of children, defining this expertise includes the assessment of specific training and skills necessary to safely render care while attending to patient factors, such as varied ages, disease states, and developmental needs. This culture depends on teamwork; shared values; the use of well-tested standardized operating procedures and prospective risk assessment, such as failure modes and effects analysis; and investment in staff training.[49]

Finally, a "learning culture" promotes an environment in which individuals have the competence and will to make the right conclusions on the basis of safety information and will implement changes when needed, supported by evidence-based guidelines whenever available.[55–57] Providers in this culture learn from mistakes through system-oriented assessments (such as root-cause analyses), share that learning throughout the whole organization, and do not hide mistakes. A culture of safety promotes a compassionate disclosure of errors to those who have suffered harm from those mistakes.[58,59]

These cultures interact to create an informed system that perpetuates safety independent from individual personalities or external forces and provide a set of principles that promote a common culture of safety across our complex medical system. The Agency for Healthcare Research and Quality (AHRQ) has developed safety culture surveys for the hospital and office settings that may be useful to identify specific gaps and monitor improvements.[60]

PATIENT SAFETY STRATEGIES

Despite best efforts by health care providers, active error detection, and an ideal safety culture, errors will inevitably occur in systems as complex as health care. Although it was published 20 years ago, the 1999

IOM report's key safety-design concepts remain solid foundational elements to consider when striving to reduce medical errors.[1] Additional guidance on creating systems can be found in the IOM principles for the design of safety systems in health care organizations (Appendix).

Methods used to assess and resolve patient safety issues incorporate the IOM's broad key safety-design concepts to improve reliability through redundancy, simplification, and standardization.[1] Specific goals, such as accurate patient identification and the prevention of indwelling catheter infections, are amenable to the introduction of checklists, double-checks at the bedside, or forcing functions, such as mandated barcode scanning before a drug can be administered to a given patient.[61] Liquid dosing errors can be addressed with in-office videos, effective measurement devices, teach-back and show-back counseling techniques, and picture-based handouts.[62] Evidence-based clinical practice guidelines can direct care decisions both toward wanted and away from unwanted actions, resulting in reduced opportunities for harm and in improved outcomes.[57]

Other safety goals, such as the recognition of a change in a patient's status or encouraging patient and family involvement in the patient's care, require a composite of changes to health care systems and expectations of both providers and consumers. In addition to involving patients and families in family-centered rounds in all units, many institutions are encouraging families to report safety concerns to enhance the prevention and identification of problems.[63] Patient- and family-centeredness play important roles in the culture of safety, including consideration of ethnic culture and language as well as health literacy level.[64–66]

Leadership

In "To Err Is Human," the IOM addressed the need for national leaders to set goals for patient safety but also charged that "Chief Executive Officers and Boards of Trustees should be held accountable for making a serious, visible and ongoing commitment to creating safe systems of care."[1] This charge to have leaders engaged in patient safety at all levels—unit, clinic, and system—is more critical now as systems merge and affiliate, which can lead to potentially unclear lines of responsibility for quality-of-care oversight across care delivery sites. This stewardship of patient safety applies to pediatric leaders in all settings. Leaders and clinicians who strive to improve patient safety need to appraise their organizations' safety culture and advocate for the best means for implementing safety strategies.

Clinicians need to be involved to support the success of patient safety as part of larger quality-improvement efforts. Roles vary and depend on the type of clinician, practice setting, and system. In all settings, individual physician participation includes taking responsibility for ongoing knowledge and practice of patient safety principles, providing patient and parent education, actively engaging in safety efforts, and working effectively within a multidisciplinary structure.[67,68] Although financial incentives may be used to facilitate involvement, providing clinicians with data and reminders and ensuring their involvement in designing processes of care are most compelling. Group leaders can perform a physician and/or practice patient-safety assessment on topics such as medication management, clinical (eg, laceration repair), or administrative (eg, acknowledgment of laboratory results) procedures. Leaders also can initiate patient safety projects, such as creating a tracking system for high-risk pregnant teenagers or a tool for parents of children with special needs that clearly defines what changes in clinical status should prompt a call to which specific clinician (Appendix). System leaders' goals and external agency mandates may target changes with a wider impact, such as a multidisciplinary approach toward medication reconciliation.[69,70]

In community and adult settings, there is an added need to advocate for pediatric-specific issues. Physician participation on key hospital committees, such as pharmacy and therapeutics, information technology, sedation, the rapid-response team, and ambulatory clinical practice, is invaluable. The creation of a pediatric multidisciplinary safety team that reports to the hospital or larger medical group board can be a productive way to link specialists and ancillary providers to promote cross-communication on safety issues for children. Pediatric expertise can be of great value when creating diagnosis and/or treatment protocols for nonpediatric clinicians who care for children.

Role of Information Technology

Pediatric-specific technological support of safety is improving, yet most interventions are still in the development phase. Although information technology cannot be used to solve all challenges to patient safety, some issues are particularly amenable to technological solutions in hospital and ambulatory settings. Since the publication of the (now retired) AAP Policy Statement "Prevention of Medication Errors in the Pediatric Inpatient Setting,"[71] it has become more apparent that CPOE systems require robust decision support to be safe and effective.[18,72–76] Some decision-support rules for drug and dosing schedules and CPOE systems are now commercially available for children; however, most of them are still created locally. Order sets, reminders, and evidence-based clinical practice guidelines embedded within information systems increase adherence to best practices. The use of electronic equipment (specifically, programmable "smart" infusion pumps) has resulted in improved detection of medication errors and decreases in calculation and administration errors.[77]

Technological solutions to medical safety concerns mostly have been applied to pediatric inpatient settings. Barcoding has been used to compare identification bands with medications and blood products before administration.[61] These systems can also be used to identify areas for improved efficiency in time for critical medication administration. Telemedicine systems can be used within a site to allow for audiovisual team communication and enhance response to critical events; however, these systems are not yet widely available. Computers can generate code sheets for bedside posting and link to a patient's most recently updated visit list for patients within an enclosed system. Electronic patient-tracking systems and equipment linked to the EHR can assist with patient flow, the notification of abnormal study results, reduced data entry error, and the identification of changes in clinical status.[78]

Other advances apply to patients seen in varied health care settings. Visual media can be used for more than documenting improvements in examination findings. Patient body diagrams and patient photos can offer clarity when discriminating sidedness (left or right) or offer evidence of catheter locations.[79,80]

Despite noted advantages of EHRs, limitations still exist, including access to technological support, variable ease of use, physician acceptance, implementation and ongoing costs, need for continued end-user training, software integration into existing facility systems and outside providers and vendors, standardization across systems, the increase in errors after implementation, and ability to address only a subset of potential medical errors. Other examples of medical errors that currently challenge decision-support programs include inappropriate selection of medication for the condition being treated, failure to recognize a change in patient status, alarm fatigue leading to failure or delays in response, excessive data autopopulating notes, documentation copy and paste without editing, and others. The loss of or barriers to accessing information across disparate EHRs is notable at transitions of care and can lead to failures in medication reconciliation, duplicate testing, failure to act on test results, and other harms.

Patient Safety Goals and Efforts

Current national patient-safety efforts are embedded in the work of many organizations, such as the National Quality Forum, Institute for Healthcare Improvement–National Patient Safety Foundation, AHRQ, National Institute for Children's Health Quality, Institute for Safe Medication Practices, and others. The Joint Commission's national patient safety goals and campaign initiatives by the Institute for Healthcare Improvement–National Patient Safety Foundation are among the most relevant.[9] The Joint Commission (as well as other organizations, such as the AHRQ, the National Institute for Children's Health Quality, etc) required that elements for patient care include verbal, written, and electronic communication of test results; information transfer at transitions of care (handoffs); medication reconciliation; and ensuring patient and/or family understanding of care plans.[81] The Joint Commission requires hospitals to reduce the risk of health care–associated infections, such as multidrug-resistant organism infections, central line–associated bloodstream infections, and surgical-site infections, and improve the recognition of and response to changes in a patient's condition, for which many pediatric hospital rapid-response teams are using the Pediatric Early Warning System.[82] Family-centered care is of particular importance and value for children in high-risk settings, such as the ED, and for children with special needs. Patients and families ideally are able to articulate care plans and demonstrate understanding of the anticipated treatment outcome. Stress and fatigue also have been associated with errors, and national efforts focused on reducing workplace stress for physician trainees and other staff are being promoted.[83–85] Diagnostic errors are receiving more attention as well.[86] Medication management continues to be a specific focus for children because of variations in body weight, body surface area, organ system maturity, developmental stage of absorption and excretion ability, dependence on others for medication administration, and need for specially compounded formulations.[45] Accurate weight scales that only measure in metric units (kilograms or grams),[87] standardized equipment throughout a system, drug dose range limits, programmable "smart" infusion pumps for hospitals, and standardized order sets should be used.[88,89] Drug shortages have recently become an additional safety risk.[90] Clinical pharmacists who are trained in pediatrics are invaluable for medication reconciliation (especially for high-risk children) and may be integrated into inpatient rounds and used for the education of staff and families in all settings as often as possible.[80] The use of differing measurement systems (eg, teaspoon versus milliliter) also result in confusion for health care providers and the public.[91,92]

The AAP has launched webinars and Web sites and has partnered with other national leaders to offer specific tools, resources, and links to best health care safety practices for children (Appendix). Collaborative implementation and the measurement of both the process (adherence to practice) and clinical outcomes of shared strategies are necessary to track and refine care practices for all children. A network of >110 children's hospitals (Solutions for Patient Safety) has set the goal of 0 harms to children with reporting by participating institutions.[93] The realities of penalties for hospital-acquired conditions have brought attention to these events a priority for hospitals. Although clinician engagement is central to success in these endeavors, to date, there are limited pediatric-focused safety-related metrics with an impact on individual providers. However, adult providers are already having to report their individual performance on measures through the Merit-Based Incentive Payment System of the Medicare Access and Children's Health Insurance Program Reauthorization Act of 2015. It would be anticipated that some similar payment model may be implemented for the Medicaid population, which comprises a large percentage of most pediatric provider practices. It is incumbent on pediatricians to engage in safety-improvement networks and lead in identifying feasible and valid metrics for the many medical environments in which children receive care.

CONCLUSIONS

The field of pediatric patient safety has matured much in recent years; there are now more robust data on the epidemiology of errors in children, and there is a meaningful understanding of the concept and measurement of a culture of safety, clear guidance on key elements of patient safety solutions, and an introduction of successful pediatric patient safety solutions. Nonetheless, continued work is needed to infuse these data and concepts into everyday pediatric practice for all clinicians, and special attention should be paid to the training of new clinicians and integrating patient safety into ongoing medical education to help the future workforce incorporate all the tenets of pediatric patient safety as part of everyday work life. It is only through the complete incorporation of the culture of safety, assumption of personal responsibility for patient care outcomes, increasing examination of risk areas for pediatric patient safety, and deployment and rigorous evaluation of systems enhancements that the risks of medical errors to children can be reduced further.

RECOMMENDATIONS

Reducing pediatric patient harm attributable to medical care requires identifying and reporting errors and adverse events, disseminating best practices to prevent errors, and cultivating a culture of safety. Many interventions to improve the culture of safety are available and are based on principles derived from the experiences of other high-risk industries. These processes have been successful in reducing the incidence of catastrophic events, and their implementation in health care should be encouraged. The outcomes of these interventions should be rigorously measured with valid and reliable tools and monitored for their effectiveness in health care. Leadership is needed to continue to make and accelerate a transformation that acknowledges that health care providers (1) work in high-risk, complex environments; (2) are fallible humans, and therefore, medical errors will occur; (3) are independently and collectively accountable for patient safety; and (4) are integral to the success of systems change. Continuous system improvements are central to creating a culture of safety through reporting errors and adverse events, being just and flexible, and learning and implementing change on the basis of experience and rigorous science.

To help create and propel a comprehensive, accelerated approach toward pediatric patient safety, the following recommendations are made for all pediatricians and other health care providers and organizations caring for children:

1. Raise awareness and improve working knowledge of pediatric patient safety issues and best practices throughout the pediatric community.
   a. Educate and train: Expand interprofessional educational efforts to reach a broad scope of clinicians. Support structures that allow for all clinicians to identify pediatric patient safety issues and describe what they can do to improve them both individually and within systems. Include patient safety curricula for all child health trainees. Emphasize the importance of communication among teams, with patients and parents, and with referring providers.
   b. Network: Participate in available patient safety programming at national and regional meetings to encourage the sharing of patient safety issues and best practices among pediatric clinicians.
   c. Create a safety culture: Challenge all organizations, including practices of all sizes that care for children, to adopt a plan that informs, supports, and educates on pediatric patient safety. Use appropriate local examples of improvements initiated because of errors or "good catches" in which harms were avoided to create a safety culture. Strive to develop programs that support members to improve their

safety culture in their clinical care settings. Start any group meeting with a 2- to 3-minute "safety story" from your own practice that highlights "good catch" or real-harm events from which we can learn.

d. Implement and use standardized protocols of care for specific conditions, such as checklists or clinical practice guidelines, and monitor adherence.

e. Expand focus: Direct the attention of pediatric health care providers to safety in ambulatory settings, including the family-centered medical home and other locations where children receive care. Develop patient safety metrics for the ambulatory pediatric setting, including the home and school environments.

2. Act and advocate to minimize preventable pediatric medical harm by using information on pediatric-specific patient-safety risks.

   a. Develop pediatric-specific error reporting: In collaboration with governmental and private entities, develop and support broad-scale pediatric error-reporting systems and analysis of submitted events. Establish nonpunitive medical error-reporting systems in pediatric practices and on interprofessional teams to review and act on reported errors. Identify trends and areas in need of action by using these data to guide action on pediatric patient safety risks.

   b. Foster leadership: Take individual responsibility for maintaining awareness of pediatric patient safety issues. When possible, lead or participate in practice-based safety initiatives and quality or patient-safety committees in any setting, including ambulatory, hospital-based, community, or tertiary-care centers. Spread the current hospital-based focus on patient safety to the ambulatory setting through the designation of patient safety champions for practices.

   c. Enhance family-centered care, actively engage patients and families in safety at all points of care, and address issues of ethnic culture, language, and health literacy. Direct families to appropriate resources, and review patients' rights and responsibilities from the perspective of safety. Involve families in identifying, creating, and implementing patient safety best practices with attention to the medical home model in the ambulatory setting. Engage families in creating safety materials and participating in safety committees. Identify opportunities for families to aid in improvements related to health literacy, handoffs, and school and home care, among others. Leverage EHR portals and tools to directly communicate and share materials with patients and families.

3. Improve health care outcomes for children by adhering to proven best practices for improving pediatric patient safety.

   a. Adhere to best practices: Disseminate and exercise proven patient safety interventions, such as vigilant hand-washing, timeouts before procedures, and rigorous patient identification processes and medication reconciliation, particularly in ambulatory settings and for children with special health care needs. Embed safety strategies, such as redundancy, forcing functions, barcoding, standardized order sets, and evidence-based clinical practice guidelines (Appendix) whenever possible. Consider using data from national medical liability carriers to help identify areas of research regarding medical errors and patient safety.

   b. Target drug safety: In collaboration with regulatory agencies, focus efforts on medication safety by advocating for the development and study of effective and safe pediatric medications and formulations and for the withdrawal of medications with unfavorable risk/benefit ratios; promoting the standardization of concentrations in compounded medications; developing, spreading, and advocating for pediatric-specific health care information technology for drug delivery; educating providers on methods to reduce medication errors, including medication reconciliation; ensuring that providers maintain access to and proficiency in the use of a comprehensive and current pharmaceutical knowledge base; and creating policies that advocate for safe medication delivery to children in all health care settings, including effective liquid measurement devices coupled with teach-back and other advanced counseling techniques.

   c. If in a position to do so, help redesign clinical systems: Instill safety-design concepts when renovating or creating medical care systems and processes. Focus on human-factor issues in patient safety and include pediatric-specific information technological advancements whenever possible (eg, when implementing barcoding and CPOE systems). Partner with and urge government and other agencies and industries to identify, test, share, and study information systems that support the unique needs of the pediatric population. Support a change from the current "1 facility at a time," pediatric-specific EHR improvements that result in variations across organizations to meaningful vendor engagement in creating a united pediatric platform that is available equitably across care settings and users.

d. Leadership: Support and expand research to identify and refine effective pediatric patient safety interventions and study how information technology and human factors affect health care teams and the care they deliver. Motivate national health care research-funding systems to include a mandatory pediatric patient safety component.

APPENDIX: TOOLS, PROJECT GUIDES, AND CULTURE OF SAFETY INTERVENTIONS

Tools and resources from the AAP include the following.

- These are available on the AAP's Web site[94]:
    - advocacy and payment resources;
    - a searchable list of opportunities to engage in quality improvement at the AAP;
    - AAP members' activities and information; and
    - a list of AAP quality groups and programs.
- The National Center for Medical Home Implementation: The AAP's National Center for Medical Home Implementation Web site is the premier resource for improving the lives of children and youth with special health care needs and their families through a medical home. For more information, visit https://medicalhomeinfo.aap.org.
- Partnership for Policy Implementation (PPI): In June 2005, the AAP launched the PPI, a pilot program to integrate health information technology functionalities into AAP policy. The goal of the PPI is to create fundamental paradigm shifts in the development of clinical guidance and recommendations with a specific focus on developing recommendations that can easily be incorporated into clinical decision-support systems within EHRs. For more information, visit the AAP Web site.[95]

Other Web-based patient safety education, resources, and tools include the following:

- AHRQ Patient Safety Network (psnet.ahrq.gov);
- Office of the National Coordinator for Health Information Technology Safety Assurance Factors for EHR Resilience Guides, which provide strategies health care organizations can use to address EHR safety. For more information, visit HealthIT.gov[96];
- issue brief "Recent Evidence that Health IT Improves Patient Safety"[97];
- Solutions for Patient Safety (solutionsforpatientsafety.org);
- Children's Hospital Association Web site[98]; and
- Institute for Healthcare Improvement–National Patient Safety Foundation patient safety resources Web page.[99]

LEAD AUTHORS

Brigitta U. Mueller, MD, MHCM, CPPS, CPHQ, FAAP
Daniel Robert Neuspiel, MD, MPH, FAAP
Erin R. Stucky Fisher, MD, FAAP

COUNCIL ON QUALITY IMPROVEMENT AND PATIENT SAFETY EXECUTIVE COMMITTEE, 2014–2017

Wayne Franklin, MD, MPH, MMM, FAAP, Chairperson
Terry Adirim, MD, MBA, MPH, FAAP
David Gordon Bundy, MD, FAAP
Laura Elizabeth Ferguson, MD, FAAP
Sean Patrick Gleeson, MD, MBA, FAAP
Michael Leu, MD, MS, MHS, FAAP
Brigitta U. Mueller, MD, MHCM, CPPS, CPHQ, FAAP
Daniel Robert Neuspiel, MD, MPH, FAAP
Ricardo A. Quinonez, MD, FAAP
Michael L. Rinke, MD, PhD, FAAP
Richard N. Shiffman, MD, MCIS, FAAP
Elizabeth Vickers Saarel, MD, FAAP
Joel S. Tieder, MD, MPH, FAAP
H. Shonna Yin, MD, MS, FAAP

COUNCIL ON QUALITY IMPROVEMENT AND PATIENT SAFETY EXECUTIVE COMMITTEE, 2017–2018

Wayne Franklin, MD, MPH, MMM, FAAP, Chairperson
Joel S. Tieder, MD, MPH, FAAP, Vice Chairperson
Terry Adirim, MD, MBA, MPH, FAAP
Laura Elizabeth Ferguson, MD, FAAP
Michael Leu, MD, MS, MHS, FAAP
Brigitta U. Mueller, MD, MHCM, CPPS, CPHQ, FAAP
Shannon Connor Phillips, MD, MPH, FAAP
Ricardo A. Quinonez, MD, FAAP
Michael L. Rinke, MD, PhD, FAAP
Elizabeth Vickers Saarel, MD, FAAP
H. Shonna Yin, MD, MS, FAAP

COUNCIL ON QUALITY IMPROVEMENT AND PATIENT SAFETY EXECUTIVE COMMITTEE, 2018–2019

Wayne Franklin, MD, MPH, MMM, FAAP, Immediate Past Chairperson
Joel S. Tieder, MD, MPH, FAAP, Chairperson
Ricardo Quinonez, MD, FAAP, Vice Chairperson
Terry Adirim, MD, MBA, MPH, FAAP
Jeffrey M. Brown, MD, MPH, CPE, FAAP
Laura Elizabeth Ferguson, MD, FAAP
Michael Leu, MD, MS, MHS, FAAP
Brigitta U. Mueller, MD, MHCM, CPPS, CPHQ, FAAP
Shannon Connor Phillips, MD, MPH, FAAP
Michael L. Rinke, MD, PhD, FAAP
Kathleen Mack Walsh, MD, FAAP
H. Shonna Yin, MD, MS, FAAP

COUNCIL ON QUALITY IMPROVEMENT AND PATIENT SAFETY EXECUTIVE COMMITTEE, LIAISONS, 2014–2018

Scott Berns, MD, MPH, FAAP – *National Institute for Children's Health Quality*
Kamila Mistry, PhD, MPH – *Agency for Healthcare Research and Quality*
Virginia Moyer, MD, MPH, FAAP – *American Board of Pediatrics*
Suzette Olu Busola Oyeku, MD, MPH, FAAP – *National Institute for Children's Health Quality*

Mimi Saffer - *Children's Hospital Association*
Ellen Schwalenstocker, PhD, MBA - *Children's Hospital Association*

STAFF

Cathleen Guch, MPH
Lisa Krams, MS

COMMITTEE ON HOSPITAL CARE, 2017–2018

Jennifer Jewell, MD, FAAP, Chairperson
Erin R. Stucky Fisher, MD, FAAP, Past Chairperson
Kimberly Ernst, MD, MSMI, FAAP
Vanessa L. Hill, MD, FAAP
Vinh Lam, MD, FAAP, FACS
Charles Vinocur, MD, FAAP, FACS
Daniel Rauch, MD, FAAP
Benson Hsu, MD, MBA, FAAP

LIAISONS

Michael S. Leonard, MD, MS, FAAP, CPPS - *The Joint Commission*
Barbara Romito, MA, CCLS - *Association of Child Life Professionals*
Karen Castleberry - *Family Representative*

STAFF

S. Niccole Alexander, MPP

ABBREVIATIONS

AAP: American Academy of Pediatrics
AHRQ: Agency for Healthcare Research and Quality
CPOE: computerized physician order entry
ED: emergency department
EHR: electronic health record
IOM: Institute of Medicine
PPI: Partnership for Policy Implementation

PEDIATRICS (ISSN Numbers: Print, 0031-4005; Online, 1098-4275).

Copyright © 2019 by the American Academy of Pediatrics

FINANCIAL DISCLOSURE: The authors have indicated they have no financial relationships relevant to this article to disclose.

FUNDING: No external funding.

POTENTIAL CONFLICT OF INTEREST: The authors have indicated they have no potential conflicts of interest to disclose.

REFERENCES

1. Kohn LT, Corrigan JM, Donaldson MS. *To Err Is Human: Building a Safer Health Care System*. Washington, DC: National Academic Press; 2000
2. Institute of Medicine. *Crossing the Quality Chasm: A New Health System for the 21st Century*. Washington, DC: National Academy Press; 2001
3. Adelman J, Aschner J, Schechter C, et al. Use of temporary names for newborns and associated risks. *Pediatrics*. 2015;136(2):327–333
4. Balogh EP, Miller BT, Ball JR, eds; Committee on Diagnostic Error in Health Care; Board on Health Care Services; Institute of Medicine; The National Academies of Sciences, Engineering, and Medicine. *Improving Diagnosis in Health Care*. Washington, DC: National Academies Press; 2015
5. Nelson CE, Selbst SM. Electronic prescription writing errors in the pediatric emergency department. *Pediatr Emerg Care*. 2015;31(5):368–372
6. Fortescue EB, Kaushal R, Landrigan CP, et al. Prioritizing strategies for preventing medication errors and adverse drug events in pediatric inpatients. *Pediatrics*. 2003;111(4, pt 1): 722–729
7. National Quality Forum. National Quality Forum issue brief: strengthening pediatric quality measurement and reporting. *J Healthc Qual*. 2008;30(3): 51–55
8. Stockwell DC, Bisarya H, Classen DC, et al. A trigger tool to detect harm in pediatric inpatient settings. *Pediatrics*. 2015;135(6):1036–1042
9. The Joint Commission. Topic library resources. 2016. Available at: https://www.jointcommission.org/hap_2017_npsgs/. Accessed December 19, 2018
10. Landrigan CP, Parry GJ, Bones CB, Hackbarth AD, Goldmann DA, Sharek PJ. Temporal trends in rates of patient harm resulting from medical care. *N Engl J Med*. 2010;363(22):2124–2134
11. Kirkendall ES, Kloppenborg E, Papp J, et al. Measuring adverse events and levels of harm in pediatric inpatients with the Global Trigger Tool. *Pediatrics*. 2012;130(5). Available at: www.pediatrics.org/cgi/content/full/130/5/e1206
12. Walsh KE, Bundy DG, Landrigan CP. Preventing health care-associated harm in children. *JAMA*. 2014;311(17): 1731–1732
13. Santell JP, Hicks R. Medication errors involving pediatric patients. *Jt Comm J Qual Patient Saf*. 2005;31(6):348–353
14. Kaushal R, Bates DW, Landrigan C, et al. Medication errors and adverse drug events in pediatric inpatients. *JAMA*. 2001;285(16):2114–2120
15. Rinke ML, Bundy DG, Velasquez CA, et al. Interventions to reduce pediatric medication errors: a systematic review. *Pediatrics*. 2014;134(2):338–360
16. Neuspiel DR, Stubbs EH, Liggin L. Improving reporting of outpatient pediatric medical errors. *Pediatrics*. 2011;128(6). Available at: www.pediatrics.org/cgi/content/full/128/6/e1608
17. Smith MD, Spiller HA, Casavant MJ, Chounthirath T, Brophy TJ, Xiang H. Out-of-hospital medication errors among young children in the United States, 2002-2012. *Pediatrics*. 2014;134(5): 867–876
18. Han YY, Carcillo JA, Venkataraman ST, et al. Unexpected increased mortality after implementation of a commercially sold computerized physician order entry system. *Pediatrics*. 2005;116(6): 1506–1512
19. Lehmann CU; Council on Clinical Information Technology. Pediatric

aspects of inpatient health information technology systems. *Pediatrics*. 2015; 135(3). Available at: www.pediatrics.org/cgi/content/full/135/3/e756

20. Lehmann CU, O'Connor KG, Shorte VA, Johnson TD. Use of electronic health record systems by office-based pediatricians. *Pediatrics*. 2015;135(1). Available at: www.pediatrics.org/cgi/content/full/135/1/e7
21. Woods D, Thomas E, Holl J, Altman S, Brennan T. Adverse events and preventable adverse events in children. *Pediatrics*. 2005;115(1):155–160
22. Leonard MS. Patient safety and quality improvement: medical errors and adverse events. *Pediatr Rev*. 2010;31(4): 151–158
23. Landrigan CP. The safety of inpatient pediatrics: preventing medical errors and injuries among hospitalized children. *Pediatr Clin North Am*. 2005; 52(4):979–993, vii
24. Sharek PJ, Classen D. The incidence of adverse events and medical error in pediatrics. *Pediatr Clin North Am*. 2006; 53(6):1067–1077
25. Slonim AD, LaFleur BJ, Ahmed W, Joseph JG. Hospital-reported medical errors in children. *Pediatrics*. 2003;111(3):617–621
26. Chaparro JD, Classen DC, Danforth M, Stockwell DC, Longhurst CA. National trends in safety performance of electronic health record systems in children's hospitals. *J Am Med Inform Assoc*. 2017;24(2):268–274
27. Khan A, Furtak SL, Melvin P, Rogers JE, Schuster MA, Landrigan CP. Parent-reported errors and adverse events in hospitalized children. *JAMA Pediatr*. 2016;170(4):e154608
28. Ahuja N, Zhao W, Xiang H. Medical errors in US pediatric inpatients with chronic conditions. *Pediatrics*. 2012;130(4). Available at: www.pediatrics.org/cgi/content/full/130/4/e786
29. Suresh GK. Measuring patient safety in neonatology. *Am J Perinatol*. 2012;29(1): 19–26
30. Suresh G, Horbar JD, Plsek P, et al. Voluntary anonymous reporting of medical errors for neonatal intensive care. *Pediatrics*. 2004;113(6):1609–1618
31. Cottrell EK, O'Brien K, Curry M, et al. Understanding safety in prehospital emergency medical services for children. *Prehosp Emerg Care*. 2014; 18(3):350–358
32. O'Neill KA, Shinn D, Starr KT, Kelley J. Patient misidentification in a pediatric emergency department: patient safety and legal perspectives. *Pediatr Emerg Care*. 2004;20(7):487–492
33. Heilman JA, Flanigan M, Nelson A, Johnson T, Yarris LM. Adapting the I-PASS handoff program for emergency department inter-shift handoffs. *West J Emerg Med*. 2016;17(6):756–761
34. Shahian DM, McEachern K, Rossi L, Chisari RG, Mort E. Large-scale implementation of the I-PASS handover system at an academic medical centre. *BMJ Qual Saf*. 2017;26(9):760–770
35. Kozer E. Medication errors in children. *Paediatr Drugs*. 2009;11(1):52–54
36. Walsh KE, Mazor KM, Stille CJ, et al. Medication errors in the homes of children with chronic conditions. *Arch Dis Child*. 2011;96(6):581–586
37. Walsh KE, Roblin DW, Weingart SN, et al. Medication errors in the home: a multisite study of children with cancer. *Pediatrics*. 2013;131(5). Available at: www.pediatrics.org/cgi/content/full/131/5/e1405
38. Mohr JJ, Lannon CM, Thoma KA, et al. Learning from errors in ambulatory pediatrics. In: Henriksen K, Battles JB, Marks ES, Lewin DI, eds. *Advances in Patient Safety: From Research to Implementation*. Vol 1. Rockville, MD: Agency for Healthcare Research and Quality; 2005:355–368
39. Kaushal R, Goldmann DA, Keohane CA, et al. Adverse drug events in pediatric outpatients. *Ambul Pediatr*. 2007;7(5): 383–389
40. McPhillips HA, Stille CJ, Smith D, et al. Potential medication dosing errors in outpatient pediatrics. *J Pediatr*. 2005; 147(6):761–767
41. Taylor JA, Winter L, Geyer LJ, Hawkins DS. Oral outpatient chemotherapy medication errors in children with acute lymphoblastic leukemia. *Cancer*. 2006; 107(6):1400–1406
42. Carroll AE, Buddenbaum JL. Malpractice claims involving pediatricians: epidemiology and etiology. *Pediatrics*. 2007;120(1):10–17
43. Choosing Wisely; American Academy of Pediatrics. Ten things physicians and patients should question. Available at: http://www.choosingwisely.org/societies/american-academy-of-pediatrics/. Accessed December 12, 2018
44. Quinonez RA, Garber MD, Schroeder AR, et al. Choosing wisely in pediatric hospital medicine: five opportunities for improved healthcare value. *J Hosp Med*. 2013;8(9):479–485
45. The Joint Commission. Preventing pediatric medication errors. *Sentinel Event Alert*. 2008;(39):1–4
46. The Leapfrog Group. Available at: http://www.leapfroggroup.org/. Accessed December 19, 2018
47. Reason J. Human error: models and management. *BMJ*. 2000;320(7237): 768–770
48. Weick K, Sutcliffe K. *Managing the Unexpected: Sustained Performance in a Complex World*. 3rd ed. San Francisco, CA: Jossey-Bass; 2015
49. Brilli RJ, McClead RE Jr, Crandall WV, et al. A comprehensive patient safety program can significantly reduce preventable harm, associated costs, and hospital mortality. *J Pediatr*. 2013;163(6): 1638–1645
50. Pronovost PJ, Armstrong CM, Demski R, et al. Creating a high-reliability health care system: improving performance on core processes of care at Johns Hopkins Medicine. *Acad Med*. 2015;90(2): 165–172
51. Chassin MR, Loeb JM. The ongoing quality improvement journey: next stop, high reliability. *Health Aff (Millwood)*. 2011;30(4):559–568
52. Cox ED, Carayon P, Hansen KW, et al. Parent perceptions of children's hospital safety climate. *BMJ Qual Saf*. 2013;22(8): 664–671
53. Muething SE, Goudie A, Schoettker PJ, et al. Quality improvement initiative to reduce serious safety events and improve patient safety culture. *Pediatrics*. 2012;130(2). Available at: www.pediatrics.org/cgi/content/full/130/2/e423
54. Pronovost PJ, Demski R, Callender T, et al. Demonstrating high reliability on accountability measures at the Johns

Hopkins Hospital. *Jt Comm J Qual Patient Saf.* 2013;39(12):531–544

55. Runnacles J, Roueché A, Lachman P. The right care, every time: improving adherence to evidence-based guidelines. *Arch Dis Child Educ Pract Ed.* 2018; 103(1):27–33
56. Kane-Gill SL, Dasta JF, Buckley MS, et al. Clinical practice guideline: safe medication use in the ICU. *Crit Care Med.* 2017;45(9):e877–e915
57. Lugtenberg M, Burgers JS, Westert GP. Effects of evidence-based clinical practice guidelines on quality of care: a systematic review. *Qual Saf Health Care.* 2009;18(5):385–392
58. Bell SK, Mann KJ, Truog R, Lantos JD. Should we tell parents when we've made an error? *Pediatrics.* 2015;135(1): 159–163
59. Committee on Medical Liability and Risk Management; Council on Quality Improvement and Patient Safety. Disclosure of adverse events in pediatrics. *Pediatrics.* 2016;138(6): e20163215
60. Agency for Healthcare Research and Quality. Surveys on patient safety culture (SOPS). Available at: https://www.ahrq.gov/sops/index.html. Accessed December 19, 2018
61. Hayden RT, Patterson DJ, Jay DW, et al. Computer-assisted bar-coding system significantly reduces clinical laboratory specimen identification errors in a pediatric oncology hospital. *J Pediatr.* 2008;152(2):219–224
62. Yin HS, Parker RM, Sanders LM, et al. Pictograms, units and dosing tools, and parent medication errors: a randomized study. *Pediatrics.* 2017;140(1):e20163237
63. Kelly MM, Hoonakker PL, Dean SM. Using an inpatient portal to engage families in pediatric hospital care. *J Am Med Inform Assoc.* 2017;24(1):153–161
64. Benjamin JM, Cox ED, Trapskin PJ, et al. Family-initiated dialogue about medications during family-centered rounds. *Pediatrics.* 2015;135(1):94–101
65. Subramony A, Hametz PA, Balmer D. Family-centered rounds in theory and practice: an ethnographic case study. *Acad Pediatr.* 2014;14(2):200–206
66. Schonlau M, Martin L, Haas A, Derose KP, Rudd R. Patients' literacy skills: more than just reading ability. *J Health Commun.* 2011;16(10):1046–1054
67. Pronovost PJ, Wachter RM. Progress in patient safety: a glass fuller than it seems. *Am J Med Qual.* 2014;29(2): 165–169
68. Wachter RM, Pronovost P, Shekelle P. Strategies to improve patient safety: the evidence base matures. *Ann Intern Med.* 2013;158(5, pt 1): 350–352
69. Neuspiel DR, Taylor MM. Reducing the risk of harm from medication errors in children. *Health Serv Insights.* 2013;6: 47–59
70. White CM, Schoettker PJ, Conway PH, et al. Utilising improvement science methods to optimise medication reconciliation. *BMJ Qual Saf.* 2011;20(4): 372–380
71. Stucky ER; American Academy of Pediatrics Committee on Drugs; American Academy of Pediatrics Committee on Hospital Care. Prevention of medication errors in the pediatric inpatient setting. *Pediatrics.* 2003;112(2): 431–436
72. Ruano M, Villamañán E, Pérez E, Herrero A, Álvarez-Sala R. New technologies as a strategy to decrease medication errors: how do they affect adults and children differently? *World J Pediatr.* 2016;12(1):28–34
73. Sethuraman U, Kannikeswaran N, Murray KP, Zidan MA, Chamberlain JM. Prescription errors before and after introduction of electronic medication alert system in a pediatric emergency department. *Acad Emerg Med.* 2015; 22(6):714–719
74. Chapman AK, Lehmann CU, Donohue PK, Aucott SW. Implementation of computerized provider order entry in a neonatal intensive care unit: impact on admission workflow. *Int J Med Inform.* 2012;81(5):291–295
75. Abramson EL, Kaushal R. Computerized provider order entry and patient safety. *Pediatr Clin North Am.* 2012;59(6): 1247–1255
76. American Academy of Pediatrics Council on Clinical Information Technology Executive Committee, 2011–2012. Electronic prescribing in pediatrics: toward safer and more effective medication management [published correction appears in *Pediatrics.* 2013; 132(1):179]. *Pediatrics.* 2013;131(4): 824–826
77. Ohashi K, Dalleur O, Dykes PC, Bates DW. Benefits and risks of using smart pumps to reduce medication error rates: a systematic review. *Drug Saf.* 2014; 37(12):1011–1020
78. Dufendach KR, Eichenberger JA, McPheeters ML, et al. *Core Functionality in Pediatric Electronic Health Records.* Rockville, MD: Agency for Healthcare Research and Quality; 2015
79. Choi JS, Lee WB, Rhee PL. Cost-benefit analysis of electronic medical record system at a tertiary care hospital. *Healthc Inform Res.* 2013;19(3): 205–214
80. Wang JK, Herzog NS, Kaushal R, Park C, Mochizuki C, Weingarten SR. Prevention of pediatric medication errors by hospital pharmacists and the potential benefit of computerized physician order entry. *Pediatrics.* 2007;119(1). Available at: www.pediatrics.org/cgi/content/full/119/1/e77
81. Starmer AJ, Landrigan CP; I-PASS Study Group. Changes in medical errors with a handoff program. *N Engl J Med.* 2015; 372(5):490–491
82. Duncan KD, McMullan C, Mills BM. Early warning systems: the next level of rapid response. *Nursing.* 2012;42(2):38–44; quiz 45
83. Honey BL, Bray WM, Gomez MR, Condren M. Frequency of prescribing errors by medical residents in various training programs. *J Patient Saf.* 2015;11(2): 100–104
84. Starmer AJ, Spector ND, Srivastava R, et al; I-PASS Study Group. Changes in medical errors after implementation of a handoff program. *N Engl J Med.* 2014; 371(19):1803–1812
85. Typpo KV, Tcharmtchi MH, Thomas EJ, Kelly PA, Castillo LD, Singh H. Impact of resident duty hour limits on safety in the intensive care unit: a national survey of pediatric and neonatal intensivists. *Pediatr Crit Care Med.* 2012;13(5): 578–582
86. Thammasitboon S, Thammasitboon S, Singhal G. Diagnosing diagnostic error. *Curr Probl Pediatr Adolesc Health Care.* 2013;43(9):227–231

87. Institute for Safe Medication Practices. 2016-2017 targeted medication safety best practices for hospitals. 2017. Available at: https://www.ismp.org/guidelines/best-practices-hospitals. Accessed December 19, 2018

88. Guérin A, Tourel J, Delage E, et al. Accidents and incidents related to intravenous drug administration: a pre-post study following implementation of smart pumps in a teaching hospital. *Drug Saf.* 2015; 38(8):729–736

89. Manrique-Rodríguez S, Sánchez-Galindo A, Fernández-Llamazares CM, et al. Developing a drug library for smart pumps in a pediatric intensive care unit. *Artif Intell Med.* 2012;54(3):155–161

90. Hughes KM, Goswami ES, Morris JL. Impact of a drug shortage on medication errors and clinical outcomes in the pediatric intensive care unit. *J Pediatr Pharmacol Ther.* 2015;20(6):453–461

91. Yin HS, Dreyer BP, Ugboaja DC, et al. Unit of measurement used and parent medication dosing errors. *Pediatrics.* 2014;134(2). Available at: www.pediatrics.org/cgi/content/full/134/2/e354

92. Paul IM, Neville K, Galinkin JL, et al. Metric units and the preferred dosing of orally administered liquid medications. *Pediatrics.* 2015;135(4): 784–787

93. Lyren A, Brilli R, Bird M, Lashutka N, Muething S. Ohio children's hospitals' solutions for patient safety: a framework for pediatric patient safety improvement. *J Healthc Qual.* 2016;38(4):213–222

94. American Academy of Pediatrics. Quality improvement. Available at: https://www.aap.org/en-us/professional-resources/quality-improvement. Accessed December 12, 2018

95. American Academy of Pediatrics. About the Child Health Informatics Center. Available at: http://www2.aap.org/informatics/PPI.html. Accessed December 12, 2018

96. HealthIT.gov. SAFER guides. Available at: https://www.healthit.gov/topic/safety/safer-guides. Accessed December 12, 2018

97. Banger A, Graber ML. Recent evidence that health IT improves patient safety. Available at: www.healthit.gov/sites/default/files/brief_1_final_feb11t.pdf. Accessed December 19, 2018

98. Children's Hospital Association. Patient safety. Available at: https://www.childrenshospitals.org/Quality-and-Performance/Patient-Safety. Accessed December 12, 2018

99. Institute for Healthcare Improvement. Patient safety. Available at: http://www.ihi.org/Topics/PatientSafety/Pages/default.aspx. Accessed December 12, 2018

Providing Care for Children in Immigrant Families

- *Policy Statement*

POLICY STATEMENT Organizational Principles to Guide and Define the Child Health Care System and/or Improve the Health of all Children

American Academy of Pediatrics

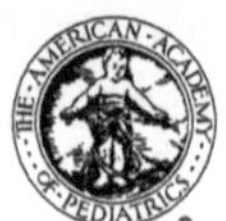

DEDICATED TO THE HEALTH OF ALL CHILDREN™

Providing Care for Children in Immigrant Families

Julie M. Linton, MD, FAAP,[a,b] Andrea Green, MDCM, FAAP,[c] COUNCIL ON COMMUNITY PEDIATRICS

Children in immigrant families (CIF), who represent 1 in 4 children in the United States, represent a growing and ever more diverse US demographic that pediatric medical providers nationwide will increasingly encounter in clinical care. Immigrant children are those born outside the United States to non–US citizen parents, and CIF are defined as those who are either foreign born or have at least 1 parent who is foreign born. Some families immigrate for economic or educational reasons, and others come fleeing persecution and seeking safe haven. Some US-born children with a foreign-born parent may share vulnerabilities with children who themselves are foreign born, particularly regarding access to care and other social determinants of health. Therefore, the larger umbrella term of CIF is used in this statement. CIF, like all children, have diverse experiences that interact with their biopsychosocial development. CIF may face inequities that can threaten their health and well-being, and CIF also offer strengths and embody resilience that can surpass challenges experienced before and during integration. This policy statement describes the evolving population of CIF in the United States, briefly introduces core competencies to enhance care within a framework of cultural humility and safety, and discusses barriers and opportunities at the practice and systems levels. Practice-level recommendations describe how pediatricians can promote health equity for CIF through careful attention to core competencies in clinical care, thoughtful community engagement, and system-level support. Advocacy and policy recommendations offer ways pediatricians can advocate for policies that promote health equity for CIF.

abstract

[a]*Departments of Pediatrics and Public Health, School of Medicine Greenville, University of South Carolina, Greenville, South Carolina;* [b]*Department of Pediatrics, School of Medicine, Wake Forest University, Winston-Salem, North Carolina; and* [c]*Larner College of Medicine, The University of Vermont, Burlington, Vermont*

Drs Linton and Green drafted, reviewed, and revised the manuscript; and both authors approved the final manuscript as submitted.

This document is copyrighted and is property of the American Academy of Pediatrics and its Board of Directors. All authors have filed conflict of interest statements with the American Academy of Pediatrics. Any conflicts have been resolved through a process approved by the Board of Directors. The American Academy of Pediatrics has neither solicited nor accepted any commercial involvement in the development of the content of this publication.

Policy statements from the American Academy of Pediatrics benefit from expertise and resources of liaisons and internal (AAP) and external reviewers. However, policy statements from the American Academy of Pediatrics may not reflect the views of the liaisons or the organizations or government agencies that they represent.

The guidance in this statement does not indicate an exclusive course of treatment or serve as a standard of medical care. Variations, taking into account individual circumstances, may be appropriate.

All policy statements from the American Academy of Pediatrics automatically expire 5 years after publication unless reaffirmed, revised, or retired at or before that time.

DOI: https://doi.org/10.1542/peds.2019-2077

Address correspondence to Julie M. Linton, MD, FAAP. E-mail: Julie.linton@prismahealth.org

PEDIATRICS (ISSN Numbers: Print, 0031-4005; Online, 1098-4275).

Copyright © 2019 by the American Academy of Pediatrics

FINANCIAL DISCLOSURE: The authors have indicated they have no financial relationships relevant to this article to disclose.

FUNDING: No external funding.

To cite: Linton JM, Green A, AAP COUNCIL ON COMMUNITY PEDIATRICS. Providing Care for Children in Immigrant Families. *Pediatrics*. 2019;144(3):e20192077

DEMOGRAPHICS

Health care of children in immigrant families (CIF) in the United States has received increasing attention over the past decade, in part because of increasing migration of children caused by conflicts globally, greater diversity among migrant populations, and divisive sociopolitical discussion regarding immigration policy. Definitions regarding immigrant children vary, but for the purposes of this policy statement, immigrant children are those born outside the United States to non–US citizen parents. The term CIF includes both those who are foreign born and those who are born in the United States and have at least 1 parent who was foreign born. In 2015, 43 million people, representing 13% of the US population, were immigrants, approaching the historic high of 14.8% in 1890.[1,2] Currently, 3% of US children are foreign born, and 25% of US children live in immigrant families.[3,4] It is projected that by 2065, 18% of the US population will be foreign born and an additional 18% will be US-born children of immigrants.[2] Immigrant children and CIF reside in all 50 states (Figs 1 and 2).

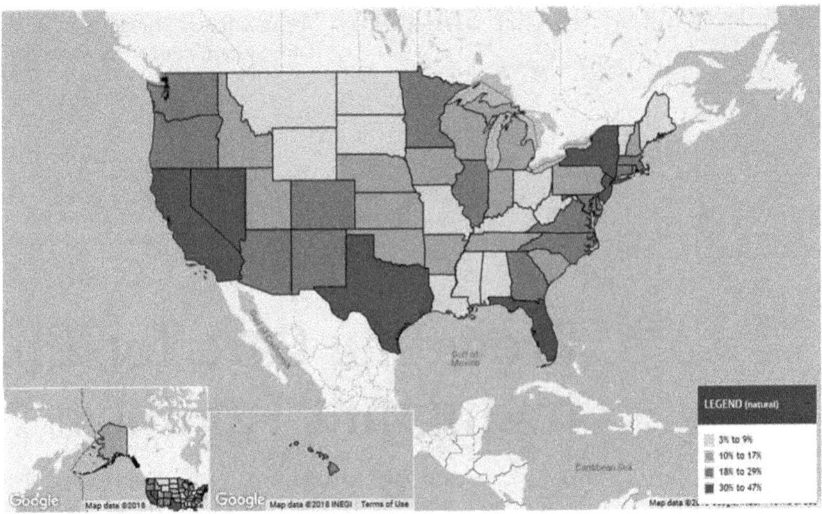

FIGURE 2
CIF, 2016. Reprinted with permission from The Annie E. Casey Foundation, KIDS COUNT Data Center, https://datacenter.kidscount.org.

Children immigrate to the United States with or without their parents for diverse and complex reasons, including, but not limited to, economic needs, educational pursuits, international adoption, human trafficking, or escape from threatening conditions in pursuit of safe haven. Immigrants may arrive with temporary visas (eg, work visa, student visa, tourist visa, J-1 classification), have or obtain permanent permission to remain in the United States (eg, lawful permanent residents [LPRs] or "green card" holders), come with refugee status, seek legal protection on arrival to the United States, or remain without legal status (Table 1). Refugees, who obtain legal status before arrival, and asylees, who can obtain legal status after arrival in the United States, must have a well-founded fear of persecution based on race, religion, nationality, sexual/gender orientation, political opinion, or membership in a particular social group.[5] LPRs and refugees can apply for citizenship after 5 years of living in the United States.[6] In addition to asylum, other forms of protection (eg, special immigrant juvenile status, T nonimmigrant status, and U nonimmigrant status) may also be available to particular children and families seeking safe haven in the United States.[7] If parents or children do not qualify for a legal form of protection, they may choose to remain in the United States without legal status. Specifically, approximately 11.1 million individuals in the United States lack current legal status,[8] and 5.1 million US children live with at least 1

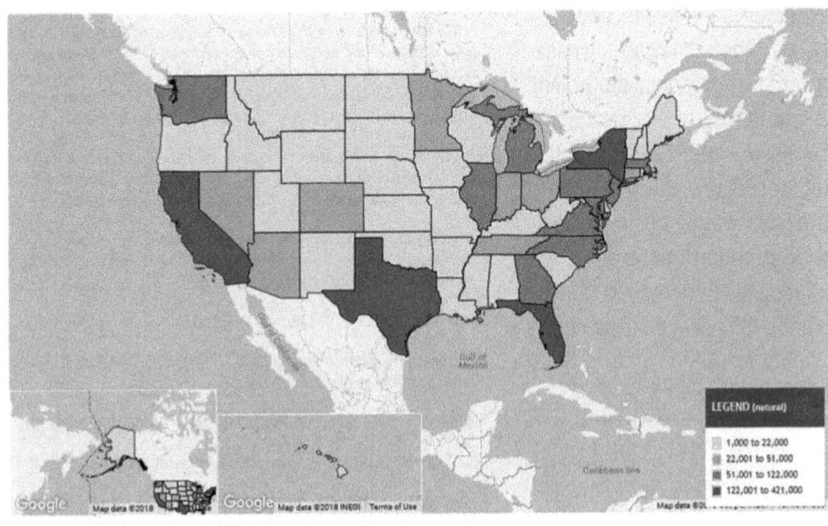

FIGURE 1
Population of immigrant children in the United States, 2017. Reprinted with permission from The Annie E. Casey Foundation, KIDS COUNT Data Center, https://datacenter.kidscount.org.

TABLE 1 Definitions

Term	Description
Children in immigrant families (CIF)	Children who are foreign born and those who are born in the United States and have at least 1 parent who was foreign born
Immigrant children	Children born outside the United States
Lawful permanent residents (LPR)	Immigrants with permission to live and work permanently in the United States
Refugee	Children or adults who fled persecution in their home countries and legally entered the United States after being screened and approved by US agencies abroad
Asylum	Status that can be granted to people already in the United States who have a well-founded fear of persecution by or permitted by their government on the basis of 1 of 5 grounds and who satisfy the requirements for refugee status
T nonimmigrant status ("T visa")	Victims of severe forms of trafficking who can demonstrate that they would suffer extreme hardship involving unusual or severe harm if removed from the United States
U nonimmigrant status ("U visa")	Victims of certain serious crimes who have cooperated with law enforcement in the investigation or prosecution of the crime
Special immigrant juvenile status (SIJS)	Noncitizen minors who were abused, neglected, or abandoned by 1 or both parents
Temporary protected status (TPS)	Status granted to individuals physically present in the United States who are from countries designated by the Secretary of the US Department of Homeland Security as unsafe to accept their return
J-1 classification (exchange visitors)	Status granted to those who intend to participate in an approved program for the purposes of teaching, instructing or lecturing, studying, observing, conducting research, consulting, demonstrating special skills, receiving training, or receiving graduate medical education or training
Deferred Action for Childhood Arrivals (DACA)	Temporary relief from deportation with strict criteria based on age of arrival to United States, whether the individual is in school or working, and whether the individual has no criminal offenses or threats
Deferred Action for Parents of Americans and Lawful Permanent Residents	Temporary relief from deportation for parents of children who are US citizens or have LPR that was never implemented

immigrant parent without legal status.[9]

In 2016, half of the 22.5 million refugees worldwide were 18 years or younger, and less than 1% are resettled annually.[10] Ongoing humanitarian needs are acutely exacerbated by global migration crises, exemplified by the displacement of nearly 12 million Syrians by the end of 2015.[10] The number of refugees entering the United States is set annually by Congress and the president and historically has fluctuated on the basis of sociopolitical events. All 50 states, with the exception of Wyoming, have refugee resettlement programs.[11]

Migration to the United States varies on the basis of global poverty, armed conflict, and exceedingly complex sociopolitical circumstances. Despite these complexities, the United Nations Convention on the Rights of the Child, endorsed by the American Academy of Pediatrics (AAP) but not ratified by the US government, is an internationally recognized legal framework for the protection of children's basic rights, regardless of the reasons children migrate.[12,13] The AAP policy statement "The Effects of Armed Conflict on Children" delineates the impact of armed conflict on children and the role of child health professionals in a global response.[14]

Responses to migration, and especially migration of children, are equally varied and complicated.[15] For instance, increasing arrivals of unaccompanied children and family units from Guatemala, Honduras, El Salvador, and Mexico at the southern US border beginning in 2014 triggered a series of governmental responses, including escalating detention of immigrant children, described in detail in the AAP policy statement "Detention of Immigrant Children."[7,16] Additionally, the Deferred Action for Childhood Arrivals (DACA) program was developed to allow young adults who had arrived in the United States as children without legal status but had grown up in the United States to apply for deportation relief and work permits.[15] A related program, Deferred Action for Parents of Americans and Lawful Permanent Residents (DAPA), would have offered similar protections for parents without legal status who have US-born children, but it was halted in federal courts and was subsequently rescinded by presidential executive order before it could be implemented.[15,17] In 2017, the president signed new executive orders focused on heightened immigration enforcement, increased border security, and limits to the US refugee program. Furthermore, changes to temporary protected status (TPS), granted to individuals physically present in the United States who are from countries designated by the secretary of the US Department of Homeland Security as unsafe to accept their return, have created uncertainty for the nearly 320 000 TPS beneficiaries and their families.[18]

In addition to changes in the numbers and demographics of immigrants and the legal protections afforded them, family immigration status represents an important and often-neglected social determinant of health. The immigration status of children and their parents relates directly to their subsequent access to and use of health care, perceived health status, and health outcomes.[7,19–26] Family immigration status is intertwined with other social determinants of health, including poverty,[27] food insecurity,[28,29] housing instability,[30,31] discrimination,[32,33] and health literacy.[34–37]

RESILIENCE AND INTEGRATION

Despite the challenges that immigrant children and families often face, many offer tremendous assets and demonstrate remarkable resilience. On first arrival in the United States, immigrant children may be healthier than native-born peers, a phenomenon often described as "the immigrant paradox" or "the healthy immigrant effect."[27,33] A strengths-based approach to immigrant child health celebrates assets of immigrant families and populations, buffers marginalization, and supports integration. Understanding cultural assets, such as ethnic-racial identity and cultural values, may offer opportunities to build resilience among immigrant children.[38–40] Furthermore, recognizing assets facilitates productive dialogue that supports immigrant families not as threats but as valuable resources to our society.[40]

CULTURAL HUMILITY AND SAFETY

When caring for CIF, health care providers must recognize the role culture plays in understanding illness without reflexively assuming that challenges are always attributable to cultural differences.[41–45] Because culture is dynamic, cultural competency is never fully realized,[46] but rather serves as a developmental process.[47] Providers bring personal cultural biases, as well as biases of biomedicine, that can implicitly or explicitly affect the provision of care.[48,49] Cultural humility is the concept of openness and respect for differences.[50–52] Cultural safety reflects the recognition of the power differences and inequities in health and the clinical encounter that result from social, historical, economic, and political circumstances.[53–55] By recognizing ourselves and others as cultural beings, by building trust through respect and awareness of power differentials and cultural beliefs, and by developing and implementing communication skills that facilitate mutual understanding, health care providers work to minimize disparities and promote equity in a health encounter.

Culturally sensitive systems of health care, ones that value cultural humility and safety, emerge when patients and families are engaged with 3 core values: curiosity, empathy, and respect.[56] Some immigrants bring with them a system of healing that, like biomedicine practiced in the United States, claims to be curative, includes interventions that can be applied by an expert practitioner, and offers a body of theory regarding disease causation, classification, and treatment.[57] With acculturation, these individuals may or may not modify their healing system to incorporate biomedical concepts. Culturally sensitive care systems have the flexibility to support health literacy, to recognize values of community and family that may supersede individual rights, to engage spirituality and respect traditions, and to include diverse perspectives in implementation and evaluation. The reciprocity of culturally sensitive health care offers us a wider lens that reduces health inequities and strengthens the practice of healing through multicultural medicine and medical practice that acknowledges nonallopathic traditions.[58,59]

CARE OF CIF: CORE COMPETENCIES

Immigrant children benefit from increased access and communication offered in a patient- and family-centered medical home with an identified primary care provider in which care "is respectful of and responsive to individual patient preferences, needs, and values."[60–64] The medical home, infused with cultural humility and safety, supports continuous, comprehensive, and compassionate care and increases collaboration with community supports, including schools, places of worship, legal agencies, and extracurricular activities. Interpreters are an essential part of the medical team to support health literacy, improve access, and ensure quality medical care.[65,66] However, disparities in access to care for CIF, and especially for those with special health care needs, have persisted.[24,25,67–72] Immigrant families, particularly those with children with special health care needs, often benefit from intensive supports in negotiating a complex medical system, special education system, and network of community resources. Pediatric providers can play a lead role for the medical home team in implementing and educating on core competencies that are meant to build health equity for CIF. Core resources for the provision of care for CIF include, but are not limited to, the AAP Immigrant Child Health Toolkit[44] and the Centers for Disease Control and Prevention Refugee Health Guidelines.[73]

Cross-cultural Approach

Rather than learning generalities of a given culture, a practical framework can guide the clinical approach.[74,75] A classic patient-based model recommends assessing for core cross-cultural issues, exploring the meaning of the illness, determining the social context, and engaging in negotiation around treatment plans.[76] Core cross-cultural issues include styles of communication, trust, family dynamics, traditions and spirituality, and sexual and gender considerations.[75] Kleinman and Benson's[45] 7 questions for cultural assessment are helpful to explore patient's perspectives; most crucially, this includes what matters most to the patient and family within the context of illness and treatment (Table 2). The efficacy of treatment may need to be understood "within the scope of cultural beliefs and not that of the scientific evidence."[77,78] Therefore, there may be need for cross-cultural negotiation facilitated through tools like "LEARN" (listen, explain, acknowledge, recommend, negotiate).[57,79]

Knowledge and skills can be developed regarding cross-cultural patient care, migration health issues, and unique vulnerabilities and strengths of immigrant families. Although all children and families are unique, origin-country profiles may be helpful to provide generalized information about immigrant groups.[80–82]

Migration Health Issues

Care of immigrant children requires knowledge of unique health issues in the child's country of origin and country or countries of refuge before arrival as well as an understanding of the challenges of resettlement and acculturation once within the United States. When taking a medical history, it is therefore necessary to elicit details of migration[73] as well as the child's birth; medical, immunization, developmental, social, and family history; and exposure to trauma and violence.[73,83] Past medical and immunization records may require translation as well as awareness and management of different global immunization schedules.[84,85] CIF often return to their families' countries of origin to visit relatives, and providers need to be familiar with travel risks, prophylactic medications, and unique vaccine needs.[86]

TABLE 2 Questions to Elicit the Patient Explanatory Model

Questions
1. What do you call this problem?
2. What do you believe is the cause of this problem?
3. What course do you expect it to take? How serious is it?
4. What do you think this problem does inside your body?
5. How does it affect your body and your mind?
6. What do you most fear about this condition?
7. What do you most fear about the treatment?

Copyright 2006 Kleinman and Benson.[45] Reprinted under the terms of the Creative Commons Attribution License.

Communicable Disease

When screening for and treating infectious diseases, a public health approach is advantageous.[44,87] For refugees, some screenings may have been performed in another country, and presumptive treatments may have been provided through the International Organization for Migration.[88] Depending on the migration history, immigrant children may need screening on arrival in the United States for infectious diseases (eg, tuberculosis; malaria; Chagas disease; intestinal parasites such as helminths, schistosomiasis, and strongyloides; chronic hepatitis B; HIV; syphilis; and other vertically and horizontally transmitted sexual infections).[44,87–94] Comprehensive reproductive and mental health services are warranted for immigrant children with a history of sexual activity, trafficking, exploitation, or victimization.

Oral Health

The global burden of oral diseases is high.[95] Caries risk varies depending on previous country of residence.[96,97] Differences in oral health may reflect cultural practices and norms related to weaning and brushing, dietary changes, and limited oral health literacy.[98–101] Access to dental services and education on oral health is essential for immigrant children.[102]

Noncommunicable Disease

The incidence of noncommunicable diseases globally has grown.[103–105] Rates of asthma, obesity, autism,[106–110] depression, anxiety, and posttraumatic stress disorder (PTSD) may be similar or disproportionately increased in immigrant children.[71,111–114] In addition, newly arrived immigrant children may present with diseases not yet diagnosed or further progressed. Examples include genetic conditions related to consanguinity. Furthermore, newborn screening for hearing loss, hypothyroidism, metabolic diseases, or hemoglobinopathies may not have been performed.[94,115] Vision problems and elevated blood lead concentrations are also common and must be considered.[94,116–120]

Nutrition and Growth

During assessment of nutrition and growth on entry into medical care, immigrant children may be recognized as wasted, having underweight, having overweight, or stunted.[97,121–124] Health care providers will need to be familiar with global diets, dietary restrictions, and vitamin and nutrient sources.[124–126] Anemia, thalassemia, glucose-6-phosphate dehydrogenase deficiency, and micronutrient deficiencies (including iron, vitamin D, and vitamin B_{12}) may exist.[97,127–129] Families can be screened for food insecurity and connected to relevant resources.[126,130,131]

Developmental and Educational Considerations

Age-appropriate developmental and behavioral screening is possible with the use of validated multilingual screening tools, such as the Ages and Stages Questionnaire[132] and the Survey of Well-being of Young Children,[133] and with historical assessment of milestones.[134,135] Care must be taken to recognize cultural bias and experiential differences in skill development.[136–139] Screening needs to be sensitive to cultural differences in parenting[140,141] and disparities in reading or sharing books with children,[142] but referral should not be delayed if screening results are concerning.[143] Age-appropriate vision and hearing screening is essential.[144] Providers' encouragement of a language-rich environment in the parent's primary language recognizes the strengths of bilingualism.[145–150]

One in 10 students from kindergarten to 12th grade in the United States is an English-language learner.[151] Dual-language learners, defined as children younger than 8 years with at least 1 parent who speaks another language in the home other than English, make up one-third of young children in the United States currently. Dual-language learners are less likely to be enrolled in high-quality early child care and preschools compared with peers, potentially limiting kindergarten readiness.[152,153]

All children are entitled to free public education and specialized educational services regardless of immigration status.[154] Immigrant children may face particular academic challenges.[155,156] Before arrival to the United States, some children may have had no opportunity for formal schooling or may have faced protracted educational interruptions. Students with interrupted or no schooling may lack strong literacy skills, age-appropriate content knowledge, and socioemotional skills; in addition, they may need to learn the English language.[157] Learning may also be affected by traumatic brain injury, cerebral malaria, malnutrition, personal trauma, in utero exposures (eg, alcohol),[94] and toxic exposures (eg, lead).[116–120] Testing for developmental and learning challenges in the school setting may result in overrepresentation of students with limited English proficiency (LEP) in special education.[158–161] Through collaboration with parents and schools, pediatricians can facilitate thoughtful consideration of learning difficulties in the setting of LEP. Supplemental anticipatory guidance may include recognition of family strengths and differences in parent-child relationships, child-rearing practices and discipline, dietary preferences, safety risks and use of car restraints and safe sleep practices, and acculturation.[162–168]

Mental Health

Many immigrant children and youth may have had disruptions to the basic experiences that allow for healthy development.[169] Immigrant children and their families may experience trauma before migration, during their journey, on arrival at our borders, and while integrating into American communities[170–176] and, as a result of their increased risk, require "health and related services of a type or amount beyond that required by children generally."[177] Trauma may include personal history of physical or sexual abuse, witnessing interpersonal violence, human trafficking, actual or threatened separation from parents, or exposure to armed conflict.[173,174,176,178] Traumatized children with traumatized parents (or, in some cases, without their parents) may be at risk for toxic stress or prolonged serious stress in the absence of buffering relationships.[179] In addition to intergenerational transfer of mental health problems, core stressors include trauma, acculturation, isolation, and resettlement.[172] In particular, acculturation includes stressors that families experience as they navigate between the culture of their country of origin and the culture in their new country.[172]

On arrival, many refugee and unaccompanied children have high levels of anxiety, depression, and PTSD.[174,180–186] Compared with US-origin youth, refugee youth have higher rates of community violence exposure, dissociative symptoms, traumatic grief, somatization, and phobic disorder.[187] Unaccompanied minors have even higher levels of PTSD compared with accompanied immigrants,[188] which may be further heightened if they are seeking asylum.[189] Immigration-related trauma history may be shared over time as a trusting relationship develops with the physician.[190] Some CIF who were born in the United States may face difficulty with emotional and behavioral problems relating to identity formation.[191] Initial and ongoing screening for mental and behavioral health problems with multiple cross-culturally validated tools (eg, the Ages and Stages Questionnaire-Social Emotional, the Survey of Well-being of Young Children, the Strengths and Difficulty Questionnaire, the Refugee Health Screener 15, and the Child Behavior Checklist) facilitates recognition of distress and concerns.[44,132,133,192–195]

By understanding the interplay of biological, social, environmental, and psychological risk and protective factors, emotional disorders can be modulated on population, community, and individual levels.[196] Protective factors and sources of resilience observed in immigrants include having a positive outlook, having strong coping skills, having positive parental coping strategies, connection to prosocial organizations such as places of worship and athletics, and cultural pride reinforcement.[32,197–200] Resilience is fostered through strong family relationships and community support.[201] Bicultural identity, a strong attachment to one's culture of origin in addition to a sense of belonging within the culture of residence, promotes resilience.[140,202]

Because of the shame and stigma associated with mental health problems, families may be reluctant to seek treatment.[203] Providers can increase access and minimize stigma by integrating culturally tailored mental health services into the medical home, in the school setting, and through engagement with community mental health resources,[78,175,204] including home visitation.[205] Community-wide strategies that foster belonging, reduce discrimination, and provide social supports can facilitate healing and reduce stigma.

Traditional Health Care and Cultural Practices

Traditional healing and cultural practices, common among some immigrant populations, warrant awareness by health care providers.[206] Patients may not disclose use of herbal and traditional treatments unless directly asked.[42,207] Some immigrant families use traditional forms of protection for vulnerable infants, such as prayer, amulets, kohl, or myrrh. Other immigrant families use traditional practices to treat illness (eg, cupping, coining, and uvulectomy), and stigmata of these traditional treatments may be observed on examination and may be misinterpreted as abuse.[208,209]

Female genital cutting or mutilation (FGC/M) is still practiced in some communities in Africa, in the Middle East, and in parts of Asia despite increased efforts to educate on risks.[210,211] Performing FGC/M is against the law in the United States and has been defined as torture by the United Nations, but foreign-born girls may have experienced this before entry into the United States.[210,212] Resources exist regarding the types of FGC/M, complications that can result, recommended documentation in the medical record, and strategies to sensitively discuss this with families.[213,214] In 2013, the United States passed the Transport for Female Genital Mutilation Act, which prohibits knowingly transporting a girl out of the United States for the purpose of "vacation cutting."[215] The need to screen for FGC/M further underscores the importance of examining the external genitalia of children at all preventive visits in addition to sensitively counseling families regarding the laws and other concerns regarding FGM/C.

PRACTICE-LEVEL BARRIERS AND POTENTIAL OPPORTUNITIES

Communication challenges between families with LEP and health care providers must be addressed to provide high-quality care. Fifty-four percent of CIF have resident parents who have difficulty speaking English.[3] Parental LEP is associated with worse health care access and quality for children.[216–220] National Standards for Culturally and Linguistically Appropriate Services in Health Care were issued by the US Department of Health and Human Services, in accordance with Title VI of the Civil Rights Act. Culturally and Linguistically Appropriate Services in Health Care Standards describe the federal expectation that health care organizations receiving federal funding must provide meaningful access to verbal and written-language services for patients with LEP.[221,222] Interpreters are an integral part of the medical home team for CIF and hold the same confidentiality standards as the physician.[67,68] Most state insurance programs and private insurers do not offer reimbursement for language services. Although teaching health care providers when and how to work with interpreters can improve care, few providers receive such training.[223,224] For these and other reasons, some providers inappropriately use family members as ad hoc interpreters.[225] However, family members, friends, and especially children are not acceptable substitutes for trained interpreters.[226,227] Trained medical interpreters, via phone or tablet or in-person, facilitate mutual understanding and a high quality of communication.[228,229] Use of trained interpreters maintains confidentiality, reduces errors and cost, and increases the quality of health care delivery.[227,228,230–232] Interpretation requires that extra time be allotted to health care encounters. Qualified bicultural and bilingual staff can receive medical interpreter training if expected to perform as interpreters, and bilingual providers can ideally demonstrate dual-language proficiency before engaging with families in their preferred language without an interpreter.[233–235] Access can be further improved by the use of multilingual signage, screening tools, handouts, and other key documents (eg, consent forms and hospital discharge summaries) that are prepared by qualified translators.

Although some immigrant families integrate without hardship, many CIF face inequities resulting from complex determinants, including poverty, immigration status, insurance status, education, and discrimination on the basis of race and/or ethnicity.[32,33] For some, fear regarding family immigration status threatens children's health, development, and access to care.[22,32,236–238] For others, growing up in 2-parent families and having environmental stimulation at home, particularly for those with low socioeconomic status, may be protective.[33,239] Screening for social determinants of health can trigger referrals to community-based supports.[240] The hallmarks of the medical home, comprehensive care and enhanced care coordination, are important supports for immigrant families. Integrated mental health, nutrition, social work, and patient navigation services allow for ease of access and for reduction in stigma and barriers. Community health workers who are members of immigrant communities have been effective in reducing disparity and improving health outcomes.[241–246]

Interagency partnerships with the local health department, home-visiting programs, community mental health providers, schools, and immigrant service organizations facilitate access to medical homes and cross-sector communication. "Warm hand-offs," or in-person transfer of care between health care team members with patients and families present, can help to ensure linkage between providers and relevant resources.[247]

SYSTEMS-LEVEL BARRIERS AND POTENTIAL OPPORTUNITIES

Health literacy challenges experienced by CIF include not only language comprehension but also the myriad of system barriers in the health care network. Limited health literacy can complicate enrollment in public benefits for CIF. Immigrant children are specifically less likely to have a medical home[67,68] and health insurance, resulting in delayed or foregone care.[248] Most immigrant children with legal status are eligible for health coverage. A majority of states have opted to allow lawfully residing immigrant children to receive Medicaid and/or Children's Health Insurance Program coverage using federal Medicaid and Children's Health Insurance Program funds without a 5-year waiting period, an option given to states by the Children's Health Insurance Program Reauthorization Act of 2009; however, 17 states have not taken the Children's Health Insurance Program Reauthorization Act of 2009 option.[249–253] Only a minority of states offer health coverage to children regardless of immigration status.[252,253] Additionally, immigrant children without legal status, including DACA youth, are excluded from eligibility for most federal programs, including health insurance, although some states have included and/or are considering inclusion of DACA youth (or, more broadly, other noncitizen children) as eligible for programs such as in-state tuition or professional licensing.[254,255] Opportunities to mitigate these literacy, access, and health insurance enrollment challenges include system-wide use and funding of interpreters and multilingual tools and use of community health workers and patient navigators to reduce barriers through facilitation, education, and advocacy.[43,58,59,256,257] For CIF without health coverage, federally qualified health centers, public health departments, free clinics, and charity care systems may offer access to consistent care. Home-visiting programs can support immigrant parents and parents with LEP who may be isolated and unable to access public services[152,258]; attention to cultural safety is particularly critical when engaging in home-based services. Quality after-school programming, with support of school social work, can also facilitate integration and build resilience for CIF.[259,260]

IMMIGRATION AND RELATED LEGAL ISSUES

Federal immigration policies can adversely affect immigrant health coverage, access, and outcomes. Immigration status of children and/or their parents continues to affect access to services and public benefits, despite some improvement.[33,261,262] Increased fears about the use of public programs and immigration status has deterred immigrants from accessing programs regardless of eligibility.[263–265] In addition, immigration enforcement activities that occur at or near sensitive locations, such as hospitals, may prevent families from accessing needed medical care.[264] Sensitive locations include medical treatment and health care facilities, places of worship, and schools, and US Immigration and Customs Enforcement actions, including apprehension, interviews, searches, or surveillance, should not occur at these locations.[266,267] Fear of immigration enforcement or discrimination may exacerbate transportation barriers and worsen perceived access to care.[23,237,268–271] Discrimination relating to immigration may intersect with religion (eg, Muslim immigrants) and race in complex ways.[264,272–274] Discrimination and immigration enforcement policies may also create fear and uncertainty, which threaten the mental health of immigrant children[275] and their families.[19,236,264,276] Families living on the US-Mexico border face particular risk of mistreatment and victimization.[277] Policies that offer protection from deportation, such as DACA, may confer large mental health benefits for youth and for the children of parenting youth.[278,279]

Immigrant children who have been detained and are in immigration proceedings face almost universal traumatic histories and ongoing stress, including actual or threatened separation from their parents at the border.[7] Immigrant children, including unaccompanied children, are not guaranteed a right to legal counsel, and as such, roughly 50% of children arriving in the United States have no one to represent them in immigration court.[280] Lack of guaranteed legal representation for immigrant children and families at risk for deportation is further complicated by funding restrictions; specifically, medical-legal partnerships receiving federal funding that operate under Legal Services Corporation guidelines cannot accept most cases related to immigration.[281] Many nongovernmental efforts have sought to address lack of legal representation for children, but opportunities remain to better provide immigration-specific legal support for immigrant families,[282,283] including novel medical-legal partnerships with different funding streams that do not exclude people without legal status and offer representation in immigration court. In addition, traumatized immigrant children can benefit from system-level supports for integration of mental health and social work supports into schools, the medical home, and protected community settings.[284]

Evidence-based programs can systematically build resilience among CIF by supporting integration into US culture while preserving home cultural heritage. Although specific evidence regarding CIF is limited, home-visiting programs offer opportunities to celebrate unique strengths and mitigate stress in a natural environment.[258,285] Programs that support literacy and encourage play, such as Reach Out and Read, can reinforce parent-child relationships, build parenting skills, support development, and prepare children for academic success.[150,286,287] For children experiencing parental reunification after prolonged separation, mental health services and educational support are particularly critical.[238] Given the strong role of communities in many cultures, community-based interventions may be particularly effective for immigrant families.

Opportunities to investigate strategies, mitigate barriers, and optimize health and well-being for CIF include research, medical education, and community engagement, including community-based participatory research and health education. Research used to examine acculturative stress and resilience of immigrant children over time is limited. Among CIF, diversity within and between racial and ethnic groups (eg, Hispanic, Asian, African, and Caribbean) and between CIF of varying socioeconomic statuses is also understudied and underappreciated.[288] Medical education has become increasingly responsive to health disparities for immigrants and to the opportunities for experiential broadening of global health. By implementing core competencies in the care of immigrant populations, trainees can learn to support a culture of health equity for CIF. Pediatricians can support families within and beyond the medical home through efforts supported by cross-sector community collaboration, including fields such as education and law, innovative research, and thoughtful advocacy, to inspire progressive policy.[171,180,289] Grants that are focused on minority and underserved pediatric populations have the potential to mitigate inequities for immigrant children.[171]

SUMMARY AND RECOMMENDATIONS

With ever-increasing levels of migration worldwide, the population of CIF residing in the United States grows. The following practice- and policy-level recommendations offer guidance for pediatricians caring for CIF. Although it is aspirational to fully implement all recommendations in all situations, most are achievable by intentionally enacting practice- and systems-based changes over time.

Practice-Level Recommendations

1. All pediatricians are encouraged to recognize their inherent biases and work to improve their skills in cultural humility and effective communication through professional development.
2. CIF benefit from comprehensive, coordinated, continuous, and culturally and linguistically effective care in a quality medical home with an identified primary care provider.
3. Co-located or integrated mental health, social work, patient navigation, and legal services are recommended to improve access and minimize barriers.
4. Trained medical interpreters, via phone or tablet or in-person, are recommended to facilitate mutual understanding and a high quality of communication. Family members, friends, and especially children are not recommended for interpretation. Materials may be translated into the patient's preferred language by qualified translators whenever possible. Consideration should be given for the extended time needed for interpretation during medical encounters.
5. It is recommended that pediatricians and staff receive training on working effectively with language services and that bilingual providers and staff demonstrate dual-language competency before interacting with patients and families without medical interpreters.
6. Pediatricians and pediatric trainees are encouraged to engage in professional development activities that include specific competencies (including immigrant health; global health, including the global burden of disease; integrative medicine; and travel medicine) and to incorporate these competencies into the evaluation and care of CIF.
7. Pediatricians caring for CIF are urged to apply a trauma-informed lens, with sensitivity to and screening for multigenerational trauma. Mental health professionals adept at treating immigrants can be integrated into the medical home or identified in the community.
8. Screening for social determinants of health, including risks and protective factors, is recommended.
9. Assessment of development, learning, and behavior is warranted for all immigrant children, regardless of age. Pediatricians can support dual language as an asset and as part of cultural pride reinforcement.

Advocacy and Policy Recommendations

1. The AAP endorses the United Nations Convention on the Rights of the Child and the principles included in this document as a legal framework for the protection of children's basic rights.
2. All US federal government, private, and community-based organizations involved with immigrant children should adopt policies that protect and prioritize their health, well-being, and safety and should consider children's best interests in all decisions by government and private actors.
3. Interagency collaboration is recommended between service providers (eg, medical, mental health, public health, legal, education, social work, and ethnic-community based) to enhance care, prevent marginalization of immigrant families, and build resilience among immigrant communities.
4. Health coverage should be provided for all children regardless of immigration status. Neither immigrant children with legal status nor their parents should be subject to a 5-year waiting period for health coverage or other federal benefits.
5. Private and public insurance payers should pay for qualified medical interpretation and translation services. Given the increased cost-effectiveness and quality of care provided with medical interpretation, payers should recognize and reimburse for the increased time needed during a medical encounter when using an interpreter.
6. Both the separation of children from their parents and the detention of children with parents as a tool of law enforcement are inhumane, counterproductive, and threatening to short- and long-term health. Immigration authorities should not separate children from their parents nor place children in detention.
7. Immigration enforcement activities should not occur at or near sensitive locations such as hospitals, health care facilities, schools (including child care and Head Start), places of worship, and other sensitive locations. Pediatricians have the right to report and protest any such enforcement. Medical records should be protected from immigration enforcement actions. Health systems can develop protocols to minimize fear and enhance trust for those seeking health care.
8. Children in immigration proceedings should have access to legal representation at no cost to the child. Medical-legal partnerships that include immigration representation (eg, Terra Firma[290]) and efforts to increase legal representation (eg, KIND,[291] the Young Center for Immigrant Children's Rights,[292] RAICES[293]) should be supported practically and financially at local, state, and federal levels.
9. Immigration policy that prioritizes children and families by ensuring access to health care and educational and economic supports, by keeping families together, and by protecting vulnerable unaccompanied children is of fundamental importance for comprehensive immigration reform. Humanitarian protection (eg, refugee resettlement and protection for victims of trafficking and asylum seekers) supports trauma-informed care of children and is an essential component of immigration policy.
10. All children with LEP merit early, intensive, and longitudinal educational support with culturally responsive teaching. Literacy skills are necessary for health literacy, an essential health need.
11. Enhanced funding is recommended to support research regarding immigrant child health, including, but not limited to, health outcomes; screening tools for development, mental health, and social determinants of health that are culturally and linguistically sensitive; developmental and/or learning difficulties in children whose home language is not English; and reduction of barriers to health access and equity.
12. Medical education can facilitate education of trainees and health care professionals through implementation of core competencies in the care of immigrant populations and through advocacy curricula that incorporate special populations, including CIF.
13. AAP chapters can work with state governments to adopt policies that protect and prioritize immigrant children's health, well-being, and safety.

CONCLUSIONS

CIF represent a growing, diverse demographic in the United States. Pediatricians play an essential role in addressing vulnerabilities, minimizing barriers to care, and supporting optimal short- and long-term health and well-being of CIF within the medical home and in communities across the nation.

With compassionate, respectful, and progressive policy, CIF can achieve their full potential for health and well-being.

LEAD AUTHORS

Julie M. Linton, MD, FAAP
Andrea Green, MD, FAAP

COUNCIL ON COMMUNITY PEDIATRICS EXECUTIVE COMMITTEE, 2017–2018

Lance A. Chilton, MD, FAAP, Chairperson
James H. Duffee, MD, MPH, FAAP, Vice-Chairperson
Kimberley J. Dilley, MD, MPH, FAAP
Andrea Green, MD, FAAP
J. Raul Gutierrez, MD, MPH, FAAP
Virginia A. Keane, MD, FAAP
Scott D. Krugman, MD, MS, FAAP
Julie M. Linton, MD, FAAP
Carla D. McKelvey, MD, MPH, FAAP
Jacqueline L. Nelson, MD, FAAP

LIAISONS

Gerri L. Mattson, MD, MPH, FAAP – *Chairperson, Public Health Special Interest Group*
Kathleen Rooney-Otero, MD, MPH – *Section on Pediatric Trainees*
Donene Feist – *Family Voices North Dakota*

STAFF

Dana Bennett-Tejes, MA, MNM
Jean Davis, MPP
Tamar Magarik Haro

ACKNOWLEDGMENT

We thank Jennifer Nagda, JD (Young Center for Immigrant Children's Rights).

ABBREVIATIONS

AAP: American Academy of Pediatrics
CIF: children in immigrant families
DACA: Deferred Action for Childhood Arrivals
FGC/M: female genital cutting or mutilation
LEP: limited English proficiency
LPR: lawful permanent resident
PTSD: posttraumatic stress disorder
TPS: temporary protected status

POTENTIAL CONFLICT OF INTEREST: The authors have indicated they have no potential conflicts of interest to disclose.

REFERENCES

1. Migration Policy Institute. Immigrant profiles and demographics. US data. Available at: https://www.migrationpolicy.org/topics/us-data. Accessed July 26, 2019
2. Pew Research Center. *Modern immigration wave brings 59 million to US, driving population growth and change through 2065: views of immigration's impact on US society mixed.* 2015. Available at: www.pewhispanic.org/2015/09/28/modern-immigration-wave-brings-59-million-to-u-s-driving-population-growth-and-change-through-2065/. Accessed August 30, 2018
3. The Annie E. Casey Foundation; Kids Count Data Center. Children in immigrant families in the United States. Available at: https://datacenter.kidscount.org/data/tables/115-children-in-immigrant-families?loc=1&loct=1#detailed/1/any/false/871,870,573,869,36,868,867,133,38,35/any/445,446. Accessed July 26, 2019
4. Urban Institute. Children of immigrants data tool. Available at: http://webapp.urban.org/charts/datatool/pages.cfm. Accessed August 30, 2018
5. United Nations Office of the High Commissioner for Refugees. Convention and protocol relating to the status of refugees. 2010. Available at: www.unhcr.org/en-us/protection/basic/3b66c2aa10/convention-protocol-relating-status-refugees.html. Accessed August 30, 2018
6. The National Child Traumatic Stress Network. Bridging refugee youth and children's services. Refugee 101. Available at: https://www.nctsn.org/resources/bridging-refugee-youth-and-childrens-services-refugee-101. Accessed August 30, 2018
7. Linton JM, Griffin M, Shapiro AJ; Council on Community Pediatrics. Detention of immigrant children. *Pediatrics.* 2017;139(5):e20170483
8. Passel JS, Cohn D. Overall number of US unauthorized immigrants holds steady since 2009. 2016. Available at: www.pewhispanic.org/2016/09/20/overall-number-of-u-s-unauthorized-immigrants-holds-steady-since-2009/. Accessed December 27, 2017
9. Capps R, Fix M, Zong J. A profile of U.S. children with unauthorized immigrant parents. Available at: https://www.migrationpolicy.org/research/profile-us-children-unauthorized-immigrant-parents. Accessed December 27, 2017
10. United Nations Office of the High Commissioner for Refugees. *Global Trends: Forced Displacement in 2015.* Geneva, Switzerland: United Nations Office of the High Commissioner for Refugees; 2016
11. Administration for Children and Families. Office of refugee resettlement. 2017. Available at: https://www.acf.hhs.gov/orr. Accessed June 12, 2017
12. Haggerty RJ. The convention on the rights of the child: it's time for the United States to ratify. *Pediatrics.* 1994;94(5):746–747
13. United Nations General Assembly. Convention on the rights of the child. 1989. Available at: www.ohchr.org/Documents/ProfessionalInterest/crc.pdf. Accessed April 8, 2016
14. Shenoda S, Kadir A, Pitterman S, Goldhagen J; Section on International Child Health. The effects of armed conflict on children. *Pediatrics.* 2018;142(6):e20182585
15. Cohn D. *How U.S. Immigration Laws and Rules Have Changed through History.* Washington, DC: Pew Research Center; 2015. Available at: www.pewresearch.

org/fact-tank/2015/09/30/how-u-s-immigration-laws-and-rules-have-changed-through-history/. Accessed June 16, 2017

16. US Customs and Border Protection. United States border patrol southwest family unit subject and unaccompanied alien children apprehensions fiscal year 2016. Available at: https://www.cbp.gov/newsroom/stats/southwest-border-unaccompanied-children/fy-2016. Accessed December 26, 2016

17. US Department of Homeland Security. Frequently asked questions: rescission of memorandum providing for Deferred Action for Parents of Americans and Lawful Permanent Residents ("DAPA"). 2017. Available at: https://www.dhs.gov/news/2017/06/15/frequently-asked-questions-rescission-memorandum-providing-deferred-action-parents. Accessed June 15, 2017

18. Cohn D, Passel JS, Bialik K. Many Immigrants With Temporary Protected Status Face Uncertain Future in U.S. 2017. Available at: www.pewresearch.org/fact-tank/2017/11/08/more-than-100000-haitian-and-central-american-immigrants-face-decision-on-their-status-in-the-u-s/. Accessed December 27, 2017

19. Martinez O, Wu E, Sandfort T, et al. Evaluating the impact of immigration policies on health status among undocumented immigrants: a systematic review [published correction appears in *J Immigr Minor Health*. 2016;18(1):288]. *J Immigr Minor Health*. 2015;17(3):947–970

20. Novak NL, Geronimus AT, Martinez-Cardoso AM. Change in birth outcomes among infants born to Latina mothers after a major immigration raid. *Int J Epidemiol*. 2017;46(3):839–849

21. Hardy LJ, Getrich CM, Quezada JC, Guay A, Michalowski RJ, Henley E. A call for further research on the impact of state-level immigration policies on public health. *Am J Public Health*. 2012;102(7): 1250–1254

22. Vargas ED, Ybarra VD. U.S. citizen children of undocumented parents: the link between state immigration policy and the health of Latino children. *J Immigr Minor Health*. 2017;19(4): 913–920

23. Lopez WD, Kruger DJ, Delva J, et al. Health implications of an immigration raid: findings from a Latino community in the midwestern United States. *J Immigr Minor Health*. 2017;19(3): 702–708

24. Yun K, Fuentes-Afflick E, Curry LA, Krumholz HM, Desai MM. Parental immigration status is associated with children's health care utilization: findings from the 2003 new immigrant survey of US legal permanent residents. *Matern Child Health J*. 2013;17(10): 1913–1921

25. Javier JR, Huffman LC, Mendoza FS, Wise PH. Children with special health care needs: how immigrant status is related to health care access, health care utilization, and health status. *Matern Child Health J*. 2010;14(4): 567–579

26. Siddiqi A, Zuberi D, Nguyen QC. The role of health insurance in explaining immigrant versus non-immigrant disparities in access to health care: comparing the United States to Canada. *Soc Sci Med*. 2009;69(10):1452–1459

27. Child Trends. Immigrant children. 2017. Available at: https://www.childtrends.org/indicators/immigrant-children. Accessed August 27, 2018

28. Chilton M, Black MM, Berkowitz C, et al. Food insecurity and risk of poor health among US-born children of immigrants. *Am J Public Health*. 2009;99(3):556–562

29. Walsemann KM, Ro A, Gee GC. Trends in food insecurity among California residents from 2001 to 2011: inequities at the intersection of immigration status and ethnicity. *Prev Med*. 2017; 105(1):142–148

30. Koball H, Capps R, Perrera K, et al. *Health and Social Service Needs of US-Citizen Children With Detained or Deported Immigrant Parents*. Washington, DC: Urban Institute, Migration Policy Institute; 2015, Available at: https://www.urban.org/research/publication/health-and-social-service-needs-us-citizen-children-detained-or-deported-immigrant-parents/view/full_report. Accessed December 27, 2017

31. Hooper K, Zong J, Capps R, Fix M. *Young Children of Refugees in the United States: Integration Successes and Challenges*. Washington, DC: Migration Policy Institute; 2016, Available at: https://www.migrationpolicy.org/research/young-children-refugees-united-states-integration-successes-and-challenges. Accessed August 27, 2018

32. Brown CS. *The Educational, Psychological, and Social Impact of Discrimination on the Immigrant Child*. Washington, DC: Migration Policy Institute; 2015, Available at: https://www.migrationpolicy.org/research/educational-psychological-and-social-impact-discrimination-immigrant-child. Accessed August 27, 2018

33. Singh GK, Rodriguez-Lainz A, Kogan MD. Immigrant health inequalities in the United States: use of eight major national data systems. *ScientificWorldJournal*. 2013;2013: 512313

34. Braveman P, Barclay C. Health disparities beginning in childhood: a life-course perspective. *Pediatrics*. 2009;124(suppl 3):S163–S175

35. Braveman P, Egerter S, Williams DR. The social determinants of health: coming of age. *Annu Rev Public Health*. 2011;32: 381–398

36. Simich L. Health literacy and immigrant populations. Public Health Agency of Canada and Metropolis Canada, Ottawa, Canada. 2009. Available at: http://www.metropolis.net/pdfs/health_literacy_policy_brief_jun15_e.pdf. Accessed August 27, 2018

37. Lee HY, Rhee TG, Kim NK, Ahluwalia JS. Health literacy as a social determinant of health in Asian American immigrants: findings from a population-based survey in California. *J Gen Intern Med*. 2015;30(8):1118–1124

38. Rivas-Drake D, Stein GL. Multicultural developmental experiences: implications for resilience in transitional age youth. *Child Adolesc Psychiatr Clin N Am*. 2017;26(2):271–281

39. US Department of Health and Human Services, Office of Minority Health. *National Standards for Culturally and Linguistically Appropriate Services in Health Care*. Washington, DC: US Department of Health and Human Services; 2001

40. Baran M, Kendall-Taylor N, Lindland E, O'Neil M, Haydon A. Getting to "we":

mapping the gaps between expert and public understandings of immigration and immigration reform. Available at: www.frameworksinstitute.org/assets/files/Immigration/immigration_mtg.pdf. Accessed December 28, 2017

41. Kodjo C. Cultural competence in clinician communication. *Pediatr Rev.* 2009;30(2):57–63; quiz 64

42. Brach C, Fraser I. Can cultural competency reduce racial and ethnic health disparities? A review and conceptual model. *Med Care Res Rev.* 2000;57(suppl 1):181–217

43. Committee on Pediatric Workforce. Enhancing pediatric workforce diversity and providing culturally effective pediatric care: implications for practice, education, and policy making. *Pediatrics.* 2013;132(4). Available at: www.pediatrics.org/cgi/content/full/132/4/e1105

44. American Academy of Pediatrics. Immigrant Child Health Toolkit. 2015. Available at: https://www.aap.org/en-us/advocacy-and-policy/aap-health-initiatives/Immigrant-Child-Health-Toolkit/Pages/Immigrant-Child-Health-Toolkit.aspx. Accessed October 29, 2018

45. Kleinman A, Benson P. Anthropology in the clinic: the problem of cultural competency and how to fix it. *PLoS Med.* 2006;3(10):e294

46. Kirmayer LJ. Rethinking cultural competence. *Transcult Psychiatry.* 2012; 49(2):149–164

47. Cross T, Bazron BJ, Dennis KW, Isaacs MR. *Towards a Culturally Competent System of Care: A Monograph on Effective Services for Minority Children Who Are Severely Emotionally Disturbed.* Washington, DC: Georgetown University Child Development Center, CASSP Technical Assistance Center; 1989

48. Project Implicit. About us. Available at: https://implicit.harvard.edu/implicit/aboutus.html. Accessed September 17, 2018

49. Blair IV, Steiner JF, Fairclough DL, et al. Clinicians' implicit ethnic/racial bias and perceptions of care among Black and Latino patients. *Ann Fam Med.* 2013; 11(1):43–52

50. Tervalon M, Murray-García J. Cultural humility versus cultural competence: a critical distinction in defining physician training outcomes in multicultural education. *J Health Care Poor Underserved.* 1998;9(2):117–125

51. Hook JN, Davis DE, Owen J, Worthington EL, Utsey SO. Cultural humility: measuring openness to culturally diverse clients. *J Couns Psychol.* 2013; 60(3):353–366

52. Yeager KA, Bauer-Wu S. Cultural humility: essential foundation for clinical researchers. *Appl Nurs Res.* 2013;26(4):251–256

53. Papps E, Ramsden I. Cultural safety in nursing: the New Zealand experience. *Int J Qual Health Care.* 1996;8(5): 491–497

54. Darroch F, Giles A, Sanderson P, et al. The United States does CAIR about cultural safety: examining cultural safety within indigenous health contexts in Canada and the United States. *J Transcult Nurs.* 2017;28(3): 269–277

55. Bozorgzad P, Negarandeh R, Raiesifar A, Poortaghi S. Cultural safety: an evolutionary concept analysis. *Holist Nurs Pract.* 2016;30(1):33–38

56. Green AR, Betancourt JR, Carillo JE. Cultural competence: a patient-based approach to caring for immigrants. In: Walker PF, Barnett ED, eds. *Immigrant Medicine.* 1st ed. Philadelphia, PA: Elsevier Health Sciences; 2007:83–97

57. Culhane-Pera KA, Borkan JM. Multicultural medicine. In: Walker PF, Barnett ED, eds. *Immigrant Medicine.* 1st ed. Philadelphia, PA: Elsevier Health Sciences; 2007:69–82

58. McPhail-Bell K, Bond C, Brough M, Fredericks B. 'We don't tell people what to do': ethical practice and Indigenous health promotion. *Health Promot J Austr.* 2015;26(3):195–199

59. Swota AH, Hester DM. Ethics for the pediatrician: providing culturally effective health care. *Pediatr Rev.* 2011; 32(3):e39–e43

60. American Academy of Pediatrics. National center for patient/family-centered medical home. Available at: https://medicalhomeinfo.aap.org/Pages/default.aspx. Accessed October 29, 2018

61. Medical Home Initiatives for Children With Special Needs Project Advisory Committee; American Academy of Pediatrics. The medical home. *Pediatrics.* 2002;110(1, pt 1):184–186

62. Barry MJ, Edgman-Levitan S. Shared decision making–pinnacle of patient-centered care. *N Engl J Med.* 2012; 366(9):780–781

63. Bennett AC, Rankin KM, Rosenberg D. Does a medical home mediate racial disparities in unmet healthcare needs among children with special healthcare needs? *Matern Child Health J.* 2012; 16(suppl 2):330–338

64. Okumura MJ, Van Cleave J, Gnanasekaran S, Houtrow A. Understanding factors associated with work loss for families caring for CSHCN. *Pediatrics.* 2009;124(suppl 4): S392–S398

65. Hsieh E, Ju H, Kong H. Dimensions of trust: the tensions and challenges in provider–interpreter trust. *Qual Health Res.* 2010;20(2):170–181

66. Hsieh E, Kramer EM. Medical interpreters as tools: dangers and challenges in the utilitarian approach to interpreters' roles and functions. *Patient Educ Couns.* 2012;89(1):158–162

67. Raphael JL, Guadagnolo BA, Beal AC, Giardino AP. Racial and ethnic disparities in indicators of a primary care medical home for children. *Acad Pediatr.* 2009;9(4):221–227

68. Kan K, Choi H, Davis M. Immigrant families, children with special health care needs, and the medical home. *Pediatrics.* 2016;137(1):e20153221

69. Mendoza FS. Health disparities and children in immigrant families: a research agenda. *Pediatrics.* 2009; 124(suppl 3):S187–S195

70. Yu SM, Huang ZJ, Kogan MD. State-level health care access and use among children in US immigrant families. *Am J Public Health.* 2008;98(11):1996–2003

71. Javier JR, Wise PH, Mendoza FS. The relationship of immigrant status with access, utilization, and health status for children with asthma. *Ambul Pediatr.* 2007;7(6):421–430

72. Health Resources and Services Administration Maternal and Child Health. Children with special health

care needs. Available at: https://mchb.hrsa.gov/maternal-child-health-topics/children-and-youth-special-health-needs. Accessed January 9, 2018

73. Centers for Disease Control and Prevention. Domestic examination for newly arrived refugees: guidelines and discussion of the history and physical examination. Available at: https://www.cdc.gov/immigrantrefugeehealth/guidelines/domestic/guidelines-history-physical.html. Accessed August 14, 2018

74. Betancourt JR. Cultural competence and medical education: many names, many perspectives, one goal. *Acad Med.* 2006;81(6):499–501

75. Epner DE, Baile WF. Patient-centered care: the key to cultural competence. *Ann Oncol.* 2012;23(suppl 3):33–42

76. Carrillo JE, Green AR, Betancourt JR. Cross-cultural primary care: a patient-based approach. *Ann Intern Med.* 1999;130(10):829–834

77. Kleinman A, Eisenberg L, Good B. Culture, illness, and care: clinical lessons from anthropologic and cross-cultural research. *Ann Intern Med.* 1978;88(2):251–258

78. Roldán-Chicano MT, Fernández-Rufete J, Hueso-Montoro C, García-López MDM, Rodríguez-Tello J, Flores-Bienert MD. Culture-bound syndromes in migratory contexts: the case of Bolivian immigrants. *Rev Lat Am Enfermagem.* 2017;25:e2915

79. Berlin EA, Fowkes WC Jr. A teaching framework for cross-cultural health care. Application in family practice. *West J Med.* 1983;139(6):934–938

80. Centers for Disease Control and Prevention. Refugee health profiles. Available at: https://www.cdc.gov/immigrantrefugeehealth/profiles/index.html. Accessed August 14, 2018

81. Cultural Orientation Resource Center. Refugee backgrounders. Available at: www.culturalorientation.net/learning/backgrounders. Accessed August 14, 2018

82. EthnoMed. Clinical topics. Available at: https://ethnomed.org/clinical. Accessed August 14, 2018

83. Centers for Disease Control and Prevention. Immigrant and refugee health. Available at: https://www.cdc.gov/immigrantrefugeehealth/index.html. Accessed August 14, 2018

84. Centers for Disease Control and Prevention. Catch-up immunization schedule for persons aged 4 months-18 years who start late or who are more than 1 month behind—United States. 2019. Available at: https://www.cdc.gov/vaccines/schedules/hcp/imz/catchup.html. Accessed July 26, 2019

85. World Health Organization. WHO Vaccine-preventable diseases monitoring system. 2019 Global Summary. Available at: https://apps.who.int/immunization_monitoring/globalsummary. Accessed July 29, 2019

86. Centers for Disease Control and Prevention. Travelers' health. Available at: https://wwwnc.cdc.gov/travel/destinations/list/. Accessed August 24, 2018

87. Centers for Disease Control and Prevention. Refugee health guidelines: guidelines for pre-departure and post-arrival medical screening and treatment of U.S.-bound refugees. Available at: https://www.cdc.gov/immigrantrefugeehealth/guidelines/refugee-guidelines.html. Accessed July 26, 2019

88. Centers for Disease Control and Prevention. Guidelines for overseas presumptive treatment of strongyloidiasis, schistosomiasis, and soil-transmitted helminth infections. 2018. Available at: https://www.cdc.gov/immigrantrefugeehealth/guidelines/overseas/intestinal-parasites-overseas.html. Accessed August 14, 2018

89. Seery T, Boswell H, Lara A. Caring for refugee children. *Pediatr Rev.* 2015;36(8):323–338

90. Haber BA, Block JM, Jonas MM, et al; Hepatitis B Foundation. Recommendations for screening, monitoring, and referral of pediatric chronic hepatitis B. *Pediatrics.* 2009;124(5). Available at: www.pediatrics.org/cgi/content/full/124/5/e1007

91. Ciaccia KA, John RM. Unaccompanied immigrant minors: where to begin. *J Pediatr Health Care.* 2016;30(3):231–240

92. Muennig P, Pallin D, Sell RL, Chan MS. The cost effectiveness of strategies for the treatment of intestinal parasites in immigrants. *N Engl J Med.* 1999;340(10):773–779

93. Centers for Disease Control and Prevention. Domestic intestinal parasite guidelines. Available at: https://www.cdc.gov/immigrantrefugeehealth/guidelines/domestic/intestinal-parasites-domestic.html. Accessed July 17, 2017

94. Jones VF, Schulte EE; Council on Foster Care, Adoption, and Kinship Care. Comprehensive health evaluation of the newly adopted child. *Pediatrics.* 2019;143(5):e20190657

95. Petersen PE, Bourgeois D, Ogawa H, Estupinan-Day S, Ndiaye C. The global burden of oral diseases and risks to oral health. *Bull World Health Organ.* 2005;83(9):661–669

96. Cote S, Geltman P, Nunn M, Lituri K, Henshaw M, Garcia RI. Dental caries of refugee children compared with US children. *Pediatrics.* 2004;114(6). Available at: www.pediatrics.org/cgi/content/full/114/6/e733

97. Shah AY, Suchdev PS, Mitchell T, et al. Nutritional status of refugee children entering DeKalb County, Georgia. *J Immigr Minor Health.* 2014;16(5):959–967

98. Finnegan DA, Rainchuso L, Jenkins S, Kierce E, Rothman A. Immigrant caregivers of young children: oral health beliefs, attitudes, and early childhood caries knowledge. *J Community Health.* 2016;41(2):250–257

99. Davidson N, Skull S, Calache H, Murray SS, Chalmers J. Holes a plenty: oral health status a major issue for newly arrived refugees in Australia. *Aust Dent J.* 2006;51(4):306–311

100. Butani Y, Weintraub JA, Barker JC. Oral health-related cultural beliefs for four racial/ethnic groups: assessment of the literature. *BMC Oral Health.* 2008;8:26

101. Riggs E, Gibbs L, Kilpatrick N, et al. Breaking down the barriers: a qualitative study to understand child oral health in refugee and migrant communities in Australia. *Ethn Health.* 2015;20(3):241–257

102. Nicol P, Al-Hanbali A, King N, Slack-Smith L, Cherian S. Informing a culturally appropriate approach to oral health and dental care for pre-school refugee

children: a community participatory study. *BMC Oral Health.* 2014;14:69

103. Beaglehole R, Horton R. Chronic diseases: global action must match global evidence. *Lancet.* 2010;376(9753): 1619–1621

104. United Nations General Assembly. Political declaration of the high-level meeting of the General Assembly on the prevention and control of non-communicable diseases. Available at: www.who.int/nmh/events/un_ncd_summit2011/political_declaration_en.pdf. Accessed August 14, 2018

105. World Health Organization. Noncommunicable diseases and mental health. Global status report on noncommunicable diseases 2014. 2014. Available at: www.who.int/nmh/publications/ncd-status-report-2014/en/. Accessed August 14, 2018

106. Pondé MP, Rousseau C. Immigrant children with autism spectrum disorder: the relationship between the perspective of the professionals and the parents' point of view. *J Can Acad Child Adolesc Psychiatry.* 2013;22(2): 131–138

107. Lin SC, Yu SM, Harwood RL. Autism spectrum disorders and developmental disabilities in children from immigrant families in the United States. *Pediatrics.* 2012;130(suppl 2):S191–S197

108. Becerra TA, von Ehrenstein OS, Heck JE, et al. Autism spectrum disorders and race, ethnicity, and nativity: a population-based study. *Pediatrics.* 2014;134(1). Available at: www.pediatrics.org/cgi/content/full/134/1/e63

109. Croen LA, Grether JK, Selvin S. Descriptive epidemiology of autism in a California population: who is at risk? *J Autism Dev Disord.* 2002;32(3): 217–224

110. Schieve LA, Boulet SL, Blumberg SJ, et al. Association between parental nativity and autism spectrum disorder among US-born non-Hispanic white and Hispanic children, 2007 National Survey of Children's Health. *Disabil Health J.* 2012;5(1):18–25

111. Akbulut-Yuksel M, Kugler AD. Intergenerational persistence of health: do immigrants get healthier as they remain in the U.S. for more generations? *Econ Hum Biol.* 2016;23: 136–148

112. Bischoff A, Schneider M, Denhaerynck K, Battegay E. Health and ill health of asylum seekers in Switzerland: an epidemiological study. *Eur J Public Health.* 2009;19(1):59–64

113. Perreira KM, Ornelas IJ. The physical and psychological well-being of immigrant children. *Future Child.* 2011; 21(1):195–218

114. Centers for Disease Control and Prevention. Non-communicable diseases (NCDs). Central American refugee health profile. Available at: https://www.cdc.gov/immigrantrefugeehealth/profiles/central-american/health-information/chronic-disease/index.html. Accessed August 14, 2018

115. Hamdoun E, Karachunski P, Nathan B, et al. Case report: the specter of untreated congenital hypothyroidism in immigrant families. *Pediatrics.* 2016; 137(5):e20153418

116. Minnesota Department of Health. Lead poisoning prevention programs biennial report to the Minnesota legislature 2019. Available at: https://www.health.state.mn.us/communities/environment/lead/docs/reports/bienniallegrept.pdf. Accessed July 29, 2019

117. Centers for Disease Control and Prevention. Managing elevated blood lead levels among children: recommendations from the Advisory Committee on Childhood Lead Poisoning Prevention. Available at: https://www.cdc.gov/nceh/lead/casemanagement/casemanage_main.htm. Accessed August 30, 2018

118. Centers for Disease Control and Prevention (CDC). Elevated blood lead levels in refugee children–New Hampshire, 2003-2004 [published correction appears in *MMWR Morb Mortal Wkly Rep.* 2005;54(3):76]. *MMWR Morb Mortal Wkly Rep.* 2005;54(2): 42–46

119. Geltman PL, Brown MJ, Cochran J. Lead poisoning among refugee children resettled in Massachusetts, 1995 to 1999. *Pediatrics.* 2001;108(1):158–162

120. Centers for Disease Control and Prevention. Screening for lead during the domestic medical examination for newly arrived refugees. 2013. Available at: www.cdc.gov/immigrantrefugeehealth/guidelines/lead-guidelines.html. Accessed July 16, 2017

121. Yun K, Matheson J, Payton C, et al. Health profiles of newly arrived refugee children in the United States, 2006-2012. *Am J Public Health.* 2016;106(1):128–135

122. Dawson-Hahn EE, Pak-Gorstein S, Hoopes AJ, Matheson J. Comparison of the nutritional status of overseas refugee children with low income children in Washington state. *PLoS One.* 2016;11(1):e0147854

123. Dawson-Hahn E, Pak-Gorstein S, Matheson J, et al. Growth trajectories of refugee and nonrefugee children in the United States. *Pediatrics.* 2016; 138(6):e20160953

124. Centers for Disease Control and Prevention. Guidelines for evaluation of the nutritional status and growth in refugee children during the domestic medical screening examination. 2012. Available at: https://www.cdc.gov/immigrantrefugeehealth/pdf/nutrition-growth.pdf. Accessed August 14, 2018

125. Oldways. Inspiring good health through cultural food traditions. Available at: https://oldwayspt.org. Accessed July 6, 2017

126. Centers for Disease Control and Prevention. Guidelines for evaluation of the nutritional status and growth in refugee children during the domestic medical screening examination. 2013. Available at: www.cdc.gov/immigrantrefugeehealth/guidelines/domestic/nutrition-growth.html. Accessed July 6, 2017

127. Centers for Disease Control and Prevention (CDC). Vitamin B12 deficiency in resettled Bhutanese refugees–United States, 2008-2011. *MMWR Morb Mortal Wkly Rep.* 2011; 60(11):343–346

128. Hintzpeter B, Scheidt-Nave C, Müller MJ, Schenk L, Mensink GB. Higher prevalence of vitamin D deficiency is associated with immigrant background among children and adolescents in Germany. *J Nutr.* 2008;138(8):1482–1490

129. Penrose K, Hunter Adams J, Nguyen T, Cochran J, Geltman PL. Vitamin D

deficiency among newly resettled refugees in Massachusetts. *J Immigr Minor Health*. 2012;14(6):941–948

130. Council on Community Pediatrics; Committee on Nutrition. Promoting food security for all children. *Pediatrics*. 2015;136(5). Available at: www.pediatrics.org/cgi/content/full/136/5/e1431
131. Food Research and Action Center. Addressing food insecurity: a toolkit for pediatricians. Available at: http://frac.org/aaptoolkit. Accessed August 14, 2018
132. Ages and Stages Questionnaires. Social-emotional health: look to ASQ:SE-2 for truly accurate screening. 2018. Available at: http://agesandstages.com/products-services/asqse-2/. Accessed August 14, 2018
133. Floating Hospital for Children at Tufts Medical Center. The survey of well-being of young children. Available at: https://www.floatinghospital.org/The-Survey-of-Wellbeing-of-Young-Children/Overview.aspx. Accessed August 14, 2018
134. Kroening AL, Moore JA, Welch TR, Halterman JS, Hyman SL. Developmental screening of refugees: a qualitative study. *Pediatrics*. 2016;138(3):e20160234
135. Martin-Herz SP, Kemper T, Brownstein M, McLaughlin JF. Developmental screening with recent immigrant and refugee children: a preliminary report. 2012. Available at: http://ethnomed.org/clinical/pediatrics/developmental-screening-with-recent-immigrant-and-refugee-children. Accessed August 14, 2018
136. Rogoff B. *The Cultural Nature of Human Development*. New York, NY: Oxford University Press; 2003
137. Cowden JD, Kreisler K. Development in children of immigrant families. *Pediatr Clin North Am*. 2016;63(5):775–793
138. Pachter LM, Dworkin PH. Maternal expectations about normal child development in 4 cultural groups. *Arch Pediatr Adolesc Med*. 1997;151(11):1144–1150
139. Stein MT, Flores G, Graham EA, Magana L, Willies-Jacobo L, Gulbronson M. Cultural and linguistic determinants in the diagnosis and management of developmental delay in a 4-year-old. *Pediatrics*. 2004;114(suppl 6):1442–1447
140. Johnson L, Radesky J, Zuckerman B. Cross-cultural parenting: reflections on autonomy and interdependence. *Pediatrics*. 2013;131(4):631–633
141. deVries MW, deVries MR. Cultural relativity of toilet training readiness: a perspective from East Africa. *Pediatrics*. 1977;60(2):170–177
142. Festa N, Loftus PD, Cullen MR, Mendoza FS. Disparities in early exposure to book sharing within immigrant families. *Pediatrics*. 2014;134(1). Available at: www.pediatrics.org/cgi/content/full/134/1/e162
143. Toppelberg CO, Collins BA. Language, culture, and adaptation in immigrant children. *Child Adolesc Psychiatr Clin N Am*. 2010;19(4):697–717
144. Hagan JF Jr, Shaw JS, Duncan PM, eds. *Bright Futures: Guidelines for Health Supervision of Infants, Children, and Adolescents*. 4th ed. Elk Grove Village, IL: American Academy of Pediatrics; 2017
145. Adesope OO, Lavin T, Thompson T, Ungerleider C. A systematic review and meta-analysis on the cognitive correlates of bilingualism. *Rev Educ Res*. 2010;80(2):207–245
146. Feliciano C. The benefits of biculturalism: exposure to immigrant culture and dropping out of school among Asian and Latino youths. *Soc Sci Q*. 2001;82(4):865–879
147. Zhou M. Growing up American: the challenge confronting immigrant children and children of immigrants. *Annu Rev Sociol*. 1997;23(1):63–95
148. Engel de Abreu PM, Cruz-Santos A, Tourinho CJ, Martin R, Bialystok E. Bilingualism enriches the poor: enhanced cognitive control in low-income minority children. *Psychol Sci*. 2012;23(11):1364–1371
149. Bialystok E. Reshaping the mind: the benefits of bilingualism. *Can J Exp Psychol*. 2011;65(4):229–235
150. High PC, Klass P; Council on Early Childhood. Literacy promotion: an essential component of primary care pediatric practice. *Pediatrics*. 2014;134(2):404–409
151. Education Commission of the States. English language learners. The progress of education reform. 2013. Available at: https://www.rwjf.org/en/library/research/2011/11/caring-across-communities–.html. Accessed July 26, 2019
152. Park M, O'Toole A, Katsiaficas C. *Dual Language Learners: A National Demographic and Policy Profile*. Washington, DC: Migration Policy Institute; 2017
153. Morland L, Ives N, McNeely C, Allen C. Providing a head start: improving access to early childhood education for refugees. Migration Policy Institute. 2016. Available at: https://www.migrationpolicy.org/research/providing-head-start-improving-access-early-childhood-education-refugees. Accessed August 30, 2018
154. Plyler v Doe, 457 US 202 (1982)
155. Graham HR, Minhas RS, Paxton G. Learning problems in children of refugee background: a systematic review. *Pediatrics*. 2016;137(6):e20153994
156. Walker SP, Wachs TD, Gardner JM, et al; International Child Development Steering Group. Child development: risk factors for adverse outcomes in developing countries. *Lancet*. 2007;369(9556):145–157
157. DeCapua A. Reaching students with limited or interrupted formal education through culturally responsive teaching. *Lang Linguist Compass*. 2016;10(5):225–237
158. Macswan J, Rolstad K. How language proficiency tests mislead us about ability: implications for English language learner placement in special education. *Teach Coll Rec (1970)*. 2006;108(11):2304–2328
159. Wagner RK, Francis DJ, Morris RD. Identifying English language learners with learning disabilities: key challenges and possible approaches. *Learn Disabil Res Pract*. 2005;20(1):6–15
160. McCardle P, Mele-McCarthy J, Cutting L, Leos K, D'Emilio T. Learning disabilities in English language learners: identifying the issues. *Learn Disabil Res Pract*. 2005;20(1):1–5
161. Figueroa RA, Newsome P. The diagnosis of LD in English learners: is it

nondiscriminatory? *J Learn Disabil.* 2006;39(3):206–214

162. Lara M, Gamboa C, Kahramanian MI, Morales LS, Bautista DE. Acculturation and Latino health in the United States: a review of the literature and its sociopolitical context. *Annu Rev Public Health.* 2005;26:367–397

163. Bornstein MH, Cote LR, eds. *Acculturation and Parent–Child Relationships: Measurement and Development.* Mahwah, NJ: Lawrence Erlbaum Associates, Inc; 2006

164. Antecol H, Bedard K. Unhealthy assimilation: why do immigrants converge to American health status levels? *Demography.* 2006;43(2): 337–360

165. Zamboanga BL, Schwartz SJ, Jarvis LH, Van Tyne K. Acculturation and substance use among Hispanic early adolescents: investigating the mediating roles of acculturative stress and self-esteem. *J Prim Prev.* 2009; 30(3–4):315–333

166. Myers R, Chou CP, Sussman S, Baezconde-Garbanati L, Pachon H, Valente TW. Acculturation and substance use: social influence as a mediator among Hispanic alternative high school youth. *J Health Soc Behav.* 2009;50(2):164–179

167. Ho J, Birman D. Acculturation gaps in Vietnamese immigrant families: impact on family relationships. *Int J Intercult Relat.* 2010;34(1):22–23

168. Birman D, Taylor-Ritzler T. Acculturation and psychological distress among adolescent immigrants from the former Soviet Union: exploring the mediating effect of family relationships. *Cultur Divers Ethnic Minor Psychol.* 2007;13(4): 337–346

169. Refugee Health Technical Assistance Center. Youth and mental health. Available at: http://refugeehealthta.org/physical-mental-health/mental-health/youth-and-mental-health/. Accessed August 30, 2018

170. The National Child Traumatic Stress Network. Learning center for child and adolescent trauma. Refugee Services Toolkit (RST). 2012. Available at: https://www.nctsn.org/resources/refugee-services-core-stressor-assessment-tool. Accessed July 26, 2019

171. Sawyer CB, Márquez J. Senseless violence against Central American unaccompanied minors: historical background and call for help. *J Psychol.* 2017;151(1):69–75

172. The National Child Traumatic Stress Network. Refugee trauma. 2017. Available at: http://nctsn.org/trauma-types/refugee-trauma/learn-about-refugee-core-stressors. Accessed August 14, 2017

173. United Nations Office of the High Commissioner for Refugees. Children on the run. Available at: www.unhcr.org/en-us/about-us/background/56fc266f4/children-on-the-run-full-report.html. Accessed August 30, 2018

174. Cleary SD, Snead R, Dietz-Chavez D, Rivera I, Edberg MC. Immigrant trauma and mental health outcomes among Latino youth. *J Immigr Minor Health.* 2018;20(5):1053–1059

175. Isakson BL, Legerski JP, Layne CM. Adapting and implementing evidence-based interventions for trauma-exposed refugee youth and families. *J Contemp Psychother.* 2015;45(4): 245–253

176. Greenbaum J, Bodrick N; Committee on Child Abuse and Neglect; Section on International Child Health. Global human trafficking and child victimization. *Pediatrics.* 2017;140(6): e20173138

177. McPherson M, Arango P, Fox H, et al. A new definition of children with special health care needs. *Pediatrics.* 1998; 102(1, pt 1):137–140

178. Dreby J. U.S. immigration policy and family separation: the consequences for children's well-being. *Soc Sci Med.* 2015;132:245–251

179. Garner AS, Shonkoff JP; Committee on Psychosocial Aspects of Child and Family Health; Committee on Early Childhood, Adoption, and Dependent Care; Section on Developmental and Behavioral Pediatrics. Early childhood adversity, toxic stress, and the role of the pediatrician: translating developmental science into lifelong health. *Pediatrics.* 2012;129(1). Available at: www.pediatrics.org/cgi/content/full/129/1/e224

180. Lustig SL, Kia-Keating M, Knight WG, et al. Review of child and adolescent refugee mental health. *J Am Acad Child Adolesc Psychiatry.* 2004;43(1):24–36

181. Savin D, Seymour DJ, Littleford LN, Bettridge J, Giese A. Findings from mental health screening of newly arrived refugees in Colorado. *Public Health Rep.* 2005;120(3):224–229

182. Allwood MA, Bell-Dolan D, Husain SA. Children's trauma and adjustment reactions to violent and nonviolent war experiences. *J Am Acad Child Adolesc Psychiatry.* 2002;41(4):450–457

183. Jaycox LH, Stein BD, Kataoka SH, et al. Violence exposure, posttraumatic stress disorder, and depressive symptoms among recent immigrant schoolchildren. *J Am Acad Child Adolesc Psychiatry.* 2002;41(9): 1104–1110

184. Fazel M, Wheeler J, Danesh J. Prevalence of serious mental disorder in 7000 refugees resettled in western countries: a systematic review. *Lancet.* 2005;365(9467):1309–1314

185. Weine SM, Vojvoda D, Becker DF, et al. PTSD symptoms in Bosnian refugees 1 year after resettlement in the United States. *Am J Psychiatry.* 1998;155(4): 562–564

186. Sack WH, Clarke GN, Seeley J. Multiple forms of stress in Cambodian adolescent refugees. *Child Dev.* 1996; 67(1):107–116

187. Betancourt TS, Newnham EA, Birman D, Lee R, Ellis BH, Layne CM. Comparing trauma exposure, mental health needs, and service utilization across clinical samples of refugee, immigrant, and U.S.-origin children. *J Trauma Stress.* 2017;30(3):209–218

188. Hodes M, Jagdev D, Chandra N, Cunniff A. Risk and resilience for psychological distress amongst unaccompanied asylum seeking adolescents. *J Child Psychol Psychiatry.* 2008;49(7):723–732

189. Jakobsen M, Meyer DeMott MA, Wentzel-Larsen T, Heir T. The impact of the asylum process on mental health: a longitudinal study of unaccompanied refugee minors in Norway. *BMJ Open.* 2017;7(6):e015157

190. Majumder P, O'Reilly M, Karim K, Vostanis P. 'This doctor, I not trust him, I'm not safe': the perceptions of mental health and services by unaccompanied

refugee adolescents. *Int J Soc Psychiatry.* 2015;61(2):129–136

191. Belhadj Kouider E, Koglin U, Petermann F. Emotional and behavioral problems in migrant children and adolescents in American countries: a systematic review. *J Immigr Minor Health.* 2015; 17(4):1240–1258

192. Youthinmind. SDQ: Information for researchers and professionals about the Strengths & Difficulties Questionnaires. Available at: www.sdqinfo.com. Accessed September 17, 2018

193. Refugee Health Technical Assistance Center. Refugee Health Screener-15 (RHS-15) packet. Available at: http://refugeehealthta.org/2012/07/31/refugee-health-screener-15-rhs-15-packet/. Accessed August 30, 2018

194. Achenbach System of Empirically Based Assessment. Multicultural applications. Available at: https://aseba.org/multicultural-applications/. Accessed July 29, 2019

195. Fazel M, Betancourt TS. Preventive mental health interventions for refugee children and adolescents in high-income settings. *Lancet Child Adolesc Health.* 2018;2(2):121–132

196. Institute of Medicine. *Preventing Mental, Emotional, and Behavioral Disorders Among Young People: Progress and Possibilities.* Washington, DC: The National Academies Press; 2009

197. Carlson BE, Cacciatore J, Klimek B. A risk and resilience perspective on unaccompanied refugee minors. *Soc Work.* 2012;57(3):259–269

198. Eide K, Hjern A. Unaccompanied refugee children–vulnerability and agency. *Acta Paediatr.* 2013;102(7):666–668

199. Timshel I, Montgomery E, Dalgaard NT. A systematic review of risk and protective factors associated with family related violence in refugee families. *Child Abuse Negl.* 2017;70:315–330

200. Anderson AT, Jackson A, Jones L, Kennedy DP, Wells K, Chung PJ. Minority parents' perspectives on racial socialization and school readiness in the early childhood period. *Acad Pediatr.* 2015;15(4):405–411

201. Ellis BH, Hulland EN, Miller AB, Bixby CB, Cardozo BL, Betancourt TS. Mental health risks and resilience among Somali and Bhutanese refugee parents. 2016. Available at: https://www.migrationpolicy.org/research/mental-health-risks-and-resilience-among-somali-and-bhutanese-refugee-parents. Accessed August 30, 2018

202. Rothe EM, Tzuang D, Pumariega AJ. Acculturation, development, and adaptation. *Child Adolesc Psychiatr Clin N Am.* 2010;19(4):681–696

203. Geltman PL, Augustyn M, Barnett ED, Klass PE, Groves BM. War trauma experience and behavioral screening of Bosnian refugee children resettled in Massachusetts. *J Dev Behav Pediatr.* 2000;21(4):255–261

204. Caballero TM, DeCamp LR, Platt RE, et al. Addressing the mental health needs of Latino children in immigrant families. *Clin Pediatr (Phila).* 2017;56(7): 648–658

205. De Milto L. National program executive summary report—caring across communities: addressing mental health needs of diverse children and youth. Available at: https://www.rwjf.org/en/library/research/2011/11/caring-across-communities–.html. Accessed July 26, 2019

206. Al-Rawi SN, Fetters MD. Traditional Arabic & Islamic medicine: a conceptual model for clinicians and researchers. *Glob J Health Sci.* 2012; 4(3):164–169

207. Pachter LM. Culture and clinical care. Folk illness beliefs and behaviors and their implications for health care delivery. *JAMA.* 1994;271(9):690–694

208. Risser AL, Mazur LJ. Use of folk remedies in a Hispanic population. *Arch Pediatr Adolesc Med.* 1995;149(9): 978–981

209. EthnoMed. Ethnic medicine information from Harborview Medical Center. Available at: https://depts.washington.edu/ethnomed/HMCproject/hmcproject_talk_0302/F_EthnoMed%20Home%20Page.htm. Accessed August 30, 2018

210. World Health Organization. *Eliminating Female Genital Mutilation. An Interagency Statement.* Geneva, Switzerland: World Health Organization; 2008. Available at: www.un.org/womenwatch/daw/csw/csw52/statements_missions/Interagency_Statement_on_Eliminating_FGM.pdf. Accessed August 30, 2018

211. United Nations Children's Fund. Female genital mutilation/cutting: a statistical overview and exploration of the dynamics of change. 2013. Available at: https://www.unicef.org/publications/index_69875.html. Accessed August 30, 2018

212. Refugee Legal Aid Information for Lawyers Representing Refugees Globally Rights in Exile Programme. United States. Available at: www.refugeelegalaidinformation.org/united-states-america-fgm. Accessed August 30, 2018

213. Hearst AA, Molnar AM. Female genital cutting: an evidence-based approach to clinical management for the primary care physician. *Mayo Clin Proc.* 2013; 88(6):618–629

214. Vissandjée B, Denetto S, Migliardi P, Proctor J. Female genital cutting (FGC) and the ethics of care: community engagement and cultural sensitivity at the interface of migration experiences. *BMC Int Health Hum Rights.* 2014;14:13

215. National Defense Authorization Act for Fiscal Year 2013, HR 4310, 112th Cong, 2nd Sess (2012). Available at: https://www.gpo.gov/fdsys/pkg/BILLS-112hr4310enr/pdf/BILLS-112hr4310enr.pdf. Accessed August 30, 2018

216. Eneriz-Wiemer M, Sanders LM, Barr DA, Mendoza FS. Parental limited English proficiency and health outcomes for children with special health care needs: a systematic review. *Acad Pediatr.* 2014; 14(2):128–136

217. Arthur KC, Mangione-Smith R, Meischke H, et al. Impact of English proficiency on care experiences in a pediatric emergency department. *Acad Pediatr.* 2015;15(2):218–224

218. Jimenez N, Jackson DL, Zhou C, Ayala NC, Ebel BE. Postoperative pain management in children, parental English proficiency, and access to interpretation. *Hosp Pediatr.* 2014;4(1): 23–30

219. Levas MN, Cowden JD, Dowd MD. Effects of the limited English proficiency of parents on hospital length of stay and home health care referral for their home health care-eligible children with

infections. *Arch Pediatr Adolesc Med.* 2011;165(9):831–836

220. Gallagher RA, Porter S, Monuteaux MC, Stack AM. Unscheduled return visits to the emergency department: the impact of language. *Pediatr Emerg Care.* 2013; 29(5):579–583

221. Title VI of the Civil Rights Act of 1964, 42 USC §2000d-1–2000d-7 (2009). Available at: http://uscode.house.gov/view.xhtml?path=%2Fprelim%40title42%2Fchapter21&req=granuleid%3AUSC-prelim-title42-chapter21&f=&fq=&num=0&hl=false&edition=prelim. Accessed November 15, 2018

222. Office of the Surgeon General; Center for Mental Health Services; National Institute of Mental Health. *Mental Health: Culture, Race, and Ethnicity: A Supplement to Mental Health: A Report of the Surgeon General.* Rockville, MD: Substance Abuse and Mental Health Services Administration; 2001. Available at: https://www.ncbi.nlm.nih.gov/books/NBK44243/. Accessed August 30, 2018

223. Flores G, Torres S, Holmes LJ, Salas-Lopez D, Youdelman MK, Tomany-Korman SC. Access to hospital interpreter services for limited English proficient patients in New Jersey: a statewide evaluation. *J Health Care Poor Underserved.* 2008;19(2):391–415

224. Jacobs EA, Diamond LC, Stevak L. The importance of teaching clinicians when and how to work with interpreters. *Patient Educ Couns.* 2010; 78(2):149–153

225. DeCamp LR, Kuo DZ, Flores G, O'Connor K, Minkovitz CS. Changes in language services use by US pediatricians. *Pediatrics.* 2013;132(2). Available at: www.pediatrics.org/cgi/content/full/132/2/e396

226. Flores G, Laws MB, Mayo SJ, et al. Errors in medical interpretation and their potential clinical consequences in pediatric encounters. *Pediatrics.* 2003; 111(1):6–14

227. Flores G, Abreu M, Barone CP, Bachur R, Lin H. Errors of medical interpretation and their potential clinical consequences: a comparison of professional versus ad hoc versus no interpreters. *Ann Emerg Med.* 2012; 60(5):545–553

228. Juckett G, Unger K. Appropriate use of medical interpreters. *Am Fam Physician.* 2014;90(7):476–480

229. Hsieh E. Not just "getting by": factors influencing providers' choice of interpreters. *J Gen Intern Med.* 2015; 30(1):75–82

230. Jacobs EA, Shepard DS, Suaya JA, Stone EL. Overcoming language barriers in health care: costs and benefits of interpreter services. *Am J Public Health.* 2004;94(5):866–869

231. Johnstone MJ, Kanitsaki O. Culture, language, and patient safety: making the link. *Int J Qual Health Care.* 2006; 18(5):383–388

232. Flores G. The impact of medical interpreter services on the quality of health care: a systematic review. *Med Care Res Rev.* 2005;62(3):255–299

233. Moreno MR, Otero-Sabogal R, Newman J. Assessing dual-role staff-interpreter linguistic competency in an integrated healthcare system. *J Gen Intern Med.* 2007;22(suppl 2):331–335

234. Tang G, Lanza O, Rodriguez FM, Chang A. The Kaiser Permanente Clinician Cultural and Linguistic Assessment Initiative: research and development in patient-provider language concordance. *Am J Public Health.* 2011;101(2):205–208

235. Lion KC, Thompson DA, Cowden JD, et al. Impact of language proficiency testing on provider use of Spanish for clinical care. *Pediatrics.* 2012;130(1). Available at: www.pediatrics.org/cgi/content/full/130/1/e80

236. Dreby J. The burden of deportation on children in Mexican immigrant families. *J Marriage Fam.* 2012;74(4):829–845

237. Rhodes SD, Mann L, Simán FM, et al. The impact of local immigration enforcement policies on the health of immigrant Hispanics/Latinos in the United States. *Am J Public Health.* 2015; 105(2):329–337

238. Suârez-Orozco C, Todorova IL, Louie J. Making up for lost time: the experience of separation and reunification among immigrant families. *Fam Process.* 2002; 41(4):625–643

239. Crosnoe R, Leventhal T, Wirth RJ, Pierce KM, Pianta RC; NICHD Early Child Care Research Network. Family socioeconomic status and consistent environmental stimulation in early childhood. *Child Dev.* 2010;81(3): 972–987

240. Council on Community Pediatrics. Poverty and child health in the United States. *Pediatrics.* 2016;137(4): e20160339

241. Singh P, Chokshi DA. Community health workers–a local solution to a global problem. *N Engl J Med.* 2013;369(10): 894–896

242. Postma J, Karr C, Kieckhefer G. Community health workers and environmental interventions for children with asthma: a systematic review. *J Asthma.* 2009;46(6):564–576

243. Coker TR, Chacon S, Elliott MN, et al. A parent coach model for well-child care among low-income children: a randomized controlled trial. *Pediatrics.* 2016;137(3):e20153013

244. Enard KR, Ganelin DM. Reducing preventable emergency department utilization and costs by using community health workers as patient navigators. *J Healthc Manag.* 2013; 58(6):412–427; discussion 428

245. Pati S, Ladowski KL, Wong AT, Huang J, Yang J. An enriched medical home intervention using community health workers improves adherence to immunization schedules. *Vaccine.* 2015; 33(46):6257–6263

246. Anugu M, Braksmajer A, Huang J, Yang J, Ladowski KL, Pati S. Enriched medical home intervention using community health worker home visitation and ED use. *Pediatrics.* 2017;139(5):e20161849

247. Agency for Healthcare Research and Quality. Design guide for implementing warm handoffs. 2017. Available at: https://www.ahrq.gov/sites/default/files/wysiwyg/professionals/quality-patient-safety/patient-family-engagement/pfeprimarycare/warmhandoff-designguide.pdf. Accessed August 30, 2018

248. Blewett LA, Johnson PJ, Mach AL. Immigrant children's access to health care: differences by global region of birth. *J Health Care Poor Underserved.* 2010;21(suppl 2):13–31

249. National Immigration Law Center. Overview of immigrant eligibility for federal programs. 2015. Available at: https://www.nilc.org/issues/economic-

support/overview-immeligfedprograms/. Accessed August 30, 2018

250. National Immigration Law Center. Table: medical assistance programs for immigrants in various states. 2018. Available at: https://www.nilc.org/wp-content/uploads/2015/11/med-services-for-imms-in-states.pdf. Accessed November 14, 2018

251. Georgetown University Health Policy Institute Center for Children and Families. Health coverage for lawfully residing children. 2018. Available at: https://ccf.georgetown.edu/wp-content/uploads/2018/05/ichia_fact_sheet.pdf. Accessed August 30, 2018

252. Brooks T, Wagnerman K, Artiga S, Cornachione E, Ubri P. Medicaid and CHIP eligibility, enrollment, renewal, and cost sharing policies as of January 2017: findings from a 50-state survey. 2017. Available at: https://www.kff.org/medicaid/report/medicaid-and-chip-eligibility-enrollment-renewal-and-cost-sharing-policies-as-of-january-2017-findings-from-a-50-state-survey/. Accessed August 30, 2018

253. National Immigration Law Center. Health care coverage maps. 2018. Available at: https://www.nilc.org/issues/health-care/healthcoveragemaps/. Accessed July 26, 2019

254. Flores SM. State dream acts: the effect of in-state resident tuition polices and undocumented Latino students. *Rev High Ed.* 2010;33(2):239–283

255. New American Economy. Removing barriers: expanding in-state tuition for Dreamers in South Carolina. 2019. Available at: https://www.newamericaneconomy.org/wp-content/uploads/2019/04/SC_InState_Tuition.pdf. Accessed April 4, 2019

256. Mirza M, Luna R, Mathews B, et al. Barriers to healthcare access among refugees with disabilities and chronic health conditions resettled in the US Midwest. *J Immigr Minor Health.* 2014;16(4):733–742

257. National Immigration Law Center. Know your rights: Is it safe to apply for health insurance or seek health care? Available at: https://www.nilc.org/issues/health-care/health-insurance-and-care-rights/. Accessed July 26, 2019

258. Duffee JH, Mendelsohn AL, Kuo AA, Legano LA, Earls MF; Council on Community Pediatrics; Council on Early Childhood; Committee on Child Abuse and Neglect. Early childhood home visiting. *Pediatrics.* 2017;140(3):e20172150

259. Greenberg JP. Determinants of after-school programming for school-age immigrant children. *Child Sch.* 2013;35(2):101–111

260. Greenberg JP. Significance of after-school programming for immigrant children during middle childhood: opportunities for school social work. *Soc Work.* 2014;59(3):243–251

261. Jarlenski M, Baller J, Borrero S, Bennett WL. Trends in disparities in low-income children's health insurance coverage and access to care by family immigration status. *Acad Pediatr.* 2016;16(2):208–215

262. Avila RM, Bramlett MD. Language and immigrant status effects on disparities in Hispanic children's health status and access to health care. *Matern Child Health J.* 2013;17(3):415–423

263. Artiga S. Immigration reform and access to health coverage: key issues to consider. 2013. Available at: https://www.kff.org/uninsured/issue-brief/immigration-reform-and-access-to-health-coverage-key-issues-to-consider/. Accessed July 29, 2019

264. Artiga S, Ubri P. *Living in an immigrant family in America: How fear and toxic stress are affecting daily life, well-being, and health.* 2017. Available at: https://www.kff.org/disparities-policy/issue-brief/living-in-an-immigrant-family-in-america-how-fear-and-toxic-stress-are-affecting-daily-life-well-being-health. Accessed August 30, 2018

265. Artiga S, Garfield R, Damico A. Estimated impacts of the proposed public charge rule on immigrants and Medicaid. 2018. Available at: https://www.cmhnetwork.org/wp-content/uploads/2018/10/Issue-Brief-Estimated-Impacts-of-the-Proposed-Public-Charge-Rule-on-Immigrants-and-Medicaid.pdf. Accessed July 30, 2019

266. US Immigration and Customs Enforcement. FAQ on sensitive locations and courthouse arrests. 2018. Available at: https://www.ice.gov/ero/enforcement/sensitive-loc. Accessed April 3, 2019

267. National Immigration Law Center. Health care providers and immigration enforcement: know your rights, know your patients' rights. Available at: https://www.nilc.org/issues/immigration-enforcement/healthcare-provider-and-patients-rights-imm-enf/. Accessed April 5, 2019

268. Mann L, Simán FM, Downs M, et al. Reducing the impact of immigration enforcement policies to ensure the health of North Carolinians: statewide community-level recommendations. *N C Med J.* 2016;77(4):240–246

269. Hacker K, Chu J, Leung C, et al. The impact of Immigration and Customs Enforcement on immigrant health: perceptions of immigrants in Everett, Massachusetts, USA. *Soc Sci Med.* 2011;73(4):586–594

270. Montealegre JR, Selwyn BJ. Healthcare coverage and use among undocumented Central American immigrant women in Houston, Texas. *J Immigr Minor Health.* 2014;16(2):204–210

271. Raymond-Flesch M, Siemons R, Pourat N, Jacobs K, Brindis CD. "There is no help out there and if there is, it's really hard to find": a qualitative study of the health concerns and health care access of Latino "DREAMers". *J Adolesc Health.* 2014;55(3):323–328

272. Giuliani C, Tagliabue S, Regalia C. Psychological well-being, multiple identities, and discrimination among first and second generation immigrant Muslims. *Eur J Psychol.* 2018;14(1):66–87

273. Suleman S, Garber J, Rutkow L. Xenophobia as a determinant of health: an integrative review. *J Public Health Policy.* 2018;39(4):407–423

274. Budhwani H, Hearld KR, Chavez-Yenter D. Depression in racial and ethnic minorities: the impact of nativity and discrimination. *J Racial Ethn Health Disparities.* 2015;2(1):34–42

275. Davis AN, Carlo G, Schwartz SJ, et al. The longitudinal associations between discrimination, depressive symptoms, and prosocial behaviors in U.S. Latino/a recent immigrant adolescents. *J Youth Adolesc.* 2016;45(3):457–470

276. Gulbas LE, Zayas LH, Yoon H, Szlyk H, Aguilar-Gaxiola S, Natera G. Deportation experiences and depression among U.S. citizen-children with undocumented Mexican parents. *Child Care Health Dev.* 2016;42(2):220–230

277. Sabo S, Shaw S, Ingram M, et al. Everyday violence, structural racism and mistreatment at the US-Mexico border. *Soc Sci Med.* 2014;109:66–74

278. Venkataramani AS, Shah SJ, O'Brien R, Kawachi I, Tsai AC. Health consequences of the US Deferred Action for Childhood Arrivals (DACA) immigration programme: a quasi-experimental study [published correction appears in *Lancet Public Health.* 2017;2(5):e213]. *Lancet Public Health.* 2017;2(4): e175–e181

279. Hainmueller J, Lawrence D, Martén L, et al. Protecting unauthorized immigrant mothers improves their children's mental health. *Science.* 2017; 357(6355):1041–1044

280. Kids in Need of Defense. *No Child Should Appear in Immigration Court Alone.* Washington, DC: Kids in Need of Defense; 2018. Available at: https://supportkind.org/wp-content/uploads/2018/01/General-KIND-Fact-Sheet_January-2018.pdf. Accessed August 30, 2018

281. Houseman AW. Civil legal aid in the United States: an update for 2013. 2013. www.clasp.org/resources-and-publications/publication-1/CIVIL-LEGAL-AID-IN-THE-UNITED-STATES-3.pdf. Accessed August 30, 2018

282. Kids in Need of Defense. *Improving the Protection and Fair Treatment of Unaccompanied Children.* Washington, DC: Kids in Need of Defense; 2016. Available at: https://supportkind.org/wp-content/uploads/2016/09/KIND-Protection-and-Fair-Treatment-Report_September-2016-FINAL.pdf. Accessed August 30, 2018

283. National Immigrant Justice Center. *Justice for Unaccompanied Immigrant Children: An Advocacy Best Practices Manual for Legal Service Providers.* Chicago, IL: National Immigrant Justice Center; 2016. Available at: https://www.americanbar.org/content/dam/aba/administrative/probono_public_service/ls_pb_uac_doc_uic_best_practices_4_27_16.pdf. Accessed August 30, 2018

284. Portes A, Rivas A. The adaptation of migrant children. *Future Child.* 2011; 21(1):219–246

285. Avellar S, Paulsell D, Sama-Miller E, Del Grosso P, Akers L, Kleinman R. *Home Visiting Evidence of Effectiveness Review: Executive Summary.* Washington, DC: Office of Planning, Research, and Evaluation, Administration for Children and Families, US Department of Health and Human Services; 2016, Available at: https://homvee.acf.hhs.gov/HomVEE-Executive-Summary-2016_Compliant.pdf. Accessed August 30, 2018

286. Yogman M, Garner A, Hutchinson J, Hirsh-Pasek K, Golinkoff RM; Committee on Psychosocial Aspects of Child and Family Health; Council on Communications and Media. The power of play: a pediatric role in enhancing development in young children. *Pediatrics.* 2018;142(3):e20182058

287. Weisleder A, Cates CB, Dreyer BP, et al. Promotion of positive parenting and prevention of socioemotional disparities. *Pediatrics.* 2016;137(2): e20153239

288. Katigbak C, Foley M, Robert L, Hutchinson MK. Experiences and lessons learned in using community-based participatory research to recruit Asian American immigrant research participants. *J Nurs Scholarsh.* 2016; 48(2):210–218

289. Huemer J, Karnik NS, Voelkl-Kernstock S, et al. Mental health issues in unaccompanied refugee minors. *Child Adolesc Psychiatry Ment Health.* 2009; 3(1):13

290. Terra Firma. Supporting Resilience for Immigrant Children. Available at: http://www.terrafirma.nyc. Accessed July 30, 2019

291. Kids in Need of Defense. Legal services. Available at: Available at: https://supportkind.org/our-work/legal-services-2/. Accessed July 30, 2019

292. Young Center for Immigrant Children's Rights. The Goal. Available at: https://www.theyoungcenter.org/big-picture. Accessed July 30, 2019

293. RAICES. Services. Available at: https://www.raicestexas.org/services/. Accessed July 30, 2019

Psychosocial Factors in Children and Youth With Special Health Care Needs and Their Families

- *Clinical Report*

CLINICAL REPORT Guidance for the Clinician in Rendering Pediatric Care

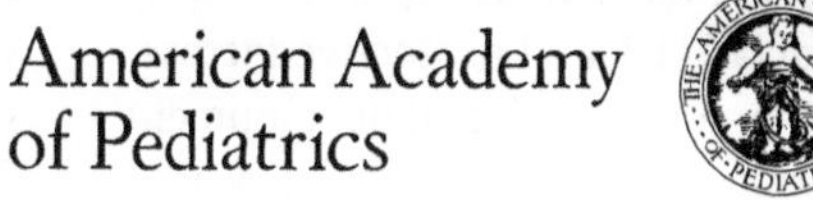

DEDICATED TO THE HEALTH OF ALL CHILDREN™

Psychosocial Factors in Children and Youth With Special Health Care Needs and Their Families

Gerri Mattson, MD, MSPH, FAAP,[a] Dennis Z. Kuo, MD, MHS, FAAP,[b] COMMITTEE ON PSYCHOSOCIAL ASPECTS OF CHILD AND FAMILY HEALTH, COUNCIL ON CHILDREN WITH DISABILITIES

abstract

Children and youth with special health care needs (CYSHCN) and their families may experience a variety of internal (ie, emotional and behavioral) and external (ie, interpersonal, financial, housing, and educational) psychosocial factors that can influence their health and wellness. Many CYSHCN and their families are resilient and thrive. Medical home teams can partner with CYSHCN and their families to screen for, evaluate, and promote psychosocial health to increase protective factors and ameliorate risk factors. Medical home teams can promote protective psychosocial factors as part of coordinated, comprehensive chronic care for CYSHCN and their families. A team-based care approach may entail collaboration across the care spectrum, including youth, families, behavioral health providers, specialists, child care providers, schools, social services, and other community agencies. The purpose of this clinical report is to raise awareness of the impact of psychosocial factors on the health and wellness of CYSHCN and their families. This clinical report provides guidance for pediatric providers to facilitate and coordinate care that can have a positive influence on the overall health, wellness, and quality of life of CYSHCN and their families.

[a]Children and Youth Branch, Division of Public Health, North Carolina Department of Health and Human Services, Raleigh, North Carolina; and [b]Department of Pediatrics, University at Buffalo, Buffalo, New York

Drs Mattson and Kuo conceptualized, designed, drafted, reviewed, and revised the manuscript, approved the final manuscript as submitted, and agree to be accountable for all aspects of the work.

This document is copyrighted and is property of the American Academy of Pediatrics and its Board of Directors. All authors have filed conflict of interest statements with the American Academy of Pediatrics. Any conflicts have been resolved through a process approved by the Board of Directors. The American Academy of Pediatrics has neither solicited nor accepted any commercial involvement in the development of the content of this publication.

Clinical reports from the American Academy of Pediatrics benefit from expertise and resources of liaisons and internal (AAP) and external reviewers. However, clinical reports from the American Academy of Pediatrics may not reflect the views of the liaisons or the organizations or government agencies that they represent.

The guidance in this report does not indicate an exclusive course of treatment or serve as a standard of medical care. Variations, taking into account individual circumstances, may be appropriate.

All clinical reports from the American Academy of Pediatrics automatically expire 5 years after publication unless reaffirmed, revised, or retired at or before that time.

DOI: https://doi.org/10.1542/peds.2018-3171

Address correspondence to Gerri Mattson, MD, MSPH, FAAP. E-mail: gerri.mattson@dhhs.nc.gov

To cite: Mattson G, Kuo DZ, AAP COMMITTEE ON PSYCHOSOCIAL ASPECTS OF CHILD AND FAMILY HEALTH, AAP COUNCIL ON CHILDREN WITH DISABILITIES. Psychosocial Factors in Children and Youth With Special Health Care Needs and Their Families. *Pediatrics.* 2019;143(1):e20183171

INTRODUCTION

Children and youth with special health care needs (CYSHCN) are "those who have or are at increased risk for a chronic physical, developmental, behavioral, or emotional condition and who also require health and related services of a type or amount beyond that required for children generally."[1] This definition has been used to guide the development of family-centered, coordinated systems of care for children with special needs and families who are served by many public and private health systems, most notably by state Title V block programs administered by the federal Maternal and Child Health Bureau. This report highlights psychosocial internal (emotional or behavioral) and external (interpersonal, housing, and financial) risk and protective factors that impact growth and development, health and wellness, and quality of life for CYSHCN and their families.[2] The report offers guidance for pediatric providers to address psychosocial risk and protective factors as part of comprehensive, coordinated care within the medical home. Such care should be delivered in partnership with families, mental and behavioral health providers, child care settings, schools, social services, and other professionals and community agencies across the care spectrum. This report complements other pediatric literature in which screening and surveillance, discussion, and the management of threats to social, behavioral, emotional, and mental health in all children are addressed.[3–7]

CHANGING EPIDEMIOLOGY OF CYSHCN

According to the 2016 National Survey of Children's Health (NSCH), 19.4% of children and youth have special health care needs.[8] This is an increase from 15.1% found in the 2009–2010 National Survey of Children with Special Health Care Needs.[9] Racial and ethnic disparities are seen in prevalence, resource use, and survival rates between children who have more medically complex and less complex physical, mental health, and developmental conditions.[10–16] Studies reveal that families caring for CYSHCN experience more significant financial and caregiving demands than families of children without special health care needs.[8,9,17] Few CYSHCN (3.8%) were reported to be uninsured on the 2016 NSCH, but 29.6% of parents of CYSHCN reported inadequate insurance coverage, compared with 23.6% of parents of children without special health care needs.[8]

National surveys have shown a significant increase in the overall prevalence and severity of specific chronic conditions, including asthma, diabetes mellitus, and obesity.[11,18–22] The 2015 data from the National Health Interview Survey of the Centers for Disease Control and Prevention show a current overall asthma prevalence of 8.4% among children younger than 18 years. However, there is racial disparity, as non-Hispanic African American children have a 13.4% prevalence of asthma.[18] There have been disproportionate increases in the prevalence of obesity and severe obesity among Hispanic, non-Hispanic African American, and American Indian and/or Alaskan native children.[20,21,23] There is also a disproportionate increase in type 2 diabetes mellitus, which is believed to be related to increasing rates of obesity,[24,25] especially in African American and American Indian and/or Alaskan native children.[22–25]

The prevalence of children with medical complexity (CMC), who represent the most resource-intensive subset of CYSHCN, is also increasing. CMC typically include children with congenital, genetic, or acquired multisystem conditions who have multiple subspecialty needs as well as children with a dependence on technology for daily needs.[17,26,27] The increase in CMC is possibly related to advances in neonatal care and additional life-saving technologies.[28–30] Despite being a small subset of CYSHCN, CMC account for an increasing proportion of pediatric inpatient admissions, with hospitalization rates that doubled between 1991 and 2005.[31,32]

The overall prevalence of children with a behavioral, mental health, learning, or developmental disability as their primary chronic health condition is increasing in the United States.[6,7] Parent surveys indicate that the prevalence of attention-deficit/hyperactivity disorder (ADHD) (currently 8.9% of children),[8] autism spectrum disorders (2.5% of children),[8] and bipolar disorders (2.2% among youth)[33] have increased over the last 2 decades.[6,7,34] ADHD has been found to be highest in the non-Hispanic multiracial group and lowest among Hispanic children. Behavioral or conduct problems are highest among non-Hispanic African American children, and autism spectrum disorders tend to be higher among non-Hispanic white children.[7] Speech disorders, ADHD, and learning disabilities are among the leading causes of limitations in play or school for children attributable to a chronic condition, and there has been a receding in importance between 1979 and 2009 in the numbers of respiratory, eye, ear, and orthopedic conditions that cause limitations for children.[35]

According to the 2016 NSCH, 42.4% of CYSHCN were reported to have an emotional, developmental, or behavioral issue.[8] Behavioral health can strongly influence health and wellness outcomes for all children and especially for CYSHCN.[36] Reviews of the literature have shown that children with chronic physical health and developmental conditions are at an increased risk for having co-occurring mental health or behavioral problems or conditions.[37,38] Internalizing problems and conditions, ranging from low self-esteem and worry to depression and anxiety, can occur in CYSHCN. CYSHCN also can experience externalizing problems and conditions, ranging from attention problems and defiant and aggressive behaviors to ADHD, conduct disorder, and oppositional defiant disorder.[38–40]

Associations of chronic illnesses with psychological and behavioral conditions, such as anxiety and depression, are well described. Such associations may be explained by biological causes, such as inflammatory processes with asthma or diabetes, and psychological causes, such as the stress of living with an adverse and potentially life-threatening condition.[36,41,42] Studies in adults reveal that comorbid mental and physical illnesses can result in more health care service needs, functional impairment, and higher medical costs compared with similar physical illnesses without the co-occurring mental health condition.[43] Fewer studies have been conducted in children, but 1 study suggests that mental health encounters may encompass a large proportion of outpatient use for some CMC.[44] A focus on psychosocial factors and wellness would appear to be an important addition to the overall chronic care model for CYSHCN.[36]

IMPACT OF PSYCHOSOCIAL FACTORS ON OVERALL HEALTH AND WELLNESS FOR CYSHCN AND THEIR FAMILIES

The biological, physical, emotional, and social environments strongly affect the capacity for children to be healthy over their life course trajectory.[45] External psychosocial factors include social determinants of health (SDH), which are defined by the Kaiser Family Foundation and World Health Organization as the "conditions in which people are born, grow, live, work and age."[46] The Centers for Disease Control and Prevention Essentials for Childhood initiative emphasizes that "[s]afe, stable, nurturing relationships and environments are essential to prevent child maltreatment…and to assure that children reach their full potential" over their lives.[47] SDH, such as housing stability and food security, have a positive influence on the health of all children and are recommended to be addressed during well-child visits.[5,46,48] Studies suggest that poor housing and neighborhood quality are associated with a greater risk for some CYSHCN experiencing a poorer quality of life.[49,50] Food insecurity may also impact CYSHCN specifically if they have increased or specialized nutritional needs or dietary restrictions.[51]

CYSHCN have higher rates of exposure to adverse childhood experiences (ACEs) or toxic stress (eg, abuse and domestic violence).[8] According to the 2016 NSCH, 37% of CYSHCN had 2 or more ACEs, compared with 18% of children without special health care needs.[9] These ACEs are often internalized, but the negative effects may be mitigated over time by protective factors.[52–54] In addition, children with 2 or more ACEs are significantly more likely to be considered CYSHCN compared with children with no exposure to ACEs.[53] The presence of 2 or more ACEs can be linked to exacerbations of their chronic conditions, an increased risk of developing secondary conditions, poor school engagement, and even an increased risk of repeating a grade in school.[52,53] Exposure to 2 or more ACEs may be associated with smoking, using drugs, participating in earlier sexual activity, and performing violent or antisocial acts.[53,54] If CYSHCN engage in these risky behaviors, there may be an increased risk for additional short- and long-term physical and mental health problems and difficulties with following treatment recommendations as well as an increased risk for poorer health care outcomes.[50,55,56] However, studies show that CYSHCN who learn and show resilience may be able to reduce the negative effects of some ACEs. This mitigation of risk occurs especially when supports are provided for key transition points, such as starting child care, school, and work.[52,53]

Children with intellectual or developmental disabilities may be at an increased risk for physical, emotional, and sexual abuse and neglect. The reasons may include inadequate social skills, limited capacity to find help or report abuse, lack of strategies to defend against abuse, or increased exposure to multiple caregivers and settings.[57,58] Additional challenges can occur if parents of children with disabilities lack respite, coping skills, or adequate social and community support. These stressors can put some children at risk for failing to receive needed medications or adequate medical care and can lead to abuse or neglect.[59]

Additional family stressors not considered ACEs can still negatively affect the health of some CYSHCN. These stressors include, but are not limited to, caregiver burden, poor coping skills, inadequate sleep, limited interactions with extended family and friends, reductions or loss of parental employment, and financial problems.[60–65] Family conflict, in particular, can be associated with a greater number of hospitalizations, as seen in 1 study for children with asthma.[41] Financial problems may result from multiple and costly medications, equipment, therapies or specialty appointments, and loss of income from taking time off work to care for CYSHCN.[17,66] Limited English proficiency in parents and lack of insurance are 2 stressors that may disproportionately affect the health and well-being of some immigrant families of CYSHCN.[67] Parenting stress may increase if negative perceptions of their child's illness occur, potentially leading to additional mental and physical health problems in the parents of some CYSHCN.[68] Siblings of some CYSHCN with developmental disabilities and cancer may be at risk for emotional and behavioral problems, difficulties with interpersonal relationships and functioning at school, and psychiatric conditions.[69,70] The effects on caregiver and family stress can be even greater in families with children who have higher medical complexity.[17,71]

Child care and school settings may struggle to accommodate the needs of CYSHCN, leading to increased stress, poor socialization, and poor school performance.[49,50,72–75] Some CYSHCN may lose motivation to do well in school, resulting in lower academic achievement and increased school absences.[75] Some CYSHCN may experience bullying, stereotyping, prejudice, or stigmatization from peers or others in their schools or communities. This negative experiences may lead to difficulties in school, including school avoidance.[50,76,77] Children with intellectual and developmental disabilities, seizure disorders, and other conditions affecting the central nervous system are at particular risk for school problems because of impairments in brain growth and development[78–80] with resultant effects on executive functioning skills.[38,78,80,81] Problems with attention, memory, language, and understanding social processes place some CYSHCN at an increased risk for academic failure, poor interpersonal skills, and low self-esteem.[38,78,80–82] Negative school experiences may also further exacerbate problems with adherence to medications, therapies, or other health recommendations at school.[83]

The cumulative effects of living with and managing a chronic condition may evolve further over the life span of a child.[84,85] Certain chronic physical and mental health conditions and treatments, particularly those affecting the central nervous system, may affect neurologic and cognitive function, social development, emotional regulation and awareness, and expressive and receptive communication. These effects may not be readily apparent to families, caregivers, teachers, and health care providers.[84–86] Developmental, social, and behavioral problems may be observed when age-appropriate and interpersonal competencies, abilities, and skills are not achieved.[38,78,87–90] Escalation in levels of needed medical care can increase the development of additional mental or behavioral health problems or social concerns in children. These developments can present additional challenges in the home and in child care and school settings.[38,78,87,88,91,92]

A negative illness perception, low self-esteem, and a belief of a lack of control can increase the risk of a co-occurring mental health concern or diagnosis in some children.[93,94] Stress from unrecognized and/or untreated mental health concerns can result in increased cortisol levels, which can negatively affect physiology and metabolism and exacerbate chronic conditions, such as asthma or diabetes.[87] Unrecognized and untreated chronic complications among CYSHCN can increase the risk of developing internalizing or externalizing behavioral problems or conditions.[95,96] For example, chronic nocturnal symptoms with uncontrolled asthma or undiagnosed sleep apnea with Down syndrome can negatively affect behavioral health and quality of life.[97] Co-occurring chronic physical and mental health conditions are associated with an attempted suicide risk in excess of that predicted by the chronic mental health condition alone.[98] A focus on behavioral health and wellness as part of chronic care may help improve health outcomes for some CYSHCN and their families.[36]

SUPPORTING PSYCHOSOCIAL PROTECTIVE FACTORS FOR CYSHCN AND THEIR FAMILIES

Psychosocial protective factors can be supported at the individual, interpersonal, and community levels. Supportive and stable relationships, processes, and policies that promote resilience benefit children and can buffer against ACEs.[99–103] Developmentally appropriate and supported cognitive, language, and communication skills and abilities may be associated with calmer temperament and higher levels of self-esteem, which can aid in coping with a chronic illness.[40,104–106] Skills for social competence have been taught by caregivers to encourage cooperation, self-control, assertion, and self-responsibility in children with mobility disorders.[99] Protective factors in some children with malignancies include comparing themselves with other children with malignancies instead of healthy peers, using positive reappraisal, spiritual or religious coping, and future-oriented thinking.[107–109]

Studies now show the importance of supporting families and communities that help CYSHCN to have positive relationships and interactions.[103] Healthy and well-functioning families may offer coping assistance for some CYSHCN.[108,110] Cohesive and connected families with stable family structures seem to be most functional.[60,110] Studies of children with autism, asthma, and diabetes suggest that instilling positive parenting beliefs helps engage parents in appropriate care.[111–114] Education of community members about a child or youth's medical condition may increase coping and resilience in some families.[110] A father's involvement in the care of a child with a chronic disease has been associated with higher treatment adherence, better psychological adjustment, and improved health for the child.[115] Higher social support for caregivers of CYSHCN has been associated with decreased psychological distress in the child and decreased risks for stress, loneliness, depression, and anxiety in caregivers.[116]

Schools can be a source of strength when there are positive parent-school partnerships and a supportive, coordinated early intervention system.[73–75] Health care providers and schools can collaborate with families on monitoring changes in health status, developing the treatment plan, and ensuring appropriate school staffing.[117,118] Schools, in partnership with families and health care providers, can play a significant role in supporting self-management of care for CYSHCN and other elements of health care transition.[119] Families, youth, providers, and school and child care staff can develop and modify an Individualized Family Service Plan, Individualized Education Program, 504 plan, or individualized health plan on the basis of medical and psychosocial needs and supports. These supports may include self-management of care and transition to adult health care systems.[117,119–122]

Fully supporting protective factors involves the development of community-based systems of care for CYSHCN that address psychosocial aspects of care.[123,124] A system of care represents a coordinated network of community-based services and supports, including the family, the medical home, child care providers, and schools. The core values include building on the strengths and needs of the youth and family. This approach has resulted in improvements in multiple domains of individual and family functioning, including the reduction of family stress and strain and increased behavioral and emotional strengths in children.[125]

ADDRESSING PSYCHOSOCIAL FACTORS IN THE MEDICAL HOME

The pediatric medical home is an ideal setting to address psychosocial factors that impact wellness and resilience for CYSHCN and their families. The medical home can conduct ongoing surveillance and screening for psychosocial factors and promote care coordination of needed services and supports.[126,127] Longitudinal, relationship-centered care may facilitate discussions about psychosocial factors, address symptoms, and increase adherence to recommendations.[127–130] Pediatric primary care and specialty providers can promote team-based care with partners from multiple disciplines by coordinating psychosocial screening, care planning, and interventions. Additional key partners may include care managers, family navigators, social workers, psychologists, professional interpreters, and public health and social service agencies.[131] Access to comprehensive care for CYSHCN through a medical home is associated with improvements in health status, access to care, and family satisfaction. Use of a medical home approach is also associated with fewer missed school days for children, issues with child care, missed days of work, and out-of-pocket costs for families.[8,9,126,132–134]

In the 2017 *Bright Futures: Guidelines for Health Supervision of Infants, Children, and Adolescents, Fourth Edition,* the American Academy of Pediatrics (AAP) emphasizes a strength-based approach to comprehensive care and wellness for all children. The need to particularly focus on health and wellness for CYSHCN is also recognized.[5] AAP *Bright Futures* recommendations for preventive pediatric health care include developmental surveillance, general developmental screening, and screening for autism at specific ages during well-child visits.[5,135–136] Recommended surveillance and screenings are important even in the presence of an existing chronic physical or mental health condition, a developmental delay, or a disability, when appropriate.

The AAP *Bright Futures* recommendations include a psychosocial and behavioral assessment at every well-child visit that is "family centered and may include an assessment of child social emotional health, caregiver depression, and social determinants."[5,135] *Bright Futures* and the US Preventive Services Task Force recommend screening for both postpartum depression and depression in adolescents at specified well-child visits.[5,137–139] Surveillance or screening for parental socioemotional well-being and SDH outside of the postpartum period may identify additional psychosocial risk factors for CYSHCN.[19,50,53,54,60,61,63–65] The AAP policy statement "Poverty and Child Health in the United States"[48] and an additional article about redesigning health care to address poverty[140] provide recommendations and resources for screening tools for SDH (eg, Safe Environment for Every Kid [SEEK]).

A variety of resources can help pediatric medical home providers address psychosocial risk factors using a team-based approach. These include the AAP Mental Health Initiatives Web site (https://www.aap.org/en-us/advocacy-and-policy/aap-health-initiatives/Mental-Health/Pages/Primary-Care-Tools.aspx), a tool kit called Mental Health Screening and Assessment Tools for Primary Care,[141] articles and resources from the AAP Task Force on Mental Health published in a June 2010 supplement to *Pediatrics*,[142] and a recent clinical report ("Promoting Optimal Development: Screening for Behavioral and Emotional Problems"[4]) that provides resources about specific behavioral and emotional tools and processes. The AAP Screening, Technical Assistance, and Resource Center provides a variety of resources about screening, discussion, management, and referral in primary care around child development, maternal depression, and SDH for young children (https://www.aap.org/en-us/advocacy-and-policy/aap-health-initiatives/Screening/Pages/default.aspx). These developmental, autism, and social-emotional screening tools were validated in the general population and normalized for typically developing children.[4,5,139,141,143,144] Validated quality-of-life screening questions have been used across several conditions, although more in research settings than in primary care.[145] Standardized care approaches and tools can be used to facilitate self-management that addresses psychosocial needs, adherence to treatment plans, and leverage of supportive community resources.[146,147]

Pediatric providers are encouraged to develop mental health competencies for direct patient care and for coordination with community resources.[3] Pediatric providers can use evidence-based techniques (eg, motivational interviewing) to address mental health concerns and social determinants identified with screening in the medical home setting. Such approaches may be used by providers while waiting for further evaluation of the child and even while a child is receiving treatment by a mental health provider.[3,130] Interventions may include counseling about family-focused physical activity guidelines, good nutrition, and improved sleep routines.[36,131] Common elements among psychosocial interventions include the use of motivational interviewing strategies to communicate hope, empathy, and loyalty; use of plain language; asking permission to ask questions or share information; and partnering with families.[130] Such elements have been found to be effective in building alliances, increasing disclosure, and facilitating discussions about psychosocial strengths and concerns.[129,130] Pediatric providers on the care team may not serve as the primary provider to deliver mental health counseling and interventions, but they can support integrated interdisciplinary efforts and partnerships.[36] A team-based approach may include the use of designated staff for wellness promotion, collocation of services (eg, social workers and psychologists), or referrals to community services for mental health assessment, counseling, and interventions.[131]

Behavioral health integration has been described as a useful "approach and model of delivering care that comprehensively addresses the primary care, behavioral health, specialty care, and social support needs of children and youth with behavioral health issues in a manner that is continuous and family-centered."[148] Behavioral health integration can aid the medical home as needs occur from infancy through adolescence and into young adulthood.[149] Practices with collocated behavioral health providers or real-time access to short-term mental health support have seen improved timely evaluations of child and family functioning, increased referrals for more specialized evaluations, and improved access to direct behavioral health services for CYSHCN.[3,150] Mindfulness and relaxation training may also be effective with stress and can be taught to parents and children.[151] However, not all practices have collocated or integrated behavioral health providers; therefore, pediatric providers are encouraged, as mentioned earlier, to develop some mental health competencies for use in primary care to enhance their delivery of direct patient care and coordination with community resources.[3] Formal care coordinators, as part of the medical home team, can assist with identifying and strengthening protective relationships to help support and monitor strategies and interventions with child care providers, schools, home health agencies, behavioral health providers, social service workers, and a variety of other professionals.[152] Care coordinators can be employed by the practice or another entity and can help facilitate management and referral and follow-up related to community resources.[3,140,152]

These community relationships can help increase awareness, communication, and transparency of the care directed by the medical home.[152] The medical home, in partnership with care coordinators and community partners, may promote planned transition from pediatric to adult health care that addresses psychosocial risk and protective factors. Planned transition includes structured assessments and planning (beginning in early adolescence) addressing SDH as well as guardianship and other legal issues. The goal is to minimize breaks in continuous care and lessen parental concern, particularly for chronic conditions accompanied by cognitive impairment.[119]

Implementation of the medical home model entails a quality improvement approach and practice transformation activities. Such activities may include a patient registry, care tracking, team-based care, and special care protocols. Strategies could include a previsit process that may include routine psychosocial screening, scheduling additional time during appointments, and identifying a team member and/or care coordinator. Additional efforts include electronic health record integration and workflow changes to incorporate screening, discussion, referrals, and follow-up as part of a comprehensive, integrated plan of care. Such a plan of care includes patient- and family-identified psychosocial goals and priorities.[48,124,153]

Individual provider and practice challenges to the medical home include time, training, and lack of knowledge about available resources.[4,154] Community and system barriers include inadequate payments, a shortage of pediatric psychiatrists and developmental-behavioral pediatricians,[155] limited community mental health resources, and limited services and abilities in communities to address SDH (eg, housing).[48,149] Flexible population-based payment models and the use of payment incentives could help to encourage increased management of psychosocial health and well-being as part of care for chronic conditions and could help to increase the use of more screening tools.[48,153]

ADDITIONAL STRATEGIES TO SUPPORT SYSTEMS ADDRESSING PSYCHOSOCIAL FACTORS

Pediatricians represent only 1 stakeholder interested in the comprehensive system of care for CYSHCN and their families. Title V Maternal and Child Health programs, health plans, insurers, state Medicaid and Children's Health Insurance Program agencies, children's hospitals, health services researchers, families, and consumers developed national standards for a system of care for CYSHCN in 2014 and then updated these standards in 2017.[124]

Recommendations for pediatric medical home teams include developing processes and protocols in collaboration with other community agencies (eg, Part C early intervention and home health) and professionals. These agencies may also perform psychosocial screenings and refer CYSHCN for further assessment of concerns. Collaboration could allow the medical home team to reduce duplication of efforts and ensure referred services regardless of who conducted the screening. Service linkage, timely communication, and appropriate data sharing can be used to promote an integrated plan of care that includes psychosocial goals and priorities from CSYHCN and their families.[124] The resource titled *Managing Chronic Health Needs in Child Care and Schools*[72] and the AAP policy statement on the role of school nurses and the medical home[117] offer collaborative strategies to support social-emotional health, which influences health, school attendance, and academic performance.[117,118]

Pediatric medical home providers and parents can learn about and be linked to several home- and community-based services and supports to help assess and address psychosocial needs for CYSHCN and their families. Respite care, palliative care, and hospice care and home-based services are examples of these services.[124] Parents may be supported through home visiting and parenting support programs regardless of whether they are specific for CYSHCN.[156–158] One parenting program, called the Positive Parenting Program or Triple P, offers a series of parenting modules called Stepping Stones, which was developed specifically for use with parents of children with developmental disabilities. Stepping Stones modules address self-efficacy, self-sufficiency, self-management, personal agency, and problem solving with parents of children with developmental disabilities. However, not all states offer Triple P Stepping Stones modules, and some states that do offer it have limited access to these modules.[159,160] Parent-to-parent support groups may help some families of CYSHCN share a social identity, experience personal growth, and learn coping strategies.[161]

Several programs serve as clearinghouses about services and supports for families. One example is the early childhood coordinated referral and system building programs called Help Me Grow (www.helpmegrownational.org/). Help Me Grow is now available in 26 states to help connect providers and families to developmental screening and services.[140] The Community Services Locator (https://www.ncemch.org/knowledge/community.php) is another clearinghouse of information that provides Web sites and phone numbers that can be used to assist with accessing national, state, and local resources for child care, early childhood education, special education services, family support, financial support, health and wellness, and parenting programs.[140] A third example is the United Way 211 line (http://www.211.org/pages/about), which is a telephone and Internet-based resource that is available 24 hours a day, 7 days a week, throughout most of the United States.[140] The 211 line can provide information about a wide variety of resources in multiple languages about housing, food pantries, and utilities in addition to child care, early education, and many other services to address SDH.[140]

RECOMMENDATIONS

Health and wellness for CYSHCN are particularly sensitive to psychosocial risk and protective factors. Pediatric providers, particularly from the primary care–based medical home, are in the position to screen for, manage, and coordinate longitudinal care in which psychosocial factors of health among CYSHCN and their families are addressed. The following suggestions are offered to pediatricians involved in caring for CYSHCN:

1. Follow *Bright Futures* recommendations and guidance for CYSHCN and their families. Recommendations include the promotion of health and wellness as well as timely assessments of child social-emotional health, parental and/or caregiver depression, and SDH.
2. Use practice transformation strategies, such as quality improvement, patient registries, and previsit planning, to promote psychosocial screening and assessment, referrals, and follow-up among CYSHCN and their families. A good resource is the AAP Practice Transformation site (https://www.aap.org/en-us/

professional-resources/practice-Transformation/Pages/practice-transformation.aspx).

3. Use team-based care strategies, care protocols, and dedicated care coordinators (if available) to recognize psychosocial protective factors and ameliorate risk factors. This strategy may involve collocation, consultation, comanagement, and/or integration with behavioral health specialists as part of medical home and specialty care teams.
4. Consider strategies for working with child care and school staff to monitor progress, reduce absences, and improve learning experiences and academic performance for CYSHCN.
5. Advocate for flexible payment redesign with Medicaid and other insurers. Payment redesign may better support wellness and chronic care management for CYSHCN and their families. Flexible payment redesign may include payments for mental health treatment, care coordination, and collocation or comanagement with behavioral health and other specialists or disciplines.
6. Promote evidence-based interventions and strategies in the medical home and subspecialty settings to support psychosocial development of CYSHCN, parenting competencies, and family resilience.
7. Advocate for research on adaptions of existing psychosocial screening tools and interventions for CYSHCN.
8. Advocate for community-based resources and strategies to address SDH and the reduction of disparities for CYSHCN and their families.
9. Pediatric providers and state AAP chapters can partner with Title V Maternal and Child Health CYSHCN programs in supporting implementation of the Association of Maternal and Child Health Program's Standards for Systems of Care for CYSHCN. These standards include increasing access for CYSHCN to quality medical homes, ease of use of community services, and transitioning across the life span.

LEAD AUTHORS

Gerri Mattson, MD, MSPH, FAAP
Dennis Z. Kuo, MD, MHS, FAAP

COMMITTEE ON PSYCHOSOCIAL ASPECTS OF CHILD AND FAMILY HEALTH, 2017–2018

Michael Yogman, MD, FAAP, Chairperson
Rebecca Baum, MD, FAAP
Thresia B. Gambon, MD, FAAP
Arthur Lavin, MD, FAAP
Gerri Mattson, MD, FAAP
Raul Montiel Esparza, MD
Arwa A. Nasir, MBBS, MSc, MPH, FAAP
Lawrence Sagin Wissow, MD, MPH, FAAP

LIAISONS

Amy Starin, PhD – *National Association of Social Workers*
Edward Christophersen, PhD, FAAP – *Society of Pediatric Psychology*
Sharon Berry, PhD, LP – *Society of Pediatric Psychology*
Norah L. Johnson, PhD, RN, CPNP-PC – *National Association of Pediatric Nurse Practitioners*
Abigail B. Schlesinger, MD – *American Academy of Child and Adolescent Psychiatry*
Aaron Pikcilingis – *Family Partnerships Network*

STAFF

Karen Smith
Tamar Magarik Haro

COUNCIL ON CHILDREN WITH DISABILITIES EXECUTIVE COMMITTEE, 2017–2018

Dennis Z. Kuo, MD, MHS, FAAP, Chairperson
Susan Apkon, MD, FAAP
Timothy J. Brei, MD, FAAP
Lynn F. Davidson, MD, FAAP
Beth Ellen Davis, MD, MPH, FAAP
Kathryn A. Ellerbeck, MD, FAAP
Susan L. Hyman, MD, FAAP
Mary O'Connor Leppert, MD, FAAP
Garey H. Noritz, MD, FAAP
Christopher J. Stille, MD, MPH, FAAP
Larry Yin, MD, MSPH, FAAP

FORMER COUNCIL ON CHILDREN WITH DISABILITIES EXECUTIVE COMMITTEE MEMBERS

Amy J. Houtrow, MD, PhD, MPH, FAAP
Kenneth W. Norwood Jr, MD, FAAP, Immediate Past Chairperson

LIAISONS

Peter J. Smith, MD, MA, FAAP – *Section on Developmental and Behavioral Pediatrics*
Edwin Simpser, MD, FAAP – *Section on Home Care*
Georgina Peacock, MD, MPH, FAAP – *Centers for Disease Control and Prevention*
Marie Mann, MD, MPH, FAAP – *Maternal and Child Health Bureau*
Cara Coleman, JD, MPH – *Family Voices*

STAFF

Alexandra Kuznetsov, RD

ABBREVIATIONS

AAP: American Academy of Pediatrics
ACE: adverse childhood experience
ADHD: attention-deficit/hyperactivity disorder
CMC: children with medical complexity
CYSHCN: children and youth with special health care needs
NSCH: National Survey of Children's Health
SDH: social determinants of health

PEDIATRICS (ISSN Numbers: Print, 0031-4005; Online, 1098-4275).

Copyright © 2019 by the American Academy of Pediatrics

FINANCIAL DISCLOSURE: The authors have indicated they have no financial relationships relevant to this article to disclose.

FUNDING: No external funding.

POTENTIAL CONFLICT OF INTEREST: The authors have indicated they have no potential conflicts of interest to disclose.

REFERENCES

1. McPherson M, Arango P, Fox H, et al. A new definition of children with special health care needs. *Pediatrics.* 1998;102(1 pt 1):137–140
2. Fee RJ, Hinton VJ. Resilience in children diagnosed with a chronic neuromuscular disorder. *J Dev Behav Pediatr.* 2011;32(9):644–650
3. Committee on Psychosocial Aspects of Child and Family Health; Task Force on Mental Health. Policy statement–the future of pediatrics: mental health competencies for pediatric primary care. *Pediatrics.* 2009;124(1):410–421
4. Weitzman C, Wegner L; Section on Developmental and Behavioral Pediatrics; Committee on Psychosocial Aspects of Child and Family Health; Council on Early Childhood; Society for Developmental and Behavioral Pediatrics; American Academy of Pediatrics. Promoting optimal development: screening for behavioral and emotional problems [published correction appears in *Pediatrics.* 2015;135(5):946]. *Pediatrics.* 2015;135(2):384–395
5. Hagan JF, Shaw JS, Duncan PM, eds. *Bright Futures: Guidelines for Health Supervision of Infants, Children, and Adolescents.* 4th ed. Elk Grove Village, IL: American Academy of Pediatrics; 2017
6. Boyle CA, Boulet S, Schieve LA, et al. Trends in the prevalence of developmental disabilities in US children, 1997-2008. *Pediatrics.* 2011;127(6):1034–1042
7. Perou R, Bitsko RH, Blumberg SJ, et al; Centers for Disease Control and Prevention (CDC). Mental health surveillance among children–United States, 2005-2011. *MMWR Suppl.* 2013;62(2):1–35
8. Child and Adolescent Health Measurement Initiative; Data Resource Center for Child and Adolescent Health. 2016 National Survey of Children's Health (NSCH) data query. Available at: http://childhealthdata.org/browse/survey/results?q=4562&r. Accessed March 5, 2018
9. US Department of Health and Human Services; Health Resources and Services Administration; Maternal and Child Health Bureau. *The National Survey of Children With Special Health Care Needs Chartbook 2009–2010.* Rockville, MD: US Department of Health and Human Services; 2013
10. Berry JG, Bloom S, Foley S, Palfrey JS. Health inequity in children and youth with chronic health conditions. *Pediatrics.* 2010;126(suppl 3):S111–S119
11. Akinbami LJ, Moorman JE, Garbe PL, Sondik EJ. Status of childhood asthma in the United States, 1980-2007. *Pediatrics.* 2009;123(suppl 3):S131–S145
12. Wu YW, Croen LA, Shah SJ, Newman TB, Najjar DV. Cerebral palsy in a term population: risk factors and neuroimaging findings. *Pediatrics.* 2006;118(2):690–697
13. Lipton R, Good G, Mikhailov T, Freels S, Donoghue E. Ethnic differences in mortality from insulin-dependent diabetes mellitus among people less than 25 years of age. *Pediatrics.* 1999;103(5 pt 1):952–956
14. Centers for Disease Control and Prevention (CDC). Racial disparities in median age at death of persons with Down syndrome–United States, 1968-1997. *MMWR Morb Mortal Wkly Rep.* 2001;50(22):463–465
15. Boneva RS, Botto LD, Moore CA, Yang Q, Correa A, Erickson JD. Mortality associated with congenital heart defects in the United States: trends and racial disparities, 1979-1997. *Circulation.* 2001;103(19):2376–2381
16. Linabery AM, Ross JA. Childhood and adolescent cancer survival in the US by race and ethnicity for the diagnostic period 1975-1999. *Cancer.* 2008;113(9):2575–2596
17. Kuo DZ, Cohen E, Agrawal R, Berry JG, Casey PH. A national profile of caregiver challenges among more medically complex children with special health care needs. *Arch Pediatr Adolesc Med.* 2011;165(11):1020–1026
18. Centers for Disease Control and Prevention. Most recent asthma data. Available at: https://www.cdc.gov/asthma/most_recent_data.htm. Accessed April 3, 2017
19. Perrin JM, Bloom SR, Gortmaker SL. The increase of childhood chronic conditions in the United States. *JAMA.* 2007;297(24):2755–2759
20. Kelly AS, Barlow SE, Rao G, et al; American Heart Association; Atherosclerosis, Hypertension, and Obesity in the Young Committee of the Council on Cardiovascular Disease in the Young; Council on Nutrition, Physical Activity and Metabolism; Council on Clinical Cardiology. Severe obesity in children and adolescents: identification, associated health risks, and treatment approaches: a scientific statement from the American Heart Association. *Circulation.* 2013;128(15):1689–1712
21. Skinner AC, Skelton JA. Prevalence and trends in obesity and severe obesity among children in the United States, 1999-2012. *JAMA Pediatr.* 2014;168(6):561–566
22. Dabelea D, Mayer-Davis EJ, Saydah S, et al; SEARCH for Diabetes in Youth Study. Prevalence of type 1 and type 2 diabetes among children and adolescents from 2001 to 2009. *JAMA.* 2014;311(17):1778–1786
23. Adams AK, Quinn RA, Prince RJ. Low recognition of childhood overweight and disease risk among Native-American caregivers. *Obes Res.* 2005;13(1):146–152
24. Reinehr T. Type 2 diabetes mellitus in children and adolescents. *World J Diabetes.* 2013;4(6):270–281
25. Goran MI, Ball GD, Cruz ML. Obesity and risk of type 2 diabetes and cardiovascular disease in children and adolescents. *J Clin Endocrinol Metab.* 2003;88(4):1417–1427
26. Cohen E, Kuo DZ, Agrawal R, et al. Children with medical complexity: an emerging population for clinical and research initiatives. *Pediatrics.* 2011;127(3):529–538
27. Berry JG, Hall M, Neff J, et al. Children with medical complexity and Medicaid: spending and cost savings. *Health Aff (Millwood).* 2014;33(12):2199–2206
28. van der Lee JH, Mokkink LB, Grootenhuis MA, Heymans HS, Offringa M. Definitions and measurement of chronic health conditions in

childhood: a systematic review. *JAMA*. 2007;297(24):2741–2751

29. Stiller C. Epidemiology of cancer in adolescents. *Med Pediatr Oncol*. 2002;39(3):149–155
30. van der Veen WJ. The small epidemiologic transition: further decrease in infant mortality due to medical intervention during pregnancy and childbirth, yet no decrease in childhood disabilities [in Dutch]. *Ned Tijdschr Geneeskd*. 2003;147(9):378–381
31. Simon TD, Berry J, Feudtner C, et al. Children with complex chronic conditions in inpatient hospital settings in the United States. *Pediatrics*. 2010;126(4):647–655
32. Burns KH, Casey PH, Lyle RE, Bird TM, Fussell JJ, Robbins JM. Increasing prevalence of medically complex children in US hospitals. *Pediatrics*. 2010;126(4):638–646
33. Merikangas KR, Cui L, Kattan G, Carlson GA, Youngstrom EA, Angst J. Mania with and without depression in a community sample of US adolescents. *Arch Gen Psychiatry*. 2012;69(9):943–951
34. Visser SN, Danielson ML, Bitsko RH, et al. Trends in the parent-report of health care provider-diagnosed and medicated attention-deficit/hyperactivity disorder: United States, 2003-2011. *J Am Acad Child Adolesc Psychiatry*. 2014;53(1):34–46.e2
35. Halfon N, Houtrow A, Larson K, Newacheck PW. The changing landscape of disability in childhood. *Future Child*. 2012;22(1):13–42
36. Boat TF, Filigno S, Amin RS. Wellness for families of children with chronic health disorders. *JAMA Pediatr*. 2017;171(9):825–826
37. Hysing M, Elgen I, Gillberg C, Lie SA, Lundervold AJ. Chronic physical illness and mental health in children. Results from a large-scale population study. *J Child Psychol Psychiatry*. 2007;48(8):785–792
38. Pinquart M, Shen Y. Behavior problems in children and adolescents with chronic physical illness: a meta-analysis. *J Pediatr Psychol*. 2011;36(9):1003–1016
39. Inkelas M, Raghavan R, Larson K, Kuo AA, Ortega AN. Unmet mental health need and access to services for children with special health care needs and their families. *Ambul Pediatr*. 2007;7(6):431–438
40. Theunissen SC, Rieffe C, Netten AP, et al. Self-esteem in hearing-impaired children: the influence of communication, education, and audiological characteristics. *PLoS One*. 2014;9(4):e94521
41. Goodwin RD, Bandiera FC, Steinberg D, Ortega AN, Feldman JM. Asthma and mental health among youth: etiology, current knowledge and future directions. *Expert Rev Respir Med*. 2012;6(4):397–406
42. Hood KK, Beavers DP, Yi-Frazier J, et al. Psychosocial burden and glycemic control during the first 6 years of diabetes: results from the SEARCH for Diabetes in Youth study. *J Adolesc Health*. 2014;55(4):498–504
43. Melek S, Norris D. *Chronic Conditions and Comorbid Psychological Disorders*. Seattle, WA: Milliman; 2008
44. Kuo DZ, Melguizo-Castro M, Goudie A, Nick TG, Robbins JM, Casey PH. Variation in child health care utilization by medical complexity. *Matern Child Health J*. 2015;19(1):40–48
45. Fine A, Kotelchuck M, Adess N, Pies C. *Policy Brief. A New Agenda for MCH Policy and Programs: Integrating a Life Course Perspective*. Martinez, CA: Contra Costa Health Services; 2009
46. Heiman HJ, Artigo S. *Beyond Health Care: The Role of Social Determinants in Promoting Health and Health Equity*. San Francisco, CA: Kaiser Family Foundation; 2015. Available at: https://www.issuelab.org/resources/22899/22899.pdf. Accessed October 24, 2018
47. Centers for Disease Control and Prevention, National Center for Injury Prevention and Control, Division of Violence Prevention. Essentials for childhood: steps to create safe, stable, nurturing relationships and environments. Available at: https://www.cdc.gov/violenceprevention/pdf/essentials_for_childhood_framework.pdf. Accessed November 4, 2017
48. Council on Community Pediatrics. Poverty and child health in the United States. *Pediatrics*. 2016;137(4):e20160339
49. Coutinho MT, McQuaid EL, Koinis-Mitchell D. Contextual and cultural risks and their association with family asthma management in urban children. *J Child Health Care*. 2013;17(2):138–152
50. Atkinson M, Rees D, Davis L. Disability and economic disadvantage: facing the facts. *Arch Dis Child*. 2015;100(4):305–307
51. Rose-Jacobs R, Fiore JG, de Cuba SE, et al. Children with special health care needs, supplemental security income, and food insecurity. *J Dev Behav Pediatr*. 2016;37(2):140–147
52. Bethell CD, Newacheck PW, Fine A, et al. Optimizing health and health care systems for children with special health care needs using the life course perspective. *Matern Child Health J*. 2014;18(2):467–477
53. Bethell CD, Newacheck P, Hawes E, Halfon N. Adverse childhood experiences: assessing the impact on health and school engagement and the mitigating role of resilience. *Health Aff (Millwood)*. 2014;33(12):2106–2115
54. Anda RF, Felitti VJ, Bremner JD, et al. The enduring effects of abuse and related adverse experiences in childhood. A convergence of evidence from neurobiology and epidemiology. *Eur Arch Psychiatry Clin Neurosci*. 2006;256(3):174–186
55. Bonnie RJ, Stratton K, Kwan LY, eds; Committee on the Public Health Implications of Raising the Minimum Age for Purchasing Tobacco Products; Board on Population Health and Public Health Practice; Institute of Medicine. *Public Health Implications of Raising the Minimum Age of Legal Access to Tobacco Products*. Washington, DC: National Academies Press; 2015
56. Weitzman ER, Ziemnik RE, Huang Q, Levy S. Alcohol and marijuana use and treatment nonadherence among medically vulnerable youth. *Pediatrics*. 2015;136(3):450–457
57. Murphy NA, Elias ER. Sexuality of children and adolescents with developmental disabilities. *Pediatrics*. 2006;118(1):398–403

58. Martinello E. Reviewing risks factors of individuals with intellectual disabilities as perpetrators of sexually abusive behaviors. *Sex Disabil.* 2015;33(2):269–278

59. Hibbard RA, Desch LW; American Academy of Pediatrics Committee on Child Abuse and Neglect; American Academy of Pediatrics Council on Children With Disabilities. Maltreatment of children with disabilities. *Pediatrics.* 2007;119(5):1018–1025

60. Churchill SS, Villareale NL, Monaghan TA, Sharp VL, Kieckhefer GM. Parents of children with special health care needs who have better coping skills have fewer depressive symptoms. *Matern Child Health J.* 2010;14(1):47–57

61. Hatzmann J, Peek N, Heymans H, Maurice-Stam H, Grootenhuis M. Consequences of caring for a child with a chronic disease: employment and leisure time of parents. *J Child Health Care.* 2014;18(4):346–357

62. Meltzer LJ, Booster GD. Sleep disturbance in caregivers of children with respiratory and atopic disease. *J Pediatr Psychol.* 2016;41(6): 643–650

63. Siden H, Steele R. Charting the territory: children and families living with progressive life-threatening conditions [published correction appears in *Paediatr Child Health.* 2015;20(8):466–467]. *Paediatr Child Health.* 2015;20(3):139–144

64. Fedele DA, Grant DM, Wolfe-Christensen C, Mullins LL, Ryan JL. An examination of the factor structure of parenting capacity measures in chronic illness populations. *J Pediatr Psychol.* 2010;35(10):1083–1092

65. Cidav Z, Marcus SC, Mandell DS. Implications of childhood autism for parental employment and earnings. *Pediatrics.* 2012;129(4):617–623

66. Romley JA, Shah AK, Chung PJ, Elliott MN, Vestal KD, Schuster MA. Family-provided health care for children with special health care needs. *Pediatrics.* 2017;139(1):e20161287

67. Singh GK, Yu SM, Kogan MD. Health, chronic conditions, and behavioral risk disparities among U.S. immigrant children and adolescents. *Public Health Rep.* 2013;128(6):463–479

68. Cousino MK, Hazen RA. Parenting stress among caregivers of children with chronic illness: a systematic review. *J Pediatr Psychol.* 2013;38(8):809–828

69. Goudie A, Havercamp S, Jamieson B, Sahr T. Assessing functional impairment in siblings living with children with disability. *Pediatrics.* 2013;132(2). Available at: www.pediatrics.org/cgi/content/full/132/2/e476

70. Houtzager BA, Oort FJ, Hoekstra-Weebers JE, Caron HN, Grootenhuis MA, Last BF. Coping and family functioning predict longitudinal psychological adaptation of siblings of childhood cancer patients. *J Pediatr Psychol.* 2004;29(8):591–605

71. Rehm RS. Nursing's contribution to research about parenting children with complex chronic conditions: an integrative review, 2002 to 2012. *Nurs Outlook.* 2013;61(5):266–290

72. Donoghue EA, Kraft CA, eds. *Managing Chronic Health Needs in Child Care and Schools.* Elk Grove Village, IL: American Academy of Pediatrics; 2010

73. Murdock KK, Robinson EM, Adams SK, Berz J, Rollock MJ. Family-school connections and internalizing problems among children living with asthma in urban, low-income neighborhoods. *J Child Health Care.* 2009;13(3):275–294

74. O'Connor M, Howell-Meurs S, Kvalsvig A, Goldfeld S. Understanding the impact of special health care needs on early school functioning: a conceptual model. *Child Care Health Dev.* 2015;41(1):15–22

75. Forrest CB, Bevans KB, Riley AW, Crespo R, Louis TA. School outcomes of children with special health care needs. *Pediatrics.* 2011;128(2): 303–312

76. Vranda MN, Mothi SN. Psychosocial issues of children infected with HIV/AIDS. *Indian J Psychol Med.* 2013;35(1):19–22

77. Van Cleave J, Davis MM. Bullying and peer victimization among children with special health care needs. *Pediatrics.* 2006;118(4). Available at: www.pediatrics.org/cgi/content/full/118/4/e1212

78. Pinquart M, Teubert D. Academic, physical, and social functioning of children and adolescents with chronic physical illness: a meta-analysis. *J Pediatr Psychol.* 2012;37(4):376–389

79. Leitner Y. The co-occurrence of autism and attention deficit hyperactivity disorder in children - what do we know? *Front Hum Neurosci.* 2014;8:268

80. Liogier d'Ardhuy X, Edgin JO, Bouis C, et al. Assessment of cognitive scales to examine memory, executive function and language in individuals with Down syndrome: implications of a 6-month observational study. *Front Behav Neurosci.* 2015;9:300

81. Schott N, Holfelder B. Relationship between motor skill competency and executive function in children with Down's syndrome. *J Intellect Disabil Res.* 2015;59(9):860–872

82. Hajek CA, Yeates KO, Anderson V, et al. Cognitive outcomes following arterial ischemic stroke in infants and children. *J Child Neurol.* 2014;29(7):887–894

83. Gidman W, Cowley J, Mullarkey C, Gibson L. Barriers to medication adherence in adolescents within a school environment [abstract]. *Arch Dis Child.* 2011;96(suppl 1):A64

84. Berg AT. Epilepsy, cognition, and behavior: the clinical picture. *Epilepsia.* 2011;52(suppl 1):7–12

85. Packer RJ, Gurney JG, Punyko JA, et al. Long-term neurologic and neurosensory sequelae in adult survivors of a childhood brain tumor: childhood cancer survivor study. *J Clin Oncol.* 2003;21(17):3255–3261

86. Reiter-Purtill J, Vannatta K, Gerhardt CA, Correll J, Noll RB. A controlled longitudinal study of the social functioning of children who completed treatment of cancer. *J Pediatr Hematol Oncol.* 2003;25(6):467–473

87. Cottrell D. Prevention and treatment of psychiatric disorders in children with chronic physical illness. *Arch Dis Child.* 2015;100(4):303–304

88. Hocking MC, McCurdy M, Turner E, et al. Social competence in pediatric brain tumor survivors: application of a model from social neuroscience and

developmental psychology. *Pediatr Blood Cancer.* 2015;62(3):375–384

89. Walterfang M, Bonnot O, Mocellin R, Velakoulis D. The neuropsychiatry of inborn errors of metabolism. *J Inherit Metab Dis.* 2013;36(4):687–702

90. Rantanen K, Eriksson K, Nieminen P. Social competence in children with epilepsy--a review. *Epilepsy Behav.* 2012;24(3):295–303

91. Ingerski LM, Modi AC, Hood KK, et al. Health-related quality of life across pediatric chronic conditions. *J Pediatr.* 2010;156(4):639–644

92. Kirk S, Glendinning C. Developing services to support parents caring for a technology-dependent child at home. *Child Care Health Dev.* 2004;30(3):209–218; discussion 219

93. Zeltner NA, Huemer M, Baumgartner MR, Landolt MA. Quality of life, psychological adjustment, and adaptive functioning of patients with intoxication-type inborn errors of metabolism - a systematic review. *Orphanet J Rare Dis.* 2014;9:159

94. Rizou I, De Gucht V, Papavasiliou A, Maes S. Illness perceptions determine psychological distress and quality of life in youngsters with epilepsy. *Epilepsy Behav.* 2015;46:144–150

95. May ME, Kennedy CH. Health and problem behavior among people with intellectual disabilities. *Behav Anal Pract.* 2010;3(2):4–12

96. Sivertsen B, Hysing M, Elgen I, Stormark KM, Lundervold AJ. Chronicity of sleep problems in children with chronic illness: a longitudinal population-based study. *Child Adolesc Psychiatry Ment Health.* 2009;3(1):22

97. Boergers J, Koinis-Mitchell D. Sleep and culture in children with medical conditions. *J Pediatr Psychol.* 2010;35(9):915–926

98. Barnes AJ, Eisenberg ME, Resnick MD. Suicide and self-injury among children and youth with chronic health conditions. *Pediatrics.* 2010;125(5):889–895

99. Alriksson-Schmidt AI, Wallander J, Biasini F. Quality of life and resilience in adolescents with a mobility disability. *J Pediatr Psychol.* 2007;32(3):370–379

100. McLeroy KR, Bibeau D, Steckler A, Glanz K. An ecological perspective on health promotion programs. *Health Educ Q.* 1988;15(4):351–377

101. Barros L, Gaspar de Matos M, Batista-Foguet JM. Chronic diseases, social context and adolescent health. *Revista Brasileira de Terapias Cognitivas.* 2008;4(1):123–141

102. Rutter M. Psychosocial resilience and protective mechanisms. *Am J Orthopsychiatry.* 1987;57(3):316–331

103. Sege R, Bethell C, Linkenbach J, Jones JA, Klika B, Pecora PJ. *Balancing Adverse Childhood Experiences With HOPE: New Insights Into the Role of Positive Experience on Child and Family Development.* Boston, MA: The Medical Foundation; 2017. Available at: www.cssp.org. Accessed November 4, 2017

104. Blackman JA, Conaway MR. Developmental, emotional and behavioral co-morbidities across the chronic health condition spectrum. *J Pediatr Rehabil Med.* 2013;6(2):63–71

105. Hintermair M. Self-esteem and satisfaction with life of deaf and hard-of-hearing people–a resource-oriented approach to identity work. *J Deaf Stud Deaf Educ.* 2008;13(2):278–300

106. Pinquart M. Self-esteem of children and adolescents with chronic illness: a meta-analysis. *Child Care Health Dev.* 2013;39(2):153–161

107. Harter S. *The Construction of the Self: A Developmental Perspective.* New York, NY: The Guilford Press; 1999

108. Hildenbrand AK, Alderfer MA, Deatrick JA, Marsac ML. A mixed methods assessment of coping with pediatric cancer. *J Psychosoc Oncol.* 2014;32(1):37–58

109. Sansom-Daly UM, Wakefield CE. Distress and adjustment among adolescents and young adults with cancer: an empirical and conceptual review. *Transl Pediatr.* 2013;2(4):167–197

110. Hall HR, Neely-Barnes SL, Graff JC, Krcek TE, Roberts RJ, Hankins JS. Parental stress in families of children with a genetic disorder/disability and the resiliency model of family stress, adjustment, and adaptation. *Issues Compr Pediatr Nurs.* 2012;35(1):24–44

111. Bekhet AK, Johnson NL, Zauszniewski JA. Effects on resilience of caregivers of persons with autism spectrum disorder: the role of positive cognitions. *J Am Psychiatr Nurses Assoc.* 2012;18(6):337–344

112. Johnson N, Frenn M, Feetham S, Simpson P. Autism spectrum disorder: parenting stress, family functioning and health-related quality of life. *Fam Syst Health.* 2011;29(3):232–252

113. Idalski Carcone A, Ellis DA, Weisz A, Naar-King S. Social support for diabetes illness management: supporting adolescents and caregivers. *J Dev Behav Pediatr.* 2011;32(8):581–590

114. Ellis DA, King P, Naar-King S, Lam P, Cunningham PB, Secord E. Effects of family treatment on parenting beliefs among caregivers of youth with poorly controlled asthma. *J Dev Behav Pediatr.* 2014;35(8):486–493

115. Wysocki T, Gavin L. Psychometric properties of a new measure of fathers' involvement in the management of pediatric chronic diseases. *J Pediatr Psychol.* 2004;29(3):231–240

116. Morelli SA, Lee IA, Arnn ME, Zaki J. Emotional and instrumental support provision interact to predict well-being. *Emotion.* 2015;15(4):484–493

117. Council on School Health. Role of the school nurse in providing school health services. *Pediatrics.* 2016;137(6):e20160852

118. Perrin JM, Anderson LE, Van Cleave J. The rise in chronic conditions among infants, children, and youth can be met with continued health system innovations. *Health Aff (Millwood).* 2014;33(12):2099–2105

119. Cooley WC, Sagerman PJ; American Academy of Pediatrics; American Academy of Family Physicians; American College of Physicians; Transitions Clinical Report Authoring Group. Supporting the health care transition from adolescence to adulthood in the medical home. *Pediatrics.* 2011;128(1):182–200

120. Lipkin PH, Okamoto J; Council on Children With Disabilities; Council on School Health. The individuals with disabilities education act (IDEA) for

children with special educational needs. *Pediatrics*. 2015;136(6). Available at: www.pediatrics.org/cgi/content/full/136/6/e1650

121. Adams RC, Tapia C; Council on Children With Disabilities. Early intervention, IDEA part C services, and the medical home: collaboration for best practice and best outcomes. *Pediatrics*. 2013;132(4). Available at: www.pediatrics.org/cgi/content/full/132/4/e1073
122. Cartwright JD; American Academy of Pediatrics Council on Children With Disabilities. Provision of educationally related services for children and adolescents with chronic diseases and disabling conditions. *Pediatrics*. 2007;119(6):1218–1223
123. Stroul BA, Blau GM, Friedman RM. *Updating the System of Care Concept and Philosophy*. Washington, DC: National Technical Assistance Center for Children's Mental Health, Georgetown University Center for Child and Human Development; 2010. Available at: https://gucchdtacenter.georgetown.edu/resources/Call%20Docs/2010Calls/SOC_Brief2010.pdf. Accessed March 7, 2018
124. Association of Maternal and Child Health Programs; Lucile Packard Foundation for Children's Health. *Standards for Systems of Care for Children and Youth With Special Health Care Needs Version 2.0*. Washington, DC: Association of Maternal and Child Health Programs;2017 . Available at: http://www.amchp.org/programsandtopics/CYSHCN/Documents/Standards for Systems of Care for Children and Youth with Special Health Care Needs Version 2.0.pdf. Accessed September 15, 2017
125. Texas System of Care. A better future for Texas children: the impact of system of care. Available at: www.txsystemofcare.org/wp-content/uploads/2013/02/TXSOC_outcomes.pdf. Accessed March 7, 2018
126. Turchi RM, Berhane Z, Bethell C, Pomponio A, Antonelli R, Minkovitz CS. Care coordination for CSHCN: associations with family-provider relations and family/child outcomes. *Pediatrics*. 2009;124(suppl 4):S428–S434
127. Little P, Everitt H, Williamson I, et al. Observational study of effect of patient centredness and positive approach on outcomes of general practice consultations. *BMJ*. 2001;323(7318):908–911
128. Thom DH, Kravitz RL, Bell RA, Krupat E, Azari R. Patient trust in the physician: relationship to patient requests. *Fam Pract*. 2002;19(5):476–483
129. Wissow LS, Larson SM, Roter D, et al; SAFE Home Project. Longitudinal care improves disclosure of psychosocial information. *Arch Pediatr Adolesc Med*. 2003;157(5):419–424
130. Wissow L, Anthony B, Brown J, et al. A common factors approach to improving the mental health capacity of pediatric primary care. *Adm Policy Ment Health*. 2008;35(4):305–318
131. Katkin JP, Kressly SJ, Edwards AR, et al; Task Force on Pediatric Practice Change. Guiding principles for team-based pediatric care. *Pediatrics*. 2017;140(2):e20171489
132. Kuhlthau KA, Bloom S, Van Cleave J, et al. Evidence for family-centered care for children with special health care needs: a systematic review. *Acad Pediatr*. 2011;11(2):136–143
133. Cooley WC, McAllister JW, Sherrieb K, Kuhlthau K. Improved outcomes associated with medical home implementation in pediatric primary care. *Pediatrics*. 2009;124(1):358–364
134. Arauz Boudreau AD, Van Cleave JM, Gnanasekaran SK, Kurowski DS, Kuhlthau KA. The medical home: relationships with family functioning for children with and without special health care needs. *Acad Pediatr*. 2012;12(5):391–398
135. Committee on Practice and Ambulatory Medicine; Bright Futures Periodicity Schedule Workgroup. 2017 recommendations for preventive pediatric health care. *Pediatrics*. 2017;139(4):e20170254
136. Myers SM, Johnson CP; American Academy of Pediatrics Council on Children With Disabilities. Management of children with autism spectrum disorders. *Pediatrics*. 2007;120(5):1162–1182
137. Earls MF; Committee on Psychosocial Aspects of Child and Family Health; American Academy of Pediatrics. Incorporating recognition and management of perinatal and postpartum depression into pediatric practice. *Pediatrics*. 2010;126(5):1032–1039
138. O'Connor E, Rossom RC, Henninger M, Groom HC, Burda BU. Primary care screening for and treatment of depression in pregnant and postpartum women: evidence report and systematic review for the US Preventive Services Task Force. *JAMA*. 2016;315(4):388–406
139. Forman-Hoffman V, McClure E, McKeeman J, et al. Screening for major depressive disorder in children and adolescents: a systematic review for the U.S. Preventive Services Task Force. *Ann Intern Med*. 2016;164(5):342–349
140. Fierman AH, Beck AF, Chung EK, et al. Redesigning health care practices to address childhood poverty. *Acad Pediatr*. 2016;16(suppl 3):S136–S146
141. American Academy of Pediatrics. Mental health screening and assessment tools for primary care. In: *Addressing Mental Health Concerns in Primary Care: A Clinician's Toolkit*. Elk Grove Village, IL: American Academy of Pediatrics; 2012
142. Foy JM, Perrin J; American Academy of Pediatrics Task Force on Mental Health. Enhancing pediatric mental health care: strategies for preparing a community. *Pediatrics*. 2010;125(suppl 3):S75–S86
143. Council on Children With Disabilities; Section on Developmental Behavioral Pediatrics; Bright Futures Steering Committee; Medical Home Initiatives for Children With Special Needs Project Advisory Committee. Identifying infants and young children with developmental disorders in the medical home: an algorithm for developmental surveillance and screening [published correction appears in *Pediatrics*. 2006;118(4):1808–1809]. *Pediatrics*. 2006;118(1):405–420
144. Johnson CP, Myers SM; American Academy of Pediatrics Council on Children With Disabilities. Identification and evaluation of children with autism spectrum disorders. *Pediatrics*. 2007;120(5):1183–1215

145. Varni JW, Limbers CA, Burwinkle TM. Impaired health-related quality of life in children and adolescents with chronic conditions: a comparative analysis of 10 disease clusters and 33 disease categories/severities utilizing the PedsQL 4.0 Generic Core Scales. *Health Qual Life Outcomes*. 2007;5:43

146. Modi AC, Pai AL, Hommel KA, et al. Pediatric self-management: a framework for research, practice, and policy. *Pediatrics*. 2012;129(2). Available at: www.pediatrics.org/cgi/content/full/129/2/e473

147. Lozano P, Houtrow A. Supporting self-management in children and adolescents with complex chronic conditions. *Pediatrics*. 2018;141(suppl 3):S233–S241

148. Substance Abuse and Mental Health Services Administration and Health Resources and Services Administration Center for Integrated Health Solutions. *Integrating Behavioral Health and Primary Care for Children and Youth: Concepts and Strategies*. Washington, DC: Substance Abuse and Mental Health Services Administration and Health Resources and Services Administration Center for Integrated Health Solutions; 2013. Available at: https://static1.squarespace.com/static/545cdfcce4b0a64725b9f65a/t/553e7ef4e4b09e24c5c935db/1430159092492/13_June_CIHS_Integrated_Care_System_for_Children_final.pdf. Accessed November 11, 2017

149. Tyler ET, Hulkower RL, Kaminski JW. Behavioral health integration in pediatric primary care: considerations and opportunities for policymakers, planners, and providers. 2017. Available at: https://www.milbank.org/wp-content/uploads/2017/03/MMF_BHI_REPORT_FINAL.pdf. Accessed November 11, 2017

150. Kuehn BM. Pediatrician-psychiatrist partnerships expand access to mental health care. *JAMA*. 2011;306(14):1531–1533

151. Fjorback LO, Arendt M, Ornbøl E, Fink P, Walach H. Mindfulness-based stress reduction and mindfulness-based cognitive therapy: a systematic review of randomized controlled trials. *Acta Psychiatr Scand*. 2011;124(2):102–119

152. Council on Children With Disabilities; Medical Home Implementation Project Advisory Committee. Patient- and family-centered care coordination: a framework for integrating care for children and youth across multiple systems. *Pediatrics*. 2014;133(5). Available at: www.pediatrics.org/cgi/content/full/133/5/e1451

153. Landon BE. Structuring payments to patient-centered medical homes. *JAMA*. 2014;312(16):1633–1634

154. Hochstein M, Sareen H, Olson L, O'Connor K, Inkelas M, Halfon N. *Periodic Survey #46. A Comparison of Barriers to the Provision of Developmental Assessments and Psychosocial Screenings During Pediatric Health Supervision*. Elk Grove Village, IL: American Academy of Pediatrics; 2001. Available at: https://www.aap.org/en-us/professional-resources/Research/Pages/PS46_AcomparisonofBarrierstotheProvisionofDevelopmentalAssessmentsandpsychosocialscreeningsduringpediatrichealthsupervision.aspx. Accessed March 7, 2018

155. Bridgemohan C, Bauer NS, Nielsen BA, et al. A workforce survey on developmental-behavioral pediatrics. *Pediatrics*. 2018;141(3):e20172164

156. Tschudy MM, Toomey SL, Cheng TL. Merging systems: integrating home visitation and the family-centered medical home. *Pediatrics*. 2013;132(suppl 2):S74–S81

157. Jones K, Daley D, Hutchings J, Bywater T, Eames C. Efficacy of the Incredible Years Basic parent training programme as an early intervention for children with conduct problems and ADHD. *Child Care Health Dev*. 2007;33(6):749–756

158. Sanders MR, Turner KM, Markie-Dadds C. The development and dissemination of the Triple P-Positive Parenting Program: a multilevel, evidence-based system of parenting and family support. *Prev Sci*. 2002;3(3):173–189

159. Mazzucchelli TG, Sanders MR. *Stepping Stones Triple P: A Population Approach to the Promotion of Competent Parenting of Children With Disability*. Queensland, Australia: University of Queensland; 2012

160. Tellegen C. *Outcomes From a Randomised Controlled Trial Evaluating a Brief Parenting Intervention With Parents of Children With an Autism Spectrum Disorder*. Queensland, Australia: University of Queensland; 2012

161. Shilling V, Morris C, Thompson-Coon J, Ukoumunne O, Rogers M, Logan S. Peer support for parents of children with chronic disabling conditions: a systematic review of quantitative and qualitative studies. *Dev Med Child Neurol*. 2013;55(7):602–609

Public Policies to Reduce Sugary Drink Consumption in Children and Adolescents

- *Policy Statement*

POLICY STATEMENT Organizational Principles to Guide and Define the Child Health Care System and/or Improve the Health of all Children

American Academy of Pediatrics

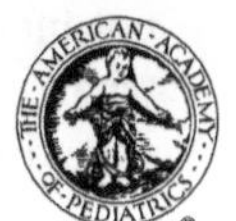

DEDICATED TO THE HEALTH OF ALL CHILDREN™

Public Policies to Reduce Sugary Drink Consumption in Children and Adolescents

Natalie D. Muth, MD, MPH, RDN, FAAP,[a,b] William H. Dietz, MD, PhD, FAAP,[c] Sheela N. Magge, MD, MSCE, FAAP,[d] Rachel K. Johnson, PhD, MPH, RD, FAHA,[e] AMERICAN ACADEMY OF PEDIATRICS, SECTION ON OBESITY, COMMITTEE ON NUTRITION, AMERICAN HEART ASSOCIATION

abstract

Excess consumption of added sugars, especially from sugary drinks, poses a grave health threat to children and adolescents, disproportionately affecting children of minority and low-income communities. Public policies, such as those detailed in this statement, are needed to decrease child and adolescent consumption of added sugars and improve health.

[a]Children's Primary Care Medical Group, Carlsbad, California; [b]Department of Community Health Sciences, Fielding School of Public Health, University of California, Los Angeles, Los Angeles, California; [c]Sumner M. Redstone Global Center for Prevention and Wellness, Milken Institute School of Public Health, The George Washington University, Washington, District of Columbia; [d]Division of Pediatric Endocrinology and Diabetes, School of Medicine, Johns Hopkins University, Baltimore, Maryland; and [e]Department of Nutrition and Food Sciences, University of Vermont, Burlington, Vermont

Dr Muth conceptualized the report; and all authors wrote and revised this statement, are jointly responsible for its content, and approved the final manuscript as submitted.

This document is copyrighted and is property of the American Academy of Pediatrics and its Board of Directors. All authors have filed conflict of interest statements with the American Academy of Pediatrics. Any conflicts have been resolved through a process approved by the Board of Directors. The American Academy of Pediatrics has neither solicited nor accepted any commercial involvement in the development of the content of this publication.

Policy statements from the American Academy of Pediatrics benefit from expertise and resources of liaisons and internal (AAP) and external reviewers. However, policy statements from the American Academy of Pediatrics may not reflect the views of the liaisons or the organizations or government agencies that they represent.

The guidance in this statement does not indicate an exclusive course of treatment or serve as a standard of medical care. Variations, taking into account individual circumstances, may be appropriate.

To cite: Muth ND, Dietz WH, Magge SN, et al. AAP AMERICAN ACADEMY OF PEDIATRICS, AAP SECTION ON OBESITY, AAP COMMITTEE ON NUTRITION, AAP AMERICAN HEART ASSOCIATION. Public Policies to Reduce Sugary Drink Consumption in Children and Adolescents. *Pediatrics.* 2019;143(4):e20190282

STATEMENT OF THE PROBLEM

Excess consumption of added sugars, especially from sugary drinks, contributes to the high prevalence of childhood and adolescent obesity,[1–3] especially among children and adolescents who are socioeconomically vulnerable.[4] It also increases the risk for dental decay,[5] cardiovascular disease,[6] hypertension,[7,8] dyslipidemia,[9,10] insulin resistance,[11,12] type 2 diabetes mellitus,[13] fatty liver disease,[14] and all-cause mortality.[15] The 2015–2020 Dietary Guidelines for Americans recommend that added sugars contribute less than 10% of total calories consumed, yet US children and adolescents report consuming 17% of their calories from added sugars, nearly half of which are from sugary drinks.[16,17] Decreasing sugary drink consumption is of particular importance because sugary drinks are the leading source of added sugars in the US diet,[18] provide little to no nutritional value, are high in energy density, and do little to increase feelings of satiety.[19,20] To protect child and adolescent health, broad implementation of policy strategies to reduce sugary drink consumption in children and adolescents is urgently needed.

DEFINITIONS

- Added sugars: sugars added to foods and beverages during processing or at the table, including, but not limited to, sucrose, glucose, high-fructose corn syrup, and processed, refined fruit juice added to beverages and foods as a sweetener. Added sugars do not include fructose and lactose when present naturally in fruits, vegetables, and unsweetened milk.

- Sugary drink, sugar-sweetened beverage, sugar drink: all terms that refer to beverages containing added sugars. Such beverages include, but are not limited to, regular soda, fruit drinks, sports and energy drinks, and sweetened coffees and teas. In most studies, diet drinks (defined as <40 kcal per 8 oz), 100% fruit juice, and flavored milks are not considered to be sugary drinks.
- Excise tax: tax imposed on product manufacturers or distributors (which often is passed down to retailers and ultimately consumers) that increases prices of products at the shelf or for distributors, in contrast to a sales tax in which the tax is added at the register.

BACKGROUND

In its scientific statement on the role of added sugars and cardiovascular disease risk in children, the American Heart Association (AHA) concluded that strong evidence supports the association of added sugars with increased cardiovascular disease risk through increased caloric intake, increased adiposity, and dyslipidemia.[6] The 2015 Dietary Guidelines Advisory Committee drew similar conclusions and advised that public health strategies are needed to reduce consumption of sugary drinks, the leading source of added sugars in the diets of US children and adolescents.[21] Highlighting the global problem of excess sugar intake and the international urgency to act, the European Society for Paediatric Gastroenterology, Hepatology and Nutrition called on national authorities to adopt policies aimed at reducing free sugar intake in infants, children, and adolescents.[22]

The World Health Organization recommends limiting added sugars intake to less than 10% of total calories, with increased benefits of reducing intake to less than 5% of calories.[23] The 2015–2020 Dietary Guidelines for Americans also recommends that less than 10% of calories consumed be from added sugars.[16] The AHA recommends that children 2 years and older consume ≤25 g (6.25 teaspoons) of added sugars per day and no more than 8 oz of sugary drinks per week. Added sugars should not be in the habitual diet of children younger than 2 years.[6] Despite these recommendations, US children and adolescents report consuming 17% of their calories from added sugars, nearly half of which are from sugary drinks. Those at the highest quintile report consuming 620 kcal daily from added sugars, of which nearly 300 kcal (equivalent to 75 g or 18.75 teaspoons) are from sugary drinks.[17] Many of these high consumers are adolescent boys, who report drinking, on average, 278 kcal of added sugars per day.[24]

Previous American Academy of Pediatrics (AAP) publications have stressed the important role that pediatricians play in the early identification, prevention, and treatment of obesity.[25] The AAP also recommends that pediatric health care providers become more involved in schools, advocating for healthier foods and activities.[26] In its 2017 statement, "Fruit Juice in Infants, Children, and Adolescents: Current Recommendations," the AAP advised pediatricians to support policies that seek to limit the consumption of fruit juice (ie, no juice in children younger than 1 year, no more than 4 oz per day in children ages 1–3 years, no more than 4–6 oz per day in children ages 4–6 years, and no more than 8 oz per day in children ages 7–18 years), including children participating in the Special Supplemental Nutrition Program for Women, Infants, and Children (WIC).[27] In its 2011 statement on sports and energy drinks, the AAP recommended that children and adolescents avoid all energy drinks and the routine consumption of carbohydrate-containing sports drinks and instead drink water.[28]

On the basis of lessons learned from tobacco-control efforts (1 of the greatest public health successes of the United States) the AAP and AHA offer additional policy recommendations targeted at federal, state, and local policy makers to improve child nutrition through reduced sugary drink intake. These policies are best implemented in conjunction with local pediatrician support to respond to the urgent need to reduce added sugars consumption in children and adolescents.

PUBLIC POLICY RECOMMENDATIONS

1. Local, state, and/or national policies intended to reduce consumption of added sugars should include the consideration of approaches that increase the price of sugary drinks, such as an excise tax. Such taxes should be accompanied by education of all stakeholders on the rationale and benefits of the tax before implementation. Tax revenues should be allocated, at least in part, to reducing health and socioeconomic disparities.

Price increases are associated with a decrease in consumption. For example, as tobacco prices increased, cigarette consumption dropped precipitously, particularly among youth and people of lower socioeconomic status.[29] Strong evidence indicates that alcohol excise taxes reduce excessive alcohol consumption and its associated harmful consequences, such as motor vehicle collisions.[30] In the case of sugary drinks, a systematic review revealed that each 10% increase in price, such as a tax, reduced sugary drink consumption by 7%.[31] The World Health Organization suggests that a higher tax of 20% would most likely have the greatest effect on reducing consumption.[32] The Childhood Obesity Intervention Cost-Effectiveness Study (CHOICES), a modeling study aimed at identifying the most cost-effective interventions to reduce childhood obesity, found implementation of a sugary drink tax to be the most cost-effective strategy to address childhood obesity, leading to prevention of 575 000 cases of childhood obesity and a health care savings of $30.78 per dollar spent over 10 years.[33] Such taxes are most effective when accompanied by a broad education campaign to help stakeholders understand the risks of sugary drink consumption and the rationale and benefits of the tax.[34]

Several countries have implemented these types of taxes. In 2014, Chile raised the tax on drinks containing more than 6.25 g of added sugars per 100 mL from 13% to 18% and lowered the tax on drinks with under 6.25 g of added sugars per 100 mL from 13% to 10%. Researchers found that sugary drink purchases decreased 21% in the year after the tax took effect.[35] The most rigorously evaluated sugary drink tax is Mexico's 2014 implementation of a nationwide 10% excise tax (1 peso per liter) on sugary drinks. The successful passage and implementation of the tax resulted from a broad education campaign organized by tax proponents that included coalition building, lobbying, media advocacy, public demonstrations, multiple forums, drafting of a legislative proposal, and public opinion polling.[36] As a result of the tax, the average volume of taxed beverages purchased was 5.5% lower in 2014 than expected without the tax, with a 9% decrease in sales to lower-income households.[37] A follow-up study of the second year of the tax (2015) revealed that consumption decreased 9.7% from baseline. Thus, over the 2 years after the tax was implemented, the net decrease in sugary drinks was 7.6%. Purchases of untaxed beverages, such as water, increased 2.1%.[38] This tax alone is projected to prevent nearly 200 000 cases of obesity and save $980 million in direct health care costs from 2013 to 2022, with the majority of benefits afforded to young adults.[39]

Berkeley, California, was the first US city to levy a relatively large tax ($0.01 per oz) on sugary drinks, effective March 2015. A study of the impact of the tax (comparing pre- and 1-year posttax beverage prices at 26 Berkeley stores; point-of-sale scanner data on 15.5 million checkouts for beverage prices, sales, and store revenue for 2 supermarket chains in 3 Berkeley and 6 nearby control non-Berkeley large supermarkets; and a representative telephone survey of 957 adult Berkeley residents) revealed that approximately 67% of the tax was passed on to consumers. Sales of sugary drinks fell 9.6%, whereas sales of untaxed beverages, such as water and milk, increased 3.5%. There was no increase in grocery bills for consumers or loss of revenue or decrease in beverage sales for stores.[40] Other studies of the Berkeley tax have found similar results,[41,42] although 1 study[43] found that the tax had minimal impact. The authors of that study cited a low pass-through rate and, thus, limited sugary drink price increase to the consumer. However, results may have been skewed because in the evaluation, national chains that were covered by the law in the first year were combined with small stores that were only covered by the law in the second year.

Other US locales, including San Francisco, Oakland, and Albany, California; Philadelphia, Pennsylvania; Boulder, Colorado; and Seattle, Washington, have implemented an excise tax on sugary drinks. Cook County, Illinois (Chicago), which did not have a high degree of buy-in from stakeholders before implementation and was associated with substantial industry resistance, briefly implemented a sales tax on sugary drinks but then repealed it.[44] Some states have passed preemption laws that prohibit local municipalities from implementing a tax on sugary drinks. In June 2018, California lawmakers passed a law prohibiting any new local sugary drink taxes until 2031 in response to threats from the American Beverage Association, which funded a likely-to-pass ballot measure that would require a two-thirds majority of voters to approve any local tax increase. In exchange, the American Beverage Association dropped the ballot measure. These laws stifle local innovation to meet the health and fiscal needs of constituents and are counter to a 2011 report from the Institute of Medicine (now the National Academy of Medicine), in which federal and state legislators were urged to "avoid framing preemptive legislation in a way that hinders public action."[45]

Although people of lower socioeconomic status bear a greater burden from taxation, they also disproportionately benefit from the health and economic benefits from prevention of cardiovascular disease and type 2 diabetes mellitus.[39] Moreover, if the tax revenue is allocated to decrease health disparities or provide other services that promote health in these specific groups, the tax ultimately may be progressive.[46,47] For example, the Philadelphia tax has been used to fund prekindergarten programs that are of direct benefit to underserved communities.

Given the success of tobacco and alcohol taxes in reducing adolescent use and consumption of these products, policy makers should consider enacting policies that raise the price of sugary drinks. A portion of tax revenues could be used to subsidize healthier options, such as water, milk, fruits, and vegetables, and/or child health or obesity and diabetes prevention programs.

2. The federal and state governments should support efforts to decrease sugary drink marketing to children and adolescents.

Similar to tobacco companies, sugary drink manufacturers aim to appeal to children and adolescents by associating their product with celebrity, glamour, and coolness. Despite the existence of the Children's Food and Beverage Advertising Initiative, an industry-initiated, self-regulatory body designed to limit marketing of unhealthful food and beverage products to children younger than 12 years, children and adolescents are frequently exposed to sugary drink advertisements. In 2009, carbonated beverage companies reported $395 million in youth-directed expenditures, approximately 97% of which were directed at teenagers.[48] According to recent Nielsen data reported by the University of Connecticut Rudd Center, children's exposure to advertisements for carbonated beverages increased 19% and their exposure to advertisements for juice, fruit drinks, and sports drinks increased 38% from 2015 to 2016. Overall, advertisements for sugary drinks have increased substantially since 2007.[49] Beverages are more heavily promoted to adolescents than to younger children,[48] who may only see 1 beverage advertisement per day on children's programs.[50] An online survey of US adolescents ages 12 to 17 years (n = 847) revealed that almost half of the adolescents reported daily sugary drink advertising exposure.[51] Among survey respondents, 14- to 15-year-old, African American male adolescents whose parents had a high school education or less (factors associated with increased sugary drink consumption[52]) reported the highest exposure to advertising of soda, fruit drinks, sports drinks, and energy drinks.[51] Because children tend to consume the beverages promoted on television and because African American children are exposed to the most sugary drink advertisements, the disparity in sugary drink advertising exposure may contribute to the disproportionate rates of obesity among African American children.

Stronger measures are needed to curtail advertising of sugary drinks to children and adolescents on television, on the Internet, and in places frequented by children, such as movie theaters, concerts, and sporting events. Although companies are protected by commercial free speech rights and may not be mandated to stop advertising to children and adolescents, other methods to reduce advertising of unhealthful food and beverages to children and adolescents could be used. For example, businesses are permitted to deduct costs of advertising as a business expense. Modeling by the CHOICES study suggests that eliminating the advertising subsidy for nutritionally poor foods and beverages marketed to children would prevent approximately 129 000 cases of obesity over a decade at a cost $0.66 for each unit of BMI reduced. The additional benefit of this approach is that it would generate approximately $80 million annually in tax revenue.[33] The US Congress should consider this and other allowable measures to reduce advertising of sugary drinks to children and adolescents.

State governments should implement the US Department of Agriculture's (USDA) local school wellness policy final rule under the Healthy, Hunger-Free Kids Act of 2010, which requires that only foods and beverages meeting the Smart Snacks standards may be marketed on school campuses during the school day.[53] State governments should also consider additional strategies to reduce sugary drink marketing and advertising to children and adolescents through measures such as prohibitions on coupons, sales, and advertising in and around schools and on school buses as well as sugary drink–branded sponsorship of youth sporting events.

3. Federal nutrition assistance programs should aim to ensure access to healthful food and beverages and discourage consumption of sugary drinks.

Several federal nutrition programs direct taxpayer dollars toward reducing food insecurity and supporting healthful nutrition for children and families of low income.

WIC

WIC provided nutritious foods to nearly 1.9 million infants and 4 million children ages 1 to 5 years in fiscal year 2016. WIC provides a supplemental package of healthful foods and beverages and offers a robust nutrition education program. Although 100% juice is allowed, sugary drinks are not included in the WIC package.

Child and Adult Food Care Program

More than 3 million children are served by the Child and Adult Care Food Program (CACFP) (a program administered by the USDA), which provides cash assistance to states to provide healthful food to children and adults in child and adult care institutions. Sugary drinks are noncreditable items in the CACFP (ie, they may be served but do not count toward meeting the meal pattern requirements for a meal to be reimbursed). Flavored milks are not creditable for children ages 2 to 5 years but are creditable for children and adults older than 6 years if they contain no more than 22 g of total sugars per 8 oz. The CACFP best practices advise early care and education centers to avoid serving noncreditable sugary drinks in their facilities.[54] However, few states currently have any provisions prohibiting access to sugary drinks in these settings. Because most early care and education centers are regulated at the state, rather than federal, level, states should adopt policies that restrict early care and education centers from serving children sugary drinks.

School Breakfast Program, School Lunch Program, and Competitive Foods

The Healthy, Hunger-Free Kids Act of 2010 required the USDA to establish national nutrition standards for all foods sold in schools at any time, including foods sold for school breakfast and school lunch and competitive foods sold outside meal programs (Smart Snacks standards). The adopted standards do not allow sugary drinks in elementary or middle school and only allow drinks other than 100% fruit juice, milk, or approved milk alternatives if they contain less than 40 kcal per 8 oz or less than 60 kcal per 12 oz for high schools. A 2018 final rule allows states flexibility to include flavored low-fat milk, in addition to flavored nonfat milk, as long as school meals stay within calorie requirements.[55] The CHOICES modeling study predicts that nutrition standards for all school meals will likely prevent 1.8 million cases of childhood obesity from 2015 to 2025 and save $0.42 per dollar spent and that including nutrition standards for all competitive foods and beverages will prevent 345 000 cases of childhood obesity and save $4.56 per dollar spent.[33] Additional evidence indicates that adolescents drink fewer sugary drinks when standards such as these are implemented.[56–59] Ultimately, the Healthy, Hunger-Free Kids Act and Smart Snacks standards improved children's nutrition and reduced intake of added sugars,[60–62] although additional technical assistance and supports are needed to increase compliance.[61,63,64] These policies should be implemented, enforced, and enhanced to further promote a healthy school environment. The policies also should be accompanied by a robust nutrition education program to help children and adolescents understand how to make healthy food and beverage choices, including information on how to identify and respond to marketing messages and how to read nutrition labels.

Supplemental Nutrition Assistance Program

The Supplemental Nutrition Assistance Program (SNAP), a vital safety net program that provides food for 45 million families, including 23 million children, is the nation's largest child nutrition program, serving approximately 1 in 4 US children.[65] Although SNAP has proven successful at addressing undernutrition and food insecurity, it is the only government feeding program that does not have nutrition standards to address diet quality. In the 2015 Dietary Guidelines Advisory Committee report, it was advised that changes be made to align WIC and SNAP with the Dietary Guidelines for Americans, including encouraging the purchase of healthful foods and discouraging the purchase and consumption of sugary drinks.[21] Additionally, the Dietary Guidelines Advisory Committee suggested that efforts are necessary to reduce access to sugary drinks in community settings and that they should be seamlessly integrated with food assistance programs, including SNAP.[21] Each day, SNAP dollars pay for 20 million servings of sugary drinks at an annual cost of $4 billion.[66] If sugary drinks were not included as a SNAP benefit, estimates suggest that 510 000 type 2 diabetes mellitus person-years and 52 000 deaths could be averted, with a savings of $2900 per quality-adjusted life-years saved.[67] Quality-adjusted life-years is an economic measure of the state of health of a person that combines quality of life and longevity.

The public and SNAP participants support both improved access to healthful foods within SNAP and removal of SNAP benefits for sugary drinks.[68,69] States cannot make changes to SNAP benefits without a waiver from the USDA. Nonetheless, the USDA has repeatedly rejected states' requests for waivers and pilot studies that would eliminate sugary drinks from SNAP. The USDA has cited concerns related to retailer implementation as well as the need for a robust evaluation framework. Moreover, the USDA and antihunger organizations have raised many concerns about the consequences of such a restriction, leading to a clear need to evaluate such a policy and gain public support before its implementation.[70] There is concern that a restriction might increase stigma and embarrassment and subsequently deter SNAP participation if a SNAP participant attempts to purchase a sugary drink with SNAP benefits and is denied at the counter. A robust information campaign detailing the benefits of change might counter, but would not eliminate, this risk, and policies should be sensitive to this issue. Some have also questioned the restriction of sugary drinks from SNAP whereas other highly processed, nonnutritious foods containing substantial amounts of added sugars (eg, snack cakes, cookies, etc) are still allowed. There is also concern that any change to SNAP may prompt cuts to the food benefits that participants receive.[71] Because the current SNAP benefit amounts to an average of $1.40 per person per meal, it is imperative that SNAP benefits and eligibility not only remain intact but also increase to provide families with the resources they need to obtain an adequate, healthful diet throughout the month.

The Healthy Incentives Pilot offers a model to evaluate the effects of making a change to SNAP. In 2008, Congress directed $20 million to fund a pilot project to subsidize fruit and vegetable purchases within SNAP. The Healthy Incentives Pilot demonstrated that providing a 30-cent incentive for every SNAP dollar spent on fruits and vegetables increased purchases of fruits and vegetables by 26%.[72] A randomized controlled trial conducted in Minnesota revealed that a food benefit program that paired incentives to eat healthful foods, such as fruits and vegetables, with restrictions on sweet baked goods, candies, and sugary drinks decreased caloric intake and improved the nutritional quality of participants' diets, compared with no change, incentive only, or restriction only.[73] A survey of SNAP participants and SNAP-eligible nonparticipants revealed support for policies that provided an incentive to purchase healthful foods and imposed restrictions on sugary drinks.[74] Congress could authorize the USDA to conduct a study to evaluate a fruit and vegetable incentive combined with restriction of sugary drinks. Such a study may help clarify the effects on consumer purchasing and SNAP participant perspectives, including real or perceived stigma, dietary quality, and retailer implementation. In addition, SNAP Education, the nutrition education component of the program, provides a mechanism to develop and test policy, system, and environmental changes to promote fruit and vegetable consumption and reduce sugary drink intake.[75] SNAP Education should be expanded and further developed so as to further emphasize the health benefits of fruits and vegetables and the health risks of sugary drinks and added sugars. Retailer incentives and new retail stocking standards could be used to reduce purchase of sugary drinks and increase purchase of healthier foods. It is critical that any change to SNAP preserves and enhances access to healthful foods and the integrity of this vital nutrition program with no decrease in the benefits to participants.

4. Children, adolescents, and their families should have ready access to credible nutrition information, including on nutrition labels, restaurant menus, and advertisements.

Whether nutrition labels help improve health is unclear.[76] However, just as consumers are advised of the health risks of nicotine and carcinogens when purchasing tobacco products, they also should be advised of nutritional risks when making purchases of sugary drinks, giving them the opportunity to use this information to make healthier choices. Encouraging policy changes include implementation of the regulations that require added sugars content to be included on the nutrition facts panel and on restaurant menus. Consumers support such measures. In 1 survey, 84% of adults believed "the government should require nutrition information labels on all packaged food sold in grocery stores," and 64% wanted similar requirements for restaurants.[77] Consumer education on how to read and use nutrition labels may help increase label effectiveness in changing behavior. For example, a study of 34 adolescents revealed that students significantly increased their ability to read and understand a nutrition label after a brief school-based educational intervention.[78] Additionally, a systematic review of 16 studies found that increased nutrition knowledge and education was associated with nutrition label use in college students.[79]

Front-of-package labels, including warning labels of the health harms of consumption of added sugars, could serve to further empower families to make healthier choices. For example, a randomized trial of 2000 adolescents revealed that those who were exposed to a health warning label chose fewer sugary drinks and believed that sugary drinks were less likely to help them lead a healthy life.[80] When parents were exposed to a warning label, they chose significantly fewer sugary drinks, believed that sugary drinks were less healthful for their children, and were less likely to intend to purchase sugary drinks.[81] The constitutionality of warning labels has been challenged by industry.[82] The controversy was prompted by a 2015 San Francisco ordinance that required advertisements for sugary drinks to include a disclaimer that says "WARNING: Drinking beverages with added sugar(s) contributes to obesity, type 2 diabetes, and tooth decay." In 2019, the Ninth Circuit Court of Appeals blocked the law, ruling that it "unduly burdens and chills protected commercial speech" and is not purely factual because the US Food and Drug Administration has stated that added sugars are "generally recognized as safe" and "can be part of a healthy dietary pattern when not consumed in excess amounts."[83]

5. Policies that make healthy beverages the default should be widely adopted and followed.

Policies and incentives should support decreased consumption of sugary drinks through environmental changes, such as promoting healthier options (like water and milk) and decreasing access to and portion sizes of sugary drinks in all locations where children and adolescents are present. For example, current standard beverage policy for federal agencies requires that 50% of beverages contain ≤40 kcal per 8 oz except for 100% juice or unsweetened fat-free or 1% milk.[84] For all vending machines contracted by New York City agencies, policy prohibits advertisements, limits high-calorie beverages to 12 oz and a maximum of 2 slots in the vending machine, requires the provision of water in 2 slots at eye level, and requires that all other beverages other than milk contain ≤25 kcal per 8 oz.[85] Several cities, states, and state parks have implemented food service guidelines, including the provision of healthful beverages.[86–88] In August 2018, California became the first state to pass a law requiring restaurants to serve water or milk as the default beverage in kids' meals. Hawaii, Vermont, Connecticut, Rhode Island, and New York City are considering similar bills, and several cities in California; Baltimore, Maryland; Louisville, Kentucky; and Lafayette, Colorado have already passed "healthy-by-default" city ordinances.[89] Some restaurants have voluntarily changed the default beverage choice on the children's menu from soda and other sugary drinks to water or milk, although more than 75% of the 50 largest chain restaurants have not.[89] A few restaurants have gone further and eliminated sugary drinks from children's menus altogether.[90] Although data on the effects of these types of changes are limited, some evidence suggests when the healthier choice is the easier or default choice, people are more likely to make it.[91–93]

6. Hospitals should serve as a model and implement policies to limit or disincentivize purchase of sugary drinks.

One of the less recognized contributors to the reduction in cigarette smoking is the role that physicians and hospitals played in changing social norms regarding tobacco use. Before the 1950s, physicians and their choice of cigarette brands featured prominently in cigarette advertising.[94] In the 1960s, hospital grand rounds were conducted in smoke-filled rooms, and doctors who smoked were less likely to counsel regarding the adverse health effects of smoking. However, as awareness of the medical consequences of tobacco use grew, physicians stopped smoking, and hospitals eliminated cigarette vending machines and the sale of cigarettes in hospital gift shops.[94–96] Although tobacco use remains a pressing threat to public health, the ongoing obesity epidemic and high consumption of added sugars has led to epidemics of type 2 diabetes mellitus and metabolic disease that require increased action by physicians and other health care providers, hospitals, and many other members of civil society.[6,97,98]

As with the ban on tobacco, leadership by hospitals and health plans to eliminate the sale of sugary drinks can improve the health of their employees, increase public awareness about the contribution of sugary drinks to obesity, and thereby change social norms regarding sugary drinks. For example, the Boston Public Health Commission engaged with 10 medical centers in Boston to reduce sugary drink consumption using a variety of strategies. Massachusetts General Hospital labeled drinks with red, yellow, or green stickers to indicate their calorie content and made the high-calorie drinks less accessible. Over 2 years, consumption of healthier products increased, consumption of high-calorie beverages decreased, and there was a modest increase in revenue from beverage sales.[99] A second hospital found that increased prices of high-calorie beverages reduced their sales.[100] Many hospitals have stopped selling sugary drinks entirely. In 2010, the Cleveland Clinic eliminated the sale of sugary drinks, extending previous efforts to improve community health through hospital practices by banning smoking on campus and eliminating the use of trans fats.[101] In 2011, Nationwide Children's Hospital eliminated all sugary drinks in all food establishments within the hospital, with no loss of revenue.[102] In 2018, Geisinger eliminated sales of sugary drinks from all campuses.[103] More than 30 health systems comprising more than 250 hospitals are participating in the Healthier Hospital Initiative, which includes a pledge to increase healthful beverages to 80% of total beverage purchases in patient care, retail, vending, and catering.[104] In 2017, the American Medical Association passed a resolution that "encourages hospitals and medical facilities to offer healthier beverages, such as water, unflavored milk, coffee, and unsweetened tea, for purchase in place of SSBs [sugar-sweetened beverages]."[97] A useful guide for the development of healthful beverage programs has been published by the Public Health Law Center and the Centers for Disease Control and Prevention.[105,106]

Decisions to reduce promotion and sale of sugary drinks in hospitals may appear to be a distraction from hospitals' core efforts to provide medical care or appear to be ineffective given that most sugary drink consumption does not occur in hospitals. The same arguments could have been made about hospitals' efforts to reduce the promotion and sale of tobacco. A well-publicized effort to reduce sugary drink consumption among hospital patients, visitors, and staff could help build public awareness of the links between sugary drink consumption, obesity, and diabetes. These efforts could also signal to employers and leaders in other settings that reducing sugary drink sales and promotion in worksites and public spaces is an important and feasible approach to improving population health.

CONCLUSIONS

Consumption of added sugars, particularly those in sugary drinks, pose a significant health risk to children and adolescents. Pediatricians are encouraged to routinely counsel children and families to decrease sugary drink consumption and increase water consumption. Pediatricians can also advocate for policy change through school boards, school health councils, hospital and medical group boards and committees, outreach to elected representatives, and public comment opportunities. Policy targets, such as those discussed in this report and summarized below, are needed to reduce sugary drink consumption in children and adolescents and subsequently improve child health.

1. Local, state, and/or national policies to reduce added sugars consumption should include policies that raise the price of sugary drinks, such as an excise tax. Such taxes should be accompanied by an education campaign on the risks of sugary drinks and on the rationale and benefits of the tax and should be supported by stakeholders. Tax revenues should be allocated, at least in part, to reducing health and socioeconomic disparities. Metrics should be established to evaluate the impact of such a tax.
2. The federal and state governments should support efforts to decrease sugary drink marketing to children and adolescents.
3. Federal nutrition assistance programs should ensure access to healthful foods and beverages and discourage consumption of sugary drinks.
4. Children, adolescents, and their families should have ready access to credible nutrition information, including on the nutrition facts panel, restaurant menus, and advertisements.
5. Policies that make healthful beverages the default choice should be widely adopted and followed.
6. Hospitals should serve as a model and implement policies to limit or disincentivize the purchase of sugary drinks.

Although the strength and availability of evidence supporting the policy recommendations addressed in this report vary and although there may be significant barriers or considerations in implementation of some or all of these recommendations, pediatricians may tailor their advocacy efforts to approaches that are most likely to lead to decreased access to and consumption of sugary drinks in the children and families they serve, whether on a local, state, or federal level.

LEAD AUTHORS

Natalie D. Muth, MD, MPH, RDN, FAAP
William H. Dietz, MD, PhD, FAAP
Sheela N. Magge, MD, MSCE, FAAP
Rachel K. Johnson, PhD, MPH, RD, FAHA

AAP SECTION ON OBESITY EXECUTIVE COMMITTEE, 2017–2018

Christopher F. Bolling, MD, FAAP, Chairperson
Sarah C. Armstrong, MD, FAAP
Matthew Allen Haemer, MD, MPH, FAAP
Natalie D. Muth, MD, MPH, RDN, FAAP
John Conrad Rausch, MD, MPH, FAAP
Victoria Weeks Rogers, MD, FAAP

LIAISONS

Marc Michalsky, MD, FACS, FAAP – *American Academy of Pediatrics Section on Surgery*

CONSULTANT

Stephanie Walsh, MD, FAAP

STAFF

Mala Thapar, MPH

AAP COMMITTEE ON NUTRITION, 2017–2018

Steven A. Abrams, MD, FAAP, Chairperson
Jae Hong Kim, MD, PhD, FAAP
Sarah Jane Schwarzenberg, MD, FAAP
George Joseph Fuchs III, MD, FAAP
Sheela N. Magge, MD, MSCE, FAAP
C. Wesley Lindsey, MD, FAAP
Ellen S. Rome, MD, MPH, FAAP

LIAISONS

Cria G. Perrine, PhD – *Centers for Disease Control and Prevention*
Andrea Lotze, MD, FAAP – *US Food and Drug Administration*
Janet M. de Jesus, MS, RD – *National Institutes of Health*
Valery Soto, MS, RD, LD – *US Department of Agriculture*

STAFF

Debra L. Burrowes, MHA
Tamar Haro

AHA STAFF

Laurie Whitsel, PhD, FAHA

ABBREVIATIONS

AAP: American Academy of Pediatrics
AHA: American Heart Association
CACFP: Child and Adult Care Food Program
CHOICES: Childhood Obesity Intervention Cost-Effectiveness Study
SNAP: Supplemental Nutrition Assistance Program
USDA: US Department of Agriculture
WIC: Special Supplemental Nutrition Program for Women, Infants, and Children

All policy statements from the American Academy of Pediatrics automatically expire 5 years after publication unless reaffirmed, revised, or retired at or before that time.

DOI: https://doi.org/10.1542/peds.2019-0282

Address correspondence to Natalie D. Muth, MD, MPH, RDN, FAAP. E-mail: nmuth@rchsd.org

PEDIATRICS (ISSN Numbers: Print, 0031-4005; Online, 1098-4275).

Copyright © 2019 by the American Academy of Pediatrics

FINANCIAL DISCLOSURE: The authors have indicated they have no financial relationships relevant to this article to disclose.

FUNDING: No external funding.

POTENTIAL CONFLICT OF INTEREST: The authors have indicated they have no potential conflicts of interest to disclose.

REFERENCES

1. de Ruyter JC, Olthof MR, Seidell JC, Katan MB. A trial of sugar-free or sugar-sweetened beverages and body weight in children. *N Engl J Med*. 2012; 367(15):1397–1406
2. Ebbeling CB, Feldman HA, Chomitz VR, et al. A randomized trial of sugar-sweetened beverages and adolescent body weight. *N Engl J Med*. 2012; 367(15):1407–1416
3. Luger M, Lafontan M, Bes-Rastrollo M, Winzer E, Yumuk V, Farpour-Lambert N. Sugar-sweetened beverages and weight gain in children and adults: a systematic review from 2013 to 2015 and a comparison with previous studies. *Obes Facts*. 2017;10(6): 674–693
4. Ogden CL, Carroll MD, Lawman HG, et al. Trends in obesity prevalence among children and adolescents in the United States, 1988-1994 through 2013-2014. *JAMA*. 2016;315(21): 2292–2299
5. Moynihan P, Petersen PE. Diet, nutrition and the prevention of dental diseases. *Public Health Nutr*. 2004;7 (1A):201–226
6. Vos MB, Kaar JL, Welsh JA, et al; American Heart Association Nutrition Committee of the Council on Lifestyle and Cardiometabolic Health; Council on Clinical Cardiology; Council on Cardiovascular Disease in the Young; Council on Cardiovascular and Stroke Nursing; Council on Epidemiology and Prevention; Council on Functional Genomics and Translational Biology; Council on Hypertension. Added sugars and cardiovascular disease risk in children: a scientific statement from the American Heart Association. *Circulation*. 2017;135(19):e1017–e1034
7. Chen L, Caballero B, Mitchell DC, et al. Reducing consumption of sugar-sweetened beverages is associated with reduced blood pressure: a prospective study among United States adults [published correction appears in *Circulation*. 2010;122(4): e408]. *Circulation*. 2010;121(22): 2398–2406
8. Perez-Pozo SE, Schold J, Nakagawa T, Sánchez-Lozada LG, Johnson RJ, Lillo JL. Excessive fructose intake induces the features of metabolic syndrome in healthy adult men: role of uric acid in the hypertensive response. *Int J Obes (Lond)*. 2010;34(3):454–461
9. Lee AK, Binongo JN, Chowdhury R, et al. Consumption of less than 10% of total energy from added sugars is associated with increasing HDL in females during adolescence: a longitudinal analysis. *J Am Heart Assoc*. 2014;3(1):e000615
10. Lustig RH, Mulligan K, Noworolski SM, et al. Isocaloric fructose restriction and metabolic improvement in children with obesity and metabolic syndrome. *Obesity (Silver Spring)*. 2016;24(2): 453–460
11. Wang JW, Mark S, Henderson M, et al. Adiposity and glucose intolerance exacerbate components of metabolic syndrome in children consuming sugar-sweetened beverages: QUALITY cohort study. *Pediatr Obes*. 2013;8(4):284–293
12. Welsh JA, Sharma A, Cunningham SA, Vos MB. Consumption of added sugars and indicators of cardiovascular disease risk among US adolescents. *Circulation*. 2011;123(3):249–257
13. Malik VS, Popkin BM, Bray GA, Després JP, Willett WC, Hu FB. Sugar-sweetened beverages and risk of metabolic syndrome and type 2 diabetes: a meta-analysis. *Diabetes Care*. 2010;33(11): 2477–2483
14. O'Sullivan TA, Oddy WH, Bremner AP, et al. Lower fructose intake may help protect against development of nonalcoholic fatty liver in adolescents with obesity. *J Pediatr Gastroenterol Nutr*. 2014;58(5):624–631
15. Shah NS, Leonard D, Finley CE, et al. Dietary patterns and long-term survival: a retrospective study of healthy primary care patients. *Am J Med*. 2018; 131(1):48–55
16. US Department of Health and Human Services; US Department of Agriculture. 2015–2020 dietary guidelines for Americans. 2015. Available at: http://health.gov/dietaryguidelines/2015/guidelines/. Accessed September 17, 2017
17. Powell ES, Smith-Taillie LP, Popkin BM. Added sugars intake across the distribution of US children and adult consumers: 1977-2012. *J Acad Nutr Diet*. 2016;116(10):1543–1550.e1
18. Drewnowski A, Rehm CD. Consumption of added sugars among US children and adults by food purchase location and food source. *Am J Clin Nutr*. 2014; 100(3):901–907
19. Pan A, Hu FB. Effects of carbohydrates on satiety: differences between liquid and solid food. *Curr Opin Clin Nutr Metab Care*. 2011;14(4):385–390
20. Shearrer GE, O'Reilly GA, Belcher BR, et al. The impact of sugar sweetened beverage intake on hunger and satiety in minority adolescents [published correction appears in *Appetite*. 2016; 100:272]. *Appetite*. 2016;97:43–48
21. Dietary Guidelines Advisory Committee. *Scientific Report of the 2015 Dietary Guidelines Advisory Committee: Advisory Report to the Secretary of Health and Human Services and the Secretary of Agriculture*. Washington, DC: US Department of Agriculture, Agricultural Research Service; 2015
22. Fidler Mis N, Braegger C, Bronsky J, et al; ESPGHAN Committee on Nutrition. Sugar in infants, children and adolescents: a position paper of the European Society for Paediatric Gastroenterology, Hepatology and Nutrition Committee on Nutrition. *J Pediatr Gastroenterol Nutr*. 2017; 65(6):681–696
23. World Health Organization. Sugar intake for adults and children. 2015. Available at: www.who.int/nutrition/publications/guidelines/sugars_intake/en/. Accessed September 17, 2017
24. Kit BK, Fakhouri TH, Park S, Nielsen SJ, Ogden CL. Trends in sugar-sweetened beverage consumption among youth and adults in the United States: 1999-

2010. *Am J Clin Nutr.* 2013;98(1): 180–188

25. Daniels SR, Hassink SG; Committee on Nutrition. The role of the pediatrician in primary prevention of obesity. *Pediatrics.* 2015;136(1). Available at: www.pediatrics.org/cgi/content/full/136/1/e275
26. Council on School Health; Committee on Nutrition. Snacks, sweetened beverages, added sugars, and schools. *Pediatrics.* 2015;135(3):575–583
27. Heyman MB, Abrams SA; Section on Gastroenterology, Hepatology, and Nutrition; Committee on Nutrition. Fruit juice in infants, children, and adolescents: current recommendations. *Pediatrics.* 2017;139(6):e20170967
28. Committee on Nutrition; Council on Sports Medicine and Fitness. Sports drinks and energy drinks for children and adolescents: are they appropriate? *Pediatrics.* 2011;127(6):1182–1189
29. Bader P, Boisclair D, Ferrence R. Effects of tobacco taxation and pricing on smoking behavior in high risk populations: a knowledge synthesis. *Int J Environ Res Public Health.* 2011;8(11): 4118–4139
30. Elder RW, Lawrence B, Ferguson A, et al; Task Force on Community Preventive Services. The effectiveness of tax policy interventions for reducing excessive alcohol consumption and related harms. *Am J Prev Med.* 2010;38(2): 217–229
31. Afshin A, Peñalvo JL, Del Gobbo L, et al. The prospective impact of food pricing on improving dietary consumption: a systematic review and meta-analysis. *PLoS One.* 2017;12(3):e0172277
32. World Health Organization. Fiscal policies for diet and the prevention of noncommunicable diseases. 2016. Available at: www.who.int/dietphysicalactivity/publications/fiscal-policies-diet-prevention/en/. Accessed October 10, 2017
33. Gortmaker SL, Wang YC, Long MW, et al. Three interventions that reduce childhood obesity are projected to save more than they cost to implement. *Health Aff (Millwood).* 2015;34(11): 1932–1939
34. Action for Healthy Food. *A Roadmap for Successful Sugary Drink Tax Campaigns.* Seattle WA: Action for Healthy Food; 2015
35. Nakamura R, Mirelman AJ, Cuadrado C, Silva-Illanes N, Dunstan J, Suhrcke M. Evaluating the 2014 sugar-sweetened beverage tax in Chile: an observational study in urban areas. *PLoS Med.* 2018; 15(7):e1002596
36. Donaldson E. *Advocating for Sugar-Sweetened Beverage Taxation: A Case Study of Mexico.* Baltimore, MD: Johns Hopkins Bloomberg School of Public Health; 2015
37. Colchero MA, Popkin BM, Rivera JA, Ng SW. Beverage purchases from stores in Mexico under the excise tax on sugar sweetened beverages: observational study. *BMJ.* 2016;352:h6704
38. Colchero MA, Rivera-Dommarco J, Popkin BM, Ng SW. In Mexico, evidence of sustained consumer response two years after implementing a sugar-sweetened beverage tax. *Health Aff (Millwood).* 2017;36(3):564–571
39. Sánchez-Romero LM, Penko J, Coxson PG, et al. Projected impact of Mexico's sugar-sweetened beverage tax policy on diabetes and cardiovascular disease: a modeling study. *PLoS Med.* 2016; 13(11):e1002158
40. Silver LD, Ng SW, Ryan-Ibarra S, et al. Changes in prices, sales, consumer spending, and beverage consumption one year after a tax on sugar-sweetened beverages in Berkeley, California, US: a before-and-after study. *PLoS Med.* 2017;14(4):e1002283
41. Falbe J, Rojas N, Grummon AH, Madsen KA. Higher retail prices of sugar-sweetened beverages 3 months after implementation of an excise tax in Berkeley, California. *Am J Public Health.* 2015;105(11):2194–2201
42. Cawley J, Frisvold DE. The pass-through of taxes on sugar-sweetened beverages to retail prices: the case of Berkeley, California. *J Policy Anal Manage.* 2017; 36(2):303–326
43. Bollinger B, Sexton SE. Local excise taxes, sticky prices, and spillovers: evidence from Berkeley's soda tax. 2018. Available at: https://ssrn.com/abstract=3087966. Accessed February 1, 2019
44. Dewey C. Why Chicago's soda tax fizzled after two months – and what it means for the anti-soda movement. *The Washington Post.* October 10, 2017. Available at: https://www.washingtonpost.com/news/wonk/wp/2017/10/10/why-chicagos-soda-tax-fizzled-after-two-months-and-what-it-means-for-the-anti-soda-movement/?noredirect=on&utm_term=.a5285122edcb. Accessed February 1, 2019
45. Institute of Medicine. *For the Public's Health: Revitalizing Law and Policy to Meet New Challenges.* Washington, DC: The National Academies Press; 2011
46. Langellier BA, Lê-Scherban F, Purtle J. Funding quality pre-kindergarten slots with Philadelphia's new 'sugary drink tax': simulating effects of using an excise tax to address a social determinant of health. *Public Health Nutr.* 2017;20(13):2450–2458
47. Hashem K, Rosborough J. Why tax sugar sweetened beverages? *J Pediatr Gastroenterol Nutr.* 2017;65(4):358–359
48. Federal Trade Commission. A review of food marketing to children and adolescents: follow-up report. 2012. Available at: https://www.ftc.gov/sites/default/files/documents/reports/review-food-marketing-children-and-adolescents-follow-report/121221foodmarketingreport.pdf. Accessed July 25, 2017
49. Frazier WC III, Harris JL. Trends in television food advertising to young people: 2016 update. 2017. Available at: http://uconnruddcenter.org/files/TVAdTrends2017.pdf. Accessed October 1, 2017
50. Powell LM, Schermbeck RM, Chaloupka FJ. Nutritional content of food and beverage products in television advertisements seen on children's programming. *Child Obes.* 2013;9(6): 524–531
51. Kumar G, Onufrak S, Zytnick D, Kingsley B, Park S. Self-reported advertising exposure to sugar-sweetened beverages among US youth. *Public Health Nutr.* 2015;18(7):1173–1179
52. Han E, Powell LM. Consumption patterns of sugar-sweetened beverages in the United States. *J Acad Nutr Diet.* 2013;113(1):43–53
53. Food and Nutrition Service, United States Department of Agriculture. Final

rule: local school wellness policy implementation under the Healthy, Hunger-Free Kids Act of 2010. 2016. Available at: https://www.gpo.gov/fdsys/pkg/FR-2016-07-29/pdf/2016-17230.pdf. Accessed July 30, 2018

54. Food and Nutrition Service, USDA. Child and Adult Care Food Program: meal pattern revisions related to the Healthy, Hunger-Free Kids Act of 2010. Final rule. *Fed Regist.* 2016;81(79):24347–24383

55. United States Department of Agriculture. *Interim Final Rule: Child Nutrition Program Flexibilities for Milk, Whole Grains, and Sodium Requirements.* Washington, DC: United States Department of Agriculture; 2017

56. Cradock AL, McHugh A, Mont-Ferguson H, et al. Effect of school district policy change on consumption of sugar-sweetened beverages among high school students, Boston, Massachusetts, 2004-2006. *Prev Chronic Dis.* 2011;8(4):A74

57. Chriqui JF, Pickel M, Story M. Influence of school competitive food and beverage policies on obesity, consumption, and availability: a systematic review. *JAMA Pediatr.* 2014;168(3):279–286

58. Hood NE, Colabianchi N, Terry-McElrath YM, O'Malley PM, Johnston LD. School wellness policies and foods and beverages available in schools. *Am J Prev Med.* 2013;45(2):143–149

59. Foster GD, Linder B, Baranowski T, et al; HEALTHY Study Group. A school-based intervention for diabetes risk reduction. *N Engl J Med.* 2010;363(5):443–453

60. Wang YC, Hsiao A, Chamberlin P, et al. Nutrition quality of US school snack foods: a first look at 2011-2014 bid records in 8 school districts. *J Sch Health.* 2017;87(1):29–35

61. Johnson DB, Podrabsky M, Rocha A, Otten JJ. Effect of the Healthy Hunger-Free Kids Act on the nutritional quality of meals selected by students and school lunch participation rates. *JAMA Pediatr.* 2016;170(1):e153918

62. Micha R, Karageorgou D, Bakogianni I, et al. Effectiveness of school food environment policies on children's dietary behaviors: a systematic review and meta-analysis. *PLoS One.* 2018; 13(3):e0194555

63. Chriqui JF, Piekarz E, Chaloupka FJ. USDA snack food and beverage standards: how big of a stretch for the states? *Child Obes.* 2014;10(3):234–240

64. Asada Y, Chriqui J, Chavez N, Odoms-Young A, Handler A. USDA snack policy implementation: best practices from the front lines, United States, 2013-2014. *Prev Chronic Dis.* 2016;13:E79

65. Gray KF, Fisher S, Lauffer S. *Characteristics of Supplemental Nutrition Assistance Program Households: Fiscal Year 2015.* Alexandria, VA: US Department of Agriculture, Food and Nutrition Service, Office of Policy Support; 2016

66. Shenkin JD, Jacobson MF. Using the Food Stamp Program and other methods to promote healthy diets for low-income consumers. *Am J Public Health.* 2010;100(9):1562–1564

67. Basu S, Seligman H, Bhattacharya J. Nutritional policy changes in the supplemental nutrition assistance program: a microsimulation and cost-effectiveness analysis. *Med Decis Making.* 2013;33(7):937–948

68. Blumenthal SJ, Hoffnagle EE, Leung CW, et al. Strategies to improve the dietary quality of Supplemental Nutrition Assistance Program (SNAP) beneficiaries: an assessment of stakeholder opinions. *Public Health Nutr.* 2014;17(12):2824–2833

69. Long MW, Leung CW, Cheung LW, Blumenthal SJ, Willett WC. Public support for policies to improve the nutritional impact of the Supplemental Nutrition Assistance Program (SNAP). *Public Health Nutr.* 2014;17(1):219–224

70. Schwartz MB. Moving beyond the debate over restricting sugary drinks in the Supplemental Nutrition Assistance Program. *Am J Prev Med.* 2017;52(2S2):S199–S205

71. Pomeranz JL, Chriqui JF. The Supplemental Nutrition Assistance Program: analysis of program administration and food law definitions. *Am J Prev Med.* 2015;49(3):428–436

72. United States Department of Agriculture. Healthy incentives pilot final evaluation report. 2014. Available at: https://www.fns.usda.gov/snap/healthy-incentives-pilot-final-evaluation-report. Accessed October 7, 2017

73. Harnack L, Oakes JM, Elbel B, Beatty T, Rydell S, French S. Effects of subsidies and prohibitions on nutrition in a food benefit program: a randomized clinical trial [published correction appears in *JAMA Intern Med.* 2017;177(1):144]. *JAMA Intern Med.* 2016;176(11): 1610–1618

74. Leung CW, Musicus AA, Willett WC, Rimm EB. Improving the nutritional impact of the Supplemental Nutrition Assistance Program: perspectives from the participants. *Am J Prev Med.* 2017;52 (2S2):S193–S198

75. United States Department of Agriculture. FY 2019 SNAP-Ed plan guidance. 2018. Available at: https://snaped.fns.usda.gov/snap/Guidance/FY2019SNAPEdPlanGuidanceFULL.pdf. Accessed February 1, 2019

76. Afshin A, Penalvo J, Del Gobbo L, et al. CVD prevention through policy: a review of mass media, food/menu labeling, taxation/subsidies, built environment, school procurement, worksite wellness, and marketing standards to improve diet. *Curr Cardiol Rep.* 2015;17(11):98

77. Prentice C, Kahn C. Americans want required food labels even if they don't read them. *Reuters.* October 2, 2017. Available at: https://www.reuters.com/article/us-usa-foodlabels-poll/americans-want-required-food-labels-even-if-they-dont-read-them-idUSKCN1C71F5. Accessed February 1, 2019

78. Hawthorne KM, Moreland K, Griffin IJ, Abrams SA. An educational program enhances food label understanding of young adolescents. *J Am Diet Assoc.* 2006;106(6):913–916

79. Christoph MJ, An R, Ellison B. Correlates of nutrition label use among college students and young adults: a review. *Public Health Nutr.* 2016;19(12): 2135–2148

80. VanEpps EM, Roberto CA. The influence of sugar-sweetened beverage warnings: a randomized trial of adolescents' choices and beliefs. *Am J Prev Med.* 2016;51(5):664–672

81. Roberto CA, Wong D, Musicus A, Hammond D. The influence of sugar-sweetened beverage health warning labels on parents' choices. *Pediatrics.* 2016;137(2):e20153185

82. Pomeranz JL, Mozaffarian D, Micha R. Can the government require health warnings on sugar-sweetened beverage advertisements? *JAMA.* 2018;319(3): 227–228

83. *American Beverage Association v City and County of San Francisco,* No 16-16072 D.C. No. 3:15-cv-03415-EMC (9th Cir 2019). Available at: https://cspinet.org/sites/default/files/attachment/SF%20Warning_Ninth%20Circuit%20En%20Banc.pdf. Accessed February 1, 2019

84. Food Service Guidelines Federal Workgroup. Food service guidelines for federal facilities. 2017. Available at: https://www.cdc.gov/obesity/downloads/guidelines_for_federal_concessions_and_vending_operations.pdf. Accessed July 29, 2017

85. City of New York. New York city food standards: beverage vending machines. Available at: https://www1.nyc.gov/assets/doh/downloads/pdf/cardio/cardio-vending-machines-bev-standards.pdf. Accessed October 7, 2017

86. Centers for Disease Control and Prevention. Food service guidelines: case studies from states and communities. 2015. Available at: https://www.cdc.gov/obesity/downloads/fsg_casestudies_508.pdf. Accessed August 1, 2017

87. City of New York. Procurement: standards for meals and snacks. Available at: http://www1.nyc.gov/site/foodpolicy/initiatives/procurement.page. Accessed October 7, 2017

88. Cradock AL, Kenney EL, McHugh A, et al. Evaluating the impact of the healthy beverage executive order for city agencies in Boston, Massachusetts, 2011-2013. *Prev Chronic Dis.* 2015;12: E147

89. Wootan, MG. California becomes first state to pass healthy restaurant kids' meal bill. 2018. Available at: https://cspinet.org/news/california-becomes-first-state-pass-healthy-restaurant-kids%E2%80%99-meal-bill-20180822. Accessed August 26, 2018

90. Ribakove S, Almy J, Wootan, MG. Soda on the menu: improvements seen but more change needed for beverages on restaurant children's menus. 2017. Available at: https://cspinet.org/kidsbeveragestudy. Accessed October 10, 2017

91. Hanks AS, Just DR, Smith LE, Wansink B. Healthy convenience: nudging students toward healthier choices in the lunchroom. *J Public Health (Oxf).* 2012; 34(3):370–376

92. Loeb KL, Radnitz C, Keller K, et al. The application of defaults to optimize parents' health-based choices for children. *Appetite.* 2017;113:368–375

93. Peters J, Beck J, Lande J, et al. Using healthy defaults in Walt Disney World restaurants to improve nutritional choices. *J Assoc Consum Res.* 2016;1(1): 92–103

94. Gardner MN, Brandt AM. "The doctors' choice is America's choice": the physician in US cigarette advertisements, 1930-1953. *Am J Public Health.* 2006;96(2): 222–232

95. New York Times. Hospitals act to curb cigarette sales, smoking. *New York Times.* February 9, 1964. Available at: https://www.nytimes.com/1964/02/09/archives/hospitals-act-to-curb-cigarette-sales-smoking.html. Accessed August 27, 2018

96. Smith DR, Leggat PA. The historical decline of tobacco smoking among Australian physicians: 1964-1997. *Tob Induc Dis.* 2008;4:13

97. American Medical Association. *AMA Adopts Policy to Reduce Consumption of Sugar-Sweetened Beverages.* Chicago, IL: American Medical Association; 2017

98. Yang Q, Zhang Z, Gregg EW, Flanders WD, Merritt R, Hu FB. Added sugar intake and cardiovascular diseases mortality among US adults. *JAMA Intern Med.* 2014;174(4):516–524

99. Thorndike AN, Sonnenberg L, Riis J, Barraclough S, Levy DE. A 2-phase labeling and choice architecture intervention to improve healthy food and beverage choices [published correction appears in *Am J Public Health.* 2012;102(4):584]. *Am J Public Health.* 2012;102(3):527–533

100. Block JP, Chandra A, McManus KD, Willett WC. Point-of-purchase price and education intervention to reduce consumption of sugary soft drinks. *Am J Public Health.* 2010;100(8):1427–1433

101. Spector K. Sugar-sweetened food, beverages will no longer be sold at the Cleveland Clinic. 2010. Available at: https://www.cleveland.com/healthfit/index.ssf/2010/07/sugar-sweetened_food_beverages.html. Accessed August 26, 2018

102. Eneli IU, Oza-Frank R, Grover K, Miller R, Kelleher K. Instituting a sugar-sweetened beverage ban: experience from a children's hospital. *Am J Public Health.* 2014;104(10):1822–1825

103. Geisinger. *Geisinger Eliminates Sugar-Sweetened Beverages.* Danville, PA: Geisinger; 2018

104. Public Health Law Center. Food and beverage pledges for hospitals and healthcare systems. Available at: www.publichealthlawcenter.org/sites/default/files/resources/KS%20Beverage%20Pledge%20Chart%204.28.14.pdf. Accessed July 31, 2017

105. Public Health Law Center. Building blocks for success: a guide for developing healthy beverage programs. Available at: www.publichealthlawcenter.org/sites/default/files/resources/phlc-fs-building-blocks-healthy-beverages-2013.pdf. Accessed July 31, 2017

106. Centers for Disease Control and Prevention. Creating healthier hospital food, beverage, and physical activity environments: forming teams, engaging stakeholders, conducting assessments and evaluations. Available at: https://www.cdc.gov/obesity/hospital-toolkit/pdf/creating-healthier-hospital-food-beverage-pa.pdf. Accessed July 31, 2017

Recommendations for Prevention and Control of Influenza in Children, 2019–2020

- *Policy Statement*
  - *PPI: AAP Partnership for Policy Implementation*
    See Appendix 1 for more information.

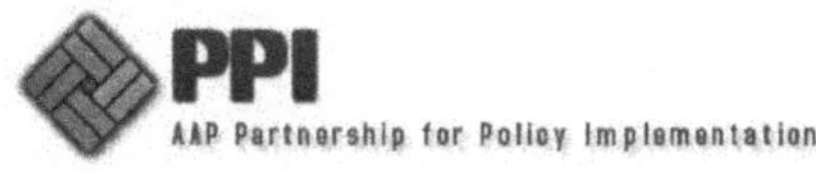

POLICY STATEMENT Organizational Principles to Guide and Define the Child Health Care System and/or Improve the Health of all Children

American Academy of Pediatrics

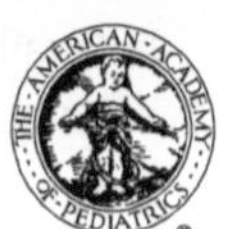

DEDICATED TO THE HEALTH OF ALL CHILDREN™

Recommendations for Prevention and Control of Influenza in Children, 2019–2020

COMMITTEE ON INFECTIOUS DISEASES

abstract

This statement updates the recommendations of the American Academy of Pediatrics for the routine use of influenza vaccines and antiviral medications in the prevention and treatment of influenza in children during the 2019–2020 season. The American Academy of Pediatrics continues to recommend routine influenza immunization of all children without medical contraindications, starting at 6 months of age. Any licensed, recommended, age-appropriate vaccine available can be administered, without preference of one product or formulation over another. Antiviral treatment of influenza with any licensed, recommended, age-appropriate influenza antiviral medication continues to be recommended for children with suspected or confirmed influenza, particularly those who are hospitalized, have severe or progressive disease, or have underlying conditions that increase their risk of complications of influenza.

The following updates for the 2019–2020 influenza season are discussed in this document:

1. Both inactivated influenza vaccine (IIV) and live attenuated influenza vaccine (LAIV) are options for influenza vaccination in children, with no preference.
2. The composition of the influenza vaccines for 2019–2020 has been updated. The A(H1N1)pdm09 and A(H3N2) components of the vaccine are new for this season. The B strains are unchanged from the previous season.
3. All pediatric influenza vaccines will be quadrivalent vaccines. The age indication for some pediatric vaccines has been expanded; therefore, there are now 4 egg-based quadrivalent inactivated influenza vaccines (IIV4s) licensed by the US Food and Drug Administration (FDA) for administration to children 6 months and older, 1 inactivated cell-based quadrivalent inactivated influenza vaccine (cIIV4) for children 4 years and older, and 1 quadrivalent live attenuated influenza vaccine (LAIV4)

Policy statements from the American Academy of Pediatrics benefit from expertise and resources of liaisons and internal (AAP) and external reviewers. However, policy statements from the American Academy of Pediatrics may not reflect the views of the liaisons or the organizations or government agencies that they represent.

The guidance in this statement does not indicate an exclusive course of treatment or serve as a standard of medical care. Variations, taking into account individual circumstances, may be appropriate.

All policy statements from the American Academy of Pediatrics automatically expire 5 years after publication unless reaffirmed, revised, or retired at or before that time.

This document is copyrighted and is property of the American Academy of Pediatrics and its Board of Directors. All authors have filed conflict of interest statements with the American Academy of Pediatrics. Any conflicts have been resolved through a process approved by the Board of Directors. The American Academy of Pediatrics has neither solicited nor accepted any commercial involvement in the development of the content of this publication.

DOI: https://doi.org/10.1542/peds.2019-2478

Address correspondence to Xxx. E-mail: xxx

PEDIATRICS (ISSN Numbers: Print, 0031-4005; Online, 1098-4275).

Copyright © 2019 by the American Academy of Pediatrics

To cite: COMMITTEE ON INFECTIOUS DISEASES. Recommendations for Prevention and Control of Influenza in Children, 2019–2020. *Pediatrics*. 2019;144(4): e20192478 for children 2 years and older. No trivalent vaccines are expected to be available for children this season.

4. New formulations of licensed influenza vaccines with a volume of 0.5 mL per dose have been approved for children 6 through 36 months of age. Children 6 through 35 months of age may now receive either the 0.25- or 0.5-mL dose, with no preference, and children ≥36 months of age (3 years and older) continue to receive a 0.5-mL dose.
5. Children 6 months through 8 years of age who are receiving influenza vaccine for the first time or who have received only 1 dose before July 1, 2019, should receive 2 doses of influenza vaccine ideally by the end of October, and vaccines should be offered as soon as they become available. Children needing only 1 dose of influenza vaccine, regardless of age, should also receive vaccination ideally by the end of October.
6. A new antiviral medication has been licensed for treatment of influenza in children.

Children often have the highest attack rates of influenza in the community during seasonal influenza epidemics. They play a pivotal role in the transmission of influenza virus infection to household and other close contacts and can experience morbidity, including severe or fatal complications from influenza infection.[1] Children younger than 5 years, especially those younger than 2 years, and children with certain underlying medical conditions are at increased risk of hospitalization and complications attributable to influenza.[1] School-aged children bear a large influenza disease burden and are more likely to seek influenza-related medical care compared with healthy adults.[1,2] Reducing influenza virus transmission among children decreases the burden of childhood influenza and transmission of influenza virus to household contacts and community members of all ages.[1,2] Routine influenza vaccination and antiviral agents for the treatment and prevention of influenza are recommended for children.[1,2]

SUMMARY OF RECENT INFLUENZA ACTIVITY IN THE UNITED STATES

2017–2018 Influenza Season

The 2017–2018 influenza season was the first classified as a high-severity season for all age groups, with high levels of outpatient clinic and emergency department visits for influenzalike illness, high influenza-related hospitalization rates, and high numbers of deaths.[3–5] Influenza A(H3N2) viruses predominated through February 2018; influenza B viruses predominated from March 2018 onward. Although hospitalization rates for children that season did not exceed those reported during the 2009 pandemic, they did surpass rates reported in previous high-severity A(H3N2)-predominant seasons. Excluding the 2009 pandemic, the 186 pediatric deaths reported during the 2017–2018 season (approximately half of which occurred in otherwise healthy children) were the highest reported since influenza-associated pediatric mortality became a nationally notifiable condition in 2004.[3–5] Among pediatric deaths of children 6 months and older who were eligible for vaccination and for whom vaccination status was known, approximately 80% had not received the influenza vaccine during the 2017–2018 season.[3]

Overall vaccine effectiveness (VE) against both influenza A and B viruses during the 2017–2018 season was estimated to be 38%, with higher VE (64%) in children 6 months to 8 years of age compared with those 9 to 17 years of age (28%).[4] Overall VE against influenza A(H1N1) was 65% (87% in those 6 months through 8 years of age; 70% in those 9 through 17 years of age), 25% against A(H3N2) (54% in those 6 months through 8 years of age; 18% in those 9 through 17 years of age), and 48% against influenza B (B/Yamagata predominant) (77% in those 6 months through 8 years of age; 28% in those 9 through 17 years of age).

2018–2019 Influenza Season

The 2018–2019 influenza season was the longest-lasting season reported in the United States in the past decade, with elevated levels of influenzalike illness activity for a total duration of 21 consecutive weeks (compared to the average duration of 16 weeks).[6] Influenza A(H1N1)pdm09 viruses predominated from October to mid-February, and influenza A(H3N2) viruses were identified more frequently from February to May. Influenza B (B/Victoria lineage predominant) represented approximately 5% of circulating strains. The majority of characterized influenza A(H1N1)pdm09 and influenza B viruses were antigenically similar to the viruses included in the 2018–2019 influenza vaccine, but most characterized influenza A(H3N2) viruses were antigenically distinct from the A(H3N2) component of the 2018–2019 vaccine. Co-circulation of multiple genetically diverse clades and/or subclades of A(H3N2) was documented. Circulating viruses identified belonged to clade 3C.2a, subclade 3C.2a1, or clade 3C.3a, with 3C.3a viruses accounting for >70% of the A(H3N2) in the United States. The 2018–2019 vaccine's A(H3N2) virus belonged to subclade 3C.2a1. This likely contributed to an overall lower VE against influenza A(H3N2) for that influenza season and supported the recommendation to change the A(H3N2) virus strain for the upcoming season's vaccine.

The 2018–2019 season was of moderate severity, with similar

hospitalization rates in children as seen during the 2017–2018 season, which were higher than in those observed in previous seasons from 2013–2014 to 2016–2017. The cumulative hospitalization rates per 100 000 population were 72.0 among children 0 through 4 years old and 20.4 among children 5 through 17 years old.[6] Among 1132 children hospitalized with influenza and for whom data were available, 45% had no recorded underlying condition, and 55% had at least 1 underlying medical condition; the most commonly reported underlying conditions were asthma or reactive airway disease (27.1%), neurologic disorders (17.7%), and obesity (11.4%).[7]

As of June 21, 2019, the following data were reported by the Centers for Disease Control and Prevention (CDC):

- There were 116 laboratory-confirmed influenza-associated pediatric deaths. Most (66%) of those children died after being admitted to the hospital. The median age of the pediatric deaths was 6.1 years (range: 2 months–17 years).
    - A total of 107 were associated with influenza A viruses: 43 with influenza A(H1N1)pdm09, 25 with A(H3N2), and 39 with an influenza A virus for which no subtyping was available.
    - Eight were associated with influenza B viruses.
    - One was associated with an undetermined type of influenza virus.
- Among the 104 children with known medical history, 51% of deaths occurred in children who had at least 1 underlying medical condition recognized by the Advisory Committee on Immunization Practices (ACIP) to increase the risk of influenza-attributable disease severity. Therefore, nearly half had no known underlying medical conditions.
- Among 89 children who were 6 months or older at the time of illness onset and, therefore, would have been eligible for vaccination and for whom vaccination status was known, most (70%) were unvaccinated. Only 30 (34%) had received at least 1 dose of influenza vaccine (25 had complete vaccination, and 5 had received 1 of 2 ACIP-recommended doses).

Preliminary estimates of the VE of the 2018–2019 seasonal influenza vaccines (not based on specific products) against medically attended influenza illness from the US Influenza VE Network reveal an overall adjusted VE of 47% (95% confidence interval [CI], 34% to 57%) for people of all ages against any type of influenza (A or B).[7] The overall VE against any type of influenza for children 6 months through 17 years was 61% (95% CI, 44% to 73%). Virus-specific preliminary VE data available for influenza A(H1N1) viruses reveal overall VE of 45% (95% CI, 30% to 58%) in people of all ages and 63% (95% CI, 40% to 75%) for children 6 months to 17 years. Preliminary VE for influenza A(H3N2) in people of all ages is 44% (95% CI, 13% to 64%). No data are yet available for children within this network for A(H3N2) or B strains.

Preliminary estimates of influenza VE against hospitalization in children, from the CDC's New Vaccine Surveillance Network, which is focused on surveillance in children, reveal an overall adjusted (for age, site, and month) VE in children of 31% (95% CI, 5% to 51%) against any influenza A or B virus, with 26% (95% CI, −6% to 49%) in children 6 months through 8 years of age and 53% (95% CI, 5% to 77%) among those 9 through 17 years of age.[1] The overall adjusted VE against pediatric hospitalization by virus subtype was 48% (95% CI, 14% to 68%) for A(H1N1)pdm09 and 13% (95% CI, −31% to 43%) for A(H3N2). These are preliminary data and not vaccine specific.

INFLUENZA MORBIDITY AND MORTALITY IN CHILDREN

Pediatric hospitalizations and deaths caused by influenza vary from one season to the next. Historically, up to 80% of pediatric deaths have occurred in unvaccinated children 6 months and older. Influenza vaccination is associated with reduced risk of laboratory-confirmed influenza-related pediatric death.[8] In 1 case-cohort analysis comparing vaccination uptake among laboratory-confirmed influenza-associated pediatric deaths with estimated vaccination coverage among pediatric cohorts in the United States from 2010 to 2014, Flannery et al[8] found that only 26% of children had received the vaccine before illness onset compared to an average vaccination coverage of 48%. Overall VE against influenza-associated death in children was 65% (95% CI, 54% to 74%). More than half of children in this study who died of influenza had ≥1 underlying medical condition associated with increased risk of severe influenza-related complications; only 1 in 3 of these at-risk children had been vaccinated; yet, VE against death in children with underlying conditions was 51% (95% CI, 31% to 67%). Similarly, influenza vaccination reduces by three quarters the risk of severe, life-threatening laboratory-confirmed influenza in children requiring admission to the ICU.[9] The rates of influenza-associated hospitalization for children younger than 5 years exceed the rates for children 5 through 17 years of age. The influenza virus type might also affect the severity of disease. In a recent study of hospitalizations for influenza A versus B, the odds of mortality were significantly greater with influenza B than with influenza A and not entirely explained by underlying health conditions.[10]

HIGH-RISK GROUPS IN PEDIATRICS

Children and adolescents with certain underlying medical conditions have a high risk of complications from influenza, as described in Table 1. Although universal influenza vaccination is recommended for everyone starting at 6 months of age, emphasis should be placed on ensuring that people in high-risk groups and their household contacts and caregivers receive an annual influenza vaccine.[11]

SEASONAL INFLUENZA VACCINES

Table 2 summarizes information on the types of influenza vaccines licensed for children and adults during the 2019–2020 season. More than 1 product may be appropriate for a given patient, and vaccination should not be delayed to obtain a specific product.

All 2019–2020 seasonal influenza vaccines contain the same influenza strains as recommended by the World Health Organization (WHO) as well as the FDA Vaccines and Related Biological Products Advisory Committee for the Northern Hemisphere[6,14]:

1. Trivalent vaccines contain the following:
   a. A/Brisbane/02/2018 (H1N1) pdm09-like virus (new this season);
   b. A/Kansas/14/2017 (H3N2)-like virus (new this season); and
   c. B/Colorado/60/2017-like virus (B/Victoria/2/87 lineage) (unchanged).
2. Quadrivalent vaccines contain a second B virus:
   a. B/Phuket/3073/2013-like virus (B/Yamagata/16/88 lineage) (unchanged).

IIV

For the 2019–2020 season, all IIVs for children in the United States will be quadrivalent vaccines, with specific age indications for available formulations (Table 2). All licensed inactivated vaccines for children in the United States are unadjuvanted; 4 are egg-based (seed strains grown in eggs), 1 is cell culture-based (seed strains grown in Madin-Darby canine kidney cells), and all are available in single-dose, thimerosal-free prefilled syringes as well multidose vial presentations. With the FDA approval of the expansion of the age indication for Afluria Quadrivalent[15] to children 6 months and older (previously approved for children 5 years and older) in October 2018, all egg-based IIV4s (Afluria, Fluarix, Flulaval, and Fluzone) are now licensed for children 6 months and older, and the cell culture–based vaccine (Flucelvax) is licensed for children 4 years and older.

The licensure of the expanded age indication for Afluria quadrivalent was supported by a single randomized, double-blind safety and immunogenicity study in children 6 through 59 months of age who received Afluria quadrivalent or a comparator licensed quadrivalent vaccine.[15] The vaccine was found to have a similar safety profile and noninferior immunogenicity as the comparator vaccine. Importantly, there were no febrile seizures in the 7 days after vaccination. The trivalent formulation is no longer expected to be available. The dose volume for Afluria quadrivalent is 0.25 mL for children 6 through 35 months of age and 0.5 mL for those 36 months and older. This vaccine should only be administered by needle and syringe in children, whereas administration via jet injector is an option for individuals 18 through 64 years of age.

A quadrivalent recombinant baculovirus-expressed hemagglutinin influenza vaccine (RIV4; Flublok) is licensed only for people 18 years and older. The high-dose trivalent inactivated influenza vaccine (IIV3; Fluzone High-Dose), containing 4 times the amount of antigen for each virus strain than the standard-dose vaccines, is licensed only for people 65 years and older. A trivalent MF59 adjuvanted IIV (Fluad) licensed

TABLE 1 Persons at High Risk of Influenza Complications

Children <5 years and especially those <2 years,[a] regardless of the presence of underlying medical conditions
Adults ≥50 years and especially those ≥65 years
Children and adults with chronic pulmonary (including asthma and cystic fibrosis), hemodynamically significant cardiovascular disease (except hypertension alone), or renal, hepatic, hematologic (including sickle cell disease and other hemoglobinopathies), or metabolic disorders (including diabetes mellitus)
Children and adults with immunosuppression attributable to any cause, including that caused by medications or by HIV infection
Children and adults with neurologic and neurodevelopment conditions (including disorders of the brain, spinal cord, peripheral nerve, and muscle such as cerebral palsy, epilepsy, stroke, intellectual disability, moderate-to-severe developmental delay, muscular dystrophy, or spinal cord injury)
Children and adults with conditions that compromise respiratory function or handling of secretions (including tracheostomy and mechanical ventilation)[12]
Women who are pregnant or postpartum during the influenza season
Children and adolescents <19 years who are receiving long-term aspirin therapy or salicylate-containing medications (including those with Kawasaki disease and rheumatologic conditions) because of increased risk of Reye syndrome
American Indian and Alaskan native people
Children and adults with extreme obesity (ie, BMI ≥40 for adults and based on age for children)
Residents of chronic care facilities and nursing homes

[a] The 2019–2020 CDC recommendations state that "Although all children younger than 5 years old are considered at higher risk for complications from influenza, the highest risk is for those younger than 2 years old, with the highest hospitalization and death rates among infants younger than 6 months old."

TABLE 2 Recommended Seasonal Influenza Vaccines for Different Age Groups: United States, 2019–2020 Influenza Season

Vaccine	Trade Name	Manufacturer	Presentation HA Antigen Content (IIVs and RIV4) or Virus Count (LAIV4) per Dose for Each Vaccine Virus	Thimerosal Mercury Content, µg of Hg/0.5-mL Dose	Age Group	CPT Code
Inactivated						
Trivalent						
IIV3	Fluzone High-Dose	Sanofi Pasteur	0.5-mL prefilled syringe (60 µg/0.5 mL)	0	≥65 y	90662
aIIV3	Fluad MF59 adjuvanted	Seqirus	0.5-mL prefilled syringe (15 µg/0.5 mL)	0	≥65 y	90653
Quadrivalent						
Egg based						
IIV4	Fluzone Quadrivalent	Sanofi Pasteur	0.25-mL prefilled syringe (7.5 µg/0.25 mL)	0	6–35 mo	90685
			0.5-mL prefilled syringe (15 µg/0.5 mL)	0	≥6 mo	90686
			0.5-mL single-dose vial (15 µg/0.5 mL)	0	≥6 mo	90686
			5.0-mL multidose vial[a] (7.5 µg/0.25 mL) (15 µg/0.5 mL)	25	≥6 mo	90687, 90688
IIV4	Fluarix Quadrivalent	GlaxoSmithKline	0.5-mL prefilled syringe (15 µg/0.5 mL)	0	≥6 mo	90686
IIV4	FluLaval Quadrivalent	ID Biomedical Corporation of Quebec (distributed by GlaxoSmithKline)	0.5-mL prefilled syringe (15 µg/0.5 mL)	0	≥6 mo	90686
			5.0-mL multidose vial (15 µg/0.5 mL)	<25	≥6 mo	90688
IIV4	Afluria Quadrivalent	Seqirus	0.25-mL prefilled syringe (7.5 µg/0.25 mL)	0	6–35 mo	90685
			0.5-mL prefilled syringe (15 µg/0.5 mL)	0	≥36 mo	90686
			5.0-mL multidose vial[a] (7.5 µg/0.25 mL) (15 µg/0.5 mL)	24.5	≥6 mo (needle/syringe) 18–64 y (jet injector)	90687, 90688
Cell based						
ccIIV4	Flucelvax Quadrivalent	Seqirus	0.5-mL prefilled syringe (15 µg/0.5 mL)	0	≥4 y	90674
			5.0 mL multidose vial (15 µg/0.5 mL)	25	≥4 y	90756
Recombinant						
RIV4	Flublok Quadrivalent	Protein Sciences Corporation (distributed by Sanofi Pasteur)	0.5-mL prefilled syringe (45 µg/0.5 mL)	0	≥18 y	90682
Live attenuated						
LAIV4	FluMist Quadrivalent	AstraZeneca	0.2-mL prefilled intranasal sprayer (virus dose: $10^{6.5-7.5}$ FFU/0.2 mL)	0	2–49 y	90672

Implementation guidance on supply, pricing, payment, CPT coding, and liability issues can be found at www.aapredbook.org/implementation. Data sources are from references[1] and[13]. aIIV3, adjuvanted trivalent inactivated influenza vaccine; ccIIV4, quadrivalent cell culture–based inactivated influenza vaccine; CPT, *Current Procedural Terminology*; FFU, focus-forming unit; —, not applicable.

[a] For vaccines that include a multidose vial presentation and a 0.25-mL dose, a maximum of 10 doses can be drawn from a multidose vial.

for people 65 years and older is the first adjuvanted influenza vaccine marketed in the United States. Adjuvants may be included in a vaccine to elicit a more robust immune response, which could lead to a reduction in the number of doses required for children. In a study in children, the relative vaccine efficacy of an MF59 adjuvanted influenza vaccine was significantly greater than nonadjuvanted vaccine in the 6- through 23-month age group.[16] Adjuvanted seasonal influenza vaccines are not licensed for children at this time.

Children 36 months (3 years) and older can receive any age-appropriate licensed IIV, administered at a 0.5-mL dose and containing 15 µg of hemagglutinin (HA) from each strain in the vaccine. Children 6 through 35 months of age may receive any licensed IIV at either 0.25 or 0.5 mL per dose, without preference over one or the other.

The only IIV products licensed for children 6 through 35 months of age before 2016 were the 0.25-mL (containing 7.5 µg of HA for each vaccine virus) dose formulations of Fluzone (IIV3) and Fluzone Quadrivalent (IIV4). The recommendation for use of a reduced dose and volume for children in this age group (half that recommended for people 3 years and older) was based on increased reactogenicity noted among younger children after receipt of whole-virus inactivated vaccines, which have since been replaced with split virus and subunit IIV. Several vaccines have been licensed for children 6 through 35 months of age since 2017, which are less reactogenic (Table 2).[17,18] All are quadrivalent, but the dose volume and, therefore, the antigen content vary among different IIV products. In addition to the 0.25-mL (7.5 μg of HA per vaccine virus) Fluzone Quadrivalent vaccine, Fluzone Quadrivalent containing 15 μg of HA per vaccine virus per 0.5-mL dose was licensed in January 2019[19,20] after these 2 formulations were compared in a single randomized, multicenter safety and immunogenicity study. Both products are expected to be available this season because no direct comparison data are available to demonstrate superiority of one over the other. In addition, 2 other vaccines, Fluarix Quadrivalent[21] and FluLaval Quadrivalent,[22] have been licensed for a 0.5-mL dose in children 6 through 35 months of age. These 2 vaccines do not have a 0.25-mL dose formulation.

Given that different formulations of IIV for children 6 through 35 months of age are available, care should be taken to administer the appropriate volume and dose for each product. In each instance, the recommended volume may be administered from an appropriate prefilled syringe, a single-dose vial, or multidose vial, as supplied by the manufacturer. For vaccines that include a multidose vial presentation and a 0.25-mL dose, a maximum of 10 doses can be drawn from a multidose vial. Importantly, dose volume is different from the number of doses needed to complete vaccination. Children 6 months through 8 years of age who require 2 doses of vaccine for the 2019–2020 season should receive 2 separate doses at the recommended dose volume specified for each product.

IIVs can be used in healthy children as well as those with underlying chronic medical conditions. IIV is well tolerated in children. The most common injection-site adverse reactions after administration of IIV in children are injection-site pain, redness, and swelling. The most common systemic adverse events are drowsiness, irritability, loss of appetite, fatigue, muscle aches, headache, arthralgia, and gastrointestinal tract symptoms.

IIV can be administered concomitantly with other inactivated or live vaccines. During the 2 influenza seasons spanning 2010–2012, there were increased reports of febrile seizures in the United States in young children who received IIV3 and the 13-valent pneumococcal conjugate vaccine (PCV13) concomitantly. Subsequent retrospective analyses of past seasons revealed a slight increase in the risk of febrile seizures in children 6 through 23 months of age when PCV13s were administered concomitantly with IIV.[23] The concomitant administration of IIV3, PCV13, and diphtheria-tetanus-acellular pertussis vaccine was associated with the greatest relative risk estimate, corresponding to a maximum additional 30 febrile seizure cases per 100 000 children vaccinated compared to the administration of the vaccines on separate days. In contrast, data from the Post-Licensure Rapid Immunization Safety Monitoring program of the FDA, the largest vaccine safety active surveillance program in the United States, revealed that there was no significant increase in febrile seizures associated with concomitant administration of these 3 vaccines in children 6 through 59 months of age during the 2010–2011 season.[24] In a subsequent sentinel Center for Biologics Evaluation and Research–Post-Licensure Rapid Immunization Safety Monitoring surveillance report evaluating influenza vaccines and febrile seizures in the 2013–2014 and 2014–2015 influenza seasons, there was no evidence of an elevated risk of febrile seizures in children 6 through 23 months of age after IIV administration during the 2013–2014 and 2014–2015 seasons. It was concluded that the risk of seizures after PCV13 or concomitant PCV13 and IIV is low compared to a child's lifetime risk of febrile seizures from other causes.[25] Although the possibility of increased risk for febrile seizures cannot be ruled out, simultaneous administration of IIV with PCV13 and/or other vaccines for the 2019–2020 influenza season continues to be recommended when these vaccines are indicated. Overall, the benefits of timely vaccination with same-day administration of IIV and PCV13 or diphtheria-tetanus-acellular pertussis vaccine outweigh the risk of febrile seizures. Vaccine-proximate febrile seizures rarely have any long-term sequelae, similar to non–vaccine-proximate febrile seizures.

Thimerosal-containing vaccines are not associated with an increased risk of autism spectrum disorder in children.[1] Thimerosal from vaccines has not been linked to any neurologic condition. The American Academy of Pediatrics (AAP) supports the current WHO recommendations for use of thimerosal as a preservative in multiuse vials in the global vaccine supply. Concerns about the residual, trace amount of thimerosal in some IIV formulations may arise. Despite the lack of evidence of harm, some states, including California, Delaware, Illinois, Missouri, New York, and Washington, have legislation restricting the use of vaccines that contain even trace amounts of thimerosal. The benefits of protecting children against the known risks of influenza are clear. Therefore, to the extent permitted by state law, children should receive any available formulation of IIV rather than delaying vaccination while waiting for reduced thimerosal-content or thimerosal-free vaccines. IIV formulations that are free of even trace amounts of thimerosal are widely available (Table 2).

Live Attenuated (Intranasal) Influenza Vaccine

The intranasal LAIV was initially licensed in the United States in 2003 for people 5 through 49 years of age as a trivalent live attenuated influenza vaccine (LAIV3) formulation. The approved age group was extended to 2 years of age in 2007. The quadrivalent formulation (LAIV4) has been licensed in the United States since 2012 and was first available during the 2013–2014 influenza season, replacing the LAIV3. The most commonly reported reactions in children are runny nose or nasal congestion, headache, decreased activity or lethargy, and sore throat. The safety of LAIV in people with a history of asthma, diabetes mellitus, or other high-risk medical conditions associated with an elevated risk of complications from influenza (see Contraindications and Precautions) has not been firmly established. In postlicensure surveillance of LAIV (including LAIV3 and LAIV4), the Vaccine Adverse Event Reporting System, jointly sponsored by the FDA and CDC, did not identify any new or unexpected safety concerns, including in people with a contraindication or precaution. Although the use of LAIV in young children with chronic medical conditions, including asthma, has been implemented outside of the United States, data are considered insufficient to support an expanded recommendation in the United States.

The CDC conducted a systematic review of published studies evaluating the effectiveness of LAIV3 and LAIV4 in children from the 2010–2011 to the 2016–2017 seasons, including data from US and European studies.[1,26] The data suggested that the effectiveness of LAIV3 or LAIV4 for influenza strain A(H1N1) was lower than that of IIV in children 2 through 17 years of age. LAIV was similarly effective against influenza B and A(H3N2) strains in some age groups compared to IIV.

For the 2017–2018 season, a new A(H1N1)pdm09-like virus (A/Slovenia/2903/2015) was included in LAIV4, replacing A/Bolivia/559/2013. A study conducted by the LAIV4 manufacturer evaluated viral shedding and immunogenicity associated with the LAIV4 formulation containing the new A(H1N1)pdm09-like virus among US children 24 months through 3 years of age.[27] Shedding and immunogenicity data provided by the manufacturer suggested that the new influenza A(H1N1)pdm09-like virus included in its latest formulation had improved replicative fitness over previous LAIV4 influenza A(H1N1) pdm09-like vaccine strains, resulting in an improved immune response comparable to that of LAIV3 available before the 2009 pandemic. Shedding and replicative fitness are not known to correlate with efficacy, and no published effectiveness estimates for this revised formulation of the vaccine against influenza A(H1N1) pdm09 viruses were available before the start of the 2018–2019 influenza season because influenza A(H3N2) and influenza B viruses predominated during the 2017–2018 northern hemisphere season. Therefore, for the 2018–2019 season, the AAP recommended IIV4 or IIV3 as the primary choice for influenza vaccination in children, with LAIV4 use reserved for children who would not otherwise receive an influenza vaccine and for whom LAIV use was appropriate for age (2 years and older) and health status (ie, healthy, without any underlying chronic medical condition).

After the ACIP meeting in February 2019, the AAP convened a meeting of its Committee on Infectious Diseases to discuss the influenza vaccination recommendations for the 2019–2020 season. The group reviewed available data on influenza epidemiology and VE for the 2018–2019 season and agreed that harmonizing recommendations between the AAP and CDC for the use of LAIV in the 2019–2020 season is appropriate as more information becomes available. Despite the early predominance of A(H1N1) circulation, low use of LAIV4 in the US population limited evaluation of product-specific VE, and no additional US data on LAIV4 VE was anticipated at the end of the 2018–2019 season. The information reviewed by the Committee on Infectious Diseases included the following:

- The epidemiology of the 2018–2019 influenza season in the United States and worldwide, showing an early predominance of A(H1N1)pdm09 virus circulation, followed by A(H3N2) (https://www.cdc.gov/flu/weekly/index.htm).
- Interim VE for 2018–2019 influenza season showing overall influenza VE against medically attended illness for influenza A(H1N1)pdm09 in children of approximately 60% (not product specific, but most vaccine used was IIV), approximately 40% for influenza A(H3N2) overall (given small numbers of H3N2 cases, no pediatric data), and no data for influenza B.[28]
- Influenza vaccine coverage rates in children, demonstrating an increase to ~45% compared with ~38% at the same time point in 2017–2018 season (interim estimate in November 2018; https://www.cdc.gov/flu/fluvaxview/nifs-estimates-nov2018.htm).
- VE data from the European surveillance networks for which uninterrupted use of LAIV continued during the 2016–2017 and 2017–2018 seasons (when it was not used in the United States) and through the 2018–2019 season. In this network, the only country with interim estimates, the United Kingdom, reported VE against medically attended influenza in children and adolescents 2 through 17 years of age for 2017–2018 and 2018–2019 (same vaccine formulation) of >85% for A(H1N1)pdm09. Estimates were based on a small number of cases and were preliminary but consistent with the previous season.[29]
- Other countries that use LAIV (Canada, Finland) may have LAIV4-

specific VE at the end of the season, but this is not certain. Small case numbers and low LAIV use may also limit accurate VE calculations in these countries. In general, as long as use of LAIV is low relative to IIV, it will be difficult to estimate LAIV VE accurately. Furthermore, variability in VE for other strains (A [H3N2] and B strains) remains for both IIV and LAIV.

- The committee noted that LAIV is licensed in the United States and recommended by the CDC.

Influenza VE varies from season to season and is affected by many factors, including age and health status of the recipient, influenza type and subtype, existing immunity from previous infection or vaccination, and degree of antigenic match between vaccine and circulating virus strains. It is possible that VE also differs among individual vaccine products; however, product-specific comparative effectiveness data are lacking for most vaccines. Additional experience spanning multiple influenza seasons will help to determine optimal use of the available vaccine formulations in children. The AAP will continue to monitor annual influenza surveillance and VE reports to update influenza vaccine recommendations if necessary.

CONTRAINDICATIONS AND PRECAUTIONS

Children who have had an allergic reaction after a previous dose of any influenza vaccine should be evaluated by an allergist to determine whether future receipt of the vaccine is appropriate. An anaphylaxis reaction after receipt of any influenza vaccine (IIV or LAIV) may be a contraindication to influenza vaccination. LAIV has specific contraindications (see below). Minor illnesses, with or without fever, are not contraindications to the use of influenza vaccines, including among children with mild upper respiratory infection symptoms or allergic rhinitis. In children with a moderate-to-severe febrile illness (eg, high fever, active infection, requiring hospitalization, etc), on the basis of the judgment of the clinician, vaccination should be deferred until resolution of the illness. Similarly, children with an amount of nasal congestion that would notably impede vaccine delivery into the nasopharyngeal mucosa should have LAIV vaccination deferred until resolution.

History of Guillain-Barré syndrome (GBS) after influenza vaccine is considered a precaution for the administration of influenza vaccines. Data on the risk of GBS after vaccination with seasonal influenza vaccine are variable and have been inconsistent across seasons. If there is an increased risk, it is likely small and primarily in adult patients. GBS is rare, especially in children, and there is a lack of evidence on risk of GBS after influenza vaccine in children. Nonetheless, regardless of age, a history of GBS <6 weeks after a previous dose of influenza vaccine is a precaution for administration of influenza vaccine. The benefits of influenza vaccination might outweigh the risks for certain people who have a history of GBS (particularly if not associated with previous influenza vaccination) and who also are at high risk for severe complications from influenza. Additional precautions for LAIV include a diagnosis of asthma in children older than 5 years and the presence of an underlying medical condition that increases the risk to severe illness with wild-type influenza virus (Table 1). Persons who should not receive LAIV are listed below.

Persons in Whom LAIV Is Contraindicated

- children younger than 2 years;
- children 2 through 4 years of age with a diagnosis of asthma or history of recurrent wheezing or a medically attended wheezing episode in the previous 12 months because of the potential for increased wheezing after immunization. In this age range, many children have a history of wheezing with respiratory tract illnesses and are eventually diagnosed with asthma;
- children who have known or suspected immunodeficiency disease or who are receiving immunosuppressive or immunomodulatory therapies;
- close contacts and caregivers of those who are severely immunocompromised and require a protected environment;
- children and adolescents receiving aspirin or salicylate-containing medications;
- children who have received other live-virus vaccines within the previous 4 weeks (except for rotavirus vaccine); however, LAIV can be administered on the same day with other live-virus vaccines if necessary;
- children taking an influenza antiviral medication and until 48 hours (oseltamivir, zanamivir, peramivir) and up to 2 weeks (baloxavir) after stopping the influenza antiviral therapy. If a child recently received LAIV but has an influenza illness for which antiviral agents are appropriate, the antiviral agents should be given. If antiviral agents are necessary for treatment within 5 to 7 days of LAIV immunization, reimmunization is indicated because of the potential effects of antiviral medications on LAIV replication and immunogenicity; and
- pregnant women.

The safety of LAIV in some high-risk populations has not been definitively established. These conditions are not contraindications but are listed under the "Warnings and Precautions" section of the LAIV package insert, including metabolic disease, diabetes mellitus, other chronic disorders of the pulmonary or cardiovascular systems, renal dysfunction, or hemoglobinopathies. A precaution is a condition in a recipient that might increase the risk or seriousness of an adverse reaction or complicate making another diagnosis because of a possible vaccine-related reaction. A precaution also may exist for conditions that might compromise the ability of the vaccine to produce immunity. Vaccination may be recommended in the presence of a precaution if the benefit of protection from the vaccine outweighs the risk.

LAIV and Immunocompromised Hosts

IIV is the vaccine of choice for anyone in close contact with a subset of severely immunocompromised people (ie, those in a protected environment). IIV is preferred over LAIV for contacts of severely immunocompromised people because of a theoretical risk of infection attributable to LAIV strain in an immunocompromised contact of an LAIV-immunized person. Available data indicate a low risk of transmission of the virus from both children and adults vaccinated with LAIV. Health care personnel (HCP) immunized with LAIV may continue to work in most units of a hospital, including the NICU and general oncology ward, using standard infection control techniques. As a precautionary measure, people recently vaccinated with LAIV should restrict contact with severely immunocompromised patients for 7 days after immunization, although there have been no reports of LAIV transmission from a vaccinated person to an immunocompromised person. In the theoretical scenario in which symptomatic LAIV infection develops in an immunocompromised host, LAIV strains are susceptible to antiviral medications.

INFLUENZA VACCINES AND EGG ALLERGY

There is strong evidence that egg-allergic individuals can safely receive influenza vaccine without any additional precautions beyond those recommended for any vaccine.[1,30,31] The presence of egg allergy in an individual is not a contraindication to receive IIV or LAIV. Vaccine recipients with egg allergy are at no greater risk for a systemic allergic reaction than those without egg allergy. Therefore, precautions such as choice of a particular vaccine, special observation periods, or restriction of administration to particular medical settings are not warranted and constitute an unnecessary barrier to immunization. It is not necessary to inquire about egg allergy before the administration of any influenza vaccine, including on screening forms. Routine prevaccination questions regarding anaphylaxis after receipt of any vaccine are appropriate. Standard vaccination practice for all vaccines in children should include the ability to respond to rare acute hypersensitivity reactions. Children who have had a previous allergic reaction to the influenza vaccine should be evaluated by an allergist to determine whether future receipt of the vaccine is appropriate.

INFLUENZA VACCINES DURING PREGNANCY AND BREASTFEEDING

Influenza vaccine is recommended by the ACIP, the American College of Obstetrics and Gynecology, and the American Academy of Family Physicians for all women during any trimester of gestation for the protection of mothers against influenza and its complications.[1,32] Substantial evidence has accumulated regarding the efficacy of maternal influenza immunization in preventing laboratory-confirmed influenza disease and its complications in both mothers and their infants in the first 2 to 6 months of life.[14,32–37] Pregnant women who are immunized against influenza at any time during their pregnancy provide protection to their infants during their first 6 months of life (when they are too young to receive influenza vaccine themselves) through transplacental passage of antibodies.[38,39] Infants born to women who receive influenza vaccination during pregnancy can have a risk reduction of 72% (95% CI, 39% to 87%) for laboratory-confirmed influenza hospitalization in the first few months of life.[40]

It is safe to administer IIV to pregnant women during any trimester of gestation and postpartum. Any licensed, recommended, and age-appropriate influenza vaccine may be used, although experience with the use of RIV4 in pregnant women is limited. LAIV is contraindicated during pregnancy. Data on the safety of influenza vaccination at any time during pregnancy continues to accumulate and support the safety of influenza immunization during pregnancy. In a 5-year retrospective cohort study from 2003 to 2008 with more than 10 000 women, influenza vaccination in the first trimester was not associated with an increase in the rates of major congenital malformations.[41] Similarly, a systematic review and meta-analysis of studies of congenital anomalies after vaccination during pregnancy, including data from 15 studies (14 cohort studies and 1 case-control study), did not show any association between congenital defects and influenza vaccination in any trimester, including the first trimester of gestation.[42] Assessments of any association with influenza vaccination and preterm birth and infants who are small for gestational age have yielded inconsistent results, with most studies reporting a protective effect or no association against these outcomes. Authors of a cohort study from the Vaccines and Medications in Pregnancy Surveillance System of vaccine exposure during the 2010–2011 through 2013–2014 seasons found no significant association of spontaneous abortion with influenza vaccine exposure in the first trimester or within the first 20 weeks of gestation.[43] One recent observational Vaccine Safety Datalink study conducted during the 2010–2011 and 2011–2012 seasons noted an association between receipt of IIV containing H1N1pdm09 and risk of spontaneous abortion when an H1N1pdm-09-containing vaccine had also been received the previous season.[44] A follow-up study conducted by the same investigators with a larger population did not reveal this association and further supported the safety of influenza vaccine during pregnancy.

Postpartum women who did not receive influenza vaccination during pregnancy should be encouraged to discuss with their obstetrician, family physician, nurse midwife, or other trusted provider receipt of the vaccine before discharge from the hospital. Vaccination during breastfeeding is safe for mothers and their infants.

Breastfeeding is strongly recommended to protect infants against influenza viruses by activating innate antiviral mechanisms, specifically type 1 interferons. Human milk from mothers vaccinated during the third trimester also contains higher levels of influenza-specific immunoglobulin A.[45] Greater exclusivity of breastfeeding in the first 6 months of life decreases the episodes of respiratory illness with fever in infants of vaccinated mothers. For infants born to mothers with confirmed influenza illness at delivery, breastfeeding is encouraged, and guidance on breastfeeding practices can be found at https://www.cdc.gov/breastfeeding/breastfeeding-special-circumstances/maternal-or-infant-illnesses/influenza.html and https://www.cdc.gov/flu/professionals/infectioncontrol/peri-post-settings.htm. Breastfeeding should be encouraged even if the mother or infant has influenza. The mother should pump and feed expressed milk if she or her infant are too sick to breastfeed. If the breastfeeding mother requires antiviral agents, treatment with oral oseltamivir is preferred. The CDC does not recommend use of baloxavir for treatment of pregnant women or breastfeeding mothers. There are no available efficacy or safety data in pregnant women, and there are no available data on the presence of baloxavir in human milk, the effects on the breastfed infant, or the effects on milk production.

VACCINE STORAGE AND ADMINISTRATION

The AAP Vaccine Storage and Handling Tip Sheet provides resources for practices to develop comprehensive vaccine management protocols to keep the temperature for vaccine storage constant during a power failure or other disaster (https://www.aap.org/en-us/Documents/immunization_disasterplanning.pdf). The AAP recommends the development of a written disaster plan for all practice settings. Additional information is available at www.aap.org/disasters.

IIVs

IIVs for intramuscular injection are shipped and stored at 2°C to 8°C (36°F–46°F); vaccines that are inadvertently frozen should not be used. These vaccines are administered intramuscularly into the anterolateral thigh of infants and young children and into the deltoid muscle of older children and adults. Given that various IIVs are available, careful attention should be used to ensure that each product is used for its approved age indication, dosing, and volume of administration (Table 2). A 0.5-mL unit dose of any IIV should not be split into 2 separate 0.25-mL doses. If a lower dose than recommended is inadvertently administered to a child 36 months or older (eg, 0.25 mL), an additional 0.25-mL dose should be administered to provide a full dose of 0.5 mL as soon as possible. The total number of full doses appropriate for age should be administered. If a child is inadvertently vaccinated with a formulation approved for adults, the dose should be counted as valid.

LAIV

The cold-adapted, temperature-sensitive LAIV4 formulation currently licensed in the United States is shipped and stored at 2°C to 8°C (35°F–46°F) and administered intranasally in a prefilled, single-use sprayer containing 0.2 mL of vaccine. A removable dose-divider clip is attached to the sprayer to facilitate administration of 0.1 mL separately into each nostril. If the child sneezes immediately after administration, the dose should not be repeated.

VACCINE DOSING RECOMMENDATIONS

The number of seasonal influenza vaccine doses recommended for children during the 2019–2020 influenza season depends on the child's age at the time of the first administered dose and vaccine history. The recommendations are unchanged from previous years, as shown in Fig 1.

1. Influenza vaccines are not licensed for administration to infants younger than 6 months and should not be used in this age group.
2. Children 9 years and older need only 1 dose, regardless of previous vaccination history.
3. Children 6 months through 8 years of age:
   a. Need 2 doses if they have received fewer than 2 doses of any trivalent or quadrivalent influenza vaccine (IIV or LAIV) before July 1, 2019. The interval between the 2 doses should be at least 4 weeks. Two

doses should be administered to children who receive their first dose before their ninth birthday, even when they turn 9 years old during the same season.

b. Require only 1 dose if they have previously received 2 or more total doses of any trivalent or quadrivalent influenza vaccine (IIV or LAIV) before July 1, 2019. The 2 previous doses do not need to have been received during the same influenza season or consecutive influenza seasons.

TIMING OF VACCINATION AND DURATION OF PROTECTION

Although peak influenza activity in the United States tends to occur from January through March, influenza can circulate from early fall (October) to late spring (May), with 1 or more disease peaks. Predicting the onset and duration or the severity of the influenza season is impossible. It is also challenging to balance public health strategies needed to achieve high vaccination coverage with achieving optimal individual immunity for protection against influenza at the peak of seasonal activity, knowing that the duration of immunity after vaccination can wane over time. Initiation of influenza vaccination before influenza is circulating in the community and continuing to vaccinate throughout the influenza season are important components of an effective influenza vaccination strategy.

Complete influenza vaccination by the end of October is recommended by the CDC and AAP. Children who need 2 doses of vaccine should receive their first dose as soon as possible when the vaccine becomes available to allow sufficient time for receipt of the second dose ≥4 weeks after the first before the onset of the influenza season. Children who require only 1 dose of influenza vaccine should also ideally be vaccinated by end of October; however, recent data (mostly in adults) suggest that early vaccination (July or August) might be associated with suboptimal immunity before the end of the influenza season.

Although the evidence is limited that waning immunity from early administration of the vaccine increases the risk of infection in children, authors of recent reports raise the possibility that early vaccination might contribute to reduced protection later in the influenza season.[46–55] These observational studies and a post hoc analysis from a randomized controlled trial (RCT) were reviewed by the ACIP influenza working group and are summarized in the CDC recommendations for 2019–2020 influenza prevention.[1] In these studies, VE decreased within a single influenza season, and this decrease was correlated with increasing time after vaccination. However, this decay in VE was not consistent across different age groups and varied by season and virus subtypes. In some studies, waning VE was more evident among older adults and younger children,[47,49] and with influenza A(H3N2) viruses more than influenza A(H1N1) or B viruses.[48,51,53] A multiseason analysis from the US Influenza VE Network found that VE declined by approximately 7% per month for influenza A(H3N2) and influenza B and by 6% to 11% per month for influenza A(H1N1)pdm09 in individuals 9 years and older.[46] VE remained greater than 0 for at least 5 to 6 months after vaccination. A more recent study including children older than 2 years of age also found evidence of declining VE with an odds ratio increasing approximately 16% with each additional 28 days from vaccine administration.[52] Another study evaluating VE from the 2011–2012 through the 2013–2014 seasons demonstrated 54% to 67% protection from 0 to 180 days after vaccination.[50] Finally, a multiseason study in Europe from 2011–2012 through 2014–2015 revealed a steady decline in VE down to 0% protection by 111 days after vaccination.[48,53]

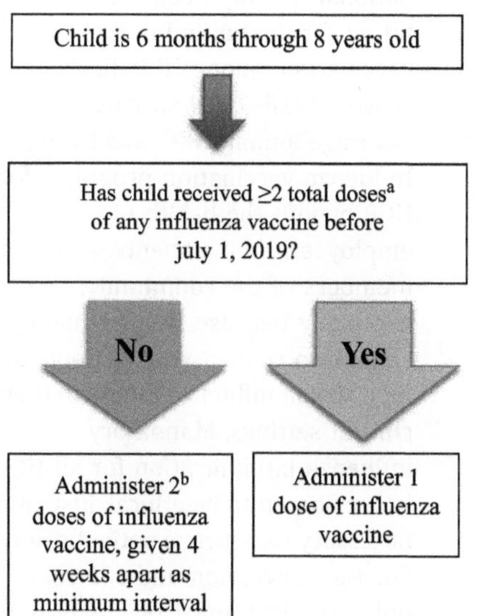

FIGURE 1
Number of 2019–2020 seasonal influenza vaccine doses for children based on age and previous vaccination history and recommendations for prevention and control of influenza in children, 2019–2020. [a] The 2 doses need not have been received during the same season or consecutive seasons. [b] Administer 2 doses based on age at receipt of the first dose of influenza vaccine during the season. Children who receive the first dose before their ninth birthday should receive 2 doses, even if they turn 9 years old during the same season.

Further evaluation is needed before any policy change in timing of influenza administration is made. An early onset of the influenza season is a concern when considering delaying vaccination. Until there are definitive data that determine if waning immunity influences VE in children, administration of influenza vaccine should not be delayed to a later date because this increases the likelihood of missing influenza vaccination altogether.[56,57] Providers may continue to offer the vaccine until June 30 of each year when the seasonal influenza vaccine expires because the duration of influenza circulation is unpredictable. Although influenza activity in the United States is typically low during the summer, influenza cases and outbreaks can occur, particularly among international travelers, who may be exposed to influenza year-round, depending on the destination.

VACCINE IMPLEMENTATION

The AAP Partnership for Policy Implementation has developed a series of definitions using accepted health information technology standards to assist in the implementation of vaccine recommendations in computer systems and quality measurement efforts. This document is available at www2.aap.org/informatics/PPI.html. In addition, the AAP has developed implementation guidance on supply, payment, coding, and liability issues; these documents can be found at www.aapredbook.org/implementation.

HCP, influenza campaign organizers, and public health agencies are encouraged to collaborate to develop improved strategies for planning, distribution, communication, and administration of vaccines.

- Plan to make influenza vaccine easily accessible for all children. Examples include sending alerts to families that the vaccine is available (eg, e-mails, texts, letters, patient portals, practice-specific websites or social media platforms); creating walk-in influenza vaccination clinics; extending hours beyond routine times during peak vaccination periods; administering the influenza vaccine during both well-child examinations and sick visits as well as in hospitalized patients, especially those at high risk of influenza complications, before hospital discharge (unless medically contraindicated); implementing standing orders for influenza vaccination; considering how to immunize parents, adult caregivers, and siblings (see risk management guidance associated with adult immunizations at http://pediatrics.aappublications.org/content/129/1/e247) at the same time as children; and working with other institutions (eg, schools, child care programs, local public health departments, and religious organizations) or alternative care sites, such as pharmacies and hospital emergency departments, to expand venues for administering vaccine. If a child receives influenza vaccine outside of his or her medical home, such as at a pharmacy, retail-based clinic, or another practice setting, appropriate documentation of vaccination should be provided to the patient to be shared with his or her medical home and entered into the state or regional immunization information system (ie, registry).
- Concerted efforts among the aforementioned groups, plus vaccine manufacturers, distributors, and payers, are necessary to prioritize distribution appropriately to the primary care office setting and patient-centered medical home before other venues, especially when vaccine supplies are delayed or limited. Similar efforts should be made to mitigate the vaccine supply discrepancy between privately insured patients and those eligible for vaccination through the Vaccines for Children program.
- Population health can benefit from pediatricians' discussions about vaccine safety and effectiveness. Pediatricians and their office staff can influence vaccine acceptance by explaining the importance of annual influenza vaccination for children and emphasizing when a second dose of vaccine is indicated. The AAP and CDC have created communication resources to convey these important messages and to help the public understand influenza recommendations. Resources will be available on *Red Book Online* (https://redbook.solutions.aap.org/selfserve/ssPage.aspx?SelfServeContentId=influenza-resources).
- The AAP supports mandatory influenza vaccination programs for all HCP in all settings, including outpatient settings.[58] Optimal prevention of influenza in the health care setting depends on the vaccination of at least 90% of HCP, which is consistent with the national Healthy People 2020 target for annual influenza vaccination among HCP. Early-season 2018–2019 vaccine coverage among HCP was 67.6%. Influenza vaccination programs for HCP benefit the health of employees, their patients, and members of the community, especially because HCP frequently come into contact with patients at high risk of influenza illness in their clinical settings. Mandatory influenza immunization for all HCP is considered to be ethical, just, and necessary to improve patient safety. For the prevention and control of influenza, HCP must prioritize the health and safety of their patients, honor the requirement of causing no harm, and act as role models for both their patients and colleagues by receiving influenza vaccination annually.

INFLUENZA VACCINE COVERAGE

Although national influenza vaccination coverage among children has not declined in the past 3 seasons, overall vaccination coverage remains suboptimal. Additional options for vaccination of children may provide a means to improve coverage, particularly in pharmacies and child care and school-based settings. Achieving high coverage rates of influenza vaccine in infants and children is a priority to protect them against influenza disease and its complications.

Children's likelihood of being immunized according to recommendations appears to be associated with the immunization practices of their parents.[59–63] Authors of 1 study found that children were 2.77 times (95% CI, 2.74 to 2.79) more likely to be immunized against seasonal influenza if their parents were immunized.[33] When parents who were previously not immunized had received immunization for seasonal influenza, their children were 5.44 times (95% CI, 5.35 to 5.53) more likely to receive influenza vaccine.

Pediatric offices may choose to serve as a venue for providing influenza vaccination for parents and other care providers of children if the practice is acceptable to both pediatricians and the adults who are to be vaccinated. Medical liability issues and medical record documentation requirements need to be considered before a pediatrician begins immunizing adults (see risk management guidance associated with adult immunizations at http://pediatrics.aappublications.org/content/129/1/e247). Pediatric practices should be aware of payment implications, including nonpayment or having the parent inappropriately attributed by a payer as a patient of the pediatrician's office. The AAP supports efforts to overcome these payment barriers with insurance payers to maximize influenza immunization rates. To avoid errors in claims processing and payment and in the exchange of immunization data, pediatricians are reminded that parents should have their own basic medical record in which their influenza vaccination should be documented. Adults should be encouraged to have a medical home and communicate their vaccination status to their primary care provider. Offering adult vaccinations in the pediatric practice setting should not undermine the adult medical home model. Vaccination of close contacts of children at high risk of influenza-related complications (Table 1) is intended to reduce children's risk of exposure to influenza (ie, "cocooning"). The practice of cocooning also may help protect infants younger than 6 months who are too young to be immunized with influenza vaccine.

SURVEILLANCE

Information about influenza surveillance is available through the CDC Voice Information System (influenza update at 1-800-232-4636) or at www.cdc.gov/flu/index.htm. Although current influenza season data on circulating strains do not necessarily predict which and in what proportion strains will circulate in the subsequent season, it is instructive to be aware of 2018–2019 influenza surveillance data and use them as a guide to empirical therapy until current seasonal data are available from the CDC. Information is posted weekly on the CDC Web site (www.cdc.gov/flu/weekly/fluactivitysurv.htm). The AAP offers "What's the Latest with the Flu" (https://www.aap.org/en-us/advocacy-and-policy/aap-health-initiatives/Pages/What's-the-Latest-with-the-Flu.aspx) messages to highlight those details most relevant for AAP members and child care providers on a monthly basis during influenza season.

INFLUENZA VACCINATION RECOMMENDATIONS

1. The AAP recommends annual influenza vaccination for everyone 6 months and older, including children and adolescents, during the 2019–2020 influenza season.
2. For the 2019–2020 season, the AAP recommends that any licensed influenza vaccine appropriate for age and health status can be used for influenza vaccination in children. IIV and LAIV are options for children for whom these vaccines are appropriate. This recommendation is based on review of current available data on LAIV and IIV VE. The AAP will continue to review VE data as they become available and update these recommendations if necessary.
3. The AAP does not have a preference for any influenza vaccine product over another for children who have no contraindication to influenza vaccination and for whom more than 1 licensed product appropriate for age and health status is available. Pediatricians should administer whichever formulation is available in their communities to achieve the highest possible coverage this influenza season.
4. Children 6 through 35 months of age may receive either a 0.25- or 0.5-mL dose of the licensed, age-appropriate IIVs available this season. No product or formulation is preferred over another for this age group. Children 36 months (3 years) and older should receive a 0.5-mL dose of any available, licensed, age-appropriate inactivated vaccine.
5. The number of seasonal influenza vaccine doses recommended to

be administered to children in the 2019–2020 influenza season remains unchanged and depends on the child's age at the time of the first administered dose and vaccine history (Fig 1).

6. Children 6 months through 8 years of age who are receiving the influenza vaccine for the first time or who have received only 1 dose before July 1, 2019, should receive 2 doses of influenza vaccine ideally by the end of October, and vaccines should be offered as soon as they become available. Children needing only 1 dose of influenza vaccine, regardless of age, should also receive the vaccination ideally by the end of October.
7. Efforts should be made to ensure vaccination for children in high-risk groups (Table 1) and their contacts unless contraindicated.
8. Product-specific contraindications must be considered when selecting the type of vaccine to administer. Children who have had an allergic reaction after a previous dose of any influenza vaccine should be evaluated by an allergist to determine whether future receipt of the vaccine is appropriate.
9. Children with egg allergy can receive influenza vaccine without any additional precautions beyond those recommended for all vaccines.
10. Pregnant women may receive IIV at any time during pregnancy to protect themselves and their infants who benefit from the transplacental transfer of antibodies. Postpartum women who did not receive vaccination during pregnancy should be encouraged to receive influenza vaccine before discharge from the hospital. Influenza vaccination during breastfeeding is safe for mothers and their infants.
11. The AAP supports mandatory vaccination of HCP as a crucial element in preventing influenza and reducing health care–associated influenza infections because HCP often care for individuals at high risk for influenza-related complications.

INFLUENZA ANTIVIRALS

Antiviral agents available for both influenza treatment and chemoprophylaxis in children of all ages can be found in Table 3 (including doses for preterm infants that have not been evaluated by the FDA) and on the CDC Web site (www.cdc.gov/flu/professionals/antivirals/index.htm). These include the neuraminidase inhibitors (NAIs) (oseltamivir, zanamivir, peramivir) and a selective inhibitor of influenza cap-dependent endonuclease (baloxavir),[64] all of which have activity against influenza A and B viruses.

Oral oseltamivir remains the antiviral drug of choice for the management of illness caused by influenza virus infections. Although more difficult to administer, inhaled zanamivir (Relenza) is an equally acceptable alternative for patients who do not have chronic respiratory disease. Options are limited for children who cannot absorb orally or enterally administered oseltamivir or tolerate inhaled zanamivir. Intravenous (IV) peramivir (Rapivab), a third NAI, was approved in September 2017 as treatment of acute uncomplicated influenza in nonhospitalized children 2 years and older who have been symptomatic for no more than 2 days. The efficacy of peramivir in patients with serious influenza requiring hospitalization has not been established.[65] A prospective, open-label pediatric clinical trial was conducted to investigate pharmacokinetics and the clinical and virological response to treatment with IV zanamivir for children aged 6 months or older with severe influenza and who could not tolerate oral or inhaled NAIs.[66] IV zanamivir is not approved in the United States. IV zanamivir for compassionate use has not been available in the United States since the 2017–2018 season.[67] The FDA licensed baloxavir marboxil in 2018 for the early treatment of uncomplicated influenza in outpatients 12 years and older who have been ill for no more than 2 days. This antiviral agent for influenza works by a different mechanism than NAIs and requires only a single oral dose for treatment of uncomplicated influenza.[68] A clinical trial of baloxavir treatment of influenza in hospitalized patients is ongoing (https://clinicaltrials.gov/ct2/show/NCT03684044?cond=baloxavir&rank=6).

INFLUENZA TREATMENT

In RCTs conducted to date to evaluate the efficacy of influenza antiviral medications among outpatients with uncomplicated influenza, researchers have found that timely treatment can reduce the duration of influenza symptoms and fever, as well as the risk of certain complications, including hospitalization and death in pediatric and adult populations.[30,31,41,42,45,69,70] The number of published RCTs in children is limited, and interpretation of the results of these studies needs to take into consideration the size of the study (the number of events might not be sufficient to assess specific outcomes in small studies), the variations in the case definition of influenza illness (clinically diagnosed versus laboratory confirmed), the time of treatment administration in relation to the onset of illness, and the child's age and health status as important variables. A Cochrane review of 6 RCTs[2,3,71] involving treatment of 2356 children with clinical influenza,[1,2,72] of whom 1255

TABLE 3 Recommended Dosage and Schedule of Influenza Antiviral Medications for Treatment and Chemoprophylaxis in Children for the 2019–2020 Influenza Season: United States

Medication	Treatment (5 d)	Chemoprophylaxis (10 d)[a]
Oseltamivir[b]		
Adults	75 mg, twice daily	75 mg, once daily
Children ≥12 mo (based on body wt)		
≤15 kg (≤33 lb)	30 mg, twice daily	30 mg, once daily
>15–23 kg (33–51 lb)	45 mg, twice daily	45 mg, once daily
>23–40 kg (>51–88 lb)	60 mg, twice daily	60 mg, once daily
>40 kg (>88 lb)	75 mg, twice daily	75 mg, once daily
Infants 9–11 mo[c]	3.5 mg/kg per dose, twice daily	3.5 mg/kg per dose, once daily
Term infants 0–8 mo[c]	3 mg/kg per dose, twice daily	3 mg/kg per dose, once daily for infants 3–8 mo Not recommended for infants <3 mo old because of limited safety and efficacy data in this age group
Preterm infants[d]		
<38 wk' postmenstrual age	1.0 mg/kg per dose, twice daily	—
38 through 40 wk' postmenstrual age	1.5 mg/kg per dose, twice daily	—
>40 wk' postmenstrual age	3.0 mg/kg per dose, twice daily	—
Zanamivir[e]		
Adults	10 mg (two 5-mg inhalations), twice daily	10 mg (two 5-mg inhalations), once daily
Children ≥7 y for treatment ≥5 y for chemoprophylaxis	10 mg (two 5-mg inhalations), twice daily	10 mg (two 5-mg inhalations), once daily
Peramivir		
Adults	One 600-mg IV infusion, given over 15–30 min	Not recommended
Children (2–12 y)	One 12 mg/kg dose, up to 600 mg maximum, via IV infusion for 15–30 min	Not recommended
Children (13–17 y)	One 600 mg dose, via IV infusion for 15–30 min	Not recommended
Baloxavir		
People ≥12 y who weigh more than 40 kg	40–80 kg: one 40-mg dose, orally ≥80 kg: one 80-mg dose, orally	Not recommended

Sources: 2018 IDSA Guidelines[65] and https://www.cdc.gov/flu/professionals/antivirals/summary-clinicians.htm. —, not applicable.

[a] CDC recommends for 7 days and 10 days only if part of institutional outbreak (https://www.cdc.gov/flu/professionals/antivirals/summary-clinicians.htm).

[b] Oseltamivir is administered orally without regard to meals, although administration with meals may improve gastrointestinal tolerability. Oseltamivir is available as Tamiflu in 30-, 45-, and 75-mg capsules and as a powder for oral suspension that is reconstituted to provide a final concentration of 6 mg/mL. For the 6-mg/mL suspension, a 30-mg dose is given with 5 mL of oral suspension, a 45-mg dose is given with 7.5 mL of oral suspension, a 60-mg dose is given with 10 mL of oral suspension, and a 75-mg dose is given with 12.5 mL of oral suspension. If the commercially manufactured oral suspension is not available, a suspension can be compounded by retail pharmacies (final concentration also 6 mg/mL) on the basis of instructions contained in the package label. In patients with renal insufficiency, the dose should be adjusted on the basis of creatinine clearance. For treatment of patients with creatinine clearance 10–30 mL/min: 75 mg, once daily, for 5 d. For chemoprophylaxis of patients with creatinine clearance 10–30 mL/min: 30 mg, once daily, for 10 d after exposure or 75 mg, once every other day, for 10 d after exposure (5 doses). See https://www.cdc.gov/flu/professionals/antivirals/summary-clinicians.htm and IDSA guidelines.[65]

[c] Approved by the FDA for children as young as 2 wk of age. Given preliminary pharmacokinetic data and limited safety data, oseltamivir can be used to treat influenza in both term and preterm infants from birth because benefits of therapy are likely to outweigh possible risks of treatment. Of note, the CDC recommends a 3 mg/kg per dose, twice daily, for all infants <12 mo old; the IDSA guidelines[65] include both AAP and CDC recommendations.

[d] Oseltamivir dosing for preterm infants. The wt-based dosing recommendation for preterm infants is lower than for term infants. Preterm infants may have lower clearance of oseltamivir because of immature renal function, and doses recommended for term infants may lead to high drug concentrations in this age group. Limited data from the National Institute of Allergy and Infectious Diseases Collaborative Antiviral Study Group provides the basis for dosing preterm infants using their postmenstrual age (gestational age + chronologic age). For extremely preterm infants (<28 wk), please consult a pediatric infectious disease physician.

[e] Zanamivir is administered by inhalation using a proprietary "Diskhaler" device distributed together with the medication. Zanamivir is a dry powder, not an aerosol, and should not be administered using nebulizers, ventilators, or other devices typically used for administering medications in aerosolized solutions. Zanamivir is not recommended for people with chronic respiratory diseases, such as asthma or chronic obstructive pulmonary disease, which increase the risk of bronchospasm.

had laboratory-confirmed influenza, revealed that in children with laboratory-confirmed influenza, oral oseltamivir and inhaled zanamivir reduced the median duration of illness by 36 hours (26%; $P < .001$) and 1.3 days (24%, $P < .001$), respectively.[68] Among the studies reviewed, 1 trial of oseltamivir in children with asthma who had laboratory-confirmed influenza revealed only a nonsignificant reduction in illness duration (10.4 hours; 8%; $P = .542$). Oseltamivir significantly reduced acute otitis media in children 1 through 5 years of age with laboratory-confirmed influenza (risk difference, −0.14; 95% CI, −0.24 to −0.04).[73] Authors of another Cochrane review of RCTs in adults and children, which included 20 oseltamivir (9623 participants) and 26 zanamivir trials (14 628 participants),[74] found no effect of oseltamivir in reducing the duration of illness in asthmatic children, but in otherwise healthy children, there was a reduction by a mean difference of 29 hours (95% CI, 12 to 47 hours; *P* = .001). No significant effect was observed with zanamivir. Regarding complications, the authors of this review did not find a significant effect of NAIs on reducing hospitalizations, pneumonia, bronchitis, otitis media, or sinusitis in children.[75] More recently, a meta-analysis of 5 new RCTs that included 1598 children with laboratory-confirmed influenza revealed that treatment with oseltamivir significantly reduced the duration of illness in this population by 17.6 hours (95% CI, −34.7 to −0.62 hours), and when children with asthma were excluded, this difference was larger (−29.9 hours; 95% CI, −53.9 to −5.8 hours). The risk of otitis media was 34% lower in this group as well.[31] Overall, efficacy outcomes are best demonstrated in patients with laboratory-confirmed influenza. All these studies confirmed vomiting as an occasional side effect of oseltamivir, occurring in approximately 5% of treated patients. The balance between benefits and harms should be considered when making decisions about the use of NAIs for either treatment or chemoprophylaxis of influenza.

Although prospective comparative studies used to determine the efficacy of influenza antiviral medications in hospitalized patients or pediatric patients with comorbidities have not been conducted, and prospectively collected data used to determine the role of antiviral agents in treating severe influenza are limited, on the basis of information obtained from retrospective observational studies and meta-analyses conducted to date in both adults and children, most experts support the use of antiviral medications as soon as possible to treat pediatric patients with severe influenza, including hospitalized patients.[76–79] In an observational epidemiological study conducted in adult patients hospitalized with severe laboratory-confirmed influenza in Spain spanning 6 influenza seasons (2010–2016), authors evaluated the effectiveness of NAIs, concluding that when started early after the onset of symptoms (≤48 hours or ≤5 days), NAI treatment was associated with a reduction in influenza-associated deaths (adjusted odds ratio, 0.37; 95% CI, 0.22 to 0.63l, and adjusted odds ratio, 0.50; 95% CI, 0.32 to 0.79, respectively).[80,81] However, treatment initiation more than 5 days after the onset of influenza symptoms was not associated with reduction in mortality in hospitalized adults.

Importantly, and despite limited evidence for efficacy, treatment with oseltamivir for children with serious, complicated, or progressive disease presumptively or definitively caused by influenza, irrespective of influenza vaccination status (the circulating strains may not be well matched with vaccine strains) or whether illness began greater than 48 hours before admission, continues to be recommended by the AAP, CDC, Infectious Diseases Society of America (IDSA),[65] and Pediatric Infectious Diseases Society (PIDS). Earlier treatment provides better clinical responses. However, treatment after 48 hours of symptoms in adults and children with moderate-to-severe disease or with progressive disease has been shown to provide some benefit and should be offered. No benefit exists for double-dose NAI therapy, compared to standard-dose therapy, on the basis of published data from a randomized prospective trial enrolling 75% of subjects younger than 15 years.[1]

Children younger than 2 years are at an increased risk of hospitalization and complications attributable to influenza. The FDA has approved oseltamivir for treatment of children as young as 2 weeks. Given preliminary pharmacokinetic data and limited safety data, the CDC and AAP support the use of oseltamivir to treat influenza in both term and preterm infants from birth because the benefits of therapy of neonatal influenza are likely to outweigh the possible risks of treatment.

Oseltamivir is available in capsule and oral suspension formulations. The available capsule doses are 30, 45, and 75 mg, and the commercially manufactured liquid formulation has a concentration of 6 mg/mL in a 60-mL bottle. If the commercially manufactured oral suspension is not available, the capsule may be opened and the contents mixed with simple syrup or Ora-Sweet SF (sugar free) by retail pharmacies to a final concentration of 6 mg/mL.

In adverse event data collected systematically in prospective trials, vomiting was the only adverse effect reported more often with oseltamivir compared to placebo when studied in children 1 through 12 years of age (ie, 15% of treated children vs 9% receiving placebo). In addition, after reports from Japan of oseltamivir-attributable neuropsychiatric adverse effects, authors of a review of controlled clinical trial data and ongoing surveillance have failed to establish a link between this drug and neurologic or psychiatric events.[66,82]

Clinical judgment (based on underlying conditions, disease severity, time since symptom onset, and local influenza activity) is an important factor in treatment decisions for pediatric patients who present with influenzalike illness. Antiviral treatment should be started as soon as possible after illness onset and should not be delayed while waiting for a definitive influenza test result because early therapy provides the best outcomes. Influenza diagnostic tests vary by method, availability, processing time, sensitivity, and cost (Table 4), all of which should be considered in making the best clinical decision. Positive and negative predictive values of influenza test results are influenced by the level of influenza activity in the population being tested, the characteristics of a test compared to a gold standard, pretest probability, whether the influenza virus is actively replicating in the person, proper collection and transport of specimens, and proper test procedures. Testing should be performed when timely results will be available to influence clinical management or infection control measures. Although decisions on treatment and infection control can be made on the basis of positive rapid antigen test results, negative results should not always be used in a similar fashion because of the suboptimal sensitivity and potential for false-negative results. Positive results of rapid influenza tests are helpful, because they may reduce additional testing to identify the cause of the child's influenzalike illness and promote appropriate antimicrobial stewardship. Available FDA-approved rapid molecular assays are highly sensitive and specific in diagnostic tests performed in <20 minutes using RNA detection. These and other FDA-approved influenza molecular assays or reverse transcription polymerase chain reaction (RT-PCR) test confirmation are preferred in hospitalized patients because they are more sensitive compared to antigen detection. Early detection, prompt antiviral treatment, and infection control interventions can lead to improved individual patient outcomes and allow for effective cohorting and disease containment.

People with suspected influenza who are at higher risk of influenza complications should be offered treatment with antiviral medications (Table 1). Efforts should be made to minimize treatment of patients who are not infected with influenza. Otherwise healthy children who have suspected influenza with an uncomplicated presentation should be considered for antiviral medication, particularly if they are in contact with other children who either are younger than 6 months (because they are not able to receive influenza vaccine) or have high-risk conditions (including young age) that predispose them to complications of influenza, when influenza viruses are known to be circulating in the community. If there is a local shortage of antiviral medications, local public health authorities should be consulted to provide additional guidance about testing and treatment. In previous years, local shortages of oseltamivir suspension have occurred because of uneven drug distribution, although national shortages have not occurred since 2009, particularly given the availability of the capsule formulation that can be made into a suspension for young children if needed (Table 3).

INFLUENZA CHEMOPROPHYLAXIS

Randomized placebo-controlled studies revealed that oral oseltamivir and inhaled zanamivir were efficacious when administered as chemoprophylaxis to household contacts after a family member had laboratory-confirmed influenza.[1,41] There are no data on IV peramivir or oral baloxavir for chemoprophylaxis. During the 2009 pandemic, the emergence of oseltamivir resistance was noted rarely among people receiving postexposure chemoprophylaxis, highlighting the need to be aware of the possibility of emerging resistance in this population. Decisions on whether to administer antiviral chemoprophylaxis should take into

TABLE 4 Comparison of Types of Influenza Diagnostic Tests

Testing Category	Method	Influenza Viruses Detected	Distinguishes Influenza A Virus Subtypes	Time to Results	Performance
Rapid molecular assay	Nucleic acid amplification	Influenza A or B viral RNA	No	15–30 min	High sensitivity; high specificity
Rapid influenza diagnostic test	Antigen detection	Influenza A or B virus antigens	No	10–15 min	Low-to-moderate sensitivity (higher with analyzer devise); high specificity
Direct and indirect immunofluorescence assays	Antigen detection	Influenza A or B virus antigens	No	1–4 h	Moderate sensitivity; high specificity
Molecular assays (including RT-PCR)	Nucleic acid amplification	Influenza A or B viral RNA	Yes, if subtype primers are used	1–8 h	High sensitivity; high specificity
Multiplex molecular assays	Nucleic acid amplification	Influenza A or B viral RNA, other viral or bacterial targets (RNA or DNA)	Yes, if subtype primers are used	1–2 h	High sensitivity; high specificity
Rapid cell culture (shell vial and cell mixtures)	Virus isolation	Influenza A or B virus	Yes	1–3 d	High sensitivity; high specificity
Viral culture (tissue cell culture)	Virus isolation	Influenza A or B virus	Yes	3–10 d	High sensitivity; high specificity

Negative test results may not rule out influenza. Respiratory tract specimens should be collected as close to illness onset as possible for testing. Clinicians should consult the manufacturer's package insert for the specific test for the approved respiratory specimen(s). Specificities are generally high (>95%) for all tests compared to RT-PCR. FDA-cleared rapid influenza diagnostic tests are waived by the Clinical Laboratory Improvement Amendments of 1988; most FDA-cleared rapid influenza molecular assays are waived by the Clinical Laboratory Improvement Amendments of 1988, depending on the specimen. Adapted from Uyeki TM, Bernstein HH, Bradley JS, et al. Clinical practice guidelines by the Infectious Diseases Society of America: 2018 update on diagnosis, treatment, chemoprophylaxis, and institutional outbreak management of seasonal influenza. *Clin Infect Dis.* 2019;68(6):e13.

account the exposed person's risk of influenza complications, vaccination status, the type and duration of contact, recommendations from local or public health authorities, and clinical judgment. Optimally, postexposure chemoprophylaxis should only be used when antiviral agents can be started within 48 hours of exposure; the lower once-daily dosing for chemoprophylaxis with oral oseltamivir or inhaled zanamivir should not be used for the treatment of children symptomatic with influenza. Early, full treatment doses (rather than chemoprophylaxis doses) should be used in high-risk symptomatic patients without waiting for laboratory confirmation.

Chemoprophylaxis should not be considered a substitute for vaccination. Influenza vaccine should always be offered before and throughout the influenza season when not contraindicated. Antiviral medications are important adjuncts to influenza vaccination for the control and prevention of influenza disease. Toxicities may be associated with antiviral agents, and indiscriminate use might limit availability. Pediatricians should inform recipients of antiviral chemoprophylaxis that the risk of influenza is lowered but still remains while taking the medication, and susceptibility to influenza returns when the medication is discontinued. Oseltamivir use is not a contraindication to vaccination with IIV, although LAIV effectiveness will be decreased for the child receiving oseltamivir.[66] No data are available on the impact of inhaled zanamivir or oral baloxavir on the effectiveness of LAIV, but it is likely that all antiviral medication will have some impact on effectiveness of LAIV. Among some high-risk people, both vaccination with IIV and antiviral chemoprophylaxis may be considered. Updates will be available at www.aapredbook.org/flu and www.cdc.gov/flu/professionals/antivirals/index.htm.

ANTIVIRAL RESISTANCE

Antiviral resistance to any drug can emerge, necessitating continuous population-based assessment that is conducted by the CDC. During the 2018–2019 season, >99% of influenza A(/H1N1)pdm09 viruses tested were susceptible to oseltamivir and peramivir, and all of the tested influenza virus strains were susceptible to zanamivir. All tested influenza A(H3N2) viruses were susceptible to oseltamivir, zanamivir, and peramivir. Influenza B virus strains were all susceptible to oseltamivir and zanamivir, and >99% were susceptible to peramivir. Decreased susceptibility to baloxavir has been reported in Japan where use has been more common,[83–85] and surveillance for resistance among circulating influenza viruses is ongoing in the United States.[83,86] In contrast, high levels of resistance to amantadine and rimantadine persist among the influenza A viruses currently circulating. Adamantane medications are not recommended for use against influenza unless resistance patterns change.[1]

Recent viral surveillance and resistance data from the CDC and WHO indicate that the majority of currently circulating influenza viruses likely to cause influenza in North America during the 2019–2020 season continue to be susceptible to oseltamivir, zanamivir, peramivir, and baloxavir.[1] If a newly emergent oseltamivir- or peramivir-resistant virus is a concern, recommendations for alternative treatment, such as use of IV zanamivir,[87,88] will be available from the CDC and AAP. Resistance characteristics can change for an individual child over the duration of a treatment course, especially in those who are severely immunocompromised and may receive extended courses of antiviral medications because of prolonged viral shedding. Up-to-date information on current recommendations and therapeutic options can be found on the AAP Web site (www.aap.org or www.aapredbook.org/flu), through state-specific AAP chapter websites, or on the CDC Web site (www.cdc.gov/flu/).

INFLUENZA ANTIVIRALS RECOMMENDATIONS

Treatment recommendations for antiviral medications for the 2019–2020 season are applicable to infants and children with suspected influenza when influenza viruses are known to be circulating in the community or when infants or children are tested and confirmed to have influenza. Continuous monitoring of the epidemiology, change in severity, and resistance patterns of influenza virus strains by the CDC may lead to new guidance. Oseltamivir (oral), zanamivir (inhaled), peramivir (IV), and baloxavir (oral) are FDA approved for treatment of uncomplicated influenza virus infection in pediatric outpatients; published data exist to support the use of oseltamivir (oral) for hospitalized children and children at high risk. For more serious influenza virus infections, particularly in immune compromised children, seeking the advice of an infectious diseases specialist is suggested.

ANTIVIRAL TREATMENT RECOMMENDATIONS

Regardless of influenza vaccination status, antiviral treatment should be offered as early as possible to the following individuals:

- any hospitalized child with suspected or confirmed influenza disease, regardless of the duration of symptoms;
- any child, inpatient or outpatient, with severe, complicated, or progressive illness attributable to

influenza, regardless of the duration of symptoms; and

- children with influenza virus infection of any severity who are at high risk of complications of influenza, as listed in Table 1, regardless of the duration of symptoms.

Antiviral treatment may be considered for the following individuals:

- any previously healthy, symptomatic outpatient not at high risk for influenza complications who is diagnosed with confirmed or suspected influenza, on the basis of clinical judgment, if treatment can be initiated within 48 hours of illness onset; and
- children with suspected or confirmed influenza disease whose siblings or household contacts either are younger than 6 months or have a high-risk condition that predisposes them to complications of influenza as listed in Table 1.

Efforts should be made to minimize treatment of patients who are not infected with influenza viruses.

ANTIVIRAL CHEMOPROPHYLAXIS RECOMMENDATIONS

Although vaccination is the preferred approach to prevention of infection, chemoprophylaxis during an influenza season, as defined by the CDC (https://www.cdc.gov/flu/professionals/antivirals/summary-clinicians.htm), is recommended in the following situations:

- for children at high risk of complications from influenza for whom influenza vaccine is contraindicated;
- for children at high risk during the 2 weeks after IIV influenza vaccination, before optimal immunity is achieved (prophylaxis after LAIV may decrease vaccine efficacy);
- for family members or HCP who are unvaccinated and are likely to have ongoing, close exposure to the following:
  - unvaccinated children at high risk; or
  - unvaccinated infants and toddlers who are younger than 24 months;
- for control of influenza outbreaks for unvaccinated staff and children in a closed institutional setting with children at high risk (eg, extended-care facilities);
- as a supplement to IIV vaccination among children at high risk, including children who are immunocompromised and may not respond with sufficient protective immune responses after influenza vaccination;
- as postexposure antiviral chemoprophylaxis for family members and close contacts of an infected person if those people are at high risk of complications from influenza; and
- for children at high risk of complications and their family members and close contacts, as well as HCP, when circulating strains of influenza virus in the community are not well matched by seasonal influenza vaccine virus strains on the basis of current data from the CDC and state or local health departments.

These recommendations apply to routine circumstances, but it should be noted that guidance may change on the basis of updated recommendations from the CDC in concert with antiviral availability, local resources, clinical judgment, recommendations from local or public health authorities, risk of influenza complications, type and duration of exposure contact, and change in epidemiology (resistance, antigenic shift) or severity of influenza. Chemoprophylaxis is not routinely recommended for infants younger than 3 months given limited safety and efficacy data in this age group.

FUTURE DIRECTIONS

Safety and effectiveness data for influenza vaccines used during the 2019–2020 season will be analyzed as they become available and reported by the CDC as they are each season.[89] Continued evaluation of the safety, immunogenicity, and effectiveness of influenza vaccine, especially for at-risk populations, is important. The duration of protection and the potential role of previous influenza vaccination on overall VE and VE by vaccine formulation, virus strain, timing of vaccination, and subject age and health status in preventing outpatient medical visits, hospitalizations, and deaths continue to be evaluated. Research to better understand how to educate parents about influenza symptoms and how to recognize when to seek medical attention would be informative. Additionally, with limited data on the use of antiviral agents in hospitalized children and in children with underlying medical conditions, prospective clinical trials to inform optimal timing and efficacy of antiviral treatment and in these populations are warranted.

There is also a need for more systematic health services research on influenza vaccine uptake and refusal as well as identification of methods to enhance uptake. Further investigation is needed about vaccine acceptance and hesitancy and methods to overcome parental concerns and improve coverage. This may include evaluating the strategy of offering to immunize parents and adult child care providers in the pediatric office setting and understanding the level of family contact satisfaction with this approach; how practices handle the logistic, liability, legal, and financial barriers that limit or complicate this service; and most importantly, how this practice may affect disease rates in children and adults. Furthermore, ongoing efforts should include broader implementation and evaluation of mandatory HCP vaccination programs in both inpatient and outpatient settings.

Efforts should be made to create adequate outreach and infrastructure to facilitate the optimal distribution of vaccine so that more people are immunized. Pediatricians should consider becoming more involved in pandemic preparedness and disaster planning efforts (especially in collaboration with schools and child care programs). A bidirectional partner dialogue between pediatricians and public health decision makers assists efforts to address children's issues during the initial state, regional, and local plan development stages. Pandemic influenza preparedness of directors of child care centers also needs to improve. Additional information can be found at www.aap.org/disasters/resourcekit and https://pediatrics.aappublications.org/content/pediatrics/early/2017/05/11/peds.2016-3690.full.pdf.

Pandemic influenza preparedness is of particular interest because of the increase in the number of human infections with Asian H7N9 virus reported in China (updates available at https://www.cdc.gov/flu/avianflu/h7n9-virus.htm). All cases of H7N0 virus infection identified outside of mainland China (eg, Taiwan, Malaysia, Canada) had exposure and were infected in China and were identified outside China after becoming ill. Although the current risk to the public's health from this virus is low, Asian H7N9 virus is among the nonhuman influenza viruses that are most concerning to public health officials because of their pandemic potential and ability to cause severe disease in infected humans. The current risk to public health from the virus remains low; however, the CDC is monitoring the situation carefully and taking routine preparedness measures, including testing candidate vaccines.

With the increased demand for vaccination during each influenza season, the AAP and CDC recommend vaccine administration at any visit to the medical home during influenza season when it is not contraindicated, at specially arranged vaccine-only sessions, and through cooperation with community sites, schools, and Head Start and child care facilities to provide influenza vaccine. It is important that the annual delivery of influenza vaccine to primary care medical homes should be timely to avoid missed opportunities. If alternate venues, including pharmacies and other retail-based clinics, are used for vaccination, a system of patient record transfer is beneficial in maintaining the accuracy of immunization records. Immunization information systems should be used whenever available and prioritized to document influenza vaccination. Two-dimensional barcodes have been used to facilitate more efficient and accurate documentation of vaccine administration with limited experience to date. Additional information concerning current vaccines shipped with two-dimensional barcodes can be found at www.cdc.gov/vaccines/programs/iis/2d-vaccine-barcodes/.

Access to care issues, lack of immunization records, and questions regarding who can provide consent may be addressed by linking children (eg, those in foster care or a juvenile justice system or refugee, immigrant, or homeless children) with a medical home, using all health care encounters as vaccination opportunities and more consistently using immunization registry data.

Development efforts continue for a universal influenza vaccine that induces broader protection and eliminates the need for annual vaccination. In addition, understanding the establishment of immunity against influenza in early life and developing a safe, immunogenic vaccine for infants younger than 6 months are essential. Studies on the effectiveness and safety of influenza vaccines containing adjuvants that enhance immune responses to influenza vaccines or that use novel routes of administration (such as microneedle patch) are ongoing.[90] Efforts to improve the vaccine development process to allow for a shorter interval between identification of vaccine strains and vaccine production continue. Many antiviral drugs are in various development phases, given the need to improve options for the treatment and chemoprophylaxis of influenza. Finally, pediatricians should remain informed during the influenza season by following the CDC influenza page (www.cdc/gov/flu) and the AAP *Red Book Online* Influenza Resource Page (www.aapredbook.org/flu).

SUMMARY OF RECOMMENDATIONS

1. The AAP recommends annual influenza vaccination for everyone 6 months and older, including children and adolescents, during the 2019–2020 influenza season.
2. For the 2019–2020 season, the AAP recommends that any licensed influenza vaccine appropriate for age and health status can be used for influenza vaccination in children. IIV and LAIV are options for children for whom these vaccines are appropriate. This recommendation is based on review of current available data on LAIV and IIV VE. The AAP will continue to review VE data as they become available and update these recommendations if necessary.
3. The AAP does not have a preference for any influenza vaccine product over another for children who have no

contraindication to influenza vaccination and for whom more than one licensed product appropriate for age and health status is available. Pediatricians should administer whichever formulation is available in their communities to achieve the highest possible coverage this influenza season.

4. Children 6 through 35 months of age may receive either a 0.25- or 0.5-mL dose of the licensed, age-appropriate IIVs available this season. No product or formulation is preferred over another for this age group. Children 36 months (3 years) and older should receive a 0.5-mL dose of any available, licensed, age-appropriate inactivated vaccine.
5. The number of seasonal influenza vaccine doses recommended to be administered to children in the 2019–2020 influenza season remains unchanged and depends on the child's age at the time of the first administered dose and vaccine history (Fig 1).
6. Children 6 months through 8 years of age who are receiving an influenza vaccine for the first time or who have received only 1 dose before July 1, 2019, should receive 2 doses of influenza vaccine ideally by the end of October, and vaccines should be offered as soon as they become available. Children needing only 1 dose of influenza vaccine, regardless of age, should also receive vaccination ideally by the end of October.
7. Efforts should be made to ensure vaccination for children in high-risk groups (Table 1) and their contacts, unless contraindicated.
8. Product-specific contraindications must be considered when selecting the type of vaccine to administer. Children who have had an allergic reaction after a previous dose of any influenza vaccine should be evaluated by an allergist to determine whether future receipt of the vaccine is appropriate.
9. Children with egg allergy can receive influenza vaccine without any additional precautions beyond those recommended for all vaccines.
10. Pregnant women may receive an IIV at any time during pregnancy to protect themselves and their infants who benefit from the transplacental transfer of antibodies. Postpartum women who did not receive vaccination during pregnancy should be encouraged to receive an influenza vaccine before discharge from the hospital. Influenza vaccination during breastfeeding is safe for mothers and their infants.
11. The AAP supports mandatory vaccination of HCP as a crucial element in preventing influenza and reducing health care–associated influenza infections because HCP often care for individuals at high risk for influenza-related complications.
12. Antiviral medications are important in the control of influenza but are not a substitute for influenza vaccination. Pediatricians should promptly identify their patients suspected of having influenza infection for timely initiation of antiviral treatment, when indicated and based on shared decision-making between the pediatrician and child's caregiver, to reduce morbidity and mortality. Although the best results are observed when the child is treated within 48 hours of symptom onset, antiviral therapy should still be considered beyond 48 hours of symptom onset in children with severe disease or those at high risk of complications.
13. Antiviral treatment should be offered as early as possible to the following individuals, regardless of influenza vaccination status:
   - any hospitalized child with suspected or confirmed influenza disease, regardless of the duration of symptoms;
   - any child, inpatient or outpatient, with severe, complicated, or progressive illness attributable to influenza, regardless of the duration of symptoms; and
   - children with influenza infection of any severity who are at high risk of complications of influenza infection (Table 1), regardless of the duration of symptoms.
14. Treatment may be considered for the following individuals:
   - any previously healthy, symptomatic outpatient not at high risk for influenza complications who is diagnosed with confirmed or suspected influenza, on the basis of clinical judgment, if treatment can be initiated within 48 hours of illness onset; and
   - children with suspected or confirmed influenza disease whose siblings or household contacts either are younger than 6 months or have a high-risk condition that predisposes them to complications of influenza (Table 1).
15. Antiviral chemoprophylaxis is recommended in the following situations:
   - for children at high risk of complications from influenza for whom influenza vaccine is contraindicated.
   - for children at high risk during the 2 weeks after influenza vaccination, before optimal immunity is achieved.
   - for family members or HCP who are unvaccinated and are

likely to have ongoing, close exposure to the following:

unvaccinated children at high risk; or

unvaccinated infants and toddlers who are younger than 24 months.

- for the control of influenza outbreaks for unvaccinated staff and children in a closed institutional setting with children at high risk (eg, extended-care facilities);
- as a supplement to vaccination among children at high risk, including children who are immunocompromised and may not respond with sufficient protective immune responses after influenza vaccination;
- as postexposure antiviral chemoprophylaxis for family members and close contacts of an infected person if those people are at high risk of complications from influenza; and
- for children at high risk of complications and their family members and close contacts, as well as HCP, when circulating strains of influenza virus in the community are not well matched by seasonal influenza vaccine virus strains on the basis of current data from the CDC and state or local health departments.

COMMITTEE ON INFECTIOUS DISEASES, 2019–2020

Yvonne A. Maldonado, MD, FAAP, Chairperson
Theoklis E. Zaoutis, MD, MSCE, FAAP, Vice Chairperson
Ritu Banerjee, MD, PhD, FAAP
Elizabeth D. Barnett, MD, FAAP, Red Book Associate Editor
James D. Campbell, MD, MS, FAAP
Mary T. Caserta, MD, FAAP
Jeffrey S. Gerber, MD, PhD, FAAP
Athena P. Kourtis, MD, PhD, MPH
Ruth Lynfield, MD, FAAP, Red Book Associate Editor
Flor M. Munoz, MD, MSc, FAAP
Dawn Nolt, MD, MPH, FAAP
Ann-Christine Nyquist, MD, MSPH, FAAP
Sean T. O'Leary, MD, MPH, FAAP
William J. Steinbach, MD, FAAP
Ken Zangwill, MD, FAAP

EX OFFICIO

Henry H. Bernstein, DO, MHCM, FAAP, Red Book Online Associate Editor
David W. Kimberlin, MD, FAAP, Red Book Editor
H. Cody Meissner, MD, FAAP, Visual Red Book Associate Editor
Mark H. Sawyer, MD, FAAP, Red Book Associate Editor

CONTRIBUTORS

Stuart T. Weinberg, MD, FAAP – *Partnership for Policy Implementation*
John M. Kelso, MD, FAAP – *Scripps Clinic*
John S. Bradley, MD, FAAP – *University of California, San Diego/Rady Children's Hospital*
Tim Uyeki, MD – *Centers for Disease Control and Prevention*

LIAISONS

Amanda C. Cohn, MD, FAAP – *Centers for Disease Control and Prevention*
Tammy R. Beckman, DVM, PhD, *National Vaccine Advisory Committee*
Jamie Deseda-Tous, MD – *Sociedad Latinoamericana de Infectologia Pediatrica*
Karen M. Farizo, MD – *US Food and Drug Administration*
Marc Fischer, MD, FAAP – *Centers for Disease Control and Prevention*
Natasha B. Halasa, MD, MPH, FAAP – *Pediatric Infectious Diseases Society*
Nicole Le Saux, MD, FRCP(C) – *Canadian Pediatric Society*
Scot Moore, MD, FAAP – *Committee on Practice Ambulatory Medicine*
Neile S. Silverman, MD – *American College of Obstetricians and Gynecologists*
Jeffrey R. Starke, MD, FAAP – *American Thoracic Society*
James J. Stevermer, MD, MSPH, FAAFP – *American Academy of Family Physicians*
Kay M. Tomashek, MD, MPH, DTM, – *National Institutes of Health*

STAFF

Jennifer M. Frantz, MPH

ACKNOWLEDGMENTS

This AAP policy statement was prepared in parallel with CDC recommendations and reports. This statement is based on literature reviews, analyses of unpublished data, and deliberations with the ACIP Influenza Work Group, with liaison from the AAP.

ABBREVIATIONS

AAP: American Academy of Pediatrics
ACIP: Advisory Committee on Immunization Practices
CDC: Centers for Disease Control and Prevention
CI: confidence interval
FDA: US Food and Drug Administration
GBS: Guillain-Barré syndrome
HA: hemagglutinin
HCP: health care personnel
IDSA: Infectious Diseases Society of America
IIV: inactivated influenza vaccine
IIV3: trivalent inactivated influenza vaccine
IIV4: quadrivalent inactivated influenza vaccine
IV: intravenous
LAIV: live attenuated influenza vaccine
LAIV3: trivalent live attenuated influenza vaccine
LAIV4: quadrivalent live attenuated influenza vaccine
NAI: neuraminidase inhibitor
PCV13: 13-valent pneumococcal conjugate vaccine
RCT: randomized controlled trial
RIV4: quadrivalent recombinant influenza vaccine
RT-PCR: reverse transcription polymerase chain reaction
VE: vaccine effectiveness
WHO: World Health Organization

REFERENCES

1. Centers for Disease Control and Prevention. Prevention and control of influenza with vaccines: recommendations of the Advisory Committee on Immunization Practices, United States, 2019–20 influenza

season. *MMWR Recomm Rep.* 2019; 68(3):1–21

2. Shope TR, Walker BH, Aird LD, et al. Pandemic influenza preparedness among child care center directors in 2008 and 2016. *Pediatrics.* 2017;139(6): e20163690
3. Garten R, Blanton L, Elal AIA, et al. Update: influenza activity in the United States during the 2017-18 season and composition of the 2018-19 influenza vaccine. *MMWR Morb Mortal Wkly Rep.* 2018;67(22):634–642
4. Centers for Disease Control and Prevention. Seasonal influenza vaccine effectiveness, 2017-2018. Available at: https://www.cdc.gov/flu/vaccines-work/2017-2018.html. Accessed May 31, 2019
5. Biggerstaff M, Kniss K, Jernigan DB, et al. Systematic assessment of multiple routine and near real-time indicators to classify the severity of influenza seasons and pandemics in the United States, 2003-2004 through 2015-2016. *Am J Epidemiol.* 2018;187(5): 1040–1050
6. Xu X, Blanton L, Elal AIA, et al. Update: influenza activity in the United States during the 2018-19 season and composition of the 2019-20 influenza vaccine. *MMWR Morb Mortal Wkly Rep.* 2019;68(24):544–551
7. Centers for Disease Control and Prevention. Weekly U.S. influenza surveillance report (FluView). Available at: https://www.cdc.gov/flu/weekly/. Accessed May 31, 2019
8. Flannery B, Reynolds SB, Blanton L, et al. Influenza vaccine effectiveness against pediatric deaths: 2010-2014. *Pediatrics.* 2017;139(5):e20164244
9. Ferdinands JM, Olsho LE, Agan AA, et al; Pediatric Acute Lung Injury and Sepsis Investigators (PALISI) Network. Effectiveness of influenza vaccine against life-threatening RT-PCR-confirmed influenza illness in US children, 2010-2012. *J Infect Dis.* 2014; 210(5):674–683
10. Tran D, Vaudry W, Moore D, et al; members of the Canadian Immunization Monitoring Program Active. Hospitalization for influenza A versus B. *Pediatrics.* 2016;138(3):e20154643
11. Lessin HR, Edwards KM; Committee on Practice and Ambulatory Medicine; Committee on Infectious Diseases. Immunizing parents and other close family contacts in the pediatric office setting. *Pediatrics.* 2012;129(1). Available at: www.pediatrics.org/cgi/content/full/129/1/e247
12. Miyakawa R, Barreto NB, Kato RM, Neely MN, Russell CJ. Early use of anti-influenza medications in hospitalized children with tracheostomy. *Pediatrics.* 2019;143(3):e20182608
13. Grohskopf LA, Sokolow LZ, Broder KR, et al. Prevention and control of seasonal influenza with vaccines: recommendations of the Advisory Committee on Immunization Practices —United States, 2019–20 influenza season. *MMWR Recomm Rep.* 2019
14. World Health Organization. Recommended composition of influenza virus vaccines for use in the 2019-2020 northern hemisphere influenza season. Available at: https://www.who.int/influenza/vaccines/virus/recommendations/2019_20_north/en/. Accessed March 21, 2019
15. US Food and Drug Administration. Afluria quadrivalent. 2018. Available at: https://www.fda.gov/vaccines-blood-biologics/vaccines/afluria-quadrivalent. Accessed June 24, 2019
16. Vesikari T, Kirstein J, Devota Go G, et al. Efficacy, immunogenicity, and safety evaluation of an MF59-adjuvanted quadrivalent influenza virus vaccine compared with non-adjuvanted influenza vaccine in children: a multicentre, randomised controlled, observer-blinded, phase 3 trial. *Lancet Respir Med.* 2018;6(5):345–356
17. Groothuis JR, Levin MJ, Rabalais GP, Meiklejohn G, Lauer BA. Immunization of high-risk infants younger than 18 months of age with split-product influenza vaccine. *Pediatrics.* 1991; 87(6):823–828
18. Halasa NB, Gerber MA, Berry AA, et al. Safety and immunogenicity of full-dose trivalent inactivated influenza vaccine (TIV) compared with half-dose TIV administered to children 6 through 35 months of age. *J Pediatric Infect Dis Soc.* 2015;4(3):214–224
19. US Food and Drug Administration. Fluzone quadrivalent. 2018. Available at: https://www.fda.gov/vaccines-blood-biologics/vaccines/fluzone-quadrivalent. Accessed June 24, 2019
20. Robertson CA, Mercer M, Selmani A, et al. Safety and immunogenicity of a full-dose, split-virion, inactivated, quadrivalent influenza vaccine in healthy children 6-35 months of age: a randomized controlled clinical trial. *Pediatr Infect Dis J.* 2019;38(3):323–328
21. Claeys C, Zaman K, Dbaibo G, et al; Flu4VEC Study Group. Prevention of vaccine-matched and mismatched influenza in children aged 6-35 months: a multinational randomised trial across five influenza seasons. *Lancet Child Adolesc Health.* 2018;2(5):338–349
22. Jain VK, Domachowske JB, Wang L, et al. Time to change dosing of inactivated quadrivalent influenza vaccine in young children: evidence from a phase III, randomized, controlled trial. *J Pediatric Infect Dis Soc.* 2017;6(1):9–19
23. Duffy J, Weintraub E, Hambidge SJ, et al; Vaccine Safety Datalink. Febrile seizure risk after vaccination in children 6 to 23 months. *Pediatrics.* 2016;138(1): e20160320
24. Thompson CA. Vaccine safety signal from spontaneous system not supported by active surveillance. *Am J Health Syst Pharm.* 2014;71(17): 1432–1433
25. Sentinel. Sentinel CBER/PRISM surveillance report: influenza vaccines and febrile seizures in the 2013-2014 and 2014-2015 influenza seasons. 2017. Available at: https://www.sentinelinitiative.org/sites/default/files/vaccines-blood-biologics/assessments/Influenza-Vaccines-Febrile-Seizures-Final-Report.pdf. Accessed June 24, 2019
26. Grohskopf LA, Sokolow LZ, Fry AM, Walter EB, Jernigan DB. Update: ACIP recommendations for the use of quadrivalent live attenuated influenza vaccine (LAIV4) - United States, 2018-19 influenza season. *MMWR Morb Mortal Wkly Rep.* 2018;67(22):643–645
27. Rondy M, Kissling E, Emborg HD, et al; I-MOVE/I-MOVE+ group. Interim 2017/18 influenza seasonal vaccine effectiveness: combined results from five European studies. *Euro Surveill.* 2018;23(9):18–00086

28. Blanton L, Dugan VG, Abd Elal AI, et al. Update: influenza activity - United States, September 30, 2018-February 2, 2019. *MMWR Morb Mortal Wkly Rep.* 2019;68(6):125–134

29. Kissling E, Rose A, Emborg HD, et al; European IVE Group. Interim 2018/19 influenza vaccine effectiveness: six European studies, October 2018 to January 2019. *Euro Surveill.* 2019;24(8): 1900121

30. Kelso JM, Greenhawt MJ, Li JT; Joint Task Force on Practice Parameters (JTFPP). Update on influenza vaccination of egg allergic patients. *Ann Allergy Asthma Immunol.* 2013;111(4): 301–302

31. Greenhawt M, Turner PJ, Kelso JM. Administration of influenza vaccines to egg allergic recipients: a practice parameter update 2017. *Ann Allergy Asthma Immunol.* 2018;120(1):49–52

32. American College of Obstetricians and Gynecologists. ACOG committee opinion no. 732: influenza vaccination during pregnancy. *Obstet Gynecol.* 2018;131(4): e109–e114

33. Robison SG, Osborn AW. The concordance of parent and child immunization. *Pediatrics.* 2017;139(5): e2016883

34. Zaman K, Roy E, Arifeen SE, et al. Effectiveness of maternal influenza immunization in mothers and infants [published correction appears in *N Engl J Med.* 2009;360(6):648]. *N Engl J Med.* 2008;359(15):1555–1564

35. Tapia MD, Sow SO, Tamboura B, et al. Maternal immunisation with trivalent inactivated influenza vaccine for prevention of influenza in infants in Mali: a prospective, active-controlled, observer-blind, randomised phase 4 trial. *Lancet Infect Dis.* 2016;16(9): 1026–1035

36. Madhi SA, Cutland CL, Kuwanda L, et al; Maternal Flu Trial (Matflu) Team. Influenza vaccination of pregnant women and protection of their infants. *N Engl J Med.* 2014;371(10):918–931

37. Steinhoff MC, Katz J, Englund JA, et al. Year-round influenza immunisation during pregnancy in Nepal: a phase 4, randomised, placebo-controlled trial. *Lancet Infect Dis.* 2017;17(9):981–989

38. Shakib JH, Korgenski K, Presson AP, et al. Influenza in infants born to women vaccinated during pregnancy. *Pediatrics.* 2016;137(6):e20152360

39. Nunes MC, Madhi SA. Influenza vaccination during pregnancy for prevention of influenza confirmed illness in the infants: a systematic review and meta-analysis. *Hum Vaccin Immunother.* 2018;14(3):758–766

40. Thompson MG, Kwong JC, Regan AK, et al; PREVENT Workgroup. Influenza vaccine effectiveness in preventing influenza-associated hospitalizations during pregnancy: a multi-country retrospective test negative design study, 2010-2016. *Clin Infect Dis.* 2019; 68(9):1444–1453

41. Sheffield JS, Greer LG, Rogers VL, et al. Effect of influenza vaccination in the first trimester of pregnancy. *Obstet Gynecol.* 2012;120(3):532–537

42. Polyzos KA, Konstantelias AA, Pitsa CE, Falagas ME. Maternal influenza vaccination and risk for congenital malformations: a systematic review and meta-analysis. *Obstet Gynecol.* 2015; 126(5):1075–1084

43. Nunes MC, Madhi SA. Prevention of influenza-related illness in young infants by maternal vaccination during pregnancy. *F1000 Res.* 2018;7:122

44. Omer SB, Clark DR, Aqil AR, et al; for BMGF Supported Maternal Influenza Immunization Trials Investigators Group. Maternal influenza immunization and prevention of severe clinical pneumonia in young infants: analysis of randomized controlled trials conducted in Nepal, Mali and South Africa. *Pediatr Infect Dis J.* 2018;37(5): 436–440

45. Schlaudecker EP, Steinhoff MC, Omer SB, et al. IgA and neutralizing antibodies to influenza a virus in human milk: a randomized trial of antenatal influenza immunization. *PLoS One.* 2013;8(8):e70867

46. Ferdinands JM, Fry AM, Reynolds S, et al. Intraseason waning of influenza vaccine protection: evidence from the US Influenza Vaccine Effectiveness Network, 2011-12 through 2014-15. *Clin Infect Dis.* 2017;64(5):544–550

47. Castilla J, Martínez-Baz I, Martínez-Artola V, et al; Primary Health Care Sentinel Network; Network for Influenza Surveillance in Hospitals of Navarre. Decline in influenza vaccine effectiveness with time after vaccination, Navarre, Spain, season 2011/12. *Euro Surveill.* 2013;18(5):20388

48. Kissling E, Valenciano M, Larrauri A, et al. Low and decreasing vaccine effectiveness against influenza A(H3) in 2011/12 among vaccination target groups in Europe: results from the I-MOVE multicentre case-control study. *Euro Surveill.* 2013;18(5):20390

49. Belongia EA, Sundaram ME, McClure DL, et al. Waning vaccine protection against influenza A (H3N2) illness in children and older adults during a single season. *Vaccine.* 2015;33(1):246–251

50. Radin JM, Hawksworth AW, Myers CA, et al. Influenza vaccine effectiveness: maintained protection throughout the duration of influenza seasons 2010-2011 through 2013-2014. *Vaccine.* 2016; 34(33):3907–3912

51. Puig-Barberà J, Mira-Iglesias A, Tortajada-Girbés M, et al; Valencia Hospital Network for the Study of Influenza and other Respiratory Viruses (VAHNSI, Spain). Waning protection of influenza vaccination during four influenza seasons, 2011/2012 to 2014/ 2015. *Vaccine.* 2017;35(43):5799–5807

52. Ray GT, Lewis N, Klein NP, et al. Intraseason waning of influenza vaccine effectiveness. *Clin Infect Dis.* 2019; 68(10):1623–1630

53. Kissling E, Nunes B, Robertson C, et al; I-MOVE Case–control study team. I-MOVE multicentre case-control study 2010/11 to 2014/15: is there within-season waning of influenza type/subtype vaccine effectiveness with increasing time since vaccination? *Euro Surveill.* 2016;21(16):30201

54. Pebody R, Andrews N, McMenamin J, et al. Vaccine effectiveness of 2011/12 trivalent seasonal influenza vaccine in preventing laboratory-confirmed influenza in primary care in the United Kingdom: evidence of waning intra-seasonal protection. *Euro Surveill.* 2013; 18(5):20389

55. Petrie JG, Ohmit SE, Truscon R, et al. Modest waning of influenza vaccine efficacy and antibody titers during the 2007-2008 influenza season. *J Infect Dis.* 2016;214(8):1142–1149

56. Ferdinands JM, Patel MM, Foppa IM, Fry AM. Influenza vaccine effectiveness. *Clin Infect Dis.* 2019;69(1):190–191

57. Doll MK, Winters N, Boikos C, et al. Safety and effectiveness of neuraminidase inhibitors for influenza treatment, prophylaxis, and outbreak control: a systematic review of systematic reviews and/or meta-analyses. *J Antimicrob Chemother.* 2017;72(11):2990–3007

58. Committee on Infectious Diseases. Influenza immunization for all health care personnel: keep it mandatory. *Pediatrics.* 2015;136(4):809–818

59. Frush K; American Academy of Pediatrics, Committee on Pediatric Emergency Medicine. Preparation for emergencies in the offices of pediatricians and pediatric primary care providers. *Pediatrics.* 2007;120(1): 200–212

60. Committee on Practice and Ambulatory Medicine; Committee on Infectious Diseases; Committee on State Government Affairs; Council on School Health; Section on Administration and Practice Management. Medical versus nonmedical immunization exemptions for child care and school attendance. *Pediatrics.* 2016;138(3):e20162145

61. Edwards KM, Hackell JM; Committee on Infectious Diseases, The Committee on Practice and Ambulatory Medicine. Countering vaccine hesitancy. *Pediatrics.* 2016;138(3):e20162146

62. Markenson D, Reynolds S; American Academy of Pediatrics Committee on Pediatric Emergency Medicine; Task Force on Terrorism. The pediatrician and disaster preparedness. *Pediatrics.* 2006;117(2). Available at: www.pediatrics.org/cgi/content/full/117/2/e340

63. American Academy of Pediatrics. Influenza. In: Kimberlin DW, Brady MT, Jackson MA, Long SS, eds. *Red Book: 2018 Report of the Committee on Infectious Diseases,* 31st ed. Elk Grove Village, IL: American Academy of Pediatrics; 2018:pp 476–489

64. Heo YA. Baloxavir: first global approval. *Drugs.* 2018;78(6):693–697

65. Uyeki TM, Bernstein HH, Bradley JS, et al. Clinical practice guidelines by the Infectious Diseases Society of America: 2018 update on diagnosis, treatment, chemoprophylaxis, and institutional outbreak management of seasonal influenza. *Clin Infect Dis.* 2019;68(6): e1–e47

66. Bradley JS, Blumer JL, Romero JR, et al. Intravenous zanamivir in hospitalized patients with influenza. *Pediatrics.* 2017;140(5):e20162727

67. Chan-Tack KM, Kim C, Moruf A, Birnkrant DB. Clinical experience with intravenous zanamivir under an Emergency IND program in the United States (2011-2014). *Antivir Ther.* 2015;20(5):561–564

68. Wang K, Shun-Shin M, Gill P, Perera R, Harnden A. Neuraminidase inhibitors for preventing and treating influenza in children (published trials only). *Cochrane Database Syst Rev.* 2012;(4): CD002744

69. Howard A, Uyeki TM, Fergie J. Influenza-associated acute necrotizing encephalopathy in siblings. *J Pediatric Infect Dis Soc.* 2018;7(3):e172–e177

70. Dobson J, Whitley RJ, Pocock S, Monto AS. Oseltamivir treatment for influenza in adults: a meta-analysis of randomised controlled trials [published correction appears in *Lancet.* 2015; 385(9979):1728]. *Lancet.* 2015;385(9979): 1729–1737

71. Koszalka P, Tilmanis D, Roe M, Vijaykrishna D, Hurt AC. Baloxavir marboxil susceptibility of influenza viruses from the Asia-Pacific, 2012-2018. *Antiviral Res.* 2019;164:91–96

72. Gubareva LV, Mishin VP, Patel MC, et al. Assessing baloxavir susceptibility of influenza viruses circulating in the United States during the 2016/17 and 2017/18 seasons. *Euro Surveill.* 2019; 24(3):1800666

73. Malosh RE, Martin ET, Heikkinen T, et al. Efficacy and safety of oseltamivir in children: systematic review and individual patient data meta-analysis of randomized controlled trials. *Clin Infect Dis.* 2018;66(10):1492–1500

74. Hsu J, Santesso N, Mustafa R, et al. Antivirals for treatment of influenza: a systematic review and meta-analysis of observational studies. *Ann Intern Med.* 2012;156(7):512–524

75. Jefferson T, Jones MA, Doshi P, et al. Neuraminidase inhibitors for preventing and treating influenza in healthy adults and children. *Cochrane Database Syst Rev.* 2014;(4):CD008965

76. Venkatesan S, Myles PR, Leonardi-Bee J, et al. Impact of outpatient neuraminidase inhibitor treatment in patients infected with influenza A(H1N1) pdm09 at high risk of hospitalization: an individual participant data metaanalysis. *Clin Infect Dis.* 2017; 64(10):1328–1334

77. Muthuri SG, Venkatesan S, Myles PR, et al; PRIDE Consortium Investigators. Effectiveness of neuraminidase inhibitors in reducing mortality in patients admitted to hospital with influenza A H1N1pdm09 virus infection: a meta-analysis of individual participant data. *Lancet Respir Med.* 2014;2(5):395–404

78. Dawood FS, Jara J, Gonzalez R, et al. A randomized, double-blind, placebo-controlled trial evaluating the safety of early oseltamivir treatment among children 0-9 years of age hospitalized with influenza in El Salvador and Panama. *Antiviral Res.* 2016;133:85–94

79. Uyeki TM. Oseltamivir treatment of influenza in children. *Clin Infect Dis.* 2018;66(10):1501–1503

80. Domínguez A, Romero-Tamarit A, Soldevila N, et al; Surveillance of Hospitalized Cases of Severe Influenza in Catalonia Working Group. Effectiveness of antiviral treatment in preventing death in severe hospitalised influenza cases over six seasons. *Epidemiol Infect.* 2018;146(7):799–808

81. South East Asia Infectious Disease Clinical Research Network. Effect of double dose oseltamivir on clinical and virological outcomes in children and adults admitted to hospital with severe influenza: double blind randomised controlled trial. *BMJ.* 2013;346:f3039

82. Takeuchi S, Tetsuhashi M, Sato D. Oseltamivir phosphate-lifting the restriction on its use to treat teenagers with influenza in Japan. *Pharmacoepidemiol Drug Saf.* 2019; 28(4):434–436

83. Takashita E, Kawakami C, Ogawa R, et al. Influenza A(H3N2) virus exhibiting reduced susceptibility to baloxavir due to a polymerase acidic subunit I38T substitution detected from a hospitalised child without prior

baloxavir treatment, Japan, January 2019. *Euro Surveill.* 2019;24(12):1900170

84. Hayden FG, Sugaya N, Hirotsu N, et al; Baloxavir Marboxil Investigators Group. Baloxavir marboxil for uncomplicated influenza in adults and adolescents. *N Engl J Med.* 2018;379(10):913–923

85. Omoto S, Speranzini V, Hashimoto T, et al. Characterization of influenza virus variants induced by treatment with the endonuclease inhibitor baloxavir marboxil. *Sci Rep.* 2018;8(1):9633

86. Takashita E, Kawakami C, Morita H, et al; On Behalf of the Influenza Virus Surveillance Group of Japan. Detection of influenza A(H3N2) viruses exhibiting reduced susceptibility to the novel cap-dependent endonuclease inhibitor baloxavir in Japan, December 2018. *Euro Surveill.* 2019; 24(3):1800698

87. Chambers CD, Johnson DL, Xu R, et al; OTIS Collaborative Research Group. Safety of the 2010-11, 2011-12, 2012-13, and 2013-14 seasonal influenza vaccines in pregnancy: birth defects, spontaneous abortion, preterm delivery, and small for gestational age infants, a study from the cohort arm of VAMPSS. *Vaccine.* 2016;34(37): 4443–4449

88. Donahue JG, Kieke BA, King JP, et al. Association of spontaneous abortion with receipt of inactivated influenza vaccine containing H1N1pdm09 in 2010-11 and 2011-12. *Vaccine.* 2017;35(40): 5314–5322

89. Flannery B, Chung JR, Belongia EA, et al. Interim estimates of 2017-18 seasonal influenza vaccine effectiveness - United States, February 2018. *MMWR Morb Mortal Wkly Rep.* 2018;67(6): 180–185

90. Rouphael NG, Paine M, Mosley R, et al; TIV-MNP 2015 Study Group. The safety, immunogenicity, and acceptability of inactivated influenza vaccine delivered by microneedle patch (TIV-MNP 2015): a randomised, partly blinded, placebo-controlled, phase 1 trial. *Lancet.* 2017; 390(10095):649–658

Recommended Childhood and Adolescent Immunization Schedule: United States, 2020

- *Policy Statement*

POLICY STATEMENT Organizational Principles to Guide and Define the Child Health Care System and/or Improve the Health of all Children

American Academy of Pediatrics

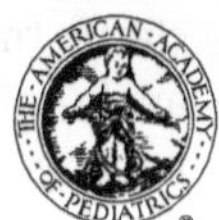

DEDICATED TO THE HEALTH OF ALL CHILDREN™

Recommended Childhood and Adolescent Immunization Schedule: United States, 2020

COMMITTEE ON INFECTIOUS DISEASES

The 2020 recommended childhood and adolescent immunization schedules have been approved by the American Academy of Pediatrics, the Advisory Committee on Immunization Practices of the Centers for Disease Control and Prevention (CDC), the American Academy of Family Physicians, and the American College of Obstetricians and Gynecologists. The schedules are revised annually to reflect current recommendations for the use of vaccines licensed by the US Food and Drug Administration.

The 2020 childhood and adolescent immunization schedule has been updated to ensure consistency between the format of the childhood and adolescent and adult immunization schedules. Similar to last year, the cover page includes a table with an alphabetical list of vaccines, approved abbreviations for each vaccine, and vaccine trade names. The American College of Nurse-Midwives has been added to the list of approving organizations.

Table 1 contains the recommended immunization schedule from birth to 18 years of age. The row for hepatitis A vaccine has been changed to a solid green bar from age 2 to 18 years to reflect routine catch-up vaccination for all children through 18 years of age. The row for meningococcal serogroups A, C, W, Y vaccine (MenACWY) was moved down in the table to appear just above the row for meningococcal serogroup B vaccine. For the label legend, the blue box legend definition, which formerly said, "Range of recommended ages for non-high-risk groups that may receive vaccine, subject to individual clinical decision-making" was changed to "Recommended based on shared clinical decision-making," with an asterisk for human papillomavirus vaccine at ages 9 and 10 years ("*can be used in this age group"). The gray box label for "no recommendation" was updated to include "not applicable."

Table 2 is the catch-up immunization schedule for persons 4 months to 18 years of age who start late or who are more than 1 month behind the recommended age for vaccine administration. The only change to table 2

Policy statements from the American Academy of Pediatrics benefit from expertise and resources of liaisons and internal (AAP) and external reviewers. However, policy statements from the American Academy of Pediatrics may not reflect the views of the liaisons or the organizations or government agencies that they represent.

The guidance in this statement does not indicate an exclusive course of treatment or serve as a standard of medical care. Variations, taking into account individual circumstances, may be appropriate.

All policy statements from the American Academy of Pediatrics automatically expire 5 years after publication unless reaffirmed, revised, or retired at or before that time.

This document is copyrighted and is property of the American Academy of Pediatrics and its Board of Directors. All authors have filed conflict of interest statements with the American Academy of Pediatrics. Any conflicts have been resolved through a process approved by the Board of Directors. The American Academy of Pediatrics has neither solicited nor accepted any commercial involvement in the development of the content of this publication.

DOI: https://doi.org/10.1542/peds.2019-3995

Copyright © 2020 by the American Academy of Pediatrics

FINANCIAL DISCLOSURE: The authors have indicated no financial relationships relevant to this article to disclose.

FUNDING: No external funding.

POTENTIAL CONFLICT OF INTEREST: The author has indicated he has no potential conflicts of interest to disclose.

To cite: COMMITTEE ON INFECTIOUS DISEASES. Recommended Childhood and Adolescent Immunization Schedule: United States, 2020. *Pediatrics.* 2020;145(3):e20193995

was that "ACWY" was added to "Meningococcal" in relevant rows to clarify that these recommendations apply to MenACWY only and not meningococcal serogroup B vaccine.

Table 3 lists the vaccines that may be indicated for children and adolescents 18 years of age or younger on the basis of medical conditions. All boxes in the hepatitis A vaccine row were changed to yellow to denote that it is a routine vaccination for all children, including those with medical indications. The pregnancy box in the MenACWY row has been changed to yellow because pregnancy is not considered an indication to withhold routine adolescent vaccination. The red box in the label legend has been updated to "Not recommended/Contraindicated—vaccine should not be administered" (from "Contraindicated or use not recommended—vaccine should not be administered because of risk for serious adverse reaction"). The gray box label for "no recommendation" was updated to include "not applicable."

Similar to the 2019 schedule, the notes are presented in alphabetical order. The following changes to individual footnotes have been made to the 2020 schedule:

- Diphtheria-tetanus-acellular pertussis (DTaP) vaccine
  - A clarification was added to the catch-up recommendation that dose 5 is not necessary if dose 4 was administered at age 4 years or older and was administered at least 6 months after dose 3.
- *Haemophilus influenzae* type b vaccine
  - A bullet was added to clarify that catch-up vaccination is not recommended for children 5 years and older who are not at high risk.
- Hepatitis A vaccine
  - A note was added to reflect the recommendation for routine catch-up vaccination through 18 years of age.
- Hepatitis B vaccine
  - A "Special Situations" section was added containing recommendations for revaccination and a link to the Advisory Committee on Immunization Practices hepatitis B recommendations. The new language states "revaccination is not generally recommended for persons with a normal immune status who were vaccinated as infants, children, adolescents or adults. Revaccination may be recommended for certain populations, including infants born to HBsAg-positive [hepatitis B surface antigen–positive] mothers, hemodialysis patients, or other immunocompromised persons."
- Influenza vaccines
  - The routine recommendations section was reformatted to more clearly outline circumstances under which 1 or 2 doses of influenza vaccine are recommended.
  - The situations under which live attenuated influenza vaccine (LAIV) should not be used was reformatted to a bulleted list instead of a paragraph.
- Poliovirus vaccine
  - The note was moved to the appropriate place alphabetically (from "I" to "P").
  - The title was changed from "Inactivated poliovirus vaccination" to "Poliovirus vaccination," and information was added regarding which doses of trivalent oral poliovirus vaccine (OPV) may be counted as valid, now reading, "Only trivalent OPV (tOPV) counts toward the US vaccination requirements. Doses of OPV administered before April 1, 2016, should be counted (unless specifically noted as administered during a campaign). Doses of OPV administered on or after April 1, 2016, should not be counted.
- MenACWY
  - Guidance was added regarding adolescent revaccination for children who received the vaccine before age 10 years. Adolescent vaccination of children who received MenACWY before age 10 years:
    - "Children in whom boosters are not recommended due to an ongoing increased risk of meningococcal disease (eg, a healthy child who traveled to a country where meningococcal disease is endemic): administer MenACWY according to the recommended adolescent schedule with dose 1 at age 11–12 years and dose 2 at age 16 years."
    - "Children in whom boosters are recommended due to an ongoing increased risk of meningococcal disease (eg, those with complement deficiency, HIV, or asplenia): follow the booster schedule for persons at increased risk."
- Meningococcal serogroup B vaccines
  - The heading that formerly read, "Clinical Discretion" was changed to "Shared Clinical Decision-Making."
  - A reference link was provided to booster dose guidance to mirror similar language in the MenACWY note.
- Tetanus toxoid, reduced diphtheria toxoid, and acellular pertussis, adsorbed (Tdap) vaccine
  - Tdap was added as an option for booster doses and remaining doses of the catch-up series.

- Guidance also was added for DTaP and Tdap doses received at 7 to 10 years of age.
  - "Tdap administered at 7–10 years:
    - Children age 7–9 years who receive Tdap should receive the routine Tdap dose at age 11–12 years.
    - Children age 10 years who receive Tdap do not need to receive the routine Tdap dose at age 11–12 years.
  - DTaP inadvertently administered after the seventh birthday:
    - Children age 7–9 years: DTaP may count as part of catch-up series. Administer routine Tdap dose at age 11–12 years.
    - Children age 10–18 years: Count dose of DTaP as the adolescent Tdap booster."

The 2020 version of tables 1 through 3 and the notes are available on the American Academy of Pediatrics Web site (https://redbook.solutions.aap.org/SS/Immunization_Schedules.aspx) and the CDC Web site (www.cdc.gov/vaccines/schedules/hcp/child-adolescent.html). A parent-friendly vaccine schedule for children and adolescents is available at www.cdc.gov/vaccines/schedules/index.html. An adult immunization schedule is published in February of each year and is available at www.cdc.gov/vaccines/schedules/hcp/adult.html.

Clinically significant adverse events that follow immunization should be reported to the Vaccine Adverse Event Reporting System. Guidance about how to obtain and complete a Vaccine Adverse Event Reporting System form can be obtained at www.vaers.hhs.gov or by calling 800-822-7967. Additional information can be found in the *Red Book* and at *Red Book* Online (http://aapredbook.aappublications.org/). Statements from the ACIP and the CDC that contain detailed recommendations for individual vaccines, including recommendations for children with high-risk conditions, are available at www.cdc.gov/vaccines/hcp/acip-recs/index.html. Information on new vaccine releases, vaccine supplies, and interim recommendations resulting from vaccine shortages and statements on specific vaccines can be found at www.aapredbook.org/news/vaccstatus.shtml.

COMMITTEE ON INFECTIOUS DISEASES, 2019–2020

Yvonne A. Maldonado, MD, FAAP, Chairperson
Theoklis E. Zaoutis, MD, MSCE, FAAP, Vice Chairperson
Ritu Banerjee, MD, PhD, FAAP
Elizabeth D. Barnett, MD, FAAP
James D. Campbell, MD, MS, FAAP
Mary T. Caserta, MD, FAAP
Jeffrey S. Gerber, MD, PhD, FAAP
Athena P. Kourtis, MD, PhD, MPH, FAAP
Ruth Lynfield, MD, FAAP
Flor M. Munoz, MD, MSc, FAAP
Dawn Nolt, MD, MPH, FAAP
Ann-Christine Nyquist, MD, MSPH, FAAP
Sean T. O'Leary, MD, MPH, FAAP
William J. Steinbach, MD, FAAP
Ken Zangwill, MD, FAAP

EX OFFICIO

David W. Kimberlin, MD, FAAP - *Red Book* Editor
Mark H. Sawyer, MD, FAAP - *Red Book* Associate Editor
Henry H. Bernstein, DO, MHCM, FAAP - *Red Book* Online Associate Editor
H. Cody Meissner, MD, FAAP - Visual *Red Book* Associate Editor

LIAISONS

Amanda C. Cohn, MD, FAAP, *Centers for Disease Control and Prevention*
David Kim, MD, HHS, *Office of Infectious Disease and HIV/AIDS Policy*
Karen M. Farizo, MD, *US Food and Drug Administration*
Marc Fischer, MD, FAAP, *Centers for Disease Control and Prevention*
Natasha B. Halasa, MD, MPH, FAAP, *Pediatric Infectious Diseases Society*
Nicole Le Saux, MD, FRCP(C), *Canadian Paediatric Society*
Eduardo Lopez, MD, *Sociedad Latinoamericana de Infectologia Pediatrica*
Scot B. Moore, MD, FAAP, *Committee on Practice Ambulatory Medicine*
Neil S. Silverman, MD, *American College of Obstetricians and Gynecologists*
Jeffrey R. Starke, MD, FAAP, *American Thoracic Society*
James J. Stevermer, MD, MSPH, FAAFP, *American Academy of Family Physicians*
Kay M. Tomashek, MD, MPH, DTM, *National Institutes of Health*

STAFF

Jennifer M. Frantz, MPH

ABBREVIATIONS

CDC: Centers for Disease Control and Prevention
DTaP: diphtheria-tetanus-acellular pertussis
MenACWY: meningococcal serogroups A, C, W, Y vaccine
OPV: oral poliovirus vaccine
Tdap: tetanus toxoid, reduced diphtheria toxoid, and acellular pertussis, adsorbed

School Readiness

- *Technical Report*

TECHNICAL REPORT

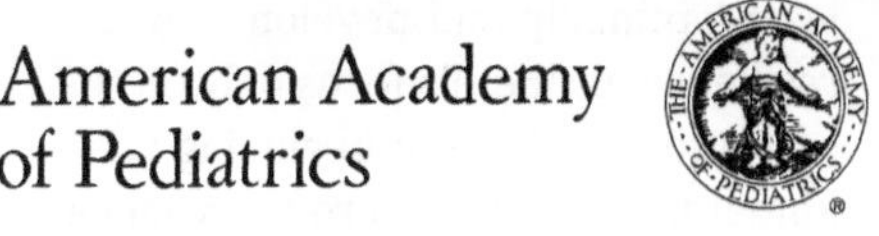

DEDICATED TO THE HEALTH OF ALL CHILDREN™

School Readiness

P. Gail Williams, MD, FAAP,[a] Marc Alan Lerner, MD, FAAP,[b] COUNCIL ON EARLY CHILDHOOD, COUNCIL ON SCHOOL HEALTH

School readiness includes the readiness of the individual child, the school's readiness for children, and the ability of the family and community to support optimal early child development. It is the responsibility of schools to meet the needs of all children at all levels of readiness. Children's readiness for kindergarten should become an outcome measure for a coordinated system of community-based programs and supports for the healthy development of young children. Our rapidly expanding insights into early brain and child development have revealed that modifiable factors in a child's early experience can greatly affect that child's health and learning trajectories. Many children in the United States enter kindergarten with limitations in their social, emotional, cognitive, and physical development that might have been significantly diminished or eliminated through early identification and attention to child and family needs. A strong correlation between social-emotional development and school and life success, combined with alarming rates of preschool expulsion, point toward the urgency of leveraging opportunities to support social-emotional development and address behavioral concerns early. Pediatric primary care providers have access to the youngest children and their families. Pediatricians can promote and use community supports, such as home visiting programs, quality early care and education programs, family support programs and resources, early intervention services, children's museums, and libraries, which are important for addressing school readiness and are too often underused by populations who can benefit most from them. When these are not available, pediatricians can support the development of such resources. The American Academy of Pediatrics affords pediatricians many opportunities to improve the physical, social-emotional, and educational health of young children, in conjunction with other advocacy groups. This technical report provides an updated version of the previous iteration from the American Academy of Pediatrics published in 2008.

EARLY EXPERIENCE MATTERS

All of a child's early experiences, whether at home, in child care, or in other preschool settings, are educational. When early experiences are

abstract

[a]*Department of Pediatrics, Weisskopf Child Evaluation Center, University of Louisville, Louisville, Kentucky; and* [b]*Center for Autism and Neurodevelopmental Disorders, University of California, Irvine, Irvine, California*

Drs Williams and Lerner were responsible for conceptualizing, writing, and revising the manuscript and for considering input from reviewers and the Board of Directors; and all authors approved the final manuscript as submitted and take responsibility for the manuscript in its final form.

This document is copyrighted and is property of the American Academy of Pediatrics and its Board of Directors. All authors have filed conflict of interest statements with the American Academy of Pediatrics. Any conflicts have been resolved through a process approved by the Board of Directors. The American Academy of Pediatrics has neither solicited nor accepted any commercial involvement in the development of the content of this publication.

Technical reports from the American Academy of Pediatrics benefit from expertise and resources of liaisons and internal (AAP) and external reviewers. However, technical reports from the American Academy of Pediatrics may not reflect the views of the liaisons or the organizations or government agencies that they represent.

The guidance in this report does not indicate an exclusive course of treatment or serve as a standard of medical care. Variations, taking into account individual circumstances, may be appropriate.

All technical reports from the American Academy of Pediatrics automatically expire 5 years after publication unless reaffirmed, revised, or retired at or before that time.

DOI: https://doi.org/10.1542/peds.2019-1766

Address correspondence to P. Gail Williams, MD, FAAP. E-mail: patricia.williams@louisville.edu

PEDIATRICS (ISSN Numbers: Print, 0031-4005; Online, 1098-4275).

Copyright © 2019 by the American Academy of Pediatrics

FINANCIAL DISCLOSURE: The authors have indicated they have no financial relationships relevant to this article to disclose.

FUNDING: No external funding.

To cite: Williams PG, Lerner MA, AAP COUNCIL ON EARLY CHILDHOOD, AAP COUNCIL ON SCHOOL HEALTH. School Readiness. *Pediatrics.* 2019;144(2):e20191766

consistent, developmentally sound, and emotionally supportive, children learn optimally and develop resilience for life. To focus only on the education of children beginning with kindergarten is to ignore the science of early development and to deny the importance of early experiences. Our current understanding of the importance of experiences in early brain development and in cognitive and social-emotional outcomes for children converge in our contemporary conceptualization of school readiness. Children who enter school ready to learn are expected to achieve more academically. Academic success has been linked to improved social, economic, and health outcomes.[1–3]

The Adverse Childhood Experiences Study revealed that multiple factors can cause toxic stress that results in changes in brain circuitry with subsequent negative effects on physical and mental health.[4,5] Toxic stress occurs when a child experiences strong, frequent, and/or prolonged adversity, such as physical or emotional abuse, chronic neglect, caregiver substance abuse or mental illness, exposure to violence, and/or the accumulated burdens of family economic hardship, without adequate adult support.[6]

According to data from the National Child Abuse and Neglect Data System, 12.5% of all US children have had a documented episode of child abuse or neglect reported by 18 years of age.[7,8] According to data from the National Survey of Children's Health, 48% of US children have had at least 1 of the 9 key adverse childhood experiences, and 22.6% of children between 0 and 17 years of age had experienced 2 or more of the experiences, although the data exhibit considerable variability across states.[9]

Authors of a recent study used 2011–2012 data from the National Survey of Children's Health to examine the impact of adverse childhood experiences on school success.[10] Data analysis revealed that children with 2 or more adverse childhood experiences were 2.67 times more likely to repeat a grade in school compared with children without any adverse experiences. Children without adverse childhood experiences were 2.59 times more likely to be usually or always engaged in school compared with their peers with 2 or more adverse experiences.[10] Resilience, defined in that study as "staying calm and in control when faced with a challenge," ameliorated these effects. Clearly, there is a role for minimizing toxic stress and building resilience in children as a way of promoting school readiness.

One of the most widely recognized risk factors for school readiness is poverty. Fewer than half (48%) of poor children are ready for school at 5 years of age as compared with 75% of children from moderate- or high-income households.[11] Poverty affects school readiness across racial and ethnic divisions, likely because of both lack of financial resources and parents having less education, higher rates of single and teenage parenthood, poorer health, etc. When family demographics are controlled for factors such as single parenthood and maternal education the poverty-related gap decreases; differences in parent characteristics and parent-child interactions account for much of the gap and have the potential for remediation to break the cycle of negative relationships that often impact 1 generation to the next.[12] Children in foster or kinship care or otherwise involved with child welfare may be less ready for school for several reasons: the impact of childhood trauma and loss on the developing brain (cognitive and emotional) and less access to early childhood education and programs that may help to remediate losses. Children in foster care are at particular risk, especially if their placement is unstable. These children demonstrate higher rates of internalizing problems, such as depression, poorer social skills, lower adaptive functioning, and more externalizing behavioral problems such as aggression and impulsivity.[13] Furthermore, there is evidence that the foster care experience itself (eg, instability of placements) may be further damaging to the developmental outcomes of children who are maltreated.[14] Other risk factors that have been shown to have an effect on school readiness are prenatal exposure to tobacco and alcohol, low birth weight, developmental disability, and maternal depression.[15] Interventions such as home visitation programs, smoking cessation programs, and preschool programs have the potential of ameliorating these negative factors and creating more positive early childhood experiences that may translate into improved school readiness.[16,17] Pediatric primary care has recently been shown to have potential to facilitate school readiness through both primary prevention programs that seek to prevent disparities by working directly with parents to enhance interactions (eg, within the context of reading, talking, and play) and through referral to secondary and/or tertiary prevention programs that identify and treat families at increased risk (eg, maternal depression) or children with already existing difficulties in 1 or more school readiness domains (behavioral health or education).[18]

HOW HAS SCHOOL READINESS BEEN DEFINED?

"Ready to Learn" became a national mantra in 1991 when the National Education Goals Panel adopted as its first goal that "by the year 2000, all children will enter school ready to learn."[19] This panel identified readiness in the child as determined by a set of interdependent developmental trajectories. Three components of school readiness were broadly described as follows:

1. readiness in the child, defined by the following:
   - physical well-being and sensory motor development, including health status and growth;
   - social and emotional development, including self-regulation, attention, impulse control, capacity to limit aggressive and disruptive behaviors, turn-taking, cooperation, empathy, and the ability to communicate one's own emotions; identification of feelings facilitates accurate communication of these feelings;
   - approaches to learning, including enthusiasm, curiosity, temperament, culture, and values;
   - language development, including listening, speaking, and vocabulary, as well as literacy skills, including print awareness, story sense, and writing and drawing processes; and
   - general knowledge and cognition, including early literacy and math skills;
2. schools' readiness for children, illustrated by the following:
   - smooth transition between home and school, including cultural sensitivity;
   - opportunities for parent engagement with schools;
   - understanding of early child development and that children learn through play and natural experiences;
   - continuity between early care, intervention, and education programs and elementary school;
   - use of high-quality instruction, provided within the context of relationships and at a rate designed to challenge but not overwhelm a child;
   - demonstration of commitment to the success of every child through awareness of the needs of individual children, including the effects of adverse childhood experiences, including poverty and racial discrimination, and trying to meet special needs within the regular classroom; implementation of individualized education programs that include adaptations to support children with disabilities;
   - demonstration of commitment to the success of every teacher in providing effective instruction to children;
   - introduction of approaches that raise achievement, such as parent involvement and early intervention for children falling behind;
   - alteration of practices and programs if they do not benefit children;
   - provision of services to children in their communities within the context of a safe, secure, and inclusive environment that supports student health and wellness and promotes learning;
   - willingness to take responsibility for results; and
   - strong leadership; and
3. family and community supports that contribute to child readiness:
   - excellent prenatal care and ongoing primary care within a medical home setting that is comprehensive, compassionate, and family centered;
   - optimal nutrition and daily physical activity so that children arrive at school with healthy minds and bodies;
   - access to high-quality preschool and child care for all children; and
   - time set aside daily for parents to help their child learn along with the supports that allow parents to be effective teachers.

WHAT DETERMINES SCHOOL READINESS?

An individual child's school readiness is determined in large measure by the environment in which he or she lives and grows. The Child Welfare League of America described a vision for the United States in which every child is healthy and safe and develops to his or her full capacity.[20] Five universal needs of all children were described. First, children need the basics of proper nutrition, economic security, adequate clothing and shelter, appropriate education, and primary and preventive physical and mental health services. Second, children need strong nurturing relationships within their families, their communities, and their peer groups. Third, children need opportunities to develop their talents and skills and to contribute to their communities. Children with indications of disability need early assessment and intervention to prevent later, more serious problems. Fourth, children need protection from injury, abuse, and neglect as well as from exposure to violence and discrimination. Fifth, children have a basic need for healing. When caregivers and providers have not been able to protect them, children need us to ease the effects of any harm they have suffered by providing emotional support, by addressing physical and mental health care needs, and by sometimes making amends through restorative judicial practices. Meeting these needs builds resilience and requires collaborative comprehensive approaches so that children become a priority at the levels of the family, the community, and the nation.[20]

Although various constructs of school readiness have been proposed in the past, the conceptualization of school readiness that is widely accepted at present is an "interactional relational" model. This model is focused on the ongoing interaction between the child and the environment. The model suggests that school readiness is "the product of a set of educational decisions that are differentially shaped by the skills, experiences and learning opportunities the child has had and the perspectives and goals of the community, classroom and teacher." This construct suggests that readiness assessments "can only be done over time and in context" rather than by means of a 1-time screening test.[21] This conceptualization is most consistent with the current understanding of the importance of early experiences and early relationships at home and in community and early education settings in promoting child development.[22]

SCHOOL READINESS TESTING

Six fundamental misconceptions prevalent regarding school readiness are as follows: (1) learning happens only at school; (2) readiness is a specific condition within each child; (3) readiness can be measured easily; (4) readiness is mostly a function of time (maturation), and some children need a little more; (5) children are ready to learn when they can sit quietly at a desk and listen; and (6) children who are not ready do not belong in school.[23]

An emphasis on kindergarten readiness that only considers the skills of a child places an undue burden of proof of readiness on that child and is particularly unfair because of economic, experiential, and cultural inequities in our society. Typical or normal development in 4- and 5-year-old children is highly variable, so labeling children as not being school ready at such an early age may cause them to be isolated from a more appropriate learning environment. In a 1988 national survey, 10% to 50% of children in various states who were eligible to enter kindergarten on the basis of age did not enter because of readiness test scores.[24] A follow-up survey in 1996[25] revealed a response to growing concerns about misuse of these kinds of data. Since that time, there has been increased recognition that school readiness assessment should not be used to exclude age-eligible children from kindergarten. In 2010, only 6% of children in kindergarten were delayed entry.[26]

Although the use of readiness assessments to restrict kindergarten entry has markedly decreased, a growing number of states are using readiness assessments for other purposes. At least 25 states in 2010 reported mandatory kindergarten assessments. These assessments varied significantly in scope: 11 evaluated between 5 and 9 domains of school readiness, 4 evaluated only reading readiness, 2 evaluated math and reading, and 2 evaluated unspecified domains. Of the states that assessed multiple domains, 7 used a state-created assessment instrument and 4 used a commercial instrument. Authors of a technical report from the National Conference of State Legislatures (NCSL) noted that although state-created instruments are less costly and better reflect state-specific learning requirements, they need to meet standards for reliability and validity.[27] Most state readiness assessments used single teacher checklists completed on the basis of child observation; these can be inaccurate because of rater bias and can have problems with reliability between raters and consistent over- or underrating on the basis of a general impression of the child.

Reported use of assessments included guidance for planning, curriculum, and instruction (18 states), informing policy decisions or tracking kindergarten readiness at the state level (12 states), feedback to parents (4 states), and evaluation of the readiness of schools to receive incoming students (2 states). Of the 25 states that required kindergarten assessment, 12 did not publish any results. Of the 13 that published results, 4 published only state-level data, and 7 reported results by geographic region. In general, these data were much less detailed than student performance results required for later grades by the No Child Left Behind Act, which was in place from 2002 to 2015. Of concern is the fact that only 22 states in 2010 had a formal definition of school readiness.[28]

Recent federal initiatives have bolstered funding for state early childhood assessments. The federal Race to the Top Early Learning Challenge allowed 9 states to put sizeable funding from their grant into development and implementation of kindergarten entry assessment. Other states received funding through the federal Enhanced Assessment Grants program to develop comprehensive kindergarten through third-grade assessment systems. An update by the NCSL in 2014 documented an additional 14 states that established or amended school readiness assessments of young children, yielding a total of 34 states and the District of Columbia, which now use a state-approved assessment for children entering kindergarten.[29] Approaches to school readiness testing are subject to frequent change. The most recent information on state laws is available through the American Academy of Pediatrics (AAP) Division of State Government Affairs (https://www.aap.org/en-us/advocacy-and-policy/state-advocacy/Pages/State-Advocacy.aspx).

A position paper by the Early Childhood Education State Collaborative on Assessment and Student Standards in 2011 stated that kindergarten readiness assessments can be helpful if used to directly support children's developmental and academic achievement to improve educational outcomes.[30] Such assessment efforts should (1) use multiple tools for multiple purposes, (2) address multiple developmental domains and diverse cultural contexts, (3) align with early learning guidelines, (4) collect information from multiple sources, (5) implement a systems-based approach, and (6) avoid inappropriate use of assessment, such as labeling children, restricting kindergarten entry, and predicting children's future academic success.

As the NCSL data from 2010 reveal, there is considerable variability in the approach taken to kindergarten readiness on the state and national level, both with regard to assessment tools and use of test results. One effort at standardizing results for state reporting is the Early Development Instrument created by Transforming Early Childhood Community Systems, a collaboration between the University of California, Los Angeles Center for Healthier Children, Families, and Communities and the United Way Worldwide.[31] This initiative currently operates in more than 40 communities across the country and reports the percentage of children who are developmentally vulnerable in 5 areas (physical health and well-being, social competence, emotional maturity, language and cognitive development, and communication and child knowledge). Transforming Early Childhood Community Systems states that the reports help guide community efforts to help children reach school healthy and ready to succeed. To the extent that such efforts decrease the disparity between school and child readiness by using the assessments as a tool to help schools prepare for the children they will be serving and promote opportunities for early childhood experiences leading to educational success, readiness assessments can be highly useful.

SCHOOLS' READINESS FOR CHILDREN

The current disparity between school and child readiness may be attributable to schools not being prepared to offer the necessary and appropriate educational setting for age-eligible children, not because children cannot learn in an appropriate educational setting. If there is a predetermined set of skills necessary for school enrollment, then commitment to promoting universal readiness must address early-life inequities in experience. Promoting universal readiness may be accomplished by providing access to opportunities that promote educational success, recognizing and supporting individual differences among children, and establishing reasonable and appropriate expectations of children's capabilities at school entry for all children.[32] The data gained from testing children at kindergarten entry need to be interpreted carefully. Ideally, data can be used as a tool to help prepare schools for the diverse group of children they will be serving. It is the responsibility of the schools to be ready for all children and to work with families to make the school experience positive for all children, even those who may be at varying stages of readiness. School programs should be flexible and adaptable to each child's level of readiness.

One example of schools seeking to address the school readiness needs of low-income and ethnically diverse populations is the Boston Public School System. In 2006, this school system implemented full-day preschool programming for 25% of 4-year-old children in the city and identified key elements of a successful prekindergarten program: a strong curriculum with focus on language, social skills, and concept development (manuals); significant educational supports for teachers in implementing the curriculum; adequate staffing; coaching and training of preschool teachers; and ongoing, independent assessment of instruction and children's skills.[33] The results of this effort were significant: participants in the prekindergarten program scored higher on third-grade language arts tests than did nonparticipants, and the African American–white achievement gap was one-third smaller among prekindergarten participants than among nonparticipants. In addition, the prekindergarten program was able to close the gap between children from low-income and affluent families by more than half. The authors of *Restoring Opportunity: The Crisis of Inequality and the Challenge for American Education* conclude that "well-designed and well-implemented pre-K programs have the potential to be a vital component of a strategy to improve the life chances of children from low income families."[33]

HOW READY ARE CHILDREN IN THE UNITED STATES AS THEY ENTER KINDERGARTEN?

A landmark study by the National Center for Education and Statistics (NCES) (1998–1999) surveyed a nationally representative sample of 22 000 first-time kindergarten students and their schools, classroom teachers, and families.[34,35] The Early Childhood Longitudinal Study (ECLS) was designed to gather information about the entry status of the nation's kindergarteners. Progress of this cohort is still being monitored to inform educational policy and practice. Information was obtained regarding children's cognitive, emotional, social, and physical development as well as their family interactions and home literacy environment. In the study, children "at risk for school difficulty" were defined as children whose mothers had less than a high school education, children who were being raised by single mothers, children whose families had received public assistance, and children in families whose primary language was not English.[34,35]

Fifty-one percent of parents of children who entered kindergarten for the first time in 1998 rated their child's general health as excellent, and 32% rated it as very good.[34,35] Kindergarteners whose mothers had higher levels of education, who were from 2-parent families, whose families had not used public assistance, and who were of white non-Hispanic descent were rated as having generally better health by their parents. Six percent of first-time kindergartners were experiencing vision problems, and 3% were identified as having hearing problems. In that study, 12% of boys and 11% of girls were at risk for overweight, defined as BMI at or above age- and sex-specific guidelines. The risk was greater for children whose mothers had not attained a bachelor's degree and for children from homes in which the primary language spoken was not English.[34,35]

The study attempted to examine the social and emotional status of first-time kindergartners. Teachers reported that 10% to 11% of children often argued or fought with others or were angered easily. Single parents were more likely to report behavior problems, such as fighting, arguing, and getting angry. Parents with partners, those with higher education, and those who had not received public assistance were more likely to have kindergartners with prosocial behaviors, such as often forming friendships. Teachers were less likely than parents to report that children were eager to learn (75% vs 92%). Children with lower maternal education, those from single-mother homes, and those whose families had received public assistance were less likely to be viewed as eager to learn by their teachers.[34,35]

Variability also was seen in home literacy environments and in family interactions for first-time kindergartners. Forty-five percent of all parents reported reading with their child every day, and this value decreased to 36% if mothers had less than a high school education, 38% if English was not the primary language spoken at home, 35% for African American non-Hispanic children, and 39% for Hispanic children. Almost three-fourths of parents reported having more than 25 children's books at home, but this was true for only 38% of kindergartners whose mothers had not graduated from high school and only 35% of those from homes where English was not the primary language spoken. Approximately half of kindergartners from African American non-Hispanic, Hispanic, or American Indian or Alaskan native families had more than 25 children's books at home.[34,35]

Early academic competencies were also surveyed in the study. In 1998 in the United States, as children entered kindergarten for the first time, two-thirds recognized their letters, and 29% also recognized beginning sounds; 94% recognized single numerals and shapes and could count to 10, and 58% could count beyond 10, recognize sequence patterns, and use nonstandard units of length to compare objects. Of those children, 37% demonstrated strong print familiarity skills, including knowing that print reads from left to right and knowing where to go when a line of print ends. Kindergartners' performance on math, reading, and general knowledge items increased with the level of their mothers' education and was higher for children from 2-parent families.[34,35]

Overall, children with few risk factors were more likely to have attained these various proficiencies and were in better general health than were children at risk. Follow-up evaluation of the same children in the spring of first grade revealed that children who demonstrated early literacy skills and who came from a positive literacy environment, who possessed a positive approach to learning, and who enjoyed very good or excellent general health at kindergarten entry performed better in both reading and mathematics after 2 years of formal schooling than did children who did not have these resources. The relationships between the resources children possessed at kindergarten entry and their reading and mathematics performance in the spring of first grade remained significant after controlling for the influence of children's poverty status and their race and/or ethnicity.[36]

When these children were evaluated after 4 years of education, in the spring of third grade, children with more family risk factors (eg, living below the poverty level, primary language spoken in the home was not English, mother had not completed high school, and single-parent home) demonstrated lower mean achievement scores in reading, mathematics, and science. Over that time, children with more family risk factors made smaller gains in math and reading, so the achievement gaps between disadvantaged and more advantaged children grew wider over the first 4 years of school. The third-graders also completed self-descriptive questionnaires evaluating internalizing (eg, shy, withdrawn, or sad) and externalizing (eg, fighting, arguing, or distractibility) behavior problems. Overall, problem behavior scores were low; however, children with lower achievement and more family risk factors tended to rate themselves higher on both of the problem behavior scales.[37]

These findings, although they are disturbing, are not surprising to pediatricians, who have long been advocates for underserved pediatric populations. This inequity in school readiness, which is apparent at school entry and is associated with persistent academic underachievement and social-emotional risk, points to a need to address these differences before children enter kindergarten, especially for families and children at risk.

More recent studies have also addressed school readiness. Data from the 2007 National Household Education Surveys Program of the NCES were used to look at how parents perceived the school readiness of their young children.[38] Among the findings were that 58% of children 3 to 6 years of age and not yet in kindergarten were reported to be attending preschool or a child care center. Eighty-nine percent of children's parents planned to enroll them into kindergarten on time; 7% planned delayed enrollment. A higher percentage of boys (9% vs 4%) had parents who planned to delay kindergarten entry. When surveyed about literacy issues, 55% of children were read to every day, 28% were read to 3 or more times in the past week, 13% were read to once or twice a week, and 3% were not read to at all in the past week; mean daily reading time was 21 minutes. A lower percentage of children residing in poor households (40%) were read to every day compared with children residing in households living above the poverty level (60%).

Average television or video time for those who watched was 2.6 hours daily. Television time was somewhat longer for children of mothers who worked 35 hours or more (3 hours daily) as compared with mothers who worked less than 35 hours weekly (2.5 hours daily) or were not in the labor force (2.4 hours). With regard to school readiness skills, 93% of parents reported that their child had speech that was understandable to a stranger, 87% of children could hold a pencil, 63% could count to 20 or higher, 60% could write their first name, 32% could recognize all the letters of the alphabet, and 8% could read written words in books. Alphabet recognition varied by age, with only 13% of 3-year-olds, 38% of 4-year-olds, and 59% of 5- and 6-year-olds not enrolled in kindergarten recognizing all letters. When parents were surveyed regarding essential skills needed to prepare for kindergarten, 62% reported that sharing was essential, 56% reported that teaching the alphabet was essential, 54% reported that teaching numbers was essential, 45% reported reading was essential, and 41% reported holding a pencil was a needed skill.[38]

Child Trends analysis of the National Household Education Surveys data in 2015 indicates an increase in early literacy skills over time.[38] The percentage of 3- to 6-year-old children able to recognize all letters increased from 21% in 1993 to 38% in 2012, and those able to count to 20 or higher increased from 52% to 68% during that period. Between 1999 and 2007, the percentage of these young children who read words in a book increased from 8% to 22%. Significant discrepancies exist between early childhood readiness skills on the basis of factors such as poverty status, parents' educational status, and race and/or ethnicity. In 2007, only 21% of children living below the poverty level were able to recognize all letters of the alphabet compared with 35% of those living above the poverty level; similarly, counting to 20 was a skill that 49% of poor children at this age achieved compared with 67% of those above poverty.[39] In 2012, only 15% of children between 3 and 6 years of age (not yet in kindergarten) whose parents had not completed high school could recognize all letters of the alphabet and only 38% could count to 20, which is between 46% and 142% lower than for children whose parents had completed some college. Young Hispanic children were less likely to demonstrate the ability to recognize all letters (27%) than white (41%) or African American (44%) children in 2012; Asian American and Pacific Islander children had the highest rate of letter recognition (58%). The sex gap in readiness skills has disappeared; although girls in 1999 were significantly more likely to have achieved skills for letter recognition and counting than boys, there were no such differences by 2012. These data reflect improvement in overall readiness skills of young children from earlier studies, but gaps in achievement based on poverty and race and/or ethnicity are still readily apparent.[39]

THE RELATIONSHIP BETWEEN EARLY CHILDHOOD EDUCATION AND SCHOOL READINESS

Measurements from 2016 of the benefits of early childhood education vary depending on the type of program studied and educational outcomes tracked. In general, benefits on standardized academic achievement tests are higher for model programs (0.57 SD; 95% confidence interval [CI], 0.24 to 0.81) than for those organized at the district, state (0.32 SD; 95% CI, 0.25 to 0.38), or federal (Head Start; 0.17 SD; 95% CI, 0.12 to 0.23) levels.[40] Model programs, such as the Abecedarian Project and Perry Preschool Program, have generally been implemented as part of well-funded research projects and are closely monitored for fidelity of implementation and staffed by highly trained individuals. Evaluation of programs at the school district and state level found a statistically significant positive effect on student self-regulation (0.23 SD; 95% CI, 0.12 to 0.33), whereas a nonsignificant benefit was shown for Head Start (0.16 SD; 95% CI, −0.09 to 0.41). Long-term follow-up of participants in Head Start revealed a positive effect on high school graduation rate (0.18 SD; 95% CI, 0.03 to 0.33). Nonsignificant beneficial effects are also reported on measures of grade retention, assignment to special education, teenage birth rates, and criminality.[16]

A study from 2005 that evaluated the economic features of investing in a 1-year, high-quality, universal, preschool education in California estimated a $7000 net present-value benefit per child. This benefit equaled a return of $2.62 for every $1 invested, with an annual return rate of 10% over 60 years. This model did not include other benefits to society, such as the improved health and well-being of participating children and the potential intergenerational transmission of favorable benefits.[41,42] Economists at the Federal Reserve Bank of Minneapolis examined the rate of return on investment for early education. When considering the Perry Preschool Program, conducted in Michigan in the 1960s, which provided high-quality preschool to 3- and 4-year-old children in poverty, along with home visitation to involve parents, the economists found a "real" return on investment, adjusted for inflation, of 16%, with at least 75% of those benefits going to the general public.[43,44] The benefit/cost ratio (the ratio of the aggregate program benefits over the life of the child to the input of costs) was found to be greater than 8:1.[41] These benefits persisted to age 40, at which time more of the program group were employed than the nonprogram group (76% vs 56%), more earned over $20 000 dollars per year (60% vs 40%), and fewer were arrested more than 5 times (36% vs 55%).[45] The Carolina Abecedarian Project conducted in 1972 provides data that support the developmental and behavioral benefits of quality education provided within the context of day care programs into adulthood.[46] Economic benefits were reported in maternal earnings, decreased schooling costs from kindergarten through grade 12, increased lifetime earnings, and decreased costs related to smoking. A position paper by the National Institute for Early Education Research was published in 2013, concluding that expanding access to quality prekindergarten programs is sound public policy.[47] That authors pointed to a meta-analysis that summarizes the effects of preschool programs, the results of which pointed to 2 basic findings: (1) state and local prekindergarten programs, almost without exception, improve academic readiness for school; and (2) there are persistent impacts on achievement well beyond school entry, even though these are somewhat smaller than short-term impacts.

Enrollment of children in state-funded preschool programs nationwide doubled from 2001 to 2016, with states serving nearly 33% of 4-year-old children in 2016.[47] However, enrollment of 3-year-old children has changed little (5% total of 3-year-old children served in public preschools in 2016). Those numbers improve when looking at all public preschool programs (including special education and Head Start) to 43% of 4-year-old and 16% of 3-year-old children. Provision of preschool services is highly variable from state to state, with some states offering nearly universal services at 4 years of age and others having no programs. A negative trend of decreased state expenditure per child occurred from 2008 to 2014, but that trend has reversed from 2014 to 2016, with total state funding for preschool programs increasing to almost 7.4 billion dollars. There has also been a positive move toward improvement in developing and implementing early learning standards and developing quality standards.[48] Benchmarks need to be applied to preschool programs, including teacher training requirements, rules on class size and staff/child ratios, adequate teacher compensation, adherence to early learning standards, provision of comprehensive services, provision of at least 1 meal, and monitoring quality of sites. In 2016, many states met fewer than half of the current quality standards benchmarks, and charter schools are not required to meet these benchmarks.[47]

The data are not as clear-cut for the benefits of child care programs. Approximately 58% of children 4 and 5 years of age received center-based care in 2012, 13% received home-based relative care, and 19% had no early childhood education arrangement on a regular basis.[49] The National Institute of Child Health and Human Development Study of Early Child Care and Youth Development (2006) found that children in higher-quality nonmaternal child care had somewhat better language and cognitive development during the first 4.5 years of life but that those children with high number of hours in child care demonstrated more behavior problems; parent and family characteristics were more associated with developmental outcome than were facility features.[50]

In general, school readiness appears to have improved over the past 2 decades. The NCES tracked 2 large, nationally representative cohorts of children entering kindergarten through its ECLS.[51] The study compared school readiness in the 1998 kindergarten cohort versus the 2010 cohort. Children in the 2010 cohort were more proficient across a variety of math and reading skills, regardless of race or socioeconomic status, with particularly large gains in math and literacy proficiency among African American children. The authors suggested that early achievement gaps are narrowing and that the skills and knowledge children possess when entering school are increasing. However, they also noted that teachers rated the 2010 cohort somewhat less favorably with respect to their "approaches to learning," a measure that encompasses eagerness to learn, ability to work independently, persistence, and attention. Authors of another study using the same ECLS data concluded that "despite widening income inequality, increasing income segregation, and growing disparities in parental spending on children, disparities in school readiness narrowed from 1998 to 2010."[52] The authors hypothesized that the narrowing of the disparity was attributable to a relatively rapid increase in overall school readiness levels among poor and Hispanic children, along with less rapid increases in readiness among high-income and white children. Although these findings are encouraging, there is still reason for concern. Authors of a previously mentioned article on school readiness in poor children noted that preschool programs offer the best chance to increase school readiness in this population.[11] Although investment in early childhood education programs increased for most states from 2001 to 2009, that trend has changed since the recession in 2008. Early childhood programs receive much less funding than public education and are often at greater risk for federal and state budget cuts. Continued recognition of the importance of quality early childhood programs and the need for adequate funding will be critical.

CHILDREN WITH SPECIAL EDUCATIONAL NEEDS

Children with developmental disabilities are particularly at risk for deficits in school readiness. The Individuals with Disabilities Education Act (IDEA) of 2004 was enacted to ensure that children with special needs have access to a free and appropriate education in the least restrictive environment with adequate supports and services. Part B of the IDEA covers children with developmental disabilities from 3 to 21 years of age, and Part C addresses the need for early intervention services for children from birth to 3 years of age with qualifying conditions.

Approximately 6% of children between 3 and 5 years of age in the United States are served under Part B of IDEA with significant variability among states (4% in AL to 14% in WY).[53] The majority of these children are served under a speech and language delay category (3.1%). The second largest category is developmental delay (2.5%), and the third largest category is autism (0.6%). White children account for 52% of this population with special needs, Hispanic children represent 25%, and African American children account for 13%. This disparity of services among ethnic minority groups likely represents underidentification of minority children with disabilities at an early age, especially given the fact that African American children represent a higher percentage (15%) than do white children (13%) when evaluating the number of children in special education services between 3 and 21 years of age.[53]

With regard to early intervention services covered under Part C of IDEA, approximately 3% of children 0 to 3 years of age are served, with boys accounting for 64% of children.[54] The categories under which children received services were not available, but white children accounted for 52.6%, Hispanic children accounted for 25.9%, and African American children accounted for 12.4%. The majority (approximately 86%) of these developmental intervention services were provided in home settings. Approximately 8% of children receiving Part C services were no longer eligible for Part B services at 3 years of age, perhaps reflecting the effectiveness of early intervention.

These data seem to reflect an underrepresentation of minorities in early childhood intervention programs. Pediatricians, through developmental surveillance and screening, play an important role in identifying all children with developmental disabilities at an early age. It also appears from the data that autism spectrum disorders may be underrecognized at an early age. The prevalence of autism spectrum disorders has increased drastically, and there is evidence that intensive early intervention makes a positive impact in school readiness.[43–57] Addressing the needs of children with developmental disabilities in a timely fashion with appropriate educational services and family resources improves potential outcomes.[58]

HOW SCHOOLS AND COMMUNITIES PROMOTE SCHOOL READINESS

Limited research is available regarding readiness of schools and communities to meet the needs of the diverse population of children. One approach to identifying and tracking indicators of school and community preparedness is the School Readiness Indicators: Making Progress for Young Children program, a partnership of 16 states funded by the David and Lucile Packard Foundation, the Ford Foundation, and the Ewing Marion Kauffman Foundation.[59] This initiative has 3 goals: (1) to create a set of measurable indicators related to and defining school readiness that can be tracked at the state and local levels; (2) to have states adopt this indicator-based definition of school readiness, to fill in gaps in data, to track data, and to report findings to their citizens; and (3) to stimulate policies, programs, and other actions to improve the ability of children to read at grade level by third grade. Sample system indicators tracked by this group include (1) the proportion of children with health coverage; (2) the proportion of 3- and 4-year-old children enrolled in high-quality early education and child care programs; (3) the proportion of schools offering universal access to full-day kindergarten; (4) the proportion of children with hearing, vision, or dental problems not detected at school entry; (5) the number of adults enrolled in adult education programs or programs teaching English as a second language per 100 adults seeking those services; (6) the proportion of births to mothers with less than a 12th-grade education; and (7) the proportion of children younger than 6 years in foster care who have had more than 2 placements in 24 months. The complete set of indicators selected by each state is available online (http://www.rikidscount.org/IssueAreas/EarlyLearningampDevelopment/GettingReady.aspx). It is the belief of those investigators that this work will play an important role in shaping the educational agenda for young children and their families across the country.[60,61]

Evidence-based interventions with substantial effects on school readiness include early intervention programs for formerly preterm infants, which have been shown to prevent developmental delay, to improve grade retention, and to accelerate placement into special education.[62–64] Food supplement programs, such as the Supplemental Nutrition Program for Women, Infants, and Children, have been shown to reduce rates of low birth weight[65] and iron deficiency.[66,67] Children attending schools with school nutrition programs have improved scores on standardized academic tests.[68] Home visiting by nurses has been shown consistently to reduce rates of childhood injury, to increase fathers' involvement, to reduce family welfare dependency, and to improve school readiness.[69,70] Housing subsidies have resulted in improved neighborhood safety and reduced exposure to violence.[71,72]

In addition, there are numerous pediatric primary care programs that have been shown to have impacts across varying domains of school readiness.[73] These programs include both primary prevention programs (which seek to prevent gaps in readiness before they emerge) as well as secondary and/or tertiary prevention programs (which seek to provide additional services for families at increased risk and/or for children with observed gaps in child school readiness); these target early literacy and/or social-emotional development. All of these programs capitalize on the unique reach of pediatric well-child visits for families with young children, especially from birth to 3 years of age, and facilitate population-level intervention at a low cost. The most studied and scaled primary prevention program is Reach Out and Read (http://www.reachoutandread.org/), which impacts more than 25% of all children in low-income families by improving child language skills and increasing reading aloud activities, according to more than 15 published studies.[74] An enhancement to Reach Out and Read, the Video Interaction Project, promotes parental self-reflection and positive actions through review of videotaped parent-child interactions and was recently found to have positive impact on child social-emotional development.[75] HealthySteps uses a specialist who facilitates the delivery of well-child care on the basis of the standards in *Bright Futures: Guidelines for Health Supervision of Infants, Children, and Adolescents, Fourth Edition*, and provides primary prevention through enhanced parenting and secondary prevention through appropriate screening and referral for services.[76,77] A primary care adaptation of The Incredible Years has been shown to promote effective parenting and improve child behavior for families with children with behavior problems.[78] Two additional programs, Assuring Better Child Health and Development and Help Me Grow, provide effective secondary prevention by linking families with appropriate community services.[79,80]

WHAT PEDIATRICIANS DO TO SUPPORT SCHOOL READINESS

The role of the pediatrician in promoting school readiness was previously delineated in a recent AAP policy statement, "The Pediatrician's Role in Optimizing School Readiness."[81] It is clear that pediatric health care providers promote school readiness in the children they serve in many ways. In their office practices, they provide medical homes that promote optimal nutrition, growth, development, and physical health as part of health maintenance. Full implementation of the recommendations in *Bright Futures: Guidelines for Health Supervision of Infants, Children, and Adolescents, Fourth Edition*, includes not only provision of immunizations in a timely manner but also anticipatory guidance regarding nutrition, safety issues, vision and hearing screening, lead and anemia screening, advice regarding dental needs, and developmental surveillance and/or screening.[77] By providing ongoing surveillance and information regarding injury prevention, pediatric providers help protect children from injury and abuse.

Pediatric health care providers promote positive parent-child relationships by screening for psychosocial risks, such as parental mental illness, substance abuse, family violence, poverty, and lack of connection to community and family supports, and then identifying appropriate community resources for families.[82] The AAP Web site on social determinants of health offers numerous screening and toolkit resources for pediatric primary care providers (https://www.aap.org/en-us/advocacy-and-policy/aap-health-initiatives/Screening/Pages/Social-Determinants-of-Health.aspx). Modeling appropriate interactions in the office and providing materials and educational opportunities that promote parental knowledge of child development enhance parent-child interactions. Ongoing assessment of the interactions between the parent and child and guidance regarding behavior, temperament, and development facilitate parent understanding of child differences. Primary care parenting models such as HealthySteps, Very Important Parenting, and colocated behavioral health models have been found to be effective in supporting positive parent-child relationships and model appropriate disciplinary strategies. For families whose children present with significant behavior concerns, use of evidence-based models, such as the Positive Parenting Program and Circle of Security, and referral to appropriate behavioral health resources provide assistance to families. The Positive Parenting Program is designed to prevent and treat behavioral and emotional problems in children and teenagers by equipping parents with skills and confidence to address these problems. The Circle of Security seeks to support secure parent-child relationships by helping parents read their child's emotional needs, enhance the child's self-esteem, and support the child's ability to manage emotions.[83] Resources available to pediatricians in promoting early literacy include such evidenced-based programs as Reach Out and Read and the AAP Books Build Connections Toolkit, as well as community libraries and early childhood education programs. Pediatricians often provide guidance to parents regarding quality early child care and child education programs, including information from the National Association for the Education of Young Children, Children's Home Society, Child Care and Resource and Referral Centers, and Help Me Grow. Pediatricians also encourage communication between parents and early learning centers.[84] Pediatric health care providers identify children with delays in their development by integrating regular, systematic, developmental screening and surveillance into their practices. Children identified as having delays and children at risk for delays can then be referred to community-based services, such as early intervention programs, home visitation programs, Head Start, and special education programs available through school departments.[85]

Many pediatricians take an active role in advocating for those evidence-based practices that promote optimal early brain and child development. Some examples include (1) access to health care, including mental health services, for all children; (2) standards for state Medicaid and Early and Periodic Screening, Diagnosis, and Treatment programs that conform, at a minimum, to AAP policy recommendations[86]; (3) universal funding for clinic-based early literacy programs such as Reach Out and Read; (4) Head Start and Early Head Start programs; and (5) federal child care subsidies. AAP chapters can be centers for advocacy because they have experience, resources, and established relationships with policy makers who will be making decisions at the state level. The AAP offers opportunities to effect these policies through their state AAP chapters and in collaboration with state early childhood comprehensive systems. On a national level, the Federal Advocacy Action Network provides an additional avenue of advocacy for interested pediatricians.

Pediatricians, in their work with young children and families, provide the skills and expertise that promote not only physical health but also social-emotional health and guidance with regard to development. Their partnership with families allows for ongoing assessment of strengths and stressors and the development of collaborative strategies and interventions, which support optimal child well-being.[82,87] Pediatricians, in collaboration with school, community, and national agencies, contribute to the school readiness of young children.[81]

CONCLUSIONS

Knowledge of early brain and child development has revealed that modifiable factors in a child's early experience can greatly affect that child's learning trajectory. Several qualities that are necessary for children to be ready for school are physical and nutritional well-being, intellectual skills, motivation to learn, and strong social-emotional capacity and supports. These qualities are influenced by the health and well-being of the families and neighborhoods in which children are raised. Many US children enter kindergarten with limitations in their social-emotional, physical, and cognitive development that might have been significantly diminished or eliminated through early recognition of and attention to child and family needs. School readiness testing, when used appropriately, can yield helpful information regarding the progress of communities and states in meeting the needs of young children. Early childhood education programs can lessen the disparity in school readiness created by poverty and other toxic stressors. Community and national programs that support young children and their families also play a significant role in optimizing school readiness. Pediatricians, by the nature of their work with young children and families, are at the forefront of the effort to promote school readiness. Pediatric primary care providers can both model and promote effective early childhood practices and interventions to promote school readiness and collaborate with communities and schools to ensure their implementation.

LEAD AUTHORS

P. Gail Williams, MD, FAAP
Marc Alan Lerner, MD, FAAP

COUNCIL ON EARLY CHILDHOOD EXECUTIVE COMMITTEE, 2017–2018

Jill Sells, MD, Chairperson
Sherri L. Alderman, MD, MPH, IMH-E, FAAP
Andrew Hashikawa, MD, MPH, FAAP
Alan Mendelsohn, MD, FAAP
Terri McFadden, MD, FAAP
Dipesh Navsaria, MD, MPH, MSILS, FAAP
Georgina Peacock, MD, MPH, FAAP
Seth Scholer, MD, MPH, FAAP
Jennifer Takagishi, MD, FAAP
Douglas Vanderbilt, MD, FAAP
P. Gail Williams, MD, FAAP

LIAISONS

Lynette Fraga, PhD – *Child Care Aware*
Rebecca Parlakian, MS – *Zero To Three*
Katiana Garagozlo, MD – *American Academy of Pediatrics Section on Pediatric Trainees*
Dina Lieser, MD, FAAP – *Maternal and Child Health Bureau*
Alecia Stephenson – *National Association for the Education of Young Children*

STAFF

Charlotte O. Zia, MPH, CHES

COUNCIL ON SCHOOL HEALTH EXECUTIVE COMMITTEE, 2017–2018

Marc Alan Lerner, MD, FAAP, Chairperson
Cheryl L. De Pinto, MD, MPH, FAAP, Chairperson Elect
Elliott Attisha, DO, FAAP
Nathaniel Beers, MD, MPA, FAAP
Erica Gibson, MD, FAAP
Peter Gorski, MD, MPA, FAAP
Chris Kjolhede, MD, MPH, FAAP
Sonja C. O'Leary, MD, FAAP
Heidi K. Schumacher, MD, FAAP
Adrienne Weiss-Harrison, MD, FAAP

LIAISONS

Susan Hocevar Adkins, MD, FAAP – *Centers for Disease Control and Prevention*
Laurie G. Combe, MN, RN, NCSN – *National Association of School Nurses*
Veda Johnson, MD, FAAP – *School-Based Health Alliance*

STAFF

Madra Guinn-Jones, MPH
Stephanie Domain, MS

ABBREVIATIONS

AAP: American Academy of Pediatrics
CI: confidence interval
ECLS: Early Childhood Longitudinal Study
IDEA: Individuals with Disabilities Education Act
NCES: National Center for Education and Statistics
NCSL: National Conference of State Legislatures

POTENTIAL CONFLICT OF INTEREST: The authors have indicated they have no potential conflicts of interest to disclose.

REFERENCES

1. Knudsen EI, Heckman JJ, Cameron JL, Shonkoff JP. Economic, neurobiological, and behavioral perspectives on building America's future workforce. *Proc Natl Acad Sci USA*. 2006;103(27): 10155–10162
2. Heckman JJ. The economics, technology, and neuroscience of human capability formation. *Proc Natl Acad Sci USA*. 2007;104(33):13250–13255
3. Zuckerman B, Halfon N. School readiness: an idea whose time has arrived. *Pediatrics*. 2003;111(6 pt 1): 1433–1436
4. Fellitti VJ, Anda RF. The relationship of adverse childhood experiences to adult medical disease, psychiatric disorders and sexual behavior: implication for health care. In: Lanius R, Vermetten E, eds. *The Hidden Epidemic: The Impact of Early Life Trauma and Health and Disease*. 1st ed. Cambridge, United Kingdom: Cambridge University Press; 2010:77–87
5. National Scientific Council on the Developing Child. Excessive stress disrupts the architecture of the developing brain. Working paper 3. 2014. Available at: https://developingchild.harvard.edu/wp-content/uploads/2005/05/Stress_Disrupts_Architecture_Developing_Brain-1.pdf. Accessed September 18, 2018
6. National Scientific Council on the Developing Child, Center on the Developing Child at Harvard University. Toxic stress. Available at: https://developingchild.harvard.edu/science/key-concepts/toxic-stress/. Accessed September 18, 2018
7. Stambaugh LF, Ringeisen H, Casanueva CC, Tueller S, Smith KE, Dolan M. *Adverse Childhood Experiences in NSCAW: OPRE Report #2013-66*. Washington, DC: Office of Planning, Research and Evaluation, Administration for Children and Families, US Department of Health and Human Services; 2013
8. Wildeman C, Emanuel N, Leventhal JM, Putnam-Hornstein E, Waldfogel J, Lee H. The prevalence of confirmed maltreatment among US children, 2004 to 2011. *JAMA Pediatr*. 2014;168(8): 706–713
9. Child and Adolescent Health Measures Initiative. Overview of adverse child and family experiences among US children. 2013. Available at: www.childhealthdata.org/docs/drc/aces-data-brief_version-1-0.pdf. Accessed September 18, 2018
10. Bethell CD, Newacheck P, Hawes E, Halfon N. Adverse childhood experiences: assessing the impact on health and school engagement and the mitigating role of resilience. *Health Aff (Millwood)*. 2014;33(12):2106–2115
11. Isaacs J. *Starting School at a Disadvantage: The School Readiness of Poor Children*. Washington, DC: Center on Children and Families at Brookings; 2012
12. Brooks-Gunn J, Markman LB. The contribution of parenting to ethnic and racial gaps in school readiness. *Future Child*. 2005;15(1):139–168

13. Webb M, Dowd K, Harden BJ, Landsverk J, Testa M. *Child Welfare and Child Well-Being: New Perspectives for the National Survey of Child and Adolescent Well-Being.* Oxford, England: Oxford Press; 2009

14. Casanueva C, Dozier M, Tueller S, Jones Harden B, Dolan M, Smith D. *Instability and Early Life Changes Among Children in the Child Welfare System: OPRE Report No. 2012.* Washington, DC: Office of Planning, Research and Evaluation, Administration for Children and Families, US Department of Health and Human Services; 2012

15. World Health Organization. *Early Childhood Development and Disability: A Discussion Paper.* Geneva, Switzerland: World Health Organization; 2012

16. Weitzman M, Lee L; Encyclopedia of Early Childhood Development. Low income and pregnancy: low income and its impact on psychosocial child development. Available at: http://www.child-encyclopedia.com/sites/default/files/textes-experts/en/794/low-income-and-its-impact-on-psychosocial-child-development.pdf. Accessed September 18, 2018

17. Weitzman M, Byrd RS, Aligne CA, Moss M. The effects of tobacco exposure on children's behavioral and cognitive functioning: implications for clinical and public health policy and future research. *Neurotoxicol Teratol.* 2002; 24(3):397–406

18. Cates CB, Weisleder A, Mendelsohn AL. Mitigating the effects of family poverty on early child development through parenting interventions in primary care. *Acad Pediatr.* 2016;16(suppl 3): S112–S120

19. National Education Goals Panel. *The Goal 1 Technical Planning Subgroup Report on School Readiness.* Washington, DC: National Education Goals Panel; 1991

20. Morgan LJ, Spears LS, Kaplan C. *Making Children a National Priority: A Framework for Community Action.* Washington, DC: Child Welfare League of America; 2003

21. Meisels SJ. Assessing readiness. In: Planta RC, Cox MJ, eds. *The Transition to Kindergarten.* Baltimore, MD: National Center for Early Development and Learning; 1999:39–66

22. National Research Council, Institute of Medicine. In: Shonkoff JP, Phillips DA, eds. *From Neurons to Neighborhoods: The Science of Early Childhood Development.* Washington, DC: National Academies Press; 2000

23. Willer B, Bredekamp S. Public policy report: redefining readiness: an essential requisite for educational reform. *Young Children.* 1990;45(5): 22–24

24. Gnedza MT, Bolig R. *A National Survey of Public School of Public School Testing of Prekindergarten and Kindergarten Children.* Alexandria, VA: National Academy of Sciences; 1988

25. Shepard LA, Taylor GA, Kagan SL. *Trends in Early Childhood Assessment Policies and Practices.* Washington, DC: US Department of Education; 1996

26. National Center for Educational Statistics. Kindergarten entry status: on-time, delayed-entry, and repeating kindergartners. 2013. Available at: https://nces.ed.gov/programs/coe/indicator_tea.asp. Accessed September 18, 2018

27. Stedron JM, Berger A. *NCSL Technical Report: State Approaches to School Readiness Update, 2010.* Denver, CO: National Conference of State Legislatures; 2010. Accessed September 18, 2018

28. National Conference of State Legislatures. *NCSL Technical Report: State Approaches to School Readiness Update, 2014.* Denver, CO: National Conference of State Legislatures;

29. Howard EC. *Moving Forward with Kindergarten Readiness Assessments: A Position Paper on the Early Childhood Education State Collaborative on Association and Student Standards.* Washington, DC: Council of Chief State School Officers; 2011

30. National Association for the Education of Young Children, National Association of Early Childhood Specialists in State Departments of Education. *Early Learning Standards: Creating the Conditions for Success: A Joint Statement of the National Association for the Education of Young Children (NAEYC) and the National Association of Early Childhood Specialists in State Departments of Education (NAECS/SDE).* Washington, DC: National Association for the Education of Young Children; 2002

31. Transforming Early Childhood Community Systems. What is TECCS? Available at: www.teccs.net. Accessed September 18, 2018

32. West J, Denton K, Germino-Hausken E. *America's Kindergartners: Early Childhood Longitudinal Study, Kindergarten Class of 1998-99.* Washington, DC: National Center for Education Statistics, US Department of Education; 2001

33. Duncan GJ, Murnane RJ. *Restoring Opportunity: The Crisis of Inequality and the Challenge for American Education.* New York, NY: Harvard Press; 2014:58–69

34. Zill N, West J. *Findings From the Condition of Education 2000: Entering Kindergarten.* Washington, DC: National Center for Education Statistics, US Department of Education; 2001

35. Denton K, West J. *Children's Reading and Mathematics Achievement in Kindergarten and First Grade.* Washington, DC: National Center for Education Statistics, US Department of Education; 2002

36. Rathburn A, West J. *From Kindergarten Through Third Grade: Children's Beginning School Experiences.* Washington, DC: National Center for Education Statistics, US Department of Education; 2004

37. O'Donnell K, Mulligan G. *Parents' Reports of the School Readiness of Young Children. National Household Education Surveys Program of 2007, First Look.* Washington, DC: National Center for Educational Statistics, US Department of Education; 2008

38. Child Trends. Early school readiness. 2012. Available at: https://www.childtrends.org/?indicators=early-childhood-readiness. Accessed June 26, 2019

39. Guide to Community Preventive Services. Why link to the community guide? Available at: https://www.thecommunityguide.org/about/link-to-us. Accessed September 18, 2018

40. Hahn RA, Barnett WS, Knopf JA, et al; Community Preventive Services Task Force. Early childhood education to promote health equity: a community guide systematic review. *J Public Health Manag Pract.* 2016;22(5):E1–E8

41. Karoly LA, Bigelow JH. *The Economics of Investing in Universal Preschool Education in California.* Santa Monica, CA: Rand Corporation; 2005

42. Currie J. Early childhood education programs. *J Econ Perspect.* 2001;15(2): 213–238

43. Rolnick AJ, Grunewald R. *Technical Report: Early Childhood Development: Economic Development With a High Public Return.* Minneapolis, MN: Federal Reserve Bank of Minneapolis; 2003

44. Friedman-Krauss A, Barnett WS. Early childhood education: pathways to better health. Available at: http://nieer.org/wp-content/uploads/2016/08/health20brief.pdf. Accessed September 18, 2018

45. Schweinhart LJ, Montie J, Xiang Z, et al. *The High/Scope Perry Preschool Study Through Age 40: Summary, Conclusions and Frequently Asked Questions.* Ypsilanti, MI: High/Scope Educational Research Foundation; 2005

46. Campbell FA, Ramey CT, Pungello E, Sparling J, Miller-Johnson S. Early childhood education: young adult outcomes from the Abecedarian Project. *Appl Dev Sci.* 2002;6(1):42–57

47. Barnett WS, Friedman-Krauss AH, Weisenfeld GG, Horowitz M, Kasmin R, Squires JH. *The State of Preschool 2016: State Preschool Yearbook.* New Brunswick, NJ: National Institute for Early Education Research; 2017

48. National Center for Education Statistics. *The Condition of Education: Children and Youth with Disabilities.* Washington, DC: National Center for Education Statistics, US Department of Education; 2016

49. National Center for Education Statistics. *Fast Facts for Child Care, Primary Early Care and Education Arrangements, and Achievement at Kindergarten Entry. Publication No. NCES 2016-070.* Washington, DC: National Center for Education Statistics, US Department of Education; 2016

50. The National Institute of Child Health and Human Development Study of Early Child Care and Youth Development. *Findings for Children up to Age 4 1/2 Years.* Washington, DC: National Institute of Child Health and Human Development, US Department of Health and Human Services; 2006

51. Bassok D, Latham S; EdPolicyWorks. Kids today: changes in school-readiness in an early childhood era. 2014. Available at: https://curry.virginia.edu/uploads/resourceLibrary/35_Kids_Today.pdf. Accessed June 26, 2019

52. Reardon SF, Portilla XA. Recent trends in income, racial, and ethnic school readiness gaps at kindergarten entry. *AERA Open.* 2016;2(3):1–8

53. US Department of Education. IDEA section 618 data products: statistic tables. Available at: https://www2.ed.gov/programs/osepidea/618-data/index.html. Accessed June 26, 2019

54. Dawson G, Jones EJ, Merkle K, et al. Early behavioral intervention is associated with normalized brain activity in young children with autism. *J Am Acad Child Adolesc Psychiatry.* 2012;51(11):1150–1159

55. Centers for Disease Control and Prevention. Autism spectrum disorders: data & statistics on autism spectrum disorder. Available at: https://www.cdc.gov/ncbddd/autism/data.html. Accessed September 18, 2018

56. Marsh A, Spagnol V, Grove R, Eapen V. Transition to school for children with autism spectrum disorder: a systematic review. *World J Psychiatry.* 2017;7(3):184–196

57. Sussman A. *Summary of Autism Spectrum Disorders Research FY 2006 - FY 2015.* Washington, DC: National Center for Special Education Research, Institute of Education Sciences; 2016

58. Dreyer BP. Early childhood stimulation in the developing and developed world: if not now, when? *Pediatrics.* 2011; 127(5):975–977

59. Zaff J, Calkins J. Background for community-level work on mental health and externalizing disorders in adolescence: reviewing the literature on contributing factors. Available at: https://www.researchgate.net/publication/237619644_Background_for_Community-Level_Work_on_Mental_Health_and_Externalizing_Disorders_in_Adolescence_Reviewing_the_Literature_on_Contributing_Factors. Accessed June 26, 2019

60. Bryant EB, Walsh CB. *States Use Indicators of School Readiness to Improve Public Policies for Young Children.* New York, NY: National Center for Children in Poverty; 2005

61. Rhode Island Kids Count. The school readiness indicators initiative: a 17 state partnership. 2005.. Available at: www.rikidscount.org/IssueAreas/EarlyLearningampDevelopment/GettingReady.aspx. Accessed September 18, 2018

62. Brooks-Gunn J, McCarton CM, Casey PH, et al. Early intervention in low-birth-weight premature infants. Results through age 5 years from the Infant Health and Development Program. *JAMA.* 1994;272(16):1257–1262

63. McCormick MC, McCarton C, Tonascia J, Brooks-Gunn J. Early educational intervention for very low birth weight infants: results from the Infant Health and Development Program. *J Pediatr.* 1993;123(4):527–533

64. Kotelchuck M, Schwartz JB, Anderka MT, Finison KS. WIC participation and pregnancy outcomes: Massachusetts Statewide Evaluation Project. *Am J Public Health.* 1984;74(10):1086–1092

65. Rush D, Leighton J, Sloan NL, et al. The National WIC Evaluation: evaluation of the Special Supplemental Food Program for Women, Infants, and Children. VI. Study of infants and children. *Am J Clin Nutr.* 1988;48(suppl 2):484–511

66. Vazquez-Seoane P, Windom R, Pearson HA. Disappearance of iron-deficiency anemia in a high-risk infant population given supplemental iron. *N Engl J Med.* 1985;313(19):1239–1240

67. Yip R, Binkin NJ, Fleshood L, Trowbridge FL. Declining prevalence of anemia among low-income children in the United States. *JAMA.* 1987;258(12): 1619–1623

68. Meyers AF, Sampson AE, Weitzman M, Rogers BL, Kayne H. School Breakfast Program and school performance. *Am J Dis Child.* 1989;143(10):1234–1239

69. Olds DL, Henderson CR Jr, Kitzman HJ, Eckenrode JJ, Cole RE, Tatelbaum RC. Prenatal and infancy home visitation by nurses: recent findings. *Future Child.* 1999;9(1):44–65, 190–191

70. Peacock S, Konrad S, Watson E, Nickel D, Muhajarine N. Effectiveness of home visiting programs on child outcomes: a systematic review. *BMC Public Health.* 2013;13:17

71. Anderson LM, Shinn C, St CJ, et al; Centers for Disease Control and Prevention. Community interventions to promote healthy social environments: early childhood development and family housing. A report on recommendations of the Task Force on Community Preventive Services. *MMWR Recomm Rep.* 2002;51(RR-1):1–8

72. Office of Policy Development and Research. Housing's and neighborhoods' role in shaping children's future. 2014. Available at: https://www.huduser.gov/portal/periodicals/em/fall14/highlight1.html. Accessed June 26, 2019

73. Cates CB, Weisleder A, Dreyer BP, et al. Leveraging healthcare to promote responsive parenting: impacts of the video interaction project on parenting stress. *J Child Fam Stud.* 2016;25(3): 827–835

74. Mendelsohn AL, Mogilner LN, Dreyer BP, et al. The impact of a clinic-based literacy intervention on language development in inner-city preschool children. *Pediatrics.* 2001;107(1): 130–134

75. Weisleder A, Cates CB, Dreyer BP, et al. Promotion of positive parenting and prevention of socioemotional disparities. *Pediatrics.* 2016;137(2): e20153239

76. Minkovitz CS, Strobino D, Mistry KB, et al. Healthy steps for young children: sustained results at 5.5 years. *Pediatrics.* 2007;120(3). Available at: www.pediatrics.org/cgi/content/full/120/3/e658

77. Hagan JF Jr, Shaw JS, Duncan PM, eds. *Bright Futures: Guidelines for Health Supervision of Infants, Children, and Adolescents.* 4th ed. Elk Grove Village, IL: American Academy of Pediatrics; 2017

78. Perrin EC, Sheldrick RC, McMenamy JM, Henson BS, Carter AS. Improving parenting skills for families of young children in pediatric settings: a randomized clinical trial. *JAMA Pediatr.* 2014;168(1):16–24

79. Earls MF, Hay SS. Setting the stage for success: implementation of developmental and behavioral screening and surveillance in primary care practice--the North Carolina Assuring Better Child Health and Development (ABCD) project. *Pediatrics.* 2006;118(1). Available at: www.pediatrics.org/cgi/content/full/118/1/e183

80. HelpMeGrow National Center. Latest resources. Available at: https://www.helpmegrownational.org. Accessed June 26, 2019

81. Council on Early Childhood; Council on School Health. The pediatrician's role in optimizing school readiness. *Pediatrics.* 2016;138(3):e20162293

82. Shonkoff JP, Garner AS; Committee on Psychosocial Aspects of Child and Family Health; Committee on Early Childhood, Adoption, and Dependent Care; Section on Developmental and Behavioral Pediatrics. The lifelong effects of early childhood adversity and toxic stress. *Pediatrics.* 2012;129(1). Available at: www.pediatrics.org/cgi/content/full/129/1/e232

83. Gleason MM, Goldson E, Yogman MW; Council on Early Childhood; Committee on Psychosocial Aspects of Child and Family Health; Section on Developmental and Behavioral Pediatrics. Addressing early childhood emotional and behavioral problems. *Pediatrics.* 2016;138(6):e20163025

84. American Academy of Pediatrics. Healthy child care. Available at: https://www.aap.org/en-us/advocacy-and-policy/aap-health-initiatives/healthy-child-care/Pages/default.aspx. Accessed September 18, 2018

85. Developmental surveillance and screening of infants and young children. *Pediatrics.* 2001;108(1): 192–196

86. Schor EL, Abrams M, Shea K. Medicaid: health promotion and disease prevention for school readiness. *Health Aff (Millwood).* 2007;26(2):420–429

87. Committee on Early Childhood, Adoption, and Dependent Care. The pediatrician's role in family support and family support programs. *Pediatrics.* 2011;128(6). Available at: www.pediatrics.org/cgi/content/full/128/6/e1680

School-Aged Children Who Are Not Progressing Academically: Considerations for Pediatricians

• *Clinical Report*

CLINICAL REPORT Guidance for the Clinician in Rendering Pediatric Care

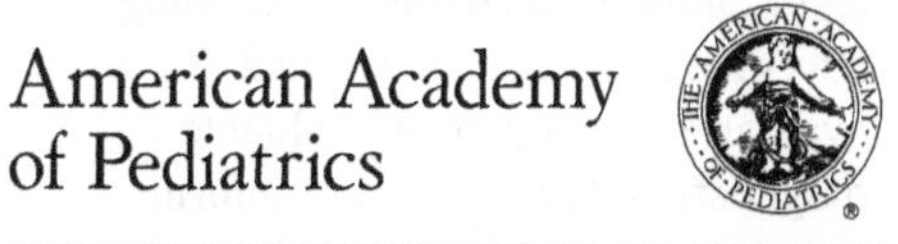

School-aged Children Who Are Not Progressing Academically: Considerations for Pediatricians

Celiane Rey-Casserly, PhD,[a] Laura McGuinn, MD, FAAP,[b] Arthur Lavin, MD, FAAP,[c] COMMITTEE ON PSYCHOSOCIAL ASPECTS OF CHILD AND FAMILY HEALTH,SECTION ON DEVELOPMENTAL AND BEHAVIORAL PEDIATRICS

abstract

Pediatricians and other pediatric primary care providers may be consulted when families have concerns that their child is not making expected progress in school. Pediatricians care not only for an increasingly diverse population of children who may have behavioral, psychological, and learning difficulties but also for increasing numbers of children with complex and chronic medical problems that can affect the development of the central nervous system and can present with learning and academic concerns. In many instances, pediatric providers require additional information about the nature of cognitive, psychosocial, and educational difficulties that affect their school-aged patients. Our purpose for this report is to describe the current state of the science regarding educational achievement to inform pediatricians' decisions regarding further evaluation of a child's challenges. In this report, we review commonly available options for psychological evaluation and/or treatment, medical referrals, and/or recommendations for referral for eligibility determinations at school and review strategies for collaborating with families, schools, and specialists to best serve children and families.

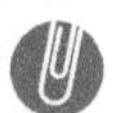

[a]Department of Psychiatry, Boston Children's Hospital and Harvard Medical School, Boston, Massachusetts; [b]Division of Developmental-Behavioral Pediatrics, Department of Pediatrics, University of Alabama, Birmingham, and Children's of Alabama, Birmingham, Alabama; and [c]Advanced Pediatrics, Beachwood, Ohio

All authors participated substantially in the concept, design, drafting, and revising of the manuscript, and all authors approved the final manuscript as submitted.

Clinical reports from the American Academy of Pediatrics benefit from expertise and resources of liaisons and internal (AAP) and external reviewers. However, clinical reports from the American Academy of Pediatrics may not reflect the views of the liaisons or the organizations or government agencies that they represent.

The guidance in this report does not indicate an exclusive course of treatment or serve as a standard of medical care. Variations, taking into account individual circumstances, may be appropriate.

All clinical reports from the American Academy of Pediatrics automatically expire 5 years after publication unless reaffirmed, revised, or retired at or before that time.

This document is copyrighted and is property of the American Academy of Pediatrics and its Board of Directors. All authors have filed conflict of interest statements with the American Academy of Pediatrics. Any conflicts have been resolved through a process approved by the Board of Directors. The American Academy of Pediatrics has neither solicited nor accepted any commercial involvement in the development of the content of this publication.

DOI: https://doi.org/10.1542/peds.2019-2520

To cite: Rey-Casserly C, McGuinn L, Lavin A, AAP COMMITTEE ON PSYCHOSOCIAL ASPECTS OF CHILD AND FAMILY HEALTH,SECTION ON DEVELOPMENTAL AND BEHAVIORAL PEDIATRICS. School-aged Children Who Are Not Progressing Academically: Considerations for Pediatricians. *Pediatrics.* 2019;144(4):e20192520

INTRODUCTION

Pediatricians and other pediatric primary care providers may be the first to be consulted when families have concerns that their child is not making expected progress in school. Furthermore, pediatricians are confronted with an increasingly diverse population of children who may have behavioral, psychological, and learning difficulties. They also provide care to increasing numbers of children with complex and chronic medical problems that affect the development of the central nervous system and have the potential to derail or divert the acquisition of behavioral capacities. In some cases, the problem can be sorted out through history and interventions conducted in a clinical visit. In other instances, pediatric providers require additional information about the nature of cognitive, psychosocial, and educational difficulties that affect their school-aged patients' academic functioning. Psychological and educational evaluations can provide valuable diagnostic information and inform strategies for intervention that address cognitive, psychosocial, and learning needs. Evaluation of these domains is accomplished in a variety of health care, community-based, and school settings. Assessment information may exist from previous evaluations, in which case the pediatrician's role is one of review and analysis of results as they relate to intervention planning and ongoing medical management. In other cases, the pediatrician will refer a child for additional evaluation. With the information from in-depth assessments, pediatricians are strategically positioned to work in partnership with families and help them in collaborating with schools and other health care specialists.

Our purpose for this clinical report is to present a clinical approach to school-aged children who are not progressing academically. It complements existing American Academy of Pediatrics (AAP) clinical reports, practice guidelines, policy statements, tool kits, books, and case presentations that provide guidance regarding the early childhood age group as well as specific issues such as learning disabilities, mental health concerns, youth violence prevention, and foster care.[1–21] In this clinical report, we first provide a clinical overview of school-aged children with academic progress problems, including the epidemiology, presentation, and differential diagnosis, and discuss the pediatrician's role in identification and management. A more detailed review follows, with strategies pediatricians can use to clarify why, when, how, and to whom to refer for further evaluation as well as guidance on how to understand evaluation results, communicate findings with families, and integrate the information into clinical management. The clinical report is guided by the AAP's medical home care-coordination framework[22] and supports the pediatrician's collaboration and consultation across service system sectors. The Supplemental Information provides resources for this collaboration, including coding and billing strategies to address the resource requirements for this type of collaboration.

It is important to acknowledge that the additional evaluation services for children can vary widely in how they are organized and funded across communities. Therefore, the content in this report does not indicate an exclusive course of treatment nor serve as a standard of care and may not be applicable to every professional situation. The suggestions are not definitive and are not intended to take precedence over the clinical judgment of pediatricians. Variations, taking into account individual circumstances, will be appropriate.

BACKGROUND

Failing to progress academically is a nonspecific symptom with many possible etiologies and forms of presentation. Problems may involve only 1 area or many aspects of academic functioning. Onset and expression of the symptom are highly variable. Some children have accompanying behavioral problems, and others do not. The severity of the problem lies on a continuum and is dependent on characteristics of the child, the school, the family, and the community and its various cultures as well as the interplay of each of these factors. Furthermore, the problem likely will vary over time as children progress in age.

Magnitude of the Problem

Estimating the prevalence of academic progress problems in school-aged children is challenging given the heterogeneity of the problem and the lack of a universally agreed on definition. In regard to neurodevelopmental and health disorders associated with academic dysfunction, statistics regarding provision of special education services offer proxy indicators (note that these numbers likely underestimate the magnitude because the Individuals with Disabilities Education Act [IDEA],[23] the US federal law mandating provision of special education services that was originally passed in 1975, requires a diagnosis, and a child's underachievement may be significant before one can be made). Data used to monitor the compliance with IDEA have been collected since 1976. In 2014–2015, the most recent school year for which analysis is available, the number of children 3 to 21 years of age served by federally supported special education programs in the United States was estimated to be 6.6 million or 13% of the total public school enrollment.[24] The distribution by disability type revealed that the highest percentage of children (35%) were qualified as having a specific learning disability (note that the IDEA defines a specific learning disability as "a disorder in one or more of the basic psychological processes involved in understanding or using language, spoken or written, that may manifest itself in an imperfect ability to listen, think, speak, read, write, spell, or do mathematical calculations"). The next largest category of children included those with speech or language impairment (20%), followed by those with other health impairments (13%), which included children with "limited strength, vitality, or alertness due to chronic or acute health problems such as a heart condition, tuberculosis, rheumatic fever, nephritis, asthma, sickle cell anemia, hemophilia, epilepsy, lead poisoning, leukemia, or diabetes." Children with autism spectrum disorder represented 9% of the distribution,

TABLE 1 Differential Diagnoses for Failing to Progress Academically, Organized by Category

Category	Example Diagnoses or Conditions and Relevant Past, Family, or Social History
Vascular	Prematurity with intraventricular hemorrhage
	Ruptured aneurysm with brain injury
	Stroke
	Congenital heart disease
	Clotting disorders
Infectious	Meningitis or encephalitis, perinatal infections
Trauma	Head trauma with brain injury
	Exposure to child abuse and neglect
	Traumatic stress
Toxic exposure	Prenatal exposure to alcohol
	Lead and/or other environmental toxicants
	Substance use by child
Attention deficits	ADHD
Affective disorders	Depression
Adjustment disorders	Adjustment disorders
Anxiety disorders	Generalized anxiety, separation anxiety, school phobia
Autism spectrum disorder	Autism
Metabolic	Inborn errors of metabolism
Iatrogenic	Medication adverse effects
Idiopathic	Despite thorough workup, cause cannot be determined
Neurologic	Intellectual disabilities
	Absence seizures
	Motor coordination disorders
	Tourette's syndrome
Neoplastic or hematologic	New onset neoplasms
	Neurologic effects of previous chemotherapy or radiotherapy
	Sickle cell anemia
	Iron deficiency anemia
Social	Inadequate financial and/or material resources, poverty
	Hunger
	Frequent school absences, truancy
	Parental or family mental health problems, substance use, domestic violence
	Separation and divorce, death of a loved one, foster care
	Poor school- or teacher-child fit
	Bullying, ostracism, cyberbullying
	Military deployment of a family member or loved one
Sensory	Visual impairment
	Hearing loss
Sleep	Sleep hygiene problems
	Obstructive sleep apnea
Speech and language	Receptive expressive language disorders
	Articulation disorders
	Learning English as a second language
	Social communication disorder
Specific learning disabilities	Reading, math, and writing learning disabilities
Congenital	Genetic disorders with associated developmental delays
	Congenital brain malformations
Chronic diseases	Asthma
	Eczema
	Diabetes
	Failure to thrive
	Chronic pain
	Dental caries
Degenerative	Neurodegenerative disorders (mitochondrial disorders, leukodystrophies, etc)
Endocrine	Type 1 diabetes mellitus
	Thyroid disease

and those with intellectual disability and developmental delay represented 6% each. Children with multiple disabilities, hearing impairments, orthopedic impairments, visual impairments, traumatic brain injuries, and deaf-blindness each accounted for ≤2% of those served under IDEA.[25] The IDEA monitoring statistics are similar to those in other national surveys that reveal that ~20% of US children have a special health care need.[26,27] These figures provide an approximate estimate of the degree of likelihood to which pediatricians will encounter patients with problems progressing academically and the relative frequency of specific etiologies.

Presentation of Academic Progress Problems

Timing of the onset of academic progress problems may provide clues to the type of underlying learning dysfunction present. In some cases, children's academic problems come to attention before they are fully manifested because of a developmental or medical condition that leads to them being more closely monitored. For example, cancer survival, prematurity, traumatic brain injury, seizures, language delays, or other conditions might place the child in contact with the health care and/or public education systems at an earlier age. In that context, risks for or problems with their academic functioning might come to recognition at an earlier stage of problem emergence through screening or evaluations conducted in those systems.

In school-aged children who have had no reason to be monitored similarly, academic progress problems often become apparent when classroom demands exceed an individual child's capacity. Therefore, timing of onset varies in relation to the progression of demands in successive school years. For example, reading decoding problems may become evident in the early elementary years, whereas reading comprehension problems and mathematic learning disabilities may not be apparent until the middle-elementary years. Children who have problems inferring from reading material and those who have written language disabilities may go unrecognized until the later elementary years, when those skills are expected regularly in the classroom. A common adage is that children learn to read before third grade and read to learn from third grade on. Some learning problems may escape detection until middle school. At that point, the increased demands to organize and prioritize materials for learning, to read larger volumes of material, or to complete long-term assignments may exceed the abilities of a child with subtler learning disabilities. Some individuals with learning disabilities who have been able to compensate throughout school years may not be recognized even until adulthood.

Whether the onset of the academic underperformance is acute or chronic may also help in determining etiology. For example, children with learning disabilities may chronically underperform academically because of their neurologically based learning differences. On the other hand, acute academic decline in a child who previously was performing well may indicate onset of a physical condition or an acute stressor (eg, bullying, ostracization, change in teachers or schools, family concerns, death of a close friend or relative, substance use, etc).

Alternatively, behavioral or emotional challenges may present concerns before the neurodevelopmental disability that is causing the academic problem is discovered. Challenging behaviors may include hyperactivity, inattention, anxiety, irritability, sadness, aggression, oppositionality, and/or social isolation. Identification of the academic difficulty as the cause of the behavioral challenge allows for optimal management of the behavior. A thorough evaluation is important in determining if behavioral and emotional challenges are co-occurring or the principal reason for the child's concerns.

The location of where a behavioral problem occurs can also provide important clues to etiology for academic underachievement. A child who displays oppositional behavior only at school but is compliant at home, where parents are not placing academic demands, may have an undiagnosed learning disability. Another child might behave well in the classroom but decompensate emotionally or behaviorally at home while completing homework.

Differential Diagnosis of Academic Progress Problems

There are many conditions that can lead to the symptoms of academic dysfunction. Disorders can involve neurologic, emotional, or behavioral functioning abnormalities alone or in various combinations. In Table 1, we offer a list of such conditions, organized into a set of categories for consideration of the range of such causes. As with any differential diagnosis of a set of symptoms, multiple etiologies may be present in an individual child.

THE PEDIATRICIAN'S ROLE

Although the majority of the responsibility for evaluation and management of children who are failing to progress academically traditionally lies with the school system, as advocates for child health and well-being, pediatricians contribute importantly. In this section, we describe the pediatrician's roles, which include prevention, early recognition, diagnosis of underlying medical conditions, referral, treatment, advocacy, and monitoring. The Medical Evaluation section that follows includes a more in-depth exploration of the role along with tools and strategies feasible for use in primary care settings when pediatricians encounter a school-aged child who is failing to progress academically.

Prevention

The pediatrician's role in preventing academic underachievement includes contributing to protecting children from brain injury. Performing immunizations; monitoring growth and nutrition; screening for anemia and lead exposure; encouraging the use of helmets, car seats, and seat belts; preventing alcohol, tobacco, nicotine, cannabis, and other substance use (including for female patients of childbearing age); and identifying and addressing psychosocial risks are just some of the tools that pediatricians employ on a regular basis that contribute to preventing brain injury in children. *Bright Futures: Guidelines for Health Supervision of Infants, Children, and Adolescents, Fourth Edition*, offers extensive resources to the pediatrician who is considering the approaches to anticipatory guidance relevant to addressing possibly emerging difficulties children face when performing schoolwork.[28]

Early Recognition

Although the primary focus of this report is school-aged children, it is important to mention the role pediatricians have in early detection throughout childhood. Surveillance of all children, beginning in infancy, for risk factors with the potential to interfere with typical academic progress can lead to earlier identification and intervention. Practice guidelines and policy statements are available to help pediatricians systematically monitor developmental progress, screen for risk, and identify preschool-aged children who warrant early intervention.[2–4,6–9,16] Surveillance for early warning signs of language-based learning disabilities in the preschool age group is warranted and can be facilitated by asking about

TABLE 2 Selected Relevant Screening Tools Feasible for Use in Pediatric Primary Care

Screening Tool	Screening Purpose	Available Forms and Languages[a]	Approximate Time to Complete	Ages	Notes and Link or Source
AAP Guide to Learning Disabilities for Primary Care, Appendix B[19]	Learning disabilities, language disabilities, motor coordination problems	Parent, teenager	5 min	Preschool to high school	Psychometrics not evaluated (meant to be checklist inventories of skills acquired at various ages not an instrument); AAP bookstore (available as an e-book at https://shop.aap.org/)
Einstein Evaluation of School-Related Skills[47]	Academic problems	Child	7–10 min	5–10 y	https://marketplace.unl.edu/buros/einstein-assessment-of-school-related-skills.html
The Brief Impairment Scale[48]	Interpersonal relations (with parents, siblings, peers, teachers, and other adults), school and/or work (attendance, performance, responsibility), and self-fulfillment (sports participation, hobbies, self-care, enjoyment)	Layperson with minimal training (possibly adaptable for completion by parent)	3–5 min	4–17 y	http://www.heardalliance.org/wp-content/uploads/2011/04/Brief-Impairment-Scale-English.pdf
Screen for Child Anxiety Related Emotional Disorders[49]	Anxiety disorders	Parent, child; 10 languages	5 min	8–18 y	http://pediatricbipolar.pitt.edu/resources/instruments
Mood and Feelings Questionnaire[50,51]	Depression	Parent, child	5 min	8–18 y	https://devepi.duhs.duke.edu/measures/the-mood-and-feelings-questionnaire-mfq/
PHQ-2[52,53]	Depression risk	Adolescent	3 min	10–21 y	http://www.cqaimh.org/pdf/tool_phq2.pdf; scoring instructions available at: https://brightfutures.aap.org/Bright%20Futures%20Documents/PHQ-2%20Instructions%20for%20Use.pdf
The Patient Health Questionnaire-9: Modified for Teens[54]	Major depression, suicidality; this tool can follow a positive PHQ-2 result	Parent, adolescent	5 min	10–21 y	https://www.aacap.org/App_Themes/AACAP/docs/member_resources/toolbox_for_clinical_practice_and_outcomes/symptoms/GLAD-PC_PHQ-9.pdf; scoring instructions available at: http://www.thereachinstitute.org/images/phq_9_teens_scoring.pdf
Pediatric Symptom Checklist[55,56]	Internalizing, externalizing, and attention problems	Parent, child, teacher; 24 languages	10–15 min	3–16 y	https://brightfutures.aap.org/materials-and-tools/tool-and-resource-kit/Pages/Developmental-Behavioral-Psychosocial-Screening-and-Assessment-Forms.aspx
Strengths and Difficulties Questionnaire[57]	Emotional symptoms, conduct problems, hyperactivity and/or inattention, peer relationships, prosocial behavior	Parent, adolescent, teacher; 49 languages	5–15 min	4–17 y	www.sdqinfo.com; sdq@youthinmind.net
Vanderbilt Rating Scales[58]	ADHD, ODD, conduct disorder, anxiety and/or depression	Parent, teacher; Spanish	5 min	6–12 y	https://www.nichq.org/sites/default/files/resource-file/NICHQ_Vanderbilt_Assessment_Scales.pdf
Bullying[20,59]	Bullying; numerous screening tools exist, but feasibility in primary care has not been established	Various	N/A	Various	See references (both articles are available electronically at no charge, and the CDC article has numerous bullying screening tools)
Screening to Brief Intervention[60]	Adolescent tobacco, alcohol, and drug use (used as part of SBIRT)[46,60]	Adolescent	3 min	14–21 y	https://www.mcpap.com/pdf/S2BI_postcard.pdf
Child and Adolescent Trauma Screen [61]	Posttraumatic stress disorder symptoms	Parent, youth	10 min	2–18 y	https://depts.washington.edu/hcsats/PDF/TF-%20CBT/pages/assessment.html

TABLE 2 Continued

Screening Tool	Screening Purpose	Available Forms and Languages[a]	Approximate Time to Complete	Ages	Notes and Link or Source
Child Stress Disorders Checklist-Short Form, 4-question version[62]	Stress symptoms in children who have experienced trauma (including medical trauma)	Parent	3 min	6–18 y	https://www.nctsn.org/measures/child-stress-disorders-checklist
Childhood Autism Spectrum Test[63]	Autism spectrum disorder	Parent; Spanish	5–10 min	4–11 y	https://psychology-tools.com/cast/

This list is not meant to be exhaustive but representative of a range of screening instruments suitable for primary care that are in the public domain (with the exception of the AAP Guide to Learning Disabilities, which is published in book format, and the Einstein Evaluation of School-Related Skills). Psychometric properties of the included measures vary on the basis of the findings of different studies; included are those for which evaluated psychometric properties indicate acceptable reliability and validity. The measures included in this table are presented to help pediatricians make informed decisions when choosing tools to use in their work. Several relevant proprietary online screening, monitoring, and decision-support platforms for use in primary care are available (eg, Child Health and Development Inventory System[64] and TriVox Health[65]) but are not free of charge for use and, therefore, are not included in this table. CDC, Centers for Disease Control and Prevention; N/A, not applicable; ODD, oppositional defiant disorder; PHQ-2, Patient Health Questionnaire-2.

a If the number of languages or additional languages is not listed in this column, the tool or instrument is available in English only.

achievement of prereading language milestones (see Table 2 for a list of suggested questions to ask). Another surveillance strategy includes focusing on sociodemographic variables at 2 years of age that are risk factors for low academic scores and problem behaviors in kindergarten in children without developmental delay.[28] Important risk factors include parental level of education below a bachelor's degree, little or no shared reading at home, food insecurity, family history, medical risk factors, and fair or poor parental health. Attention to the value of protective factors is also a helpful approach in surveillance strategy. Clinical strategies and psychometrically sound tools feasible for use in busy primary care settings are available to identify frequently occurring risk factors in academic underachievement and are discussed further in the Medical Evaluation section (Table 2 contains a selected list of relevant screening tools).

Diagnosis

An important aspect of the pediatrician's role in caring for children who experience challenges with academic progress is to identify what conditions are contributing to the child's difficulties. Table 1 offers a resource to help the pediatrician consider the range of conditions and situations that can lead to academic challenges. Many of the screening instruments listed in Table 2 can help with differential diagnosis and identification of the comorbidity. Pediatricians already routinely screen for hearing and vision problems in the course of providing health supervision,[29] which remains an important part of the comprehensive diagnostic workup for any child who is not progressing academically.

Referral

When additional information is required to clarify the etiology of the child's academic progress problem, the pediatrician's role is to refer the child, as available in the community, for evaluation to 1 or more of a number of subspecialists, such as child psychologists, neuropsychologists, speech or language pathologists, occupational therapists, physical therapists, developmental-behavioral pediatricians, child neurologists, and/or child psychiatrists for further consultation. Pediatricians also may care for children with medical or neurologic conditions who require referral for serial reassessments every few years to measure progress and identify emerging issues.

When applicable, pediatricians also have a role in helping families navigate the school-based evaluation

TABLE 3 Prereading Skills (in Native English Speakers)

	By Approximate Mean Age
Says first words	12 mo
Follows 1-part directions	15 mo
Uses 2- to 3-word phrases or sentences	2 y
Can speak many words, uses prepositions	2–3 y
Begins to sing the ABC song (as a string of connected letters)	3 y
Begins to enjoy rhyming games[41]	3 y, 4 mo
Can name parts of words that rhyme[41]	3 y, 6 mo
Recognizes and names written letters	4 y
Pronounces new words with little difficulty	4 y
Begins to learn the sounds that letters make	5 y
Masters the sounds of all letters	5 y (early in kindergarten)
Recognizes most or all lower- and upper-case letters	5 y (end of kindergarten)

and intervention services available in the education system. Familiarity with special education legal rights allows pediatricians to support families effectively in advocating for their child who is not progressing as expected academically. The AAP Council on Children With Disabilities and the Council on School Health jointly published a clinical report in 2015 detailing the IDEA concept and process that contains key information and guidance for pediatricians.[30]

Treatment

When co-occurring mental or behavioral health concerns are present or suspected, the pediatrician's role is to help the family initiate appropriate therapies. They can fulfill this role by either referring to individual and/or family counseling, initiating medication therapy, or referring for initiation of medication therapy, as indicated.[13,31,32] Collaborating with schools on medication management is a common activity expected of pediatricians. For treatments that occur in the school setting or the community, for example, reading tutoring for children with learning disabilities, classroom modifications for children with attention-deficit/hyperactivity disorder (ADHD), etc, the pediatrician's role is one of helping families locate services and ensure their quality and effectiveness with periodic monitoring of the child's progress.

Advocacy and Monitoring

The factors discovered to be contributing to the child's academic progress problems will guide the pediatrician's role in advocacy and monitoring. When a psychological evaluation reveals the presence of neurodevelopmental disorders, such as language disorders, learning disabilities, intellectual disabilities, or emotional health issues, advocacy roles for the pediatrician include the following: (1) ensuring that the family understands the results and recommendations after consultation visits (see Template for Referral Letter From Pediatrician to Allied Health and/or Subspecialist for Additional Evaluation in the Supplemental Information for help with understanding standardized test scores); (2) helping the family make a request for an evaluation at the public school to determine the child's eligibility for an Individualized Education Program (IEP) or 504 plan (example letters, Template for Letter Requesting Initiating School Evaluation Written by Parent(s) and Template for Referral Letter for School Evaluation Written by Pediatrician, in the Supplemental Information); (3) providing guidance to the family regarding the goals and objectives in the child's IEP (see the 2015 AAP guidance on special education[30] for additional information); (4) helping families advocate for the most appropriate IEP for the child, including the initially formulated one and subsequent renditions; (4) periodically monitoring the child's academic progress; and (5) facilitating referrals for repeated evaluation when indicated.

A key advocacy role for the pediatrician caring for a child discovered to have a neurodevelopmental or mental health disorder is helping adults involved in the child's life view the child's strengths and challenges appropriately. Children with these disorders may be perceived as lazy or willfully oppositional rather than as having neurocognitive deficits that preclude typical academic progress.

Advocacy roles for pediatricians to improve the educational system at the community, state, and federal levels abound but are beyond the scope of this report. These roles are exemplified in publications from the AAP and other organizations.[33–36]

MEDICAL EVALUATION

The diagnostic workup starts with a detailed history. To determine why academic progress is not occurring, information needed to characterize the nature, chronology, and context of the problem dictates what pertinent history should be obtained. Given that a comprehensive history is likely to be required to characterize the source and nature of the child's academic progress problem and because obtaining a comprehensive history is relatively time consuming, appropriate documentation supports billing for the additional time needed to evaluate the problem.

Perinatal History

Prenatal and perinatal events may be relevant to the child's cognitive, emotional, and behavioral functioning later in life. As part of the evaluation of the child who is not progressing academically, obtaining the history of pregnancy, labor, and delivery can be helpful. Of concern are complications of previous pregnancies; history of prenatal exposures to alcohol, drugs, and medications; malnutrition; maternal medical conditions; maternal emotional and mental health challenges; prematurity and fetal growth difficulties; and complications of labor and delivery.

Results of a newborn hearing screening and metabolic screening should be obtained, if possible.

Past Medical History

The presence of medical conditions associated with neurologic dysfunction (eg, meningitis, traumatic brain injury or loss of consciousness, seizures, anemia, lead intoxication, chronic illness, etc) is important to elicit in the past medical history. To increase pediatricians' awareness of issues regarding monitoring, assessing, and reducing children's exposure to neurotoxic chemicals and environmental pollutants, the reader is referred to the 2015 consensus statement, "Project TENDR: Targeting Environmental Neuro-Developmental Risks."[37] The authors pointed out that "communities of color and socioeconomically stressed communities face disproportionately high exposures and health impacts,"[38–40] which emphasizes the need to keep a higher index of suspicion for toxin contribution in children with these factors in their history.

Developmental and Behavioral History

The child's developmental history is also critical to assessing academic progress problems. Any delays in achieving developmental milestones or the presence of atypical behavior as an infant or young child should be recorded. Any regression in milestones should be noted. A history of late-normal or mildly delayed onset of early speech and language milestones raises the suspicion for underlying language-based learning disabilities (see Table 3).

The child's motor coordination (eg, ability to ride a tricycle or bicycle, tie shoes, fasten clothing, use utensils and writing instruments, etc) should be noted because children with learning disabilities may have associated subtle delays in the development of motor coordination.[42]

The behavioral history obtained through discussion can be supplemented with and/or guided by structured questionnaires when indicated. See Table 2 for a list of selected tools relevant to assessments of school-aged children who are not progressing academically. The strategies for history-taking and questionnaires should include noting the presence of any symptoms of hyperactivity, impulsivity, inattention, and/or tics along with the child's predominant mood, ability to self-regulate, any anxiety or exaggerated normal childhood fears, and the presence or absence of perseverative or stereotypical behaviors. The child's play behaviors and interaction with peers are also useful details to elicit.

Regarding the screening tools selected for inclusion in Table 2, rather than create a comprehensive list of the many questionnaires and screening tools available, included are ones that (1) screen for academic dysfunction in school-aged children; (2) screen for some of the more common reasons for academic progress problems, such as learning disabilities, mental health disorders, etc; (3) are feasible for use in primary care settings (ie, are brief, have questionnaire forms that can be completed by children and/or caregivers, and can be scored quickly, etc); (4) have sound psychometric properties (ie, acceptable validity and reliability); and (5) are available in the public domain (ie, at no cost to the pediatrician). Factors that will impact decision-making regarding screening tool selection include, for example, the unique characteristics of the population of children in a pediatrician's practice, such as age groups, literacy levels, staffing considerations, and payer reimbursement policies.

Regarding inclusion of the Screening to Brief Intervention in Table 2, it is a public domain tool that can be used to screen for substance use of school-aged children who are not progressing academically, especially those who may have been performing well previously and then stopped progressing suddenly. The AAP and other organizations have recommended the screening, brief intervention, and referral to treatment (SBIRT) strategies to provide an organizing framework to assist primary care providers with this task.[43–46] For alcohol use screening, SBIRT includes asking 2 questions: 1 about friends' drinking and 1 about the child or teenager's drinking.

The screening tools listed in Table 2 are meant to serve as a reference for tools general pediatricians might use as they deem useful. This is presented as a resource, not a list of tools that need to be used in every instance.

Sleep History

Assessing the child's sleep patterns is important.[66] Along with other health and mental health problems, causes of academic dysfunction, including the symptoms of ADHD, have been linked with inadequate sleep duration and quality.[67–72] Alternately, anxiety associated with academic problems may interfere with sleep onset or maintenance.[73] Growing evidence reveals that average sleep time per night for children has gradually been decreasing over the recent decades.[74] Assessing adequacy of sleep hygiene, including screen use in the child's bedroom, sleep duration, and symptoms of obstructive sleep apnea (excessive snoring, pauses in breathing) and parasomnias (night terrors or nightmares, sleep walking, sleep talking), is important. The AAP has endorsed[75] the 2016 consensus guidelines from the American Academy of Sleep Medicine and the Sleep Research Society for the recommended sleep duration for children from infancy to adolescence.[76] The guidelines recommend that school-aged children (6–12 years) sleep 9 to 12 hours per night on a regular basis and that teenagers (13–18 years) sleep 8 to 10 hours to promote optimal health. Additionally, the AAP suggests that all screens be turned off 30 minutes before bedtime and that televisions, computers, and other screens not be allowed in children's bedrooms. The AAP also has advocated for later school start times for adolescents.[77]

Family and Social History

Eliciting information about relatives' level of education completed, problems with early speech or language development, learning problems, attention and/or hyperactivity problems, anxiety symptoms, affective disorders, social interaction differences, substance use problems, seizures, and hearing or vision loss may provide information regarding possible etiologies for the child's academic progress problems.

Social history, including household composition and adequacy of housing, family income sources and adequacy, transportation, food security, social network and/or degree of social support, and interpersonal violence or personal trauma history, can help to identify social determinants of health and well-being that may be contributory to the academic functioning problems. When obtaining history of this nature, a thoughtful, family-centered approach that identifies not only risks but also resiliency factors is warranted.[78]

Children with a history of adversity and/or trauma (eg, poverty, homelessness, abuse, neglect, parental mental health issues, etc) deserve special consideration. Sometimes their historical or ongoing emotional trauma and anxiety may be interfering with learning. In other cases, children with these histories may also have specific learning issues related to the impact of trauma on the developing brain.[16,17] When a child has this history, it is not a reason to automatically expect them to do poorly, so if they are struggling academically, they warrant additional evaluation. It is important to consider that children in foster care or kinship care or children who have had involvement with child welfare not only have experienced trauma but also have possibly had multiple school changes. Each school change can essentially result in a loss of 4 months of academic skills.[21] For these children, making sure that basic supports are in place, such as corrective lenses and hearing aids that may have been lost during a move from one home to the next, is important. Assessing whether an existing IEP was transferred with the child to a new school is important. Awareness of the ongoing social trauma for children in foster care can help to unravel why a child might be struggling academically or emotionally. Examples of such traumatic situations include visits with biological parents, entering a new school in the middle of the year, and trying to fit into established social groups.

Physical Examination

The physical examination should be thorough. Growth percentiles in children with academic progress problems should be recorded. Obtaining head circumference percentiles can aid in differential diagnosis. For example, microcephaly may reveal a previously unrecognized congenital or acquired structural brain difference as a potential source of the child's academic progress problems. Measuring it even in children older than 3 years can be helpful. Observing carefully for the presence or absence of any neurocutaneous markers, dysmorphic features (eg, shortened palpebral fissures, flattened philtrum, and thinned upper lip when exposure to alcohol prenatally is known or suspected), and neurologic abnormalities, especially in tone, coordination, and symmetry, can contribute to the etiologic determination.

Behavioral Observation

Observe the child's language, affect, and social interaction skills. A child's behavior in the clinic may not be representative of their predominant behavioral, mood, or communicative repertoire, and asking parents whether they correlate is important. If adolescents' behavior observed when talking with them privately differs from that observed in the presence of their parents or caregivers, it reveals potential sources of academic dysfunction (eg, parent-child conflict) that need further historical exploration.

Imaging and Laboratory Tests

Generally, additional imaging and laboratory workups are unnecessary. However, in some children, history and physical findings reveal the need for additional testing, such as EEG, neuroimaging, and genetic and/or metabolic testing.

Referral for Additional Evaluations

Clarifying the nature and etiology of academic progress problems may require referral for testing to assess cognitive abilities, adaptive functioning, academic achievement, communication abilities, motor functioning, behavior, and/or emotional status. Various professionals perform these assessments. The child's specific concerns as well as his or her source of health insurance, resources available in the community, and family preference will affect the decisions the pediatrician and family make together regarding whether and where additional referrals are made. Given that not all children referred to mental health specialists follow through with an initial appointment, engaging parents in the decision-making regarding referrals is important.[79] Motivational interviewing and shared decision-making are family-centered strategies that pediatricians can use that hold potential to improve the effectiveness of making referrals.[80–83]

In some settings, the pediatrician is colocated with allied health professionals (audiologists, speech pathologists, occupational therapists, and physical therapists) and/or mental health professionals qualified to conduct additional assessments.[84] In other situations, these additional evaluations are conducted in non-colocated offices or in the public school. When a child has a complex medical condition involving the structure or function of the nervous system (eg, surviving childhood cancer, traumatic brain injury, etc), the pediatrician may elect to consult a neuropsychologist to conduct the testing. Some children with these types of issues are already part of a condition-specific clinic or program (eg, sickle cell disease, neuromuscular disorders, autism, etc) that is organized as a multidisciplinary team that includes a psychologist or neuropsychologist. Pediatricians can enhance their ability to provide comprehensive, coordinated, and collaborative care by developing familiarity with some of the relevant resources in their local community.

Creating a well-crafted referral is also of key importance to its success. An effective referral question includes brief but detailed-enough information to facilitate the evaluation by other specialists. Including any relevant clinic visit notes, in-office screening results, previous standardized testing results, and school documentation, such as report cards or IEPs, if available, is helpful to guide the specialist's decisions regarding what to prioritize in the child's assessment. A template for a referral letter is in the Supplemental Information (see Template for Letter Requesting Initiating School Evaluation Written by Parent[s]). Appendix S1 in the AAP clinical report on strategies for preparing a primary care practice to enhance mental health care[12] contains a table used to summarize sources of specialty services to help pediatricians locate and catalog relevant professional resources in their community.

Insurance coverage for psychological and neuropsychological testing is a key driver in deciding to whom to refer an individual patient. The level of complexity involved in ascertaining the level of coverage for the various evaluation services required for a child has been documented to be daunting.[85,86] When making decisions to refer, it is important to understand that insurers may cover the cost of testing when they judge that the results will influence clinical decision-making but may restrict coverage if they judge that the purpose is to evaluate or determine educational interventions. Some policies cover testing through the child's medical benefits, and others cover it through mental health benefits. Insurance companies also vary on the type of professional training a clinician performing the testing must have. Some companies allow master's level clinicians to perform the testing, others require that a psychologist or neuropsychologist with a doctoral degree conduct the testing personally, and others will pay for a graduate trainee to administer the testing if they are supervised by a PhD or PsyD. A template for a letter of medical necessity is included in the Supplemental Information (see Template for Referral Letter for School Evaluation Written by Pediatrician). Additionally, billing and coding strategies that may offset some portion of the time and cost needed to conduct referrals are discussed in more detail in the Supplemental Information (see Letter of Medical Necessity for Psychological or Neuropsychological Evaluation from Pediatrician to Insurance Company).

Requests for School Evaluations and Ongoing Collaboration and/or Communication

With respect to testing performed through the school, it is important to understand that these evaluations are conducted for a different purpose from those performed by psychologists and neuropsychologists in health care settings. Traditionally, private psychologists and neuropsychologists perform testing to make diagnoses and recommendations. In contrast, in school settings, school psychologists perform testing as part of a team to determine eligibility for special education. Public schools in different states and districts vary in their capacity to complete more complex evaluations. Some schools have clinical psychologists and/or neuropsychologists on staff; others may contract with private psychologists or neuropsychologists to conduct evaluations. Another important resource in the school setting is the school nurse, who can serve as an important coordinator between the school and the medical home. Furthermore, although pediatricians may be familiar with making referrals for additional evaluations to private or university-based colleagues and therapy agencies, in the case of public schools, the referral communication process is different. Although a letter from a pediatrician can be helpful, ultimately, it does not require the school to perform an evaluation. Pediatricians can help families by providing a letter template (Template for Referral Letter for School Evaluation Written by Pediatrician in the Supplemental Information) that families can use to request the school to evaluate their child. The Template for Referral Letter From Pediatrician to Allied Health and/or Subspecialist for Additional Evaluation in the Supplemental Information is a sample letter template that pediatricians can use to communicate with schools in support of parents' requests for school evaluations. Another option is for the pediatrician to write a letter on behalf of the family and have the parents cosign it.

In some states and communities, school districts may have a physician who can be available to attend IEP meetings. Pediatricians can make families aware of the fact that parents can request the presence of the physician member of the committee on special education with at least 72 hours' notice to the school. It can be helpful for pediatricians to ask their local public schools if the committee includes a physician and, if so, develop a relationship with that physician. Pediatricians also can help families seeking special education resources for their child by providing them with information on state advocacy organizations and Web sites.

An understanding of federal privacy laws governing the exchange of information is necessary.

Pediatricians are likely most familiar with those governing the release of health information, namely the Health Insurance Portability and Accountability Act of 1996 (HIPAA), but may have less familiarity with similar rules that protect the privacy of student public education records in the Family Educational Rights and Privacy Act (FERPA). HIPAA also governs the exchange of mental health information separately from physical health information, but only regarding psychotherapy counseling session notes and substance use, not results of clinical tests such as IQ and academic achievement testing.[87] Despite common misperceptions, HIPAA actually allows health care providers involved in the care of a mutual patient to exchange information, with the exception of psychotherapy and substance use records, without requiring patient consent. The US Department of Health and Human Services and the US Department of Education have guidance clarifying how HIPAA and FERPA apply in educational and health settings.[88] It is also important to understand that regulations across states vary and may be more restrictive than federal guidelines. Familiarity with specific state regulations is important to ensure compliance.[89] A strategy to foster bidirectional exchange of information that can be initiated in the medical home is to have families sign forms permitting bidirectional release of information at the time a referral is initiated. Supplemental Fig 2 includes example HIPAA and FERPA release-of-information forms in English and Spanish.

After appropriate permissions are secured and consultation results are received, another strategy to enhance collaboration with evaluators includes contacting the outside clinician directly to clarify any information in the report before discussing the findings with families. For both before- and after-referral communication purposes, innovative, secure Web-based platforms that facilitate meaningful interprofessional dialogues exist. However, significant barriers, such as proprietary protections, cost, and lack of interoperability with 1 or more electronic health records, can limit their widespread use. Regardless of the channel used, repeated episodes of communication with psychologists and neuropsychologists serves to strengthen collaborations and, in turn, improve the quality of care pediatricians provide to their patients who are not progressing academically.

Similarly, ongoing dialogue between pediatricians and schools that occurs in the course of providing care for children with academic progress problems strengthens collaborative relationships on behalf of children. As noted, pediatricians can provide letters to accompany parents' letters requesting school evaluations. Pediatricians regularly are called on to communicate with schools, for example, in the course of providing care for children with chronic health conditions or special health care needs, for medication management and monitoring, and for other issues.

Testing Assessments and Who Conducts Them

Structured instruments and questionnaires are used to measure the child's cognitive and adaptive functioning, speech and language, behavioral and emotional status, fine motor skills, and coordination in assessments. Psychologists and neuropsychologists typically measure overall cognitive function (ie, IQ) and specific aspects of cognitive ability (eg, attention, working memory, and verbal comprehension), adaptive functioning, and behavioral and emotional capacities and challenges. Psychologists also may observe a child's behavior informally in the classroom.

The child's academic achievement is assessed by using standard measures of reading decoding, reading fluency, and reading comprehension; writing (handwriting and composition); and math reasoning and calculation ability to better understand what, if any, difficulties the child is experiencing. Sometimes psychologists conduct these evaluations, and in other situations, educators perform academic achievement assessments.

In some cases, psychologists and/or speech language pathologists may assess speech and language skills as part of a neuropsychological evaluation. Regardless of who conducts the speech and language evaluations, aspects of communication that may be assessed include receptive and expressive vocabulary, speech sound production (articulation and phonology), language usage, pragmatics, discourse, and social interaction.

Having an audiologist conduct a formal hearing assessment is important when a child who is not progressing academically fails a hearing screen conducted in the pediatrician's office or at the child's school.

Occupational therapists assess fine motor abilities and gauge the degree of developmental coordination the child has attained to see whether coordination problems could be contributing to the academic problems.

Physical therapists may also be involved in evaluating a child who is not progressing academically, especially in cases in which a motor disability is known or suspected (eg, hemiplegia, cerebral palsy, etc).

In some communities, developmental-behavioral pediatricians, neurodevelopmental disabilities pediatricians, neurologists, pediatric physiatrists, and/or child and adolescent psychiatrists may conduct some or all of the assessments.

Reviewing Consultants' Reports

Consultants' reports vary in what is included depending on the purpose of the evaluation. The purpose of a school psychology evaluation is to contribute to the determination of the child's eligibility for special education. As such, reports typically do not contain a diagnosis or recommendations. Those are instead included in the child's IEP as educational categories (akin to diagnoses in medical reports) and goals and objectives (akin to the recommendations in medical notes).

Psychological and neuropsychological evaluations, on the other hand, are designed not only to address the child's school curricular needs but also to provide a comprehensive conceptualization of the child's cognitive, emotional, and learning strengths and challenges. In contrast to school psychologists' reports, psychologists' and neuropsychologists' evaluation reports typically include not only cognitive and academic testing results but also assessments of mental health diagnoses, such as anxiety or depression, if relevant, along with diagnostic formulations and recommendations. These reports usually include details of the feedback provided to families and other recommended community and educational services that families can access. For information on understanding test scores, see Understanding Test Scores in the Supplemental Information.

Treatment

The ultimate goal of treatment is to allow the child to achieve his or her maximum potential. Once the reason for the child's failure to proceed academically has been diagnosed, the pediatrician's role in management of the problem is to ensure the family's understanding of the problem conceptualization, assist the family in obtaining comprehensive individualized educational intervention strategies, monitor for and identify any secondary morbidities (eg, depression and/or anxiety because of the child's inability to meet expectations that exceed his or her neurologic capacity), prescribe medication and/or behavioral therapy when indicated, and initiate appropriate referral when deemed necessary.

Pediatricians can help parents interpret diagnostic results to ensure accurate parental understanding of the source of their child's learning difficulties. Parents may believe that they have done something to cause their child's problem or that their child is lazy. Pediatricians can help parents reframe their understanding of the problem as one arising instead from the child's neurologic functioning. Parents may benefit from an opportunity to discuss their feelings, including identifying their grief over the loss of their idealized version of their child's future. Helping families to problem solve how they can adapt daily routines to help their child succeed and helping families to understand their educational rights so they can advocate effectively on behalf of their child are also important roles for pediatricians. A list of national support resources is available in Supplemental Table 4.

Pediatricians can help families advocate for appropriate educational supports to be included in their child's IEP. Educational supports can include accommodations and modifications. Accommodations change how the material is delivered to a child, how they demonstrate their learning and understanding, and the settings where they learn. Accommodations can include those for presentation of material (eg, listening to audio recordings or watching a video, reading larger print, etc), those for responses (eg, dictate answers to a scribe, use a calculator or table of math facts, etc), those for settings (eg, work in a smaller room, sit close to the teacher, etc), those for organizational skills (eg, have work broken down into smaller increments, be allowed frequent breaks, use a highlighter or an alarm, etc), and those for extended time for homework, other assignments, and testing sessions. Accommodations offered for instruction can be different from those used for testing. Modifications change what a child is taught or what a child is expected to learn (eg, allowed to complete every other problem on a worksheet, continue working on addition while classmates move on to subtraction, etc). As mentioned previously, these supports are provided through either an IEP or a 504 plan, which are described in the AAP clinical report on the IDEA concept and process.[30] For children with dyslexia as the source of their academic progress problems, effective treatments are focused on remediation of phonologic deficits early on through emphasis on teaching sound recognition and sound-symbol relationships. In junior high and high school, the focus shifts from remediation to providing accommodations.[90,91]

It is important to note that the preponderance of evidence reveals that having a child repeat a grade is not an effective strategy to help a child with academic difficulties meet his or her maximum potential.[92,93]

For children with learning disorders whose problems are based in language centers rather than in the visual cortex, no evidence supports interventions that are focused on improving visual-pathway functioning. Nonsupported treatments include eye muscle exercises, ocular pursuits, training with or without bifocals, balance-board training, crawling exercises, and tinted (Irlen) lenses. These treatments, at best, provide no benefit and, at worst, may delay receipt of effective evidence-based treatments and require significant out-of-pocket costs for the family.[15]

Ongoing monitoring is an important role for the pediatrician. Children with learning disabilities or other sources of academic progress problems are at risk for discouragement, withdrawal, eroded self-esteem, and lack of sense of efficacy; they may develop or have co-occurring depression and/or anxiety.[94,95]

Periodically monitoring children (eg, at annually scheduled health supervision visits or targeted follow-up visits) can contribute to early identification and treatment of co-occurring mental health and behavioral problems and, in turn, can help children meet their maximum potential. Given that the academic demands on children increase over time, assessing the appropriateness of the supports as children progress through successive school years is important to ensure that adequate resources are available to the child.

SUMMARY AND RECOMMENDATIONS

When children struggle academically, they typically turn to the adults in their life for help. Evaluation of the difficulty is key to ultimately responding to the needs of these children. Pediatricians play an important part in affecting children's academic progress, including prevention and early detection of problems, diagnosis of contributory medical conditions and/or other psychosocial contributors, referral for additional evaluation, assisting families with navigating school evaluations, treatment, medication management, and ongoing progress monitoring. The ultimate goal is to identify reasons why the child is struggling in school and to provide the child and family with realistic opportunities to improve the child's education. The process of achieving a good evaluation is complicated by the range of reasons children struggle, the range of professionals available to provide evaluation, the variability in insurance coverage for evaluation, and the resources needed to address the complex biopsychosocial issues. In this clinical report, we offer guidance to the pediatrician to help families achieve a good evaluation for their child who is struggling in school while facilitating the feasibility for the pediatrician to provide this support.

Recommendations are as follows:

1. Pediatricians should take an active role in the prevention, early identification, diagnosis, and treatment of academic progress problems. To this end, pediatricians should be knowledgeable of relevant AAP resources that allow them to effectively manage the care of school-aged children who are not progressing academically.
2. Care coordination for children who are not progressing academically should take place in the context of the child's medical home. Team-based care must include the pediatrician, specialists, and other health and human services professionals and families, regardless of the location of, or source of payment for, these services.
3. Payment for all the activities, including non–face-to-face visits and coordination required to provide high-quality care to children who are not progressing academically, should be considered by payers.
4. Pediatricians need to understand the rights that all children in the United States have to receive a free and appropriate public education, including those with learning disabilities, developmental disabilities, and chronic health conditions. Understanding these rights allows pediatricians to most effectively support families as they advocate for evaluations and interventions in the public school.
5. Pediatricians should be familiar with the AAP clinical report on IDEA[30] so that they are familiar with the law, the processes, and the challenges of the IDEA and Section 504 of the Rehabilitation Act of 1973.
6. Considerations when choosing an approach to evaluation need to include the depth of evaluation necessary, the complexity of the intervention that will be required, the resource costs to families for the various options, and the level of coverage by insurance plan(s) for the recommended evaluations.
7. Pediatricians can most effectively serve their patients by establishing relationships with colleagues who can conduct further diagnostic evaluations when a school-aged child is not progressing academically, including subspecialists (such as developmental-behavioral pediatricians, neurologists, physiatrists, and child and adolescent psychiatrists), psychologists, neuropsychologists, allied health professionals (such as occupational, physical, and speech therapists), and school nurses.
8. Pediatricians can develop an understanding of the different goals of evaluations to guide families to the most appropriate resources. Pediatricians should understand that the purpose of school psychology evaluations is to determine eligibility for education supports, and the purpose of evaluations by psychologists and neuropsychologists is to determine diagnoses and interventions. In schools, interventions are determined by the goals and objectives written in IEPs or 504 plans.
9. Pediatricians may take an active role in the initiation, development, and implementation of IEPs and 504 plans when applicable.

LEAD AUTHORS

Celiane Rey-Casserly, PhD
Laura Joan McGuinn, MD, FAAP
Arthur Lavin, MD, FAAP

COMMITTEE ON PSYCHOSOCIAL ASPECTS OF CHILD AND FAMILY HEALTH, 2018–2019

Arthur Lavin, MD, FAAP, Chairperson
George LaMonte Askew, MD, FAAP
Rebecca Baum, MD, FAAP
Evelyn Berger-Jenkins, MD, FAAP
Thresia B. Gambon, MD, FAAP
Arwa Abdulhaq Nasir, MBBS, MSc, MPH, FAAP
Lawrence Sagin Wissow, MD, MPH, FAAP

FORMER COMMITTEE ON PSYCHOSOCIAL ASPECTS OF CHILD AND FAMILY HEALTH MEMBERS

Michael Yogman, MD, FAAP, Former Chairperson
Keith M. Lemmon, MD, FAAP
Gerri Mattson, MD, FAAP
Jason Richard Rafferty, MD, MPH, EdM, FAAP

LIAISONS

Sharon Berry, PhD, ABPP, LP – *Society of Pediatric Psychology*
Edward R. Christophersen, PhD, FAAP – *Society of Pediatric Psychology*
Norah L. Johnson, PhD, RN, CPNP-BC – *National Association of Pediatric Nurse Practitioners*
Abigail Boden Schlesinger, MD – *American Academy of Child and Adolescent Psychiatry*
Rachel Shana Segal, MD – *Section on Pediatric Trainees*
Amy Starin, PhD – *National Association of Social Workers*

STAFF

Carolyn L. McCarty, PhD

SECTION ON DEVELOPMENTAL AND BEHAVIORAL PEDIATRICS EXECUTIVE COMMITTEE, 2018–2019

Carol C. Weitzman, MD, FAAP, Chairperson
Nathan Jon Blum, MD, FAAP, Immediate Past Chairperson
David Omer Childers Jr, MD, FAAP
Jack M. Levine, MD, FAAP
Ada Myriam Peralta-Carcelen, MD, MPH, FAAP
Jennifer K. Poon, MD, FAAP
Peter Joseph Smith, MD, MA, FAAP
John Ichiro Takayama, MD, MPH, FAAP, Web site Editor
Robert G. Voigt, MD, FAAP, Newsletter Editor
Carolyn Bridgemohan, MD, FAAP, Program Chairperson

FORMER SECTION ON DEVELOPMENTAL AND BEHAVIORAL PEDIATRICS EXECUTIVE COMMITTEE

Nerissa S. Bauer, MD, MPH, FAAP
Nathan J. Blum, MD, FAAP
Edward Goldson, MD, FAAP
Michelle M. Macias, MD, FAAP
Laura Joan McGuinn, MD, FAAP

LIAISONS

Marilyn Christine Augustyn, MD, FAAP – *Society for Developmental and Behavioral Pediatrics*
Beth Ellen Davis, MD, MPH, FAAP – *Council on Children With Disabilities*
Alice Meng, MD – *Section on Pediatric Trainees*

STAFF

Carolyn L. McCarty, PhD

ABBREVIATIONS

AAP: American Academy of Pediatrics
ADHD: attention-deficit/hyperactivity disorder
FERPA: Family Educational Rights and Privacy Act
HIPAA: Health Insurance Portability and Accountability Act of 1996
IDEA: Individuals with Disabilities Education Act
IEP: Individualized Education Program
SBIRT: screening
brief intervention: and referral to treatment

Address correspondence to Arthur Lavin, MD, FAAP. Email: alavin@aap.net

PEDIATRICS (ISSN Numbers: Print, 0031-4005; Online, 1098-4275).

Copyright © 2019 by the American Academy of Pediatrics

FINANCIAL DISCLOSURE: The authors have indicated they have no financial relationships relevant to this article to disclose.

FUNDING: No external funding.

POTENTIAL CONFLICT OF INTEREST: The authors have indicated they have no potential conflicts of interest to disclose.

REFERENCES

1. American Academy of Pediatrics. *Caring for Children With ADHD: A Resource Toolkit for Clinicians*. 3rd ed. Itasca, IL: American Academy of Pediatrics; 2019
2. Council on Early Childhood; Council on School Health. The pediatrician's role in optimizing school readiness. *Pediatrics*. 2016;138(3):e20162293
3. Council on Children With Disabilities; Section on Developmental Behavioral Pediatrics; Bright Futures Steering Committee; Medical Home Initiatives for Children With Special Needs Project Advisory Committee. Identifying infants and young children with developmental disorders in the medical home: an algorithm for developmental surveillance and screening [published correction appears in *Pediatrics*. 2006;118(4):1808–1809]. *Pediatrics*. 2006;118(1):405–420
4. Johnson CP, Myers SM; American Academy of Pediatrics Council on Children With Disabilities. Identification and evaluation of children with autism spectrum disorders. *Pediatrics*. 2007;120(5):1183–1215
5. Myers SM, Johnson CP; American Academy of Pediatrics Council on Children With Disabilities. Management of children with autism spectrum disorders. *Pediatrics*. 2007;120(5):1162–1182

6. Earls MF, Yogman MW, Mattson G, Rafferty J; Committee on Psychosocial Aspects of Child and Family Health. Incorporating recognition and management of perinatal depression into pediatric practice. *Pediatrics*. 2019; 143(1):e20183259
7. Weitzman C, Wegner L; Section on Developmental and Behavioral Pediatrics; Committee on Psychosocial Aspects of Child and Family Health; Council on Early Childhood; Society for Developmental and Behavioral Pediatrics; American Academy of Pediatrics. Promoting optimal development: screening for behavioral and emotional problems [published correction appears in *Pediatrics*. 2015; 135(5):946]. *Pediatrics*. 2015;135(2): 384–395
8. Noritz GH, Murphy NA; Neuromotor Screening Expert Panel. Motor delays: early identification and evaluation [published correction appears in *Pediatrics*. 2017;140(3):e20172081]. *Pediatrics*. 2013;131(6). Available at: www.pediatrics.org/cgi/content/full/131/6/e2016
9. Noritz G, Murphy N; Neuromotor Screening Expert Panel. Authors' response: Re: my concerns about the American Academy of Pediatrics clinical report on "Motor delays: early identification and evaluation". *Pediatrics*. 2013;132(5). Available at: www.pediatrics.org/cgi/content/full/132/5/e1450.2
10. Foy JM; American Academy of Pediatrics Task Force on Mental Health. Enhancing pediatric mental health care: report from the American Academy of Pediatrics Task Force on Mental Health. Introduction. *Pediatrics*. 2010;125(suppl 3):S69–S74
11. Foy JM, Perrin J; American Academy of Pediatrics Task Force on Mental Health. Enhancing pediatric mental health care: strategies for preparing a community. *Pediatrics*. 2010;125(suppl 3):S75–S86
12. Foy JM, Kelleher KJ, Laraque D; American Academy of Pediatrics Task Force on Mental Health. Enhancing pediatric mental health care: strategies for preparing a primary care practice. *Pediatrics*. 2010;125(suppl 3):S87–S108
13. Foy JM; American Academy of Pediatrics Task Force on Mental Health. Enhancing pediatric mental health care: algorithms for primary care. *Pediatrics*. 2010;125(suppl 3):S109–S125
14. American Academy of Pediatrics. *Addressing Mental Health Concerns in Primary Care: A Clinician's Toolkit*. 1st ed. Elk Grove Village, IL: American Academy of Pediatrics; 2010
15. American Academy of Pediatrics, Section on Ophthalmology, Council on Children with Disabilities; American Academy of Ophthalmology; American Association for Pediatric Ophthalmology and Strabismus; American Association of Certified Orthoptists. Joint statement–learning disabilities, dyslexia, and vision. *Pediatrics*. 2009; 124(2):837–844
16. Garner AS, Shonkoff JP; Committee on Psychosocial Aspects of Child and Family Health; Committee on Early Childhood, Adoption, and Dependent Care; Section on Developmental and Behavioral Pediatrics. Early childhood adversity, toxic stress, and the role of the pediatrician: translating developmental science into lifelong health. *Pediatrics*. 2012;129(1). Available at: www.pediatrics.org/cgi/content/full/129/1/e224
17. Shonkoff JP, Garner AS; Committee on Psychosocial Aspects of Child and Family Health; Committee on Early Childhood, Adoption, and Dependent Care; Section on Developmental and Behavioral Pediatrics. The lifelong effects of early childhood adversity and toxic stress. *Pediatrics*. 2012;129(1). Available at: www.pediatrics.org/cgi/content/full/129/1/e232
18. A child with a learning disability: navigating school-based services. *Pediatrics*. 2004;114(suppl 6):1432–1436
19. Silver LB, Silver DL. *Guide to Learning Disabilities for Primary Care: How to Screen, Identify, Manage, and Advocate for Children With Learning Disabilities*. Elk Grove Village, IL: American Academy of Pediatrics; 2010
20. Committee on Injury, Violence, and Poison Prevention. Policy statement–role of the pediatrician in youth violence prevention. *Pediatrics*. 2009;124(1):393–402
21. Szilagyi MA, Rosen DS, Rubin D, Zlotnik S; Council on Foster Care, Adoption, and Kinship Care; Committee on Adolescence; Council on Early Childhood. Health care issues for children and adolescents in foster care and kinship care. *Pediatrics*. 2015; 136(4). Available at: www.pediatrics.org/cgi/content/full/136/4/e1142
22. Council on Children With Disabilities; Medical Home Implementation Project Advisory Committee. Patient- and family-centered care coordination: a framework for integrating care for children and youth across multiple systems. *Pediatrics*. 2014;133(5). Available at: www.pediatrics.org/cgi/content/full/133/5/e1451
23. Individuals With Disabilities Education Improvement Act, 20 USC §1400 et seq (2004)
24. Institute of Education Sciences, National Center for Education Statistics. Fast facts: students with disabilities. 2016. Available at: https://nces.ed.gov/fastfacts/display.asp?id=64. Accessed September 4, 2019
25. Institute of Education Sciences, National Center for Education Statistics. The condition of education. 2016. Available at: https://nces.ed.gov/programs/coe/indicator_cgg.asp. Accessed September 4, 2019
26. Data Resource Center for Child and Adolescent Health. 2016-2017 National Survey of Children's Health. Available at: https://www.childhealthdata.org/browse/survey/results?q=5355&r=1. Accessed July 29, 2019
27. Boyle CA, Boulet S, Schieve LA, et al. Trends in the prevalence of developmental disabilities in US children, 1997-2008. *Pediatrics*. 2011; 127(6):1034–1042
28. Nelson BB, Dudovitz RN, Coker TR, et al. Predictors of poor school readiness in children without developmental delay at age 2. *Pediatrics*. 2016;138(2): e20154477
29. Hagan JF Jr, Shaw JS, Duncan PM, eds. *Bright Futures: Guidelines for Health Supervision of Infants, Children, and Adolescents*. 4th ed. Elk Grove Village, IL: American Academy of Pediatrics; 2017
30. Lipkin PH, Okamoto J; Council on Children with Disabilities; Council on School Health. The Individuals With Disabilities Education Act (IDEA) for children with special educational

needs. *Pediatrics.* 2015;136(6). Available at: www.pediatrics.org/cgi/content/full/136/6/e1650

31. Appendix S1: sources of specialty services for children with mental health problems and their families. *Pediatrics.* 2010;125(suppl 3): S126–S127

32. Wolraich M, Brown L, Brown RT, et al; Subcommittee on Attention-Deficit/Hyperactivity Disorder; Steering Committee on Quality Improvement and Management. ADHD: clinical practice guideline for the diagnosis, evaluation, and treatment of attention-deficit/hyperactivity disorder in children and adolescents. *Pediatrics.* 2011;128(5): 1007–1022

33. Devore CD, Wheeler LS; Council on School Health; American Academy of Pediatrics. Role of the school physician. *Pediatrics.* 2013;131(1):178–182

34. Gereige RS,Zenni EA, eds; American Academy of Pediatrics Council on School Health. *School Health Policy and Practice.* 7th ed. Elk Grove Village, IL: American Academy of Pediatrics; 2016

35. Council on Community Pediatrics. Community pediatrics: navigating the intersection of medicine, public health, and social determinants of children's health. *Pediatrics.* 2013;131(3):623–628

36. Kuo AA, Etzel RA, Chilton LA, Watson C, Gorski PA. Primary care pediatrics and public health: meeting the needs of today's children. *Am J Public Health.* 2012;102(12):e17–e23

37. Bennett D, Bellinger DC, Birnbaum LS, et al; American College of Obstetricians and Gynecologists (ACOG); Child Neurology Society; Endocrine Society; International Neurotoxicology Association; International Society for Children's Health and the Environment; International Society for Environmental Epidemiology; National Council of Asian Pacific Islander Physicians; National Hispanic Medical Association; National Medical Association. Project TENDR: targeting environmental neuro-developmental risks the TENDR consensus statement. *Environ Health Perspect.* 2016;124(7):A118–A122

38. Adamkiewicz G, Zota AR, Fabian MP, et al. Moving environmental justice indoors: understanding structural influences on residential exposure patterns in low-income communities. *Am J Public Health.* 2011;101(suppl 1): S238–S245

39. Engel SM, Bradman A, Wolff MS, et al. Prenatal organophosphorus pesticide exposure and child neurodevelopment at 24 months: an analysis of four birth cohorts. *Environ Health Perspect.* 2016; 124(6):822–830

40. Zota AR, Adamkiewicz G, Morello-Frosch RA. Are PBDEs an environmental equity concern? Exposure disparities by socioeconomic status. *Environ Sci Technol.* 2010;44(15):5691–5692

41. National Institute on Deafness and Other Communication Disorders. Speech and language developmental milestones. 2017. Available at: https://www.nidcd.nih.gov/health/speech-and-language. Accessed May 22, 2019

42. Sugden D, Kirby A, Dunford C. Issues surrounding children with developmental coordination disorder. *Int J Disabil Dev Educ.* 2008;55(2): 173–187

43. Committee on Substance Use and Prevention. Substance use screening, brief intervention, and referral to treatment. *Pediatrics.* 2016;138(1): e20161210

44. Quigley J; Committee on Substance Use and Prevention. Alcohol use by youth. *Pediatrics.* 2019;144(1):e20191356

45. National Institute on Alcohol Abuse and Alcoholism. Alcohol screening and brief intervention for youth: a practitioner's guide. Available at: www.integration.samhsa.gov/clinical-practice/sbirt/Guide_for_Youth_Screening_and_Brief_Intervention.pdf. Accessed September 4, 2019

46. Substance Abuse and Mental Health Services Administration. About screening, brief intervention, and referral to treatment (SBIRT). 2015. Available at: www.samhsa.gov/sbirt/about. Accessed September 4, 2019

47. Gottesman RL, Cerullo FM. The development and preliminary evaluation of a screening test to detect school learning problems. *J Dev Behav Pediatr.* 1989;10(2):68–74

48. Bird HR, Canino GJ, Davies M, et al. The Brief Impairment Scale (BIS): a multidimensional scale of functional impairment for children and adolescents. *J Am Acad Child Adolesc Psychiatry.* 2005;44(7):699–707

49. Birmaher B, Brent DA, Chiappetta L, Bridge J, Monga S, Baugher M. Psychometric properties of the Screen for Child Anxiety Related Emotional Disorders (SCARED): a replication study. *J Am Acad Child Adolesc Psychiatry.* 1999;38(10):1230–1236

50. Angold A, Costello EJ, Messer SC, Pickles A. Development of a short questionnaire for use in epidemiological studies of depression in children and adolescents. *Int J Methods Psychiatr Res.* 1995;5(4): 237–249

51. Rhew IC, Simpson K, Tracy M, et al. Criterion validity of the Short Mood and Feelings Questionnaire and one- and two-item depression screens in young adolescents. *Child Adolesc Psychiatry Ment Health.* 2010;4(1):8

52. Kroenke K, Spitzer RL, Williams JB. The Patient Health Questionnaire-2: validity of a two-item depression screener. *Med Care.* 2003;41(11):1284–1292

53. Richardson LP, Rockhill C, Russo JE, et al. Evaluation of the PHQ-2 as a brief screen for detecting major depression among adolescents. *Pediatrics.* 2010; 125(5). Available at: www.pediatrics.org/cgi/content/full/125/5/e1097

54. Richardson LP, McCauley E, Grossman DC, et al. Evaluation of the Patient Health Questionnaire-9 Item for detecting major depression among adolescents. *Pediatrics.* 2010;126(6): 1117–1123

55. Gardner W, Murphy M, Childs G, et al. The PSC-17: a brief pediatric symptom checklist with psychosocial problem subscales. A report from PROS and ASPN. *Ambulatory Child Health.* 1999; 5(3):225–236

56. Murphy JM, Bergmann P, Chiang C, et al. The PSC-17: subscale scores, reliability, and factor structure in a new national sample. *Pediatrics.* 2016; 138(3):e20160038

57. Bourdon KH, Goodman R, Rae DS, Simpson G, Koretz DS. The Strengths and Difficulties Questionnaire: U.S. normative data and psychometric properties. *J Am Acad Child Adolesc Psychiatry.* 2005;44(6):557–564

58. Wolraich ML, Lambert W, Doffing MA, Bickman L, Simmons T, Worley K. Psychometric properties of the Vanderbilt ADHD diagnostic parent rating scale in a referred population. *J Pediatr Psychol.* 2003;28(8):559–567

59. Hamburger ME, Basile K,C Vivolo AM. *Measuring Bullying Victimization, Perpetration, and Bystander Experiences: A Compendium of Assessment Tools.* Atlanta, GA: Centers for Disease Control and Prevention, National Center for Injury Prevention and Control; 2011

60. Kelly SM, Gryczynski J, Mitchelle SG, Kirk A, O'Grady KE, Schwartz RP. Validity of brief screening instrument for adolescent tobacco, alcohol, and drug use. *Pediatrics.* 2014;133(5):819–826

61. Sachser C, Berliner L, Holt T, et al. International development and psychometric properties of the Child and Adolescent Trauma Screen (CATS). *J Affect Disord.* 2017;210:189–195

62. Bosquet Enlow M, Kassam-Adams N, Saxe G. The Child Stress Disorders Checklist-Short Form: a four-item scale of traumatic stress symptoms in children. *Gen Hosp Psychiatry.* 2010; 32(3):321–327

63. Williams J, Scott F, Stott C, et al. The CAST (Childhood Asperger Syndrome Test): test accuracy. *Autism.* 2005;9(1): 45–68

64. CHADIS-Child Health and Development Inventory System. Questionnaires. Available at: https://www.site.chadis.com/questionnaires. Accessed September 4, 2019

65. Boston Children's Hospital. TriVox Health: improving care through shared online tracking. Available at: https://vector.childrenshospital.org/2015/11/trivox-health-improving-care-through-shared-online-tracking/. Accessed September 4, 2019

66. Grandner MA, Malhotra A. Sleep as a vital sign: why medical practitioners need to routinely ask their patients about sleep. *Sleep Health.* 2015;1(1): 11–12

67. Wolfson AR, Carskadon MA. Sleep schedules and daytime functioning in adolescents. *Child Dev.* 1998;69(4): 875–887

68. Dahl RE, Lewin DS. Pathways to adolescent health sleep regulation and behavior. *J Adolesc Health.* 2002; 31(suppl 6):175–184

69. Curcio G, Ferrara M, De Gennaro L. Sleep loss, learning capacity and academic performance. *Sleep Med Rev.* 2006;10(5):323–337

70. Baum KT, Desai A, Field J, Miller LE, Rausch J, Beebe DW. Sleep restriction worsens mood and emotion regulation in adolescents. *J Child Psychol Psychiatry.* 2014;55(2):180–190

71. Short MA, Gradisar M, Lack LC, Wright HR. The impact of sleep on adolescent depressed mood, alertness and academic performance. *J Adolesc.* 2013; 36(6):1025–1033

72. Shochat T, Cohen-Zion M, Tzischinsky O. Functional consequences of inadequate sleep in adolescents: a systematic review. *Sleep Med Rev.* 2014;18(1):75–87

73. Sarchiapone M, Mandelli L, Carli V, et al. Hours of sleep in adolescents and its association with anxiety, emotional concerns, and suicidal ideation. *Sleep Med.* 2014;15(2):248–254

74. Blunden S, Hoban TF, Chervin RD. Sleepiness in children. *Sleep Med Clin.* 2006;1(1):105–118

75. Recommended amount of sleep for pediatric populations. *Pediatrics.* 2016; 138(2):e20161601

76. Paruthi S, Brooks LJ, D'Ambrosio C, et al. Recommended amount of sleep for pediatric populations: a consensus statement of the American Academy of Sleep Medicine. *J Clin Sleep Med.* 2016; 12(6):785–786

77. Adolescent Sleep Working Group; Committee on Adolescence; Council on School Health. School start times for adolescents. *Pediatrics.* 2014;134(3): 642–649

78. Garg A, Boynton-Jarrett R, Dworkin PH. Avoiding the unintended consequences of screening for social determinants of health. *JAMA.* 2016;316(8):813–814

79. Joost JC, Chessare JB, Schaeufele J, Link D, Weaver MT. Compliance with a prescription for psychotherapeutic counseling in childhood. *J Dev Behav Pediatr.* 1989;10(2):98–102

80. Howard BJ. The referral role of pediatricians. *Pediatr Clin North Am.* 1995;42(1):103–118

81. Wyatt KD, List B, Brinkman WB, et al. Shared decision making in pediatrics: a systematic review and meta-analysis. *Acad Pediatr.* 2015; 15(6):573–583

82. Miller WR, Rollnick S. *Motivational Interviewing: Helping People Change.* 3rd ed. New York, NY: The Guilford Press; 2012

83. American Academy of Pediatrics. Motivational interviewing. Available at: https://www.aap.org/en-us/advocacy-and-policy/aap-health-initiatives/Mental-Health/Pages/motivational-interviewing.aspx. Accessed September 4, 2019

84. Ginsburg S. Commonwealth fund issue brief: co-locating health services: a way to improve coordination of children's health care? 2008. Available at: https://www.commonwealthfund.org/publications/issue-briefs/2008/jul/colocating-health-services-way-improve-coordination-childrens. Accessed September 4, 2019

85. UnitedHealthcare. Commercial medical policy: neuropsychological testing under the medical benefit. Policy Number: 2019T0152T. 2019. Available at: https://www.uhcprovider.com/content/dam/provider/docs/public/policies/comm-medical-drug/neuropsychological-testing-under-medical-benefit.pdf. Accessed September 4, 2019

86. Aetna. Neuropsychological and psychological testing. 2017. Available at: www.aetna.com/cpb/medical/data/100_199/0158.html. Accessed September 4, 2019

87. US Department of Health and Human Services. HIPAA privacy rule and sharing information related to mental health. 2014. Available at: https://www.hhs.gov/sites/default/files/ocr/privacy/hipaa/understanding/special/mhguidancepdf.pdf. Accessed September 4, 2019

88. US Department of Health and Human Services; US Department of Education. Joint guidance on the application of the Family Educational Rights and Privacy Act (FERPA) and the Health Insurance Portability and Accountability Act of

1996 (HIPAA) to student health records. 2008. Available at: https://www2.ed.gov/policy/gen/guid/fpco/doc/ferpa-hipaa-guidance.pdf. Accessed September 4, 2019

89. American Academy of Pediatrics. HIPAA privacy rule and provider to provider communication. Available at: https://www.aap.org/en-us/advocacy-and-policy/aap-health-initiatives/Mental-Health/Pages/HIPAA-Privacy-Rule-and-Provider-to-Provider-Communication.aspx. Accessed September 4, 2019

90. Shaywitz S. *Overcoming Dyslexia: A New and Complete Science-Based Program for Reading Problems at Any Level.* New York, NY: Vintage Books; 2003

91. National Reading Panel. *Teaching Children to Read: An Evidence-Based Assessment of the Scientific Research Literature and Its Implications for Reading Instruction.* Washington, DC: US Department of Health and Human Services, Public Health Service, National Institutes of Health, National Institute of Child Health and Human Development; 2000

92. David JL. What research says about grade retention. *Educ Leadersh.* 2008; 65(6):83–84

93. Krier J; National Center for Mental Health in Schools at University of California, Los Angeles. Information resource: grade retention in elementary schools: policies, practices, results, and proposed new directions. 2012. Available at: http://smhp.psych.ucla.edu/pdfdocs/graderet.pdf. Accessed September 4, 2019

94. Willcutt EG, Pennington BF. Psychiatric comorbidity in children and adolescents with reading disability. *J Child Psychol Psychiatry.* 2000;41(8):1039–1048

95. Deighton J, Humphrey N, Belsky J, Boehnke J, Vostanis P, Patalay P. Longitudinal pathways between mental health difficulties and academic performance during middle childhood and early adolescence. *Br J Dev Psychol.* 2018; 36(1):110–126

Selecting Appropriate Toys for Young Children in the Digital Era

• *Clinical Report*

CLINICAL REPORT Guidance for the Clinician in Rendering Pediatric Care

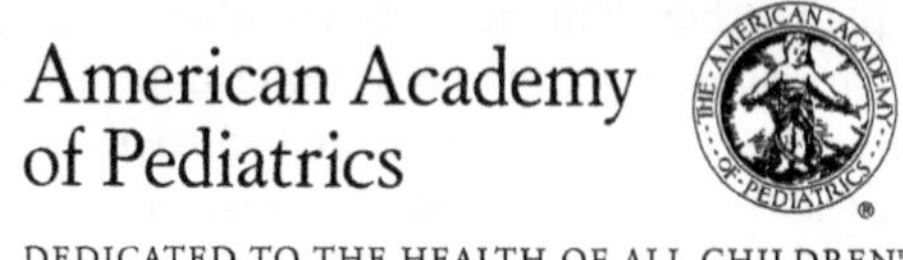

Selecting Appropriate Toys for Young Children in the Digital Era

Aleeya Healey, MD, FAAP,[a,b] Alan Mendelsohn, MD, FAAP,[a,c] COUNCIL ON EARLY CHILDHOOD

abstract

Play is essential to optimal child development because it contributes to the cognitive, physical, social, and emotional well-being of children and youth. It also offers an ideal and significant opportunity for parents and other caregivers to engage fully with children using toys as an instrument of play and interaction. The evolution of societal perceptions of toys from children's playthings to critical facilitators of early brain and child development has challenged caregivers in deciding which toys are most appropriate for their children. This clinical report strives to provide pediatric health care providers with evidence-based information that can be used to support caregivers as they choose toys for their children. The report highlights the broad definition of a toy; consideration of potential benefits and possible harmful effects of toy choices on child development; and the promotion of positive caregiving and development when toys are used to engage caregivers in play-based interactions with their children that are rich in language, pretending, problem-solving, and creativity. The report aims to address the evolving replacement of more traditional toys with digital media–based virtual "toys" and the lack of evidence for similar benefits in child development. Furthermore, this report briefly addresses the role of toys in advertising and/or incentive programs and aims to bring awareness regarding safety and health hazards associated with toy availability and accessibility in public settings, including some health care settings.

[a]New York University Langone Health, New York City, New York; [b]Bernard and Millie Duker Children's Hospital at Albany Medical Center, Albany, New York; and [c]Bellevue Hospital Center, New York City, New York

Drs Healey and Mendelsohn conducted a thorough literature review on all topics, integrated the most up-to-date data, and synthesized this evidence to create an original authorship with cited references of recommendations for the use of toys in promoting optimal child development; and all authors approved the final manuscript as submitted.

This document is copyrighted and is property of the American Academy of Pediatrics and its Board of Directors. All authors have filed conflict of interest statements with the American Academy of Pediatrics. Any conflicts have been resolved through a process approved by the Board of Directors. The American Academy of Pediatrics has neither solicited nor accepted any commercial involvement in the development of the content of this publication.

Clinical reports from the American Academy of Pediatrics benefit from expertise and resources of liaisons and internal (AAP) and external reviewers. However, clinical reports from the American Academy of Pediatrics may not reflect the views of the liaisons or the organizations or government agencies that they represent.

The guidance in this report does not indicate an exclusive course of treatment or serve as a standard of medical care. Variations, taking into account individual circumstances, may be appropriate.

All clinical reports from the American Academy of Pediatrics automatically expire 5 years after publication unless reaffirmed, revised, or retired at or before that time.

DOI: https://doi.org/10.1542/peds.2018-3348

Address correspondence to Alan Mendelsohn, MD, FAAP. E-mail: alm5@nyu.edu

PEDIATRICS (ISSN Numbers: Print, 0031-4005; Online, 1098-4275).

Copyright © 2019 by the American Academy of Pediatrics

To cite: Healey A, Mendelsohn A, AAP COUNCIL ON EARLY CHILDHOOD. Selecting Appropriate Toys for Young Children in the Digital Era. *Pediatrics.* 2019;143(1):e20183348

RATIONALE FOR CLINICAL REPORT

The last 20 years have brought a shift in parental and societal perception of toys, with parents and other caregivers increasingly likely to view toys as being important for children's development, self-regulation, and executive functioning.[1,2] A number of interrelated underlying factors have contributed to this shift, including: (1) increased recognition of early brain and child development as critical to educational success; (2) increased recognition of early experiences in the home and in child care settings as facilitating early brain and child development[3]; (3) increased marketing of so-called "educational" toys as critical for enhancing early experiences; (4) the perception (perhaps misperception) of toy play rather than interaction with caregivers around toys as important for the child's development, inclusive of self-regulation[3]; and (5) increasing sophistication of digital media–based virtual "toys" replacing physical toys and often incorrectly perceived by caregivers as having educational benefit.[4,5]

Although high-quality toys facilitate child development when they lead to the engagement of caregivers in play-based interactions that are rich in language, pretending, problem-solving, reciprocity, cooperation, and creativity[4] (and potentially for older children in solitary play[1]), many of the claims advertised for toys are not based on scientific evidence. Additionally, there has been increasing recognition of potential for harm in the context of exposure to electronic media, environmental toxins, and safety hazards. In particular, electronic media have been associated with displacement of play-based caregiver-child interactions and reductions in cognitive and/or language[6–10] and gross motor activities,[11] with implications for child development[7] and health outcomes (eg, obesity).[11]

This clinical report addresses the pediatric health care providers' role in advising caregivers about toys in the context of changes in caregivers' perceptions of toys and the evolution of what now constitutes a toy. It complements existing policy from the American Academy of Pediatrics related to play,[4] media,[12,13] school readiness,[14] toxic stress,[15,16] injury prevention,[17] toxicology,[18] and poverty.[4]

AN EVOLVING DEFINITION OF TOYS

In this report, a toy is defined as an object (whether made, purchased, or found in nature) intended for children's play. Developmentally, the importance of toys is strongly supported by the large body of research documenting the role of play in fostering development across all domains (including cognitive, language, social-emotional, and physical).[1,4,19] Although the concept of play has not changed over time, what constitutes a toy at the time of this report is substantially different than what it was during the previous century.[20] This difference is attributable in part to the proliferation of electronic, sensory-stimulating noise and light toys and digital media–based platforms with child-oriented software and mobile applications[1,21] that can be perceived by parents as necessary for developmental progress despite the lack of supporting evidence and, perhaps most importantly, with the potential for the disruption of caregiver-child interactions.[22]

Traditional (physical) toys can be categorized in a variety of ways: (1) symbolic and/or pretend (eg, dolls, action figures, cars, cooking and/or feeding implements, etc); (2) fine motor, adaptive, and/or manipulative (eg, blocks, shapes, puzzles, trains, etc); (3) art (eg, clay and coloring); (4) language and/or concepts (eg, card games, toy letters, and board games); and (5) gross motor and/or physical (eg, large toy cars, tricycles, and push and pull toys).[23] High-quality toys in each of these categories can facilitate caregiver-child interactions, peer play, and the growth of imagination. It should be emphasized that high-quality toys need not be expensive. For example, toy blocks, in addition to household objects, can be interesting for a child to examine and explore, especially if the child observes adults using them. Unfortunately, many caregivers believe that expensive electronic toys (eg, sensory-stimulating noise and light toys for infants and toddlers) and tablet-based toys are essential for their children's healthy development[2]; however, evidence suggests that core elements of such toys (eg, lights and sounds emanating from a robot) detract from social engagement that might otherwise take place through facial expressions, gestures, and vocalizations and that may be important for social development.[24,25]

Over the past 2 decades, a number of core elements of traditional toys have been adapted to electronic (virtual) versions, such as laptops, tablets, phones, other mobile devices, and stand-alone electronic game devices, and to toys that substitute for human interaction (eg, toy bear that can read a story aloud).[2,5] In many cases, these have been integrated with new elements not previously available within traditional toys, such as sensory-stimulating toys (especially for infants, for whom the strong visual engagement and neurodevelopmental consequences are not presently known[2]). This blurring of the line between physical and virtual toys has greatly complicated caregiver decision-making when selecting toys, especially because mobile device applications for children have proliferated at an extraordinary pace.[1,21] As a result, pediatric health care providers have an important role in providing guidance for selecting appropriate applications[21] and toys.

TOYS AND CHILD DEVELOPMENT

General Considerations

Toys are important in early child development in relation to their facilitation of cognitive development, language interactions, symbolic and pretend play, problem-solving, social interactions, and physical activity, with increasing importance as children move from infancy into toddlerhood.[1] Pretending through toy characters (eg, dolls, animals, and figures) and associated toy objects (eg, food, utensils, cars, planes, and buildings) can promote the use of words and narratives to imitate, describe, and cope with actual circumstances and feelings. Such imaginative play ultimately facilitates language development, self-regulation, symbolic thinking, and social-emotional development.[26] Problem-solving through play with the "traditional favorites," such as blocks and puzzles, can support fine motor skills and language and cognitive development and predicts both spatial and early mathematics skills.[27,28] The use of toys in physical activity (such as playing with balls) has the potential to facilitate gross motor development together with self-regulation and peer interaction because of the negotiations regarding rules that typically take place. The aforementioned are only a few examples of skill development associated with toy play. Play with caregivers is most likely necessary to support skill development. However, solitary play can also have a role (especially for older children, for whom exploration and play with toys on their own time and pace can foster their independent creativity, investigation, and assimilation skills[1]).

In general, the best toys are those that match children's developmental skills and abilities and further encourage the development of new skills. Developmentally advanced toys can be appropriate too, especially when caregivers scaffold (eg, setting up a storyline for pretending together or providing support for the child's learning of a new skill) children in their play. Some toys have the ability to "grow" with the child, in that they can be used differently as children advance developmentally. For example, an 18-month-old child might try to use blocks functionally (eg, stack them), whereas a 2-year-old might use the same blocks to engage in sophisticated symbolic play (eg, by feeding the doll with a block that represents a bottle[1]) or use the same blocks to construct a bridge, demonstrating the development of spatial awareness.

Notably, data in support of a developmental role for toys primarily come from studies of activities in which children play with caregivers[3] rather than alone.[4,27,29] In particular, toys that are most likely to facilitate development are those that are most enjoyably and productively used for play together with an engaged caregiver, because in such contexts play with toys is likely to include rich language experiences, reciprocal ("serve and return"[15,16]) verbal interactions, and scaffolding. Toys can play an especially important role in the promotion of learning and discovery in "guided play," in which children take the lead, but caregivers support their exploration in the context of learning goals.[1,30] The idea that play with toys is enriched by use with a caregiver is consistent with the many studies of early childhood documenting that learning takes place optimally in the context of serve-and-return conversations that build on the child's focus[31] (and are analogous to shared book reading). In general, toys that facilitate imaginative play and problem-solving are most likely to enable such engagement by caregivers, whereas toys that are electronically based (whether traditional or media based) are less likely to do so.[10,32] Therefore, when pediatric health care providers advise parents and caregivers, it is important to stress that toys can serve an important but supportive role in enhancing a child's social development in addition to other domains, such as language, primarily through engaging caregivers in responsive interactions[3] and pretend play. The pace of life in today's society provides limited time available to many caregivers, and solitary play with toys should not be a substitute for caregiver-child interactions during play or other contexts, such as reading aloud. Electronic toys by themselves will not provide children with the interaction and parental engagement that are critical for the healthy development.

Appropriateness of Toys for Children With Special Needs

Children with developmental delays or disabilities may face a variety of difficulties or obstacles in their play because of factors such as intellectual limitations or physical restrictions. One of the greatest difficulties is when the play itself becomes atypical in nature. For example, they may play with objects repetitively (eg, stacking blocks in the same way over and over again but not constructing anything per se) or nonfunctionally (eg, tapping a toy phone on the floor versus talking into it) or engage with toys at a significantly different developmental level than that of peers of a similar age (eg, 3 toddlers are having their toy dinosaurs chase one another, whereas a fourth is standing aside chewing on the toy dinosaur's tail). Furthermore, atypical behaviors among children with disabilities may themselves disrupt social interactions in addition to the play itself. These differences in developmental capacities are exhibited across domains,[3] and in turn, how children play with their toys may limit their ability to learn and develop maximally from parent-child and peer play opportunities.

The choice of toys may be especially complex for children with special needs given that recommendations on packaging are usually based on age and not developmental capacities. For instance, caregivers of children with special needs may be more likely to choose functional toys (eg, toys that are easily activated and often respond with lights and sounds)[33] over symbolic toys that encourage pretend play, creativity, and interactions (eg, toy animal farm).[34] Thus, caregivers of children with special needs may benefit from additional guidance from specialty therapists (eg, speech, occupational, or physical therapists) in choosing which toys, activities, and interactions are most appropriate for the developmental age of their child to ensure continued growth and skill mastery.

Adaptations of toys to accommodate a motor, visual, or other disability can be important for children with special needs. This can be accomplished by combining easy access with multisensory feedback,[35] such as light and sound when a toy is powered on. Examples of adaptations in design include Velcro strips to help a child hold a toy,[36] adding a piece of foam around a marker or paintbrush to make the art utensil easier to hold for a child with an inability to grasp the utensil independently,[37] and the use of a larger push button to activate a toy for a child with fine motor difficulties who cannot easily manipulate a small switch.[35] Technology has played a particularly important role in supporting the use of toys, and it is anticipated that the role of technology in addressing developmental interventions will increase over time with the guidance of research. As with children who are typically developing, children with special needs maximally benefit from play with toys in the context of caregiver interaction.

Toys can be used as a mode of incentive in the context of early intervention services and physical therapy more generally. For example, therapists often use toys to stimulate the use of a nondominant hand by placing the toy on that side of the body. Alternatively, using a toy as a reward may help elicit verbalizations in a child with a language disability. Novel or preferred toys can be held near an adult's face to encourage eye contact for a child with autism spectrum disorder.[38,39]

Toys and the Promotion of Parenting, Positive Caregiving, and Child Development

There has been a broad range of scientific- and policy-based efforts to enhance early development by promoting caregivers and children to play together with toys. These efforts are especially important for children growing up in poverty, for whom there is both reduced access to developmentally appropriate toys and barriers to caregiver-child interaction.[4,14,15] Such initiatives complement existing programs seeking to enhance early literacy within the pediatric medical home (eg, Reach Out and Read[40]). Efforts to promote play with toys have taken place across diverse platforms, including in (1) preschools (eg, Tools of the Mind[41]), (2) home visiting (eg, Parent-Child Home Program and Play and Learning Strategies[42]), (3) public health (eg, Building Blocks[29] and Blocktivities[43]), and (4) pediatric primary care (eg, Video Interaction Project[29]), to name a few. Findings from these programs strongly suggest that toys are most likely to facilitate developmental advances in the context of interactions[3] with and support by caregivers (including scaffolding and guided play rather than as a result of the toy itself[31]), early childhood educators, and other providers.[44] Pediatric health care providers' knowledge and awareness of these programs can inform anticipatory guidance to parents, provide opportunities for integration within the medical home enhancement, and function as potential sources of referral depending on availability within the communities they serve. Furthermore, the selection of toys offered to children should reflect the diverse and multicultural world we live in (ie, selecting dolls of various ethnicities in the pediatric office waiting area).[45]

ELECTRONIC MEDIA EXPOSURE AND PLAY WITH TOYS

A 2013 study revealed that 38% of US children younger than 2 years and 80% of 2 to 4 year-old children[11,46] have used a mobile electronic media device; this has more than doubled when compared with data collected in 2011.[4,11,32] More recent data presented in 2015 suggests that 96.9% of children have used mobile devices, and most started using them before 1 year of age.[47] For young children, the increase in screen time, which has evolved over the past decade, has taken place in association with a decrease in play, including both active play and play with toys.[11] This is especially significant for young children's development because screen time directly interferes with both play activities and parent-child interactions,[48] and even educational media is typically watched without caregiver input.[11,21,48] Furthermore, virtual toys (ie, screen games and/or applications) are increasingly designed to emulate and even replace physical toys. This potentially increases known risks of electronic media exposure, such as the promotion of aggressive behavior[49] and obesity.[50] The potential for these risks is especially great in the context of violence portrayed as humorous or justified, which can reinforce aggressive behavior and desensitize children to violence and its consequences.[51] Although it has been suggested that there may be learning benefits in association with interactive media,[46,52,53] there is presently no evidence to suggest that possible benefits of interactive media match those of active, creative, hands-on, and pretend play with more traditional toys.[4,9] In particular, children need to use their hands to explore and manipulate to strengthen those areas in the brain associated with spatial and mathematical learning.[54,55] Recent investigations have revealed that during children's play with electronic toys, there were fewer adult words, fewer conversational turns, fewer parental responses, and fewer productions of content-specific words than during play with traditional toys or books. Children, themselves vocalized less during play with electronic toys than with books.[8] Newer smartphone applications are focused on addressing the lack of social and physical interactivity; however, long-term risk and benefit studies are necessary to determine their actual impact and sustainability.[56] It is ironic that at a time when psychologists and other developmental scientists are recognizing the role of the body in learning, toys for children are becoming increasingly two-dimensional.[57]

ADVERTISING AND TOYS

A great deal of marketing in both traditional and new media is used to encourage caregivers to view technologically driven toys as critical for development. Such marketing has led to increasing exposure by children to enrichment videos, computer programs, specialized books with voice-recorded reading, and "developmental" toys beginning in early infancy.[4,58] It is important to note that claims for such toys on packaging and advertising are largely unsubstantiated[59–61] by credible studies, and thus, it is important for pediatric health care providers to aid caregivers in deciphering such advertisements.

Toys are also used extensively as a mechanism for marketing. For example, there has been a trend over the past decade of coupling food consumption with a toy incentive. Many fast food restaurants offer a toy incentive with particular meal purchases (many of which are energy dense and nutrient poor) to increase sales; such incentives are thought to have contributed to childhood obesity.[62] Promotions and incentives are an especially important consideration for children younger than 8 years, who are unaware that promotions and advertisements are actually designed to persuade them to have their caregivers buy specific products.[59] Recent initiatives at the federal (Federal Communications Commission and Federal Trade Commission) and local levels have sought and continue to develop regulations to guide and reduce such suggestive content in advertisements. One example is the US toy ordinance piloted in Santa Clara County, California, which prohibited the distribution of toys and other incentives to children in conjunction with meals, foods, or beverages that do not meet minimal nutritional criteria. This ordinance, in turn, positively influenced the marketing of healthful menu items with the toy incentive, and children then requested their parents to purchase the healthier meal options. The trial period provided data revealing the effects of marketing through toy incentives on children's food choices and, furthermore, the effects of their requests on the parental purchase of the meal.[62] The initiative was later expanded to similar changes in a number of major US cities (San Francisco and New York City).

TOY SAFETY CONSIDERATIONS

Government regulations, improved safety standards for the manufacture and use of toys, and product testing have made most toys safe when used appropriately for recommended ages and stages of development. However, just because a product is on the market does not mean that it is safe. In determining toy safety, the characteristics of the toy should be considered as well as how the toy might be used or abused and the amount of supervision or help needed for safe play. In a recent example of potential dangers, ingestion of high-powered magnetic objects (eg, rare earth magnets and strong permanent magnets) sometimes used in toys resulted in significant child morbidity.[63] Button batteries are ubiquitous as energy sources in electronic toys and have been associated with gastrointestinal hemorrhage and death when ingested.[60] The US Consumer Product Safety Commission (CPSC) Web site (www.cpsc.gov/) contains information regarding toy safety and can be a resource for pediatric providers and caregivers.[17,64] Two CPSC initiatives of particular relevance are SaferProducts (www.saferproducts.gov/), which allows anyone to report safety concerns, and the Recalls.gov Web site (www.recalls.gov), which provides information about safety recalls. In addition to physical safety characteristics, close attention should be paid to a toy's contact with harmful substances that may be used to treat its materials (eg, arsenic used to treat some wood products, lead paint, or chemicals such as bisphenol A[18]). *Caring for Our Children, Third Edition*, includes detailed information regarding potential hazards.[65]

TOYS AND THE OUTPATIENT PEDIATRIC SETTING

Toys provided in the waiting rooms of pediatric offices and other medical settings can serve as a model for caregivers and thereby aid in their decision-making about toys. Such toys can also help reduce child anxiety regarding visits and procedures. However, toys in pediatric settings also have the potential to become a vehicle for transmitting viruses and other pathogens among pediatric patients. Clear, easy-to-follow recommendations for the use and cleaning of toys in the pediatric office have been made by the Centers for Disease Control and Prevention and others.[66–69] For example, the sanitization of toys can be safely accomplished by washing with soap and water and then disinfecting by using a freshly prepared solution (1:100 dilution of household bleach; soak for at least 2 minutes) or by using an Environmental Protection Agency–registered sanitizing solution (according to the manufacturer's instructions) and then rinsing and air drying.[66–68] Toys should be cleaned between uses to avoid the transfer of infectious agents.[67] Also, caregivers can be given the option to bring their child's own toys for office visits to minimize the sharing and transmission of infectious disease. Although some available toys are marketed as incorporating antibacterial agents in their construction, it is important to note that such construction is currently unproven to be "antibacterial."[66] Further guidance of cleaning and disinfecting toys can be found in *Caring For Our Children, Third Edition*.[65] Although adequate infection control measures may seem daunting, recommendations tend to be straightforward to implement and should not be considered a barrier to the use of toys in the outpatient setting.

CONSIDERATIONS FOR PEDIATRIC HEALTH CARE PROVIDERS IN THE OFFICE SETTING

1. Advice regarding toys and/or play with toys can be offered together with guidance in 5 related areas: social-emotional development through social interactions, literacy promotion, block and puzzle play in relation to science and/or math and spatial skills, imaginative and creative play in relation to make-believe and/or free play, and electronic media exposure.
2. Pediatric health care providers can advise parents and caregivers regarding toys that are appropriate for young children in terms of stage of development, learning opportunities, and safety. For families for whom the literacy level of the caregivers is of concern, handouts with example toy pictures may be created by the practitioner.
3. If toys are available for children in waiting and examination rooms, they may be viewed as models for toys that are appropriate for the home.
4. Pediatric health care providers may choose to give parents information about developmentally appropriate toys, which are those that promote language-rich caregiver-child interactions, pretend play, physically active play, problem-solving, and creativity. Lists of appropriate toys can be found through many resources, including books, pamphlets from organizations such as Zero to Three, and instruments for assessment of the provision of toys in the home. Pediatric health care providers can also recommend books that provide guidance about interacting with children, including in the context of toy play to encourage language development (see Resources).
5. If pediatric health care providers make toys available in the office, they may consider whether they are safe for all children of all ages according to the following recommendations:
    - do not provide small toys or toys with easily dislodged parts that fit in an infant's or toddler's mouth;
    - do not provide toys with loose string, rope, ribbons, or cord;
    - do not provide toys with sharp edges;
    - do not provide toys that make loud or shrill noises;
    - provide only toys made of nontoxic materials;
    - always store toys safely and avoid toy chests with lids; and
    - be extremely cautious of toys with button batteries; ensure that they are not accessible to children so that they cannot be accidentally ingested.
6. Although pediatric health care providers can make toys available in their offices, those who do so should choose toys that are easily and routinely cleaned. When possible, each time a toy has been in contact with saliva or other bodily fluids, it should be sanitized.
7. Displaying notices in the office about product recalls of toys is important to inform parents of product dangers.
8. Take available opportunities to counsel caregivers regarding dangers associated with high-powered magnet toys as well as button batteries that are ubiquitous in electronic toys.

ADVICE FOR PARENTS AND CAREGIVERS

1. Recognize that one of the most important purposes of play with toys throughout childhood, and especially in infancy, is not educational at all but rather to facilitate warm, supportive interactions and relationships.
2. Scientific studies supporting a developmental role for toys primarily come from studies of activities in which children play with caregivers rather than alone. The most educational toy is one that fosters interactions between caregivers and children in supportive, unconditional play.
3. Provide children with safe, affordable toys that are developmentally appropriate. Include toys that promote learning and growth in all areas of development. Choose toys that are not overstimulating and encourage children to use their imaginations. Social-emotional and cognitive skills are developed and enhanced as children use play to work out real-life problems (see Zero to

Three: Tips for Choosing Toys for Toddlers in Resources).

4. Make a thoughtful selection of toys and remember that a good toy does not have to be trendy or expensive. Indeed, sometimes the simplest toys may be the best, in that they provide opportunities for children to use their imagination to create the toy use, not the other way around. Choose toys that will grow with the child, foster interactions with caregivers, encourage exploration and problem-solving, and spark the child's imagination.
5. Use children's books to develop ideas for pretending together while playing with toys; use of the library should be routine for all parents regardless of socioeconomic status. A list of community library locations for the office should be considered.
6. Keep in mind that toys are not a substitute for warm, loving, dependable relationships. Use toys to enhance interactions between the caregiver and child rather than to direct children's play.
7. Seek the pediatric health care provider's advice in distinguishing between safe and unsafe toys (see Resources).
8. Be aware of the potential for toys to promote race- or gender-based stereotypes.
9. Limit video game and computer game use. Total screen time, including television and computer use, should be less than 1 hour per day for children 2 years or older and avoided in children 18 to 24 months of age. Children younger than 5 years should play with computer or video games only if they are developmentally appropriate, and they should be accompanied by the parent or caregiver. The use of media together with caregiver interaction is essential to minimizing adverse media effects on the young mind.
10. Seek out toys that encourage the child to be both mentally and physically active.

RESOURCES

• For information on toy safety concerns or questions, refer to the US Consumer Product Safety Commission Web site (www.cpsc.gov) and *Caring for Our Children, Third Edition.*

• For questions or concerns regarding infection control guidelines, refer to Centers for Disease Control and Prevention guidelines (http://www.cdc.gov).

• For guidance in identifying appropriate toys for young children, refer to the following resources:

1. Zero to Three, "Tips for Choosing Toys for Toddlers" (https://www.zerotothree.org/resources/1076-tips-for-choosing-toys-for-toddlers);
2. The National Association for the Education for Young Children (NAEYC) (http://www.naeyc.org/ecp/resources/goodtoys); and
3. StimQ (http://www.med.nyu.edu/pediatrics/developmental/research/belle-project/stimq-cognitive-home-environment).

• For suggestions on how caregivers can use toys, play, and other activities to encourage language development, refer to the following Web sites:

1. Too Small to Fail (http://toosmall.org/), and
2. Bridging the Word Gap (http://bwgresnet.ku.edu/).

• For a resource list of suggestions on toys, play, and recreation for children with disabilities, refer to the following Web sites:

1. The Northwest Access Fund Web site (http://washingtonaccessfund.org/toys-play-for-children-with-disabilities-resource-list/), and
2. How We Play! A Guidebook for Parents and Early Intervention Professionals. Birth through Two (https://eric.ed.gov/?id=ED447660).

• For information regarding the promotion of physical activity, refer to the following resources:

1. Let's Move (https://letsmove.obamawhitehouse.archives.gov/get-active), and
2. National Resource Center for Health and Safety in Child Care and Early Education (http://nrckids.org/index.cfm/products/videos11/motion-moments1/).

LEAD AUTHORS

Aleeya Healey, MD, FAAP
Alan Mendelsohn, MD, FAAP

COUNCIL ON EARLY CHILDHOOD EXECUTIVE COMMITTEE, 2017–2018

Jill M. Sells, MD, FAAP, Chairperson
Sherri L. Alderman, MD, MPH, IMH-E, FAAP
Andrew Hashikawa, MD, MPH, FAAP
Alan Mendelsohn, MD, FAAP
Terri McFadden, MD, FAAP
Dipesh Navsaria, MD, MPH, MSILS, FAAP
Georgina Peacock, MD, MPH, FAAP
Seth Scholer, MD, MPH, FAAP
Jennifer Takagishi, MD, FAAP
Douglas Vanderbilt, MD, MS, FAAP
P. Gail Williams, MD, FAAP

FORMER COMMITTEE MEMBERS

Marian Earls, MD, MTS, FAAP
Elaine Donoghue, MD, FAAP

CONSULTANTS

Kathy Hirsh-Pasek, PhD
Roberta Golinkoff, PhD

LIAISONS

Lynette Fraga, PhD – *Child Care Aware*
Katiana Garagozlo, MD – *AAP Section on Pediatric Trainees*
Dina Lieser, MD, FAAP – *Maternal and Child Health Bureau*
Rebecca Parlakian, MA, Ed – *Zero to Three*
Alecia Stephenson and Lucy Recio – *National Association for the Education of Young Children*

FORMER LIAISONS

David Willis, MD, FAAP – *(Formerly with the Maternal and Child Health Bureau)*
Barbary Sargent, PNP – *National Association of Pediatric Nurse Practitioners*
Laurel Hoffmann, MD – *AAP Section on Medical Students, Residents, and Fellows in Training*

STAFF

Charlotte O. Zia, MPH, CHES

ABBREVIATION

CPSC: Consumer Product Safety Commission

FINANCIAL DISCLOSURE: The authors have indicated they have no financial relationships relevant to this article to disclose.

FUNDING: No external funding.

POTENTIAL CONFLICT OF INTEREST: The authors have indicated they have no potential conflicts of interest to disclose.

REFERENCES

1. Goldstein J. *Play in Children's Development, Health and Well-Being.* Brussels, Belgium: Toy Industries of Europe; 2012. Available at: www.ornes.nl/wp-content/uploads/2010/08/Play-in-children-s-development-health-and-well-being-feb-2012.pdf. Accessed February 13, 2018
2. Levin DE, Rosenquest B. The increasing role of electronic toys in the lives of infants and toddlers: should we be concerned? *Contemporary Issues in Early Childhood.* 2001;2(2):242–247
3. Greenspan SI. Levels of infant-caregiver interactions and the DIR model: implications for the development of signal affects, the regulation of mood and behavior, the formation of a sense of self, the creation of internal representation, and the construction of defenses and character structure. *J Infant Child Adolesc Psychother.* 2007;6(3):174–210
4. Milteer RM, Ginsburg KR; Council on Communications and Media; Committee on Psychosocial Aspects of Child and Family Health. The importance of play in promoting healthy child development and maintaining strong parent-child bond: focus on children in poverty. *Pediatrics.* 2012;129(1). Available at: www.pediatrics.org/cgi/content/full/129/1/e204
5. Clifford S. Go directly, digitally to jail? Classic toys learn new clicks. *The New York Times.* February 25, 2012. Available at https://www.livemint.com/Industry/tfpaBedcGvvWtXSbSCgHVI/Go-directly-digitally-to-jail-classic-toys-learn-new-click.html. Accessed November 26, 2018
6. Christakis DA, Gilkerson J, Richards JA, et al. Audible television and decreased adult words, infant vocalizations, and conversational turns: a population-based study. *Arch Pediatr Adolesc Med.* 2009;163(6):554–558
7. Zimmerman FJ, Christakis DA. Children's television viewing and cognitive outcomes: a longitudinal analysis of national data. *Arch Pediatr Adolesc Med.* 2005;159(7):619–625
8. Sosa AV. Association of the type of toy used during play with the quantity and quality of parent-infant communication. *JAMA Pediatr.* 2016;170(2):132–137
9. Parish-Morris J, Mahajan N, Hirsh-Pasek K, Golinkoff RM, Collins MF. Once upon a time: parent–child dialogue and storybook reading in the electronic era. *Mind Brain Educ.* 2013;7(3):200–211
10. Zosh JM, Verdine BN, Filipowicz A, Golinkoff RM, Hirsh-Pasek K, Newcombe NS. Talking shape: parental language with electronic versus traditional shape sorters. *Mind Brain Educ.* 2015;9(3):136–144
11. Common Sense Media. *Zero to Eight: Children's Media Use in America 2013.* San Francisco, CA: Common Sense Media; 2013. Available at: www.commonsensemedia.org/research/zero-to-eight-childrens-media-use-in-america-2013. Accessed February 13, 2018
12. Council on Communications and Media. Children, adolescents, and the media. *Pediatrics.* 2013;132(5):958–961
13. Brown A; Council on Communications and Media. Media use by children younger than 2 years. *Pediatrics.* 2011;128(5):1040–1045
14. High PC; American Academy of Pediatrics; Committee on Early Childhood, Adoption, and Dependent Care; Council on School Health. School readiness. *Pediatrics.* 2008;121(4). Available at: www.pediatrics.org/cgi/content/full/121/4/e1008
15. Garner AS, Shonkoff JP; Committee on Psychosocial Aspects of Child and Family Health; Committee on Early Childhood, Adoption, and Dependent Care; Section on Developmental and Behavioral Pediatrics. Early childhood adversity, toxic stress, and the role of the pediatrician: translating developmental science into lifelong health. *Pediatrics.* 2012;129(1). Available at: www.pediatrics.org/cgi/content/full/129/1/e224
16. Shonkoff JP, Garner AS; Committee on Psychosocial Aspects of Child and Family Health; Committee on Early Childhood, Adoption, and Dependent Care; Section on Developmental and Behavioral Pediatrics. The lifelong effects of early childhood adversity and toxic stress. *Pediatrics.* 2012;129(1). Available at: www.pediatrics.org/cgi/content/full/129/1/e232
17. Gardner HG; American Academy of Pediatrics Committee on Injury, Violence, and Poison Prevention. Office-based counseling for unintentional injury prevention. *Pediatrics.* 2007;119(1):202–206
18. Karr C. Addressing environmental contaminants in pediatric practice. *Pediatr Rev.* 2011;32(5):190–200; quiz 200

19. Fisher K, Hirsh-Pasek K, Golinkoff RM, Singer DG, Berk L. Playing around in school: implications for learning and educational policy. In: Nathan P, Pellegrini AD, eds. *The Oxford Handbook of the Development of Play.* Oxford, UK: Oxford University Press; 2010

20. Fisher KR, Hirsh-Pasek K, Golinkoff RM, Gryfe SG. Conceptual split? Parents' and experts' perceptions of play in the 21st century. *J Appl Dev Psychol.* 2008;29(4):305–316

21. Hirsh-Pasek K, Zosh JM, Golinkoff RM, Gray JH, Robb MB, Kaufman J. Putting education in "educational" apps: lessons from the science of learning. *Psychol Sci Public Interest.* 2015;16(1):3–34

22. Schore AN. Effects of a secure attachment relationship on right brain development, affect regulation, and infant mental health. *Infant Ment Health J.* 2001;22(1–2):7–66

23. Dreyer BP, Mendelsohn AL, Tamis-LeMonda CS. StimQ cognitive home environment. Available at: www.med.nyu.edu/pediatrics/developmental/research/belle-project/stimq-cognitive-home-environment. Accessed February 14, 2018

24. Klin A, Jones W, Schultz R, Volkmar F. The enactive mind, or from actions to cognition: lessons from autism. *Philos Trans R Soc Lond B Biol Sci.* 2003;358(1430):345–360

25. Zero to Three. Early development & well-being. Available at: www.zerotothree.org/child-development/. Accessed February 14, 2018

26. Weisleder A, Cates CB, Dreyer BP, et al. Promotion of positive parenting and prevention of socioemotional disparities. *Pediatrics.* 2016;137(2):e20153239

27. Weisberg DS, Hirsh-Pasek K, Golinkoff RM. Guided play: where curricular goals meet a playful pedagogy. *Mind Brain Educ.* 2013;7(2):104–112

28. Ferrara K, Hirsh-Pasek K, Newcombe NS, Golinkoff RM, Lam WS. Block talk: spatial language during block play. *Mind Brain Educ.* 2011;5(3):143–151

29. Mendelsohn A, Huberman HS, Berkule SB, Brockmeyer CA, Morrow LM, Dreyer BP. Primary care strategies for promoting parent-child interactions and school readiness in at-risk families: the Bellevue project for early language, literacy, and education success. *Arch Pediatr Adolesc Med.* 2011;165(1):33–41

30. Weisberg DS, Hirsh-Pasek K, Golinkoff RM, Kittredge AK, Klahr D. Guided play: principles and practices. *Curr Dir Psychol Sci.* 2016;25(3):177–182

31. Hirsh-Pasek K, Golinkoff R. Kathy Hirsh-Pasek and Roberta Michnick Golinkoff: how and how much we talk to children matters. *The Dallas Morning News.* June 12, 2015. Available at: www.dallasnews.com/opinion/latest-columns/20150612-kathy-hirsh-pasek-and-roberta-michnick-golinkoff-how-and-how-much-we-talk-to-children-matters.ece. Accessed February 14, 2018

32. Shifrin D, Brown A, Hill D, Jana L, Flinn SK. *Growing Up Digital: Media Research Symposium.* Elk Grove Village, IL: American Academy of Pediatrics; 2015. Available at: https://www.aap.org/en-us/Documents/digital_media_symposium_proceedings.pdf. Accessed February 14, 2018

33. Patrizia M, Claudio M, Leonardo G, Alessandro P. A robotic toy for children with special needs: from requirements to design. In: *2009 Institute of Electronical and Electronics Engineers 11th International Conference on Rehabilitation Robotics*; June 23–26, 2009; Kyoto, Japan

34. Hamm EM, Mistrett SG, Ruffino AG. Play outcomes and satisfaction with toys and technology of young children with special needs. *J Spec Educ Technol.* 2005;21(1):29–35

35. University at Buffalo Center for Assistive Technology. Guidelines to promote play opportunities for children with disabilities. Available at: https://familydaycare.com/wp-content/uploads/pop_pt2_Guidelines-to-Promote-Play-Opportunities-for-Children-with-Disabilities.pdf. Accessed February 20, 2018

36. Hsieh HC. Effects of ordinary and adaptive toys on pre-school children with developmental disabilities. *Res Dev Disabil.* 2008;29(5):459–466

37. Early Childhood Learning and Knowledge Center. Children with disabilities. Available at: https://eclkc.ohs.acf.hhs.gov/children-disabilities. Accessed February 14, 2018

38. Nwokah E. The toy bag: an examination of its history and use in early intervention for infants and toddlers with special needs. In: Clark CD, ed. *Transactions at Play: Play and Culture Studies.* Vol 9. Lanham, MD: University Press of America; 2009:166–182

39. Guyton G. Using toys to support infant-toddler learning and development. *Young Child.* 2011;66(5):50–54, 56

40. High PC, Klass P; Council on Early Childhood. Literacy promotion: an essential component of primary care pediatric practice. *Pediatrics.* 2014;134(2):404–409

41. Bodrova E, Leong DJ. Tools of the mind: the Vygotskian approach to early childhood education. In: Rooparine JL, Johnson JE, eds. *Approaches to Early Childhood Education.* 6th ed. Columbus, OH: Merrill/Prentice Hall; 2012:241–260

42. Parent-Child Home Program. Available at: www.parent-child.org/. Accessed February 14, 2018

43. Christakis DA, Zimmerman FJ, Garrison MM. Effect of block play on language acquisition and attention in toddlers: a pilot randomized controlled trial. *Arch Pediatr Adolesc Med.* 2007;161(10):967–971

44. Tomopoulos S, Dreyer BP, Tamis-LeMonda C, et al. Books, toys, parent-child interaction, and development in young Latino children. *Ambul Pediatr.* 2006;6(2):72–78

45. Clark KB, Clark MK. Skin color as a factor in racial identification of Negro preschool children. *Journal of Social Psychology.* 1940;11:159–169

46. Christakis DA. Interactive media use at younger than the age of 2 years: time to rethink the American Academy of Pediatrics guideline? *JAMA Pediatr.* 2014;168(5):399–400

47. Kabali HK, Irigoyen MM, Nunez-Davis R, et al. Exposure and use of mobile media devices by young children. *Pediatrics.* 2015;136(6):1044–1050

48. Pagani LS, Fitzpatrick C, Barnett TA, Dubow E. Prospective associations between early childhood television

exposure and academic, psychosocial, and physical well-being by middle childhood. *Arch Pediatr Adolesc Med.* 2010;164(5):425–431

49. Anderson CA, Bushman BJ. Effects of violent video games on aggressive behavior, aggressive cognition, aggressive affect, physiological arousal, and prosocial behavior: a meta-analytic review of the scientific literature. *Psychol Sci.* 2001;12(5):353–359
50. Jackson DM, Djafarian K, Stewart J, Speakman JR. Increased television viewing is associated with elevated body fatness but not with lower total energy expenditure in children. *Am J Clin Nutr.* 2009;89(4): 1031–1036
51. American Academy of Pediatrics. Available at: https://healthychildren.org/English. Accessed February 14, 2018
52. Li X, Atkins MS. Early childhood computer experience and cognitive and motor development. *Pediatrics.* 2004;113(6):1715–1722
53. Baydar N, Kağitçibaşi Ç, Küntay AC, Gökşen F. Effects of an educational television program on preschoolers: variability in benefits. *J Appl Dev Psychol.* 2008;29(5):349–360
54. Greaves S, Imms C, Krumlinde-Sundholm L, Dodd K, Eliasson AC. Bimanual behaviours in children aged 8-18 months: a literature review to select toys that elicit the use of two hands. *Res Dev Disabil.* 2012;33(1):240–250
55. Lillard AS, Peterson J. The immediate impact of different types of television on young children's executive function. *Pediatrics.* 2011;128(4):644–649
56. LeBlanc AG, Chaput JP. Pokémon Go: a game changer for the physical inactivity crisis? *Prev Med.* 2017;101:235–237
57. Hastings EC, Karas TL, Winsler A, Way E, Madigan A, Tyler S. Young children's video/computer game use: relations with school performance and behavior. *Issues Ment Health Nurs.* 2009;30(10):638–649
58. Fletcher R, Nielsen M. Product-based television and young children's pretend play in Australia. *J Child Media.* 2012;6(1):5–17
59. Calvert SL. Children as consumers: advertising and marketing. *Future Child.* 2008;18(1):205–234
60. Common Sense Media. *Advertising to Children and Teens: Current Practices.* San Francisco, CA: Common Sense Media; 2014. Available at: https://www.commonsensemedia.org/research/advertising-to-children-and-teens-current-practices. Accessed February 14, 2018
61. Vaala S, Ly A, Levine MH. *Getting a Read on the App Stores: A Market Scan and Analysis of Children's Literacy Apps.* New York, NY: The Joan Ganz Cooney Center at Sesame Workshop; 2015
62. Otten JJ, Hekler EB, Krukowski RA, et al. Food marketing to children through toys: response of restaurants to the first U.S. toy ordinance. *Am J Prev Med.* 2012;42(1):56–60
63. Brown JC, Otjen JP, Drugas GT. Pediatric magnet ingestions: the dark side of the force. *Am J Surg.* 2014;207(5):754–759; discussion 759
64. Goodson B, Bronson M. *Which Toy for Which Child: A Consumer's Guide for Selecting Suitable Toys, Ages Birth Through Five.* Bethesda, MD: US Consumer Product Safety Commission; 2003
65. American Academy of Pediatrics; American Public Health Association; National Resource Center for Health and Safety in Child Care and Early Education. *Caring for Our Children: National Health and Safety Performance Standards; Guidelines for Early Care and Education Programs.* 3rd ed. Elk Grove Village, IL: American Academy of Pediatrics; 2011
66. Centers for Disease Control and Prevention, Healthcare Infection Control Practices Advisory Committee. Guideline for isolation precautions: preventing transmission of infectious agents in healthcare settings. 2007. Available at: www.cdc.gov/ncidod/dhqp/pdf/isolation2007.pdf. Accessed February 14, 2018
67. Rathore MH, Jackson MA; Committee on Infectious Diseases. Infection prevention and control in pediatric ambulatory settings. *Pediatrics.* 2017;140(5):e20172857
68. Martínez-Bastidas T, Castro-del Campo N, Mena KD, et al. Detection of pathogenic micro-organisms on children's hands and toys during play. *J Appl Microbiol.* 2014;116(6):1668–1675
69. Merriman E, Corwin P, Ikram R. Toys are a potential source of cross-infection in general practitioners' waiting rooms. *Br J Gen Pract.* 2002;52(475):138–140

Soccer Injuries in Children and Adolescents

- *Clinical Report*

CLINICAL REPORT Guidance for the Clinician in Rendering Pediatric Care

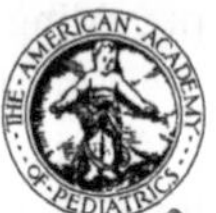

American Academy of Pediatrics

DEDICATED TO THE HEALTH OF ALL CHILDREN™

Soccer Injuries in Children and Adolescents

Andrew Watson, MD, MS, FAAP,[a] Jeffrey M. Mjaanes, MD, FAAP,[b] COUNCIL ON SPORTS MEDICINE AND FITNESS

abstract

Participation in youth soccer in the United States continues to increase steadily, with a greater percentage of preadolescent participants than perhaps any other youth sport. Despite the wide-ranging health benefits of participation in organized sports, injuries occur and represent a threat to the health and performance of young athletes. Youth soccer has a greater reported injury rate than many other contact sports, and recent studies suggest that injury rates are increasing. Large increases in the incidence of concussions in youth soccer have been reported, and anterior cruciate ligament injuries remain a significant problem in this sport, particularly among female athletes. Considerable new research has identified a number of modifiable risk factors for lower-extremity injuries and concussion, and several prevention programs have been identified to reduce the risk of injury. Rule enforcement and fair play also serve an important role in reducing the risk of injury among youth soccer participants. This report provides an updated review of the relevant literature as well as recommendations to promote the safe participation of children and adolescents in soccer.

Soccer is the most popular youth sport in the world and is 1 of the most popular team sports in the United States.[1] It is estimated that 3.9 million children and adolescents participate in soccer annually,[2] and from 1990 to 2014, the number of youth officially registered with US youth soccer programs increased by almost 90%.[3] Despite the wide-ranging health benefits of participation in organized sports, injuries occur and represent a threat to both athlete health and performance.[4] Unfortunately, recent studies suggest that injury rates in youth soccer may be increasing. Sports-related injuries represent a significant and increasing economic burden to the health care system, and the prevention of sports-related injuries in children has far-reaching health and economic benefits to the patient, the family, and the health care system as a whole. Given the number of children and youth participating in youth soccer, reducing the risk of injury among such a large group of participants has the potential to reduce attrition rates, promote lifelong participation in sport, and facilitate the

[a]*Department of Orthopedics and Rehabilitation, School of Medicine and Public Health, University of Wisconsin–Madison, Madison, Wisconsin; and* [b]*Department of Orthopedic Surgery, Feinberg School of Medicine, Northwestern University, Chicago, Illinois*

Drs Watson and Mjaanes served as coauthors of the manuscript, contributed substantial input into the content and revision, and approved the final manuscript as submitted.

This document is copyrighted and is property of the American Academy of Pediatrics and its Board of Directors. All authors have filed conflict of interest statements with the American Academy of Pediatrics. Any conflicts have been resolved through a process approved by the Board of Directors. The American Academy of Pediatrics has neither solicited nor accepted any commercial involvement in the development of the content of this publication.

Clinical reports from the American Academy of Pediatrics benefit from expertise and resources of liaisons and internal (AAP) and external reviewers. However, clinical reports from the American Academy of Pediatrics may not reflect the views of the liaisons or the organizations or government agencies that they represent.

The guidance in this report does not indicate an exclusive course of treatment or serve as a standard of medical care. Variations, taking into account individual circumstances, may be appropriate.

All clinical reports from the American Academy of Pediatrics automatically expire 5 years after publication unless reaffirmed, revised, or retired at or before that time.

DOI: https://doi.org/10.1542/peds.2019-2759

Address correspondence to Andrew Watson, MD, MS, FAAP. E-mail: watson@ortho.wisc.edu

PEDIATRICS (ISSN Numbers: Print, 0031-4005; Online, 1098-4275).

Copyright © 2019 by the American Academy of Pediatrics

FINANCIAL DISCLOSURE: The authors have indicated they have no financial relationships relevant to this article to disclose.

FUNDING: No external funding.

To cite: Watson A, Mjaanes JM, AAP COUNCIL ON SPORTS MEDICINE AND FITNESS. Soccer Injuries in Children and Adolescents. *Pediatrics.* 2019;144(5):e20192759

improvements in public health associated with regular exercise. By providing this updated clinical report, the American Academy of Pediatrics (AAP) intends to familiarize pediatric health care providers with current information regarding the risk of injury in youth sport participation, strategies for injury prevention, legislative changes aimed at reducing injury risk in youth soccer, and important concepts with which pediatricians can guide families and sport governing bodies to reduce risk and facilitate participation

INJURY INCIDENCE IN YOUTH SOCCER

Injury incidence rates in youth soccer vary considerably between studies and have been reported to be anywhere from 2.0 to 19.4 injuries per 1000 hours of exposure.[5–7] Injury incidence has been consistently documented to be much greater during games than during training in adolescents[5,8] as well as 7- to 12-year-olds.[5] In a recent systematic review of injury incidence in male soccer players, injury rates among adolescent athletes was found to range from 3.7 to 11.1 injuries per 1000 hours in training but 9.5 to 48.7 injuries per 1000 hours during games.[5] Injury incidence appears to increase with age, such that injuries to players younger than 12 years have been reported to be 1.0 to 1.6 per 1000 hours, whereas adolescents have demonstrated an injury rate of 2.6 to 15.3 per 1000 hours.[6,7,9] Incidence rates may vary depending on the specific reporting mechanism, however, and self-reporting mechanisms may identify an even greater proportion of injuries than those identified through traditional injury reporting mechanisms involving a health care provider.[4,9]

Despite ongoing efforts to reduce the risk of injury in youth sports, injury rates among youth soccer participants may be increasing and are greater than those for a number of other team and individual sports (see Table 1). In a recent retrospective study of 25 years of emergency department visits, Smith et al[10] found that the annual number of soccer-related injuries among 7- to 17-year-olds per 10 000 soccer participants increased 111% from 1990 to 2014. Although it is unclear whether this increase is attributable to greater incidence, increased recognition, or both; a considerable portion of this increase was attributed to a greater number of concussions, with a relatively higher overall injury incidence among girls and adolescent athletes. A similar study also revealed a significant increase in pediatric soccer-related injuries evaluated in the emergency department between 2000 and 2012, with significantly greater numbers of injuries for male youth soccer participants throughout the study.[11]

As observed with other sports, many young athletes now play soccer year-round, including indoor soccer. Indoor soccer involves essentially the same rules as outdoor soccer but is played on a covered field of artificial turf with walls. Futsal is a derivative of indoor soccer but is played on a smaller indoor court with only 5 players to a side and a ball smaller in diameter. Most studies involving the epidemiology of indoor soccer injuries originate in Europe or Asia and involve adult professional teams.[13] Despite early evidence that indoor soccer carried a higher risk of injury than outdoor soccer, a more recent study involving adolescent soccer players revealed no significant differences in overall injury rates by sex or age for indoor compared with outdoor soccer.[14]

INJURY TYPES AND MECHANISMS

The majority of youth soccer injuries are acute events resulting from player-to-player contact, with a considerably greater proportion of injuries occurring during competition than practice.[5,15,16] With respect to severe injuries (time loss >21 days), incidence remains considerably higher during games than practice, and girls demonstrate a greater incidence than boys (3.3 vs 2.5 per 1000 athletic exposures).[17] In fact, the incidence of injuries among high school soccer players that resulted in medical disqualification (career- or season-ending injuries) between 2005 and 2014 was found to be 0.17 and 0.10 per 1000 athletic exposures for girls and boys, respectively.[16] Among the 11 sports evaluated, the injury rate for soccer for boys was lower only than those for football, ice hockey, and lacrosse, and for girls, only gymnastics had a greater rate of disqualifying injury. Although not as common, youth soccer players are also at risk for overuse injuries, with a recent study identifying injury rates of 0.15 and 0.20 injuries per 10 000 athletic exposures among high school male and female soccer players, respectively, with knees and lower legs being the most common locations of injury.[18] Although data are limited, a single study revealed that tendinitis, patellofemoral pain, and Osgood-Schlatter disease were the most common overuse injuries in youth soccer players.[19]

Although rates of soccer injuries evaluated in the emergency department appear to be lower among younger soccer athletes compared with older players,[10] the types of injuries differ by age. A prospective study of emergency department visits for soccer-related injuries between 1990 and 2003 suggested that 5- to 14-year-old athletes were more likely to suffer upper-extremity injuries than high school athletes, and high school athletes were more likely to suffer a concussion.[20] More recently, a similar study of soccer-related injuries presented to emergency departments between 1990 and 2014 revealed lower overall injury rates among 7- to 11-year-olds compared with 12- to 17-year-olds, with younger athletes more likely to suffer

TABLE 1 Rates of Severe Injuries, Fractures, and Season-Ending Injuries in High School Sports

Injury Type	Sport	Rate per 1000 AEs
Severe[a]		
Boys		
	Football	0.69
	Wrestling	0.52
	Basketball	0.24
	Baseball	0.19
	Soccer	0.25
Girls		
	Basketball	0.34
	Soccer	0.33
	Volleyball	0.15
	Softball	0.18
Fracture		
Boys		
	Football	0.44
	Ice hockey	0.31
	Lacrosse	0.26
	Wrestling	0.23
	Soccer	0.20
	Basketball	0.16
	Baseball	0.15
	Track and field	0.02
	Swimming or diving	0.00
Girls		
	Lacrosse	0.26
	Basketball	0.16
	Softball	0.15
	Gymnastics	0.15
	Soccer	0.14
	Field hockey	0.14
	Cheerleading	0.07
	Volleyball	0.06
	Track and field	0.03
	Swimming or diving	0.003
Season ending		
Boys		
	Football	0.26
	Wrestling	0.17
	Lacrosse	0.16
	Ice hockey	0.12
	Soccer	0.10
	Basketball	0.069
	Baseball	0.056
	Cross country	0.021
	Track and field	0.018
	Volleyball	0.018
	Swimming or diving	0.002
Girls		
	Soccer	0.16
	Basketball	0.11
	Lacrosse	0.093
	Softball	0.068
	Field hockey	0.061
	Cross country	0.056
	Track and field	0.048
	Volleyball	0.040
	Cheerleading	0.033
	Gymnastics	0.019
	Swimming or diving	0.005

Adapted from Darrow et al[17]; Swenson et al[12]; and Tirabassi et al.[16] AE, athletic exposure.
[a] Severe injury is defined as any injury resulting in ≥21 days of time lost from sport.

a fracture and less likely to suffer a concussion (see Table 2).[10] Nonetheless, the differences between these age groups appear to be relatively small, and the types of injuries suffered by both groups appear to be similar overall.

Lower Extremities

The majority of injuries among youth soccer players involve the lower extremities. The ankles and knees are the most commonly injured body parts, whereas sprains and/or strains and contusions are the most commonly reported injury types.[5,8,9,21,22] Fractures represent only approximately 3% to 10% of all injuries but up to 28% of soccer-related injuries seen in emergency departments.[7,8,10,23] Younger athletes tend to have a lower overall injury incidence but typically demonstrate similar injury locations. In a study of time-loss injuries among 417 soccer players ages 5 to 17 over a 2-year period, ankles and knees were the most commonly injured body parts (20.9% and 16.3% of all injuries, respectively), whereas sprains, contusions, and muscle injuries were the most common diagnoses (20.6%, 22.5%, and 20.6% of all injuries, respectively). Although overuse injuries are less common, they appear to be more common among female youth soccer players, with feet and/or ankles and lower legs being the most commonly injured areas among boys and girls.[18] Among high school athletes, the majority of overuse injuries were less severe, with only 7.7% resulting in time loss greater than 21 days.[18] Although the majority of overuse injuries involve apophysitis and tendinopathy, stress fractures are another important consideration for youth soccer athletes.

With respect to severe injuries, player-to-player contact is the most common mechanism for injuries resulting in significant time loss (>21 days)[24] as well as medical

TABLE 2 Soccer-Related Injuries Among Children 7 to 17 Years of Age Evaluated in US Emergency Departments by Age Group, From 1990 to 2014

	7–11 y, *n* (%)	12–17 y, *n* (%)
Body region injured		
Upper extremity	222 833 (27.3)	396 813 (18.2)
Ankle	99 479 (12.2)	432 344 (19.9)
Head or neck	124 239 (15.2)	404 356 (18.6)
Knee	75 038 (9.2)	260 526 (12.0)
Foot or toe	87 483 (10.7)	204 786 (9.4)
Hand or finger	113 490 (13.9)	174 373 (8.0)
Upper or lower leg	46 379 (5.7)	151 743 (7.0)
Trunk	42 992 (5.3)	141 842 (6.5)
Other	4471 (0.5)	10 990 (0.5)
Subtotal	816 404 (100.0)	2 177 773 (100.0)
Diagnosis		
Sprain or strain	242 814 (29.8)	793 437 (36.5)
Fracture	231 776 (28.4)	461 611 (21.2)
Soft tissue injury	192 396 (23.6)	463 469 (21.3)
Concussion or CHI	45 016 (5.5)	172 346 (7.9)
Other	56 598 (6.9)	139 166 (6.4)
Laceration	40 339 (4.9)	102 626 (4.7)
Dislocation	6793 (0.8)	43 747 (2.0)
Subtotal	815 732 (100.0)	2 176 402 (100.0)

Adapted from Smith et al.[10] CHI, closed head injury.

disqualification.[16] The knees are the most commonly affected body part in season-ending injuries, and player-to-player contact is the most common mechanism for both boys and girls.[16] Anterior cruciate ligament (ACL) rupture remains a significant lower-extremity injury among youth soccer players, with noncontact valgus hyperextension during rapid change of direction or deceleration as the most common mechanism.[25,26] Female soccer players appear to be at an increased risk for ACL injury compared with their male counterparts, and this has been attributed to a number of factors, including lower-limb anatomy, hormonal influences, and neuromuscular activation patterns.[25,27]

Concussion

Recent data suggest that concussion rates may be increasing among youth soccer athletes, and concussion remains more common among girls than boys.[28–30] In a recent 9-year study of high school soccer players, concussion incidence was found to be 0.28 and 0.45 per 1000 athletic exposures for boys and girls, respectively. For both sexes, concussion incidence has been found to be greater during games than during practice, and concussion rates during both practices and games increased significantly during the study period.[30] Finally, a recent study of soccer-related injuries among 7- to 17-year-old children presenting to the emergency department revealed that concussion incidence increased nearly 1600% between 1990 and 2014.[10] It is unclear, however, whether this increase in concussion rates is the result of a greater number of concussions sustained or of increased recognition and diagnosis of concussions as a result of previous education efforts.

Heading is the most common sport-specific activity during which concussions occur, although the majority of injuries are attributable to contact with another player while heading rather than contact with the ball itself.[30,31] Concussions are a result of brain acceleration after contact. Theoretically, concussion incidence could be reduced if the magnitude of horizontal head acceleration could be reduced. In addition to the mass and velocity of the player, factors that affect horizontal acceleration include the mass, size, speed, and inflation pressure of the ball. Therefore, balls that are overinflated or inappropriately large for the age and size of the athletes may increase the risk of head injury in young soccer players.[32] Data are insufficient to determine if concussions or subconcussive impacts (repetitive heading or blows to the head that do not result in concussive symptoms) result in potentially detrimental long-term cognitive effects.[33]

Facial and Ocular Injury

Although there are limited data regarding ocular injuries in youth soccer, a recent 10-year study among soccer players identified the incidence of eye injuries to be 1.0 and 0.8 per 100 000 athletic exposures for boys and girls, respectively.[34] The incidence of eye injuries was found to be higher than that in a number of other sports but lower than in wrestling, basketball, and baseball for boys and lower than in field hockey and softball for girls. The use of appropriate protective eyewear can substantially decrease the risk of ocular injuries in athletes. A recent 5-year study has revealed that among youth soccer players, lacerations were the most common facial injury, followed by contusion and fracture. The nose was the most common site of injury, and contact with an opposing player's head or upper extremity was the most common mechanism.[35] Dental injuries also occur with a frequency similar to eye injuries (1.1 per 100 000 athletic exposures), with injuries occurring more commonly during competition (3.2 per 100 000) than during practice (0.3 per 100 000).[36]

Environmental Injuries

As an outdoor sport, soccer also carries a potential risk for dehydration, exertional heat illness, and other environmental dangers. Heat illness encompasses a variety of conditions and can range from heat cramps and heat exhaustion to life-threatening heat stroke.[37] Although these issues may occur at any ambient temperature, the incidence increases with increasing temperature and humidity. Heat cramps are painful involuntary muscle contractions that usually occur during preseason conditioning and are treated with stretching the muscle, rest, and rehydration. Heat exhaustion is a moderate heat illness characterized by the inability to continue exercising because of cardiovascular insufficiency resulting from strenuous exercise, environmental heat stress, dehydration, and energy depletion.[37] Heat exhaustion typically manifests as a headache, nausea, profuse sweating, incoordination, weakness, syncope, and mildly elevated core body temperature. Heat stroke is a life-threatening condition characterized by elevated core body temperature >104°F (>40°C) resulting in central nervous system dysfunction, circulatory failure, and potential multiorgan failure.[37] Initial treatment of heat stroke includes immediate cooling via whole body immersion, if available, and transfer to the nearest emergency department. Guidelines to minimize risk of exertional heat illness in youth sports are applicable to soccer, particularly during hotter months and the early part of the season, when players may not be sufficiently acclimatized.[37]

Another potential hazard for those engaging in outdoor activities is lightning. According to the National Oceanic and Atmospheric Association, lightning strikes an average of 400 people and kills 49 of these victims every year in the United States.[38] Although there are no specific data with respect to youth soccer, this remains a risk in all outdoor physical activities, and careful monitoring during inclement weather can identify potentially dangerous conditions so prevention strategies can be implemented.

Fatalities in Soccer

Fatalities in youth soccer are rare and have historically been attributable to blunt trauma with goalposts.[39,40] A previous study of 1.6 million emergency department visits attributable to soccer injuries from 1990 to 2003 identified 2 fatalities resulting from a brain hemorrhage and a ruptured spleen caused by blunt trauma.[20] The US Consumer Product Safety Commission has reported 36 previous fatalities in soccer as a result of falling goalposts since 1979 and has published specific recommendations regarding proper installation, use, and storage of goalposts to reduce the risk of injury.[41]

Footwear and Playing Surface

Footwear type and playing surface may affect lower-extremity injury rates. Outdoor soccer shoes are cleated and have either bladed studs or a combination of bladed and conical studs. Generally, bladed studs afford greater traction and speed; however, they may be associated with increased rates of injury. In a systematic review of 23 studies investigating the relationship between cleat-surface interaction and injury rates, Silva et al[42] found that bladed studs were associated with an increased risk of injury related to higher pressure on the lateral foot border when compared with rounded studs. Conical studs allow for quicker release and provide a greater degree of stability because they offer more points of contact with the playing surface. Although this stabilizing feature may translate to a lower risk of injury, more in vivo studies are needed. The pattern of stud placement on cleated shoes may also affect injury rates. A study on American football revealed that shoes with longer irregular cleats placed at the peripheral margin of the sole and a number of smaller pointed cleats positioned interiorly were associated with a higher risk of ACL injuries than flat, soccer-style cleats on which the studs on the forefoot were the same height, shape, and diameter.[43]

When artificial turf debuted, an increase in lower-extremity injuries was noted.[44] Authors of initial studies postulated that increased shoe-surface friction produced increased torque at the knee and ankle.[42] The most recent third generation of artificial turf has longer grass-like fibers embedded in granules of sand, rubber, and/or silica and more closely mimics natural grass. Several recent studies reveal no difference in injury rates during games played on grass or turf but higher injury rates during training on grass.[45,46] In youth soccer specifically, a 2016 study revealed that players who suffered a lower-extremity injury were 2.83-fold more likely to have played on a grass surface and were 2.40-fold more likely to have worn cleats on grass in practice (versus cleats on artificial turf) compared with players who were uninjured. These researchers also found that training on grass was associated with a 2.8-fold increased risk of lower-extremity injury, but game injuries did not vary significantly when comparing artificial turf with grass.[46] This finding mirrors a similar study in adults that revealed no significant differences in the incidence of lower-extremity injuries on artificial turf or grass for male and female elite soccer players in games.[45]

In the last few years, media reports have surfaced suggesting a possible relationship between playing on synthetic turf and the development of certain childhood cancers, particularly leukemia and lymphoma.[47] The basis for these media reports has been anecdotal, and to date, no epidemiological or longitudinal research regarding a causative relationship between artificial turf and neoplasia has been published.[48]

INJURY RISK FACTORS

Considerable recent research has undertaken the goal of identifying modifiable risk factors for injury in youth soccer, specifically related to lower-limb injuries and concussions. A number of neuromuscular imbalances have been suggested as risk factors for injury, including quadriceps dominance, leg dominance, dynamic instability, and neuromuscular activation patterns.[49] In previous research of biomechanical risk factors for overuse injuries in youth soccer players, increased quadriceps, hamstring, and hip flexor strength were found to be protective, but increased knee valgus was found to increase risk.[19] In a single prospective study of 11- to 15-year-old female soccer players, low normalized knee separation during drop-jump testing was found to be a significant predictor of subsequent lower-limb injury.[50] All of these risk factors may be exacerbated by fatigue because injury risk appears to be greater during the later portions of practices and games[51,52] as well as among players with decreased levels of aerobic fitness.[53] In addition, previous lower-extremity injury has been consistently identified as an important risk factor that may reduce strength and alter neuromuscular recruitment patterns.[49,54,55] Although this has not been studied in youth soccer specifically, history of previous concussion may also increase the risk of subsequent lower-limb injury among collegiate athletes and represents an important area of future investigation.[56,57]

Sport participation history and training loads may also influence the risk of injury in youth athletes,[58–60] but further information is needed to guide recommendations for soccer players specifically. Injury risk does seem to increase with age, but the relationship with competition level is unclear.[61–64] A single study of youth soccer players revealed that children in higher skill-level leagues had reduced injuries per 1000 hours compared with age-matched counterparts, although players at a higher competition level had a much higher participation volume, leading to a similar number of absolute injuries per year.[65] Early sport specialization has been shown to be associated with an increased risk of overuse injury across a number of youth sports.[59,66–68] There are few data regarding sport specialization and injury risk specifically among soccer players, with a single recent study of elite male adolescent soccer athletes revealing that specialization was associated with a decreased risk of previous injury overall and was not related to previous overuse injury.[69] Inadequate sleep and fatigue have been shown to be risk factors for injury in youth athletes,[60,70] although this has not been specifically studied in soccer. Finally, overtraining is considered an important risk factor for injury in a number of sports, and acute increases in training load have been shown to be an independent risk factor for injury in youth soccer players, perhaps as a result of impairments in sleep and subjective well-being, which serve as early indicators of overtraining.[58,71,72]

An often overlooked risk factor for injury is illegal play.[73] Collins et al[73] analyzed data regarding rates of injury attributable to activity that was deemed to be a violation of the rules of the game in high school athletes involved in various sports. Soccer had the highest rates of injury related to illegal activity, and a greater proportion of injuries related to illegal activity involved the head and neck, including concussion, compared with injuries from legal activities.[73]

INJURY PREVENTION

Injury prevention involves the identification of risk factors and subsequent modification of those factors to decrease the likelihood of injury. Risk factors can be proper to the athlete, also called intrinsic factors (such as anatomy or emotional well-being), or can originate outside the athlete, also called extrinsic factors (such as environmental conditions or playing surface).[74] Injury prevention can be classified as primary or secondary. With primary prevention, the aim is to prevent injuries before they occur, whereas the goal for secondary intervention is to reduce the impact of an injury once it has occurred.[74] Most of the strategies discussed in this report will be focused on the primary prevention of injuries in youth soccer through modification of both intrinsic and extrinsic modifiable risk factors.

Preparticipation Physical Examination

The preparticipation evaluation (PPE) is a critical opportunity for primary prevention and takes place before the athlete even touches the soccer field. Although few concrete data exist to validate its use as a screening tool, a uniformly applied PPE is generally believed to be the optimal opportunity to detect any medical conditions that may be potentially life-threatening or disabling or that may predispose the athlete to injury.[75] The PPE monograph is a collaborative effort among several national medical organizations, including the AAP, and serves as a useful tool for pediatricians regarding best practices for performing the examination.[76]

For soccer players, noting any previous musculoskeletal injuries, especially lower-extremity injuries such as ankle sprains, knee injuries, or groin strains, as well as a detailed history of previous concussions or head injuries allows for rehabilitation if deficits are identified. Given that cardiac etiologies account for 56% of nontraumatic causes of sudden death in collegiate athletes,[77] noting the presence of any cardiac-related symptoms as well as a detailed family history of any cardiac conditions, especially hypertrophic cardiomyopathy, allows for further workup. As part of a complete physical examination for sport, critical areas of focus include assessment of the cardiovascular system, a baseline ocular examination, and a thorough musculoskeletal examination with special attention to the weight-bearing joints of the lower extremities.[75]

Neuromuscular and Biomechanical Training

As previously mentioned, ACL injuries represent a source of significant morbidity for youth soccer players, especially girls. The reasons for the relatively high prevalence of ACL injuries in girls are likely multifactorial.[25] Most noncontact ACL injuries occur when landing from a jump, stopping abruptly, or quickly changing direction during deceleration. Compared with boys, girls tend to have a higher degree of internal rotation at the hip and external rotation of the tibia when decelerating or landing. Girls also have a higher tendency to land with insufficient knee and hip flexion.[78] Additionally, girls tend to have a greater degree of quadriceps activation and differences in muscle recruitment, timing, and strength, which appear to increase the risk for ACL injury. Given that these biomechanical factors represent a potentially modifiable risk factor for ACL injuries, authors of multiple studies have investigated the effectiveness of teaching proper landing and deceleration techniques, muscle strengthening and recruitment, neuromuscular warm-up, proprioception, and plyometrics.[79–81] Mandelbaum et al[79] studied the effectiveness of such a program and demonstrated a 74% to 88% reduction in ACL injury. In 2011, LaBella et al[81] investigated the effects of a neuromuscular warm-up program in female athletes in Chicago public high schools and showed a 56% reduction in noncontact lower-extremity injuries and a lower ACL injury rate in the intervention group. General recommendations for strengthening programs include an emphasis on gluteal and hamstring strength and recruitment as well as core strength and trunk stabilization.[82] Pediatricians can access a video demonstration of such ACL injury prevention exercises on the AAP Web site (https://www.aap.org/en-us/about-the-aap/aap-press-room/aap-press-room-media-center/Pages/preventingACLinjury.aspx). The Fédération Internationale de Football Association (FIFA) developed a warm-up program called "FIFA 11+" that consisted of 10 strengthening, plyometric, and proprioceptive exercises designed to decrease the frequency and severity of injuries in soccer.[83] Multiple studies have revealed the program to be significantly effective at decreasing the incidence of injury in male and female youth players.[80,83–86]

Individual Player Monitoring

Overtraining, stress, and inadequate rest may individually or jointly contribute to risk of injuries among athletes in soccer and other youth sports.[58,87,88] As previously mentioned, an acute increase in training load has been shown to be an independent risk factor for injury in youth soccer players. Spurred by advances in development of wearable technology, individual player monitoring has exploded in popularity in the last few years.[24,89–91] Although not as prevalent as in collegiate or professional teams, youth teams, especially elite club and travel teams, are beginning to employ user-friendly wearable technologies to measure training loads, accelerations, and decelerations as well as heart rate. Many training staffs use such technologies to adjust the design, pace, and components of practice sessions in an effort to maximize performance and reduce injuries; however, there is limited research regarding the effectiveness of such technology in achieving these aims.

Because fatigue and inadequate sleep may be risk factors for injury,[60,70] multiple technologies exist for monitoring sleep, such as sensor-embedded wristbands and smart phone applications; however, there is a paucity of medical literature regarding their effectiveness, particularly in young athletes. Various studies have revealed an inverse relationship between psychological well-being and risk of injury. Steffen et al[92] discovered that in female youth soccer players ages 14 to 16 years, the risk of injury was 70% greater among players with a high degree of perceived life stress. Many professional and collegiate programs are now using athlete self-report measures to gauge their athletes' response to training with respect to mood, motivation, perception of well-being, and stress levels. In addition, programs are also training athletes in mindfulness skills, coping mechanisms, and stress-reduction strategies in an attempt to mitigate the effects of negative self-perception and stress. Swedish investigators conducted a randomized study in junior elite soccer players and found that 67%

of the players in the intervention group who received mindfulness-based training remained injury free at the end of the season, compared with 40% in the control group.[93]

Concussion

Eliminating all concussions from soccer is unattainable; however, implementation of prevention strategies may reduce the number and severity of concussive injuries.

All 50 states and the District of Columbia have passed concussion legislation mandating schools to develop concussion protocols and restrict participation after suffering a head injury.[33] Most are modeled after Washington State's Lystedt Law, which mandates automatic removal from play for any suspected concussion, medical clearance before returning to sport, and education for parents, athletes, and coaches. Pediatricians and other health care providers are encouraged to familiarize themselves with the precise language and requirements in the legislation regarding concussion in their individual states.

As mentioned previously, the majority of concussions in soccer occur during the act of heading but are attributable to player-player contact, not player-ball contact.[30] In a recent study, contact with another player was the most common mechanism of injury in heading-related concussions among boys (68.8%) and girls (51.3%).[28] Because of concerns regarding heading, the US Soccer Federation unveiled an initiative aimed at reducing concussions by banning heading for children 10 years and younger and limiting the amount of heading in practice for children between the ages of 11 and 13 years.[94] More research is needed to evaluate whether this program will reduce the number of concussions in these age groups. Instructing young soccer players in proper heading techniques once the athletes demonstrate body awareness and visual tracking skills and have developed the requisite core and cervical strength is imperative. Following manufacturer recommendations for proper ball inflation and size for the age of the players also is recommended. Finally, adherence to fair-play practice and enforcement of rules may reduce the number of foul plays and dangerous contacts and may therefore reduce the risk of concussive injuries.[30]

Current evidence is insufficient to support the uniform use of headgear or mouth guards to prevent concussion.[95,96] Mouth guards have been shown to prevent orofacial injuries; however, evidence is mixed regarding risk reduction in sports-related concussion.[95,97] The use of soft headgear has been studied more extensively in rugby, in which it has been shown to reduce superficial abrasions but not affect the overall rate of concussion.[98] In laboratory testing, by using head forms, soccer headgear has not been shown to attenuate the head impacts during simulated soccer ball heading.[99] Although Delaney et al[100] concluded that headgear use in youth soccer players may reduce the risk of concussion, the national governing body for soccer in the United States does not permit its members or affiliates to require the use of headgear by players.[101] Use of padded headgear is controversial because of the paucity of rigorous medical studies as well as concern for possible increased risk of injury resulting from a false sense of security.[96]

Fair Play and Rule Enforcement

Foul play, or actions that violate the rules of the game, has been associated with an increased incidence of injuries in various levels of many sports, including soccer. In a study of professional soccer players, foul play was found to be involved in 14% to 37% of all injuries.[102] Peterson et al[65] studied soccer injuries over a 1-year period in different age groups and skill levels and found that 82% of players suffered at least 1 injury. Forty-six percent of the injuries were attributable to contact, and almost half of these were associated with foul play.[65] With respect purely to youth soccer, Emery et al[103] discovered that direct contact was involved in 46.2% of all injuries. Limiting foul play, penalizing dangerous behavior, and properly enforcing the rules are generally believed to reduce the risk of injury in sport. Referees, players, and spectators all have a responsibility to advocate for fair play and sportsmanship.

Protective Equipment

Shin guards are the only protective devices that are required by FIFA, the National Collegiate Athletic Association, and the US Soccer Federation.[104–106] Currently, shin guards are typically made of polypropylene and plastic composites, although some also contain fiberglass, para-aramid synthetic fibers, or copper. Although they certainly protect against leg abrasions and contusions, the role of shin guards in reducing the risk of fractures has not been fully demonstrated to date.[107,108] Nevertheless, laboratory studies indicate that shin guards significantly dissipate the forces and strain on the tibia that could cause fracture.[109,110] Appropriately sized shin guards should cover most of the anterior tibia, and the National Operating Committee for Standards in Athletic Equipment has established standards for function.[111]

Dental injuries can occur in all contact sports, and soccer is no exception. Two older studies revealed that dental injuries account for 0.2% of all high school athletic injuries,[112,113] and more recent data suggest an overall incidence rate of 0.06 and 0.11 dental injuries per 10 000 athletic exposures in boys' and girls' high school soccer, respectively.[36] In all of these studies, the rate of dental injuries appears to be lower for soccer than for many other contact sports.[36,112,113] Although most studies affirm that custom-made mouth guards confer better protection than the more common "boil and bite" type, a vast majority of studies reveal that simply by wearing mouth guards, athletes can significantly decrease the frequency and severity of orofacial injuries in contact sports.[114–116]

Injuries to the eye and surrounding orbit can occur in any contact or projectile sport. Traumatic ocular injuries have the potential for significant long-term morbidity. Boys account for a significantly greater proportion of injuries than girls, and the peak incidence occurs in mid-to-late adolescence. A recent study revealed that soccer accounted for almost 7% of all ocular trauma.[117] Approximately 90% of serious eye injuries are preventable through use of appropriate protective eyewear.[118] The AAP and the American Academy of Ophthalmology classify soccer as a moderate-risk sport and strongly recommend that all young participants wear eye protection that meets the American Society for Testing and Materials standard F803,[119] which specifies that protective eyewear be made of polycarbonate, impact-resistant plastic and be worn by all athletes who are functionally monocular or who have a history of major eye surgery or trauma.[119]

Given that sudden cardiac arrest is the leading cause of nonaccidental death in youth and can occur with athletic activity, physicians involved with soccer organizations are encouraged to advocate for basic life-support training of coaches as well as placement of automated external defibrillators at practice and competition sites.[120]

Environmental Safety

Heat and lightning pose an extrinsic risk to participants in outdoor sports. The number of heat-related injuries increased 133% from 1997 to 2006, and youth accounted for the largest proportion of those injuries.[121] Additionally, recent evidence suggests that heat-related illness may be increasing with climate change.[122,123] Every year, lightning accounts for dozens of deaths in the United States, although data regarding the incidence among youth soccer participants are not available.[124] Precautions and simple strategies may reduce the risk of injury due to adverse environmental conditions.

Heat

Some primary prevention strategies for heat illness include acclimatization, activity modification, development of an emergency action plan, and hydration.[37] The risk of heat illness appears to be highest in deconditioned athletes at the start of the season.[37] Allowing athletes 7 to 14 days to acclimate their bodies to heat is essential. Several state high school organizations have formal policies regarding heat acclimatization. It is recommended that all youth teams and institutions have a policy regarding heat that incorporates an emergency action plan that addresses properly monitoring ambient weather conditions, ideally with a wet-bulb globe temperature device, and modifying training sessions in certain hot and humid conditions.[37] Some activity-modification strategies include limiting warm-ups, scheduling hydration and rest breaks, shortening sessions or holding them earlier or later in the day, and canceling events in case of dangerous conditions.[37] Although the incidence of heat illness has not been directly compared between artificial turf and natural grass surfaces, significantly elevated surface temperatures have been reported on in-filled turf fields,[125] and this may need to be considered for soccer played on turf.

Ensuring proper hydration before starting a workout and replacing fluids lost through sweating during and after exercise are important considerations for athletes.[37,126] Although fluid requirements will vary between individuals and environmental conditions, fluid intake of 300 to 750 mL/hour for 9- to 12-year-olds and 1.0 to 1.5 L/hour for adolescents is typically sufficient to offset sweat losses and reduce the risk of dehydration during intense exercise in hot conditions.[37] Water is generally sufficient for hydration during soccer competition, although sports drinks that contain additional electrolytes and carbohydrates may be considered during periods of prolonged, intense activity.[127] In general, caffeine and energy drinks do not play a role in proper hydration during exercise and are not recommended in children and adolescents.[127]

Lightning

Primary prevention of lightning injuries requires careful monitoring of weather conditions. Strategies for prevention of lightning injuries by the Centers for Disease Control and Prevention include having venue-specific emergency action plans, suspending activities when thunder and lightning are present (typically within 6 miles), and moving athletes and spectators to shelters designated specifically for lightning.[128] Activities may resume 30 minutes after the last strike of lightning is seen (or at least 5 miles away) and after the last sound of thunder is heard.[38,128,129]

Footwear, Playing Surface, and Field Conditions

Some studies in soccer athletes indicate that shoes with bladed cleats improve performance during changes of direction but may increase the torque and rotational movements on the ankle and knee joints, which may theoretically lead to injury; however, most studies reveal no increased rate of injury when comparing cleat type.[42] General recommendations for soccer footwear include ensuring that the shoe fits properly, that the laces are fastened completely, and that the cleat type is appropriate for the surface of play. Although practicing on artificial turf may be associated with a decreased injury risk compared with natural grass, injury rates during games appear to be similar between the 2 surfaces.[45,46] Regardless of the playing field type, players as well as coaches and referees may consider checking the condition of the field before playing to identify potential hazards, remove any debris, fill any divots or holes, and assess for areas of poor water drainage. The US Consumer Product Safety Commission recommends that movable soccer goals be securely anchored to the ground and only used on level playing fields and that no one climbs or hangs from a post.[41]

CONCLUSIONS AND GUIDANCE FOR PEDIATRICIANS

1. Soccer remains the most popular youth sport in the United States, with a relatively large proportion of preadolescent participants. Although injuries occur in soccer, injury rates appear lower than those for many other contact sports and are particularly low in soccer players younger than 12 years of age. Pediatric health care providers can feel comfortable with advocating for participation in soccer as a means of promoting physical fitness and the wide-ranging benefits of exercise.
2. Soccer is associated with certain types of injuries that commonly present to pediatric offices, school-based health clinics, and emergency departments. These injuries include lower-extremity sprains, strains, fractures, and concussions. Familiarity with the management of these injuries will aid the pediatrician in the care of this large and growing population of young athletes.
3. ACL tears are a significant cause of morbidity in young soccer players, especially girls. Neuromuscular training programs have been shown to reduce the risk of injury by teaching proper landing and stopping techniques and developing strength and balance. Pediatricians can access a video demonstration of such ACL injury prevention exercises on the AAP Web site (https://www.aap.org/en-us/about-the-aap/aap-press-room/aap-press-room-media-center/Pages/preventingACLinjury.aspx).
4. Concussions are relatively common in soccer. Data are insufficient regarding the long-term effects of repetitive heading in youth soccer. Further research is needed regarding the potential protective effect of headgear or intervention programs on reducing the risk of concussion. The majority of concussions occur as a result of contact with an opposing player rather than the ball; however, an emphasis on fair play, rule enforcement, and proper age-appropriate heading techniques may reduce the risk of concussion in youth soccer participants. Encouraging athletes to report subjective symptoms facilitates proper diagnosis and management.
5. Other injury reduction strategies for soccer include completion of a PPE before the start of the season to identify any risk factors for injury, proper hydration and rest, modification of activities in hot and humid weather, use of appropriately sized shin guards and mouth guards, and use of proper protective eyewear, especially for athletes who are functionally one-eyed.
6. Adherence to fair-play rules may reduce injuries. Physicians who work with soccer organizations are encouraged to advocate for enforcement of rules and promotion of fair play at all levels of the game. Parents, spectators, and coaches can assist referees by honoring and promoting the spirit of fair play with young athletes.

RECOMMENDED RESOURCES

The US Consumer Product Safety Commission guidelines for movable goals[41]: www.cpsc.gov/safety-education/safety-guides/sports-fitness-and-recreation/guidelines-movable-soccer-goals

The Centers for Disease Control and Prevention lightning safety tips[128]: www.cdc.gov/disasters/lightning/safetytips.html

The AAP ACL injury prevention video demonstration: https://www.aap.org/en-us/about-the-aap/aap-press-room/aap-press-room-media-center/Pages/preventingACLinjury.aspx

The AAP climatic heat stress policy statement.[37]: http://pediatrics.aappublications.org/content/128/3/e741

LEAD AUTHORS

Andrew Watson, MD, MS, FAAP
Jeffrey M. Mjaanes, MD, FAAP

COUNCIL ON SPORTS MEDICINE AND FITNESS EXECUTIVE COMMITTEE, 2017–2018

Cynthia R. LaBella, MD, FAAP, Chairperson
M. Alison Brooks, MD, FAAP
Greg Canty, MD, FAAP
Alex B. Diamond, DO, MPH, FAAP
William Hennrikus, MD, FAAP
Kelsey Logan, MD, MPH, FAAP
Kody Moffatt, MD, FAAP
Blaise A. Nemeth, MD, MS, FAAP
K. Brooke Pengel, MD, FAAP

Andrew R. Peterson, MD, MSPH, FAAP
Paul R. Stricker, MD, FAAP

LIAISONS

Donald W. Bagnall – *National Athletic Trainers' Association*
Mark E. Halstead, MD, FAAP – *American Medical Society for Sports Medicine*

CONSULTANTS

Nicholas M. Edwards, MD, MPH, FAAP
Avery D. Faigenbaum, EdD, FACSM
Chris G. Koutures, MD, FAAP
J. Terry Parker, PhD, ATC

STAFF

Anjie Emanuel, MPH

ABBREVIATIONS

AAP: American Academy of Pediatrics
ACL: anterior cruciate ligament
FIFA: Fédération Internationale de Football Association
PPE: preparticipation evaluation

POTENTIAL CONFLICT OF INTEREST: The authors have indicated they have no potential conflicts of interest to disclose.

REFERENCES

1. Hulteen RM, Smith JJ, Morgan PJ, et al. Global participation in sport and leisure-time physical activities: a systematic review and meta-analysis. *Prev Med.* 2017;95:14–25
2. FIFA. Big count 2006: statistical summary report by association. Available at: http://resources.fifa.com/mm/document/fifafacts/bcoffsurv/statsumrepassoc_10342.pdf. Accessed February 10, 2018
3. US Youth Soccer. Media kit. Available at: www.usyouthsoccer.org/media_kit/keystatistics/. Accessed February 10, 2018
4. Nilstad A, Bahr R, Andersen TE. Text messaging as a new method for injury registration in sports: a methodological study in elite female football. *Scand J Med Sci Sports.* 2014;24(1):243–249
5. Pfirrmann D, Herbst M, Ingelfinger P, Simon P, Tug S. Analysis of injury incidences in male professional adult and elite youth soccer players: a systematic review. *J Athl Train.* 2016;51(5):410–424
6. Froholdt A, Olsen OE, Bahr R. Low risk of injuries among children playing organized soccer: a prospective cohort study. *Am J Sports Med.* 2009;37(6):1155–1160
7. Rössler R, Junge A, Chomiak J, Dvorak J, Faude O. Soccer injuries in players aged 7 to 12 years: a descriptive epidemiological study over 2 seasons. *Am J Sports Med.* 2016;44(2):309–317
8. Le Gall F, Carling C, Reilly T. Injuries in young elite female soccer players: an 8-season prospective study. *Am J Sports Med.* 2008;36(2):276–284
9. Clausen MB, Zebis MK, Møller M, et al. High injury incidence in adolescent female soccer. *Am J Sports Med.* 2014;42(10):2487–2494
10. Smith NA, Chounthirath T, Xiang H. Soccer-related injuries treated in emergency departments: 1990-2014. *Pediatrics.* 2016;138(4):e20160346
11. Esquivel AO, Bruder A, Ratkowiak K, Lemos SE. Soccer-related injuries in children and adults aged 5 to 49 years in US emergency departments from 2000 to 2012. *Sports Health.* 2015;7(4):366–370
12. Swenson DM, Henke NM, Collins CL, Fileds SK. Epidemiology of United States high school sports-related fractures, 2008-09 to 2010-11. *Am J Sports Med.* 2012;40(9):2078–2084
13. Lindenfeld TN, Schmitt DJ, Hendy MP, Mangine RE, Noyes FR. Incidence of injury in indoor soccer. *Am J Sports Med.* 1994;22(3):364–371
14. Emery CA, Meeuwisse WH. Risk factors for injury in indoor compared with outdoor adolescent soccer. *Am J Sports Med.* 2006;34(10):1636–1642
15. Kerr ZY, Collins CL, Fields SK, Comstock RD. Epidemiology of player–player contact injuries among US high school athletes, 2005-2009. *Clin Pediatr (Phila).* 2011;50(7):594–603
16. Tirabassi J, Brou L, Khodaee M, et al. Epidemiology of high school sports-related injuries resulting in medical disqualification: 2005-2006 through 2013-2014 academic years. *Am J Sports Med.* 2016;44(11):2925–2932
17. Darrow CJ, Collins CL, Yard EE, Comstock RD. Epidemiology of severe injuries among United States high school athletes: 2005-2007. *Am J Sports Med.* 2009;37(9):1798–1805
18. Roos KG, Marshall SW, Kerr ZY, et al. Epidemiology of overuse injuries in collegiate and high school athletics in the United States. *Am J Sports Med.* 2015;43(7):1790–1797
19. O'Kane JW, Neradilek M, Polissar N, Sabado L, Tencer A, Schiff MA. Risk factors for lower extremity overuse injuries in female youth soccer players. *Orthop J Sports Med.* 2017;5(10):2325967117733963
20. Leininger RE, Knox CL, Comstock RD. Epidemiology of 1.6 million pediatric soccer-related injuries presenting to US emergency departments from 1990 to 2003. *Am J Sports Med.* 2007;35(2):288–293
21. Kakavelakis KN, Vlazakis S, Vlahakis I, Charissis G. Soccer injuries in childhood. *Scand J Med Sci Sports.* 2003;13(3):175–178
22. Wong P, Hong Y. Soccer injury in the lower extremities. *Br J Sports Med.* 2005;39(8):473–482
23. Kerr ZY, Pierpont LA, Currie DW, Wasserman EB, Comstock RD. Epidemiologic comparisons of soccer-related injuries presenting to emergency departments and reported within high school and collegiate settings. *Inj Epidemiol.* 2017;4(1):19
24. Alexandre D, da Silva CD, Hill-Haas S, et al. Heart rate monitoring in soccer: interest and limits during competitive match play and training, practical application. *J Strength Cond Res.* 2012;26(10):2890–2906

25. Hewett TE, Myer GD, Ford KR. Anterior cruciate ligament injuries in female athletes: part 1, mechanisms and risk factors. *Am J Sports Med.* 2006;34(2): 299–311

26. Arendt EA, Agel J, Dick R. Anterior cruciate ligament injury patterns among collegiate men and women. *J Athl Train.* 1999;34(2):86–92

27. LaBella CR, Hennrikus W, Hewett TE; Council on Sports Medicine and Fitness; Section on Orthopaedics. Anterior cruciate ligament injuries: diagnosis, treatment, and prevention. *Pediatrics.* 2014;133(5). Available at: www.pediatrics.org/cgi/content/full/133/5/e1437

28. Khodaee M, Currie DW, Asif IM, Comstock RD. Nine-year study of US high school soccer injuries: data from a national sports injury surveillance programme. *Br J Sports Med.* 2017; 51(3):185–193

29. Kerr ZY, Pierpoint LA, Currie DW, Wasserman EB, Comstock RD. Epidemiologic comparisons of soccer-related injuries presenting to emergency departments and reported within high school and collegiate settings. *Inj Epidemiol.* 2017;4(1):19

30. Comstock RD, Currie DW, Pierpoint LA, Grubenhoff JA, Fields SK. An evidence-based discussion of heading the ball and concussions in high school soccer. *JAMA Pediatr.* 2015;169(9):830–837

31. O'Kane JW, Spieker A, Levy MR, et al. Concussion among female middle-school soccer players. *JAMA Pediatr.* 2014;168(3):258–264

32. Babbs CF. Biomechanics of heading a soccer ball: implications for player safety. *ScientificWorldJournal.* 2001;1: 281–322

33. Halstead ME, Walter KD, Moffatt K; Council on Sports Medicine and Fitness. Sport-related concussion in children and adolescents. *Pediatrics.* 2018; 142(6):e20183074

34. Boden BP, Pierpoint LA, Boden RG, Comstock RD, Kerr ZY. Eye injuries in high school and collegiate athletes. *Sports Health.* 2017;9(5):444–449

35. Bobian MR, Hanba CJ, Svider PF, et al. Soccer-related facial trauma: a nationwide perspective. *Ann Otol Rhinol Laryngol.* 2016;125(12):992–996

36. Collins CL, McKenzie LB, Ferketich AK, et al. Dental injuries sustained by high school athletes in the United States, from 2008/2009 through 2013/2014 academic years. *Dent Traumatol.* 2016; 32(2):121–127

37. Bergeron MF, Devore C, Rice SG; Council on Sports Medicine and Fitness; Council on School Health; American Academy of Pediatrics. Policy statement—climatic heat stress and exercising children and adolescents. *Pediatrics.* 2011;128(3). Available at: www.pediatrics.org/cgi/content/full/128/3/e741

38. National Weather Service. Lightning safety tips and resources. Available at: https://www.weather.gov/safety/lightning. Accessed October 11, 2019

39. Janda DH, Bir C, Wild B, Olson S, Hensinger RN. Goal post injuries in soccer. A laboratory and field testing analysis of a preventive intervention. *Am J Sports Med.* 1995;23(3):340–344

40. Koutures CG, Gregory AJ; American Academy of Pediatrics. Council on Sports Medicine and Fitness. Injuries in youth soccer. *Pediatrics.* 2010;125(2): 410–414

41. US Consumer Product Safety Commission. Guidelines for movable soccer goals. Available at: https://www.cpsc.gov/safety-education/safety-guides/sports-fitness-and-recreation/guidelines-movable-soccer-goals. Accessed March 23, 2018

42. Silva DCF, Santos R, Vilas-Boas JP, et al. Influence of cleats-surface interaction on the performance and risk of injury in soccer: a systematic review. *Appl Bionics Biomech.* 2017;2017:1305479

43. Lambson RB, Barnhill BS, Higgins RW. Football cleat design and its effect on anterior cruciate ligament injuries. A three-year prospective study. *Am J Sports Med.* 1996;24(2):155–159

44. Powell JW, Schootman M. A multivariate risk analysis of selected playing surfaces in the National Football League: 1980 to 1989. An epidemiologic study of knee injuries. *Am J Sports Med.* 1992;20(6):686–694

45. Ekstrand J, Hägglund M, Fuller CW. Comparison of injuries sustained on artificial turf and grass by male and female elite football players. *Scand J Med Sci Sports.* 2011;21(6):824–832

46. O'Kane JW, Gray KE, Levy MR, et al. Shoe and field surface risk factors for acute lower extremity injuries among female youth soccer players. *Clin J Sport Med.* 2016;26(3):245–250

47. Bleyer A. Synthetic turf fields, crumb rubber, and alleged cancer risk. *Sports Med.* 2017;47(12):2437–2441

48. Watterson A. Artificial turf: contested terrains for precautionary public health with particular reference to Europe? *Int J Environ Res Public Health.* 2017;14(9): E1050

49. Read PJ, Oliver JL, De Ste Croix MB, Myer GD, Lloyd RS. Neuromuscular risk factors for knee and ankle ligament injuries in male youth soccer players. *Sports Med.* 2016;46(8):1059–1066

50. O'Kane JW, Tencer A, Neradilek M, et al. Is knee separation during a drop jump associated with lower extremity injury in adolescent female soccer players? *Am J Sports Med.* 2016;44(2):318–323

51. Nagle K, Johnson B, Brou L, et al. Timing of lower extremity injuries in competition and practice in high school sports. *Sports Health.* 2017;9(3): 238–246

52. Price RJ, Hawkins RD, Hulse MA, Hodson A. The Football Association medical research programme: an audit of injuries in academy youth football. *Br J Sports Med.* 2004;38(4):466–471

53. Watson A, Brickson S, Brooks MA, Dunn W. Preseason aerobic fitness predicts in-season injury and illness in female youth athletes. *Orthop J Sports Med.* 2017;5(9):2325967117726976

54. Steffen K, Myklebust G, Andersen TE, Holme I, Bahr R. Self-reported injury history and lower limb function as risk factors for injuries in female youth soccer. *Am J Sports Med.* 2008;36(4): 700–708

55. Kucera KL, Marshall SW, Kirkendall DT, Marchak PM, Garrett WE Jr. Injury history as a risk factor for incident injury in youth soccer. *Br J Sports Med.* 2005;39(7):462

56. Herman DC, Jones D, Harrison A, et al. Concussion may increase the risk of subsequent lower extremity musculoskeletal injury in collegiate athletes. *Sports Med.* 2017;47(5): 1003–1010

57. Brooks MA, Peterson K, Biese K, et al. Concussion increases odds of sustaining a lower extremity musculoskeletal injury after return to play among collegiate athletes. *Am J Sports Med.* 2016;44(3):742–747

58. Watson A, Brickson S, Brooks A, Dunn W. Subjective well-being and training load predict in-season injury and illness risk in female youth soccer players. *Br J Sports Med.* 2017;51(3): 194–199

59. McGuine TA, Post EG, Hetzel SJ, et al. A prospective study on the effect of sport specialization on lower extremity injury rates in high school athletes. *Am J Sports Med.* 2017;45(12):2706–2712

60. von Rosen P, Frohm A, Kottorp A, Fridén C, Heijne A. Multiple factors explain injury risk in adolescent elite athletes: applying a biopsychosocial perspective. *Scand J Med Sci Sports.* 2017;27(12): 2059–2069

61. Read PJ, Oliver JL, De Ste Croix MBA, Myer GD, Lloyd RS. A prospective investigation to evaluate risk factors for lower extremity injury risk in male youth soccer players. *Scand J Med Sci Sports.* 2018;28(3):1244–1251

62. Schwebel DC, Banaszek MM, McDaniel M. Brief report: behavioral risk factors for youth soccer (football) injury. *J Pediatr Psychol.* 2007;32(4):411–416

63. Inklaar H, Bol E, Schmikli SL, Mosterd WL. Injuries in male soccer players: team risk analysis. *Int J Sports Med.* 1996;17(3):229–234

64. Poulsen TD, Freund KG, Madsen F, Sandvej K. Injuries in high-skilled and low-skilled soccer: a prospective study. *Br J Sports Med.* 1991;25(3):151–153

65. Peterson L, Junge A, Chomiak J, Graf-Baumann T, Dvorak J. Incidence of football injuries and complaints in different age groups and skill-level groups. *Am J Sports Med.* 2000;28(5 suppl):S51–S57

66. Post EG, Trigsted SM, Riekena JW, et al. The association of sport specialization and training volume with injury history in youth athletes. *Am J Sports Med.* 2017;45(6):1405–1412

67. Post EG, Bell DR, Trigsted SM, et al. Association of competition volume, club sports, and sport specialization with sex and lower extremity injury history in high school athletes. *Sports Health.* 2017;9(6):518–523

68. Jayanthi NA, LaBella CR, Fischer D, Pasulka J, Dugas LR. Sports-specialized intensive training and the risk of injury in young athletes: a clinical case-control study. *Am J Sports Med.* 2015; 43(4):794–801

69. Frome D, Rychlik K, Fokas J, et al. Sports specialization is not associated with greater odds of previous injury in elite male youth soccer players. *Clin J Sport Med.* 2019;29(5):368–373

70. Milewski MD, Skaggs DL, Bishop GA, et al. Chronic lack of sleep is associated with increased sports injuries in adolescent athletes. *J Pediatr Orthop.* 2014;34(2):129–133

71. Watson A, Brickson S. Impaired sleep mediates the negative effects of training load on subjective well-being in female youth athletes. *Sports Health.* 2018;10(3):244–249

72. Bowen L, Gross AS, Gimpel M, Li FX. Accumulated workloads and the acute: chronic workload ratio relate to injury risk in elite youth football players. *Br J Sports Med.* 2017;51(5): 452–459

73. Collins CL, Fields SK, Comstock RD. When the rules of the game are broken: what proportion of high school sports-related injuries are related to illegal activity? *Inj Prev.* 2008;14(1):34–38

74. Meeuwisse WH, Tyreman H, Hagel B, Emery C. A dynamic model of etiology in sport injury: the recursive nature of risk and causation. *Clin J Sport Med.* 2007;17(3):215–219

75. LaBotz M, Bernhardt D. Preparticipation physical evaluation. *Adolesc Med State Art Rev.* 2015;26(1):18–38

76. American Academy of Family Physicians; American Academy of Pediatrics; American College of Sports Medicine; American Medical Society for Sports Medicine; American Orthopaedic Society for Sports Medicine; American Osteopathic Academy of Sports Medicine. In: Bernhardt DT, Roberts WO, eds. *Preparticipation Physical Evaluation*, 4th ed. Elk Grove Village, IL: American Academy of Pediatrics; 2010

77. Harmon KG, Asif IM, Klossner D, Drezner JA. Incidence of sudden cardiac death in National Collegiate Athletic Association athletes. *Circulation.* 2011; 123(15):1594–1600

78. Voskanian N. ACL injury prevention in female athletes: review of the literature and practical considerations in implementing an ACL prevention program. *Curr Rev Musculoskelet Med.* 2013;6(2):158–163

79. Mandelbaum BR, Silvers HJ, Watanabe DS, et al. Effectiveness of a neuromuscular and proprioceptive training program in preventing anterior cruciate ligament injuries in female athletes: 2-year follow-up. *Am J Sports Med.* 2005;33(7):1003–1010

80. Silvers-Granelli H, Mandelbaum B, Adeniji O, et al. Efficacy of the FIFA 11+ injury prevention program in the collegiate male soccer player. *Am J Sports Med.* 2015;43(11):2628–2637

81. LaBella CR, Huxford MR, Grissom J, et al. Effect of neuromuscular warm-up on injuries in female soccer and basketball athletes in urban public high schools: cluster randomized controlled trial. *Arch Pediatr Adolesc Med.* 2011; 165(11):1033–1040

82. Myer GD, Chu DA, Brent JL, Hewett TE. Trunk and hip control neuromuscular training for the prevention of knee joint injury. *Clin Sports Med.* 2008;27(3): 425–448, ix

83. Owoeye OB, Akinbo SR, Tella BA, Olawale OA. Efficacy of the FIFA 11+ warm-up programme in male youth football: a cluster randomised controlled trial. *J Sports Sci Med.* 2014;13(2):321–328

84. Soligard T, Myklebust G, Steffen K, et al. Comprehensive warm-up programme to prevent injuries in young female footballers: cluster randomised controlled trial. *BMJ.* 2008;337:a2469

85. Steffen K, Emery CA, Romiti M, et al. High adherence to a neuromuscular injury prevention programme (FIFA 11+) improves functional balance and reduces injury risk in Canadian youth female football players: a cluster randomised trial. *Br J Sports Med.* 2013;47(12):794–802

86. Rossler R, Verhagen E, Rommers N, et al. Comparison of the '11+ Kids' injury prevention programme and a regular warmup in children's football (soccer): a cost effectiveness analysis. *Br J Sports Med.* 2019;53(5):309–314

87. Gabbett TJ, Whyte DG, Hartwig TB, Wescombe H, Naughton GA. The relationship between workloads, physical performance, injury and illness in adolescent male football players. *Sports Med.* 2014;44(7): 989–1003

88. von Rosen P, Frohm A, Kottorp A, Fridén C, Heijne A. Too little sleep and an unhealthy diet could increase the risk of sustaining a new injury in adolescent elite athletes. *Scand J Med Sci Sports.* 2017;27(11):1364–1371

89. Brink MS, Visscher C, Arends S, et al. Monitoring stress and recovery: new insights for the prevention of injuries and illnesses in elite youth soccer players. *Br J Sports Med.* 2010;44(11): 809–815

90. Djaoui L, Haddad M, Chamari K, Dellal A. Monitoring training load and fatigue in soccer players with physiological markers. *Physiol Behav.* 2017;181:86–94

91. Halson SL. Monitoring training load to understand fatigue in athletes. *Sports Med.* 2014;44(2 suppl):S139–S147

92. Steffen K, Pensgaard AM, Bahr R. Self-reported psychological characteristics as risk factors for injuries in female youth football. *Scand J Med Sci Sports.* 2009;19(3):442–451

93. Ivarsson A, Johnson U, Andersen MB, Fallby J, Altemyr M. It pays to pay attention: a mindfulness-based program for injury prevention with soccer players. *J Appl Sport Psychol.* 2015;27(3):319–334

94. US Soccer Federation. Recognize to recover. US soccer concussion guidelines. Available at: http://www.recognizetorecover.org/head-and-brain#concussions. Accessed October 11, 2019

95. McCrory P. Do mouthguards prevent concussion? *Br J Sports Med.* 2001; 35(2):81–82

96. Niedfeldt MW. Head injuries, heading, and the use of headgear in soccer. *Curr Sports Med Rep.* 2011;10(6):324–329

97. McCrory P, Meeuwisse W, Dvořák J, et al. Consensus statement on concussion in sport-the 5th international conference on concussion in sport held in Berlin, October 2016. *Br J Sports Med.* 2017;51(11):838–847

98. Pettersen JA. Does rugby headgear prevent concussion? Attitudes of Canadian players and coaches. *Br J Sports Med.* 2002;36(1):19–22

99. Naunheim RS, Ryden A, Standeven J, et al. Does soccer headgear attenuate the impact when heading a soccer ball? *Acad Emerg Med.* 2003;10(1):85–90

100. Delaney JS, Al-Kashmiri A, Drummond R, Correa JA. The effect of protective headgear on head injuries and concussions in adolescent football (soccer) players. *Br J Sports Med.* 2008; 42(2):110–115; discussion 115

101. US Soccer Federation. Soccer on head injuries and padded headgear. Available at: https://www.usyouthsoccer.org/news/us_soccer_federation_statement_on_head_injuries_in_soccer_and_padded_headgear/. Accessed October 11, 2019

102. Ryynänen J, Junge A, Dvorak J, et al. Foul play is associated with injury incidence: an epidemiological study of three FIFA World Cups (2002-2010). *Br J Sports Med.* 2013;47(15):986–991

103. Emery CA, Meeuwisse WH, Hartmann SE. Evaluation of risk factors for injury in adolescent soccer: implementation and validation of an injury surveillance system. *Am J Sports Med.* 2005;33(12): 1882–1891

104. International Football Association Board. Laws of the game. Available at: https://www.fifa.com/development/education-and-technical/referees/laws-of-the-game.html. Accessed February 7, 2019

105. National Collegiate Athletic Association. Soccer rules of the game. Available at: www.ncaa.org/playing-rules/soccer-rules-game. Accessed February 7, 2019

106. US Soccer Federation. Laws of the game.. Available at: https://www.ussoccer.com/referees/laws-of-the-game. Accessed February 7, 2019

107. Ankrah S, Mills NJ. Performance of football shin guards for direct stud impacts. *Sports Engineering.* 2003;6:207

108. Arnason A, Sigurdsson SB, Gudmundsson A, et al. Risk factors for injuries in football. *Am J Sports Med.* 2004;32(1 suppl):5S–16S

109. Francisco AC, Nightingale RW, Guilak F, Glisson RR, Garrett WE Jr. Comparison of soccer shin guards in preventing tibia fracture. *Am J Sports Med.* 2000; 28(2):227–233

110. Tatar Y, Ramazanoglu N, Camliguney AF, Saygi EK, Cotuk HB. The effectiveness of shin guards used by football players. *J Sports Sci Med.* 2014;13(1):120–127

111. National Operating Committee on Standards for Athletic Equipment. Standard test method and performance specification for newly manufactured soccer shin guards. Available at: https://nocsae.org/wp-content/uploads/2018/05/1521574443ND09006m18MfrdSoccerShinGuardsStdperformance.pdf. Accessed February 14, 2019

112. Huffman EA, Yard EE, Fields SK, Collins CL, Comstock RD. Epidemiology of rare injuries and conditions among United States high school athletes during the 2005-2006 and 2006-2007 school years. *J Athl Train.* 2008;43(6):624–630

113. Beachy G. Dental injuries in intermediate and high school athletes: a 15-year study at Punahou School. *J Athl Train.* 2004;39(4):310–315

114. Mueller FO, Marshall SW, Kirby DP. Injuries in little league baseball from 1987 through 1996: implications for prevention. *Phys Sportsmed.* 2001; 29(7):41–48

115. Kerr IL. Mouth guards for the prevention of injuries in contact sports. *Sports Med.* 1986;3(6):415–427

116. Newsome PR, Tran DC, Cooke MS. The role of the mouthguard in the prevention of sports-related dental injuries: a review. *Int J Paediatr Dent.* 2001;11(6):396–404

117. Haring RS, Sheffield ID, Canner JK, Schneider EB. Epidemiology of sports-related eye injuries in the United States. *JAMA Ophthalmol.* 2016;134(12): 1382–1390

118. Rodriguez JO, Lavina AM, Agarwal A. Prevention and treatment of common eye injuries in sports. *Am Fam Physician.* 2003;67(7):1481–1488

119. American Academy of Pediatrics Committee on Sports Medicine and Fitness. Protective eyewear for young athletes. *Pediatrics.* 2004;113(3, pt 1): 619–622

120. Markenson D; American Academy of Pediatrics Committee on Pediatric Emergency Medicine; American Academy of Pediatrics Section on Cardiology and Cardiac Surgery. Ventricular fibrillation and the use of automated external defibrillators on children. *Pediatrics*. 2007;120(5): 1159–1161

121. Nelson NG, Collins CL, Comstock RD, McKenzie LB. Exertional heat-related injuries treated in emergency departments in the U.S., 1997-2006. *Am J Prev Med*. 2011;40(1):54–60

122. Nichols AW. Heat-related illness in sports and exercise. *Curr Rev Musculoskelet Med*. 2014;7(4):355–365

123. Sarofim MC, Saha S, Hawkins MD, et al. Ch. 2: Temperature-Related Death and Illness. In: Crimmins A, Balbus J, Gamble JL, eds. *The Impacts of Climate Change on Human Health in the United States: A Scientific Assessment*. Washington, DC: US Global Change Research Program; 2016. Available at: https://health2016.globalchange.gov/

124. National Oceanic and Atmospheric Administration. National Weather Service lightning fatalities in 2019:13. Available at: https://www.weather.gov/safety/lightning-fatalities. Accessed January 31, 2019

125. Thoms AW, Brosnan JT, Zidek JM, Sorochan JC. Models for predicting surface temperatures on synthetic turf playing surfaces. *Procedia Eng*. 2014;72: 895–900

126. Casa DJ, DeMartini JK, Bergeron MF, et al. National Athletic Trainers' Association position statement: exertional heat illnesses [published correction appears in *J Athl Train*. 2017; 52(4):401]. *J Athl Train*. 2015;50(9): 986–1000

127. Committee on Nutrition; Council on Sports Medicine and Fitness. Sports drinks and energy drinks for children and adolescents: are they appropriate? *Pediatrics*. 2011;127(6):1182–1189

128. Centers for Disease Control and Prevention. Lightning: lightning safety tips. Available at: https://www.cdc.gov/disasters/lightning/safetytips.html. Accessed August 1, 2018

129. Walsh KM, Cooper MA, Holle R, et al; National Athletic Trainers' Association. National Athletic Trainers' Association position statement: lightning safety for athletics and recreation. *J Athl Train*. 2013;48(2):258–270

Transporting Children With Special Health Care Needs

- *Policy Statement*

POLICY STATEMENT Organizational Principles to Guide and Define the Child Health Care System and/or Improve the Health of all Children

American Academy of Pediatrics

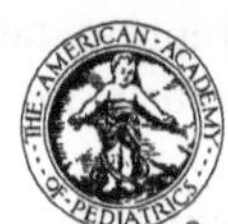

DEDICATED TO THE HEALTH OF ALL CHILDREN™

Transporting Children With Special Health Care Needs

Joseph O'Neil, MD, MPH, FAAP,[a] Benjamin Hoffman, MD, FAAP,[b] COUNCIL ON INJURY, VIOLENCE, AND POISON PREVENTION

abstract

Children with special health care needs should have access to proper resources for safe transportation as do typical children. This policy statement reviews important considerations for transporting children with special health care needs and provides current guidance for the protection of children with specific health care needs, including those with airway obstruction, orthopedic conditions or procedures, developmental delays, muscle tone abnormalities, challenging behaviors, and gastrointestinal disorders.

[a]Department of Clinical Pediatrics, Riley Children's Health, Indiana University Health and School of Medicine, Indiana University, Indianapolis, Indiana; and [b]Department of Pediatrics, School of Medicine, Oregon Health and Science University, Portland, Oregon

Dr O'Neil wrote and revised the draft with the help of Council on Injury, Violence, and Poison Prevention chair Dr Hoffman.

This document is copyrighted and is property of the American Academy of Pediatrics and its Board of Directors. All authors have filed conflict of interest statements with the American Academy of Pediatrics. Any conflicts have been resolved through a process approved by the Board of Directors. The American Academy of Pediatrics has neither solicited nor accepted any commercial involvement in the development of the content of this publication.

Policy statements from the American Academy of Pediatrics benefit from expertise and resources of liaisons and internal (AAP) and external reviewers. However, policy statements from the American Academy of Pediatrics may not reflect the views of the liaisons or the organizations or government agencies that they represent.

The guidance in this statement does not indicate an exclusive course of treatment or serve as a standard of medical care. Variations, taking into account individual circumstances, may be appropriate.

All policy statements from the American Academy of Pediatrics automatically expire 5 years after publication unless reaffirmed, revised, or retired at or before that time.

DOI: https://doi.org/10.1542/peds.2019-0724

Address correspondence to Joseph O'Neil, MD, MPH, FAAP. E-mail: joeoneil@iu.edu

PEDIATRICS (ISSN Numbers: Print, 0031-4005; Online, 1098-4275).

Copyright © 2019 by the American Academy of Pediatrics

FINANCIAL DISCLOSURE: The authors have indicated they have no financial relationships relevant to this article to disclose.

FUNDING: No external funding.

To cite: O'Neil J, Hoffman B, AAP COUNCIL ON INJURY, VIOLENCE, AND POISON PREVENTION. Transporting Children With Special Health Care Needs. *Pediatrics.* 2019;143(5): e20190724

All children, including those with special health care needs, should have access to proper resources for safe transportation. The purpose of this policy statement is to assist caregivers and health care providers in ensuring that children with special health care needs travel in appropriate restraints and are properly positioned and secured in the vehicles in which they ride. This statement supplements the current American Academy of Pediatrics policy statements "Child Passenger Safety" and "School Transportation Safety."[1,2] Primary care providers and subspecialists caring for children with special health care needs as well as parents should be aware of the resources available for proper restraint during travel so that the most appropriate and protective resources are selected for the child each and every ride. This guidance may be used to help parents, caregivers, and others responsible for the safe transportation of a child to avoid products that are inappropriate or incorrectly used, avoid discomfort, and avoid increased injury risk to children transported in motor vehicles.

For many children with special health care needs, a standard car safety seat (CSS) provides the best protection for most travel needs. Federal Motor Vehicle Safety Standard (FMVSS) 213 regulates the design and performance of child restraint systems for children weighing up to 80 lb.[3] Some children with special health care needs will need to use an occupant restraint system beyond 80 lb, and some manufacturers have tested their restraints for weights beyond those regulated by FMVSS 213.

Unfortunately, the biomechanical effects of a crash on test dummies representative of children with special medical needs in any restraint system have not been adequately studied. Further research is needed, including development of such test dummies by the National Highway Traffic Safety Administration (NHTSA), to address these concerns.

In March 2014, the "Hospital Discharge Recommendations for Safe Transportation of Children" was published by an expert working group convened by the NHTSA.[4] This policy was endorsed by the National Child Passenger Safety Board, the Children's Hospital Association, and the National Safety Council. It recommends that hospitals that discharge children should have a hospital-based, multidisciplinary child passenger safety program. Hospital discharge policies and programs should be based on best practice recommendations by the American Academy of Pediatrics and NHTSA. Development and implementation of these policies requires planning, collaboration with appropriate staff, proper training, ongoing competency assessment, and the ability to secure funds and resources to sustain the program. Hospitals should consider having resources for conventional CSSs as well as child passenger safety restraints for children with special transportation needs related to their medical condition. All pertinent interactions between primary care providers, therapists, and child passenger safety technicians (CPSTs) should be documented in the child's medical record. The ideal child passenger safety programs should maintain an inventory of necessary child passenger restraints, have access to custom medical transportation products, and conduct program evaluations to ensure alignment with both patient needs and best practice guidelines.[4] Pediatricians should consider advocating within their local health care community to promote policies so that all children have access to an appropriate, correctly used CSS. In addition, assessment of transportation needs, procurement of the most appropriate restraint, and training for the proper use of the device and its installation in the vehicle may be incorporated into hospital discharge planning for all children with special needs.[4] Any child with a medical condition should have a special care plan that includes what to do during transport if a medical emergency occurs. The individual or group responsible for disseminating emergency plans can be determined at the time the child's individualized education program is developed. Plans should be shared with all individuals who have responsibility for the safety and welfare of the child during transport.

Children with special needs should not be exempt from the requirements of each state's laws regarding child restraint and seat belt use. Pediatricians can serve as resources for information to legislators, policy makers, and law enforcement professionals, as well as to school officials, who may be less familiar with the importance and availability of occupant protection systems for children with special needs.

GENERAL GUIDANCE FOR SAFE TRANSPORTATION OF CHILDREN WITH SPECIAL HEALTH CARE NEEDS

1. All child restraint systems should meet FMVSS 213.[3] Standard child restraint devices may be used for many children with special health care needs, and whenever possible, a standard child restraint is preferable. Use of a custom or "special" child restraint system for a child with special health care needs often may be postponed until a child exceeds the physical limitations of a standard CSS. CSSs with 5-point harnesses can be adjusted to provide good upper torso support for many children with special needs. American Academy of Pediatrics recommendations state that all children should ride rear facing in a CSS as long as possible until they exceed the weight, length, and/or height of that seat as recommended by the seat's manufacturer. These recommendations are based on expert opinion, highway crash data analysis, and sled crash tests.[1,5,6] Objective data from crash tests have shown that a rear-facing CSS provides support to the head and spine that significantly reduces neck loading in crashes that have a frontal component. By extension, small children with neuromuscular conditions will likely be at increased injury risk if forward facing. Thus, riding in a rear-facing CSS should be strongly encouraged as long as possible for these children until they exceed the weight and length limits of the device.
2. When a child has outgrown the length or weight limits of a conventional CSS with an internal 5-point harness, other resources are available for proper and secure occupant restraint. Some systems provide full support for the child's head, neck, and back, accommodate children up to 115 lb, and may be customized to meet a child's particular needs. Others, such as the conventional travel vests or specialized medical seating systems, can be used to provide additional trunk support for a child who already has stable neck control. Tethers, additional lap seat belts, or appropriate tie-down systems are required for some of these devices and may be considerations for selection and proper use.[7,8]
   a. Large medical CSSs are an option for occupants who

require additional positioning support once they exceed the manufacturer's weight and length recommendations of standard CSSs. Positioning accessories, such as abductor wedges, support pads, and seat depth extenders, are available to provide a child with a more customized fit.

b. Some older children with disabilities who have poor trunk control can be transported in a special needs belt-positioning booster or a conventional belt-positioning booster with trunk support. These booster seats help ensure proper positioning of the vehicle shoulder and the lap belt across the child's chest and pelvis. Depending on the type of booster seat, positioning accessories may be available to help maintain posture and comfort. A CPST with additional training in the transportation of children and adolescents with special health care needs could be a resource to the providers and family in choosing the most appropriate vehicle occupant restraint system. Resources to locate local CPST support are located at the end of this policy statement.[7]

c. Many older children and adolescents can be safely transported by using conventional lap-and-shoulder belt systems. Lap-and-shoulder belts should be used properly; the lap belt should be low and flat across the child's hips, and the shoulder belt should be snug across the chest. If the lap belt lies on the child's abdomen or the shoulder belt rests on the child's neck, the child must use either a belt-positioning booster or a different CSS. The shoulder belt should never be placed underneath the child's arms or behind the child's back.[9]

3. Vehicle passengers should never be transported in a reclined vehicle seat. During a crash, the lap-and-shoulder belt system will not be positioned properly, thus imperiling the occupant.[9]
4. The rear seat is the safest place for all children, and children should never ride in the front seat until they are at least 13 years of age.[1] A rear-facing CSS may never be placed in the front seat of a vehicle that has a front passenger air bag. The impact of a deploying air bag can severely injure or kill an infant or small child.[1,9] Children may also be at risk for injury if they are out of position or lie against the door of a vehicle with a side air bag. For specific information, consult both the vehicle operator's manual and CSS manual.
5. Car restraint systems should not be modified or used in a manner other than that specified by the manufacturer unless the modified restraint system has been crash tested and has met all applicable FMVSSs approved by the NHTSA.[9]
6. For a child with special health care needs who requires frequent observation during travel and for whom no adult is available to accompany the child in the back seat, seating in the front seat may be considered; however, an air bag on-off switch should be considered for the vehicle. This can only be considered after the NHTSA approves a petition to disable the air bag.[10]
7. Recommendations and guidelines provided by the manufacturer of the vehicle and the manufacturer of the CSS should always be followed.[1,9]
8. Parents, health care providers, and educators should be encouraged to incorporate a child's special transportation needs into his or her individualized education program developed with the school.
9. For additional information on transporting low birth weight or preterm infants, refer to the appropriate policy statements by the American Academy of Pediatrics.[11]
10. Children with special health care needs may travel on commercial airlines. Each airline has its own policies in accordance with Federal Aviation Administration regulations regarding the use of assistive devices on a commercial aircraft. The use of medical assistive devices is allowed under the Air Carrier Access Act (14 CFR §382).[12] Caregivers may be advised to refer to the Federal Aviation Administration Web site for regulations regarding air travel for individuals with disabilities (www.transportation.gov/airconsumer/disability).

GUIDANCE FOR SAFE TRANSPORTATION OF CHILDREN WITH SPECIFIC MEDICAL CONDITIONS

Although research has been limited, current information suggests the following guidance when selecting an appropriate occupant protection system and positioning a child with special needs properly in the vehicle.

Airway Obstruction

Airway obstruction may occur in infants, children, or adolescents for many reasons. Conditions encountered may include hypotonia, craniofacial abnormalities, or primary airway problems. There are many ways to maintain a stable airway during the vehicle transport of an affected child. If there is any concern about airway or respiratory compromise during vehicle transport, an evaluation should be performed before the child is discharged.[11] This evaluation should include a multidisciplinary team, including someone with advanced training in the transportation of children with special health care needs. For infants and young children, a car seat study using the child's CSS at the angle recommended for use in the vehicle seat during travel should be performed.[11] Abnormal results need to be addressed by the care team and may require coordination with the child's medical home. CSSs that are only rear facing with multiple recline options are useful for infants with many medical problems, especially respiratory conditions. Sometimes a firm, lightweight object such as a rolled towel or Styrofoam pool noodle can be placed in the vehicle seat crease to adjust the angle in accordance with manufacturers' instructions.[9] Convertible CSSs also can be used in the rear-facing position for children and can accommodate weights up to approximately 50 lb. These restraints may be especially useful for children with poor head and neck control. If a child has a specific medical condition such as Pierre Robin sequence and requires prone positioning for transport, the infant will need to be placed in a car bed and must be tested in the car bed before discharge.

Infants and children with a tracheostomy tube should not use child restraint systems with a harness or seat belts that could make contact with the tube and cause it to dislodge. An occupational therapist or CPST with training and experience in the safe transportation of children with special needs could provide guidance for best seat selection. Even with typically developing children, the risk of airway obstruction exists[13]; therefore, all children should use their CSSs only for travel and should not be left in the CSSs outside of the vehicle.[9] Children with significant airway obstruction or who have a tracheostomy should have a trained person with them at all times who can relieve the obstruction and monitor the airway. These caregivers should be trained in the emergency replacement of the tracheostomy tube if it comes out during travel.[7,8]

Muscle Tone Abnormalities

Muscle tone abnormalities, including both hypo- and hypertonia, can affect infants, children, or adolescents for many reasons. Muscle tone varies with each child and can fluctuate during the day. Airway issues in children with abnormal muscle tone may lead to airway obstruction. (Please refer to the previous section on airway obstruction for guidance.) For most situations, the infant or toddler with hypotonia will be safest in the rear-facing orientation within the vehicle as long as the height and weight of the patient does not exceed the CSS manufacturer's recommendations. Some manufacturers allow their forward-facing CSSs to be used in a semireclined position; these can be useful for larger toddlers with poor head control. Crotch rolls, made with a rolled towel or a diaper, may be added between the child's legs and the crotch strap to keep the hips against the back of the seat and prevent the child from slumping forward in the seat.[9] Lateral support may be provided with rolled blankets, towels, or foam rolls to ensure proper upright positioning of the child. However, padding should never be placed between the child and the CSS.[9] Soft padding (such as blankets, pillows, or soft foam) compresses on impact and prevents harness straps from maintaining a secure, tight fit on a child's body. Only products that come with the seat or are sold by the manufacturer for use with the specific seat should be used.[9] Also, head bands or stiff cervical collars may not be used to restrain the child's head. For children with increased muscle tone whose opisthotonic posturing makes sitting in a CSS difficult, a foam roll or rolled blanket under the child's knees may help with positioning.[14] Children with cerebral palsy or spina bifida may have scoliosis that makes it difficult to be seated in a conventional CSS. A large medical seat or an adaptive restraint may need to be obtained. Large medical seats can be customized to suit the individual needs of occupants who require positioning support beyond that offered by a conventional restraint system. For children who have sufficient head, neck, and trunk support to sit upright during travel but need supplemental support, adaptive belt-positioning booster seats may suffice. Like all belt-positioning booster seats, these seats must be used only with both the lap-and-shoulder belt system of the vehicle.[9] These adaptive boosters are easier to transfer between vehicles and may be an option for children who often ride in many vehicles. Use of car beds, large medical seats, and adaptive boosters may require an order by a physician and a letter of medical necessity. It is important that a rehabilitation therapist with training in the safe transportation of children with special health care needs be included in the evaluation, ordering, and implementation of the seat.[7]

Gastrointestinal Issues

Many children with special health care needs suffer from emesis or severe gastroesophageal reflux or have gastrostomy feeding tubes. The angle at which the infant or child sits in the CSS may increase the intra-abdominal pressure and aggravate the reflux.[15–17] Solutions to addressing these issues can include waiting a period of time after feeding before traveling, optimizing the medical management of reflux, changing the angle that the infant or child travels with a CSS that allows multiple options for angle of recline, or using a car bed. Because there is potential for increased gastroesophageal reflux during the time the child is in the CSS, the restraint device should only be used for travel, and the infant or child should be removed from the CSS when at the destination. Gastrostomy tubes may affect the CSS harness fit. It is important to select a CSS that does not have a harness that rubs against the feeding tube. Families should have an emergency plan to be able to replace the tube or to cover the stoma if the tube comes out during travel.

Casts

Casts are often applied to a patient for a variety of circumstances, whether to maintain a bony alignment postoperatively or to allow a bone to heal after trauma. For most situations, the cast will not interfere with the use of a CSS. However, there are circumstances when a cast interferes with positioning the child in a CSS.

For children with spica casts, frequently the side of the CSS prevents proper positioning because of the fixed flexion and abduction of the femurs. Consultation with occupational therapists specially trained in the transportation requirements of children with special health care needs could be helpful in the selection of a CSS or an alternative that will provide protection and comfort during motor vehicle transportation. Availability of specialty CSSs can be labile, as new models are introduced and existing products are removed from the marketplace, and consultation with individuals familiar with current products will be helpful. Consideration of hospital-based loaner programs that obtain and maintain specialty seating systems should be considered to provide appropriate CSSs as needed.[4] Planning for the transportation needs of the child before discharge may help prevent delays in leaving the facility.

Many older children and youth in body or hip spica casts have limited resources available for safe transport in motor vehicles. Often, these children have outgrown the weight and height limits or simply do not fit into a conventional seat. Older children who might be able to correctly use the vehicle seat belt may not be able sit upright as required. A travel vest or harness can be a reasonable alternative for many such children. Such vests can accommodate a child sitting in a vehicle seat from 2 years of age and from 20 to 168 lb. This restraint system will not be appropriate for children with poor head, neck, or trunk control.

Another vest-style option for a child who must travel lying down is available commercially. The child must be able to fit lengthwise on a vehicle bench seat perpendicular to the direction of the vehicle. These vests are available for children 1 to 12 years of age who weigh between 20 and 100 lb. Two sets of seat belts are routed through the vest to secure the child at his or her side against the vehicle seat. An ancillary belt loops around the casted leg or legs at the knees and is routed through the other seat belt. When it is not possible to fit a child onto a vehicle seat, use of an ambulance for transport is recommended.

Challenging Behavior

Children may exhibit behaviors that preclude safe use of a particular CSS, are distracting to the driver, or otherwise place the child or passengers at risk. Although challenging behaviors can be observed among typical children, these behaviors can also be seen in children with developmental delay (or intellectual disability), autism, or emotional problems and may include impulsive, hyperactive, aggressive, and noncompliant behaviors in the vehicle, making transportation dangerous. In-depth discussions with parents or caregivers, teachers, therapists, or psychologists may be helpful to identify triggers and develop strategies to possibly avoid inappropriate behavior. Monitors or aides trained in behavioral techniques and both qualified and capable of meeting the child's specific needs may be needed to help ensure safe transport. Although many of these children can be safely transported in standard CSSs, children with severe behavioral challenges may require specialized restraints during travel. Use of standard CSSs with higher-weight internal harnesses or large medical seats may be useful for some older and larger children who will not remain seated in a booster seat or seat belt. Families should never modify the CSS to make it more difficult to escape.[9] In addition, travel vests with rear back closure and a floor mount tether also may be helpful for use with children who have behavioral problems that interfere with safe travel.

Wheelchair Transportation

Any child who can assist with transfer, be reasonably moved from a wheelchair, stroller, or special seating or mobility device to the forward-facing vehicle seat equipped with dynamically tested occupant restraints or be reasonably moved to a child restraint system complying with FMVSS 213 requirement should be transferred accordingly for transportation. In these cases, "reasonably" implies that the child can be moved from the wheelchair to the bus seat or occupant restraint without significant discomfort or risk of injury to either the child or caregiver. The unoccupied wheelchair also should be secured adequately in the vehicle to prevent it from becoming a dangerous projectile in the event of a sudden stop or crash.[18]

If the child must travel in a wheelchair, it should be secured in a forward-facing position. It is also recommended that the child or adolescent be transported in a transit option wheelchair. Transit option wheelchairs have been specifically designed for vehicle transport and are thus safer to use in a vehicle than a wheelchair without a transit option.[18] Transit option wheelchairs should comply with American National Standards Institute/Rehabilitation Engineering and Assistive Technology Society of North America WC19, a voluntary standard to ensure that the design and performance requirements for use in motor vehicles are met.[19] If a transit option wheelchair is not available, the wheelchair should have a metal frame to which tie-down straps and hooks can be attached at frame junctions. Tie-down straps, restraint belts, and wheelchairs that meet current standards should be used during transport.[20] Any occupied wheelchair should be secured with 4-point tie-down devices. Lap boards or metal or plastic trays attached to the wheelchair or to adaptive equipment should be removed and secured separately for transport.[21] An occupant restraint system that includes upper torso restraint (ie, shoulder harness) and lower torso restraint (ie, a lap belt over the pelvis) should be provided for each wheelchair-seated occupant. Head bands or stiff cervical collars may not be used to restrain the child's head separately from the torso or support the head.

EQUIPMENT TRANSPORTATION

1. When transporting a child with special needs, ancillary pieces of medical equipment (eg, walkers, ventilators, pumps, oxygen tanks, monitors) should be secured on the vehicle floor or, if allowed by the vehicle manufacturer, underneath a vehicle seat or wheelchair or below the window line. These devices can become projectiles during a crash and can strike an occupant, making safe storage a critical consideration. In most passenger vehicles, the safest option is the vehicle trunk. The driver or caregiver should refer to the vehicle owner's manual or consult the vehicle manufacturer to identify proper locations and methods for the safe storage of equipment.[14]
2. Children who require electricity-powered medical equipment for use during transit should have portable self-contained power for twice the expected duration of the trip as well as a fully charged backup system with them. Additionally, the child's medical equipment should include a connector to attach medical equipment to the vehicle power source in case of an emergency. The caregiver should contact the vendor, medical equipment provider, or manufacturer for the appropriate equipment. For improved safety, lead acid batteries, electricity-powered wheelchairs, or other mobile seating devices and respiratory systems should be converted, when possible, to gel-cell or dry-cell batteries. To house and protect batteries during everyday use, transportation, and collision, the use of external battery boxes is recommended.[21]

CONCLUSIONS

It is essential that all children have the opportunity to be transported in the safest possible way. For children with special health care needs, life includes all the components that any other child enjoys. It must be ensured that they have access to the expertise and means to travel safely to help them achieve their greatest potential.

RESOURCE AVAILABILITY

Resources can be found at the National Center for Transportation of Children with Special Health Care Needs, Riley Hospital for Children, Indiana University School of Medicine (1-800-755-0912), or https://preventinjury.pediatrics.iu.edu/special-needs/, which includes photographs of specialized products for children with special needs.

Additional resources can be found at the Rehabilitation Engineering Research Center on Wheelchair Transportation Safety and the University of Michigan Transportation Research Institute. A detailed brochure on the use of a wheelchair as a transportation device on the bus or the family vehicle is available at http://www.travelsafer.org.

LEAD AUTHORS

Joseph O'Neil, MD, MPH
Benjamin Hoffman, MD

COUNCIL ON INJURY, VIOLENCE, AND POISON PREVENTION, 2018–2019

Benjamin Hoffman, MD, Chairperson
Phyllis F. Agran, MD, MPH
Sarah A. Denny, MD
Michael Hirsh, MD
Brian Johnston, MD, MPH
Lois K. Lee, MD, MPH
Kathy Monroe, MD
Judy Schaechter, MD, MBA
Milton Tenenbein, MD
Mark R. Zonfrillo, MD, MSCE
Kyran Quinlan, MD, MPH, Immediate Past Chairperson

LIAISONS

Lynne Janecek Haverkos, MD, MPH – *National Institute of Child Health and Human Development*
Jonathan D. Midgett, PhD – *Consumer Product Safety Commission*
Alexander W. (Sandy) Sinclair – *National Highway Traffic Safety Administration*
Richard Stanwick, MD – *Canadian Pediatric Society*

STAFF

Bonnie Kozial

ABBREVIATIONS

CPST: child passenger safety technician
CSS: car safety seat
FMVSS: Federal Motor Vehicle Safety Standard
NHTSA: National Highway Traffic Safety Administration

POTENTIAL CONFLICT OF INTEREST: The authors have indicated they have no potential conflicts of interest to disclose.

REFERENCES

1. Durbin DR, Hoffman BD; Council on Injury, Violence, and Poison Prevention. Child passenger safety. *Pediatrics*. 2018; 142(5):e20182460
2. Agran PF; American Academy of Pediatrics Committee on Injury, Violence, and Poison Prevention; American Academy of Pediatrics Council on School Health. School transportation safety. *Pediatrics*. 2007; 120(1):213–220
3. National Highway Traffic Safety Administration. Federal Motor Vehicle Safety Standards: child restraint systems, child restraint anchorage systems. Available at: www.gpo.gov/fdsys/pkg/CFR-2011-title49-vol6/pdf/CFR-2011-title49-vol6-sec571-213.pdf. Accessed July 25, 2018
4. National Child Passenger Safety Board. Hospital discharge recommendations for safe transportation of children. Available at: http://cpsboard.org/cps/wp-content/uploads/2014/02/FINAL_dischargeprotocol_7_3_20141.pdf. Accessed July 25, 2018
5. McMurry TL, Arbogast KB, Sherwood CP, et al. Rear-facing versus forward-facing child restraints: an updated assessment. *Inj Prev*. 2018;24(1):55–59
6. Sherwood CP, Crandall JR. Frontal sled tests comparing rear and forward facing child restraints with 1-3 year old dummies. *Annu Proc Assoc Adv Automot Med*. 2007;51:169–180
7. Bull MJ. Safe transportation of children with special healthcare needs. *Pediatr Ann*. 2008;37(9):624–631
8. National Center for Safe Transportation of Children with Special Healthcare Needs. Special needs transportation. Available at: https://preventinjury.pediatrics.iu.edu/special-needs/. Accessed February 8, 2019
9. National Child Passenger Safety Board. National child passenger safety certificate training. Available at: http://cpsboard.org/2014-tg. Accessed July 25, 2018
10. Department of Transportation, National Highway Traffic Safety Administration. 49 CFR Part 595 (Docket No. 74-14; Notice 107) RIN 2127 - AG61. Air Bag Deactivation. Available at: www.nhtsa.gov/cars/rules/rulings/deactnpr.n21.html. Accessed March 18, 2019
11. Bull MJ, Engle WA; Committee on Injury, Violence, and Poison Prevention and Committee on Fetus and Newborn; American Academy of Pediatrics. Safe transportation of preterm and low birth weight infants at hospital discharge. *Pediatrics*. 2009;123(5): 1424–1429
12. US Department of Transportation Office of the Secretary. Air carrier access act. 14 CFR-P §382. Available at: https://www.transportation.gov/airconsumer/passengers-disabilities. Accessed March 18, 2019
13. Merchant JR, Worwa C, Porter S, Coleman JM, deRegnier RA. Respiratory instability of term and near-term healthy newborn infants in car safety seats. *Pediatrics*. 2001;108(3):647–652
14. O'Neil J, Bull MJ, Sobus K. Issues and approaches to safely transporting children with special healthcare needs. *J Pediatr Rehabil Med*. 2011;4(4): 279–288
15. Orenstein SR, Whitington PF. Positioning for prevention of infant gastroesophageal reflux. *J Pediatr*. 1983;103(4):534–537
16. Orenstein SR, Whitington PF, Orenstein DM. The infant seat as treatment for gastroesophageal reflux. *N Engl J Med*. 1983;309(13):760–763
17. Lightdale JR, Gremse DA; Section on Gastroenterology, Hepatology, and Nutrition. Gastroesophageal reflux: management guidance for the pediatrician. *Pediatrics*. 2013;131(5). Available at: www.pediatrics.org/cgi/content/full/131/5/e1684
18. University of Michigan Transportation Research Institute. Ride safe: information to help you travel more safely in motor vehicles while seated in your wheelchair. Available at: https://docs.google.com/viewer?a=v&pid=sites&srcid=dW1pY2guZWR1fHdjLXRyYW5zcG9ydGF0aW9uLXNhZmV0eXxneDoyYjBjOGMxYmM1M2RkNTNm. Accessed August 7, 2018
19. American National Standards Institute; Rehabilitation Engineering and Assistive Technology Society of North America . *Wheelchairs Used as Seats in Motor Vehicles*. Arlington, VA: American National Standards Institute/Rehabilitation Engineering and Assistive Technology Society of North America; 2000
20. American National Standards Institute; Rehabilitation Engineering and Assistive Technology Society of North America . *Wheelchair Tiedown and Occupant Restraint Systems for Use in Motor Vehicles*. Arlington, VA: American National Standards Institute/Rehabilitation Engineering and Assistive Technology Society of North America; 2013
21. Snell MA. Guidelines for safely transporting wheelchair users. *OT Pract*. 1999;4(5):35–38

Understanding Liability Risks and Protections for Pediatric Providers During Disasters

- *Policy Statement*

POLICY STATEMENT Organizational Principles to Guide and Define the Child Health Care System and/or Improve the Health of all Children

American Academy of Pediatrics 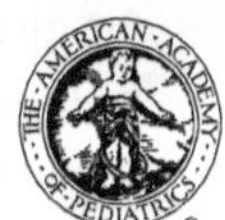

DEDICATED TO THE HEALTH OF ALL CHILDREN™

Understanding Liability Risks and Protections for Pediatric Providers During Disasters

Robin L. Altman, MD, FAAP,[a] Karen A. Santucci, MD, FAAP,[b] Michael R. Anderson, MD, MBA, FAAP,[c] William M. McDonnell, MD, JD, FAAP,[d] COMMITTEE ON MEDICAL LIABILITY AND RISK MANAGEMENT

abstract

Although most health care providers will go through their careers without experiencing a major disaster in their local communities, if one does occur, it can be life and career altering. The American Academy of Pediatrics has been at the forefront of providing education and advocacy on the critical importance of disaster preparedness. From experiences over the past decade, new evidence and analysis have broadened our understanding that the concept of preparedness is also applicable to addressing the unique professional liability risks that can occur when caring for patients and families during a disaster. In our recommendations in this policy statement, we target pediatric health care providers, advocates, and policy makers and address how individuals, institutions, and government can work together to strengthen the system of liability protections during disasters so that appropriate and timely care can be delivered with minimal fear of legal reprisal or confusion.

[a]Department of Pediatrics, New York Medical College of Touro University System and Maria Fareri Children's Hospital of Westchester Medical Center Health Network, Valhalla, New York; [b]Department of Pediatrics, School of Medicine, Yale University and Children's Emergency Department, Yale-New Haven Hospital, New Haven, Connecticut; [c]UCSF Benioff Children's Hospital, San Francisco, California; and [d]Department of Pediatrics, University of Nebraska Medical Center, Omaha, Nebraska

Drs Santucci and Anderson substantially contributed to the conception and design of the policy statement and technical report, analysis and interpretation of information and references, writing of specific portions of the manuscripts, critical review, and revisions; Dr McDonnell substantially contributed to refining the conception and design of the policy statement and technical report, analysis and interpretation of information, critical review, and revisions; Dr Altman was responsible for the original ideas, conception, and design of the policy statement and technical report, acquisition and analysis of information and references, design of articles, outline of topics, draft of both manuscripts and writing of specific portions, compilation of other authors' contributions, editing, critical review and revisions, and response to American Academy of Pediatrics reviewers; and all authors approved final manuscripts as submitted.

This document is copyrighted and is property of the American Academy of Pediatrics and its Board of Directors. All authors have filed conflict of interest statements with the American Academy of Pediatrics. Any conflicts have been resolved through a process approved by the Board of Directors. The American Academy of Pediatrics has neither solicited nor accepted any commercial involvement in the development of the content of this publication.

Policy statements from the American Academy of Pediatrics benefit from expertise and resources of liaisons and internal (AAP) and external reviewers. However, policy statements from the American Academy of Pediatrics may not reflect the views of the liaisons or the organizations or government agencies that they represent.

To cite: Altman RL, Santucci KA, Anderson MR, et al. AAP COMMITTEE ON MEDICAL LIABILITY AND RISK MANAGEMENT. Understanding Liability Risks and Protections for Pediatric Providers During Disasters. *Pediatrics.* 2019;143(3):e20183892

INTRODUCTION

The purpose of this policy statement is to educate and raise awareness for providers and policy makers about the current state of liability risk and protection for health care providers who are caring for children during disasters. The goal is to equip and encourage pediatric providers to respond to disasters without fear of unanticipated legal issues. It also provides advocacy recommendations to strengthen liability protections. Detailed information forming the basis of the recommendations in this policy statement is found in the accompanying technical report.[1]

RECOMMENDATIONS

1. Pediatric leaders should continue to emphasize and promote the American Academy of Pediatrics' expanding drive to educate pediatric

providers and patients' families on the importance of preparedness for disasters.

2. Pediatricians should continue to promote leadership at the federal, state, and local levels to:
   a. ensure that children's needs in disasters are adequately addressed; and
   b. ascertain status of the most current disaster liability-related laws applicable in each state; and advocate accordingly.
3. The US Department of Health and Human Services should conduct a review, potentially through its Federal Advisory Committee processes, of current state and federal liability laws and issue recommendations for Congress to enact laws that address:
   a. disaster-response liability protections for nonvolunteer clinicians affected by conditions and decisions outside of their control;
   b. timing of declarations and how affected clinicians are covered;
   c. inconsistency in state malpractice liability protections for volunteer physicians able and willing to care for patients and nonvolunteer physicians performing in their usual capacity;
   d. a renewed assessment of vulnerable patients' rights, protections, and access to health care during disasters as related to provider liability protections; and
   e. an updated assessment of liability coverage needs during times of "crisis standards of care."
4. Pediatric providers should strive to understand their own liability risks, protections, and limitations during disasters and take steps to mitigate them by developing a disaster readiness plan, including:
   a. education of self and staff on providing medical care during disasters and how to best document clinical decisions made in an altered health care environment;
   b. proactive identification of obstacles to providing care during disasters, using an all-hazards approach, with the goal of maintaining continuity of operations throughout;
   c. education of patients and their families before and during disasters;
   d. use of the American Academy of Pediatrics Department of State Government Affairs as a resource for current information on disaster liability laws in their respective states;
   e. understanding of potential limits to their professional malpractice insurance coverage during disasters and, if possible, taking steps to add additional coverage for identified gaps;
   f. advocating for their hospitals to have active disaster plans that address the unique needs of children and conduct disaster drills that test pediatric capabilities; and
   g. for any provider whose personal circumstances would allow, consideration of registering and training with a volunteer organization.
5. Health care institutions and employers should provide appropriate disaster liability protections for employed health care workers through:
   a. offering disaster preparedness programs;
   b. providing adequate professional malpractice insurance coverage that explicitly includes conditions that may occur during disasters while performing one's job; and
   c. developing policies to allow and support their employees to volunteer.
6. Medical liability insurers should reduce gaps in coverage for insured individuals providing necessary health care services in good faith in response to disasters.

LEAD AUTHORS

Robin L. Altman, MD, FAAP
Karen A. Santucci, MD, FAAP
Michael R. Anderson, MD, MBA, FAAP
William M. McDonnell, MD, JD, FAAP

COMMITTEE ON MEDICAL LIABILITY AND RISK MANAGEMENT, 2017–2018

Jon Mark Fanaroff, MD, JD, FAAP, Chairperson
Robin L. Altman, MD, FAAP
Steven A. Bondi, JD, MD, FAAP
Sandeep K. Narang, MD, JD, FAAP
Richard L. Oken, MD, FAAP
John W. Rusher, MD, JD, FAAP
Karen A. Santucci, MD, FAAP
James P. Scibilia, MD, FAAP
Susan M. Scott, MD, JD, FAAP
Laura J. Sigman, MD, JD, FAAP

FORMER COMMITTEE MEMBER

William M. McDonnell, MD, JD, FAAP

CONSULTANT

Michael R. Anderson, MD, MBA, FAAP

STAFF

Julie Kersten Ake

ACKNOWLEDGMENT

We extend our appreciation to Jay Goldsmith, MD, FAAP, for his review and technical advice.

The guidance in this statement does not indicate an exclusive course of treatment or serve as a standard of medical care. Variations, taking into account individual circumstances, may be appropriate.

All policy statements from the American Academy of Pediatrics automatically expire 5 years after publication unless reaffirmed, revised, or retired at or before that time.

DOI: https://doi.org/10.1542/peds.2018-3892

Address correspondence to Robin L. Altman, MD, FAAP. Email: robin_altman@nymc.edu.

PEDIATRICS (ISSN Numbers: Print, 0031-4005; Online, 1098-4275).

Copyright © 2019 by the American Academy of Pediatrics

FINANCIAL DISCLOSURE: The authors have indicated they have no financial relationships relevant to this article to disclose.

FUNDING: No external funding.

POTENTIAL CONFLICT OF INTEREST: The authors have indicated they have no potential conflicts of interest to disclose.

REFERENCE

1. Altman RL, Santucci KA, Anderson MR, McDonnell WM; American Academy of Pediatrics, Committee on Medical Liability and Risk Management. Technical report: understanding liability risks and protections for pediatric providers during disasters. *Pediatrics*. 2019;143(3):e20183893

Understanding Liability Risks and Protections for Pediatric Providers During Disasters

- *Technical Report*

TECHNICAL REPORT

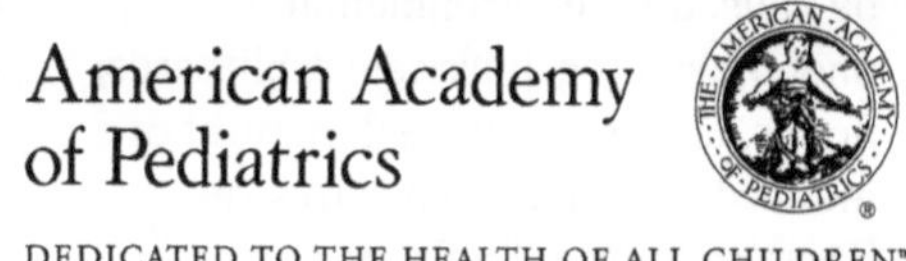

Understanding Liability Risks and Protections for Pediatric Providers During Disasters

Robin L. Altman, MD, FAAP,[a] Karen A. Santucci, MD, FAAP,[b] Michael R. Anderson, MD, MBA, FAAP,[c] William M. McDonnell, MD, JD, FAAP,[d] COMMITTEE ON MEDICAL LIABILITY AND RISK MANAGEMENT

abstract

Although most health care providers will go through their careers without experiencing a major disaster in their local communities, if one does occur, it can be life and career altering. The American Academy of Pediatrics has been in the forefront of providing education and advocacy on the critical importance of disaster preparedness. From experiences over the past decade, new evidence and analysis have broadened our understanding that the concept of preparedness is also applicable to addressing the unique professional liability risks that can occur when caring for patients and families during a disaster. Concepts explored in this technical report will help to inform pediatric health care providers, advocates, and policy makers about the complexities of how providers are currently protected, with a focus on areas of unappreciated liability. The timeliness of this technical report is emphasized by the fact that during the time of its development (ie, late summer and early fall of 2017), the United States went through an extraordinary period of multiple, successive, and overlapping disasters within a concentrated period of time of both natural and man-made causes. In a companion policy statement (www.pediatrics.org/cgi/doi/10.1542/peds.2018-3892), recommendations are offered on how individuals, institutions, and governments can work together to strengthen the system of liability protections during disasters so that appropriate and timely care can be delivered with minimal fear of legal reprisal or confusion.

[a]Department of Pediatrics, New York Medical College of Touro University and Maria Fareri Children's Hospital of Westchester Medical Center Health Network, Valhalla, New York; [b]Department of Pediatrics, School of Medicine, Yale University and Children's Emergency Department, Yale-New Haven Hospital, New Haven, Connecticut; [c]UCSF Benioff Children's Hospital, San Francisco, California; and [d]Department of Pediatrics, University of Nebraska Medical Center, Omaha, Nebraska

Drs Santucci and Anderson substantially contributed to the conception and design of the policy statement and technical report, analysis and interpretation of information and references, writing of specific portions of the manuscripts, critical review, and revisions; Dr McDonnell substantially contributed to refining the conception and design of the policy statement and technical report, analysis and interpretation of information, critical review, and revisions; Dr Altman was responsible for the original ideas, conception, and design of the policy statement and technical report, acquisition and analysis of information and references, design of articles, outline of topics, draft of both manuscripts and writing of specific portions, compilation of other authors' contributions, editing, critical review and revisions, and response to American Academy of Pediatrics reviewers; and all authors approved final manuscripts as submitted.

This document is copyrighted and is property of the American Academy of Pediatrics and its Board of Directors. All authors have filed conflict of interest statements with the American Academy of Pediatrics. Any conflicts have been resolved through a process approved by the Board of Directors. The American Academy of Pediatrics has neither solicited nor accepted any commercial involvement in the development of the content of this publication.

Technical reports from the American Academy of Pediatrics benefit from expertise and resources of liaisons and internal (AAP) and external reviewers. However, technical reports from the American Academy of Pediatrics may not reflect the views of the liaisons or the organizations or government agencies that they represent.

To cite: Altman RL, Santucci KA, Anderson MR, et al. AAP COMMITTEE ON MEDICAL LIABILITY AND RISK MANAGEMENT. Understanding Liability Risks and Protections for Pediatric Providers During Disasters. *Pediatrics.* 2019;143(3):e20183893

INTRODUCTION

A disaster, simply defined, is when community resources are challenged by an evolving circumstance, usually an acute event of unpredictable impact that has the potential for health effects, property damage, and disruption of services.[1] The timing of a disaster can be sudden and unexpected, or it can be slow and continual, each process having the potential of building up to the point of resource exhaustion.[2] In general, disasters may be caused by environmental phenomena (eg, hurricanes, blizzards, floods, and earthquakes), natural or induced infectious exposures (eg, H1N1 influenza, Ebola, and bioterrorism), or man-made hazards (eg, industrial accidents and terrorism).[3,4] Although many pediatricians and health care entities take disaster preparedness seriously, the ability to withstand the demands of a disaster is directly linked to how well an individual or a practice and/or entity prepares.[3,5] Disaster preparedness takes many forms, such as training oneself and staff, securing supplies, conducting drills, learning the local disaster command structure, understanding one's potential role as a provider or practice, determining how to receive and disseminate communications, and identifying locations of stockpiles, to name a few. In this technical report, we examine the important elements surrounding preparing for the liability issues facing pediatric providers who are involved in responding to a disaster.

The terrorist attack on September 11, 2001, and the subsequent anthrax bioterrorism scare riveted the nation, and the attention of public health officials was focused on the importance of health care provider preparedness.[6–9] Four years later, Hurricane Katrina directed national focus to the response side and the unique challenges of caring for children during disasters.[1,10–12] Countless children, many displaced from families, received medical care during Hurricane Katrina and in the days to weeks after its devastation.[6,13] Over the past decade, that experience has been memorialized to help us understand how disaster conditions alter the provision of medical care and create liability risks for providers who are working in those conditions.[6,14–24]

Society benefits when pediatric providers move quickly to address the emergency needs of children during disasters, regardless of the circumstances.[4,25] For providers who live and work within harm's way of a disaster, this would mean reporting to work despite likely personal obstacles.[26–28] Such providers would be followed and augmented by additional volunteer providers, as needed, to assist in the disaster's wake. Ideally, all providers functioning during crisis situations when resources may be scarce and demands for health care may exceed capacity would be able to care for patients without fear of facing unreasonable liability risks. Evidence reveals that concern or confusion about various legal protections during public health emergencies may interfere with providers' responsiveness and willingness to volunteer.[2,7,11,26,29–35] Ethically, providing necessary medical care should not be hampered by legal considerations.

Our purpose for this technical report is to educate and raise awareness for providers and policy makers about the current state of liability risk and protection for health care providers who are caring for children during disasters. The goal is to equip and encourage pediatric providers to respond to disasters without fear of unanticipated legal issues. This technical report also supports and is accompanied by a policy statement of the same title in which advocacy recommendations are provided to strengthen liability protections.[36]

ALTERED HEALTH CARE ENVIRONMENT AND PRACTICE DURING A DISASTER

Disaster response has been described as an "imperfect process fraught with unpredictable dynamics and countless decisions."[37] Unpredictable dynamics relate to the interplay of 3 forces: the magnitude of the health care needs of the population affected by the disaster (ie, demand), the levels of resilience and preparedness of the health care providers responding to the disaster, and the rate at which available resources become overwhelmed. Resilience and preparedness refer not only to the ability to ramp up space, staff, and supplies but also to the strength of individual and institutional training and the presence of predetermined strategies, such as emergency operations plans. The relative weight of each of the intersecting forces influences medical decision-making, which drives actions.[1,13,38,39]

If demand is matched by readiness and adequate resources, providers may not be faced with an environment of care that is different from that under normal conditions.[14] For example, health care entities with policies for addressing times of extreme surges in patient volume, such as during an infectious disease epidemic or after a single, contained community event (such as a train crash), have a better ability to scale up operations as needed.[3,30] On this end of the disaster spectrum, health care entities and providers who are prepared for potential disasters are likely able to use standard methods of triage and have access to usual diagnostic and therapeutic modalities.[35,38] Staffing may be extremely taxed, but decision-making is less likely to be altered.

However, if demand begins to outpace readiness and/or resources, such as during a major natural event (such as an earthquake), health care processes can be disrupted.[37] Providers may have to reallocate shrinking resources between patients or locations, assume new tasks outside their usual practice or location because of staff shortages, and provide care in temporary areas that might not have conventional capabilities because usual clinical areas are full or not available.[2,5,38,40–43] These changes can include, although are not limited to, providing critical care outside of critical care units or using alternate care sites, such as mobile or community-based sites, for screening and delivering urgent care. Under these conditions, space, staffing, and supplies may not be consistent with daily practice, but medical decision-making and care provided may remain functionally equivalent to usual practice.[35]

If resources become inadequate during sustained overwhelming demand, such as in the aftermath of Hurricane Sandy (with widespread damage), providers may face caring for patients in an environment that makes it increasingly difficult to use traditional decision-making processes.[17,18,44] Faced with severe shortages of staff, space, supplies, equipment, and medication, health care providers will have to make difficult decisions about how to allocate limited resources and may not be able to provide care that is functionally equivalent to usual practice.[35,45,46] An example of this is when triaging is shifted to addressing patients with the best potential outcomes first because that is a more effective use of resources and time.[14,39] This approach has been described as shifting from individual-based care to population-based care, a trade-off to do the greatest good for the most people.[14,25,39,43]

At the extreme end of the continuum is the catastrophic disaster that causes devastation beyond the primary event, such as varying degrees of collapse of societal infrastructure, as happened after Hurricane Katrina and the resulting flooding.[38] There may be staff fear and confusion, people not showing up for work, lack of medications, lack of laboratory facilities, families separated, children displaced, lack of power, no access to clean water, loss of communication, loss of transportation, and lack of security.[3,13,14,35] Under these extreme circumstances when resources are surpassed, providers may face withholding or withdrawing life-sustaining treatment so it can be redirected to a more salvageable patient because no other treatment option is available.[6,24,31,35,38,40]

Although the focus during disasters is typically on the role of the hospital as the center of disaster management, in fact, office-based providers can be faced with perilous conditions, limited or nonexistent resources, and challenges that may alter medical decision-making. These providers, whose practice locations may vary widely throughout a community, may have a small safety net for their practices during major catastrophes and may quickly become overwhelmed by a disaster's impact while being called on to serve vital community functions.[19,23] Conditions may result in the inability to get to the office because of impassable roads, inability to instruct patients because of disrupted telephone lines, and lack of access to medical records as well as loss or damage to equipment or medical supplies, such as medications or vaccines, because of power outages.[16] Patients in need of higher-level care may receive treatment in an ambulatory setting because emergency transfer services are not functioning, modes of communication between providers and hospitals are interrupted, or a receiving hospital is not responding.[20] In a catastrophic disaster, an outpatient facility may, by necessity, become a site of triage and urgent care because a devastated hospital may be forced to divert patients.[9] In these conditions, it is likely that local pharmacies and patient information and/or insurance systems are inoperable as well.[20] When a community is crippled, patients who would normally seek basic information and guidance from authorities regarding conditions and expectations may instead turn to their primary care provider(s) as a trusted source.

LIABILITY RISKS DURING A DISASTER

Liability risk exists with all medical care scenarios, especially when there is a less-than-optimal or unanticipated outcome. Disaster circumstances can devolve into an environment of limited choices for both patients and providers.[35] Patient preference for health care options may necessarily carry less weight, and providers may have fewer treatment options available to them. Denial of treatment that would have been provided in a routine health care environment may increase the chance of a provider facing a lawsuit. It is important to note that malpractice claims after disasters are infrequent. However, there is evidence that the health care providers at greatest risk of being sued are those who live and work in the disaster-affected area and report to work instead of evacuating.[11,14]

Generally during disasters, the 3 broad categories of potential liability claims have been described as the following: suboptimal medical care, such as negligence; a regulatory or administrative breach, such as violating the Emergency Medical Treatment and Labor Act (EMTALA); and wanton behavior, such as criminal acts. Other types of potential claims, less discussed in the pediatric literature but nevertheless still possible, include constitutional violations and lack of preparedness.

Claims Arising From Alleged Suboptimal Medical Care

Several types of potential claims can arise from conduct during direct patient care in a disaster. Three commonly described examples are negligence, abandonment, and lack of informed consent.[2,47]

Negligence

During a disaster, a provider may be forced to modify treatment of a particular patient because of limited supplies of medicine, vaccines, or equipment.[45] This has the potential to increase risk of being accused of negligence if the patient's outcome is negatively affected by the modified treatment.[48] A court may find liability against the provider if it determines that the provider had a duty to treat, that the duty was breached, that the breach resulted in harm, and that the harm can be linked to damages.[49] To determine that a breach occurred, the court must find that the provider failed to deliver care that a reasonable individual would have provided under similar circumstances.[2]

When a disaster progresses to overwhelming conditions, practitioners face increased chances of an altered health care environment that will demand nonroutine actions.[45] Nonroutine actions may include diagnosing without laboratories or radiology, treating without medications or equipment, managing without consultative expertise from specialists, assessing symptoms and diseases outside the scope of a provider's training, or having fewer to no actual treatment options to consider. Providing evidence that a reasonable practitioner would have made similar decisions becomes more difficult in a disaster environment for many reasons. For example, contemporaneous documentation of medical decision-making, a primary defense for one's actions, may be compromised because lack of electricity renders the electronic health record inoperable.[45] Medical records for past medical history may not be available, which may affect the appropriateness of care provided. In addition, conditions may be changing so rapidly that it is virtually impossible to maintain the usual levels of information sharing, communication, and collaboration with patients or parents when medical care decisions must be made.[45] All of these factors can contribute to the perception of suboptimal care.

Abandonment

In extreme conditions, providers may cease treating some patients entirely so they can focus their time and resources elsewhere, including potentially withholding or withdrawing life support for patients with a lower expected chance of survival.[2,7,39,50] These actions can increase the chance of a potential claim of abandonment, that is, the unilateral termination of a physician-patient relationship by the health care provider (without proper notice to the patient) when there is still the necessity of continuing medical attention.[2] During chaotic conditions and desperate circumstances, provider communication with patients may not keep pace with real-time decision-making, sowing seeds of dissatisfaction.[45] This dissatisfaction can occur around publicly visible decisions regarding the transfer of patients to another facility or general evacuation of people to other locations. Determining whom to transfer or evacuate can ignite potentially violent conflict with those remaining behind.[14]

Lack of Informed Consent

Another liability risk is providing care without proper informed consent or, in the case of a child, without adequate parental consent.[11] Although the elements of what constitutes informed consent may vary between states, it generally means reviewing risks, benefits, and alternatives and receiving consent before starting a course of treatment. Unlike competent adults, minor children (with some exceptions, such as emancipated adolescents) lack the legal authority to provide informed consent for medical care, placing that responsibility on parents or legal guardians.[5] During disasters, families may be separated, and children may be displaced from parents, some of whom may themselves be injured, making it impossible to obtain consent for necessary treatment.[6,51,52]

The primary exception to the legal requirement for informed consent before treating an unaccompanied minor is a medical emergency that a provider determines requires immediate action and the absence of any indication that the parent(s) would refuse consent.[51] In addition, EMTALA, described more in the next section, both empowers and requires providers in emergency departments to perform medical screening examinations and provide necessary stabilizing treatment of emergency conditions in the absence of express informed consent.[52] However, during a disaster, if a separated child presents for medical treatment of a nonemergency condition or at an alternative medical facility, these exceptions may not apply.[53] Unaccompanied children with preexisting but stable health conditions, who may be technology or medication dependent, are particularly vulnerable during disasters and may create legal challenges for health care providers.[12,51]

Courts generally allow considerable leeway in the likely scenario of implied consent, that is, a parent separated from a child would likely consent to treatment of an active medical condition.[11] However, if the provider is forced by disaster conditions to depart from routine medical practices, treatment without express informed consent could create an increased liability risk.[2,11] In addition, even when a parent is present, there may not be time to obtain informed consent for nontraditional care or for care by providers exceeding their usual scope of expertise.[45]

Claims Arising From Administrative or Regulatory Breach

Claims that can arise from a regulatory or administrative breach relate to actions taken as real-time demands are unfolding on the frontlines in the changing health care environment during a disaster, often during early stages. Providers may breach state regulation if they rush to where the need is regardless of whether they are properly licensed in that state. Overwhelmed hospitals and providers may violate EMTALA requirements if they are forced to turn away patients in need of emergency treatment because they lack the resources or the space to treat them. Providers may face a breakdown in their systems of documentation and communication, resulting in potential exposure of individually identifiable health information and a breach of the Health Insurance Portability and Accountability Act (HIPAA) privacy rule.[45]

Practicing Without Proper State Licensure or Privileges

A potential regulatory breach during a disaster is practicing without a properly recognized state license or assisting at a facility without proper privileges. This can occur when an out-of-state provider shows up at, or an in-state provider is reassigned to, an unfamiliar facility perceived to be in need of emergency manpower.[2] Spontaneous volunteers, although typically acting in good faith and out of a desire to help, create liability risks for themselves, for the institution, and for their full-time employer.[54]

EMTALA Violation

Under EMTALA, hospital emergency departments and physicians are obligated to provide medical screening and treatment of patients at a level consistent with the institution's capabilities. Providers in the emergency department or inpatient units are required to treat a patient until the condition has been resolved or stabilized.[55] During a disaster, hospitals may not be able to provide care in line with their usual services for many reasons, such as insufficient staff or space, lack of electricity, or destroyed equipment.[53] Providers may be forced to refuse to treat patients outright, may refer patients to alternative community locations, or may transfer patients to facilities with less specialized capabilities but adequate power to function.[41,50] These actions can expose a hospital and its providers to sanctions under EMTALA, with further liability exposure if a diverted patient suffers an adverse outcome.

HIPAA Privacy Rule Breach

Another regulatory breach can occur when a patient's protected health information is compromised. During the chaotic conditions of a disaster, lack of electricity or destroyed equipment may render normally protected modes of communication and documentation inoperable, increasing the chances of unintentional leaks or public exposure of private health information.[45] Moments vulnerable to potential privacy breaches are those involving rationing resources, arranging transportation, or making evacuation decisions, especially for patients with special needs.[12,13,34]

Claims Arising From Alleged Wanton Behavior

In truly extreme conditions, providers can face claims of gross negligence or actual criminal conduct while providing care.[48] Gross negligence is when negligent behavior is particularly egregious or reckless and closer to willful or wanton misconduct.[53] A criminal act can be practicing without a license (in addition to being a regulatory breach) or wantonly withholding or withdrawing treatment, thereby causing injury or death.* These types of allegations may arise in situations that are so extreme that providers facing them have no other available recourse when making decisions that would never be made under normal circumstances.[2] Examples of such situations are when providers are forced to remove a ventilator from 1 patient to give it to a patient who is more salvageable or to escalate parenteral pain medication for a patient who is critical with severe pain but has a high risk of respiratory depression.[24,45,48] These situations can occur because the environment of care is extremely compromised or has collapsed, giving providers no other options. Although less likely than other types of claims to arise from care provided during an extreme disaster, criminal claims are also less likely to be covered or indemnified by malpractice insurance. Furthermore, these types of claims are excluded from legislation that provides immunity during disasters.[48]

* This is to be distinguished from careful, sensitive, and deliberative decisions regarding do-not-resuscitate status or foregoing nonbeneficial treatment in a patient who is terminally ill.

Other Potential Claims

Constitutional Violations

Discrimination claims may arise from medical care decisions that appear to affect, either negatively or favorably, specific populations, including people with disabilities, minorities, and those with limited English proficiency.[7] In addition, equal protection claims may arise from individuals who believe they received inferior services because of their race, ethnicity, or socioeconomic class.[29,48]

Failure to Prepare

Health care entities have an obligation to prepare for emergencies, and lawsuits against hospitals and other health care entities alleging liability for patient harms are brought and settled routinely in the United States.[30,56,57] When patient harms can be linked to an entity's failure to prepare sufficiently for emergencies, defending the claims can be difficult because emergency preparedness is mandated by law, endorsed by practice, and ultimately beneficial to patients.[57,58] These factors and others create a strong legal presumption that health care entities are obligated to avert preventable patient harms through emergency planning and preparedness.[7]

Multiple federal and state laws and agencies mandate or encourage hospital emergency planning and preparedness; furthermore, the US Department of Homeland Security requires funded hospitals to adopt its standards within their emergency plans.[57] State laws and licensing provisions also call for preparedness for catastrophic events, and The Joint Commission requires accredited hospitals to demonstrate levels of emergency preparedness.[59–61] The US Department of Health and Human Services has allocated hundreds of millions of dollars to hospitals to improve emergency preparedness by mandating the development of comprehensive emergency response plans and withholding funds from hospitals that do not meet certain benchmarks.[9,62–64] In 2016, the Centers for Medicare and Medicaid Services (CMS) issued new emergency preparedness requirements for facilities to develop and implement emergency continuity of operations plans that contain core elements of predisaster risk assessment, maintenance of communication, and regular training and testing of policies and procedures.[65]

LEGISLATION PROVIDING PROTECTIONS FROM CIVIL LIABILITY DURING A DISASTER

Overview

State tort law defines the rights and liabilities arising out of an injury and the framework through which damages are recoverable.[66] Tort law seeks accountability and aims to compensate victims when providers engage in negligent conduct. As noted earlier, the legal basis for accountability in medical negligence is based on determining duty, breach, causation, and harm. Once determined, those responsible can be found liable for damages in a court of law.

Legislation can provide a powerful shield of liability protection to health care providers through either limiting the degree a provider could be held liable or by establishing an absolute prohibition on any liability. In the former case, laws can create limitations to personal liability for individual providers through processes such as reducing statutes of limitations, establishing caps on damage awards, or creating a victims' injury fund. In the latter, a different and arguably more controversial type of shield, legislation can provide immunity against any liability under certain conditions. This means that an individual provider who meets those conditions would either not be sued or ultimately be dropped as a defendant if a malpractice case arose.

There are no comprehensive national liability protections for all health care providers during disasters.[10,25] Rather, many laws exist at the federal and state levels to reduce civil liability for certain health care practitioner categories by providing immunity against certain types of claims.[34,48] Table 1 provides a summary of existing federal legislation, and the following sections provide basic highlights of these laws and regulations. Important references and informational Web sites are provided for a more in-depth discussion. These laws are described as "patchwork" with wide variability and important exclusions.[11,35,47,48] Protections only apply to providers acting in good faith and without willful misconduct, gross negligence, or recklessness.[2]

Government Declarations and Waivers

Most of the laws providing liability protections are triggered once an emergency is declared by the government.[2,9,35] Under the Robert T. Stafford Disaster Relief and Emergency Assistance Act, a governor may request a presidential declaration of a major disaster or emergency.[67] In addition, the US Secretary of Health and Human Services can declare a public health emergency under section 319 of the Public Health Service Act. Government declarations activate emergency management systems that provide a wide range of federal assistance programs to the affected area(s) and trigger emergency liability protections for certain health care providers, especially volunteers.[68] If a disaster is beyond the combined response capabilities of state and local governments, section 1135 of the Social Security Act additionally authorizes the US Secretary of Health and Human Services to temporarily waive or modify certain Medicare, Medicaid, Children's Health Insurance Program, and HIPAA requirements, as determined necessary by CMS.[69]

The purpose of waivers is to ensure that sufficient health care supplies and services are available in the emergency areas during the emergency time periods to meet the needs of individuals enrolled in Social Security Act programs and that providers who provide such services in good faith can be reimbursed and exempted from sanctions (absent any determination of fraud or abuse). Examples of 1135 waivers include the following: program certification requirements; preapproval requirements; state licensure for interstate volunteers, as long as the provider has equivalent licensure in another state; EMTALA sanctions, such as for the transfer of an individual who has not been stabilized or the redirection of an individual to receive medical screening; and penalties for noncompliance with

TABLE 1 Survey of State and Federal Laws Providing Limited Immunity From Civil Liability for Health Care Providers During Disasters

Law or Act	Federal or State	Year First Enacted	Individuals Protected	Conditions
Tort Claims Act	Federal, State	1946	Government employees	Government consents to substitute as defendant
Good Samaritan laws	State	1980	Volunteers	Rendering aid at scene of emergency
Emergency Management Assistance Compact	State	1996	Volunteers	Rendering care as an agent of the requesting state
Volunteer Protection Act	Federal	1997	Volunteers	Serving nonprofit organization or government entity
Model State Emergency Health Powers Act	State	2001	All providers	Rendering care under contract with or at request of a state
Model Intrastate Mutual Aid Legislation	State	2004	Volunteers	Rendering care as an employee of the state
Public Readiness and Emergency Preparedness Act	Federal	2005	All providers	When dispensing a countermeasure
Uniform Emergency Volunteer Health Practitioners Act	State	2007	Volunteers	Rendering care under host entity at direction of requesting state

Adapted from Pope TM, Palazzo MF. Legal briefing: crisis standards of care and legal protections during disasters and emergencies. *J Clin Ethics.* 2010;21(4):358–367; Hodge JG Jr, Garcia AM, Anderson ED, Kaufman T. Emergency legal preparedness for hospitals and health care personnel. Disaster Med Public Health Prep. 2009;3(suppl 2):S37–S44; Hodge JG Jr. The evolution of law in biopreparedness. Biosecur Bioterror. 2012;10(1):38–48; Courtney B, Hodge JG Jr; Task Force for Pediatric Emergency Mass Critical Care. Legal considerations during pediatric emergency mass critical care events. *Pediatr Crit Care Med.* 2011;12(suppl 6):S152–S156; Burkle FM Jr, Williams A, Kissoon N; Task Force for Pediatric Emergency Mass Critical Care. Pediatric emergency mass critical care: the role of community preparedness in conserving critical care resources. *Pediatr Crit Care Med.* 2011;12(suppl 6):S141–S151; Rothstein MA. Currents in contemporary ethics. Malpractice immunity for volunteer physicians in public health emergencies: adding insult to injury. *J Law Med Ethics.* 2010;38(1):149–153; Rosenbaum S, Harty MB, Sheer J. State laws extending comprehensive legal liability protections for professional health-care volunteers during public health emergencies. *Public Health Rep.* 2008;123(2):238–241; Hanfling D, Altevogt BM, Viswanathan K, Gostin LO, eds; Committee on Guidance for Establishing Crisis Standards of Care for Use in Disaster Situations; Institute of Medicine. *Crisis Standards of Care: A Systems Framework for Catastrophic Disaster Response.* Washington, DC: The National Academies Press; 2012. Available at: https://www.ncbi.nlm.nih.gov/books/NBK201063/pdf/Bookshelf_NBK201063.pdf. Accessed July 24, 2017; Barnett DJ, Taylor HA, Hodge JG Jr, Links JM. Resource allocation on the frontlines of public health preparedness and response: report of a summit on legal and ethical issues. *Public Health Rep.* 2009;124(2):295–303; Eddy A. First responder and physician liability during an emergency. *Am J Disaster Med.* 2013;8(4):267–272; Hoffman S, Goodman RA, Stier DD. Law, liability, and public health emergencies. *Disaster Med Public Health Prep.* 2009;3(2):117–125; Rutkow L, Vernick JS, Wissow LS, Tung GJ, Marum F, Barnett DJ. Legal issues affecting children with preexisting conditions during public health emergencies. *Biosecur Bioterror.* 2013;11(2):89–95; Foltin GL, Lucky C, Portelli I, et al. Overcoming legal obstacles involving the voluntary care of children who are separated from their legal guardians during a disaster. *Pediatr Emerg Care.* 2008;24(6):392–398; Sauer LM, Catlett C, Tosatto R, Kirsch TD. The utility of and risks associated with the use of spontaneous volunteers in disaster response: a survey. *Disaster Med Public Health Prep.* 2014;8(1):65–69; Pandemic and All-Hazards Preparedness Act, 42 §USC 300hh et seq (2006); and Cole C, Marzen C. A review of state sovereign immunity statutes and the management of liability risks by states. *Journal of Insurance Regulation.* 2013;32:45–82; and Lopez W, Kershner SP, Penn MS. EMAC volunteers: liability and workers' compensation. *Biosecur Bioterror.* 2013;11(3):217–225.

certain patient privacy provisions of HIPAA.[7,35]

A significant limitation of 1135 waivers and other liability protections triggered by declarations is that they commence on the date of the declaration, which may lag from the start of the disaster, and end when the declaration is terminated, which may precede conditions returning to normal operations.[30,41] This can potentially leave responders whose efforts precede or exceed the time period of the formal declaration unprotected.[70] Waivers may be granted retrospectively to the start of a disaster, but that is not guaranteed.[42,53] Waivers must be pursuant to a state emergency preparedness plan, must be necessitated by the circumstances of the disaster, must be linked to implementation of a hospital disaster protocol, and do not apply to hospitals nearby but outside of the disaster declaration that may experience surge conditions from receiving diverted patients. In addition, waivers are not automatic.[2,42] Once 1135 waiver authority has been invoked, governors and individual hospitals must submit requests to CMS, after which need is determined. Depending on the scope, severity, and duration of the disaster, CMS may grant "blanket" waivers to all similarly impacted providers in the disaster area. Of note, 1135 waiver authority applies only to federal program requirements. State law and gubernatorial authority determine state modifications to requirements for professional licensure, credentialing or privileging at certain facilities, and authorization of emergency liability protections for certain health care providers.

Tort Claims Act and Government Employees

An exception to tort law accountability is the doctrine of sovereign immunity. Sovereign immunity is a legal doctrine that protects a sovereign body (ie, federal or state government and their agencies) from being held liable for civil wrongs committed by its employees.[66] The Federal Tort Claims Act, enacted in 1946, limits this immunity by allowing the federal government to incur liability for injuries caused by the negligent acts of a federal employee acting within the scope and course of their employment.[71] Under the Federal Tort Claims Act, the government waives its sovereign immunity by allowing itself to be sued and giving plaintiffs the option of suing the government instead of an individual employee (ie, defendant substitution). As long as the government employee commits the tort within the scope and course of employment, the employee cannot incur personal liability.[71] A majority of states have enacted similar statutes. Federal and state tort claims acts give government-employed health care providers a unique shield from liability and relatively more protection against medical negligence lawsuits than private clinicians.

With narrow exceptions, government-employed health care providers working at a public facility and performing their official duties during a public health emergency will have immunity from liability for negligence.[48] However, the exceptions can be important. For instance, there must be a credible connection between the provider's activities and the government's interest, and the government must consent to be substituted as the defendant. If these conditions do not apply, the individual physician can be exposed to major liability.[66]

Under the tort claims acts, discretionary decisions by government officials are immune. Therefore, nonmedical government employees have immunity for discretionary actions during a disaster. Nonmedical government employees may include public health officials, law enforcement officers, or agency managers who may make decisions regarding evacuation of patients or staff, resource allocation, or interstate patient transfers to institutions outside of the disaster zone. Each of these decisions may directly and profoundly influence management options available for the frontline medical providers, thereby shifting potential liability risks to providers without the same level of immunity.[48]

Volunteers

After September 11, 2001, and Hurricane Katrina, legislative focus has been to create improved systems to streamline processes to facilitate the movement of volunteers between states during emergencies. In addition to liability concerns, out-of-state volunteers are faced with the need for rapid licensing and privileging.[2,30,72,73]

Liability Protections

Under the federal provisions listed in Table 1, volunteers will receive immunity from claims of negligence if they are properly licensed in the state where care is rendered, are working for a nonprofit or government entity or through an established response system, and are not compensated.[48,74]

In addition to federal laws, all states and the District of Columbia have enacted statutes extending qualified immunity protections to volunteers who provide emergency-related health care. The vast majority of states stipulate immunity for care provided at the scene of an emergency in good faith, without expectation of compensation, and absent of gross negligence or wanton misconduct. These Good Samaritan laws are intended to permit physicians to render emergency aid without fear of malpractice claims stemming from that care.[†] These statutes do not block the provider from being sued, but act as a defense from liability if invoked during a malpractice trial.[34] However, there is much variability and ambiguity between states. For instance, state laws vary on whether protection applies only for care provided at the scene of an isolated emergency, such as a car crash, and may not extend to other locations, including a hospital, during a disaster.[47] Furthermore, state laws vary considerably on what constitutes "good faith" and "without compensation," that is, whether protection applies for a provider who is otherwise salaried in a regular job.[2,48,53,75]

[†] It should be noted that Good Samaritan laws differ from laws that address administration of opioid antagonist drugs for the treatment of overdose or that shield lay people who render aid or assist overdose victims to reach the emergency department from drug possession charges, which are also often referred to as Good Samaritan laws.

Licensing and Privileging

Regarding licensing, states' emergency laws recognize out-of-state health care licenses for the duration of a declared emergency through licensure reciprocity provisions.[48] These provisions allow for the interstate sharing of out-of-state health care personnel whose licenses are viewed as in-state licenses for the duration of the declared emergency.[76] In 2007, the Uniform Emergency Volunteer Health Practitioners Act established a system whereby health professionals may register either in advance of or during an emergency to provide volunteer services in another state.[35,51,77,78] Registration may occur in any state by using governmentally established registration systems, such as the federally funded Emergency System for Advance Registration of Volunteer Health Professionals.[30,33,72] These national systems allow states to verify an out-of-state volunteer's identity, licensing, and credentialing.[79] The Emergency Management Assistance Compact authorizes license reciprocity between states for health care practitioners during a declared state of emergency.[35]

Providers of telemedicine not themselves experiencing technological failures can assist with patient monitoring and online consultations during a disaster. Interstate providers temporarily volunteering their services via telemedicine must have an appropriate state license, be part of a multistate reciprocal or compact license, or obtain a temporary practice permit.[80] Information is available from the respective licensing boards.

The National Disaster Medical System

The National Disaster Medical System (NDMS) and the Medical Reserve Corp are responsible, during declared emergencies, for the mobilization and assignment of trained volunteers who are considered federal employees during their deployment.[10,41,53,81] The role of the NDMS is to provide civilian medical support to state and local governments for disaster victims through a national network of rapidly deployable medical teams.[41] The NDMS teams that provide general medical care are disaster medical assistance teams. Under these systems, out-of-state volunteers are considered to be either federal or state government agents and receive liability protections accordingly. For a volunteer who is not registered with such a system to receive liability protection, the volunteer must work either through another established response system, for a designated "host entity," or at the direction of the requesting state.[35,48,77,82]

Private Sector Providers

In contrast to volunteers and government employees, private sector providers performing in their regular job capacity during a disaster are generally not provided immunity for negligence by any legislation.[2] A notable exception in some states is the Model State Emergency Health Powers Act, which may provide immunity for negligence if the private provider is rendering care under contract with or at the request of a state. However, a private provider who runs to his or her office or a local hospital to help will not receive protection through any of these laws. Even Good Samaritan laws, considered to be the safety net of protection from claims of negligence for some actions taken during a disaster, may not apply unless care is rendered at the scene of an emergency.[83] Another exception is the Public Readiness and Emergency Preparedness Act, which provides immunity for all providers from claims that may arise from dispensing a specific medical countermeasure during a declared public health emergency.[35] Examples of medical countermeasures, many of which would require consent before distribution to children, are medications, vaccines, medical devices, or lifesaving equipment required to protect or treat children for possible chemical, biological, or nuclear threats.[84]

Health care providers in the private sector are likely to bear the brunt of the burden of a disaster, especially in the early stages, as hundreds or thousands of patients rush to emergency departments, clinics, and physicians' offices to receive care.[10] Yet, legislation does not address the associated disproportionate liability risk burden of this large percentage of crucial frontline providers.[7]

A small number of states have attempted to bridge this gap by enacting laws that provide immunity more broadly for health care providers, regardless of volunteer or compensation status.[35] Elements of the laws‡ of these few states include acting in response to a declared emergency or disaster, in which there is a recognized depletion of resources attributable to the disaster, at express or implied request of government and consistent with emergency plans.

ROLE OF MALPRACTICE INSURANCE

For health care practitioners who are not protected through federal or state legislation that provides immunity or a shield against claims, malpractice insurance would be the next layer of protection for defense and potential indemnification if necessary. Malpractice insurance coverage differs across states and is dependent on the specific insurance policy language. Many providers receive professional malpractice insurance through an employer and may have little input into the scope of coverage. Providers in the private sector may obtain their own malpractice insurance. In either case, there might be need for supplemental coverage for care provided out of state during a disaster.

Most, but not all, malpractice coverage is limited to the provider's usual practice scope in his or her usual practice setting and may not cross over state lines. Plans may not cover a practitioner's actions during an emergency if the actions fall outside the individual's normal scope of activity or location. This may leave the provider completely unprotected if, for instance, a Good Samaritan law in that state does not apply to the circumstances giving rise to a claim.

Insurance coverage does not prevent litigation, which can cause emotional stress, a damaged reputation, and increased insurance premiums. Furthermore, there is a distinction between a malpractice insurance carrier's role in providing legal advice and defense against a claim and providing indemnification for damages that are based on a monetary award by a jury verdict. Typical insurance plans provide both defense and indemnification for negligence up to a specified cap in award payments. However, most malpractice carriers will defend against claims but not indemnify for verdicts of gross negligence, willful or wanton misconduct, or crimes, which leaves the individual practitioner at risk for payment of monetary awards for these types of judgments.[2,14]

MITIGATING LIABILITY RISKS DURING A DISASTER

At the heart of mitigating liability risks during a disaster is being prepared. Being prepared is not just learning about disaster medicine. It necessitates taking steps in advance

‡ On file with the American Medical Association Advocacy Resource Center and available via e-mail at ARC@amaassn.org.

of a crisis to have a strategy that can be implemented as a disaster unfolds.[9] An all-hazards approach to emergency planning for disasters can identify many different types of potential threats with varied approaches to management and mitigation.[85] In general, a disaster preparedness strategy can have 3 overlapping components: educating self and personnel, securing the physical aspects of the health care environment, and creating a framework through which the provision of care may be sustained during and after a disaster.

Education

For all providers, a disaster strategy starts with training and preparing themselves and their staff for possible contingencies.[5,86,87] The American Academy of Pediatrics (AAP) Disaster Preparedness Advisory Council has established a strategic plan for disaster preparedness in which a roadmap for the advocacy of children as well as preparedness for pediatricians is outlined.[88] Addressing pediatric readiness is especially important because the majority of children in the United States who go to emergency departments are seen in community hospitals with a low pediatric volume.[89] The AAP has many readily available resources, including a preparedness checklist, for pediatric providers to keep themselves and their patients informed and to play a key role for families, schools, and communities.[86,90–92]

Securing the Health Care Environment

This mitigation strategy involves proactively assigning contingency staff roles and lines of communication; identifying transportation obstacles; exploring back-up energy sources or alternate locations to provide services; creating temporary medical records; protecting valuable equipment or medical supplies, such as vaccines and medication; identifying how to receive accurate information and up-to-date instructions from authorities; and considering the impact on patients with special needs, especially those who are technology dependent.[8,93]

Framework for Sustained Provision of Care

Liability risk mitigation also includes taking steps to improve the likelihood that provision of care will not be interrupted. This involves developing methods for keeping patients and families informed during prolonged periods of relentless and unpredictable change. Cultural sensitivity during disasters is especially important because beliefs about disasters may make communication even more difficult and add to confusion.[94] Liability risk mitigation also includes understanding how to tap into local resources, such as emergency rescue services, nearby hospitals, and the local disaster command center. For providers affiliated with hospitals or other health care entities, it necessitates being familiar with the institution's crisis management plan. In considering one's support network, providers need to be prepared for the possibility of having to care for patients or conditions beyond their training, such as caring for adult family members. Disaster preparedness training that includes the potential lack of other specialists when urgent treatment is needed during disasters can mitigate the liability risk associated with this situation.

Although documentation is not a priority during a disaster, accurate documentation that reflects and memorializes the reasoning behind decision-making in an altered environment could mitigate liability risk.[45] Documentation could also improve postdisaster care and patient outcomes. Accordingly, it behooves providers to consider including relevant information about resource limitations in the medical record if such limitations influence decision-making. However, there are currently no guidelines or consensus on the best way to achieve the most efficient, appropriate, and transparent medical chart during a disaster.

National recognition for the need to better elucidate how medical care delivery changes under disaster-response conditions and the resulting liability risks led the US Department of Health and Human Services to engage with the National Academy of Sciences' Institute of Medicine (now the National Academy of Medicine) to issue reports in 2009 and 2012. A key element of the Institute of Medicine analysis is that the best outcomes during a disaster occur with integration of all components of the health care system (hospitals, emergency medical services, government agencies, and community providers).[39] A second key element is that effective crisis-level preparation requires anticipating and preparing for how a disaster can alter delivery of health care services (ie, "crisis standards of care"[3,35]). It is through development and implementation of effective disaster planning that providers can take active steps to reduce their liability risks during disasters.[25]

THE BRIDGE BETWEEN LIABILITY CONCERNS AND PATIENTS' RIGHTS

It is important to understand how laws providing immunity for health care providers may negatively affect some segments of the population. In the years since September 11, 2001, and Hurricane Katrina, a prominent concern among public health officials has been ensuring the presence of adequate health care providers during a public health emergency.[27] One way of preventing a shortage is to encourage providers from outside the affected areas to volunteer their services, and laws that provide volunteers with immunity can remove potential obstacles for volunteers. However, experience has shown that when large numbers of volunteers have been needed after a disaster, the predominant populations served were those without health insurance or those too poor to evacuate.[27] Therefore, legislation providing immunity only for volunteer health care providers may have the unintentional impact of creating a system of unequal patients' rights and a distinction between nonvolunteer and volunteer physicians.[3,27] During some disasters, patients in specific at-risk populations, such as the elderly, racial minorities, and those of lower socioeconomic status, may suffer disproportionately relative to others. Therefore, any laws offering immunity from liability for health care workers may have a disproportionate effect if they deny certain patient populations the right to seek recourse for injuries caused by negligent acts.[35]

The extremely important role of the pediatric provider through the entire spectrum of disaster preparedness and response has been well described.[50,84,87] Infants, children, adolescents, and young adults have unique physical, emotional, behavioral, developmental, communication, therapeutic, and social needs that make them particularly vulnerable during disasters.[50,56,95] Pediatric providers are best positioned to address those vulnerabilities.[25,96] Being an active participant in the analysis and discussion of liability risks and protection during disasters serves to advance the important advocacy role of the pediatrician.[97]

OVERSIGHT OF PEDIATRIC MEDICAL RESPONSE DURING DISASTERS

Oversight and direction of medical assets during times of crisis are complicated. Local jurisdictions maintain control of their assets and personnel during times of crisis (ie, local hospitals, emergency medical services, etc). When a governor declares a disaster, state agencies can then mobilize assets and augment local medical responses.[74] For instance, the State of California engages the Emergency Medical Services Authority, which can send medical response teams and emergency medical services equipment to bolster the on-site responses. Each state has unique approaches and possesses different types of assets.

The federal oversight of disaster medical response is housed within the National Disaster Framework (Federal Emergency Management Agency in 2016) under the Emergency Services Framework 8.[98] The lead federal agency for the Emergency Services Framework 8 is the Department of Health and Human Services, under the guidance of the Assistant Secretary of Preparedness and Response (ASPR). Formed under the Pandemic and All-Hazards Preparedness Act of 2006, the ASPR is charged with the massive responsibility of preparing for and responding to the health needs of Americans during times of disasters.[64] The Pandemic All-Hazards Preparedness Reauthorization Act of 2013 reaffirmed consideration for children in disaster preparedness and response.[99]

The ASPR has been key in assessing and implementing needed changes for children affected by disasters. In response to the 2011 final report of the National Commission on Children and Disasters, the ASPR established a multiagency work group on children's needs and subsequently housed the National Advisory Committee on Children and Disasters, supported by federal and nonfederal disaster experts.[100] The formation of the National Advisory Committee on Children and Disasters was due, in large part, to the legislative and advocacy leadership of the AAP and embodied in the language of the Pandemic All-Hazards Preparedness Reauthorization Act. A second advisory committee, the National Biodefense Science Board, is currently charged with assessing the science and data supporting current disaster planning.[101] Other key federal partners in assuring that children's unique needs in disasters are being addressed include the Centers for Disease Control and Prevention and the Federal Emergency Management Agency. Since Hurricane Katrina, these agencies have formed important relationships with the AAP and other advocacy organizations.

This complicated federal structure is important for ensuring adequate pediatric response. Only through federal collaboration with states and regions can the nation be truly prepared.

CONCLUSIONS

National experiences over the past 15 years have revealed that preparing for and responding to disasters are national security concerns.[102–104] Health care providers typically occupy critically important roles in leadership and the implementation of frontline responses. Children and infants are likely to be victims in a disaster and are more vulnerable than adults.[73] Specialized resources needed to care for children who are ill and injured vary widely by geographical region. In a disaster, pediatric centers may be overwhelmed or rendered inoperable, and many children may be taken to hospitals that cannot provide specialized pediatric care. Developing prehospital pediatric protocols and transfer agreements are of paramount importance.[21,25,30,73]

Because of the vulnerabilities of children during disasters, pediatric health care providers play a uniquely important role.[13,25] History has revealed that pediatricians and other pediatric providers are eager to help children affected by major disasters.[1,13,14,39,56] Although much progress has been made in addressing the needs of children affected by disasters, work remains to protect the risk of liability for those health care providers who step up to help the most vulnerable among us.[11]

Areas of liability protection inequity deserve attention. Although all providers responding to a disaster will face similar conditions, arguably, the frontline nonvolunteers will be faced with unfolding conditions with an uncertain end point and a higher chance of exposure to the kinds of liability risks explored in this report. In addition, government agents and law enforcement officials who are responsible for discretionary decisions, such as evacuation, are usually protected for those decisions, whereas the providers left to care for patients affected by those decisions are not.[7,48] Liability protection that is linked to a government-declared emergency might not completely reflect, in timeliness or scope, the conditions being faced by providers on the front lines.

There are increased potential risks for liability amid attempting to treat patients with limited resources in difficult conditions.[10,30,53] The better prepared health care providers, institutions, volunteers, and communities are to care for children and families during disasters, the better the outcomes will be and the smaller the chances of unintended harm.[105] With that in mind, the most important step to reducing liability risk for providers during a disaster, regardless of type and location of health care practice, is to remain informed and prepared for a potential disaster. Expanding the pool of properly trained pediatric volunteers who can be quickly mobilized remains a national priority.

The time has long passed when health care providers can think that it will never happen to them. In 2000, the AAP Committee on Pediatric Emergency Medicine and the AAP Committee on Medical Liability issued a joint statement on the need for professional liability insurance coverage for pediatricians volunteering during disasters.[106] Since that time, considerably more information has become available to broaden the understanding of the scope of this issue, allowing for it to be addressed more fully[§] Reducing liability risks for health care providers delivering essential medical care amid disasters requires a multilayered, coordinated approach through education, preparation, and, when appropriate, legislative protections. Recommendations related to this technical report are found in the accompanying policy statement of the same title (www.pediatrics.org/cgi/doi/10.1542/peds.2018-3892).[36]

LEAD AUTHORS

Robin L. Altman, MD, FAAP
Karen A. Santucci, MD, FAAP
Michael R. Anderson, MD, MBA, FAAP
William M. McDonnell, MD, JD, FAAP

[§] State laws are amended on a frequent basis. For information about current laws addressing medical liability in your state, please contact the AAP Division of State Government Affairs at stgov@aap.org.

COMMITTEE ON MEDICAL LIABILITY AND RISK MANAGEMENT, 2017–2018

Jon Mark Fanaroff, MD, JD, FAAP, Chairperson
Robin L. Altman, MD, FAAP
Steven A. Bondi, JD, MD, FAAP
Sandeep K. Narang, MD, JD, FAAP
Richard L. Oken, MD, FAAP
John W. Rusher, MD, JD, FAAP
Karen A. Santucci, MD, FAAP
James P. Scibilia, MD, FAAP
Susan M. Scott, MD, JD, FAAP
Laura J. Sigman, MD, JD, FAAP

FORMER COMMITTEE MEMBER

William M. McDonnell, MD, JD, FAAP

CONSULTANT

Michael R. Anderson, MD, MBA, FAAP

STAFF

Julie Kersten Ake

ACKNOWLEDGMENT

We extend our appreciation to Jay Goldsmith, MD, FAAP, for his review and technical advice.

ABBREVIATIONS

AAP: American Academy of Pediatrics
ASPR: Assistant Secretary of Preparedness and Response
CMS: Centers for Medicare and Medicaid Services
EMTALA: Emergency Medical Treatment and Labor Act
HIPAA: Health Insurance Portability and Accountability Act
NDMS: National Disaster Medical System

The guidance in this report does not indicate an exclusive course of treatment or serve as a standard of medical care. Variations, taking into account individual circumstances, may be appropriate.

All technical reports from the American Academy of Pediatrics automatically expire 5 years after publication unless reaffirmed, revised, or retired at or before that time.

DOI: https://doi.org/10.1542/peds.2018-3893

Address correspondence to Robin L. Altman, MD, FAAP. Email: robin_altman@nymc.edu.

PEDIATRICS (ISSN Numbers: Print, 0031-4005; Online, 1098-4275).

Copyright © 2019 by the American Academy of Pediatrics

FINANCIAL DISCLOSURE: The authors have indicated they have no financial relationships relevant to this article to disclose.

FUNDING: No external funding.

POTENTIAL CONFLICT OF INTEREST: The authors have indicated they have no potential conflicts of interest to disclose.

REFERENCES

1. Kelly F. Keeping PEDIATRICS in pediatric disaster management: before, during, and in the aftermath of complex emergencies. *Crit Care Nurs Clin North Am.* 2010;22(4):465–480
2. Pope TM, Palazzo MF. Legal briefing: crisis standards of care and legal protections during disasters and emergencies. *J Clin Ethics.* 2010;21(4):358–367
3. Hanfling D. When the bells toll: engaging healthcare providers in catastrophic disaster response planning. *South Med J.* 2013;106(1):7–12
4. Brandenburg MA, Arneson WL. Pediatric disaster response in developed countries: ten guiding principles. *Am J Disaster Med.* 2007;2(3):151–162
5. Tegtmeyer K, Conway EE Jr, Upperman JS, Kissoon N; Task Force for Pediatric Emergency Mass Critical Care. Education in a pediatric emergency mass critical care setting. *Pediatr Crit Care Med.* 2011;12(suppl 6):S135–S140
6. Sirbaugh PE. Katrina changed us (and me) in so many ways. *Pediatrics.* 2011;128(suppl 1):S20–S22
7. Hodge JG Jr, Garcia AM, Anderson ED, Kaufman T. Emergency legal preparedness for hospitals and health care personnel. *Disaster Med Public Health Prep.* 2009;3(suppl 2):S37–S44
8. American Academy of Pediatrics Committee on Pediatric Emergency Medicine; American Academy of Pediatrics Committee on Medical Liability; Task Force on Terrorism. The pediatrician and disaster preparedness. *Pediatrics.* 2006;117(2):560–565
9. Markenson D, Reynolds S; American Academy of Pediatrics Committee on Pediatric Emergency Medicine; Task Force on Terrorism. The pediatrician and disaster preparedness. *Pediatrics.* 2006;117(2). Available at: www.pediatrics.org/cgi/content/full/117/2/e340
10. Hodge JG Jr. The evolution of law in biopreparedness. *Biosecur Bioterror.* 2012;10(1):38–48
11. Courtney B, Hodge JG Jr; Task Force for Pediatric Emergency Mass Critical Care. Legal considerations during pediatric emergency mass critical care events. *Pediatr Crit Care Med.* 2011;12(suppl 6):S152–S156
12. Mace SE, Sharieff G, Bern A, et al. Pediatric issues in disaster management, part 3: special healthcare needs patients and mental health issues. *Am J Disaster Med.* 2010;5(5):261–274
13. Garrett AL, Grant R, Madrid P, Brito A, Abramson D, Redlener I. Children and megadisasters: lessons learned in the new millennium. *Adv Pediatr.* 2007;54:189–214
14. Pou AM. Ethical and legal challenges in disaster medicine: are you ready? *South Med J.* 2013;106(1):27–30
15. VanDevanter N, Kovner CT, Raveis VH, McCollum M, Keller R. Challenges of nurses' deployment to other New York City hospitals in the aftermath of Hurricane Sandy. *J Urban Health.* 2014;91(4):603–614
16. Gruich M Jr. Life-changing experiences of a private practicing pediatrician: perspectives from a private pediatric practice. *Pediatrics.* 2006;117(5, pt 3):S359–S364
17. Barkemeyer BM. Practicing neonatology in a blackout: the University Hospital NICU in the midst of Hurricane Katrina: caring for children without power or water. *Pediatrics.* 2006;117(5, pt 3):S369–S374
18. Spedale SB. Opening our doors for all newborns: caring for displaced neonates: intrastate. *Pediatrics.* 2006;117(5, pt 3):S389–S395
19. Thomas DE, Gordon ST, Melton JA, Funes CM, Collinsworth HJ, Vicari RC. Pediatricians' experiences 80 miles up the river: Baton Rouge pediatricians' experiences meeting the health needs of evacuated children. *Pediatrics.* 2006;117(5, pt 3):S396–S401
20. Shapiro A, Seim L, Christensen RC, et al. Chronicles from out-of-state professionals: providing primary care to underserved children after a disaster: a national organization response. *Pediatrics.* 2006;117(5, pt 3):S412–S415
21. Baldwin S, Robinson A, Barlow P, Fargason CA Jr. Moving hospitalized children all over the southeast: interstate transfer of pediatric patients during Hurricane Katrina. *Pediatrics.* 2006;117(5, pt 3):S416–S420
22. Sirbaugh PE, Gurwitch KD, Macias CG, Ligon BL, Gavagan T, Feigin RD. Caring for evacuated children housed in the Astrodome: creation and implementation of a mobile pediatric emergency response team: regionalized caring for displaced children after a disaster. *Pediatrics.* 2006;117(5, pt 3):S428–S438
23. Madrid PA, Schacher SJ. A critical concern: pediatrician self-care after disasters [published correction appears in *Pediatrics.* 2006;118(5):2271]. *Pediatrics.* 2006;117(5, pt 3):S454–S457
24. Fink S. The deadly choices at memorial. *The New York Times.* August 25, 2009. Available at: www.nytimes.com/2009/08/30/magazine/30doctors.html?pagewanted=all. Accessed July 24, 2017
25. Burkle FM Jr, Williams A, Kissoon N; Task Force for Pediatric Emergency Mass Critical Care. Pediatric emergency mass critical care: the role of community preparedness in conserving

critical care resources. *Pediatr Crit Care Med.* 2011;12(suppl 6):S141–S151

26. Watson CM, Barnett DJ, Thompson CB, et al. Characterizing public health emergency perceptions and influential modifiers of willingness to respond among pediatric healthcare staff. *Am J Disaster Med.* 2011;6(5):299–308
27. Rothstein MA. Currents in contemporary ethics. Malpractice immunity for volunteer physicians in public health emergencies: adding insult to injury. *J Law Med Ethics.* 2010; 38(1):149–153
28. Iserson KV, Heine CE, Larkin GL, Moskop JC, Baruch J, Aswegan AL. Fight or flight: the ethics of emergency physician disaster response. *Ann Emerg Med.* 2008;51(4):345–353
29. Jacobson PD, Wasserman J, Botoseneanu A, Silverstein A, Wu HW. The role of law in public health preparedness: opportunities and challenges. *J Health Polit Policy Law.* 2012;37(2):297–328
30. Courtney B, Hodge JG Jr, Toner ES, et al; Task Force for Mass Critical Care. Legal preparedness: care of the critically ill and injured during pandemics and disasters: CHEST consensus statement. *Chest.* 2014;146(suppl 4):e134S–e144S
31. Qureshi K, Gershon RM, Conde F. Factors that influence Medical Reserve Corps recruitment. *Prehosp Disaster Med.* 2008;23(3):s27–s34
32. Rutkow L, Vernick JS, Thompson CB, Piltch-Loeb R, Barnett DJ. Legal protections to promote response willingness among the local public health workforce. *Disaster Med Public Health Prep.* 2015;9(2):98–102
33. Weiss RI, McKie KL, Goodman RA. The law and emergencies: surveillance for public health-related legal issues during Hurricanes Katrina and Rita. *Am J Public Health.* 2007;97(suppl 1): S73–S81
34. Rosenbaum S, Harty MB, Sheer J. State laws extending comprehensive legal liability protections for professional health-care volunteers during public health emergencies. *Public Health Rep.* 2008;123(2):238–241
35. Hanfling D, Altevogt BM, Viswanathan K, Gostin LO, eds; Committee on Guidance for Establishing Crisis Standards of Care for Use in Disaster Situations; Institute of Medicine. *Crisis Standards of Care: A Systems Framework for Catastrophic Disaster Response.* Washington, DC: The National Academies Press; 2012. Available at: https://www.ncbi.nlm.nih.gov/books/NBK201063/pdf/Bookshelf_NBK201063.pdf. Accessed July 24, 2017
36. Altman RL, Santucci KA, Anderson MR, McDonnell WM; Committee on Medical Liability and Risk Management. Understanding liability risks and protections for pediatric providers during disasters. *Pediatrics.* 2019; 143(3):e20183892
37. Barnett DJ, Taylor HA, Hodge JG Jr, Links JM. Resource allocation on the frontlines of public health preparedness and response: report of a summit on legal and ethical issues. *Public Health Rep.* 2009;124(2):295–303
38. Antommaria AH, Kaziny BD. Ethical issues in pediatric emergency medicine's preparation for and response to disasters. *Virtual Mentor.* 2012;14(10):801–804
39. Altevogt BM, Stroud C, Hanson SL, Hanfling D, Gostin LO, eds; Committee on Guidance for Establishing Standards of Care for Use in Disaster Situations; Institute of Medicine. *Guidance for Establishing Crisis Standards of Care for Use in Disaster Situations: A Letter Report.* Washington, DC: The National Academies Press; 2009. Available at: https://www.ncbi.nlm.nih.gov/books/NBK219958/pdf/Bookshelf_NBK219958.pdf. Accessed July 24, 2017
40. Mace SE, Sharieff G, Bern A, et al. Pediatric issues in disaster management, part 2: evacuation centers and family separation/reunification. *Am J Disaster Med.* 2010; 5(3):149–161
41. Weiner DL, Manzi SF, Waltzman ML, Morin M, Meginniss A, Fleisher GR. FEMA's organized response with a pediatric subspecialty team: the National Disaster Medical System response: a pediatric perspective. *Pediatrics.* 2006;117(5, pt 3):S405–S411
42. Roszak AR, Jensen FR, Wild RE, Yeskey K, Handrigan MT. Implications of the Emergency Medical Treatment and Labor Act (EMTALA) during public health emergencies and on alternate sites of care. *Disaster Med Public Health Prep.* 2009;3(suppl 2):S172–S175
43. Iserson KV, Moskop JC. Triage in medicine, part I: concept, history, and types. *Ann Emerg Med.* 2007;49(3): 275–281
44. Markovitz BP. Pediatric critical care surge capacity. *J Trauma.* 2009;67(suppl 2):S140–S142
45. Zoraster RM, Burkle CM. Disaster documentation for the clinician. *Disaster Med Public Health Prep.* 2013; 7(4):354–360
46. Cohen R, Murphy B, Ahern T, Hackel A. Regional disaster planning for neonatology. *J Perinatol.* 2010;30(11): 709–711
47. Eddy A. First responder and physician liability during an emergency. *Am J Disaster Med.* 2013;8(4):267–272
48. Hoffman S, Goodman RA, Stier DD. Law, liability, and public health emergencies. *Disaster Med Public Health Prep.* 2009; 3(2):117–125
49. Williams SP, Boyd HS. Is there much limited legal liability protection for physicians in crisis standards of care in SC? *J S C Med Assoc.* 2011;107(3): 96–98
50. Schonfeld DJ, Demaria T; Disaster Preparedness Advisory Council; Committee on Psychosocial Aspects of Child and Family Health. Providing psychosocial support to children and families in the aftermath of disasters and crises. *Pediatrics.* 2015;136(4). Available at: www.pediatrics.org/cgi/content/full/136/4/e1120
51. Rutkow L, Vernick JS, Wissow LS, Tung GJ, Marum F, Barnett DJ. Legal issues affecting children with preexisting conditions during public health emergencies. *Biosecur Bioterror.* 2013; 11(2):89–95
52. Fanaroff JM; Committee on Medical Liability and Risk Management. Consent by proxy for nonurgent pediatric care. *Pediatrics.* 2017;139(2):e20163911
53. Foltin GL, Lucky C, Portelli I, et al. Overcoming legal obstacles involving the voluntary care of children who are separated from their legal guardians during a disaster. *Pediatr Emerg Care.* 2008;24(6):392–398

54. Sauer LM, Catlett C, Tosatto R, Kirsch TD. The utility of and risks associated with the use of spontaneous volunteers in disaster response: a survey. *Disaster Med Public Health Prep.* 2014;8(1): 65–69

55. Bailey PV. A crisis in the ED: liability protection needed STAT. *Bull Am Coll Surg.* 2012;97(3):19–22

56. Thompson T, Lyle K, Mullins SH, Dick R, Graham J. A state survey of emergency department preparedness for the care of children in a mass casualty event. *Am J Disaster Med.* 2009;4(4):227–232

57. Hodge JG Jr, Brown EF. Assessing liability for health care entities that insufficiently prepare for catastrophic emergencies. *JAMA.* 2011;306(3): 308–309

58. Chokshi NK, Behar S, Nager AL, Dorey F, Upperman JS. Disaster management among pediatric surgeons: preparedness, training and involvement. *Am J Disaster Med.* 2008; 3(1):5–14

59. Maldin B, Lam C, Franco C, et al. Regional approaches to hospital preparedness. *Biosecur Bioterror.* 2007; 5(1):43–53

60. The Joint Commission. Surge hospitals: providing safe care in emergencies. 2006. Available at: https://www.jointcommission.org/assets/1/18/surge_hospital.pdf. Accessed July 24, 2017

61. Ferrer RR, Balasuriya D, Iverson E, Upperman JS. Pediatric disaster preparedness of a hospital network in a large metropolitan region. *Am J Disaster Med.* 2010;5(1):27–34

62. Public Health Service Act, 42 USC §247d-6d (2006)

63. Fink S. Trial to open in lawsuit connected to hospital deaths after Katrina. *The New York Times.* March 20, 2011. Available at: www.nytimes.com/2011/03/21/us/21hospital.html?r=1&ref=tenethealthcarecorporation. Accessed July 24, 2017

64. US Department of Health and Human Services. Pandemic and All-Hazards Preparedness Act, 42 §USC 300hh et seq (2006). Available at: https://www.phe.gov/preparedness/legal/pahpa/pages/default.aspx. Accessed January 29, 2019

65. Centers for Medicare and Medicaid Services. Emergency preparedness rule. Available at: https://www.cms.gov/Medicare/Provider-Enrollment-and-Certification/SurveyCertEmergPrep/Emergency-Prep-Rule.html. Accessed July 24, 2017

66. Suk M. Sovereign immunity: principles and application in medical malpractice. *Clin Orthop Relat Res.* 2012;470(5): 1365–1369

67. Federal Emergency Management Agency. The disaster declaration process. Available at: https://www.fema.gov/disaster-declaration-process. Accessed July 24, 2017

68. Hodge JG, Anderson ED. Principles and practice of legal triage during public health emergencies. *Annu Surv Am Law.* 2008;64:249–291

69. US Department of Health and Human Services, Office of the Assistant Secretary for Preparedness and Response. 1135 waivers. Available at: https://www.phe.gov/Preparedness/legal/Pages/1135-waivers.aspx. Accessed July 24, 2017

70. Hershey TB, Van Nostrand E, Sood RK, Potter M. Legal considerations for health care practitioners after Superstorm Sandy. *Disaster Med Public Health Prep.* 2016;10(3):518–524

71. Cole C, Marzen C. A review of state sovereign immunity statutes and the management of liability risks by states. *Journal of Insurance Regulation.* 2013; 32:45–82

72. Stier DD, Goodman RA. Mutual aid agreements: essential legal tools for public health preparedness and response. *Am J Public Health.* 2007;97 (suppl 1):S62–S68

73. Mace SE, Sharieff G, Bern A, et al. Pediatric issues in disaster management, part 1: the emergency medical system and surge capacity. *Am J Disaster Med.* 2010;5(2):83–93

74. Lopez W, Kershner SP, Penn MS. EMAC volunteers: liability and workers' compensation. *Biosecur Bioterror.* 2013; 11(3):217–225

75. Hanna J. Good Samaritan Act doesn't shield on-duty emergency doctors. *Ill Bar J.* 2014;102(5):214

76. Hodge JG Jr, Pepe RP, Henning WH. Voluntarism in the wake of Hurricane Katrina: the uniform emergency volunteer health practitioners act. *Disaster Med Public Health Prep.* 2007; 1(1):44–50

77. Foxhall K. License to serve: a model law could make it easier for medical volunteers to respond immediately during emergencies. *State Legis.* 2008; 34(4):27–28

78. Uniform Law Commission. Emergency volunteer health practitioners. Available at: https://www.facs.org/advocacy/state/uevhpa. Accessed July 24, 2017

79. Hodge JG Jr, Gable LA, Cálves SH. Volunteer health professionals and emergencies: assessing and transforming the legal environment. *Biosecur Bioterror.* 2005;3(3):216–223

80. American Telemedicine Association. Disaster relief center: resources to prepare for and respond to natural disasters. Available at: http://www.americantelemed.org/main/policy-page/state-policy-resource-center. Accessed July 24, 2017

81. Hoard ML, Tosatto RJ. Medical Reserve Corps: strengthening public health and improving preparedness. *Disaster Manag Response.* 2005;3(2):48–52

82. Orenstein DG. When law is not law: setting aside legal provisions during declared emergencies. *J Law Med Ethics.* 2013;41(suppl 1):73–76

83. The Network for Public Health Law. Legal liability protections for emergency medical/public health responses. Available at: https://www.networkforphl.org/_asset/xbt7sg/Liability-Protections-for-Emergency-Response.pdf. Accessed July 24, 2017

84. Disaster Preparedness Advisory Council. Medical countermeasures for children in public health emergencies, disasters, or terrorism. *Pediatrics.* 2016;137(2):e20154273

85. US Department of Homeland Security. Planning. Available at: https://www.ready.gov/planning. Accessed July 24, 2017

86. Disaster Preparedness Advisory Council; Committee on Pediatric Emergency Medicine. Ensuring the health of children in disasters. *Pediatrics.* 2015;136(5). Available at:

www.pediatrics.org/cgi/content/full/136/5/e1407

87. Krug SE, Needle S, Schonfeld D, Aird L, Hurley H. Improving pediatric preparedness performance through strategic partnerships. *Disaster Med Public Health Prep.* 2012;6(2):94–96

88. American Academy of Pediatrics. Strategic plan for disaster preparedness. Available at: www.aap.org/disasters/strategicplan. Accessed July 24, 2017

89. Emergency Medical Services for Children Innovation and Improvement Center. National pediatric readiness project. Available at: https://emscimprovement.center/projects/pediatricreadiness/. Accessed July 24, 2017

90. Krug SE, Tait VF, Aird L. Helping the helpers to help children: advances by the American Academy of Pediatrics. *Pediatrics.* 2011;128(suppl 1):S37–S39

91. American Academy of Pediatrics. Children and disasters. Available at: www.aap.org/disasters. Accessed July 24, 2017

92. American Academy of Pediatrics. Preparedness checklist for pediatric practices. 2013. Available at: www.aap.org/disasters/checklist. Accessed July 24, 2017

93. American Academy of Pediatrics. Children and youth with special needs. Available at: www.aap.org/disasters/cyshcn. Accessed July 24, 2017

94. US Department of Health and Human Services, Office of the Assistant Secretary for Preparedness and Response. Cultural and linguistic competency for disaster preparedness planning and crisis response. Available at: https://www.phe.gov/Preparedness/planning/abc/Pages/linguistic.aspx. Accessed July 24, 2017

95. Stankovic C, Mahajan P, Ye H, Dunne RB, Knazik SR. Bioterrorism: evaluating the preparedness of pediatricians in Michigan. *Pediatr Emerg Care.* 2009;25(2):88–92

96. Branson RD. Disaster planning for pediatrics. *Respir Care.* 2011;56(9):1457–1463; discussion 1463–1465

97. Allen GM, Parrillo SJ, Will J, Mohr JA. Principles of disaster planning for the pediatric population. *Prehosp Disaster Med.* 2007;22(6):537–540

98. Federal Emergency Management Agency; US Department of Homeland Security. National response framework. 2016. Available at: https://www.fema.gov/media-library-data/20130726-1914-25045-1246/final_national_response_framework_20130501.pdf. Accessed July 24, 2017

99. US Department of Health and Human Services, Office of the Assistant Secretary for Preparedness and Response. Pandemic and All-Hazards Preparedness Reauthorization Act. Available at: https://www.phe.gov/preparedness/legal/pahpa/pages/pahpra.aspx. Accessed July 24, 2017

100. US Department of Health and Human Services, Office of the Assistant Secretary for Preparedness and Response. National advisory committee on children and disasters. Available at: https://www.phe.gov/Preparedness/legal/boards/naccd/Pages/default.aspx. Accessed July 24, 2017

101. US Department of Health and Human Services, Office of the Assistant Secretary for Preparedness and Response. National biodefense science board. Available at: https://www.phe.gov/nprsb. Accessed July 24, 2017

102. Benjamin GC, Moulton AD. Public health legal preparedness: a framework for action. *J Law Med Ethics.* 2008;36(suppl 1):13–17

103. Gausche-Hill M. Pediatric disaster preparedness: are we really prepared? *J Trauma.* 2009;67(suppl 2):S73–S76

104. Dunlop AL, Logue KM, Isakov AP. The engagement of academic institutions in community disaster response: a comparative analysis. *Public Health Rep.* 2014;129(suppl 4):87–95

105. Fitch E. Managing the risks of incorporating volunteers into public health emergency response: the other side of the liability issue. *Disaster Med Public Health Prep.* 2010;4(3):252–254

106. Committee on Pediatric Emergency Medicine; Committee on Medical Liability. Pediatricians' liability during disasters. *Pediatrics.* 2000;106(6):1492–1493

Unique Needs of the Adolescent

- *Policy Statement*

POLICY STATEMENT Organizational Principles to Guide and Define the Child Health Care System and/or Improve the Health of all Children

American Academy of Pediatrics

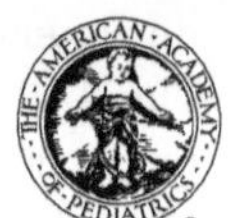

DEDICATED TO THE HEALTH OF ALL CHILDREN™

Unique Needs of the Adolescent

Elizabeth M. Alderman, MD, FSAHM, FAAP,[a] Cora C. Breuner, MD, MPH, FAAP,[b] COMMITTEE ON ADOLESCENCE

abstract

Adolescence is the transitional bridge between childhood and adulthood; it encompasses developmental milestones that are unique to this age group. Healthy cognitive, physical, sexual, and psychosocial development is both a right and a responsibility that must be guaranteed for all adolescents to successfully enter adulthood. There is consensus among national and international organizations that the unique needs of adolescents must be addressed and promoted to ensure the health of all adolescents. This policy statement outlines the special health challenges that adolescents face on their journey and transition to adulthood and provides recommendations for those who care for adolescents, their families, and the communities in which they live.

[a]Division of Adolescent Medicine, Department of Pediatrics, Albert Einstein College of Medicine and The Children's Hospital at Montefiore, Bronx, New York; and [b]Division of Adolescent Medicine, Departments of Pediatrics and Orthopedics and Sports Medicine, University of Washington and Seattle Children's Hospital, Seattle, Washington

Policy statements from the American Academy of Pediatrics benefit from expertise and resources of liaisons and internal (AAP) and external reviewers. However, policy statements from the American Academy of Pediatrics may not reflect the views of the liaisons or the organizations or government agencies that they represent.

Drs Alderman and Breuner were equally responsible for writing and revising this policy statement with input from various internal and external reviewers as well as the Board of Directors, and both authors approved the final manuscript as submitted.

The guidance in this statement does not indicate an exclusive course of treatment or serve as a standard of medical care. Variations, taking into account individual circumstances, may be appropriate.

All policy statements from the American Academy of Pediatrics automatically expire 5 years after publication unless reaffirmed, revised, or retired at or before that time.

This document is copyrighted and is property of the American Academy of Pediatrics and its Board of Directors. All authors have filed conflict of interest statements with the American Academy of Pediatrics. Any conflicts have been resolved through a process approved by the Board of Directors. The American Academy of Pediatrics has neither solicited nor accepted any commercial involvement in the development of the content of this publication.

DOI: https://doi.org/10.1542/peds.2019-3150

Address correspondence to Elizabeth M. Alderman, MD, FSAHM, FAAP. Email: ealderma@montefiore.org

PEDIATRICS (ISSN Numbers: Print, 0031-4005; Online, 1098-4275).

Copyright © 2019 by the American Academy of Pediatrics

FINANCIAL DISCLOSURE: The authors have indicated they have no financial relationships relevant to this article to disclose.

FUNDING: No external funding.

To cite: Alderman EM, Breuner CC, AAP COMMITTEE ON ADOLESCENCE. Unique Needs of the Adolescent. *Pediatrics*. 2019;144(6):e20193150

Adolescence, defined as 11 through 21 years of age,[1] is a critical period of development in a young person's life, one filled with distinctive and pivotal biological, cognitive, emotional, and social changes.[2] The World Health Organization[3]; the Office of Adolescent Health of the US Department of Health and Human Services[4]; the Health and Medicine Division of the National Academies of Sciences, Engineering, and Medicine (formerly the Institute of Medicine)[5,6]; the *Lancet*,[7] with 4 international academic institutions[8]; and the Society for Adolescent Health and Medicine[9] have called for a closer examination of the unique health needs of adolescents. In 2018, *Nature* devoted an issue to the advances in the science of adolescence and called for ongoing further study of this important population.[10] As a leader in adolescent health care, the American Academy of Pediatrics (AAP) is motivated to describe why adolescents are a unique and vulnerable population and why it is crucial that the AAP focus on adolescents' health concerns to optimize healthy development during the transition to adulthood. Addressing the unique needs of adolescents with disabilities is outside the scope of this statement; several statements specific to this population are available at https://pediatrics.aappublications.org/collection/council-children-disabilities. In addition, specific guidance around the transition to adult health care is not covered in this statement; please refer to the list of transition resources at the end of this document.

The need for comprehensive health services for teenagers has been well documented since the 1990s.[11–13] The AAP advocates for the pediatrician to provide the medical home for adolescent primary care.[14] Other professional societies, such as the Society for Adolescent Health and Medicine, the American Academy of Family Physicians, and the American College of Obstetricians and Gynecologists and school-based health initiatives (https://www.sbh4all.org/), recognize the unique needs of adolescents. These organizations recommend an increase in adolescent medicine training, along with the Accreditation Committee for Graduate Medical Education. The Accreditation Committee for Graduate Medical Education currently requires only 1 month of adolescent medicine training from a board-certified adolescent medicine specialist for all pediatric residency programs (adolescent medicine; [Core] IV.A.6.[b].[3].[a].[i]); there must be one educational unit).[15] The importance of addressing the physical and mental health of adolescents has become more evident, with investigators in recent studies pointing to the fact that unmet health needs during adolescence and in the transition to adulthood predict not only poor health outcomes as adults but also lower quality of life in adulthood.[16]

HEALTH RISKS IN ADOLESCENCE

A hallmark of adolescence is a gradual development toward autonomy and individual adult decision-making. However, adolescents are often faced with situations for which they may not be prepared, and many are likely to be involved in risk-taking behaviors, such as use of alcohol, tobacco, and other drugs and engaging in unprotected sex. Most recently, there is increased concern about the rise in electronic cigarette use among adolescence.[17] In fact, most health care visits by adolescents to their pediatricians or other health care providers are to seek treatment of conditions or injuries that could have been prevented if screened for and addressed at an earlier comprehensive visit.[18] Although some risk-taking behavior is considered normal in adolescence, engaging in certain types of risky behavior can have adverse and potentially long-term health consequences. The majority of mortality and morbidity during adolescence, which can be prevented, is attributable to unintentional injuries, suicide, and homicide.[19] Approximately 72% of deaths among adolescents are attributable to injuries from motor vehicle crashes, other unintentional and intentional injuries, injuries caused by firearms, injuries influenced by use of alcohol and illicit substances, homicide, or suicide.[20,21] These causes of death greatly surpass medical etiologies such as cancer, HIV infection, and heart disease in the United States and other industrialized nations.[21]

The AAP *Bright Futures: Guidelines for Health Supervision of Infants, Children, and Adolescents* recommends a strength-based approach to screening and counseling around these behaviors that lead to mortality and morbidity in adolescents.[1,22] However, according to the National Ambulatory Medical Care Survey and the National Hospital Ambulatory Medical Care Survey, only 39% of adolescents received any type of preventive counseling during ambulatory visits.[23] Seventy-one percent of teenagers reported at least 1 potential health risk, yet only 37% of these teenagers reported discussing any of these risks with their pediatrician or primary care physician. Clearly, screening for and counseling around these high-risk behaviors needs to be improved.[24]

New screening codes for depression, substance use, and alcohol and tobacco use as well as brief intervention services may provide opportunities to receive payment for the services pediatricians are providing to adolescents. These include 96127, brief emotional and behavioral assessment (eg, depression inventory, attention-deficit/hyperactivity disorder scale) with scoring and documentation, per standardized instrument, and 96150, health and behavior assessment (eg, health-focused clinical interview, behavioral observations, psychophysiological monitoring, health-oriented questionnaires).[25] However, it is important to recognize that coding for specific diagnoses may be challenging if the patient does not want his or her parent(s) to know the reasons for the clinical visit. Adolescent visits and documentation of visits are confidential to promote better access and to protect the rights of adolescents.[26]

Another trend in the health status of adolescents (reflecting technological advances in pediatric medical care) is the increasing number of pediatric patients with chronic medical conditions and developmental challenges who enter adolescence. Adolescents with chronic conditions face developmental challenges similar to their healthy peers but may have special educational, vocational, and transitional concerns because of their medical issues.[27]

The prevalence of chronic medical conditions and developmental and physical disabilities in adolescents is difficult to assess because of the variation of study methodologies and categorical versus noncategorical approaches to the epidemiology of chronic illness.[28] According to the National Survey of Children's Health, funded by the US Department of Health and Human Services, almost 31% of adolescents have 1 moderate to severe chronic illness, such as asthma or a mental health condition.[29] Other common chronic illnesses include obesity, cancer, cardiac disease, HIV infection, spastic quadriplegia, and developmental disabilities.[30–32] One in 4 adolescents with chronic illness has at least 1 unmet health need that may affect physical growth and development, including puberty and overall health status as well as future adult health.[33]

Within pediatric practice, integrating adolescent-centered, family-involved approaches into the care of adolescents as well as culturally competent and effective approaches (as outlined in *Bright Futures: Guidelines for Health Supervision of Infants, Children, and Adolescents*) has the potential not only to identify threats to well-being but also to create a space to work with families to bolster opportunities for optimal development of all children.[1] When considering the health challenges adolescents face, it is imperative to take into account not only the ethnic and racial diversity of the adolescent population in the United States but also the social and ecologic factors (eg, socioeconomic status, family composition, parental education and engagement, neighborhood and school environment, religion, earlier childhood trauma and toxic stress, and access to health care).

The Search Foundation has conducted research that suggests that for minority youth, a positive ethnic identity is a critical spark for emergence of the required developmental assets to enable adolescents to develop into successful and contributing adults.[34,35] This theory is supported by a recent study in *The Journal of Pediatrics* that suggests minority youth are still prone to depression because of isolation and discrimination faced during adolescence while navigating neighborhood and school environments, even when they have educated and supportive parents.[36] African American male adolescents have the highest rates of mortality, followed by American Indian, white, Hispanic, and Asian American or Pacific Islander male adolescents, pointing to racial and ethnic disparities in adolescent health and the potential to achieve a healthy adulthood.[37]

The AAP has previously published policy statements addressing the unique strengths and health disparities that exist for specific groups of adolescents, such as lesbian, gay, bisexual, and transgender youth and those in the juvenile justice system, foster care, and the military.[38–42] Pediatricians must pay attention to how care is delivered to the increasingly diverse adolescent populations to prevent a decline in health status and increase in health care disparities.

UNIQUE BIOLOGICAL AND PSYCHOSOCIAL CHANGES OCCURRING DURING ADOLESCENCE

Biological and psychosocial changes that occur during adolescence make this age group unique. Research describing the timing and physiology of puberty has been invaluable in revealing not only differences between racial groups but also between adolescents with different chronic conditions.[43–46]

Puberty

Puberty is the hallmark of physiologic progression from child to adult body habitus. Chronic conditions, such as obesity and intracranial lesions, or trauma may cause early puberty, which may put the adolescent at risk for engagement in higher-risk behaviors at an earlier age.[44] Delayed puberty is often a variant of normal development but may also be seen in adolescents with inflammatory bowel disease, eating disorders, and chronic conditions that create malnutrition as well as adolescents who have undergone treatment of malignancies. Comorbid mental disease (eg, an eating disorder that causes delayed puberty) or medication for psychiatric illness that causes obesity, which may cause early puberty, can complicate optimal adolescent psychosocial development.

Brain Development

The work of Giedd[47] and others shows that brain development during adolescence is ongoing and affects behavior and health. Because of changes in signaling that relate to the reward system in which the brain motivates behavior and the continuing maturation of the parts of the brain that regulate impulse control, adolescents may have a propensity to be involved with high-risk behaviors and have heightened response to emotionally loaded situations. In addition, adverse childhood experiences can have an impact on brain development, affecting behaviors and health during adolescence.[48] During adolescence, there is a "pruning" of gray matter and synapses, which makes the brain more efficient.[47] White matter increases throughout adolescence, which allows the older adolescent and adult brain to conduct more-complex cognitive tasks and adaptive behavior.[49]

Increasingly, studies show that the adolescent brain responds to alcohol and illicit substances differently than adults.[50,51] This difference may explain the increased risk of binge drinking as well as greater untoward cognitive effects of alcohol and marijuana.

Sexual Orientation and Gender Identification

Sexual (and gender) development is a process that starts early in childhood and involves negotiating and experimenting with identity, relationships, and roles. In early adolescence, people begin to recognize or become aware of their sexual orientation.[52,53]

However, some adolescents are still unsure of their sexual attractions, and others struggle with their known sexual attraction. Adolescence is a time of identity formation and experimentation, so labels that one uses for their sexual orientation (eg, gay, straight, bisexual, etc) often do not correlate to actual sexual behaviors and partners. Sexual orientation and behaviors should be assessed by the pediatrician without making assumptions. Adolescents should be allowed to apply and explain the labels they choose to use for sexuality and gender using open-ended questions.[54–56]

Sexual minority adolescents may engage in heterosexual practices, and heterosexual adolescents may engage in same-sex sexual activity. Depending on their specific behaviors and the gender of various partners, all sexually active adolescents may be at risk for sexually transmitted infections and unplanned pregnancy. Sexual minority youth are at higher risk of sexually transmitted infections and unplanned pregnancy, often because they do not receive education that applies to their sexual behaviors and are less likely to be screened appropriately (http://www.cdc.gov/healthyyouth/disparities/smy.htm).[57,58]

Sexual minority and transgender youth, because of the stigma they face, are also at higher risk of mental health problems, including depression and suicidality, altered body image, and substance use.[38]

There is strong evidence that when sexual minority and transgender youth feel they cannot express their true selves, they go underground by either hiding or denying their attractions and identity.[59] When this is combined with reinforcing parental rejection, bullying, etc, it is believed to lead to internalization, low self-esteem, and ultimately, depression and suicide.[59] Using an explanation like this places the problem on the societal context, not the adolescent or his or her identity.[38,39,60,61]

A relatively higher proportion of homeless adolescents are lesbian, gay, bisexual, transgender, and queer or questioning youth.[61] They leave their family homes because of abuse or having been thrown out. These adolescents are at high risk for victimization and often need to engage in unsafe sexual practices to provide themselves food and shelter.[61]

Mental health problems may become more pronounced when sexual minority teenagers come out during adolescence to unsupportive family members and friends or health care providers.[38] These youth are more likely to experience violence both in their homes and in their schools and communities. Studies have shown that sexual minority youth reveal higher rates of tobacco, alcohol, marijuana, and other illicit substance use.[62]

Most adolescents identify by and express a gender that conforms to their anatomic sex. However, some adolescents experience gender dysphoria with their anatomic sex when entering puberty. As they consider transgender options, they are at an increased risk of mental or emotional health problems, including depression and suicidality, victimization and violence, eating disorders, substance use, and unaccepting or intolerant family members and peers. Crucial to the successful navigation of gender dysphoria issues are health care providers who can assist transgender youth and families to achieve safe, healthy transitioning both in the postponement of puberty, when indicated, and in transitioning to preferred gender with psychosocial and behavioral support.[59]

Legal Status

Adolescence heralds a change of legal status, in which the age of 18 or 19 years transforms legal status from minors to adults with full legal privileges and obligations related to health care. However, certain states afford minors the right to confidentiality and consent to or for reproductive and mental health and substance use treatment confidential health services.[26,63] Generally, minors may receive confidential screening and care for sexually transmitted infections in all 50 states and the District of Columbia. However, accessing contraception to prevent unwanted pregnancy as well as the ability to self-consent to pregnancy options counseling, prenatal care, and termination of pregnancy vary between states.[64] These discrepancies also exist in accessing outpatient mental health and substance use services. Many adolescents in need of these services do not know they may have the right to access them on their own and may avoid interaction with the health care system to assist with reproductive and mental health concerns.[16] Delaying such care leads to adverse health outcomes.[16] A recent survey confirms that adolescents value private time with their health care providers, with confidentiality assurances by health care providers.[65] The need for office policies in negotiating private time was suggested. Moreover, health care providers reported needing more education in the provision of confidential services.[66] Adolescents in foster care may also be limited in their autonomous access to confidential services, which varies state to state.[41] In certain states, pregnant and parenting adolescents may have the right to consent for their care and the care of their child (https://www.guttmacher.org/state-policy/explore/minors-rights-parents, https://www.schoolhouseconnection.org/state-laws-on-minor-consent-for-routine-medical-care/). Few adolescents are considered emancipated minors and, thereby, entitled to all legal privileges of adults.[67]

Mental Health and Emotional Well-being

Mental health and emotional well-being, in combination with issues pertaining to sexual and reproductive health, violence and unintentional injury, substance use, eating disorders, and obesity, create potential challenges to adolescents' healthy emotional and physical development.[68] Approximately 20% of adolescents have a diagnosable mental health disorder.[69] Many mental health disorders present initially during adolescence. Twenty-five percent of adults with mood disorder had their first major depressive episode during adolescence.[70]

Suicide is the second leading cause of death in adolescents, resulting in more than 5700 deaths in 2016.[71] Between 2007 and 2016, the overall suicide rate for children and adolescents ages 10 to 19 years increased by 56%.[71] Older adolescents (15–19 years of age) are at an increased risk of suicide, with a rate of 5 in 100 000 for girls and 20 in 100 000 for boys.[71] According to the 2017 Youth Risk Behavior Survey of high school students, 7.4% of high school students attempted suicide in the last 12 months, and 13.6% made a suicide plan.[72] Adolescents with parents in the military were at increased risk of suicidal ideation (odds ratio [OR]: 1.43; 95% confidence interval [CI]: 1.37–1.49), making a plan to harm themselves (OR: 1.19; 95% CI: 1.06–1.34), attempting suicide (OR: 1.67; 95% CI: 1.43–1.95), and an attempted suicide that required medical treatment.[73]

Eating disorders typically present in the adolescent years. Although the incidence of eating disorders is low compared with depression, anxiety, and other mental health problems, these problems are often comorbid with eating disorders.[74] Moreover, the incidence of anorexia nervosa, bulimia nervosa, and other disordered eating is becoming more prevalent in formerly obese teenagers, male teenagers, and teenagers from lower socioeconomic groups.[75–77]

Teenagers with mental health issues may have subsequent poor school performance, school dropout, difficult family relationships, involvement in the juvenile justice system, substance use, and high-risk sexual behaviors.[78] Almost 70% of youth in the juvenile justice system have a diagnosed mental health disorder.[79,80]

Rates of serious mental health disorders among homeless youth range from 19% to 50%.[81,82] Homeless youth have a high need for treatment but rarely use formal treatment programs for medical, mental, and substance use services.[81] Confidentiality is also an issue for adolescents, as evidenced by the fact that in adolescents to whom confidentiality is not assured, there is a higher prevalence of depressive symptoms, suicidal thoughts, and suicide attempts.[83] There is a paucity of adequately trained mental health professionals to care for adolescents with these mental health challenges.[84] In addition, coverage for mental health services by insurance plans can be variable.[78]

Morbidity From High-Risk Sexual Activity

Multiple factors, including the increase in use of long-acting reversible contraception, have resulted in the teenage pregnancy rate decreasing in the United States over the past 20 years.[85,86] However, pregnancy still contributes to delays in educational and career success for adolescents. Moreover, pregnant teenagers are more likely to delay seeking medical care, putting them at risk for pregnancy-related health problems and putting their children at risk for prematurity and other negative birth outcomes.[87]

Adolescents continue to have the highest rates of sexually transmitted infections (eg, gonorrhea and *Chlamydia*).[88] Although screening most sexually active adolescents for *Chlamydia* infection is covered by the Patient Protection and Affordable Care Act (Pub L No. 111–148 [2010]) and recommended by the AAP *Bright Futures: Guidelines for Health Supervision of Infants, Children, and Adolescents*, adolescent concerns about billing and confidentiality are obstacles to medical screening.[1,89] Pediatricians can refer to AAP guidance to find appropriate codes for payment for providing adolescent health services (https://www.aap.org/en-us/Documents/coding_factsheet_adolescenthealth.pdf).

THE ADOLESCENT MEDICAL HOME

Consideration of the unique health risks as well as the biological and psychosocial elements of adolescence allows the AAP-endorsed patient-centered medical home (PCMH) to serve as an ideal conceptual framework by which a primary care practice can maximize the quality, efficiency, and patient experience of care. In 2007, the AAP joined the American Academy of Family Physicians, the American College of Physicians, and the American Osteopathic Association to endorse the "Joint Principals of the Patient-Centered Medical Home," which describes 7 core characteristics: (1) personal physician for every patient; (2) physician-directed medical practice; (3) whole person orientation; (4) care is coordinated and/or integrated; (5) quality and safety are hallmarks of PCMH care; (6)

enhanced access to care; and (7) appropriate payment for providing PCMH care.[90] The AAP, American Academy of Family Physicians, and American College of Physicians assert that optimal health care is achieved when each person, at every age, receives developmentally appropriate care.[91] Pediatricians provide quality adolescent care when they maintain relationships with families and with their patients and, thus, help patients develop autonomy, responsibility, and an adult identity.[92] Issues unique to adolescence to consider within the PCMH model include the following: adolescent-oriented developmentally appropriate care, which may require longer appointment times; confidentiality of health care visits, health records, billing, and the location where adolescents receive care; providers who offer such care; and the transition to adult care.[91,93] Moreover, using a strengths-based approach in the care of adolescents, as well as capitalizing on resiliency, is instrumental to maintaining the health of the individual adolescent.[94]

Schools have an important role for adolescents who either do not have access to a PCMH or do not use their access to receive recommended preventive services. School-based health centers and school-based mental health services can meet the needs of adolescents who do not have a PCMH or can coordinate school-based health services with the PCMH if the student has one. School nurses can help identify and refer adolescents who need these services.[95]

Financing health care of the adolescent can be challenging. Please see the detailed AAP policy statement on reforms in health care financing with the ultimate goal to improve the health care of all adolescents.[92]

RECOMMENDATIONS

On the basis of the unique biological and psychosocial aspects of adolescence, the AAP supports the following:

1. continued recognition by international and national organizations, including the AAP, the Society for Adolescent Health and Medicine, the American College of Obstetricians and Gynecologists, the North American Society for Pediatric and Adolescent Gynecology, and the American Academy of Family Physicians, of the need for policies and advocacy related to adolescent health and well-being;
2. sustained funding for research to further elucidate the biological basis of the growth and development of adolescents and how they affect adolescent behavior;
3. educational programs and adequate financial compensation for pediatricians and other health care professionals to support them in providing evidence-based, quality primary care for adolescents;
4. pediatricians receiving training on how to maintain the clinical setting as a "safe space," particularly in terms of confidentiality, especially when working with lesbian, gay, bisexual, transgender, and queer or questioning adolescents;
5. the role of schools, including school nurses and school-based health centers, and their role in promoting healthy adolescent development and providing access to health care;
6. further education, training, and advocacy for mental health care services that specifically address the needs of adolescents, preferably as part of a medical home model, stressing the importance of mental health for all youth;
7. federal confidentiality protection for mental health and reproductive services, as is currently provided in many states;
8. innovative postresidency training programs to increase the number of adolescent-trained pediatric providers in the workforce;
9. improved access to medical homes for all adolescents to ensure access to preventive medical care;
10. affiliation of middle and high schools with a physician trained to care for adolescents, unless the student already has access to comprehensive adolescent health services;
11. education for pediatricians so that they are aware of the laws regarding confidential care of adolescents in their states; and
12. familiarity with community resources for confidential reproductive and mental health care if they cannot provide confidential care themselves. Pediatricians who are unable to provide these services should learn about local community resources that provide confidential reproductive and mental health care.

The AAP recommends the following strategies targeted at improving financing for the health care of adolescents:

1. Federal and state agencies should increase their efforts to further reduce the number of adolescents who are not insured or who lack comprehensive and affordable health insurance.
2. The Centers for Medicare and Medicaid Services should implement its regulatory authority to update its standards for essential health benefits, as defined in the Patient Protection

and Affordable Care Act, in the 2 categories of mental and behavioral health services and pediatric services. These essential health benefits should be consistent with the full scope of benefits outlined in *Bright Futures: Guidelines for Health Supervision of Infants, Children, and Adolescents* (including health supervision visits, recommended immunizations, screening for high-risk conditions, and adequate counseling and treatment of conditions related to sexual, reproductive, mental, and behavioral health and substance use disorder). In this way, all adolescents can access the full range of services needed during this developmentally critical period to secure optimal physical and mental health on entry into midadulthood.

3. All health plans should provide preventive services without member cost sharing. In addition, to reduce financial barriers to care for adolescents, payers should limit the burden on families by reducing or eliminating copayments and eliminating coinsurance for visits related to anticipatory guidance and/or treatment of sexual and reproductive health, behavioral health, and immunization visits.
4. To provide sufficient payment to physicians and other health care providers for medical services to adolescents, insurers' claims systems should recognize and pay for all preventive medicine *Current Procedural Terminology* codes related to services for health and behavior assessment, counseling, risk screening, and/or appropriate interventions recommended in *Bright Futures*: *Guidelines for Health Supervision of Infants, Children, and Adolescents.* These services should not be bundled under a single health maintenance *Current Procedural Terminology* code.
5. Government and private insurance payers should increase the relative value unit allocation and level of payment for pediatricians delivering care and clinical preventive services to adolescents to a level that is commensurate with the time and effort expended, including health maintenance services, screening, and counseling.
6. The Centers for Medicare and Medicaid Services should mandate that payers provide enhanced access to cost-effective and clinically sound behavioral health services for adolescents, ensure that payment for all mental health services is more equitable with payment provided for medical and surgical services, and ensure that pediatricians are paid for mental health services provided during health maintenance and follow-up visits.

APPENDIX: ONLINE RESOURCES

AMERICAN ACADEMY OF PEDIATRICS

- Confidentiality Protections for Adolescents and Young Adults in the Health Care Billing and Insurance Claims Process: http://pediatrics.aappublications.org/content/137/5/e20160593
- Office-Based Care for Lesbian, Gay, Bisexual, Transgender, and Questioning Youth: http://pediatrics.aappublications.org/content/pediatrics/132/1/e297.full.pdf

SOCIETY FOR ADOLESCENT HEALTH AND MEDICINE

Resources for adolescents and parents are online resources aimed specifically at adolescents and their parents. Health care providers and youth-serving professionals can offer these additional resources or print a 1-page reference sheet (PDF) for adolescents and parents looking for additional information, including support groups, peer networks, helplines, treatment locators, and advocacy opportunities.

- Mental Health Resources for Adolescents: http://www.adolescenthealth.org/Topics-in-Adolescent-Health/Mental-Health/Mental-Health-Resources-For-Adolesc.aspx
- Mental Health Resources for Parents of Adolescents: http://www.adolescenthealth.org/Topics-in-Adolescent-Health/Mental-Health/Mental-Health-Resources-For-Parents-of-Adolescents.aspx
- Substance Use Resources for Adolescents: http://www.adolescenthealth.org/Topics-in-Adolescent-Health/Substance-Use/Substance-Use-Resources-For-Adolesc.aspx
- Substance Use Resources for Parents of Adolescents: http://www.adolescenthealth.org/Topics-in-Adolescent-Health/Substance-Use/Substance-Use-Resources-For-Parents-of-Adolesc.aspx
- Confidentiality in Health Care Resources for Adolescents and Parents of Adolescents: http://www.adolescenthealth.org/Topics-in-Adolescent-Health/Confidentiality/Confidentiality-Resources-For-Adolesc.aspx
- Sexual and Reproductive Health Resources for Adolescents: http://www.adolescenthealth.org/Topics-in-Adolescent-Health/Sexual-Reproductive-Health/Sexual-Reproductive-Health-Resources-For-Adolesc.aspx
- Sexual and Reproductive Health Resources for Parents of Adolescents: http://www.adolescenthealth.org/Topics-in-Adolescent-Health/Sexual-Reproductive-Health/SandRH-Resources-For-Parents-of-Adolesc.aspx
- Physical and Psychosocial Development Resources for

Adolescents: http://www.adolescenthealth.org/Topics-in-Adolescent-Health/Physical-and-Psychosocial-Development/Physical-Pschosocial-Develop-Resources-For-Adolesc.aspx

- Physical and Psychosocial Development Resources for Parents of Adolescents: http://www.adolescenthealth.org/Topics-in-Adolescent-Health/Physical-and-Psychosocial-Development/Physical-Psych-Resources-For-Parents-of-Adolesc.aspx

TRANSITION RESOURCES

General Resources

- National Health Care Transition Center (www.gottransition.org)
- Family Voices, Inc (www.familyvoices.org)
- National Alliance to Advance Adolescent Health (www.thenationalalliance.org)

Transition Care Plans

- AAP/National Center for Medical Home Implementation (www.medicalhomeinfo.org/how/care_delivery/transitions.aspx)
- British Columbia Ministry of Children and Family Development, "Transition Planning for Youth With Special Needs" (www.mcf.gov.bc.ca/spec_needs/pdf/support_guide.pdf)
- University of Washington, Adolescent Health Transition Project (http://depts.washington.edu/healthtr)

Transition Assessment and Evaluation Tools

- AAP/National Center for Medical Home Implementation (www.medicalhomeinfo.org/health/trans.html)
- JaxHATS, evaluation tools for youth and caregivers and training materials for medical providers (www.jaxhats.ufl.edu/docs)
- Texas Children's Hospital transition template (http://leah.mchtraining.net/bcm/resources/tracs)
- Carolina Health and Transition Project (www.mahec.net/quality/chat.aspx?a=10)
- University of Washington, Adolescent Health Transition Project (http://depts.washington.edu/healthtr)
- Wisconsin Community of Practice on Transition (www.waisman.wisc.edu/wrc/pdf/pubs/THCL.pdf)

NATIONAL ALLIANCE TO END HOMELESSNESS

- http://www.endhomelessness.org/

LEAD AUTHORS

Elizabeth M. Alderman, MD, FSAHM, FAAP
Cora C. Breuner, MD, MPH, FAAP

COMMITTEE ON ADOLESCENCE, 2017–2018

Cora Breuner, MD, MPH, FAAP, Chairperson
Elizabeth M. Alderman, MD, FSAHM, FAAP
Laura K. Grubb, MD, MPH, FAAP
Makia E. Powers, MD, MPH, FAAP
Krishna Upadhya, MD, FAAP
Stephenie B. Wallace, MD, FAAP

LIAISONS

Laurie Hornberger, MD, MPH, FAAP – *Section on Adolescent Health*
Liwei L. Hua, MD, PhD – *American Academy of Child and Adolescent Psychiatry*
Margo A. Lane, MD, FRCPC, FAAP – *Canadian Paediatric Society*
Meredith Loveless, MD, FACOG – *American College of Obstetricians and Gynecologists*
Seema Menon, MD – *North American Society of Pediatric and Adolescent Gynecology*
CDR Lauren B. Zapata, PhD, MSPH – *Centers for Disease Control and Prevention*

STAFF

Karen S. Smith
James D. Baumberger, MPP

ABBREVIATIONS

AAP: American Academy of Pediatrics
CI: confidence interval
OR: odds ratio
PCMH: Patient-Centered Medical Home

POTENTIAL CONFLICT OF INTEREST: The authors have indicated they have no potential conflicts of interest to disclose.

REFERENCES

1. Hagan JF, Shaw JS, Duncan PM, eds. *Bright Futures: Guidelines for Health Supervision of Infants, Children, and Adolescents*, 4th ed. Elk Grove Village, IL: American Academy of Pediatrics; 2017
2. Shlafer R, Hergenroeder AC, Jean Emans S, et al. Adolescence as a critical stage in the MCH Life Course Model: commentary for the Leadership Education in Adolescent Health (LEAH) interdisciplinary training program projects. *Matern Child Health J*. 2014; 18(2):462–466
3. World Health Organization. *Health for the World's Adolescents: A Second Chance for a Second Decade*. Geneva, Switzerland: World Health Organization; 2014. Available at: www.who.int/maternal_child_adolescent/documents/second-decade/en/. Accessed March 27, 2017
4. United States Department of Health and Human Services. About the office of adolescent health. Available at: www.hhs.gov/ash/oah/about-us/index.html. Accessed March 27, 2017
5. Institute of Medicine. *Child and Adolescent Health and Health Care Quality: Measuring What Matters*. Washington, DC: National Academies Press; 2011. Available at: http://nationalacademies.org/hmd/reports/2011/child-and-adolescent-health-and-health-care-quality.aspx. Accessed March 27, 2017

6. Institute of Medicine. *Adolescent Health Services: Missing Opportunities.* Washington, DC: National Academies Press; 2008. Available at: http://nationalacademies.org/hmd/reports/2008/adolescent-health-services-missing-opportunities.aspx. Accessed March 27, 2017
7. Patton GC, Sawyer SM, Santelli JS, et al. Our future: a *Lancet* commission on adolescent health and wellbeing. *Lancet.* 2016;387(10036):2423–2478
8. Patton GC, Ross DA, Santelli JS, et al. Next steps for adolescent health: a Lancet Commission. *Lancet.* 2014; 383(9915):385–386
9. English A, Park MJ, Shafer MA, Kreipe RE, D'Angelo LJ. Health care reform and adolescents-an agenda for the lifespan: a position paper of the Society for Adolescent Medicine. *J Adolesc Health.* 2009;45(3):310–315
10. Special issue: adolescence. *Nature.* 2018;554(7693):403–561
11. Elster AB. Comparison of recommendations for adolescent clinical preventive services developed by national organizations. *Arch Pediatr Adolesc Med.* 1998;152(2): 193–198
12. Ressel G; American Academy of Family Physicians. Introduction to AAFP summary of recommendations for periodic health examinations. *Am Fam Physician.* 2002;65(7):1467
13. Blum RW, Bastos FI, Kabiru CW, Le LC. Adolescent health in the 21st century. *Lancet.* 2012;379(9826):1567–1568
14. American Academy of Pediatrics Ad Hoc Task Force on Definition of the Medical Home: the medical home. *Pediatrics.* 1992;90(5):774
15. Accreditation Council on Graduate Medical Education. ACGME program requirements for graduate medical education in pediatrics. 2013. Available at: https://www.acgme.org/Specialties/Program-Requirements-and-FAQs-and-Applications/pfcatid/16/Pediatrics. Accessed March 27, 2017
16. Hargreaves DS, Elliott MN, Viner RM, Richmond TK, Schuster MA. Unmet health care need in US adolescents and adult health outcomes. *Pediatrics.* 2015; 136(3):513–520
17. Jenssen BP, Walley SC; Section on Tobacco Control. E-cigarettes and similar devices. *Pediatrics.* 2019;143(2): e20183652
18. Nordin JD, Solberg LI, Parker ED. Adolescent primary care visit patterns. *Ann Fam Med.* 2010;8(6):511–516
19. Heron M; Centers for Disease Control and Prevention. Deaths: leading causes for 2013. *Natl Vital Stat Rep.* 2016;65(2): 1–95
20. Centers for Disease Control and Prevention. National Center for Health Statistics Compressed mortality rate 1999-2010. 2012. Available at: http://wonder.cdc.gov/ucd-icd10.html. Accessed March 27, 2017
21. Murphy SL, Xu J, Kochanek KD, Curtin SC, Arias E. Deaths: final data for 2015. *Natl Vital Stat Rep.* 2017;66(6): 1–75
22. American Academy of Pediatrics. Bright futures. Adolescence Tools. Available at: https://brightfutures.aap.org/materials-and-tools/tool-and-resource-kit/Pages/adolescence-tools.aspx. Accessed March 27, 2017
23. Ma J, Wang Y, Stafford RSUS. U.S. adolescents receive suboptimal preventive counseling during ambulatory care. *J Adolesc Health.* 2005;36(5):441
24. Chung PJ, Lee TC, Morrison JL, Schuster MA. Preventive care for children in the United States: quality and barriers. *Annu Rev Public Health.* 2006;27: 491–515
25. American Academy of Pediatrics. *Coding for Pediatrics 2016: A Manual for Pediatric Documentation and Payment.* Elk Grove Village, IL: American Academy of Pediatrics; 2016
26. Society for Adolescent Health and Medicine; American Academy of Pediatrics. Confidentiality protections for adolescents and young adults in the health care billing and insurance claims process. *J Adolesc Health.* 2016; 58(3):374–377
27. Hale DR, Bevilacqua L, Viner RM. Adolescent health and adult education and employment: a systematic review. *Pediatrics.* 2015;136(1):128–140
28. Michaud PA, Suris JC, Viner R. *The Adolescent with a Chronic Condition: Epidemiology, Developmental Issues and Health Care Provision.* Geneva, Switzerland: World Health Organization; 2007. Available at http://apps.who.int/iris/bitstream/10665/43775/1/9789241595704_eng.pdf. Accessed March 27, 2017
29. Child and Adolescent Health Measurement Initiative. Data Resource Center for Child and Adolescent Health: 2016 National Survey of Children's Health data query. Available at: www.childhealthdata.org. Accessed March 27, 2017
30. Newacheck PW, McManus MA, Fox HB. Prevalence and impact of chronic illness among adolescents. *Am J Dis Child.* 1991;145(12):1367–1373
31. Denny S, de Silva M, Fleming T, et al. The prevalence of chronic health conditions impacting on daily functioning and the association with emotional well-being among a national sample of high school students. *J Adolesc Health.* 2014; 54(4):410–415
32. Compas BE, Jaser SS, Dunn MJ, Rodriguez EM. Coping with chronic illness in childhood and adolescence. *Annu Rev Clin Psychol.* 2012;8: 455–480
33. Child and Adolescent Health Measurement Initiative, Data Resource Center for Child and Adolescent Health. *National Survey of Children's Health (2016–2017).* Portland, OR: Child and Adolescent Health Measurement Initiative, the Data Resource Center for Child and Adolescent Health; 2009–2010. Available at: http://childhealthdata.org/browse/survey/results?q=1624&r=1&g=86. Accessed March 27, 2017
34. Search Foundation. Relationships that matter to America's teens. Available at: www.search-institute.org/sites/default/files/a/TeenVoice2010.pdf. Accessed March 27, 2017
35. Search Institute. Developmental assets. Available at: www.search-institute.org/research/developmental-assets. Accessed March 27, 2017
36. Cheng ER, Cohen A, Goodman E. The role of perceived discrimination during

childhood and adolescence in understanding racial and socioeconomic influences on depression in young adulthood. *J Pediatr.* 2015;166(2):370–377.e1

37. Centers for Disease Control and Prevention, National Center for Health Statistics. Vital statistics online data portal. Available at: www.cdc.gov/nchs/data_access/Vitalstatsonline.htm. Accessed March 27, 2017
38. Committee On Adolescence. Office-based care for lesbian, gay, bisexual, transgender, and questioning youth. *Pediatrics.* 2013;132(1):198–203
39. Levine DA; Committee On Adolescence. Office-based care for lesbian, gay, bisexual, transgender, and questioning youth. *Pediatrics.* 2013;132(1). Available at: www.pediatrics.org/cgi/content/full/132/1/e297
40. Committee on Adolescence. Health care for youth in the juvenile justice system. *Pediatrics.* 2011;128(6):1219–1235
41. Council on Foster Care, Adoption, and Kinship Care; Committee on Adolescence; Council on Early Childhood. Health care issues for children and adolescents in foster care and kinship care. *Pediatrics.* 2015;136(4). Available at: www.pediatrics.org/cgi/content/full/136/4/e1131
42. Siegel BS, Davis BE; Committee on Psychosocial Aspects of Child and Family Health and Section on Uniformed Services. Health and mental health needs of children in US military families. *Pediatrics.* 2013;131(6). Available at: www.pediatrics.org/cgi/content/full/131/6/e2002
43. Herman-Giddens ME, Slora EJ, Wasserman RC, et al. Secondary sexual characteristics and menses in young girls seen in office practice: a study from the Pediatric Research in Office Settings network. *Pediatrics.* 1997;99(4):505–512
44. Suris JC, Michaud PA, Viner R. The adolescent with a chronic condition. Part I: developmental issues. *Arch Dis Child.* 2004;89(10):938–942
45. Romer D, Reyna VF, Satterthwaite TD. Beyond stereotypes of adolescent risk taking: placing the adolescent brain in developmental context. *Dev Cogn Neurosci.* 2017;27:19–34
46. Suleiman AB, Dahl RE. Leveraging neuroscience to inform adolescent health: the need for an innovative transdisciplinary developmental science of adolescence. *J Adolesc Health.* 2017;60(3):240–248
47. Giedd JN. Structural magnetic resonance imaging of the adolescent brain. *Ann N Y Acad Sci.* 2004;1021(1):77–85
48. Hughes K, Bellis MA, Hardcastle KA, et al. The effect of multiple adverse childhood experiences on health: a systematic review and meta-analysis. *Lancet Public Health.* 2017;2(8):e356–e366
49. Giedd JN. The teen brain: insights from neuroimaging. *J Adolesc Health.* 2008;42(4):335–343
50. Bava S, Tapert SF. Adolescent brain development and the risk for alcohol and other drug problems. *Neuropsychol Rev.* 2010;20(4):398–413
51. Spear LP. The adolescent brain and age-related behavioral manifestations. *Neurosci Biobehav Rev.* 2000;24(4):417–463
52. Frankowski BL; American Academy of Pediatrics Committee on Adolescence. Sexual orientation and adolescents. *Pediatrics.* 2004;113(6):1827–1832
53. Spigarelli MG. Adolescent sexual orientation. *Adolesc Med State Art Rev.* 2007;18(3):508–518, vii
54. Zimmerman MA. Resiliency theory: a strengths-based approach to research and practice for adolescent health. *Health Educ Behav.* 2013;40(4):381–383
55. Duncan PM, Garcia AC, Frankowski BL, et al. Inspiring healthy adolescent choices: a rationale for and guide to strength promotion in primary care. *J Adolesc Health.* 2007;41(6):525–535
56. Benson PL, Scales PC, Hamilton SF, Sesma A Jr. Positive Youth Development: Theory, Research and Applications. In: Damon W, Lerner R, eds. *Handbook of Child Psychology.* Hoboken, NJ: John Wiley & Sons; 2007:894–941
57. Igartua K, Thombs BD, Burgos G, Montoro R. Concordance and discrepancy in sexual identity, attraction, and behavior among adolescents. *J Adolesc Health.* 2009;45(6):602–608
58. Goodenow C, Szalacha LA, Robin LE, Westheimer K. Dimensions of sexual orientation and HIV-related risk among adolescent females: evidence from a statewide survey. *Am J Public Health.* 2008;98(6):1051–1058
59. Rafferty J; Committee on Psychosocial Aspects of Child and Family Health; Committee on Adolescence; Section on Lesbian, Gay, Bisexual, and Transgender Health and Wellness. Ensuring comprehensive care and support for transgender and gender-diverse children and adolescents. *Pediatrics.* 2018;142(4):e20182162
60. Kitts RL. Gay adolescents and suicide: understanding the association. *Adolescence.* 2005;40(159):621–628
61. Keuroghlian AS, Shtasel D, Bassuk EL. Out on the street: a public health and policy agenda for lesbian, gay, bisexual, and transgender youth who are homeless. *Am J Orthopsychiatry.* 2014;84(1):66–72
62. Parsons JT, Kelly BC, Weiser JD. Initiation into methamphetamine use for young gay and bisexual men. *Drug Alcohol Depend.* 2007;90(2–3):135–144
63. Alan Guttmacher Institute. An overview of consent to reproductive health services by young people. Available at: https://www.guttmacher.org/state-policy/explore/overview-minors-consent-law. Accessed August 13, 2018
64. Alan Guttmacher Institute. State policies on teens. Available at: https://www.guttmacher.org/united-states/teens/state-policies-teens. Accessed March 27, 2017
65. Song X, Klein JD, Yan H, et al. Parent and adolescent attitudes toward preventive care and confidentiality. *J Adolesc Health.* 2019;64(2):235–241
66. World Health Organization. *Global Standards for Quality Health-Care Services for Adolescents: A Guide to Implement A Standards-Driven Approach to Improve the Quality of Health Care Services for Adolescents.*

Geneva, Switzerland: World Health Organization; 2015

67. American Academy of Pediatrics, Committee on Medical Liability and Risk Management. In: Donn SM, McAbee GN, eds. *Medicolegal Issues in Pediatrics*, 7th ed. Elk Grove Village, IL: American Academy of Pediatrics; 2005

68. National Research Council and Institute of Medicine. *A Study of Interactions: Emerging Issues in the Science of Adolescence: Workshop Summary.* Washington, DC: The National Academies Press; 2006

69. Kessler RC, Berglund P, Demler O, et al. Lifetime prevalence and age-of-onset distributions of DSM-IV disorders in the National Comorbidity Survey Replication [published correction appears in *Arch Gen Psychiatry.* 2005;62(7):768]. *Arch Gen Psychiatry.* 2005;62(6):593–602

70. Rushton JL, Forcier M, Schectman RM. Epidemiology of depressive symptoms in the National Longitudinal Study of Adolescent Health. *J Am Acad Child Adolesc Psychiatry.* 2002;41(2): 199–205

71. Curtain SC, Heron M, Minino AM, Warner M. Recent increases in injury mortality among children and adolescents aged 10-19 years in the United States: 1999-2016. *Natl Vit Stat Rep.* 2018;67(4):1–16

72. Centers for Disease Control and Prevention. Trends in the prevalence of suicide-related behaviors. National YRBS: 1991–2017. Available at: https://www.cdc.gov/healthyyouth/data/yrbs/pdf/trends/2017_suicide_trend_yrbs.pdf. Accessed June 26, 2018

73. Gilreath TD, Wrabel SL, Sullivan KS, et al. Suicidality among military-connected adolescents in California schools. *Eur Child Adolesc Psychiatry.* 2016;25(1): 61–66

74. Rosen DS; American Academy of Pediatrics Committee on Adolescence. Identification and management of eating disorders in children and adolescents. *Pediatrics.* 2010;126(6): 1240–1253

75. Robinson TN, Killen JD, Litt IF, et al. Ethnicity and body dissatisfaction: are Hispanic and Asian girls at increased risk for eating disorders? *J Adolesc Health.* 1996;19(6):384–393

76. Crago M, Shisslak CM, Estes LS. Eating disturbances among American minority groups: a review. *Int J Eat Disord.* 1996; 19(3):239–248

77. Gard MC, Freeman CP. The dismantling of a myth: a review of eating disorders and socioeconomic status. *Int J Eat Disord.* 1996;20(1):1–12

78. Kapphahn CJ, Morreale MC, Rickert VI, Walker LR; Society for Adolescent Medicine. Financing mental health services for adolescents: a position paper of the Society for Adolescent Medicine. *J Adolesc Health.* 2006;39(3): 456–458

79. Skowyra KR, Cocozza JJ. *Blueprint for Change: A Comprehensive Model for the Identification and Treatment of Youth with Mental Health Needs in Contact with the Juvenile Justice System.* Delmar, NY: The National Center for Mental Health and Juvenile Justice Policy Research Associates, Inc; 2007

80. Teplin LA, Abram KM, McClelland GM, Dulcan MK, Mericle AA. Psychiatric disorders in youth in juvenile detention. *Arch Gen Psychiatry.* 2002;59(12): 1133–1143

81. Toro PA, Dworsky A, Fowler PJ. *Toward Understanding Homelessness: The 2007 National Symposium on Homelessness Research.* Washington, DC: US Department of Health and Human Services; 2007

82. Baird M, Blount A, Brungardt S, et al; Working Party Group on Integrated Behavioral Healthcare. Joint principles: integrating behavioral health care into the patient-centered medical home. *Ann Fam Med.* 2014;12(2): 183–185

83. Lehrer JA, Pantell R, Tebb K, Shafer MA. Forgone health care among U.S. adolescents: associations between risk characteristics and confidentiality concern. *J Adolesc Health.* 2007;40(3): 218–226

84. Kulik DM, Gaetz S, Crowe C, Ford-Jones EL. Homeless youth's overwhelming health burden: a review of the literature. *Paediatr Child Health.* 2011; 16(6):e43–e47

85. Secura GM, Madden T, McNicholas C, et al. Provision of no-cost, long-acting contraception and teenage pregnancy. *N Engl J Med.* 2014; 371(14):1316–1323

86. Baldwin MK, Edelman AB. The effect of long-acting reversible contraception on rapid repeat pregnancy in adolescents: a review. *J Adolesc Health.* 2013;52(suppl 4): S47–S53

87. Chen XK, Wen SW, Fleming N, et al. Teenage pregnancy and adverse birth outcomes: a large population based retrospective cohort study. *Int J Epidemiol.* 2007;36(2): 368–373

88. Centers for Disease Control and Prevention. *Sexually Transmitted Disease Surveillance 2016.* Atlanta, GA: US Department of Health and Human Services; 2017

89. McKee MD, Rubin SE, Campos G, O'Sullivan LF. Challenges of providing confidential care to adolescents in urban primary care: clinician perspectives. *Ann Fam Med.* 2011;9(1): 37–43

90. American Academy of Family Physicians, American Academy of Pediatrics, American College of Physicians, American Osteopathic Association. Joint Principles of the patient-centered medical home. 2007. Available at: https://www.aafp.org/dam/AAFP/documents/practice_management/pcmh/initiatives/PCMHJoint.pdf. Accessed March 27, 2017

91. Cooley WC, Sagerman PJ; American Academy of Pediatrics; American Academy of Family Physicians; American College of Physicians; Transitions Clinical Report Authoring Group. Supporting the health care transition from adolescence to adulthood in the medical home. *Pediatrics.* 2011;128(1): 182–200

92. Committee on Adolescence American Academy of Pediatrics. Achieving quality health services for adolescents. *Pediatrics.* 2008;121(6): 1263–1270

93. Agency for Healthcare Research and Quality. *2006 National*

Healthcare Quality Report. Rockville, MD: US Department of Health and Human Services, Agency for Healthcare Research and Quality; 2006

94. Ginsburg KR, Alexander PM, Hunt J, et al. Enhancing their likelihood for a positive future: the perspective of inner-city youth. *Pediatrics*. 2002;109(6):1136–1142

95. Arenson M, Hudson PJ, Lai B. The evidence on school-based health centers: a review. *Glob Pediatr Health*. 2019;6:2333794X19828745

Updates on an At-Risk Population: Late-Preterm and Early-Term Infants

- *Clinical Report*

CLINICAL REPORT Guidance for the Clinician in Rendering Pediatric Care

American Academy of Pediatrics

DEDICATED TO THE HEALTH OF ALL CHILDREN™

Updates on an At-Risk Population: Late-Preterm and Early-Term Infants

Dan L. Stewart, MD, FAAP,[a] Wanda D. Barfield, MD, MPH, FAAP, RADM, USPHS,[b] COMMITTEE ON FETUS AND NEWBORN

abstract

The American Academy of Pediatrics published a clinical report on late-preterm (LPT) infants in 2007 that was largely based on a summary of a 2005 workshop convened by the *Eunice Kennedy Shriver* National Institute of Child Health and Human Development, at which a change in terminology from "near term" to "late preterm" was proposed. This paradigm-shifting recommendation had a remarkable impact: federal agencies (the Centers for Disease Control and Prevention), professional societies (the American Academy of Pediatrics and American College of Obstetricians and Gynecologists), and organizations (March of Dimes) initiated nationwide monitoring and educational plans that had a significant effect on decreasing the rates of iatrogenic LPT deliveries. However, there is now an evolving concern. After nearly a decade of steady decreases in the LPT birth rate that largely contributed to the decline in total US preterm birth rates, the birth rate in LPT infants has been inching upward since 2015. In addition, evidence revealed by strong population health research demonstrates that being born as an early-term infant poses a significant risk to an infant's survival, growth, and development. In this report, we summarize the initial progress and discuss the potential reasons for the current trends in LPT and early-term birth rates and propose research recommendations.

[a]*School of Medicine, University of Louisville, Louisville, Kentucky; and* [b]*Centers for Disease Control and Prevention, Atlanta, Georgia*

Clinical reports from the American Academy of Pediatrics benefit from expertise and resources of liaisons and internal (AAP) and external reviewers. However, clinical reports from the American Academy of Pediatrics may not reflect the views of the liaisons or the organizations or government agencies that they represent.

Dr Stewart and the members of the Committee on Fetus and Newborn conceived the concept of updating the previous American Academy of Pediatrics publication on late-preterm infants, collaborated with Drs Barfield and Raju, and reviewed the manuscript; Drs Barfield and Raju collaborated with Dr Stewart and members of the Committee on Fetus and Newborn and reviewed the manuscript; and both authors approved the final manuscript as submitted and agree to be accountable for all aspects of the work.

The guidance in this report does not indicate an exclusive course of treatment or serve as a standard of medical care. Variations, taking into account individual circumstances, may be appropriate.

All clinical reports from the American Academy of Pediatrics automatically expire 5 years after publication unless reaffirmed, revised, or retired at or before that time.

The findings and conclusions in this article are those of the authors and do not necessarily represent the official position of the Centers for Disease Control and Prevention.

This document is copyrighted and is property of the American Academy of Pediatrics and its Board of Directors. All authors have filed conflict of interest statements with the American Academy of Pediatrics. Any conflicts have been resolved through a process approved by the Board of Directors. The American Academy of Pediatrics has neither solicited nor accepted any commercial involvement in the development of the content of this publication.

DOI: https://doi.org/10.1542/peds.2019-2760

Address correspondence to Dan L. Stewart, MD, FAAP. E-mail: dan.stewart@louisville.edu

To cite: Stewart DL, Barfield WD, AAP COMMITTEE ON FETUS AND NEWBORN. Updates on an At-Risk Population: Late-Preterm and Early-Term Infants. *Pediatrics.* 2019;144(5): e20192760

INTRODUCTION

The American Academy of Pediatrics (AAP) published a clinical report on late-preterm (LPT) infants (born between 34 0/7 weeks' gestation and 36 6/7 weeks' gestation; Fig 1) in 2007[1] that was largely based on a summary of the 2005 workshop convened by the *Eunice Kennedy Shriver* National Institute of Child Health and Human Development.[2] At this workshop, a change in terminology from "near term" to "late preterm" was proposed. This shift in the paradigm recommendation led to a remarkable impact: federal agencies (the Centers for Disease Control and Prevention), professional societies (the AAP and American College of Obstetrics and Gynecology), and organizations (March of Dimes) initiated nationwide monitoring and educational plans that had a significant effect on decreasing the rates of iatrogenic LPT deliveries, as noted in numerous publications.

Evidence revealed by strong population health research demonstrated that LPT or early-term (ET) births (between 37 0/7 weeks' gestation and 38 6/7 weeks' gestation; Fig 1) pose a significant risk to an infant's survival, growth, and development because of increased morbidities and mortality in these at-risk groups (Fig 2). The 2007 AAP clinical report on LPT births was an important milestone in helping health care providers understand the magnitude of these untimely births and their relative contribution to overall preterm birth and disparities. Neonatologists and pediatricians should be aware of the current and ongoing challenges infants face after being born LPT or ET. Understanding the current terminology, factors contributing to these early deliveries, and long-term implications for growth and development will help in prevention, clinical management, and population-based quality-improvement efforts.

Because LPT infants account for approximately 70% of preterm births in the United States, this is a costly and important public health matter.[3] LPTs represent 7% of all live births; ET infants represent 26% of all live births and 29% of all term infants[4] (Fig 3). Recognition of these at-risk subsets of preterm and term infants has affected perinatal care and launched a robust research endeavor to decrease the number of nonmedically indicated deliveries of infants born LPT and ET[5] while seeking methods to optimize care provided to these patients. There have been more than 500 publications investigating the reasons for LPT and ET while recognizing that there are a number of maternal, fetal, and placental complications for which either LPT or ET birth is warranted.[5]

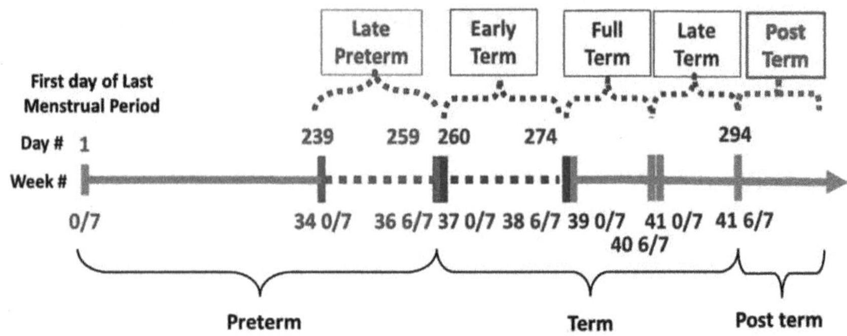

FIGURE 1
Definitions of gestational age periods from LPT to postterm. (Reprinted with permission from Engle WA, Kominiarek M. Late preterm infants, early term infants, and timing of elective deliveries. *Clin Perinatol.* 2008;35(2):325–341.)

After reaching a nadir of 9.57% in 2014, the preterm birth rate increased to 9.97% in quarter 3 of 2018 (Fig 4).[6] This report shows an emerging concern. After nearly a decade of steady decreases, the preterm birth rate is inching upward again. These trends are largely attributable to increases in the rate of LPT births, predominantly among non-Hispanic black and Hispanic women.[4,7] In 2018, the LPT birth rate rose to 7.28% (Fig 5). These trends must be continually monitored with an exploration of causality.[8] In this report, the initial progress is summarized, the potential reasons for the current trends in LPT birth rates are discussed, and practice

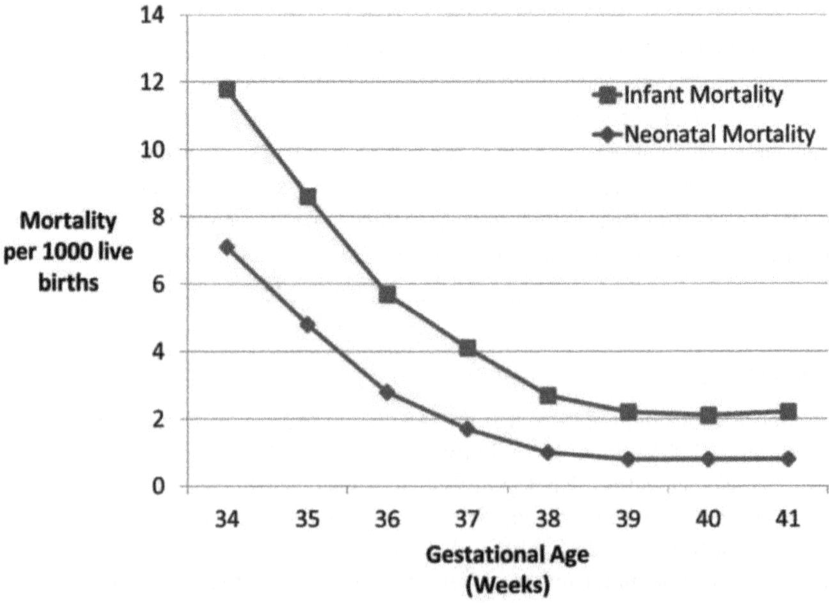

FIGURE 2
Neonatal and infant mortality by gestational age. Adapted from Reddy UM, Ko CW, Raju TN, Willinger M. Delivery indications at late-preterm gestations and infant mortality rates in the United States. *Pediatrics.* 2009;124(1):234–240. (Reprinted with permission from Kardatzke MA, Rose RS, Engle WA. Late preterm and early term birth: at-risk populations and targets for reducing such early births. *NeoReviews.* 2017;18(5):e265–e276.)

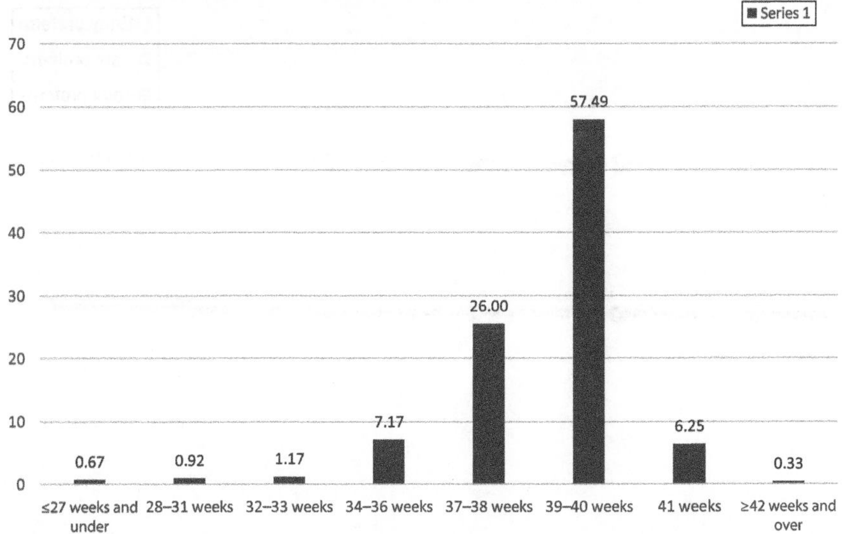

FIGURE 3

Percentage of births by gestational age at birth: United States 2017. (Adapted from Martin JA, Hamilton BE, Osterman MJ, Driscoll AK, Drake P. Births: final data for 2017. *Natl Vital Stat Rep*. 2018; 67:8.)

and research recommendations are proposed.

CURRENT DEFINITIONS

The national emphasis on reducing preterm births and the increase in scheduled deliveries has created confusion around the definition of term gestation.[9] The concept of "term" gestation provides guidance to clinicians and influences the public's perceptions about the optimal timing of delivery for a healthy pregnancy.[9] This nomenclature acknowledged that fetal maturation is a continuum, yet the use of the label of term for pregnancies spanning 37 weeks' 0 days gestation through 41 weeks 6 days' gestation remained unchanged. Recent data demonstrate that maternal and neonatal adverse outcome rates are not the same across the 5-week gestational age range that constitutes term.[9] Rather, the frequency distribution of adverse outcomes is U shaped, with the nadir being between 39 weeks 0 days' gestation and 40 weeks 6 days' gestation.[9] The Defining "Term" Pregnancy workshop recommended that births occurring between 37 weeks 0 days' gestation and 38 weeks 6 days' gestation be designated as ET, those between 39 weeks 0 days' gestation and 40 weeks 6 days' gestation be designated as term, and those occurring at 41 weeks 0 days' gestation through 41 weeks 6 days' gestation be designated as late term.[9,10]

According to the American College of Obstetricians and Gynecologists (ACOG), accurate dating of pregnancy is important to improve outcomes and is a research and public health imperative. As soon as data from the last menstrual period, the first accurate ultrasound examination, or both are obtained, the gestational age and the estimated due date should be determined, discussed with the patient, and documented clearly in the medical record. A pregnancy without an ultrasound examination that confirms or revises the estimated due date before 22 0/7 weeks' gestation should be considered suboptimally dated. For the purposes of research and surveillance, the best obstetric estimate, rather than estimates based on the last menstrual period alone, should be used as the measure for gestational age.[11]

"Implicit in any definition or subclassification of preterm or term birth is the need for accurate dating, which would likely lead to a lower proportion of deliveries categorized as postterm or early term."[8] The ACOG considers first-trimester ultrasonography to be the most accurate method to establish or confirm gestational age. Pregnancies without an ultrasonographic examination confirming or revising the estimated due date before 22 0/7 weeks' gestation should be considered suboptimally dated. There is no role for elective delivery in a woman with a suboptimally dated pregnancy. Although guidelines for indicated LPT and ET deliveries depend on an accurate determination of gestational age, women with suboptimally dated pregnancies should be managed according to these same guidelines because of the lack of a superior alternative.[12]

After the 2005 *Eunice Kennedy Shriver* National Institute of Child Health and Human Development workshop, there were concerns about unintended consequences, including an increase in stillbirths[13] and increasing the risks for the mother and her fetus by the avoidance of indicated LPT deliveries. Current ACOG and Society for Maternal-Fetal Medicine recommendations state that there are a number of maternal, fetal, and placental complications for which either an LPT or ET delivery is warranted. The timing of delivery in such cases must balance the maternal and newborn risks of LPT and ET delivery with the risks associated with further continuation of pregnancy. Deferring delivery to the 39th week is not recommended if there is a medical or obstetric indication for earlier delivery.

PATHOGENESIS OF PRETERM BIRTHS

The pathogenesis of preterm birth is not completely understood. Two-thirds of preterm deliveries occur as

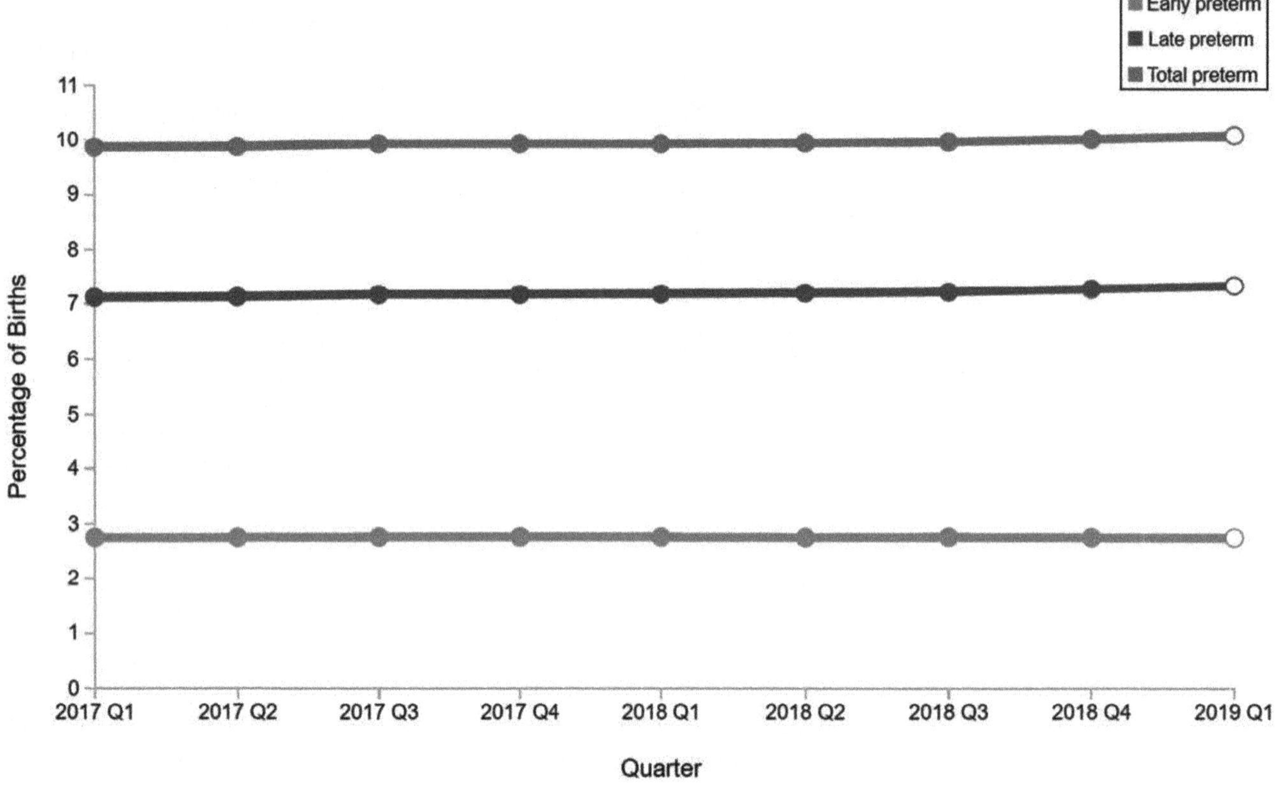

FIGURE 4
Quarterly preterm birth rates 2017 to quarter 1 of 2019. (Adapted from Rossen LM, Osterman MJK, Hamilton BE, Martin JA. Quarterly Provisional Estimates for Selected Birth Indicators, 2017–quarter 1, 2019. Hyattsville, MD: National Center for Health Statistics NVSS, Vital Statistics Rapid Release Program; 2019.)

a result of spontaneous preterm labor and/or premature rupture of membranes.[14] Risk factors that may contribute to these events include a history of a previous preterm delivery (risk is 1.5–2.0 times higher)[15]; infection; inflammation; maternal stress (acute and/or chronic); uterine, placental, and/or fetal anomalies; short cervix; as well as multifetal pregnancies.[16] Newnham et al[17] recently reviewed current strategies for prevention of preterm birth, which include decreasing smoking during pregnancy, cervical cerclage, judicious use of fertility treatments, prevention of nonmedically indicated deliveries, and the establishment of high-risk obstetric clinics. Public health efforts also contributed, using the Collaboration on Innovation and Improvement Network to reduce infant mortality. In these efforts, states focused on policies and practices to reduce tobacco use in pregnancy and reduce nonindicated preterm delivery.[18,19] State perinatal quality collaboratives, which consisted of teams of clinical and public health members, have also helped to reduce the rates of nonmedically indicated LPT and ET births.[20] Progress has been made in the rate for triplet and higher-order–multiple births, which has been on the decline since 1998 and presently is the lowest in more than 2 decades.[3,21–23] In part from the efforts from the March of Dimes program that no infant be delivered electively before 39 weeks' gestation, the cesarean delivery rate is down 3% from a peak of 32.9% in 2009.[3]

In a large randomized controlled trial, the benefits of a single course of antenatal betamethasone was investigated in women anticipated to deliver between 34 and 37 weeks of pregnancy.[24] Infants of women treated had significantly lower rates of respiratory complications. However, 35 women needed to be treated to improve outcomes in 1 infant, and 24% of steroid-exposed infants developed hypoglycemia compared with 14.9% of those in the placebo group. Thus, despite endorsements by the obstetric professional societies,[25–27] several experts have raised concerns about the routine use of antenatal steroids in women during LPT gestations.[27–29] Pediatric providers, too, need to review a history of antenatal steroid exposure while evaluating LPT infants, including checking for neonatal hypoglycemia.

Use of progesterone for women with a previous history of spontaneous

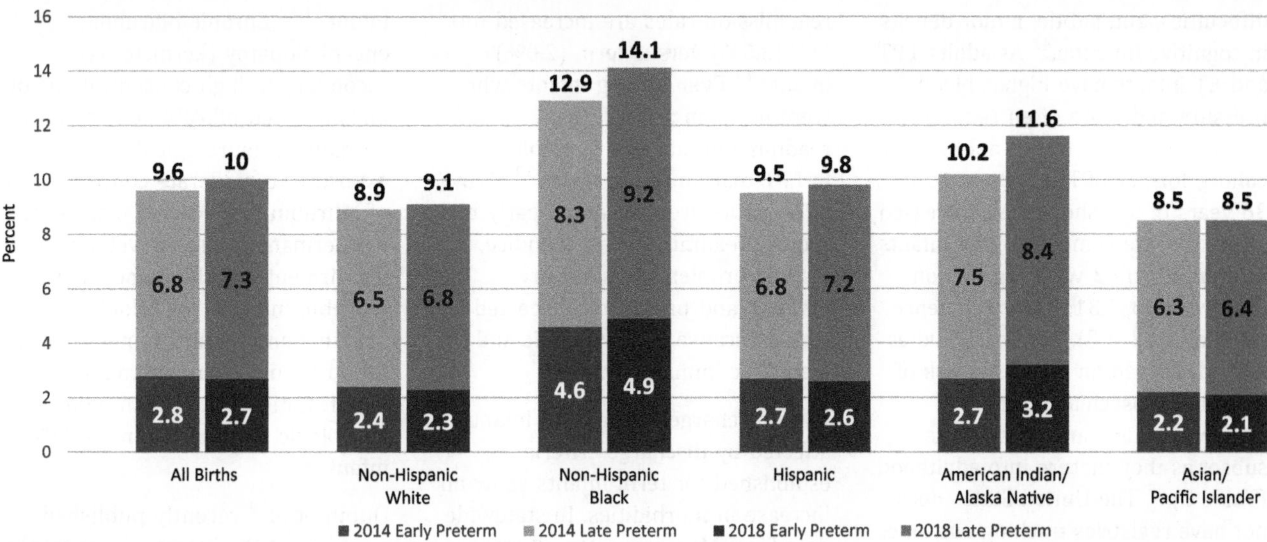

FIGURE 5
Preterm birth rates: United States, overall and by race and ethnicity, 2014 and 2018. Source: National Center for Health Statistics, National Vital Statistics System–Natality.

preterm birth decreases mortality and the need for admission to the NICU. Unfortunately, this improvement is limited to singleton pregnancies, not multiples.[15,30,31] Likewise, 17-hydroxyprogesterone has shown efficacy in women with a short cervix documented by ultrasonography.[32] Screening of women with a previous preterm birth at less than 34 weeks' gestation may identify women with a cervical length <25 mm before 24 weeks' gestation who might potentially benefit from a cervical cerclage.[33,34] Variable access to 17-hydroxyprogesterone, antenatal steroids, prenatal ultrasonography, and early treatment and/or management of preterm prolonged rupture of membranes and/or signs of infection may be contributing to racial disparities in preterm birth rates.[35,36] In addition, lack of adequate prenatal care may delay appropriate management of conditions that develop before and during pregnancies, such as diabetes, hypertension, preeclampsia, and others.[23]

Since the birth of the first US infant conceived with assisted reproductive technology (ART) in 1981, the use of advanced technologies to overcome infertility has resulted in millions of pregnancies and subsequent live births.[37] Since 1995, the number of ART procedures performed in the United States and the number of infants born as a result of these procedures have nearly tripled.[22] Because many ART procedures involve transferring multiple embryos, ART results in multiple-gestation pregnancies and multiple births. The percentage of infants born preterm and very preterm is higher among ART-conceived infants than among infants in the total birth population even with elective single-embryo transfers, which involves the transfer of a single embryo. The contribution of ART to preterm births, the majority of which are also low birth weight, is a factor in the increases observed in the LPT and ET population (Table 1).[38,39]

SHORT- AND LONG-TERM MEDICAL AND NEURODEVELOPMENTAL SEQUELAE FOR LPT AND ET INFANTS

LPT infants are at increased risk for a number of adverse events, including respiratory distress, hypoglycemia, feeding difficulties, hypothermia, hyperbilirubinemia, apnea, seizures, and a higher rate of readmission after initial discharge.[40,41] In addition, LPT infants have higher rates of pulmonary disorders during childhood and adolescence, learning

TABLE 1 The Percentage of Preterm Births by Gestational Age Groups Attributable to ART, 2015

Region	Preterm (<37 wk) Births Attributable to ART, %	Very Preterm (<32 wk) Births Attributable to ART, %	LPT Births (34 + 0/7–36 + 6/7 wk) Attributable to ART, %	ET Births (37 + 0/7–38 + 6/7 wk) Attributable to ART, %
United States and Puerto Rico	5.3	5.4	5.0	2.1

Preterm: <37 wk; very preterm: <32 wk; LPT: 34 0/7–36 6/7 wk; ET: 37 0/7–38 6/7 wk. Source: Analyses of the National ART Surveillance System (NASS) data. Written communication with the Division of Reproductive Health, National Center for Chronic Disease Prevention and Health Promotion, Centers for Disease Control and Prevention, April 19, 2018.

difficulties, and subtle, minor deficits in cognitive function.[42] As adults, LPT and ET infants have higher blood pressure and more often require treatment of diabetes.[43] In a Swedish cohort, former LPT infants at 18 to 36 years of age showed an increased mortality rate compared with infants born at 37 to 42 weeks' gestation (hazard ratio, 1.31; 95% confidence interval, 1.13–1.5).[44] Several studies have described an increased risk of neurologic, psychiatric, and developmental conditions in this subset as they mature into adulthood (Table 2).[45] The United States does not have registries tracking outcomes of infants born at LPT gestations into adult age groups. However, on the basis of its national registry, the Swedish National Cohort Study reported a stepwise increase in disability rates in young adulthood, which increased with the degree of preterm birth.[46]

LENGTH OF STAY AND DISCHARGE CRITERIA

The duration of birth hospitalization correlates with gestational age at birth.[47,48] Among 235 LPTs at 1 birth center, the length of the birth hospitalization (mean ± SD) was 12.6 ± 10.6 days at 34 weeks' gestation, 6.1 ± 5.8 days at 35 weeks' gestation, and 3.8 ± 3.6 days at 36 weeks' gestation. The usual hospital stay for a term infant is 2 days for a vaginal delivery and 3 days for a cesarean delivery. In addition, hospital readmission rates are increased for LPT (3.5%) versus term (2.0%) infants.[49] Even among infants who were never in a NICU, the readmission rate was threefold higher in LPT than in term infants.[50] Many LPT infants are discharged early but require readmission for jaundice, feeding problems, respiratory distress, and proven or suspected sepsis because of physiologic and metabolic immaturity.

Early discharge among LPT infants affected by discharge criteria established for term infants show an increase in morbidities. In statewide data from Massachusetts, all state-resident infants discharged after a hospital stay of less than 2 nights were analyzed. In the LPT group (1004 infants), 4.3% were readmitted or required an observational stay versus 2.7% of the term infants (n = 24 320). LPT infants were also 1.5 times more likely to require hospital-related care. This study suggested that LPT infants discharged early experience significantly more neonatal morbidity than term infants; however, this may be true only for breastfed infants. The authors concluded that evidence-based recommendations for appropriate discharge timing and postdischarge follow-up are needed.[49]

Moderately preterm infants are also at increased risk for acute bilirubin encephalopathy. Clinical manifestations may be more subtle in the LPT infant versus the term infant.[51,52] Chronic bilirubin encephalopathy (kernicterus) secondary to high concentrations of unconjugated bilirubin can result in permanent neurologic damage. Even exposure to moderate concentrations of bilirubin may lead to more subtle yet permanent neurodevelopmental impairment, which is labeled as bilirubin-induced neurologic dysfunction.[51] Auditory neuropathy spectrum disorder is a common manifestation of bilirubin-induced neurologic dysfunction in the LPT infant.[53]

Quinn et al[54] recently published a review of the literature concerning discharge criteria for the LPT infant. They found few differences in discharge criteria between infants in the newborn nursery and those in the NICU.[55] Previously published discharge criteria from the AAP evolved over time and include physiologic stability and completed screenings for hearing loss, hyperbilirubinemia, car seat safety, hypoglycemia, critical congenital heart disease, and sepsis. Parental education was also a major component of discharge planning, including umbilical cord care, feeding, voiding and/or stooling, and weight gain. In addition, Quinn et al[54] recommended maternal screening assessments for depression, drug use, a safe home environment, and the existence of a support system.

A major difference between newborn discharge and discharge criteria for the LPT infant is the transition to safe sleep before discharge (supine position). Given that LPT and ET infants are at an increased risk of morbidity and mortality, greater efforts are needed to ensure safe and healthy posthospitalization and home care practices for these vulnerable infants.[56] Finally, standardized criteria for discharge may improve outcomes and reduce maternal stress in these high-risk groups.

TABLE 2 Neurologic, Psychiatric, and Developmental Disorders in LPT Infants as Adults

Neurologic and Psychiatric Conditions	Relative Risk of LPT Versus Term (95% CI)
Attention-deficit/hyperactivity disorder	1.7 (1.2–2.5)
Any psychiatric disorder	3.74 (1.59–8.78)
Any anxiety disorder	3.85 (1.52–9.52)
Cerebral palsy	2.7 (2.2–3.3)
Cognitive disability	1.6 (1.4–1.8)
Schizophrenia	1.3 (1.0–1.7)
Any disorder of psychological development, behavior, and emotion	1.4 (1.3–1.5)

Adapted from Moster D, Lie RT, Markestad T. Long-term medical and social consequences of preterm birth. *N Engl J Med.* 2008;359(3):262–273; and Kardatzke MA, Rose RS, Engle WA. Late preterm and early term birth: at-risk populations and targets for reducing such early births. *NeoReviews.* 2017;18(5):e265–2376. CI, confidence interval.

Evaluating 161 804 infants in Florida between 34 and 41 weeks' gestation with a length of stay of ≤72 hours revealed that LPT infants, compared with term infants, had a 36% higher risk for developmental delay or disability and a 19% higher risk of suspension in kindergarten after adjustment for 15 potential confounders. Disability in prekindergarten at 3 and 4 years of age, exceptional student education, and retention in kindergarten all carried a 10% to 13% increased risk among LPT infants. "Not ready to start school" was borderline significant. The authors concluded that healthy LPT infants have a greater risk for developmental delay and school problems than term infants through the first 5 years of life.[57]

School performance is also a concern in LPT and ET infants. School performance in this group was evaluated in a cohort study at 7 years of age in the population-based prospective UK Millennium Cohort Study with >6000 children. This study used the statutory key stage 1 teacher assessment performed in the third school year in England. The primary outcome was not achieving the expected level (≥2) in reading, writing, and mathematics. There was a statistically significant increased risk of poor performance in those born LPT (adjusted relative risk, 1.36; 95% confidence interval, 1.09–1.68). ET infants performed statistically significantly worse than the term children in 4 of 5 individual subject domains but not in the primary outcome. This study concluded that LPT, and to a lesser extent ET, birth negatively affected academic outcomes at 7 years of age as measured by key stage 1 assessments.[58]

After review of 126 publications, Raju et al concluded that the overwhelming majority of adults born at preterm gestation remain healthy and well, but adult outcomes in a small but significant fraction of infants born preterm are concerning. This population is at a slightly higher risk for neuropsychological and behavioral problems, hypertensive disorders and metabolic syndrome, and developing at an earlier age when compared with term infants. Preterm birth should be considered a chronic condition, and the primary care physician should glean this information; this would potentiate early diagnoses and timely intervention.[59] Because of the research gaps that exist, the US National Institutes of Health convened a multidisciplinary conference with experts on adult diseases in infants born preterm and proposed a research agenda.[60]

PRACTICAL CONSIDERATIONS

Acceptance that early birth is not an inevitable and natural feature of human reproduction is the first step in ameliorating the societal burden of LPT and ET births.[17] LPT and ET births are not caused by a single entity but are the result of a heterogeneous group of conditions that affect the mother and/or fetus.[61] Potential interventions to reduce LPT births include the following:

1. prevention of exposure of pregnant women to cigarette smoke,[19]
2. judicious use of non-ART fertility treatments and ART treatments (eg, elective single-embryo transfer),[39]
3. improvement of preconception health to reduce chronic medical conditions such as diabetes, obesity, and poor nutrition,[15] and
4. encouragement of longer interpregnancy interval because a short interpregnancy interval of <6 months poses a higher risk of LPT delivery.[62–64]

Further success can be anticipated in the future as other research discoveries are translated into clinical practice, including new approaches to treating intrauterine infection, improving maternal nutrition, and lifestyle modifications to decrease stress.[17]

RECOMMENDATIONS

Accounting for approximately 32% of nearly 4 million live births annually, LPT and ET births remain a challenge, with a recent increase seen in rates in the United States. Pediatricians can continue to play an important role in the reduction of these at-risk births.

1. LPT and ET infants have increased risks of adverse medical, neurodevelopmental, behavioral, and social sequelae into and through adulthood. Neonatologists and pediatricians can continue to understand these risks and inform parents, educators, and adult care clinicians.
2. Continued use of population data within hospitals, states, regions, and networks will help to monitor rates of LPT and ET births for trends, changes in practice, and need for intervention.
3. Promising interventions exist to prevent LPT and ET births, but these interventions need to be adopted and disseminated equitably and financed by payers adequately to reduce disparities.
4. Multidisciplinary discussions and planning with obstetric providers will improve the understanding of the causes of and indications for LPT and ET deliveries with the intention of preventing iatrogenic deliveries.[18, 65]
5. Health care providers for all age groups should consider obtaining a patient's birth history to include gestational age as a comprehensive means of evaluating and predicting current and future health.[48,49]
6. Because these at-risk populations of LPT and ET infants are at risk

for adverse health outcomes, these groups should be added to payment models that better finance practitioners who have to increase their outreach, screening, and treatment to provide appropriate care to these patients.

LEAD AUTHORS

Dan L. Stewart, MD, FAAP
Wanda D. Barfield, MD, MPH, FAAP, RADM USPHS

COMMITTEE ON FETUS AND NEWBORN, 2018–2019

James J. Cummings, MD, FAAP, Chairperson
Ira S. Adams-Chapman, MD, FAAP
Susan Wright Aucott, MD, FAAP
Jay P. Goldsmith, MD, FAAP
Ivan L. Hand, MD, FAAP
Sandra E. Juul, MD, PhD, FAAP
Brenda Bradley Poindexter, MD, MS, FAAP
Karen Marie Puopolo, MD, PhD, FAAP
Dan L. Stewart, MD, FAAP

LIAISONS

Wanda D. Barfield, MD, MPH, FAAP, RADM USPHS
Yasser El-Sayed, MD
Erin L. Keels, DNP, APRN, NNP-BC – *National Association of Neonatal Nurses*
Meredith Mowitz, MD, MS, FAAP
Michael Ryan Narvey, MD, FAAP – *Canadian Paediatric Society*
Tonse N. K. Raju, MD, DCH, FAAP – *National Institutes of Health*
Kasper S. Wang, MD, FACS, FAAP – *Section on Surgery*

STAFF

Jim Couto, MA

ABBREVIATIONS

AAP: American Academy of Pediatrics
ACOG: American College of Obstetricians and Gynecologists
ART: assisted reproductive technology
ET: early-term
LPT: late-preterm

PEDIATRICS (ISSN Numbers: Print, 0031-4005; Online, 1098-4275).

Copyright © 2019 by the American Academy of Pediatrics

FINANCIAL DISCLOSURE: The authors have indicated they have no financial relationships relevant to this article to disclose.

FUNDING: No external funding.

POTENTIAL CONFLICT OF INTEREST: The authors have indicated they have no potential conflicts of interest to disclose.

REFERENCES

1. Engle WA, Tomashek KM, Wallman C; Committee on Fetus and Newborn, American Academy of Pediatrics. "Late-preterm" infants: a population at risk. *Pediatrics*. 2007;120(6):1390–1401
2. Raju TN, Higgins RD, Stark AR, Leveno KJ. Optimizing care and outcome for late-preterm (near-term) infants: a summary of the workshop sponsored by the National Institute of Child Health and Human Development. *Pediatrics*. 2006;118(3):1207–1214
3. Martin JA, Hamilton BE, Osterman MJK. Births in the United States, 2018. *NCHS Data Brief*. 2019;(346):1–8
4. Martin JA, Hamilton BE, Osterman MJ. Births: final data for 2017. *Natl Vital Stat Rep*. 2018;67(8):1–50
5. ACOG Committee Opinion No. ACOG committee opinion No. 764: medically indicated late-preterm and early-term deliveries. *Obstet Gynecol*. 2019;133(2): e151–e155
6. Rossen LM, Osterman MJK, Hamilton BE, Martin JA. *Quarterly Provisional Estimates for Selected Birth Indicators, 2017-Quarter 3, 2018*. Hyattsville, MD: National Center for Health Statistics NVSS, Vital Statistics Rapid Release Program; 2019
7. Shapiro-Mendoza CK, Lackritz EM. Epidemiology of late and moderate preterm birth. *Semin Fetal Neonatal Med*. 2012;17(3):120–125
8. Raju TNKR. The "late preterm" birth-ten years later. *Pediatrics*. 2017;139(3): e20163331
9. Spong CY. Defining "term" pregnancy: recommendations from the defining "term" pregnancy workgroup. *JAMA*. 2013;309(23):2445–2446
10. ACOG committee opinion No 579: definition of term pregnancy. *Obstet Gynecol*. 2013;122(5):1139–1140
11. ACOG. Committee opinion No. 700 summary: methods for estimating the due date. *Obstet Gynecol*. 2017;129(5): 967–968
12. Committee opinion No. 688 summary: management of suboptimally dated pregnancies. *Obstet Gynecol*. 2017; 129(3):591–592
13. MacDorman MF, Reddy UM, Silver RM. Trends in stillbirth by gestational age in the United States, 2006-2012. *Obstet Gynecol*. 2015;126(6):1146–1150
14. Ananth CV, Joseph KS, Oyelese Y, Demissie K, Vintzileos AM. Trends in preterm birth and perinatal mortality among singletons: United States, 1989 through 2000. *Obstet Gynecol*. 2005; 105(5, pt 1):1084–1091
15. Shapiro-Mendoza CK, Barfield WD, Henderson Z, et al. CDC grand rounds: public health strategies to prevent preterm birth. *MMWR Morb Mortal Wkly Rep*. 2016;65(32):826–830
16. Committee on Practice Bulletins—Obstetrics, The American College of Obstetricians and Gynecologists. Practice bulletin no. 130: prediction and prevention of preterm birth. *Obstet Gynecol*. 2012;120(4):964–973
17. Newnham JP, Dickinson JE, Hart RJ, et al. Strategies to prevent preterm birth. *Front Immunol*. 2014;5:584
18. Hirai AH, Sappenfield WM, Ghandour RM, et al. The Collaborative

Improvement and Innovation Network (CoIIN) to reduce infant mortality: an outcome evaluation from the US South, 2011 to 2014. *Am J Public Health.* 2018; 108(6):815–821

19. Dietz PM, England LJ, Shapiro-Mendoza CK, et al. Infant morbidity and mortality attributable to prenatal smoking in the U.S. *Am J Prev Med.* 2010;39(1):45–52
20. ACOG. ACOG committee opinion no. 765: avoidance of nonmedically indicated early-term deliveries and associated neonatal morbidities. *Obstet Gynecol.* 2019;133(2):e156–e163
21. Martin JA, Osterman MJ, Thoma ME. Declines in triplet and higher-order multiple births in the United States, 1998-2014. *NCHS Data Brief.* 2016;(243): 1–8
22. Sunderam S, Kissin DM, Crawford SB, et al. Assisted reproductive technology surveillance - United States, 2015. *MMWR Surveill Summ.* 2018;67(3): 1–28
23. Robbins C, Boulet SL, Morgan I, et al. Disparities in preconception health indicators - behavioral risk factor surveillance system, 2013-2015, and pregnancy risk assessment monitoring system, 2013-2014. *MMWR Surveill Summ.* 2018;67(1):1–16
24. Gyamfi-Bannerman C, Thom EA. Antenatal betamethasone for women at risk for late preterm delivery. *N Engl J Med.* 2016;375(5):486–487
25. American College of Obstetricians and Gynecologists' Committee on Obstetric Practice; Society for Maternal– Fetal Medicine. Committee opinion No.677: antenatal corticosteroid therapy for fetal maturation. *Obstet Gynecol.* 2016; 128(4):e187–e194
26. Committee on Obstetric Practice. Committee opinion No. 713: antenatal corticosteroid therapy for fetal maturation. *Obstet Gynecol.* 2017; 130(2):e102–e109
27. Kamath-Rayne BD, Rozance PJ, Goldenberg RL, Jobe AH. Antenatal corticosteroids beyond 34 weeks gestation: what do we do now? *Am J Obstet Gynecol.* 2016;215(4):423–430
28. Jobe AH, Goldenberg RL. Antenatal corticosteroids: an assessment of anticipated benefits and potential risks. *Am J Obstet Gynecol.* 2018;219(1):62–74
29. Kaempf JW, Suresh G. Antenatal corticosteroids for the late preterm infant and agnotology. *J Perinatol.* 2017; 37(12):1265–1267
30. Dodd JM, Jones L, Flenady V, Cincotta R, Crowther CA. Prenatal administration of progesterone for preventing preterm birth in women considered to be at risk of preterm birth. *Cochrane Database Syst Rev.* 2013;(7):CD004947
31. Iams JD, Applegate MS, Marcotte MP, et al. A statewide progestogen promotion program in Ohio. *Obstet Gynecol.* 2017;129(2):337–346
32. Romero R, Nicolaides K, Conde-Agudelo A, et al. Vaginal progesterone in women with an asymptomatic sonographic short cervix in the midtrimester decreases preterm delivery and neonatal morbidity: a systematic review and metaanalysis of individual patient data. *Am J Obstet Gynecol.* 2012;206(2):124.e1–124.e19
33. Owen J, Hankins G, Iams JD, et al. Multicenter randomized trial of cerclage for preterm birth prevention in high-risk women with shortened midtrimester cervical length. *Am J Obstet Gynecol.* 2009;201(4):375.e1–375.e8
34. Berghella V, Rafael TJ, Szychowski JM, Rust OA, Owen J. Cerclage for short cervix on ultrasonography in women with singleton gestations and previous preterm birth: a meta-analysis. *Obstet Gynecol.* 2011;117(3):663–671
35. Braveman P, Heck K, Egerter S, et al. Worry about racial discrimination: a missing piece of the puzzle of Black-White disparities in preterm birth? *PLoS One.* 2017;12(10):e0186151
36. Profit J, Gould JB, Bennett M, et al. Racial/ethnic disparity in NICU quality of care delivery. *Pediatrics.* 2017;140(3): e20170918
37. American College of Obstetricians and Gynecologists' Committee on Obstetric Practice; Committee on Genetics; U.S. Food and Drug Administration. Committee opinion No 671: perinatal risks associated with assisted reproductive technology. *Obstet Gynecol.* 2016;128(3):e61–e68
38. Analyses of the National ART Surveillance System (NASS) data. Written communication with the Division of Reproductive Health, National Center for Chronic Disease Prevention and Health Promotion, Centers for Disease Control and Prevention. 2018
39. Sunderam S, Kissin DM, Zhang Y, et al. Assisted reproductive technology surveillance - United States, 2016. *MMWR Surveill Summ.* 2019;68(4):1–23
40. Institute of Medicine (US); Committee on Understanding Premature Birth and Assuring Healthy Outcomes. The National Academies Collection: Reports Funded by National Institutes of Health. In: Behrman RE, Butler AS, eds. *Preterm Birth: Causes, Consequences, and Prevention.* Washington, DC: National Academies Press (US); 2007
41. Hibbard JU, Wilkins I, Sun L, et al; Consortium on Safe Labor. Respiratory morbidity in late preterm births. *JAMA.* 2010;304(4):419–425
42. Vohr B. Long-term outcomes of moderately preterm, late preterm, and early term infants. *Clin Perinatol.* 2013; 40(4):739–751
43. Gunay F, Alpay H, Gokce I, Bilgen H. Is late-preterm birth a risk factor for hypertension in childhood? *Eur J Pediatr.* 2014;173(6):751–756
44. Crump C, Sundquist K, Winkleby MA, Sundquist J. Preterm birth and risk of epilepsy in Swedish adults. *Neurology.* 2011;77(14):1376–1382
45. Moster D, Lie RT, Markestad T. Long-term medical and social consequences of preterm birth. *N Engl J Med.* 2008; 359(3):262–273
46. Lindström K, Winbladh B, Haglund B, Hjern A. Preterm infants as young adults: a Swedish national cohort study. *Pediatrics.* 2007;120(1):70–77
47. Laughon SK, Reddy UM, Sun L, Zhang J. Precursors for late preterm birth in singleton gestations. *Obstet Gynecol.* 2010;116(5):1047–1055
48. Pulver LS, Denney JM, Silver RM, Young PC. Morbidity and discharge timing of late preterm newborns. *Clin Pediatr (Phila).* 2010;49(11):1061–1067
49. Tomashek KM, Shapiro-Mendoza CK, Weiss J, et al. Early discharge among late preterm and term newborns and risk of neonatal morbidity. *Semin Perinatol.* 2006;30(2):61–68
50. Escobar GJ, Greene JD, Hulac P, et al. Rehospitalisation after birth

hospitalisation: patterns among infants of all gestations. *Arch Dis Child.* 2005; 90(2):125–131

51. Wallenstein MB, Bhutani VK. Jaundice and kernicterus in the moderately preterm infant. *Clin Perinatol.* 2013; 40(4):679–688
52. Bhutani VK, Johnson L. Kernicterus in late preterm infants cared for as term healthy infants. *Semin Perinatol.* 2006; 30(2):89–97
53. Saluja S, Agarwal A, Kler N, Amin S. Auditory neuropathy spectrum disorder in late preterm and term infants with severe jaundice. *Int J Pediatr Otorhinolaryngol.* 2010;74(11):1292–1297
54. Quinn JM, Sparks M, Gephart SM. Discharge criteria for the late preterm infant: a review of the literature. *Adv Neonatal Care.* 2017;17(5):362–371
55. Benitz WE; Committee on Fetus and Newborn, American Academy of Pediatrics. Hospital stay for healthy term newborn infants. *Pediatrics.* 2015; 135(5):948–953
56. Hwang SS, Barfield WD, Smith RA, et al. Discharge timing, outpatient follow-up, and home care of late-preterm and early-term infants. *Pediatrics.* 2013; 132(1):101–108
57. Morse SB, Zheng H, Tang Y, Roth J. Early school-age outcomes of late preterm infants. *Pediatrics.* 2009;123(4). Available at: www.pediatrics.org/cgi/content/full/123/4/e622
58. Chan E, Quigley MA. School performance at age 7 years in late preterm and early term birth: a cohort study. *Arch Dis Child Fetal Neonatal Ed.* 2014;99(6):F451–F457
59. Raju TNK, Buist AS, Blaisdell CJ, Moxey-Mims M, Saigal S. Adults born preterm: a review of general health and system-specific outcomes. *Acta Paediatr.* 2017; 106(9):1409–1437
60. Raju TNK, Pemberton VL, Saigal S, et al; Adults Born Preterm Conference Speakers and Discussants. Long-term healthcare outcomes of preterm birth: an executive summary of a conference sponsored by the National Institutes of Health. *J Pediatr.* 2017;181:309–318.e1
61. Holland MG, Refuerzo JS, Ramin SM, Saade GR, Blackwell SC. Late preterm birth: how often is it avoidable? *Am J Obstet Gynecol.* 2009;201(4): 404.e1–404.e4
62. Klebanoff MA. Interpregnancy interval and pregnancy outcomes: causal or not? *Obstet Gynecol.* 2017;129(3): 405–407
63. Ball SJ, Pereira G, Jacoby P, de Klerk N, Stanley FJ. Re-evaluation of link between interpregnancy interval and adverse birth outcomes: retrospective cohort study matching two intervals per mother. *BMJ.* 2014;349:g4333
64. Hanley GE, Hutcheon JA, Kinniburgh BA, Lee L. Interpregnancy interval and adverse pregnancy outcomes: an analysis of successive pregnancies. *Obstet Gynecol.* 2017;129(3):408–415
65. Donovan EF, Lannon C, Bailit J, et al; Ohio Perinatal Quality Collaborative Writing Committee. A statewide initiative to reduce inappropriate scheduled births at 36(0/7)-38(6/7) weeks' gestation [published correction appears in *Am J Obstet Gynecol.* 2010; 202(6):603]. *Am J Obstet Gynecol.* 2010; 202(3):243.e1–243.e8

The Use of Nonnutritive Sweeteners in Children

- *Policy Statement*

POLICY STATEMENT Organizational Principles to Guide and Define the Child Health Care System and/or Improve the Health of all Children

American Academy of Pediatrics

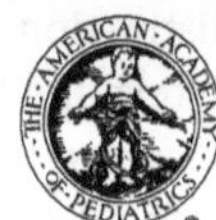

DEDICATED TO THE HEALTH OF ALL CHILDREN™

The Use of Nonnutritive Sweeteners in Children

Carissa M. Baker-Smith, MD, MPH, FAAP,[a] Sarah D. de Ferranti, MD, MPH, FAAP,[b] William J. Cochran, MD, FAAP,[c] COMMITTEE ON NUTRITION, SECTION ON GASTROENTEROLOGY, HEPATOLOGY, AND NUTRITION

abstract

The prevalence of nonnutritive sweeteners (NNSs) in the food supply has increased over time. Not only are more children and adolescents consuming NNSs, but they are also consuming a larger quantity of NNSs in the absence of strong scientific evidence to refute or support the safety of these agents. This policy statement from the American Academy of Pediatrics is intended to provide the pediatric provider with a review of (1) previous steps taken for approved use of NNSs, (2) existing data regarding the safety of NNS use in the general pediatric population, (3) what is known regarding the potential benefits and/or adverse effects of NNS use in children and adolescents, (4) identified gaps in existing knowledge and potential areas of future research, and (5) suggested talking points that pediatricians may use when discussing NNS use with families

[a]School of Medicine, University of Maryland, Baltimore, Maryland; [b]Boston Children's Hospital, Boston, Massachusetts; and [c]Geisinger Medical Center, Danville, Pennsylvania

Dr Baker-Smith is the primary author and drafted this policy statement, conducted the literature search and literature review, created the evidence table used to support the content of this policy statement, and assisted with final revisions and review of the document; Dr de Ferranti reviewed the literature, assisted with the drafting and editing of the policy statement, and conducted final revisions and review; Dr Cochran assisted with literature review, contributed to the creation of the evidence table used to support the content of this policy statement, and assisted with the final review of the document; and all authors approved the final version of the manuscript as submitted.

Policy statements from the American Academy of Pediatrics benefit from expertise and resources of liaisons and internal (AAP) and external reviewers. However, policy statements from the American Academy of Pediatrics may not reflect the views of the liaisons or the organizations or government agencies that they represent.

This document is copyrighted and is property of the American Academy of Pediatrics and its Board of Directors. All authors have filed conflict of interest statements with the American Academy of Pediatrics. Any conflicts have been resolved through a process approved by the Board of Directors. The American Academy of Pediatrics has neither solicited nor accepted any commercial involvement in the development of the content of this publication.

The guidance in this statement does not indicate an exclusive course of treatment or serve as a standard of medical care. Variations, taking into account individual circumstances, may be appropriate.

All policy statements from the American Academy of Pediatrics automatically expire 5 years after publication unless reaffirmed, revised, or retired at or before that time.

DOI: https://doi.org/10.1542/peds.2019-2765

To cite: Baker-Smith CM, de Ferranti SD, Cochran WJ, AAP COMMITTEE ON NUTRITION, SECTION ON GASTROENTEROLOGY, HEPATOLOGY, AND NUTRITION. The Use of Nonnutritive Sweeteners in Children. *Pediatrics.* 2019;144(5):e20192765

INTRODUCTION

Nonnutritive sweeteners (NNSs), also known as noncaloric artificial sweeteners or high-intensity sweeteners, were first introduced into the food supply in the late 1800s (eg, saccharin) and were first approved for use as a food additive under the Food Additives Amendment of the Federal Food, Drug, and Cosmetic Act of 1958.[1,2] NNSs increase the palatability of food and beverages without increasing caloric content. It has been proposed that the lack of caloric content of the sweeteners may contribute to weight loss. To date, however, there has been no consistent or conclusive evidence that NNS use lends to a reduction in total caloric intake and thereby to weight loss in humans[3–8] or in animal physiology models.[9] Questions regarding the long-term safety of these agents also remain.[3] Most NNSs, including saccharin, aspartame, acesulfame potassium, sucralose, and neotame, have been approved by the US Food and Drug Administration (FDA) for use as food additives and, as such, have undergone premarket review and approval (https://www.fda.gov/food/food-ingredients-packaging/overview-food-ingredients-additives-colors). Other agents such as stevia and luo han guo have been approved by the FDA under the "generally recognized as safe" (GRAS) distinction, a distinction that has been determined to be insufficient for ensuring the safety of food additives without specific protections against conflict of interest and without mechanisms to ensure ongoing acquisition of safety data.[10,11]

Concerns regarding the safety of NNSs were initially related to their potential carcinogenic effects. Cyclamate, first approved for use in 1958, was later removed from the list of approved food additives in 1969 because of concerns regarding an association between cyclamate use and the development of bladder cancer.[1,2,10,12] The relationship between cyclamate and cancer was later refuted on the basis of additional scientific data in rats, mice, dogs, hamsters, and monkeys.

Cyclamate was not the only NNS initially suspected of an associated cancer risk. Beginning in the 1970s and 1980s, animal studies suggested an association between saccharin intake and the development of bladder cancer in rodents.[3,13,14] This association was later refuted because it was determined that the "cancer-causing mechanisms in rodents are not applicable to humans."[3,14] Furthermore, human studies evaluating the relationship between saccharin intake and stomach, pancreatic, and endometrial cancer have not identified a relationship between the consumption of saccharin and cancer.[2,3,15,16] Overall, it appears that science does not support a potential carcinogenic effect of cyclamate, saccharin, or sucralose in humans.[3,17–19] The relationship between aspartame and the development of attention-deficit disorders, birth defects, diabetes, and lupus has also been refuted.[3]

A number of health organizations have supported the use of NNSs but within an acceptable dietary intake (ADI) level.[20–25] Despite this, studies conclusively demonstrating the long-term safety and efficacy of NNS agents are lacking.[3,26] Also lacking is published evidence of parental confidence in the safety of NNSs. Despite FDA assurances, published data reveal that parents continue to have questions about the safety of NNSs. For instance, in a single-site study, only 16% of parents responded in the affirmative to the statement, "Nonnutritive sweeteners (ie, Splenda, Sweet'N Low, and Equal) are safe for my child to use."[27] Knowledge of how to identify products containing NNSs remains poor because only 23% of parents were able to correctly identify food products that contain NNSs. In fact, 53% of parents stated they seek items labeled "reduced sugar," but most did not recognize that the sweet taste was instead being provided by an NNS,[27] and only one-quarter of youth were able to distinguish the taste of NNS from sucrose.[28]

Estimating total content of NNS in manufactured products has been challenging. Manufactured products containing NNSs are not required to specify the content of NNS in a product. However, the consumption of NNSs among children has increased.[29,30] The long-term safety or potential benefit of the growing prevalence of NNS use in children has not been systematically reviewed.[31] One barrier to better understanding the health effects of NNS is the difficulty inherent in measuring the amount of NNS consumed at the individual and population levels. The FDA designation of a food item as an additive or GRAS means that although manufacturers must report that a particular product contains a sweetener, there is no obligation to state the amount of sweetener a product contains,[1] making it difficult to estimate how much NNS the average American consumes per day. This is compounded by the fact that NNS can also be found in our drinking water.[32] Thus, even those who do not believe that they have been exposed to NNSs have detectable levels of NNS in their urine.[32,33]

Estimates of consumption are largely based on dietary recall[12,29,30,34,35]; however, such studies are fraught with inaccuracies and thus may result in underestimates of true intake.[29] Ideally, intake of NNS remains within the ADI level. Studies from the late 1990s and early 2000s, including studies in children, had suggested that intake of intense sweeteners was substantially below the ADI.[34–36] Contemporary data addressing total daily intake of NNS in adults and children are limited. According to select studies, intake of particular NNSs (eg, acesulfame potassium or cyclamate) may exceed the ADI.[37] Historically, carbonated beverages have contributed the greatest milligram dosage to total daily intake of NNS (eg, saccharin).[12,38] However, there is a growing and widening variety of food, drink, and consumer products that contain NNSs (eg, chewing gum, oral rehydration solutions, mouthwash, etc; Table 1).[10] Therefore, estimates of intake would be difficult to capture given current methods of reporting.

Ongoing questions also exist regarding the benefits of NNSs. Added sugars are known to have detrimental effects,[39,40] including an association between sugar intake and increased body mass, dyslipidemia, and blood pressure.[40] Recommendations to promote cardiovascular health in children include limiting the total intake of sugar-sweetened beverages (SSBs) to 4 to 6 oz per day in children 1 to 6 years of age and limiting the total intake of SSBs to 8 to 12 oz per day in children 7 to 18 years of age.[41] NNSs have been considered for use among those aiming to reduce their total SSB intake while still preserving the sweet taste. In particular, NNS use has been proposed among individuals with diabetes and among those aiming to lose or maintain weight.

TABLE 1 Commercial Products Reported to Contain NNS

NNS	No. Products	Product Examples
Saccharin	100	Smucker's Low Sugar Reduced Sugar Sweet Orange Marmalade, Bubble Yum Sugarless chewing gum, diet sodas (Tab), yogurt
Aspartame	2307	Jell-O, diet sodas (Diet Coke, Coke Zero, Diet Dr Pepper, Fresca, Tab), Country Time Sugar Free lemonade
Acesulfame potassium	3882	SlimFast, Werther's Original Sugar Free hard candies, Del Monte Mandarin Oranges No Sugar Added, Pedialyte, diet sodas (Pepsi One, Sprite Zero, Fresca)
Sucralose	5148	Lean Pockets, diet sodas (Diet Mountain Dew)
Neotame	114	Sunny D, protein shakes, chewing gum
Stevia	642	Some Muscle Milk products
Advantame	0	N/A
Luo han guo	98	Some Celestial Seasonings products

Adapted from FoodFacts.com (accessed July 12, 2015); Franz M. Amounts of sweeteners in popular sodas. Available at: https://static.diabetesselfmanagement.com/pdfs/DSM0310_012.pdf. Accessed April 28, 2019; and Food Standards New Zealand Australia. Sweeteners. 2018. Available at: www.foodstandards.gov.au/consumer/additives/Pages/Sweeteners.aspx. Accessed April 28, 2019. N/A, not applicable.

However, concerns have arisen that NNS use in animals may alter gut microbiota in such a way that there is an enhanced risk for glucose intolerance, insulin resistance, diabetes, and increased weight.[42,43]

This report summarizes the available literature regarding NNS use in children and adolescents, including the penetrance of these agents into the pediatric food chain and effects on taste preferences in children. This statement also addresses proposed potential benefits of NNSs in specific pediatric populations (ie, those with obesity, diabetes, etc). Consideration of the strength of the data was also included. Our purpose with this statement is not to provide specific clinical guidance regarding the use of NNSs in children but rather to provide a summary of the existing data. Finally, recommendations are made for future directions in research and policy.

METHODS

A systematic review was beyond the scope of this publication; however, the authors used a common search strategy to identify relevant publications. A literature review was conducted regarding the use and safety of NNSs in the pediatric population (ie, 0–18 years of age) in 2011. The search was updated on October 15, 2014, and then again on May 25, 2018, because of delays in publication related to a lengthy review process. A final selection of references was performed by August 20, 2018, resulting in 40 additional references.

The following search terms were used in PubMed (www.pubmed.gov): "nonnutritive sweetener" or the name of each individual FDA-approved nonnutritive sweetener (ie, "aspartame," "neotame," "saccharin," "sucralose," "advantame," or "acesulfame"). "Stevia" also was included in the search because this agent received the designation of GRAS. The search was limited to studies published within the previous 10 years (before the initial search) in human subjects and written in the English language. Eighty-three studies were identified. Studies that did not pertain to the use, safety, potential benefits, or associated risks of NNS use in children were excluded (n = 31). Studies addressing the use of NNSs in pain control were excluded. The reference lists of selected articles were reviewed, and relevant cited references were also included. Additional searches were performed to fill in identified knowledge gaps (n = 30). Finally, policy statements of other organizations on NNS use, including the Academy of Nutrition and Dietetics (AND),[21–23] American Diabetes Association (ADA),[44] and American Heart Association (AHA),[12] were reviewed (n = 4). It should be stated that the highest-quality evidence is derived from randomized controlled trials (RCTs) within the population of interest. To date, however, few such studies exist (n = 6).[4,45–49]

SWEETENERS AND NNSS

Sweeteners can be classified as sugars (ie, brown sugar, cane sugar, fructose, and high-fructose corn syrup), alcohol sugars (ie, isomalt, maltitol, mannitol, sorbitol, and xylitol), and NNSs (ie, saccharin, aspartame, acesulfame potassium, sucralose, stevia, neotame, and advantame). NNSs are high-intensity sweeteners that provide a sweet taste with little to no glycemic response and few to no calories.[1]

Eight NNSs are currently approved by the FDA,[1] and their levels of sweetness range from 180 to 20 000 times sweeter than sucrose (ie, table sugar). Each NNS possesses varying properties; some are stable when heated. Some are contraindicated for use in particular patient populations, such as aspartame use in people with phenylketonuria (Table 2). Most have been approved for use as a food additive and, as such, have undergone a premarket approval process in accordance with stipulations made by

TABLE 2 FDA-Approved NNSs

Type (Approval Distinction)	Commercial Name	Kcal/g	Sweetness Compared With Sucrose	Introduction and/or FDA Approval	Heating Reduces Sweetness	Contraindication and/or Safety Issues
Saccharin (1,2- benzisothiazolin-3-1, 1,1-dioxide) (food additive)	Sweet'N Low, Sugar Twin, Necta Sweet	0	200–700	Introduced in 1879; FDA approved for use	No	None
Aspartame (N-[l-α- Aspartyl]-L-phe, 1-methyl ester) (food additive)	NutraSweet, Equal, Sugar Twin	4[a]	180	Approved for limited use (ie, tabletop sweetener) by the FDA in 1981 and approved for general use in 1996	Yes	Phenylketonuria; reported cases of thrombocytopenia (78)[50]
Acesulfame potassium and/or acelsulfame potassium (potassium 6–methyl-2,2-dioxo-oxathiazin-4-folate) (food additive)	Sunett, Sweet One	0	300	Discovered 1967; FDA approved limited use 1988 and general use (exceptions: meat and poultry) in 2003	No	Associated with cancer in animals at high dose; no known association in humans
Sucralose (1,6- Dichloro-1, 6-dideoxy-β-D- fructofuranosyl-4-chloro-4-deoxy-α-D-galactopyranoside) (food additive)	Splenda	0	600	Discovered in 1976; FDA approved for limited use in 1998 and for general use in 1999	No	None
Neotame (N-[N-(3,3-dimethylbutyl)-L-α-aspartyl-L-phe 1-methyl ester]) (food additive)	Newtame	0	7000–13 000	FDA approved for general use 2002 (exceptions: meat and poultry)	No	Contains phe and asp and is therefore contraindicated in those with phenylketonuria
Stevia (1,1-dioxo-1,2-benzothiazol-3-1), GRAS	Truvia, Pure Via, Enliten	0	200–400	Accepted as GRAS April 20, 2015	Yes	None
Advantame ([N-(3-(3-hydroxy-4-methoxyphenyl))-propyl-α-aspartyl]-L-phe 1-methyl ester)	None	3.85	20 000	FDA approved for general use 2014 (exceptions: meat and poultry)	No	Determined to be safe for use in children
Luo han guo fruit extract (GRAS)	Monk Fruit in the Raw, PureLo Lo Han Sweetener	Unknown	600	GRAS January 15, 2010; intended for use as a tabletop sweetener, food ingredient, and additional sweetening agent	Unknown	None

Adapted from AND. Scientific opinion on the safety of advantame for the proposed uses as a food additive. *EFSA J.* 2013;11(7):3301; Fitch C, Keim KS; Academy of Nutrition and Dietetics. Position of the Academy of Nutrition and Dietetics: use of nutritive and nonnutritive sweeteners. *J Acad Nutr Diet.* 2012;112(5):739–758; Renwick AG. Postscript on advantame–a novel high-potency low-calorie sweetener. *Food Chem Toxicol.* 2011;49(suppl 1):S1; Kroger M, Meister K, Kava R. Low-calorie sweeteners and other sugar substitutes: a review of the safety issues. *Compr Rev Food Sci Food Saf.* 2006;5:35–47; and Magnuson BA, Roberts A, Nestmann ER. Critical review of the current literature on the safety of sucralose. *Food Chem Toxicol.* 2017;106(pt A):324–355.

[a] Although aspartame contains 4 kcal/g, little is used, and therefore, it essentially provides no extra calories.[51]

the 1958 Food Additives Amendment to the Federal Food, Drug, and Cosmetic Act.

Under the 1958 Food Additive Amendment to the Federal Food, Drug, and Cosmetic Act, only substances with GRAS designation do not require premarket approval. Although the market studies for aspartame, acesulfame potassium, sucralose, advantame (an N-substituted analog of aspartame), saccharin, and neotame are not widely available, these NNSs have been studied for safety.[1] Studies number more than 100 for aspartame, nearly 100 for acesulfame potassium, approximately 110 for neotame (in animals and humans), and 37 for advantame (in animals and humans), the NNS food additive most recently approved by the FDA.[1,52,53] Only 2 approved NNSs, *Stevia rebaudiana* and luo han guo (or monk fruit), have been approved under the GRAS notification process. After the passage of the 1958 Food Additives Amendment, President Nixon ordered an evaluation of GRAS substances, largely in response to concerns raised about some of the substances with GRAS designation, including cyclamate. After this order in the 1970s, the FDA hired the Life Sciences Research Office, which then selected qualified scientists (ie, the Select Committee on GRAS Substances) as consultants to review and evaluate the available information on each of the GRAS substances. The select committee's evaluations were made independently of the FDA or any other governmental or nongovernmental group. In 1972, a GRAS affirmation process began. The FDA established procedures (21 Code of Federal Regulations 170.35) that it would then use to affirm the GRAS status of substances. The GRAS notification process began in 1997. By the end of 2006, 193 GRAS notices were filed, and the glycoside isolated from the plant *S rebaudiana Bertoni* and luo han guo were accepted as GRAS for use in baked foods and soft drinks.[1,3] Additional information regarding NNSs can be found in previously published review articles.[10,21,22,38,43,51–61]

PENETRANCE OF NNSS INTO THE NORTH AMERICAN DIET: HOW MUCH NNS DO CHILDREN ACTUALLY CONSUME?

Information about NNS consumption by children and adolescents is mostly derived from dietary recall[12,62–69] and cross-sectional analysis,[29,30] which limits the ability to estimate the quantity of NNS consumed because the quantity of NNS per serving of any given food is not publicly available and because dietary recall is prone to error. Early studies found that approximately 15% of the population older than 2 years old consumes some type of NNS per year (eg, 2003–2004).[70] Older review articles concluded that pediatric NNS intake was within the ADI level.[34,62,63] Still others have found, on the basis of estimated intake from 24-hour dietary recall, that intake of cyclamate and saccharin may exceed the ADI for some youth.[69] Regardless, intake of NNS among children tends to exceed NNS intake for adults when assessed as milligrams per kilogram of body weight.[12]

The prevalence of NNS use is increasing, and inclusion of NNSs in daily food products is more pervasive.[10,70,71] A single prospective study of youth with diabetes mellitus (n = 227) estimated, on the basis of a 5-day food diary, that the theoretical maximum daily intake of saccharin, acesulfame potassium, and aspartame did not exceed ADI but varied between 5% and 94% of the ADI.[36] According to Web sites such as FoodFacts.com, the number of foods and consumer products that include at least 1 NNS as an ingredient has tripled within the last 4 to 5 years. In 2010, Yang[72] found that according to FoodFacts.com, 3648 products contained at least 1 NNS.[10] As of July 12, 2015, approximately 12 291 products contained at least 1 NNS.[10]

People are not always aware of their intake of NNS. Some artificial sweeteners can be found in groundwater and drinking water, although at magnitudes below the ADI level.[32] Furthermore, people inadvertently consume NNS, according to a recent study of 18 reported "nonconsumers," 44% of whom had sucralose in their urine that was unexplained by the trivial amounts of sucralose that are sometimes reported in the water supply.[32,33]

The majority of NNS intake is derived from intake of NNS-containing beverages (~11%), followed by food (~4%) and individual NNS packets (~1%).[38] Data from the NHANES 1999–2000 to 2007–2008 show that the percentage of children consuming NNS-containing beverages increased from <1% to >7%.[29] More recent NHANES cross-sectional data analysis (2009–2012) revealed that 25.1% of children, compared with 44% of adults, reported consumption of NNSs.[30] Most reported daily use (80% of children and 56% of adults). Analysis of the 2009–2012 NHANES data suggests that NNS intake is higher in women and girls, individuals with obesity (versus those with overweight or normal weight), non-Hispanic white individuals (versus non-Hispanic African American or Hispanic individuals), and individuals in the highest tertile of income.[30] Between 4% and 18% of carbonated beverages consumed by children contain NNSs.[71] Household purchase of NNS-containing beverages has also increased at the same time that the purchase of SSBs has decreased: between 2003 and 2010.[73]

International recommendations have established an ADI (per kilogram) for NNSs. The ADI is typically 100 times lower than the dose of the sweetener known to cause toxicity in animals.[71] The concept of the ADI was established by an international scientific committee and the Joint Food and Agriculture Organization of the United Nations–World Health Organization Expert Committee on Food Additives. Other organizations have reported ADI levels for various NNSs, including the European Food Safety Authority and the Danish Veterinary and Food Administration (Table 3).[70] US federal regulations (FDA Code 21 Code of Federal Regulations 170) do not require that the amount of NNS in a food item be listed on the product label if it has been determined to be safe for use in a particular food.[1] However, without proper knowledge of true content, it is difficult to know whether intake of a particular sweetener is within the ADI level.

It is also difficult to know whether intake of a particular NNS by a child is within the ADI level, but it is worth noting that there have been few cases of reported adverse events related to NNS intake.[50] Proponents of NNS use argue that safety information can be assumed on the basis of more than 30 years of use of these agents with relatively few reported adverse effects. However, it is also true that there has been no systematic or formal method for capturing and recording adverse effects related to the use of these agents.

Given the proliferation of products containing NNSs in the food supply, which may lead to both increased consumption and combined use of NNSs, there is a need for contemporary peer-reviewed studies

TABLE 3 ADI Level

Sweetener	JECFA ADI, mg/kg	EFSA ADI, mg/kg	DVFA ADI, mg/kg	FDA ADI, mg/kg	Number of Packets Equivalent to ADI (Based on a 68-kg Person)
Saccharin (Sweet'N Low)	5	5	5	15	250
Aspartame (NutraSweet and Equal)	40	40	15	50	165
Acesulfame potassium (Sweet One)	15	9	40	15	165
Sucralose (Splenda)	15	15	15	5	165
Neotame	0–2	1	Unknown	0.3	200
Stevia	4	4	Unknown	12	30
Advantame	0–5	5	4000	33	4000

Adapted from US Food and Drug Administration. Food additives and ingredients. Available at: www.fda.gov/food/ingredientspackaginglabeling/foodadditivesingredients. Accessed March 26, 2019; Gardner C, Wylie-Rosett J, Gidding SS, et al; American Heart Association Nutrition Committee of the Council on Nutrition, Physical Activity and Metabolism, Council on Arteriosclerosis, Thrombosis and Vascular Biology, Council on Cardiovascular Disease in the Young, and the American Diabetes Association. Nonnutritive sweeteners: current use and health perspectives: a scientific statement from the American Heart Association and the American Diabetes Association. *Circulation*. 2012;126(4):509–519; and Mattes RD, Popkin BM. Nonnutritive sweetener consumption in humans: effects on appetite and food intake and their putative mechanisms. *Am J Clin Nutr*. 2009;89(1):1–14. DVFA, Danish Veterinary and Food Administration; EFSA, European Food and Safety Agency; JECFA, Joint Food and Agriculture Organization of the United Nations–World Health Organization Expert Committee on Food Additives.

to estimate the current prevalence of NNS use, amounts consumed by children, and any potential adverse effects.

IMPACT OF NNSS ON APPETITE AND TASTE PREFERENCE

Studies regarding the potential impact of NNS intake on appetite and taste preference can be divided into animal studies and human studies. Animal models have shown that nutritive sweeteners activate the sweet-taste receptors (ie, T1R family and α-gustducin receptors).[74,75] According to animal studies, saccharin intake weakens the ability of Sprague Dawley rats to signal the caloric "postingestive consequences of eating" so that if saccharin is administered, rats did not regulate their intake of sugar-sweetened food and/or beverages after saccharin-sweetened solution intake.[76] This study suggests that NNS intake may affect normal responses to caloric intake such that overeating may be more likely if the diet after NNS administration is a sweeter diet.[76]

In children, the taste receptors are located in the lingual taste buds and along the intestinal mucosa.[77] Activation of the sweet-taste receptors results in stimulus to the pleasure-generating loci of the brain,[77] triggering glucose uptake and appetite regulation. Individuals vary in their ability to perceive taste, and thus, individuals differ in their potential "gain" achieved from various sweet stimuli.[78,79] It was once believed that only nutritive sweeteners activate the sweet-taste receptors; however, it is now known that NNSs, which are several hundred times sweeter than table sugar, also activate these receptors.[70] The effect of NNS activation on taste preference, food intake, the activation of metabolic pathways, and appetite is not well understood.[80,81]

Human studies have been inconsistent in their reporting of the potential impact of NNS use on appetite and taste preferences. Furthermore, genetic differences in taste perception may also exist and influence study results.[82] A small study of 10 healthy adults given 1 of 4 drinks that contained either glucose alone or glucose plus 1 of 3 sweeteners (eg, 45 g glucose and 150 mg aspartame, 45 g glucose and 20 mg saccharin, or 45 g glucose and 85 mg acesulfame potassium in 250 mL of water) did not report differences in hunger or fullness within 60 minutes of ingestion.[83] In contrast, a single study of 115 college students 18 to 22 years of age given either Sprite Zero (NNS-containing beverage), mineral water, or regular Sprite reported that those who consumed NNS (ie, Sprite Zero) were more likely to subsequently choose a bag of chocolate M&M's (43%), whereas those who consumed a nutritive sweetener (eg, regular Sprite) or water were more likely to select a less-sweet snack, such as water or chewing gum (41% and 33%, respectively).[84] The authors concluded that participants who consumed NNSs felt less satisfied with what they had drunk compared with those who consumed a sugar-sweetened or an unsweetened beverage (P = .004).[84] As for assessing how intake of NNS influenced preference for sweet food, researchers found in this study of 115 college students that participants who consumed NNS were more likely to provide the names of high-calorie food items compared with those who consumed a sugar-sweetened or an unsweetened drink (P = .001)[84] after consumption of the NNS-containing beverage.

NNS use in children may be associated with a greater preference for sweet foods[77]; however, the effect of NNSs on taste preference is not well understood. Humans have an innate preference for sweet foods, and children in particular prefer high levels of sweetness.[77] Children who consume large amounts of SSBs may tend to prefer foods that are richer in both sugar and calories. The American Academy of Pediatrics (AAP) recognizes the detrimental effect of high sugar content on the health of children and the propensity that high sugar content has for promoting obesity in childhood.[6,39,85–87] The AAP recommends against routine consumption of sports and energy drinks because of their high sugar content.[39] A single, small population study found that adults who consumed NNSs tend to prefer a sweet versus salty and/or savory snack after this ingestion. The authors suggest that NNS intake can increase the motivation for one to access sweet relative to savory snacks[88] and thereby alter energy balance in such a way that children who consume these agents are more likely to consume sugary food and drinks.[84] The temporal correlation between the increase in childhood overweight and obesity and the increase in intake of NNS-containing beverages is suggestive of a relationship.[38] However, the relationship may be one of reverse causality, whereby children who have obesity (or their parents) may be substituting food or beverages sweetened with NNSs for those containing sugar in an attempt to limit caloric intake.

In summary, increasing trends in NNS use are coincident with an increase in the prevalence of childhood obesity. Data suggest but do not conclusively demonstrate that NNS use may promote the intake of sugary food and drink by affecting taste preferences. It has been demonstrated that excessive intake of SSBs (and increased calories) has been associated with childhood obesity. Additional information regarding the effects of NNS use on taste preferences and caloric intake and comparison of the long-term effect of NNS-containing versus SSBs is needed.

SAFETY AND NNS USE

Most NNSs have been approved by the FDA for use as a food additive; 2 NNSs were approved under the GRAS distinction for a particular intended use.[1] Reviews and investigative studies discussing and evaluating the safety of NNSs, including sucralose,[19] have been published. Studies investigating the potential toxic effects of NNSs have been performed in animals[55–58] and humans.[51,59] Results from these more recent studies have concluded that there are no potential teratogenic effects or negative effects of NNS use on weight or development in animals. However, cases of aspartame-induced thrombocytopenia have been reported.[50] Furthermore, aspartame is uniformly contraindicated in people with phenylketonuria.

NNS USE AND CANCER RISK

Concerns regarding a potential relationship between NNSs and cancer were raised shortly after the introduction of NNS into the food supply.[1,10] Cyclamate was first approved for use in humans in the 1950s[89]; however, concerns arose regarding a potential increased risk for bladder cancer after use of cyclamate in rats.[89] It was also proposed that the metabolism of cyclamate to cyclohexylamine, which is toxic to rats and dogs, caused testicular atrophy and impaired spermatogenesis.[89] When administered to nonhuman primates, 3 of 14 monkeys given cyclamate developed neoplasms versus 0 of 16 controls. The 3 tumors, developed after receipt of "the equivalent of ~30 calorie-reduced drinks" (containing cyclamate), were a metastatic adenocarcinoma of the colon, a metastatic hepatocellular carcinoma, and a papillary adenocarcinoma of the prostate. The authors concluded that there was "no evidence for carcinogenicity of sodium cyclamate because the tumors in the treatment group were of different histologies and the tumors occurred at a rate frequently observed in monkeys."[89] To date, there have been no case control studies of cyclamate, particularly related to tumor formation in humans.[89] The relationship between cyclamate and cancer was later refuted, and permissions for use of cyclamate were thus reinstated in 1992.[2]

A study of Sprague Dawley rats fed diets supplemented with 0%, 5%, and 7.5% (of the total diet) saccharin experienced differences in the proliferation of the epithelial cells (used as a marker of cancer risk) by diet and concentration of saccharin.[14] However, this study was not deemed to be relevant to humans because the form of saccharin used, sodium-saccharin, is considered "representative of a large group of sodium salts known to act as tumor promoters in the male rat urinary bladder when high doses (of saccharin) are administered."[14] The FDA reports that a total of 30 human studies have been conducted to date and have not found an association between saccharin use and cancer of any type.[1] A large case control study of people with bladder cancer (n = 3010) and controls (n = 5783) found no association between self-reported past NNS use and bladder cancer.[66] However, not all studies have agreed with this conclusion.[16] A number of observational studies later determined that the relationship between saccharin and bladder cancer was specific to rodents.[17] Saccharin was removed from the list of potential carcinogens in 2001 by the National Toxicology Program of the National Institutes of Health.[10]

A case control study of adults with incident neoplasia (eg, stomach, pancreas, and endometrium) versus unaffected controls did not find greater odds of cancer among those exposed to NNSs.[90] However, 1 of the limitations of this case control study was low NNS use among participants and potentially insufficient sample size to detect even weak associations between NNS use and cancer.[90]

A systematic review of the safety and potential carcinogenic effect of aspartame in mice found no association between aspartame administration and risk of cancer.[91] A meta-analysis of studies of aspartame in rats showed no association between aspartame and cancer.[92] A review of human (adult) cohort and case control studies showed no relationship between most types of cancer and aspartame use.[18,51,92,93]

Newer data have failed to demonstrate an association between NNS use and cancer.[90] The long latency period, the penetrance of NNSs into the food supply (making it difficult to isolate an adequate unexposed control group), and the diversity of potential mechanisms have made it difficult to definitively exclude potential carcinogenic properties of NNSs but also make it difficult to conclude that there is any such association. The type of research that would more definitively address the effects of NNS intake over the long-term and across the life span (for example, long-term randomized clinical trials or prospective cohorts with well-defined measures of exposure over multiple time points) is not likely to occur.

In summary, observational data in adult-human studies show no association between NNS use and cancer. There are no long-term studies in children. Studies have been limited to animal and adult-human studies, and the long-term risk of cancer and other conditions among children who use NNSs is not known and is likely to be difficult to obtain.

NNS USE IN SELECT PEDIATRIC POPULATIONS

It can be reasonably argued that certain subpopulations of children might benefit from the use of NNSs. For example, children and adolescents who have obesity might benefit from lower total caloric intake. Children who have type 1 or 2 diabetes mellitus might also benefit from the lack of a glycemic response while enjoying the sweet taste of NNSs. Similarly, those with multiple metabolic or cardiovascular disease risk factors also might experience a benefit because excess carbohydrate intake is likely a factor contributing to their health risk.[94–96]

NNS USE AND CHILDREN WITH OBESITY

NNSs pass through the human gastrointestinal tract without being digested, providing sweet taste without added calories, a property that is potentially advantageous for preventing and controlling obesity given the association between sugary beverage consumption and obesity.[6,64,87,97] However, the data are conflicting as to whether consuming NNSs leads to weight loss or weight gain.[6,87]

Swithers et al[98] also provided animal studies reporting that use of artificial sweeteners may increase weight gain. Observational studies in adults show that NNS intake is associated with increased BMI. Analysis of the San Antonio Heart Study, an adult prospective cohort study, showed a dose-response adverse effect of NNS intake on overweight and obesity status over 7 to 8 years of follow-up.[99] However, these data are vulnerable to reverse causality because it has been demonstrated that individuals who are attempting to lose weight are more likely to use NNSs.[26] Additionally, the San Antonio analysis is subject to the same vulnerabilities regarding the accuracy of estimated NNS intake, particularly because the baseline data were collected decades before the current era and estimates were reliant on dietary recall.

Several cross-sectional studies in children and adolescents have also reported positive associations between NNS intake and BMI (ie, high NNS intake is associated with higher BMI).[64,100] However, results from longitudinal follow-up are conflicting, with a few studies supporting these findings[6,86,87] and others suggesting either no relationship[101] or a small beneficial effect of NNS intake on BMI.[97]

A double-blind RCT from the Netherlands found that replacement of SSB intake with NNS intake in school-aged children was associated with reduced weight gain (not weight loss) during an 18-month period.[4] A study of aspartame use in adults with overweight (eg, mean age 19 years) was associated with greater weight reduction than among the control population.[102] Similarly, a study from South Africa found that intake of 25 mg of sucralose per day by youth 6 to 11 years of age was associated with a lower BMI-for-age *z* score (control and nutritive sweetener of 7.1 and micronutrient and NNS of 6 versus control and sucrose of 10.8 and micronutrient and NNS of 10.9) compared with sugar intake. In contrast, a higher weight-for-age *z* score change was associated with NNS use in a separate study.[5] Prospective studies have revealed mixed results: Newby et al[103] did not identify an association between NNS intake and weight change in a prospective cohort study of 2- to 5-year-olds (n = 1345) but reported that intake of diet soda was low (<5 oz per day), with poor correlation seen between estimated beverage intake at the time of the first visit compared with at the second visit. A prospective study investigating the effect of intake of SSBs and NNSs on weight among school-aged youth (n = 164) found that for each 12 oz of diet soda consumed per day, there was a 2-year BMI *z* score that was 0.156 higher than predicted on the basis of baseline-BMI *z* score.[6] A prospective cohort study of 4746 youth found that consumption of low-calorie soft drinks (positive association; $P = .002$) was associated with weight gain, whereas consumption of white milk (inverse association; $P = .03$) was associated with weight loss.[104] Analysis of the relationship between NNS use and weight gain, however, did not control for parental weight and other important confounders.[104] Limitations of prospective cohort studies include failure to control for other dietary and lifestyle factors[105] and shorter long-term follow-up. Interpretations of the relationship between NNS use and BMI are limited by the inability to determine causality because of cross-sectional study design as well as reverse causality and inaccurate dietary recording in prospective cohort study design.[105] Youth who consume NNSs may have different food consumption patterns and a variety and parental and environmental factors not adjusted for in the prospective studies that may affect the relationship between NNS use and BMI.

Meta-analysis of 15 RCTs examining the relationship between NNS use and BMI in adults and youth (ages 10–65 years) reported that intake of NNS is associated with modestly reduced body weight, BMI, fat mass, and waist circumference (WC) with a mean reduction in weight of 0.8 kg.[105] However, RCTs suggest that substituting NNSs for SSBs is associated with a modest reduction in body weight for youth with the highest baseline BMI but not for all youth. Ebbeling et al reported results from a pilot study for an RCT evaluating the potential impact of replacement of SSBs with NNSs on body weight in youth and found that change in BMI, adjusted for sex and age, was 0.07 ± 0.14 (mean ± SE) for the intervention group and 0.21 ± 0.15 for the control group with a net difference of –0.14 ± 0.21, which was not significant. Baseline BMI was a significant effect modifier such that youth in the upper baseline-BMI tertile experienced a significant reduction in BMI between the intervention (–0.63 ± 0.23) and control (+0.12 ± 0.26) groups.[47] A systematic review and meta-analysis of NNS use and cardiometabolic health evaluating change in BMI among NNS consumers 12 years and older from 7 RCTs and 30 observational studies reported mixed results. Analysis of data from 2 of the 7 selected RCTs found that use of NNS was not associated with a significant effect on BMI over a 6- to 24-month period (–0.37; 95% confidence interval [CI]: −1.10 to 0.36; I^2: 9%).[8] Two cohort studies showed a possible correlation between NNS use and BMI over a 3- to 13-year period, and a third cohort study found that participants who consumed NNSs daily had a greater increase in BMI during an 8-year follow-up period.[8] As highlighted in the systematic review, overall, data suggest an increase in BMI with NNS use over the long-term without confirmation of these findings via RCTs.[8]

Controlled experimental studies have tried to better address the question of the effect of NNS on weight by giving controlled meals and measuring caloric intake after the controlled meals. Some studies show lower calorie consumption after foods containing NNSs compared with calorically sweetened foods,[106] but other studies support the phenomenon of "make-up" calorie consumption, showing higher intake[107–110] immediately after NNS intake. The make-up theory has not been proven conclusively[81] and represents only the immediate postprandial effects of NNS intake.

Most short-term studies support a beneficial role of NNS in weight loss.[111] A patient-blinded prospective cohort study in adults comparing satiety, energy intake, and body weight during a 10-week supplementation with either sucrose or artificial sweetener found a significant but modest reduction in fat mass and body weight with artificial sweetener use.[112] A randomized 25-week intervention study of 103 adolescents 13 to 18 years of age that included home delivery of noncaloric beverages (4 servings per day for the adolescent and 2 servings per day for each additional household member) revealed an additional BMI decrease of 0.08 for every 1 at baseline. This study found that the effect of NNS use on BMI in adolescents was most significant for adolescents with a baseline BMI >30.[10,47] A different RCT in children that combined NNS use with total caloric restriction did not find an association between NNS use and weight loss.[102] Given the multitude of factors affecting weight, including high-fat- and low-water-intake diets and the complex behavioral interactions related to response to use of NNS, some have argued that NNS use alone may not be an effective remedy for weight loss.[113]

The long-term effect of NNS use on weight remains poorly defined, and thus far, data suggest the benefits are limited.[69,114] A prospective double-blind study showed that children 4 to 11 years of age with normal weight who consume a beverage containing NNS per day experience less weight gain over an 18-month period compared with those who consume sugar-containing beverages[4]; the change in weight between the 2 cohorts differed by 2.2 lb (1 kg). The America On the Move study found that, combined with additional changes in lifestyle, use of NNSs may contribute to slowed weight gain in overweight and at-risk children[46] over a 6-month study period. A study in children with obesity showed that use of NNSs contributed to slowed weight gain over the first year, but the difference in weight was not maintained during the subsequent year even when controlling for confounders such as screen time, parental BMI, energy intake, physical activity, and fat consumption.[45] In that study, Ebbeling et al found that NNS use did not result in a significant change in BMI after 2 years of replacement of SSBs with NNSs. Systematic reviews of the existing data concluded that in children, NNS use may prevent excess weight gain over a period of 6 to 18 months but that, in general, studies evaluating the relationship between NNS intake and obesity are lacking rigor.[26] According to 1 published systematic review, use of NNSs in place of sugar, in children and adults, leads to reduced energy intake and a small reduction in body weight (on average, 1.3 kg).[115] Finally, a Cochrane Review reported that NNS use was associated with a significantly reduced body weight (−1.07 kg [95% CI: 0.41 to 1.72]), and among people younger than18 years, the NNS group demonstrated a significant reduction in body weight (1.18 kg [95% CI: 0.34 to 1.04]), an association that was not demonstrated for adults.[116]

In summary, the preponderance of data suggests that the use of NNSs can lead to weight stabilization or a small degree of weight loss by helping lower total caloric intake, especially among children and adolescents with obesity. Studies suggest that NNSs may be considered part of a comprehensive program and a substitute for foods and beverages containing caloric sweeteners for weight loss or weight maintenance. The current data would suggest that depending on baseline BMI and without easily taking into account what else is being consumed or substituted for, NNS use is associated with a modest improvement in weight. However, the long-term effects of NNS use in children and adolescents, including use pertaining to weight loss or weight management, are currently unknown.[31,106]

NNS USE AND EFFECTS ON METABOLIC SYNDROME AND DIABETES

Observational and experimental data in adults suggest that the use of NNSs may alter glucose metabolism in the presence of obesity, although these studies are subject to the same vulnerabilities as described above with regard to obesity.[8] Cross-sectional analysis of 2856 adults participating in the NHANES demonstrated that aspartame intake affects the association between BMI and glucose tolerance (interaction: $P = .004$), showing worse glucose tolerance with increasing BMI in those reporting consumption of aspartame.[117] Similarly, cross-sectional analysis of the Framingham Offspring Cohort showed an association between diet soda consumption, as assessed by a food frequency questionnaire, and metabolic syndrome.[7]

Prospective cohort data from the Coronary Artery Risk Development in Young Adults (CARDIA) study of the evolution of cardiovascular disease risk showed that among young adult NNS consumers 18 to 45 years of age, consumers of NNS were more likely to have metabolic syndrome and a higher WC. In comparing those who consumed a Western diet and NNSs versus individuals who consumed a Western diet but not NNSs, there was no significant difference in WC, the presence of high fasting glucose, low low-density lipoprotein concentration, high triglycerides, high blood pressure, or overall metabolic syndrome. However, young adults who consumed a prudent diet and NNSs (prudent consumers) were less likely to have a high fasting glucose (hazard ratio [HR]: 0.75; 95% CI: 0.57 to 0.99) and a low high-density lipoprotein concentration (HR: 0.69; 95% CI: 0.54 to 0.87). There was no significant difference in the presence of metabolic syndrome among consumers of the Western diet and prudent diet consumers of NNSs. However, prudent diet nonconsumers of NNSs were less likely to have metabolic syndrome (HR: 0.64; 95% CI: 0.5 to 82) compared with consumers of a Western diet. Results from this study suggest that a prudent dietary pattern is consistently associated with lower risk for metabolic syndrome, but being a nonconsumer of NNSs is not.[118] Use of NNSs can be associated with a lower likelihood of high fasting glucose and of low high-density lipoprotein but did not significantly affect WC (prudent nonconsumers were actually less likely to have a high WC [HR: 0.78; 95% CI: 0.62 to 0.97]), the likelihood of high triglycerides, or metabolic syndrome.[7,118] Findings from the CARDIA study were also observed in other prospective cohorts. A prospective analysis of the association between beverage consumption (SSBs and NNS soda intake) found that intake of greater than or equal to 1 soft drink per day (regular or diet) was associated with a higher prevalence of metabolic syndrome.[7] Again, given the cross-sectional and observational design of these studies, causality cannot be determined; nonetheless, data suggest that there is a correlation between NNS use and metabolic syndrome.

The Multi-Ethnic Study of Atherosclerosis cohort study showed that daily consumption of diet soda was associated with a 36% higher relative risk of metabolic syndrome and a 67% higher relative risk of type 2 diabetes mellitus.[68] However, once adjustments were made to account for baseline measures of adiposity, the association between diet soda consumption and metabolic syndrome was no longer significant, but the association between diet soda consumption and diabetes remained.[119] Findings suggest that additional factors among those who consume diet sodas may be associated with a greater risk for diabetes mellitus and metabolic syndrome. Analysis of the Framingham study stopped short of reporting an association between NNSs and WC but did find that prudent nonconsumers of NNSs were less likely to have a higher WC.

In the Atherosclerosis Risk in Communities Study, diet soda consumption was associated with incident metabolic syndrome ($P <$ .001 for trend).[120] Again, causality cannot be determined in observational study designs, and there are likely significant confounding factors, but longitudinal cohort studies show that there is an association between NNS use and abnormal glucose metabolism in adults.[7,118–120]

Few data exist regarding the role of NNSs in children and youth with diabetes, insulin resistance, or metabolic syndrome. One small study of youth and young adults 12 to 25 years of age with type 1 (n = 9) and type 2 (n = 10) diabetes mellitus compared the effect of drinking carbonated water versus carbonated beverages with NNSs on glucose tolerance (with a 75 g oral glucose tolerance test) using a crossover design.[121] According to this study, there were no differences in glucose or C-peptide secretion in people with either type 1 or type 2 diabetes mellitus after NNS consumption. Youth with type 1 diabetes mellitus released more glucagonlike peptide 1 after they consumed NNS-containing carbonated beverages versus carbonated water; no differences were seen in youth with type 2 diabetes mellitus.

A systematic review of the evidence from prospective studies evaluating the association between early life NNS exposure on long-term metabolic health identified conflicting results from 2 RCTs and 6 prospective cohort studies.[122] Studies selected included a total of more than 15 000 children exposed to NNS for >6 months.[122] The Growing Up Today Study, a prospective cohort study that relied on questionnaires administered between 1996 and 1998 to examine the relationship between beverage intake and change in BMI among >10 000 boys and girls ages 9 to 17 years, demonstrated a relationship between diet soda consumption and increased BMI over 2 years' follow-up in boys (P = .016) but not girls (P = .152).[87,122] Data from the Framingham Children's Study[46,122] among 3- to 15-year-olds revealed that although there was no consistent trend in body fat associated with intake of SSBs or NNS-containing beverages, the highest NNS intake was associated with increased body fat, as measured by skinfolds.[111]

The mechanism by which NNSs might adversely affect body weight, insulin resistance, and long-term metabolic risk is unknown, but 1 hypothesis is that it results in adverse effects on the gut microbiome. Alterations in microbiota structure and function have been associated with a greater propensity for developing metabolic syndrome.[123] Suez et al[42] published a small but frequently cited study in rodents with some human data comparing the effects of NNSs (eg, saccharin, sucralose, and aspartame) on glucose tolerance in mice and changes in the intestinal microbiota.[43] The animal data showed that NNS intake, particularly saccharin, leads to a change in the structure and function of the microbiota. A small study in human volunteers (who did not previously consume NNSs) showed that receipt of saccharin within ADI levels for 5 days was associated with the development of glucose intolerance.[42] The findings from these animal data and the small, single, human (adult) study suggest a detrimental effect of NNS use on gut metabolism, whereas a systematic review suggests that NNS use does not alter blood glucose levels over time.[124] In adults, observational data from the CARDIA study show that adults who consume diet soda beverages at baseline, regardless of whether they followed a "prudent" (eg, fruit, fish, and whole grains) or Western dietary pattern (eg, fast foods, refined grains, and sugar-sweetened soda), had higher rates of metabolic syndrome compared with those who did not consume diet soda beverages.[94,118]

Better understanding is needed concerning the effects of NNSs on metabolism and risk of diabetes,[125] including whether NNS intake is merely correlated with a higher risk of metabolic syndrome and diabetes or there is a causal and harmful relationship mediated through the gut microbiome or other as-yet-unidentified pathways.

NNS USE AND CARDIOVASCULAR DISEASE RISK FACTORS

Greater sweetened beverage use has been associated with increase obesity, increased central obesity, and abnormal perturbations in the lipid profile, all of which are risk factors for premature cardiovascular disease.[40] Although consumption of added sugars is known to cause detrimental effects on lipid concentrations,[94,96] no clinical trials have addressed the effects of NNSs on lipid concentrations in childhood.

Current data regarding the potential benefit of NNSs in modifying cardiovascular disease risk factors are limited but suggest an association between NNS consumption and metabolic syndrome, an association that may be limited by reverse causation. There are no conclusive data regarding the risk of cardiovascular disease events and NNS intake.

NNS USE AND ATTENTION-DEFICIT/HYPERACTIVITY DISORDER AND AUTISM

The lay press has raised the concern that NNS use is associated with behavior, cognition, hyperactivity, and attention issues. Two RCTs show no relationship between NNS use and behavior and cognition among school-aged children.[48,126] Several review articles regarding the potential impact of NNS use on behavior have been published.[114,127,128] Some data in adults also suggest an association between short-term aspartame consumption and more irritable mood, depression, and poorer performance in spatial orientation.[129] To date, however, there have been no studies to conclude that there is an association between attention-deficit/hyperactivity disorder (ADHD) and NNS use.[128] No literature was found to support a relationship between NNS use and autism.[130]

At the present time, there are no data to support an association between NNS use and the development of ADHD or autism in children or worsening of ADHD symptoms.[48]

OTHER POTENTIAL HEALTH EFFECTS

With the exception of the use of aspartame and neotame in children with phenylketonuria, there are no absolute contraindications to NNS use in children. NNSs may help to reduce the incidence of dental caries in children.[131]

PUBLISHED GUIDANCE AND RECOMMENDATIONS

Several organizations have published summary statements regarding the use of NNSs, including the AND, ADA, and AHA.[21–23,41] The AND states that "consumers can safely enjoy a range of nutritive and nonnutritive sweeteners when consumed in a diet that is guided by current federal nutrition recommendations, such as the *Dietary Guidelines for Americans and the Dietary References Intakes*."[21,22] With regard to the potential benefit of NNSs on weight loss, the AND states that there is a good level of evidence to conclude that NNS use, as part of a comprehensive weight loss or maintenance program, may be associated with weight loss and lead to improved weight management over time in adults; the statements for children were less definitive because of a lack of data. Information regarding use, safety, effect on taste preferences, and potential benefits in special populations was either limited or not available for other NNSs.

The ADA and AHA published a joint summary statement on NNSs in 2012 supporting the position that NNSs are safe when consumed within the ADI levels established by the FDA. Furthermore, the ADA and AHA have argued that NNSs may be helpful in reducing weight gain by limiting caloric intake if used in such a way that total diet caloric intake is reduced. The statement specifically did not address NNS use in children.[38]

RESEARCH GAPS

Gaps remain regarding our knowledge of the impact on NNS use on energy sensing and effects on glycemic control, appetite, and dietary intake for >6 months, and even fewer data exist specifically addressing the pediatric population.[132] Future research should explore novel approaches to assessing the long-term effects of NNS use in children (both type and amount), the effect of age of exposure to NNSs and the development of taste preferences, and the effects of age of exposure to NNSs on the development of diabetes mellitus, obesity, early cardiovascular disease, and the developing brain. Research should explore these topics across the age continuum: toddlers, children, and adolescents. Comparisons should be made with nutritive sweeteners and other beverages (eg, water and milk). Additional research is needed regarding genetic differences that may affect a child's response to a particular NNS and to determine if various NNSs differ in their benefits or risks. Approaches should take into consideration the need for long-term follow-up, adjust for multiple exposures, and account for imprecise exposure measures.

SUMMARY AND RECOMMENDATIONS

NNSs were introduced into the food supply to provide a noncaloric, sweet-tasting alternative to caloric sweeteners, which is useful for those with diabetes mellitus or who are avoiding sweet calories for other reasons, including obesity prevention and reduction. Concerns were initially raised about an association with cancer, but research in animal models and adult-human populations has shown no association between NNS use and cancer.[133] Some observational data in cross-sectional and prospective cohort studies in adults suggest that NNSs may promote obesity and metabolic syndrome but are subject to confounding and reverse causation.[26] Food challenge studies and short- and medium-term interventional data support a small benefit in weight maintenance or reduction in adults and children when NNSs are used as a substitute for caloric sweeteners. However, work remains to better understand the use of NNSs in toddlers, children, and adolescents in the general population and in at-risk populations (eg, diabetes, obesity, etc). Because of the ubiquitous presence of NNSs in everyday products and foods, it is unknown how much NNSs youth are consuming. Contemporary intake of NNSs (type and amount) and how they relate to ADI levels, specifically with regard to younger children, requires better and more detailed data. More information about the type and quantity of NNSs contained in various foods, beverages, and other products is recommended to better understand pediatric exposures. In particular, not only should the particular NNS contained in a product be noted as an ingredient, but the exact amount of any NNS within a particular food item should also be included in the nutrition facts label.

KEY FINDINGS AND RECOMMENDATIONS

Findings and recommendations are as follows.

1. Current FDA-approved NNSs include saccharin, aspartame, acesulfame potassium, sucralose, neotame, stevia, and advantame. These agents are 180 to 20 000 times sweeter than sugar, potentially affecting preferences for sweet taste.
2. NNSs are designated either as food additives or as GRAS; the long-term safety of NNSs in childhood has not been assessed in humans.
3. No advice can be provided on the use of NNS in children younger than 2 years old given the absence of data on this age group.
4. The number of consumer products containing NNSs has quadrupled over the past several years; manufacturers must list NNSs in the ingredient list but are not required to indicate the amount per serving.
5. When substituted for caloric-sweetened foods or beverages, NNSs can reduce weight gain or promote small amounts of weight loss (~1 kg) in children (and adults); however, data are limited, and use of NNSs in isolation is unlikely to lead to substantial weight loss.
6. Individuals affected by certain conditions (eg, obesity and type 1 or 2 diabetes mellitus) may benefit from the use of NNSs if substituted for caloric sweeteners. However, health care providers should be aware that NNS use in isolation is unlikely to result in important weight loss, that observational studies show that NNS intake is associated with higher rates of metabolic syndrome and diabetes, and that a better understanding is needed about whether NNS use has a causal and harmful effect on metabolism and the risk of diabetes mediated through the gut microbiome or other as-yet-unidentified pathways.
7. To better inform the public about consumption of NNSs, the FDA should require products marketed in the United States to include labels that list the type and quantity of any NNS contained per serving of a product.
8. Funding should be allocated to encourage researchers to conduct high-quality research on the use of NNSs in childhood, focusing on age of exposure and taste preferences, neurodevelopment, and effect on the microbiome and its relevance to obesity, metabolic syndrome, and diabetes.
9. Health care providers are encouraged to remain alert to new information and sensitive to patient and family preferences.
10. With the exception of aspartame and neotame in children with phenylketonuria, there are no absolute contraindications to use of NNSs by children.
11. Use of NNSs has been associated with a reduced presence of dental caries.

GUIDANCE FOR PEDIATRICIANS

Primary health care providers should discuss with parents and patients (as appropriate) the available evidence regarding the benefits and harms of NNS use in children and adolescents. The AAP recommends that pediatricians discuss the following points with families.

1. NNSs are FDA approved for use in humans or are GRAS and, thereby, approved for use under the GRAS designation.
2. The GRAS designation is based on consumption of NNSs within an ADI level; it is not possible to measure an individual's daily intake of NNSs at this time.
3. Higher-quality data suggest that NNS use is associated with weight stabilization and/or weight loss in the short-term. Currently, there is a paucity of long-term data.
4. High-quality evidence, including meta-analysis and data from RCTs, suggests that there is no association between hyperactivity and NNS use in children.
5. There are limited data regarding the effect of NNS use on appetite change and taste preference.

AUTHORS

Carissa M. Baker-Smith, MD, MPH, FAAP, General Pediatrics and Pediatric Cardiology

Sarah D. de Ferranti, MD, MPH, FAAP, General and Preventive Pediatric Cardiology

William J. Cochran, MD, FAAP, Pediatric Gastroenterology

COMMITTEE ON NUTRITION, 2018–2019

Steven A. Abrams, MD, FAAP, Chair

George J. Fuchs III, MD, FAAP

Jae Hong Kim, MD, PhD, FAAP

C. Wesley Lindsey, MD, FAAP

Sheela N. Magge, MD, FAAP

Ellen S. Rome, MD, MPH, FAAP

Sarah Jane Schwarzenberg, MD, FAAP

PAST COMMITTEE MEMBERS

Jatinder J.S. Bhatia, MD, FAAP, Past Chair

Mark R. Corkins, MD, FAAP

Stephen R. Daniels, MD, PhD, FAAP, Immediate Past Chair

Sarah D. de Ferranti, MD, MPH, FAAP

Neville H. Golden, MD, FAAP

LIAISONS

Jeff Critch, MD – *Canadian Pediatric Society*

Cria G. Perrine, PhD – *Centers for Disease Control and Prevention*

Janet M. de Jesus, MS, RD – *National Institutes of Health*

Andrea Lotze, MD, FAAP – *US Food and Drug Administration*

Valery Soto, MS, RD, LD – *US Department of Agriculture*

SECTION ON GASTROENTEROLOGY, HEPATOLOGY, AND NUTRITION EXECUTIVE COMMITTEE, 2018–2019

Jenifer R. Lightdale, MD, MPH, FAAP, Chair

David Brumbaugh, MD, FAAP

Mitchell B. Cohen, MD, FAAP

Jennifer L. Dotson, MD, MPH, FAAP

Sanjiv Harpavat, MD, PhD, FAAP

Maria M. Oliva-Hemker, MD, FAAP

Leo A. Heitlinger, MD, FAAP, Immediate Past Chair

PAST COMMITTEE MEMBERS

Michael deCastro Cabana, MD, MPH, FAAP

Mark A. Gilger, MD, FAAP

Roberto Gugig, MD, FAAP

Melvin B. Heyman, MD, FAAP, Past Chair

Ivor D. Hill, MD, FAAP

STAFF

Debra L. Burrowes, MHA

ABBREVIATIONS

AAP: American Academy of Pediatrics
ADA: American Diabetes Association
ADHD: attention-deficit/hyperactivity disorder
ADI: acceptable dietary intake
AHA: American Heart Association
AND: Academy of Nutrition and Dietetics
CARDIA: Coronary Artery Risk Development in Young Adults
CI: confidence interval
FDA: US Food and Drug Administration
GRAS: generally recognized assafe
HR: hazardratio
NNS: nonnutritive sweetener
RCT: randomized controlledtrial
SSB: sugar-sweetened beverage
WC: waist circumference

Address correspondence to: Carissa Baker-Smith, MD, MPH, FAAP. Email: cbaker-smith@som.umaryland.edu

PEDIATRICS (ISSN Numbers: Print, 0031-4005; Online, 1098-4275).

Copyright © 2019 by the American Academy of Pediatrics

FINANCIAL DISCLOSURE: The authors have indicated they have no financial relationships relevant to this article to disclose.

FUNDING: No external funding.

POTENTIAL CONFLICT OF INTEREST: The authors have indicated they have no potential conflicts of interest to disclose.

REFERENCES

1. US Food and Drug Administration. Food additives and ingredients. Available at: www.fda.gov/food/ingredientspackaginglabeling/foodadditivesingredients. Accessed March 26, 2019
2. Kroger M, Meister K, Kava R. Low-calorie sweeteners and other sugar substitutes: a review of the safety issues. *Compr Rev Food Sci Food Saf.* 2006;5:35–47
3. Shankar P, Ahuja S, Sriram K. Non-nutritive sweeteners: review and update. *Nutrition.* 2013;29(11–12):1293–1299
4. de Ruyter JC, Olthof MR, Seidell JC, Katan MB. A trial of sugar-free or sugar-sweetened beverages and body weight in children. *N Engl J Med.* 2012;367(15):1397–1406
5. Taljaard C, Covic NM, van Graan AE, et al. Effects of a multi-micronutrient-fortified beverage, with and without sugar, on growth and cognition in South African schoolchildren: a randomised, double-blind, controlled intervention. *Br J Nutr.* 2013;110(12):2271–2284
6. Blum JW, Jacobsen DJ, Donnelly JE. Beverage consumption patterns in elementary school aged children across a two-year period. *J Am Coll Nutr.* 2005;24(2):93–98
7. Dhingra R, Sullivan L, Jacques PF, et al. Soft drink consumption and risk of developing cardiometabolic risk factors and the metabolic syndrome in middle-aged adults in the community. *Circulation.* 2007;116(5):480–488
8. Azad MB, Abou-Setta AM, Chauhan BF, et al. Nonnutritive sweeteners and cardiometabolic health: a systematic review and meta-analysis of randomized controlled trials and prospective cohort studies. *CMAJ.* 2017;189(28):E929–E939
9. Swithers SE, Martin AA, Davidson TL. High-intensity sweeteners and energy balance. *Physiol Behav.* 2010;100(1):55–62
10. Food Standards New Zealand Australia. Intense sweeteners. 2018. Available at: www.foodstandards.gov.au/consumer/

additives/Pages/Sweeteners.aspx. Accessed April 28, 2019

11. Trasande L, Shaffer RM, Sathyanarayana S; Council on Environmental Health. Food additives and child health. *Pediatrics*. 2018; 142(2):e20181408
12. Morgan KJ, Stults VJ, Zabik ME. Amount and dietary sources of caffeine and saccharin intake by individuals ages 5 to 18 years. *Regul Toxicol Pharmacol*. 1982;2(4):296–307
13. US Department of Health and Human Services, National Toxicology Program. 14th report on carcinogens. 2016. Available at: https://ntp.niehs.nih.gov/pubhealth/roc/index-1.html. Accessed April 28, 2019
14. Garland EM, Sakata T, Fisher MJ, Masui T, Cohen SM. Influences of diet and strain on the proliferative effect on the rat urinary bladder induced by sodium saccharin. *Cancer Res*. 1989;49(14): 3789–3794
15. Elcock M, Morgan RW. Update on artificial sweeteners and bladder cancer. *Regul Toxicol Pharmacol*. 1993; 17(1):35–43
16. Sullivan JW. Epidemiologic survey of bladder cancer in greater New Orleans. *J Urol*. 1982;128(2):281–283
17. Morgan RW, Wong O. A review of epidemiological studies on artificial sweeteners and bladder cancer. *Food Chem Toxicol*. 1985;23(4–5):529–533
18. Marinovich M, Galli CL, Bosetti C, Gallus S, La Vecchia C. Aspartame, low-calorie sweeteners and disease: regulatory safety and epidemiological issues. *Food Chem Toxicol*. 2013;60:109–115
19. Magnuson BA, Roberts A, Nestmann ER. Critical review of the current literature on the safety of sucralose. *Food Chem Toxicol*. 2017;106(pt A):324–355
20. European Food Safety Authority. Neotame as a sweetener and flavour enhancer – scientific opinion of the Panel on Food Additives, Flavourings, Processing Aids and Materials in Contact with Food. *EFSA J*. 2007;581: 1–43
21. Academy of Nutrition and Dietetics. Scientific opinion on the safety of advantame for the proposed uses as a food additive. *EFSA J*. 2013;11(7):3301
22. Fitch C, Keim KS; Academy of Nutrition and Dietetics. Position of the Academy of Nutrition and Dietetics: use of nutritive and nonnutritive sweeteners. *J Acad Nutr Diet*. 2012;112(5):739–758
23. Academy of Nutrition and Dietetics. Position and practice paper update for 2014. *J Acad Nutr Diet*. 2014;114(2): 297–298
24. American Dietetic Association. Position of the American Dietetic Association: use of nutritive and nonnutritive sweeteners. *J Am Diet Assoc*. 2004; 104(2):255–275
25. National Cancer Institute. Artificial sweeteners and cancer. Available at: www.cancer.gov/cancertopics/factsheet/Risk/artificial-sweeteners. Accessed March 26, 2019
26. Pereira MA. Diet beverages and the risk of obesity, diabetes, and cardiovascular disease: a review of the evidence. *Nutr Rev*. 2013;71(7):433–440
27. Sylvetsky AC, Greenberg M, Zhao X, Rother KI. What parents think about giving nonnutritive sweeteners to their children: a pilot study. *Int J Pediatr*. 2014;2014:819872
28. de Ruyter JC, Katan MB, Kas R, Olthof MR. Can children discriminate sugar-sweetened from non-nutritively sweetened beverages and how do they like them? *PLoS One*. 2014;9(12):e115113
29. Sylvetsky AC, Welsh JA, Brown RJ, Vos MB. Low-calorie sweetener consumption is increasing in the United States. *Am J Clin Nutr*. 2012;96(3): 640–646
30. Sylvetsky AC, Jin Y, Clark EJ, et al. Consumption of low-calorie sweeteners among children and adults in the United States. *J Acad Nutr Diet*. 2017; 117(3):441–448.e2
31. Archibald AJ, Dolinsky VW, Azad MB. Early-life exposure to non-nutritive sweeteners and the developmental origins of childhood obesity: global evidence from human and rodent studies. *Nutrients*. 2018;10(2):e194
32. Lange FT, Scheurer M, Brauch HJ. Artificial sweeteners–a recently recognized class of emerging environmental contaminants: a review. *Anal Bioanal Chem*. 2012;403(9): 2503–2518
33. Sylvetsky AC, Walter PJ, Garraffo HM, Robien K, Rother KI. Widespread sucralose exposure in a randomized clinical trial in healthy young adults. *Am J Clin Nutr*. 2017;105(4):820–823
34. Butchko HH, Kotsonis FN. Acceptable daily intake vs actual intake: the aspartame example. *J Am Coll Nutr*. 1991;10(3):258–266
35. Bär A, Biermann C. Intake of intense sweeteners in Germany. *Z Ernahrungswiss*. 1992;31(1):25–39
36. Garnier-Sagne I, Leblanc JC, Verger P. Calculation of the intake of three intense sweeteners in young insulin-dependent diabetics. *Food Chem Toxicol*. 2001;39(7):745–749
37. Dewinter L, Casteels K, Corthouts K, et al. Dietary intake of non-nutritive sweeteners in type 1 diabetes mellitus children. *Food Addit Contam Part A Chem Anal Control Expo Risk Assess*. 2016;33(1):19–26
38. Gardner C, Wylie-Rosett J, Gidding SS, et al; American Heart Association Nutrition Committee of the Council on Nutrition, Physical Activity and Metabolism, Council on Arteriosclerosis, Thrombosis and Vascular Biology, Council on Cardiovascular Disease in the Young, and the American D. Nonnutritive sweeteners: current use and health perspectives: a scientific statement from the American Heart Association and the American Diabetes Association. *Circulation*. 2012;126(4):509–519
39. Committee on Nutrition, Council on Sports Medicine and Fitness. Sports drinks and energy drinks for children and adolescents: are they appropriate? *Pediatrics*. 2011;127(6):1182–1189. Reaffirmed July 2017
40. Vos MB, Kaar JL, Welsh JA, et al; American Heart Association Nutrition Committee of the Council on Lifestyle and Cardiometabolic Health; Council on Clinical Cardiology; Council on Cardiovascular Disease in the Young; Council on Cardiovascular and Stroke Nursing; Council on Epidemiology and Prevention; Council on Functional Genomics and Translational Biology; and Council on Hypertension. Added sugars and cardiovascular disease risk in children: a scientific statement from

the American Heart Association. *Circulation.* 2017;135(19):e1017–e1034

41. Gidding SS, Dennison BA, Birch LL, et al; American Heart Association; American Academy of Pediatrics. Dietary recommendations for children and adolescents: a guide for practitioners: consensus statement from the American Heart Association [published correction appears in *Circulation.* 2006; 113(23):e857]. *Circulation.* 2005;112(13): 2061–2075
42. Suez J, Korem T, Zeevi D, et al. Artificial sweeteners induce glucose intolerance by altering the gut microbiota. *Nature.* 2014;514(7521):181–186
43. Abbott A. Sugar substitutes linked to obesity. *Nature.* 2014;513(7518):290
44. American Diabetes Association. Type 2 diabetes in children and adolescents. *Pediatrics.* 2000;105(3, pt 1):671–680
45. Ebbeling CB, Feldman HA, Chomitz VR, et al. A randomized trial of sugar-sweetened beverages and adolescent body weight. *N Engl J Med.* 2012; 367(15):1407–1416
46. Rodearmel SJ, Wyatt HR, Stroebele N, et al. Small changes in dietary sugar and physical activity as an approach to preventing excessive weight gain: the America on the Move family study. *Pediatrics.* 2007;120(4). Available at: www.pediatrics.org/cgi/content/full/120/4/e869
47. Ebbeling CB, Feldman HA, Osganian SK, et al. Effects of decreasing sugar-sweetened beverage consumption on body weight in adolescents: a randomized, controlled pilot study. *Pediatrics.* 2006;117(3):673–680
48. Wolraich ML, Lindgren SD, Stumbo PJ, et al. Effects of diets high in sucrose or aspartame on the behavior and cognitive performance of children. *N Engl J Med.* 1994;330(5):301–307
49. Williams CL, Strobino BA, Brotanek J. Weight control among obese adolescents: a pilot study. *Int J Food Sci Nutr.* 2007;58(3):217–230
50. Roberts HJ. Aspartame-induced thrombocytopenia. *South Med J.* 2007; 100(5):543
51. Butchko HH, Stargel WW, Comer CP, et al. Aspartame: review of safety. *Regul Toxicol Pharmacol.* 2002;35(2 pt 2): S1–S93
52. Ubukata K, Nakayama A, Mihara R. Pharmacokinetics and metabolism of N-[N-[3-(3-hydroxy-4-methoxyphenyl) propyl]-α-aspartyl]-L-phenylalanine 1-methyl ester, monohydrate (advantame) in the rat, dog, and man. *Food Chem Toxicol.* 2011;49(suppl 1): S8–S29
53. Otabe A, Fujieda T, Masuyama T, Ubukata K, Lee C. Advantame–an overview of the toxicity data. *Food Chem Toxicol.* 2011;49(suppl 1):S2–S7
54. Renwick AG. Postscript on advantame–a novel high-potency low-calorie sweetener. *Food Chem Toxicol.* 2011; 49(suppl 1):S1
55. Otabe A, Fujieda T, Masuyama T. Evaluation of the teratogenic potential of N-[N-[3-(3-hydroxy-4-methoxyphenyl) propyl]-α-aspartyl]-L-phenylalanine 1-methyl ester, monohydrate (advantame) in the rat and rabbit. *Food Chem Toxicol.* 2011;49(suppl 1):S60–S69
56. Otabe A, Fujieda T, Masuyama T. Chronic toxicity and carcinogenicity of N-[N-[3-(3-hydroxy-4-methoxyphenyl) propyl]-α-aspartyl]-L-phenylalanine 1-methyl ester, monohydrate (advantame) in the rat. *Food Chem Toxicol.* 2011;49(suppl 1):S35–S48
57. Otabe A, Fujieda T, Masuyama T. In vitro and in vivo assessment of the mutagenic activity of N-[N-[3-(3-hydroxy-4-methoxyphenyl) propyl]-α-aspartyl]-L-phenylalanine 1-methyl ester, monohydrate (advantame). *Food Chem Toxicol.* 2011;49(suppl 1):S30–S34
58. Otabe A, Fujieda T, Masuyama T. A two-generation reproductive toxicity study of the high-intensity sweetener advantame in CD rats. *Food Chem Toxicol.* 2011;49(suppl 1):S70–S76
59. Ulbricht C, Isaac R, Milkin T, et al. An evidence-based systematic review of stevia by the Natural Standard Research Collaboration. *Cardiovasc Hematol Agents Med Chem.* 2010;8(2): 113–127
60. Renwick AG. Acceptable daily intake and the regulation of intense sweeteners. *Food Addit Contam.* 1990;7(4):463–475
61. Kauffman GB, Priebe PM. The discovery of saccharin: a centennial retrospect. *Ambix.* 1978;25(3):191–207
62. Renwick AG. The intake of intense sweeteners - an update review. *Food Addit Contam.* 2006;23(4):327–338
63. Arcella D, Le Donne C, Piccinelli R, Leclercq C. Dietary estimated intake of intense sweeteners by Italian teenagers. Present levels and projections derived from the INRAN-RM-2001 food survey. *Food Chem Toxicol.* 2004;42(4):677–685
64. Giammattei J, Blix G, Marshak HH, Wollitzer AO, Pettitt DJ. Television watching and soft drink consumption: associations with obesity in 11- to 13-year-old schoolchildren. *Arch Pediatr Adolesc Med.* 2003;157(9):882–886
65. Ilbäck NG, Alzin M, Jahrl S, Enghardt-Barbieri H, Busk L. Estimated intake of the artificial sweeteners acesulfame-K, aspartame, cyclamate and saccharin in a group of Swedish diabetics. *Food Addit Contam.* 2003;20(2):99–114
66. Hoover RN, Strasser PH. Artificial sweeteners and human bladder cancer. Preliminary results. *Lancet.* 1980; 1(8173):837–840
67. Leth T, Jensen U, Fagt S, Andersen R. Estimated intake of intense sweeteners from non-alcoholic beverages in Denmark, 2005. *Food Addit Contam Part A Chem Anal Control Expo Risk Assess.* 2008;25(6):662–668
68. Nettleton JA, Lutsey PL, Wang Y, et al. Diet soda intake and risk of incident metabolic syndrome and type 2 diabetes in the Multi-Ethnic Study of Atherosclerosis (MESA). *Diabetes Care.* 2009;32(4):688–694
69. Garavaglia MB, Rodríguez García V, Zapata ME, et al. Non-nutritive sweeteners: children and adolescent consumption and food sources. *Arch Argent Pediatr.* 2018;116(3):186–191
70. Mattes RD, Popkin BM. Nonnutritive sweetener consumption in humans: effects on appetite and food intake and their putative mechanisms. *Am J Clin Nutr.* 2009;89(1):1–14
71. Sylvetsky A, Rother KI, Brown R. Artificial sweetener use among children: epidemiology, recommendations, metabolic outcomes, and future directions. *Pediatr Clin North Am.* 2011;58(6):1467–1480, xi
72. Yang Q. Gain weight by "going diet?" Artificial sweeteners and the

neurobiology of sugar cravings: neuroscience 2010. *Yale J Biol Med.* 2010;83(2):101–108

73. Piernas C, Ng SW, Popkin B. Trends in purchases and intake of foods and beverages containing caloric and low-calorie sweeteners over the last decade in the United States. *Pediatr Obes.* 2013;8(4):294–306
74. Nelson G, Hoon MA, Chandrashekar J, et al. Mammalian sweet taste receptors. *Cell.* 2001;106(3):381–390
75. Fernstrom JD, Munger SD, Sclafani A, et al. Mechanisms for sweetness. *J Nutr.* 2012;142(6):1134S–1141S
76. Davidson TL, Martin AA, Clark K, Swithers SE. Intake of high-intensity sweeteners alters the ability of sweet taste to signal caloric consequences: implications for the learned control of energy and body weight regulation. *Q J Exp Psychol (Hove).* 2011;64(7): 1430–1441
77. Ventura AK, Mennella JA. Innate and learned preferences for sweet taste during childhood. *Curr Opin Clin Nutr Metab Care.* 2011;14(4):379–384
78. Freeman RP, Booth DA. Users of 'diet' drinks who think that sweetness is calories. *Appetite.* 2010;55(1):152–155
79. Green BG, George P. 'Thermal taste' predicts higher responsiveness to chemical taste and flavor. *Chem Senses.* 2004;29(7):617–628
80. Pepino MY, Bourne C. Non-nutritive sweeteners, energy balance, and glucose homeostasis. *Curr Opin Clin Nutr Metab Care.* 2011;14(4):391–395
81. Anton SD, Martin CK, Han H, et al. Effects of stevia, aspartame, and sucrose on food intake, satiety, and postprandial glucose and insulin levels. *Appetite.* 2010;55(1):37–43
82. Reed DR, Tanaka T, McDaniel AH. Diverse tastes: genetics of sweet and bitter perception. *Physiol Behav.* 2006;88(3): 215–226
83. Bryant CE, Wasse LK, Astbury N, Nandra G, McLaughlin JT. Non-nutritive sweeteners: no class effect on the glycaemic or appetite responses to ingested glucose. *Eur J Clin Nutr.* 2014; 68(5):629–631
84. Hill SE, Prokosch ML, Morin A, Rodeheffer CD. The effect of non-caloric sweeteners on cognition, choice, and post-consumption satisfaction. *Appetite.* 2014;83:82–88
85. Libuda L, Alexy U, Sichert-Hellert W, et al. Pattern of beverage consumption and long-term association with body-weight status in German adolescents–results from the DONALD study. *Br J Nutr.* 2008;99(6):1370–1379
86. Striegel-Moore RH, Thompson D, Affenito SG, et al. Correlates of beverage intake in adolescent girls: the National Heart, Lung, and Blood Institute Growth and Health Study. *J Pediatr.* 2006;148(2):183–187
87. Berkey CS, Rockett HR, Field AE, Gillman MW, Colditz GA. Sugar-added beverages and adolescent weight change. *Obes Res.* 2004;12(5):778–788
88. Casperson SL, Johnson L, Roemmich JN. The relative reinforcing value of sweet versus savory snack foods after consumption of sugar- or non-nutritive sweetened beverages. *Appetite.* 2017; 112:143–149
89. Weihrauch MR, Diehl V. Artificial sweeteners–do they bear a carcinogenic risk? *Ann Oncol.* 2004; 15(10):1460–1465
90. Bosetti C, Gallus S, Talamini R, et al. Artificial sweeteners and the risk of gastric, pancreatic, and endometrial cancers in Italy. *Cancer Epidemiol Biomarkers Prev.* 2009;18(8):2235–2238
91. Haighton L, Roberts A, Walters B, Lynch B. Systematic review and evaluation of aspartame carcinogenicity bioassays using quality criteria. *Regul Toxicol Pharmacol.* 2019;103:332–344
92. Mallikarjun S, Sieburth RM. Aspartame and risk of cancer: a meta-analytic review. *Arch Environ Occup Health.* 2015;70(3):133–141
93. Magnuson BA, Burdock GA, Doull J, et al. Aspartame: a safety evaluation based on current use levels, regulations, and toxicological and epidemiological studies. *Crit Rev Toxicol.* 2007;37(8): 629–727
94. Welsh JA, Sharma A, Abramson JL, et al. Caloric sweetener consumption and dyslipidemia among US adults. *JAMA.* 2010;303(15):1490–1497
95. Fernandes J, Arts J, Dimond E, Hirshberg S, Lofgren IE. Dietary factors are associated with coronary heart disease risk factors in college students. *Nutr Res.* 2013;33(8):647–652
96. Welsh JA, Sharma A, Cunningham SA, Vos MB. Consumption of added sugars and indicators of cardiovascular disease risk among US adolescents. *Circulation.* 2011;123(3):249–257
97. Ludwig DS, Peterson KE, Gortmaker SL. Relation between consumption of sugar-sweetened drinks and childhood obesity: a prospective, observational analysis. *Lancet.* 2001;357(9255): 505–508
98. Swithers SE, Martin AA, Clark KM, Laboy AF, Davidson TL. Body weight gain in rats consuming sweetened liquids. Effects of caffeine and diet composition. *Appetite.* 2010;55(3):528–533
99. Fowler SP, Williams K, Resendez RG, et al. Fueling the obesity epidemic? Artificially sweetened beverage use and long-term weight gain. *Obesity (Silver Spring).* 2008;16(8):1894–1900
100. Forshee RA, Storey ML. Total beverage consumption and beverage choices among children and adolescents. *Int J Food Sci Nutr.* 2003;54(4):297–307
101. Laska MN, Murray DM, Lytle LA, Harnack LJ. Longitudinal associations between key dietary behaviors and weight gain over time: transitions through the adolescent years. *Obesity (Silver Spring).* 2012;20(1):118–125
102. Knopp RH, Brandt K, Arky RA. Effects of aspartame in young persons during weight reduction. *J Toxicol Environ Health.* 1976;2(2):417–428
103. Newby PK, Peterson KE, Berkey CS, et al. Beverage consumption is not associated with changes in weight and body mass index among low-income preschool children in North Dakota. *J Am Diet Assoc.* 2004;104(7):1086–1094
104. Vanselow MS, Pereira MA, Neumark-Sztainer D, Raatz SK. Adolescent beverage habits and changes in weight over time: findings from Project EAT. *Am J Clin Nutr.* 2009;90(6):1489–1495
105. Miller PE, Perez V. Low-calorie sweeteners and body weight and composition: a meta-analysis of randomized controlled trials and prospective cohort studies. *Am J Clin Nutr.* 2014;100(3):765–777

106. Foreyt J, Kleinman R, Brown RJ, Lindstrom R. The use of low-calorie sweeteners by children: implications for weight management. *J Nutr.* 2012; 142(6):1155S–1162S

107. Birch LL, Deysher M. Caloric compensation and sensory specific satiety: evidence for self regulation of food intake by young children. *Appetite.* 1986;7(4):323–331

108. Birch LL, McPhee L, Sullivan S. Children's food intake following drinks sweetened with sucrose or aspartame: time course effects. *Physiol Behav.* 1989;45(2):387–395

109. Kral TV, Allison DB, Birch LL, et al. Caloric compensation and eating in the absence of hunger in 5- to 12-y-old weight-discordant siblings. *Am J Clin Nutr.* 2012;96(3):574–583

110. Anderson GH, Saravis S, Schacher R, Zlotkin S, Leiter LA. Aspartame: effect on lunch-time food intake, appetite and hedonic response in children. *Appetite.* 1989;13(2):93–103

111. Hasnain SR, Singer MR, Bradlee ML, Moore LL. Beverage intake in early childhood and change in body fat from preschool to adolescence. *Child Obes.* 2014;10(1):42–49

112. Raben A, Vasilaras TH, Møller AC, Astrup A. Sucrose compared with artificial sweeteners: different effects on ad libitum food intake and body weight after 10 wk of supplementation in overweight subjects. *Am J Clin Nutr.* 2002;76(4):721–729

113. Benton D. Can artificial sweeteners help control body weight and prevent obesity? *Nutr Res Rev.* 2005;18(1):63–76

114. Millichap JG, Yee MM. The diet factor in attention-deficit/hyperactivity disorder. *Pediatrics.* 2012;129(2):330–337

115. Rogers PJ, Hogenkamp PS, de Graaf C, et al. Does low-energy sweetener consumption affect energy intake and body weight? A systematic review, including meta-analyses, of the evidence from human and animal studies. *Int J Obes.* 2016;40(3):381–394

116. Chen C. Non-calorie artificial sweeteners affect body weight: a meta-analysis of randomised controlled trials. In: Proceedings from the Challenges to Evidence-Based Health Care and Cochrane. Abstracts of the 24th Cochrane Colloquium; October 23–27, 2016; Seoul, Korea

117. Kuk JL, Brown RE. Aspartame intake is associated with greater glucose intolerance in individuals with obesity. *Appl Physiol Nutr Metab.* 2016;41(7): 795–798

118. Duffey KJ, Steffen LM, Van Horn L, Jacobs DR Jr., Popkin BM. Dietary patterns matter: diet beverages and cardiometabolic risks in the longitudinal Coronary Artery Risk Development in Young Adults (CARDIA) study. *Am J Clin Nutr.* 2012;95(4): 909–915

119. Nettleton JA, Polak JF, Tracy R, Burke GL, Jacobs DR Jr.. Dietary patterns and incident cardiovascular disease in the Multi-Ethnic Study of Atherosclerosis. *Am J Clin Nutr.* 2009;90(3):647–654

120. Lutsey PL, Steffen LM, Stevens J. Dietary intake and the development of the metabolic syndrome: the Atherosclerosis Risk in Communities study. *Circulation.* 2008;117(6):754–761

121. Brown RJ, Walter M, Rother KI. Effects of diet soda on gut hormones in youths with diabetes. *Diabetes Care.* 2012; 35(5):959–964

122. Reid AE, Chauhan BF, Rabbani R, et al. Early exposure to nonnutritive sweeteners and long-term metabolic health: a systematic review. *Pediatrics.* 2016;137(3):e20153603

123. Hartstra AV, Bouter KE, Bäckhed F, Nieuwdorp M. Insights into the role of the microbiome in obesity and type 2 diabetes. *Diabetes Care.* 2015;38(1): 159–165

124. Nichol AD, Holle MJ, An R. Glycemic impact of non-nutritive sweeteners: a systematic review and meta-analysis of randomized controlled trials. *Eur J Clin Nutr.* 2018;72(6):796–804

125. Brown RJ, de Banate MA, Rother KI. Artificial sweeteners: a systematic review of metabolic effects in youth. *Int J Pediatr Obes.* 2010;5(4):305–312

126. Shaywitz BA, Sullivan CM, Anderson GM, et al. Aspartame, behavior, and cognitive function in children with attention deficit disorder. *Pediatrics.* 1994;93(1):70–75

127. Wolraich ML, Wilson DB, White JW. The effect of sugar on behavior or cognition in children. A meta-analysis. *JAMA.* 1995;274(20):1617–1621

128. Kanarek RB. Does sucrose or aspartame cause hyperactivity in children? *Nutr Rev.* 1994;52(5):173–175

129. Lindseth GN, Coolahan SE, Petros TV, Lindseth PD. Neurobehavioral effects of aspartame consumption. *Res Nurs Health.* 2014;37(3):185–193

130. Whitehouse CR, Boullata J, McCauley LA. The potential toxicity of artificial sweeteners. *AAOHN J.* 2008;56(6): 251–259; quiz 260–261

131. Roberts MW, Wright JT. Nonnutritive, low caloric substitutes for food sugars: clinical implications for addressing the incidence of dental caries and overweight/obesity. *Int J Dent.* 2012; 2012:625701

132. Wang DD, Shams-White M, Bright OJ, Parrott JS, Chung M. Creating a literature database of low-calorie sweeteners and health studies: evidence mapping. *BMC Med Res Methodol.* 2016;16:1

133. Lohner S, Toews I, Meerpohl JJ. Health outcomes of non-nutritive sweeteners: analysis of the research landscape. *Nutr J.* 2017;16(1):55

SECTION 4

Current Policies

From the American Academy of Pediatrics

• •

(Through December 31, 2019)

- ***Policy Statements***
  ORGANIZATIONAL PRINCIPLES TO GUIDE AND DEFINE THE CHILD HEALTH CARE SYSTEM AND TO IMPROVE THE HEALTH OF ALL CHILDREN
- ***Clinical Reports***
  GUIDANCE FOR THE CLINICIAN IN RENDERING PEDIATRIC CARE
- ***Technical Reports***
  BACKGROUND INFORMATION TO SUPPORT AMERICAN ACADEMY OF PEDIATRICS POLICY

American Academy of Pediatrics

Policy Statements, Clinical Reports, Technical Reports

Current through December 31, 2019
The companion *Pediatric Clinical Practice Guidelines & Policies* eBook points to the full text of all titles listed herein.

2019 RECOMMENDATIONS FOR PREVENTIVE PEDIATRIC HEALTH CARE

Committee on Practice and Ambulatory Medicine and Bright Futures Periodicity Schedule Workgoup

ABSTRACT. The 2019 Recommendations for Preventive Pediatric Health Care (Periodicity Schedule) have been approved by the American Academy of Pediatrics (AAP) and represent a consensus of AAP and the Bright Futures Periodicity Schedule Workgroup. Each child and family is unique; therefore, these recommendations are designed for the care of children who are receiving competent parenting, have no manifestations of any important health problems, and are growing and developing in a satisfactory fashion. Developmental, psychosocial, and chronic disease issues for children and adolescents may require frequent counseling and treatment visits separate from preventive care visits. Additional visits also may become necessary if circumstances suggest variations from the normal.

The AAP continues to emphasize the great importance of continuity of care in comprehensive health supervision and the need to avoid fragmentation of care.

The Periodicity Schedule will not be published in *Pediatrics*. Readers are referred to the AAP Web site (www.aap.org/periodicityschedule) for the most recent version of the Periodicity Schedule and the full set of footnotes. This process will ensure that health care professionals have the most current recommendations. The Periodicity Schedule will be reviewed and revised annually to reflect current recommendations. (2/19)

See full text on page 545.

https://pediatrics.aappublications.org/content/143/3/e20183971

AAP DIVERSITY AND INCLUSION STATEMENT

American Academy of Pediatrics

ABSTRACT. The vision of the American Academy of Pediatrics (AAP) is that all children have optimal health and well-being and are valued by society and that AAP members practice the highest quality health care and experience professional satisfaction and personal well-being. From the founding of the AAP, pursuing this vision has included treasuring the uniqueness of each child and fostering a profession, health care system, and communities that celebrate all aspects of the diversity of each child and family. (3/18)

http://pediatrics.aappublications.org/content/141/4/e20180193

ABUSIVE HEAD TRAUMA IN INFANTS AND CHILDREN

Cindy W. Christian, MD; Robert Block, MD; and Committee on Child Abuse and Neglect

ABSTRACT. Shaken baby syndrome is a term often used by physicians and the public to describe abusive head trauma inflicted on infants and young children. Although the term is well known and has been used for a number of decades, advances in the understanding of the mechanisms and clinical spectrum of injury associated with abusive head trauma compel us to modify our terminology to keep pace with our understanding of pathologic mechanisms. Although shaking an infant has the potential to cause neurologic injury, blunt impact or a combination of shaking and blunt impact cause injury as well. Spinal cord injury and secondary hypoxic ischemic injury can contribute to poor outcomes of victims. The use of broad medical terminology that is inclusive of all mechanisms of injury, including shaking, is required. The American Academy of Pediatrics recommends that pediatricians develop skills in the recognition of signs and symptoms of abusive head injury, including those caused by both shaking and blunt impact, consult with pediatric subspecialists when necessary, and embrace a less mechanistic term, abusive head trauma, when describing an inflicted injury to the head and its contents. (4/09, reaffirmed 3/13, 4/17)

http://pediatrics.aappublications.org/content/123/5/1409

ACCESS TO OPTIMAL EMERGENCY CARE FOR CHILDREN

Committee on Pediatric Emergency Medicine

ABSTRACT. Millions of pediatric patients require some level of emergency care annually, and significant barriers limit access to appropriate services for large numbers of children. The American Academy of Pediatrics has a strong commitment to identifying barriers to access to emergency care, working to surmount these obstacles, and encouraging, through education and system changes, improved levels of emergency care available to all children. (1/07, reaffirmed 8/10, 7/14)

http://pediatrics.aappublications.org/content/119/1/161

ACHIEVING QUALITY HEALTH SERVICES FOR ADOLESCENTS

Committee on Adolescence

ABSTRACT. This update of the 2008 statement from the American Academy of Pediatrics redirects the discussion of quality health care from the theoretical to the practical within the medical home. This statement reviews the evolution of the medical home concept and challenges the provision of quality adolescent health care within the patient-centered medical home. Areas of attention for quality adolescent health care are reviewed, including developmentally appropriate care, confidentiality, location of adolescent care, providers who offer such care, the role of research in advancing care, and the transition to adult care. (7/16)

http://pediatrics.aappublications.org/content/138/2/e20161347

ACHIEVING THE PEDIATRIC MENTAL HEALTH COMPETENCIES (TECHNICAL REPORT)

Cori M. Green, MD, MS, FAAP; Jane Meschan Foy, MD, FAAP; Marian F. Earls, MD, FAAP; Committee on Psychosocial Aspects of Child and Family Health; and Mental Health Leadership Work Group

ABSTRACT. Mental health disorders affect 1 in 5 children; however, the majority of affected children do not receive appropriate services, leading to adverse adult outcomes. To meet the needs of children, pediatricians need to take on a larger role in addressing mental health problems. The accompanying policy statement, "Mental Health Competencies for Pediatric Practice," articulates mental health competencies pediatricians could achieve to improve the mental health care of children; yet, the majority of pediatricians do not feel prepared to do so. In this technical report, we summarize current initiatives and resources that exist for trainees and practicing pediatricians across the training continuum. We also identify gaps in mental health clinical experience and training and suggest areas in which education can be strengthened. With this report, we aim to stimulate efforts to address gaps by summarizing educational strategies that have been applied and could be applied to undergraduate medical education, residency and fellowship training, continuing medical education, maintenance of certification, and practice quality improvement activities to achieve the pediatric mental health competencies. In this report, we also articulate the research questions important to the future of pediatric mental health training and practice. (10/19)

See full text on page 549.

https://pediatrics.aappublications.org/content/144/5/e20192758

ADDRESSING EARLY CHILDHOOD EMOTIONAL AND BEHAVIORAL PROBLEMS

Council on Early Childhood, Committee on Psychosocial Aspects of Child and Family Health, and Section on Developmental and Behavioral Pediatrics

ABSTRACT. Emotional, behavioral, and relationship problems can develop in very young children, especially those living in high-risk families or communities. These early problems interfere with the normative activities of young children and their families and predict long-lasting problems across multiple domains. A growing evidence base demonstrates the efficacy of specific family-focused therapies in reducing the symptoms of emotional, behavioral, and relationship symptoms, with effects lasting years after the therapy has ended. Pediatricians are usually the primary health care providers for children with emotional or behavioral difficulties, and awareness of emerging research about evidence-based treatments will enhance this care. In most communities, access to these interventions is insufficient. Pediatricians can improve the care of young children with emotional, behavioral, and relationship problems by calling for the following: increased access to care; increased research identifying alternative approaches, including primary care delivery of treatments; adequate payment for pediatric providers who serve these young children; and improved education for pediatric providers about the principles of evidence-based interventions. (11/16)

http://pediatrics.aappublications.org/content/138/6/e20163023

ADDRESSING EARLY CHILDHOOD EMOTIONAL AND BEHAVIORAL PROBLEMS (TECHNICAL REPORT)

Mary Margaret Gleason, MD, FAAP; Edward Goldson, MD, FAAP; Michael W. Yogman, MD, FAAP; Council on Early Childhood; Committee on Psychosocial Aspects of Child and Family Health; and Section on Developmental and Behavioral Pediatrics

ABSTRACT. More than 10% of young children experience clinically significant mental health problems, with rates of impairment and persistence comparable to those seen in older children. For many of these clinical disorders, effective treatments supported by rigorous data are available. On the other hand, rigorous support for psychopharmacologic interventions is limited to 2 large randomized controlled trials. Access to psychotherapeutic interventions is limited. The pediatrician has a critical role as the leader of the medical home to promote well-being that includes emotional, behavioral, and relationship health. To be effective in this role, pediatricians promote the use of safe and effective treatments and recognize the limitations of psychopharmacologic interventions. This technical report reviews the data supporting treatments for young children with emotional, behavioral, and relationship problems and supports the policy statement of the same name. (11/16)

http://pediatrics.aappublications.org/content/138/6/e20163025

ADMISSION AND DISCHARGE GUIDELINES FOR THE PEDIATRIC PATIENT REQUIRING INTERMEDIATE CARE (CLINICAL REPORT)

Committee on Hospital Care and Section on Critical Care (joint with Society of Critical Care Medicine)

ABSTRACT. During the past 3 decades, the specialty of pediatric critical care medicine has grown rapidly, leading to a number of pediatric intensive care units opening across the country. Many patients who are admitted to the hospital require a higher level of care than routine inpatient general pediatric care, yet not to the degree of intensity of pediatric critical care; therefore, an intermediate care level has been developed in institutions providing multidisciplinary subspecialty pediatric care. These patients may require frequent monitoring of vital signs and nursing interventions, but usually they do not require invasive monitoring. The admission of the pediatric intermediate care patient is guided by physiologic parameters depending on the respective organ system involved relative to an institution's resources and capacity to care for a patient in a general care environment. This report provides admission and discharge guidelines for intermediate pediatric care. Intermediate care promotes greater flexibility in patient triage and provides a cost-effective alternative to admission to a pediatric intensive care unit. This level of care may enhance the efficiency of care and make health care more affordable for patients receiving intermediate care. (5/04, reaffirmed 2/08, 5/17)

http://pediatrics.aappublications.org/content/113/5/1430

ADOLESCENT AND YOUNG ADULT TATTOOING, PIERCING, AND SCARIFICATION (CLINICAL REPORT)

Cora C. Breuner, MD, MPH; David A. Levine, MD; and Committee on Adolescence

ABSTRACT. Tattoos, piercing, and scarification are now commonplace among adolescents and young adults. This first clinical report from the American Academy of Pediatrics on voluntary body modification will review the methods used to perform the modifications. Complications resulting from body modification methods, although not common, are discussed to provide the pediatrician with management information. Body modification will be contrasted with nonsuicidal self-injury. When available, information also is presented on societal perceptions of body modification. (9/17)

http://pediatrics.aappublications.org/content/140/4/e20163494

ADOLESCENT DRUG TESTING POLICIES IN SCHOOLS

Sharon Levy, MD, MPH, FAAP; Miriam Schizer, MD, MPH, FAAP; and Committee on Substance Abuse

ABSTRACT. School-based drug testing is a controversial approach to preventing substance use by students. Although school drug testing has hypothetical benefits, and studies have noted modest reductions in self-reported student drug use, the American Academy of Pediatrics opposes widespread implementation of these programs because of the lack of solid evidence for their effectiveness. (3/15)

http://pediatrics.aappublications.org/content/135/4/782

ADOLESCENT DRUG TESTING POLICIES IN SCHOOLS (TECHNICAL REPORT)

Sharon Levy, MD, MPH, FAAP; Miriam Schizer, MD, MPH, FAAP; and Committee on Substance Abuse

ABSTRACT. More than a decade after the US Supreme Court established the legality of school-based drug testing, these programs remain controversial, and the evidence evaluating efficacy and risks is inconclusive. The objective of this technical report is to review the relevant literature that explores the benefits, risks, and costs of these programs. (3/15)

http://pediatrics.aappublications.org/content/135/4/e1107

ADOLESCENT PREGNANCY: CURRENT TRENDS AND ISSUES (CLINICAL REPORT)

Jonathan D. Klein, MD, MPH, and Committee on Adolescence

ABSTRACT. The prevention of unintended adolescent pregnancy is an important goal of the American Academy of Pediatrics and our society. Although adolescent pregnancy and birth rates have been steadily decreasing, many adolescents still become pregnant. Since the last statement on adolescent pregnancy was issued by the Academy in 1998, efforts to prevent adolescent pregnancy have increased, and new observations, technologies, and prevention effectiveness data have emerged. The purpose of this clinical report is to review current trends and issues related to adolescent pregnancy, update practitioners on this topic, and review legal and policy implications of concern to pediatricians. (7/05)

http://pediatrics.aappublications.org/content/116/1/281

ADOLESCENT PREGNANCY: CURRENT TRENDS AND ISSUES—ADDENDUM

Committee on Adolescence

INTRODUCTION. The purpose of this addendum is to update pediatricians and other professionals on recent research and data regarding adolescent sexuality, contraceptive use, and childbearing since publication of the original 2005 clinical report, "Adolescent Pregnancy: Current Trends and Issues." There has been a trend of decreasing sexual activity and teen births and pregnancies since 1991, except between the years of 2005 and 2007, when there was a 5% increase in birth rates. Currently, teen birth rates in the United States are at a record low secondary to increased use of contraception at first intercourse and use of dual methods of condoms and hormonal contraception among sexually active teenagers. Despite these data, the United States continues to lead other industrialized countries in having unacceptably high rates of adolescent pregnancy, with over 700 000 pregnancies per year, the direct health consequence of unprotected intercourse. Importantly, the 2006–2010 National Survey of Family Growth (NSFG) revealed that less than one-third of 15- to 19-year-old female subjects consistently used contraceptive methods at last intercourse. (4/14)

http://pediatrics.aappublications.org/content/133/5/954

ADOLESCENTS AND HIV INFECTION: THE PEDIATRICIAN'S ROLE IN PROMOTING ROUTINE TESTING

Committee on Pediatric AIDS

ABSTRACT. Pediatricians can play a key role in preventing and controlling HIV infection by promoting risk-reduction counseling and offering routine HIV testing to adolescent and young adult patients. Most sexually active youth do not feel that they are at risk of contracting HIV and have never been tested. Obtaining a sexual history and creating an atmosphere that promotes nonjudgmental risk counseling is a key component of the adolescent visit. In light of increasing numbers of people with HIV/AIDS and missed opportunities for HIV testing, the Centers for Disease Control and Prevention recommends universal and routine HIV testing for all patients seen in health care settings who are 13 to 64 years of age. There are advances in diagnostics and treatment that help support this recommendation. This policy statement reviews the epidemiologic data and recommends that routine screening be offered to all adolescents at least once by 16 to 18 years of age in health care settings when the prevalence of HIV in the patient population is more than 0.1%. In areas of lower community HIV prevalence, routine HIV testing is encouraged for all sexually active adolescents and those with other risk factors for HIV. This statement addresses many of the real and perceived barriers that pediatricians face in promoting routine HIV testing for their patients. (10/11, reaffirmed 9/15)

http://pediatrics.aappublications.org/content/128/5/1023

THE ADOLESCENT'S RIGHT TO CONFIDENTIAL CARE WHEN CONSIDERING ABORTION

Committee on Adolescence

ABSTRACT. In this statement, the American Academy of Pediatrics reaffirms its position that the rights of adolescents to confidential care when considering abortion should be protected. Adolescents should be encouraged to involve their parents and other trusted adults in decisions regarding pregnancy termination, and most do so voluntarily. The majority of states require that minors have parental consent for an abortion. However, legislation mandating parental involvement does not achieve the intended benefit of promoting family communication, and it increases the risk of harm to the adolescent by delaying access to appropriate medical care. This statement presents a summary of pertinent current information related to the benefits and risks of legislation requiring mandatory parental involvement in an adolescent's decision to obtain an abortion. (1/17)

http://pediatrics.aappublications.org/content/139/2/e20163861

ADVANCED PRACTICE IN NEONATAL NURSING

Committee on Fetus and Newborn

ABSTRACT. The participation of advanced practice registered nurses in neonatal care continues to be accepted and supported by the American Academy of Pediatrics. Recognized categories of advanced practice neonatal nursing are the neonatal clinical nurse specialist and the neonatal nurse practitioner. (5/09, reaffirmed 1/14)

http://pediatrics.aappublications.org/content/123/6/1606

ADVOCACY FOR IMPROVING NUTRITION IN THE FIRST 1000 DAYS TO SUPPORT CHILDHOOD DEVELOPMENT AND ADULT HEALTH

Sarah Jane Schwarzenberg, MD, FAAP; Michael K. Georgieff, MD, FAAP; and Committee on Nutrition

ABSTRACT. Maternal prenatal nutrition and the child's nutrition in the first 2 years of life (1000 days) are crucial factors in a child's neurodevelopment and lifelong mental health. Child and adult health risks, including obesity, hypertension, and diabetes, may be programmed by nutritional status during this period. Calories are essential for growth of both fetus and child but are not sufficient for normal brain development. Although all nutrients are necessary for brain growth, key nutrients that support neurodevelopment include protein; zinc; iron; choline; folate; iodine; vitamins A, D, B_6, and B_{12}; and long-chain polyunsaturated fatty acids. Failure to provide key nutrients during this critical period of brain development may result in lifelong deficits in brain function despite subsequent nutrient repletion. Understanding the complex interplay of micro- and macronutrients and neurodevelopment is key to moving beyond simply recommending a "good diet" to optimizing nutrient delivery for the developing child. Leaders in pediatric health and policy makers must be aware of this research given its implications for public policy at the federal and state level. Pediatricians should refer to existing services for nutrition support for pregnant and breastfeeding women, infants, and toddlers. Finally, all providers caring for children can advocate for healthy diets for mothers, infants, and young children in the first 1000 days. Prioritizing public policies that ensure the provision of adequate nutrients and healthy eating during this crucial time would ensure that all children have an early foundation for optimal neurodevelopment, a key factor in long-term health. (1/18)

http://pediatrics.aappublications.org/content/141/2/e20173716

ADVOCATING FOR LIFE SUPPORT TRAINING OF CHILDREN, PARENTS, CAREGIVERS, SCHOOL PERSONNEL, AND THE PUBLIC

James M. Callahan, MD, FAAP; Susan M. Fuchs, MD, FAAP; and Committee on Pediatric Emergency Medicine

ABSTRACT. Out-of-hospital cardiac arrest occurs frequently among people of all ages, including more than 6000 children annually. Pediatric cardiac arrest in the out-of-hospital setting is a stressful event for family, friends, caregivers, classmates, school personnel, and witnesses. Immediate bystander cardiopulmonary resuscitation and the use of automated external defibrillators are associated with improved survival in adults. There is some evidence in which improved survival in children who receive immediate bystander cardiopulmonary resuscitation is shown. Pediatricians, in their role as advocates to improve the health of all children, are uniquely positioned to strongly encourage the training of children, parents, caregivers, school personnel, and the lay public in the provision of basic life support, including pediatric basic life support, as well as the appropriate use of automated external defibrillators. (5/18)

http://pediatrics.aappublications.org/content/141/6/e20180704

ADVOCATING FOR LIFE SUPPORT TRAINING OF CHILDREN, PARENTS, CAREGIVERS, SCHOOL PERSONNEL, AND THE PUBLIC (TECHNICAL REPORT)

Susan M. Fuchs, MD, FAAP, and Committee on Pediatric Emergency Medicine

ABSTRACT. Pediatric cardiac arrest in the out-of-hospital setting is a traumatic event for family, friends, caregivers, classmates, and school personnel. Immediate bystander cardiopulmonary resuscitation and the use of automatic external defibrillators have been shown to improve survival in adults. There is some evidence to show improved survival in children who receive immediate bystander cardiopulmonary resuscitation. Pediatricians, in their role as advocates to improve the health of all children, are uniquely positioned to strongly encourage the training of children, parents, caregivers, school personnel, and the lay public in the provision of basic life support, including pediatric basic life support, as well as the appropriate use of automated external defibrillators. (5/18)

http://pediatrics.aappublications.org/content/141/6/e20180705

AGE LIMIT OF PEDIATRICS

Amy Peykoff Hardin, MD, FAAP; Jesse M. Hackell, MD, FAAP; and Committee on Practice and Ambulatory Medicine

ABSTRACT. Pediatrics is a multifaceted specialty that encompasses children's physical, psychosocial, developmental, and mental health. Pediatric care may begin periconceptionally and continues through gestation, infancy, childhood, adolescence, and young adulthood. Although adolescence and young adulthood are recognizable phases of life, an upper age limit is not easily demarcated and varies depending on the individual patient. The establishment of arbitrary age limits on pediatric care by health care providers should be discouraged. The decision to continue care with a pediatrician or pediatric medical or surgical subspecialist should be made solely by the patient (and family, when appropriate) and the physician and must take into account the physical and psychosocial needs of the patient and the abilities of the pediatric provider to meet these needs. (8/17)

http://pediatrics.aappublications.org/content/140/3/e20172151

AGE TERMINOLOGY DURING THE PERINATAL PERIOD

Committee on Fetus and Newborn

ABSTRACT. Consistent definitions to describe the length of gestation and age in neonates are needed to compare neurodevelopmental, medical, and growth outcomes. The purposes of this policy statement are to review conventional definitions of age during the perinatal period and to recommend use of standard terminology including gestational age, postmenstrual age, chronological age, corrected age, adjusted age, and estimated date of delivery. (11/04, reaffirmed 10/07, 11/08, 7/14)

http://pediatrics.aappublications.org/content/114/5/1362

ALCOHOL USE BY YOUTH

Joanna Quigley, MD, FAAP, and Committee on Substance Use and Prevention

ABSTRACT. Alcohol use continues to be problematic for youth and young adults in the United States. Understanding of neurobiology and neuroplasticity continues to highlight the potential adverse impact of underage drinking on the developing brain. This policy statement provides the position of the American Academy of Pediatrics on the issue of alcohol and is supported by an accompanying technical report. (6/19)

See full text on page 565.

https://pediatrics.aappublications.org/content/144/1/e20191356

ALCOHOL USE BY YOUTH (TECHNICAL REPORT)

Sheryl A. Ryan, MD, FAAP; Patricia Kokotailo, MD, MPH, FAAP; and Committee on Substance Use and Prevention

ABSTRACT. Alcohol use continues to be a major concern from preadolescence through young adulthood in the United States. Results of recent neuroscience research have helped to elucidate neurobiological models of addiction, substantiated the deleterious effects of alcohol on adolescent brain development, and added additional evidence to support the call to prevent and reduce underage drinking. This technical report reviews the relevant literature and supports the accompanying policy statement in this issue of *Pediatrics*. (6/19)

See full text on page 573.

https://pediatrics.aappublications.org/content/144/1/e20191357

ALLERGY TESTING IN CHILDHOOD: USING ALLERGEN-SPECIFIC IGE TESTS (CLINICAL REPORT)

Scott H. Sicherer, MD; Robert A. Wood, MD; and Section on Allergy and Immunology

ABSTRACT. A variety of triggers can induce common pediatric allergic diseases which include asthma, allergic rhinitis, atopic dermatitis, food allergy, and anaphylaxis. Allergy testing serves to confirm an allergic trigger suspected on the basis of history. Tests for allergen-specific immunoglobulin E (IgE) are performed by in vitro assays or skin tests. The tests are excellent for identifying a sensitized state in which allergen-specific IgE is present, and may identify triggers to be eliminated and help guide immunotherapy treatment. However, a positive test result does not always equate with clinical allergy. Newer enzymatic assays based on anti-IgE antibodies have supplanted the radioallergosorbent test (RAST). This clinical report focuses on allergen-specific IgE testing, emphasizing that the medical history and knowledge of disease characteristics are crucial for rational test selection and interpretation. (12/11)

http://pediatrics.aappublications.org/content/129/1/193

ALL-TERRAIN VEHICLE INJURY PREVENTION: TWO-, THREE-, AND FOUR-WHEELED UNLICENSED MOTOR VEHICLES

Committee on Injury and Poison Prevention

ABSTRACT. Since 1987, the American Academy of Pediatrics (AAP) has had a policy about the use of motorized cycles and all-terrain vehicles (ATVs) by children. The purpose of this policy statement is to update and strengthen previous policy. This statement describes the various kinds of motorized cycles and ATVs and outlines the epidemiologic characteristics of deaths

and injuries related to their use by children in light of the 1987 consent decrees entered into by the US Consumer Product Safety Commission and the manufacturers of ATVs. Recommendations are made for public, patient, and parent education by pediatricians; equipment modifications; the use of safety equipment; and the development and improvement of safer off-road trails and responsive emergency medical systems. In addition, the AAP strengthens its recommendation for passage of legislation in all states prohibiting the use of 2- and 4-wheeled off-road vehicles by children younger than 16 years, as well as a ban on the sale of new and used 3-wheeled ATVs, with a recall of all used 3-wheeled ATVs. (6/00, reaffirmed 5/04, 1/07, 5/13)
http://pediatrics.aappublications.org/content/105/6/1352

ALUMINUM EFFECTS IN INFANTS AND CHILDREN

Mark R. Corkins, MD, FAAP, and Committee on Nutrition

ABSTRACT. Aluminum has no known biological function; however, it is a contaminant present in most foods and medications. Aluminum is excreted by the renal system, and patients with renal diseases should avoid aluminum-containing medications. Studies demonstrating long-term toxicity from the aluminum content in parenteral nutrition components led the US Food and Drug Administration to implement rules for these solutions. Large-volume ingredients were required to reduce the aluminum concentration, and small-volume components were required to be labeled with the aluminum concentration. Despite these rules, the total aluminum concentration from some components continues to be above the recommended final concentration. The concerns about toxicity from the aluminum present in infant formulas and antiperspirants have not been substantiated but require more research. Aluminum is one of the most effective adjuvants used in vaccines, and a large number of studies have documented minimal adverse effects from this use. Long-term, high-concentration exposure to aluminum has been linked in meta-analyses with the development of Alzheimer disease. (11/19)

See full text on page 589.
https://pediatrics.aappublications.org/content/144/6/e20193148

AMBIENT AIR POLLUTION: HEALTH HAZARDS TO CHILDREN

Committee on Environmental Health

ABSTRACT. Ambient (outdoor) air pollution is now recognized as an important problem, both nationally and worldwide. Our scientific understanding of the spectrum of health effects of air pollution has increased, and numerous studies are finding important health effects from air pollution at levels once considered safe. Children and infants are among the most susceptible to many of the air pollutants. In addition to associations between air pollution and respiratory symptoms, asthma exacerbations, and asthma hospitalizations, recent studies have found links between air pollution and preterm birth, infant mortality, deficits in lung growth, and possibly, development of asthma. This policy statement summarizes the recent literature linking ambient air pollution to adverse health outcomes in children and includes a perspective on the current regulatory process. The statement provides advice to pediatricians on how to integrate issues regarding air quality and health into patient education and children's environmental health advocacy and concludes with recommendations to the government on promotion of effective air-pollution policies to ensure protection of children's health. (12/04, reaffirmed 4/09)
http://pediatrics.aappublications.org/content/114/6/1699

ANTENATAL COUNSELING REGARDING RESUSCITATION AND INTENSIVE CARE BEFORE 25 WEEKS OF GESTATION (CLINICAL REPORT)

James Cummings, MD, FAAP, and Committee on Fetus and Newborn

ABSTRACT. The anticipated birth of an extremely low gestational age (<25 weeks) infant presents many difficult questions, and variations in practice continue to exist. Decisions regarding care of periviable infants should ideally be well informed, ethically sound, consistent within medical teams, and consonant with the parents' wishes. Each health care institution should consider having policies and procedures for antenatal counseling in these situations. Family counseling may be aided by the use of visual materials, which should take into consideration the intellectual, cultural, and other characteristics of the family members. Although general recommendations can guide practice, each situation is unique; thus, decision-making should be individualized. In most cases, the approach should be shared decision-making with the family, guided by considering both the likelihood of death or morbidity and the parents' desires for their unborn child. If a decision is made not to resuscitate, providing comfort care, encouraging family bonding, and palliative care support are appropriate. (8/15)
http://pediatrics.aappublications.org/content/136/3/588

ANTERIOR CRUCIATE LIGAMENT INJURIES: DIAGNOSIS, TREATMENT, AND PREVENTION (CLINICAL REPORT)

Cynthia R. LaBella, MD, FAAP; William Hennrikus, MD, FAAP; Timothy E. Hewett, PhD, FACSM; Council on Sports Medicine and Fitness; and Section on Orthopaedics

ABSTRACT. The number of anterior cruciate ligament (ACL) injuries reported in athletes younger than 18 years has increased over the past 2 decades. Reasons for the increasing ACL injury rate include the growing number of children and adolescents participating in organized sports, intensive sports training at an earlier age, and greater rate of diagnosis because of increased awareness and greater use of advanced medical imaging. ACL injury rates are low in young children and increase sharply during puberty, especially for girls, who have higher rates of noncontact ACL injuries than boys do in similar sports. Intrinsic risk factors for ACL injury include higher BMI, subtalar joint overpronation, generalized ligamentous laxity, and decreased neuromuscular control of knee motion. ACL injuries often require surgery and/or many months of rehabilitation and substantial time lost from school and sports participation. Unfortunately, regardless of treatment, athletes with ACL injuries are up to 10 times more likely to develop degenerative arthritis of the knee. Safe and effective surgical techniques for children and adolescents continue to evolve. Neuromuscular training can reduce risk of ACL injury in adolescent girls. This report outlines the current state of knowledge on epidemiology, diagnosis, treatment, and prevention of ACL injuries in children and adolescents. (4/14, reaffirmed 7/18)
http://pediatrics.aappublications.org/content/133/5/e1437

THE APGAR SCORE

Committee on Fetus and Newborn (joint with American College of Obstetricians and Gynecologists Committee on Obstetric Practice)

ABSTRACT. The Apgar score provides an accepted and convenient method for reporting the status of the newborn infant immediately after birth and the response to resuscitation if needed. The Apgar score alone cannot be considered as evidence of, or a consequence of, asphyxia; does not predict individual neonatal mortality or neurologic outcome; and should not be used for that purpose. An Apgar score assigned during resuscitation is not equivalent to a score assigned to a spontaneously breathing infant. The American Academy of Pediatrics and the

American College of Obstetricians and Gynecologists encourage use of an expanded Apgar score reporting form that accounts for concurrent resuscitative interventions. (9/15)
http://pediatrics.aappublications.org/content/136/4/819

APNEA OF PREMATURITY (CLINICAL REPORT)

Eric C. Eichenwald, MD, FAAP, and Committee on Fetus and Newborn

ABSTRACT. Apnea of prematurity is one of the most common diagnoses in the NICU. Despite the frequency of apnea of prematurity, it is unknown whether recurrent apnea, bradycardia, and hypoxemia in preterm infants are harmful. Research into the development of respiratory control in immature animals and preterm infants has facilitated our understanding of the pathogenesis and treatment of apnea of prematurity. However, the lack of consistent definitions, monitoring practices, and consensus about clinical significance leads to significant variation in practice. The purpose of this clinical report is to review the evidence basis for the definition, epidemiology, and treatment of apnea of prematurity as well as discharge recommendations for preterm infants diagnosed with recurrent apneic events. (12/15)
http://pediatrics.aappublications.org/content/137/1/e20153757

ASSESSMENT AND MANAGEMENT OF INGUINAL HERNIA IN INFANTS (CLINICAL REPORT)

Kasper S. Wang, MD; Committee on Fetus and Newborn; and Section on Surgery

ABSTRACT. Inguinal hernia repair in infants is a routine surgical procedure. However, numerous issues, including timing of the repair, the need to explore the contralateral groin, use of laparoscopy, and anesthetic approach, remain unsettled. Given the lack of compelling data, consideration should be given to large, prospective, randomized controlled trials to determine best practices for the management of inguinal hernias in infants. (9/12)
http://pediatrics.aappublications.org/content/130/4/768

ATOPIC DERMATITIS: SKIN-DIRECTED MANAGEMENT (CLINICAL REPORT)

Megha M. Tollefson, MD; Anna L. Bruckner, MD, FAAP; and Section on Dermatology

ABSTRACT. Atopic dermatitis is a common inflammatory skin condition characterized by relapsing eczematous lesions in a typical distribution. It can be frustrating for pediatric patients, parents, and health care providers alike. The pediatrician will treat the majority of children with atopic dermatitis as many patients will not have access to a pediatric medical subspecialist, such as a pediatric dermatologist or pediatric allergist. This report provides up-to-date information regarding the disease and its impact, pathogenesis, treatment options, and potential complications. The goal of this report is to assist pediatricians with accurate and useful information that will improve the care of patients with atopic dermatitis. (11/14)
http://pediatrics.aappublications.org/content/134/6/e1735

ATTENTION-DEFICIT/HYPERACTIVITY DISORDER AND SUBSTANCE ABUSE (CLINICAL REPORT)

Elizabeth Harstad, MD, MPH, FAAP; Sharon Levy, MD, MPH, FAAP; and Committee on Substance Abuse

ABSTRACT. Attention-deficit/hyperactivity disorder (ADHD) and substance use disorders are inextricably intertwined. Children with ADHD are more likely than peers to develop substance use disorders. Treatment with stimulants may reduce the risk of substance use disorders, but stimulants are a class of medication with significant abuse and diversion potential. The objectives of this clinical report were to present practical strategies for reducing the risk of substance use disorders in patients with ADHD and suggestions for safe stimulant prescribing. (6/14)
http://pediatrics.aappublications.org/content/134/1/e293

BASEBALL AND SOFTBALL

Council on Sports Medicine and Fitness

ABSTRACT. Baseball and softball are among the most popular and safest sports in which children and adolescents participate. Nevertheless, traumatic and overuse injuries occur regularly, including occasional catastrophic injury and even death. Safety of the athlete is a constant focus of attention among those responsible for modifying rules. Understanding the stresses placed on the arm, especially while pitching, led to the institution of rules controlling the quantity of pitches thrown in youth baseball and established rest periods between pitching assignments. Similarly, field maintenance and awareness of environmental conditions as well as equipment maintenance and creative prevention strategies are critically important in minimizing the risk of injury. This statement serves as a basis for encouraging safe participation in baseball and softball. This statement has been endorsed by the Canadian Paediatric Society. (2/12, reaffirmed 7/15)
http://pediatrics.aappublications.org/content/129/3/e842

BEST PRACTICES FOR IMPROVING FLOW AND CARE OF PEDIATRIC PATIENTS IN THE EMERGENCY DEPARTMENT (TECHNICAL REPORT)

Isabel A. Barata, MD, FACEP; Kathleen M. Brown, MD, FACEP; Laura Fitzmaurice, MD, FACEP, FAAP; Elizabeth Stone Griffin, RN; Sally K. Snow, BSN, RN; and Committee on Pediatric Emergency Medicine (joint with American College of Emergency Physicians Pediatric Emergency Medicine Committee and Emergency Nurses Association Pediatric Committee)

ABSTRACT. This report provides a summary of best practices for improving flow, reducing waiting times, and improving the quality of care of pediatric patients in the emergency department. (12/14)
http://pediatrics.aappublications.org/content/135/1/e273

BICYCLE HELMETS

Committee on Injury and Poison Prevention

ABSTRACT. Bicycling remains one of the most popular recreational sports among children in America and is the leading cause of recreational sports injuries treated in emergency departments. An estimated 23 000 children younger than 21 years sustained head injuries (excluding the face) while bicycling in 1998. The bicycle helmet is a very effective device that can prevent the occurrence of up to 88% of serious brain injuries. Despite this, most children do not wear a helmet each time they ride a bicycle, and adolescents are particularly resistant to helmet use. Recently, a group of national experts and government agencies renewed the call for all bicyclists to wear helmets. This policy statement describes the role of the pediatrician in helping attain universal helmet use among children and teens for each bicycle ride. (10/01, reaffirmed 1/05, 2/08, 11/11)
http://pediatrics.aappublications.org/content/108/4/1030

BINGE DRINKING (CLINICAL REPORT)

Lorena Siqueira, MD, MSPH, FAAP; Vincent C. Smith, MD, MPH, FAAP; and Committee on Substance Abuse

ABSTRACT. Alcohol is the substance most frequently abused by children and adolescents in the United States, and its use is associated with the leading causes of death and serious injury at this age (ie, motor vehicle accidents, homicides, and suicides). Among youth who drink, the proportion who drink heavily is higher than among adult drinkers, increasing from approximately 50% in those 12 to 14 years of age to 72% among those 18 to 20 years of age. In this clinical report, the definition, epidemiology, and risk factors for binge drinking; the neurobiology of intoxication, blackouts, and hangovers; genetic considerations; and adverse outcomes are discussed. The report offers guidance for the pediatrician. As with any high-risk behavior, prevention plays a more important role than later intervention and has been

shown to be more effective. In the pediatric office setting, it is important to ask every adolescent about alcohol use. (8/15)
http://pediatrics.aappublications.org/content/136/3/e718

BONE DENSITOMETRY IN CHILDREN AND ADOLESCENTS (CLINICAL REPORT)

Laura K. Bachrach, MD; Catherine M. Gordon, MD, MS; and Section on Endocrinology

ABSTRACT. Concerns about bone health and potential fragility in children and adolescents have led to a high interest in bone densitometry. Pediatric patients with genetic and acquired chronic diseases, immobility, and inadequate nutrition may fail to achieve expected gains in bone size, mass, and strength, leaving them vulnerable to fracture. In older adults, bone densitometry has been shown to predict fracture risk and reflect response to therapy. The role of densitometry in the management of children at risk of bone fragility is less clear. This clinical report summarizes current knowledge about bone densitometry in the pediatric population, including indications for its use, interpretation of results, and risks and costs. The report emphasizes updated consensus statements generated at the 2013 Pediatric Position Development Conference of the International Society of Clinical Densitometry by an international panel of bone experts. Some of these recommendations are evidence-based, whereas others reflect expert opinion, because data are sparse on many topics. The statements from this and other expert panels provide general guidance to the pediatrician, but decisions about ordering and interpreting bone densitometry still require clinical judgment. The interpretation of bone densitometry results in children differs from that in older adults. The terms "osteopenia" and "osteoporosis" based on bone densitometry findings alone should not be used in younger patients; instead, bone mineral content or density that falls >2 SDs below expected is labeled "low for age." Pediatric osteoporosis is defined by the Pediatric Position Development Conference by using 1 of the following criteria: ≥1 vertebral fractures occurring in the absence of local disease or high-energy trauma (without or with densitometry measurements) or low bone density for age and a significant fracture history (defined as ≥2 long bone fractures before 10 years of age or ≥3 long bone fractures before 19 years of age). Ongoing research will help define the indications and best methods for assessing bone strength in children and the clinical factors that contribute to fracture risk. The Pediatric Endocrine Society affirms the educational value of this publication. (9/16)
http://pediatrics.aappublications.org/content/138/4/e20162398

BOXING PARTICIPATION BY CHILDREN AND ADOLESCENTS

Council on Sports Medicine and Fitness (joint with Canadian Paediatric Society Healthy Active Living and Sports Medicine Committee)

ABSTRACT. Thousands of boys and girls younger than 19 years participate in boxing in North America. Although boxing provides benefits for participants, including exercise, self-discipline, and self-confidence, the sport of boxing encourages and rewards deliberate blows to the head and face. Participants in boxing are at risk of head, face, and neck injuries, including chronic and even fatal neurologic injuries. Concussions are one of the most common injuries that occur with boxing. Because of the risk of head and facial injuries, the American Academy of Pediatrics and the Canadian Paediatric Society oppose boxing as a sport for children and adolescents. These organizations recommend that physicians vigorously oppose boxing in youth and encourage patients to participate in alternative sports in which intentional head blows are not central to the sport. (8/11, reaffirmed 2/15)
http://pediatrics.aappublications.org/content/128/3/617

BREASTFEEDING AND THE USE OF HUMAN MILK

Section on Breastfeeding

ABSTRACT. Breastfeeding and human milk are the normative standards for infant feeding and nutrition. Given the documented short- and long-term medical and neurodevelopmental advantages of breastfeeding, infant nutrition should be considered a public health issue and not only a lifestyle choice. The American Academy of Pediatrics reaffirms its recommendation of exclusive breastfeeding for about 6 months, followed by continued breastfeeding as complementary foods are introduced, with continuation of breastfeeding for 1 year or longer as mutually desired by mother and infant. Medical contraindications to breastfeeding are rare. Infant growth should be monitored with the World Health Organization (WHO) Growth Curve Standards to avoid mislabeling infants as underweight or failing to thrive. Hospital routines to encourage and support the initiation and sustaining of exclusive breastfeeding should be based on the American Academy of Pediatrics-endorsed WHO/UNICEF "Ten Steps to Successful Breastfeeding." National strategies supported by the US Surgeon General's Call to Action, the Centers for Disease Control and Prevention, and The Joint Commission are involved to facilitate breastfeeding practices in US hospitals and communities. Pediatricians play a critical role in their practices and communities as advocates of breastfeeding and thus should be knowledgeable about the health risks of not breastfeeding, the economic benefits to society of breastfeeding, and the techniques for managing and supporting the breastfeeding dyad. The "Business Case for Breastfeeding" details how mothers can maintain lactation in the workplace and the benefits to employers who facilitate this practice. (2/12)
http://pediatrics.aappublications.org/content/129/3/e827

THE BREASTFEEDING-FRIENDLY PEDIATRIC OFFICE PRACTICE (CLINICAL REPORT)

Joan Younger Meek, MD, MS, RD, FAAP, IBCLC; Amy J. Hatcher, MD, FAAP; and Section on Breastfeeding

ABSTRACT. The landscape of breastfeeding has changed over the past several decades as more women initiate breastfeeding in the postpartum period and more hospitals are designated as Baby-Friendly Hospitals by following the evidence-based Ten Steps to Successful Breastfeeding. The number of births in such facilities has increased more than sixfold over the past decade. With more women breastfeeding and stays in the maternity facilities lasting only a few days, the vast majority of continued breastfeeding support occurs in the community. Pediatric care providers evaluate breastfeeding infants and their mothers in the office setting frequently during the first year of life. The office setting should be conducive to providing ongoing breastfeeding support. Likewise, the office practice should avoid creating barriers for breastfeeding mothers and families or unduly promoting infant formula. This clinical report aims to review practices shown to support breastfeeding that can be implemented in the outpatient setting, with the ultimate goal of increasing the duration of exclusive breastfeeding and the continuation of any breastfeeding. (4/17)
http://pediatrics.aappublications.org/content/139/5/e20170647

THE BUILT ENVIRONMENT: DESIGNING COMMUNITIES TO PROMOTE PHYSICAL ACTIVITY IN CHILDREN

Committee on Environmental Health

ABSTRACT. An estimated 32% of American children are overweight, and physical inactivity contributes to this high prevalence of overweight. This policy statement highlights how the built environment of a community affects children's opportunities for physical activity. Neighborhoods and communities can provide opportunities for recreational physical activity with parks and open spaces, and policies must support this capacity. Children can engage in physical activity as a part of their

daily lives, such as on their travel to school. Factors such as school location have played a significant role in the decreased rates of walking to school, and changes in policy may help to increase the number of children who are able to walk to school. Environment modification that addresses risks associated with automobile traffic is likely to be conducive to more walking and biking among children. Actions that reduce parental perception and fear of crime may promote outdoor physical activity. Policies that promote more active lifestyles among children and adolescents will enable them to achieve the recommended 60 minutes of daily physical activity. By working with community partners, pediatricians can participate in establishing communities designed for activity and health. (5/09, reaffirmed 1/13)
http://pediatrics.aappublications.org/content/123/6/1591

CALCIUM AND VITAMIN D REQUIREMENTS OF ENTERALLY FED PRETERM INFANTS (CLINICAL REPORT)

Steven A. Abrams, MD, and Committee on Nutrition

ABSTRACT. Bone health is a critical concern in managing preterm infants. Key nutrients of importance are calcium, vitamin D, and phosphorus. Although human milk is critical for the health of preterm infants, it is low in these nutrients relative to the needs of the infants during growth. Strategies should be in place to fortify human milk for preterm infants with birth weight <1800 to 2000 g and to ensure adequate mineral intake during hospitalization and after hospital discharge. Biochemical monitoring of very low birth weight infants should be performed during their hospitalization. Vitamin D should be provided at 200 to 400 IU/day both during hospitalization and after discharge from the hospital. Infants with radiologic evidence of rickets should have efforts made to maximize calcium and phosphorus intake by using available commercial products and, if needed, direct supplementation with these minerals. (4/13)
http://pediatrics.aappublications.org/content/131/5/e1676

CARDIOVASCULAR MONITORING AND STIMULANT DRUGS FOR ATTENTION-DEFICIT/HYPERACTIVITY DISORDER

James M. Perrin, MD; Richard A. Friedman, MD; Timothy K. Knilans, MD; Black Box Working Group; and Section on Cardiology and Cardiac Surgery

ABSTRACT. A recent American Heart Association (AHA) statement recommended electrocardiograms (ECGs) routinely for children before they start medications to treat attention-deficit/hyperactivity disorder (ADHD). The AHA statement reflected the thoughtful work of a group committed to improving the health of children with heart disease. However, the recommendation to obtain an ECG before starting medications for treating ADHD contradicts the carefully considered and evidence-based recommendations of the American Academy of Child and Adolescent Psychiatry and the American Academy of Pediatrics (AAP). These organizations have concluded that sudden cardiac death (SCD) in persons taking medications for ADHD is a very rare event, occurring at rates no higher than those in the general population of children and adolescents. Both of these groups also noted the lack of any evidence that the routine use of ECG screening before beginning medication for ADHD treatment would prevent sudden death. The AHA statement pointed out the importance of detecting silent but clinically important cardiac conditions in children and adolescents, which is a goal that the AAP shares. The primary purpose of the AHA statement is to prevent cases of SCD that may be related to stimulant medications. The recommendations of the AAP and the rationale for these recommendations are the subject of this statement. (8/08)
http://pediatrics.aappublications.org/content/122/2/451

CARE OF ADOLESCENT PARENTS AND THEIR CHILDREN (CLINICAL REPORT)

Jorge L. Pinzon, MD; Veronnie F. Jones, MD; Committee on Adolescence; and Committee on Early Childhood

ABSTRACT. Teen pregnancy and parenting remain an important public health issue in the United States and the world, and many children live with their adolescent parents alone or as part of an extended family. A significant proportion of teen parents reside with their family of origin, significantly affecting the multigenerational family structure. Repeated births to teen parents are also common. This clinical report updates a previous policy statement on care of the adolescent parent and their children and addresses medical and psychosocial risks specific to this population. Challenges unique to teen parents and their children are reviewed, along with suggestions for the pediatrician on models for intervention and care. (11/12, reaffirmed 7/16)
http://pediatrics.aappublications.org/content/130/6/e1743

THE CARE OF CHILDREN WITH CONGENITAL HEART DISEASE IN THEIR PRIMARY MEDICAL HOME

M. Regina Lantin-Hermoso, MD, FAAP, FACC; Stuart Berger, MD, FAAP; Ami B. Bhatt, MD, FACC; Julia E. Richerson, MD, FAAP; Robert Morrow, MD, FAAP; Michael D. Freed, MD, FAAP, FACC; Robert H. Beekman III, MD, FAAP, FACC; and Section on Cardiology and Cardiac Surgery

ABSTRACT. Congenital heart disease (CHD) is the most common birth anomaly. With advances in repair and palliation of these complex lesions, more and more patients are surviving and are discharged from the hospital to return to their families. Patients with CHD have complex health care needs that often must be provided for or coordinated for by the primary care provider (PCP) and medical home. This policy statement aims to provide the PCP with general guidelines for the care of the child with congenital heart defects and outlines anticipated problems, serving as a repository of current knowledge in a practical, readily accessible format. A timeline approach is used, emphasizing the role of the PCP and medical home in the management of patients with CHD in their various life stages. (10/17)
http://pediatrics.aappublications.org/content/140/5/e20172607

CARE OF THE ADOLESCENT AFTER AN ACUTE SEXUAL ASSAULT (CLINICAL REPORT)

James E. Crawford-Jakubiak, MD, FAAP; Elizabeth M. Alderman, MD, FAAP, SAHM; John M. Leventhal, MD, FAAP; Committee on Child Abuse and Neglect; and Committee on Adolescence

ABSTRACT. *Sexual violence* is a broad term that encompasses a wide range of sexual victimizations. Since the American Academy of Pediatrics published its last policy statement on sexual assault in 2008, additional information and data have emerged about sexual violence affecting adolescents and the treatment and management of the adolescent who has been a victim of sexual assault. This report provides new information to update physicians and focuses on the acute assessment and care of adolescent victims who have experienced a recent sexual assault. Follow-up of the acute assault, as well as prevention of sexual assault, are also discussed. (2/17)
http://pediatrics.aappublications.org/content/139/3/e20164243

CAREGIVER-FABRICATED ILLNESS IN A CHILD: A MANIFESTATION OF CHILD MALTREATMENT (CLINICAL REPORT)

Emalee G. Flaherty, MD, FAAP; Harriet L. MacMillan, MD; and Committee on Child Abuse and Neglect

ABSTRACT. Caregiver-fabricated illness in a child is a form of child maltreatment caused by a caregiver who falsifies and/or induces a child's illness, leading to unnecessary and potentially harmful medical investigations and/or treatment. This condi-

tion can result in significant morbidity and mortality. Although caregiver-fabricated illness in a child has been widely known as Munchausen syndrome by proxy, there is ongoing discussion about alternative names, including pediatric condition falsification, factitious disorder (illness) by proxy, child abuse in the medical setting, and medical child abuse. Because it is a relatively uncommon form of maltreatment, pediatricians need to have a high index of suspicion when faced with a persistent or recurrent illness that cannot be explained and that results in multiple medical procedures or when there are discrepancies between the history, physical examination, and health of a child. This report updates the previous clinical report "Beyond Munchausen Syndrome by Proxy: Identification and Treatment of Child Abuse in the Medical Setting." The authors discuss the need to agree on appropriate terminology, provide an update on published reports of new manifestations of fabricated medical conditions, and discuss approaches to assessment, diagnosis, and management, including how best to protect the child from further harm. (8/13, reaffirmed 8/18)
http://pediatrics.aappublications.org/content/132/3/590

CHEERLEADING INJURIES: EPIDEMIOLOGY AND RECOMMENDATIONS FOR PREVENTION

Council on Sports Medicine and Fitness

ABSTRACT. Over the last 30 years, cheerleading has increased dramatically in popularity and has evolved from leading the crowd in cheers at sporting events into a competitive, year-round sport involving complex acrobatic stunts and tumbling. Consequently, cheerleading injuries have steadily increased over the years in both number and severity. Sprains and strains to the lower extremities are the most common injuries. Although the overall injury rate remains relatively low, cheerleading has accounted for approximately 66% of all catastrophic injuries in high school girl athletes over the past 25 years. Risk factors for injuries in cheerleading include higher BMI, previous injury, cheering on harder surfaces, performing stunts, and supervision by a coach with low level of training and experience. This policy statement describes the epidemiology of cheerleading injuries and provides recommendations for injury prevention. (10/12, reaffirmed 7/15)
http://pediatrics.aappublications.org/content/130/5/966

CHEMICAL-BIOLOGICAL TERRORISM AND ITS IMPACT ON CHILDREN

Committee on Environmental Health and Committee on Infectious Diseases

ABSTRACT. Children remain potential victims of chemical or biological terrorism. In recent years, children have even been specific targets of terrorist acts. Consequently, it is necessary to address the needs that children would face after a terrorist incident. A broad range of public health initiatives have occurred since September 11, 2001. Although the needs of children have been addressed in many of them, in many cases, these initiatives have been inadequate in ensuring the protection of children. In addition, public health and health care system preparedness for terrorism has been broadened to the so-called all-hazards approach, in which response plans for terrorism are blended with plans for a public health or health care system response to unintentional disasters (eg, natural events such as earthquakes or pandemic flu or manmade catastrophes such as a hazardous-materials spill). In response to new principles and programs that have appeared over the last 5 years, this policy statement provides an update of the 2000 policy statement. The roles of both the pediatrician and public health agencies continue to be emphasized; only a coordinated effort by pediatricians and public health can ensure that the needs of children, including emergency protocols in schools or child care centers, decontamination protocols, and mental health interventions, will be successful. (9/06, reaffirmed 12/16)
http://pediatrics.aappublications.org/content/118/3/1267

CHEMICAL-MANAGEMENT POLICY: PRIORITIZING CHILDREN'S HEALTH

Council on Environmental Health

ABSTRACT. The American Academy of Pediatrics recommends that chemical-management policy in the United States be revised to protect children and pregnant women and to better protect other populations. The Toxic Substance Control Act (TSCA) was passed in 1976. It is widely recognized to have been ineffective in protecting children, pregnant women, and the general population from hazardous chemicals in the marketplace. It does not take into account the special vulnerabilities of children in attempting to protect the population from chemical hazards. Its processes are so cumbersome that in its more than 30 years of existence, the TSCA has been used to regulate only 5 chemicals or chemical classes of the tens of thousands of chemicals that are in commerce. Under the TSCA, chemical companies have no responsibility to perform premarket testing or postmarket follow-up of the products that they produce; in fact, the TSCA contains disincentives for the companies to produce such data. Voluntary programs have been inadequate in resolving problems. Therefore, chemical-management policy needs to be rewritten in the United States. Manufacturers must be responsible for developing information about chemicals before marketing. The US Environmental Protection Agency must have the authority to demand additional safety data about a chemical and to limit or stop the marketing of a chemical when there is a high degree of suspicion that the chemical might be harmful to children, pregnant women, or other populations. (4/11, reaffirmed 9/16)
http://pediatrics.aappublications.org/content/127/5/983

CHILD ABUSE, CONFIDENTIALITY, AND THE HEALTH INSURANCE PORTABILITY AND ACCOUNTABILITY ACT

Committee on Child Abuse and Neglect

ABSTRACT. The federal Health Insurance Portability and Accountability Act (HIPAA) of 1996 has significantly affected clinical practice, particularly with regard to how patient information is shared. HIPAA addresses the security and privacy of patient health data, ensuring that information is released appropriately with patient or guardian consent and knowledge. However, when child abuse or neglect is suspected in a clinical setting, the physician may determine that release of information without consent is necessary to ensure the health and safety of the child. This policy statement provides an overview of HIPAA regulations with regard to the role of the pediatrician in releasing or reviewing patient health information when the patient is a child who is a suspected victim of abuse or neglect. This statement is based on the most current regulations provided by the US Department of Health and Human Services and is subject to future changes and clarifications as updates are provided. (12/09, reaffirmed 1/14)
http://pediatrics.aappublications.org/content/125/1/197

CHILD FATALITY REVIEW

Cindy W. Christian, MD; Robert D. Sege, MD, PhD; Committee on Child Abuse and Neglect; Committee on Injury, Violence, and Poison Prevention; and Council on Community Pediatrics

ABSTRACT. Injury remains the leading cause of pediatric mortality and requires public health approaches to reduce preventable deaths. Child fatality review teams, first established to review suspicious child deaths involving abuse or neglect, have expanded toward a public health model of prevention of child fatality through systematic review of child deaths from birth through adolescence. Approximately half of all states report reviewing child deaths from all causes, and the process of fatality review has identified effective local and state prevention strategies for reducing child deaths. This expanded approach can be a powerful tool in understanding the epidemiology and preventability of child death locally, regionally, and nationally; improving accuracy of vital statistics data; and identifying public health and legislative strategies for reducing preventable child fatalities. The American Academy of Pediatrics supports the development of federal and state legislation to enhance the child fatality review process and recommends that pediatricians become involved in local and state child death reviews. (8/10, reaffirmed 5/14)

http://pediatrics.aappublications.org/content/126/3/592

CHILD LIFE SERVICES

Committee on Hospital Care and Child Life Council

ABSTRACT. Child life programs are an important component of pediatric hospital–based care to address the psychosocial concerns that accompany hospitalization and other health care experiences. Child life specialists focus on the optimal development and well-being of infants, children, adolescents, and young adults while promoting coping skills and minimizing the adverse effects of hospitalization, health care, and/or other potentially stressful experiences. Using therapeutic play, expressive modalities, and psychological preparation as primary tools, in collaboration with the entire health care team and family, child life interventions facilitate coping and adjustment at times and under circumstances that might otherwise prove overwhelming for the child. Play and developmentally appropriate communication are used to: (1) promote optimal development; (2) educate children and families about health conditions; (3) prepare children and families for medical events or procedures; (4) plan and rehearse useful coping and pain management strategies; (5) help children work through feelings about past or impending experiences; and (6) establish therapeutic relationships with patients, siblings, and parents to support family involvement in each child's care. (4/14, reaffirmed 2/18)

http://pediatrics.aappublications.org/content/133/5/e1471

CHILD PASSENGER SAFETY

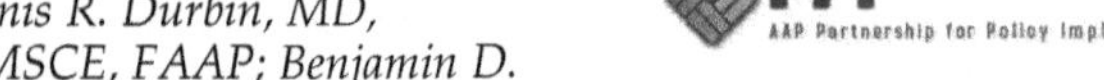

Dennis R. Durbin, MD, MSCE, FAAP; Benjamin D. Hoffman, MD, FAAP; and Council on Injury, Violence, and Poison Prevention

ABSTRACT. Child passenger safety has dramatically evolved over the past decade; however, motor vehicle crashes continue to be the leading cause of death for children 4 years and older. This policy statement provides 4 evidence-based recommendations for best practices in the choice of a child restraint system to optimize safety in passenger vehicles for children from birth through adolescence: (1) rear-facing car safety seats as long as possible; (2) forward-facing car safety seats from the time they outgrow rear-facing seats for most children through at least 4 years of age; (3) belt-positioning booster seats from the time they outgrow forward-facing seats for most children through at least 8 years of age; and (4) lap and shoulder seat belts for all who have outgrown booster seats. In addition, a fifth evidence-based recommendation is for all children younger than 13 years to ride in the rear seats of vehicles. It is important to note that every transition is associated with some decrease in protection; therefore, parents should be encouraged to delay these transitions for as long as possible. These recommendations are presented in the form of an algorithm that is intended to facilitate implementation of the recommendations by pediatricians to their patients and families and should cover most situations that pediatricians will encounter in practice. The American Academy of Pediatrics urges all pediatricians to know and promote these recommendations as part of child passenger safety anticipatory guidance at every health supervision visit. (10/18)

http://pediatrics.aappublications.org/content/142/5/e20182460

CHILD PASSENGER SAFETY (TECHNICAL REPORT)

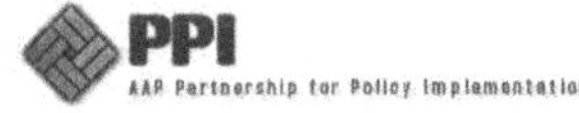

Dennis R. Durbin, MD, MSCE, FAAP; Benjamin D. Hoffman, MD, FAAP; and Council on Injury, Violence, and Poison Prevention

ABSTRACT. Despite significant reductions in the number of children killed in motor vehicle crashes over the past decade, crashes continue to be the leading cause of death to children 4 years and older. Therefore, the American Academy of Pediatrics continues to recommend the inclusion of child passenger safety anticipatory guidance at every health supervision visit. This technical report provides a summary of the evidence in support of 5 recommendations for best practices to optimize safety in passenger vehicles for children from birth through adolescence that all pediatricians should know and promote in their routine practice. These recommendations are presented in the revised policy statement on child passenger safety in the form of an algorithm that is intended to facilitate their implementation by pediatricians with their patients and families. The algorithm is designed to cover the majority of situations that pediatricians will encounter in practice. In addition, a summary of evidence on a number of additional issues affecting the safety of children in motor vehicles, including the proper use and installation of child restraints, exposure to air bags, travel in pickup trucks, children left in or around vehicles, and the importance of restraint laws, is provided. Finally, this technical report provides pediatricians with a number of resources for additional information to use when providing anticipatory guidance to families. (10/18)

http://pediatrics.aappublications.org/content/142/5/e20182461

CHILD SEX TRAFFICKING AND COMMERCIAL SEXUAL EXPLOITATION: HEALTH CARE NEEDS OF VICTIMS (CLINICAL REPORT)

Jordan Greenbaum, MD; James E. Crawford-Jakubiak, MD, FAAP; and Committee on Child Abuse and Neglect

ABSTRACT. Child sex trafficking and commercial sexual exploitation of children (CSEC) are major public health problems in the United States and throughout the world. Despite large numbers of American and foreign youth affected and a plethora of serious physical and mental health problems associated with CSEC, there is limited information available to pediatricians regarding the nature and scope of human trafficking and how pediatricians and other health care providers may help protect children. Knowledge of risk factors, recruitment practices, possible indicators of CSEC, and common medical and behavioral health problems experienced by victims will help pediatricians recognize potential victims and respond appropriately. As health care providers, educators, and leaders in child advocacy, pediatricians play an essential role in addressing the public health issues faced by child victims of CSEC. Their roles can include working to increase recognition of CSEC, providing direct care and anticipatory guidance related to CSEC, engaging in collaborative efforts with medical and nonmedical colleagues to provide for the complex needs of youth, and educating child-serving professionals and the public. (2/15)

http://pediatrics.aappublications.org/content/135/3/566

THE CHILD WITNESS IN THE COURTROOM

Robert H. Pantell, MD, FAAP, and Committee on Psychosocial Aspects of Child and Family Health

ABSTRACT. Beginning in the 1980s, children have increasingly served as witnesses in the criminal, civil, and family courts; currently, >100 000 children appear in court each year. This statement updates the 1992 American Academy of Pediatrics (AAP)

policy statement "The Child as a Witness" and the subsequent 1999 "The Child in Court: A Subject Review." It also builds on existing AAP policy on adverse life events affecting children and resources developed to understand and address childhood trauma. The purpose of this policy statement is to provide background information on some of the legal issues involving children testifying in court, including the accuracy and psychological impact of child testimony; to provide suggestions for how pediatricians can support patients who will testify in court; and to make recommendations for policy improvements to minimize the adverse psychological consequences for child witnesses. These recommendations are, for the most part, based on studies on the psychological and physiologic consequences of children witnessing and experiencing violence, as well as appearing in court, that have emerged since the previous AAP publications on the subject. The goal is to reduce the secondary traumatization of and long-term consequences for children providing testimony about violence they have experienced or witnessed. This statement primarily addresses children appearing in court as victims of physical or sexual abuse or as witnesses of violent acts; most of the scientific literature addresses these specific situations. It may apply, in certain situations, to children required to provide testimony in custody disputes, child welfare proceedings, or immigration court. It does not address children appearing in court as offenders or as part of juvenile justice proceedings. (2/17)
http://pediatrics.aappublications.org/content/139/3/e20164008

CHILDREN, ADOLESCENTS, AND THE MEDIA

Council on Communications and Media

ABSTRACT. Media, from television to the "new media" (including cell phones, iPads, and social media), are a dominant force in children's lives. Although television is still the predominant medium for children and adolescents, new technologies are increasingly popular. The American Academy of Pediatrics continues to be concerned by evidence about the potential harmful effects of media messages and images; however, important positive and prosocial effects of media use should also be recognized. Pediatricians are encouraged to take a media history and ask 2 media questions at every well-child visit: How much recreational screen time does your child or teenager consume daily? Is there a television set or Internet-connected device in the child's bedroom? Parents are encouraged to establish a family home use plan for all media. Media influences on children and teenagers should be recognized by schools, policymakers, product advertisers, and entertainment producers. (10/13)
http://pediatrics.aappublications.org/content/132/5/958

CHILDREN AND ADOLESCENTS AND DIGITAL MEDIA (TECHNICAL REPORT)

Yolanda (Linda) Reid Chassiakos, MD, FAAP; Jenny Radesky, MD, FAAP; Dimitri Christakis, MD, FAAP; Megan A. Moreno, MD, MSEd, MPH, FAAP; Corinn Cross, MD, FAAP; and Council on Communications and Media

ABSTRACT. Today's children and adolescents are immersed in both traditional and new forms of digital media. Research on traditional media, such as television, has identified health concerns and negative outcomes that correlate with the duration and content of viewing. Over the past decade, the use of digital media, including interactive and social media, has grown, and research evidence suggests that these newer media offer both benefits and risks to the health of children and teenagers. Evidence-based benefits identified from the use of digital and social media include early learning, exposure to new ideas and knowledge, increased opportunities for social contact and support, and new opportunities to access health promotion messages and information. Risks of such media include negative health effects on sleep, attention, and learning; a higher incidence of obesity and depression; exposure to inaccurate, inappropriate, or unsafe content and contacts; and compromised privacy and confidentiality. This technical report reviews the literature regarding these opportunities and risks, framed around clinical questions, for children from birth to adulthood. To promote health and wellness in children and adolescents, it is important to maintain adequate physical activity, healthy nutrition, good sleep hygiene, and a nurturing social environment. A healthy Family Media Use Plan (www.healthychildren.org/MediaUsePlan) that is individualized for a specific child, teenager, or family can identify an appropriate balance between screen time/online time and other activities, set boundaries for accessing content, guide displays of personal information, encourage age-appropriate critical thinking and digital literacy, and support open family communication and implementation of consistent rules about media use. (10/16)
http://pediatrics.aappublications.org/content/138/5/e20162593

CHILDREN'S HEALTH INSURANCE PROGRAM (CHIP): ACCOMPLISHMENTS, CHALLENGES, AND POLICY RECOMMENDATIONS

Committee on Child Health Financing

ABSTRACT. Sixteen years ago, the 105th Congress, responding to the needs of 10 million children in the United States who lacked health insurance, created the State Children's Health Insurance Program (SCHIP) as part of the Balanced Budget Act of 1997. Enacted as Title XXI of the Social Security Act, the Children's Health Insurance Program (CHIP; or SCHIP as it has been known at some points) provided states with federal assistance to create programs specifically designed for children from families with incomes that exceeded Medicaid thresholds but that were insufficient to enable them to afford private health insurance. Congress provided $40 billion in block grants over 10 years for states to expand their existing Medicaid programs to cover the intended populations, to erect new stand-alone SCHIP programs for these children, or to effect some combination of both options. Congress reauthorized CHIP once in 2009 under the Children's Health Insurance Program Reauthorization Act and extended its life further within provisions of the Patient Protection and Affordable Care Act of 2010. The purpose of this statement is to review the features of CHIP as it has evolved over the 16 years of its existence; to summarize what is known about the effects that the program has had on coverage, access, health status, and disparities among participants; to identify challenges that remain with respect to insuring this group of vulnerable children, including the impact that provisions of the new Affordable Care Act will have on the issue of health insurance coverage for near-poor children after 2015; and to offer recommendations on how to expand and strengthen the national commitment to provide health insurance to all children regardless of means. (2/14)
http://pediatrics.aappublications.org/content/133/3/e784

CIRCUMCISION POLICY STATEMENT

Task Force on Circumcision

ABSTRACT. Male circumcision is a common procedure, generally performed during the newborn period in the United States. In 2007, the American Academy of Pediatrics (AAP) formed a multidisciplinary task force of AAP members and other stakeholders to evaluate the recent evidence on male circumcision and update the Academy's 1999 recommendations in this area. Evaluation of current evidence indicates that the health benefits of newborn male circumcision outweigh the risks and that the procedure's benefits justify access to this procedure for families who choose it. Specific benefits identified included prevention of urinary tract infections, penile cancer, and transmission of some sexually transmitted infections, including HIV. The American

College of Obstetricians and Gynecologists has endorsed this statement. (8/12)
http://pediatrics.aappublications.org/content/130/3/585

CLIMATIC HEAT STRESS AND EXERCISING CHILDREN AND ADOLESCENTS

Council on Sports Medicine and Fitness and Council on School Health

ABSTRACT. Results of new research indicate that, contrary to previous thinking, youth do not have less effective thermoregulatory ability, insufficient cardiovascular capacity, or lower physical exertion tolerance compared with adults during exercise in the heat when adequate hydration is maintained. Accordingly, besides poor hydration status, the primary determinants of reduced performance and exertional heat-illness risk in youth during sports and other physical activities in a hot environment include undue physical exertion, insufficient recovery between repeated exercise bouts or closely scheduled same-day training sessions or rounds of sports competition, and inappropriately wearing clothing, uniforms, and protective equipment that play a role in excessive heat retention. Because these known contributing risk factors are modifiable, exertional heat illness is usually preventable. With appropriate preparation, modifications, and monitoring, most healthy children and adolescents can safely participate in outdoor sports and other physical activities through a wide range of challenging warm to hot climatic conditions. (8/11, reaffirmed 2/15)
http://pediatrics.aappublications.org/content/128/3/e741

CLINICAL CONSIDERATIONS RELATED TO THE BEHAVIORAL MANIFESTATIONS OF CHILD MALTREATMENT (CLINICAL REPORT)

Robert D. Sege, MD, PhD, FAAP; Lisa Amaya-Jackson, MD, MPH, FAACAP; Committee on Child Abuse and Neglect; and Council on Foster Care, Adoption, and Kinship Care (joint with American Academy of Child and Adolescent Psychiatry Committee on Child Maltreatment and Violence and National Center for Child Traumatic Stress)

ABSTRACT. Children who have suffered early abuse or neglect may later present with significant health and behavior problems that may persist long after the abusive or neglectful environment has been remediated. Neurobiological research suggests that early maltreatment may result in an altered psychological and physiologic response to stressful stimuli, a response that deleteriously affects the child's subsequent development. Pediatricians can assist caregivers by helping them recognize the abused or neglected child's emotional and behavioral responses associated with child maltreatment and guide them in the use of positive parenting strategies, referring the children and families to evidence-based therapeutic treatment and mobilizing available community resources. (3/17)
http://pediatrics.aappublications.org/content/139/4/e20170100

CLINICAL GENETIC EVALUATION OF THE CHILD WITH MENTAL RETARDATION OR DEVELOPMENTAL DELAYS (CLINICAL REPORT)

John B. Moeschler, MD; Michael Shevell, MD; and Committee on Genetics

ABSTRACT. This clinical report describes the clinical genetic evaluation of the child with developmental delays or mental retardation. The purpose of this report is to describe the optimal clinical genetics diagnostic evaluation to assist pediatricians in providing a medical home for children with developmental delays or mental retardation and their families. The literature supports the benefit of expert clinical judgment by a consulting clinical geneticist in the diagnostic evaluation. However, it is recognized that local factors may preclude this particular option. No single approach to the diagnostic process is supported by the literature. This report addresses the diagnostic importance of clinical history, 3-generation family history, dysmorphologic examination, neurologic examination, chromosome analysis (≥650 bands), fragile X molecular genetic testing, fluorescence in situ hybridization studies for subtelomere chromosome rearrangements, molecular genetic testing for typical and atypical presentations of known syndromes, computed tomography and/or magnetic resonance brain imaging, and targeted studies for metabolic disorders. (6/06, reaffirmed 5/12)
http://pediatrics.aappublications.org/content/117/6/2304

CLINICAL PRACTICE POLICY TO PROTECT CHILDREN FROM TOBACCO, NICOTINE, AND TOBACCO SMOKE

Section on Tobacco Control

ABSTRACT. Tobacco dependence starts in childhood. Tobacco exposure of children is common and causes illness and premature death in children and adults, with adverse effects starting in the womb. There is no safe level of tobacco smoke exposure. Pediatricians should screen for use of tobacco and other nicotine delivery devices and provide anticipatory guidance to prevent smoking initiation and reduce tobacco smoke exposure. Pediatricians need to be aware of the different nicotine delivery systems marketed and available.

Parents and caregivers are important sources of children's tobacco smoke exposure. Because tobacco dependence is a severe addiction, to protect children's health, caregiver tobacco dependence treatment should be offered or referral for treatment should be provided (such as referral to the national smoker's quitline at 1-800-QUIT-NOW). If the source of tobacco exposure cannot be eliminated, counseling about reducing exposure to children should be provided.

Health care delivery systems should facilitate the effective prevention, identification, and treatment of tobacco dependence in children and adolescents, their parents, and other caregivers. Health care facilities should protect children from tobacco smoke exposure and tobacco promotion. Tobacco dependence prevention and treatment should be part of medical education, with knowledge assessed as part of board certification examinations. (10/15)
http://pediatrics.aappublications.org/content/136/5/1008

CLINICAL TOOLS TO ASSESS ASTHMA CONTROL IN CHILDREN (CLINICAL REPORT)

Chitra Dinakar, MD, FAAP; Bradley E. Chipps, MD, FAAP; Section on Allergy and Immunology; and Section on Pediatric Pulmonology and Sleep Medicine

ABSTRACT. Asthma affects an estimated 7 million children and causes significant health care and disease burden. The most recent iteration of the National Heart, Lung and Blood Institute asthma guidelines, the Expert Panel Report 3, emphasizes the assessment and monitoring of asthma control in the management of asthma. Asthma control refers to the degree to which the manifestations of asthma are minimized by therapeutic interventions and the goals of therapy are met. Although assessment of asthma severity is used to guide initiation of therapy, monitoring of asthma control helps determine whether therapy should be maintained or adjusted. The nuances of estimation of asthma control include understanding concepts of current impairment and future risk and incorporating their measurement into clinical practice. Impairment is assessed on the basis of frequency and intensity of symptoms, variations in lung function, and limitations of daily activities. "Risk" refers to the likelihood of exacerbations, progressive loss of lung function, or adverse effects from medications. Currently available ambulatory tools to measure asthma control range are subjective measures, such as patient-reported composite asthma control score instruments or objective measures of lung function, airway hyperreactivity, and biomarkers. Because asthma control exhibits short- and long-term variability, health care providers need to be vigilant regarding the fluctuations in the factors that can create discordance between subjective and objective assessment of asthma control. Familiarity with the properties, application, and relative value of these measures will enable health care providers to choose the optimal set of measures that will adhere to national standards of care and ensure delivery of high-quality care customized to their patients. (12/16)

http://pediatrics.aappublications.org/content/139/1/e20163438

COCHLEAR IMPLANTS IN CHILDREN: SURGICAL SITE INFECTIONS AND PREVENTION AND TREATMENT OF ACUTE OTITIS MEDIA AND MENINGITIS

Lorry G. Rubin, MD; Blake Papsin, MD; Committee on Infectious Diseases; and Section on Otolaryngology—Head and Neck Surgery

ABSTRACT. The use of cochlear implants is increasingly common, particularly in children younger than 3 years. Bacterial meningitis, often with associated acute otitis media, is more common in children with cochlear implants than in groups of control children. Children with profound deafness who are candidates for cochlear implants should receive all age-appropriate doses of pneumococcal conjugate and Haemophilus influenzae type b conjugate vaccines and appropriate annual immunization against influenza. In addition, starting at 24 months of age, a single dose of 23-valent pneumococcal polysaccharide vaccine should be administered. Before implant surgery, primary care providers and cochlear implant teams should ensure that immunizations are up-to-date, preferably with completion of indicated vaccines at least 2 weeks before implant surgery. Imaging of the temporal bone/inner ear should be performed before cochlear implantation in all children with congenital deafness and all patients with profound hearing impairment and a history of bacterial meningitis to identify those with inner-ear malformations/cerebrospinal fluid fistulas or ossification of the cochlea. During the initial months after cochlear implantation, the risk of complications of acute otitis media may be higher than during subsequent time periods. Therefore, it is recommended that acute otitis media diagnosed during the first 2 months after implantation be initially treated with a parenteral antibiotic (eg, ceftriaxone or cefotaxime). Episodes occurring 2 months or longer after implantation can be treated with a trial of an oral antimicrobial agent (eg, amoxicillin or amoxicillin/clavulanate at a dose of approximately 90 mg/kg per day of amoxicillin component), provided the child does not appear toxic and the implant does not have a spacer/positioner, a wedge that rests in the cochlea next to the electrodes present in certain implant models available between 1999 and 2002. "Watchful waiting" without antimicrobial therapy is inappropriate for children with implants with acute otitis media. If feasible, tympanocentesis should be performed for acute otitis media, and the material should be sent for culture, but performance of this procedure should not result in an undue delay in initiating antimicrobial therapy. For patients with suspected meningitis, cerebrospinal fluid as well as middle-ear fluid, if present, should be sent for culture. Empiric antimicrobial therapy for meningitis occurring within 2 months of implantation should include an agent with broad activity against Gram-negative bacilli (eg, meropenem) plus vancomycin. For meningitis occurring 2 months or longer after implantation, standard empiric antimicrobial therapy for meningitis (eg, ceftriaxone plus vancomycin) is indicated. For patients with meningitis, urgent evaluation by an otolaryngologist is indicated for consideration of imaging and surgical exploration. (7/10, reaffirmed 1/18)

http://pediatrics.aappublications.org/content/126/2/381

CODEINE: TIME TO SAY "NO" (CLINICAL REPORT)

Joseph D. Tobias, MD, FAAP; Thomas P. Green, MD, FAAP; Charles J. Coté, MD, FAAP; Section on Anesthesiology and Pain Medicine; and Committee on Drugs

ABSTRACT. Codeine has been prescribed to pediatric patients for many decades as both an analgesic and an antitussive agent. Codeine is a prodrug with little inherent pharmacologic activity and must be metabolized in the liver into morphine, which is responsible for codeine's analgesic effects. However, there is substantial genetic variability in the activity of the responsible hepatic enzyme, *CYP2D6*, and, as a consequence, individual patient response to codeine varies from no effect to high sensitivity. Drug surveillance has documented the occurrence of unanticipated respiratory depression and death after receiving codeine in children, many of whom have been shown to be ultrarapid metabolizers. Patients with documented or suspected obstructive sleep apnea appear to be at particular risk because of opioid sensitivity, compounding the danger among rapid metabolizers in this group. Recently, various organizations and regulatory bodies, including the World Health Organization, the US Food and Drug Administration, and the European Medicines Agency, have promulgated stern warnings regarding the occurrence of adverse effects of codeine in children. These and other groups have or are considering a declaration of a contraindication for the use of codeine for children as either an analgesic or an antitussive. Additional clinical research must extend the understanding of the risks and benefits of both opioid and nonopioid alternatives for orally administered, effective agents for acute and chronic pain. (9/16)

http://pediatrics.aappublications.org/content/138/4/e20162396

COLLABORATIVE ROLE OF THE PEDIATRICIAN IN THE DIAGNOSIS AND MANAGEMENT OF BIPOLAR DISORDER IN ADOLESCENTS (CLINICAL REPORT)

Benjamin N. Shain, MD, PhD, and Committee on Adolescence

ABSTRACT. Despite the complexity of diagnosis and management, pediatricians have an important collaborative role in referring and partnering in the management of adolescents with bipolar disorder. This report presents the classification of bipolar disorder as well as interviewing and diagnostic guidelines. Treatment options are described, particularly focusing on medication management and rationale for the common practice of multiple, simultaneous medications. Medication adverse effects may be problematic and better managed with collaboration between mental health professionals and pediatricians. Case examples illustrate a number of common diagnostic and management issues. (11/12)

http://pediatrics.aappublications.org/content/130/6/e1725

COMMUNICATING WITH CHILDREN AND FAMILIES: FROM EVERYDAY INTERACTIONS TO SKILL IN CONVEYING DISTRESSING INFORMATION (TECHNICAL REPORT)

Marcia Levetown, MD, and Committee on Bioethics

ABSTRACT. Health care communication is a skill that is critical to safe and effective medical practice; it can and must be taught. Communication skill influences patient disclosure, treatment adherence and outcome, adaptation to illness, and bereavement. This article provides a review of the evidence regarding clinical communication in the pediatric setting, covering the spectrum from outpatient primary care consultation to death notification, and provides practical suggestions to improve communication with patients and families, enabling more effective, efficient, and empathic pediatric health care. (5/08, reaffirmed 12/16)

http://pediatrics.aappublications.org/content/121/5/e1441

COMMUNITY PEDIATRICS: NAVIGATING THE INTERSECTION OF MEDICINE, PUBLIC HEALTH, AND SOCIAL DETERMINANTS OF CHILDREN'S HEALTH

Council on Community Pediatrics

ABSTRACT. This policy statement provides a framework for the pediatrician's role in promoting the health and well-being of all children in the context of their families and communities. It offers pediatricians a definition of community pediatrics, emphasizes the importance of recognizing social determinants of health, and delineates the need to partner with public health to address population-based child health issues. It also recognizes the importance of pediatric involvement in child advocacy at local, state, and federal levels to ensure all children have access to a high-quality medical home and to eliminate child health disparities. This statement provides a set of specific recommendations that underscore the critical nature of this dimension of pediatric practice, teaching, and research. (2/13, reaffirmed 10/16)

http://pediatrics.aappublications.org/content/131/3/623

COMPREHENSIVE EVALUATION OF THE CHILD WITH INTELLECTUAL DISABILITY OR GLOBAL DEVELOPMENTAL DELAYS (CLINICAL REPORT)

John B. Moeschler, MD, MS, FAAP, FACMG; Michael Shevell, MDCM, FRCP; and Committee on Genetics

ABSTRACT. Global developmental delay and intellectual disability are relatively common pediatric conditions. This report describes the recommended clinical genetics diagnostic approach. The report is based on a review of published reports, most consisting of medium to large case series of diagnostic tests used, and the proportion of those that led to a diagnosis in such patients. Chromosome microarray is designated as a first-line test and replaces the standard karyotype and fluorescent in situ hybridization subtelomere tests for the child with intellectual disability of unknown etiology. Fragile X testing remains an important first-line test. The importance of considering testing for inborn errors of metabolism in this population is supported by a recent systematic review of the literature and several case series recently published. The role of brain MRI remains important in certain patients. There is also a discussion of the emerging literature on the use of whole-exome sequencing as a diagnostic test in this population. Finally, the importance of intentional comanagement among families, the medical home, and the clinical genetics specialty clinic is discussed. (8/14)

http://pediatrics.aappublications.org/content/134/3/e903

COMPREHENSIVE HEALTH EVALUATION OF THE NEWLY ADOPTED CHILD (CLINICAL REPORT)

Veronnie Faye Jones, MD, PhD, MSPH, FAAP; Elaine E. Schulte, MD, MPH, FAAP; and Council on Foster Care, Adoption, and Kinship Care

ABSTRACT. Children who join families through the process of adoption, whether through a domestic or international route, often have multiple health care needs. Pediatricians and other health care personnel are in a unique position to guide families in achieving optimal health for the adopted children as families establish a medical home. Shortly after placement in an adoptive home, it is recommended that children have a timely comprehensive health evaluation to provide care for known medical needs and identify health issues that are unknown. It is important to begin this evaluation with a review of all available medical records and pertinent verbal history. A complete physical examination then follows. The evaluation should also include diagnostic testing based on findings from the history and physical examination as well as the risks presented by the child's previous living conditions. Age-appropriate screenings may include, but are not limited to, newborn screening panels and hearing, vision, dental, and formal behavioral and/or developmental screenings. The comprehensive assessment may occur at the time of the initial visit to the physician after adoptive placement or can take place over several visits. Adopted children can be referred to other medical specialists as deemed appropriate. The Council on Adoption, Foster Care, and Kinship Care is a resource within the American Academy of Pediatrics for physicians providing care for children who are being adopted. (4/19)

See full text on page 597.

https://pediatrics.aappublications.org/content/143/5/e20190657

CONDOM USE BY ADOLESCENTS

Committee on Adolescence

ABSTRACT. Rates of sexual activity, pregnancies, and births among adolescents have continued to decline during the past decade to historic lows. Despite these positive trends, many adolescents remain at risk for unintended pregnancy and sexually transmitted infections (STIs). This policy statement has been developed to assist the pediatrician in understanding and supporting the use of condoms by their patients to prevent unintended pregnancies and STIs and address barriers to their use. When used consistently and correctly, male latex condoms reduce the risk of pregnancy and many STIs, including HIV. Since the last policy statement published 12 years ago, there is an increased evidence base supporting the protection provided by condoms against STIs. Rates of acquisition of STIs/HIV among adolescents remain unacceptably high. Interventions that increase availability or accessibility to condoms are most efficacious when combined with additional individual, small-group, or community-level activities that include messages about safer sex. Continued research is needed to inform public health interventions for adolescents that increase the consistent and correct use of condoms and promote dual protection of condoms for STI prevention with other effective methods of contraception. (10/13)

http://pediatrics.aappublications.org/content/132/5/973

CONFLICTS BETWEEN RELIGIOUS OR SPIRITUAL BELIEFS AND PEDIATRIC CARE: INFORMED REFUSAL, EXEMPTIONS, AND PUBLIC FUNDING

Committee on Bioethics

ABSTRACT. Although respect for parents' decision-making authority is an important principle, pediatricians should report suspected cases of medical neglect, and the state should, at times, intervene to require medical treatment of children. Some parents' reasons for refusing medical treatment are based on their religious or spiritual beliefs. In cases in which treatment is likely to prevent death or serious disability or relieve severe pain, children's health and future autonomy should be protected. Because religious exemptions to child abuse and neglect laws do not equally protect all children and may harm some children by causing confusion about the duty to provide medical treatment, these exemptions should be repealed. Furthermore, public health care funds should not cover alternative unproven religious or spiritual healing practices. Such payments may inappropriately legitimize these practices as appropriate medical treatment. (10/13, reaffirmed 12/16, 11/17)

http://pediatrics.aappublications.org/content/132/5/962

CONGENITAL BRAIN AND SPINAL CORD MALFORMATIONS AND THEIR ASSOCIATED CUTANEOUS MARKERS (CLINICAL REPORT)

Mark Dias, MD, FAANS, FAAP; Michael Partington, MD, FAANS, FAAP; and Section on Neurologic Surgery

ABSTRACT. The brain, spinal cord, and skin are all derived from the embryonic ectoderm; this common derivation leads to a high association between central nervous system dysraphic malformations and abnormalities of the overlying skin. A myelomeningocele is an obvious open malformation, the identification of which is not usually difficult. However, the relationship between congenital spinal cord malformations and other cutaneous malformations, such as dimples, vascular anomalies (including infantile hemangiomata and other vascular malformations), congenital pigmented nevi or other hamartomata, or midline hairy patches may be less obvious but no less important. Pediatricians should be aware of these associations, recognize the cutaneous markers associated with congenital central nervous system malformations, and refer children with such markers to the appropriate specialist in a timely fashion for further evaluation and treatment. (9/15)

http://pediatrics.aappublications.org/content/136/4/e1105

CONSENT BY PROXY FOR NONURGENT PEDIATRIC CARE (CLINICAL REPORT)

Jonathan M. Fanaroff, MD, JD, FAAP, FCLM, and Committee on Medical Liability and Risk Management

ABSTRACT. Minor-aged patients are often brought to the pediatrician for nonurgent acute medical care, physical examinations, or health supervision visits by someone other than their legally authorized representative, which, in most situations, is a parent. These surrogates or proxies can be members of the child's extended family, such as a grandparent, adult sibling, or aunt/uncle; a noncustodial parent or stepparent in cases of divorce and remarriage; an adult who lives in the home but is not biologically or legally related to the child; or even a child care provider (eg, au pair, nanny, private-duty nurse/nurse's aide, group home supervisor). This report identifies common situations in which pediatricians may encounter "consent by proxy" for nonurgent medical care for minors, including physical examinations, and explains the potential for liability exposure associated with these circumstances. The report suggests practical steps that balance the need to minimize the physician's liability exposure with the patient's access to health care. Key issues to be considered when creating or updating office policies for obtaining and documenting consent by proxy are offered. (1/17)

http://pediatrics.aappublications.org/content/139/2/e20163911

CONSENT FOR EMERGENCY MEDICAL SERVICES FOR CHILDREN AND ADOLESCENTS

Committee on Pediatric Emergency Medicine and Committee on Bioethics

ABSTRACT. Parental consent generally is required for the medical evaluation and treatment of minor children. However, children and adolescents might require evaluation of and treatment for emergency medical conditions in situations in which a parent or legal guardian is not available to provide consent or conditions under which an adolescent patient might possess the legal authority to provide consent. In general, a medical screening examination and any medical care necessary and likely to prevent imminent and significant harm to the pediatric patient with an emergency medical condition should not be withheld or delayed because of problems obtaining consent. The purpose of this policy statement is to provide guidance in those situations in which parental consent is not readily available, in which parental consent is not necessary, or in which parental refusal of consent places a child at risk of significant harm. (7/11, reaffirmed 9/15)

http://pediatrics.aappublications.org/content/128/2/427

CONSUMPTION OF RAW OR UNPASTEURIZED MILK AND MILK PRODUCTS BY PREGNANT WOMEN AND CHILDREN

Committee on Infectious Diseases and Committee on Nutrition

ABSTRACT. Sales of raw or unpasteurized milk and milk products are still legal in at least 30 states in the United States. Raw milk and milk products from cows, goats, and sheep continue to be a source of bacterial infections attributable to a number of virulent pathogens, including *Listeria monocytogenes*, *Campylobacter jejuni*, *Salmonella* species, *Brucella* species, and *Escherichia coli* O157. These infections can occur in both healthy and immunocompromised individuals, including older adults, infants, young children, and pregnant women and their unborn fetuses, in whom life-threatening infections and fetal miscarriage can occur. Efforts to limit the sale of raw milk products have met with opposition from those who are proponents of the purported health benefits of consuming raw milk products, which contain natural or unprocessed factors not inactivated by pasteurization. However, the benefits of these natural factors have not been clearly demonstrated in evidence-based studies and, therefore, do not outweigh the risks of raw milk consumption. Substantial data suggest that pasteurized milk confers equivalent health benefits compared with raw milk, without the additional risk of bacterial infections. The purpose of this policy statement was to review the risks of raw milk consumption in the United States and to provide evidence of the risks of infectious complications associated with consumption of unpasteurized milk and milk products, especially among pregnant women, infants, and children. (12/13)

http://pediatrics.aappublications.org/content/133/1/175

CONTRACEPTION FOR ADOLESCENTS

Committee on Adolescence

ABSTRACT. Contraception is a pillar in reducing adolescent pregnancy rates. The American Academy of Pediatrics recommends that pediatricians develop a working knowledge of contraception to help adolescents reduce risks of and negative health consequences related to unintended pregnancy. Over the past 10 years, a number of new contraceptive methods have become available to adolescents, newer guidance has been issued on existing contraceptive methods, and the evidence base for contraception for special populations (adolescents who have disabilities, are obese, are recipients of solid organ transplants, or are HIV infected) has expanded. The Academy has addressed contraception since 1980, and this policy statement updates the 2007 statement on contraception and adolescents. It provides the pediatrician with a description and rationale for best practices in counseling and prescribing contraception for adolescents. It is supported by an accompanying technical report. (9/14)

http://pediatrics.aappublications.org/content/134/4/e1244

CONTRACEPTION FOR ADOLESCENTS (TECHNICAL REPORT)

Mary A. Ott, MD, MA, FAAP; Gina S. Sucato, MD, MPH, FAAP; and Committee on Adolescence

ABSTRACT. A working knowledge of contraception will assist the pediatrician in both sexual health promotion as well as treatment of common adolescent gynecologic problems. Best practices in adolescent anticipatory guidance and screening include a sexual health history, screening for pregnancy and sexually transmitted infections, counseling, and if indicated, providing access to contraceptives. Pediatricians' long-term relationships with adolescents and families allow them to help promote healthy sexual decision-making, including abstinence and contraceptive use. Additionally, medical indications for contraception, such as acne, dysmenorrhea, and heavy menstrual bleeding, are frequently uncovered during adolescent visits. This technical report provides an evidence base for the accompanying policy statement and addresses key aspects of adolescent contraceptive use, including the following: (1) sexual history taking, confidentiality, and counseling; (2) adolescent data on the use and side effects of newer contraceptive methods; (3) new data on older contraceptive methods; and (4) evidence supporting the use of contraceptives in adolescent patients with complex medical conditions. (9/14)

http://pediatrics.aappublications.org/content/134/4/e1257

CONTRACEPTION FOR HIV-INFECTED ADOLESCENTS (CLINICAL REPORT)

Athena P. Kourtis, MD, PhD, MPH, FAAP; Ayesha Mirza, MD, FAAP; and Committee on Pediatric AIDS

ABSTRACT. Access to high-quality reproductive health care is important for adolescents and young adults with HIV infection to prevent unintended pregnancies, sexually transmitted infections, and secondary transmission of HIV to partners and children. As perinatally HIV-infected children mature into adolescence and adulthood and new HIV infections among adolescents and young adults continue to occur in the United States, medical providers taking care of such individuals often face issues related to sexual and reproductive health. Challenges including drug interactions between several hormonal methods and antiretroviral agents make decisions regarding contraceptive options more complex for these adolescents. Dual protection, defined as the use of an effective contraceptive along with condoms, should be central to ongoing discussions with HIV-infected young women and couples wishing to avoid pregnancy. Last, reproductive health discussions need to be integrated with discussions on HIV care, because a reduction in plasma HIV viral load below the level of detection (an "undetectable viral load") is essential for the individual's health as well as for a reduction in HIV transmission to partners and children. (8/16)

http://pediatrics.aappublications.org/content/138/3/e20161892

CONTROVERSIES CONCERNING VITAMIN K AND THE NEWBORN

Committee on Fetus and Newborn

ABSTRACT. Prevention of early vitamin K deficiency bleeding (VKDB) of the newborn, with onset at birth to 2 weeks of age (formerly known as classic hemorrhagic disease of the newborn), by oral or parenteral administration of vitamin K is accepted practice. In contrast, late VKDB, with onset from 2 to 12 weeks of age, is most effectively prevented by parenteral administration of vitamin K. Earlier concern regarding a possible causal association between parenteral vitamin K and childhood cancer has not been substantiated. This revised statement presents updated recommendations for the use of vitamin K in the prevention of early and late VKDB. (7/03, reaffirmed 5/06, 5/09, 9/14)

http://pediatrics.aappublications.org/content/112/1/191

CORD BLOOD BANKING FOR POTENTIAL FUTURE TRANSPLANTATION

William T. Shearer, MD, PhD, FAAP; Bertram H. Lubin, MD, FAAP; Mitchell S. Cairo, MD, FAAP; Luigi D. Notarangelo, MD; Section on Hematology/Oncology; and Section on Allergy and Immunology

ABSTRACT. This policy statement is intended to provide information to guide pediatricians, obstetricians, and other medical specialists and health care providers in responding to parents' questions about cord blood donation and banking as well as the types (public versus private) and quality of cord blood banks. Cord blood is an excellent source of stem cells for hematopoietic stem cell transplantation in children with some fatal diseases. Cord blood transplantation offers another method of definitive therapy for infants, children, and adults with certain hematologic malignancies, hemoglobinopathies, severe forms of T-lymphocyte and other immunodeficiencies, and metabolic diseases. The development of universal screening for severe immunodeficiency assay in a growing number of states is likely to increase the number of cord blood transplants. Both public and private cord blood banks worldwide hold hundreds of thousands of cord blood units designated for the treatment of fatal or debilitating illnesses. The procurement, characterization, and cryopreservation of cord blood is free for families who choose public banking. However, the family cost for private banking is significant and not covered by insurance, and the unit may never be used. Quality-assessment reviews by several national and international accrediting bodies show private cord blood banks to be underused for treatment, less regulated for quality control, and more expensive for the family than public cord blood banks. There is an unquestionable need to study the use of cord blood banking to make new and important alternative means of reconstituting the hematopoietic blood system in patients with malignancies and blood disorders and possibly regenerating tissue systems in the future. Recommendations regarding appropriate ethical and operational standards (including informed consent policies, financial disclosures, and conflict-of-interest policies) are provided for physicians, institutions, and organizations that operate or have a relationship with cord blood banking programs. The information on all aspects of cord blood banking gathered in this policy statement will facilitate parental choice for public or private cord blood banking. (10/17)

http://pediatrics.aappublications.org/content/140/5/e20172695

CORPORAL PUNISHMENT IN SCHOOLS

Committee on School Health

ABSTRACT. The American Academy of Pediatrics recommends that corporal punishment in schools be abolished in all states by law and that alternative forms of student behavior management be used. (8/00, reaffirmed 6/03, 5/06, 2/12, 12/18)

http://pediatrics.aappublications.org/content/106/2/343

COUNSELING IN PEDIATRIC POPULATIONS AT RISK FOR INFERTILITY AND/OR SEXUAL FUNCTION CONCERNS (CLINICAL REPORT)

Leena Nahata, MD, FAAP; Gwendolyn P. Quinn, PhD; Amy C. Tishelman, PhD; and Section on Endocrinology

ABSTRACT. Reproductive health is an important yet often overlooked topic in pediatric health care; when addressed, the focus is generally on prevention of sexually transmitted infections and unwanted pregnancy. Two aspects of reproductive health counseling that have received minimal attention in pediatrics are fertility and sexual function for at-risk pediatric populations, and youth across many disciplines are affected. Although professional organizations, such as the American Academy of Pediatrics and the American Society of Clinical Oncology, have published recommendations about fertility preservation discussions, none of these guidelines address how to have ongoing conversations with at-risk youth and their families about the potential for future infertility and sexual dysfunction in developmentally appropriate ways. Researchers suggest many pediatric patients at risk for reproductive problems remain uncertain and confused about their fertility or sexual function status well into young adulthood. Potential infertility may cause distress and anxiety, has been shown to affect formation of romantic relationships, and may lead to unplanned pregnancy in those who incorrectly assumed they were infertile. Sexual dysfunction is also common and may lead to problems with intimacy and self-esteem; survivors of pediatric conditions consistently report inadequate guidance from clinicians in this area. Health care providers and parents report challenges in knowing how and when to discuss these issues. In this context, the goal of this clinical report is to review evidence and considerations for providers related to information sharing about impaired fertility and sexual function in pediatric patients attributable to congenital and acquired conditions or treatments. (7/18)

http://pediatrics.aappublications.org/content/142/2/e20181435

COUNSELING PARENTS AND TEENS ABOUT MARIJUANA USE IN THE ERA OF LEGALIZATION OF MARIJUANA (CLINICAL REPORT)

Sheryl A. Ryan, MD, FAAP; Seth D. Ammerman, MD, FAAP; and Committee on Substance Use and Prevention

ABSTRACT. Many states have recently made significant changes to their legislation making recreational and/or medical marijuana use by adults legal. Although these laws, for the most part, have not targeted the adolescent population, they have created an environment in which marijuana increasingly is seen as acceptable, safe, and therapeutic. This clinical report offers guidance to the practicing pediatrician based on existing evidence and expert opinion/consensus of the American Academy of Pediatrics regarding anticipatory guidance and counseling to teenagers and their parents about marijuana and its use. The recently published technical report provides the detailed evidence and references regarding the research on which the information in this clinical report is based. (2/17)

http://pediatrics.aappublications.org/content/139/3/e20164069

COUNTERING VACCINE HESITANCY (CLINICAL REPORT)

Kathryn M. Edwards, MD, FAAP; Jesse M. Hackell, MD, FAAP; Committee on Infectious Diseases; and Committee on Practice and Ambulatory Medicine

ABSTRACT. Immunizations have led to a significant decrease in rates of vaccine-preventable diseases and have made a significant impact on the health of children. However, some parents express concerns about vaccine safety and the necessity of vaccines. The concerns of parents range from hesitancy about some immunizations to refusal of all vaccines. This clinical report provides information about addressing parental concerns about vaccination. (8/16)

http://pediatrics.aappublications.org/content/138/3/e20162146

CRITICAL ELEMENTS FOR THE PEDIATRIC PERIOPERATIVE ANESTHESIA ENVIRONMENT

Section on Anesthesiology and Pain Medicine

ABSTRACT. The American Academy of Pediatrics proposes guidance for the pediatric perioperative anesthesia environment. Essential components are identified to optimize the perioperative environment for the anesthetic care of infants and children. Such an environment promotes the safety and well-being of infants and children by reducing the risk of adverse events. (11/15)

http://pediatrics.aappublications.org/content/136/6/1200

THE CRUCIAL ROLE OF RECESS IN SCHOOL

Council on School Health

ABSTRACT. Recess is at the heart of a vigorous debate over the role of schools in promoting the optimal development of the whole child. A growing trend toward reallocating time in school to accentuate the more academic subjects has put this important facet of a child's school day at risk. Recess serves as a necessary break from the rigors of concentrated, academic challenges in the classroom. But equally important is the fact that safe and well-supervised recess offers cognitive, social, emotional, and physical benefits that may not be fully appreciated when a decision is made to diminish it. Recess is unique from, and a complement to, physical education—not a substitute for it. The American Academy of Pediatrics believes that recess is a crucial and necessary component of a child's development and, as such, it should not be withheld for punitive or academic reasons. (12/12, reaffirmed 8/16)

http://pediatrics.aappublications.org/content/131/1/183

DEALING WITH THE CARETAKER WHOSE JUDGMENT IS IMPAIRED BY ALCOHOL OR DRUGS: LEGAL AND ETHICAL CONSIDERATIONS (CLINICAL REPORT)

Steven A. Bondi, JD, MD, FAAP; James Scibilia, MD, FAAP; and Committee on Medical Liability and Risk Management

ABSTRACT. An estimated 8.7 million children live in a household with a substance-using parent or guardian. Substance-using caretakers may have impaired judgment that can negatively affect their child's well-being, including his or her ability to receive appropriate medical care. Although the physician-patient relationship exists between the pediatrician and the child, obligations related to safety and confidentiality should be considered as well. In managing encounters with impaired caretakers who may become disruptive or dangerous, pediatricians should be aware of their responsibilities before acting. In addition to fulfilling the duty involved with an established physician-patient relationship, the pediatrician should take reasonable care to safeguard patient confidentiality; protect the safety of their patient, other patients in the facility, visitors, and employees; and comply with reporting mandates. This clinical report identifies and discusses the legal and ethical concepts related to these circumstances. The report offers implementation suggestions when establishing anticipatory procedures and training programs for staff in such situations to maximize the patient's well-being and safety and minimize the liability of the pediatrician. (11/19)

See full text on page 615.

https://pediatrics.aappublications.org/content/144/6/e20193153

DEATH OF A CHILD IN THE EMERGENCY DEPARTMENT

Committee on Pediatric Emergency Medicine (joint with American College of Emergency Physicians Pediatric Emergency Medicine Committee and Emergency Nurses Association Pediatric Committee)

ABSTRACT. The American Academy of Pediatrics, American College of Emergency Physicians, and Emergency Nurses Association have collaborated to identify practices and principles to guide the care of children, families, and staff in the challenging and uncommon event of the death of a child in the emergency department in this policy statement and in an accompanying technical report. (6/14)

http://pediatrics.aappublications.org/content/134/1/198

DEATH OF A CHILD IN THE EMERGENCY DEPARTMENT (TECHNICAL REPORT)

Patricia J. O'Malley, MD, FAAP; Isabel A. Barata, MD, FACEP, FAAP; Sally K. Snow, RN, BSN, CPEN, FAEN; and Committee on Pediatric Emergency Medicine (joint with American College of Emergency Physicians Pediatric Emergency Medicine Committee and Emergency Nurses Association Pediatric Committee)

ABSTRACT. The death of a child in the emergency department (ED) is one of the most challenging problems facing ED clinicians. This revised technical report and accompanying policy statement reaffirm principles of patient- and family-centered care. Recent literature is examined regarding family presence, termination of resuscitation, bereavement responsibilities of ED clinicians, support of child fatality review efforts, and other issues inherent in caring for the patient, family, and staff when a child dies in the ED. Appendices are provided that offer an approach to bereavement activities in the ED, carrying out forensic responsibilities while providing compassionate care, communicating the news of the death of a child in the acute setting, providing a closing ritual at the time of terminating resuscitation efforts, and managing the child with a terminal condition who presents near death in the ED. (6/14)

http://pediatrics.aappublications.org/content/134/1/e313

DEFINITION OF A PEDIATRICIAN

Committee on Pediatric Workforce

POLICY. The American Academy of Pediatrics (AAP) has developed the following definition of pediatrics and a pediatrician:

Pediatrics is the specialty of medical science concerned with the physical, mental, and social health of children from birth to young adulthood. Pediatric care encompasses a broad spectrum of health services ranging from preventive health care to the diagnosis and treatment of acute and chronic diseases.

Pediatrics is a discipline that deals with biological, social, and environmental influences on the developing child and with the impact of disease and dysfunction on development. Children differ from adults anatomically, physiologically, immunologically, psychologically, developmentally, and metabolically.

The pediatrician, a term that includes primary care pediatricians, pediatric medical subspecialists, and pediatric surgical specialists, understands this constantly changing functional status of his or her patients' incident to growth and development and the consequent changing standards of "normal" for age. A pediatrician is a physician who is concerned primarily with the health, welfare, and development of children and is uniquely qualified for these endeavors by virtue of interest and initial training. This training includes 4 years of medical school education, plus an additional year or years (usually at least 3) of intensive training devoted solely to all aspects of medical care for children, adolescents, and young adults. Maintenance of these competencies is achieved by experience, training, continuous education, self-assessment, and practice improvement.

A pediatrician is able to define accurately the child's health status and to serve as a consultant and make use of other specialists as consultants as needed, ideally in the context of, or in conjunction with, the physician-led medical home. Because the child's welfare is heavily dependent on the home and family, the pediatrician supports efforts to create a nurturing environment. Such support includes education about healthful living and anticipatory guidance for both patients and parents.

A pediatrician participates at the community level in preventing or solving problems in child health care and publicly advocates the causes of children. (3/15)

http://pediatrics.aappublications.org/content/135/4/780

DETENTION OF IMMIGRANT CHILDREN

Julie M. Linton, MD, FAAP; Marsha Griffin, MD, FAAP; Alan J. Shapiro, MD, FAAP; and Council on Community Pediatrics

ABSTRACT. Immigrant children seeking safe haven in the United States, whether arriving unaccompanied or in family units, face a complicated evaluation and legal process from the point of arrival through permanent resettlement in communities. The conditions in which children are detained and the support services that are available to them are of great concern to pediatricians and other advocates for children. In accordance with internationally accepted rights of the child, immigrant and refugee children should be treated with dignity and respect and should not be exposed to conditions that may harm or traumatize them. The Department of Homeland Security facilities do not meet the basic standards for the care of children in residential settings. The recommendations in this statement call for limited exposure of any child to current Department of Homeland Security facilities (ie, Customs and Border Protection and Immigration and Customs Enforcement facilities) and for longitudinal evaluation of the health consequences of detention of immigrant children in the United States. From the moment children are in the custody of the United States, they deserve health care that meets guideline-based standards, treatment that mitigates harm or traumatization, and services that support their health and well-being. This policy statement also provides specific recommendations regarding postrelease services once a child is released into communities across the country, including a coordinated system that facilitates access to a medical home and consistent access to education, child care, interpretation services, and legal services. (4/17)

http://pediatrics.aappublications.org/content/139/5/e20170483

DEVELOPMENTAL DYSPLASIA OF THE HIP PRACTICE GUIDELINE (TECHNICAL REPORT)

Harold P. Lehmann, MD, PhD; Richard Hinton, MD, MPH; Paola Morello, MD; Jeanne Santoli, MD; in conjunction with Steering Committee on Quality Improvement and Subcommittee on Developmental Dysplasia of the Hip Detention of Immigrant Children

ABSTRACT. *Objective.* To create a recommendation for pediatricians and other primary care providers about their role as screeners for detecting developmental dysplasia of the hip (DDH) in children.

Patients. Theoretical cohorts of newborns.

Method. Model-based approach using decision analysis as the foundation. Components of the approach include the following:

Perspective: Primary care provider.

Outcomes: DDH, avascular necrosis of the hip (AVN).

Options: Newborn screening by pediatric examination; orthopaedic examination; ultrasonographic examination; orthopaedic or ultrasonographic examination by risk factors. Intercurrent health supervision-based screening.

Preferences: 0 for bad outcomes, 1 for best outcomes.

Model: Influence diagram assessed by the Subcommittee and by the methodology team, with critical feedback from the Subcommittee.

Evidence Sources: Medline and EMBASE search of the research literature through June 1996. Hand search of sentinel journals from June 1996 through March 1997. Ancestor search of accepted articles.

Evidence Quality: Assessed on a custom subjective scale, based primarily on the fit of the evidence to the decision model.

Results. After discussion, explicit modeling, and critique, an influence diagram of 31 nodes was created. The computer-based and the hand literature searches found 534 articles, 101 of which were reviewed by 2 or more readers. Ancestor searches of these yielded a further 17 articles for evidence abstraction. Articles came from around the globe, although primarily Europe, British Isles, Scandinavia, and their descendants. There were 5 controlled trials, each with a sample size less than 40. The remainder were case series. Evidence was available for 17 of the desired 30 probabilities. Evidence quality ranged primarily between one third and two thirds of the maximum attainable score (median: 10–21; interquartile range: 8–14). Based on the raw evidence and Bayesian hierarchical meta-analyses, our estimate for the incidence of DDH revealed by physical examination performed by pediatricians is 8.6 per 1000; for orthopaedic screening, 11.5; for ultrasonography, 25. The odds ratio for DDH, given breech delivery, is 5.5; for female sex, 4.1; for positive family history, 1.7, although this last factor is not statistically significant. Postneonatal cases of DDH were divided into mid-term (younger than 6 months of age) and late-term (older than 6 months of age). Our estimates for the mid-term rate for screening by pediatricians is 0.34/1000 children screened; for orthopaedists, 0.1; and for ultrasonography, 0.28. Our estimates for late-term DDH rates are 0.21/1000 newborns screened by pediatricians; 0.08, by orthopaedists; and 0.2 for ultrasonography. The rates of AVN for children referred before 6 months of age is estimated at 2.5/1000 infants referred. For those referred after 6 months of age, our estimate is 109/1000 referred infants. The decision model (reduced, based on available evidence) suggests that orthopaedic screening is optimal, but because orthopaedists in the published studies and in practice would differ, the supply of orthopaedists is relatively limited, and the difference between orthopaedists and pediatricians is statistically insignificant, we conclude that pedi-

atric screening is to be recommended. The place of ultrasonography in the screening process remains to be defined because there are too few data about postneonatal diagnosis by ultrasonographic screening to permit definitive recommendations. These data could be used by others to refine the conclusions based on costs, parental preferences, or physician style. Areas for research are well defined by our model-based approach. (4/00)
http://pediatrics.aappublications.org/content/105/4/e57

DIAGNOSIS, EVALUATION, AND MANAGEMENT OF HIGH BLOOD PRESSURE IN CHILDREN AND ADOLESCENTS (TECHNICAL REPORT)

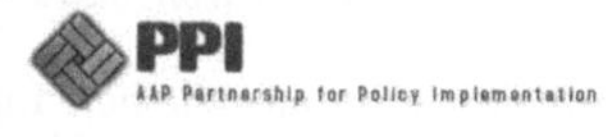

Carissa M. Baker-Smith, MD, MS, MPH, FAAP, FAHA; Susan K. Flinn, MA; Joseph T. Flynn, MD, MS, FAAP; David C. Kaelber, MD, PhD, MPH, FAAP, FACP, FACMI; Douglas Blowey, MD; Aaron E. Carroll, MD, MS, FAAP; Stephen R. Daniels, MD, PhD, FAAP; Sarah D. de Ferranti, MD, MPH, FAAP; Janis M. Dionne, MD, FRCPC; Bonita Falkner, MD; Samuel S. Gidding, MD; Celeste Goodwin; Michael G. Leu, MD, MS, MHS, FAAP; Makia E. Powers, MD, MPH, FAAP; Corinna Rea, MD, MPH, FAAP; Joshua Samuels, MD, MPH, FAAP; Madeline Simasek, MD, MSCP, FAAP; Vidhu V. Thaker, MD, FAAP; Elaine M. Urbina, MD, MS, FAAP; and Subcommittee on Screening and Management of High Blood Pressure in Children

ABSTRACT. Systemic hypertension is a major cause of morbidity and mortality in adulthood. High blood pressure (HBP) and repeated measures of HBP, hypertension (HTN), begin in youth. Knowledge of how best to diagnose, manage, and treat systemic HTN in children and adolescents is important for primary and subspecialty care providers.

Objectives: To provide a technical summary of the methodology used to generate the 2017 "Clinical Practice Guideline for Screening and Management of High Blood Pressure in Children and Adolescents," an update to the 2004 "Fourth Report on the Diagnosis, Evaluation, and Treatment of High Blood Pressure in Children and Adolescents."

Data Sources: Medline, Cochrane Central Register of Controlled Trials, and Excerpta Medica Database references published between January 2003 and July 2015 followed by an additional search between August 2015 and July 2016.

Study Selection: English-language observational studies and randomized trials.

Methods: Key action statements (KASs) and additional recommendations regarding the diagnosis, management, and treatment of HBP in youth were the product of a detailed systematic review of the literature. A content outline establishing the breadth and depth was followed by the generation of 4 patient, intervention, comparison, outcome, time questions. Key questions addressed: (1) diagnosis of systemic HTN, (2) recommended work-up of systemic HTN, (3) optimal blood pressure (BP) goals, and (4) impact of high BP on indirect markers of cardiovascular disease in youth. Once selected, references were subjected to a 2-person review of the abstract and title followed by a separate 2-person full-text review. Full citation information, population data, findings, benefits and harms of the findings, as well as other key reference information were archived. Selected primary references were then used for KAS generation. Level of evidence (LOE) scoring was assigned for each reference and then in aggregate. Appropriate language was used to generate each KAS based on the LOE and the balance of benefit versus harm of the findings. Topics that could not be researched via the stated approach were (1) definition of HTN in youth, and (2) definition of left ventricular hypertrophy. KASs related to these stated topics were generated via expert opinion.

Results: Nearly 15000 references were identified during an initial literature search. After a deduplication process, 14382 references were available for title and abstract review, and 1379 underwent full text review. One hundred twenty-four experimental and observational studies published between 2003 and 2016 were selected as primary references for KAS generation, followed by an additional 269 primary references selected between August 2015 and July 2016. The LOE for the majority of references was C. In total, 30 KASs and 27 additional recommendations were generated; 12 were related to the diagnosis of HTN, 13 were related to management and additional diagnostic testing, 3 to treatment goals, and 2 to treatment options. Finally, special additions to the clinical practice guideline included creation of new BP tables based on BP values obtained solely from children with normal weight, creation of a simplified table to enhance screening and recognition of abnormal BP, and a revision of the criteria for diagnosing left ventricular hypertrophy.

Conclusions: An extensive and detailed systematic approach was used to generate evidence-based guidelines for the diagnosis, management, and treatment of youth with systemic HTN. (8/18)
http://pediatrics.aappublications.org/content/142/3/e20182096

DIAGNOSIS, TREATMENT, AND PREVENTION OF CONGENITAL TOXOPLASMOSIS IN THE UNITED STATES (TECHNICAL REPORT)

Yvonne A. Maldonado, MD, FAAP; Jennifer S. Read, MD, MS, MPH, DTM&H, FAAP; and Committee on Infectious Diseases

ABSTRACT. Congenital toxoplasmosis (CT) is a parasitic disease that can cause significant fetal and neonatal harm. Coordinated efforts by pregnant women, researchers, physicians, and health policy makers regarding potential primary and secondary preventive measures for CT and their implementation may lead to a lower incidence of CT as well as lower morbidity and mortality rates associated with CT. The purpose of this technical report is to summarize available information regarding the diagnosis, treatment, and prevention of CT. (1/17)
http://pediatrics.aappublications.org/content/139/2/e20163860

DIAGNOSIS AND MANAGEMENT OF AN INITIAL UTI IN FEBRILE INFANTS AND YOUNG CHILDREN (TECHNICAL REPORT)

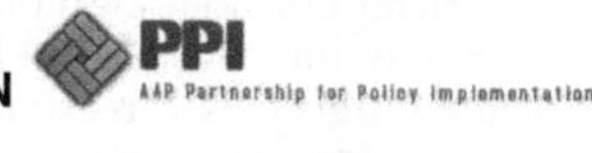

S. Maria E. Finnell, MD, MS; Aaron E. Carroll, MD, MS; Stephen M. Downs, MD, MS; Steering Committee on Quality Improvement and Management; and Subcommittee on Urinary Tract Infection

ABSTRACT. *Objectives.* The diagnosis and management of urinary tract infections (UTIs) in young children are clinically challenging. This report was developed to inform the revised, evidence-based, clinical guideline regarding the diagnosis and management of initial UTIs in febrile infants and young children, 2 to 24 months of age, from the American Academy of Pediatrics Subcommittee on Urinary Tract Infection.

Methods. The conceptual model presented in the 1999 technical report was updated after a comprehensive review of published literature. Studies with potentially new information or with evidence that reinforced the 1999 technical report were retained. Meta-analyses on the effectiveness of antimicrobial prophylaxis to prevent recurrent UTI were performed.

Results. Review of recent literature revealed new evidence in the following areas. Certain clinical findings and new urinalysis methods can help clinicians identify febrile children at very low risk of UTI. Oral antimicrobial therapy is as effective as parenteral therapy in treating UTI. Data from published, randomized controlled trials do not support antimicrobial prophylaxis to prevent febrile UTI when vesicoureteral reflux is found through voiding cystourethrography. Ultrasonography of the urinary tract after the first UTI has poor sensitivity. Early antimicrobial treatment may decrease the risk of renal damage from UTI.

Conclusions. Recent literature agrees with most of the evidence presented in the 1999 technical report, but meta-analyses of data from recent, randomized controlled trials do not support antimicrobial prophylaxis to prevent febrile UTI. This finding argues against voiding cystourethrography after the first UTI. (8/11)
http://pediatrics.aappublications.org/content/128/3/e749

DIAGNOSIS AND MANAGEMENT OF CHILDHOOD OBSTRUCTIVE SLEEP APNEA SYNDROME (TECHNICAL REPORT)

Carole L. Marcus, MBBCh; Lee J. Brooks, MD; Sally Davidson Ward, MD; Kari A. Draper, MD; David Gozal, MD; Ann C. Halbower, MD; Jacqueline Jones, MD; Christopher Lehmann, MD; Michael S. Schechter, MD, MPH; Stephen Sheldon, MD; Richard N. Shiffman, MD, MCIS; Karen Spruyt, PhD; Steering Committee on Quality Improvement and Management; and Subcommittee on Obstructive Sleep Apnea Syndrome

ABSTRACT. *Objective.* This technical report describes the procedures involved in developing recommendations on the management of childhood obstructive sleep apnea syndrome (OSAS).

Methods. The literature from 1999 through 2011 was evaluated.

Results and Conclusions. A total of 3166 titles were reviewed, of which 350 provided relevant data. Most articles were level II through IV. The prevalence of OSAS ranged from 0% to 5.7%, with obesity being an independent risk factor. OSAS was associated with cardiovascular, growth, and neurobehavioral abnormalities and possibly inflammation. Most diagnostic screening tests had low sensitivity and specificity. Treatment of OSAS resulted in improvements in behavior and attention and likely improvement in cognitive abilities. Primary treatment is adenotonsillectomy (AT). Data were insufficient to recommend specific surgical techniques; however, children undergoing partial tonsillectomy should be monitored for possible recurrence of OSAS. Although OSAS improved postoperatively, the proportion of patients who had residual OSAS ranged from 13% to 29% in low-risk populations to 73% when obese children were included and stricter polysomnographic criteria were used. Nevertheless, OSAS may improve after AT even in obese children, thus supporting surgery as a reasonable initial treatment. A significant number of obese patients required intubation or continuous positive airway pressure (CPAP) postoperatively, which reinforces the need for inpatient observation. CPAP was effective in the treatment of OSAS, but adherence is a major barrier. For this reason, CPAP is not recommended as first-line therapy for OSAS when AT is an option. Intranasal steroids may ameliorate mild OSAS, but follow-up is needed. Data were insufficient to recommend rapid maxillary expansion. (8/12)
http://pediatrics.aappublications.org/content/130/3/e714

DIAGNOSIS AND MANAGEMENT OF GASTROESOPHAGEAL REFLUX IN PRETERM INFANTS (CLINICAL REPORT)

Eric C. Eichenwald, MD, FAAP, and Committee on Fetus and Newborn

ABSTRACT. Gastroesophageal reflux (GER), generally defined as the passage of gastric contents into the esophagus, is an almost universal phenomenon in preterm infants. It is a common diagnosis in the NICU; however, there is large variation in its treatment across NICU sites. In this clinical report, the physiology, diagnosis, and symptomatology in preterm infants as well as currently used treatment strategies in the NICU are examined. Conservative measures to control reflux, such as left lateral body position, head elevation, and feeding regimen manipulation, have not been shown to reduce clinically assessed signs of GER in the preterm infant. In addition, preterm infants with clinically diagnosed GER are often treated with pharmacologic agents; however, a lack of evidence of efficacy together with emerging evidence of significant harm (particularly with gastric acid blockade) strongly suggest that these agents should be used sparingly, if at all, in preterm infants. (6/18)
http://pediatrics.aappublications.org/content/142/1/e20181061

DIAGNOSIS AND MANAGEMENT OF INFANTILE HEMANGIOMA (CLINICAL REPORT)

David H. Darrow, MD, DDS; Arin K. Greene, MD; Anthony J. Mancini, MD; Amy J. Nopper, MD; Section on Dermatology; Section on Otolaryngology—Head & Neck Surgery; and Section on Plastic Surgery

ABSTRACT. Infantile hemangiomas (IHs) are the most common tumors of childhood. Unlike other tumors, they have the unique ability to involute after proliferation, often leading primary care providers to assume they will resolve without intervention or consequence. Unfortunately, a subset of IHs rapidly develop complications, resulting in pain, functional impairment, or permanent disfigurement. As a result, the primary clinician has the task of determining which lesions require early consultation with a specialist. Although several recent reviews have been published, this clinical report is the first based on input from individuals representing the many specialties involved in the treatment of IH. Its purpose is to update the pediatric community regarding recent discoveries in IH pathogenesis, treatment, and clinical associations and to provide a basis for clinical decision-making in the management of IH. (9/15)
http://pediatrics.aappublications.org/content/136/4/e1060

DIAGNOSIS AND MANAGEMENT OF INFANTILE HEMANGIOMA: EXECUTIVE SUMMARY

David H. Darrow, MD, DDS, FAAP; Arin K. Greene, MD, FAAP; Anthony J. Mancini, MD, FAAP; Amy J. Nopper, MD, FAAP; Section on Dermatology; Section on Otolaryngology—Head & Neck Surgery; and Section on Plastic Surgery

ABSTRACT. Infantile hemangiomas (IHs) are the most common tumors of childhood. Unlike other tumors, they have the capacity to involute after proliferation, often leading primary care providers to assume they will resolve without intervention or consequence. However, a subset of IHs may be associated with complications, resulting in pain, functional impairment, or permanent disfigurement. As a result, the primary care provider is often called on to decide which lesions should be referred for early consultation with a specialist.

This document provides a summary of the guidance contained in the clinical report "Diagnosis and Management of Infantile Hemangioma," published concurrently in the online version of *Pediatrics* (*Pediatrics.* 2015;136[4]:e1060–e1104, available at: www.pediatrics.org/content/136/4/e1060). The report is uniquely based on input from the many specialties involved in the treatment of IH. Its purpose is to update the pediatric community about recent discoveries in IH pathogenesis, clinical associations, and treatment and to provide a knowledge base and framework for clinical decision-making in the management of IH. (9/15)
http://pediatrics.aappublications.org/content/136/4/786

DIAGNOSIS AND PREVENTION OF IRON DEFICIENCY AND IRON-DEFICIENCY ANEMIA IN INFANTS AND YOUNG CHILDREN (0–3 YEARS OF AGE) (CLINICAL REPORT)

Robert D. Baker, MD, PhD; Frank R. Greer, MD; and Committee on Nutrition

ABSTRACT. This clinical report covers diagnosis and prevention of iron deficiency and iron-deficiency anemia in infants (both breastfed and formula fed) and toddlers from birth through 3 years of age. Results of recent basic research support the concerns that iron-deficiency anemia and iron deficiency without anemia during infancy and childhood can have long-lasting detrimental effects on neurodevelopment. Therefore, pediatricians and other health care providers should strive to eliminate iron

deficiency and iron-deficiency anemia. Appropriate iron intakes for infants and toddlers as well as methods for screening for iron deficiency and iron-deficiency anemia are presented. (10/10)
http://pediatrics.aappublications.org/content/126/5/1040

DIAGNOSIS OF HIV-1 INFECTION IN CHILDREN YOUNGER THAN 18 MONTHS IN THE UNITED STATES (TECHNICAL REPORT)

Jennifer S. Read, MD, MS, MPH, DTM&H, and Committee on Pediatric AIDS

ABSTRACT. The objectives of this technical report are to describe methods of diagnosis of HIV-1 infection in children younger than 18 months in the United States and to review important issues that must be considered by clinicians who care for infants and young children born to HIV-1–infected women. Appropriate HIV-1 diagnostic testing for infants and children younger than 18 months differs from that for older children, adolescents, and adults because of passively transferred maternal HIV-1 antibodies, which may be detectable in the child's bloodstream until 18 months of age. Therefore, routine serologic testing of these infants and young children is generally only informative before the age of 18 months if the test result is negative. Virologic assays, including HIV-1 DNA or RNA assays, represent the gold standard for diagnostic testing of infants and children younger than 18 months. With such testing, the diagnosis of HIV-1 infection (as well as the presumptive exclusion of HIV-1 infection) can be established within the first several weeks of life among nonbreastfed infants. Important factors that must be considered when selecting HIV-1 diagnostic assays for pediatric patients and when choosing the timing of such assays include the age of the child, potential timing of infection of the child, whether the infection status of the child's mother is known or unknown, the antiretroviral exposure history of the mother and of the child, and characteristics of the virus. If the mother's HIV-1 serostatus is unknown, rapid HIV-1 antibody testing of the newborn infant to identify HIV-1 exposure is essential so that antiretroviral prophylaxis can be initiated within the first 12 hours of life if test results are positive. For HIV-1–exposed infants (identified by positive maternal test results or positive antibody results for the infant shortly after birth), it has been recommended that diagnostic testing with HIV-1 DNA or RNA assays be performed within the first 14 days of life, at 1 to 2 months of age, and at 3 to 6 months of age. If any of these test results are positive, repeat testing is recommended to confirm the diagnosis of HIV-1 infection. A diagnosis of HIV-1 infection can be made on the basis of 2 positive HIV-1 DNA or RNA assay results. In nonbreastfeeding children younger than 18 months with no positive HIV-1 virologic test results, presumptive exclusion of HIV-1 infection can be based on 2 negative virologic test results (1 obtained at ≥2 weeks and 1 obtained at ≥4 weeks of age); 1 negative virologic test result obtained at ≥8 weeks of age; or 1 negative HIV-1 antibody test result obtained at ≥6 months of age. Alternatively, presumptive exclusion of HIV-1 infection can be based on 1 positive HIV-1 virologic test with at least 2 subsequent negative virologic test results (at least 1 of which is performed at ≥8 weeks of age) or negative HIV-1 antibody test results (at least 1 of which is performed at ≥6 months of age). Definitive exclusion of HIV-1 infection is based on 2 negative virologic test results, 1 obtained at ≥1 month of age and 1 obtained at ≥4 months of age, or 2 negative HIV-1 antibody test results from separate specimens obtained at ≥6 months of age. For both presumptive and definitive exclusion of infection, the child should have no other laboratory (eg, no positive virologic test results) or clinical (eg, no AIDS-defining conditions) evidence of HIV-1 infection. Many clinicians confirm the absence of HIV-1 infection with a negative HIV-1 antibody assay result at 12 to 18 months of age. For breastfeeding infants, a similar testing algorithm can be followed, with timing of testing starting from the date of complete cessation of breastfeeding instead of the date of birth. (12/07, reaffirmed 4/10, 2/15)
http://pediatrics.aappublications.org/content/120/6/e1547

DIAGNOSIS OF PREGNANCY AND PROVIDING OPTIONS COUNSELING FOR THE ADOLESCENT PATIENT (CLINICAL REPORT)

Laurie L. Hornberger, MD, MPH, FAAP, and Committee on Adolescence

ABSTRACT. The American Academy of Pediatrics policy statement "Options Counseling for the Pregnant Adolescent Patient" recommends the basic content of the pediatrician's counseling for an adolescent facing a new diagnosis of pregnancy. However, options counseling is just one aspect of what may be one of the more challenging scenarios in the pediatric office. Pediatricians must remain alert to the possibility of pregnancy among their adolescent female patients. When discovering symptoms suggestive of pregnancy, pediatricians must obtain a relevant history, perform diagnostic testing and properly interpret the results, and understand the significance of the results from the patient perspective and reveal them to the patient in a sensitive manner. If the patient is indeed pregnant, the pediatrician, in addition to providing comprehensive options counseling, may need to help recruit adult support for the patient and should offer continued assistance to the adolescent and her family after the office visit. All pediatricians should be aware of the legal aspects of adolescent reproductive care and the resources for pregnant adolescents in their communities. This clinical report presents a more comprehensive view of the evaluation and management of pregnancy in the adolescent patient and a context for options counseling. (8/17)
http://pediatrics.aappublications.org/content/140/3/e20172273

DIAGNOSTIC IMAGING OF CHILD ABUSE

Section on Radiology

ABSTRACT. The role of imaging in cases of child abuse is to identify the extent of physical injury when abuse is present and to elucidate all imaging findings that point to alternative diagnoses. Effective diagnostic imaging of child abuse rests on high-quality technology as well as a full appreciation of the clinical and pathologic alterations occurring in abused children. This statement is a revision of the previous policy published in 2000. (4/09)
http://pediatrics.aappublications.org/content/123/5/1430

DISASTER PREPAREDNESS IN NEONATAL INTENSIVE CARE UNITS (CLINICAL REPORT)

Wanda D. Barfield, MD, MPH, FAAP, RADM USPHS; Steven E. Krug, MD, FAAP; Committee on Fetus and Newborn; and Disaster Preparedness Council

ABSTRACT. Disasters disproportionally affect vulnerable, technology-dependent people, including preterm and critically ill newborn infants. It is important for health care providers to be aware of and prepared for the potential consequences of disasters for the NICU. Neonatal intensive care personnel can provide specialized expertise for their hospital, community, and regional emergency preparedness plans and can help develop institutional surge capacity for mass critical care, including equipment, medications, personnel, and facility resources. (4/17)
http://pediatrics.aappublications.org/content/139/5/e20170507

DISCLOSURE OF ADVERSE EVENTS IN PEDIATRICS

Committee on Medical Liability and Risk Management and Council on Quality Improvement and Patient Safety

ABSTRACT. Despite increasing attention to issues of patient safety, preventable adverse events (AEs) continue to occur, causing direct and consequential injuries to patients, families, and health care providers. Pediatricians generally agree that there is

an ethical obligation to inform patients and families about preventable AEs and medical errors. Nonetheless, barriers, such as fear of liability, interfere with disclosure regarding preventable AEs. Changes to the legal system, improved communications skills, and carefully developed disclosure policies and programs can improve the quality and frequency of appropriate AE disclosure communications. (11/16)
http://pediatrics.aappublications.org/content/138/6/e20163215

DISPENSING MEDICATIONS AT THE HOSPITAL UPON DISCHARGE FROM AN EMERGENCY DEPARTMENT (TECHNICAL REPORT)

Loren G. Yamamoto, MD, MPH, MBA; Shannon Manzi, PharmD; and Committee on Pediatric Emergency Medicine

ABSTRACT. Although most health care services can and should be provided by their medical home, children will be referred or require visits to the emergency department (ED) for emergent clinical conditions or injuries. Continuation of medical care after discharge from an ED is dependent on parents or caregivers' understanding of and compliance with follow-up instructions and on adherence to medication recommendations. ED visits often occur at times when the majority of pharmacies are not open and caregivers are concerned with getting their ill or injured child directly home. Approximately one-third of patients fail to obtain priority medications from a pharmacy after discharge from an ED. The option of judiciously dispensing ED discharge medications from the ED's outpatient pharmacy within the facility is a major convenience that overcomes this obstacle, improving the likelihood of medication adherence. Emergency care encounters should be routinely followed up with primary care provider medical homes to ensure complete and comprehensive care. (1/12, reaffirmed 9/15, 7/19)
http://pediatrics.aappublications.org/content/129/2/e562

DISTINGUISHING SUDDEN INFANT DEATH SYNDROME FROM CHILD ABUSE FATALITIES (CLINICAL REPORT)

Kent P. Hymel, MD, and Committee on Child Abuse and Neglect (joint with National Association of Medical Examiners)

ABSTRACT. Fatal child abuse has been mistaken for sudden infant death syndrome. When a healthy infant younger than 1 year dies suddenly and unexpectedly, the cause of death may be certified as sudden infant death syndrome. Sudden infant death syndrome is more common than infanticide. Parents of sudden infant death syndrome victims typically are anxious to provide unlimited information to professionals involved in death investigation or research. They also want and deserve to be approached in a nonaccusatory manner. This clinical report provides professionals with information and suggestions for procedures to help avoid stigmatizing families of sudden infant death syndrome victims while allowing accumulation of appropriate evidence in potential cases of infanticide. This clinical report addresses deficiencies and updates recommendations in the 2001 American Academy of Pediatrics policy statement of the same name. (7/06, reaffirmed 4/09, 3/13, 7/17)
http://pediatrics.aappublications.org/content/118/1/421

DONOR HUMAN MILK FOR THE HIGH-RISK INFANT: PREPARATION, SAFETY, AND USAGE OPTIONS IN THE UNITED STATES

Committee on Nutrition, Section on Breastfeeding, and Committee on Fetus and Newborn

ABSTRACT. The use of donor human milk is increasing for high-risk infants, primarily for infants born weighing <1500 g or those who have severe intestinal disorders. Pasteurized donor milk may be considered in situations in which the supply of maternal milk is insufficient. The use of pasteurized donor milk is safe when appropriate measures are used to screen donors and collect, store, and pasteurize the milk and then distribute it through established human milk banks. The use of nonpasteurized donor milk and other forms of direct, Internet-based, or informal human milk sharing does not involve this level of safety and is not recommended. It is important that health care providers counsel families considering milk sharing about the risks of bacterial or viral contamination of nonpasteurized human milk and about the possibilities of exposure to medications, drugs, or herbs in human milk. Currently, the use of pasteurized donor milk is limited by its availability and affordability. The development of public policy to improve and expand access to pasteurized donor milk, including policies that support improved governmental and private financial support for donor milk banks and the use of donor milk, is important. (12/16)
http://pediatrics.aappublications.org/content/139/1/e20163440

DRINKING WATER FROM PRIVATE WELLS AND RISKS TO CHILDREN

Committee on Environmental Health and Committee on Infectious Diseases

ABSTRACT. Drinking water for approximately one sixth of US households is obtained from private wells. These wells can become contaminated by pollutant chemicals or pathogenic organisms and cause illness. Although the US Environmental Protection Agency and all states offer guidance for construction, maintenance, and testing of private wells, there is little regulation. With few exceptions, well owners are responsible for their own wells. Children may also drink well water at child care or when traveling. Illness resulting from children's ingestion of contaminated water can be severe. This policy statement provides recommendations for inspection, testing, and remediation for wells providing drinking water for children. (5/09, reaffirmed 1/13, 9/19)
http://pediatrics.aappublications.org/content/123/6/1599

DRINKING WATER FROM PRIVATE WELLS AND RISKS TO CHILDREN (TECHNICAL REPORT)

Walter J. Rogan, MD; Michael T. Brady, MD; Committee on Environmental Health; and Committee on Infectious Diseases

ABSTRACT. Drinking water for approximately one sixth of US households is obtained from private wells. These wells can become contaminated by pollutant chemicals or pathogenic organisms, leading to significant illness. Although the US Environmental Protection Agency and all states offer guidance for construction, maintenance, and testing of private wells, there is little regulation, and with few exceptions, well owners are responsible for their own wells. Children may also drink well water at child care or when traveling. Illness resulting from children's ingestion of contaminated water can be severe. This report reviews relevant aspects of groundwater and wells; describes the common chemical and microbiologic contaminants; gives an algorithm with recommendations for inspection, testing, and remediation for wells providing drinking water for children; reviews the definitions and uses of various bottled waters; provides current estimates of costs for well testing; and provides federal, national, state, and, where appropriate, tribal contacts for more information. (5/09, reaffirmed 1/13, 9/19)
http://pediatrics.aappublications.org/content/123/6/e1123

E-CIGARETTES AND SIMILAR DEVICES

Brian P. Jenssen, MD, MSHP, FAAP; Susan C. Walley, MD, FAAP; and Section on Tobacco Control

ABSTRACT. Electronic cigarettes (e-cigarettes) are the most commonly used tobacco product among youth. The 2016 US Surgeon General's Report on e-cigarette use among youth and young adults concluded that e-cigarettes are unsafe for children and adolescents. Furthermore, strong and consistent evidence finds that children and adolescents who use e-cigarettes are significantly more likely to go on to use traditional cigarettes—a product that kills half its long-term users. E-cigarette manufacturers target children with enticing candy and fruit flavors and use marketing strategies that have been previously successful with traditional cigarettes to attract youth to these products. Numerous toxicants and carcinogens have been found in e-cigarette solutions. Nonusers are involuntarily exposed to the emissions of these devices with secondhand and thirdhand aerosol. To prevent children, adolescents, and young adults from transitioning from e-cigarettes to traditional cigarettes and minimize the potential public health harm from e-cigarette use, there is a critical need for e-cigarette regulation, legislative action, and counterpromotion to protect youth. (1/19)

See full text on page 623.

https://pediatrics.aappublications.org/content/143/2/e20183652

EARLY CHILDHOOD ADVERSITY, TOXIC STRESS, AND THE ROLE OF THE PEDIATRICIAN: TRANSLATING DEVELOPMENTAL SCIENCE INTO LIFELONG HEALTH

Committee on Psychosocial Aspects of Child and Family Health; Committee on Early Childhood, Adoption, and Dependent Care; and Section on Developmental and Behavioral Pediatrics

ABSTRACT. Advances in a wide range of biological, behavioral, and social sciences are expanding our understanding of how early environmental influences (the ecology) and genetic predispositions (the biologic program) affect learning capacities, adaptive behaviors, lifelong physical and mental health, and adult productivity. A supporting technical report from the American Academy of Pediatrics (AAP) presents an integrated ecobiodevelopmental framework to assist in translating these dramatic advances in developmental science into improved health across the life span. Pediatricians are now armed with new information about the adverse effects of toxic stress on brain development, as well as a deeper understanding of the early life origins of many adult diseases. As trusted authorities in child health and development, pediatric providers must now complement the early identification of developmental concerns with a greater focus on those interventions and community investments that reduce external threats to healthy brain growth. To this end, AAP endorses a developing leadership role for the entire pediatric community—one that mobilizes the scientific expertise of both basic and clinical researchers, the family-centered care of the pediatric medical home, and the public influence of AAP and its state chapters—to catalyze fundamental change in early childhood policy and services. AAP is committed to leveraging science to inform the development of innovative strategies to reduce the precipitants of toxic stress in young children and to mitigate their negative effects on the course of development and health across the life span. (12/11, reaffirmed 7/16)

http://pediatrics.aappublications.org/content/129/1/e224

EARLY CHILDHOOD CARIES IN INDIGENOUS COMMUNITIES

Committee on Native American Child Health (joint with Canadian Paediatric Society First Nations, Inuit, and Métis Committee)

ABSTRACT. The oral health of Indigenous children of Canada (First Nations, Inuit, and Métis) and the United States (American Indian, Alaska Native) is a major child health issue: there is a high prevalence of early childhood caries (ECC) and resulting adverse health effects in this community, as well as high rates and costs of restorative and surgical treatments under general anesthesia. ECC is an infectious disease that is influenced by multiple factors, including socioeconomic determinants, and requires a combination of approaches for improvement. This statement includes recommendations for preventive oral health and clinical care for young infants and pregnant women by primary health care providers, community-based health-promotion initiatives, oral health workforce and access issues, and advocacy for community water fluoridation and fluoride-varnish program access. Further community-based research on the epidemiology, prevention, management, and microbiology of ECC in Indigenous communities would be beneficial. (5/11, reaffirmed 10/16)

http://pediatrics.aappublications.org/content/127/6/1190

EARLY CHILDHOOD HOME VISITING

James H. Duffee, MD, MPH, FAAP; Alan L. Mendelsohn, MD, FAAP; Alice A. Kuo, MD, PhD, FAAP; Lori A. Legano, MD, FAAP; Marian F. Earls, MD, MTS, FAAP; Council on Community Pediatrics; Council on Early Childhood; and Committee on Child Abuse and Neglect

ABSTRACT. High-quality home-visiting services for infants and young children can improve family relationships, advance school readiness, reduce child maltreatment, improve maternal-infant health outcomes, and increase family economic self-sufficiency. The American Academy of Pediatrics supports unwavering federal funding of state home-visiting initiatives, the expansion of evidence-based programs, and a robust, coordinated national evaluation designed to confirm best practices and cost-efficiency. Community home visiting is most effective as a component of a comprehensive early childhood system that actively includes and enhances a family-centered medical home. (8/17)

http://pediatrics.aappublications.org/content/140/3/e20172150

EARLY INTERVENTION, IDEA PART C SERVICES, AND THE MEDICAL HOME: COLLABORATION FOR BEST PRACTICE AND BEST OUTCOMES (CLINICAL REPORT)

Richard C. Adams, MD; Carl Tapia, MD; and Council on Children With Disabilities

ABSTRACT. The medical home and the Individuals With Disabilities Education Act Part C Early Intervention Program share many common purposes for infants and children ages 0 to 3 years, not the least of which is a family-centered focus. Professionals in pediatric medical home practices see substantial numbers of infants and toddlers with developmental delays and/or complex chronic conditions. Economic, health, and family-focused data each underscore the critical role of timely referral for relationship-based, individualized, accessible early intervention services and the need for collaborative partnerships in care. The medical home process and Individuals With Disabilities Education Act Part C policy both support nurturing relationships and family-centered care; both offer clear value in terms of economic and health outcomes. Best practice models for early intervention services incorporate learning in the natural environment and coaching models. Proactive medical homes provide strategies for effective developmental surveillance, family-centered resources, and tools to support high-risk groups, and comanagement of infants with special health care needs, including the monitoring of services provided and outcomes achieved. (9/13, reaffirmed 5/17)

http://pediatrics.aappublications.org/content/132/4/e1073

ECHOCARDIOGRAPHY IN INFANTS AND CHILDREN

Section on Cardiology

ABSTRACT. It is the intent of this statement to inform pediatric providers on the appropriate use of echocardiography. Although on-site consultation may be impossible, methods should be established to ensure timely review of echocardiograms by a pediatric cardiologist. With advances in data transmission, echocardiography information can be exchanged, in some cases eliminating the need for a costly patient transfer. By cooperating through training, education, and referral, complete and cost-effective echocardiographic services can be provided to all children. (6/97, reaffirmed 3/03, 3/07)

http://pediatrics.aappublications.org/content/99/6/921

EFFECTIVE DISCIPLINE TO RAISE HEALTHY CHILDREN

Robert D. Sege, MD, PhD, FAAP; Benjamin S. Siegel, MD, FAAP; Council on Child Abuse and Neglect; and Committee on Psychosocial Aspects of Child and Family Health

ABSTRACT. Pediatricians are a source of advice for parents and guardians concerning the management of child behavior, including discipline strategies that are used to teach appropriate behavior and protect their children and others from the adverse effects of challenging behavior. Aversive disciplinary strategies, including all forms of corporal punishment and yelling at or shaming children, are minimally effective in the short-term and not effective in the long-term. With new evidence, researchers link corporal punishment to an increased risk of negative behavioral, cognitive, psychosocial, and emotional outcomes for children. In this Policy Statement, the American Academy of Pediatrics provides guidance for pediatricians and other child health care providers on educating parents about positive and effective parenting strategies of discipline for children at each stage of development as well as references to educational materials. This statement supports the need for adults to avoid physical punishment and verbal abuse of children. (11/18)

http://pediatrics.aappublications.org/content/142/6/e20183112

THE EFFECTS OF ARMED CONFLICT ON CHILDREN

Sherry Shenoda, MD, FAAP; Ayesha Kadir, MD, MSc, FAAP; Shelly Pitterman, PhD; Jeffrey Goldhagen, MD, MPH, FAAP; and Section on International Child Health

ABSTRACT. Children are increasingly exposed to armed conflict and targeted by governmental and nongovernmental combatants. Armed conflict directly and indirectly affects children's physical, mental, and behavioral health. It can affect every organ system, and its impact can persist throughout the life course. In addition, children are disproportionately impacted by morbidity and mortality associated with armed conflict. A children's rights–based approach provides a framework for collaboration by the American Academy of Pediatrics, child health professionals, and national and international partners to respond in the domains of clinical care, systems development, and policy formulation. The American Academy of Pediatrics and child health professionals have critical and synergistic roles to play in the global response to the impact of armed conflict on children. (11/18)

http://pediatrics.aappublications.org/content/142/6/e20182585

THE EFFECTS OF ARMED CONFLICT ON CHILDREN (TECHNICAL REPORT)

Ayesha Kadir, MD, MSc, FAAP; Sherry Shenoda, MD, FAAP; Jeffrey Goldhagen, MD, MPH, FAAP; Shelly Pitterman, PhD; and Section on International Child Health

ABSTRACT. More than 1 in 10 children worldwide are affected by armed conflict. The effects are both direct and indirect and are associated with immediate and long-term harm. The direct effects of conflict include death, physical and psychological trauma, and displacement. Indirect effects are related to a large number of factors, including inadequate and unsafe living conditions, environmental hazards, caregiver mental health, separation from family, displacement-related health risks, and the destruction of health, public health, education, and economic infrastructure. Children and health workers are targeted by combatants during attacks, and children are recruited or forced to take part in combat in a variety of ways. Armed conflict is both a toxic stress and a significant social determinant of child health. In this Technical Report, we review the available knowledge on the effects of armed conflict on children and support the recommendations in the accompanying Policy Statement on children and armed conflict. (11/18)

http://pediatrics.aappublications.org/content/142/6/e20182586

THE EFFECTS OF EARLY NUTRITIONAL INTERVENTIONS ON THE DEVELOPMENT OF ATOPIC DISEASE IN INFANTS AND CHILDREN: THE ROLE OF MATERNAL DIETARY RESTRICTION, BREASTFEEDING, HYDROLYZED FORMULAS, AND TIMING OF INTRODUCTION OF ALLERGENIC COMPLEMENTARY FOODS (CLINICAL REPORT)

Frank R. Greer, MD, FAAP; Scott H. Sicherer, MD, FAAP; A. Wesley Burks, MD, FAAP; Committee on Nutrition; and Section on Allergy and Immunology

ABSTRACT. This clinical report updates and replaces a 2008 clinical report from the American Academy of Pediatrics, which addressed the roles of maternal and early infant diet on the prevention of atopic disease, including atopic dermatitis, asthma, and food allergy. As with the previous report, the available data still limit the ability to draw firm conclusions about various aspects of atopy prevention through early dietary interventions. Current evidence does not support a role for maternal dietary restrictions during pregnancy or lactation. Although there is evidence that exclusive breastfeeding for 3 to 4 months decreases the incidence of eczema in the first 2 years of life, there are no short- or long-term advantages for exclusive breastfeeding beyond 3 to 4 months for prevention of atopic disease. The evidence now suggests that any duration of breastfeeding ≥3 to 4 months is protective against wheezing in the first 2 years of life, and some evidence suggests that longer duration of any breastfeeding protects against asthma even after 5 years of age. No conclusions can be made about the role of breastfeeding in either preventing or delaying the onset of specific food allergies. There is a lack of evidence that partially or extensively hydrolyzed formula prevents atopic disease. There is no evidence that delaying the introduction of allergenic foods, including peanuts, eggs, and fish, beyond 4 to 6 months prevents atopic disease. There is now evidence that early introduction of peanuts may prevent peanut allergy. (3/19)

See full text on page 633.

https://pediatrics.aappublications.org/content/143/4/e20190281

ELECTRONIC COMMUNICATION OF THE HEALTH RECORD AND INFORMATION WITH PEDIATRIC PATIENTS AND THEIR GUARDIANS

Emily C. Webber, MD, FAAP, FAMIA; David Brick, MD, FAAP; James P. Scibilia, MD, FAAP; Peter Dehnel, MD, FAAP; Council on Clinical Information Technology; Committee on Medical Liability and Risk Management; and Section on Telehealth Care

ABSTRACT. Communication of health data has evolved rapidly with the widespread adoption of electronic health records (EHRs) and communication technology. What used to be sent to patients via paper mail, fax, or e-mail may now be accessed by patients via their EHRs, and patients may also communicate securely with their medical team via certified technology. Although EHR technologies have great potential, their most effective applications and uses for communication between pediatric and adolescent patients, guardians, and medical teams has not been realized. There are wide variations in available technologies, guiding policies, and practices; some physicians and patients are successful in using certified tools but others are forced to limit their patients' access to e-health data and associated communication altogether. In general, pediatric and adolescent patients are less likely than adult patients to have electronic access and the ability to exchange health data. There are several reasons for these limitations, including inconsistent standards and recommendations regarding the recommended age for independent access, lack of routine EHR support for the ability to filter or proxy such access, and conflicting laws about patients' and physicians' rights to access EHRs and ability to communicate electronically. Effective, safe electronic exchange of health data requires active collaboration between physicians, patients, policy makers, and health information technology vendors. This policy statement addresses current best practices for these stakeholders and delineates the continued gaps and how to address them. (6/19)

See full text on page 647.

https://pediatrics.aappublications.org/content/144/1/e20191359

ELECTRONIC PRESCRIBING IN PEDIATRICS: TOWARD SAFER AND MORE EFFECTIVE MEDICATION MANAGEMENT

Council on Clinical Information Technology

ABSTRACT. This policy statement identifies the potential value of electronic prescribing (e-prescribing) systems in improving quality and reducing harm in pediatric health care. On the basis of limited but positive pediatric data and on the basis of federal statutes that provide incentives for the use of e-prescribing systems, the American Academy of Pediatrics recommends the adoption of e-prescribing systems with pediatric functionality. The American Academy of Pediatrics also recommends a set of functions that technology vendors should provide when e-prescribing systems are used in environments in which children receive care. (3/13, reaffirmed 12/18)

http://pediatrics.aappublications.org/content/131/4/824

ELECTRONIC PRESCRIBING IN PEDIATRICS: TOWARD SAFER AND MORE EFFECTIVE MEDICATION MANAGEMENT (TECHNICAL REPORT)

Kevin B. Johnson, MD, MS; Christoph U. Lehmann, MD; and Council on Clinical Information Technology

ABSRACT. This technical report discusses recent advances in electronic prescribing (e-prescribing) systems, including the evidence base supporting their limitations and potential benefits. Specifically, this report acknowledges that there are limited but positive pediatric data supporting the role of e-prescribing in mitigating medication errors, improving communication with dispensing pharmacists, and improving medication adherence. On the basis of these data and on the basis of federal statutes that provide incentives for the use of e-prescribing systems, the American Academy of Pediatrics recommends the adoption of e-prescribing systems with pediatric functionality. This report supports the accompanying policy statement from the American Academy of Pediatrics recommending the adoption of e-prescribing by pediatric health care providers. (3/13, reaffirmed 12/18)

http://pediatrics.aappublications.org/content/131/4/e1350

ELIMINATION OF PERINATAL HEPATITIS B: PROVIDING THE FIRST VACCINE DOSE WITHIN 24 HOURS OF BIRTH

Committee on Infectious Diseases and Committee on Fetus and Newborn

ABSTRACT. After the introduction of the hepatitis B vaccine in the United States in 1982, a greater than 90% reduction in new infections was achieved. However, approximately 1000 new cases of perinatal hepatitis B infection are still identified annually in the United States. Prevention of perinatal hepatitis B relies on the proper and timely identification of infants born to mothers who are hepatitis B surface antigen positive and to mothers with unknown status to ensure administration of appropriate postexposure immunoprophylaxis with hepatitis B vaccine and immune globulin. To reduce the incidence of perinatal hepatitis B transmission further, the American Academy of Pediatrics endorses the recommendation of the Advisory Committee on Immunization Practices of the Centers for Disease Control and Prevention that all newborn infants with a birth weight of greater than or equal to 2000 g receive hepatitis B vaccine by 24 hours of age. (8/17)

http://pediatrics.aappublications.org/content/140/3/e20171870

EMERGENCY CONTRACEPTION

Krishna K. Upadhya, MD, MPH, FAAP, and Committee on Adolescence

ABSTRACT. Despite significant declines over the past 2 decades, the United States continues to experience birth rates among teenagers that are significantly higher than other high-income nations. Use of emergency contraception (EC) within 120 hours after unprotected or underprotected intercourse can reduce the risk of pregnancy. Emergency contraceptive methods include oral medications labeled and dedicated for use as EC by the US Food and Drug Administration (ulipristal and levonorgestrel), the "off-label" use of combined oral contraceptives, and insertion of a copper intrauterine device. Indications for the use of EC include intercourse without use of contraception; condom breakage or slippage; missed or late doses of contraceptives, including the oral contraceptive pill, contraceptive patch, contraceptive ring, and injectable contraception; vomiting after use of oral contraceptives; and sexual assault. Our aim in this updated policy statement is to (1) educate pediatricians and other physicians on available emergency contraceptive methods; (2) provide current data on the safety, efficacy, and use of EC in teenagers; and (3) encourage routine counseling and advance EC prescription as 1 public health strategy to reduce teenaged pregnancy. (11/19)

See full text on page 657.

https://pediatrics.aappublications.org/content/144/6/e20193149

EMERGENCY INFORMATION FORMS AND EMERGENCY PREPAREDNESS FOR CHILDREN WITH SPECIAL HEALTH CARE NEEDS

Committee on Pediatric Emergency Medicine and Council on Clinical Information Technology (joint with American College of Emergency Physicians Pediatric Emergency Medicine Committee)

ABSTRACT. Children with chronic medical conditions rely on complex management plans for problems that cause them to be at increased risk for suboptimal outcomes in emergency situations. The emergency information form (EIF) is a medical summary that describes medical condition(s), medications, and special health care needs to inform health care providers of a child's special health conditions and needs so that optimal emergency medical care can be provided. This statement describes updates to EIFs, including computerization of the EIF, expanding the potential benefits of the EIF, quality-improvement programs using the EIF, the EIF as a central repository, and facilitating emergency preparedness in disaster management and drills by using the EIF. (3/10, reaffirmed 7/14, 10/14)

http://pediatrics.aappublications.org/content/125/4/829

ENDORSEMENT OF HEALTH AND HUMAN SERVICES RECOMMENDATION FOR PULSE OXIMETRY SCREENING FOR CRITICAL CONGENITAL HEART DISEASE

Section on Cardiology and Cardiac Surgery Executive Committee

ABSTRACT. Incorporation of pulse oximetry to the assessment of the newborn infant can enhance detection of critical congenital heart disease (CCHD). Recently, the Secretary of Health and Human Services (HHS) recommended that screening for CCHD be added to the uniform screening panel. The American Academy of Pediatrics (AAP) has been a strong advocate of early detection of CCHD and fully supports the decision of the Secretary of HHS.

The AAP has published strategies for the implementation of pulse oximetry screening, which addressed critical issues such as necessary equipment, personnel, and training, and also provided specific recommendations for assessment of saturation by using pulse oximetry as well as appropriate management of a positive screening result. The AAP is committed to the safe and effective implementation of pulse oximetry screening and is working with other advocacy groups and governmental agencies to promote pulse oximetry and to support widespread surveillance for CCHD.

Going forward, AAP chapters will partner with state health departments to implement the new screening strategy for CCHD and will work to ensure that there is an adequate system for referral for echocardiographic/pediatric cardiac evaluation after a positive screening result. It is imperative that AAP members engage their respective policy makers in adopting and funding the recommendations made by the Secretary of HHS. (12/11)
http://pediatrics.aappublications.org/content/129/1/190

ENHANCING PEDIATRIC WORKFORCE DIVERSITY AND PROVIDING CULTURALLY EFFECTIVE PEDIATRIC CARE: IMPLICATIONS FOR PRACTICE, EDUCATION, AND POLICY MAKING

Committee on Pediatric Workforce

ABSTRACT. This policy statement serves to combine and update 2 previously independent but overlapping statements from the American Academy of Pediatrics (AAP) on culturally effective health care (CEHC) and workforce diversity. The AAP has long recognized that with the ever-increasing diversity of the pediatric population in the United States, the health of all children depends on the ability of all pediatricians to practice culturally effective care. CEHC can be defined as the delivery of care within the context of appropriate physician knowledge, understanding, and appreciation of all cultural distinctions, leading to optimal health outcomes. The AAP believes that CEHC is a critical social value and that the knowledge and skills necessary for providing CEHC can be taught and acquired through focused curricula across the spectrum of lifelong learning.

This statement also addresses workforce diversity, health disparities, and affirmative action. The discussion of diversity is broadened to include not only race, ethnicity, and language but also cultural attributes such as gender, religious beliefs, sexual orientation, and disability, which may affect the quality of health care. The AAP believes that efforts must be supported through health policy and advocacy initiatives to promote the delivery of CEHC and to overcome educational, organizational, and other barriers to improving workforce diversity. (9/13, reaffirmed 10/15)
http://pediatrics.aappublications.org/content/132/4/e1105

ENSURING COMPREHENSIVE CARE AND SUPPORT FOR TRANSGENDER AND GENDER-DIVERSE CHILDREN AND ADOLESCENTS

Jason Rafferty, MD, MPH, EdM, FAAP; Committee on Psychosocial Aspects of Child and Family Health; Committee on Adolescence; and Section on Lesbian, Gay, Bisexual, and Transgender Health and Wellness

ABSTRACT. As a traditionally underserved population that faces numerous health disparities, youth who identify as transgender and gender diverse (TGD) and their families are increasingly presenting to pediatric providers for education, care, and referrals. The need for more formal training, standardized treatment, and research on safety and medical outcomes often leaves providers feeling ill equipped to support and care for patients that identify as TGD and families. In this policy statement, we review relevant concepts and challenges and provide suggestions for pediatric providers that are focused on promoting the health and positive development of youth that identify as TGD while eliminating discrimination and stigma. (9/18)
http://pediatrics.aappublications.org/content/142/4/e20182162

ENSURING THE HEALTH OF CHILDREN IN DISASTERS

Disaster Preparedness Advisory Council and Committee on Pediatric Emergency Medicine

ABSTRACT. Infants, children, adolescents, and young adults have unique physical, mental, behavioral, developmental, communication, therapeutic, and social needs that must be addressed and met in all aspects of disaster preparedness, response, and recovery. Pediatricians, including primary care pediatricians, pediatric medical subspecialists, and pediatric surgical specialists, have key roles to play in preparing and treating families in cases of disasters. Pediatricians should attend to the continuity of practice operations to provide services in time of need and stay abreast of disaster and public health developments to be active participants in community planning efforts. Federal, state, tribal, local, and regional institutions and agencies that serve children should collaborate with pediatricians to ensure the health and well-being of children in disasters. (10/15)
http://pediatrics.aappublications.org/content/136/5/e1407

EPIDEMIOLOGY AND DIAGNOSIS OF HEALTH CARE–ASSOCIATED INFECTIONS IN THE NICU (TECHNICAL REPORT)

Committee on Fetus and Newborn and Committee on Infectious Diseases

ABSTRACT. Health care–associated infections in the NICU are a major clinical problem resulting in increased morbidity and mortality, prolonged length of hospital stays, and increased medical costs. Neonates are at high risk for health care–associated infections because of impaired host defense mechanisms, limited amounts of protective endogenous flora on skin and mucosal surfaces at time of birth, reduced barrier function of neonatal skin, the use of invasive procedures and devices, and frequent exposure to broad-spectrum antibiotics. This statement will review the epidemiology and diagnosis of health care–associated infections in newborn infants. (3/12, reaffirmed 2/16)
http://pediatrics.aappublications.org/content/129/4/e1104

EPINEPHRINE FOR FIRST-AID MANAGEMENT OF ANAPHYLAXIS (CLINICAL REPORT)

Scott H. Sicherer, MD, FAAP; F. Estelle R. Simons, MD, FAAP; and Section on Allergy and Immunology

ABSTRACT. Anaphylaxis is a severe, generalized allergic or hypersensitivity reaction that is rapid in onset and may cause death. Epinephrine (adrenaline) can be life-saving when administered as rapidly as possible once anaphylaxis is recognized. This clinical report from the American Academy of Pediatrics is an update of the 2007 clinical report on this topic. It provides information to help clinicians identify patients at risk of anaphylaxis and new information about epinephrine and epinephrine autoinjectors (EAs). The report also highlights the importance of patient and family education about the recognition and management of anaphylaxis in the community. Key points emphasized include the following: (1) validated clinical criteria are available to facilitate prompt diagnosis of anaphylaxis; (2) prompt intramuscular epinephrine injection in the mid-outer thigh reduces hospitalizations, morbidity, and mortality; (3) prescribing EAs facilitates timely epinephrine injection in community settings for patients with a history of anaphylaxis and, if specific circumstances warrant, for some high-risk patients who have not previously experienced anaphylaxis; (4) prescribing epinephrine for infants and young children weighing <15 kg, especially those who weigh 7.5 kg and under, currently presents a dilemma, because the lowest dose available in EAs, 0.15 mg, is a high dose for many infants and some young children; (5) effective management of anaphylaxis in the community requires a comprehensive approach involving children, families, preschools, schools, camps, and sports organizations; and (6) prevention of anaphy-

laxis recurrences involves confirmation of the trigger, discussion of specific allergen avoidance, allergen immunotherapy (eg, with stinging insect venom, if relevant), and a written, personalized anaphylaxis emergency action plan; and (7) the management of anaphylaxis also involves education of children and supervising adults about anaphylaxis recognition and first-aid treatment. (2/17)
http://pediatrics.aappublications.org/content/139/3/e20164006

EQUIPMENT FOR GROUND AMBULANCES

American Academy of Pediatrics (joint with American College of Emergency Physicians, American College of Surgeons Committee on Trauma, Emergency Medical Services for Children, Emergency Nurses Association, National Association of EMS Physicians, and National Association of State EMS Officials)

On January 1, 2014, the American Academy of Pediatrics, American College of Emergency Physicians, American College of Surgeons Committee on Trauma, Emergency Medical Services for Children, Emergency Nurses Association, National Association of EMS Physicians, and National Association of State EMS Officials coauthored a joint policy statement, "Equipment for Ground Ambulances" (*Prehosp Emerg Care.* 2014;19[1]:92–97). The full text of the joint policy statement is available at: http://informahealthcare.com/doi/full/10.3109/10903127.2013.851312. Copyright © 2014 Informa Plc. (8/14)
http://pediatrics.aappublications.org/content/134/3/e919

ERADICATING POLIO: HOW THE WORLD'S PEDIATRICIANS CAN HELP STOP THIS CRIPPLING ILLNESS FOREVER (CLINICAL REPORT)

Walter A. Orenstein, MD, FAAP, and Committee on Infectious Diseases

ABSTRACT. The American Academy of Pediatrics strongly supports the Polio Eradication and Endgame Strategic Plan of the Global Polio Eradication Initiative. This plan was endorsed in November 2012 by the Strategic Advisory Group of Experts on Immunization of the World Health Organization and published by the World Health Organization in April 2013. As a key component of the plan, it will be necessary to stop oral polio vaccine (OPV) use globally to achieve eradication, because the attenuated viruses in the vaccine rarely can cause polio. The plan includes procedures for elimination of vaccine-associated paralytic polio and circulating vaccine-derived polioviruses (cVDPVs). cVDPVs can proliferate when vaccine viruses are transmitted among susceptible people, resulting in mutations conferring both the neurovirulence and transmissibility characteristics of wild polioviruses. Although there are 3 different types of wild poliovirus strains, the polio eradication effort has already resulted in the global elimination of type 2 poliovirus for more than a decade. Type 3 poliovirus may be eliminated because the wild type 3 poliovirus was last detected in 2012. Thus, of the 3 wild types, only wild type 1 poliovirus is still known to be circulating and causing disease. OPV remains the key vaccine for eradicating wild polioviruses in polio-infected countries because it induces high levels of systemic immunity to prevent paralysis and intestinal immunity to reduce transmission. However, OPV is a rare cause of paralysis and the substantial decrease in wild-type disease has resulted in estimates that the vaccine is causing more polio-related paralysis annually in recent years than the wild virus. The new endgame strategic plan calls for stepwise removal of the type 2 poliovirus component from trivalent oral vaccines, because type 2 wild poliovirus appears to have been eradicated (since 1999) and yet is the main cause of cVDPV outbreaks and approximately 40% of vaccine-associated paralytic polio cases. The Endgame and Strategic Plan will be accomplished by shifting from trivalent OPV to bivalent OPV (containing types 1 and 3 poliovirus only). It will be necessary to introduce trivalent inactivated poliovirus vaccine (IPV) into routine immunization programs in all countries using OPV to provide population immunity to type 2 before the switch from trivalent OPV to bivalent OPV. The Global Polio Eradication Initiative hopes to achieve global eradication of polio by 2018 with this strategy, after which all OPV use will be stopped. Challenges expected for adding IPV into routine immunization schedules include higher cost of IPV compared with OPV, cold-chain capacity limits, more complex administration of vaccine because IPV requires injections as opposed to oral administration, and inferior intestinal immunity conferred by IPV. The goal of this report is to help pediatricians understand the change in strategy and outline ways that pediatricians can help global polio eradication efforts, including advocating for the resources needed to accomplish polio eradication and for incorporation of IPV into routine immunization programs in all countries. (12/14)
http://pediatrics.aappublications.org/content/135/1/196

ESSENTIAL CONTRACTUAL LANGUAGE FOR MEDICAL NECESSITY IN CHILDREN

Committee on Child Health Financing

ABSTRACT. The previous policy statement from the American Academy of Pediatrics, "Model Language for Medical Necessity in Children," was published in July 2005. Since that time, there have been new and emerging delivery and payment models. The relationship established between health care providers and health plans should promote arrangements that are beneficial to all who are affected by these contractual arrangements. Pediatricians play an important role in ensuring that the needs of children are addressed in these emerging systems. It is important to recognize that health care plans designed for adults may not meet the needs of children. Language in health care contracts should reflect the health care needs of children and families. Informed pediatricians can make a difference in the care of children and influence the role of primary care physicians in the new paradigms. This policy highlights many of the important elements pediatricians should assess as providers develop a role in emerging care models. (7/13, reaffirmed 9/17)
http://pediatrics.aappublications.org/content/132/2/398

ESTABLISHING A STANDARD PROTOCOL FOR THE VOIDING CYSTOURETHROGRAPHY (CLINICAL REPORT)

Dominic Frimberger, MD; Maria-Gisela Mercado-Deane, MD, FAAP; Section on Urology; and Section on Radiology

ABSTRACT. The voiding cystourethrogram (VCUG) is a frequently performed test to diagnose a variety of urologic conditions, such as vesicoureteral reflux. The test results determine whether continued observation or an interventional procedure is indicated. VCUGs are ordered by many specialists and primary care providers, including pediatricians, family practitioners, nephrologists, hospitalists, emergency department physicians, and urologists. Current protocols for performing and interpreting a VCUG are based on the International Reflux Study in 1985. However, more recent information provided by many national and international institutions suggests a need to refine those recommendations. The lead author of the 1985 study, R.L. Lebowitz, agreed to and participated in the current protocol. In addition, a recent survey directed to the chairpersons of pediatric radiology of 65 children's hospitals throughout the United States and Canada showed that VCUG protocols vary substantially. Recent guidelines from the American Academy of Pediatrics (AAP) recommend a VCUG for children between 2 and 24 months of age with urinary tract infections but did not specify how this test should be performed. To improve patient safety and to standardize the data obtained when a VCUG is performed, the AAP Section on Radiology and the AAP Section on Urology initiated the current VCUG protocol to create a consensus on how to perform this test. (10/16)
http://pediatrics.aappublications.org/content/138/5/e20162590

ETHICAL AND POLICY ISSUES IN GENETIC TESTING AND SCREENING OF CHILDREN

Committee on Bioethics and Committee on Genetics (joint with American College of Medical Genetics and Genomics)

ABSTRACT. The genetic testing and genetic screening of children are commonplace. Decisions about whether to offer genetic testing and screening should be driven by the best interest of the child. The growing literature on the psychosocial and clinical effects of such testing and screening can help inform best practices. This policy statement represents recommendations developed collaboratively by the American Academy of Pediatrics and the American College of Medical Genetics and Genomics with respect to many of the scenarios in which genetic testing and screening can occur. (2/13, reaffirmed 6/18)

http://pediatrics.aappublications.org/content/131/3/620

ETHICAL CONSIDERATIONS IN RESEARCH WITH SOCIALLY IDENTIFIABLE POPULATIONS

Committee on Native American Child Health and Committee on Community Health Services

ABSTRACT. Community-based research raises ethical issues not normally encountered in research conducted in academic settings. In particular, conventional risk-benefits assessments frequently fail to recognize harms that can occur in socially identifiable populations as a result of research participation. Furthermore, many such communities require more stringent measures of beneficence that must be applied directly to the participating communities. In this statement, the American Academy of Pediatrics sets forth recommendations for minimizing harms that may result from community-based research by emphasizing community involvement in the research process. (1/04, reaffirmed 10/07, 1/13)

http://pediatrics.aappublications.org/content/113/1/148

ETHICAL CONTROVERSIES IN ORGAN DONATION AFTER CIRCULATORY DEATH

Committee on Bioethics

ABSTRACT. The persistent mismatch between the supply of and need for transplantable organs has led to efforts to increase the supply, including controlled donation after circulatory death (DCD). Controlled DCD involves organ recovery after the planned withdrawal of life-sustaining treatment and the declaration of death according to the cardiorespiratory criteria. Two central ethical issues in DCD are when organ recovery can begin and how to manage conflicts of interests. The "dead donor rule" should be maintained, and donors in cases of DCD should only be declared dead after the permanent cessation of circulatory function. Permanence is generally established by a 2- to 5-minute waiting period. Given ongoing controversy over whether the cessation must also be irreversible, physicians should not be required to participate in DCD. Because the preparation for organ recovery in DCD begins before the declaration of death, there are potential conflicts between the donor's and recipient's interests. These conflicts can be managed in a variety of ways, including informed consent and separating the various participants' roles. For example, informed consent should be sought for premortem interventions to improve organ viability, and organ procurement organization personnel and members of the transplant team should not be involved in the discontinuation of life-sustaining treatment or the declaration of death. It is also important to emphasize that potential donors in cases of DCD should receive integrated interdisciplinary palliative care, including sedation and analgesia. (4/13, reaffirmed 12/16)

http://pediatrics.aappublications.org/content/131/5/1021

EVALUATING CHILDREN WITH FRACTURES FOR CHILD PHYSICAL ABUSE (CLINICAL REPORT)

Emalee G. Flaherty, MD, FAAP; Jeannette M. Perez-Rossello, MD; Michael A. Levine, MD; William L. Hennrikus, MD; Committee on Child Abuse and Neglect; Section on Radiology; Section on Endocrinology; and Section on Orthopaedics (joint with Society for Pediatric Radiology)

ABSTRACT. Fractures are common injuries caused by child abuse. Although the consequences of failing to diagnose an abusive injury in a child can be grave, incorrectly diagnosing child abuse in a child whose fractures have another etiology can be distressing for a family. The aim of this report is to review recent advances in the understanding of fracture specificity, the mechanism of fractures, and other medical diseases that predispose to fractures in infants and children. This clinical report will aid physicians in developing an evidence-based differential diagnosis and performing the appropriate evaluation when assessing a child with fractures. (1/14)

http://pediatrics.aappublications.org/content/133/2/e477

EVALUATING FOR SUSPECTED CHILD ABUSE: CONDITIONS THAT PREDISPOSE TO BLEEDING (TECHNICAL REPORT)

Shannon L. Carpenter, MD, MS; Thomas C. Abshire, MD; James D. Anderst, MD, MS; Section on Hematology/Oncology; and Committee on Child Abuse and Neglect

ABSTRACT. Child abuse might be suspected when children present with cutaneous bruising, intracranial hemorrhage, or other manifestations of bleeding. In these cases, it is necessary to consider medical conditions that predispose to easy bleeding/bruising. When evaluating for the possibility of bleeding disorders and other conditions that predispose to hemorrhage, the pediatrician must consider the child's presenting history, medical history, and physical examination findings before initiating a laboratory investigation. Many medical conditions can predispose to easy bleeding. Before ordering laboratory tests for a disease, it is useful to understand the biochemical basis and clinical presentation of the disorder, condition prevalence, and test characteristics. This technical report reviews the major medical conditions that predispose to bruising/bleeding and should be considered when evaluating for abusive injury. (3/13, reaffirmed 7/16)

http://pediatrics.aappublications.org/content/131/4/e1357

EVALUATION AND MANAGEMENT OF CHILDREN AND ADOLESCENTS WITH ACUTE MENTAL HEALTH OR BEHAVIORAL PROBLEMS. PART I: COMMON CLINICAL CHALLENGES OF PATIENTS WITH MENTAL HEALTH AND/OR BEHAVIORAL EMERGENCIES (CLINICAL REPORT)

Thomas H. Chun, MD, MPH, FAAP; Sharon E. Mace, MD, FAAP, FACEP; Emily R. Katz, MD, FAAP; and Committee on Pediatric Emergency Medicine (joint with American College of Emergency Physicians Pediatric Emergency Medicine Committee)

INTRODUCTION. Mental health problems are among the leading contributors to the global burden of disease. Unfortunately, pediatric populations are not spared of mental health problems. In the United States, 21% to 23% of children and adolescents have a diagnosable mental health or substance use disorder. Among patients of emergency departments (EDs), 70% screen positive for at least 1 mental health disorder, 23% meet criteria for 2 or more mental health concerns, 45% have a mental health problem resulting in impaired psychosocial functioning, and 10% of adolescents endorse significant levels of psychiatric distress at the time of their ED visit. In pediatric primary care settings, the reported prevalence of mental health and behavioral disorders is between 12% to 22% of children and adolescents.

Although the American Academy of Pediatrics (AAP) has published a policy statement on mental health competencies and a Mental Health Toolkit for pediatric primary care providers, no such guidelines or resources exist for clinicians who care for pediatric mental health emergencies. This clinical report supports the 2006 joint policy statement of the AAP and American College of Emergency Physicians (ACEP) on pediatric mental health emergencies, with the goal of addressing the knowledge gaps in this area. The report is written primarily from the perspective of ED clinicians, but it is intended for all clinicians who care for children and adolescents with acute mental health and behavioral problems.

Recent epidemiologic studies of mental health visits have revealed a rapid burgeoning of both ED and primary care visits. An especially problematic trend is the increase in "boarding" of psychiatric patients in the ED and inpatient pediatric beds (ie, extended stays lasting days or even weeks). Although investigation of boarding practices is still in its infancy, the ACEP and the American Medical Association have both expressed concern about it, because it significantly taxes the functioning and efficiency of both the ED and hospital, and mental health services may not be available in the ED.

In addition, compared with other pediatric care settings, ED patients are known to be at higher risk of mental health disorders, including depression, anxiety, posttraumatic stress disorder, and substance abuse. These mental health conditions may be unrecognized not only by treating clinicians but also by the child/adolescent and his or her parents. A similar phenomenon has been described with suicidal patients. Individuals who have committed suicide frequently visited a health care provider in the months preceding their death. Although a minority of suicidal patients present with some form of self-harm, many have vague somatic complaints (eg, headache, gastrointestinal tract distress, back pain, concern for a sexually transmitted infection) masking their underlying mental health condition.

Despite studies demonstrating moderate agreement between emergency physicians and psychiatrists in the assessment and management of patients with mental health problems, ED clinicians frequently cite lack of training and confidence in their abilities as barriers to caring for patients with mental health emergencies. Another study of emergency medicine and pediatric emergency medicine training programs found that formal training in psychiatric problems is not required nor offered by most programs. Pediatric primary care providers report similar barriers to caring for their patients with mental health problems.

Part I of this clinical report focuses on the issues relevant to patients presenting to the ED with a mental health chief complaint and covers the following topics:

- Medical clearance of pediatric psychiatric patients
- Suicidal ideation and suicide attempts
- Involuntary hospitalization
- Restraint of the agitated patient
  - Verbal restraint
  - Chemical restraint
  - Physical restraint
- Coordination with the medical home

Part II discusses challenging patients with primarily medical or indeterminate presentations, in which the contribution of an underlying mental health condition may be unclear or a complicating factor, including:

- Somatic symptom and related disorders
- Adverse effects to psychiatric medications
  - Antipsychotic adverse effects
  - Neuroleptic malignant syndrome
  - Serotonin syndrome
- Children with special needs in the ED (autism spectrum and developmental disorders)
- Mental health screening in the ED

An executive summary of this clinical report can be found at www.pediatrics.org/cgi/doi/10.1542/peds.2016-1571. (8/16)
http://pediatrics.aappublications.org/content/138/3/e20161570

EVALUATION AND MANAGEMENT OF CHILDREN AND ADOLESCENTS WITH ACUTE MENTAL HEALTH OR BEHAVIORAL PROBLEMS. PART I: COMMON CLINICAL CHALLENGES OF PATIENTS WITH MENTAL HEALTH AND/OR BEHAVIORAL EMERGENCIES—EXECUTIVE SUMMARY (CLINICAL REPORT)

Thomas H. Chun, MD, MPH, FAAP; Sharon E. Mace, MD, FAAP, FACEP; Emily R. Katz, MD, FAAP; and Committee on Pediatric Emergency Medicine (joint with American College of Emergency Physicians Pediatric Emergency Medicine Committee)

ABSTRACT. The number of children and adolescents seen in emergency departments (EDs) and primary care settings for mental health problems has skyrocketed in recent years, with up to 23% of patients in both settings having diagnosable mental health conditions. Even when a mental health problem is not the focus of an ED or primary care visit, mental health conditions, both known and occult, may challenge the treating clinician and complicate the patient's care.

Although the American Academy of Pediatrics has published a policy statement on mental health competencies and a Mental Health Toolkit for pediatric primary care providers, no such guidelines or resources exist for clinicians who care for pediatric mental health emergencies. Many ED and primary care physicians report a paucity of training and lack of confidence in caring for pediatric psychiatry patients. The 2 clinical reports (www.pediatrics.org/cgi/doi/10.1542/peds.2016-1570 and www.pediatrics.org/cgi/doi/10.1542/peds.2016-1573) support the 2006 joint policy statement of the American Academy of Pediatrics and the American College of Emergency Physicians on pediatric mental health emergencies, with the goal of addressing the knowledge gaps in this area. Although written primarily from the perspective of ED clinicians, they are intended for all clinicians who care for children and adolescents with acute mental health and behavioral problems.

The clinical reports are organized around the common clinical challenges pediatric caregivers face, both when a child or adolescent presents with a psychiatric chief complaint or emergency (part I) and also when a mental health condition may be an unclear or complicating factor in a non–mental health clinical presentation (part II). Part II of the clinical reports (www.pediatrics.org/cgi/doi/10.1542/peds.2016-1573) includes discussions of somatic symptom and related disorders, adverse effects of psychiatric medications including neuroleptic malignant syndrome and serotonin syndrome, caring for children with special needs such as autism and developmental disorders, and mental health screening. This executive summary is an overview of part I of the clinical reports. The full text of the below topics can be accessed online at (www.pediatrics.org/cgi/doi/10.1542/peds.2016-1570). (8/16)
http://pediatrics.aappublications.org/content/138/3/e20161571

EVALUATION AND MANAGEMENT OF CHILDREN WITH ACUTE MENTAL HEALTH OR BEHAVIORAL PROBLEMS. PART II: RECOGNITION OF CLINICALLY CHALLENGING MENTAL HEALTH RELATED CONDITIONS PRESENTING WITH MEDICAL OR UNCERTAIN SYMPTOMS (CLINICAL REPORT)

Thomas H. Chun, MD, MPH, FAAP; Sharon E. Mace, MD, FAAP, FACEP; Emily R. Katz, MD, FAAP; and Committee on Pediatric Emergency Medicine (joint with American College of Emergency Physicians Pediatric Emergency Medicine Committee)

INTRODUCTION. Part I of this clinical report (http://www.pediatrics.org/cgi/doi/10.1542/peds.2016-1570) discusses the common clinical issues that may be encountered in caring for children and adolescents presenting to the emergency department (ED) or primary care setting with a mental health condition or emergency and includes the following:

- Medical clearance of pediatric psychiatric patients
- Suicidal ideation and suicide attempts
- Involuntary hospitalization
- Restraint of the agitated patient
  - — Verbal restraint
  - — Chemical restraint
  - — Physical restraint
- Coordination with the medical home

Part II discusses the challenges a pediatric clinician may face when evaluating patients with a mental health condition, which may be contributing to or a complicating factor for a medical or indeterminate clinical presentation. Topics covered include the following:

- Somatic symptom and related disorders
- Adverse effects of psychiatric medications
  - — Antipsychotic adverse effects
  - — Neuroleptic malignant syndrome
  - — Serotonin syndrome
- Children with special needs (autism spectrum disorders [ASDs] and developmental disorders [DDs])
- Mental health screening

The report is written primarily from the perspective of ED clinicians, but it is intended for all clinicians who care for children and adolescents with acute mental health and behavioral problems. An executive summary of this clinical report can be found at http://www.pediatrics.org/cgi/doi/10.1542/peds.2016-1574. (8/16)

http://pediatrics.aappublications.org/content/138/3/e20161573

EVALUATION AND MANAGEMENT OF CHILDREN WITH ACUTE MENTAL HEALTH OR BEHAVIORAL PROBLEMS. PART II: RECOGNITION OF CLINICALLY CHALLENGING MENTAL HEALTH RELATED CONDITIONS PRESENTING WITH MEDICAL OR UNCERTAIN SYMPTOMS—EXECUTIVE SUMMARY (CLINICAL REPORT)

Thomas H. Chun, MD, MPH, FAAP; Sharon E. Mace, MD, FAAP, FACEP; Emily R. Katz, MD, FAAP; and Committee on Pediatric Emergency Medicine (joint with American College of Emergency Physicians Pediatric Emergency Medicine Committee)

ABSTRACT. The number of children and adolescents seen in emergency departments (EDs) and primary care settings for mental health problems has skyrocketed in recent years, with up to 23% of patients in both settings having diagnosable mental health conditions. Even when a mental health problem is not the focus of an ED or primary care visit, mental health conditions, both known and occult, may challenge the treating clinician and complicate the patient's care.

Although the American Academy of Pediatrics (AAP) has published a policy statement on mental health competencies and a Mental Health Toolkit for pediatric primary care providers, no such guidelines or resources exist for clinicians who care for pediatric mental health emergencies. Many ED and primary care physicians report paucity of training and lack of confidence in caring for pediatric psychiatry patients. The 2 clinical reports support the 2006 joint policy statement of the AAP and the American College of Emergency Physicians on pediatric mental health emergencies, with the goal of addressing the knowledge gaps in this area. Although written primarily from the perspective of ED clinicians, it is intended for all clinicians who care for children and adolescents with acute mental health and behavioral problems. They are organized around the common clinical challenges pediatric caregivers face, both when a child or adolescent presents with a psychiatric chief complaint or emergency (part I) and when a mental health condition may be an unclear or complicating factor in a non-mental health ED presentation (part II). Part I of the clinical reports includes discussions of Medical Clearance of Pediatric Psychiatric Patients; Suicide and Suicidal Ideation; Restraint of the Agitated Patient Including Verbal, Chemical, and Physical Restraint; and Coordination of Care With the Medical Home, and it can be accessed online at www.pediatrics.org/cgi/doi/10.1542/peds.2016-1570. This executive summary is an overview of part II of the clinical reports. Full text of the following topics can be accessed online at www.pediatrics.org/cgi/doi/10.1542/peds.2016-1573. (8/16)

http://pediatrics.aappublications.org/content/138/3/e20161574

EVALUATION AND MANAGEMENT OF THE INFANT EXPOSED TO HIV-1 IN THE UNITED STATES (CLINICAL REPORT)

Peter L. Havens, MD; Lynne M. Mofenson, MD; and Committee on Pediatric AIDS

ABSTRACT. The pediatrician plays a key role in the prevention of mother-to-child transmission of HIV-1 infection. For infants born to women with HIV-1 infection identified during pregnancy, the pediatrician ensures that antiretroviral prophylaxis is provided to the infant to decrease the risk of acquiring HIV-1 infection and promotes avoidance of postnatal HIV-1 transmission by advising HIV-1–infected women not to breastfeed. The pediatrician should perform HIV-1 antibody testing for infants born to women whose HIV-1 infection status was not determined during pregnancy or labor. For HIV-1–exposed infants, the pediatrician monitors the infant for early determination of HIV-1 infection status and for possible short- and long-term toxicity from antiretroviral exposures. Provision of chemoprophylaxis for *Pneumocystis jiroveci* pneumonia and support of families living with HIV-1 by providing counseling to parents or caregivers are also important components of care. (12/08, reaffirmed 8/15)

http://pediatrics.aappublications.org/content/123/1/175

EVALUATION AND MANAGEMENT OF THE INFANT EXPOSED TO HIV-1 IN THE UNITED STATES—ADDENDUM

Peter L. Havens, MD; Lynne M. Mofenson, MD; and Committee on Pediatric AIDS

The following paragraph is an addendum to the clinical report "Evaluation and Management of the Infant Exposed to HIV-1 in the United States" (*Pediatrics* 2009;123[1]:175–187). It pertains to the section with the heading "HIV-1 Testing of the Infant if the Mother's HIV-1 Infection Status Is Unknown":

For newborn infants whose mother's HIV-1 serostatus is unknown, the newborn infant's health care provider should perform rapid HIV-1 antibody testing on the mother or the infant as soon as possible after birth with appropriate consent as required by state and local law. These test results should be available as early as possible and certainly within 12 hours after birth and can be used to guide initiation of infant antiretroviral prophylaxis. Rapid HIV-1 antibody testing, by using either blood or saliva, is licensed for the diagnosis of HIV infection in adults. Rapid HIV-1 antibody testing of women in labor and delivery units at 16 US hospitals identified a prevalence of undiagnosed HIV infection of 7 of 1000 women and demonstrated a sensitivity of 100% and specificity of 99.9% by using several rapid test kits. Positive predictive value was 90% compared with 76% for enzyme immunoassay. However, the use of these tests in infants is neither well described nor licensed. Sherman et al evaluated 7 HIV-1 rapid tests on stored samples from 116 HIV-exposed infants and compared the findings to standard HIV enzyme immunoassay testing. In the youngest cohort tested (median age, 1.5 months; range, 3–7 weeks), sensitivity of rapid testing was greater than 99%. In a subsequent study using whole blood, sensitivities ranged between 93.3% and 99.3% in infants younger than 3 months by using 5 rapid tests. In both of these studies, rapid HIV-1 rapid tests failed to identify some HIV-infected infants. Oral fluid testing has been demonstrated to have a negative predictive value of >99% in HIV-exposed children older than 12 months. However, when used for screening infants with a median age of 1.5 months (range, birth to 6 months), oral fluid testing had a sensitivity less than 90% and failed to detect 14 of 63 HIV-infected infants (22.2%). On the basis of these findings, only blood should be used to perform rapid HIV-1 antibody testing in newborn infants. Furthermore, rapid testing of the mother, by using either blood or saliva, is preferred over rapid testing in her infant (blood only) because of increased sensitivity in identifying HIV-1 infection. (11/12, reaffirmed 8/15)

http://pediatrics.aappublications.org/content/130/6/64

EVALUATION AND REFERRAL FOR DEVELOPMENTAL DYSPLASIA OF THE HIP IN INFANTS (CLINICAL REPORT)

Brian A. Shaw, MD, FAAOS, FAAP; Lee S. Segal, MD, FAAOS, FAAP; and Section on Orthopaedics

ABSTRACT. Developmental dysplasia of the hip (DDH) encompasses a wide spectrum of clinical severity, from mild developmental abnormalities to frank dislocation. Clinical hip instability occurs in 1% to 2% of full-term infants, and up to 15% have hip instability or hip immaturity detectable by imaging studies. Hip dysplasia is the most common cause of hip arthritis in women younger than 40 years and accounts for 5% to 10% of all total hip replacements in the United States. Newborn and periodic screening have been practiced for decades, because DDH is clinically silent during the first year of life, can be treated more effectively if detected early, and can have severe consequences if left untreated. However, screening programs and techniques are not uniform, and there is little evidence-based literature to support current practice, leading to controversy. Recent literature shows that many mild forms of DDH resolve without treatment, and there is a lack of agreement on ultrasonographic diagnostic criteria for DDH as a disease versus developmental variations. The American Academy of Pediatrics has not published any policy statements on DDH since its 2000 clinical practice guideline and accompanying technical report. Developments since then include a controversial US Preventive Services Task Force "inconclusive" determination regarding usefulness of DDH screening, several prospective studies supporting observation over treatment of minor ultrasonographic hip variations, and a recent evidence-based clinical practice guideline from the American Academy of Orthopaedic Surgeons on the detection and management of DDH in infants 0 to 6 months of age. The purpose of this clinical report was to provide literature-based updated direction for the clinician in screening and referral for DDH, with the primary goal of preventing and/or detecting a dislocated hip by 6 to 12 months of age in an otherwise healthy child, understanding that no screening program has eliminated late development or presentation of a dislocated hip and that the diagnosis and treatment of milder forms of hip dysplasia remain controversial. (11/16)

http://pediatrics.aappublications.org/content/138/6/e20163107

EVALUATION AND REFERRAL OF CHILDREN WITH SIGNS OF EARLY PUBERTY (CLINICAL REPORT)

Paul Kaplowitz, MD, PhD, FAAP; Clifford Bloch, MD, FAAP; and Section on Endocrinology

ABSTRACT. Concerns about possible early pubertal development are a common cause for referral to pediatric medical subspecialists. Several recent studies have suggested that onset of breast and/or pubic hair development may be occurring earlier than in the past. Although there is a chance of finding pathology in girls with signs of puberty before 8 years of age and in boys before 9 years of age, the vast majority of these children with signs of apparent puberty have variations of normal growth and physical development and do not require laboratory testing, bone age radiographs, or intervention. The most common of these signs of early puberty are premature adrenarche (early onset of pubic hair and/or body odor), premature thelarche (nonprogressive breast development, usually occurring before 2 years of age), and lipomastia, in which girls have apparent breast development which, on careful palpation, is determined to be adipose tissue. Indicators that the signs of sexual maturation may represent true, central precocious puberty include progressive breast development over a 4- to 6-month period of observation or progressive penis and testicular enlargement, especially if accompanied by rapid linear growth. Children exhibiting these true indicators of early puberty need prompt evaluation by the appropriate pediatric medical subspecialist. Therapy with a gonadotropin-releasing hormone agonist may be indicated, as discussed in this report. (12/15)

http://pediatrics.aappublications.org/content/137/1/e20153732

EVALUATION FOR BLEEDING DISORDERS IN SUSPECTED CHILD ABUSE (CLINICAL REPORT)

James D. Anderst, MD, MS; Shannon L. Carpenter, MD, MS; Thomas C. Abshire, MD; Section on Hematology/Oncology; and Committee on Child Abuse and Neglect

ABSTRACT. Bruising or bleeding in a child can raise the concern for child abuse. Assessing whether the findings are the result of trauma and/or whether the child has a bleeding disorder is critical. Many bleeding disorders are rare, and not every child with bruising/bleeding concerning for abuse requires an evaluation for bleeding disorders. In some instances, however, bleeding disorders can present in a manner similar to child abuse. The history and clinical evaluation can be used to determine the necessity of an evaluation for a possible bleeding disorder, and prevalence and known clinical presentations of individual bleeding disorders can be used to guide the extent of the laboratory testing. This clinical report provides guidance to pediatricians and other clinicians regarding the evaluation for bleeding disorders when child abuse is suspected. (3/13, reaffirmed 7/16)

http://pediatrics.aappublications.org/content/131/4/e1314

THE EVALUATION OF CHILDREN IN THE PRIMARY CARE SETTING WHEN SEXUAL ABUSE IS SUSPECTED (CLINICAL REPORT)

Carole Jenny, MD, MBA, FAAP; James E. Crawford-Jakubiak, MD, FAAP; and Committee on Child Abuse and Neglect

ABSTRACT. This clinical report updates a 2005 report from the American Academy of Pediatrics on the evaluation of sexual abuse in children. The medical assessment of suspected child sexual abuse should include obtaining a history, performing a physical examination, and obtaining appropriate laboratory tests. The role of the physician includes determining the need to report suspected sexual abuse; assessing the physical, emotional, and behavioral consequences of sexual abuse; providing information to parents about how to support their child; and coordinating with other professionals to provide comprehensive

treatment and follow-up of children exposed to child sexual abuse. (7/13, reaffirmed 8/18)
http://pediatrics.aappublications.org/content/132/2/e558

THE EVALUATION OF SEXUAL BEHAVIORS IN CHILDREN (CLINICAL REPORT)

Nancy D. Kellogg, MD, and Committee on Child Abuse and Neglect

ABSTRACT. Most children will engage in sexual behaviors at some time during childhood. These behaviors may be normal but can be confusing and concerning to parents or disruptive or intrusive to others. Knowledge of age-appropriate sexual behaviors that vary with situational and environmental factors can assist the clinician in differentiating normal sexual behaviors from sexual behavior problems. Most situations that involve sexual behaviors in young children do not require child protective services intervention; for behaviors that are age-appropriate and transient, the pediatrician may provide guidance in supervision and monitoring of the behavior. If the behavior is intrusive, hurtful, and/or age-inappropriate, a more comprehensive assessment is warranted. Some children with sexual behavior problems may reside or have resided in homes characterized by inconsistent parenting, violence, abuse, or neglect and may require more immediate intervention and referrals. (8/09, reaffirmed 3/13, 10/18)
http://pediatrics.aappublications.org/content/124/3/992

THE EVALUATION OF SUSPECTED CHILD PHYSICAL ABUSE (CLINICAL REPORT)

Cindy W. Christian, MD, FAAP, and Committee on Child Abuse and Neglect

ABSTRACT. Child physical abuse is an important cause of pediatric morbidity and mortality and is associated with major physical and mental health problems that can extend into adulthood. Pediatricians are in a unique position to identify and prevent child abuse, and this clinical report provides guidance to the practitioner regarding indicators and evaluation of suspected physical abuse of children. The role of the physician may include identifying abused children with suspicious injuries who present for care, reporting suspected abuse to the child protection agency for investigation, supporting families who are affected by child abuse, coordinating with other professionals and community agencies to provide immediate and long-term treatment to victimized children, providing court testimony when necessary, providing preventive care and anticipatory guidance in the office, and advocating for policies and programs that support families and protect vulnerable children. (4/15)
http://pediatrics.aappublications.org/content/135/5/e1337

EVIDENCE FOR THE DIAGNOSIS AND TREATMENT OF ACUTE UNCOMPLICATED SINUSITIS IN CHILDREN: A SYSTEMATIC REVIEW (TECHNICAL REPORT)

Michael J. Smith, MD, MSCE

ABSTRACT. In 2001, the American Academy of Pediatrics published clinical practice guidelines for the management of acute bacterial sinusitis (ABS) in children. The technical report accompanying those guidelines included 21 studies that assessed the diagnosis and management of ABS in children. This update to that report incorporates studies of pediatric ABS that have been performed since 2001. Overall, 17 randomized controlled trials of the treatment of sinusitis in children were identified and analyzed. Four randomized, double-blind, placebo-controlled trials of antimicrobial therapy have been published. The results of these studies varied, likely due to differences in inclusion and exclusion criteria. Because of this heterogeneity, formal meta-analyses were not performed. However, qualitative analysis of these studies suggests that children with greater severity of illness at presentation are more likely to benefit from antimicrobial therapy. An additional 5 trials compared different antimicrobial therapies but did not include placebo groups. Six trials assessed a variety of ancillary treatments for ABS in children, and 3 focused on subacute sinusitis. Although the number of pediatric trials has increased since 2001, there are still limited data to guide the diagnosis and management of ABS in children. Diagnostic and treatment guidelines focusing on severity of illness at the time of presentation have the potential to identify those children most likely to benefit from antimicrobial therapy and at the same time minimize unnecessary use of antibiotics. (6/13)
http://pediatrics.aappublications.org/content/132/1/e284

EXECUTIVE SUMMARY: CRITERIA FOR CRITICAL CARE OF INFANTS AND CHILDREN: PICU ADMISSION, DISCHARGE, AND TRIAGE PRACTICE STATEMENT AND LEVELS OF CARE GUIDANCE

Benson S. Hsu, MD, MBA, FAAP; Vanessa Hill, MD, FAAP; Lorry R. Frankel, MD, FCCM; Timothy S. Yeh, MD, MCCM; Shari Simone, CRNP, DNP, FCCM, FAANP, FAAN; Marjorie J. Arca, MD, FACS, FAAP; Jorge A. Coss-Bu, MD; Mary E. Fallat, MD, FACS, FAAP; Jason Foland, MD; Samir Gadepalli, MD, MBA; Michael O. Gayle, BS, MD, FCCM; Lori A. Harmon, RRT, MBA, CPHQ; Christa A. Joseph, RN, MSN; Aaron D. Kessel, BS, MD; Niranjan Kissoon, MD, MCCM; Michele Moss, MD, FCCM; Mohan R. Mysore, MD, FAAP, FCCM; Michele C. Papo, MD, MPH, FCCM; Kari L. Rajzer-Wakeham, CCRN, MSN, PCCNP, RN; Tom B. Rice, MD; David L. Rosenberg, MD, FAAP, FCCM; Martin K. Wakeham, MD; Edward E. Conway, Jr, MD, FCCM, MS; Michael S.D. Agus, MD, FAAP, FCCM

ABSTRACT. This is an executive summary of the 2019 update of the 2004 guidelines and levels of care for PICU. Since previous guidelines, there has been a tremendous transformation of Pediatric Critical Care Medicine with advancements in pediatric cardiovascular medicine, transplant, neurology, trauma, and oncology as well as improvements of care in general PICUs. This has led to the evolution of resources and training in the provision of care through the PICU. Outcome and quality research related to admission, transfer, and discharge criteria as well as literature regarding PICU levels of care to include volume, staffing, and structure were reviewed and included in this statement as appropriate. Consequently, the purposes of this significant update are to address the transformation of the field and codify a revised set of guidelines that will enable hospitals, institutions, and individuals in developing the appropriate PICU for their community needs. The target audiences of the practice statement and guidance are broad and include critical care professionals; pediatricians; pediatric subspecialists; pediatric surgeons; pediatric surgical subspecialists; pediatric imaging physicians; and other members of the patient care team such as nurses, therapists, dieticians, pharmacists, social workers, care coordinators, and hospital administrators who make daily administrative and clinical decisions in all PICU levels of care. (9/19)

See full text on page 669.

https://pediatrics.aappublications.org/content/144/4/e20192433

EXPERT WITNESS PARTICIPATION IN CIVIL AND CRIMINAL PROCEEDINGS

Stephan R. Paul, MD, JD, FAAP; Sandeep K. Narang, MD, JD, FAAP; and Committee on Medical Liability and Risk Management

ABSTRACT. The interests of the public and both the medical and legal professions are best served when scientifically sound and unbiased expert witness testimony is readily available in civil and criminal proceedings. As members of the medical community, patient advocates, and private citizens, pediatricians have ethical and professional obligations to assist in the civil and criminal judicial processes. This policy statement offers recommendations on advocacy, education, research, qualifications,

standards, and ethical business practices all aimed at improving expert testimony. (2/17)
http://pediatrics.aappublications.org/content/139/3/e20163862

EXPERT WITNESS PARTICIPATION IN CIVIL AND CRIMINAL PROCEEDINGS (TECHNICAL REPORT)

Sandeep K. Narang, MD, JD, FAAP; Stephan R. Paul, MD, JD, FAAP; and Committee on Medical Liability and Risk Management

ABSTRACT. The interests of the public and both the medical and legal professions are best served when scientifically sound and unbiased expert witness testimony is readily available in civil and criminal proceedings. As members of the medical community, patient advocates, and private citizens, pediatricians have ethical and professional obligations to assist in the civil and criminal judicial processes. This technical report explains how the role of the expert witness differs in civil and criminal proceedings, legal and ethical standards for expert witnesses, and strategies that have been employed to deter unscientific and irresponsible testimony. A companion policy statement offers recommendations on advocacy, education, research, qualifications, standards, and ethical business practices all aimed at improving expert testimony. (2/17)
http://pediatrics.aappublications.org/content/139/3/e20164122

EXPOSURE TO NONTRADITIONAL PETS AT HOME AND TO ANIMALS IN PUBLIC SETTINGS: RISKS TO CHILDREN (CLINICAL REPORT)

Larry K. Pickering, MD; Nina Marano, DVM, MPH; Joseph A. Bocchini, MD; Frederick J. Angulo, DVM, PhD; and Committee on Infectious Diseases

ABSTRACT. Exposure to animals can provide many benefits during the growth and development of children. However, there are potential risks associated with animal exposures, including exposure to nontraditional pets in the home and animals in public settings. Educational materials, regulations, and guidelines have been developed to minimize these risks. Pediatricians, veterinarians, and other health care professionals can provide advice on selection of appropriate pets as well as prevention of disease transmission from nontraditional pets and when children contact animals in public settings. (10/08, reaffirmed 12/11, 1/15, 6/15)
http://pediatrics.aappublications.org/content/122/4/876

THE EYE EXAMINATION IN THE EVALUATION OF CHILD ABUSE (CLINICAL REPORT)

Cindy W. Christian, MD, FAAP; Alex V. Levin, MD, MHSc, FAAO, FRCSC, FAAP; Council on Child Abuse and Neglect; and Section on Ophthalmology (joint with American Association of Certified Orthoptists, American Association for Pediatric Ophthalmology and Strabismus, and American Academy of Ophthalmology)

ABSTRACT. Child abuse can cause injury to any part of the eye. The most common manifestations are retinal hemorrhages (RHs) in infants and young children with abusive head trauma (AHT). Although RHs are an important indicator of possible AHT, they are also found in other conditions. Distinguishing the number, type, location, and pattern of RHs is important in evaluating a differential diagnosis. Eye trauma can be seen in cases of physical abuse or AHT and may prompt referral for ophthalmologic assessment. Physicians have a responsibility to consider abuse in the differential diagnosis of pediatric eye trauma. Identification and documentation of inflicted ocular trauma requires a thorough examination by an ophthalmologist, including indirect ophthalmoscopy, most optimally through a dilated pupil, especially for the evaluation of possible RHs. An eye examination is helpful in detecting abnormalities that can help identify a medical or traumatic etiology for previously well young children who experience unexpected and unexplained mental status changes with no obvious cause, children with head trauma that results in significant intracranial hemorrhage and brain injury, and children with unexplained death. (7/18)
http://pediatrics.aappublications.org/content/142/2/e20181411

FACILITIES AND EQUIPMENT FOR THE CARE OF PEDIATRIC PATIENTS IN A COMMUNITY HOSPITAL (CLINICAL REPORT)

Committee on Hospital Care

ABSTRACT. Many children who require hospitalization are admitted to community hospitals that are more accessible for families and their primary care physicians but vary substantially in their pediatric resources. The intent of this clinical report is to provide basic guidelines for furnishing and equipping a pediatric area in a community hospital. (5/03, reaffirmed 5/07, 8/13, 1/17)
http://pediatrics.aappublications.org/content/111/5/1120

FALLS FROM HEIGHTS: WINDOWS, ROOFS, AND BALCONIES

Committee on Injury and Poison Prevention

ABSTRACT. Falls of all kinds represent an important cause of child injury and death. In the United States, approximately 140 deaths from falls occur annually in children younger than 15 years. Three million children require emergency department care for fall-related injuries. This policy statement examines the epidemiology of falls from heights and recommends preventive strategies for pediatricians and other child health care professionals. Such strategies involve parent counseling, community programs, building code changes, legislation, and environmental modification, such as the installation of window guards and balcony railings. (5/01, reaffirmed 10/04, 5/07, 6/10)
http://pediatrics.aappublications.org/content/107/5/1188

FAMILIES AFFECTED BY PARENTAL SUBSTANCE USE (CLINICAL REPORT)

Vincent C. Smith, MD, MPH, FAAP; Celeste R. Wilson, MD, FAAP; and Committee on Substance Use and Prevention

ABSTRACT. Children whose parents or caregivers use drugs or alcohol are at increased risk of short- and long-term sequelae ranging from medical problems to psychosocial and behavioral challenges. In the course of providing health care services to children, pediatricians are likely to encounter families affected by parental substance use and are in a unique position to intervene. Therefore, pediatricians need to know how to assess a child's risk in the context of a parent's substance use. The purposes of this clinical report are to review some of the short-term effects of maternal substance use during pregnancy and long-term implications of fetal exposure; describe typical medical, psychiatric, and behavioral symptoms of children and adolescents in families affected by substance use; and suggest proficiencies for pediatricians involved in the care of children and adolescents of families affected by substance use, including screening families, mandated reporting requirements, and directing families to community, regional, and state resources that can address needs and problems. (7/16)
http://pediatrics.aappublications.org/content/138/2/e20161575

FATHERS' ROLES IN THE CARE AND DEVELOPMENT OF THEIR CHILDREN: THE ROLE OF PEDIATRICIANS (CLINICAL REPORT)

Michael Yogman, MD, FAAP; Craig F. Garfield, MD, FAAP; and Committee on Psychosocial Aspects of Child and Family Health

ABSTRACT. Fathers' involvement in and influence on the health and development of their children have increased in a myriad of ways in the past 10 years and have been widely studied. The role of pediatricians in working with fathers has correspondingly increased in importance. This report reviews new

studies of the epidemiology of father involvement, including nonresidential as well as residential fathers. The effects of father involvement on child outcomes are discussed within each phase of a child's development. Particular emphasis is placed on (1) fathers' involvement across childhood ages and (2) the influence of fathers' physical and mental health on their children. Implications and advice for all child health providers to encourage and support father involvement are outlined. (6/16)
http://pediatrics.aappublications.org/content/138/1/e20161128

THE FEMALE ATHLETE TRIAD (CLINICAL REPORT)

Amanda K. Weiss Kelly, MD, FAAP; Suzanne Hecht, MD, FACSM; and Council on Sports Medicine and Fitness

ABSTRACT. The number of girls participating in sports has increased significantly since the introduction of Title XI in 1972. As a result, more girls have been able to experience the social, educational, and health-related benefits of sports participation. However, there are risks associated with sports participation, including the female athlete triad. The triad was originally recognized as the interrelationship of amenorrhea, osteoporosis, and disordered eating, but our understanding has evolved to recognize that each of the components of the triad exists on a spectrum from optimal health to disease. The triad occurs when energy intake does not adequately compensate for exercise-related energy expenditure, leading to adverse effects on reproductive, bone, and cardiovascular health. Athletes can present with a single component or any combination of the components. The triad can have a more significant effect on the health of adolescent athletes than on adults because adolescence is a critical time for bone mass accumulation. This report outlines the current state of knowledge on the epidemiology, diagnosis, and treatment of the triad conditions. (7/16)
http://pediatrics.aappublications.org/content/138/2/e20160922

FETAL ALCOHOL SPECTRUM DISORDERS (CLINICAL REPORT)

Janet F. Williams, MD, FAAP; Vincent C. Smith, MD, MPH, FAAP; and Committee on Substance Abuse

ABSTRACT. Prenatal exposure to alcohol can damage the developing fetus and is the leading preventable cause of birth defects and intellectual and neurodevelopmental disabilities. In 1973, fetal alcohol syndrome was first described as a specific cluster of birth defects resulting from alcohol exposure in utero. Subsequently, research unequivocally revealed that prenatal alcohol exposure causes a broad range of adverse developmental effects. Fetal alcohol spectrum disorder (FASD) is the general term that encompasses the range of adverse effects associated with prenatal alcohol exposure. The diagnostic criteria for fetal alcohol syndrome are specific, and comprehensive efforts are ongoing to establish definitive criteria for diagnosing the other FASDs. A large and growing body of research has led to evidence-based FASD education of professionals and the public, broader prevention initiatives, and recommended treatment approaches based on the following premises:

- Alcohol-related birth defects and developmental disabilities are completely preventable when pregnant women abstain from alcohol use.
- Neurocognitive and behavioral problems resulting from prenatal alcohol exposure are lifelong.
- Early recognition, diagnosis, and therapy for any condition along the FASD continuum can result in improved outcomes.
- During pregnancy:
  — no amount of alcohol intake should be considered safe;
  — there is no safe trimester to drink alcohol;
  — all forms of alcohol, such as beer, wine, and liquor, pose similar risk; and
  — binge drinking poses dose-related risk to the developing fetus. (10/15)

http://pediatrics.aappublications.org/content/136/5/e1395

FEVER AND ANTIPYRETIC USE IN CHILDREN (CLINICAL REPORT)

Janice E. Sullivan, MD; Henry C. Farrar, MD; Section on Clinical Pharmacology and Therapeutics; and Committee on Drugs

ABSTRACT. Fever in a child is one of the most common clinical symptoms managed by pediatricians and other health care providers and a frequent cause of parental concern. Many parents administer antipyretics even when there is minimal or no fever, because they are concerned that the child must maintain a "normal" temperature. Fever, however, is not the primary illness but is a physiologic mechanism that has beneficial effects in fighting infection. There is no evidence that fever itself worsens the course of an illness or that it causes long-term neurologic complications. Thus, the primary goal of treating the febrile child should be to improve the child's overall comfort rather than focus on the normalization of body temperature. When counseling the parents or caregivers of a febrile child, the general well-being of the child, the importance of monitoring activity, observing for signs of serious illness, encouraging appropriate fluid intake, and the safe storage of antipyretics should be emphasized. Current evidence suggests that there is no substantial difference in the safety and effectiveness of acetaminophen and ibuprofen in the care of a generally healthy child with fever. There is evidence that combining these 2 products is more effective than the use of a single agent alone; however, there are concerns that combined treatment may be more complicated and contribute to the unsafe use of these drugs. Pediatricians should also promote patient safety by advocating for simplified formulations, dosing instructions, and dosing devices. (2/11, reaffirmed 7/16)
http://pediatrics.aappublications.org/content/127/3/580

FINANCING GRADUATE MEDICAL EDUCATION TO MEET THE NEEDS OF CHILDREN AND THE FUTURE PEDIATRICIAN WORKFORCE

Committee on Pediatric Workforce

ABSTRACT. The American Academy of Pediatrics (AAP) believes that an appropriately financed graduate medical education (GME) system is critical to ensuring that sufficient numbers of trained pediatricians are available to provide optimal health care to all children. A shortage of pediatric medical subspecialists and pediatric surgical specialists currently exists in the United States, and this shortage is likely to intensify because of the growing numbers of children with chronic health problems and special health care needs. It is equally important to maintain the supply of primary care pediatricians. The AAP, therefore, recommends that children's hospital GME positions funded by the Health Resources and Services Administration be increased to address this escalating demand for pediatric health services. The AAP also recommends that GME funding for pediatric physician training provide full financial support for all years of training necessary to meet program requirements. In addition, all other entities that gain from GME training should participate in its funding in a manner that does not influence curriculum, requirements, or outcomes. Furthermore, the AAP supports funding for training innovations that improve the health of children. Finally, the AAP recommends that all institutional recipients of GME funding allocate these funds directly to the settings where training occurs in a transparent manner. (3/16)
http://pediatrics.aappublications.org/content/137/4/e20160211

FINANCING OF PEDIATRIC HOME HEALTH CARE

Edwin Simpser, MD, FAAP; Mark L. Hudak, MD, FAAP; Section on Home Care; and Committee on Child Health Financing

ABSTRACT. Pediatric home health care is an effective and holistic venue of treatment of children with medical complexity or developmental disabilities who otherwise may experience frequent and/or prolonged hospitalizations or who may enter chronic institutional care. Demand for pediatric home health care is increasing while the provider base is eroding, primarily because of inadequate payment or restrictions on benefits. As a result, home care responsibilities assumed by family caregivers have increased and imposed financial, physical, and psychological burdens on the family. The Patient Protection and Affordable Care Act set forth 10 mandated essential health benefits. Home care should be considered as an integral component of the habilitative and rehabilitative services and devices benefit, even though it is not explicitly recognized as a specific category of service. Pediatric-specific home health care services should be defined clearly as components of pediatric services, the 10th essential benefit, and recognized by all payers. Payments for home health care services should be sufficient to maintain an adequate provider work force with the pediatric-specific expertise and skills to care for children with medical complexity or developmental disability. Furthermore, coordination of care among various providers and the necessary direct patient care from which these care coordination plans are developed should be required and enabled by adequate payment. The American Academy of Pediatrics advocates for high-quality care by calling for development of pediatric-specific home health regulations and the licensure and certification of pediatric home health providers. (2/17)

http://pediatrics.aappublications.org/content/139/3/e20164202

FIREARM-RELATED INJURIES AFFECTING THE PEDIATRIC POPULATION

Council on Injury, Violence, and Poison Prevention Executive Committee

ABSTRACT. The absence of guns from children's homes and communities is the most reliable and effective measure to prevent firearm-related injuries in children and adolescents. Adolescent suicide risk is strongly associated with firearm availability. Safe gun storage (guns unloaded and locked, ammunition locked separately) reduces children's risk of injury. Physician counseling of parents about firearm safety appears to be effective, but firearm safety education programs directed at children are ineffective. The American Academy of Pediatrics continues to support a number of specific measures to reduce the destructive effects of guns in the lives of children and adolescents, including the regulation of the manufacture, sale, purchase, ownership, and use of firearms; a ban on semiautomatic assault weapons; and the strongest possible regulations of handguns for civilian use. (10/12, reaffirmed 12/16)

http://pediatrics.aappublications.org/content/130/5/e1416

FIREWORKS-RELATED INJURIES TO CHILDREN

Committee on Injury and Poison Prevention

ABSTRACT. An estimated 8500 individuals, approximately 45% of them children younger than 15 years, were treated in US hospital emergency departments during 1999 for fireworks-related injuries. The hands (40%), eyes (20%), and head and face (20%) are the body areas most often involved. Approximately one third of eye injuries from fireworks result in permanent blindness. During 1999, 16 people died as a result of injuries associated with fireworks. Every type of legally available consumer (so-called "safe and sane") firework has been associated with serious injury or death. In 1997, 20,100 fires were caused by fireworks, resulting in $22.7 million in direct property damage. Fireworks typically cause more fires in the United States on the Fourth of July than all other causes of fire combined on that day. Pediatricians should educate parents, children, community leaders, and others about the dangers of fireworks. Fireworks for individual private use should be banned. Children and their families should be encouraged to enjoy fireworks at public fireworks displays conducted by professionals rather than purchase fireworks for home or private use. (7/01, reaffirmed 1/05, 2/08, 10/11, 11/14)

http://pediatrics.aappublications.org/content/108/1/190

FISH, SHELLFISH, AND CHILDREN'S HEALTH: AN ASSESSMENT OF BENEFITS, RISKS, AND SUSTAINABILITY (TECHNICAL REPORT)

Aaron S. Bernstein, MD, MPH, FAAP; Emily Oken, MD, MPH; Sarah de Ferranti, MD, MPH, FAAP; Council on Environmental Health; and Committee on Nutrition

ABSTRACT. American children eat relatively little fish and shellfish in comparison with other sources of animal protein, despite the health benefits that eating fish and shellfish may confer. At the same time, fish and shellfish may be sources of toxicants. This report serves to inform pediatricians about available research that elucidates health risks and benefits associated with fish and shellfish consumption in childhood as well as the sustainability of fish and shellfish harvests. (5/19)

See full text on page 681.

https://pediatrics.aappublications.org/content/143/6/e20190999

FLUORIDE USE IN CARIES PREVENTION IN THE PRIMARY CARE SETTING (CLINICAL REPORT)

Melinda B. Clark, MD, FAAP; Rebecca L. Slayton, DDS, PhD; and Section on Oral Health

ABSTRACT. Dental caries remains the most common chronic disease of childhood in the United States. Caries is a largely preventable condition, and fluoride has proven effectiveness in the prevention of caries. The goals of this clinical report are to clarify the use of available fluoride modalities for caries prevention in the primary care setting and to assist pediatricians in using fluoride to achieve maximum protection against dental caries while minimizing the likelihood of enamel fluorosis. (8/14)

http://pediatrics.aappublications.org/content/134/3/626

FOLIC ACID FOR THE PREVENTION OF NEURAL TUBE DEFECTS

Committee on Genetics

ABSTRACT. The American Academy of Pediatrics endorses the US Public Health Service (USPHS) recommendation that all women capable of becoming pregnant consume 400 µg of folic acid daily to prevent neural tube defects (NTDs). Studies have demonstrated that periconceptional folic acid supplementation can prevent 50% or more of NTDs such as spina bifida and anencephaly. For women who have previously had an NTD-affected pregnancy, the Centers for Disease Control and Prevention (CDC) recommends increasing the intake of folic acid to 4000 µg per day beginning at least 1 month before conception and continuing through the first trimester. Implementation of these recommendations is essential for the primary prevention of these serious and disabling birth defects. Because fewer than 1 in 3 women consume the amount of folic acid recommended by the USPHS, the Academy notes that the prevention of NTDs depends on an urgent and effective campaign to close this prevention gap. (8/99, reaffirmed 9/16)

http://pediatrics.aappublications.org/content/104/2/325

FOLLOW-UP MANAGEMENT OF CHILDREN WITH TYMPANOSTOMY TUBES

Section on Otolaryngology and Bronchoesophagology

ABSTRACT. The follow-up care of children in whom tympanostomy tubes have been placed is shared by the pediatrician and the otolaryngologist. Guidelines are provided for routine follow-up evaluation, perioperative hearing assessment, and the identification of specific conditions and complications that warrant urgent otolaryngologic consultation. These guidelines have been developed by a consensus of expert opinions. (2/02)

http://pediatrics.aappublications.org/content/109/2/328

FOOD ADDITIVES AND CHILD HEALTH

Leonardo Trasande, MD, MPP, FAAP; Rachel M. Shaffer, MPH; Sheela Sathyanarayana, MD, MPH; and Council on Environmental Health

ABSTRACT. Our purposes with this policy statement and its accompanying technical report are to review and highlight emerging child health concerns related to the use of colorings, flavorings, and chemicals deliberately added to food during processing (direct food additives) as well as substances in food contact materials, including adhesives, dyes, coatings, paper, paperboard, plastic, and other polymers, which may contaminate food as part of packaging or manufacturing equipment (indirect food additives); to make reasonable recommendations that the pediatrician might be able to adopt into the guidance provided during pediatric visits; and to propose urgently needed reforms to the current regulatory process at the US Food and Drug Administration (FDA) for food additives. Concern regarding food additives has increased in the past 2 decades, in part because of studies in which authors document endocrine disruption and other adverse health effects. In some cases, exposure to these chemicals is disproportionate among minority and low-income populations. Regulation and oversight of many food additives is inadequate because of several key problems in the Federal Food, Drug, and Cosmetic Act. Current requirements for a "generally recognized as safe" (GRAS) designation are insufficient to ensure the safety of food additives and do not contain sufficient protections against conflict of interest. Additionally, the FDA does not have adequate authority to acquire data on chemicals on the market or reassess their safety for human health. These are critical weaknesses in the current regulatory system for food additives. Data about health effects of food additives on infants and children are limited or missing; however, in general, infants and children are more vulnerable to chemical exposures. Substantial improvements to the food additives regulatory system are urgently needed, including greatly strengthening or replacing the "generally recognized as safe" (GRAS) determination process, updating the scientific foundation of the FDA's safety assessment program, retesting all previously approved chemicals, and labeling direct additives with limited or no toxicity data. (7/18)

http://pediatrics.aappublications.org/content/142/2/e20181408

FOOD ADDITIVES AND CHILD HEALTH (TECHNICAL REPORT)

Leonardo Trasande, MD, MPP, FAAP; Rachel M. Shaffer, MPH; Sheela Sathyanarayana, MD, MPH; and Council on Environmental Health

ABSTRACT. Increasing scientific evidence suggests potential adverse effects on children's health from synthetic chemicals used as food additives, both those deliberately added to food during processing (direct) and those used in materials that may contaminate food as part of packaging or manufacturing (indirect). Concern regarding food additives has increased in the past 2 decades in part because of studies that increasingly document endocrine disruption and other adverse health effects. In some cases, exposure to these chemicals is disproportionate among minority and low-income populations. This report focuses on those food additives with the strongest scientific evidence for concern. Further research is needed to study effects of exposure over various points in the life course, and toxicity testing must be advanced to be able to better identify health concerns prior to widespread population exposure. The accompanying policy statement describes approaches policy makers and pediatricians can take to prevent the disease and disability that are increasingly being identified in relation to chemicals used as food additives, among other uses. (7/18)

http://pediatrics.aappublications.org/content/142/2/e20181410

FORGOING MEDICALLY PROVIDED NUTRITION AND HYDRATION IN CHILDREN (CLINICAL REPORT)

Douglas S. Diekema, MD, MPH; Jeffrey R. Botkin, MD, MPH; and Committee on Bioethics

ABSTRACT. There is broad consensus that withholding or withdrawing medical interventions is morally permissible when requested by competent patients or, in the case of patients without decision-making capacity, when the interventions no longer confer a benefit to the patient or when the burdens associated with the interventions outweigh the benefits received. The withdrawal or withholding of measures such as attempted resuscitation, ventilators, and critical care medications is common in the terminal care of adults and children. In the case of adults, a consensus has emerged in law and ethics that the medical administration of fluid and nutrition is not fundamentally different from other medical interventions such as use of ventilators; therefore, it can be forgone or withdrawn when a competent adult or legally authorized surrogate requests withdrawal or when the intervention no longer provides a net benefit to the patient. In pediatrics, forgoing or withdrawing medically administered fluids and nutrition has been more controversial because of the inability of children to make autonomous decisions and the emotional power of feeding as a basic element of the care of children. This statement reviews the medical, ethical, and legal issues relevant to the withholding or withdrawing of medically provided fluids and nutrition in children. The American Academy of Pediatrics concludes that the withdrawal of medically administered fluids and nutrition for pediatric patients is ethically acceptable in limited circumstances. Ethics consultation is strongly recommended when particularly difficult or controversial decisions are being considered. (7/09, reaffirmed 1/14)

http://pediatrics.aappublications.org/content/124/2/813

FRUIT JUICE IN INFANTS, CHILDREN, AND ADOLESCENTS: CURRENT RECOMMENDATIONS

Melvin B. Heyman, MD, FAAP; Steven A. Abrams, MD, FAAP; Section on Gastroenterology, Hepatology, and Nutrition; and Committee on Nutrition

ABSTRACT. Historically, fruit juice was recommended by pediatricians as a source of vitamin C and as an extra source of water for healthy infants and young children as their diets expanded to include solid foods with higher renal solute load. It was also sometimes recommended for children with constipation. Fruit juice is marketed as a healthy, natural source of vitamins and, in some instances, calcium. Because juice tastes good, children readily accept it. Although juice consumption has some benefits, it also has potential detrimental effects. High sugar content in juice contributes to increased calorie consumption and the risk of dental caries. In addition, the lack of protein and fiber in juice can predispose to inappropriate weight gain (too much or too little). Pediatricians need to be knowledgeable about juice to inform parents and patients on its appropriate uses. (5/17)

http://pediatrics.aappublications.org/content/139/6/e20170967

GASTROESOPHAGEAL REFLUX: MANAGEMENT GUIDANCE FOR THE PEDIATRICIAN (CLINICAL REPORT)

Jenifer R. Lightdale, MD, MPH; David A. Gremse, MD; and Section on Gastroenterology, Hepatology, and Nutrition

ABSTRACT. Recent comprehensive guidelines developed by the North American Society for Pediatric Gastroenterology, Hepatology, and Nutrition define the common entities of gastroesophageal reflux (GER) as the physiologic passage of gastric contents into the esophagus and gastroesophageal reflux disease (GERD) as reflux associated with troublesome symptoms or complications. The ability to distinguish between GER and GERD is increasingly important to implement best practices in the management of acid reflux in patients across all pediatric age groups, as children with GERD may benefit from further evaluation and treatment, whereas conservative recommendations are the only indicated therapy in those with uncomplicated physiologic reflux. This clinical report endorses the rigorously developed, well-referenced North American Society for Pediatric Gastroenterology, Hepatology, and Nutrition guidelines and likewise emphasizes important concepts for the general pediatrician. A key issue is distinguishing between clinical manifestations of GER and GERD in term infants, children, and adolescents to identify patients who can be managed with conservative treatment by the pediatrician and to refer patients who require consultation with the gastroenterologist. Accordingly, the evidence basis presented by the guidelines for diagnostic approaches as well as treatments is discussed. Lifestyle changes are emphasized as first-line therapy in both GER and GERD, whereas medications are explicitly indicated only for patients with GERD. Surgical therapies are reserved for children with intractable symptoms or who are at risk for life-threatening complications of GERD. Recent black box warnings from the US Food and Drug Administration are discussed, and caution is underlined when using promoters of gastric emptying and motility. Finally, attention is paid to increasing evidence of inappropriate prescriptions for proton pump inhibitors in the pediatric population. (4/13)

http://pediatrics.aappublications.org/content/131/5/e1684

GENERIC PRESCRIBING, GENERIC SUBSTITUTION, AND THERAPEUTIC SUBSTITUTION

Committee on Drugs

(5/87, reaffirmed 6/93, 5/96, 6/99, 5/01, 5/05, 10/08, 10/12, 9/19)

http://pediatrics.aappublications.org/content/79/5/835

GLOBAL CLIMATE CHANGE AND CHILDREN'S HEALTH

Council on Environmental Health

ABSTRACT. Rising global temperatures are causing major physical, chemical, and ecological changes in the planet. There is wide consensus among scientific organizations and climatologists that these broad effects, known as "climate change," are the result of contemporary human activity. Climate change poses threats to human health, safety, and security, and children are uniquely vulnerable to these threats. The effects of climate change on child health include: physical and psychological sequelae of weather disasters; increased heat stress; decreased air quality; altered disease patterns of some climate-sensitive infections; and food, water, and nutrient insecurity in vulnerable regions. The social foundations of children's mental and physical health are threatened by the specter of far-reaching effects of unchecked climate change, including community and global instability, mass migrations, and increased conflict. Given this knowledge, failure to take prompt, substantive action would be an act of injustice to all children. A paradigm shift in production and consumption of energy is both a necessity and an opportunity for major innovation, job creation, and significant, immediate associated health benefits. Pediatricians have a uniquely valuable role to play in the societal response to this global challenge. (10/15)

http://pediatrics.aappublications.org/content/136/5/992

GLOBAL CLIMATE CHANGE AND CHILDREN'S HEALTH (TECHNICAL REPORT)

Samantha Ahdoot, MD, FAAP; Susan E. Pacheco, MD, FAAP; and Council on Environmental Health

ABSTRACT. Rising global temperature is causing major physical, chemical, and ecological changes across the planet. There is wide consensus among scientific organizations and climatologists that these broad effects, known as climate change, are the result of contemporary human activity. Climate change poses threats to human health, safety, and security. Children are uniquely vulnerable to these threats. The effects of climate change on child health include physical and psychological sequelae of weather disasters, increased heat stress, decreased air quality, altered disease patterns of some climate-sensitive infections, and food, water, and nutrient insecurity in vulnerable regions. Prompt implementation of mitigation and adaptation strategies will protect children against worsening of the problem and its associated health effects. This technical report reviews the nature of climate change and its associated child health effects and supports the recommendations in the accompanying policy statement on climate change and children's health. (10/15)

http://pediatrics.aappublications.org/content/136/5/e1468

GLOBAL HUMAN TRAFFICKING AND CHILD VICTIMIZATION

Jordan Greenbaum, MD; Nia Bodrick, MD, MPH, FAAP; Committee on Child Abuse and Neglect; and Section on International Child Health

ABSTRACT. Trafficking of children for labor and sexual exploitation violates basic human rights and constitutes a major global public health problem. Pediatricians and other health care professionals may encounter victims who present with infections, injuries, posttraumatic stress disorder, suicidality, or a variety of other physical or behavioral health conditions. Preventing child trafficking, recognizing victimization, and intervening appropriately require a public health approach that incorporates rigorous research on the risk factors, health impact, and effective treatment options for child exploitation as well as implementation and evaluation of primary prevention programs. Health care professionals need training to recognize possible signs of exploitation and to intervene appropriately. They need to adopt a multidisciplinary, outward-focused approach to service provision, working with nonmedical professionals in the community to assist victims. Pediatricians also need to advocate for legislation and policies that promote child rights and victim services as well as those that address the social determinants of health, which influence the vulnerability to human trafficking. This policy statement outlines major issues regarding public policy, medical education, research, and collaboration in the area of child labor and sex trafficking and provides recommendations for future work. (11/17)

http://pediatrics.aappublications.org/content/140/6/e20173138

GUIDANCE FOR THE ADMINISTRATION OF MEDICATION IN SCHOOL

Council on School Health

ABSTRACT. Many children who take medications require them during the school day. This policy statement is designed to guide prescribing health care professionals, school physicians, and school health councils on the administration of medications to children at school. All districts and schools need to have policies and plans in place for safe, effective, and efficient administration of medications at school. Having full-time licensed registered nurses administering all routine and emergency medications in schools is the best situation. When a licensed registered nurse is not available, a licensed practical nurse may administer medications. When a nurse cannot administer medication in school, the American Academy of Pediatrics supports appropriate delegation of nursing services in the school setting. Delegation is a tool that may be used by the licensed registered school nurse to allow unlicensed assistive personnel to provide standardized, routine health services under the supervision of the nurse and on the basis of physician guidance and school nursing assessment of the unique needs of the individual child and the suitability of delegation of specific nursing tasks. Any delegation of nursing duties must be consistent with the requirements of state nurse practice acts, state regulations, and guidelines provided by professional nursing organizations. Long-term, emergency, and short-term medications; over-the-counter medications; alternative medications; and experimental drugs that are administered as part of a clinical trial are discussed in this statement. This statement has been endorsed by the American School Health Association. (9/09, reaffirmed 2/13)

http://pediatrics.aappublications.org/content/124/4/1244

GUIDANCE ON COMPLETING A WRITTEN ALLERGY AND ANAPHYLAXIS EMERGENCY PLAN (CLINICAL REPORT)

Julie Wang, MD, FAAP; Scott H. Sicherer, MD, FAAP; and Section on Allergy and Immunology

ABSTRACT. Anaphylaxis is a potentially life-threatening, severe allergic reaction. The immediate assessment of patients having an allergic reaction and prompt administration of epinephrine, if criteria for anaphylaxis are met, promote optimal outcomes. National and international guidelines for the management of anaphylaxis, including those for management of allergic reactions at school, as well as several clinical reports from the American Academy of Pediatrics, recommend the provision of written emergency action plans to those at risk of anaphylaxis, in addition to the prescription of epinephrine autoinjectors. This clinical report provides information to help health care providers understand the role of a written, personalized allergy and anaphylaxis emergency plan to enhance the care of children at risk of allergic reactions, including anaphylaxis. This report offers a comprehensive written plan, with advice on individualizing instructions to suit specific patient circumstances. (2/17)

http://pediatrics.aappublications.org/content/139/3/e20164005

GUIDANCE ON FORGOING LIFE-SUSTAINING MEDICAL TREATMENT

Kathryn L. Weise, MD, MA, FAAP; Alexander L. Okun, MD, FAAP; Brian S. Carter, MD, FAAP; Cindy W. Christian, MD, FAAP; Committee on Bioethics; Section on Hospice and Palliative Medicine; and Committee on Child Abuse and Neglect

ABSTRACT. Pediatric health care is practiced with the goal of promoting the best interests of the child. Treatment generally is rendered under a presumption in favor of sustaining life. However, in some circumstances, the balance of benefits and burdens to the child leads to an assessment that forgoing life-sustaining medical treatment (LSMT) is ethically supportable or advisable. Parents are given wide latitude in decision-making concerning end-of-life care for their children in most situations. Collaborative decision-making around LSMT is improved by thorough communication among all stakeholders, including medical staff, the family, and the patient, when possible, throughout the evolving course of the patient's illness. Clear communication of overall goals of care is advised to promote agreed-on plans, including resuscitation status. Perceived disagreement among the team of professionals may be stressful to families. At the same time, understanding the range of professional opinions behind treatment recommendations is critical to informing family decision-making. Input from specialists in palliative care, ethics, pastoral care, and other disciplines enhances support for families and medical staff when decisions to forgo LSMT are being considered. Understanding specific applicability of institutional, regional, state, and national regulations related to forgoing LSMT is important to practice ethically within existing legal frameworks. This guidance represents an update of the 1994 statement from the American Academy of Pediatrics on forgoing LSMT. (8/17)

http://pediatrics.aappublications.org/content/140/3/e20171905

GUIDANCE ON MANAGEMENT OF ASYMPTOMATIC NEONATES BORN TO WOMEN WITH ACTIVE GENITAL HERPES LESIONS (CLINICAL REPORT)

Committee on Infectious Diseases and Committee on Fetus and Newborn

ABSTRACT. Herpes simplex virus (HSV) infection of the neonate is uncommon, but genital herpes infections in adults are very common. Thus, although treating an infant with neonatal herpes is a relatively rare occurrence, managing infants potentially exposed to HSV at the time of delivery occurs more frequently. The risk of transmitting HSV to an infant during delivery is determined in part by the mother's previous immunity to HSV. Women with primary genital HSV infections who are shedding HSV at delivery are 10 to 30 times more likely to transmit the virus to their newborn infants than are women with recurrent HSV infection who are shedding virus at delivery. With the availability of commercial serological tests that reliably can distinguish type-specific HSV antibodies, it is now possible to determine the type of maternal infection and, thus, further refine management of infants delivered to women who have active genital HSV lesions. The management algorithm presented herein uses both serological and virological studies to determine the risk of HSV transmission to the neonate who is delivered to a mother with active herpetic genital lesions and tailors management accordingly. The algorithm does not address the approach to asymptomatic neonates delivered to women with a history of genital herpes but no active lesions at delivery. (1/13, reaffirmed 9/16)

http://pediatrics.aappublications.org/content/131/2/e635

GUIDELINES FOR DEVELOPING ADMISSION AND DISCHARGE POLICIES FOR THE PEDIATRIC INTENSIVE CARE UNIT (CLINICAL REPORT)

Committee on Hospital Care and Section on Critical Care (joint with Society of Critical Care Medicine Pediatric Section Admission Criteria Task Force)

ABSTRACT. These guidelines were developed to provide a reference for preparing policies on admission to and discharge from pediatric intensive care units. They represent a consensus opinion of physicians, nurses, and allied health care professionals. By using this document as a framework for developing multidisciplinary admission and discharge policies, use of pediatric intensive care units can be optimized and patients can receive the level of care appropriate for their condition. (4/99, reaffirmed 5/17)

http://pediatrics.aappublications.org/content/103/4/840

GUIDELINES FOR MONITORING AND MANAGEMENT OF PEDIATRIC PATIENTS BEFORE, DURING, AND AFTER SEDATION FOR DIAGNOSTIC AND THERAPEUTIC PROCEDURES

Charles J. Coté, MD, FAAP; Stephen Wilson, DMD, MA, PhD; and American Academy of Pediatrics (joint with American Academy of Pediatric Dentistry)

ABSTRACT. The safe sedation of children for procedures requires a systematic approach that includes the following: no administration of sedating medication without the safety net of medical/dental supervision, careful presedation evaluation for underlying medical or surgical conditions that would place the child at increased risk from sedating medications, appropriate fasting for elective procedures and a balance between the depth of sedation and risk for those who are unable to fast because of the urgent nature of the procedure, a focused airway examination for large (kissing) tonsils or anatomic airway abnormalities that might increase the potential for airway obstruction, a clear understanding of the medication's pharmacokinetic and pharmacodynamic effects and drug interactions, appropriate training and skills in airway management to allow rescue of the patient, age- and size-appropriate equipment for airway management and venous access, appropriate medications and reversal agents, sufficient numbers of appropriately trained staff to both carry out the procedure and monitor the patient, appropriate physiologic monitoring during and after the procedure, a properly equipped and staffed recovery area, recovery to the presedation level of consciousness before discharge from medical/dental supervision, and appropriate discharge instructions. This report was developed through a collaborative effort of the American Academy of Pediatrics and the American Academy of Pediatric Dentistry to offer pediatric providers updated information and guidance in delivering safe sedation to children. (5/19)

See full text on page 707.

https://pediatrics.aappublications.org/content/143/6/e20191000

GUIDELINES FOR PEDIATRIC CANCER CENTERS

Section on Hematology/Oncology

ABSTRACT. Since the American Academy of Pediatrics published guidelines for pediatric cancer centers in 1986 and 1997, significant changes in the delivery of health care have prompted a review of the role of tertiary medical centers in the care of pediatric patients. The potential effect of these changes on the treatment and survival rates of children with cancer led to this revision. The intent of this statement is to delineate personnel and facilities that are essential to provide state-of-the-art care for children and adolescents with cancer. This statement emphasizes the importance of board-certified pediatric hematologists/oncologists, pediatric subspecialty consultants, and appropriately qualified pediatric medical subspecialists and pediatric surgical specialists overseeing the care of all pediatric and adolescent cancer patients and the need for facilities available only at a tertiary center as essential for the initial management and much of the follow-up for pediatric and adolescent cancer patients. (6/04, reaffirmed 10/08, 10/18)

http://pediatrics.aappublications.org/content/113/6/1833

GUIDELINES FOR THE DETERMINATION OF BRAIN DEATH IN INFANTS AND CHILDREN: AN UPDATE OF THE 1987 TASK FORCE RECOMMENDATIONS (CLINICAL REPORT)

Thomas A. Nakagawa, MD; Stephen Ashwal, MD; Mudit Mathur, MD; Mohan Mysore, MD; Section on Critical Care; and Section on Neurology (joint with Society of Critical Care Medicine and Child Neurology Society)

ABSTRACT. *Objective.* To review and revise the 1987 pediatric brain death guidelines.

Methods. Relevant literature was reviewed. Recommendations were developed using the GRADE system.

Conclusions and Recommendations.

1. Determination of brain death in term newborns, infants and children is a clinical diagnosis based on the absence of neurologic function with a known irreversible cause of coma. Because of insufficient data in the literature, recommendations for preterm infants less than 37 weeks' gestational age are not included in this guideline.
2. Hypotension, hypothermia, and metabolic disturbances should be treated and corrected and medications that can interfere with the neurologic examination and apnea testing should be discontinued allowing for adequate clearance before proceeding with these evaluations.
3. Two examinations including apnea testing with each examination separated by an observation period are required. Examinations should be performed by different attending physicians. Apnea testing may be performed by the same physician. An observation period of 24 hours for term newborns (37 weeks' gestational age) to 30 days of age, and 12 hours for infants and children (> 30 days to 18 years) is recommended. The first examination determines the child has met the accepted neurologic examination criteria for brain death. The second examination confirms brain death based on an unchanged and irreversible condition. Assessment of neurologic function following cardiopulmonary resuscitation or other severe acute brain injuries should be deferred for 24 hours or longer if there are concerns or inconsistencies in the examination.
4. Apnea testing to support the diagnosis of brain death must be performed safely and requires documentation of an arterial $Paco_2$ 20 mm Hg above the baseline and ≥60 mm Hg with no respiratory effort during the testing period. If the apnea test cannot be safely completed, an ancillary study should be performed.
5. Ancillary studies (electroencephalogram and radionuclide cerebral blood flow) are not required to establish brain death and are not a substitute for the neurologic examination. Ancillary studies may be used to assist the clinician in making the diagnosis of brain death (1) when components of the examination or apnea testing cannot be completed safely due to the underlying medical condition of the patient; (2) if there is uncertainty about the results of the neurologic examination; (3) if a medication effect may be present; or (4) to reduce the inter-examination observation period. When ancillary studies are used, a second clinical examination and apnea test should be performed and components that can be completed must remain consistent with brain death. In this instance the observation interval may be shortened and the second neurologic examination and apnea test (or all components that are able to be completed safely) can be performed at any time thereafter.
6. Death is declared when the above criteria are fulfilled. (8/11, reaffirmed 1/15, 5/19)

http://pediatrics.aappublications.org/content/128/3/e720

GUIDELINES FOR THE ETHICAL CONDUCT OF STUDIES TO EVALUATE DRUGS IN PEDIATRIC POPULATIONS (CLINICAL REPORT)

Robert E. Shaddy, MD; Scott C. Denne, MD; Committee on Drugs; and Committee on Pediatric Research

ABSTRACT. The proper ethical conduct of studies to evaluate drugs in children is of paramount importance to all those involved in these types of studies. This report is an updated revision to the previously published guidelines from the American Academy of Pediatrics in 1995. Since the previous publication, there have been great strides made in the science and ethics of studying drugs in children. There have also been numerous legislative and regulatory advancements that have promoted the study of drugs in children while simultaneously allowing for the protection of this particularly vulnerable group. This report summarizes these changes and advances and provides a framework from which to guide and monitor the ethical conduct of studies to evaluate drugs in children. (3/10, reaffirmed 1/14, 2/18)

http://pediatrics.aappublications.org/content/125/4/850

GUIDING PRINCIPLES FOR MANAGED CARE ARRANGEMENTS FOR THE HEALTH CARE OF NEWBORNS, INFANTS, CHILDREN, ADOLESCENTS, AND YOUNG ADULTS

Committee on Child Health Financing

ABSTRACT. By including the precepts of primary care and the medical home in the delivery of services, managed care can be effective in increasing access to a full range of health care services and clinicians. A carefully designed and administered managed care plan can minimize patient under- and overutilization of services, as well as enhance quality of care. Therefore, the American Academy of Pediatrics urges the use of the key principles outlined in this statement in designing and implementing managed care programs for newborns, infants, children, adolescents, and young adults to maximize the positive potential of managed care for pediatrics. (10/13)

http://pediatrics.aappublications.org/content/132/5/e1452

GUIDING PRINCIPLES FOR PEDIATRIC HOSPITAL MEDICINE PROGRAMS

Section on Hospital Medicine

ABSTRACT. Pediatric hospital medicine programs have an established place in pediatric medicine. This statement speaks to the expanded roles and responsibilities of pediatric hospitalists and their integrated role among the community of pediatricians who care for children within and outside of the hospital setting. (9/13, reaffirmed 10/17)

http://pediatrics.aappublications.org/content/132/4/782

GUIDING PRINCIPLES FOR TEAM-BASED PEDIATRIC CARE

Julie P. Katkin, MD, FAAP; Susan J. Kressly, MD, FAAP; Anne R. Edwards, MD, FAAP; James M. Perrin, MD, FAAP; Colleen A. Kraft, MD, FAAP; Julia E. Richerson, MD, FAAP; Joel S. Tieder, MD, MPH, FAAP; Liz Wall; and Task Force on Pediatric Practice Change

ABSTRACT. The American Academy of Pediatrics (AAP) recognizes that children's unique and ever-changing needs depend on a variety of support systems. Key components of effective support systems address the needs of the child and family in the context of their home and community and are dynamic so that they reflect, monitor, and respond to changes as the needs of the child and family change. The AAP believes that team-based care involving medical providers and community partners (eg, teachers and state agencies) is a crucial and necessary component of providing high-quality care to children and their families. Team-based care builds on the foundation of the medical home by reaching out to a potentially broad array of participants in the life of a child and incorporating them into the care provided. Importantly, the AAP believes that a high-functioning team includes children and their families as essential partners. The overall goal of team-based care is to enhance communication and cooperation among the varied medical, social, and educational partners in a child's life to better meet the global needs of children and their families, helping them to achieve their best potential. In support of the team-based approach, the AAP urges stakeholders to invest in infrastructure, education, and privacy-secured technology to meet the needs of children. This statement includes limited specific examples of potential team members, including health care providers and community partners, that are meant to be illustrative and in no way represent a complete or comprehensive listing of all team members who may be of importance for a specific child and family. (7/17)

http://pediatrics.aappublications.org/content/140/2/e20171489

GYNECOLOGIC EXAMINATION FOR ADOLESCENTS IN THE PEDIATRIC OFFICE SETTING (CLINICAL REPORT)

Paula K. Braverman, MD; Lesley Breech, MD; and Committee on Adolescence

ABSTRACT. The American Academy of Pediatrics promotes the inclusion of the gynecologic examination in the primary care setting within the medical home. Gynecologic issues are commonly seen by clinicians who provide primary care to adolescents. Some of the most common concerns include questions related to pubertal development; menstrual disorders such as dysmenorrhea, amenorrhea, oligomenorrhea, and abnormal uterine bleeding; contraception; and sexually transmitted and non–sexually transmitted infections. The gynecologic examination is a key element in assessing pubertal status and documenting physical findings. Most adolescents do not need an internal examination involving a speculum or bimanual examination. However, for cases in which more extensive examination is needed, the primary care office with the primary care clinician who has established rapport and trust with the patient is often the best setting for pelvic examination. This report reviews the gynecologic examination, including indications for the pelvic examination in adolescents and the approach to this examination in the office setting. Indications for referral to a gynecologist are included. The pelvic examination may be successfully completed when conducted without pressure and approached as a normal part of routine young women's health care. (8/10, reaffirmed 5/13)

http://pediatrics.aappublications.org/content/126/3/583

HANDOFFS: TRANSITIONS OF CARE FOR CHILDREN IN THE EMERGENCY DEPARTMENT

Committee on Pediatric Emergency Medicine (joint with American College of Emergency Physicians Pediatric Emergency Medicine Committee and Emergency Nurses Association Pediatric Committee)

ABSTRACT. Transitions of care (ToCs), also referred to as handoffs or sign-outs, occur when the responsibility for a patient's care transfers from 1 health care provider to another. Transitions are common in the acute care setting and have been noted to be vulnerable events with opportunities for error. Health care is taking ideas from other high-risk industries, such as aerospace and nuclear power, to create models of structured transition processes. Although little literature currently exists to establish 1 model as superior, multiorganizational consensus groups agree that standardization is warranted and that additional work is needed to establish characteristics of ToCs that are associated with clinical or practice outcomes. The rationale for structuring ToCs, specifically those related to the care of children in the emergency setting, and a description of identified strategies are presented, along with resources for educating health care providers on ToCs. Recommendations for development, education, and implementation of transition models are included. (10/16)

http://pediatrics.aappublications.org/content/138/5/e20162680

HEAD LICE (CLINICAL REPORT)

Cynthia D. Devore, MD, FAAP; Gordon E. Schutze, MD, FAAP; Council on School Health; and Committee on Infectious Diseases

ABSTRACT. Head lice infestation is associated with limited morbidity but causes a high level of anxiety among parents of school-aged children. Since the 2010 clinical report on head lice was published by the American Academy of Pediatrics, newer medications have been approved for the treatment of head lice. This revised clinical report clarifies current diagnosis and treatment protocols and provides guidance for the management of children with head lice in the school setting. (4/15)

http://pediatrics.aappublications.org/content/135/5/e1355

HEALTH AND MENTAL HEALTH NEEDS OF CHILDREN IN US MILITARY FAMILIES (CLINICAL REPORT)

CDR Chadley R. Huebner, MD, MPH, FAAP; Section on Uniformed Services; and Committee on Psychosocial Aspects of Child and Family Health

ABSTRACT. Children in US military families share common experiences and unique challenges, including parental deployment and frequent relocation. Although some of the stressors of military life have been associated with higher rates of mental health disorders and increased health care use among family members, there are various factors and interventions that have been found to promote resilience. Military children often live on or near military installations, where they may attend Department of Defense–sponsored child care programs and schools and receive medical care through military treatment facilities. However, many families live in remote communities without access to these services. Because of this wide geographic distribution, military children are cared for in both military and civilian medical practices. This clinical report provides a background to military culture and offers practical guidance to assist civilian and military pediatricians caring for military children. (12/18)

See full text on page 741.

https://pediatrics.aappublications.org/content/143/1/e20183258

HEALTH CARE ISSUES FOR CHILDREN AND ADOLESCENTS IN FOSTER CARE AND KINSHIP CARE

Council on Foster Care, Adoption, and Kinship Care; Committee on Adolescence; and Council on Early Childhood

ABSTRACT. Children and adolescents who enter foster care often do so with complicated and serious medical, mental health, developmental, oral health, and psychosocial problems rooted in their history of childhood trauma. Ideally, health care for this population is provided in a pediatric medical home by physicians who are familiar with the sequelae of childhood trauma and adversity. As youth with special health care needs, children and adolescents in foster care require more frequent monitoring of their health status, and pediatricians have a critical role in ensuring the well-being of children in out-of-home care through the provision of high-quality pediatric health services, health care coordination, and advocacy on their behalves. (9/15)

http://pediatrics.aappublications.org/content/136/4/e1131

HEALTH CARE ISSUES FOR CHILDREN AND ADOLESCENTS IN FOSTER CARE AND KINSHIP CARE (TECHNICAL REPORT)

Moira A. Szilagyi, MD, PhD; David S. Rosen, MD, MPH; David Rubin, MD, MSCE; Sarah Zlotnik, MSW, MSPH; Council on Foster Care, Adoption, and Kinship Care; Committee on Adolescence; and Council on Early Childhood

ABSTRACT. Children and adolescents involved with child welfare, especially those who are removed from their family of origin and placed in out-of-home care, often present with complex and serious physical, mental health, developmental, and psychosocial problems rooted in childhood adversity and trauma. As such, they are designated as children with special health care needs. There are many barriers to providing high-quality comprehensive health care services to children and adolescents whose lives are characterized by transience and uncertainty. Pediatricians have a critical role in ensuring the well-being of children in out-of-home care through the provision of high-quality pediatric health services in the context of a medical home, and health care coordination and advocacy on their behalf. This technical report supports the policy statement of the same title. (9/15)

http://pediatrics.aappublications.org/content/136/4/e1142

HEALTH CARE OF YOUTH AGING OUT OF FOSTER CARE

Council on Foster Care, Adoption, and Kinship Care and Committee on Early Childhood

ABSTRACT. Youth transitioning out of foster care face significant medical and mental health care needs. Unfortunately, these youth rarely receive the services they need because of lack of health insurance. Through many policies and programs, the federal government has taken steps to support older youth in foster care and those aging out. The Fostering Connections to Success and Increasing Adoptions Act of 2008 (Pub L No. 110-354) requires states to work with youth to develop a transition plan that addresses issues such as health insurance. In addition, beginning in 2014, the Patient Protection and Affordable Care Act of 2010 (Pub L No. 111-148) makes youth aging out of foster care eligible for Medicaid coverage until age 26 years, regardless of income. Pediatricians can support youth aging out of foster care by working collaboratively with the child welfare agency in their state to ensure that the ongoing health needs of transitioning youth are met. (11/12, reaffirmed 7/17)

http://pediatrics.aappublications.org/content/130/6/1170

HEALTH CARE SUPERVISION FOR CHILDREN WITH WILLIAMS SYNDROME

Committee on Genetics

ABSTRACT. This set of guidelines is designed to assist the pediatrician to care for children with Williams syndrome diagnosed by clinical features and with regional chromosomal microdeletion confirmed by fluorescence in situ hybridization. (5/01, reaffirmed 5/05, 1/09)

http://pediatrics.aappublications.org/content/107/5/1192

HEALTH INFORMATION TECHNOLOGY AND THE MEDICAL HOME

Council on Clinical Information Technology

ABSTRACT. The American Academy of Pediatrics (AAP) supports development and universal implementation of a comprehensive electronic infrastructure to support pediatric information functions of the medical home. These functions include (1) timely and continuous management and tracking of health data and services over a patient's lifetime for all providers, patients, families, and guardians, (2) comprehensive organization and secure transfer of health data during patient-care transitions between providers, institutions, and practices, (3) establishment and maintenance of central coordination of a patient's health information among multiple repositories (including personal health records and information exchanges), (4) translation of evidence into actionable clinical decision support, and (5) reuse of archived clinical data for continuous quality improvement. The AAP supports universal, secure, and vendor-neutral portability of health information for all patients contained within the medical home across all care settings (ambulatory practices, inpatient settings, emergency departments, pharmacies, consultants, support service providers, and therapists) for multiple purposes including direct care, personal health records, public health, and registries. The AAP also supports financial incentives that promote the development of information tools that meet the needs of pediatric workflows and that appropriately recognize the added value of medical homes to pediatric care. (4/11, reaffirmed 7/15)

http://pediatrics.aappublications.org/content/127/5/978

HEALTH SUPERVISION FOR CHILDREN WITH ACHONDROPLASIA (CLINICAL REPORT)

Tracy L. Trotter, MD; Judith G. Hall, OC, MD; and Committee on Genetics

ABSTRACT. Achondroplasia is the most common condition associated with disproportionate short stature. Substantial information is available concerning the natural history and anticipa-

tory health supervision needs in children with this dwarfing disorder. Most children with achondroplasia have delayed motor milestones, problems with persistent or recurrent middle-ear dysfunction, and bowing of the lower legs. Less often, infants and children may have serious health consequences related to hydrocephalus, craniocervical junction compression, upper-airway obstruction, or thoracolumbar kyphosis. Anticipatory care should be directed at identifying children who are at high risk and intervening to prevent serious sequelae. This report is designed to help the pediatrician care for children with achondroplasia and their families. (9/05, reaffirmed 5/12)
http://pediatrics.aappublications.org/content/116/3/771

HEALTH SUPERVISION FOR CHILDREN WITH DOWN SYNDROME (CLINICAL REPORT)

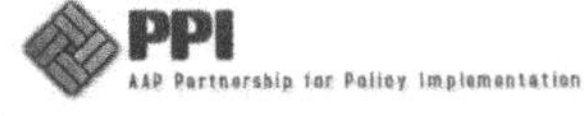

Marilyn J. Bull, MD, and Committee on Genetics
ABSTRACT. These guidelines are designed to assist the pediatrician in caring for the child in whom a diagnosis of Down syndrome has been confirmed by chromosome analysis. Although a pediatrician's initial contact with the child is usually during infancy, occasionally the pregnant woman who has been given a prenatal diagnosis of Down syndrome will be referred for review of the condition and the genetic counseling provided. Therefore, this report offers guidance for this situation as well. (7/11, reaffirmed 9/16, 1/18)
http://pediatrics.aappublications.org/content/128/2/393

HEALTH SUPERVISION FOR CHILDREN WITH FRAGILE X SYNDROME (CLINICAL REPORT)

Joseph H. Hersh, MD; Robert A. Saul, MD; and Committee on Genetics
ABSTRACT. Fragile X syndrome (an *FMR1*–related disorder) is the most commonly inherited form of mental retardation. Early physical recognition is difficult, so boys with developmental delay should be strongly considered for molecular testing. The characteristic adult phenotype usually does not develop until the second decade of life. Girls can also be affected with developmental delay. Because multiple family members can be affected with mental retardation and other conditions (premature ovarian failure and tremor/ataxia), family history information is of critical importance for the diagnosis and management of affected patients and their families. This report summarizes issues for fragile X syndrome regarding clinical diagnosis, laboratory diagnosis, genetic counseling, related health problems, behavior management, and age-related health supervision guidelines. The diagnosis of fragile X syndrome not only involves the affected children but also potentially has significant health consequences for multiple generations in each family. (4/11)
http://pediatrics.aappublications.org/content/127/5/994

HEALTH SUPERVISION FOR CHILDREN WITH MARFAN SYNDROME (CLINICAL REPORT)

Brad T. Tinkle, MD, PhD; Howard M. Saal, MD; and Committee on Genetics
ABSTRACT. Marfan syndrome is a systemic, heritable connective tissue disorder that affects many different organ systems and is best managed by using a multidisciplinary approach. The guidance in this report is designed to assist the pediatrician in recognizing the features of Marfan syndrome as well as caring for the individual with this disorder. (9/13)
http://pediatrics.aappublications.org/content/132/4/e1059

HEALTH SUPERVISION FOR CHILDREN WITH NEUROFIBROMATOSIS TYPE 1 (CLINICAL REPORT)

David T. Miller, MD, PhD, FAAP; Debra Freedenberg, MD, PhD, FAAP; Elizabeth Schorry, MD; Nicole J. Ullrich, MD, PhD; David Viskochil, MD, PhD; Bruce R. Korf, MD, PhD, FAAP; and Council on Genetics (joint with American College of Medical Genetics and Genomics)
ABSTRACT. Neurofibromatosis type 1 (NF1) is a multisystem disorder that primarily involves the skin and peripheral nervous system. Its population prevalence is approximately 1 in 3000. The condition is usually recognized in early childhood, when pigmentary manifestations emerge. Although NF1 is associated with marked clinical variability, most children affected follow patterns of growth and development within the normal range. Some features of NF1 can be present at birth, but most manifestations emerge with age, necessitating periodic monitoring to address ongoing health and developmental needs and minimize the risk of serious medical complications. In this report, we provide a review of the clinical criteria needed to establish a diagnosis, the inheritance pattern of NF1, its major clinical and developmental manifestations, and guidelines for monitoring and providing intervention to maximize the health and quality of life of a child affected. (4/19)
See full text on page 757.
https://pediatrics.aappublications.org/content/143/5/e20190660

HEALTH SUPERVISION FOR CHILDREN WITH PRADER-WILLI SYNDROME (CLINICAL REPORT)

Shawn E. McCandless, MD, and Committee on Genetics
ABSTRACT. This set of guidelines was designed to assist the pediatrician in caring for children with Prader-Willi syndrome diagnosed by clinical features and confirmed by molecular testing. Prader-Willi syndrome provides an excellent example of how early diagnosis and management can improve the long-term outcome for some genetic disorders. (12/10)
http://pediatrics.aappublications.org/content/127/1/195

HEALTH SUPERVISION FOR CHILDREN WITH SICKLE CELL DISEASE

Section on Hematology/Oncology and Committee on Genetics
ABSTRACT. Sickle cell disease (SCD) is a group of complex genetic disorders with multisystem manifestations. This statement provides pediatricians in primary care and subspecialty practice with an overview of the genetics, diagnosis, clinical manifestations, and treatment of SCD. Specialized comprehensive medical care decreases morbidity and mortality during childhood. The provision of comprehensive care is a time-intensive endeavor that includes ongoing patient and family education, periodic comprehensive evaluations and other disease-specific health maintenance services, psychosocial care, and genetic counseling. Timely and appropriate treatment of acute illness is critical, because life-threatening complications develop rapidly. It is essential that every child with SCD receive comprehensive care that is coordinated through a medical home with appropriate expertise. (3/02, reaffirmed 1/06, 1/11, 2/16)
http://pediatrics.aappublications.org/content/109/3/526

HELPING CHILDREN AND FAMILIES DEAL WITH DIVORCE AND SEPARATION (CLINICAL REPORT)

George J. Cohen, MD, FAAP; Carol C. Weitzman, MD, FAAP; Committee on Psychosocial Aspects of Child and Family Health; and Section on Developmental and Behavioral Pediatrics
ABSTRACT. For the past several years in the United States, there have been more than 800 000 divorces and parent separations annually, with over 1 million children affected. Children and their parents can experience emotional trauma before, during,

and after a separation or divorce. Pediatricians can be aware of their patients' behavior and parental attitudes and behaviors that may indicate family dysfunction and that can indicate need for intervention. Age-appropriate explanation and counseling for the child and advice and guidance for the parents, as well as recommendation of reading material, may help reduce the potential negative effects of divorce. Often, referral to professionals with expertise in the social, emotional, and legal aspects of the separation and its aftermath may be helpful for these families. (11/16)
http://pediatrics.aappublications.org/content/138/6/e20163020

HIGH-DEDUCTIBLE HEALTH PLANS

Committee on Child Health Financing

ABSTRACT. High-deductible health plans (HDHPs) are insurance policies with higher deductibles than conventional plans. The Medicare Prescription Drug Improvement and Modernization Act of 2003 linked many HDHPs with tax-advantaged spending accounts. The 2010 Patient Protection and Affordable Care Act continues to provide for HDHPs in its lower-level plans on the health insurance marketplace and provides for them in employer-offered plans. HDHPs decrease the premium cost of insurance policies for purchasers and shift the risk of further payments to the individual subscriber. HDHPs reduce utilization and total medical costs, at least in the short term. Because HDHPs require out-of-pocket payment in the initial stages of care, primary care and other outpatient services as well as elective procedures are the services most affected, whereas higher-cost services in the health care system, incurred after the deductible is met, are unaffected. HDHPs promote adverse selection because healthier and wealthier patients tend to opt out of conventional plans in favor of HDHPs. Because the ill pay more than the healthy under HDHPs, families with children with special health care needs bear an increased cost burden in this model. HDHPs discourage use of nonpreventive primary care and thus are at odds with most recommendations for improving the organization of health care, which focus on strengthening primary care.

This policy statement provides background information on HDHPs, discusses the implications for families and pediatric care providers, and suggests courses of action. (4/14, reaffirmed 10/18)
http://pediatrics.aappublications.org/content/133/5/e1461

HIV TESTING AND PROPHYLAXIS TO PREVENT MOTHER-TO-CHILD TRANSMISSION IN THE UNITED STATES

Committee on Pediatric AIDS

ABSTRACT. Universal HIV testing of pregnant women in the United States is the key to prevention of mother-to-child transmission of HIV. Repeat testing in the third trimester and rapid HIV testing at labor and delivery are additional strategies to further reduce the rate of perinatal HIV transmission. Prevention of mother-to-child transmission of HIV is most effective when antiretroviral drugs are received by the mother during her pregnancy and continued through delivery and then administered to the infant after birth. Antiretroviral drugs are effective in reducing the risk of mother-to-child transmission of HIV even when prophylaxis is started for the infant soon after birth. New rapid testing methods allow identification of HIV-infected women or HIV-exposed infants in 20 to 60 minutes. The American Academy of Pediatrics recommends documented, routine HIV testing for all pregnant women in the United States after notifying the patient that testing will be performed, unless the patient declines HIV testing ("opt-out" consent or "right of refusal"). For women in labor with undocumented HIV-infection status during the current pregnancy, immediate maternal HIV testing with opt-out consent, using a rapid HIV antibody test, is recommended. Positive HIV antibody screening test results should be confirmed with immunofluorescent antibody or Western blot assay. For women with a positive rapid HIV antibody test result, antiretroviral prophylaxis should be administered promptly to the mother and newborn infant on the basis of the positive result of the rapid antibody test without waiting for results of confirmatory HIV testing. If the confirmatory test result is negative, then prophylaxis should be discontinued. For a newborn infant whose mother's HIV serostatus is unknown, the health care professional should perform rapid HIV antibody testing on the mother or on the newborn infant, with results reported to the health care professional no later than 12 hours after the infant's birth. If the rapid HIV antibody test result is positive, antiretroviral prophylaxis should be instituted as soon as possible after birth but certainly by 12 hours after delivery, pending completion of confirmatory HIV testing. The mother should be counseled not to breastfeed the infant. Assistance with immediate initiation of hand and pump expression to stimulate milk production should be offered to the mother, given the possibility that the confirmatory test result may be negative. If the confirmatory test result is negative, then prophylaxis should be stopped and breastfeeding may be initiated. If the confirmatory test result is positive, infants should receive antiretroviral prophylaxis for 6 weeks after birth, and the mother should not breastfeed the infant. (11/08, reaffirmed 6/11, 11/14)
http://pediatrics.aappublications.org/content/122/5/1127

HOME CARE OF CHILDREN AND YOUTH WITH COMPLEX HEALTH CARE NEEDS AND TECHNOLOGY DEPENDENCIES (CLINICAL REPORT)

Ellen Roy Elias, MD; Nancy A. Murphy, MD; and Council on Children With Disabilities

ABSTRACT. Children and youth with complex medical issues, especially those with technology dependencies, experience frequent and often lengthy hospitalizations. Hospital discharges for these children can be a complicated process that requires a deliberate, multistep approach. In addition to successful discharges to home, it is essential that pediatric providers develop and implement an interdisciplinary and coordinated plan of care that addresses the child's ongoing health care needs. The goal is to ensure that each child remains healthy, thrives, and obtains optimal medical home and developmental supports that promote ongoing care at home and minimize recurrent hospitalizations. This clinical report presents an approach to discharging the child with complex medical needs with technology dependencies from hospital to home and then continually addressing the needs of the child and family in the home environment. (4/12, reaffirmed 5/17)
http://pediatrics.aappublications.org/content/129/5/996

HONORING DO-NOT-ATTEMPT-RESUSCITATION REQUESTS IN SCHOOLS

Council on School Health and Committee on Bioethics

ABSTRACT. Increasingly, children and adolescents with complex chronic conditions are living in the community. Federal legislation and regulations facilitate their participation in school. Some of these children and adolescents and their families may wish to forego life-sustaining medical treatment, including cardiopulmonary resuscitation, because they would be ineffective or because the risks outweigh the benefits. Honoring these requests in the school environment is complex because of the limited availability of school nurses and the frequent lack of supporting state legislation and regulations. Understanding and collaboration on the part of all parties is essential. Pediatricians have an important role in helping school nurses incorporate a specific action plan into the student's individualized health care plan. The action plan should include both communication and comfort-care plans. Pediatricians who work directly with schools can also help implement policies, and professional organizations can advocate for regulations and legislation that enable students

and their families to effectuate their preferences. (4/10, reaffirmed 7/13, 8/16)
http://pediatrics.aappublications.org/content/125/5/1073

HOSPITAL DISCHARGE OF THE HIGH-RISK NEONATE

Committee on Fetus and Newborn

ABSTRACT. This policy statement updates the guidelines on discharge of the high-risk neonate first published by the American Academy of Pediatrics in 1998. As with the earlier document, this statement is based, insofar as possible, on published, scientifically derived information. This updated statement incorporates new knowledge about risks and medical care of the high-risk neonate, the timing of discharge, and planning for care after discharge. It also refers to other American Academy of Pediatrics publications that are relevant to these issues. This statement draws on the previous classification of high-risk infants into 4 categories: (1) the preterm infant; (2) the infant with special health care needs or dependence on technology; (3) the infant at risk because of family issues; and (4) the infant with anticipated early death. The issues of deciding when discharge is appropriate, defining the specific needs for follow-up care, and the process of detailed discharge planning are addressed as they apply in general to all 4 categories; in addition, special attention is directed to the particular issues presented by the 4 individual categories. Recommendations are given to aid in deciding when discharge is appropriate and to ensure that all necessary care will be available and well coordinated after discharge. The need for individualized planning and physician judgment is emphasized. (11/08, reaffirmed 5/11, 11/18)
http://pediatrics.aappublications.org/content/122/5/1119

THE HOSPITAL RECORD OF THE INJURED CHILD AND THE NEED FOR EXTERNAL CAUSE-OF-INJURY CODES

Committee on Injury and Poison Prevention

ABSTRACT. Proper record-keeping of emergency department visits and hospitalizations of injured children is vital for appropriate patient management. Determination and documentation of the circumstances surrounding the injury event are essential. This information not only is the basis for preventive counseling, but also provides clues about how similar injuries in other youth can be avoided. The hospital records have an important secondary purpose; namely, if sufficient information about the cause and mechanism of injury is documented, it can be subsequently coded, electronically compiled, and retrieved later to provide an epidemiologic profile of the injury, the first step in prevention at the population level. To be of greatest use, hospital records should indicate the "who, what, when, where, why, and how" of the injury occurrence and whether protective equipment (eg, a seat belt) was used. The pediatrician has two important roles in this area: to document fully the injury event and to advocate the use of standardized external cause-of-injury codes, which allow such data to be compiled and analyzed. (2/99, reaffirmed 5/02, 5/05, 10/08, 10/13)
http://pediatrics.aappublications.org/content/103/2/524

HOSPITAL STAY FOR HEALTHY TERM NEWBORN INFANTS

William E. Benitz, MD, FAAP, and Committee on Fetus and Newborn

ABSTRACT. The hospital stay of the mother and her healthy term newborn infant should be long enough to allow identification of problems and to ensure that the mother is sufficiently recovered and prepared to care for herself and her newborn at home. The length of stay should be based on the unique characteristics of each mother-infant dyad, including the health of the mother, the health and stability of the newborn, the ability and confidence of the mother to care for herself and her newborn, the adequacy of support systems at home, and access to appropriate follow-up care in a medical home. Input from the mother and her obstetrical care provider should be considered before a decision to discharge a newborn is made, and all efforts should be made to keep a mother and her newborn together to ensure simultaneous discharge. (4/15)
http://pediatrics.aappublications.org/content/135/5/948

HUMAN EMBRYONIC STEM CELL (HESC) AND HUMAN EMBRYO RESEARCH

Committee on Pediatric Research and Committee on Bioethics

ABSTRACT. Human embryonic stem cell research has emerged as an important platform for the understanding and treatment of pediatric diseases. From its inception, however, it has raised ethical concerns based not on the use of stem cells themselves but on objections to the source of the cells—specifically, the destruction of preimplantation human embryos. Despite differences in public opinion on this issue, a large majority of the public supports continued research using embryonic stem cells. Given the possible substantial benefit of stem cell research on child health and development, the American Academy of Pediatrics believes that funding and oversight for human embryo and embryonic stem cell research should continue. (10/12, reaffirmed 7/17)
http://pediatrics.aappublications.org/content/130/5/972

HUMAN IMMUNODEFICIENCY VIRUS AND OTHER BLOOD-BORNE VIRAL PATHOGENS IN THE ATHLETIC SETTING

Committee on Sports Medicine and Fitness

ABSTRACT. Because athletes and the staff of athletic programs can be exposed to blood during athletic activity, they have a very small risk of becoming infected with human immunodeficiency virus, hepatitis B virus, or hepatitis C virus. This statement, which updates a previous position statement of the American Academy of Pediatrics, discusses sports participation for athletes infected with these pathogens and the precautions needed to reduce the risk of infection to others in the athletic setting. Each of the recommendations in this statement is dependent upon and intended to be considered with reference to the other recommendations in this statement and not in isolation. (12/99, reaffirmed 1/05, 1/09, 11/11, 2/15)
http://pediatrics.aappublications.org/content/104/6/1400

HYPOTHERMIA AND NEONATAL ENCEPHALOPATHY (CLINICAL REPORT)

Committee on Fetus and Newborn

ABSTRACT. Data from large randomized clinical trials indicate that therapeutic hypothermia, using either selective head cooling or systemic cooling, is an effective therapy for neonatal encephalopathy. Infants selected for cooling must meet the criteria outlined in published clinical trials. The implementation of cooling needs to be performed at centers that have the capability to manage medically complex infants. Because the majority of infants who have neonatal encephalopathy are born at community hospitals, centers that perform cooling should work with their referring hospitals to implement education programs focused on increasing the awareness and identification of infants at risk for encephalopathy, and the initial clinical management of affected infants. (5/14)
http://pediatrics.aappublications.org/content/133/6/1146

IDENTIFICATION AND CARE OF HIV-EXPOSED AND HIV-INFECTED INFANTS, CHILDREN, AND ADOLESCENTS IN FOSTER CARE

Committee on Pediatric AIDS

ABSTRACT. As a consequence of the expanding human immunodeficiency virus (HIV) epidemic and major advances in medical management of HIV-exposed and HIV-infected persons, revised recommendations are provided for HIV testing of infants, children, and adolescents in foster care. Updated recommendations

also are provided for the care of HIV-exposed and HIV-infected persons who are in foster care. (7/00, reaffirmed 12/16)
http://pediatrics.aappublications.org/content/106/1/149

IDENTIFICATION AND EVALUATION OF CHILDREN WITH AUTISM SPECTRUM DISORDERS (CLINICAL REPORT)

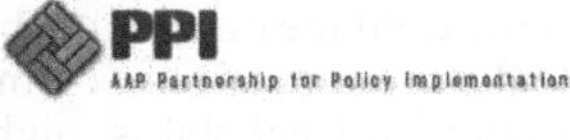

Chris Plauché Johnson, MD, MEd; Scott M. Myers, MD; and Council on Children With Disabilities

ABSTRACT. Autism spectrum disorders are not rare; many primary care pediatricians care for several children with autism spectrum disorders. Pediatricians play an important role in early recognition of autism spectrum disorders, because they usually are the first point of contact for parents. Parents are now much more aware of the early signs of autism spectrum disorders because of frequent coverage in the media; if their child demonstrates any of the published signs, they will most likely raise their concerns to their child's pediatrician. It is important that pediatricians be able to recognize the signs and symptoms of autism spectrum disorders and have a strategy for assessing them systematically. Pediatricians also must be aware of local resources that can assist in making a definitive diagnosis of, and in managing, autism spectrum disorders. The pediatrician must be familiar with developmental, educational, and community resources as well as medical subspecialty clinics. This clinical report is 1 of 2 documents that replace the original American Academy of Pediatrics policy statement and technical report published in 2001. This report addresses background information, including definition, history, epidemiology, diagnostic criteria, early signs, neuropathologic aspects, and etiologic possibilities in autism spectrum disorders. In addition, this report provides an algorithm to help the pediatrician develop a strategy for early identification of children with autism spectrum disorders. The accompanying clinical report addresses the management of children with autism spectrum disorders and follows this report on page 1162 [available at www.pediatrics.org/cgi/content/full/120/5/1162]. Both clinical reports are complemented by the toolkit titled *"Autism: Caring for Children With Autism Spectrum Disorders: A Resource Toolkit for Clinicians,"* which contains screening and surveillance tools, practical forms, tables, and parent handouts to assist the pediatrician in the identification, evaluation, and management of autism spectrum disorders in children. (11/07, reaffirmed 9/10, 8/14)
http://pediatrics.aappublications.org/content/120/5/1183

IDENTIFYING CHILD ABUSE FATALITIES DURING INFANCY (CLINICAL REPORT)

Vincent J. Palusci, MD, MS, FAAP; Amanda J. Kay, MD, MPH, FAAP; Erich Batra, MD, FAAP; Rachel Y. Moon, MD, FAAP; Council on Child Abuse and Neglect; Section on Child Death Review and Prevention; and Task Force on Sudden Infant Death Syndrome (joint with Tracey S. Corey, MD; Thomas Andrew, MD; Michael Graham, MD; and National Association of Medical Examiners)

ABSTRACT. When a healthy infant dies suddenly and unexpectedly, it is critical to correctly determine if the death was caused by child abuse or neglect. Sudden unexpected infant deaths should be comprehensively investigated, ancillary tests and forensic procedures should be used to more-accurately identify the cause of death, and parents deserve to be approached in a nonaccusatory manner during the investigation. Missing a child abuse death can place other children at risk, and inappropriately approaching a sleep-related death as maltreatment can result in inappropriate criminal and protective services investigations. Communities can learn from these deaths by using multidisciplinary child death reviews. Pediatricians can support families during investigation, advocate for and support state policies that require autopsies and scene investigation, and advocate for establishing comprehensive and fully funded child death investigation and reviews at the local and state levels. Additional funding is also needed for research to advance our ability to prevent these deaths. (8/19)

See full text on page 775.
https://pediatrics.aappublications.org/content/144/3/e20192076

IDENTIFYING INFANTS AND YOUNG CHILDREN WITH DEVELOPMENTAL DISORDERS IN THE MEDICAL HOME: AN ALGORITHM FOR DEVELOPMENTAL SURVEILLANCE AND SCREENING

Council on Children With Disabilities, Section on Developmental and Behavioral Pediatrics, Bright Futures Steering Committee, and Medical Home Initiatives for Children With Special Needs Project Advisory Committee

ABSTRACT. Early identification of developmental disorders is critical to the well-being of children and their families. It is an integral function of the primary care medical home and an appropriate responsibility of all pediatric health care professionals. This statement provides an algorithm as a strategy to support health care professionals in developing a pattern and practice for addressing developmental concerns in children from birth through 3 years of age. The authors recommend that developmental surveillance be incorporated at every well-child preventive care visit. Any concerns raised during surveillance should be promptly addressed with standardized developmental screening tests. In addition, screening tests should be administered regularly at the 9-, 18-, and 30-month visits. (Because the 30-month visit is not yet a part of the preventive care system and is often not reimbursable by third-party payers at this time, developmental screening can be performed at 24 months of age. In addition, because the frequency of regular pediatric visits decreases after 24 months of age, a pediatrician who expects that his or her patients will have difficulty attending a 30-month visit should conduct screening during the 24-month visit.) The early identification of developmental problems should lead to further developmental and medical evaluation, diagnosis, and treatment, including early developmental intervention. Children diagnosed with developmental disorders should be identified as children with special health care needs, and chronic-condition management should be initiated. Identification of a developmental disorder and its underlying etiology may also drive a range of treatment planning, from medical treatment of the child to family planning for his or her parents. (7/06, reaffirmed 12/09, 8/14)
http://pediatrics.aappublications.org/content/118/1/405

IMMERSION IN WATER DURING LABOR AND DELIVERY (CLINICAL REPORT)

Committee on Fetus and Newborn (joint with American College of Obstetricians and Gynecologists Committee on Obstetric Practice)

ABSTRACT. Immersion in water has been suggested as a beneficial alternative for labor, delivery, or both and over the past decades has gained popularity in many parts of the world. Immersion in water during the first stage of labor may be associated with decreased pain or use of anesthesia and decreased duration of labor. However, there is no evidence that immersion in water during the first stage of labor otherwise improves perinatal outcomes, and it should not prevent or inhibit other elements of care. The safety and efficacy of immersion in water during the second stage of labor have not been established, and immersion in water during the second stage of labor has not been associated with maternal or fetal benefit. Given these facts and case reports of rare but serious adverse effects in the newborn, the practice of immersion in the second stage of labor (underwater delivery) should be considered an experimental procedure

that only should be performed within the context of an appropriately designed clinical trial with informed consent. Facilities that plan to offer immersion in the first stage of labor need to establish rigorous protocols for candidate selection, maintenance and cleaning of tubs and immersion pools, infection control procedures, monitoring of mothers and fetuses at appropriate intervals while immersed, and immediately and safely moving women out of the tubs if maternal or fetal concerns develop. (3/14)
http://pediatrics.aappublications.org/content/133/4/758

IMMUNIZATION INFORMATION SYSTEMS

Committee on Practice and Ambulatory Medicine

ABSTRACT. The American Academy of Pediatrics continues to support the development and implementation of immunization information systems, previously referred to as immunization registries, and other systems for the benefit of children, pediatricians, and their communities. Pediatricians and others must be aware of the value that immunization information systems have for society, the potential fiscal influences on their practice, the costs and benefits, and areas for future improvement. (9/06, reaffirmed 10/11)
http://pediatrics.aappublications.org/content/118/3/1293

IMMUNIZING PARENTS AND OTHER CLOSE FAMILY CONTACTS IN THE PEDIATRIC OFFICE SETTING (TECHNICAL REPORT)

Herschel R. Lessin, MD; Kathryn M. Edwards, MD; Committee on Practice and Ambulatory Medicine; and Committee on Infectious Diseases

ABSTRACT. Additional strategies are needed to protect children from vaccine-preventable diseases. In particular, very young infants, as well as children who are immunocompromised, are at especially high risk for developing the serious consequences of vaccine-preventable diseases and cannot be immunized completely. There is some evidence that children who become infected with these diseases are exposed to pathogens through household contacts, particularly from parents or other close family contacts. Such infections likely are attributable to adults who are not fully protected from these diseases, either because their immunity to vaccine-preventable diseases has waned over time or because they have not received a vaccine. There are many challenges that have added to low adult immunization rates in the United States. One option to increase immunization coverage for parents and close family contacts of infants and vulnerable children is to provide alternative locations for these adults to be immunized, such as the pediatric office setting. Ideally, adults should receive immunizations in their medical homes; however, to provide greater protection to these adults and reduce the exposure of children to pathogens, immunizing parents or other adult family contacts in the pediatric office setting could increase immunization coverage for this population to protect themselves as well as children to whom they provide care. (12/11, reaffirmed 8/16)
http://pediatrics.aappublications.org/content/129/1/e247

THE IMPACT OF MARIJUANA POLICIES ON YOUTH: CLINICAL, RESEARCH, AND LEGAL UPDATE

Committee on Substance Abuse and Committee on Adolescence

ABSTRACT. This policy statement is an update of the American Academy of Pediatrics policy statement "Legalization of Marijuana: Potential Impact on Youth," published in 2004. Pediatricians have special expertise in the care of children and adolescents and may be called on to advise legislators about the potential impact of changes in the legal status of marijuana on adolescents. Parents also may look to pediatricians for advice as they consider whether to support state-level initiatives that propose to legalize the use of marijuana for medical and nonmedical purposes or to decriminalize the possession of small amounts of marijuana. This policy statement provides the position of the American Academy of Pediatrics on the issue of marijuana legalization. The accompanying technical report reviews what is currently known about the relationships of marijuana use with health and the developing brain and the legal status of marijuana and adolescents' use of marijuana to better understand how change in legal status might influence the degree of marijuana use by adolescents in the future. (2/15)
http://pediatrics.aappublications.org/content/135/3/584

THE IMPACT OF MARIJUANA POLICIES ON YOUTH: CLINICAL, RESEARCH, AND LEGAL UPDATE (TECHNICAL REPORT)

Seth Ammerman, MD, FAAP; Sheryl Ryan, MD, FAAP; William P. Adelman, MD, FAAP; Committee on Substance Abuse; and Committee on Adolescence

ABSTRACT. This technical report updates the 2004 American Academy of Pediatrics technical report on the legalization of marijuana. Current epidemiology of marijuana use is presented, as are definitions and biology of marijuana compounds, side effects of marijuana use, and effects of use on adolescent brain development. Issues concerning medical marijuana specifically are also addressed. Concerning legalization of marijuana, 4 different approaches in the United States are discussed: legalization of marijuana solely for medical purposes, decriminalization of recreational use of marijuana, legalization of recreational use of marijuana, and criminal prosecution of recreational (and medical) use of marijuana. These approaches are compared, and the latest available data are presented to aid in forming public policy. The effects on youth of criminal penalties for marijuana use and possession are also addressed, as are the effects or potential effects of the other 3 policy approaches on adolescent marijuana use. Recommendations are included in the accompanying policy statement. (2/15)
http://pediatrics.aappublications.org/content/135/3/e769

THE IMPACT OF RACISM ON CHILD AND ADOLESCENT HEALTH

Maria Trent, MD, MPH, FAAP, FSAHM; Danielle G. Dooley, MD, MPhil, FAAP; Jacqueline Dougé, MD, MPH, FAAP; Section on Adolescent Health; Council on Community Pediatrics; and Committee on Adolescence

ABSTRACT. The American Academy of Pediatrics is committed to addressing the factors that affect child and adolescent health with a focus on issues that may leave some children more vulnerable than others. Racism is a social determinant of health that has a profound impact on the health status of children, adolescents, emerging adults, and their families. Although progress has been made toward racial equality and equity, the evidence to support the continued negative impact of racism on health and well-being through implicit and explicit biases, institutional structures, and interpersonal relationships is clear. The objective of this policy statement is to provide an evidence-based document focused on the role of racism in child and adolescent development and health outcomes. By acknowledging the role of racism in child and adolescent health, pediatricians and other pediatric health professionals will be able to proactively engage in strategies to optimize clinical care, workforce development, professional education, systems engagement, and research in a manner designed to reduce the health effects of structural, personally mediated, and internalized racism and improve the health and well-being of all children, adolescents, emerging adults, and their families. (7/19)

See full text on page 787.

https://pediatrics.aappublications.org/content/144/2/e20191765

THE IMPACT OF SOCIAL MEDIA ON CHILDREN, ADOLESCENTS, AND FAMILIES (CLINICAL REPORT)

Gwenn Schurgin O'Keeffe, MD; Kathleen Clarke-Pearson, MD; and Council on Communications and Media

ABSTRACT. Using social media Web sites is among the most common activity of today's children and adolescents. Any Web site that allows social interaction is considered a social media site, including social networking sites such as Facebook, MySpace, and Twitter; gaming sites and virtual worlds such as Club Penguin, Second Life, and the Sims; video sites such as YouTube; and blogs. Such sites offer today's youth a portal for entertainment and communication and have grown exponentially in recent years. For this reason, it is important that parents become aware of the nature of social media sites, given that not all of them are healthy environments for children and adolescents. Pediatricians are in a unique position to help families understand these sites and to encourage healthy use and urge parents to monitor for potential problems with cyberbullying, "Facebook depression," sexting, and exposure to inappropriate content. (3/11)

http://pediatrics.aappublications.org/content/127/4/800

IMPROVING HEALTH AND SAFETY AT CAMP

Michael J. Ambrose, MD, FAAP; Edward A. Walton, MD, FAAP; and Council on School Health

ABSTRACT. The American Academy of Pediatrics has created recommendations for health appraisal and preparation of young people before participation in day, resident, or family camps and to guide health and safety practices at camp. These recommendations are intended for parents and families, primary health care providers, and camp administration and health center staff. Although camps have diverse environments, there are general guidelines that apply to all situations and specific recommendations that are appropriate under special conditions. This policy statement has been reviewed and is supported by the American Camp Association and Association of Camp Nursing. (6/19)

See full text on page 803.

https://pediatrics.aappublications.org/content/144/1/e20191355

INCIDENTAL FINDINGS ON BRAIN AND SPINE IMAGING IN CHILDREN (CLINICAL REPORT)

Cormac O. Maher, MD, FAAP; Joseph H. Piatt Jr, MD, FAAP; and Section on Neurologic Surgery

ABSTRACT. In recent years, the utilization of diagnostic imaging of the brain and spine in children has increased dramatically, leading to a corresponding increase in the detection of incidental findings of the central nervous system. Patients with unexpected findings on imaging are often referred for subspecialty evaluation. Even with rational use of diagnostic imaging and subspecialty consultation, the diagnostic process will always generate unexpected findings that must be explained and managed. Familiarity with the most common findings that are discovered incidentally on diagnostic imaging of the brain and spine will assist the pediatrician in providing counseling to families and in making recommendations in conjunction with a neurosurgeon, when needed, regarding additional treatments and prognosis. (3/15)

http://pediatrics.aappublications.org/content/135/4/e1084

INCORPORATING RECOGNITION AND MANAGEMENT OF PERINATAL DEPRESSION INTO PEDIATRIC PRACTICE

Marian F. Earls, MD, MTS, FAAP; Michael W. Yogman, MD, FAAP; Gerri Mattson, MD, MSPH, FAAP; Jason Rafferty, MD, MPH, EdM, FAAP; and Committee on Psychosocial Aspects of Child and Family Health

ABSTRACT. Perinatal depression (PND) is the most common obstetric complication in the United States. Even when screening results are positive, mothers often do not receive further evaluation, and even when PND is diagnosed, mothers do not receive evidence-based treatments. Studies reveal that postpartum depression (PPD), a subset of PND, leads to increased costs of medical care, inappropriate medical treatment of the infant, discontinuation of breastfeeding, family dysfunction, and an increased risk of abuse and neglect. PPD, specifically, adversely affects this critical early period of infant brain development. PND is an example of an adverse childhood experience that has potential long-term adverse health complications for the mother, her partner, the infant, and the mother-infant dyad. However, PND can be treated effectively, and the stress on the infant can be buffered. Pediatric medical homes should coordinate care more effectively with prenatal providers for women with prenatally diagnosed maternal depression; establish a system to implement PPD screening at the 1-, 2-, 4-, and 6-month well-child visits; use community resources for the treatment and referral of the mother with depression; and provide support for the maternal-child (dyad) relationship, including breastfeeding support. State chapters of the American Academy of Pediatrics, working with state departments of public health, public and private payers, and maternal and child health programs, should advocate for payment and for increased training for PND screening and treatment. American Academy of Pediatrics recommends advocacy for workforce development for mental health professionals who care for young children and mother-infant dyads, and for promotion of evidence-based interventions focused on healthy attachment and parent-child relationships. (12/18)

See full text on page 813.

https://pediatrics.aappublications.org/content/143/1/e20183259

INCORPORATING RECOGNITION AND MANAGEMENT OF PERINATAL DEPRESSION INTO PEDIATRIC PRACTICE (TECHNICAL REPORT)

Jason Rafferty, MD, MPH, EdM, FAAP; Gerri Mattson, MD, MSPH, FAAP; Marian F. Earls, MD, MTS, FAAP; Michael W. Yogman, MD, FAAP; and Committee on Psychosocial Aspects of Child and Family Health

ABSTRACT. Perinatal depression is the most common obstetric complication in the United States, with prevalence rates of 15% to 20% among new mothers. Untreated, it can adversly affect the well-being of children and families through increasing the risk for costly complications during birth and lead to deterioration of core supports, including partner relationships and social networks. Perinatal depression contributes to long-lasting, and even permanent, consequences for the physical and mental health of parents and children, including poor family functioning, increased risk of child abuse and neglect, delayed infant development, perinatal obstetric complications, challenges with breastfeeding, and costly increases in health care use. Perinatal depression can interfere with early parent-infant interaction and attachment, leading to potentially long-term disturbances in the child's physical, emotional, cognitive, and social development. Fortunately, perinatal depression is identifiable and treatable. The US Preventive Services Task Force, Centers for Medicare and Medicaid Services, and many professional organizations recommend routine universal screening for perinatal depression in women to facilitate early evidence-based treatment and referrals, if necessary. Despite significant gains in screening rates from 2004 to 2013, a minority of pediatricians routinely screen for postpartum depression, and many mothers are still not identified or treated. Pediatric primary care clinicians, with a core mission of promoting child and family health, are in an ideal position to implement routine postpartum depression screens at several well-child visits throughout infancy and to provide mental health support through referrals and/or the interdisciplinary services of a pediatric patient-centered medical home model. (12/18)

See full text on page 825.
https://pediatrics.aappublications.org/content/143/1/e20183260

INCREASING ANTIRETROVIRAL DRUG ACCESS FOR CHILDREN WITH HIV INFECTION

Committee on Pediatric AIDS and Section on International Child Health

ABSTRACT. Although there have been great gains in the prevention of pediatric HIV infection and provision of antiretroviral therapy for children with HIV infection in resource-rich countries, many barriers remain to scaling up HIV prevention and treatment for children in resource-limited areas of the world. Appropriate testing technologies need to be made more widely available to identify HIV infection in infants. Training of practitioners in the skills required to care for children with HIV infection is required to increase the number of children receiving antiretroviral therapy. Lack of availability of appropriate antiretroviral drug formulations that are easily usable and inexpensive is a major impediment to optimal care for children with HIV. The time and energy spent trying to develop liquid antiretroviral formulations might be better used in the manufacture of smaller pill sizes or crushable tablets, which are easier to dispense, transport, store, and administer to children. (4/07, reaffirmed 4/10, 4/16)
http://pediatrics.aappublications.org/content/119/4/838

INCREASING IMMUNIZATION COVERAGE

Committee on Practice and Ambulatory Medicine and Council on Community Pediatrics

ABSTRACT. In 1977, the American Academy of Pediatrics issued a statement calling for universal immunization of all children for whom vaccines are not contraindicated. In 1995, the policy statement "Implementation of the Immunization Policy" was published by the American Academy of Pediatrics, followed in 2003 with publication of the first version of this statement, "Increasing Immunization Coverage." Since 2003, there have continued to be improvements in immunization coverage, with progress toward meeting the goals set forth in *Healthy People 2010*. Data from the 2007 National Immunization Survey showed that 90% of children 19 to 35 months of age have received recommended doses of each of the following vaccines: inactivated poliovirus (IPV), measles-mumps-rubella (MMR), varicella-zoster virus (VZB), hepatitis B virus (HBV), and *Haemophilus influenzae* type b (Hib). For diphtheria and tetanus and acellular pertussis (DTaP) vaccine, 84.5% have received the recommended 4 doses by 35 months of age. Nevertheless, the *Healthy People 2010* goal of at least 80% coverage for the full series (at least 4 doses of DTaP, 3 doses of IPV, 1 dose of MMR, 3 doses of Hib, 3 doses of HBV, and 1 dose of varicella-zoster virus vaccine) has not yet been met, and immunization coverage of adolescents continues to lag behind the goals set forth in *Healthy People 2010*. Despite these encouraging data, a vast number of new challenges that threaten continued success toward the goal of universal immunization coverage have emerged. These challenges include an increase in new vaccines and new vaccine combinations as well as a significant number of vaccines currently under development; a dramatic increase in the acquisition cost of vaccines, coupled with a lack of adequate payment to practitioners to buy and administer vaccines; unanticipated manufacturing and delivery problems that have caused significant shortages of various vaccine products; and the rise of a public antivaccination movement that uses the Internet as well as standard media outlets to advance a position, wholly unsupported by any scientific evidence, linking vaccines with various childhood conditions, particularly autism. Much remains to be accomplished by physician organizations; vaccine manufacturers; third-party payers; the media; and local, state, and federal governments to ensure dependable vaccine supply and payments that are sufficient to continue to provide immunizations in public and private settings and to promote effective strategies to combat unjustified misstatements by the antivaccination movement.

Pediatricians should work individually and collectively at the local, state, and national levels to ensure that all children without a valid contraindication receive all childhood immunizations on time. Pediatricians and pediatric organizations, in conjunction with government agencies such as the Centers for Disease Control and Prevention, must communicate effectively with parents to maximize their understanding of the overall safety and efficacy of vaccines. Most parents and children have not experienced many of the vaccine-preventable diseases, and the general public is not well informed about the risks and sequelae of these conditions. A number of recommendations are included for pediatricians, individually and collectively, to support further progress toward the goal of universal immunization coverage of all children for whom vaccines are not contraindicated. (5/10)
http://pediatrics.aappublications.org/content/125/6/1295

THE INDIVIDUALS WITH DISABILITIES EDUCATION ACT (IDEA) FOR CHILDREN WITH SPECIAL EDUCATIONAL NEEDS (CLINICAL REPORT)

Paul H. Lipkin, MD, FAAP; Jeffrey Okamoto, MD, FAAP; Council on Children With Disabilities; and Council on School Health

ABSTRACT. The pediatric health care provider has a critical role in supporting the health and well-being of children and adolescents in all settings, including early intervention (EI), preschool, and school environments. It is estimated that 15% of children in the United States have a disability. The Individuals with Disabilities Education Act entitles every affected child in the United States from infancy to young adulthood to a free appropriate public education through EI and special education services. These services bolster development and learning of children with various disabilities. This clinical report provides the pediatric health care provider with a summary of key components of the most recent version of this law. Guidance is also provided to ensure that every child in need receives the EI and special education services to which he or she is entitled. (11/15)
http://pediatrics.aappublications.org/content/136/6/e1650

INDOOR ENVIRONMENTAL CONTROL PRACTICES AND ASTHMA MANAGEMENT (CLINICAL REPORT)

Elizabeth C. Matsui, MD, MHS, FAAP; Stuart L. Abramson, MD, PhD, AE-C, FAAP; Megan T. Sandel, MD, MPH, FAAP; Section on Allergy and Immunology; and Council on Environmental Health

ABSTRACT. Indoor environmental exposures, particularly allergens and pollutants, are major contributors to asthma morbidity in children; environmental control practices aimed at reducing these exposures are an integral component of asthma management. Some individually tailored environmental control practices that have been shown to reduce asthma symptoms and exacerbations are similar in efficacy and cost to controller medications. As a part of developing tailored strategies regarding environmental control measures, an environmental history can be obtained to evaluate the key indoor environmental exposures that are known to trigger asthma symptoms and exacerbations, including both indoor pollutants and allergens. An environmental history includes questions regarding the presence of pets or pests or evidence of pests in the home, as well as knowledge regarding whether the climatic characteristics in the community favor dust mites. In addition, the history focuses on sources of indoor air pollution, including the presence of smokers who live in the home or care for children and the use of gas stoves and appliances in the home. Serum allergen-specific immunoglobulin E antibody tests can be performed or the patient can be referred for allergy skin testing to identify indoor allergens that are most likely to be clinically relevant. Environmental control strategies

are tailored to each potentially relevant indoor exposure and are based on knowledge of the sources and underlying characteristics of the exposure. Strategies include source removal, source control, and mitigation strategies, such as high-efficiency particulate air purifiers and allergen-proof mattress and pillow encasements, as well as education, which can be delivered by primary care pediatricians, allergists, pediatric pulmonologists, other health care workers, or community health workers trained in asthma environmental control and asthma education. (10/16)
http://pediatrics.aappublications.org/content/138/5/e20162589

INFANT FEEDING AND TRANSMISSION OF HUMAN IMMUNODEFICIENCY VIRUS IN THE UNITED STATES

Committee on Pediatric AIDS

ABSTRACT. Physicians caring for infants born to women infected with HIV are likely to be involved in providing guidance to HIV-infected mothers on appropriate infant feeding practices. It is critical that physicians are aware of the HIV transmission risk from human milk and the current recommendations for feeding HIV-exposed infants in the United States. Because the only intervention to completely prevent HIV transmission via human milk is not to breastfeed, in the United States, where clean water and affordable replacement feeding are available, the American Academy of Pediatrics recommends that HIV-infected mothers not breastfeed their infants, regardless of maternal viral load and antiretroviral therapy. (1/13, reaffirmed 4/16)
http://pediatrics.aappublications.org/content/131/2/391

INFANT METHEMOGLOBINEMIA: THE ROLE OF DIETARY NITRATE IN FOOD AND WATER (CLINICAL REPORT)

Frank R. Greer, MD; Michael Shannon, MD; Committee on Nutrition; and Committee on Environmental Health

ABSTRACT. Infants for whom formula may be prepared with well water remain a high-risk group for nitrate poisoning. This clinical report reinforces the need for testing of well water for nitrate content. There seems to be little or no risk of nitrate poisoning from commercially prepared infant foods in the United States. However, reports of nitrate poisoning from home-prepared vegetable foods for infants continue to occur. Breastfeeding infants are not at risk of methemoglobinemia even when mothers ingest water with very high concentrations of nitrate nitrogen (100 ppm). (9/05, reaffirmed 4/09)
http://pediatrics.aappublications.org/content/116/3/784

INFECTION PREVENTION AND CONTROL IN PEDIATRIC AMBULATORY SETTINGS

Mobeen H. Rathore, MD, FAAP; Mary Anne Jackson, MD, FAAP; and Committee on Infectious Diseases

ABSTRACT. Since the American Academy of Pediatrics published its statement titled "Infection Prevention and Control in Pediatric Ambulatory Settings" in 2007, there have been significant changes that prompted this updated statement. Infection prevention and control is an integral part of pediatric practice in ambulatory medical settings as well as in hospitals. Infection prevention and control practices should begin at the time the ambulatory visit is scheduled. All health care personnel should be educated regarding the routes of transmission and techniques used to prevent the transmission of infectious agents. Policies for infection prevention and control should be written, readily available, updated every 2 years, and enforced. Many of the recommendations for infection control and prevention from the Centers for Disease Control and Prevention for hospitalized patients are also applicable in the ambulatory setting. These recommendations include requirements for pediatricians to take precautions to identify and protect employees likely to be exposed to blood or other potentially infectious materials while on the job. In addition to emphasizing the key principles of infection prevention and control in this policy, we update those that are relevant to the ambulatory care patient. These guidelines emphasize the role of hand hygiene and the implementation of diagnosis- and syndrome-specific isolation precautions, with the exemption of the use of gloves for routine diaper changes and wiping a well child's nose or tears for most patient encounters. Additional topics include respiratory hygiene and cough etiquette strategies for patients with a respiratory tract infection, including those relevant for special populations like patients with cystic fibrosis or those in short-term residential facilities; separation of infected, contagious children from uninfected children when feasible; safe handling and disposal of needles and other sharp medical devices; appropriate use of personal protective equipment, such as gloves, gowns, masks, and eye protection; and appropriate use of sterilization, disinfection, and antisepsis. Lastly, in this policy, we emphasize the importance of public health interventions, including vaccination for patients and health care personnel, and outline the responsibilities of the health care provider related to prompt public health notification for specific reportable diseases and communication with colleagues who may be providing subsequent care of an infected patient to optimize the use of isolation precautions and limit the spread of contagions. (10/17)
http://pediatrics.aappublications.org/content/140/5/e20172857

INFECTIOUS COMPLICATIONS WITH THE USE OF BIOLOGIC RESPONSE MODIFIERS IN INFANTS AND CHILDREN (CLINICAL REPORT)

H. Dele Davies, MD, FAAP, and Committee on Infectious Diseases

ABSTRACT. Biologic response modifiers (BRMs) are substances that interact with and modify the host immune system. BRMs that dampen the immune system are used to treat conditions such as juvenile idiopathic arthritis, psoriatic arthritis, or inflammatory bowel disease and often in combination with other immunosuppressive agents, such as methotrexate and corticosteroids. Cytokines that are targeted include tumor necrosis factor α; interleukins (ILs) 6, 12, and 23; and the receptors for IL-1α (IL-1A) and IL-1β (IL-1B) as well as other molecules. Although the risk varies with the class of BRM, patients receiving immune-dampening BRMs generally are at increased risk of infection or reactivation with mycobacterial infections (*Mycobacterium tuberculosis* and nontuberculous mycobacteria), some viral (herpes simplex virus, varicella-zoster virus, Epstein-Barr virus, hepatitis B) and fungal (histoplasmosis, coccidioidomycosis) infections, as well as other opportunistic infections. The use of BRMs warrants careful determination of infectious risk on the basis of history (including exposure, residence, and travel and immunization history) and selected baseline screening test results. Routine immunizations should be given at least 2 weeks (inactivated or subunit vaccines) or 4 weeks (live vaccines) before initiation of BRMs whenever feasible, and inactivated influenza vaccine should be given annually. Inactivated and subunit vaccines should be given when needed while taking BRMs, but live vaccines should be avoided unless under special circumstances in consultation with an infectious diseases specialist. If the patient develops a febrile or serious respiratory illness during BRM therapy, consideration should be given to stopping the BRM while actively searching for and treating possible infectious causes. (7/16)
http://pediatrics.aappublications.org/content/138/2/e20161209

INFECTIOUS DISEASES ASSOCIATED WITH ORGANIZED SPORTS AND OUTBREAK CONTROL (CLINICAL REPORT)

H. Dele Davies, MD, MS, MHCM, FAAP; Mary Anne Jackson, MD, FAAP; Stephen G. Rice, MD, PhD, MPH, FAAP; Committee on Infectious Diseases; and Council on Sports Medicine and Fitness

ABSTRACT. Participation in organized sports has a variety of health benefits but also has the potential to expose the athlete to a variety of infectious diseases, some of which may produce out-

breaks. Major risk factors for infection include skin-to-skin contact with athletes who have active skin infections, environmental exposures and physical trauma, and sharing of equipment and contact with contaminated fomites. Close contact that is intrinsic to team sports and psychosocial factors associated with adolescence are additional risks. Minimizing risk requires leadership by the organized sports community (including the athlete's primary care provider) and depends on outlining key hygiene behaviors, recognition, diagnosis, and treatment of common sports-related infections, and the implementation of preventive interventions. (9/17)
http://pediatrics.aappublications.org/content/140/4/e20172477

INFLUENZA IMMUNIZATION FOR ALL HEALTH CARE PERSONNEL: KEEP IT MANDATORY

Committee on Infectious Diseases

ABSTRACT. The purpose of this statement is to reaffirm the American Academy of Pediatrics' support for a mandatory influenza immunization policy for all health care personnel. With an increasing number of organizations requiring influenza vaccination, coverage among health care personnel has risen to 75% in the 2013 to 2014 influenza season but still remains below the Healthy People 2020 objective of 90%. Mandatory influenza immunization for all health care personnel is ethical, just, and necessary to improve patient safety. It is a crucial step in efforts to reduce health care–associated influenza infections. (9/15)
http://pediatrics.aappublications.org/content/136/4/809

INFORMED CONSENT IN DECISION-MAKING IN PEDIATRIC PRACTICE

Committee on Bioethics

ABSTRACT. Informed consent should be seen as an essential part of health care practice; parental permission and childhood assent is an active process that engages patients, both adults and children, in health care. Pediatric practice is unique in that developmental maturation allows, over time, for increasing inclusion of the child's and adolescent's opinion in medical decision-making in clinical practice and research. (7/16)
http://pediatrics.aappublications.org/content/138/2/e20161484

INFORMED CONSENT IN DECISION-MAKING IN PEDIATRIC PRACTICE (TECHNICAL REPORT)

Aviva L. Katz, MD, FAAP; Sally A. Webb, MD, FAAP; and Committee on Bioethics

ABSTRACT. Informed consent should be seen as an essential part of health care practice; parental permission and childhood assent is an active process that engages patients, both adults and children, in their health care. Pediatric practice is unique in that developmental maturation allows, over time, for increasing inclusion of the child's and adolescent's opinion in medical decision-making in clinical practice and research. This technical report, which accompanies the policy statement "Informed Consent in Decision-Making in Pediatric Practice," was written to provide a broader background on the nature of informed consent, surrogate decision-making in pediatric practice, information on child and adolescent decision-making, and special issues in adolescent informed consent, assent, and refusal. It is anticipated that this information will help provide support for the recommendations included in the policy statement. (7/16)
http://pediatrics.aappublications.org/content/138/2/e20161485

INJURIES ASSOCIATED WITH INFANT WALKERS

Committee on Injury and Poison Prevention

ABSTRACT. In 1999, an estimated 8800 children younger than 15 months were treated in hospital emergency departments in the United States for injuries associated with infant walkers. Thirty-four infant walker-related deaths were reported from 1973 through 1998. The vast majority of injuries occur from falls down stairs, and head injuries are common. Walkers do not help a child learn to walk; indeed, they can delay normal motor and mental development. The use of warning labels, public education, adult supervision during walker use, and stair gates have all been demonstrated to be insufficient strategies to prevent injuries associated with infant walkers. To comply with the revised voluntary standard (ASTM F977-96), walkers manufactured after June 30, 1997, must be wider than a 36-in doorway or must have a braking mechanism designed to stop the walker if 1 or more wheels drop off the riding surface, such as at the top of a stairway. Because data indicate a considerable risk of major and minor injury and even death from the use of infant walkers, and because there is no clear benefit from their use, the American Academy of Pediatrics recommends a ban on the manufacture and sale of mobile infant walkers. If a parent insists on using a mobile infant walker, it is vital that they choose a walker that meets the performance standards of ASTM F977-96 to prevent falls down stairs. Stationary activity centers should be promoted as a safer alternative to mobile infant walkers. (9/01, reaffirmed 1/05, 2/08, 10/11, 11/14)
http://pediatrics.aappublications.org/content/108/3/790

INJURY RISK OF NONPOWDER GUNS (TECHNICAL REPORT)

Committee on Injury, Violence, and Poison Prevention

ABSTRACT. Nonpowder guns (ball-bearing [BB] guns, pellet guns, air rifles, paintball guns) continue to cause serious injuries to children and adolescents. The muzzle velocity of these guns can range from approximately 150 ft/second to 1200 ft/second (the muzzle velocities of traditional firearm pistols are 750 ft/second to 1450 ft/second). Both low- and high-velocity nonpowder guns are associated with serious injuries, and fatalities can result from high-velocity guns. A persisting problem is the lack of medical recognition of the severity of injuries that can result from these guns, including penetration of the eye, skin, internal organs, and bone. Nationally, in 2000, there were an estimated 21840 (coefficient of variation: 0.0821) injuries related to nonpowder guns, with approximately 4% resulting in hospitalization. Between 1990 and 2000, the US Consumer Product Safety Commission reported 39 nonpowder gun–related deaths, of which 32 were children younger than 15 years. The introduction of high-powered air rifles in the 1970s has been associated with approximately 4 deaths per year. The advent of war games and the use of paintball guns have resulted in a number of reports of injuries, especially to the eye. Injuries associated with nonpowder guns should receive prompt medical management similar to the management of firearm-related injuries, and nonpowder guns should never be characterized as toys. (11/04, reaffirmed 2/08, 10/11)
http://pediatrics.aappublications.org/content/114/5/1357

IN-LINE SKATING INJURIES IN CHILDREN AND ADOLESCENTS

Committee on Injury and Poison Prevention and Committee on Sports Medicine and Fitness

ABSTRACT. In-line skating has become one of the fastest-growing recreational sports in the United States. Recent studies emphasize the value of protective gear in reducing the incidence of injuries. Recommendations are provided for parents and pediatricians, with special emphasis on the novice or inexperienced skater. (4/98, reaffirmed 1/02, 1/06, 1/09, 11/11)
http://pediatrics.aappublications.org/content/101/4/720

INSTITUTIONAL ETHICS COMMITTEES

Margaret Moon, MD, MPH, FAAP, and Committee on Bioethics

ABSTRACT. In hospitals throughout the United States, institutional ethics committees (IECs) have become a standard vehicle for the education of health professionals about biomedical ethics, for the drafting and review of hospital policy, and for clinical ethics case consultation. In addition, there is increasing interest in a role for the IEC in organizational ethics. Recommendations are made about the membership and structure of an IEC, and guidance is provided for those serving on an IEC. (4/19)

See full text on page 857.

https://pediatrics.aappublications.org/content/143/5/e20190659

INSUFFICIENT SLEEP IN ADOLESCENTS AND YOUNG ADULTS: AN UPDATE ON CAUSES AND CONSEQUENCES (TECHNICAL REPORT)

Judith Owens, MD, MPH, FAAP; Adolescent Sleep Working Group; and Committee on Adolescence

ABSTRACT. Chronic sleep loss and associated sleepiness and daytime impairments in adolescence are a serious threat to the academic success, health, and safety of our nation's youth and an important public health issue. Understanding the extent and potential short- and long-term repercussions of sleep restriction, as well as the unhealthy sleep practices and environmental factors that contribute to sleep loss in adolescents, is key in setting public policies to mitigate these effects and in counseling patients and families in the clinical setting. This report reviews the current literature on sleep patterns in adolescents, factors contributing to chronic sleep loss (ie, electronic media use, caffeine consumption), and health-related consequences, such as depression, increased obesity risk, and higher rates of drowsy driving accidents. The report also discusses the potential role of later school start times as a means of reducing adolescent sleepiness. (8/14)

http://pediatrics.aappublications.org/content/134/3/e921

INTENSIVE TRAINING AND SPORTS SPECIALIZATION IN YOUNG ATHLETES

Committee on Sports Medicine and Fitness

ABSTRACT. Children involved in sports should be encouraged to participate in a variety of different activities and develop a wide range of skills. Young athletes who specialize in just one sport may be denied the benefits of varied activity while facing additional physical, physiologic, and psychologic demands from intense training and competition.

This statement reviews the potential risks of high-intensity training and sports specialization in young athletes. Pediatricians who recognize these risks can have a key role in monitoring the health of these young athletes and helping reduce risks associated with high-level sports participation. (7/00, reaffirmed 11/04, 1/06, 5/09, 10/14)

http://pediatrics.aappublications.org/content/106/1/154

INTERFERON-γ RELEASE ASSAYS FOR DIAGNOSIS OF TUBERCULOSIS INFECTION AND DISEASE IN CHILDREN (TECHNICAL REPORT)

Jeffrey R. Starke, MD, FAAP, and Committee on Infectious Diseases

ABSTRACT. Tuberculosis (TB) remains an important problem among children in the United States and throughout the world. Although diagnosis and treatment of infection with *Mycobacterium tuberculosis* (also referred to as latent tuberculosis infection [LTBI] or TB infection) remain the lynchpins of TB prevention, there is no diagnostic reference standard for LTBI. The tuberculin skin test (TST) has many limitations, including difficulty in administration and interpretation, the need for a return visit by the patient, and false-positive results caused by significant cross-reaction with *Mycobacterium bovis*–bacille Calmette-Guérin (BCG) vaccines and many nontuberculous mycobacteria. Interferon-γ release assays (IGRAs) are blood tests that measure ex vivo T-lymphocyte release of interferon-γ after stimulation by antigens specific for *M tuberculosis*. Because these antigens are not found on *M bovis*–BCG or most nontuberculous mycobacteria, IGRAs are more specific tests than the TST, yielding fewer false-positive results. However, IGRAs have little advantage over the TST in sensitivity, and both methods have reduced sensitivity in immunocompromised children, including children with severe TB disease. Both methods have a higher positive predictive value when applied to children with risk factors for LTBI. Unfortunately, neither method distinguishes between TB infection and TB disease. The objective of this technical report is to review what IGRAs are most useful for: (1) increasing test specificity in children who have received a BCG vaccine and may have a false-positive TST result; (2) using with the TST to increase sensitivity for finding LTBI in patients at high risk of developing progression from LTBI to disease; and (3) helping to diagnose TB disease. (11/14, reaffirmed 7/18)

http://pediatrics.aappublications.org/content/134/6/e1763

INTERPRETATION OF DO NOT ATTEMPT RESUSCITATION ORDERS FOR CHILDREN REQUIRING ANESTHESIA AND SURGERY (CLINICAL REPORT)

Mary E. Fallat, MD, FAAP; Courtney Hardy, MD, MBA, FAAP; Section on Surgery; Section on Anesthesiology and Pain Medicine; and Committee on Bioethics

ABSTRACT. This clinical report addresses the topic of preexisting do not attempt resuscitation or limited resuscitation orders for children and adolescents undergoing anesthesia and surgery. Pertinent considerations for the clinician include the rights of children, decision-making by parents or legally approved representatives, the process of informed consent, and the roles of surgeon and anesthesiologist. A process of re-evaluation of the do not attempt resuscitation orders, called "required reconsideration," should be incorporated into the process of informed consent for surgery and anesthesia, distinguishing between goal-directed and procedure-directed approaches. The child's individual needs are best served by allowing the parent or legally approved representative and involved clinicians to consider whether full resuscitation, limitations based on procedures, or limitations based on goals is most appropriate. (4/18)

http://pediatrics.aappublications.org/content/141/5/e20180598

INTIMATE PARTNER VIOLENCE: THE ROLE OF THE PEDIATRICIAN (CLINICAL REPORT)

Jonathan D. Thackeray, MD; Roberta Hibbard, MD; M. Denise Dowd, MD, MPH; Committee on Child Abuse and Neglect; and Committee on Injury, Violence, and Poison Prevention

ABSTRACT. The American Academy of Pediatrics and its members recognize the importance of improving the physician's ability to recognize intimate partner violence (IPV) and understand its effects on child health and development and its role in the continuum of family violence. Pediatricians are in a unique position to identify abused caregivers in pediatric settings and to evaluate and treat children raised in homes in which IPV may occur. Children exposed to IPV are at increased risk of being abused and neglected and are more likely to develop adverse health, behavioral, psychological, and social disorders later in life. Identifying IPV, therefore, may be one of the most effective means of preventing child abuse and identifying caregivers and children who may be in need of treatment and/or therapy. Pediatricians should be aware of the profound effects of exposure to IPV on children. (4/10, reaffirmed 1/14, 3/19)

http://pediatrics.aappublications.org/content/125/5/1094

IODINE DEFICIENCY, POLLUTANT CHEMICALS, AND THE THYROID: NEW INFORMATION ON AN OLD PROBLEM

Council on Environmental Health

ABSTRACT. Many women of reproductive age in the United States are marginally iodine deficient, perhaps because the salt in processed foods is not iodized. Iodine deficiency, per se, can interfere with normal brain development in their offspring;

in addition, it increases vulnerability to the effects of certain environmental pollutants, such as nitrate, thiocyanate, and perchlorate. Although pregnant and lactating women should take a supplement containing adequate iodide, only about 15% do so. Such supplements, however, may not contain enough iodide and may not be labeled accurately. The American Thyroid Association recommends that pregnant and lactating women take a supplement with adequate iodide. The American Academy of Pediatrics recommends that pregnant and lactating women also avoid exposure to excess nitrate, which would usually occur from contaminated well water, and thiocyanate, which is in cigarette smoke. Perchlorate is currently a candidate for regulation as a water pollutant. The Environmental Protection Agency should proceed with appropriate regulation, and the Food and Drug Administration should address the mislabeling of the iodine content of prenatal/lactation supplements. (5/14)
http://pediatrics.aappublications.org/content/133/6/1163

LACTOSE INTOLERANCE IN INFANTS, CHILDREN, AND ADOLESCENTS (CLINICAL REPORT)

Melvin B. Heyman, MD, MPH, and Committee on Nutrition

ABSTRACT. The American Academy of Pediatrics Committee on Nutrition presents an updated review of lactose intolerance in infants, children, and adolescents. Differences between primary, secondary, congenital, and developmental lactase deficiency that may result in lactose intolerance are discussed. Children with suspected lactose intolerance can be assessed clinically by dietary lactose elimination or by tests including noninvasive hydrogen breath testing or invasive intestinal biopsy determination of lactase (and other disaccharidase) concentrations. Treatment consists of use of lactase-treated dairy products or oral lactase supplementation, limitation of lactose-containing foods, or dairy elimination. The American Academy of Pediatrics supports use of dairy foods as an important source of calcium for bone mineral health and of other nutrients that facilitate growth in children and adolescents. If dairy products are eliminated, other dietary sources of calcium or calcium supplements need to be provided. (9/06, reaffirmed 8/12)
http://pediatrics.aappublications.org/content/118/3/1279

"LATE-PRETERM" INFANTS: A POPULATION AT RISK (CLINICAL REPORT)

William A. Engle, MD; Kay M. Tomashek, MD; Carol Wallman, MSN; and Committee on Fetus and Newborn

ABSTRACT. Late-preterm infants, defined by birth at $34\frac{0}{7}$ through $36\frac{6}{7}$ weeks' gestation, are less physiologically and metabolically mature than term infants. Thus, they are at higher risk of morbidity and mortality than term infants. The purpose of this report is to define "late preterm," recommend a change in terminology from "near term" to "late preterm," present the characteristics of late-preterm infants that predispose them to a higher risk of morbidity and mortality than term infants, and propose guidelines for the evaluation and management of these infants after birth. (12/07, reaffirmed 5/10, 6/18)
http://pediatrics.aappublications.org/content/120/6/1390

LAWN MOWER-RELATED INJURIES TO CHILDREN

Committee on Injury and Poison Prevention

ABSTRACT. Lawn mower-related injuries to children are relatively common and can result in severe injury or death. Many amputations during childhood are caused by power mowers. Pediatricians have an important role as advocates and educators to promote the prevention of these injuries. (6/01, reaffirmed 10/04, 5/07, 6/10)
http://pediatrics.aappublications.org/content/107/6/1480

LAWN MOWER-RELATED INJURIES TO CHILDREN (TECHNICAL REPORT)

Committee on Injury and Poison Prevention

ABSTRACT. In the United States, approximately 9400 children younger than 18 years receive emergency treatment annually for lawn mower-related injuries. More than 7% of these children require hospitalization, and power mowers cause a large proportion of the amputations during childhood. Prevention of lawn mower-related injuries can be achieved by design changes of lawn mowers, guidelines for mower operation, and education of parents, child caregivers, and children. Pediatricians have an important role as advocates and educators to promote the prevention of these injuries. (6/01, reaffirmed 10/04, 5/07, 6/10)
http://pediatrics.aappublications.org/content/107/6/e106

LEARNING DISABILITIES, DYSLEXIA, AND VISION

Section on Ophthalmology and Council on Children With Disabilities (joint with American Academy of Ophthalmology, American Association for Pediatric Ophthalmology and Strabismus, and American Association of Certified Orthoptists)

ABSTRACT. Learning disabilities, including reading disabilities, are commonly diagnosed in children. Their etiologies are multifactorial, reflecting genetic influences and dysfunction of brain systems. Learning disabilities are complex problems that require complex solutions. Early recognition and referral to qualified educational professionals for evidence-based evaluations and treatments seem necessary to achieve the best possible outcome. Most experts believe that dyslexia is a language-based disorder. Vision problems can interfere with the process of learning; however, vision problems are not the cause of primary dyslexia or learning disabilities. Scientific evidence does not support the efficacy of eye exercises, behavioral vision therapy, or special tinted filters or lenses for improving the long-term educational performance in these complex pediatric neurocognitive conditions. Diagnostic and treatment approaches that lack scientific evidence of efficacy, including eye exercises, behavioral vision therapy, or special tinted filters or lenses, are not endorsed and should not be recommended. (7/09, reaffirmed 7/14)
http://pediatrics.aappublications.org/content/124/2/837

LEARNING DISABILITIES, DYSLEXIA, AND VISION (TECHNICAL REPORT)

Sheryl M. Handler, MD; Walter M. Fierson, MD; Section on Ophthalmology; and Council on Children With Disabilities (joint with American Academy of Ophthalmology, American Association for Pediatric Ophthalmology and Strabismus, and American Association of Certified Orthoptists)

ABSTRACT. Learning disabilities constitute a diverse group of disorders in which children who generally possess at least average intelligence have problems processing information or generating output. Their etiologies are multifactorial and reflect genetic influences and dysfunction of brain systems. Reading disability, or dyslexia, is the most common learning disability. It is a receptive language-based learning disability that is characterized by difficulties with decoding, fluent word recognition, rapid automatic naming, and/or reading-comprehension skills. These difficulties typically result from a deficit in the phonologic component of language that makes it difficult to use the alphabetic code to decode the written word. Early recognition and referral to qualified professionals for evidence-based evaluations and treatments are necessary to achieve the best possible outcome. Because dyslexia is a language-based disorder, treatment should be directed at this etiology. Remedial programs should include specific instruction in decoding, fluency training, vocabulary, and comprehension. Most programs include daily intensive individualized instruction that explicitly teaches phonemic awareness and the application of phonics. Vision problems can interfere with the process of reading, but children with dyslexia or related learning disabilities have the same visual function and ocular health as children without such conditions. Currently, there is inadequate scientific evidence to support the view that subtle eye or visual problems cause or increase the severity of learning disabilities. Because they are difficult for the public to understand and for educators to treat, learning disabilities have spawned a wide variety of scientifically unsupported vision-based diagnostic and treatment procedures. Scientific evidence does not support the claims that visual training, muscle exercises, ocular pursuit-and-tracking exercises, behavioral/perceptual vision therapy, "training" glasses, prisms, and colored lenses and filters are effective direct or indirect treatments for learning disabilities. There is no valid evidence that children who participate in vision therapy are more responsive to educational instruction than children who do not participate. (3/11)

http://pediatrics.aappublications.org/content/127/3/e818

LEVELS OF NEONATAL CARE

Committee on Fetus and Newborn

ABSTRACT. Provision of risk-appropriate care for newborn infants and mothers was first proposed in 1976. This updated policy statement provides a review of data supporting evidence for a tiered provision of care and reaffirms the need for uniform, nationally applicable definitions and consistent standards of service for public health to improve neonatal outcomes. Facilities that provide hospital care for newborn infants should be classified on the basis of functional capabilities, and these facilities should be organized within a regionalized system of perinatal care. (8/12, reaffirmed 9/15)

http://pediatrics.aappublications.org/content/130/3/587

THE LIFELONG EFFECTS OF EARLY CHILDHOOD ADVERSITY AND TOXIC STRESS (TECHNICAL REPORT)

Jack P. Shonkoff, MD; Andrew S. Garner, MD, PhD; Committee on Psychosocial Aspects of Child and Family Health; Committee on Early Childhood, Adoption, and Dependent Care; and Section on Developmental and Behavioral Pediatrics

ABSTRACT. Advances in fields of inquiry as diverse as neuroscience, molecular biology, genomics, developmental psychology, epidemiology, sociology, and economics are catalyzing an important paradigm shift in our understanding of health and disease across the lifespan. This converging, multidisciplinary science of human development has profound implications for our ability to enhance the life prospects of children and to strengthen the social and economic fabric of society. Drawing on these multiple streams of investigation, this report presents an ecobiodevelopmental framework that illustrates how early experiences and environmental influences can leave a lasting signature on the genetic predispositions that affect emerging brain architecture and long-term health. The report also examines extensive evidence of the disruptive impacts of toxic stress, offering intriguing insights into causal mechanisms that link early adversity to later impairments in learning, behavior, and both physical and mental well-being. The implications of this framework for the practice of medicine, in general, and pediatrics, specifically, are potentially transformational. They suggest that many adult diseases should be viewed as developmental disorders that begin early in life and that persistent health disparities associated with poverty, discrimination, or maltreatment could be reduced by the alleviation of toxic stress in childhood. An ecobiodevelopmental framework also underscores the need for new thinking about the focus and boundaries of pediatric practice. It calls for pediatricians to serve as both front-line guardians of healthy child development and strategically positioned, community leaders to inform new science-based strategies that build strong foundations for educational achievement, economic productivity, responsible citizenship, and lifelong health. (12/11, reaffirmed 7/16)

http://pediatrics.aappublications.org/content/129/1/e232

THE LINK BETWEEN SCHOOL ATTENDANCE AND GOOD HEALTH

Mandy A. Allison, MD, MSPH, FAAP; Elliott Attisha, DO, FAAP; and Council on School Health

ABSTRACT. More than 6.5 million children in the United States, approximately 13% of all students, miss 15 or more days of school each year. The rates of chronic absenteeism vary between states, communities, and schools, with significant disparities based on income, race, and ethnicity. Chronic school absenteeism, starting as early as preschool and kindergarten, puts students at risk for poor school performance and school dropout, which in turn, put them at risk for unhealthy behaviors as adolescents and young adults as well as poor long-term health outcomes. Pediatricians and their colleagues caring for children in the medical setting have opportunities at the individual patient and/or family, practice, and population levels to promote school attendance and reduce chronic absenteeism and resulting health disparities. Although this policy statement is primarily focused on absenteeism related to students' physical and mental health, pediatricians may play a role in addressing absenteeism attributable to a wide range of factors through individual interactions with patients and their parents and through community-, state-, and federal-level advocacy. (1/19)

See full text on page 867.

https://pediatrics.aappublications.org/content/143/2/e20183648

LITERACY PROMOTION: AN ESSENTIAL COMPONENT OF PRIMARY CARE PEDIATRIC PRACTICE

Council on Early Childhood

ABSTRACT. Reading regularly with young children stimulates optimal patterns of brain development and strengthens parent-child relationships at a critical time in child development, which, in turn, builds language, literacy, and social-emotional skills that last a lifetime. Pediatric providers have a unique opportunity to encourage parents to engage in this important and enjoyable activity with their children beginning in infancy. Research has revealed that parents listen and children learn as a result of literacy promotion by pediatricians, which provides a practical and evidence-based opportunity to support early brain development in primary care practice. The American Academy of Pediatrics (AAP) recommends that pediatric providers promote early literacy development for children beginning in infancy and continuing at least until the age of kindergarten entry by (1) advising all parents that reading aloud with young children can enhance parent-child relationships and prepare young minds to learn language and early literacy skills; (2) counseling all parents about developmentally appropriate shared-reading activities that are enjoyable for children and their parents and offer language-rich exposure to books, pictures, and the written word; (3) providing developmentally appropriate books given at health supervision visits for all high-risk, low-income young children; (4) using a robust spectrum of options to support and promote these efforts; and (5) partnering with other child advocates to influence national messaging and policies that support and promote these key early shared-reading experiences. The AAP supports federal and state funding for children's books to be provided at pediatric health supervision visits to children at high risk living at or near the poverty threshold and the integration of literacy promotion, an essential component of pediatric primary care, into pediatric resident education. This policy statement is supported by the AAP technical report "School Readiness" and supports the AAP policy statement "Early Childhood Adversity, Toxic Stress, and the Role of the Pediatrician: Translating Developmental Science Into Lifelong Health." (7/14)

http://pediatrics.aappublications.org/content/134/2/404

LONG-TERM FOLLOW-UP CARE FOR PEDIATRIC CANCER SURVIVORS (CLINICAL REPORT)

Section on Hematology/Oncology (joint with Children's Oncology Group)

ABSTRACT. Progress in therapy has made survival into adulthood a reality for most children, adolescents, and young adults diagnosed with cancer today. Notably, this growing population remains vulnerable to a variety of long-term therapy-related sequelae. Systematic ongoing follow-up of these patients, therefore, is important for providing for early detection of and intervention for potentially serious late-onset complications. In addition, health counseling and promotion of healthy lifestyles are important aspects of long-term follow-up care to promote risk reduction for health problems that commonly present during adulthood. Both general and subspecialty pediatric health care providers are playing an increasingly important role in the ongoing care of childhood cancer survivors, beyond the routine preventive care, health supervision, and anticipatory guidance provided to all patients. This report is based on the guidelines that have been developed by the Children's Oncology Group to facilitate comprehensive long-term follow-up of childhood cancer survivors (www.survivorshipguidelines.org). (3/09, reaffirmed 4/13, 8/17)

http://pediatrics.aappublications.org/content/123/3/906

MAINTAINING AND IMPROVING THE ORAL HEALTH OF YOUNG CHILDREN

Section on Oral Health

ABSTRACT. Oral health is an integral part of the overall health of children. Dental caries is a common and chronic disease process with significant short- and long-term consequences. The prevalence of dental caries for the youngest of children has not decreased over the past decade, despite improvements for older children. As health care professionals responsible for the overall health of children, pediatricians frequently confront morbidity associated with dental caries. Because the youngest children visit the pediatrician more often than they visit the dentist, it is important that pediatricians be knowledgeable about the disease process of dental caries, prevention of the disease, and interventions available to the pediatrician and the family to maintain and restore health. (11/14, reaffirmed 1/19)

http://pediatrics.aappublications.org/content/134/6/1224

MALE ADOLESCENT SEXUAL AND REPRODUCTIVE HEALTH CARE (CLINICAL REPORT)

Arik V. Marcell, MD, MPH; Charles Wibbelsman, MD; Warren M. Seigel, MD; and Committee on Adolescence

ABSTRACT. Male adolescents' sexual and reproductive health needs often go unmet in the primary care setting. This report discusses specific issues related to male adolescents' sexual and reproductive health care in the context of primary care, including pubertal and sexual development, sexual behavior, consequences of sexual behavior, and methods of preventing sexually transmitted infections (including HIV) and pregnancy. Pediatricians are encouraged to address male adolescent sexual and reproductive health on a regular basis, including taking a sexual history, performing an appropriate examination, providing patient-centered and age-appropriate anticipatory guidance, and delivering appropriate vaccinations. Pediatricians should provide these services to male adolescent patients in a confidential and culturally appropriate manner, promote healthy sexual relationships and responsibility, and involve parents in age-appropriate discussions about sexual health with their sons. (11/11, reaffirmed 5/15)

http://pediatrics.aappublications.org/content/128/6/e1658

MALE CIRCUMCISION (TECHNICAL REPORT)

Task Force on Circumcision

ABSTRACT. Male circumcision consists of the surgical removal of some, or all, of the foreskin (or prepuce) from the penis. It is one of the most common procedures in the world. In the United States, the procedure is commonly performed during the newborn period. In 2007, the American Academy of Pediatrics (AAP) convened a multidisciplinary workgroup of AAP members and other stakeholders to evaluate the evidence regarding male circumcision and update the AAP's 1999 recommendations in this area. The Task Force included AAP representatives from specialty areas as well as members of the AAP Board of Directors and liaisons representing the American Academy of Family Physicians, the American College of Obstetricians and Gynecologists, and the Centers for Disease Control and Prevention. The Task Force members identified selected topics relevant to male circumcision and conducted a critical review of peer-reviewed literature by using the American Heart Association's template for evidence evaluation.

Evaluation of current evidence indicates that the health benefits of newborn male circumcision outweigh the risks; furthermore, the benefits of newborn male circumcision justify access to this procedure for families who choose it. Specific benefits from male circumcision were identified for the prevention of urinary tract infections, acquisition of HIV, transmission of some sexually transmitted infections, and penile cancer. Male circumcision does not appear to adversely affect penile sexual function/sensitivity or sexual satisfaction. It is imperative that those providing circumcision are adequately trained and that both sterile techniques and effective pain management are used. Significant acute complications are rare. In general, untrained providers who perform circumcisions have more complications than well-trained providers who perform the procedure, regardless of whether the former are physicians, nurses, or traditional religious providers.

Parents are entitled to factually correct, nonbiased information about circumcision and should receive this information from clinicians before conception or early in pregnancy, which is when parents typically make circumcision decisions. Parents should determine what is in the best interest of their child. Physicians who counsel families about this decision should provide assistance by explaining the potential benefits and risks and ensuring that parents understand that circumcision is an elective procedure. The Task Force strongly recommends the creation, revision, and enhancement of educational materials to assist parents of male infants with the care of circumcised and uncircumcised penises. The Task Force also strongly recommends the development of educational materials for providers to enhance practitioners' competency in discussing circumcision's benefits and risks with parents.

The Task Force made the following recommendations:

- Evaluation of current evidence indicates that the health benefits of newborn male circumcision outweigh the risks, and the benefits of newborn male circumcision justify access to this procedure for those families who choose it.
- Parents are entitled to factually correct, nonbiased information about circumcision that should be provided before conception and early in pregnancy, when parents are most likely to be weighing the option of circumcision of a male child.
- Physicians counseling families about elective male circumcision should assist parents by explaining, in a nonbiased manner, the potential benefits and risks and by ensuring that they understand the elective nature of the procedure.
- Parents should weigh the health benefits and risks in light of their own religious, cultural, and personal preferences, as the medical benefits alone may not outweigh these other considerations for individual families.

- Parents of newborn boys should be instructed in the care of the penis, regardless of whether the newborn has been circumcised or not.
- Elective circumcision should be performed only if the infant's condition is stable and healthy.
- Male circumcision should be performed by trained and competent practitioners, by using sterile techniques and effective pain management.
- Analgesia is safe and effective in reducing the procedural pain associated with newborn circumcision; thus, adequate analgesia should be provided whenever newborn circumcision is performed.
  - Nonpharmacologic techniques (eg, positioning, sucrose pacifiers) alone are insufficient to prevent procedural and postprocedural pain and are not recommended as the sole method of analgesia. They should be used only as analgesic adjuncts to improve infant comfort during circumcision.
  - If used, topical creams may cause a higher incidence of skin irritation in low birth weight infants, compared with infants of normal weight; penile nerve block techniques should therefore be chosen for this group of newborns.
- Key professional organizations (AAP, the American Academy of Family Physicians, the American College of Obstetricians and Gynecologists, the American Society of Anesthesiologists, the American College of Nurse Midwives, and other midlevel clinicians such as nurse practitioners) should work collaboratively to:
  - Develop standards of trainee proficiency in the performance of anesthetic and procedure techniques, including suturing;
  - Teach the procedure and analgesic techniques during postgraduate training programs;
  - Develop educational materials for clinicians to enhance their own competency in discussing the benefits and risks of circumcision with parents;
  - Offer educational materials to assist parents of male infants with the care of both circumcised and uncircumcised penises.
- The preventive and public health benefits associated with newborn male circumcision warrant third-party reimbursement of the procedure.

The American College of Obstetricians and Gynecologists has endorsed this technical report. (8/12)
http://pediatrics.aappublications.org/content/130/3/e756

MALTREATMENT OF CHILDREN WITH DISABILITIES (CLINICAL REPORT)

Roberta A. Hibbard, MD; Larry W. Desch, MD; Committee on Child Abuse and Neglect; and Council on Children With Disabilities

ABSTRACT. Widespread efforts are being made to increase awareness and provide education to pediatricians regarding risk factors of child abuse and neglect. The purpose of this clinical report is to ensure that children with disabilities are recognized as a population that is also at risk of maltreatment. Some conditions related to a disability can be confused with maltreatment. The need for early recognition and intervention of child abuse and neglect in this population, as well as the ways that a medical home can facilitate the prevention and early detection of child maltreatment, are the subject of this report. (5/07, reaffirmed 1/11, 4/16)
http://pediatrics.aappublications.org/content/119/5/1018

MANAGEMENT OF CHILDREN WITH AUTISM SPECTRUM DISORDERS (CLINICAL REPORT)

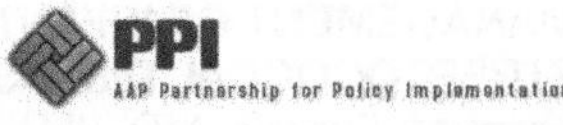

Scott M. Myers, MD; Chris Plauché Johnson, MD, MEd; and Council on Children With Disabilities

ABSTRACT. Pediatricians have an important role not only in early recognition and evaluation of autism spectrum disorders but also in chronic management of these disorders. The primary goals of treatment are to maximize the child's ultimate functional independence and quality of life by minimizing the core autism spectrum disorder features, facilitating development and learning, promoting socialization, reducing maladaptive behaviors, and educating and supporting families. To assist pediatricians in educating families and guiding them toward empirically supported interventions for their children, this report reviews the educational strategies and associated therapies that are the primary treatments for children with autism spectrum disorders. Optimization of health care is likely to have a positive effect on habilitative progress, functional outcome, and quality of life; therefore, important issues, such as management of associated medical problems, pharmacologic and nonpharmacologic intervention for challenging behaviors or coexisting mental health conditions, and use of complementary and alternative medical treatments, are also addressed. (11/07, reaffirmed 9/10, 8/14)
http://pediatrics.aappublications.org/content/120/5/1162

MANAGEMENT OF DENTAL TRAUMA IN A PRIMARY CARE SETTING (CLINICAL REPORT)

Martha Ann Keels, DDS, PhD, and Section on Oral Health

ABSTRACT. The American Academy of Pediatrics and its Section on Oral Health have developed this clinical report for pediatricians and primary care physicians regarding the diagnosis, evaluation, and management of dental trauma in children aged 1 to 21 years. This report was developed through a comprehensive search and analysis of the medical and dental literature and expert consensus. Guidelines published and updated by the International Association of Dental Traumatology (www.dentaltraumaguide.com) are an excellent resource for both dental and nondental health care providers. (1/14)
http://pediatrics.aappublications.org/content/133/2/e466

MANAGEMENT OF FOOD ALLERGY IN THE SCHOOL SETTING (CLINICAL REPORT)

Scott H. Sicherer, MD; Todd Mahr, MD; and Section on Allergy and Immunology

ABSTRACT. Food allergy is estimated to affect approximately 1 in 25 school-aged children and is the most common trigger of anaphylaxis in this age group. School food-allergy management requires strategies to reduce the risk of ingestion of the allergen as well as procedures to recognize and treat allergic reactions and anaphylaxis. The role of the pediatrician or pediatric health care provider may include diagnosing and documenting a potentially life-threatening food allergy, prescribing selfinjectable epinephrine, helping the child learn how to store and use the medication in a responsible manner, educating the parents of their responsibility to implement prevention strategies within and outside the home environment, and working with families, schools, and students in developing written plans to reduce the risk of anaphylaxis and to implement emergency treatment in the event of a reaction. This clinical report highlights the role of the pediatrician and pediatric health care provider in managing students with food allergies. (11/10)
http://pediatrics.aappublications.org/content/126/6/1232

MANAGEMENT OF INFANTS AT RISK FOR GROUP B STREPTOCOCCAL DISEASE (CLINICAL REPORT)

Karen M. Puopolo, MD, PhD, FAAP; Ruth Lynfield, MD, FAAP; James J. Cummings, MD, MS, FAAP; Committee on Fetus and Newborn; and Committee on Infectious Diseases

ABSTRACT. Group B streptococcal (GBS) infection remains the most common cause of neonatal early-onset sepsis and a significant cause of late-onset sepsis among young infants. Administration of intrapartum antibiotic prophylaxis is the only currently available effective strategy for the prevention of perinatal GBS early-onset disease, and there is no effective approach for the prevention of late-onset disease. The American Academy of Pediatrics joins with the American College of Obstetricians and Gynecologists to reaffirm the use of universal antenatal microbiologic-based testing for the detection of maternal GBS colonization to facilitate appropriate administration of intrapartum antibiotic prophylaxis. The purpose of this clinical report is to provide neonatal clinicians with updated information regarding the epidemiology of GBS disease as well current recommendations for the evaluation of newborn infants at risk for GBS disease and for treatment of those with confirmed GBS infection. This clinical report is endorsed by the American College of Obstetricians and Gynecologists (ACOG), July 2019, and should be construed as ACOG clinical guidance. (7/19)

See full text on page 883.

https://pediatrics.aappublications.org/content/144/2/e20191881

MANAGEMENT OF NEONATES BORN AT ≥35 0/7 WEEKS' GESTATION WITH SUSPECTED OR PROVEN EARLY-ONSET BACTERIAL SEPSIS (CLINICAL REPORT)

Karen M. Puopolo, MD, PhD, FAAP; William E. Benitz, MD, FAAP; Theoklis E. Zaoutis, MD, MSCE, FAAP; Committee on Fetus and Newborn; and Committee on Infectious Diseases

ABSTRACT. The incidence of neonatal early-onset sepsis (EOS) has declined substantially over the last 2 decades, primarily because of the implementation of evidence-based intrapartum antimicrobial therapy. However, EOS remains a serious and potentially fatal illness. Laboratory tests alone are neither sensitive nor specific enough to guide EOS management decisions. Maternal and infant clinical characteristics can help identify newborn infants who are at risk and guide the administration of empirical antibiotic therapy. The incidence of EOS, the prevalence and implications of established risk factors, the predictive value of commonly used laboratory tests, and the uncertainties in the risk/benefit balance of antibiotic exposures all vary significantly with gestational age at birth. Our purpose in this clinical report is to provide a summary of the current epidemiology of neonatal sepsis among infants born at ≥35 0/7 weeks' gestation and a framework for the development of evidence-based approaches to sepsis risk assessment among these infants. (11/18)

http://pediatrics.aappublications.org/content/142/6/e20182894

MANAGEMENT OF NEONATES BORN AT ≤34 6/7 WEEKS' GESTATION WITH SUSPECTED OR PROVEN EARLY-ONSET BACTERIAL SEPSIS (CLINICAL REPORT)

Karen M. Puopolo, MD, PhD, FAAP; William E. Benitz, MD, FAAP; Theoklis E. Zaoutis, MD, MSCE, FAAP; Committee on Fetus and Newborn; and Committee on Infectious Diseases

ABSTRACT. Early-onset sepsis (EOS) remains a serious and often fatal illness among infants born preterm, particularly among newborn infants of the lowest gestational age. Currently, most preterm infants with very low birth weight are treated empirically with antibiotics for risk of EOS, often for prolonged periods, in the absence of a culture-confirmed infection. Retrospective studies have revealed that antibiotic exposures after birth are associated with multiple subsequent poor outcomes among preterm infants, making the risk/benefit balance of these antibiotic treatments uncertain. Gestational age is the strongest single predictor of EOS, and the majority of preterm births occur in the setting of other factors associated with risk of EOS, making it difficult to apply risk stratification strategies to preterm infants. Laboratory tests alone have a poor predictive value in preterm EOS. Delivery characteristics of extremely preterm infants present an opportunity to identify those with a lower risk of EOS and may inform decisions to initiate or extend antibiotic therapies. Our purpose for this clinical report is to provide a summary of the current epidemiology of preterm neonatal sepsis and provide guidance for the development of evidence-based approaches to sepsis risk assessment among preterm newborn infants. (11/18)

http://pediatrics.aappublications.org/content/142/6/e20182896

MANAGEMENT OF PEDIATRIC TRAUMA

Committee on Pediatric Emergency Medicine; Council on Injury, Violence, and Poison Prevention; Section on Critical Care; Section on Orthopaedics; Section on Surgery; and Section on Transport Medicine (joint with Pediatric Trauma Society and Society of Trauma Nurses Pediatric Committee)

ABSTRACT. Injury is still the number 1 killer of children ages 1 to 18 years in the United States (http://www.cdc.gov/nchs/fastats/children.htm). Children who sustain injuries with resulting disabilities incur significant costs not only for their health care but also for productivity lost to the economy. The families of children who survive childhood injury with disability face years of emotional and financial hardship, along with a significant societal burden. The entire process of managing childhood injury is enormously complex and varies by region. Only the comprehensive cooperation of a broadly diverse trauma team will have a significant effect on improving the care of injured children. (7/16)

http://pediatrics.aappublications.org/content/138/2/e20161569

MANAGEMENT OF TYPE 2 DIABETES MELLITUS IN CHILDREN AND ADOLESCENTS (TECHNICAL REPORT)

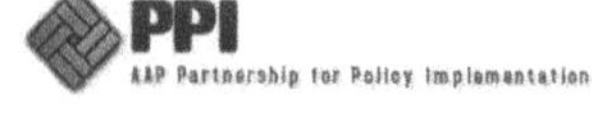

Shelley C. Springer, MD, MBA, MSc, JD, FAAP; Janet Silverstein, MD, FAAP; Kenneth Copeland, MD, FAAP; Kelly R. Moore, MD, FAAP; Greg E. Prazar, MD, FAAP; Terry Raymer, MD, CDE; Richard N. Shiffman, MD, FAAP; Vidhu V. Thaker, MD, FAAP; Meaghan Anderson, MS, RD, LD, CDE; Stephen J. Spann, MD, MBA, FAAFP; and Susan K. Flinn, MA

ABSTRACT. *Objective.* Over the last 3 decades, the prevalence of childhood obesity has increased dramatically in North America, ushering in a variety of health problems, including type 2 diabetes mellitus (T2DM), which previously was not typically seen until much later in life. This technical report describes, in detail, the procedures undertaken to develop the recommendations given in the accompanying clinical practice guideline, "Management of Type 2 Diabetes Mellitus in Children and Adolescents," and provides in-depth information about the rationale for the recommendations and the studies used to make the clinical practice guideline's recommendations.

Methods. A primary literature search was conducted relating to the treatment of T2DM in children and adolescents, and a secondary literature search was conducted relating to the screening and treatment of T2DM's comorbidities in children and adolescents. Inclusion criteria were prospectively and unanimously agreed on by members of the committee. An article was eligible for inclusion if it addressed treatment (primary search) or 1 of 4 comorbidities (secondary search) of T2DM, was published in 1990 or later, was written in English, and included an abstract. Only primary research inquiries were considered; review articles were considered if they included primary data or opinion. The research population had to constitute children and/or adolescents with an existing diagnosis of T2DM; studies of adult patients were considered if at least 10% of the study population was younger than 35 years. All retrieved titles, abstracts, and articles were reviewed by the consulting epidemiologist.

Results. Thousands of articles were retrieved and considered in both searches on the basis of the aforementioned criteria. From those, in the primary search, 199 abstracts were identified for possible inclusion, 58 of which were retained for systematic review. Five of these studies were classified as grade A studies, 1 as grade B, 20 as grade C, and 32 as grade D. Articles regarding treatment of T2DM selected for inclusion were divided into 4 major subcategories on the basis of type of treatment being discussed: (1) medical treatments (32 studies); (2) nonmedical treatments (9 studies); (3) provider behaviors (8 studies); and (4) social issues (9 studies). From the secondary search, an additional 336 abstracts relating to comorbidities were identified for possible inclusion, of which 26 were retained for systematic review. These articles included the following: 1 systematic review of literature regarding comorbidities of T2DM in adolescents; 5 expert opinions presenting global recommendations not based on evidence; 5 cohort studies reporting natural history of disease and comorbidities; 3 with specific attention to comorbidity patterns in specific ethnic groups (case-control, cohort, and clinical report using adult literature); 3 reporting an association between microalbuminuria and retinopathy (2 case-control, 1 cohort); 3 reporting the prevalence of nephropathy (cohort); 1 reporting peripheral vascular disease (case series); 2 discussing retinopathy (1 case-control, 1 position statement); and 3 addressing hyperlipidemia (American Heart Association position statement on cardiovascular risks; American Diabetes Association consensus statement; case series). A breakdown of grade of recommendation shows no grade A studies, 10 grade B studies, 6 grade C studies, and 10 grade D studies. With regard to screening and treatment recommendations for comorbidities, data in children are scarce, and the available literature is conflicting. Therapeutic recommendations for hypertension, dyslipidemia, retinopathy, microalbuminuria, and depression were summarized from expert guideline documents and are presented in detail in the guideline. The references are provided, but the committee did not independently assess the supporting evidence. Screening tools are provided in the Supplemental Information. (1/13)

http://pediatrics.aappublications.org/content/131/2/e648

MARIJUANA USE DURING PREGNANCY AND BREASTFEEDING: IMPLICATIONS FOR NEONATAL AND CHILDHOOD OUTCOMES (CLINICAL REPORT)

Sheryl A. Ryan, MD, FAAP; Seth D. Ammerman, MD, FAAP, FSAHM, DABAM; Mary E. O'Connor, MD, MPH, FAAP; Committee on Substance Use and Prevention; and Section on Breastfeeding

ABSTRACT. Marijuana is one of the most widely used substances during pregnancy in the United States. Emerging data on the ability of cannabinoids to cross the placenta and affect the development of the fetus raise concerns about both pregnancy outcomes and long-term consequences for the infant or child. Social media is used to tout the use of marijuana for severe nausea associated with pregnancy. Concerns have also been raised about marijuana use by breastfeeding mothers. With this clinical report, we provide data on the current rates of marijuana use among pregnant and lactating women, discuss what is known about the effects of marijuana on fetal development and later neurodevelopmental and behavioral outcomes, and address implications for education and policy. (8/18)

http://pediatrics.aappublications.org/content/142/3/e20181889

MATERNAL-FETAL INTERVENTION AND FETAL CARE CENTERS (CLINICAL REPORT)

Committee on Bioethics (joint with American College of Obstetricians and Gynecologists Committee on Ethics)

ABSTRACT. The past 2 decades have yielded profound advances in the fields of prenatal diagnosis and fetal intervention. Although fetal interventions are driven by a beneficence-based motivation to improve fetal and neonatal outcomes, advancement in fetal therapies raises ethical issues surrounding maternal autonomy and decision-making, concepts of innovation versus research, and organizational aspects within institutions in the development of fetal care centers. To safeguard the interests of both the pregnant woman and the fetus, the American College of Obstetricians and Gynecologists and the American Academy of Pediatrics make recommendations regarding informed consent, the role of research subject advocates and other independent advocates, the availability of support services, the multidisciplinary nature of fetal intervention teams, the oversight of centers, and the need to accumulate maternal and fetal outcome data. (7/11, reaffirmed 2/18)

http://pediatrics.aappublications.org/content/128/2/e473

MEDIA AND YOUNG MINDS

Council on Communications and Media

ABSTRACT. Infants, toddlers, and preschoolers are now growing up in environments saturated with a variety of traditional and new technologies, which they are adopting at increasing rates. Although there has been much hope for the educational potential of interactive media for young children, accompanied by fears about their overuse during this crucial period of rapid brain development, research in this area still remains limited. This policy statement reviews the existing literature on television, videos, and mobile/interactive technologies; their potential for educational benefit; and related health concerns for young children (0 to 5 years of age). The statement also highlights areas in which pediatric providers can offer specific guidance to families in managing their young children's media use, not only in terms of content or time limits, but also emphasizing the importance of parent-child shared media use and allowing the child time to take part in other developmentally healthy activities. (10/16)

http://pediatrics.aappublications.org/content/138/5/e20162591

MEDIA EDUCATION

Committee on Communications and Media

ABSTRACT. The American Academy of Pediatrics recognizes that exposure to mass media (eg, television, movies, video and computer games, the Internet, music lyrics and videos, newspapers, magazines, books, advertising) presents health risks for children and adolescents but can provide benefits as well. Media education has the potential to reduce the harmful effects of media and accentuate the positive effects. By understanding and supporting media education, pediatricians can play an important role in reducing harmful effects of media on children and adolescents. (9/10)

http://pediatrics.aappublications.org/content/126/5/1012

MEDIA USE IN SCHOOL-AGED CHILDREN AND ADOLESCENTS

Council on Communications and Media

ABSTRACT. This policy statement focuses on children and adolescents 5 through 18 years of age. Research suggests both benefits and risks of media use for the health of children and teenagers. Benefits include exposure to new ideas and knowledge acquisition, increased opportunities for social contact and support, and new opportunities to access health-promotion messages and information. Risks include negative health effects on weight and sleep; exposure to inaccurate, inappropriate, or

unsafe content and contacts; and compromised privacy and confidentiality. Parents face challenges in monitoring their children's and their own media use and in serving as positive role models. In this new era, evidence regarding healthy media use does not support a one-size-fits-all approach. Parents and pediatricians can work together to develop a Family Media Use Plan (www.healthychildren.org/MediaUsePlan) that considers their children's developmental stages to individualize an appropriate balance for media time and consistent rules about media use, to mentor their children, to set boundaries for accessing content and displaying personal information, and to implement open family communication about media. (10/16)
http://pediatrics.aappublications.org/content/138/5/e20162592

MEDIATORS AND ADVERSE EFFECTS OF CHILD POVERTY IN THE UNITED STATES (TECHNICAL REPORT)

John M. Pascoe, MD, MPH, FAAP; David L. Wood, MD, MPH, FAAP; James H. Duffee, MD, MPH, FAAP; Alice Kuo, MD, PhD, MEd, FAAP; Committee on Psychosocial Aspects of Child and Family Health; and Council on Community Pediatrics

ABSTRACT. The link between poverty and children's health is well recognized. Even temporary poverty may have an adverse effect on children's health, and data consistently support the observation that poverty in childhood continues to have a negative effect on health into adulthood. In addition to childhood morbidity being related to child poverty, epidemiologic studies have documented a mortality gradient for children aged 1 to 15 years (and adults), with poor children experiencing a higher mortality rate than children from higher-income families. The global great recession is only now very slowly abating for millions of America's children and their families. At this difficult time in the history of our nation's families and immediately after the 50th anniversary year of President Lyndon Johnson's War on Poverty, it is particularly germane for the American Academy of Pediatrics, which is "dedicated to the health of all children," to publish a research-supported technical report that examines the mediators associated with the long-recognized adverse effects of child poverty on children and their families. This technical report draws on research from a number of disciplines, including physiology, sociology, psychology, economics, and epidemiology, to describe the present state of knowledge regarding poverty's negative impact on children's health and development. Children inherit not only their parents' genes but also the family ecology and its social milieu. Thus, parenting skills, housing, neighborhood, schools, and other factors (eg, medical care) all have complex relations to each other and influence how each child's genetic canvas is expressed. Accompanying this technical report is a policy statement that describes specific actions that pediatricians and other child advocates can take to attenuate the negative effects of the mediators identified in this technical report and improve the well-being of our nation's children and their families. (3/16)
http://pediatrics.aappublications.org/content/137/4/e20160340

MEDICAID POLICY STATEMENT

Committee on Child Health Financing

ABSTRACT. Medicaid insures 39% of the children in the United States. This revision of the 2005 Medicaid Policy Statement of the American Academy of Pediatrics reflects opportunities for changes in state Medicaid programs resulting from the 2010 Patient Protection and Affordable Care Act as upheld in 2012 by the Supreme Court. Policy recommendations focus on the areas of benefit coverage, financing and payment, eligibility, outreach and enrollment, managed care, and quality improvement. (4/13, reaffirmed 3/19)
http://pediatrics.aappublications.org/content/131/5/e1697

MEDICAL COUNTERMEASURES FOR CHILDREN IN PUBLIC HEALTH EMERGENCIES, DISASTERS, OR TERRORISM

Disaster Preparedness Advisory Council

ABSTRACT. Significant strides have been made over the past 10 to 15 years to develop medical countermeasures (MCMs) to address potential disaster hazards, including chemical, biological, radiologic, and nuclear threats. Significant and effective collaboration between the pediatric health community, including the American Academy of Pediatrics, and federal partners, such as the Office of the Assistant Secretary for Preparedness and Response, Centers for Disease Control and Prevention, Federal Emergency Management Agency, National Institutes of Health, Food and Drug Administration, and other federal agencies, over the past 5 years has resulted in substantial gains in addressing the needs of children related to disaster preparedness in general and MCMs in particular. Yet, major gaps still remain related to MCMs for children, a population highly vulnerable to the effects of exposure to such threats, because many vaccines and pharmaceuticals approved for use by adults as MCMs do not yet have pediatric formulations, dosing information, or safety information. As a result, the nation's stockpiles and other caches (designated supply of MCMs) where pharmacotherapeutic and other MCMs are stored are less prepared to address the needs of children compared with those of adults in the event of a disaster. This policy statement provides recommendations to close the remaining gaps for the development and use of MCMs in children during public health emergencies or disasters. The progress made by federal agencies to date to address the needs of children and the shared commitment of collaboration that characterizes the current relationship between the pediatric health community and the federal agencies responsible for MCMs should encourage all child advocates to invest the necessary energy and resources now to complete the process of remedying the remaining significant gaps in preparedness. (1/16)
http://pediatrics.aappublications.org/content/137/2/e20154273

MEDICAL EMERGENCIES OCCURRING AT SCHOOL

Council on School Health

ABSTRACT. Children and adults might experience medical emergency situations because of injuries, complications of chronic health conditions, or unexpected major illnesses that occur in schools. In February 2001, the American Academy of Pediatrics issued a policy statement titled "Guidelines for Emergency Medical Care in Schools" (available at: http://aappolicy.aappublications.org/cgi/content/full/pediatrics;107/2/435). Since the release of that statement, the spectrum of potential individual student emergencies has changed significantly. The increase in the number of children with special health care needs and chronic medical conditions attending schools and the challenges associated with ensuring that schools have access to on-site licensed health care professionals on an ongoing basis have added to increasing the risks of medical emergencies in schools. The goal of this statement is to increase pediatricians' awareness of schools' roles in preparing for individual student emergencies and to provide recommendations for primary care and school physicians on how to assist and support school personnel. (10/08, reaffirmed 9/11, 4/17)
http://pediatrics.aappublications.org/content/122/4/887

MEDICAL STAFF APPOINTMENT AND DELINEATION OF PEDIATRIC PRIVILEGES IN HOSPITALS (CLINICAL REPORT)

Daniel A. Rauch, MD; Committee on Hospital Care; and Section on Hospital Medicine

ABSTRACT. The review and verification of credentials and the granting of clinical privileges are required of every hospital to ensure that members of the medical staff are competent and qualified to provide specified levels of patient care. The credentialing process involves the following: (1) assessment of the professional

and personal background of each practitioner seeking privileges; (2) assignment of privileges appropriate for the clinician's training and experience; (3) ongoing monitoring of the professional activities of each staff member; and (4) periodic reappointment to the medical staff on the basis of objectively measured performance. We examine the essential elements of a credentials review for initial and renewed medical staff appointments along with suggested criteria for the delineation of clinical privileges. Sample forms for the delineation of privileges can be found on the American Academy of Pediatrics Committee on Hospital Care Web site (http://www.aap.org/visit/cmte19.htm). Because of differences among individual hospitals, no 1 method for credentialing is universally applicable. The medical staff of each hospital must, therefore, establish its own process based on the general principles reviewed in this report. The issues of medical staff membership and credentialing have become very complex, and institutions and medical staffs are vulnerable to legal action. Consequently, it is advisable for hospitals and medical staffs to obtain expert legal advice when medical staff bylaws are constructed or revised. (3/12, reaffirmed 2/16)
http://pediatrics.aappublications.org/content/129/4/797

MEDICAL VERSUS NONMEDICAL IMMUNIZATION EXEMPTIONS FOR CHILD CARE AND SCHOOL ATTENDANCE

Committee on Practice and Ambulatory Medicine, Committee on Infectious Diseases, Committee on State Government Affairs, Council on School Health, and Section on Administration and Practice Management

ABSTRACT. Routine childhood immunizations against infectious diseases are an integral part of our public health infrastructure. They provide direct protection to the immunized individual and indirect protection to children and adults unable to be immunized via the effect of community immunity. All 50 states, the District of Columbia, and Puerto Rico have regulations requiring proof of immunization for child care and school attendance as a public health strategy to protect children in these settings and to secondarily serve as a mechanism to promote timely immunization of children by their caregivers. Although all states and the District of Columbia have mechanisms to exempt school attendees from specific immunization requirements for medical reasons, the majority also have a heterogeneous collection of regulations and laws that allow nonmedical exemptions from childhood immunizations otherwise required for child care and school attendance. The American Academy of Pediatrics (AAP) supports regulations and laws requiring certification of immunization to attend child care and school as a sound means of providing a safe environment for attendees and employees of these settings. The AAP also supports medically indicated exemptions to specific immunizations as determined for each individual child. The AAP views nonmedical exemptions to school-required immunizations as inappropriate for individual, public health, and ethical reasons and advocates for their elimination. (8/16)
http://pediatrics.aappublications.org/content/138/3/e20162145

MEDICATION-ASSISTED TREATMENT OF ADOLESCENTS WITH OPIOID USE DISORDERS

Committee on Substance Use and Prevention

ABSTRACT. Opioid use disorder is a leading cause of morbidity and mortality among US youth. Effective treatments, both medications and substance use disorder counseling, are available but underused, and access to developmentally appropriate treatment is severely restricted for adolescents and young adults. Resources to disseminate available therapies and to develop new treatments specifically for this age group are needed to save and improve lives of youth with opioid addiction. (8/16)
http://pediatrics.aappublications.org/content/138/3/e20161893

MENSTRUAL MANAGEMENT FOR ADOLESCENTS WITH DISABILITIES (CLINICAL REPORT)

Elisabeth H. Quint, MD; Rebecca F. O'Brien, MD; and Committee on Adolescence (joint with North American Society for Pediatric and Adolescent Gynecology)

ABSTRACT. The onset of menses for adolescents with physical or intellectual disabilities can affect their independence and add additional concerns for families at home, in schools, and in other settings. The pediatrician is the primary health care provider to explore and assist with the pubertal transition and menstrual management. Menstrual management of both normal and abnormal cycles may be requested to minimize hygiene issues, premenstrual symptoms, dysmenorrhea, heavy or irregular bleeding, contraception, and conditions exacerbated by the menstrual cycle. Several options are available for menstrual management, depending on the outcome that is desired, ranging from cycle regulation to complete amenorrhea. The use of medications or the request for surgeries to help with the menstrual cycles in teenagers with disabilities has medical, social, legal, and ethical implications. This clinical report is designed to help guide pediatricians in assisting adolescent females with intellectual and/or physical disabilities and their families in making decisions related to successfully navigating menarche and subsequent menstrual cycles. (6/16)
http://pediatrics.aappublications.org/content/138/1/e20160295

MENTAL HEALTH COMPETENCIES FOR PEDIATRIC PRACTICE

Jane Meschan Foy, MD, FAAP; Cori M. Green, MD, MS, FAAP; Marian F. Earls, MD, MTS, FAAP; Committee on Psychosocial Aspects of Child and Family Health; and Mental Health Leadership Work Group

ABSTRACT. Pediatricians have unique opportunities and an increasing sense of responsibility to promote healthy social-emotional development of children and to prevent and address their mental health and substance use conditions. In this report, the American Academy of Pediatrics updates its 2009 policy statement, which proposed competencies for providing mental health care to children in primary care settings and recommended steps toward achieving them. This 2019 policy statement affirms the 2009 statement and expands competencies in response to science and policy that have emerged since: the impact of adverse childhood experiences and social determinants on mental health, trauma-informed practice, and team-based care. Importantly, it also recognizes ways in which the competencies are pertinent to pediatric subspecialty practice. Proposed mental health competencies include foundational communication skills, capacity to incorporate mental health content and tools into health promotion and primary and secondary preventive care, skills in the psychosocial assessment and care of children with mental health conditions, knowledge and skills of evidence-based psychosocial therapy and psychopharmacologic therapy, skills to function as a team member and comanager with mental health specialists, and commitment to embrace mental health practice as integral to pediatric care. Achievement of these competencies will necessarily be incremental, requiring partnership with fellow advocates, system changes, new payment mechanisms, practice enhancements, and decision support for pediatricians in their expanded scope of practice. (10/19)

See full text on page 903.

https://pediatrics.aappublications.org/content/144/5/e20192757

METABOLIC AND BARIATRIC SURGERY FOR PEDIATRIC PATIENTS WITH SEVERE OBESITY (TECHNICAL REPORT)

Christopher F. Bolling, MD, FAAP; Sarah C. Armstrong, MD, FAAP; Kirk W. Reichard, MD, MBA, FAAP; Marc P. Michalsky, MD, FACS, FAAP, FASMBS; Section on Obesity; and Section on Surgery

ABSTRACT. Severe obesity affects the health and well-being of millions of children and adolescents in the United States and is widely considered to be an "epidemic within an epidemic" that poses a major public health crisis. Currently, few effective treatments for severe obesity exist. Metabolic and bariatric surgery are existing but underuse treatment options for pediatric patients with severe obesity. Roux-en-Y gastric bypass and vertical sleeve gastrectomy are the most commonly performed metabolic and bariatric procedures in the United States and have been shown to result in sustained short-, mid-, and long-term weight loss, with associated resolution of multiple obesity-related comorbid diseases. Substantial evidence supports the safety and effectiveness of surgical weight loss for children and adolescents, and robust best practice guidelines for these procedures exist. (11/19)

See full text on page 921.

https://pediatrics.aappublications.org/content/144/6/e20193224

THE METABOLIC SYNDROME IN CHILDREN AND ADOLESCENTS: SHIFTING THE FOCUS TO CARDIOMETABOLIC RISK FACTOR CLUSTERING (CLINICAL REPORT)

Sheela N. Magge, MD, MSCE, FAAP; Elizabeth Goodman, MD, MBA, FAAP; Sarah C. Armstrong, MD, FAAP; Committee on Nutrition; Section on Endocrinology; and Section on Obesity

ABSTRACT. Metabolic syndrome (MetS) was developed by the National Cholesterol Education Program Adult Treatment Panel III, identifying adults with at least 3 of 5 cardiometabolic risk factors (hyperglycemia, increased central adiposity, elevated triglycerides, decreased high-density lipoprotein cholesterol, and elevated blood pressure) who are at increased risk of diabetes and cardiovascular disease. The constellation of MetS component risk factors has a shared pathophysiology and many common treatment approaches grounded in lifestyle modification. Several attempts have been made to define MetS in the pediatric population. However, in children, the construct is difficult to define and has unclear implications for clinical care. In this Clinical Report, we focus on the importance of screening for and treating the individual risk factor components of MetS. Focusing attention on children with cardiometabolic risk factor clustering is emphasized over the need to define a pediatric MetS. (7/17)

http://pediatrics.aappublications.org/content/140/2/e20171603

METRIC UNITS AND THE PREFERRED DOSING OF ORALLY ADMINISTERED LIQUID MEDICATIONS

Committee on Drugs

ABSTRACT. Medication overdoses are a common, but preventable, problem among children. Volumetric dosing errors and the use of incorrect dosing delivery devices are 2 common sources of these preventable errors for orally administered liquid medications. To reduce errors and increase precision of drug administration, milliliter-based dosing should be used exclusively when prescribing and administering liquid medications. Teaspoon- and tablespoon-based dosing should not be used. Devices that allow for precise dose administration (preferably syringes with metric markings) should be used instead of household spoons and should be distributed with the medication. (3/15)

http://pediatrics.aappublications.org/content/135/4/784

MIND-BODY THERAPIES IN CHILDREN AND YOUTH (CLINICAL REPORT)

Section on Integrative Medicine

ABSTRACT. Mind-body therapies are popular and are ranked among the top 10 complementary and integrative medicine practices reportedly used by adults and children in the 2007–2012 National Health Interview Survey. A growing body of evidence supports the effectiveness and safety of mind-body therapies in pediatrics. This clinical report outlines popular mind-body therapies for children and youth and examines the best-available evidence for a variety of mind-body therapies and practices, including biofeedback, clinical hypnosis, guided imagery, meditation, and yoga. The report is intended to help health care professionals guide their patients to nonpharmacologic approaches to improve concentration, help decrease pain, control discomfort, or ease anxiety. (8/16)

http://pediatrics.aappublications.org/content/138/3/e20161896

MINORS AS LIVING SOLID-ORGAN DONORS (CLINICAL REPORT)

Lainie Friedman Ross, MD, PhD; J. Richard Thistlethwaite Jr, MD, PhD; and Committee on Bioethics

ABSTRACT. In the past half-century, solid-organ transplantation has become standard treatment for a variety of diseases in children and adults. The major limitation for all transplantation is the availability of donors, and the gap between demand and supply continues to grow despite the increase in living donors. Although rare, children do serve as living donors, and these donations raise serious ethical issues. This clinical report includes a discussion of the ethical considerations regarding minors serving as living donors, using the traditional benefit/burden calculus from the perspectives of both the donor and the recipient. The report also includes an examination of the circumstances under which a minor may morally participate as a living donor, how to minimize risks, and what the informed-consent process should entail. The American Academy of Pediatrics holds that minors can morally serve as living organ donors but only in exceptional circumstances when specific criteria are fulfilled. (8/08, reaffirmed 5/11)

http://pediatrics.aappublications.org/content/122/2/454

MODEL CONTRACTUAL LANGUAGE FOR MEDICAL NECESSITY FOR CHILDREN

Committee on Child Health Financing

ABSTRACT. The term "medical necessity" is used by Medicare and Medicaid and in insurance contracts to refer to medical services that are generally recognized as appropriate for the diagnosis, prevention, or treatment of disease and injury. There is no consensus on how to define and apply the term and the accompanying rules and regulations, and as a result there has been substantial variation in medical-necessity definitions and interpretations. With this policy statement, the American Academy of Pediatrics hopes to encourage insurers to adopt more consistent medical-necessity definitions that take into account the needs of children. (7/05, reaffirmed 10/11)

http://pediatrics.aappublications.org/content/116/1/261

MOTOR DELAYS: EARLY IDENTIFICATION AND EVALUATION (CLINICAL REPORT)

Garey H. Noritz, MD; Nancy A. Murphy, MD; and Neuromotor Screening Expert Panel

ABSTRACT. Pediatricians often encounter children with delays of motor development in their clinical practices. Earlier identification of motor delays allows for timely referral for developmental interventions as well as diagnostic evaluations and treatment planning. A multidisciplinary expert panel developed an algorithm for the surveillance and screening of children for motor delays within the medical home, offering guidance for the initial workup and referral of the child with possible delays in motor development. Highlights of this clinical report include suggestions for formal developmental screening at the 9-, 18-, 30-, and 48-month well-child visits; approaches to the neurologic examination, with emphasis on the assessment of muscle tone; and initial diagnostic approaches for medical home providers. Use of diagnostic tests to evaluate children with motor delays are described, including brain MRI for children with high muscle tone, and measuring serum creatine kinase concentration of those with decreased muscle tone. The importance of pursuing diagnostic tests while concurrently referring patients to early intervention programs is emphasized. (5/13, reaffirmed 5/17)

http://pediatrics.aappublications.org/content/131/6/e2016

THE NEED TO OPTIMIZE ADOLESCENT IMMUNIZATION (CLINICAL REPORT)

Henry H. Bernstein, DO, MHCM, FAAP; Joseph A. Bocchini Jr, MD, FAAP; and Committee on Infectious Diseases

ABSTRACT. The adolescent period heralds the pediatric patient's transition into adulthood. It is a time of dynamic development during which effective preventive care measures can promote safe behaviors and the development of lifelong health habits. One of the foundations of preventive adolescent health care is timely vaccination, and every visit can be viewed as an opportunity to update and complete an adolescent's immunizations.

In the past decade, the adolescent immunization schedule has expanded to include 2 doses of quadrivalent meningococcal conjugate vaccine; 1 dose of tetanus, diphtheria, acellular pertussis, absorbed vaccine; 2 or 3 doses of human papillomavirus vaccine, depending on the child's age; and an annual influenza vaccine. In addition, during adolescent visits, health care providers can determine whether catch-up vaccination is needed to meet early childhood recommendations for hepatitis B; hepatitis A; measles, mumps, rubella; poliovirus; and varicella vaccines. New serogroup B meningococcal vaccines are now available for those at increased risk for meningococcal disease; in addition, these serogroup B meningococcal vaccines received a Category B recommendation for healthy adolescents, where individual counseling and risk–benefit evaluation based on health care provider judgements and patient preferences are indicated. This clinical report focuses on the epidemiology of adolescent vaccine-preventable diseases by reviewing the rationale for the annual universally recommended adolescent immunization schedule of the American Academy of Pediatrics, the American Academy of Family Physicians, the Centers for Disease Control and Prevention, and the American Congress of Obstetricians and Gynecologists. In addition, the barriers that negatively influence adherence to this current adolescent immunization schedule will be highlighted. (2/17)

http://pediatrics.aappublications.org/content/139/3/e20164186

NEEDS OF KINSHIP CARE FAMILIES AND PEDIATRIC PRACTICE

David Rubin, MD, FAAP; Sarah H. Springer, MD, FAAP; Sarah Zlotnik, MSW, MSPH; Christina D. Kang-Yi, PhD; and Council on Foster Care, Adoption, and Kinship Care

ABSTRACT. As many as 3% of children in the United States live in kinship care arrangements with caregivers who are relatives but not the biological parents of the child. A growing body of evidence suggests that children who cannot live with their biological parents fare better, overall, when living with extended family than with nonrelated foster parents. Acknowledging this, federal laws and public policies increasingly favor kinship care over nonrelative foster care when children are unable to live with their biological parents. Despite overall better outcomes, families providing kinship care experience many hardships, and the children experience many of the same adversities of children in traditional foster care. This policy statement reviews both the strengths and vulnerabilities of kinship families and suggests strategies for pediatricians to use to address the needs of individual patients and families. Strategies are also outlined for community, state, and federal advocacy on behalf of these children and their families. (3/17)

http://pediatrics.aappublications.org/content/139/4/e20170099

NEONATAL DRUG WITHDRAWAL (CLINICAL REPORT)

Mark L. Hudak, MD; Rosemarie C. Tan, MD, PhD; Committee on Drugs; and Committee on Fetus and Newborn

ABSTRACT. Maternal use of certain drugs during pregnancy can result in transient neonatal signs consistent with withdrawal or acute toxicity or cause sustained signs consistent with a lasting drug effect. In addition, hospitalized infants who are treated with opioids or benzodiazepines to provide analgesia or sedation may be at risk for manifesting signs of withdrawal. This statement updates information about the clinical presentation of infants exposed to intrauterine drugs and the therapeutic options for treatment of withdrawal and is expanded to include evidence-based approaches to the management of the hospitalized infant who requires weaning from analgesics or sedatives. (1/12, reaffirmed 2/16)

http://pediatrics.aappublications.org/content/129/2/e540

NEONATAL PROVIDER WORKFORCE (TECHNICAL REPORT)

Erin L. Keels, DNP, APRN-CNP, NNP-BC; Jay P. Goldsmith, MD, FAAP; and Committee on Fetus and Newborn

ABSTRACT. This technical report reviews education, training, competency requirements, and scopes of practice of the different neonatal care providers who work to meet the special needs of neonatal patients and their families in the NICU. Additionally, this report examines the current workforce issues of NICU providers, offers suggestions for establishing and monitoring quality and safety of care, and suggests potential solutions to the NICU provider workforce shortages now and in the future. (11/19)

See full text on page 933.

https://pediatrics.aappublications.org/content/144/6/e20193147

A NEW ERA IN QUALITY MEASUREMENT: THE DEVELOPMENT AND APPLICATION OF QUALITY MEASURES

Terry Adirim, MD, MPH, FAAP; Kelley Meade, MD, FAAP; Kamila Mistry, PhD, MPH; Council on Quality Improvement and Patient Safety; and Committee on Practice and Ambulatory Medicine

ABSTRACT. Quality measures are used for a variety of purposes in health care, including clinical care improvement, regulation, accreditation, public reporting, surveillance, and maintenance of certification. Most quality measures are 1 of 3 types: structure, process, or outcome. Health care quality measures should address the domains of quality across the continuum of care and reflect patient and family experience. Measure development for pediatric health care has a number of important challenges, including gaps in the evidence base; the fact that measures for most conditions must be age-specific; the long, resourceintensive development process; and the national focus on measure development for adult conditions. Numerous national organizations focus on the development and application of quality measures, including the Pediatric Quality Measures Program, which is focused solely on the development and implementation of pediatric-specific measures. Once a quality measure is developed for use in national measurement programs, the organization that develops and/or "stewards" the measure may submit the measure or set of measures for endorsement, which is recognition of the scientific soundness, usability, and relevance of the measure. Quality measures must then be disseminated and applied to improve care. Although pediatric health care providers and child health care institutions alike must continually balance time and resources needed to address multiple reporting requirements, quality measurement is an important tool for advancing high-quality and safe health care for children. This policy statement provides an overview of quality measurement and describes the opportunities for pediatric health care providers to apply quality measures to improve clinical quality and performance in the delivery of pediatric health care services. (12/16)

http://pediatrics.aappublications.org/content/139/1/e20163442

NEWBORN SCREENING EXPANDS: RECOMMENDATIONS FOR PEDIATRICIANS AND MEDICAL HOMES—IMPLICATIONS FOR THE SYSTEM (CLINICAL REPORT)

PPI AAP Partnership for Policy Implementation

Newborn Screening Authoring Committee

ABSTRACT. Advances in newborn screening technology, coupled with recent advances in the diagnosis and treatment of rare but serious congenital conditions that affect newborn infants, provide increased opportunities for positively affecting the lives of children and their families. These advantages also pose new challenges to primary care pediatricians, both educationally and in response to the management of affected infants. Primary care pediatricians require immediate access to clinical and diagnostic information and guidance and have a proactive role to play in supporting the performance of the newborn screening system. Primary care pediatricians must develop office policies and procedures to ensure that newborn screening is conducted and that results are transmitted to them in a timely fashion; they must also develop strategies to use should these systems fail. In addition, collaboration with local, state, and national partners is essential for promoting actions and policies that will optimize the function of the newborn screening systems and ensure that families receive the full benefit of them. (1/08, reaffirmed 9/16)

http://pediatrics.aappublications.org/content/121/1/192

NEWBORN SCREENING FOR BILIARY ATRESIA (TECHNICAL REPORT)

Kasper S. Wang, MD, FAAP, FACS; Section on Surgery; and Committee on Fetus and Newborn (joint with Childhood Liver Disease Research Network)

ABSTRACT. Biliary atresia is the most common cause of pediatric end-stage liver disease and the leading indication for pediatric liver transplantation. Affected infants exhibit evidence of biliary obstruction within the first few weeks after birth. Early diagnosis and successful surgical drainage of bile are associated with greater survival with the child's native liver. Unfortunately, because noncholestatic jaundice is extremely common in early infancy, it is difficult to identify the rare infant with cholestatic jaundice who has biliary atresia. Hence, the need for timely diagnosis of this disease warrants a discussion of the feasibility of screening for biliary atresia to improve outcomes. Herein, newborn screening for biliary atresia in the United States is assessed by using criteria established by the Discretionary Advisory Committee on Heritable Disorders in Newborns and Children. Published analyses indicate that newborn screening for biliary atresia by using serum bilirubin concentrations or stool color cards is potentially life-saving and cost-effective. Further studies are necessary to evaluate the feasibility, effectiveness, and costs of potential screening strategies for early identification of biliary atresia in the United States. (11/15)

http://pediatrics.aappublications.org/content/136/6/e1663

NICOTINE AND TOBACCO AS SUBSTANCES OF ABUSE IN CHILDREN AND ADOLESCENTS (TECHNICAL REPORT)

Lorena M. Siqueira, MD, MSPH, FAAP, FSAHM, and Committee on Substance Use and Prevention

ABSTRACT. Nicotine is the primary pharmacologic component of tobacco, and users of tobacco products seek out its effects. The highly addictive nature of nicotine is responsible for its widespread use and difficulty with quitting. This technical report focuses on nicotine and discusses the stages of use in progression to dependence on nicotine-containing products; the physiologic characteristics, neurobiology, metabolism, pharmacogenetics, and health effects of nicotine; and acute nicotine toxicity. Finally, some newer approaches to cessation are noted. (12/16)

http://pediatrics.aappublications.org/content/139/1/e20163436

NONDISCRIMINATION IN PEDIATRIC HEALTH CARE

Committee on Pediatric Workforce

ABSTRACT. This policy statement is a revision of a 2001 statement and articulates the positions of the American Academy of Pediatrics on nondiscrimination in pediatric health care. It addresses both pediatricians who provide health care and the infants, children, adolescents, and young adults whom they serve. (10/07, reaffirmed 6/11, 1/15)

http://pediatrics.aappublications.org/content/120/4/922

NONEMERGENCY ACUTE CARE: WHEN IT'S NOT THE MEDICAL HOME

Gregory P. Conners, MD, MPH, MBA, FAAP; Susan J. Kressly, MD, FAAP; James M. Perrin, MD, FAAP; Julia E. Richerson, MD, FAAP; Usha M. Sankrithi, MBBS, MPH, FAAP; Committee on Practice and Ambulatory Medicine; Committee on Pediatric Emergency Medicine; Section on Telehealth Care; Section on Emergency Medicine; Subcommittee on Urgent Care; and Task Force on Pediatric Practice Change

ABSTRACT. The American Academy of Pediatrics (AAP) affirms that the optimal location for children to receive care for acute, nonemergency health concerns is the medical home. The medical home is characterized by the AAP as a care model that "must be accessible, family centered, continuous, comprehensive, coordinated, compassionate, and culturally effective." However, some children and families use acute care services outside the medical home because there is a perceived or real benefit related to accessibility, convenience, or cost of care. Examples of such acute care entities include urgent care facilities, retail-based clinics, and commercial telemedicine services. Children deserve high-quality, appropriate, and safe acute care services wherever they access the health care system, with timely and complete communication with the medical home, to ensure coordinated and continuous care. Treatment of children under established, new, and evolving practice arrangements in acute care entities should adhere to the core principles of continuity of care and communication, best practices within a defined scope of services, pediatric-trained staff, safe transitions of care, and continuous improvement. In support of the medical home, the AAP urges stakeholders, including payers, to avoid any incentives (eg, reduced copays) that encourage visits to external entities for acute issues as a preference over the medical home. (4/17)

http://pediatrics.aappublications.org/content/139/5/e20170629

NONINITIATION OR WITHDRAWAL OF INTENSIVE CARE FOR HIGH-RISK NEWBORNS

Committee on Fetus and Newborn

ABSTRACT. Advances in medical technology have led to dilemmas in initiation and withdrawal of intensive care of newborn infants with a very poor prognosis. Physicians and parents together must make difficult decisions guided by their understanding of the child's best interest. The foundation for these decisions consists of several key elements: (1) direct and open

communication between the health care team and the parents of the child with regard to the medical status, prognosis, and treatment options; (2) inclusion of the parents as active participants in the decision process; (3) continuation of comfort care even when intensive care is not being provided; and (4) treatment decisions that are guided primarily by the best interest of the child. (2/07, reaffirmed 5/10, 6/15)
http://pediatrics.aappublications.org/content/119/2/401

NONINVASIVE RESPIRATORY SUPPORT (CLINICAL REPORT)

James J. Cummings, MD, FAAP; Richard A. Polin, MD, FAAP; and Committee on Fetus and Newborn

ABSTRACT. Mechanical ventilation is associated with increased survival of preterm infants but is also associated with an increased incidence of chronic lung disease (bronchopulmonary dysplasia) in survivors. Nasal continuous positive airway pressure (nCPAP) is a form of noninvasive ventilation that reduces the need for mechanical ventilation and decreases the combined outcome of death or bronchopulmonary dysplasia. Other modes of noninvasive ventilation, including nasal intermittent positive pressure ventilation, biphasic positive airway pressure, and high-flow nasal cannula, have recently been introduced into the NICU setting as potential alternatives to mechanical ventilation or nCPAP. Randomized controlled trials suggest that these newer modalities may be effective alternatives to nCPAP and may offer some advantages over nCPAP, but efficacy and safety data are limited. (12/15)
http://pediatrics.aappublications.org/content/137/1/e20153758

NONORAL FEEDING FOR CHILDREN AND YOUTH WITH DEVELOPMENTAL OR ACQUIRED DISABILITIES (CLINICAL REPORT)

Richard C. Adams, MD, FAAP; Ellen Roy Elias, MD, FAAP; and Council on Children With Disabilities

ABSTRACT. The decision to initiate enteral feedings is multifaceted, involving medical, financial, cultural, and emotional considerations. Children who have developmental or acquired disabilities are at risk for having primary and secondary conditions that affect growth and nutritional well-being. This clinical report provides (1) an overview of clinical issues in children who have developmental or acquired disabilities that may prompt a need to consider nonoral feedings, (2) a systematic way to support the child and family in clinical decisions related to initiating nonoral feeding, (3) information on surgical options that the family may need to consider in that decision-making process, and (4) pediatric guidance for ongoing care after initiation of nonoral feeding intervention, including care of the gastrostomy tube and skin site. Ongoing medical and psychosocial support is needed after initiation of nonoral feedings and is best provided through the collaborative efforts of the family and a team of professionals that may include the pediatrician, dietitian, social worker, and/or therapists. (11/14, reaffirmed 6/19)
http://pediatrics.aappublications.org/content/134/6/e1745

NONTHERAPEUTIC USE OF ANTIMICROBIAL AGENTS IN ANIMAL AGRICULTURE: IMPLICATIONS FOR PEDIATRICS (TECHNICAL REPORT)

Jerome A. Paulson, MD, FAAP; Theoklis E. Zaoutis, MD, MSCE, FAAP; Council on Environmental Health; and Committee on Infectious Diseases

ABSTRACT. Antimicrobial resistance is one of the most serious threats to public health globally and threatens our ability to treat infectious diseases. Antimicrobial-resistant infections are associated with increased morbidity, mortality, and health care costs. Infants and children are affected by transmission of susceptible and resistant food zoonotic pathogens through the food supply, direct contact with animals, and environmental pathways. The overuse and misuse of antimicrobial agents in veterinary and human medicine is, in large part, responsible for the emergence of antibiotic resistance. Approximately 80% of the overall tonnage of antimicrobial agents sold in the United States in 2012 was for animal use, and approximately 60% of those agents are considered important for human medicine. Most of the use involves the addition of low doses of antimicrobial agents to the feed of healthy animals over prolonged periods to promote growth and increase feed efficiency or at a range of doses to prevent disease. These nontherapeutic uses contribute to resistance and create new health dangers for humans. This report describes how antimicrobial agents are used in animal agriculture, reviews the mechanisms of how such use contributes to development of resistance, and discusses US and global initiatives to curb the use of antimicrobial agents in agriculture. (11/15)
http://pediatrics.aappublications.org/content/136/6/e1670

OFFICE-BASED CARE FOR LESBIAN, GAY, BISEXUAL, TRANSGENDER, AND QUESTIONING YOUTH

Committee on Adolescence

ABSTRACT. The American Academy of Pediatrics issued its last statement on homosexuality and adolescents in 2004. Although most lesbian, gay, bisexual, transgender, and questioning (LGBTQ) youth are quite resilient and emerge from adolescence as healthy adults, the effects of homophobia and heterosexism can contribute to health disparities in mental health with higher rates of depression and suicidal ideation, higher rates of substance abuse, and more sexually transmitted and HIV infections. Pediatricians should have offices that are teen-friendly and welcoming to sexual minority youth. Obtaining a comprehensive, confidential, developmentally appropriate adolescent psychosocial history allows for the discovery of strengths and assets as well as risks. Referrals for mental health or substance abuse may be warranted. Sexually active LGBTQ youth should have sexually transmitted infection/HIV testing according to recommendations of the Sexually Transmitted Diseases Treatment Guidelines of the Centers for Disease Control and Prevention based on sexual behaviors. With appropriate assistance and care, sexual minority youth should live healthy, productive lives while transitioning through adolescence and young adulthood. (6/13)
http://pediatrics.aappublications.org/content/132/1/198

OFFICE-BASED CARE FOR LESBIAN, GAY, BISEXUAL, TRANSGENDER, AND QUESTIONING YOUTH (TECHNICAL REPORT)

David A. Levine, MD, and Committee on Adolescence

ABSTRACT. The American Academy of Pediatrics issued its last statement on homosexuality and adolescents in 2004. This technical report reflects the rapidly expanding medical and psychosocial literature about sexual minority youth. Pediatricians should be aware that some youth in their care may have concerns or questions about their sexual orientation or that of siblings, friends, parents, relatives, or others and should provide factual, current, nonjudgmental information in a confidential manner. Although most lesbian, gay, bisexual, transgender, and questioning (LGBTQ) youth are quite resilient and emerge from adolescence as healthy adults, the effects of homophobia and heterosexism can contribute to increased mental health issues for sexual minority youth. LGBTQ and MSM/WSW (men having sex with men and women having sex with women) adolescents, in comparison with heterosexual adolescents, have higher rates of depression and suicidal ideation, higher rates of substance abuse, and more risky sexual behaviors. Obtaining a comprehensive, confidential, developmentally appropriate adolescent psychosocial history allows for the discovery of strengths and assets as well as risks. Pediatricians should have offices that are teen-friendly and welcoming to sexual minority youth. This includes having supportive, engaging office staff members who ensure that there are no barriers to care. For transgender youth, pediatricians should provide the opportunity to acknowledge and affirm their feelings of gender dysphoria and desires to transition to the opposite gender. Referral of transgender youth to a qualified mental health professional is critical to assist with the dysphoria, to educate them, and to assess their readiness for transition. With appropriate assistance and care, sexual minority youth should live healthy, productive lives while transitioning through adolescence and young adulthood. (6/13)

http://pediatrics.aappublications.org/content/132/1/e297

OFFICE-BASED COUNSELING FOR UNINTENTIONAL INJURY PREVENTION (CLINICAL REPORT)

H. Garry Gardner, MD, and Committee on Injury, Violence, and Poison Prevention

ABSTRACT. Unintentional injuries are the leading cause of death for children older than 1 year. Pediatricians should include unintentional injury prevention as a major component of anticipatory guidance for infants, children, and adolescents. The content of injury-prevention counseling varies for infants, preschool-aged children, school-aged children, and adolescents. This report provides guidance on the content of unintentional injury-prevention counseling for each of those age groups. (1/07)

http://pediatrics.aappublications.org/content/119/1/202

OFF-LABEL USE OF DRUGS IN CHILDREN

Committee on Drugs

ABSTRACT. The passage of the Best Pharmaceuticals for Children Act and the Pediatric Research Equity Act has collectively resulted in an improvement in rational prescribing for children, including more than 500 labeling changes. However, off-label drug use remains an important public health issue for infants, children, and adolescents, because an overwhelming number of drugs still have no information in the labeling for use in pediatrics. The purpose of off-label use is to benefit the individual patient. Practitioners use their professional judgment to determine these uses. As such, the term "off-label" does not imply an improper, illegal, contraindicated, or investigational use. Therapeutic decision-making must always rely on the best available evidence and the importance of the benefit for the individual patient. (2/14)

http://pediatrics.aappublications.org/content/133/3/563

OFF-LABEL USE OF MEDICAL DEVICES IN CHILDREN

Section on Cardiology and Cardiac Surgery and Section on Orthopaedics

ABSTRACT. Despite widespread therapeutic needs, the majority of medical and surgical devices used in children do not have approval or clearance from the Food and Drug Administration (FDA) for use in pediatric populations. The clinical need for devices to diagnose and treat diseases or conditions occurring in children has led to the widespread and necessary practice in pediatric medicine and surgery of using approved devices for "off-label" or "physician-directed" applications that are not included in FDA-approved labeling. This practice is common and often appropriate, even with the highest-risk (class III) devices. The legal and regulatory framework used by the FDA for devices is complex, and economic or market barriers to medical and surgical device development for children are significant. Given the need for pediatric medical and surgical devices and the challenges to pediatric device development, off-label use is a necessary and appropriate part of care. In addition, because of the relatively uncommon nature of pediatric conditions, FDA clearance or approval often requires other regulatory pathways (eg, Humanitarian Device Exemption), which can cause confusion among pediatricians and payers about whether a specific use, even of an approved device, is considered experimental. This policy statement describes the appropriateness of off-label use of devices in children; the use of devices approved or cleared through the FDA regulatory processes, including through the Humanitarian Device Exemption; and the important need to increase pediatric device labeling information for all devices and especially those that pose the highest risk to children. (12/16)

http://pediatrics.aappublications.org/content/139/1/e20163439

ONGOING PEDIATRIC HEALTH CARE FOR THE CHILD WHO HAS BEEN MALTREATED (CLINICAL REPORT)

Emalee Flaherty, MD, FAAP; Lori Legano, MD, FAAP; Sheila Idzerda, MD, FAAP; and Council on Child Abuse and Neglect

ABSTRACT. Pediatricians provide continuous medical care and anticipatory guidance for children who have been reported to state child protection agencies, including tribal child protection agencies, because of suspected child maltreatment. Because families may continue their relationships with their pediatricians after these reports, these primary care providers are in a unique position to recognize and manage the physical, developmental, academic, and emotional consequences of maltreatment and exposure to childhood adversity. Substantial information is available to optimize follow-up medical care of maltreated children. This new clinical report will provide guidance to pediatricians about how they can best oversee and foster the optimal physical health, growth, and development of children who have been maltreated and remain in the care of their biological family or are returned to their care by Child Protective Services agencies. The report describes the pediatrician's role in helping to strengthen families' and caregivers' capabilities and competencies and in promoting and maximizing high-quality services for their families in their community. Pediatricians should refer to other reports and policies from the American Academy of Pediatrics for more information about the emotional and behavioral consequences of child maltreatment and the treatment of these consequences. (3/19)

See full text on page 949.

https://pediatrics.aappublications.org/content/143/4/e20190284

OPHTHALMOLOGIC EXAMINATIONS IN CHILDREN WITH JUVENILE RHEUMATOID ARTHRITIS (CLINICAL REPORT)

James Cassidy, MD; Jane Kivlin, MD; Carol Lindsley, MD; James Nocton, MD; Section on Rheumatology; and Section on Ophthalmology

ABSTRACT. Unlike the joints, ocular involvement with juvenile rheumatoid arthritis is most often asymptomatic; yet, the inflammation can cause serious morbidity with loss of vision. Scheduled slit-lamp examinations by an ophthalmologist at specific intervals can detect ocular disease early, and prompt treatment can prevent vision loss. (5/06, reaffirmed 10/12, 7/18)

http://pediatrics.aappublications.org/content/117/5/1843

OPTIMIZING BONE HEALTH IN CHILDREN AND ADOLESCENTS (CLINICAL REPORT)

Neville H. Golden, MD; Steven A. Abrams, MD; and Committee on Nutrition

ABSTRACT. The pediatrician plays a major role in helping optimize bone health in children and adolescents. This clinical report reviews normal bone acquisition in infants, children, and adolescents and discusses factors affecting bone health in this age group. Previous recommended daily allowances for calcium and vitamin D are updated, and clinical guidance is provided regarding weight-bearing activities and recommendations for calcium and vitamin D intake and supplementation. Routine calcium supplementation is not recommended for healthy children and adolescents, but increased dietary intake to meet daily requirements is encouraged. The American Academy of Pediatrics endorses the higher recommended dietary allowances for vitamin D advised by the Institute of Medicine and supports testing for vitamin D deficiency in children and adolescents with conditions associated with increased bone fragility. Universal screening for vitamin D deficiency is not routinely recommended in healthy children or in children with dark skin or obesity because there is insufficient evidence of the cost–benefit of such a practice in reducing fracture risk. The preferred test to assess bone health is dual-energy x-ray absorptiometry, but caution is advised when interpreting results in children and adolescents who may not yet have achieved peak bone mass. For analyses, z scores should be used instead of T scores, and corrections should be made for size. Office-based strategies for the pediatrician to optimize bone health are provided. This clinical report has been endorsed by American Bone Health. (9/14)

http://pediatrics.aappublications.org/content/134/4/e1229

OPTIONS COUNSELING FOR THE PREGNANT ADOLESCENT PATIENT

Laurie L. Hornberger, MD, MPH, FAAP, and Committee on Adolescence

ABSTRACT. Each year, more than 500000 girls and young women younger than 20 years become pregnant. It is important for pediatricians to have the ability and the resources in their offices to make a timely pregnancy diagnosis in their adolescent patients and provide them with nonjudgmental pregnancy options counseling. Counseling includes an unbiased discussion of the adolescent's legal options to either continue or terminate her pregnancy, supporting the adolescent in the decision-making process, and referring the adolescent to appropriate resources and services. Pediatricians who choose not to provide such discussions should promptly refer pregnant adolescent patients to a health care professional who will offer developmentally appropriate pregnancy options counseling. This approach to pregnancy options counseling has not changed since the original 1989 American Academy of Pediatrics statement on this issue. (8/17)

http://pediatrics.aappublications.org/content/140/3/e20172274

ORAL AND DENTAL ASPECTS OF CHILD ABUSE AND NEGLECT (CLINICAL REPORT)

Susan A. Fisher-Owens, MD, MPH, FAAP; James L. Lukefahr, MD, FAAP; Anupama Rao Tate, DMD, MPH; Section on Oral Health; and Committee on Child Abuse and Neglect (joint with American Academy of Pediatric Dentistry Council on Clinical Affairs, Council on Scientific Affairs, and Ad Hoc Work Group on Child Abuse and Neglect)

ABSTRACT. In all 50 states, health care providers (including dentists) are mandated to report suspected cases of abuse and neglect to social service or law enforcement agencies. The purpose of this report is to review the oral and dental aspects of physical and sexual abuse and dental neglect in children and the role of pediatric care providers and dental providers in evaluating such conditions. This report addresses the evaluation of bite marks as well as perioral and intraoral injuries, infections, and diseases that may raise suspicion for child abuse or neglect. Oral health issues can also be associated with bullying and are commonly seen in human trafficking victims. Some medical providers may receive less education pertaining to oral health and dental injury and disease and may not detect the mouth and gum findings that are related to abuse or neglect as readily as they detect those involving other areas of the body. Therefore, pediatric care providers and dental providers are encouraged to collaborate to increase the prevention, detection, and treatment of these conditions in children. (7/17)

http://pediatrics.aappublications.org/content/140/2/e20171487

ORAL HEALTH CARE FOR CHILDREN WITH DEVELOPMENTAL DISABILITIES (CLINICAL REPORT)

Kenneth W. Norwood Jr, MD; Rebecca L. Slayton, DDS, PhD; Council on Children With Disabilities; and Section on Oral Health

ABSTRACT. Children with developmental disabilities often have unmet complex health care needs as well as significant physical and cognitive limitations. Children with more severe conditions and from low-income families are particularly at risk with high dental needs and poor access to care. In addition, children with developmental disabilities are living longer, requiring continued oral health care. This clinical report describes the effect that poor oral health has on children with developmental disabilities as well as the importance of partnerships between the pediatric medical and dental homes. Basic knowledge of the oral health risk factors affecting children with developmental disabilities is provided. Pediatricians may use the report to guide their incorporation of oral health assessments and education into their well-child examinations for children with developmental disabilities. This report has medical, legal, educational, and operational implications for practicing pediatricians. (2/13, reaffirmed 6/18)

http://pediatrics.aappublications.org/content/131/3/614

ORGANIC FOODS: HEALTH AND ENVIRONMENTAL ADVANTAGES AND DISADVANTAGES (CLINICAL REPORT)

Joel Forman, MD; Janet Silverstein, MD; Committee on Nutrition; and Council on Environmental Health

ABSTRACT. The US market for organic foods has grown from $3.5 billion in 1996 to $28.6 billion in 2010, according to the Organic Trade Association. Organic products are now sold in specialty stores and conventional supermarkets. Organic products contain numerous marketing claims and terms, only some of which are standardized and regulated.

In terms of health advantages, organic diets have been convincingly demonstrated to expose consumers to fewer pesticides associated with human disease. Organic farming has been demonstrated to have less environmental impact than conventional approaches. However, current evidence does not support any meaningful nutritional benefits or deficits from eating organic compared with conventionally grown foods, and there are no well-powered human studies that directly demonstrate health benefits or disease protection as a result of consuming an organic diet. Studies also have not demonstrated any detrimental or disease-promoting effects from an organic diet. Although organic foods regularly command a significant price premium, well-designed farming studies demonstrate that costs can be competitive and yields comparable to those of conventional farming techniques. Pediatricians should incorporate this evidence when discussing the health and environmental impact of organic foods and organic farming while continuing to encourage all patients and their families to attain optimal nutrition and dietary variety consistent with the US Department of Agriculture's MyPlate recommendations.

This clinical report reviews the health and environmental issues related to organic food production and consumption. It defines the term "organic," reviews organic food-labeling standards, describes organic and conventional farming practices, and explores the cost and environmental implications of organic production techniques. It examines the evidence available on nutritional quality and production contaminants in conventionally produced and organic foods. Finally, this report provides guidance for pediatricians to assist them in advising their patients regarding organic and conventionally produced food choices. (10/12)

http://pediatrics.aappublications.org/content/130/5/e1406

ORGANIZED SPORTS FOR CHILDREN, PREADOLESCENTS, AND ADOLESCENTS (CLINICAL REPORT)

Kelsey Logan, MD, MPH, FAAP; Steven Cuff, MD, FAAP; and Council on Sports Medicine and Fitness

ABSTRACT. Interest and participation in organized sports for children, preadolescents, and adolescents continue to grow. Because of increased participation, and younger entry age, in organized sports, appropriate practice, game schedules, and content become more important, taking into account athlete developmental stage and skills. Parental support for organized sports in general, with focus on development and fun instead of winning, has emerged as a key factor in the athlete's enjoyment of sports. Schools and community sports organizations who support multiple levels of sport (eg, recreational, competitive, elite) can include more youth who want to play sports and combat sport dropout. This report reviews the benefits and risks of organized sports as well as the roles of schools, community organizations, parents, and coaches in organized sports. It is designed to complement the American Academy of Pediatrics clinical reports "Physical Activity Assessment and Counseling in Pediatric Clinical Settings" and "Sports Specialization and Intensive Training in Young Athletes" by reviewing relevant literature on healthy organized sports for youth and providing guidance on organized sport readiness and entry. The report also provides guidance for pediatricians on counseling parents and advocating for healthy organized sports participation. (5/19)

See full text on page 967.

https://pediatrics.aappublications.org/content/143/6/e20190997

OUT-OF-HOME PLACEMENT FOR CHILDREN AND ADOLESCENTS WITH DISABILITIES (CLINICAL REPORT)

Sandra L. Friedman, MD, MPH, FAAP; Miriam A. Kalichman, MD, FAAP; and Council on Children With Disabilities

ABSTRACT. The vast majority of children and youth with chronic and complex health conditions who also have intellectual and developmental disabilities are cared for in their homes. Social, legal, policy, and medical changes through the years have allowed for an increase in needed support within the community. However, there continues to be a relatively small group of children who live in various types of congregate care settings. This clinical report describes these settings and the care and services that are provided in them. The report also discusses reasons families choose out-of-home placement for their children, barriers to placement, and potential effects of this decision on family members. We examine the pediatrician's role in caring for children with severe intellectual and developmental disabilities and complex medical problems in the context of responding to parental inquiries about out-of-home placement and understanding factors affecting these types of decisions. Common medical problems and care issues for children residing outside the family home are reviewed. Variations in state and federal regulations, challenges in understanding local systems, and access to services are also discussed. (9/14, reaffirmed 2/19)

http://pediatrics.aappublications.org/content/134/4/836

OUT-OF-HOME PLACEMENT FOR CHILDREN AND ADOLESCENTS WITH DISABILITIES—ADDENDUM: CARE OPTIONS FOR CHILDREN AND ADOLESCENTS WITH DISABILITIES AND MEDICAL COMPLEXITY (CLINICAL REPORT)

Sandra L. Friedman, MD, MPH, FAAP; Kenneth W. Norwood Jr, MD, FAAP; and Council on Children With Disabilities

ABSTRACT. Children and adolescents with significant intellectual and developmental disabilities and complex medical problems require safe and comprehensive care to meet their medical and psychosocial needs. Ideally, such children and youth should be cared for by their families in their home environments. When this type of arrangement is not possible, there should be exploration of appropriate, alternative noncongregate community-based settings, especially alternative family homes. Government funding sources exist to support care in the community, although there is variability among states with regard to the availability of community programs and resources. It is important that families are supported in learning about options of care. Pediatricians can serve as advocates for their patients and their families to access community-based services and to increase the availability of resources to ensure that the option to live in a family home is available to all children with complex medical needs. (11/16, reaffirmed 2/19)

http://pediatrics.aappublications.org/content/138/6/e20163216

OUT-OF-SCHOOL SUSPENSION AND EXPULSION

Council on School Health

ABSTRACT. The primary mission of any school system is to educate students. To achieve this goal, the school district must maintain a culture and environment where all students feel safe, nurtured, and valued and where order and civility are expected standards of behavior. Schools cannot allow unacceptable behavior to interfere with the school district's primary mission. To this end, school districts adopt codes of conduct for expected behaviors and policies to address unacceptable behavior. In developing these policies, school boards must weigh the severity of the offense and the consequences of the punishment and the balance between individual and institutional rights and responsibilities. Out-of-school suspension and expulsion are the most severe consequences that a school district can impose for unacceptable behavior. Traditionally, these consequences have been reserved for offenses deemed especially severe or dangerous and/or for recalcitrant offenders. However, the implications and consequences of out-of-school suspension and expulsion and "zero-tolerance" are of such severity that their application and appropriateness for a developing child require periodic review. The indications and effectiveness of exclusionary discipline policies that demand automatic or rigorous application are increasingly questionable. The impact of these policies on offenders, other children, school districts, and communities is broad. Periodic scrutiny of policies should be placed not only on the need for a better understanding of the educational, emotional, and social impact of out-of-school suspension and expulsion on the individual student but also on the greater societal costs of such rigid policies. Pediatricians should be prepared to assist students and families affected by out-of-school suspension and expulsion and should be willing to guide school districts in their communities to find more effective and appropriate alternatives to exclusionary discipline policies for the developing child. A discussion of preventive strategies and alternatives to out-of-school suspension and expulsion, as well as recommendations for the role of the physician in matters of out-of-school suspension and expulsion are included. School-wide positive behavior support/positive behavior intervention and support is discussed as an effective alternative. (2/13)

http://pediatrics.aappublications.org/content/131/3/e1000

OVERCROWDING CRISIS IN OUR NATION'S EMERGENCY DEPARTMENTS: IS OUR SAFETY NET UNRAVELING?

Committee on Pediatric Emergency Medicine

ABSTRACT. Emergency departments (EDs) are a vital component in our health care safety net, available 24 hours a day, 7 days a week, for all who require care. There has been a steady increase in the volume and acuity of patient visits to EDs, now with well over 100 million Americans (30 million children) receiving emergency care annually. This rise in ED utilization has effectively saturated the capacity of EDs and emergency medical services in many communities. The resulting phenomenon, commonly referred to as ED overcrowding, now threatens access to emer-

gency services for those who need them the most. As managers of the pediatric medical home and advocates for children and optimal pediatric health care, there is a very important role for pediatricians and the American Academy of Pediatrics in guiding health policy decision-makers toward effective solutions that promote the medical home and timely access to emergency care. (9/04, reaffirmed 5/07, 6/11, 7/16)
http://pediatrics.aappublications.org/content/114/3/878

OVERUSE INJURIES, OVERTRAINING, AND BURNOUT IN CHILD AND ADOLESCENT ATHLETES (CLINICAL REPORT)

Joel S. Brenner, MD, MPH, and Council on Sports Medicine and Fitness

ABSTRACT. Overuse is one of the most common etiologic factors that lead to injuries in the pediatric and adolescent athlete. As more children are becoming involved in organized and recreational athletics, the incidence of overuse injuries is increasing. Many children are participating in sports year-round and sometimes on multiple teams simultaneously. This overtraining can lead to burnout, which may have a detrimental effect on the child participating in sports as a lifelong healthy activity. One contributing factor to overtraining may be parental pressure to compete and succeed. The purpose of this clinical report is to assist pediatricians in identifying and counseling at-risk children and their families. This report supports the American Academy of Pediatrics policy statement on intensive training and sport specialization. (6/07, reaffirmed 3/11, 6/14)
http://pediatrics.aappublications.org/content/119/6/1242

OXYGEN TARGETING IN EXTREMELY LOW BIRTH WEIGHT INFANTS (CLINICAL REPORT)

James J. Cummings, MD, FAAP; Richard A. Polin, MD, FAAP; and Committee on Fetus and Newborn

ABSTRACT. The use of supplemental oxygen plays a vital role in the care of the critically ill preterm infant, but the unrestricted use of oxygen can lead to unintended harms, such as chronic lung disease and retinopathy of prematurity. An overly restricted use of supplemental oxygen may have adverse effects as well. Ideally, continuous monitoring of tissue and cellular oxygen delivery would allow clinicians to better titrate the use of supplemental oxygen, but such monitoring is not currently feasible in the clinical setting. The introduction of pulse oximetry has greatly aided the clinician by providing a relatively easy and continuous estimate of arterial oxygen saturation, but pulse oximetry has several practical, technical, and physiologic limitations. Recent randomized clinical trials comparing different pulse oximetry targets have been conducted to better inform the practice of supplemental oxygen use. This clinical report discusses the benefits and limitations of pulse oximetry for assessing oxygenation, summarizes randomized clinical trials of oxygen saturation targeting, and addresses implications for practice. (7/16)
http://pediatrics.aappublications.org/content/138/2/e20161576

PAIN ASSESSMENT AND TREATMENT IN CHILDREN WITH SIGNIFICANT IMPAIRMENT OF THE CENTRAL NERVOUS SYSTEM (CLINICAL REPORT)

Julie Hauer, MD, FAAP; Amy J. Houtrow, MD, PhD, MPH, FAAP; Section on Hospice and Palliative Medicine; and Council on Children With Disabilities

ABSTRACT. Pain is a frequent and significant problem for children with impairment of the central nervous system, with the highest frequency and severity occurring in children with the greatest impairment. Despite the significance of the problem, this population remains vulnerable to underrecognition and undertreatment of pain. Barriers to treatment may include uncertainty in identifying pain along with limited experience and fear with the use of medications for pain treatment. Behavioral pain-assessment tools are reviewed in this clinical report, along with other strategies for monitoring pain after an intervention. Sources of pain in this population include acute-onset pain attributable to tissue injury or inflammation resulting in nociceptive pain, with pain then expected to resolve after treatment directed at the source. Other sources can result in chronic intermittent pain that, for many, occurs on a weekly to daily basis, commonly attributed to gastroesophageal reflux, spasticity, and hip subluxation. Most challenging are pain sources attributable to the impaired central nervous system, requiring empirical medication trials directed at causes that cannot be identified by diagnostic tests, such as central neuropathic pain. Interventions reviewed include integrative therapies and medications, such as gabapentinoids, tricyclic antidepressants, α-agonists, and opioids. This clinical report aims to address, with evidence-based guidance, the inherent challenges with the goal to improve comfort throughout life in this vulnerable group of children. (5/17)
http://pediatrics.aappublications.org/content/139/6/e20171002

PARENTAL LEAVE FOR RESIDENTS AND PEDIATRIC TRAINING PROGRAMS

Section on Medical Students, Residents, and Fellowship Trainees and Committee on Early Childhood

ABSTRACT. The American Academy of Pediatrics (AAP) is committed to the development of rational, equitable, and effective parental leave policies that are sensitive to the needs of pediatric residents, families, and developing infants and that enable parents to spend adequate and good-quality time with their young children. It is important for each residency program to have a policy for parental leave that is written, that is accessible to residents, and that clearly delineates program practices regarding parental leave. At a minimum, a parental leave policy for residents and fellows should conform legally with the Family Medical Leave Act as well as with respective state laws and should meet institutional requirements of the Accreditation Council for Graduate Medical Education for accredited programs. Policies should be well formulated and communicated in a culturally sensitive manner. The AAP advocates for extension of benefits consistent with the Family Medical Leave Act to all residents and interns beginning at the time that pediatric residency training begins. The AAP recommends that regardless of gender, residents who become parents should be guaranteed 6 to 8 weeks, at a minimum, of parental leave with pay after the infant's birth. In addition, in conformance with federal law, the resident should be allowed to extend the leave time when necessary by using paid vacation time or leave without pay. Coparenting, adopting, or fostering of a child should entitle the resident, regardless of gender, to the same amount of paid leave (6–8 weeks) as a person who takes maternity/paternity leave. Flexibility, creativity, and advanced planning are necessary to arrange schedules that optimize resident education and experience, cultivate equity in sharing workloads, and protect pregnant residents from overly strenuous work experiences at critical times of their pregnancies. (1/13, reaffirmed 4/19)
http://pediatrics.aappublications.org/content/131/2/387

PARENTAL PRESENCE DURING TREATMENT OF EBOLA OR OTHER HIGHLY CONSEQUENTIAL INFECTION (CLINICAL REPORT)

H. Dele Davies, MD, MS, MHCM, FAAP; Carrie L. Byington, MD, FAAP; and Committee on Infectious Diseases

ABSTRACT. This clinical report offers guidance to health care providers and hospitals on options to consider regarding parental presence at the bedside while caring for a child with suspected or proven Ebola virus disease (Ebola) or other highly consequential infection. Options are presented to help meet the needs of the patient and the family while also posing the least risk to providers and health care organizations. The optimal way to minimize

risk is to limit contact between the person under investigation or treatment and family members/caregivers whenever possible while working to meet the emotional support needs of both patient and family. At times, caregiver presence may be deemed to be in the best interest of the patient, and in such situations, a strong effort should be made to limit potential risks of exposure to the caregiver, health care providers, and the community. The decision to allow parental/caregiver presence should be made in consultation with a team including an infectious diseases expert and state and/or local public health authorities and should involve consideration of many factors, depending on the stage of investigation and management, including (1) a careful history, physical examination, and investigations to elucidate the likelihood of the diagnosis of Ebola or other highly consequential infection; (2) ability of the facility to offer appropriate isolation for the person under investigation and family members and to manage Ebola; (3) ability to recognize and exclude people at increased risk of worse outcomes (eg, pregnant women); and (4) ability of parent/caregiver to follow instructions, including appropriate donning and doffing of personal protective equipment. (8/16)
http://pediatrics.aappublications.org/content/138/3/e20161891

PARENT-PROVIDER-COMMUNITY PARTNERSHIPS: OPTIMIZING OUTCOMES FOR CHILDREN WITH DISABILITIES (CLINICAL REPORT)

Nancy A. Murphy, MD; Paul S. Carbone, MD; and Council on Children With Disabilities

ABSTRACT. Children with disabilities and their families have multifaceted medical, developmental, educational, and habilitative needs that are best addressed through strong partnerships among parents, providers, and communities. However, traditional health care systems are designed to address acute rather than chronic conditions. Children with disabilities require high-quality medical homes that provide care coordination and transitional care, and their families require social and financial supports. Integrated community systems of care that promote participation of all children are needed. The purpose of this clinical report is to explore the challenges of developing effective community-based systems of care and to offer suggestions to pediatricians and policy-makers regarding the development of partnerships among children with disabilities, their families, and health care and other providers to maximize health and well-being of these children and their families. (9/11, reaffirmed 5/17)
http://pediatrics.aappublications.org/content/128/4/795

PATENT DUCTUS ARTERIOSUS IN PRETERM INFANTS (CLINICAL REPORT)

William E. Benitz, MD, FAAP, and Committee on Fetus and Newborn

ABSTRACT. Despite a large body of basic science and clinical research and clinical experience with thousands of infants over nearly 6 decades, there is still uncertainty and controversy about the significance, evaluation, and management of patent ductus arteriosus in preterm infants, resulting in substantial heterogeneity in clinical practice. The purpose of this clinical report is to summarize the evidence available to guide evaluation and treatment of preterm infants with prolonged ductal patency in the first few weeks after birth. (12/15)
http://pediatrics.aappublications.org/content/137/1/e20153730

PATIENT- AND FAMILY-CENTERED CARE AND THE PEDIATRICIAN'S ROLE

Committee on Hospital Care and Institute for Patient- and Family-Centered Care

ABSTRACT. Drawing on several decades of work with families, pediatricians, other health care professionals, and policy makers, the American Academy of Pediatrics provides a definition of patient- and family-centered care. In pediatrics, patient- and family-centered care is based on the understanding that the family is the child's primary source of strength and support. Further, this approach to care recognizes that the perspectives and information provided by families, children, and young adults are essential components of high-quality clinical decision-making, and that patients and family are integral partners with the health care team. This policy statement outlines the core principles of patient- and family-centered care, summarizes some of the recent literature linking patient- and family-centered care to improved health outcomes, and lists various other benefits to be expected when engaging in patient- and family-centered pediatric practice. The statement concludes with specific recommendations for how pediatricians can integrate patient- and family-centered care in hospitals, clinics, and community settings, and in broader systems of care, as well. (1/12, reaffirmed 2/18)
http://pediatrics.aappublications.org/content/129/2/394

PATIENT- AND FAMILY-CENTERED CARE AND THE ROLE OF THE EMERGENCY PHYSICIAN PROVIDING CARE TO A CHILD IN THE EMERGENCY DEPARTMENT

Committee on Pediatric Emergency Medicine (joint with American College of Emergency Physicians)

ABSTRACT. Patient- and family-centered care is an approach to health care that recognizes the role of the family in providing medical care; encourages collaboration between the patient, family, and health care professionals; and honors individual and family strengths, cultures, traditions, and expertise. Although there are many opportunities for providing patient- and family-centered care in the emergency department, there are also challenges to doing so. The American Academy of Pediatrics and the American College of Emergency Physicians support promoting patient dignity, comfort, and autonomy; recognizing the patient and family as key decision-makers in the patient's medical care; recognizing the patient's experience and perspective in a culturally sensitive manner; acknowledging the interdependence of child and parent as well as the pediatric patient's evolving independence; encouraging family-member presence; providing information to the family during interventions; encouraging collaboration with other health care professionals; acknowledging the importance of the patient's medical home; and encouraging institutional policies for patient- and family-centered care. (11/06, reaffirmed 6/09, 10/11, 9/15)
http://pediatrics.aappublications.org/content/118/5/2242

PATIENT- AND FAMILY-CENTERED CARE COORDINATION: A FRAMEWORK FOR INTEGRATING CARE FOR CHILDREN AND YOUTH ACROSS MULTIPLE SYSTEMS

Council on Children With Disabilities and Medical Home Implementation Project Advisory Committee

ABSTRACT. Understanding a care coordination framework, its functions, and its effects on children and families is critical for patients and families themselves, as well as for pediatricians, pediatric medical subspecialists/surgical specialists, and anyone providing services to children and families. Care coordination is an essential element of a transformed American health care delivery system that emphasizes optimal quality and cost outcomes, addresses family-centered care, and calls for partnership across various settings and communities. High-quality, cost-effective health care requires that the delivery system include elements for the provision of services supporting the coordination of care across settings and professionals. This requirement of supporting coordination of care is generally true for health systems providing care for all children and youth but especially for those with special health care needs. At the foundation of an efficient and effective system of care delivery is the patient-/family-centered medical home. From its inception, the medical home has had care coordination as a core element. In general, optimal outcomes for children and youth, especially those with special health care needs, require interfacing among multiple care systems and individuals, including the following: medical, social, and behavioral professionals; the educational system; payers; medical equipment providers; home care agencies; advocacy groups; needed supportive therapies/services; and families. Coordination of care across settings permits an integration of services that is centered on the comprehensive needs of the patient and family, leading to decreased health care costs, reduction in fragmented care, and improvement in the patient/family experience of care. (4/14, reaffirmed 4/18)

http://pediatrics.aappublications.org/content/133/5/e1451

PATIENT- AND FAMILY-CENTERED CARE OF CHILDREN IN THE EMERGENCY DEPARTMENT (TECHNICAL REPORT)

Nanette Dudley, MD, FAAP; Alice Ackerman, MD, MBA, FAAP; Kathleen M. Brown, MD, FACEP; Sally K. Snow, BSN, RN, CPEN, FAEN; and Committee on Pediatric Emergency Medicine (joint with American College of Emergency Physicians Pediatric Emergency Medicine Committee and Emergency Nurses Association Pediatric Committee)

ABSTRACT. Patient- and family-centered care is an approach to the planning, delivery, and evaluation of health care that is grounded in a mutually beneficial partnership among patients, families, and health care professionals. Providing patient- and family-centered care to children in the emergency department setting presents many opportunities and challenges. This revised technical report draws on previously published policy statements and reports, reviews the current literature, and describes the present state of practice and research regarding patient- and family-centered care for children in the emergency department setting as well as some of the complexities of providing such care. (12/14)

http://pediatrics.aappublications.org/content/135/1/e255

PATIENT SAFETY IN THE PEDIATRIC EMERGENCY CARE SETTING

Committee on Pediatric Emergency Medicine

ABSTRACT. Patient safety is a priority for all health care professionals, including those who work in emergency care. Unique aspects of pediatric care may increase the risk of medical error and harm to patients, especially in the emergency care setting. Although errors can happen despite the best human efforts, given the right set of circumstances, health care professionals must work proactively to improve safety in the pediatric emergency care system. Specific recommendations to improve pediatric patient safety in the emergency department are provided in this policy statement. (12/07, reaffirmed 6/11, 7/14)

http://pediatrics.aappublications.org/content/120/6/1367

PEDESTRIAN SAFETY

Committee on Injury, Violence, and Poison Prevention

ABSTRACT. Each year, approximately 900 pediatric pedestrians younger than 19 years are killed. In addition, 51000 children are injured as pedestrians, and 5300 of them are hospitalized because of their injuries. Parents should be warned that young children often do not have the cognitive, perceptual, and behavioral abilities to negotiate traffic independently. Parents should also be informed about the danger of vehicle back-over injuries to toddlers playing in driveways. Because posttraumatic stress syndrome commonly follows even minor pedestrian injury, pediatricians should screen and refer for this condition as necessary. The American Academy of Pediatrics supports community- and school-based strategies that minimize a child's exposure to traffic, especially to high-speed, high-volume traffic. Furthermore, the American Academy of Pediatrics supports governmental and industry action that would lead to improvements in vehicle design, driver manuals, driver education, and data collection for the purpose of reducing pediatric pedestrian injury. (7/09, reaffirmed 8/13, 5/19)

http://pediatrics.aappublications.org/content/124/2/802

PEDIATRIC AND ADOLESCENT MENTAL HEALTH EMERGENCIES IN THE EMERGENCY MEDICAL SERVICES SYSTEM (TECHNICAL REPORT)

Margaret A. Dolan, MD; Joel A. Fein, MD, MPH; and Committee on Pediatric Emergency Medicine

ABSTRACT. Emergency department (ED) health care professionals often care for patients with previously diagnosed psychiatric illnesses who are ill, injured, or having a behavioral crisis. In addition, ED personnel encounter children with psychiatric illnesses who may not present to the ED with overt mental health symptoms. Staff education and training regarding identification and management of pediatric mental health illness can help EDs overcome the perceived limitations of the setting that influence timely and comprehensive evaluation. In addition, ED physicians can inform and advocate for policy changes at local, state, and national levels that are needed to ensure comprehensive care of children with mental health illnesses. This report addresses the roles that the ED and ED health care professionals play in emergency mental health care of children and adolescents in the United States, which includes the stabilization and management of patients in mental health crisis, the discovery of mental illnesses and suicidal ideation in ED patients, and approaches to advocating for improved recognition and treatment of mental illnesses in children. The report also addresses special issues related to mental illness in the ED, such as minority populations, children with special health care needs, and children's mental health during and after disasters and trauma. (4/11, reaffirmed 7/14)

http://pediatrics.aappublications.org/content/127/5/e1356

PEDIATRIC ANTHRAX CLINICAL MANAGEMENT (CLINICAL REPORT)

John S. Bradley, MD, FAAP, FIDSA, FPIDS; Georgina Peacock, MD, MPH, FAAP; Steven E. Krug, MD, FAAP; William A. Bower, MD, FIDSA; Amanda C. Cohn, MD; Dana Meaney-Delman, MD, MPH, FACOG; Andrew T. Pavia, MD, FAAP, FIDSA; Committee on Infectious Diseases; and Disaster Preparedness Advisory Council

ABSTRACT. Anthrax is a zoonotic disease caused by *Bacillus anthracis*, which has multiple routes of infection in humans, manifesting in different initial presentations of disease. Because *B anthracis* has the potential to be used as a biological weapon and can rapidly progress to systemic anthrax with high mortality in those who are exposed and untreated, clinical guidance that can be quickly implemented must be in place before any intentional release of the agent. This document provides clinical guidance for the prophylaxis and treatment of neonates, infants, children, adolescents, and young adults up to the age of 21 (referred to as "children") in the event of a deliberate *B anthracis* release and offers guidance in areas where the unique characteristics of children dictate a different clinical recommendation from adults. (4/14)

http://pediatrics.aappublications.org/content/133/5/e1411

PEDIATRIC ANTHRAX CLINICAL MANAGEMENT: EXECUTIVE SUMMARY

John S. Bradley, MD, FAAP, FIDSA, FPIDS; Georgina Peacock, MD, MPH, FAAP; Steven E. Krug, MD, FAAP; William A. Bower, MD, FIDSA; Amanda C. Cohn, MD; Dana Meaney-Delman, MD, MPH, FACOG; Andrew T. Pavia, MD, FAAP, FIDSA; Committee on Infectious Diseases; and Disaster Preparedness Advisory Council

The use of *Bacillus anthracis* as a biological weapon is considered a potential national security threat by the US government. *B anthracis* has the ability to be used as a biological weapon and to cause anthrax, which can rapidly progress to systemic disease with high mortality in those who are untreated. Therefore, clear plans for managing children after a *B anthracis* bioterror exposure event must be in place before any intentional release of the agent. This document provides a summary of the guidance contained in the clinical report (appendices cited in this executive summary refer to those in the clinical report) for diagnosis and management of anthrax, including antimicrobial treatment and postexposure prophylaxis (PEP), use of antitoxin, and recommendations for use of anthrax vaccine in neonates, infants, children, adolescents, and young adults up to the age of 21 years (referred to as "children"). (4/14)

http://pediatrics.aappublications.org/content/133/5/940

PEDIATRIC APPLICATION OF CODING AND VALUATION SYSTEMS

David M. Kanter, MD, MBA, FAAP; Richard Lander, MD, FAAP, CIC; Richard A. Molteni, MD, FAAP; Committee on Coding and Nomenclature; and Private Payer Advocacy Advisory Committee

ABSTRACT. The American Academy of Pediatrics provides this revised policy statement to address health care changes that impact procedural and visit coding and valuation as well as the incorporation of coding principles into innovative, newer payment models. This policy statement focuses solely on recommendations, and an accompanying technical report provides supplemental coding and valuation background. (9/19)

See full text on page 989.

https://pediatrics.aappublications.org/content/144/4/e20192496

PEDIATRIC APPLICATION OF CODING AND VALUATION SYSTEMS (TECHNICAL REPORT)

David M. Kanter, MD, MBA, FAAP; Richard A. Molteni, MD, FAAP; and Committee on Coding and Nomenclature

ABSTRACT. The American Academy of Pediatrics provides this technical report as supplemental background to the accompanying coding and valuation system policy statement. The rapid evolution in health care payment modeling requires that clinicians have a current appreciation of the mechanics of service representation and valuation. The accompanying policy statement provides recommendations relevant to this area, and this technical report provides a format to outline important concepts that allow for effective translation of bedside clinical events into physician payment. (9/19)

See full text on page 999.

https://pediatrics.aappublications.org/content/144/4/e20192498

PEDIATRIC ASPECTS OF INPATIENT HEALTH INFORMATION TECHNOLOGY SYSTEMS (TECHNICAL REPORT)

Christoph U. Lehmann, MD, FAAP, FACMI, and Council on Clinical Information Technology

ABSTRACT. In the past 3 years, the Health Information Technology for Economic and Clinical Health Act accelerated the adoption of electronic health records (EHRs) with providers and hospitals, who can claim incentive monies related to meaningful use. Despite the increase in adoption of commercial EHRs in pediatric settings, there has been little support for EHR tools and functionalities that promote pediatric quality improvement and patient safety, and children remain at higher risk than adults for medical errors in inpatient environments. Health information technology (HIT) tailored to the needs of pediatric health care providers can improve care by reducing the likelihood of errors through information assurance and minimizing the harm that results from errors. This technical report outlines pediatric-specific concepts, child health needs and their data elements, and required functionalities in inpatient clinical information systems that may be missing in adult-oriented HIT systems with negative consequences for pediatric inpatient care. It is imperative that inpatient (and outpatient) HIT systems be adapted to improve their ability to properly support safe health care delivery for children. (2/15)

http://pediatrics.aappublications.org/content/135/3/e756

PEDIATRIC CONSIDERATIONS BEFORE, DURING, AND AFTER RADIOLOGICAL OR NUCLEAR EMERGENCIES

Jerome A. Paulson, MD, FAAP and AAP Council on Environmental Health

ABSTRACT. Infants, children, and adolescents can be exposed unexpectedly to ionizing radiation from nuclear power plant events, improvised nuclear or radiologic dispersal device explosions, or inappropriate disposal of radiotherapy equipment. Children are likely to experience higher external and internal radiation exposure levels than adults because of their smaller body and organ size and other physiologic characteristics, by picking up contaminated items, and through consumption of contaminated milk or foodstuffs. This policy statement and accompanying technical report update the 2003 American Academy of Pediatrics policy statement on pediatric radiation emergencies by summarizing newer scientific knowledge from studies of the Chernobyl and Fukushima Daiichi nuclear power plant events, use of improvised radiologic dispersal devices, exposures from inappropriate disposal of radiotherapy equipment, and potential health effects from residential proximity to nuclear plants. Policy recommendations are made for providers and governments to improve future responses to these types of events. (11/18)

http://pediatrics.aappublications.org/content/142/6/e20183000

PEDIATRIC CONSIDERATIONS BEFORE, DURING, AND AFTER RADIOLOGICAL OR NUCLEAR EMERGENCIES (TECHNICAL REPORT)

Martha S. Linet, MD, MPH; Ziad Kazzi, MD; Jerome A. Paulson, MD, FAAP; AAP Council on Environmental Health

ABSTRACT. Infants, children, and adolescents can be exposed unexpectedly to ionizing radiation from nuclear power plant events, improvised nuclear or radiologic dispersal device explosions, or inappropriate disposal of radiotherapy equipment. Children are likely to experience higher external and internal radiation exposure levels than adults because of their smaller body and organ size and other physiologic characteristics as well as their tendency to pick up contaminated items and consume contaminated milk or foodstuffs. This technical report accompanies the revision of the 2003 American Academy of Pediatrics policy statement on pediatric radiation emergencies by summarizing newer scientific data from studies of the Chernobyl and the Fukushima Daiichi nuclear power plant events, use of improvised radiologic dispersal devices, exposures from inappropriate disposal of radiotherapy equipment, and potential health effects from residential proximity to nuclear plants. Also included are recommendations from epidemiological studies and biokinetic models to address mitigation efforts. The report includes major emphases on acute radiation syndrome, acute and long-term psychological effects, cancer risks, and other late tissue reactions after low-to-high levels of radiation exposure. Results, along with public health and clinical implications, are described from studies of the Japanese atomic bomb survivors, nuclear plant accidents (eg, Three Mile Island, Chernobyl, and Fukushima), improper disposal of radiotherapy equipment in Goiania, Brazil, and residence in proximity to nuclear plants. Measures to reduce radiation exposure in the immediate aftermath of a radiologic or nuclear disaster are described, including the diagnosis and management of external and internal contamination, use of potassium iodide, and actions in relation to breastfeeding. (11/18)

http://pediatrics.aappublications.org/content/142/6/e20183001

PEDIATRIC INTEGRATIVE MEDICINE (CLINICAL REPORT)

Hilary McClafferty, MD, FAAP; Sunita Vohra, MD, FAAP; Michelle Bailey, MD, FAAP; Melanie Brown, MD, MSE, FAAP; Anna Esparham, MD, FAAP; Dana Gerstbacher, MD, FAAP; Brenda Golianu, MD, FAAP; Anna-Kaisa Niemi, MD, PhD, FAAP, FACMG; Erica Sibinga, MD, FAAP; Joy Weydert, MD, FAAP; Ann Ming Yeh, MD; and Section on Integrative Medicine

ABSTRACT. The American Academy of Pediatrics is dedicated to optimizing the well-being of children and advancing family-centered health care. Related to this mission, the American Academy of Pediatrics recognizes the increasing use of complementary and integrative therapies for children and the subsequent need to provide reliable information and high-quality clinical resources to support pediatricians. This Clinical Report serves as an update to the original 2008 statement on complementary medicine. The range of complementary therapies is both extensive and diverse. Therefore, in-depth discussion of each therapy or product is beyond the scope of this report. Instead, our intentions are to define terms; describe epidemiology of use; outline common types of complementary therapies; review medicolegal, ethical, and research implications; review education and training for select providers of complementary therapies; provide educational resources; and suggest communication strategies for discussing complementary therapies with patients and families. (8/17)

http://pediatrics.aappublications.org/content/140/3/e20171961

PEDIATRIC MEDICATION SAFETY IN THE EMERGENCY DEPARTMENT

Lee Benjamin, MD, FAAP, FACEP; Karen Frush, MD, FAAP; Kathy Shaw, MD, MSCE, FAAP; Joan E. Shook, MD, MBA, FAAP; Sally K. Snow, BSN, RN, CPEN, FAEN; and Committee on Pediatric Emergency Medicine (joint with American College of Emergency Physicians Pediatric Emergency Medicine Committee and Emergency Nurses Association Pediatric Emergency Medicine Committee)

ABSTRACT. Pediatric patients cared for in emergency departments (EDs) are at high risk of medication errors for a variety of reasons. A multidisciplinary panel was convened by the Emergency Medical Services for Children program and the American Academy of Pediatrics Committee on Pediatric Emergency Medicine to initiate a discussion on medication safety in the ED. Top opportunities identified to improve medication safety include using kilogram-only weight-based dosing, optimizing computerized physician order entry by using clinical decision support, developing a standard formulary for pediatric patients while limiting variability of medication concentrations, using pharmacist support within EDs, enhancing training of medical professionals, systematizing the dispensing and administration of medications within the ED, and addressing challenges for home medication administration before discharge. (2/18)

http://pediatrics.aappublications.org/content/141/3/e20174066

PEDIATRIC MENTAL HEALTH EMERGENCIES IN THE EMERGENCY MEDICAL SERVICES SYSTEM

Committee on Pediatric Emergency Medicine (joint with American College of Emergency Physicians)

ABSTRACT. Emergency departments are vital in the management of pediatric patients with mental health emergencies. Pediatric mental health emergencies are an increasing part of emergency medical practice because emergency departments have become the safety net for a fragmented mental health infrastructure that is experiencing critical shortages in services in all sectors. Emergency departments must safely, humanely, and in a culturally and developmentally appropriate manner manage pediatric patients with undiagnosed and known mental illnesses, including those with mental retardation, autistic spectrum disorders, and attention-deficit/hyperactivity disorder and those experiencing a behavioral crisis. Emergency departments also manage patients with suicidal ideation, depression, escalating aggression, substance abuse, posttraumatic stress disorder, and maltreatment and those exposed to violence and unexpected deaths. Emergency departments must address not only the physical but also the mental health needs of patients during and after mass-casualty incidents and disasters. The American Academy of Pediatrics and the American College of Emergency Physicians support advocacy for increased mental health resources, including improved pediatric mental health tools for the emergency department, increased mental health insurance coverage, and adequate reimbursement at all levels; acknowledgment of the importance of the child's medical home; and promotion of education and research for mental health emergencies. (10/06, reaffirmed 6/09, 4/13)

http://pediatrics.aappublications.org/content/118/4/1764

PEDIATRIC METABOLIC AND BARIATRIC SURGERY: EVIDENCE, BARRIERS, AND BEST PRACTICES

Sarah C. Armstrong, MD, FAAP; Christopher F. Bolling, MD, FAAP; Marc P. Michalsky, MD, FACS, FAAP, FASMBS; Kirk W. Reichard, MD, MBA, FAAP, FACS; Section on Obesity; and Section on Surgery

ABSTRACT. Severe obesity among youth is an "epidemic within an epidemic" and portends a shortened life expectancy for today's children compared with those of their parents' generation. Severe obesity has outpaced less severe forms of childhood obesity in prevalence, and it disproportionately affects adolescents. Emerging evidence has linked severe obesity to the development and progression of multiple comorbid states, including increased cardiometabolic risk resulting in end-organ damage in adulthood. Lifestyle modification treatment has achieved moderate short-term success among young children and those with less severe forms of obesity, but no studies to date demonstrate significant and durable weight loss among youth with severe obesity. Metabolic and bariatric surgery has emerged as an important treatment for adults with severe obesity and, more recently, has been shown to be a safe and effective strategy for groups of youth with severe obesity. However, current data suggest that youth with severe obesity may not have adequate access to metabolic and bariatric surgery, especially among underserved populations. This report outlines the current evidence regarding adolescent bariatric surgery, provides recommendations for practitioners and policy makers, and serves as a companion to an accompanying technical report, "Metabolic and Bariatric Surgery for Pediatric Patients With Severe Obesity," which provides details and supporting evidence. (11/19)

See full text on page 1009.

https://pediatrics.aappublications.org/content/144/6/e20193223

PEDIATRIC OBSERVATION UNITS (CLINICAL REPORT)

Gregory P. Conners, MD, MPH, MBA; Sanford M. Melzer, MD, MBA; Committee on Hospital Care; and Committee on Pediatric Emergency Medicine

ABSTRACT. Pediatric observation units (OUs) are hospital areas used to provide medical evaluation and/or management for health-related conditions in children, typically for a well-defined, brief period. Pediatric OUs represent an emerging alternative site of care for selected groups of children who historically may have received their treatment in an ambulatory setting, emergency department, or hospital-based inpatient unit. This clinical report provides an overview of pediatric OUs, including the definitions and operating characteristics of different types of OUs, quality considerations and coding for observation services, and the effect of OUs on inpatient hospital utilization. (6/12, reaffirmed 9/15)

http://pediatrics.aappublications.org/content/130/1/172

PEDIATRIC ORGAN DONATION AND TRANSPLANTATION

Committee on Hospital Care, Section on Surgery, and Section on Critical Care

ABSTRACT. Pediatric organ donation and organ transplantation can have a significant life-extending benefit to the young recipients of these organs and a high emotional impact on donor and recipient families. Pediatricians, pediatric medical specialists, and pediatric transplant surgeons need to be better acquainted with evolving national strategies that involve organ procurement and organ transplantation to help acquaint families with the benefits and risks of organ donation and transplantation. Efforts of pediatric professionals are needed to shape public policies to provide a system in which procurement, distribution, and cost are fair and equitable to children and adults. Major issues of concern are availability of and access to donor organs; oversight and control of the process; pediatric medical and surgical consultation and continued care throughout the organ-donation and transplantation process; ethical, social, financial, and follow-up issues; insurance-coverage issues; and public awareness of the need for organ donors of all ages. (3/10, reaffirmed 3/14, 4/19)

http://pediatrics.aappublications.org/content/125/4/822

PEDIATRIC PALLIATIVE CARE AND HOSPICE CARE COMMITMENTS, GUIDELINES, AND RECOMMENDATIONS

Section on Hospice and Palliative Medicine and Committee on Hospital Care

ABSTRACT. Pediatric palliative care and pediatric hospice care (PPC-PHC) are often essential aspects of medical care for patients who have life-threatening conditions or need end-of-life care. PPC-PHC aims to relieve suffering, improve quality of life, facilitate informed decision-making, and assist in care coordination between clinicians and across sites of care. Core commitments of PPC-PHC include being patient centered and family engaged; respecting and partnering with patients and families; pursuing care that is high quality, readily accessible, and equitable; providing care across the age spectrum and life span, integrated into the continuum of care; ensuring that all clinicians can provide basic palliative care and consult PPC-PHC specialists in a timely manner; and improving care through research and quality improvement efforts. PPC-PHC guidelines and recommendations include ensuring that all large health care organizations serving children with life-threatening conditions have dedicated interdisciplinary PPC-PHC teams, which should develop collaborative relationships between hospital- and community-based teams; that PPC-PHC be provided as integrated multimodal care and practiced as a cornerstone of patient safety and quality for patients with life-threatening conditions; that PPC-PHC teams should facilitate clear, compassionate, and forthright discussions about medical issues and the goals of care and support families, siblings, and health care staff; that PPC-PHC be part of all pediatric education and training curricula, be an active area of research and quality improvement, and exemplify the highest ethical standards; and that PPC-PHC services be supported by financial and regulatory arrangements to ensure access to high-quality PPC-PHC by all patients with life-threatening and life-shortening diseases. (10/13)

http://pediatrics.aappublications.org/content/132/5/966

PEDIATRIC PRIMARY HEALTH CARE

Committee on Pediatric Workforce

ABSTRACT. Primary health care is described as accessible and affordable, first contact, continuous and comprehensive, and coordinated to meet the health needs of the individual and the family being served.

Pediatric primary health care encompasses health supervision and anticipatory guidance; monitoring physical and psychosocial growth and development; age-appropriate screening; diagnosis and treatment of acute and chronic disorders; management of serious and life-threatening illness and, when appropriate, referral of more complex conditions; and provision of first contact care as well as coordinated management of health problems requiring multiple professional services.

Pediatric primary health care for children and adolescents is family centered and incorporates community resources and strengths, needs and risk factors, and sociocultural sensitivities into strategies for care delivery and clinical practice. Pediatric primary health care is best delivered within the context of a "medical home," where comprehensive, continuously accessible and affordable care is available and delivered or supervised by qualified child health specialists.

The pediatrician, because of training (which includes 4 years of medical school education, plus an additional 3 or more years of intensive training devoted solely to all aspects of medical care for children and adolescents), coupled with the demonstrated interest in and total professional commitment to the health care of infants, children, adolescents, and young adults, is the most appropriate provider of pediatric primary health care. (1/11, reaffirmed 10/13, 5/17)

http://pediatrics.aappublications.org/content/127/2/397

PEDIATRIC READINESS IN THE EMERGENCY DEPARTMENT

Katherine Remick, MD, FAAP, FACEP, FAEMS; Marianne Gausche-Hill, MD, FAAP, FACEP, FAEMS; Madeline M. Joseph, MD, FAAP, FACEP; Kathleen Brown, MD, FAAP, FACEP; Sally K. Snow, BSN, RN, CPEN, FAEN; Joseph L. Wright, MD, MPH, FAAP; Committee on Pediatric Emergency Medicine; and Section on Surgery (joint with American College of Emergency Physicians Pediatric Emergency Medicine Committee and Emergency Nurses Association Pediatric Committee)

ABSTRACT. This is a revision of the previous joint Policy Statement titled "Guidelines for Care of Children in the Emergency Department." Children have unique physical and psychosocial needs that are heightened in the setting of serious or life-threatening emergencies. The majority of children who are ill and injured are brought to community hospital emergency departments (EDs) by virtue of proximity. It is therefore imperative that all EDs have the appropriate resources (medications, equipment, policies, and education) and capable staff to provide effective emergency care for children. In this Policy Statement, we outline the resources necessary for EDs to stand ready to care for children of all ages. These recommendations are consistent with the recommendations of the Institute of Medicine (now called the National Academy of Medicine) in its report "The Future of Emergency Care in the US Health System." Although resources within emergency and trauma care systems vary locally, regionally, and nationally, it is essential that ED staff, administrators, and medical directors seek to meet or exceed these recommendations to ensure that high-quality emergency care is available for all children. These updated recommendations are intended to serve as a resource for clinical and administrative leadership in EDs as they strive to improve their readiness for children of all ages. (10/18)

http://pediatrics.aappublications.org/content/142/5/e20182459

PEDIATRIC SUDDEN CARDIAC ARREST

Section on Cardiology and Cardiac Surgery

ABSTRACT. Pediatric sudden cardiac arrest (SCA), which can cause sudden cardiac death if not treated within minutes, has a profound effect on everyone: children, parents, family members, communities, and health care providers. Preventing the tragedy of pediatric SCA, defined as the abrupt and unexpected loss of heart function, remains a concern to all. The goal of this statement is to increase the knowledge of pediatricians (including primary care providers and specialists) of the incidence of pediatric SCA, the spectrum of causes of pediatric SCA, disease-

specific presentations, the role of patient and family screening, the rapidly evolving role of genetic testing, and finally, important aspects of secondary SCA prevention. This statement is not intended to address sudden infant death syndrome or sudden unexplained death syndrome, nor will specific treatment of individual cardiac conditions be discussed. This statement has been endorsed by the American College of Cardiology, the American Heart Association, and the Heart Rhythm Society. (3/12)
http://pediatrics.aappublications.org/content/129/4/e1094

PEDIATRICIAN WORKFORCE POLICY STATEMENT

Committee on Pediatric Workforce

ABSTRACT. This policy statement reviews important trends and other factors that affect the pediatrician workforce and the provision of pediatric health care, including changes in the pediatric patient population, pediatrician workforce, and nature of pediatric practice. The effect of these changes on pediatricians and the demand for pediatric care are discussed. The American Academy of Pediatrics (AAP) concludes that there is currently a shortage of pediatric medical subspecialists in many fields, as well as a shortage of pediatric surgical specialists. In addition, the AAP believes that the current distribution of primary care pediatricians is inadequate to meet the needs of children living in rural and other underserved areas, and more primary care pediatricians will be needed in the future because of the increasing number of children who have significant chronic health problems, changes in physician work hours, and implementation of current health reform efforts that seek to improve access to comprehensive patient- and family-centered care for all children in a medical home. The AAP is committed to being an active participant in physician workforce policy development with both professional organizations and governmental bodies to ensure a pediatric perspective on health care workforce issues. The overall purpose of this statement is to summarize policy recommendations and serve as a resource for the AAP and other stakeholders as they address pediatrician workforce issues that ultimately influence the quality of pediatric health care provided to children in the United States. (7/13)
http://pediatrics.aappublications.org/content/132/2/390

PEDIATRICIAN-FAMILY-PATIENT RELATIONSHIPS: MANAGING THE BOUNDARIES

Committee on Bioethics

ABSTRACT. All professionals are concerned about maintaining the appropriate limits in their relationships with those they serve. Pediatricians should be aware that, under normal circumstances, caring for one's own children presents significant ethical issues. Pediatricians also must strive to maintain appropriate professional boundaries in their relationships with the family members of their patients. Pediatricians should avoid behavior that patients and parents might misunderstand as having sexual or inappropriate social meaning. Romantic and sexual involvement between physicians and patients is unacceptable. The acceptance of gifts or nonmonetary compensation for medical services has the potential to affect the professional relationship adversely. (11/09, reaffirmed 1/14)
http://pediatrics.aappublications.org/content/124/6/1685

THE PEDIATRICIAN'S ROLE IN CHILD MALTREATMENT PREVENTION (CLINICAL REPORT)

Emalee G. Flaherty, MD; John Stirling Jr, MD; and Committee on Child Abuse and Neglect

ABSTRACT. It is the pediatrician's role to promote the child's well-being and to help parents raise healthy, well-adjusted children. Pediatricians, therefore, can play an important role in the prevention of child maltreatment. Previous clinical reports and policy statements from the American Academy of Pediatrics have focused on improving the identification and management of child maltreatment. This clinical report outlines how the pediatrician can help to strengthen families and promote safe, stable, nurturing relationships with the aim of preventing maltreatment. After describing some of the triggers and factors that place children at risk for maltreatment, the report describes how pediatricians can identify family strengths, recognize risk factors, provide helpful guidance, and refer families to programs and other resources with the goal of strengthening families, preventing child maltreatment, and enhancing child development. (9/10, reaffirmed 1/14)
http://pediatrics.aappublications.org/content/126/4/833

THE PEDIATRICIAN'S ROLE IN FAMILY SUPPORT AND FAMILY SUPPORT PROGRAMS

Committee on Early Childhood, Adoption, and Dependent Care

ABSTRACT. Children's social, emotional, and physical health; their developmental trajectory; and the neurocircuits that are being created and reinforced in their developing brains are all directly influenced by their relationships during early childhood. The stresses associated with contemporary American life can challenge families' abilities to promote successful developmental outcomes and emotional health for their children. Pediatricians are positioned to serve as partners with families and other community providers in supporting the well-being of children and their families. The structure and support of families involve forces that are often outside the agenda of the usual pediatric health supervision visits. Pediatricians must ensure that their medical home efforts promote a holistically healthy family environment for all children. This statement recommends opportunities for pediatricians to develop their expertise in assessing the strengths and stresses in families, in counseling families about strategies and resources, and in collaborating with others in their communities to support family relationships. (11/11, reaffirmed 12/16)
http://pediatrics.aappublications.org/content/128/6/e1680

THE PEDIATRICIAN'S ROLE IN OPTIMIZING SCHOOL READINESS

Council on Early Childhood and Council on School Health

ABSTRACT. School readiness includes not only the early academic skills of children but also their physical health, language skills, social and emotional development, motivation to learn, creativity, and general knowledge. Families and communities play a critical role in ensuring children's growth in all of these areas and thus their readiness for school. Schools must be prepared to teach all children when they reach the age of school entry, regardless of their degree of readiness. Research on early brain development emphasizes the effects of early experiences, relationships, and emotions on creating and reinforcing the neural connections that are the basis for learning. Pediatricians, by the nature of their relationships with families and children, may significantly influence school readiness. Pediatricians have a primary role in ensuring children's physical health through the provision of preventive care, treatment of illness, screening for sensory deficits, and monitoring nutrition and growth. They can promote and monitor the social-emotional development of children by providing anticipatory guidance on development and behavior, by encouraging positive parenting practices, by modeling reciprocal and respectful communication with adults and children, by identifying and addressing psychosocial risk factors, and by providing community-based resources and referrals when warranted. Cognitive and language skills are fostered through timely identification of developmental problems and appropriate referrals for services, including early intervention and special education services; guidance regarding safe and stimulating early education and child care programs; and promotion of early literacy by encouraging language-rich activities such as reading together, telling stories, and playing games.

Pediatricians are also well positioned to advocate not only for children's access to health care but also for high-quality early childhood education and evidence-based family supports such as home visits, which help provide a foundation for optimal learning. (8/16)

http://pediatrics.aappublications.org/content/138/3/e20162293

THE PEDIATRICIAN'S ROLE IN SUPPORTING ADOPTIVE FAMILIES (CLINICAL REPORT)

Veronnie F. Jones, MD, PhD, MSPH; Elaine E. Schulte, MD, MPH; Committee on Early Childhood; and Council on Foster Care, Adoption, and Kinship Care

ABSTRACT. Each year, more children join families through adoption. Pediatricians have an important role in assisting adoptive families in the various challenges they may face with respect to adoption. The acceptance of the differences between families formed through birth and those formed through adoption is essential in promoting positive emotional growth within the family. It is important for pediatricians to be aware of the adoptive parents' need to be supported in their communication with their adopted children. (9/12, reaffirmed 12/16)

http://pediatrics.aappublications.org/content/130/4/e1040

THE PEDIATRICIAN'S ROLE IN THE EVALUATION AND PREPARATION OF PEDIATRIC PATIENTS UNDERGOING ANESTHESIA

Section on Anesthesiology and Pain Medicine

ABSTRACT. Pediatricians play a key role in helping prepare patients and families for anesthesia and surgery. The questions to be answered by the pediatrician fall into 2 categories. The first involves preparation: is the patient in optimal medical condition for surgery, and are the patient and family emotionally and cognitively ready for surgery? The second category concerns logistics: what communication and organizational needs are necessary to enable safe passage through the perioperative process? This revised statement updates the recommendations for the pediatrician's role in the preoperative preparation of patients. (8/14)

http://pediatrics.aappublications.org/content/134/3/634

THE PEDIATRICIAN'S ROLE IN THE PREVENTION OF MISSING CHILDREN (CLINICAL REPORT)

Committee on Psychosocial Aspects of Child and Family Health

ABSTRACT. In 2002, the *Second National Incidence Studies of Missing, Abducted, Runaway, and Thrownaway Children* report was released by the US Department of Justice, providing new data on a problem that our nation continues to face. This clinical report describes the categories of missing children, the prevalence of each, and prevention strategies that primary care pediatricians can share with parents to increase awareness and education about the safety of their children. (10/04, reaffirmed 1/15)

http://pediatrics.aappublications.org/content/114/4/1100

PEDIATRICIANS AND PUBLIC HEALTH: OPTIMIZING THE HEALTH AND WELL-BEING OF THE NATION'S CHILDREN

Alice A. Kuo, MD, PhD, FAAP; Pauline A. Thomas, MD, FAAP; Lance A. Chilton, MD, FAAP; Laurene Mascola, MD, MPH; Council on Community Pediatrics; and Section on Epidemiology, Public Health, and Evidence

ABSTRACT. Ensuring optimal health for children requires a population-based approach and collaboration between pediatrics and public health. The prevention of major threats to children's health (such as behavioral health issues) and the control and management of chronic diseases, obesity, injury, communicable diseases, and other problems cannot be managed solely in the pediatric office. The integration of clinical practice with public health actions is necessary for multiple levels of disease prevention that involve the child, family, and community. Although pediatricians and public health professionals interact frequently to the benefit of children and their families, increased integration of the 2 disciplines is critical to improving child health at the individual and population levels. Effective collaboration is necessary to ensure that population health activities include children and that the child health priorities of the American Academy of Pediatrics (AAP), such as poverty and child health, early brain and child development, obesity, and mental health, can engage federal, state, and local public health initiatives. In this policy statement, we build on the 2013 AAP Policy Statement on community pediatrics by identifying specific opportunities for collaboration between pediatricians and public health professionals that are likely to improve the health of children in communities. In the statement, we provide recommendations for pediatricians, public health professionals, and the AAP and its chapters. (1/18)

http://pediatrics.aappublications.org/content/141/2/e20173848

PERSONAL WATERCRAFT USE BY CHILDREN AND ADOLESCENTS

Committee on Injury and Poison Prevention

ABSTRACT. The use of personal watercraft (PWC) has increased dramatically during the past decade as have the speed and mobility of the watercraft. A similar dramatic increase in PWC-related injury and death has occurred simultaneously. No one younger than 16 years should operate a PWC. The operator and all passengers must wear US Coast Guard-approved personal flotation devices. Other safety recommendations are suggested for parents and pediatricians. (2/00, reaffirmed 5/04, 1/07, 6/10)

http://pediatrics.aappublications.org/content/105/2/452

PESTICIDE EXPOSURE IN CHILDREN

Council on Environmental Health

ABSTRACT. This statement presents the position of the American Academy of Pediatrics on pesticides. Pesticides are a collective term for chemicals intended to kill unwanted insects, plants, molds, and rodents. Children encounter pesticides daily and have unique susceptibilities to their potential toxicity. Acute poisoning risks are clear, and understanding of chronic health implications from both acute and chronic exposure are emerging. Epidemiologic evidence demonstrates associations between early life exposure to pesticides and pediatric cancers, decreased cognitive function, and behavioral problems. Related animal toxicology studies provide supportive biological plausibility for these findings. Recognizing and reducing problematic exposures will require attention to current inadequacies in medical training, public health tracking, and regulatory action on pesticides. Ongoing research describing toxicologic vulnerabilities and exposure factors across the life span are needed to inform regulatory needs and appropriate interventions. Policies that promote integrated pest management, comprehensive pesticide labeling, and marketing practices that incorporate child health considerations will enhance safe use. (11/12)

http://pediatrics.aappublications.org/content/130/6/e1757

PESTICIDE EXPOSURE IN CHILDREN (TECHNICAL REPORT)

James R. Roberts, MD, MPH; Catherine J. Karr, MD, PhD; and Council on Environmental Health

ABSTRACT. Pesticides are a collective term for a wide array of chemicals intended to kill unwanted insects, plants, molds, and rodents. Food, water, and treatment in the home, yard, and school are all potential sources of children's exposure. Exposures to pesticides may be overt or subacute, and effects range from acute to chronic toxicity. In 2008, pesticides were the ninth most common substance reported to poison control centers, and approximately 45% of all reports of pesticide poisoning were for children. Organophosphate and carbamate poisoning are perhaps the most widely known acute poisoning syndromes, can be diagnosed by depressed red blood cell cholinesterase levels, and have available antidotal therapy. However, numerous other pesticides that may cause acute toxicity, such as pyrethroid and neonicotinoid insecticides, herbicides, fungicides, and rodenticides, also have specific toxic effects; recognition of these effects may help identify acute exposures. Evidence is increasingly emerging about chronic health implications from both acute and chronic exposure. A growing body of epidemiological evidence demonstrates associations between parental use of pesticides, particularly insecticides, with acute lymphocytic leukemia and brain tumors. Prenatal, household, and occupational exposures (maternal and paternal) appear to be the largest risks. Prospective cohort studies link early-life exposure to organophosphates and organochlorine pesticides (primarily DDT) with adverse effects on neurodevelopment and behavior. Among the findings associated with increased pesticide levels are poorer mental development by using the Bayley index and increased scores on measures assessing pervasive developmental disorder, inattention, and attention-deficit/hyperactivity disorder. Related animal toxicology studies provide supportive biological plausibility for these findings. Additional data suggest that there may also be an association between parental pesticide use and adverse birth outcomes including physical birth defects, low birth weight, and fetal death, although the data are less robust than for cancer and neurodevelopmental effects. Children's exposures to pesticides should be limited as much as possible. (11/12)

http://pediatrics.aappublications.org/content/130/6/e1765

PHOTOTHERAPY TO PREVENT SEVERE NEONATAL HYPERBILIRUBINEMIA IN THE NEWBORN INFANT 35 OR MORE WEEKS OF GESTATION (TECHNICAL REPORT)

Vinod K. Bhutani, MD, and Committee on Fetus and Newborn

ABSTRACT. *Objective.* To standardize the use of phototherapy consistent with the American Academy of Pediatrics clinical practice guideline for the management of hyperbilirubinemia in the newborn infant 35 or more weeks of gestation.

Methods. Relevant literature was reviewed. Phototherapy devices currently marketed in the United States that incorporate fluorescent, halogen, fiber-optic, or blue light-emitting diode light sources were assessed in the laboratory.

Results. The efficacy of phototherapy units varies widely because of differences in light source and configuration. The following characteristics of a device contribute to its effectiveness: (1) emission of light in the blue-to-green range that overlaps the in vivo plasma bilirubin absorption spectrum (~460–490 nm); (2) irradiance of at least 30 µW·cm–2·nm–1 (confirmed with an appropriate irradiance meter calibrated over the appropriate wavelength range); (3) illumination of maximal body surface; and (4) demonstration of a decrease in total bilirubin concentrations during the first 4 to 6 hours of exposure.

Recommendations. The intensity and spectral output of phototherapy devices is useful in predicting potential effectiveness in treating hyperbilirubinemia (group B recommendation). Clinical effectiveness should be evaluated before and monitored during use (group B recommendation). Blocking the light source or reducing exposed body surface should be avoided (group B recommendation). Standardization of irradiance meters, improvements in device design, and lower-upper limits of light intensity for phototherapy units merit further study. Comparing the in vivo performance of devices is not practical, in general, and alternative procedures need to be explored. (9/11, reaffirmed 7/14)

http://pediatrics.aappublications.org/content/128/4/e1046

PHYSICIAN HEALTH AND WELLNESS (CLINICAL REPORT)

Hilary McClafferty, MD, FAAP; Oscar W. Brown, MD, FAAP; Section on Integrative Medicine; and Committee on Practice and Ambulatory Medicine

ABSTRACT. Physician health and wellness is a critical issue gaining national attention because of the high prevalence of physician burnout. Pediatricians and pediatric trainees experience burnout at levels equivalent to other medical specialties, highlighting a need for more effective efforts to promote health and well-being in the pediatric community. This report will provide an overview of physician burnout, an update on work in the field of preventive physician health and wellness, and a discussion of emerging initiatives that have potential to promote health at all levels of pediatric training.

Pediatricians are uniquely positioned to lead this movement nationally, in part because of the emphasis placed on wellness in the Pediatric Milestone Project, a joint collaboration between the Accreditation Council for Graduate Medical Education and the American Board of Pediatrics. Updated core competencies calling for a balanced approach to health, including focus on nutrition, exercise, mindfulness, and effective stress management, signal a paradigm shift and send the message that it is time for pediatricians to cultivate a culture of wellness better aligned with their responsibilities as role models and congruent with advances in pediatric training.

Rather than reviewing programs in place to address substance abuse and other serious conditions in distressed physicians, this article focuses on forward progress in the field, with an emphasis on the need for prevention and anticipation of predictable stressors related to burnout in medical training and practice. Examples of positive progress and several programs designed to promote physician health and wellness are reviewed. Areas where more research is needed are highlighted. (9/14)

http://pediatrics.aappublications.org/content/134/4/830

PHYSICIAN REFUSAL TO PROVIDE INFORMATION OR TREATMENT ON THE BASIS OF CLAIMS OF CONSCIENCE

Committee on Bioethics

ABSTRACT. Health care professionals may have moral objections to particular medical interventions. They may refuse to provide or cooperate in the provision of these interventions. Such objections are referred to as conscientious objections. Although it may be difficult to characterize or validate claims of conscience, respecting the individual physician's moral integrity is important. Conflicts arise when claims of conscience impede a patient's access to medical information or care. A physician's conscientious objection to certain interventions or treatments may be constrained in some situations. Physicians have a duty to disclose to prospective patients treatments they refuse to perform. As part of informed consent, physicians also have a duty to inform their patients of all relevant and legally available treatment options, including options to which they object. They have a moral obligation to refer patients to other health care professionals who are willing to provide those services when failing to do so would cause harm to the patient, and they have a duty to treat patients in emergencies when referral would significantly increase the probability of mortality or serious morbidity. Conversely, the health care system should make reasonable accommodations for physicians with conscientious objections. (11/09, reaffirmed 1/14, 6/18)

http://pediatrics.aappublications.org/content/124/6/1689

PHYSICIAN'S ROLE IN COORDINATING CARE OF HOSPITALIZED CHILDREN (CLINICAL REPORT)

Daniel A. Rauch, MD, FAAP; Committee on Hospital Care; and Section on Hospital Medicine

ABSTRACT. The hospitalization of a child is a stressful event for the child and family. The physician responsible for the admission has an important role in directing the care of the child, communicating with the child's providers (medical and primary caregivers), and advocating for the safety of the child during the hospitalization and transition out of the hospital. These challenges remain constant across the varied facilities in which children are hospitalized. The purpose of this revised clinical report is to update pediatricians about principles to improve the coordination of care and review expectations and practice. (7/18)

http://pediatrics.aappublications.org/content/142/2/e20181503

PLANNED HOME BIRTH

Committee on Fetus and Newborn

ABSTRACT. The American Academy of Pediatrics concurs with the recent statement of the American College of Obstetricians and Gynecologists affirming that hospitals and birthing centers are the safest settings for birth in the United States while respecting the right of women to make a medically informed decision about delivery. This statement is intended to help pediatricians provide supportive, informed counsel to women considering home birth while retaining their role as child advocates and to summarize the standards of care for newborn infants born at home, which are consistent with standards for infants born in a medical care facility. Regardless of the circumstances of his or her birth, including location, every newborn infant deserves health care that adheres to the standards highlighted in this statement, more completely described in other publications from the American Academy of Pediatrics, including *Guidelines for Perinatal Care*. The goal of providing high-quality care to all newborn infants can best be achieved through continuing efforts by all participating health care providers and institutions to develop and sustain communications and understanding on the basis of professional interaction and mutual respect throughout the health care system. (4/13, reaffirmed 12/16)

http://pediatrics.aappublications.org/content/131/5/1016

POINT-OF-CARE ULTRASONOGRAPHY BY PEDIATRIC EMERGENCY MEDICINE PHYSICIANS

Committee on Pediatric Emergency Medicine (joint with Society for Academic Emergency Medicine Academy of Emergency Ultrasound, American College of Emergency Physicians Pediatric Emergency Medicine Committee, and World Interactive Network Focused on Critical Ultrasound)

ABSTRACT. Point-of-care ultrasonography is increasingly being used to facilitate accurate and timely diagnoses and to guide procedures. It is important for pediatric emergency medicine (PEM) physicians caring for patients in the emergency department to receive adequate and continued point-of-care ultrasonography training for those indications used in their practice setting. Emergency departments should have credentialing and quality assurance programs. PEM fellowships should provide appropriate training to physician trainees. Hospitals should provide privileges to physicians who demonstrate competency in point-of-care ultrasonography. Ongoing research will provide the necessary measures to define the optimal training and competency assessment standards. Requirements for credentialing and hospital privileges will vary and will be specific to individual departments and hospitals. As more physicians are trained and more research is completed, there should be one national standard for credentialing and privileging in point-of-care ultrasonography for PEM physicians. (3/15)

http://pediatrics.aappublications.org/content/135/4/e1097

POINT-OF-CARE ULTRASONOGRAPHY BY PEDIATRIC EMERGENCY MEDICINE PHYSICIANS (TECHNICAL REPORT)

Jennifer R. Marin, MD, MSc; Resa E. Lewiss, MD; and Committee on Pediatric Emergency Medicine (joint with Society for Academic Emergency Medicine Academy of Emergency Ultrasound, American College of Emergency Physicians Pediatric Emergency Medicine Committee, and World Interactive Network Focused on Critical Ultrasound)

ABSTRACT. Emergency physicians have used point-of-care ultrasonography since the 1990s. Pediatric emergency medicine physicians have more recently adopted this technology. Point-of-care ultrasonography is used for various scenarios, particularly the evaluation of soft tissue infections or blunt abdominal trauma and procedural guidance. To date, there are no published statements from national organizations specifically for pediatric emergency physicians describing the incorporation of point-of-care ultrasonography into their practice. This document outlines how pediatric emergency departments may establish a formal point-of-care ultrasonography program. This task includes appointing leaders with expertise in point-of-care ultrasonography, effectively training and credentialing physicians in the department, and providing ongoing quality assurance reviews.

Point-of-care ultrasonography (US) is a bedside technology that enables clinicians to integrate clinical examination findings with real-time sonographic imaging. General emergency physicians and other specialists have used point-of-care US for many years, and more recently, pediatric emergency medicine (PEM) physicians have adopted point-of-care US as a diagnostic and procedural adjunct. This technical report and accompanying policy statement provide a framework for point-of-care US training and point-of-care US integration into pediatric care by PEM physicians. (3/15)

http://pediatrics.aappublications.org/content/135/4/e1113

POSTDISCHARGE FOLLOW-UP OF INFANTS WITH CONGENITAL DIAPHRAGMATIC HERNIA (CLINICAL REPORT)

Section on Surgery and Committee on Fetus and Newborn

ABSTRACT. Infants with congenital diaphragmatic hernia often require intensive treatment after birth, have prolonged hospitalizations, and have other congenital anomalies. After discharge from the hospital, they may have long-term sequelae such as respiratory insufficiency, gastroesophageal reflux, poor growth, neurodevelopmental delay, behavior problems, hearing loss, hernia recurrence, and orthopedic deformities. Structured follow-up for these patients facilitates early recognition and treatment of these complications. In this report, follow-up of infants with congenital diaphragmatic hernia is outlined. (3/08, reaffirmed 5/11)

http://pediatrics.aappublications.org/content/121/3/627

POSTNATAL CORTICOSTEROIDS TO PREVENT OR TREAT BRONCHOPULMONARY DYSPLASIA

Kristi L. Watterberg, MD, and Committee on Fetus and Newborn

ABSTRACT. The purpose of this revised statement is to review current information on the use of postnatal glucocorticoids to prevent or treat bronchopulmonary dysplasia in the preterm infant and to make updated recommendations regarding their use. High-dose dexamethasone (0.5 mg/kg per day) does not seem to confer additional therapeutic benefit over lower doses and is not recommended. Evidence is insufficient to make a recommendation regarding other glucocorticoid doses and preparations. The clinician must use clinical judgment when attempting to balance the potential adverse effects of glucocorticoid treatment with those of bronchopulmonary dysplasia. (9/10, reaffirmed 1/14)

http://pediatrics.aappublications.org/content/126/4/800

POSTNATAL GLUCOSE HOMEOSTASIS IN LATE-PRETERM AND TERM INFANTS (CLINICAL REPORT)

David H. Adamkin, MD, and Committee on Fetus and Newborn

ABSTRACT. This report provides a practical guide and algorithm for the screening and subsequent management of neonatal hypoglycemia. Current evidence does not support a specific concentration of glucose that can discriminate normal from abnormal or can potentially result in acute or chronic irreversible neurologic damage. Early identification of the at-risk infant and institution of prophylactic measures to prevent neonatal hypoglycemia are recommended as a pragmatic approach despite the absence of a consistent definition of hypoglycemia in the literature. (3/11, reaffirmed 6/15)

http://pediatrics.aappublications.org/content/127/3/575

POVERTY AND CHILD HEALTH IN THE UNITED STATES

Council on Community Pediatrics

ABSTRACT. Almost half of young children in the United States live in poverty or near poverty. The American Academy of Pediatrics is committed to reducing and ultimately eliminating child poverty in the United States. Poverty and related social determinants of health can lead to adverse health outcomes in childhood and across the life course, negatively affecting physical health, socioemotional development, and educational achievement. The American Academy of Pediatrics advocates for programs and policies that have been shown to improve the quality of life and health outcomes for children and families living in poverty. With an awareness and understanding of the effects of poverty on children, pediatricians and other pediatric health practitioners in a family-centered medical home can assess the financial stability of families, link families to resources, and coordinate care with community partners. Further research, advocacy, and continuing education will improve the ability of pediatricians to address the social determinants of health when caring for children who live in poverty. Accompanying this policy statement is a technical report that describes current knowledge on child poverty and the mechanisms by which poverty influences the health and well-being of children. (3/16)

http://pediatrics.aappublications.org/content/137/4/e20160339

THE POWER OF PLAY: A PEDIATRIC ROLE IN ENHANCING DEVELOPMENT IN YOUNG CHILDREN (CLINICAL REPORT)

Michael Yogman, MD, FAAP; Andrew Garner, MD, PhD, FAAP; Jeffrey Hutchinson, MD, FAAP; Kathy Hirsh-Pasek, PhD; Roberta Michnick Golinkoff, PhD; Committee on Psychosocial Aspects of Child and Family Health; and Council on Communications and Media

ABSTRACT. Children need to develop a variety of skill sets to optimize their development and manage toxic stress. Research demonstrates that developmentally appropriate play with parents and peers is a singular opportunity to promote the social-emotional, cognitive, language, and self-regulation skills that build executive function and a prosocial brain. Furthermore, play supports the formation of the safe, stable, and nurturing relationships with all caregivers that children need to thrive.

Play is not frivolous: it enhances brain structure and function and promotes executive function (ie, the process of learning, rather than the content), which allow us to pursue goals and ignore distractions.

When play and safe, stable, nurturing relationships are missing in a child's life, toxic stress can disrupt the development of executive function and the learning of prosocial behavior; in the presence of childhood adversity, play becomes even more important. The mutual joy and shared communication and attunement (harmonious serve and return interactions) that parents and children can experience during play regulate the body's stress response. This clinical report provides pediatric providers with the information they need to promote the benefits of play and to write a prescription for play at well visits to complement reach out and read. At a time when early childhood programs are pressured to add more didactic components and less playful learning, pediatricians can play an important role in emphasizing the role of a balanced curriculum that includes the importance of playful learning for the promotion of healthy child development. (8/18)

http://pediatrics.aappublications.org/content/142/3/e20182058

PRACTICAL APPROACHES TO OPTIMIZE ADOLESCENT IMMUNIZATION (CLINICAL REPORT)

Henry H. Bernstein, DO, MHCM, FAAP; Joseph A. Bocchini Jr, MD, FAAP; and Committee on Infectious Diseases

ABSTRACT. With the expansion of the adolescent immunization schedule during the past decade, immunization rates notably vary by vaccine and by state. Addressing barriers to improving adolescent vaccination rates is a priority. Every visit can be viewed as an opportunity to update and complete an adolescent's immunizations. It is essential to continue to focus and refine the appropriate techniques in approaching the adolescent patient and parent in the office setting. Health care providers must continuously strive to educate their patients and develop skills that can help parents and adolescents overcome vaccine hesitancy. Research on strategies to achieve higher vaccination rates is ongoing, and it is important to increase the knowledge and implementation of these strategies. This clinical report focuses on increasing adherence to the universally recommended vaccines in the annual adolescent immunization schedule of the American Academy of Pediatrics, the American Academy of Family Physicians, the Centers for Disease Control and Prevention, and the American Congress of Obstetricians and Gynecologists. This will be accomplished by (1) examining strategies that heighten confidence in immunizations and address patient and parental concerns to promote adolescent immunization and (2) exploring how best to approach the adolescent and family to improve immunization rates. (2/17)

http://pediatrics.aappublications.org/content/139/3/e20164187

PREMEDICATION FOR NONEMERGENCY ENDOTRACHEAL INTUBATION IN THE NEONATE (CLINICAL REPORT)

Praveen Kumar, MD; Susan E. Denson, MD; Thomas J. Mancuso, MD; Committee on Fetus and Newborn; and Section on Anesthesiology and Pain Medicine

ABSTRACT. Endotracheal intubation is a common procedure in newborn care. The purpose of this clinical report is to review currently available evidence on use of premedication for intubation, identify gaps in knowledge, and provide guidance for making decisions about the use of premedication. (2/10, reaffirmed 8/13, 5/18)

http://pediatrics.aappublications.org/content/125/3/608

THE PRENATAL VISIT (CLINICAL REPORT)

Michael Yogman, MD, FAAP; Arthur Lavin, MD, FAAP; George Cohen, MD, FAAP; and Committee on Psychosocial Aspects of Child and Family Health

ABSTRACT. A pediatric prenatal visit during the third trimester is recommended for all expectant families as an important first step in establishing a child's medical home, as recommended by *Bright Futures: Guidelines for Health Supervision of Infants, Children, and Adolescents, Fourth Edition.* As advocates for children and their families, pediatricians can support and guide expectant parents in the prenatal period. Prenatal visits allow general pediatricians to establish a supportive and trusting relationship with both parents, gather basic information from expectant parents, offer information and advice regarding the infant, and may identify psychosocial risks early and high-risk conditions that may require special care. There are several possible formats for this first visit. The one used depends on the experience and

preference of the parents, the style of the pediatrician's practice, and pragmatic issues of payment. (6/18)
http://pediatrics.aappublications.org/content/142/1/e20181218

PREPARATION FOR EMERGENCIES IN THE OFFICES OF PEDIATRICIANS AND PEDIATRIC PRIMARY CARE PROVIDERS

Committee on Pediatric Emergency Medicine

ABSTRACT. High-quality pediatric emergency care can be provided only through the collaborative efforts of many health care professionals and child advocates working together throughout a continuum of care that extends from prevention and the medical home to prehospital care, to emergency department stabilization, to critical care and rehabilitation, and finally to a return to care in the medical home. At times, the office of the pediatric primary care provider will serve as the entry site into the emergency care system, which comprises out-of-hospital emergency medical services personnel, emergency department nurses and physicians, and other emergency and critical care providers. Recognizing the important role of pediatric primary care providers in the emergency care system for children and understanding the capabilities and limitations of that system are essential if pediatric primary care providers are to offer the best chance at intact survival for every child who is brought to the office with an emergency. Optimizing pediatric primary care provider office readiness for emergencies requires consideration of the unique aspects of each office practice, the types of patients and emergencies that might be seen, the resources on site, and the resources of the larger emergency care system of which the pediatric primary care provider's office is a part. Parent education regarding prevention, recognition, and response to emergencies, patient triage, early recognition and stabilization of pediatric emergencies in the office, and timely transfer to an appropriate facility for definitive care are important responsibilities of every pediatric primary care provider. In addition, pediatric primary care providers can collaborate with out-of-hospital and hospital-based providers and advocate for the best-quality emergency care for their patients. (7/07, reaffirmed 6/11, 11/18)
http://pediatrics.aappublications.org/content/120/1/200

PREPARING FOR PEDIATRIC EMERGENCIES: DRUGS TO CONSIDER (CLINICAL REPORT)

Mary A. Hegenbarth, MD, and Committee on Drugs

ABSTRACT. This clinical report provides current recommendations regarding the selection and use of drugs in preparation for pediatric emergencies. It is not intended to be a comprehensive list of all medications that may be used in all emergencies. When possible, dosage recommendations are consistent with those used in current emergency references such as the *Advanced Pediatric Life Support and Pediatric Advanced Life Support* textbooks and the recently revised American Heart Association resuscitation guidelines. (2/08, reaffirmed 10/11, 2/16)
http://pediatrics.aappublications.org/content/121/2/433

PRESCRIBING ASSISTIVE-TECHNOLOGY SYSTEMS: FOCUS ON CHILDREN WITH IMPAIRED COMMUNICATION (CLINICAL REPORT)

Larry W. Desch, MD; Deborah Gaebler-Spira, MD; and Council on Children With Disabilities

ABSTRACT. This clinical report defines common terms of use and provides information on current practice, research, and limitations of assistive technology that can be used in systems for communication. The assessment process to determine the best devices for use with a particular child (ie, the best fit of a device) is also reviewed. The primary care pediatrician, as part of the medical home, plays an important role in the interdisciplinary effort to provide appropriate assistive technology and may be asked to make a referral for assessment or prescribe a particular device. This report provides resources to assist pediatricians in this role and reviews the interdisciplinary team functional evaluation using standardized assessments; the multiple funding opportunities available for obtaining devices and ways in which pediatricians can assist families with obtaining them; the training necessary to use these systems once the devices are procured; the follow-up evaluation to ensure that the systems are meeting their goals; and the leadership skills needed to advocate for this technology. The American Academy of Pediatrics acknowledges the need for key resources to be identified in the community and recognizes that these resources are a shared medical, educational, therapeutic, and family responsibility. Although this report primarily deals with assistive technology specific for communication impairments, many of the details in this report also can aid in the acquisition and use of other types of assistive technology. (6/08, reaffirmed 1/12, 6/18)
http://pediatrics.aappublications.org/content/121/6/1271

PRESCRIBING PHYSICAL, OCCUPATIONAL, AND SPEECH THERAPY SERVICES FOR CHILDREN WITH DISABILITIES (CLINICAL REPORT)

Amy Houtrow, MD, PhD, MPH, FAAP, FAAPMR; Nancy Murphy, MD, FAAP, FAAPMR; and Council on Children With Disabilities

ABSTRACT. Pediatric health care providers are frequently responsible for prescribing physical, occupational, and speech therapies and monitoring therapeutic progress for children with temporary or permanent disabilities in their practices. This clinical report will provide pediatricians and other pediatric health care providers with information about how best to manage the therapeutic needs of their patients in the medical home by reviewing the International Classification of Functioning, Disability and Health; describing the general goals of habilitative and rehabilitative therapies; delineating the types, locations, and benefits of therapy services; and detailing how to write a therapy prescription and include therapists in the medical home neighborhood. (3/19)
See full text on page 1019.
https://pediatrics.aappublications.org/content/143/4/e20190285

PREVENTING OBESITY AND EATING DISORDERS IN ADOLESCENTS (CLINICAL REPORT)

Neville H. Golden, MD, FAAP; Marcie Schneider, MD, FAAP; Christine Wood, MD, FAAP; Committee on Nutrition; Committee on Adolescence; and Section on Obesity

ABSTRACT. Obesity and eating disorders (EDs) are both prevalent in adolescents. There are concerns that obesity prevention efforts may lead to the development of an ED. Most adolescents who develop an ED did not have obesity previously, but some teenagers, in an attempt to lose weight, may develop an ED. This clinical report addresses the interaction between obesity prevention and EDs in teenagers, provides the pediatrician with evidence-informed tools to identify behaviors that predispose to both obesity and EDs, and provides guidance about obesity and ED prevention messages. The focus should be on a healthy lifestyle rather than on weight. Evidence suggests that obesity prevention and treatment, if conducted correctly, do not predispose to EDs. (8/16)
http://pediatrics.aappublications.org/content/138/3/e20161649

PREVENTION AND MANAGEMENT OF PROCEDURAL PAIN IN THE NEONATE: AN UPDATE

Committee on Fetus and Newborn and Section on Anesthesiology and Pain Medicine

ABSTRACT. The prevention of pain in neonates should be the goal of all pediatricians and health care professionals who work with neonates, not only because it is ethical but also because

repeated painful exposures have the potential for deleterious consequences. Neonates at greatest risk of neurodevelopmental impairment as a result of preterm birth (ie, the smallest and sickest) are also those most likely to be exposed to the greatest number of painful stimuli in the NICU. Although there are major gaps in knowledge regarding the most effective way to prevent and relieve pain in neonates, proven and safe therapies are currently underused for routine minor, yet painful procedures. Therefore, every health care facility caring for neonates should implement (1) a pain-prevention program that includes strategies for minimizing the number of painful procedures performed and (2) a pain assessment and management plan that includes routine assessment of pain, pharmacologic and nonpharmacologic therapies for the prevention of pain associated with routine minor procedures, and measures for minimizing pain associated with surgery and other major procedures. (1/16)
http://pediatrics.aappublications.org/content/137/2/e20154271

PREVENTION OF AGRICULTURAL INJURIES AMONG CHILDREN AND ADOLESCENTS

Committee on Injury and Poison Prevention and Committee on Community Health Services

ABSTRACT. Although the annual number of farm deaths to children and adolescents has decreased since publication of the 1988 American Academy of Pediatrics statement, "Rural Injuries," the rate of nonfatal farm injuries has increased. Approximately 100 unintentional injury deaths occur annually to children and adolescents on US farms, and an additional 22 000 injuries to children younger than 20 years occur on farms. Relatively few adolescents are employed on farms compared with other types of industry, yet the proportion of fatalities in agriculture is higher than that for any other type of adolescent employment. The high mortality and severe morbidity associated with farm injuries require continuing and improved injury-control strategies. This statement provides recommendations for pediatricians regarding patient and community education as well as public advocacy related to agricultural injury prevention in childhood and adolescence. (10/01, reaffirmed 1/07, 11/11)
http://pediatrics.aappublications.org/content/108/4/1016

PREVENTION OF CHILDHOOD LEAD TOXICITY

Council on Environmental Health

ABSTRACT. Blood lead concentrations have decreased dramatically in US children over the past 4 decades, but too many children still live in housing with deteriorated lead-based paint and are at risk for lead exposure with resulting lead-associated cognitive impairment and behavioral problems. Evidence continues to accrue that commonly encountered blood lead concentrations, even those below 5 µg/dL (50 ppb), impair cognition; there is no identified threshold or safe level of lead in blood. From 2007 to 2010, approximately 2.6% of preschool children in the United States had a blood lead concentration ≥5 µg/dL (≥50 ppb), which represents about 535 000 US children 1 to 5 years of age. Evidence-based guidance is available for managing increased lead exposure in children, and reducing sources of lead in the environment, including lead in housing, soil, water, and consumer products, has been shown to be cost-beneficial. Primary prevention should be the focus of policy on childhood lead toxicity. (6/16)
http://pediatrics.aappublications.org/content/138/1/e20161493

PREVENTION OF CHOKING AMONG CHILDREN

Committee on Injury, Violence, and Poison Prevention

ABSTRACT. Choking is a leading cause of morbidity and mortality among children, especially those aged 3 years or younger. Food, coins, and toys are the primary causes of choking-related injury and death. Certain characteristics, including shape, size, and consistency, of certain toys and foods increase their potential to cause choking among children. Childhood choking hazards should be addressed through comprehensive and coordinated prevention activities. The US Consumer Product Safety Commission (CPSC) should increase efforts to ensure that toys that are sold in retail store bins, vending machines, or on the Internet have appropriate choking-hazard warnings; work with manufacturers to improve the effectiveness of recalls of products that pose a choking risk to children; and increase efforts to prevent the resale of these recalled products via online auction sites. Current gaps in choking-prevention standards for children's toys should be reevaluated and addressed, as appropriate, via revisions to the standards established under the Child Safety Protection Act, the Consumer Product Safety Improvement Act, or regulation by the CPSC. Prevention of food-related choking among children in the United States has been inadequately addressed at the federal level. The US Food and Drug Administration should establish a systematic, institutionalized process for examining and addressing the hazards of food-related choking. This process should include the establishment of the necessary surveillance, hazard evaluation, enforcement, and public education activities to prevent food-related choking among children. While maintaining its highly cooperative arrangements with the CPSC and the US Department of Agriculture, the Food and Drug Administration should have the authority to address choking-related risks of all food products, including meat products that fall under the jurisdiction of the US Department of Agriculture. The existing National Electronic Injury Surveillance System–All Injury Program of the CPSC should be modified to conduct more-detailed surveillance of choking on food among children. Food manufacturers should design new foods and redesign existing foods to avoid shapes, sizes, textures, and other characteristics that increase choking risk to children, to the extent possible. Pediatricians, dentists, and other infant and child health care providers should provide choking-prevention counseling to parents as an integral part of anticipatory guidance activities. (2/10)
http://pediatrics.aappublications.org/content/125/3/601

PREVENTION OF DROWNING

Sarah A. Denny, MD, FAAP; Linda Quan, MD, FAAP; Julie Gilchrist, MD, FAAP; Tracy McCallin, MD, FAAP; Rohit Shenoi, MD, FAAP; Shabana Yusuf, MD, Med, FAAP; Benjamin Hoffman, MD, FAAP; Jeffrey Weiss, MD, FAAP; and Council on Injury, Violence, and Poison Prevention

ABSTRACT. Drowning is a leading cause of injury-related death in children. In 2017, drowning claimed the lives of almost 1000 US children younger than 20 years. A number of strategies are available to prevent these tragedies. As educators and advocates, pediatricians can play an important role in the prevention of drowning. (4/19)

See full text on page 1035.

https://pediatrics.aappublications.org/content/143/5/e20190850

PREVENTION OF SEXUAL HARASSMENT IN THE WORKPLACE AND EDUCATIONAL SETTINGS

Committee on Pediatric Workforce

ABSTRACT. The American Academy of Pediatrics is committed to working to ensure that workplaces and educational settings in which pediatricians spend time are free of sexual harassment. The purpose of this statement is to heighten awareness and sensitivity to this important issue, recognizing that institutions, clinics, and office-based practices may have existing policies. (10/06, reaffirmed 5/09, 1/12, 10/14)
http://pediatrics.aappublications.org/content/118/4/1752

THE PREVENTION OF UNINTENTIONAL INJURY AMONG AMERICAN INDIAN AND ALASKA NATIVE CHILDREN: A SUBJECT REVIEW (CLINICAL REPORT)

Committee on Native American Child Health and Committee on Injury and Poison Prevention

ABSTRACT. Among ethnic groups in the United States, American Indian and Alaska Native (AI/AN) children experience the highest rates of injury mortality and morbidity. Injury mortality rates for AI/AN children have decreased during the past quarter century, but remain almost double the rate for all children in the United States. The Indian Health Service (IHS), the federal agency with the primary responsibility for the health care of AI/AN people, has sponsored an internationally recognized injury prevention program designed to reduce the risk of injury death by addressing community-specific risk factors. Model programs developed by the IHS and tribal governments have led to successful outcomes in motor vehicle occupant safety, drowning prevention, and fire safety. Injury prevention programs in tribal communities require special attention to the sovereignty of tribal governments and the unique cultural aspects of health care and communication. Pediatricians working with AI/AN children on reservations or in urban environments are strongly urged to collaborate with tribes and the IHS to create community-based coalitions and develop programs to address highly preventable injury-related mortality and morbidity. Strong advocacy also is needed to promote childhood injury prevention as an important priority for federal agencies and tribes. (12/99, reaffirmed 12/02 COIVPP, 5/03 CONACH, 1/06, 9/08)

http://pediatrics.aappublications.org/content/104/6/1397

THE PRIMARY CARE PEDIATRICIAN AND THE CARE OF CHILDREN WITH CLEFT LIP AND/OR CLEFT PALATE (CLINICAL REPORT)

PPI AAP Partnership for Policy Implementation

Charlotte W. Lewis, MD, MPH, FAAP; Lisa S. Jacob, DDS, MS; Christoph U. Lehmann, MD, FAAP, FACMI; and Section on Oral Health

ABSTRACT. Orofacial clefts, specifically cleft lip and/or cleft palate (CL/P), are among the most common congenital anomalies. CL/P vary in their location and severity and comprise 3 overarching groups: cleft lip (CL), cleft lip with cleft palate (CLP), and cleft palate alone (CP). CL/P may be associated with one of many syndromes that could further complicate a child's needs. Care of patients with CL/P spans prenatal diagnosis into adulthood. The appropriate timing and order of specific cleft-related care are important factors for optimizing outcomes; however, care should be individualized to meet the specific needs of each patient and family. Children with CL/P should receive their specialty cleft-related care from a multidisciplinary cleft or craniofacial team with sufficient patient and surgical volume to promote successful outcomes. The primary care pediatrician at the child's medical home has an essential role in making a timely diagnosis and referral; providing ongoing health care maintenance, anticipatory guidance, and acute care; and functioning as an advocate for the patient and a liaison between the family and the craniofacial/cleft team. This document provides background on CL/P and multidisciplinary team care, information about typical timing and order of cleft-related care, and recommendations for cleft/craniofacial teams and primary care pediatricians in the care of children with CL/P. (4/17)

http://pediatrics.aappublications.org/content/139/5/e20170628

PRINCIPLES OF CHILD HEALTH CARE FINANCING

Mark L. Hudak, MD, FAAP; Mark E. Helm, MD, MBA, FAAP; Patience H. White, MD, MA, FAAP, FACP; and Committee on Child Health Financing

ABSTRACT. After passage of the Patient Protection and Affordable Care Act, more children and young adults have become insured and have benefited from health care coverage than at any time since the creation of the Medicaid program in 1965. From 2009 to 2015, the uninsurance rate for children younger than 19 years fell from 9.7% to 5.3%, whereas the uninsurance rate for young adults 19 to 25 years of age declined from 31.7% to 14.5%. Nonetheless, much work remains to be done. The American Academy of Pediatrics (AAP) believes that the United States can and should ensure that all children, adolescents, and young adults from birth through the age of 26 years who reside within its borders have affordable access to high-quality and comprehensive health care, regardless of their or their families' incomes. Public and private health insurance should safeguard existing benefits for children and take further steps to cover the full array of essential health care services recommended by the AAP. Each family should be able to afford the premiums, deductibles, and other cost-sharing provisions of the plan. Health plans providing these benefits should ensure, insofar as possible, that families have a choice of professionals and facilities with expertise in the care of children within a reasonable distance of their residence. Traditional and innovative payment methodologies by public and private payers should be structured to guarantee the economic viability of the pediatric medical home and of other pediatric specialty and subspecialty practices to address developing shortages in the pediatric specialty and subspecialty workforce, to promote the use of health information technology, to improve population health and the experience of care, and to encourage the delivery of evidence-based and quality health care in the medical home, as well as in other outpatient, inpatient, and home settings. All current and future health care insurance plans should incorporate the principles for child health financing outlined in this statement. Espousing the core principle to do no harm, the AAP believes that the United States must not sacrifice any of the hard-won gains for our children. Medicaid, as the largest single payer of health care for children and young adults, should remain true to its origins as an entitlement program; in other words, future fiscal or regulatory reforms of Medicaid should not reduce the eligibility and scope of benefits for children and young adults below current levels nor jeopardize children's access to care. Proposed Medicaid funding "reforms" (eg, institution of block grant, capped allotment, or per-capita capitation payments to states) will achieve their goal of securing cost savings but will inevitably compel states to reduce enrollee eligibility, trim existing benefits (such as Early and Periodic Screening, Diagnostic, and Treatment), and/or compromise children's access to necessary and timely care through cuts in payments to providers and delivery systems. In fact, the AAP advocates for increased Medicaid funding to improve access to essential care for existing enrollees, fund care for eligible but uninsured children once they enroll, and accommodate enrollment growth that will occur in states that choose to expand Medicaid eligibility. The AAP also calls for Congress to extend funding for the Children's Health Insurance Program, a plan vital to the 8.9 million children it covered in fiscal year 2016, for a minimum of 5 years. (8/17)

http://pediatrics.aappublications.org/content/140/3/e20172098

PRINCIPLES OF PEDIATRIC PATIENT SAFETY: REDUCING HARM DUE TO MEDICAL CARE

Brigitta U. Mueller, MD, MHCM, CPPS, CPHQ, FAAP; Daniel Robert Neuspiel, MD, MPH, FAAP; Erin R. Stucky Fisher, MD, FAAP; Council on Quality Improvement and Patient Safety; and Committee on Hospital Care

ABSTRACT. Pediatricians render care in an increasingly complex environment, which results in multiple opportunities to cause unintended harm. National awareness of patient safety risks has grown since the National Academy of Medicine (formerly the Institute of Medicine) published its report "To Err Is Human: Building a Safer Health System" in 1999. Patients and society as a whole continue to challenge health care providers to examine their practices and implement safety solutions. The depth and breadth of harm incurred by the practice of medicine is still being defined as reports continue to reveal a variety of avoidable errors, from those that involve specific high-risk medications to those that are more generalizable, such as patient misidentification and diagnostic error. Pediatric health care providers in all practice environments benefit from having a working knowledge of patient safety language. Pediatric providers should serve as advocates for best practices and policies with the goal of attending to risks that are unique to children, identifying and supporting a culture of safety, and leading efforts to eliminate avoidable harm in any setting in which medical care is rendered to children. In this Policy Statement, we provide an update to the 2011 Policy Statement "Principles of Pediatric Patient Safety: Reducing Harm Due to Medical Care." (1/19)

See full text on page 1049.

https://pediatrics.aappublications.org/content/143/2/e20183649

PROBIOTICS AND PREBIOTICS IN PEDIATRICS (CLINICAL REPORT)

Dan W. Thomas, MD; Frank R. Greer, MD; Committee on Nutrition; and Section on Gastroenterology, Hepatology, and Nutrition

ABSTRACT. This clinical report reviews the currently known health benefits of probiotic and prebiotic products, including those added to commercially available infant formula and other food products for use in children. Probiotics are supplements or foods that contain viable microorganisms that cause alterations of the microflora of the host. Use of probiotics has been shown to be modestly effective in randomized clinical trials (RCTs) in (1) treating acute viral gastroenteritis in healthy children; and (2) preventing antibiotic-associated diarrhea in healthy children. There is some evidence that probiotics prevent necrotizing enterocolitis in very low birth weight infants (birth weight between 1000 and 1500 g), but more studies are needed. The results of RCTs in which probiotics were used to treat childhood *Helicobacter pylori* gastritis, irritable bowel syndrome, chronic ulcerative colitis, and infantile colic, as well as in preventing childhood atopy, although encouraging, are preliminary and require further confirmation. Probiotics have not been proven to be beneficial in treating or preventing human cancers or in treating children with Crohn disease. There are also safety concerns with the use of probiotics in infants and children who are immunocompromised, chronically debilitated, or seriously ill with indwelling medical devices.

Prebiotics are supplements or foods that contain a nondigestible food ingredient that selectively stimulates the favorable growth and/or activity of indigenous probiotic bacteria. Human milk contains substantial quantities of prebiotics. There is a paucity of RCTs examining prebiotics in children, although there may be some long-term benefit of prebiotics for the prevention of atopic eczema and common infections in healthy infants. Confirmatory well-designed clinical research studies are necessary. (11/10)

http://pediatrics.aappublications.org/content/126/6/1217

PROCEDURES FOR THE EVALUATION OF THE VISUAL SYSTEM BY PEDIATRICIANS (CLINICAL REPORT)

Sean P. Donahue, MD, PhD, FAAP; Cynthia N. Baker, MD, FAAP; Committee on Practice and Ambulatory Medicine; and Section on Ophthalmology (joint with American Association of Certified Orthoptists, American Association for Pediatric Ophthalmology and Strabismus, and American Academy of Ophthalmology)

ABSTRACT. Vision screening is crucial for the detection of visual and systemic disorders. It should begin in the newborn nursery and continue throughout childhood. This clinical report provides details regarding methods for pediatricians to use for screening. (12/15)

http://pediatrics.aappublications.org/content/137/1/e20153597

PROFESSIONALISM IN PEDIATRICS (TECHNICAL REPORT)

Mary E. Fallat, MD; Jacqueline Glover, PhD; and Committee on Bioethics

ABSTRACT. The purpose of this report is to provide a concrete overview of the ideal standards of behavior and professional practice to which pediatricians should aspire and by which students and residents can be evaluated. Recognizing that the ideal is not always achievable in the practical sense, this document details the key components of professionalism in pediatric practice with an emphasis on core professional values for which pediatricians should strive and that will serve as a moral compass needed to provide quality care for children and their families. (10/07, reaffirmed 5/11)

http://pediatrics.aappublications.org/content/120/4/e1123

PROFESSIONALISM IN PEDIATRICS: STATEMENT OF PRINCIPLES

Committee on Bioethics

ABSTRACT. The purpose of this statement is to delineate the concept of professionalism within the context of pediatrics and to provide a brief statement of principles to guide the behavior and professional practice of pediatricians. (10/07, reaffirmed 5/11)

http://pediatrics.aappublications.org/content/120/4/895

PROMOTING EDUCATION, MENTORSHIP, AND SUPPORT FOR PEDIATRIC RESEARCH

Committee on Pediatric Research

ABSTRACT. Pediatricians play a key role in advancing child health research to best attain and improve the physical, mental, and social health and well-being of all infants, children, adolescents, and young adults. Child health presents unique issues that require investigators who specialize in pediatric research. In addition, the scope of the pediatric research enterprise is transdisciplinary and includes the full spectrum of basic science, translational, community-based, health services, and child health policy research. Although most pediatricians do not directly engage in research, knowledge of research methodologies and approaches promotes critical evaluation of scientific literature, the practice of evidence-based medicine, and advocacy for evidence-based child health policy. This statement includes specific recommendations to promote further research education and support at all levels of pediatric training, from premedical to continuing medical education, as well as recommendations to increase support and mentorship for research activities. Pediatric research is crucial to the American Academy of Pediatrics' goal of improving the health of all children. The American Academy of Pediatrics continues to promote and encourage efforts to facilitate the creation of new knowledge and ways to reduce barriers experienced by trainees, practitioners, and academic faculty pursuing research. (4/14, reaffirmed 2/18)

http://pediatrics.aappublications.org/content/133/5/943

PROMOTING FOOD SECURITY FOR ALL CHILDREN

Council on Community Pediatrics and Committee on Nutrition

ABSTRACT. Sixteen million US children (21%) live in households without consistent access to adequate food. After multiple risk factors are considered, children who live in households that are food insecure, even at the lowest levels, are likely to be sick more often, recover from illness more slowly, and be hospitalized more frequently. Lack of adequate healthy food can impair a child's ability to concentrate and perform well in school and is linked to higher levels of behavioral and emotional problems from preschool through adolescence. Food insecurity can affect

children in any community, not only traditionally underserved ones. Pediatricians can play a central role in screening and identifying children at risk for food insecurity and in connecting families with needed community resources. Pediatricians should also advocate for federal and local policies that support access to adequate healthy food for an active and healthy life for all children and their families. (10/15)
http://pediatrics.aappublications.org/content/136/5/e1431

PROMOTING OPTIMAL DEVELOPMENT: SCREENING FOR BEHAVIORAL AND EMOTIONAL PROBLEMS (CLINICAL REPORT)

Carol Weitzman, MD, FAAP; Lynn Wegner, MD, FAAP; Section on Developmental and Behavioral Pediatrics; Committee on Psychosocial Aspects of Child and Family Health; and Council on Early Childhood (joint with Society for Developmental and Behavioral Pediatrics)

ABSTRACT. By current estimates, at any given time, approximately 11% to 20% of children in the United States have a behavioral or emotional disorder, as defined in the *Diagnostic and Statistical Manual of Mental Disorders, Fifth Edition*. Between 37% and 39% of children will have a behavioral or emotional disorder diagnosed by 16 years of age, regardless of geographic location in the United States. Behavioral and emotional problems and concerns in children and adolescents are not being reliably identified or treated in the US health system. This clinical report focuses on the need to increase behavioral screening and offers potential changes in practice and the health system, as well as the research needed to accomplish this. This report also (1) reviews the prevalence of behavioral and emotional disorders, (2) describes factors affecting the emergence of behavioral and emotional problems, (3) articulates the current state of detection of these problems in pediatric primary care, (4) describes barriers to screening and means to overcome those barriers, and (5) discusses potential changes at a practice and systems level that are needed to facilitate successful behavioral and emotional screening. Highlighted and discussed are the many factors at the level of the pediatric practice, health system, and society contributing to these behavioral and emotional problems. (1/15)
http://pediatrics.aappublications.org/content/135/2/384

PROMOTING THE PARTICIPATION OF CHILDREN WITH DISABILITIES IN SPORTS, RECREATION, AND PHYSICAL ACTIVITIES (CLINICAL REPORT)

Nancy A. Murphy, MD; Paul S. Carbone, MD; and Council on Children With Disabilities

ABSTRACT. The benefits of physical activity are universal for all children, including those with disabilities. The participation of children with disabilities in sports and recreational activities promotes inclusion, minimizes deconditioning, optimizes physical functioning, and enhances overall well-being. Despite these benefits, children with disabilities are more restricted in their participation, have lower levels of fitness, and have higher levels of obesity than their peers without disabilities. Pediatricians and parents may overestimate the risks or overlook the benefits of physical activity in children with disabilities. Well-informed decisions regarding each child's participation must consider overall health status, individual activity preferences, safety precautions, and availability of appropriate programs and equipment. Health supervision visits afford pediatricians, children with disabilities, and parents opportunities to collaboratively generate goal-directed activity "prescriptions." Child, family, financial, and societal barriers to participation need to be directly identified and addressed in the context of local, state, and federal laws. The goal is inclusion for all children with disabilities in appropriate activities. This clinical report discusses the importance of physical activity, recreation, and sports participation for children with disabilities and offers practical suggestions to pediatric health care professionals for the promotion of participation. (5/08, reaffirmed 1/12, 6/18)
http://pediatrics.aappublications.org/content/121/5/1057

PROMOTING THE WELL-BEING OF CHILDREN WHOSE PARENTS ARE GAY OR LESBIAN

Committee on Psychosocial Aspects of Child and Family Health

ABSTRACT. To promote optimal health and well-being of all children, the American Academy of Pediatrics (AAP) supports access for all children to (1) civil marriage rights for their parents and (2) willing and capable foster and adoptive parents, regardless of the parents' sexual orientation. The AAP has always been an advocate for, and has developed policies to support, the optimal physical, mental, and social health and well-being of all infants, children, adolescents, and young adults. In so doing, the AAP has supported families in all their diversity, because the family has always been the basic social unit in which children develop the supporting and nurturing relationships with adults that they need to thrive. Children may be born to, adopted by, or cared for temporarily by married couples, nonmarried couples, single parents, grandparents, or legal guardians, and any of these may be heterosexual, gay or lesbian, or of another orientation. Children need secure and enduring relationships with committed and nurturing adults to enhance their life experiences for optimal social-emotional and cognitive development. Scientific evidence affirms that children have similar developmental and emotional needs and receive similar parenting whether they are raised by parents of the same or different genders. If a child has 2 living and capable parents who choose to create a permanent bond by way of civil marriage, it is in the best interests of their child(ren) that legal and social institutions allow and support them to do so, irrespective of their sexual orientation. If 2 parents are not available to the child, adoption or foster parenting remain acceptable options to provide a loving home for a child and should be available without regard to the sexual orientation of the parent(s). (3/13)
http://pediatrics.aappublications.org/content/131/4/827

PROMOTING THE WELL-BEING OF CHILDREN WHOSE PARENTS ARE GAY OR LESBIAN (TECHNICAL REPORT)

Ellen C. Perrin, MD, MA; Benjamin S. Siegel, MD; and Committee on Psychosocial Aspects of Child and Family Health

ABSTRACT. Extensive data available from more than 30 years of research reveal that children raised by gay and lesbian parents have demonstrated resilience with regard to social, psychological, and sexual health despite economic and legal disparities and social stigma. Many studies have demonstrated that children's well-being is affected much more by their relationships with their parents, their parents' sense of competence and security, and the presence of social and economic support for the family than by the gender or the sexual orientation of their parents. Lack of opportunity for same-gender couples to marry adds to families' stress, which affects the health and welfare of all household members. Because marriage strengthens families and, in so doing, benefits children's development, children should not be deprived of the opportunity for their parents to be married. Paths to parenthood that include assisted reproductive techniques, adoption, and foster parenting should focus on competency of the parents rather than their sexual orientation. (3/13)
http://pediatrics.aappublications.org/content/131/4/e1374

PROMOTION OF HEALTHY WEIGHT-CONTROL PRACTICES IN YOUNG ATHLETES (CLINICAL REPORT)

Rebecca L. Carl, MD, MS, FAAP; Miriam D. Johnson, MD, FAAP; Thomas J. Martin, MD, FAAP; and Council on Sports Medicine and Fitness

ABSTRACT. Children and adolescents may participate in sports that favor a particular body type. Some sports, such as gymnastics, dance, and distance running, emphasize a slim or lean physique for aesthetic or performance reasons. Participants in weight-class sports, such as wrestling and martial arts, may attempt weight loss so they can compete at a lower weight class. Other sports, such as football and bodybuilding, highlight a muscular physique; young athletes engaged in these sports may desire to gain weight and muscle mass. This clinical report describes unhealthy methods of weight loss and gain as well as policies and approaches used to curb these practices. The report also reviews healthy strategies for weight loss and weight gain and provides recommendations for pediatricians on how to promote healthy weight control in young athletes. (8/17)

http://pediatrics.aappublications.org/content/140/3/e20171871

PROTECTING CHILDREN FROM SEXUAL ABUSE BY HEALTH CARE PROVIDERS

Committee on Child Abuse and Neglect

ABSTRACT. Sexual abuse or exploitation of children is never acceptable. Such behavior by health care providers is particularly concerning because of the trust that children and their families place on adults in the health care profession. The American Academy of Pediatrics strongly endorses the social and moral prohibition against sexual abuse or exploitation of children by health care providers. The academy opposes any such sexual abuse or exploitation by providers, particularly by the academy's members. Health care providers should be trained to recognize and abide by appropriate provider-patient boundaries. Medical institutions should screen staff members for a history of child abuse issues, train them to respect and maintain appropriate boundaries, and establish policies and procedures to receive and investigate concerns about patient abuse. Each person has a responsibility to ensure the safety of children in health care settings and to scrupulously follow appropriate legal and ethical reporting and investigation procedures. (6/11, reaffirmed 10/14)

http://pediatrics.aappublications.org/content/128/2/407

PROTECTING CHILDREN FROM TOBACCO, NICOTINE, AND TOBACCO SMOKE (TECHNICAL REPORT)

Harold J. Farber, MD, MSPH, FAAP; Judith Groner, MD, FAAP; Susan Walley, MD, FAAP; Kevin Nelson, MD, PhD, FAAP; and Section on Tobacco Control

ABSTRACT. This technical report serves to provide the evidence base for the American Academy of Pediatrics' policy statements "Clinical Practice Policy to Protect Children From Tobacco, Nicotine, and Tobacco Smoke" and "Public Policy to Protect Children From Tobacco, Nicotine, and Tobacco Smoke." Tobacco use and involuntary exposure are major preventable causes of morbidity and premature mortality in adults and children. Tobacco dependence almost always starts in childhood or adolescence. Electronic nicotine delivery systems are rapidly gaining popularity among youth, and their significant harms are being documented. In utero tobacco smoke exposure, in addition to increasing the risk of preterm birth, low birth weight, stillbirth, placental abruption, and sudden infant death, has been found to increase the risk of obesity and neurodevelopmental disorders. Actions by pediatricians can help to reduce children's risk of developing tobacco dependence and reduce children's involuntary tobacco smoke exposure. Public policy actions to protect children from tobacco are essential to reduce the toll that the tobacco epidemic takes on our children. (10/15)

http://pediatrics.aappublications.org/content/136/5/e1439

PROVIDING A PRIMARY CARE MEDICAL HOME FOR CHILDREN AND YOUTH WITH CEREBRAL PALSY (CLINICAL REPORT)

Gregory S. Liptak, MD, MPH; Nancy A. Murphy, MD; and Council on Children With Disabilities

ABSTRACT. All primary care providers will care for children with cerebral palsy in their practice. In addition to well-child and acute illness care, the role of the medical home in the management of these children includes diagnosis, planning for interventions, authorizing treatments, and follow-up. Optimizing health and well-being for children with cerebral palsy and their families entails family-centered care provided in the medical home; comanagement is the most common model. This report reviews the aspects of care specific to cerebral palsy that a medical home should provide beyond the routine health care needed by all children. (10/11, reaffirmed 11/14, 8/18)

http://pediatrics.aappublications.org/content/128/5/e1321

PROVIDING A PRIMARY CARE MEDICAL HOME FOR CHILDREN AND YOUTH WITH SPINA BIFIDA (CLINICAL REPORT)

Robert Burke, MD, MPH; Gregory S. Liptak, MD, MPH; and Council on Children With Disabilities

ABSTRACT. The pediatric primary care provider in the medical home has a central and unique role in the care of children with spina bifida. The primary care provider addresses not only the typical issues of preventive and acute health care but also the needs specific to these children. Optimal care requires communication and comanagement with pediatric medical and developmental subspecialists, surgical specialists, therapists, and community providers. The medical home provider is essential in supporting the family and advocating for the child from the time of entry into the practice through adolescence, which includes transition and transfer to adult health care. This report reviews aspects of care specific to the infant with spina bifida (particularly myelomeningocele) that will facilitate optimal medical, functional, and developmental outcomes. (11/11, reaffirmed 2/15, 7/18)

http://pediatrics.aappublications.org/content/128/6/e1645

PROVIDING CARE FOR CHILDREN AND ADOLESCENTS FACING HOMELESSNESS AND HOUSING INSECURITY

Council on Community Pediatrics

ABSTRACT. Child health and housing security are closely intertwined, and children without homes are more likely to suffer from chronic disease, hunger, and malnutrition than are children with homes. Homeless children and youth often have significant psychosocial development issues, and their education is frequently interrupted. Given the overall effects that homelessness can have on a child's health and potential, it is important for pediatricians to recognize the factors that lead to homelessness, understand the ways that homelessness and its causes can lead to poor health outcomes, and when possible, help children and families mitigate some of the effects of homelessness. Through practice change, partnership with community resources, awareness, and advocacy, pediatricians can help optimize the health and well-being of children affected by homelessness. (5/13, reaffirmed 10/16)

http://pediatrics.aappublications.org/content/131/6/1206

PROVIDING CARE FOR CHILDREN IN IMMIGRANT FAMILIES

Julie M. Linton, MD, FAAP; Andrea Green, MDCM, FAAP; and Council on Community Pediatrics

ABSTRACT. Children in immigrant families (CIF), who represent 1 in 4 children in the United States, represent a growing and ever more diverse US demographic that pediatric medical providers nationwide will increasingly encounter in clinical care.

Immigrant children are those born outside the United States to non–US citizen parents, and CIF are defined as those who are either foreign born or have at least 1 parent who is foreign born. Some families immigrate for economic or educational reasons, and others come fleeing persecution and seeking safe haven. Some US-born children with a foreign-born parent may share vulnerabilities with children who themselves are foreign born, particularly regarding access to care and other social determinants of health. Therefore, the larger umbrella term of CIF is used in this statement. CIF, like all children, have diverse experiences that interact with their biopsychosocial development. CIF may face inequities that can threaten their health and well-being, and CIF also offer strengths and embody resilience that can surpass challenges experienced before and during integration. This policy statement describes the evolving population of CIF in the United States, briefly introduces core competencies to enhance care within a framework of cultural humility and safety, and discusses barriers and opportunities at the practice and systems levels. Practice-level recommendations describe how pediatricians can promote health equity for CIF through careful attention to core competencies in clinical care, thoughtful community engagement, and system-level support. Advocacy and policy recommendations offer ways pediatricians can advocate for policies that promote health equity for CIF. (8/19)

See full text on page 1065.

https://pediatrics.aappublications.org/content/144/3/e20192077

PROVIDING PSYCHOSOCIAL SUPPORT TO CHILDREN AND FAMILIES IN THE AFTERMATH OF DISASTERS AND CRISES (CLINICAL REPORT)

David J. Schonfeld, MD, FAAP; Thomas Demaria, PhD; Disaster Preparedness Advisory Council; and Committee on Psychosocial Aspects of Child and Family Health

ABSTRACT. Disasters have the potential to cause short- and long-term effects on the psychological functioning, emotional adjustment, health, and developmental trajectory of children. This clinical report provides practical suggestions on how to identify common adjustment difficulties in children in the aftermath of a disaster and to promote effective coping strategies to mitigate the impact of the disaster as well as any associated bereavement and secondary stressors. This information can serve as a guide to pediatricians as they offer anticipatory guidance to families or consultation to schools, child care centers, and other child congregate care sites. Knowledge of risk factors for adjustment difficulties can serve as the basis for mental health triage. The importance of basic supportive services, psychological first aid, and professional self-care are discussed. Stress is intrinsic to many major life events that children and families face, including the experience of significant illness and its treatment. The information provided in this clinical report may, therefore, be relevant for a broad range of patient encounters, even outside the context of a disaster. Most pediatricians enter the profession because of a heartfelt desire to help children and families most in need. If adequately prepared and supported, pediatricians who are able to draw on their skills to assist children, families, and communities to recover after a disaster will find the work to be particularly rewarding. (9/15)

http://pediatrics.aappublications.org/content/136/4/e1120

PSYCHOLOGICAL MALTREATMENT (CLINICAL REPORT)

Roberta Hibbard, MD; Jane Barlow, DPhil; Harriet MacMillan, MD; Committee on Child Abuse and Neglect (joint with American Academy of Child and Adolescent Psychiatry Child Maltreatment and Violence Committee)

ABSTRACT. Psychological or emotional maltreatment of children may be the most challenging and prevalent form of child abuse and neglect. Caregiver behaviors include acts of omission (ignoring need for social interactions) or commission (spurning, terrorizing); may be verbal or nonverbal, active or passive, and with or without intent to harm; and negatively affect the child's cognitive, social, emotional, and/or physical development. Psychological maltreatment has been linked with disorders of attachment, developmental and educational problems, socialization problems, disruptive behavior, and later psychopathology. Although no evidence-based interventions that can prevent psychological maltreatment have been identified to date, it is possible that interventions shown to be effective in reducing overall types of child maltreatment, such as the Nurse Family Partnership, may have a role to play. Furthermore, prevention before occurrence will require both the use of universal interventions aimed at promoting the type of parenting that is now recognized to be necessary for optimal child development, alongside the use of targeted interventions directed at improving parental sensitivity to a child's cues during infancy and later parent-child interactions. Intervention should, first and foremost, focus on a thorough assessment and ensuring the child's safety. Potentially effective treatments include cognitive behavioral parenting programs and other psychotherapeutic interventions. The high prevalence of psychological abuse in advanced Western societies, along with the serious consequences, point to the importance of effective management. Pediatricians should be alert to the occurrence of psychological maltreatment and identify ways to support families who have risk indicators for, or evidence of, this problem. (7/12, reaffirmed 4/16)

http://pediatrics.aappublications.org/content/130/2/372

PSYCHOSOCIAL FACTORS IN CHILDREN AND YOUTH WITH SPECIAL HEALTH CARE NEEDS AND THEIR FAMILIES (CLINICAL REPORT)

Gerri Mattson, MD, MSPH, FAAP; Dennis Z. Kuo, MD, MHS, FAAP; Committee on Psychosocial Aspects of Child and Family Health; and Council on Children With Disabilities

ABSTRACT. Children and youth with special health care needs (CYSHCN) and their families may experience a variety of internal (ie, emotional and behavioral) and external (ie, interpersonal, financial, housing, and educational) psychosocial factors that can influence their health and wellness. Many CYSHCN and their families are resilient and thrive. Medical home teams can partner with CYSHCN and their families to screen for, evaluate, and promote psychosocial health to increase protective factors and ameliorate risk factors. Medical home teams can promote protective psychosocial factors as part of coordinated, comprehensive chronic care for CYSHCN and their families. A team-based care approach may entail collaboration across the care spectrum, including youth, families, behavioral health providers, specialists, child care providers, schools, social services, and other community agencies. The purpose of this clinical report is to raise awareness of the impact of psychosocial factors on the health and wellness of CYSHCN and their families. This clinical report provides guidance for pediatric providers to facilitate and coordinate care that can have a positive influence on the overall health, wellness, and quality of life of CYSHCN and their families. (12/18)

See full text on page 1089.

https://pediatrics.aappublications.org/content/143/1/e20183171

PSYCHOSOCIAL SUPPORT FOR YOUTH LIVING WITH HIV (CLINICAL REPORT)

Jaime Martinez, MD, FAAP; Rana Chakraborty, MD, FAAP; and Committee on Pediatric AIDS

ABSTRACT. This clinical report provides guidance for the pediatrician in addressing the psychosocial needs of adolescents and young adults living with HIV, which can improve linkage to care and adherence to life-saving antiretroviral (ARV) therapy.

Recent national case surveillance data for youth (defined here as adolescents and young adults 13 to 24 years of age) revealed that the burden of HIV/AIDS fell most heavily and disproportionately on African American youth, particularly males having sex with males. To effectively increase linkage to care and sustain adherence to therapy, interventions should address the immediate drivers of ARV compliance and also address factors that provide broader social and structural support for HIV-infected adolescents and young adults. Interventions should address psychosocial development, including lack of future orientation, inadequate educational attainment and limited health literacy, failure to focus on the long-term consequences of near-term risk behaviors, and coping ability. Associated challenges are closely linked to the structural environment. Individual case management is essential to linkage to and retention in care, ARV adherence, and management of associated comorbidities. Integrating these skills into pediatric and adolescent HIV practice in a medical home setting is critical, given the alarming increase in new HIV infections in youth in the United States. (2/14)
http://pediatrics.aappublications.org/content/133/3/558

A PUBLIC HEALTH RESPONSE TO OPIOID USE IN PREGNANCY

Stephen W. Patrick, MD, MPH, MS, FAAP; Davida M. Schiff, MD, FAAP; and Committee on Substance Use and Prevention

ABSTRACT. The use of opioids during pregnancy has grown rapidly in the past decade. As opioid use during pregnancy increased, so did complications from their use, including neonatal abstinence syndrome. Several state governments responded to this increase by prosecuting and incarcerating pregnant women with substance use disorders; however, this approach has no proven benefits for maternal or infant health and may lead to avoidance of prenatal care and a decreased willingness to engage in substance use disorder treatment programs. A public health response, rather than a punitive approach to the opioid epidemic and substance use during pregnancy, is critical, including the following: a focus on preventing unintended pregnancies and improving access to contraception; universal screening for alcohol and other drug use in women of childbearing age; knowledge and informed consent of maternal drug testing and reporting practices; improved access to comprehensive obstetric care, including opioid-replacement therapy; gender-specific substance use treatment programs; and improved funding for social services and child welfare systems. The American College of Obstetricians and Gynecologists supports the value of this clinical document as an educational tool (December 2016). (2/17)
http://pediatrics.aappublications.org/content/139/3/e20164070

PUBLIC POLICIES TO REDUCE SUGARY DRINK CONSUMPTION IN CHILDREN AND ADOLESCENTS

Natalie D. Muth, MD, MPH, RDN, FAAP; William H. Dietz, MD, PhD, FAAP; Sheela N. Magge, MD, MSCE, FAAP; Rachel K. Johnson, PhD, MPH, RD, FAHA; Section on Obesity; and Committee on Nutrition (joint with American Heart Association)

ABSTRACT. Excess consumption of added sugars, especially from sugary drinks, poses a grave health threat to children and adolescents, disproportionately affecting children of minority and low-income communities. Public policies, such as those detailed in this statement, are needed to decrease child and adolescent consumption of added sugars and improve health. (3/19)

See full text on page 1105.

https://pediatrics.aappublications.org/content/143/4/e20190282

PUBLIC POLICY TO PROTECT CHILDREN FROM TOBACCO, NICOTINE, AND TOBACCO SMOKE

Section on Tobacco Control

ABSTRACT. Tobacco use and tobacco smoke exposure are among the most important health threats to children, adolescents, and adults. There is no safe level of tobacco smoke exposure. The developing brains of children and adolescents are particularly vulnerable to the development of tobacco and nicotine dependence. Tobacco is unique among consumer products in that it causes disease and death when used exactly as intended. Tobacco continues to be heavily promoted to children and young adults. Flavored and alternative tobacco products, including little cigars, chewing tobacco, and electronic nicotine delivery systems, are gaining popularity among youth. This statement describes important evidence-based public policy actions that, when implemented, will reduce tobacco product use and tobacco smoke exposure among youth and, by doing so, improve the health of children and young adults. (10/15)
http://pediatrics.aappublications.org/content/136/5/998

QUALITY EARLY EDUCATION AND CHILD CARE FROM BIRTH TO KINDERGARTEN

Elaine A. Donoghue, MD, FAAP, and Council on Early Childhood

ABSTRACT. High-quality early education and child care for young children improves physical and cognitive outcomes for the children and can result in enhanced school readiness. Preschool education can be viewed as an investment (especially for at-risk children), and studies show a positive return on that investment. Barriers to high-quality early childhood education include inadequate funding and staff education as well as variable regulation and enforcement. Steps that have been taken to improve the quality of early education and child care include creating multidisciplinary, evidence-based child care practice standards; establishing state quality rating and improvement systems; improving federal and state regulations; providing child care health consultation; and initiating other innovative partnerships. Pediatricians have a role in promoting quality early education and child care for all children not only in the medical home but also at the community, state, and national levels. (7/17)
http://pediatrics.aappublications.org/content/140/2/e20171488

RACE, ETHNICITY, AND SOCIOECONOMIC STATUS IN RESEARCH ON CHILD HEALTH

Tina L. Cheng, MD, MPH, FAAP; Elizabeth Goodman, MD, FAAP; and Committee on Pediatric Research

ABSTRACT. An extensive literature documents the existence of pervasive and persistent child health, development, and health care disparities by race, ethnicity, and socioeconomic status (SES). Disparities experienced during childhood can result in a wide variety of health and health care outcomes, including adult morbidity and mortality, indicating that it is crucial to examine the influence of disparities across the life course. Studies often collect data on the race, ethnicity, and SES of research participants to be used as covariates or explanatory factors. In the past, these variables have often been assumed to exert their effects through individual or genetically determined biologic mechanisms. However, it is now widely accepted that these variables have important social dimensions that influence health. SES, a multidimensional construct, interacts with and confounds analyses of race and ethnicity. Because SES, race, and ethnicity are often difficult to measure accurately, leading to the potential for misattribution of causality, thoughtful consideration should be given to appropriate measurement, analysis, and interpretation of such factors. Scientists who study child and adolescent health and development should understand the multiple measures used to assess race, ethnicity, and SES, including their validity and shortcomings and potential confounding of race and ethnicity with

SES. The American Academy of Pediatrics (AAP) recommends that research on eliminating health and health care disparities related to race, ethnicity, and SES be a priority. Data on race, ethnicity, and SES should be collected in research on child health to improve their definitions and increase understanding of how these factors and their complex interrelationships affect child health. Furthermore, the AAP believes that researchers should consider both biological and social mechanisms of action of race, ethnicity, and SES as they relate to the aims and hypothesis of the specific area of investigation. It is important to measure these variables, but it is not sufficient to use these variables alone as explanatory for differences in disease, morbidity, and outcomes without attention to the social and biologic influences they have on health throughout the life course. The AAP recommends more research, both in the United States and internationally, on measures of race, ethnicity, and SES and how these complex constructs affect health care and health outcomes throughout the life course. (12/14)

http://pediatrics.aappublications.org/content/135/1/e225

RADIATION RISK TO CHILDREN FROM COMPUTED TOMOGRAPHY (CLINICAL REPORT)

Alan S. Brody, MD; Donald P. Frush, MD; Walter Huda, PhD; Robert L. Brent, MD, PhD; and Section on Radiology

ABSTRACT. Imaging studies that use ionizing radiation are an essential tool for the evaluation of many disorders of childhood. Ionizing radiation is used in radiography, fluoroscopy, angiography, and computed tomography scanning. Computed tomography is of particular interest because of its relatively high radiation dose and wide use. Consensus statements on radiation risk suggest that it is reasonable to act on the assumption that low-level radiation may have a small risk of causing cancer. The medical community should seek ways to decrease radiation exposure by using radiation doses as low as reasonably achievable and by performing these studies only when necessary. There is wide agreement that the benefits of an indicated computed tomography scan far outweigh the risks. Pediatric health care professionals' roles in the use of computed tomography on children include deciding when a computed tomography scan is necessary and discussing the risk with patients and families. Radiologists should be a source of consultation when forming imaging strategies and should create specific protocols with scanning techniques optimized for pediatric patients. Families and patients should be encouraged to ask questions about the risks and benefits of computed tomography scanning. The information in this report is provided to aid in decision-making and discussions with the health care team, patients, and families. (9/07)

http://pediatrics.aappublications.org/content/120/3/677

RECOGNITION AND MANAGEMENT OF IATROGENICALLY INDUCED OPIOID DEPENDENCE AND WITHDRAWAL IN CHILDREN (CLINICAL REPORT)

Jeffrey Galinkin, MD, FAAP; Jeffrey Lee Koh, MD, FAAP; Committee on Drugs; and Section on Anesthesiology and Pain Medicine

ABSTRACT. Opioids are often prescribed to children for pain relief related to procedures, acute injuries, and chronic conditions. Round-the-clock dosing of opioids can produce opioid dependence within 5 days. According to a 2001 consensus paper from the American Academy of Pain Medicine, American Pain Society, and American Society of Addiction Medicine, dependence is defined as "a state of adaptation that is manifested by a drug class specific withdrawal syndrome that can be produced by abrupt cessation, rapid dose reduction, decreasing blood level of the drug, and/or administration of an antagonist." Although the experience of many children undergoing iatrogenically induced withdrawal may be mild or goes unreported, there is currently no guidance for recognition or management of withdrawal for this population. Guidance on this subject is available only for adults and primarily for adults with substance use disorders. The guideline will summarize existing literature and provide readers with information currently not available in any single source specific for this vulnerable pediatric population. (12/13)

http://pediatrics.aappublications.org/content/133/1/152

RECOGNITION AND MANAGEMENT OF MEDICAL COMPLEXITY (CLINICAL REPORT)

Dennis Z. Kuo, MD, MHS, FAAP; Amy J. Houtrow, MD, PhD, MPH, FAAP; and Council on Children With Disabilities

ABSTRACT. Children with medical complexity have extensive needs for health services, experience functional limitations, and are high resource utilizers. Addressing the needs of this population to achieve high-value health care requires optimizing care within the medical home and medical neighborhood. Opportunities exist for health care providers, payers, and policy makers to develop strategies to enhance care delivery and to decrease costs. Important outcomes include decreasing unplanned hospital admissions, decreasing emergency department use, ensuring access to health services, limiting out-of-pocket expenses for families, and improving patient and family experiences, quality of life, and satisfaction with care. This report describes the population of children with medical complexity and provides strategies to optimize medical and health outcomes. (11/16)

http://pediatrics.aappublications.org/content/138/6/e20163021

RECOGNIZING AND RESPONDING TO MEDICAL NEGLECT (CLINICAL REPORT)

Carole Jenny, MD, MBA, and Committee on Child Abuse and Neglect

ABSTRACT. A caregiver may fail to recognize or respond to a child's medical needs for a variety of reasons. An effective response by a health care professional to medical neglect requires a comprehensive assessment of the child's needs, the parents' resources, the parents' efforts to provide for the needs of the child, and options for ensuring optimal health for the child. Such an assessment requires clear, 2-way communication between the family and the health care professional. Physicians should consider the least intrusive options for managing cases of medical neglect that ensure the health and safety of the child. (12/07, reaffirmed 1/11, 2/16)

http://pediatrics.aappublications.org/content/120/6/1385

RECOMMENDATIONS FOR PREVENTION AND CONTROL OF INFLUENZA IN CHILDREN, 2019–2020

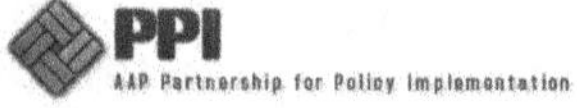

Committee on Infectious Diseases

ABSTRACT. This statement updates the recommendations of the American Academy of Pediatrics for the routine use of influenza vaccines and antiviral medications in the prevention and treatment of influenza in children during the 2019–2020 season. The American Academy of Pediatrics continues to recommend routine influenza immunization of all children without medical contraindications, starting at 6 months of age. Any licensed, recommended, age-appropriate vaccine available can be administered, without preference of one product or formulation over another. Antiviral treatment of influenza with any licensed, recommended, age-appropriate influenza antiviral medication continues to be recommended for children with suspected or confirmed influenza, particularly those who are hospitalized, have severe or progressive disease, or have underlying conditions that increase their risk of complications of influenza. (9/19)

See full text on page 1119.

https://pediatrics.aappublications.org/content/144/4/e20192478

RECOMMENDATIONS FOR SEROGROUP B MENINGOCOCCAL VACCINE FOR PERSONS 10 YEARS AND OLDER

Committee on Infectious Diseases

ABSTRACT. This policy statement provides recommendations for the prevention of serogroup B meningococcal disease through the use of 2 newly licensed serogroup B meningococcal vaccines: MenB-FHbp (Trumenba; Wyeth Pharmaceuticals, a subsidiary of Pfizer, Philadelphia, PA) and MenB-4C (Bexsero; Novartis Vaccines, Siena, Italy). Both vaccines are approved for use in persons 10 through 25 years of age. MenB-FHbp is licensed as a 2- or 3-dose series, and MenB-4C is licensed as a 2-dose series for all groups. Either vaccine is recommended for routine use in persons 10 years and older who are at increased risk of serogroup B meningococcal disease (category A recommendation). Persons at increased risk of meningococcal serogroup B disease include the following: (1) persons with persistent complement component diseases, including inherited or chronic deficiencies in C3, C5–C9, properdin, factor D, or factor H, or persons receiving eculizumab (Soliris; Alexion Pharmaceuticals, Cheshire, CT), a monoclonal antibody that acts as a terminal complement inhibitor by binding C5 and inhibiting cleavage of C5 to C5A; (2) persons with anatomic or functional asplenia, including sickle cell disease; and (3) healthy persons at increased risk because of a serogroup B meningococcal disease outbreak. Both serogroup B meningococcal vaccines have been shown to be safe and immunogenic and are licensed by the US Food and Drug Administration for individuals between the ages of 10 and 25 years. On the basis of epidemiologic and antibody persistence data, the American Academy of Pediatrics agrees with the Advisory Committee on Immunization Practices of the Centers for Disease Control and Prevention that either vaccine may be administered to healthy adolescents and young adults 16 through 23 years of age (preferred ages are 16 through 18 years) to provide short-term protection against most strains of serogroup B meningococcal disease (category B recommendation). (8/16)

http://pediatrics.aappublications.org/content/138/3/e20161890

RECOMMENDED CHILDHOOD AND ADOLESCENT IMMUNIZATION SCHEDULE: UNITED STATES, 2020

Committee on Infectious Diseases (2/20)

See full text on page 1147.

https://pediatrics.aappublications.org/content/early/2020/01/31/peds.2019-3995

REDUCING INJURY RISK FROM BODY CHECKING IN BOYS' YOUTH ICE HOCKEY

Council on Sports Medicine and Fitness

ABSTRACT. Ice hockey is an increasingly popular sport that allows intentional collision in the form of body checking for males but not for females. There is a two- to threefold increased risk of all injury, severe injury, and concussion related to body checking at all levels of boys' youth ice hockey. The American Academy of Pediatrics reinforces the importance of stringent enforcement of rules to protect player safety as well as educational interventions to decrease unsafe tactics. To promote ice hockey as a lifelong recreational pursuit for boys, the American Academy of Pediatrics recommends the expansion of nonchecking programs and the restriction of body checking to elite levels of boys' youth ice hockey, starting no earlier than 15 years of age. (5/14, reaffirmed 7/18)

http://pediatrics.aappublications.org/content/133/6/1151

REDUCING THE NUMBER OF DEATHS AND INJURIES FROM RESIDENTIAL FIRES

Committee on Injury and Poison Prevention

ABSTRACT. Smoke inhalation, severe burns, and death from residential fires are devastating events, most of which are preventable. In 1998, approximately 381 500 residential structure fires resulted in 3250 non-firefighter deaths, 17 175 injuries, and approximately $4.4 billion in property loss. This statement reviews important prevention messages and intervention strategies related to residential fires. It also includes recommendations for pediatricians regarding office anticipatory guidance, work in the community, and support of regulation and legislation that could result in a decrease in the number of fire-related injuries and deaths to children. (6/00)

http://pediatrics.aappublications.org/content/105/6/1355

REFERRAL TO PEDIATRIC SURGICAL SPECIALISTS

Surgical Advisory Panel

ABSTRACT. The American Academy of Pediatrics, with the collaboration of the Surgical Sections of the American Academy of Pediatrics, has created referral recommendations intended to serve as voluntary practice parameters to assist general pediatricians in determining when and to whom to refer their patients for pediatric surgical specialty care. It is recognized that these recommendations may be difficult to implement, because communities vary in terms of access to major pediatric medical centers. Limited access does not negate the value of the recommendations, however, because the child who needs specialized surgical and anesthetic care is best served by the skills of the appropriate pediatric surgical team. Major congenital anomalies, malignancies, major trauma, and chronic illnesses (including those associated with preterm birth) in infants and children should be managed by pediatric medical subspecialists and pediatric surgical specialists at pediatric referral centers that can provide expertise in many areas, including the pediatric medical subspecialties and surgical specialties of pediatric radiology, pediatric anesthesiology, pediatric pathology, and pediatric intensive care. The optimal management of the child with complex problems, chronic illness, or disabilities requires coordination, communication, and cooperation of the pediatric surgical specialist with the child's primary care pediatrician or physician. (1/14)

http://pediatrics.aappublications.org/content/133/2/350

RELIEF OF PAIN AND ANXIETY IN PEDIATRIC PATIENTS IN EMERGENCY MEDICAL SYSTEMS (CLINICAL REPORT)

Joel A. Fein, MD, MPH; William T. Zempsky, MD, MPH; Joseph P. Cravero, MD; Committee on Pediatric Emergency Medicine; and Section on Anesthesiology and Pain Medicine

ABSTRACT. Control of pain and stress for children is a vital component of emergency medical care. Timely administration of analgesia affects the entire emergency medical experience and can have a lasting effect on a child's and family's reaction to current and future medical care. A systematic approach to pain management and anxiolysis, including staff education and protocol development, can provide comfort to children in the emergency setting and improve staff and family satisfaction. (10/12, reaffirmed 9/15)

http://pediatrics.aappublications.org/content/130/5/e1391

RESCUE MEDICINE FOR EPILEPSY IN EDUCATION SETTINGS (CLINICAL REPORT)

Adam L. Hartman, MD, FAAP; Cynthia Di Laura Devore, MD; Section on Neurology; and Council on School Health

ABSTRACT. Children and adolescents with epilepsy may experience prolonged seizures in school-associated settings (eg, during transportation, in the classroom, or during sports activities). Prolonged seizures may evolve into status epilepticus.

Administering a seizure rescue medication can abort the seizure and may obviate the need for emergency medical services and subsequent care in an emergency department. In turn, this may save patients from the morbidity of more invasive interventions and the cost of escalated care. There are significant variations in prescribing practices for seizure rescue medications, partly because of inconsistencies between jurisdictions in legislation and professional practice guidelines among potential first responders (including school staff). There also are potential liability issues for prescribers, school districts, and unlicensed assistive personnel who might administer the seizure rescue medications. This clinical report highlights issues that providers may consider when prescribing seizure rescue medications and creating school medical orders and/or action plans for students with epilepsy. Collaboration among prescribing providers, families, and schools may be useful in developing plans for the use of seizure rescue medications. (12/15)

http://pediatrics.aappublications.org/content/137/1/e20153876

RESPIRATORY SUPPORT IN PRETERM INFANTS AT BIRTH

Committee on Fetus and Newborn

ABSTRACT. Current practice guidelines recommend administration of surfactant at or soon after birth in preterm infants with respiratory distress syndrome. However, recent multicenter randomized controlled trials indicate that early use of continuous positive airway pressure with subsequent selective surfactant administration in extremely preterm infants results in lower rates of bronchopulmonary dysplasia/death when compared with treatment with prophylactic or early surfactant therapy. Continuous positive airway pressure started at or soon after birth with subsequent selective surfactant administration may be considered as an alternative to routine intubation with prophylactic or early surfactant administration in preterm infants. (12/13)

http://pediatrics.aappublications.org/content/133/1/171

RESPONDING TO PARENTAL REFUSALS OF IMMUNIZATION OF CHILDREN (CLINICAL REPORT)

Douglas S. Diekema, MD, MPH, and Committee on Bioethics

ABSTRACT. The American Academy of Pediatrics strongly endorses universal immunization. However, for childhood immunization programs to be successful, parents must comply with immunization recommendations. The problem of parental refusal of immunization for children is an important one for pediatricians. The goal of this report is to assist pediatricians in understanding the reasons parents may have for refusing to immunize their children, review the limited circumstances under which parental refusals should be referred to child protective services agencies or public health authorities, and provide practical guidance to assist the pediatrician faced with a parent who is reluctant to allow immunization of his or her child. (5/05, reaffirmed 1/09, 11/12)

http://pediatrics.aappublications.org/content/115/5/1428

RESPONSIBLE INNOVATION IN CHILDREN'S SURGICAL CARE

Section on Surgery and Committee on Bioethics (joint with American Pediatric Surgical Association New Technology Committee)

ABSTRACT. Advances in medical care may occur when a change in practice incorporates a new treatment or methodology. In surgery, this may involve the translation of a completely novel concept into a new procedure or device or the adaptation of existing treatment approaches or technology to a new clinical application. Regardless of the specifics, innovation should have, as its primary goal, the enhancement of care leading to improved outcomes from the patient's perspective. This policy statement examines innovation as it pertains to surgical care, focusing on some of the definitions that help differentiate applied innovation or innovative therapy from research. The ethical challenges and the potential for conflict of interest for surgeons or institutions seeking to offer innovative surgical therapy are examined. The importance of engaging patients and families as "innovation partners" to ensure complete transparency of expectations from the patient's and provider's perspectives is also examined, with specific emphasis on cultural competence and mutually respectful approaches. A framework for identifying, evaluating, and safely implementing innovative surgical therapy in children is provided. (12/16)

http://pediatrics.aappublications.org/content/139/1/e20163437

RETURNING TO LEARNING FOLLOWING A CONCUSSION (CLINICAL REPORT)

Mark E. Halstead, MD, FAAP; Karen McAvoy, PsyD; Cynthia D. Devore, MD, FAAP; Rebecca Carl, MD, FAAP; Michael Lee, MD, FAAP; Kelsey Logan, MD, FAAP; Council on Sports Medicine and Fitness; and Council on School Health

ABSTRACT. Following a concussion, it is common for children and adolescents to experience difficulties in the school setting. Cognitive difficulties, such as learning new tasks or remembering previously learned material, may pose challenges in the classroom. The school environment may also increase symptoms with exposure to bright lights and screens or noisy cafeterias and hallways. Unfortunately, because most children and adolescents look physically normal after a concussion, school officials often fail to recognize the need for academic or environmental adjustments. Appropriate guidance and recommendations from the pediatrician may ease the transition back to the school environment and facilitate the recovery of the child or adolescent. This report serves to provide a better understanding of possible factors that may contribute to difficulties in a school environment after a concussion and serves as a framework for the medical home, the educational home, and the family home to guide the student to a successful and safe return to learning. (10/13, reaffirmed 7/18)

http://pediatrics.aappublications.org/content/132/5/948

RITUAL GENITAL CUTTING OF FEMALE MINORS

Board of Directors (6/10)

http://pediatrics.aappublications.org/content/126/1/191

THE ROLE OF INTEGRATED CARE IN A MEDICAL HOME FOR PATIENTS WITH A FETAL ALCOHOL SPECTRUM DISORDER (CLINICAL REPORT)

Renee M. Turchi, MD, MPH, FAAP; Vincent C. Smith, MD, MPH, FAAP; Committee on Substance Use and Prevention; and Council on Children With Disabilities

ABSTRACT. Fetal alcohol spectrum disorder (FASD) is an umbrella term used to describe preventable birth defects and intellectual and/or developmental disabilities resulting from prenatal alcohol exposure. The American Academy of Pediatrics has a previous clinical report in which diagnostic criteria for a child with an FASD are discussed and tools to assist pediatricians with its management can be found. This clinical report is intended to foster pediatrician awareness of approaches for screening for prenatal alcohol exposure in clinical practice, to guide management of a child with an FASD after the diagnosis is made, and to summarize available resources for FASD management. (9/18)

http://pediatrics.aappublications.org/content/142/4/e20182333

THE ROLE OF PEDIATRICIANS IN GLOBAL HEALTH

Parminder S. Suchdev, MD, MPH, FAAP; Cynthia R. Howard, MD, MPHTM, FAAP; Section on International Child Health

ABSTRACT. Ninety percent of the world's children live in low- and middle-income countries, where barriers to health contribute to significant child morbidity and mortality. The American

Academy of Pediatrics is dedicated to the health and well-being of *all* children. To fulfill this promise, this policy statement defines the role of the pediatrician in global health and provides a specific set of recommendations directed to all pediatricians, emphasizing the importance of global health as an integral function of the profession of pediatrics. (11/18)
http://pediatrics.aappublications.org/content/142/6/e20182997

ROLE OF PULSE OXIMETRY IN EXAMINING NEWBORNS FOR CONGENITAL HEART DISEASE: A SCIENTIFIC STATEMENT FROM THE AHA AND AAP

William T. Mahle, MD; Jane W. Newburger, MD, MPH; G. Paul Matherne, MD; Frank C. Smith, MD; Tracey R. Hoke, MD; Robert Koppel, MD; Samuel S. Gidding, MD; Robert H. Beekman III, MD; Scott D. Grosse, PhD; on behalf of Section on Cardiology and Cardiac Surgery and Committee of Fetus and Newborn (joint with American Heart Association Congenital Heart Defects Committee of the Council on Cardiovascular Disease in the Young, Council on Cardiovascular Nursing, and Interdisciplinary Council on Quality of Care and Outcomes Research)

ABSTRACT. *Background.* The purpose of this statement is to address the state of evidence on the routine use of pulse oximetry in newborns to detect critical congenital heart disease (CCHD).

Methods and Results. A writing group appointed by the American Heart Association and the American Academy of Pediatrics reviewed the available literature addressing current detection methods for CCHD, burden of missed and/or delayed diagnosis of CCHD, rationale of oximetry screening, and clinical studies of oximetry in otherwise asymptomatic newborns. MEDLINE database searches from 1966 to 2008 were done for English-language papers using the following search terms: congenital heart disease, pulse oximetry, physical examination, murmur, echocardiography, fetal echocardiography, and newborn screening. The reference lists of identified papers were also searched. Published abstracts from major pediatric scientific meetings in 2006 to 2008 were also reviewed. The American Heart Association classification of recommendations and levels of evidence for practice guidelines were used. In an analysis of pooled studies of oximetry assessment performed after 24 hours of life, the estimated sensitivity for detecting CCHD was 69.6%, and the positive predictive value was 47.0%; however, sensitivity varied dramatically among studies from 0% to 100%. False-positive screens that required further evaluation occurred in only 0.035% of infants screened after 24 hours.

Conclusions. Currently, CCHD is not detected in some newborns until after their hospital discharge, which results in significant morbidity and occasional mortality. Furthermore, routine pulse oximetry performed on asymptomatic newborns after 24 hours of life, but before hospital discharge, may detect CCHD. Routine pulse oximetry performed after 24 hours in hospitals that have on-site pediatric cardiovascular services incurs very low cost and risk of harm. Future studies in larger populations and across a broad range of newborn delivery systems are needed to determine whether this practice should become standard of care in the routine assessment of the neonate. (8/09)
http://pediatrics.aappublications.org/content/124/2/823

THE ROLE OF THE PEDIATRICIAN IN PRIMARY PREVENTION OF OBESITY (CLINICAL REPORT)

Stephen R. Daniels, MD, PhD, FAAP; Sandra G. Hassink, MD, FAAP; and Committee on Nutrition

ABSTRACT. The adoption of healthful lifestyles by individuals and families can result in a reduction in many chronic diseases and conditions of which obesity is the most prevalent. Obesity prevention, in addition to treatment, is an important public health priority. This clinical report describes the rationale for pediatricians to be an integral part of the obesity-prevention effort. In addition, the 2012 Institute of Medicine report "Accelerating Progress in Obesity Prevention" includes health care providers as a crucial component of successful weight control. Research on obesity prevention in the pediatric care setting as well as evidence-informed practical approaches and targets for prevention are reviewed. Pediatricians should use a longitudinal, developmentally appropriate life-course approach to help identify children early on the path to obesity and base prevention efforts on family dynamics and reduction in high-risk dietary and activity behaviors. They should promote a diet free of sugar-sweetened beverages, of fewer foods with high caloric density, and of increased intake of fruits and vegetables. It is also important to promote a lifestyle with reduced sedentary behavior and with 60 minutes of daily moderate to vigorous physical activity. This report also identifies important gaps in evidence that need to be filled by future research. (6/15)
http://pediatrics.aappublications.org/content/136/1/e275

THE ROLE OF THE PEDIATRICIAN IN RURAL EMERGENCY MEDICAL SERVICES FOR CHILDREN

Committee on Pediatric Emergency Medicine

ABSTRACT. In rural America, pediatricians can play a key role in the development, implementation, and ongoing supervision of emergency medical services for children (EMSC). Pediatricians may represent the only source of pediatric expertise for a large region and are a vital resource for rural physicians (eg, general and family practice, emergency medicine) and other rural health care professionals (physician assistants, nurse practitioners, and emergency medical technicians), providing education about management and prevention of pediatric illness and injury; appropriate equipment for the acutely ill or injured child; and acute, chronic, and rehabilitative care. In addition to providing clinical expertise, the pediatrician may be involved in quality assurance, clinical protocol development, and advocacy, and may serve as a liaison between emergency medical services and other entities working with children (eg, school nurses, child care centers, athletic programs, and programs for children with special health care needs). (10/12, reaffirmed 9/15)
http://pediatrics.aappublications.org/content/130/5/978

ROLE OF THE PEDIATRICIAN IN YOUTH VIOLENCE PREVENTION

Committee on Injury, Violence, and Poison Prevention

ABSTRACT. Youth violence continues to be a serious threat to the health of children and adolescents in the United States. It is crucial that pediatricians clearly define their role and develop the appropriate skills to address this threat effectively. From a clinical perspective, pediatricians should become familiar with *Connected Kids: Safe, Strong, Secure,* the American Academy of Pediatrics' primary care violence prevention protocol. Using this material, practices can incorporate preventive education, screening for risk, and linkages to community-based counseling and treatment resources. As advocates, pediatricians may bring newly developed information regarding key risk factors such as exposure to firearms, teen dating violence, and bullying to the attention of local and national policy makers. This policy statement refines the developing role of pediatricians in youth violence prevention and emphasizes the importance of this issue in the strategic agenda of the American Academy of Pediatrics. (6/09, reaffirmed 4/19)
http://pediatrics.aappublications.org/content/124/1/393

ROLE OF THE SCHOOL NURSE IN PROVIDING SCHOOL HEALTH SERVICES

Council on School Health

ABSTRACT. The American Academy of Pediatrics recognizes the important role school nurses play in promoting the optimal biopsychosocial health and well-being of school-aged children in the school setting. Although the concept of a school nurse

has existed for more than a century, uniformity among states and school districts regarding the role of a registered professional nurse in schools and the laws governing it are lacking. By understanding the benefits, roles, and responsibilities of school nurses working as a team with the school physician, as well as their contributions to school-aged children, pediatricians can collaborate with, support, and promote school nurses in their own communities, thus improving the health, wellness, and safety of children and adolescents. (5/16)
http://pediatrics.aappublications.org/content/137/6/e20160852

ROLE OF THE SCHOOL PHYSICIAN

Council on School Health

ABSTRACT. The American Academy of Pediatrics recognizes the important role physicians play in promoting the optimal biopsychosocial well-being of children in the school setting. Although the concept of a school physician has existed for more than a century, uniformity among states and school districts regarding physicians in schools and the laws governing it are lacking. By understanding the roles and contributions physicians can make to schools, pediatricians can support and promote school physicians in their communities and improve health and safety for children. (12/12, reaffirmed 1/19)
http://pediatrics.aappublications.org/content/131/1/178

SAFE SLEEP AND SKIN-TO-SKIN CARE IN THE NEONATAL PERIOD FOR HEALTHY TERM NEWBORNS (CLINICAL REPORT)

Lori Feldman-Winter, MD, MPH, FAAP; Jay P. Goldsmith, MD, FAAP; Committee on Fetus and Newborn; and Task Force on Sudden Infant Death Syndrome

ABSTRACT. Skin-to-skin care (SSC) and rooming-in have become common practice in the newborn period for healthy newborns with the implementation of maternity care practices that support breastfeeding as delineated in the World Health Organization's "Ten Steps to Successful Breastfeeding." SSC and rooming-in are supported by evidence that indicates that the implementation of these practices increases overall and exclusive breastfeeding, safer and healthier transitions, and improved maternal-infant bonding. In some cases, however, the practice of SSC and rooming-in may pose safety concerns, particularly with regard to sleep. There have been several recent case reports and case series of severe and sudden unexpected postnatal collapse in the neonatal period among otherwise healthy newborns and near fatal or fatal events related to sleep, suffocation, and falls from adult hospital beds. Although these are largely case reports, there are potential dangers of unobserved SSC immediately after birth and throughout the postpartum hospital period as well as with unobserved rooming-in for at-risk situations. Moreover, behaviors that are modeled in the hospital after birth, such as sleep position, are likely to influence sleeping practices after discharge. Hospitals and birthing centers have found it difficult to develop policies that will allow SSC and rooming-in to continue in a safe manner. This clinical report is intended for birthing centers and delivery hospitals caring for healthy newborns to assist in the establishment of appropriate SSC and safe sleep policies. (8/16)
http://pediatrics.aappublications.org/content/138/3/e20161889

SAFE TRANSPORTATION OF PRETERM AND LOW BIRTH WEIGHT INFANTS AT HOSPITAL DISCHARGE (CLINICAL REPORT)

Marilyn J. Bull, MD; William A. Engle, MD; Committee on Injury, Violence, and Poison Prevention; and Committee on Fetus and Newborn

ABSTRACT. Safe transportation of preterm and low birth weight infants requires special considerations. Both physiologic immaturity and low birth weight must be taken into account to properly position such infants. This clinical report provides guidelines for pediatricians and other caregivers who counsel parents of preterm and low birth weight infants about car safety seats. (4/09, reaffirmed 8/13, 6/18)
http://pediatrics.aappublications.org/content/123/5/1424

SCHOOL BUS TRANSPORTATION OF CHILDREN WITH SPECIAL HEALTH CARE NEEDS

Joseph O'Neil, MD, MPH, FAAP; Benjamin D. Hoffman, MD, FAAP; and Council on Injury, Violence, and Poison Prevention

ABSTRACT. School systems are responsible for ensuring that children with special needs are safely transported on all forms of federally approved transportation provided by the school system. A plan to provide the most current and proper support to children with special transportation needs should be developed by the Individualized Education Program team, including the parent, school transportation director, and school nurse, in conjunction with physician orders and recommendations. With this statement, we provide current guidance for the protection of child passengers with specific health care needs. Guidance that applies to general school transportation should be followed, inclusive of staff training, provision of nurses or aides if needed, and establishment of a written emergency evacuation plan as well as a comprehensive infection control program. Researchers provide the basis for recommendations concerning occupant securement for children in wheelchairs and children with other special needs who are transported on a school bus. Pediatricians can help their patients by being aware of guidance for restraint systems for children with special needs and by remaining informed of new resources. Pediatricians can also play an important role at the state and local level in the development of school bus specifications. (4/18)
http://pediatrics.aappublications.org/content/141/5/e20180513

SCHOOL READINESS (TECHNICAL REPORT)

P. Gail Williams, MD, FAAP; Marc Alan Lerner, MD, FAAP; Council on Early Childhood; and Council on School Health

ABSTRACT. School readiness includes the readiness of the individual child, the school's readiness for children, and the ability of the family and community to support optimal early child development. It is the responsibility of schools to meet the needs of all children at all levels of readiness. Children's readiness for kindergarten should become an outcome measure for a coordinated system of community-based programs and supports for the healthy development of young children. Our rapidly expanding insights into early brain and child development have revealed that modifiable factors in a child's early experience can greatly affect that child's health and learning trajectories. Many children in the United States enter kindergarten with limitations in their social, emotional, cognitive, and physical development that might have been significantly diminished or eliminated through early identification and attention to child and family needs. A strong correlation between social-emotional development and school and life success, combined with alarming rates of preschool expulsion, point toward the urgency of leveraging opportunities to support social-emotional development and address behavioral concerns early. Pediatric primary care providers have access to the youngest children and their families. Pediatricians can promote and use community supports, such as home visiting programs, quality early care and education programs, family support programs and resources, early intervention services, children's museums, and libraries, which are important for addressing school readiness and are too often underused by populations who can benefit most from them. When these are not available, pediatricians can support the development of such resources. The American Academy of Pediatrics affords pediatricians many opportunities to improve the physical, social-emotional, and educational health of young children, in conjunction with other advocacy groups. This technical report provides an updated version of the previous iteration from the American Academy of Pediatrics published in 2008. (7/19)

See full text on page 1153.

https://pediatrics.aappublications.org/content/144/2/e20191766

SCHOOL START TIMES FOR ADOLESCENTS

Adolescent Sleep Working Group, Committee on Adolescence, and Council on School Health

ABSTRACT. The American Academy of Pediatrics recognizes insufficient sleep in adolescents as an important public health issue that significantly affects the health and safety, as well as the academic success, of our nation's middle and high school students. Although a number of factors, including biological changes in sleep associated with puberty, lifestyle choices, and academic demands, negatively affect middle and high school students' ability to obtain sufficient sleep, the evidence strongly implicates earlier school start times (ie, before 8:30 AM) as a key modifiable contributor to insufficient sleep, as well as circadian rhythm disruption, in this population. Furthermore, a substantial body of research has now demonstrated that delaying school start times is an effective countermeasure to chronic sleep loss and has a wide range of potential benefits to students with regard to physical and mental health, safety, and academic achievement. The American Academy of Pediatrics strongly supports the efforts of school districts to optimize sleep in students and urges high schools and middle schools to aim for start times that allow students the opportunity to achieve optimal levels of sleep (8.5–9.5 hours) and to improve physical (eg, reduced obesity risk) and mental (eg, lower rates of depression) health, safety (eg, drowsy driving crashes), academic performance, and quality of life. (8/14)

http://pediatrics.aappublications.org/content/134/3/642

SCHOOL TRANSPORTATION SAFETY

Committee on Injury, Violence, and Poison Prevention and Council on School Health

ABSTRACT. This policy statement replaces the previous version published in 1996. It provides new information, studies, regulations, and recommendations related to the safe transportation of children to and from school and school-related activities. Pediatricians can play an important role at the patient/family, community, state, and national levels as child advocates and consultants to schools and early education programs about transportation safety. (7/07, reaffirmed 10/11)

http://pediatrics.aappublications.org/content/120/1/213

SCHOOL-AGED CHILDREN WHO ARE NOT PROGRESSING ACADEMICALLY: CONSIDERATIONS FOR PEDIATRICIANS (CLINICAL REPORT)

Celiane Rey-Casserly, PhD; Laura McGuinn, MD, FAAP; Arthur Lavin, MD, FAAP; Committee on Psychosocial Aspects of Child and Family Health; Section on Developmental and Behavioral Pediatrics

ABSTRACT. Pediatricians and other pediatric primary care providers may be consulted when families have concerns that their child is not making expected progress in school. Pediatricians care not only for an increasingly diverse population of children who may have behavioral, psychological, and learning difficulties but also for increasing numbers of children with complex and chronic medical problems that can affect the development of the central nervous system and can present with learning and academic concerns. In many instances, pediatric providers require additional information about the nature of cognitive, psychosocial, and educational difficulties that affect their school-aged patients. Our purpose for this report is to describe the current state of the science regarding educational achievement to inform pediatricians' decisions regarding further evaluation of a child's challenges. In this report, we review commonly available options for psychological evaluation and/or treatment, medical referrals, and/or recommendations for referral for eligibility determinations at school and review strategies for collaborating with families, schools, and specialists to best serve children and families. (9/19)

See full text on page 1171.

https://pediatrics.aappublications.org/content/144/4/e20192520

SCHOOL-BASED HEALTH CENTERS AND PEDIATRIC PRACTICE

Council on School Health

ABSTRACT. School-based health centers (SBHCs) have become an important method of health care delivery for the youth of our nation. Although they only represent 1 aspect of a coordinated school health program approach, SBHCs have provided access to health care services for youth confronted with age, financial, cultural, and geographic barriers. A fundamental principle of SBHCs is to create an environment of service coordination and collaboration that addresses the health needs and well-being of youth with health disparities or poor access to health care services. Some pediatricians have concerns that these centers are in conflict with the primary care provider's medical home. This policy provides an overview of SBHCs and some of their documented benefits, addresses the issue of potential conflict with the medical home, and provides recommendations that support the integration and coordination of SBHCs and the pediatric medical home practice. (1/12, reaffirmed 6/17)

http://pediatrics.aappublications.org/content/129/2/387

SCOPE OF HEALTH CARE BENEFITS FOR CHILDREN FROM BIRTH THROUGH AGE 26

Committee on Child Health Financing

ABSTRACT. The optimal health of all children is best achieved with access to appropriate and comprehensive health care benefits. This policy statement outlines and defines the recommended set of health insurance benefits for children through age 26. The American Academy of Pediatrics developed a set of recommendations concerning preventive care services for children, adolescents, and young adults. These recommendations are compiled in the publication *Bright Futures: Guidelines for Health Supervision of Infants, Children, and Adolescents*, third edition. The Bright Futures recommendations were referenced as a standard for access and design of age-appropriate health insurance benefits for infants, children, adolescents, and young adults in the Patient Protection and Affordable Care Act of 2010 (Pub L No. 114–148). (12/11)

http://pediatrics.aappublications.org/content/129/1/185

SCOPE OF PRACTICE ISSUES IN THE DELIVERY OF PEDIATRIC HEALTH CARE

Committee on Pediatric Workforce

ABSTRACT. The American Academy of Pediatrics (AAP) believes that optimal pediatric health care depends on a team-based approach with supervision by a physician leader, preferably a pediatrician. The pediatrician, here defined to include not only pediatric generalists but all pediatric medical subspecialists, all surgical specialists, and internal medicine/pediatric physicians, is uniquely qualified to manage, coordinate, and supervise the entire spectrum of pediatric care, from diagnosis through all stages of treatment, in all practice settings. The AAP recognizes the valuable contributions of nonphysician clinicians, including nurse practitioners and physician assistants, in delivering optimal pediatric care. However, the expansion of the scope of practice of nonphysician pediatric clinicians raises critical public policy and child health advocacy concerns. Pediatricians should

serve as advocates for optimal pediatric care in state legislatures, public policy forums, and the media and should pursue opportunities to resolve scope of practice conflicts outside state legislatures. The AAP affirms the importance of appropriate documentation and standards in pediatric education, training, skills, clinical competencies, examination, regulation, and patient care to ensure safety and quality health care for all infants, children, adolescents, and young adults. (5/13, reaffirmed 10/15)
http://pediatrics.aappublications.org/content/131/6/1211

SCREENING EXAMINATION OF PREMATURE INFANTS FOR RETINOPATHY OF PREMATURITY

Walter M. Fierson, MD, FAAP, and Section on Ophthalmology (joint with American Academy of Ophthalmology, American Association for Pediatric Ophthalmology and Strabismus, and American Association of Certified Orthoptists)

ABSTRACT. This policy statement revises a previous statement on screening of preterm infants for retinopathy of prematurity (ROP) that was published in 2013. ROP is a pathologic process that occurs in immature retinal tissue and can progress to a tractional retinal detachment, which may then result in visual loss or blindness. For more than 3 decades, treatment of severe ROP that markedly decreases the incidence of this poor visual outcome has been available. However, severe, treatment-requiring ROP must be diagnosed in a timely fashion to be treated effectively. The sequential nature of ROP requires that infants who are at-risk and preterm be examined at proper times and intervals to detect the changes of ROP before they become destructive. This statement presents the attributes of an effective program to detect and treat ROP, including the timing of initial and follow-up examinations. (11/18)
http://pediatrics.aappublications.org/content/142/6/e20183061

SCREENING FOR NONVIRAL SEXUALLY TRANSMITTED INFECTIONS IN ADOLESCENTS AND YOUNG ADULTS

Committee on Adolescence (joint with Society for Adolescent Health and Medicine)

ABSTRACT. Prevalence rates of many sexually transmitted infections (STIs) are highest among adolescents. If nonviral STIs are detected early, they can be treated, transmission to others can be eliminated, and sequelae can be averted. The US Preventive Services Task Force and the Centers for Disease Control and Prevention have published chlamydia, gonorrhea, and syphilis screening guidelines that recommend screening those at risk on the basis of epidemiologic and clinical outcomes data. This policy statement specifically focuses on these curable, nonviral STIs and reviews the evidence for nonviral STI screening in adolescents, communicates the value of screening, and outlines recommendations for routine nonviral STI screening of adolescents. (6/14)
http://pediatrics.aappublications.org/content/134/1/e302

SCREENING FOR RETINOPATHY IN THE PEDIATRIC PATIENT WITH TYPE 1 DIABETES MELLITUS (CLINICAL REPORT)

Gregg T. Lueder, MD; Janet Silverstein, MD; Section on Ophthalmology; and Section on Endocrinology (joint with American Association for Pediatric Ophthalmology and Strabismus)

ABSTRACT. Diabetic retinopathy (DR) is the leading cause of blindness in young adults in the United States. Early identification and treatment of DR can decrease the risk of vision loss in affected patients. This clinical report reviews the risk factors for the development of DR and screening guidance for pediatric patients with type 1 diabetes mellitus. (7/05, reaffirmed 1/09, 7/14)
http://pediatrics.aappublications.org/content/116/1/270

SELECTING APPROPRIATE TOYS FOR YOUNG CHILDREN IN THE DIGITAL ERA (CLINICAL REPORT)

Aleeya Healey, MD, FAAP; Alan Mendelsohn, MD, FAAP; and Council on Early Childhood

ABSTRACT. Play is essential to optimal child development because it contributes to the cognitive, physical, social, and emotional well-being of children and youth. It also offers an ideal and significant opportunity for parents and other caregivers to engage fully with children using toys as an instrument of play and interaction. The evolution of societal perceptions of toys from children's playthings to critical facilitators of early brain and child development has challenged caregivers in deciding which toys are most appropriate for their children. This clinical report strives to provide pediatric health care providers with evidence-based information that can be used to support caregivers as they choose toys for their children. The report highlights the broad definition of a toy; consideration of potential benefits and possible harmful effects of toy choices on child development; and the promotion of positive caregiving and development when toys are used to engage caregivers in play-based interactions with their children that are rich in language, pretending, problem-solving, and creativity. The report aims to address the evolving replacement of more traditional toys with digital media–based virtual "toys" and the lack of evidence for similar benefits in child development. Furthermore, this report briefly addresses the role of toys in advertising and/or incentive programs and aims to bring awareness regarding safety and health hazards associated with toy availability and accessibility in public settings, including some health care settings. (12/18)

See full text on page 1191.

https://pediatrics.aappublications.org/content/143/1/e20183348

SENSORY INTEGRATION THERAPIES FOR CHILDREN WITH DEVELOPMENTAL AND BEHAVIORAL DISORDERS

Section on Complementary and Integrative Medicine and Council on Children With Disabilities

ABSTRACT. Sensory-based therapies are increasingly used by occupational therapists and sometimes by other types of therapists in treatment of children with developmental and behavioral disorders. Sensory-based therapies involve activities that are believed to organize the sensory system by providing vestibular, proprioceptive, auditory, and tactile inputs. Brushes, swings, balls, and other specially designed therapeutic or recreational equipment are used to provide these inputs. However, it is unclear whether children who present with sensory-based problems have an actual "disorder" of the sensory pathways of the brain or whether these deficits are characteristics associated with other developmental and behavioral disorders. Because there is no universally accepted framework for diagnosis, sensory processing disorder generally should not be diagnosed. Other developmental and behavioral disorders must always be considered, and a thorough evaluation should be completed. Difficulty tolerating or processing sensory information is a characteristic that may be seen in many developmental behavioral disorders, including autism spectrum disorders, attention-deficit/hyperactivity disorder, developmental coordination disorders, and childhood anxiety disorders.

Occupational therapy with the use of sensory-based therapies may be acceptable as one of the components of a comprehensive treatment plan. However, parents should be informed that the amount of research regarding the effectiveness of sensory integration therapy is limited and inconclusive. Important roles for pediatricians and other clinicians may include discussing these limitations with parents, talking with families about a trial period of sensory integration therapy, and teaching families how to evaluate the effectiveness of a therapy. (5/12)
http://pediatrics.aappublications.org/content/129/6/1186

SEXUAL AND REPRODUCTIVE HEALTH CARE SERVICES IN THE PEDIATRIC SETTING (CLINICAL REPORT)

Arik V. Marcell, MD, MPH; Gale R. Burstein, MD, MPH; and Committee on Adolescence

ABSTRACT. Pediatricians are an important source of health care for adolescents and young adults and can play a significant role in addressing their patients' sexual and reproductive health needs, including preventing unintended pregnancies and sexually transmitted infections (STIs), including HIV, and promoting healthy relationships. STIs, HIV, and unintended pregnancy are all preventable health outcomes with potentially serious permanent sequelae; the highest rates of STIs, HIV, and unintended pregnancy are reported among adolescents and young adults. Office visits present opportunities to provide comprehensive education and health care services to adolescents and young adults to prevent STIs, HIV, and unintended pregnancies. The American Academy of Pediatrics, other professional medical organizations, and the government have guidelines and recommendations regarding the provision of sexual and reproductive health information and services. However, despite these recommendations, recent studies have revealed that there is substantial room for improvement in actually delivering the recommended services. The purpose of this clinical report is to assist pediatricians to operationalize the provision of various aspects of sexual and reproductive health care into their practices and to provide guidance on overcoming barriers to providing this care routinely while maximizing opportunities for confidential health services delivery in their offices. (10/17)

http://pediatrics.aappublications.org/content/140/5/e20172858

SEXUALITY EDUCATION FOR CHILDREN AND ADOLESCENTS (CLINICAL REPORT)

Cora C. Breuner, MD, MPH, FAAP; Gerri Mattson, MD, MSPH, FAAP; Committee on Adolescence; and Committee on Psychosocial Aspects of Child and Family Health

ABSTRACT. The purpose of this clinical report is to provide pediatricians updated research on evidence-based sexual and reproductive health education conducted since the original clinical report on the subject was published by the American Academy of Pediatrics in 2001. Sexuality education is defined as teaching about human sexuality, including intimate relationships, human sexual anatomy, sexual reproduction, sexually transmitted infections, sexual activity, sexual orientation, gender identity, abstinence, contraception, and reproductive rights and responsibilities. Developmentally appropriate and evidence-based education about human sexuality and sexual reproduction over time provided by pediatricians, schools, other professionals, and parents is important to help children and adolescents make informed, positive, and safe choices about healthy relationships, responsible sexual activity, and their reproductive health. Sexuality education has been shown to help to prevent and reduce the risks of adolescent pregnancy, HIV, and sexually transmitted infections for children and adolescents with and without chronic health conditions and disabilities in the United States. (7/16)

http://pediatrics.aappublications.org/content/138/2/e20161348

SEXUALITY OF CHILDREN AND ADOLESCENTS WITH DEVELOPMENTAL DISABILITIES (CLINICAL REPORT)

Nancy A. Murphy, MD; Ellen Roy Elias, MD; for Council on Children With Disabilities

ABSTRACT. Children and adolescents with developmental disabilities, like all children, are sexual persons. However, attention to their complex medical and functional issues often consumes time that might otherwise be invested in addressing the anatomic, physiologic, emotional, and social aspects of their developing sexuality. This report discusses issues of puberty, contraception, psychosexual development, sexual abuse, and sexuality education specific to children and adolescents with disabilities and their families. Pediatricians, in the context of the medical home, are encouraged to discuss issues of sexuality on a regular basis, ensure the privacy of each child and adolescent, promote self-care and social independence among persons with disabilities, advocate for appropriate sexuality education, and provide ongoing education for children and adolescents with developmental disabilities and their families. (7/06, reaffirmed 12/09, 7/13, 11/17)

http://pediatrics.aappublications.org/content/118/1/398

SHARED DECISION-MAKING AND CHILDREN WITH DISABILITIES: PATHWAYS TO CONSENSUS (CLINICAL REPORT)

Richard C. Adams, MD, FAAP; Susan E. Levy, MD, MPH, FAAP; and Council on Children With Disabilities

ABSTRACT. Shared decision-making (SDM) promotes family and clinician collaboration, with ultimate goals of improved health and satisfaction. This clinical report provides a basis for a systematic approach to the implementation of SDM by clinicians for children with disabilities. Often in the discussion of treatment plans, there are gaps between the child's/family's values, priorities, and understanding of perceived "best choices" and those of the clinician. When conducted well, SDM affords an appropriate balance incorporating voices of all stakeholders, ultimately supporting both the child/family and clinician. With increasing knowledge of and functional use of SDM skills, the clinician will become an effective partner in the decision-making process with families, providing family-centered care. The outcome of the process will support the beneficence of the physician, the authority of the family, and the autonomy and well-being of the child. (5/17)

http://pediatrics.aappublications.org/content/139/6/e20170956

SHOPPING CART–RELATED INJURIES TO CHILDREN

Committee on Injury, Violence, and Poison Prevention

ABSTRACT. Shopping cart–related injuries to children are common and can result in severe injury or even death. Most injuries result from falls from carts or cart tip-overs, and injuries to the head and neck represent three fourths of cases. The current US standard for shopping carts should be revised to include clear and effective performance criteria to prevent falls from carts and cart tip-overs. Pediatricians have an important role as educators, researchers, and advocates to promote the prevention of these injuries. (8/06, reaffirmed 4/09, 8/13)

http://pediatrics.aappublications.org/content/118/2/825

SHOPPING CART–RELATED INJURIES TO CHILDREN (TECHNICAL REPORT)

Gary A. Smith, MD, DrPH, for Committee on Injury, Violence, and Poison Prevention

ABSTRACT. An estimated 24 200 children younger than 15 years, 20 700 (85%) of whom were younger than 5 years, were treated in US hospital emergency departments in 2005 for shopping cart–related injuries. Approximately 4% of shopping cart–related injuries to children younger than 15 years require admission to the hospital. Injuries to the head and neck represent three fourths of all injuries. Fractures account for 45% of all hospitalizations. Deaths have occurred from falls from shopping carts and cart tip-overs. Falls are the most common mechanism of injury and account for more than half of injuries associated with shopping carts. Cart tip-overs are the second most common mechanism, responsible for up to one fourth of injuries and almost 40% of shopping cart–related injuries among children younger than 2 years. Public-awareness initiatives, education programs, and parental supervision, although important, are not enough to prevent these injuries effectively. European Standard EN 1929-1:1998 and joint Australian/New Zealand Standard

AS/NZS 3847.1:1999 specify requirements for the construction, performance, testing, and safety of shopping carts and have been implemented as national standards in 21 countries. A US performance standard for shopping carts (ASTM [American Society for Testing and Materials] F2372-04) was established in July 2004; however, it does not adequately address falls and cart tip-overs, which are the leading mechanisms of shopping cart–related injuries to children. The current US standard for shopping carts should be revised to include clear and effective performance criteria for shopping cart child-restraint systems and cart stability to prevent falls from carts and cart tip-overs. This is imperative to decrease the number and severity of shopping cart–related injuries to children. Recommendations from the American Academy of Pediatrics regarding prevention of shopping cart–related injuries are included in the accompanying policy statement. (8/06, reaffirmed 4/09, 8/13)
http://pediatrics.aappublications.org/content/118/2/e540

SIDS AND OTHER SLEEP-RELATED INFANT DEATHS: EVIDENCE BASE FOR 2016 UPDATED RECOMMENDATIONS FOR A SAFE INFANT SLEEPING ENVIRONMENT (TECHNICAL REPORT)

Rachel Y. Moon, MD, FAAP, and Task Force on Sudden Infant Death Syndrome

ABSTRACT. Approximately 3500 infants die annually in the United States from sleep-related infant deaths, including sudden infant death syndrome (SIDS), ill-defined deaths, and accidental suffocation and strangulation in bed. After an initial decrease in the 1990s, the overall sleep-related infant death rate has not declined in more recent years. Many of the modifiable and nonmodifiable risk factors for SIDS and other sleep-related infant deaths are strikingly similar. The American Academy of Pediatrics recommends a safe sleep environment that can reduce the risk of all sleep-related infant deaths. Recommendations for a safe sleep environment include supine positioning, use of a firm sleep surface, room-sharing without bed-sharing, and avoidance of soft bedding and overheating. Additional recommendations for SIDS risk reduction include avoidance of exposure to smoke, alcohol, and illicit drugs; breastfeeding; routine immunization; and use of a pacifier. New evidence and rationale for recommendations are presented for skin-to-skin care for newborn infants, bedside and in-bed sleepers, sleeping on couches/armchairs and in sitting devices, and use of soft bedding after 4 months of age. In addition, expanded recommendations for infant sleep location are included. The recommendations and strength of evidence for each recommendation are published in the accompanying policy statement, "SIDS and Other Sleep-Related Infant Deaths: Updated 2016 Recommendations for a Safe Infant Sleeping Environment," which is included in this issue. (10/16)
http://pediatrics.aappublications.org/content/138/5/e20162940

SIDS AND OTHER SLEEP-RELATED INFANT DEATHS: UPDATED 2016 RECOMMENDATIONS FOR A SAFE INFANT SLEEPING ENVIRONMENT

Task Force on Sudden Infant Death Syndrome

ABSTRACT. Approximately 3500 infants die annually in the United States from sleep-related infant deaths, including sudden infant death syndrome (SIDS; International Classification of Diseases, 10th Revision [ICD-10], R95), ill-defined deaths (ICD-10 R99), and accidental suffocation and strangulation in bed (ICD-10 W75). After an initial decrease in the 1990s, the overall death rate attributable to sleep-related infant deaths has not declined in more recent years. Many of the modifiable and nonmodifiable risk factors for SIDS and other sleep-related infant deaths are strikingly similar. The American Academy of Pediatrics recommends a safe sleep environment that can reduce the risk of all sleep-related infant deaths. Recommendations for a safe sleep environment include supine positioning, the use of a firm sleep surface, room-sharing without bed-sharing, and the avoidance of soft bedding and overheating. Additional recommendations for SIDS reduction include the avoidance of exposure to smoke, alcohol, and illicit drugs; breastfeeding; routine immunization; and use of a pacifier. New evidence is presented for skin-to-skin care for newborn infants, use of bedside and in-bed sleepers, sleeping on couches/armchairs and in sitting devices, and use of soft bedding after 4 months of age. The recommendations and strength of evidence for each recommendation are included in this policy statement. The rationale for these recommendations is discussed in detail in the accompanying technical report (www.pediatrics.org/cgi/doi/10.1542/peds.2016-2940). (10/16)
http://pediatrics.aappublications.org/content/138/5/e20162938

SKATEBOARD AND SCOOTER INJURIES

Committee on Injury, Violence, and Poison Prevention

ABSTRACT. Skateboard-related injuries account for an estimated 50 000 emergency department visits and 1500 hospitalizations among children and adolescents in the United States each year. Nonpowered scooter-related injuries accounted for an estimated 9400 emergency department visits between January and August 2000, and 90% of these patients were children younger than 15 years. Many such injuries can be avoided if children and youth do not ride in traffic, if proper protective gear is worn, and if, in the absence of close adult supervision, skateboards and scooters are not used by children younger than 10 and 8 years, respectively. (3/02, reaffirmed 5/05, 10/08, 10/13)
http://pediatrics.aappublications.org/content/109/3/542

SKIN-TO-SKIN CARE FOR TERM AND PRETERM INFANTS IN THE NEONATAL ICU (CLINICAL REPORT)

Jill Baley, MD, and Committee on Fetus and Newborn

ABSTRACT. "Kangaroo mother care" was first described as an alternative method of caring for low birth weight infants in resource-limited countries, where neonatal mortality and infection rates are high because of overcrowded nurseries, inadequate staffing, and lack of equipment. Intermittent skin-to-skin care (SSC), a modified version of kangaroo mother care, is now being offered in resource-rich countries to infants needing neonatal intensive care, including those who require ventilator support or are extremely premature. SSC significantly improves milk production by the mother and is associated with a longer duration of breastfeeding. Increased parent satisfaction, better sleep organization, a longer duration of quiet sleep, and decreased pain perception during procedures have also been reported in association with SSC. Despite apparent physiologic stability during SSC, it is prudent that infants in the NICU have continuous cardiovascular monitoring and that care be taken to verify correct head positioning for airway patency as well as the stability of the endotracheal tube, arterial and venous access devices, and other life support equipment. (8/15)
http://pediatrics.aappublications.org/content/136/3/596

SNACKS, SWEETENED BEVERAGES, ADDED SUGARS, AND SCHOOLS

Council on School Health and Committee on Nutrition

ABSTRACT. Concern over childhood obesity has generated a decade-long reformation of school nutrition policies. Food is available in school in 3 venues: federally sponsored school meal programs; items sold in competition to school meals, such as a la carte, vending machines, and school stores; and foods available in myriad informal settings, including packed meals and snacks, bake sales, fundraisers, sports booster sales, in-class parties, or other school celebrations. High-energy, low-nutrient beverages, in particular, contribute substantial calories, but little nutrient content, to a student's diet. In 2004, the American Academy of Pediatrics recommended that sweetened drinks be replaced in school by water, white and flavored milks, or 100% fruit and vegetable beverages. Since then, school nutrition has undergone a significant transformation. Federal, state, and local regulations and policies, along with alternative products developed by industry, have helped decrease the availability of nutrient-poor foods and beverages in school. However, regular access to foods of high energy and low quality remains a school issue, much of it attributable to students, parents, and staff. Pediatricians, aligning with experts on child nutrition, are in a position to offer a perspective promoting nutrient-rich foods within calorie guidelines to improve those foods brought into or sold in schools. A positive emphasis on nutritional value, variety, appropriate portion, and encouragement for a steady improvement in quality will be a more effective approach for improving nutrition and health than simply advocating for the elimination of added sugars. (2/15)

http://pediatrics.aappublications.org/content/135/3/575

SNOWMOBILING HAZARDS

Committee on Injury and Poison Prevention

ABSTRACT. Snowmobiles continue to pose a significant risk to children younger than 15 years and adolescents and young adults 15 through 24 years of age. Head injuries remain the leading cause of mortality and serious morbidity, arising largely from snowmobilers colliding, falling, or overturning during operation. Children also were injured while being towed in a variety of conveyances by snowmobiles. No uniform code of state laws governs the use of snowmobiles by children and youth. Because evidence is lacking to support the effectiveness of operator safety certification and because many children and adolescents do not have the required strength and skills to operate a snowmobile safely, the recreational operation of snowmobiles by persons younger than 16 years is not recommended. Snowmobiles should not be used to tow persons on a tube, tire, sled, or saucer. Furthermore, a graduated licensing program is advised for snowmobilers 16 years and older. Both active and passive snowmobile injury prevention strategies are suggested, as well as recommendations for manufacturers to make safer equipment for snowmobilers of all ages. (11/00, reaffirmed 5/04, 1/07, 6/10)

http://pediatrics.aappublications.org/content/106/5/1142

SOCCER INJURIES IN CHILDREN AND ADOLESCENTS (CLINICAL REPORT)

Andrew Watson, MD, MS, FAAP; Jeffrey M. Mjaanes, MD, FAAP; Council on Sports Medicine and Fitness

ABSTRACT. Participation in youth soccer in the United States continues to increase steadily, with a greater percentage of preadolescent participants than perhaps any other youth sport. Despite the wide-ranging health benefits of participation in organized sports, injuries occur and represent a threat to the health and performance of young athletes. Youth soccer has a greater reported injury rate than many other contact sports, and recent studies suggest that injury rates are increasing. Large increases in the incidence of concussions in youth soccer have been reported, and anterior cruciate ligament injuries remain a significant problem in this sport, particularly among female athletes. Considerable new research has identified a number of modifiable risk factors for lower-extremity injuries and concussion, and several prevention programs have been identified to reduce the risk of injury. Rule enforcement and fair play also serve an important role in reducing the risk of injury among youth soccer participants. This report provides an updated review of the relevant literature as well as recommendations to promote the safe participation of children and adolescents in soccer. (10/19)

See full text on page 1203.

https://pediatrics.aappublications.org/content/144/5/e20192759

SPECIAL REQUIREMENTS OF ELECTRONIC HEALTH RECORD SYSTEMS IN PEDIATRICS (CLINICAL REPORT)

S. Andrew Spooner, MD, MS, and Council on Clinical Information Technology

ABSTRACT. Some functions of an electronic health record system are much more important in providing pediatric care than in adult care. Pediatricians commonly complain about the absence of these "pediatric functions" when they are not available in electronic health record systems. To stimulate electronic health record system vendors to recognize and incorporate pediatric functionality into pediatric electronic health record systems, this clinical report reviews the major functions of importance to child health care providers. Also reviewed are important but less critical functions, any of which might be of major importance in a particular clinical context. The major areas described here are immunization management, growth tracking, medication dosing, data norms, and privacy in special pediatric populations. The American Academy of Pediatrics believes that if the functions described in this document are supported in all electronic health record systems, these systems will be more useful for patients of all ages. (3/07, reaffirmed 5/12, 5/16)

http://pediatrics.aappublications.org/content/119/3/631

SPECTRUM OF NONINFECTIOUS HEALTH EFFECTS FROM MOLDS

Committee on Environmental Health

ABSTRACT. Molds are eukaryotic (possessing a true nucleus) nonphotosynthetic organisms that flourish both indoors and outdoors. For humans, the link between mold exposure and asthma exacerbations, allergic rhinitis, infections, and toxicities from ingestion of mycotoxin-contaminated foods are well known. However, the cause-and-effect relationship between inhalational exposure to mold and other untoward health effects (eg, acute idiopathic pulmonary hemorrhage in infants and other illnesses and health complaints) requires additional investigation. Pediatricians play an important role in the education of families about mold, its adverse health effects, exposure prevention, and remediation procedures. (12/06, reaffirmed 9/16)

http://pediatrics.aappublications.org/content/118/6/2582

SPECTRUM OF NONINFECTIOUS HEALTH EFFECTS FROM MOLDS (TECHNICAL REPORT)

Lynnette J. Mazur, MD, MPH; Janice Kim, MD, PhD, MPH; and Committee on Environmental Health

ABSTRACT. Molds are multicellular fungi that are ubiquitous in outdoor and indoor environments. For humans, they are both beneficial (for the production of antimicrobial agents, chemotherapeutic agents, and vitamins) and detrimental. Exposure to mold can occur through inhalation, ingestion, and touching moldy surfaces. Adverse health effects may occur through allergic, infectious, irritant, or toxic processes. The cause-and-effect relationship between mold exposure and allergic and infectious illnesses is well known. Exposures to toxins via the gastrointestinal tract also are well described. However, the cause-and-effect relationship between inhalational exposure to mold toxins and other untoward health effects (eg, acute idiopathic pulmonary hemorrhage in infants and other illnesses and health complaints) is controversial and requires additional investigation. In this report we examine evidence of fungal-related illnesses and the unique aspects of mold exposure to children. Mold-remediation procedures are also discussed. (12/06, reaffirmed 9/16)

http://pediatrics.aappublications.org/content/118/6/e1909

SPORT-RELATED CONCUSSION IN CHILDREN AND ADOLESCENTS (CLINICAL REPORT)

Mark E. Halstead, MD, FAAP; Kevin D. Walter, MD, FAAP; Kody Moffatt, MD, FAAP; and Council on Sports Medicine and Fitness

ABSTRACT. Sport-related concussion is an important topic in nearly all sports and at all levels of sport for children and adolescents. Concussion knowledge and approaches to management have progressed since the American Academy of Pediatrics published its first clinical report on the subject in 2010. Concussion's definition, signs, and symptoms must be understood to diagnose it and rule out more severe intracranial injury. Pediatric health care providers should have a good understanding of diagnostic evaluation and initial management strategies. Effective management can aid recovery and potentially reduce the risk of long-term symptoms and complications. Because concussion symptoms often interfere with school, social life, family relationships, and athletics, a concussion may affect the emotional well-being of the injured athlete. Because every concussion has its own unique spectrum and severity of symptoms, individualized management is appropriate. The reduction, not necessarily elimination, of physical and cognitive activity is the mainstay of treatment. A full return to activity and/or sport is accomplished by using a stepwise program while evaluating for a return of symptoms. An understanding of prolonged symptoms and complications will help the pediatric health care provider know when to refer to a specialist. Additional research is needed in nearly all aspects of concussion in the young athlete. This report provides education on the current state of sport-related concussion knowledge, diagnosis, and management in children and adolescents. (11/18)

http://pediatrics.aappublications.org/content/142/6/e20183074

SPORTS DRINKS AND ENERGY DRINKS FOR CHILDREN AND ADOLESCENTS: ARE THEY APPROPRIATE? (CLINICAL REPORT)

Committee on Nutrition and Council on Sports Medicine and Fitness

ABSTRACT. Sports and energy drinks are being marketed to children and adolescents for a wide variety of inappropriate uses. Sports drinks and energy drinks are significantly different products, and the terms should not be used interchangeably. The primary objectives of this clinical report are to define the ingredients of sports and energy drinks, categorize the similarities and differences between the products, and discuss misuses and abuses. Secondary objectives are to encourage screening during annual physical examinations for sports and energy drink use, to understand the reasons why youth consumption is widespread, and to improve education aimed at decreasing or eliminating the inappropriate use of these beverages by children and adolescents. Rigorous review and analysis of the literature reveal that caffeine and other stimulant substances contained in energy drinks have no place in the diet of children and adolescents. Furthermore, frequent or excessive intake of caloric sports drinks can substantially increase the risk for overweight or obesity in children and adolescents. Discussion regarding the appropriate use of sports drinks in the youth athlete who participates regularly in endurance or high-intensity sports and vigorous physical activity is beyond the scope of this report. (5/11, reaffirmed 7/17)

http://pediatrics.aappublications.org/content/127/6/1182

SPORTS SPECIALIZATION AND INTENSIVE TRAINING IN YOUNG ATHLETES (CLINICAL REPORT)

Joel S. Brenner, MD, MPH, FAAP, and Council on Sports Medicine and Fitness

ABSTRACT. Sports specialization is becoming the norm in youth sports for a variety of reasons. When sports specialization occurs too early, detrimental effects may occur, both physically and psychologically. If the timing is correct and sports specialization is performed under the correct conditions, the athlete may be successful in reaching specific goals. Young athletes who train intensively, whether specialized or not, can also be at risk of adverse effects on the mind and body. The purpose of this clinical report is to assist pediatricians in counseling their young athlete patients and their parents regarding sports specialization and intensive training. This report supports the American Academy of Pediatrics clinical report "Overuse Injuries, Overtraining, and Burnout in Child and Adolescent Athletes." (8/16)

http://pediatrics.aappublications.org/content/138/3/e20162148

STANDARD TERMINOLOGY FOR FETAL, INFANT, AND PERINATAL DEATHS (CLINICAL REPORT)

Wanda D. Barfield, MD, MPH, FAAP, and Committee on Fetus and Newborn

ABSTRACT. Accurately defining and reporting perinatal deaths (ie, fetal and infant deaths) is a critical first step in understanding the magnitude and causes of these important events. In addition to obstetric health care providers, neonatologists and pediatricians should have easy access to current and updated resources that clearly provide US definitions and reporting requirements for live births, fetal deaths, and infant deaths. Correct identification of these vital events will improve local, state, and national data so that these deaths can be better addressed and prevented. (4/16)

http://pediatrics.aappublications.org/content/137/5/e20160551

STANDARDIZATION OF INPATIENT HANDOFF COMMUNICATION (CLINICAL REPORT)

Jennifer A. Jewell, MD, FAAP, and Committee on Hospital Care

ABSTRACT. Handoff communication is identified as an integral part of hospital care. Throughout medical communities, inadequate handoff communication is being highlighted as a significant risk to patients. The complexity of hospitals and the number of providers involved in the care of hospitalized patients place inpatients at high risk of communication lapses. This miscommunication and the potential resulting harm make effective handoffs more critical than ever. Although hospitalized patients are being exposed to many handoffs each day, this report is limited to describing the best handoff practices between providers at the time of shift change. (10/16)

http://pediatrics.aappublications.org/content/138/5/e20162681

STANDARDS FOR HEALTH INFORMATION TECHNOLOGY TO ENSURE ADOLESCENT PRIVACY

Committee on Adolescence and Council on Clinical Information Technology

ABSTRACT. Privacy and security of health information is a basic expectation of patients. Despite the existence of federal and state laws safeguarding the privacy of health information, health information systems currently lack the capability to allow for protection of this information for minors. This policy statement reviews the challenges to privacy for adolescents posed by commercial health information technology systems and recommends basic principles for ideal electronic health record systems. This policy statement has been endorsed by the Society for Adolescent Health and Medicine. (10/12, reaffirmed 12/18)

http://pediatrics.aappublications.org/content/130/5/987

STANDARDS FOR PEDIATRIC CANCER CENTERS

Section on Hematology/Oncology

ABSTRACT. Since the American Academy of Pediatrics–published guidelines for pediatric cancer centers in 1986, 1997, and 2004, significant changes in the delivery of health care have prompted a review of the role of medical centers in the care of pediatric patients. The potential effect of these changes on the treatment and survival rates of children with cancer led to this revision. The intent of this statement is to delineate personnel,

capabilities, and facilities that are essential to provide state-of-the-art care for children, adolescents, and young adults with cancer. This statement emphasizes the importance of board-certified pediatric hematologists/oncologists and appropriately qualified pediatric medical subspecialists and pediatric surgical specialists overseeing patient care and the need for specialized facilities as essential for the initial management and much of the follow-up for pediatric, adolescent, and young adult patients with cancer. For patients without practical access to a pediatric cancer center, care may be provided locally by a primary care physician or adult oncologist but at the direction of a pediatric oncologist. (7/14, reaffirmed 10/18)
http://pediatrics.aappublications.org/content/134/2/410

STIGMA EXPERIENCED BY CHILDREN AND ADOLESCENTS WITH OBESITY

Stephen J. Pont, MD, MPH, FAAP; Rebecca Puhl, PhD, FTOS; Stephen R. Cook, MD, MPH, FAAP, FTOS; Wendelin Slusser, MD, MS, FAAP; and Section on Obesity (joint with The Obesity Society)

ABSTRACT. The stigmatization of people with obesity is widespread and causes harm. Weight stigma is often propagated and tolerated in society because of beliefs that stigma and shame will motivate people to lose weight. However, rather than motivating positive change, this stigma contributes to behaviors such as binge eating, social isolation, avoidance of health care services, decreased physical activity, and increased weight gain, which worsen obesity and create additional barriers to healthy behavior change. Furthermore, experiences of weight stigma also dramatically impair quality of life, especially for youth. Health care professionals continue to seek effective strategies and resources to address the obesity epidemic; however, they also frequently exhibit weight bias and stigmatizing behaviors. This policy statement seeks to raise awareness regarding the prevalence and negative effects of weight stigma on pediatric patients and their families and provides 6 clinical practice and 4 advocacy recommendations regarding the role of pediatricians in addressing weight stigma. In summary, these recommendations include improving the clinical setting by modeling best practices for non-biased behaviors and language; using empathetic and empowering counseling techniques, such as motivational interviewing, and addressing weight stigma and bullying in the clinic visit; advocating for inclusion of training and education about weight stigma in medical schools, residency programs, and continuing medical education programs; and empowering families to be advocates to address weight stigma in the home environment and school setting. (11/17)
http://pediatrics.aappublications.org/content/140/6/e20173034

STRATEGIES FOR PREVENTION OF HEALTH CARE–ASSOCIATED INFECTIONS IN THE NICU (CLINICAL REPORT)

Richard A. Polin, MD; Susan Denson, MD; Michael T. Brady, MD; Committee on Fetus and Newborn; and Committee on Infectious Diseases

ABSTRACT. Health care–associated infections in the NICU result in increased morbidity and mortality, prolonged lengths of stay, and increased medical costs. Neonates are at high risk of acquiring health care–associated infections because of impaired host-defense mechanisms, limited amounts of protective endogenous flora on skin and mucosal surfaces at time of birth, reduced barrier function of their skin, use of invasive procedures and devices, and frequent exposure to broad-spectrum antibiotic agents. This clinical report reviews management and prevention of health care–associated infections in newborn infants. (3/12, reaffirmed 2/16)
http://pediatrics.aappublications.org/content/129/4/e1085

STRENGTH TRAINING BY CHILDREN AND ADOLESCENTS

Council on Sports Medicine and Fitness

ABSTRACT. Pediatricians are often asked to give advice on the safety and efficacy of strength-training programs for children and adolescents. This statement, which is a revision of a previous American Academy of Pediatrics policy statement, defines relevant terminology and provides current information on risks and benefits of strength training for children and adolescents. (4/08, reaffirmed 6/11, 12/16)
http://pediatrics.aappublications.org/content/121/4/835

SUBSTANCE USE SCREENING, BRIEF INTERVENTION, AND REFERRAL TO TREATMENT

Committee on Substance Use and Prevention

ABSTRACT. The enormous public health impact of adolescent substance use and its preventable morbidity and mortality show the need for the health care sector, including pediatricians and the medical home, to increase its capacity related to substance use prevention, detection, assessment, and intervention. The American Academy of Pediatrics published its policy statement "Substance Use Screening, Brief Intervention, and Referral to Treatment for Pediatricians" in 2011 to introduce the concepts and terminology of screening, brief intervention, and referral to treatment (SBIRT) and to offer clinical guidance about available substance use screening tools and intervention procedures. This policy statement is a revision of the 2011 SBIRT statement. An accompanying clinical report updates clinical guidance for adolescent SBIRT. (6/16)
http://pediatrics.aappublications.org/content/138/1/e20161210

SUBSTANCE USE SCREENING, BRIEF INTERVENTION, AND REFERRAL TO TREATMENT (CLINICAL REPORT)

Sharon J. L. Levy, MD, MPH, FAAP; Janet F. Williams, MD, FAAP; and Committee on Substance Use and Prevention

ABSTRACT. The enormous public health impact of adolescent substance use and its preventable morbidity and mortality highlight the need for the health care sector, including pediatricians and the medical home, to increase its capacity regarding adolescent substance use screening, brief intervention, and referral to treatment (SBIRT). The American Academy of Pediatrics first published a policy statement on SBIRT and adolescents in 2011 to introduce SBIRT concepts and terminology and to offer clinical guidance about available substance use screening tools and intervention procedures. This clinical report provides a simplified adolescent SBIRT clinical approach that, in combination with the accompanying updated policy statement, guides pediatricians in implementing substance use prevention, detection, assessment, and intervention practices across the varied clinical settings in which adolescents receive health care. (6/16)
http://pediatrics.aappublications.org/content/138/1/e20161211

SUICIDE AND SUICIDE ATTEMPTS IN ADOLESCENTS (CLINICAL REPORT)

Benjamin Shain, MD, PhD, and Committee on Adolescence

ABSTRACT. Suicide is the second leading cause of death for adolescents 15 to 19 years old. This report updates the previous statement of the American Academy of Pediatrics and is intended to assist pediatricians, in collaboration with other child and adolescent health care professionals, in the identification and management of the adolescent at risk for suicide. Suicide risk can only be reduced, not eliminated, and risk factors provide no more than guidance. Nonetheless, care for suicidal adolescents may be improved with the pediatrician's knowledge, skill, and comfort with the topic, as well as ready access to appropriate community resources and mental health professionals. (6/16)
http://pediatrics.aappublications.org/content/138/1/e20161420

SUPPLEMENTAL SECURITY INCOME (SSI) FOR CHILDREN AND YOUTH WITH DISABILITIES

Council on Children With Disabilities

ABSTRACT. The Supplemental Security Income (SSI) program remains an important source of financial support for low-income families of children with special health care needs and disabling conditions. In most states, SSI eligibility also qualifies children for the state Medicaid program, providing access to health care services. The Social Security Administration (SSA), which administers the SSI program, considers a child disabled under SSI if there is a medically determinable physical or mental impairment or combination of impairments that results in marked and severe functional limitations. The impairment(s) must be expected to result in death or have lasted or be expected to last for a continuous period of at least 12 months. The income and assets of families of children with disabilities are also considered when determining financial eligibility. When an individual with a disability becomes an adult at 18 years of age, the SSA considers only the individual's income and assets. The SSA considers an adult to be disabled if there is a medically determinable impairment (or combination of impairments) that prevents substantial gainful activity for at least 12 continuous months. SSI benefits are important for youth with chronic conditions who are transitioning to adulthood. The purpose of this statement is to provide updated information about the SSI medical and financial eligibility criteria and the disability-determination process. This statement also discusses how pediatricians can help children and youth when they apply for SSI benefits. (11/09, reaffirmed 2/15)

http://pediatrics.aappublications.org/content/124/6/1702

SUPPORTING THE FAMILY AFTER THE DEATH OF A CHILD (CLINICAL REPORT)

Esther Wender, MD, and Committee on Psychosocial Aspects of Child and Family Health

ABSTRACT. The death of a child can have a devastating effect on the family. The pediatrician has an important role to play in supporting the parents and any siblings still in his or her practice after such a death. Pediatricians may be poorly prepared to provide this support. Also, because of the pain of confronting the grief of family members, they may be reluctant to become involved. This statement gives guidelines to help the pediatrician provide such support. It describes the grief reactions that can be expected in family members after the death of a child. Ways of supporting family members are suggested, and other helpful resources in the community are described. The goal of this guidance is to prevent outcomes that may impair the health and development of affected parents and children. (11/12, reaffirmed 12/16)

http://pediatrics.aappublications.org/content/130/6/1164

SUPPORTING THE GRIEVING CHILD AND FAMILY (CLINICAL REPORT)

David J. Schonfeld, MD, FAAP; Thomas Demaria, PhD; Committee on Psychosocial Aspects of Child and Family Health; and Disaster Preparedness Advisory Council

ABSTRACT. The death of someone close to a child often has a profound and lifelong effect on the child and results in a range of both short- and long-term reactions. Pediatricians, within a patient-centered medical home, are in an excellent position to provide anticipatory guidance to caregivers and to offer assistance and support to children and families who are grieving. This clinical report offers practical suggestions on how to talk with grieving children to help them better understand what has happened and its implications and to address any misinformation, misinterpretations, or misconceptions. An understanding of guilt, shame, and other common reactions, as well an appreciation of the role of secondary losses and the unique challenges facing children in communities characterized by chronic trauma and cumulative loss, will help the pediatrician to address factors that may impair grieving and children's adjustment and to identify complicated mourning and situations when professional counseling is indicated. Advice on how to support children's participation in funerals and other memorial services and to anticipate and address grief triggers and anniversary reactions is provided so that pediatricians are in a better position to advise caregivers and to offer consultation to schools, early education and child care facilities, and other child congregate care sites. Pediatricians often enter their profession out of a profound desire to minimize the suffering of children and may find it personally challenging when they find themselves in situations in which they are asked to bear witness to the distress of children who are acutely grieving. The importance of professional preparation and self-care is therefore emphasized, and resources are recommended. (8/16)

http://pediatrics.aappublications.org/content/138/3/e20162147

SUPPORTING THE HEALTH CARE TRANSITION FROM ADOLESCENCE TO ADULTHOOD IN THE MEDICAL HOME (CLINICAL REPORT)

Patience H. White, MD, MA, FAAP, FACP; W. Carl Cooley, MD, FAAP; American Academy of Pediatrics (joint with Transitions Clinical Report Authoring Group, American Academy of Family Physicians, and American College of Physicians)

ABSTRACT. Risk and vulnerability encompass many dimensions of the transition from adolescence to adulthood. Transition from pediatric, parent-supervised health care to more independent, patient-centered adult health care is no exception. The tenets and algorithm of the original 2011 clinical report, "Supporting the Health Care Transition from Adolescence to Adulthood in the Medical Home," are unchanged. This updated clinical report provides more practice-based quality improvement guidance on key elements of transition planning, transfer, and integration into adult care for all youth and young adults. It also includes new and updated sections on definition and guiding principles, the status of health care transition preparation among youth, barriers, outcome evidence, recommended health care transition processes and implementation strategies using quality improvement methods, special populations, education and training in pediatric onset conditions, and payment options. The clinical report also includes new recommendations pertaining to infrastructure, education and training, payment, and research. (10/18)

http://pediatrics.aappublications.org/content/142/5/e20182587

SURFACTANT REPLACEMENT THERAPY FOR PRETERM AND TERM NEONATES WITH RESPIRATORY DISTRESS (CLINICAL REPORT)

Richard A. Polin, MD, FAAP; Waldemar A. Carlo, MD, FAAP; and Committee on Fetus and Newborn

ABSTRACT. Respiratory failure secondary to surfactant deficiency is a major cause of morbidity and mortality in preterm infants. Surfactant therapy substantially reduces mortality and respiratory morbidity for this population. Secondary surfactant deficiency also contributes to acute respiratory morbidity in late-preterm and term neonates with meconium aspiration syndrome, pneumonia/sepsis, and perhaps pulmonary hemorrhage; surfactant replacement may be beneficial for these infants. This statement summarizes the evidence regarding indications, administration, formulations, and outcomes for surfactant-replacement therapy. The clinical strategy of intubation, surfactant administration, and extubation to continuous positive airway pressure and the effect of continuous positive airway pressure on outcomes and surfactant use in preterm infants are also reviewed. (12/13)

http://pediatrics.aappublications.org/content/133/1/156

TACKLING IN YOUTH FOOTBALL

Council on Sports Medicine and Fitness

ABSTRACT. American football remains one of the most popular sports for young athletes. The injuries sustained during football, especially those to the head and neck, have been a topic of intense interest recently in both the public media and medical literature. The recognition of these injuries and the potential for long-term sequelae have led some physicians to call for a reduction in the number of contact practices, a postponement of tackling until a certain age, and even a ban on high school football. This statement reviews the literature regarding injuries in football, particularly those of the head and neck, the relationship between tackling and football-related injuries, and the potential effects of limiting or delaying tackling on injury risk. (10/15)

http://pediatrics.aappublications.org/content/136/5/e1419

TARGETED REFORMS IN HEALTH CARE FINANCING TO IMPROVE THE CARE OF ADOLESCENTS AND YOUNG ADULTS

Arik V. Marcell, MD, MPH, FAAP; Cora C. Breuner, MD, MPH, FAAP; Lawrence Hammer, MD, FAAP; Mark L. Hudak, MD, FAAP; Committee on Adolescence; and Committee on Child Health Financing

ABSTRACT. Significant changes have occurred in the commercial and government insurance marketplace after the passage of 2 federal legislation acts, the Patient Protection and Affordable Care Act of 2010 and the Paul Wellstone and Pete Domenici Mental Health Parity and Addiction Equity Act of 2008. Despite the potential these 2 acts held to improve the health care of adolescents and young adults (AYAs), including the financing of care, there are barriers to achieving this goal. In the first quarter of 2016, 13.7% of individuals 18 to 24 years of age still lacked health insurance. Limitations in the scope of benefits coverage and inadequate provider payment can curtail access to health care for AYAs, particularly care related to sexual and reproductive health and mental and behavioral health. Some health plans impose financial barriers to access because they require families to absorb high cost-sharing expenses (eg, deductibles, copayments, and coinsurance). Finally, challenges of confidentiality inherent in the billing and insurance claim practices of some health insurance plans can discourage access to health care in the absence of other obstacles and interfere with provision of confidential care. This policy statement summarizes the current state of impediments that AYA, including those with special health care needs, face in accessing timely and appropriate health care and that providers face in serving these patients. These impediments include limited scope of benefits, high cost sharing, inadequate provider payment, and insufficient confidentiality protections. With this statement, we aim to improve both access to health care by AYAs and providers' delivery of developmentally appropriate health care for these patients through the presentation of an overview of the issues, specific recommendations for reform of health care financing for AYAs, and practical actions that pediatricians and other providers can take to advocate for appropriate payments for providing health care to AYAs. (11/18)

http://pediatrics.aappublications.org/content/142/6/e20182998

THE TEEN DRIVER

Elizabeth M. Alderman, MD, FAAP, FSAHM; Brian D. Johnston, MD, MPH, FAAP; Committee on Adolescence; and Council on Injury, Violence, and Poison Prevention

ABSTRACT. For many teenagers, obtaining a driver's license is a rite of passage, conferring the ability to independently travel to school, work, or social events. However, immaturity, inexperience, and risky behavior put newly licensed teen drivers at risk. Motor vehicle crashes are the most common cause of mortality and injury for adolescents and young adults in developed countries. Teen drivers (15–19 years of age) have the highest rate of motor vehicle crashes among all age groups in the United States and contribute disproportionately to traffic fatalities. In addition to the deaths of teen drivers, more than half of 8- to 17-year-old children who die in car crashes are killed as passengers of drivers younger than 20 years of age. This policy statement, in which we update the previous 2006 iteration of this policy statement, is used to reflect new research on the risks faced by teen drivers and offer advice for pediatricians counseling teen drivers and their families. (9/18)

http://pediatrics.aappublications.org/content/142/4/e20182163

TELEMEDICINE FOR EVALUATION OF RETINOPATHY OF PREMATURITY (TECHNICAL REPORT)

Walter M. Fierson, MD, FAAP; Antonio Capone Jr, MD; and Section on Ophthalmology (joint with American Academy of Ophthalmology and American Association of Certified Orthoptists)

ABSTRACT. Retinopathy of prematurity (ROP) remains a significant threat to vision for extremely premature infants despite the availability of therapeutic modalities capable, in most cases, of managing this disorder. It has been shown in many controlled trials that application of therapies at the appropriate time is essential to successful outcomes in premature infants affected by ROP. Bedside binocular indirect ophthalmoscopy has been the standard technique for diagnosis and monitoring of ROP in these patients. However, implementation of routine use of this screening method for at-risk premature infants has presented challenges within our existing care systems, including relative local scarcity of qualified ophthalmologist examiners in some locations and the remote location of some NICUs. Modern technology, including the development of wide-angle ocular digital fundus photography, coupled with the ability to send digital images electronically to remote locations, has led to the development of telemedicine-based remote digital fundus imaging (RDFI-TM) evaluation techniques. These techniques have the potential to allow the diagnosis and monitoring of ROP to occur in lieu of the necessity for some repeated on-site examinations in NICUs. This report reviews the currently available literature on RDFI-TM evaluations for ROP and outlines pertinent practical and risk management considerations that should be used when including RDFI-TM in any new or existing ROP care structure. (12/14)

http://pediatrics.aappublications.org/content/135/1/e238

TELEMEDICINE: PEDIATRIC APPLICATIONS (TECHNICAL REPORT)

Bryan L. Burke Jr, MD, FAAP; R. W. Hall, MD, FAAP; and Section on Telehealth Care

ABSTRACT. Telemedicine is a technological tool that is improving the health of children around the world. This report chronicles the use of telemedicine by pediatricians and pediatric medical and surgical specialists to deliver inpatient and outpatient care, educate physicians and patients, and conduct medical research. It also describes the importance of telemedicine in responding to emergencies and disasters and providing access to pediatric care to remote and underserved populations. Barriers to telemedicine expansion are explained, such as legal issues, inadequate payment for services, technology costs and sustainability, and the lack of technology infrastructure on a national scale. Although certain challenges have constrained more widespread implementation, telemedicine's current use bears testimony to its effectiveness and potential. Telemedicine's widespread adoption will be influenced by the implementation of key provisions of the Patient Protection and Affordable Care Act, technological advances, and growing patient demand for virtual visits. (6/15)

http://pediatrics.aappublications.org/content/136/1/e293

TESTING FOR DRUGS OF ABUSE IN CHILDREN AND ADOLESCENTS (CLINICAL REPORT)

Sharon Levy, MD, MPH, FAAP; Lorena M. Siqueira, MD, MSPH, FAAP; and Committee on Substance Abuse

ABSTRACT. Drug testing is often used as part of an assessment for substance use in children and adolescents. However, the indications for drug testing and guidance on how to use this procedure effectively are not clear. The complexity and invasiveness of the procedure and limitations to the information derived from drug testing all affect its utility. The objective of this clinical report is to provide guidance to pediatricians and other clinicians on the efficacy and efficient use of drug testing on the basis of a review of the nascent scientific literature, policy guidelines, and published clinical recommendations. (5/14)

http://pediatrics.aappublications.org/content/133/6/e1798

TOWARD TRANSPARENT CLINICAL POLICIES

Steering Committee on Quality Improvement and Management

ABSTRACT. Clinical policies of professional societies such as the American Academy of Pediatrics are valued highly, not only by clinicians who provide direct health care to children but also by many others who rely on the professional expertise of these organizations, including parents, employers, insurers, and legislators. The utility of a policy depends, in large part, on the degree to which its purpose and basis are clear to policy users, an attribute known as the policy's transparency. This statement describes the critical importance and special value of transparency in clinical policies, guidelines, and recommendations; helps identify obstacles to achieving transparency; and suggests several approaches to overcome these obstacles. (3/08, reaffirmed 2/14)

http://pediatrics.aappublications.org/content/121/3/643

TRAMPOLINE SAFETY IN CHILDHOOD AND ADOLESCENCE

Council on Sports Medicine and Fitness

ABSTRACT. Despite previous recommendations from the American Academy of Pediatrics discouraging home use of trampolines, recreational use of trampolines in the home setting continues to be a popular activity among children and adolescents. This policy statement is an update to previous statements, reflecting the current literature on prevalence, patterns, and mechanisms of trampoline-related injuries. Most trampoline injuries occur with multiple simultaneous users on the mat. Cervical spine injuries often occur with falls off the trampoline or with attempts at somersaults or flips. Studies on the efficacy of trampoline safety measures are reviewed, and although there is a paucity of data, current implementation of safety measures have not appeared to mitigate risk substantially. Therefore, the home use of trampolines is strongly discouraged. The role of trampoline as a competitive sport and in structured training settings is reviewed, and recommendations for enhancing safety in these environments are made. (9/12, reaffirmed 7/15)

http://pediatrics.aappublications.org/content/130/4/774

THE TRANSFER OF DRUGS AND THERAPEUTICS INTO HUMAN BREAST MILK: AN UPDATE ON SELECTED TOPICS (CLINICAL REPORT)

Hari Cheryl Sachs, MD, FAAP, and Committee on Drugs

ABSTRACT. Many mothers are inappropriately advised to discontinue breastfeeding or avoid taking essential medications because of fears of adverse effects on their infants. This cautious approach may be unnecessary in many cases, because only a small proportion of medications are contraindicated in breastfeeding mothers or associated with adverse effects on their infants. Information to inform physicians about the extent of excretion for a particular drug into human milk is needed but may not be available. Previous statements on this topic from the American Academy of Pediatrics provided physicians with data concerning the known excretion of specific medications into breast milk. More current and comprehensive information is now available on the Internet, as well as an application for mobile devices, at LactMed (http://toxnet.nlm.nih.gov). Therefore, with the exception of radioactive compounds requiring temporary cessation of breastfeeding, the reader will be referred to LactMed to obtain the most current data on an individual medication. This report discusses several topics of interest surrounding lactation, such as the use of psychotropic therapies, drugs to treat substance abuse, narcotics, galactagogues, and herbal products, as well as immunization of breastfeeding women. A discussion regarding the global implications of maternal medications and lactation in the developing world is beyond the scope of this report. The World Health Organization offers several programs and resources that address the importance of breastfeeding (see http://www.who.int/topics/breastfeeding/en/). (8/13, reaffirmed 5/18)

http://pediatrics.aappublications.org/content/132/3/e796

TRANSITIONING HIV-INFECTED YOUTH INTO ADULT HEALTH CARE

Committee on Pediatric AIDS

ABSTRACT. With advances in antiretroviral therapy, most HIV-infected children survive into adulthood. Optimal health care for these youth includes a formal plan for the transition of care from primary and/or subspecialty pediatric/adolescent/family medicine health care providers (medical home) to adult health care provider(s). Successful transition involves the early engagement and participation of the youth and his or her family with the pediatric medical home and adult health care teams in developing a formal plan. Referring providers should have a written policy for the transfer of HIV-infected youth to adult care, which will guide in the development of an individualized plan for each youth. The plan should be introduced to the youth in early adolescence and modified as the youth approaches transition. Assessment of developmental milestones is important to define the readiness of the youth in assuming responsibility for his or her own care before initiating the transfer. Communication among all providers is essential and should include both personal contact and a written medical summary. Progress toward the transition should be tracked and, once completed, should be documented and assessed. (6/13, reaffirmed 4/16)

http://pediatrics.aappublications.org/content/132/1/192

TRANSPORTING CHILDREN WITH SPECIAL HEALTH CARE NEEDS

Joseph O'Neil, MD, MPH, FAAP; Benjamin Hoffman, MD, FAAP; and Council on Injury, Violence, and Poison Prevention

ABSTRACT. Children with special health care needs should have access to proper resources for safe transportation as do typical children. This policy statement reviews important considerations for transporting children with special health care needs and provides current guidance for the protection of children with specific health care needs, including those with airway obstruction, orthopedic conditions or procedures, developmental delays, muscle tone abnormalities, challenging behaviors, and gastrointestinal disorders. (4/19)

See full text on page 1221.

https://pediatrics.aappublications.org/content/143/5/e20190724

THE TREATMENT OF NEUROLOGICALLY IMPAIRED CHILDREN USING PATTERNING

Committee on Children With Disabilities

ABSTRACT. This statement reviews patterning as a treatment for children with neurologic impairments. This treatment is based on an outmoded and oversimplified theory of brain development. Current information does not support the claims of propo-

nents that this treatment is efficacious, and its use continues to be unwarranted. (11/99, reaffirmed 11/02, 1/06, 8/10, 4/14, 5/18)
http://pediatrics.aappublications.org/content/104/5/1149

ULTRAVIOLET RADIATION: A HAZARD TO CHILDREN AND ADOLESCENTS

Council on Environmental Health and Section on Dermatology

ABSTRACT. Ultraviolet radiation (UVR) causes the 3 major forms of skin cancer: basal cell carcinoma; squamous cell carcinoma; and cutaneous malignant melanoma. Public awareness of the risk is not optimal, overall compliance with sun protection is inconsistent, and melanoma rates continue to rise. The risk of skin cancer increases when people overexpose themselves to sun and intentionally expose themselves to artificial sources of UVR. Yet, people continue to sunburn, and teenagers and adults alike remain frequent visitors to tanning parlors. Pediatricians should provide advice about UVR exposure during health-supervision visits and at other relevant times. Advice includes avoiding sunburning, wearing clothing and hats, timing activities (when possible) before or after periods of peak sun exposure, wearing protective sunglasses, and applying and reapplying sunscreen. Advice should be framed in the context of promoting outdoor physical activity. Adolescents should be strongly discouraged from visiting tanning parlors. Sun exposure and vitamin D status are intertwined. Cutaneous vitamin D production requires sunlight exposure, and many factors, such as skin pigmentation, season, and time of day, complicate efficiency of cutaneous vitamin D production that results from sun exposure. Adequate vitamin D is needed for bone health. Accumulating information suggests a beneficial influence of vitamin D on many health conditions. Although vitamin D is available through the diet, supplements, and incidental sun exposure, many children have low vitamin D concentrations. Ensuring vitamin D adequacy while promoting sun-protection strategies will require renewed attention to children's use of dietary and supplemental vitamin D. (2/11, reaffirmed 9/16)
http://pediatrics.aappublications.org/content/127/3/588

ULTRAVIOLET RADIATION: A HAZARD TO CHILDREN AND ADOLESCENTS (TECHNICAL REPORT)

Sophie J. Balk, MD; Council on Environmental Health; and Section on Dermatology

ABSTRACT. Sunlight sustains life on earth. Sunlight is essential for vitamin D synthesis in the skin. The sun's ultraviolet rays can be hazardous, however, because excessive exposure causes skin cancer and other adverse health effects. Skin cancer is a major public health problem; more than 2 million new cases are diagnosed in the United States each year. Ultraviolet radiation (UVR) causes the 3 major forms of skin cancer: basal cell carcinoma; squamous cell carcinoma; and cutaneous malignant melanoma. Exposure to UVR from sunlight and artificial sources early in life elevates the risk of developing skin cancer. Approximately 25% of sun exposure occurs before 18 years of age. The risk of skin cancer is increased when people overexpose themselves to sun and intentionally expose themselves to artificial sources of UVR. Public awareness of the risk is not optimal, compliance with sun protection is inconsistent, and skin-cancer rates continue to rise in all age groups including the younger population. People continue to sunburn, and teenagers and adults are frequent visitors to tanning parlors. Sun exposure and vitamin D status are intertwined. Adequate vitamin D is needed for bone health in children and adults. In addition, there is accumulating information suggesting a beneficial influence of vitamin D on various health conditions. Cutaneous vitamin D production requires sunlight, and many factors complicate the efficiency of vitamin D production that results from sunlight exposure. Ensuring vitamin D adequacy while promoting sun-protection strategies, therefore, requires renewed attention to evaluating the adequacy of dietary and supplemental vitamin D. Daily intake of 400 IU of vitamin D will prevent vitamin D deficiency rickets in infants. The vitamin D supplementation amounts necessary to support optimal health in older children and adolescents are less clear. This report updates information on the relationship of sun exposure to skin cancer and other adverse health effects, the relationship of exposure to artificial sources of UVR and skin cancer, sun-protection methods, vitamin D, community skin-cancer–prevention efforts, and the pediatrician's role in preventing skin cancer. In addition to pediatricians' efforts, a sustained public health effort is needed to change attitudes and behaviors regarding UVR exposure. (2/11, reaffirmed 9/16)
http://pediatrics.aappublications.org/content/127/3/e791

UMBILICAL CORD CARE IN THE NEWBORN INFANT (CLINICAL REPORT)

Dan Stewart, MD, FAAP; William Benitz, MD, FAAP; and Committee on Fetus and Newborn

ABSTRACT. Postpartum infections remain a leading cause of neonatal morbidity and mortality worldwide. A high percentage of these infections may stem from bacterial colonization of the umbilicus, because cord care practices vary in reflection of cultural traditions within communities and disparities in health care practices globally. After birth, the devitalized umbilical cord often proves to be an ideal substrate for bacterial growth and also provides direct access to the bloodstream of the neonate. Bacterial colonization of the cord not infrequently leads to omphalitis and associated thrombophlebitis, cellulitis, or necrotizing fasciitis. Various topical substances continue to be used for cord care around the world to mitigate the risk of serious infection. More recently, particularly in high-resource countries, the treatment paradigm has shifted toward dry umbilical cord care. This clinical report reviews the evidence underlying recommendations for care of the umbilical cord in different clinical settings. (8/16)
http://pediatrics.aappublications.org/content/138/3/e20162149

UNDERSTANDING LIABILITY RISKS AND PROTECTIONS FOR PEDIATRIC PROVIDERS DURING DISASTERS

Robin L. Altman, MD, FAAP; Karen A. Santucci, MD, FAAP; Michael R. Anderson, MD, MBA, FAAP; William M. McDonnell, MD, JD, FAAP; and Committee on Medical Liability and Risk Management

ABSTRACT. Although most health care providers will go through their careers without experiencing a major disaster in their local communities, if one does occur, it can be life and career altering. The American Academy of Pediatrics has been at the forefront of providing education and advocacy on the critical importance of disaster preparedness. From experiences over the past decade, new evidence and analysis have broadened our understanding that the concept of preparedness is also applicable to addressing the unique professional liability risks that can occur when caring for patients and families during a disaster. In our recommendations in this policy statement, we target pediatric health care providers, advocates, and policy makers and address how individuals, institutions, and government can work together to strengthen the system of liability protections during disasters so that appropriate and timely care can be delivered with minimal fear of legal reprisal or confusion. (2/19)

See full text on page 1231.

https://pediatrics.aappublications.org/content/143/3/e20183892

UNDERSTANDING LIABILITY RISKS AND PROTECTIONS FOR PEDIATRIC PROVIDERS DURING DISASTERS (TECHNICAL REPORT)

Robin L. Altman, MD, FAAP; Karen A. Santucci, MD, FAAP; Michael R. Anderson, MD, MBA, FAAP; William M. McDonnell, MD, JD, FAAP; and Committee on Medical Liability and Risk Management

ABSTRACT. Although most health care providers will go through their careers without experiencing a major disaster in their local communities, if one does occur, it can be life and career altering. The American Academy of Pediatrics has been in the forefront of providing education and advocacy on the critical importance of disaster preparedness. From experiences over the past decade, new evidence and analysis have broadened our understanding that the concept of preparedness is also applicable to addressing the unique professional liability risks that can occur when caring for patients and families during a disaster. Concepts explored in this technical report will help to inform pediatric health care providers, advocates, and policy makers about the complexities of how providers are currently protected, with a focus on areas of unappreciated liability. The timeliness of this technical report is emphasized by the fact that during the time of its development (ie, late summer and early fall of 2017), the United States went through an extraordinary period of multiple, successive, and overlapping disasters within a concentrated period of time of both natural and man-made causes. In a companion policy statement (www.pediatrics.org/cgi/doi/10.1542/peds.2018-3892), recommendations are offered on how individuals, institutions, and governments can work together to strengthen the system of liability protections during disasters so that appropriate and timely care can be delivered with minimal fear of legal reprisal or confusion. (2/19)

See full text on page 1237.

https://pediatrics.aappublications.org/content/143/3/e20183893

UNIQUE NEEDS OF THE ADOLESCENT

Elizabeth M. Alderman, MD, FSAHM, FAAP; Cora C. Breuner, MD, MPH, FAAP; and Committee on Adolescence

ABSTRACT. Adolescence is the transitional bridge between childhood and adulthood; it encompasses developmental milestones that are unique to this age group. Healthy cognitive, physical, sexual, and psychosocial development is both a right and a responsibility that must be guaranteed for all adolescents to successfully enter adulthood. There is consensus among national and international organizations that the unique needs of adolescents must be addressed and promoted to ensure the health of all adolescents. This policy statement outlines the special health challenges that adolescents face on their journey and transition to adulthood and provides recommendations for those who care for adolescents, their families, and the communities in which they live. (11/19)

See full text on page 1255.

https://pediatrics.aappublications.org/content/144/6/e20193150

UPDATE OF NEWBORN SCREENING AND THERAPY FOR CONGENITAL HYPOTHYROIDISM (CLINICAL REPORT)

Susan R. Rose, MD; Section on Endocrinology; and Committee on Genetics (joint with Rosalind S. Brown, MD; American Thyroid Association; and Lawson Wilkins Pediatric Endocrine Society)

ABSTRACT. Unrecognized congenital hypothyroidism leads to mental retardation. Newborn screening and thyroid therapy started within 2 weeks of age can normalize cognitive development. The primary thyroid-stimulating hormone screening has become standard in many parts of the world. However, newborn thyroid screening is not yet universal in some countries. Initial dosage of 10 to 15 μg/kg levothyroxine is recommended. The goals of thyroid hormone therapy should be to maintain frequent evaluations of total thyroxine or free thyroxine in the upper half of the reference range during the first 3 years of life and to normalize the serum thyroid-stimulating hormone concentration to ensure optimal thyroid hormone dosage and compliance.

Improvements in screening and therapy have led to improved developmental outcomes in adults with congenital hypothyroidism who are now in their 20s and 30s. Thyroid hormone regimens used today are more aggressive in targeting early correction of thyroid-stimulating hormone than were those used 20 or even 10 years ago. Thus, newborn infants with congenital hypothyroidism today may have an even better intellectual and neurologic prognosis. Efforts are ongoing to establish the optimal therapy that leads to maximum potential for normal development for infants with congenital hypothyroidism.

Remaining controversy centers on infants whose abnormality in neonatal thyroid function is transient or mild and on optimal care of very low birth weight or preterm infants. Of note, thyroid-stimulating hormone is not elevated in central hypothyroidism. An algorithm is proposed for diagnosis and management.

Physicians must not relinquish their clinical judgment and experience in the face of normal newborn thyroid test results. Hypothyroidism can be acquired after the newborn screening. When clinical symptoms and signs suggest hypothyroidism, regardless of newborn screening results, serum free thyroxine and thyroid-stimulating hormone determinations should be performed. (6/06, reaffirmed 12/11)

http://pediatrics.aappublications.org/content/117/6/2290

UPDATED GUIDANCE FOR PALIVIZUMAB PROPHYLAXIS AMONG INFANTS AND YOUNG CHILDREN AT INCREASED RISK OF HOSPITALIZATION FOR RESPIRATORY SYNCYTIAL VIRUS INFECTION

PPI AAP Partnership for Policy Implementation

Committee on Infectious Diseases and Bronchiolitis Guidelines Committee

ABSTRACT. Palivizumab was licensed in June 1998 by the Food and Drug Administration for the reduction of serious lower respiratory tract infection caused by respiratory syncytial virus (RSV) in children at increased risk of severe disease. Since that time, the American Academy of Pediatrics has updated its guidance for the use of palivizumab 4 times as additional data became available to provide a better understanding of infants and young children at greatest risk of hospitalization attributable to RSV infection. The updated recommendations in this policy statement reflect new information regarding the seasonality of RSV circulation, palivizumab pharmacokinetics, the changing incidence of bronchiolitis hospitalizations, the effect of gestational age and other risk factors on RSV hospitalization rates, the mortality of children hospitalized with RSV infection, the effect of prophylaxis on wheezing, and palivizumab-resistant RSV isolates. (7/14, reaffirmed 2/19)

http://pediatrics.aappublications.org/content/134/2/415

UPDATED GUIDANCE FOR PALIVIZUMAB PROPHYLAXIS AMONG INFANTS AND YOUNG CHILDREN AT INCREASED RISK OF HOSPITALIZATION FOR RESPIRATORY SYNCYTIAL VIRUS INFECTION (TECHNICAL REPORT)

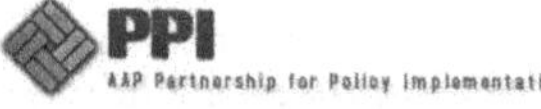

Committee on Infectious Diseases and Bronchiolitis Guidelines Committee

ABSTRACT. Guidance from the American Academy of Pediatrics (AAP) for the use of palivizumab prophylaxis against respiratory syncytial virus (RSV) was first published in a policy state-

ment in 1998. Guidance initially was based on the result from a single randomized, placebo-controlled clinical trial conducted in 1996–1997 describing an overall reduction in RSV hospitalization rate from 10.6% among placebo recipients to 4.8% among children who received prophylaxis. The results of a second randomized, placebo-controlled trial of children with hemodynamically significant heart disease were published in 2003 and revealed a reduction in RSV hospitalization rate from 9.7% in control subjects to 5.3% among prophylaxis recipients. Because no additional controlled trials regarding efficacy were published, AAP guidance has been updated periodically to reflect the most recent literature regarding children at greatest risk of severe disease. Since the last update in 2012, new data have become available regarding the seasonality of RSV circulation, palivizumab pharmacokinetics, the changing incidence of bronchiolitis hospitalizations, the effects of gestational age and other risk factors on RSV hospitalization rates, the mortality of children hospitalized with RSV infection, and the effect of prophylaxis on wheezing and palivizumab-resistant RSV isolates. These data enable further refinement of AAP guidance to most clearly focus on those children at greatest risk. (7/14)
http://pediatrics.aappublications.org/content/134/2/e620

UPDATES ON AN AT-RISK POPULATION: LATE-PRETERM AND EARLYL-TERM INFANTS (CLINICAL REPORT)

Dan L. Stewart, MD, FAAP; Wanda D. Barfield, MD, MPH, FAAP, RADM, USPHS; Committee on Fetus and Newborn

ABSTRACT. The American Academy of Pediatrics published a clinical report on late-preterm (LPT) infants in 2007 that was largely based on a summary of a 2005 workshop convened by the *Eunice Kennedy Shriver* National Institute of Child Health and Human Development, at which a change in terminology from "near term" to "late preterm" was proposed. This paradigm-shifting recommendation had a remarkable impact: federal agencies (the Centers for Disease Control and Prevention), professional societies (the American Academy of Pediatrics and American College of Obstetricians and Gynecologists), and organizations (March of Dimes) initiated nationwide monitoring and educational plans that had a significant effect on decreasing the rates of iatrogenic LPT deliveries. However, there is now an evolving concern. After nearly a decade of steady decreases in the LPT birth rate that largely contributed to the decline in total US preterm birth rates, the birth rate in LPT infants has been inching upward since 2015. In addition, evidence revealed by strong population health research demonstrates that being born as an early-term infant poses a significant risk to an infant's survival, growth, and development. In this report, we summarize the initial progress and discuss the potential reasons for the current trends in LPT and early-term birth rates and propose research recommendations. (10/19)

See full text on page 1269.

https://pediatrics.aappublications.org/content/144/5/e20192760

USE OF CHAPERONES DURING THE PHYSICAL EXAMINATION OF THE PEDIATRIC PATIENT

Committee on Practice and Ambulatory Medicine

ABSTRACT. Physicians should always communicate the scope and nature of the physical examination to be performed to the pediatric patient and his or her parent. This statement addresses the use of chaperones and issues of patient comfort, confidentiality, and privacy. The use of a chaperone should be a shared decision between the patient and physician. In some states, the use of a chaperone is mandated by state regulations. (4/11, 11/17)
http://pediatrics.aappublications.org/content/127/5/991

USE OF INHALED NITRIC OXIDE IN PRETERM INFANTS (CLINICAL REPORT)

Praveen Kumar, MD, FAAP, and Committee on Fetus and Newborn

ABSTRACT. Nitric oxide, an important signaling molecule with multiple regulatory effects throughout the body, is an important tool for the treatment of full-term and late-preterm infants with persistent pulmonary hypertension of the newborn and hypoxemic respiratory failure. Several randomized controlled trials have evaluated its role in the management of preterm infants ≤34 weeks' gestational age with varying results. The purpose of this clinical report is to summarize the existing evidence for the use of inhaled nitric oxide in preterm infants and provide guidance regarding its use in this population. (12/13)
http://pediatrics.aappublications.org/content/133/1/164

THE USE OF NONNUTRITIVE SWEETENERS IN CHILDREN

Carissa M. Baker-Smith, MD, MPH, FAAP; Sarah D. de Ferranti, MD, MPH, FAAP; William J. Cochran, MD, FAAP; Committee on Nutrition; and Section on Gastroenterology, Hepatology, and Nutrition

ABSTRACT. The prevalence of nonnutritive sweeteners (NNSs) in the food supply has increased over time. Not only are more children and adolescents consuming NNSs, but they are also consuming a larger quantity of NNSs in the absence of strong scientific evidence to refute or support the safety of these agents. This policy statement from the American Academy of Pediatrics is intended to provide the pediatric provider with a review of (1) previous steps taken for approved use of NNSs, (2) existing data regarding the safety of NNS use in the general pediatric population, (3) what is known regarding the potential benefits and/or adverse effects of NNS use in children and adolescents, (4) identified gaps in existing knowledge and potential areas of future research, and (5) suggested talking points that pediatricians may use when discussing NNS use with families. (10/19)

See full text on page 1281.

https://pediatrics.aappublications.org/content/144/5/e20192765

USE OF PERFORMANCE-ENHANCING SUBSTANCES (CLINICAL REPORT)

Michele LaBotz, MD, FAAP; Bernard A. Griesemer, MD, FAAP; and Council on Sports Medicine and Fitness

ABSTRACT. Performance-enhancing substances (PESs) are used commonly by children and adolescents in attempts to improve athletic performance. More recent data reveal that these same substances often are used for appearance-related reasons as well. PESs include both legal over-the-counter dietary supplements and illicit pharmacologic agents. This report reviews the current epidemiology of PES use in the pediatric population, as well as information on those PESs in most common use. Concerns regarding use of legal PESs include high rates of product contamination, correlation with future use of anabolic androgenic steroids, and adverse effects on the focus and experience of youth sports participation. The physical maturation and endogenous hormone production that occur in adolescence are associated with large improvements in strength and athletic performance. For most young athletes, PES use does not produce significant gains over those seen with the onset of puberty and adherence to an appropriate nutrition and training program. (6/16)
http://pediatrics.aappublications.org/content/138/1/e20161300

THE USE OF SYSTEMIC AND TOPICAL FLUOROQUINOLONES (CLINICAL REPORT)

Mary Anne Jackson, MD, FAAP; Gordon E. Schutze, MD, FAAP; and Committee on Infectious Diseases

ABSTRACT. Appropriate prescribing practices for fluoroquinolones, as well as all antimicrobial agents, are essential as evolving resistance patterns are considered, additional treatment indica-

tions are identified, and the toxicity profile of fluoroquinolones in children has become better defined. Earlier recommendations for systemic therapy remain; expanded uses of fluoroquinolones for the treatment of certain infections are outlined in this report. Prescribing clinicians should be aware of specific adverse reactions associated with fluoroquinolones, and their use in children should continue to be limited to the treatment of infections for which no safe and effective alternative exists or in situations in which oral fluoroquinolone treatment represents a reasonable alternative to parenteral antimicrobial therapy. (10/16)
http://pediatrics.aappublications.org/content/138/5/e20162706

THE USE OF TELEMEDICINE TO ADDRESS ACCESS AND PHYSICIAN WORKFORCE SHORTAGES

Committee on Pediatric Workforce

ABSTRACT. The use of telemedicine technologies by primary care pediatricians, pediatric medical subspecialists, and pediatric surgical specialists (henceforth referred to as "pediatric physicians") has the potential to transform the practice of pediatrics. The purpose of this policy statement is to describe the expected and potential impact that telemedicine will have on pediatric physicians' efforts to improve access and physician workforce shortages. The policy statement also describes how the American Academy of Pediatrics can advocate for its members and their patients to best use telemedicine technologies to improve access to care, provide more patient- and family-centered care, increase efficiencies in practice, enhance the quality of care, and address projected shortages in the clinical workforce. As the use of telemedicine increases, it is likely to impact health care access, quality, and education and costs of care. Telemedicine technologies, applied to the medical home and its collaborating providers, have the potential to improve current models of care by increasing communication among clinicians, resulting in more efficient, higher quality, and less expensive care. Such a model can serve as a platform for providing more continuous care, linking primary and specialty care to support management of the needs of complex patients. In addition, telemedicine technologies can be used to efficiently provide pediatric physicians working in remote locations with ongoing medical education, increasing their ability to care for more complex patients in their community, reducing the burdens of travel on patients and families, and supporting the medical home. On the other hand, telemedicine technologies used for episodic care by nonmedical home providers have the potential to disrupt continuity of care and to create redundancy and imprudent use of health care resources. Fragmentation should be avoided, and telemedicine, like all primary and specialty services, should be coordinated through the medical home. (6/15, reaffirmed 5/19)
http://pediatrics.aappublications.org/content/136/1/202

VIRTUAL VIOLENCE

Council on Communications and Media

ABSTRACT. In the United States, exposure to media violence is becoming an inescapable component of children's lives. With the rise in new technologies, such as tablets and new gaming platforms, children and adolescents increasingly are exposed to what is known as "virtual violence." This form of violence is not experienced physically; rather, it is experienced in realistic ways via new technology and ever more intense and realistic games. The American Academy of Pediatrics continues to be concerned about children's exposure to virtual violence and the effect it has on their overall health and well-being. This policy statement aims to summarize the current state of scientific knowledge regarding the effects of virtual violence on children's attitudes and behaviors and to make specific recommendations for pediatricians, parents, industry, and policy makers. (7/16)
http://pediatrics.aappublications.org/content/138/2/e20161298

VISUAL SYSTEM ASSESSMENT IN INFANTS, CHILDREN, AND YOUNG ADULTS BY PEDIATRICIANS

Committee on Practice and Ambulatory Medicine and Section on Ophthalmology (joint with American Association of Certified Orthoptists, American Association for Pediatric Ophthalmology and Strabismus, and American Academy of Ophthalmology)

ABSTRACT. Appropriate visual assessments help identify children who may benefit from early interventions to correct or improve vision. Examination of the eyes and visual system should begin in the nursery and continue throughout both childhood and adolescence during routine well-child visits in the medical home. Newborn infants should be examined using inspection and red reflex testing to detect structural ocular abnormalities, such as cataract, corneal opacity, and ptosis. Instrument-based screening, if available, should be first attempted between 12 months and 3 years of age and at annual well-child visits until acuity can be tested directly. Direct testing of visual acuity can often begin by 4 years of age, using age-appropriate symbols (optotypes). Children found to have an ocular abnormality or who fail a vision assessment should be referred to a pediatric ophthalmologist or an eye care specialist appropriately trained to treat pediatric patients. (12/15)
http://pediatrics.aappublications.org/content/137/1/e20153596

WITHHOLDING OR TERMINATION OF RESUSCITATION IN PEDIATRIC OUT-OF-HOSPITAL TRAUMATIC CARDIOPULMONARY ARREST

Committee on Pediatric Emergency Medicine (joint with American College of Surgeons Committee on Trauma and National Association of EMS Physicians)

ABSTRACT. This multiorganizational literature review was undertaken to provide an evidence base for determining whether recommendations for out-of-hospital termination of resuscitation could be made for children who are victims of traumatic cardiopulmonary arrest. Although there is increasing acceptance of out-of-hospital termination of resuscitation for adult traumatic cardiopulmonary arrest when there is no expectation of a good outcome, children are routinely excluded from state termination-of-resuscitation protocols. The decision to withhold resuscitative efforts in a child under specific circumstances (decapitation or dependent lividity, rigor mortis, etc) is reasonable. If there is any doubt as to the circumstances or timing of the traumatic cardiopulmonary arrest, under the current status of limiting termination of resuscitation in the field to persons older than 18 years in most states, resuscitation should be initiated and continued until arrival to the appropriate facility. If the patient has arrested, resuscitation has already exceeded 30 minutes, and the nearest facility is more than 30 minutes away, involvement of parents and family of these children in the decision-making process with assistance and guidance from medical professionals should be considered as part of an emphasis on family-centered care because the evidence suggests that either death or a poor outcome is inevitable. (3/14)
http://pediatrics.aappublications.org/content/133/4/e1104

YOUTH PARTICIPATION AND INJURY RISK IN MARTIAL ARTS (CLINICAL REPORT)

Rebecca A. Demorest, MD, FAAP; Chris Koutures, MD, FAAP; and Council on Sports Medicine and Fitness

ABSTRACT. The martial arts can provide children and adolescents with vigorous levels of physical exercise that can improve overall physical fitness. The various types of martial arts encompass noncontact basic forms and techniques that may have a lower relative risk of injury. Contact-based sparring with competitive training and bouts have a higher risk of injury. This clinical report describes important techniques and movement patterns in several types of martial arts and reviews frequently reported injuries encountered in each discipline, with focused

discussions of higher risk activities. Some of these higher risk activities include blows to the head and choking or submission movements that may cause concussions or significant head injuries. The roles of rule changes, documented benefits of protective equipment, and changes in training recommendations in attempts to reduce injury are critically assessed. This information is intended to help pediatric health care providers counsel patients and families in encouraging safe participation in martial arts. (11/16)
http://pediatrics.aappublications.org/content/138/6/e20163022

SECTION 5

Endorsed Policies

The American Academy of Pediatrics endorses and accepts as its policy the following documents from other organizations.

AMERICAN ACADEMY OF PEDIATRICS

Endorsed Policies

2015 SPCTPD/ACC/AAP/AHA TRAINING GUIDELINES FOR PEDIATRIC CARDIOLOGY FELLOWSHIP PROGRAMS (REVISION OF THE 2005 TRAINING GUIDELINES FOR PEDIATRIC CARDIOLOGY FELLOWSHIP PROGRAMS)

Robert D. Ross, MD, FAAP, FACC; Michael Brook, MD; Jeffrey A. Feinstein, MD; et al (8/15)

INTRODUCTION
Robert D. Ross, MD, FAAP, FACC; Michael Brook, MD; Peter Koenig, MD, FACC, FASE; et al (8/15)

TASK FORCE 1: GENERAL CARDIOLOGY
Alan B. Lewis, MD, FAAP, FACC; Gerard R. Martin, MD, FAAP, FACC, FAHA; Peter J. Bartz, MD, FASE; et al (8/15)

TASK FORCE 2: NONINVASIVE CARDIAC IMAGING
Shubhika Srivastava, MBBS, FAAP, FACC, FASE; Beth F. Printz, MD, PhD, FAAP, FASE; Tal Geva, MD, FACC; et al (8/15)

TASK FORCE 3: CARDIAC CATHETERIZATION
Laurie B. Armsby, MD, FAAP, FSCAI; Robert N. Vincent, MD, CM, FACC, FSCAI; Susan R. Foerster, MD, FSCAI; et al (8/15)

TASK FORCE 4: ELECTROPHYSIOLOGY
Anne M. Dubin, MD, FHRS; Edward P. Walsh, MD, FHRS; Wayne Franklin, MD, FAAP, FACC, FAHA; et al (8/15)

TASK FORCE 5: CRITICAL CARE CARDIOLOGY
Timothy F. Feltes, MD, FAAP, FACC, FAHA; Stephen J. Roth, MD, MPH, FAAP; Melvin C. Almodovar, MD; et al (8/15)

TASK FORCE 6: ADULT CONGENITAL HEART DISEASE
Karen Stout, MD, FACC; Anne Marie Valente, MD, FACC; Peter J. Bartz, MD, FASE; et al (8/15)

TASK FORCE 7: PULMONARY HYPERTENSION, ADVANCED HEART FAILURE, AND TRANSPLANTATION
Steven A. Webber, MB, ChB; Daphne T. Hsu, MD, FAAP, FACC, FAHA; D. Dunbar Ivy, MD, FAAP, FACC; et al (8/15)

TASK FORCE 8: RESEARCH AND SCHOLARLY ACTIVITY
William T. Mahle, MD, FAAP, FACC, FAHA; Anne M. Murphy, MD, FACC, FAHA; Jennifer S. Li, MD; et al (8/15)

ADVANCED PRACTICE REGISTERED NURSE: ROLE, PREPARATION, AND SCOPE OF PRACTICE

National Association of Neonatal Nurses
ABSTRACT. In recent years, the National Association of Neonatal Nurses (NANN) and the National Association of Neonatal Nurse Practitioners (NANNP) have developed several policy statements on neonatal advanced practice registered nurse (APRN) workforce, education, competency, fatigue, safety, and scope of practice. This position paper is a synthesis of previous efforts and discusses the role, preparation, and scope of practice of the neonatal APRN. (1/14)

ANTENATAL CORTICOSTEROID THERAPY FOR FETAL MATURATION

American College of Obstetricians and Gynecologists
ABSTRACT. Corticosteroid administration before anticipated preterm birth is one of the most important antenatal therapies available to improve newborn outcomes. A single course of corticosteroids is recommended for pregnant women between 24 0/7 weeks and 33 6/7 weeks of gestation who are at risk of preterm delivery within 7 days, including for those with ruptured membranes and multiple gestations. It also may be considered for pregnant women starting at 23 0/7 weeks of gestation who are at risk of preterm delivery within 7 days, based on a family's decision regarding resuscitation, irrespective of membrane rupture status and regardless of fetal number. Administration of betamethasone may be considered in pregnant women between 34 0/7 weeks and 36 6/7 weeks of gestation who are at risk of preterm birth within 7 days, and who have not received a previous course of antenatal corticosteroids. A single repeat course of antenatal corticosteroids should be considered in women who are less than 34 0/7 weeks of gestation who are at risk of preterm delivery within 7 days, and whose prior course of antenatal corticosteroids was administered more than 14 days previously. Rescue course corticosteroids could be provided as early as 7 days from the prior dose, if indicated by the clinical scenario. Continued surveillance of long-term outcomes after in utero corticosteroid exposure should be supported. Quality improvement strategies to optimize appropriate and timely antenatal corticosteroid administration are encouraged. (8/17)

APPROPRIATE USE CRITERIA FOR INITIAL TRANSTHORACIC ECHOCARDIOGRAPHY IN OUTPATIENT PEDIATRIC CARDIOLOGY

American College of Cardiology Appropriate Use Task Force
ABSTRACT. The American College of Cardiology (ACC) participated in a joint project with the American Society of Echocardiography, the Society of Pediatric Echocardiography, and several other subspecialty societies and organizations to establish and evaluate Appropriate Use Criteria (AUC) for the initial use of outpatient pediatric echocardiography. Assumptions for the AUC were identified, including the fact that all indications assumed a first-time transthoracic echocardiographic study in an outpatient setting for patients without previously known heart disease. The definitions for frequently used terminology in outpatient pediatric cardiology were established using published guidelines and standards and expert opinion. These AUC serve as a guide to help clinicians in the care of children with possible heart disease, specifically in terms of when a transthoracic echocardiogram is warranted as an initial diagnostic modality in the outpatient setting. They are also a useful tool for education and provide the infrastructure for future quality improvement initiatives as well as research in healthcare delivery, outcomes, and resource utilization.

To complete the AUC process, the writing group identified 113 indications based on common clinical scenarios and/or published clinical practice guidelines, and each indication was classified into 1 of 9 categories of common clinical presentations, including palpitations, syncope, chest pain, and murmur. A separate, independent rating panel evaluated each indication using a scoring scale of 1 to 9, thereby designating each indication as "Appropriate" (median score 7 to 9), "May Be Appropriate" (median score 4 to 6), or "Rarely Appropriate" (median score 1 to 3). Fifty-three indications were identified as Appropriate, 28 as May Be Appropriate, and 32 as Rarely Appropriate. (11/14)

CHILDREN'S SURGERY VERIFICATION PILOT DRAFT DOCUMENTS

OPTIMAL RESOURCES FOR CHILDREN'S SURGICAL CARE—DRAFT

American College of Surgeons

EXECUTIVE SUMMARY. The Task Force for Children's Surgical Care, an ad hoc multidisciplinary group of invited leaders in relevant disciplines, assembled in Rosemont, IL, initially April 30—May 1, 2012, and subsequently in 2013 and 2014 to consider approaches to optimize the delivery of children's surgical care in today's competitive national healthcare environment. Specifically, a mismatch between individual patient needs and available clinical resources for some infants and children receiving surgical care is recognized as a problem in the U.S. and elsewhere. While this phenomenon is apparent to most practitioners involved with children's surgical care, comprehensive data are not available and relevant data are imperfect. The scope of this problem is unknown at present. However, it does periodically, and possibly systematically result in suboptimal patient outcomes. The composition of the Task Force is detailed above. Support was provided by the Children's Hospital Association (CHA) and the American College of Surgeons (ACS). The group represented key disciplines and perspectives. Published literature and data were utilized when available and expert opinion when not, as the basis for these recommendations. The objective was to develop consensus recommendations that would be of use to relevant policy makers and to providers. Principles regarding resource standards, quality improvement and safety processes, data collection and a verification process were initially published in March 2014 [*J Am Coll Surg* 2014;218(3):479-487]. This document details those principles in a specific manner designed to inform and direct a verification process to be conducted by the American College of Surgeons and the ACS Committee on Children's Surgery. (11/14)

HOSPITAL PREREVIEW QUESTIONNAIRE (PRQ)—DRAFT

American College of Surgeons (11/14)

COLLABORATION IN PRACTICE: IMPLEMENTING TEAM-BASED CARE

American College of Obstetricians and Gynecologists Task Force on Collaborative Practice

INTRODUCTION. Quality, efficiency, and value are necessary characteristics of our evolving health care system. Team-based care will work toward the Triple Aim of 1) improving the experience of care of individuals and families; 2) improving the health of populations; and 3) lowering per capita costs. It also should respond to emerging demands and reduce undue burdens on health care providers. Team-based care has the ability to more effectively meet the core expectations of the health care system proposed by the Institute of Medicine. These expectations require that care be safe, effective, patient centered, timely, efficient, and equitable. This report outlines a mechanism that all specialties and practices can use to achieve these expectations.

The report was written by the interprofessional Task Force on Collaborative Practice and is intended to appeal to multiple specialties (eg, internal medicine, pediatrics, family medicine, and women's health) and professions (eg, nurse practitioners, certified nurse–midwives/certified midwives, physician assistants, physicians, clinical pharmacists, and advanced practice registered nurses). This document provides a framework for organizations or practices across all specialties to develop team-based care. In doing so, it offers a map to help practices navigate the increasingly complex and continuously evolving health care system. The guidance presented is a result of the task force's work and is based on current evidence and expert consensus. The task force challenges and welcomes all medical specialties to gather additional data on how and what types of team-based care best accomplish the Triple Aim and the Institute of Medicine's expectations of health care. (3/16)

CONFIDENTIALITY PROTECTIONS FOR ADOLESCENTS AND YOUNG ADULTS IN THE HEALTH CARE BILLING AND INSURANCE CLAIMS PROCESS

Society for Adolescent Health and Medicine

ABSTRACT. The importance of protecting confidential health care for adolescents and young adults is well documented. State and federal confidentiality protections exist for both minors and young adults, although the laws vary among states, particularly for minors. However, such confidentiality is potentially violated by billing practices and in the processing of health insurance claims. To address this problem, policies and procedures should be established so that health care billing and insurance claims processes do not impede the ability of providers to deliver essential health care services on a confidential basis to adolescents and young adults covered as dependents on a family's health insurance plan. (3/16)

CONSENSUS COMMUNICATION ON EARLY PEANUT INTRODUCTION AND THE PREVENTION OF PEANUT ALLERGY IN HIGH-RISK INFANTS

Primary contributors: David M. Fleischer, MD; Scott Sicherer, MD; Matthew Greenhawt, MD; Dianne Campbell, MB BS, FRACP, PhD; Edmond Chan, MD; Antonella Muraro, MD, PhD; Susanne Halken, MD; Yitzhak Katz, MD; Motohiro Ebisawa, MD, PhD; Lawrence Eichenfield, MD; Hugh Sampson, MD; Gideon Lack, MB, BCh; and George Du Toit, MB, BCh

INTRODUCTION AND RATIONALE. Peanut allergy is an increasingly troubling global health problem affecting between 1% and 3% of children in many westernized countries. Although multiple methods of measurement have been used and specific estimates differ, there appears to have been a sudden increase in the number of cases in the past 10- to 15-year period, suggesting that the prevalence might have tripled in some countries, such as the United States. Extrapolating the currently estimated prevalence, this translates to nearly 100000 new cases annually (in the United States and United Kingdom), affecting some 1 in 50 primary school-aged children in the United States, Canada, the United Kingdom, and Australia. A similar increase in incidence is now being noted in developing countries, such as Ghana.

The purpose of this brief communication is to highlight emerging evidence for existing allergy prevention guidelines regarding potential benefits of supporting early rather than delayed peanut introduction during the period of complementary food introduction in infants. A recent study entitled "Randomized trial of peanut consumption in infants at risk for peanut allergy" demonstrated a successful 11% to 25% absolute reduction in the risk of peanut allergy in high-risk infants (and a relative risk reduction of up to 80%) if peanut was introduced between 4 and 11 months of age. In light of the significance of these findings, this document serves to better inform the decision-making process for health care providers regarding such potential benefits of early peanut introduction. More formal guidelines regarding early-life, complementary feeding practices and the risk of allergy development will follow in the next year from the National Institute of Allergy and Infectious Diseases (NIAID)–sponsored Working Group and the European Academy of Allergy and Clinical Immunology (EAACI), and thus this document should be considered interim guidance. (8/15)

CONSENSUS STATEMENT: ABUSIVE HEAD TRAUMA IN INFANTS AND YOUNG CHILDREN

Arabinda Kumar Choudhary; Sabah Servaes; Thomas L. Slovis; Vincent J. Palusci; Gary L. Hedlund; Sandeep K. Narang; Joëlle Anne Moreno; Mark S. Dias; Cindy W. Christian; Marvin D. Nelson Jr; V. Michelle Silvera; Susan Palasis; Maria Raissaki; Andrea Rossi; and Amaka C. Offiah

ABSTRACT. Abusive head trauma (AHT) is the leading cause of fatal head injuries in children younger than 2 years. A multidisciplinary team bases this diagnosis on history, physical examination, imaging and laboratory findings. Because the etiology of the injury is multifactorial (shaking, shaking and impact, impact, etc.) the current best and inclusive term is AHT. There is no controversy concerning the medical validity of the existence of AHT, with multiple components including subdural hematoma, intracranial and spinal changes, complex retinal hemorrhages, and rib and other fractures that are inconsistent with the provided mechanism of trauma. The workup must exclude medical diseases that can mimic AHT. However, the courtroom has become a forum for speculative theories that cannot be reconciled with generally accepted medical literature. There is no reliable medical evidence that the following processes are causative in the constellation of injuries of AHT: cerebral sinovenous thrombosis, hypoxic-ischemic injury, lumbar puncture or dysphagic choking/vomiting. There is no substantiation, at a time remote from birth, that an asymptomatic birth-related subdural hemorrhage can result in rebleeding and sudden collapse. Further, a diagnosis of AHT is a medical conclusion, not a legal determination of the intent of the perpetrator or a diagnosis of murder. We hope that this consensus document reduces confusion by recommending to judges and jurors the tools necessary to distinguish genuine evidence-based opinions of the relevant medical community from legal arguments or etiological speculations that are unwarranted by the clinical findings, medical evidence and evidence-based literature. (5/18)

CONSENSUS STATEMENT: DEFINITIONS FOR CONSISTENT EMERGENCY DEPARTMENT METRICS

American Academy of Emergency Medicine, American Association of Critical Care Nurses, American College of Emergency Physicians, Association of periOperative Registered Nurses, Emergency Department Practice Management Association, Emergency Nurses Association, and National Association of EMS Physicians (2/10)

DEFINING PEDIATRIC MALNUTRITION: A PARADIGM SHIFT TOWARD ETIOLOGY-RELATED DEFINITIONS

American Society for Parenteral and Enteral Nutrition

ABSTRACT. Lack of a uniform definition is responsible for underrecognition of the prevalence of malnutrition and its impact on outcomes in children. A pediatric malnutrition definitions workgroup reviewed existing pediatric age group English-language literature from 1955 to 2011, for relevant references related to 5 domains of the definition of *malnutrition* that were *a priori* identified: anthropometric parameters, growth, chronicity of malnutrition, etiology and pathogenesis, and developmental/functional outcomes. Based on available evidence and an iterative process to arrive at multidisciplinary consensus in the group, these domains were included in the overall construct of a new definition. Pediatric malnutrition (undernutrition) is defined as an imbalance between nutrient requirements and intake that results in cumulative deficits of energy, protein, or micronutrients that may negatively affect growth, development, and other relevant outcomes. A summary of the literature is presented and a new classification scheme is proposed that incorporates chronicity, etiology, mechanisms of nutrient imbalance, severity of malnutrition, and its impact on outcomes. Based on its etiology, malnutrition is either *illness related* (secondary to 1 or more diseases/injury) or *non–illness related,* (caused by environmental/behavioral factors), or both. Future research must focus on the relationship between inflammation and illness-related malnutrition. We anticipate that the definition of malnutrition will continue to evolve with improved understanding of the processes that lead to and complicate the treatment of this condition. A uniform definition should permit future research to focus on the impact of pediatric malnutrition on functional outcomes and help solidify the scientific basis for evidence-based nutrition practices. (3/13)

DELAYED UMBILICAL CORD CLAMPING AFTER BIRTH

American College of Obstetricians and Gynecologists

ABSTRACT. Delayed umbilical cord clamping appears to be beneficial for term and preterm infants. In term infants, delayed umbilical cord clamping increases hemoglobin levels at birth and improves iron stores in the first several months of life, which may have a favorable effect on developmental outcomes. There is a small increase in jaundice that requires phototherapy in this group of infants. Consequently, health care providers adopting delayed umbilical cord clamping in term infants should ensure that mechanisms are in place to monitor for and treat neonatal jaundice. In preterm infants, delayed umbilical cord clamping is associated with significant neonatal benefits, including improved transitional circulation, better establishment of red blood cell volume, decreased need for blood transfusion, and lower incidence of necrotizing enterocolitis and intraventricular hemorrhage. Delayed umbilical cord clamping was not associated with an increased risk of postpartum hemorrhage or increased blood loss at delivery, nor was it associated with a difference in postpartum hemoglobin levels or the need for blood transfusion. Given the benefits to most newborns and concordant with other professional organizations, the American College of Obstetricians and Gynecologists now recommends a delay in umbilical cord clamping in vigorous term and preterm infants for at least 30–60 seconds after birth. The ability to provide delayed umbilical cord clamping may vary among institutions and settings; decisions in those circumstances are best made by the team caring for the mother–infant dyad. (1/17)

DIABETES CARE FOR EMERGING ADULTS: RECOMMENDATIONS FOR TRANSITION FROM PEDIATRIC TO ADULT DIABETES CARE SYSTEMS

American Diabetes Association (11/11)

DIETARY REFERENCE INTAKES FOR CALCIUM AND VITAMIN D

Institute of Medicine (2011)

EMERGENCY EQUIPMENT AND SUPPLIES IN THE SCHOOL SETTING

National Association of School Nurses (1/12)

ENHANCING THE WORK OF THE HHS NATIONAL VACCINE PROGRAM IN GLOBAL IMMUNIZATIONS

National Vaccine Advisory Committee (9/13)

EPIDEMIOLOGY IN FIREARM VIOLENCE PREVENTION

Amy B. Davis; James A. Gaudino; Colin L. Soskolne; Wael K. Al-Delaimy; and International Network for Epidemiology in Policy

INTRODUCTION. Firearm violence has reached pandemic levels, with some countries experiencing high injury and death rates from privately owned guns and firearms (hereinafter collectively referred to as 'firearms'). Significant factors in the increase in deaths and injuries from privately held firearms include the ease of obtaining these arms and, most importantly, the growing lethality of these weapons.

Society cannot be satisfied with reactive responses only in treating victims' physical and psychological wounds after these occurrences; more must be done proactively to prevent firearm violence and address societal circumstances that either facilitate or impede it. Where they exist, well-intended policies fail to adequately protect people from firearm violence, often because they mainly focus on the purchase and illegal uses of guns while neglecting underlying social determinants of the violent uses of firearms.

Laws intended to curb firearm violence are often not enforced, are inadequate or do not address local societal factors of crime, mental well-being, poverty or low education in the relevant communities. These considerations point to the need for a multisectoral approach in which the public health sciences would play a pivotal role in preventing harms relating to firearm violence with a greater focus on its causes. Evidence-based multicomponent interventions, often shown by systematic reviews to be the most effective to address complex, community-level health issues, are needed but are not well-defined to address firearm violence. To both advance understanding of and to guide community-level public health services and actions needed to prevent firearm violence, decision-makers need to rely more on surveillance, research and programme evaluation by public health organizations, schools and universities.

Epidemiologists have unique interdisciplinary tools for addressing the contributors and barriers to preventing and mitigating injury, including firearm violence. These include quantitative, qualitative and social epidemiological methods. Interventions to prevent and mitigate the problem are currently under-developed, under-funded and under-utilized, particularly in the USA. The problem could be addressed by putting in place a robust evidence base to inform policy decisions. Additionally, public health can create, scale up and evaluate interventions designed to address social and behavioural factors associated with firearm violence. We call on governments, community leaders and community members to take meaningful action to support public health in addressing the problem of firearm violence. (4/18)

ETHICAL CONSIDERATION FOR INCLUDING WOMEN AS RESEARCH PARTICIPANTS

American College of Obstetricians and Gynecologists

ABSTRACT. Inclusion of women in research studies is necessary for valid inferences about health and disease in women. The generalization of results from trials conducted in men may yield erroneous conclusions that fail to account for the biologic differences between men and women. Although significant changes in research design and practice have led to an increase in the proportion of women included in research trials, knowledge gaps remain because of a continued lack of inclusion of women, especially those who are pregnant, in premarketing research trials. This document provides a historical overview of issues surrounding women as participants in research trials, followed by an ethical framework and discussion of the issues of informed consent, contraception requirements, intimate partner consent, and the appropriate inclusion of pregnant women in research studies. (11/15)

EVIDENCE REPORT: GENETIC AND METABOLIC TESTING ON CHILDREN WITH GLOBAL DEVELOPMENTAL DELAY

American Academy of Neurology and Child Neurology Society

ABSTRACT. *Objective.* To systematically review the evidence concerning the diagnostic yield of genetic and metabolic evaluation of children with global developmental delay or intellectual disability (GDD/ID).

Methods. Relevant literature was reviewed, abstracted, and classified according to the 4-tiered American Academy of Neurology classification of evidence scheme.

Results and Conclusions. In patients with GDD/ID, microarray testing is diagnostic on average in 7.8% (Class III), G-banded karyotyping is abnormal in at least 4% (Class II and III), and subtelomeric fluorescence in situ hybridization is positive in 3.5% (Class I, II, and III). Testing for X-linked ID genes has a yield of up to 42% in males with an appropriate family history (Class III). *FMR*1 testing shows full expansion in at least 2% of patients with mild to moderate GDD/ID (Class II and III), and *MeCP*2 testing is diagnostic in 1.5% of females with moderate to severe GDD/ID (Class III). Tests for metabolic disorders have a yield of up to 5%, and tests for congenital disorders of glycosylation and cerebral creatine disorders have yields of up to 2.8% (Class III). Several genetic and metabolic screening tests have been shown to have a better than 1% diagnostic yield in selected populations of children with GDD/ID. These values should be among the many factors considered in planning the laboratory evaluation of such children. (9/11)

EVIDENCE-BASED MANAGEMENT OF SICKLE CELL DISEASE: EXPERT PANEL REPORT, 2014

National Heart, Lung, and Blood Institute (2014)

FACULTY COMPETENCIES FOR GLOBAL HEALTH

Academic Pediatric Association Global Health Task Force

International partnerships among medical professionals from different countries are an increasingly common form of clinical and academic collaboration. Global health partnerships can include a variety of activities and serve multiple purposes in the areas of research, medical education and training, health system improvement, and clinical care. Competency domains, introduced by the Accreditation Council for Graduate Medical Education and the American Board of Medical Specialties in 1999, are now widely accepted to provide an organized, structured set of interrelated competencies, mostly for medical trainees. Although there are now competency domains and specific competencies recommended for pediatric trainees pursuing further professional training in global child health, none of these addresses competencies for faculty in global health.

In 2010 the Academic Pediatric Association established a Global Health Task Force to provide a forum for communication and collaboration for diverse pediatric academic societies and groups to advance global child health. Given the burgeoning demand for global health training, and particularly in light of a new global perspective on health education, as outlined in a Lancet Commission Report: *Health Professionals for a New Century: Transforming Education to Strengthen Health Systems in an Interdependent World,* in 2012 the Global Health Task Force noted the lack of defined faculty competencies and decided to develop a set of global health competencies for pediatric faculty engaged in the teaching and practice of global health. Using some of the principles suggested by Milner, et al. to define a competency framework, four domains were chosen, adapted from existing collaborative practice competencies. A fifth domain was added to address some of the unique challenges of global health practice encountered when working outside of one's own culture and health system. The domains are described below and specific competencies are provided for faculty working in global health research, education, administration, and clinical practice. (6/14)

GUIDELINES FOR FIELD TRIAGE OF INJURED PATIENTS

Centers for Disease Control and Prevention (1/12)

IMPORTANCE AND IMPLEMENTATION OF TRAINING IN CARDIOPULMONARY RESUSCITATION AND AUTOMATED EXTERNAL DEFIBRILLATION IN SCHOOLS

American Heart Association Emergency Cardiovascular Care Committee; Council on Cardiopulmonary, Critical Care, Perioperative and Resuscitation; Council on Cardiovascular Diseases in the Young; Council on Cardiovascular Nursing; Council on Clinical Cardiology; and Advocacy Coordinating Committee

ABSTRACT. In 2003, the International Liaison Committee on Resuscitation published a consensus document on education in resuscitation that strongly recommended that "...instruction in CPR [cardiopulmonary resuscitation] be incorporated as a standard part of the school curriculum." The next year the American Heart Association (AHA) recommended that schools "...establish a goal to train every teacher in CPR and first aid and train all students in CPR" as part of their preparation for a response to medical emergencies on campus.

Since that time, there has been an increased interest in legislation that would mandate that school curricula include training in CPR or CPR and automated external defibrillation. Laws or curriculum content standards in 36 states (as of the 2009–2010 school year) now encourage the inclusion of CPR training programs in school curricula. The language in those laws and standards varies greatly, ranging from a suggestion that students "recognize" the steps of CPR to a requirement for certification in CPR. Not surprisingly, then, implementation is not uniform among states, even those whose laws or standards encourage CPR training in schools in the strongest language. This statement recommends that training in CPR and familiarization with automated external defibrillators (AEDs) should be required elements of secondary school curricula and provides the rationale for implementation of CPR training, as well as guidance in overcoming barriers to implementation. (2/11)

INTER-ASSOCIATION CONSENSUS STATEMENT ON BEST PRACTICES FOR SPORTS MEDICINE MANAGEMENT FOR SECONDARY SCHOOLS AND COLLEGES

National Athletic Trainers Association, National Interscholastic Athletic Administrators Association, College Athletic Trainers' Society, National Federation of State High School Associations, American College Health Association, American Orthopaedic Society for Sports Medicine, National Collegiate Athletic Association, American Medical Society for Sports Medicine, National Association of Collegiate Directors of Athletics, and National Association of Intercollegiate Athletics (7/13)

LONG-TERM CARDIOVASCULAR TOXICITY IN CHILDREN, ADOLESCENTS, AND YOUNG ADULTS WHO RECEIVE CANCER THERAPY: PATHOPHYSIOLOGY, COURSE, MONITORING, MANAGEMENT, PREVENTION, AND RESEARCH DIRECTIONS; A SCIENTIFIC STATEMENT FROM THE AMERICAN HEART ASSOCIATION

American Heart Association (5/13)

MEETING OF THE STRATEGIC ADVISORY GROUP OF EXPERTS ON IMMUNIZATION, APRIL 2012–CONCLUSIONS AND RECOMMENDATIONS

World Health Organization (5/12) (The AAP endorses the recommendation pertaining to the use of thimerosal in vaccines.)

MENSTRUATION IN GIRLS AND ADOLESCENTS: USING THE MENSTRUAL CYCLE AS A VITAL SIGN

American College of Obstetricians and Gynecologists Committee on Adolescent Health Care

ABSTRACT. Despite variations worldwide and within the U.S. population, median age at menarche has remained relatively stable—between 12 years and 13 years—across well-nourished populations in developed countries. Environmental factors, including socioeconomic conditions, nutrition, and access to preventive health care, may influence the timing and progression of puberty. A number of medical conditions can cause abnormal uterine bleeding, characterized by unpredictable timing and variable amount of flow. Clinicians should educate girls and their caretakers (eg, parents or guardians) about what to expect of a first menstrual period and the range for normal cycle length of subsequent menses. Identification of abnormal menstrual patterns in adolescence may improve early identification of potential health concerns for adulthood. It is important for clinicians to have an understanding of the menstrual patterns of adolescent girls, the ability to differentiate between normal and abnormal menstruation, and the skill to know how to evaluate the adolescent girl patient. By including an evaluation of the menstrual cycle as an additional vital sign, clinicians reinforce its importance in assessing overall health status for patients and caretakers. (12/15)

MULTILINGUAL CHILDREN: BEYOND MYTHS AND TOWARD BEST PRACTICES

Society for Research in Child Development

ABSTRACT. Multilingualism is an international fact of life and increasing in the United States. Multilingual families are exceedingly diverse, and policies relevant to them should take this into account. The quantity and quality of a child's exposure to responsive conversation spoken by fluent adults predicts both monolingual and multilingual language and literacy achievement. Contexts supporting optimal multilingualism involve early exposure to high quality conversation in each language, along with continued support for speaking both languages. Parents who are not fluent in English should not be told to speak English instead of their native language to their children; children require fluent input, and fluent input in another language will transfer to learning a second or third language. Messages regarding optimal multilingual practices should be made available to families using any and all available methods for delivering such information, including home visitation programs, healthcare settings, center-based early childhood programs, and mass media. (2013)

NATIONAL ADOPTION CENTER: OPEN RECORDS

National Adoption Center

The National Adoption Center believes that it is an inalienable right of all citizens, including adopted adults, to have unencumbered access to their original birth certificates. In keeping with this position, we believe that copies of both the original and the amended birth certificate should be given to the adoptive family at the time of finalization unless specifically denied by the birthparents. In any case, the National Adoption Center advocates that the adoptee, at age 18, be granted access to his/her original birth certificate. (6/00)

NEONATAL ENCEPHALOPATHY AND NEUROLOGIC OUTCOME, SECOND EDITION

American College of Obstetricians and Gynecologists Task Force on Neonatal Encephalopathy

In the first edition of this report, the Task Force on Neonatal Encephalopathy and Cerebral Palsy outlined criteria deemed essential to establish a causal link between intrapartum hypoxic events and cerebral palsy. It is now known that there are multiple potential causal pathways that lead to cerebral palsy in term infants, and the signs and symptoms of neonatal encephalopathy may range from mild to severe, depending on the nature and timing of the brain injury. Thus, for the current edition, the Task Force on Neonatal Encephalopathy determined that a broader perspective may be more fruitful. This conclusion reflects the sober recognition that knowledge gaps still preclude a definitive test or set of markers that accurately identifies, with high sensitivity and specificity, an infant in whom neonatal encephalopathy is attributable to an acute intrapartum event. The information necessary for assessment of likelihood can be derived from a comprehensive evaluation of all potential contributing factors in cases of neonatal encephalopathy. This is the broader perspective championed in the current report. If a comprehensive etiologic evaluation is not possible, the term hypoxic–ischemic encephalopathy should best be replaced by neonatal encephalopathy because neither hypoxia nor ischemia can be assumed to have been the unique initiating causal mechanism. The title of this report has been changed from *Neonatal Encephalopathy and Cerebral Palsy: Defining the Pathogenesis and Pathophysiology* to *Neonatal Encephalopathy and Neurologic Outcome* to indicate that an array of developmental outcomes may arise after neonatal encephalopathy in addition to cerebral palsy. (4/14)

NEURODEVELOPMENTAL OUTCOMES IN CHILDREN WITH CONGENITAL HEART DISEASE: EVALUATION AND MANAGEMENT; A SCIENTIFIC STATEMENT FROM THE AMERICAN HEART ASSOCIATION

American Heart Association (7/12)

THE NEUROLOGIST'S ROLE IN SUPPORTING TRANSITION TO ADULT HEALTH CARE

Lawrence W. Brown, MD; Peter Camfield, MD, FRCPC; Melissa Capers, MA; Greg Cascino, MD; Mary Ciccarelli, MD; Claudio M. de Gusmao, MD; Stephen M. Downs, MD; Annette Majnemer, PhD, FCAHS; Amy Brin Miller, MSN; Christina SanInocencio, MS; Rebecca Schultz, PhD; Anne Tilton, MD; Annick Winokur, BS; and Mary Zupanc, MD

ABSTRACT. The child neurologist has a critical role in planning and coordinating the successful transition from the pediatric to adult health care system for youth with neurologic conditions. Leadership in appropriately planning a youth's transition and in care coordination among health care, educational, vocational, and community services providers may assist in preventing gaps in care, delayed entry into the adult care system, and/or health crises for their adolescent patients. Youth whose neurologic conditions result in cognitive or physical disability and their families may need additional support during this transition, given the legal and financial considerations that may be required. Eight common principles that define the child neurologist's role in a successful transition process have been outlined by a multidisciplinary panel convened by the Child Neurology Foundation are introduced and described. The authors of this consensus statement recognize the current paucity of evidence for successful transition models and outline areas for future consideration. *Neurology*. 2016;87:1–6. (7/16)

NONINHERITED RISK FACTORS AND CONGENITAL CARDIOVASCULAR DEFECTS: CURRENT KNOWLEDGE

American Heart Association

ABSTRACT. Prevention of congenital cardiovascular defects has been hampered by a lack of information about modifiable risk factors for abnormalities in cardiac development. Over the past decade, there have been major breakthroughs in the understanding of inherited causes of congenital heart disease, including the identification of specific genetic abnormalities for some types of malformations. Although relatively less information has been available on noninherited modifiable factors that may have an adverse effect on the fetal heart, there is a growing body of epidemiological literature on this topic. This statement summarizes the currently available literature on potential fetal exposures that might alter risk for cardiovascular defects. Information is summarized for periconceptional multivitamin or folic acid intake, which may reduce the risk of cardiac disease in the fetus, and for additional types of potential exposures that may increase the risk, including maternal illnesses, maternal therapeutic and nontherapeutic drug exposures, environmental exposures, and paternal exposures. Information is highlighted regarding definitive risk factors such as maternal rubella; phenylketonuria; pregestational diabetes; exposure to thalidomide, vitamin A cogeners, or retinoids; and indomethacin tocolysis. Caveats regarding interpretation of possible exposure-outcome relationships from case-control studies are given because this type of study has provided most of the available information. Guidelines for prospective parents that could reduce the likelihood that their child will have a major cardiac malformation are given. Issues related to pregnancy monitoring are discussed. Knowledge gaps and future sources of new information on risk factors are described. (*Circulation*. 2007;115:2995–3014.) (6/07)

NUSINERSEN USE IN SPINAL MUSCULAR ATROPHY

David Michelson, MD; Emma Ciafaloni, MD; Stephen Ashwal, MD; Elliot Lewis, Pushpa Narayanaswami, MBBS; Maryam Oskoui, MD, MSc; Melissa J. Armstrong, MD, MSc; and American Academy of Neurology

ABSTRACT. *Objective*. To identify the level of evidence for use of nusinersen to treat spinal muscular atrophy (SMA) and review clinical considerations regarding use.

Methods. The author panel systematically reviewed nusinersen clinical trials for patients with SMA and assigned level of evidence statements based on the American Academy of Neurology's 2017 therapeutic classification of evidence scheme. Safety information, regulatory decisions, and clinical context were also reviewed.

Results. Four published clinical trials were identified, 3 of which were rated above Class IV. There is Class III evidence that in infants with homozygous deletions or mutations of *SMN1*, nusinersen improves the probability of permanent ventilation-free survival at 24 months vs a well-defined historical cohort. There is Class I evidence that in term infants with SMA and 2 copies of *SMN2*, treatment with nusinersen started in individuals younger than 7 months results in a better motor milestone response and higher rates of event-free survival than sham control. There is Class I evidence that in children aged 2–12 years with SMA symptom onset after 6 months of age, nusinersen results in greater improvement in motor function at 15 months than sham control. Nusinersen was safe and well-tolerated.

Clinical context. Evidence of efficacy is currently highest for treatment of infantile- and childhood-onset SMA in the early and middle symptomatic phases. While approved indications for nusinersen use in North America and Europe are broad, payer coverage for populations outside those in clinical trials remain variable. Evidence, availability, cost, and patient preferences all influence decision-making regarding nusinersen use. (10/18)

ORTHOPTISTS AS PHYSICIAN EXTENDERS

American Association for Pediatric Ophthalmology and Strabismus (5/15)

PERINATAL PALLIATIVE CARE

American College of Obstetricians and Gynecologists

ABSTRACT. Perinatal palliative care refers to a coordinated care strategy that comprises options for obstetric and newborn care that include a focus on maximizing quality of life and comfort for newborns with a variety of conditions considered to be life-limiting in early infancy. With a dual focus on ameliorating suffering and honoring patient values, perinatal palliative care can be provided concurrently with life-prolonging treatment. The focus of this document, however, involves the provision of exclusively palliative care without intent to prolong life in the context of a life-limiting condition, otherwise known as perinatal palliative comfort care. Once a life-limiting diagnosis is suspected antenatally, the tenets of informed consent require that the pregnant patient be given information of sufficient depth and breadth to make an informed, voluntary choice for her care. Health care providers are encouraged to model effective, compassionate communication that respects patient cultural beliefs and values and to promote shared decision making with patients. Perinatal palliative comfort care is one of several options along a spectrum of care, which includes pregnancy termination (abortion) and full neonatal resuscitation and treatment, that should be presented to pregnant patients faced with pregnancies complicated by life-limiting fetal conditions. If a patient opts to pursue perinatal palliative comfort care, a multidisciplinary team should be identified with the infrastructure and support to administer this care. The perinatal palliative care team should prepare families for the possibility that there may be differences of opinion between family members before and after the delivery of the infant, and that there may be differences between parents and the neonatal care providers about appropriate postnatal therapies, especially if the postnatal diagnosis and prognosis differ substantially from antenatal predictions. Procedures for resolving such differences should be discussed with families ahead of time. (8/19)

A PRACTICAL GUIDE FOR PRIMARY CARE PHYSICIANS: INSTRUMENT-BASED VISION SCREENING IN CHILDREN

Children's Eye Foundation

SUMMARY. In January 2016 a new joint policy statement from the American Academy of Pediatrics (AAP), American Academy of Ophthalmology (AAO), American Association for Pediatric Ophthalmology and Strabismus (AAPOS) and American Association of Certified Orthoptists (AACO) regarding the pediatric eye examination was published. The updated policy statement, published in the journal *Pediatrics,* incorporates earlier and routine visual assessments using instrument-based screening to help identify children who may benefit from early intervention to improve vision (or correct vision problems). Instrument-based screening technology is revolutionizing early detection and prevention of amblyopia by allowing screening of more children and at a younger age.

This guide for primary care physicians is produced by the Children's Eye Foundation of AAPOS to provide information regarding instrument-based screening. Early detection and treatment of amblyopia is key to preventing unnecessary blindness, and primary care physicians play a critical role in its detection through vision screening in the preschool and school age groups. (2016)

PREVENTION AND CONTROL OF MENINGOCOCCAL DISEASE: RECOMMENDATIONS OF THE ADVISORY COMMITTEE ON IMMUNIZATION PRACTICES (ACIP)

Centers for Disease Control and Prevention

SUMMARY. Meningococcal disease describes the spectrum of infections caused by *Neisseria meningitidis,* including meningitidis, bacteremia, and bacteremic pneumonia. Two quadrivalent meningococcal polysaccharide-protein conjugate vaccines that provide protection against meningococcal serogroups A, C, W, and Y (MenACWY-D [Menactra, manufactured by Sanofi Pasteur, Inc., Swiftwater, Pennsylvania] and MenACWY-CRM [Menveo, manufactured by Novartis Vaccines, Cambridge, Massachusetts]) are licensed in the United States for use among persons aged 2 through 55 years. MenACWY-D also is licensed for use among infants and toddlers aged 9 through 23 months. Quadrivalent meningococcal polysaccharide vaccine (MPSV4 [Menommune, manufactured by Sanofi Pasteur, Inc., Swiftwater, Pennsylvania]) is the only vaccine licensed for use among persons aged ≥56 years. A bivalent meningococcal polysaccharide protein conjugate vaccine that provides protection against meningococcal serogroups C and Y along with *Haemophilus influenzae* type b (Hib) (Hib-MenCY-TT [MenHibrix, manufactured by GlaxoSmithKline Biologicals, Rixensart, Belgium]) is licensed for use in children aged 6 weeks through 18 months.

This report compiles and summarizes all recommendations from CDC's Advisory Committee on Immunization Practices (ACIP) regarding prevention and control of meningococcal disease in the United States, specifically the changes in the recommendations published since 2005 (CDC. Prevention and control of meningococcal disease: recommendations of the Advisory Committee on Immunization Practices [ACIP]. *MMWR* 2005;54 Adobe PDF file [No. RR-7]). As a comprehensive summary of previously published recommendations, this report does not contain any new recommendations; it is intended for use by clinicians as a resource. ACIP recommends routine vaccination with a quadrivalent meningococcal conjugate vaccine (MenACWY) for adolescents aged 11 or 12 years, with a booster dose at age 16 years. ACIP also recommends routine vaccination for persons at increased risk for meningococcal disease (i.e., persons who have persistent complement component deficiencies, persons who have anatomic or functional asplenia, microbiologists who routinely are exposed to isolates of *N. meningitidis,* military recruits, and persons who travel to or reside in areas in which meningococcal disease is hyperendemic or epidemic). Guidelines for antimicrobial chemoprophylaxis and for evaluation and management of suspected outbreaks of meningococcal disease also are provided. (3/13)

PREVENTION OF GROUP B STREPTOCOCCAL EARLY-ONSET DISEASE IN NEWBORNS

American College of Obstetricians and Gynecologists Committee on Obstetric Practice

ABSTRACT. Group B streptococcus (GBS) is the leading cause of newborn infection (1). The primary risk factor for neonatal GBS early-onset disease (EOD) is maternal colonization of the genitourinary and gastrointestinal tracts. Approximately 50% of women who are colonized with GBS will transmit the bacteria to their newborns. Vertical transmission usually occurs during labor or after rupture of membranes. In the absence of intrapartum antibiotic prophylaxis, 1–2% of those newborns will develop GBS EOD. Other risk factors include gestational age of less than 37 weeks, very low birth weight, prolonged rupture of membranes, intraamniotic infection, young maternal age, and maternal black race. The key obstetric measures necessary for effective prevention of GBS EOD continue to include universal prenatal screening by vaginal–rectal culture, correct specimen collection and processing, appropriate implementation of intrapartum antibiotic prophylaxis, and coordination with pediatric care providers. The American College of Obstetricians and Gynecologists now recommends performing universal GBS screening between 36 0/7 and 37 6/7 weeks of gestation. All women whose vaginal–rectal cultures at 36 0/7 and 37 6/7 weeks of gestation are positive for GBS should receive appropriate intrapartum antibiotic prophylaxis unless a prelabor cesarean birth is performed in the setting of intact membranes. Although a shorter duration of recommended intrapartum antibiotics is less effective than 4 or more hours of prophylaxis, 2 hours of antibiotic exposure has been shown to reduce GBS vaginal colony counts and decrease the frequency of a clinical neonatal sepsis diagnosis. Obstetric interventions, when necessary, should not be delayed solely to provide 4 hours of antibiotic administration before birth. This Committee Opinion, including Table 1, Box 2, and Figures 1–3, updates and replaces the obstetric components of the CDC 2010 guidelines, "Prevention of Perinatal Group B Streptococcal Disease: Revised Guidelines From CDC, 2010." (6/19)

RECOMMENDED AMOUNT OF SLEEP FOR PEDIATRIC POPULATIONS: A CONSENSUS STATEMENT OF THE AMERICAN ACADEMY OF SLEEP MEDICINE

Shalini Paruthi, MD; Lee J. Brooks, MD; Carolyn D'Ambrosio, MD; Wendy A. Hall, PhD, RN; Suresh Kotagal, MD; Robin M. Lloyd, MD; Beth A. Malow, MD, MS; Kiran Maski, MD; Cynthia Nichols, PhD; Stuart F. Quan, MD; Carol L. Rosen, MD; Matthew M. Troester, DO; and Merrill S. Wise, MD

Background and Methodology. Healthy sleep requires adequate duration, appropriate timing, good quality, regularity, and the absence of sleep disturbances or disorders. Sleep duration is a frequently investigated sleep measure in relation to health. A panel of 13 experts in sleep medicine and research used a modified RAND Appropriateness Method to develop recommendations regarding the sleep duration range that promotes optimal health in children aged 0–18 years. The expert panel reviewed published scientific evidence addressing the relationship between sleep duration and health using a broad set of National Library of Medicine Medical Subject Headings (MeSH) terms and no date restrictions, which resulted in a total of 864 scientific articles. The process was further guided by the Oxford grading system. The panel focused on seven health categories with the best available evidence in relation to sleep duration: general health, cardiovascular health, metabolic health, mental health, immunologic function, developmental health, and human performance. Consistent with the RAND Appropriateness Method, multiple rounds of evidence review, discussion, and voting were conducted to arrive at the final recommendations. The process to develop these recommendations was conducted over a 10-month period and concluded with a meeting held February 19–21, 2016, in Chicago, Illinois. (6/16)

SCREENING CHILDREN AT RISK FOR RETINOBLASTOMA: CONSENSUS REPORT FROM THE AMERICAN ASSOCIATION OF OPHTHALMIC ONCOLOGISTS AND PATHOLOGISTS

Alison H. Skalet, MD, PhD; Dan S. Gombos, MD; Brenda L. Gallie, MD; Jonathan W. Kim, MD; Carol L. Shields, MD; Brian P. Marr, MD; Sharon E. Plon, MD, PhD; and Patricia Chévez-Barrios, MD

Purpose: To provide a set of surveillance guidelines for children at risk for development of retinoblastoma.

Design: Consensus panel.

Participants: Expert panel of ophthalmic oncologists, pathologists, and geneticists.

Methods: A group of members of the American Association of Ophthalmic Oncologists and Pathologists (AAOOP) with support of the American Association for Pediatric Ophthalmology and Strabismus and the American Academy of Pediatrics (AAP) was convened. The panel included representative ophthalmic oncologists, pathologists, and geneticists from retinoblastoma referral centers located in various geographic regions who met and discussed screening approaches for retinoblastoma. A patient "at risk" was defined as a person with a family history of retinoblastoma in a parent, sibling, or first- or second-degree relative.

Main Outcome Measures: Screening recommendations for children at risk for retinoblastoma.

Results: Consensus statement from the panel: (1) Dedicated ophthalmic screening is recommended for all children at risk for retinoblastoma above the population risk. (2) Frequency of examinations is adjusted on the basis of expected risk for *RB1* mutation. (3) Genetic counseling and testing clarify the risk for retinoblastoma in children with a family history of the disease. (4) Examination schedules are stratified on the basis of high-, intermediate-, and low-risk children. (5) Children at high risk for retinoblastoma require more frequent screening, which may preferentially be examinations under anesthesia.

Conclusions: Risk stratification including genetic testing and counseling serves as the basis for screening of children at elevated risk for development of retinoblastoma. (10/17)

SCREENING FOR IDIOPATHIC SCOLIOSIS IN ADOLESCENTS—POSITION STATEMENT

American Academy of Orthopedic Surgeons, Scoliosis Research Society, and Pediatric Orthopedic Society of North America

ABSTRACT. The Scoliosis Research Society (SRS), American Academy of Orthopedic Surgeons (AAOS), Pediatric Orthopedic Society of North America (POSNA), and American Academy of Pediatrics (AAP) believe that there has been additional useful research in the early detection and management of adolescent idiopathic scoliosis (AIS) since the review performed by the United States Preventive Services Task Force (USPSTF) in 2004. This information should be available for use by patients, treating health care providers, and policy makers in assessing the relative risks and benefits of the early identification and management of AIS.

The AAOS, SRS, POSNA, and AAP believe that there are documented benefits of earlier detection and non-surgical management of AIS, earlier identification of severe deformities that are surgically treated, and of incorporating screening of children for AIS by knowledgeable health care providers as a part of their care. (9/15)

SKIING AND SNOWBOARDING INJURY PREVENTION

Canadian Paediatric Society

ABSTRACT. Skiing and snowboarding are popular recreational and competitive sport activities for children and youth. Injuries associated with both activities are frequent and can be serious. There is new evidence documenting the benefit of wearing helmets while skiing and snowboarding, as well as data refuting suggestions that helmet use may increase the risk of neck injury. There is also evidence to support using wrist guards while snowboarding. There is poor uptake of effective preventive measures such as protective equipment use and related policy. Physicians should have the information required to counsel children, youth and families regarding safer snow sport participation, including helmet use, wearing wrist guards for snowboarding, training and supervision, the importance of proper equipment fitting and binding adjustment, sun safety and avoiding substance use while on the slopes. (1/12)

SPINAL MOTION RESTRICTION IN THE TRAUMA PATIENT—A JOINT POSITION STATEMENT

Peter E. Fischer, MD, MS; Debra G. Perina, MD; Theodore R. Delbridge, MD, MPH; Mary E. Fallat, MD; Jeffrey P. Salomone, MD; Jimm Dodd, MS, MA; Eileen M. Bulger, MD; and Mark L. Gestring, MD

ABSTRACT. The American College of Surgeons Committee on Trauma (ACS-COT), American College of Emergency Physicians (ACEP), and the National Association of EMS Physicians (NAEMSP) have previously offered varied guidance on the role of backboards and spinal immobilization in out-of-hospital situations. This updated consensus statement on spinal motion restriction in the trauma patient represents the collective positions of the ACS-COT, ACEP and NAEMSP. It has further been formally endorsed by a number of national stakeholder organizations. This updated uniform guidance is intended for use by emergency medical services (EMS) personnel, EMS medical directors, emergency physicians, trauma surgeons, and nurses as they strive to improve the care of trauma victims within their respective domains. (8/18)

SUPPLEMENT TO THE JCIH 2007 POSITION STATEMENT: PRINCIPLES AND GUIDELINES FOR EARLY INTERVENTION AFTER CONFIRMATION THAT A CHILD IS DEAF OR HARD OF HEARING

Joint Committee on Infant Hearing

PREFACE. This document is a supplement to the recommendations in the year 2007 position statement of the Joint Committee on Infant Hearing (JCIH) and provides comprehensive guidelines for early hearing detection and intervention (EHDI) programs on establishing strong early intervention (EI) systems with appropriate expertise to meet the needs of children who are deaf or hard of hearing (D/HH).

EI services represent the purpose and goal of the entire EHDI process. Screening and confirmation that a child is D/HH are largely meaningless without appropriate, individualized, targeted and high-quality intervention. For the infant or young child who is D/HH to reach his or her full potential, carefully designed individualized intervention must be implemented promptly, utilizing service providers with optimal knowledge and skill levels and providing services on the basis of research, best practices, and proven models.

The delivery of EI services is complex and requires individualization to meet the identified needs of the child and family. Because of the diverse needs of the population of children who are D/HH and their families, well-controlled intervention studies are challenging. At this time, few comparative effectiveness studies have been conducted. Randomized controlled trials are particularly difficult for ethical reasons, making it challenging to establish causal links between interventions and outcomes. EI systems must partner with colleagues in research to document what works for children and families and to strengthen the evidence base supporting practices.

Despite limitations and gaps in the evidence, the literature does contain research studies in which all children who were D/HH had access to the same well-defined EI service. These studies indicate that positive outcomes are possible, and they provide guidance about key program components that appear to promote these outcomes. This EI services document, drafted by teams of professionals with extensive expertise in EI programs for children who are D/HH and their families, relied on literature searches, existing systematic reviews, and recent professional consensus statements in developing this set of guidelines.

Terminology presented a challenge throughout document development. The committee noted that many of the frequently occurring terms necessary within the supplement may not reflect the most contemporary understanding and/or could convey inaccurate meaning. Rather than add to the lack of clarity or consensus and to avoid introducing new terminology to stakeholders, the committee opted to use currently recognized terms consistently herein and will monitor the emergence and/or development of new descriptors before the next JCIH consensus statement.

For purposes of this supplement:

- *Language* refers to all spoken and signed languages.
- *Early intervention* (EI), according to part C of the Individuals with Disabilities Education Improvement Act (IDEA) of 2004, is the process of providing services, education, and support to young children who are deemed to have an established condition, those who are evaluated and deemed to have a diagnosed physical or mental condition (with a high probability of resulting in a developmental delay), those who have an existing delay, or those who are at risk of developing a delay or special need that may affect their development or impede their education.
- *Communication* is used in lieu of terms such as communication options, methods, opportunities, approaches, etc.
- *Deaf or hard of hearing* (D/HH) is intended to be inclusive of all children with congenital and acquired hearing loss, unilateral and bilateral hearing loss, all degrees of hearing loss from minimal to profound, and all types of hearing loss (sensorineural, auditory neuropathy spectrum disorder, permanent conductive, and mixed).
- *Core knowledge and skills* is used to describe the expertise needed to provide appropriate EI that will optimize the development and well-being of infants/children and their families. Core knowledge and skills will differ according to the roles of individuals within the EI system (eg, service coordinator or EI provider).

This supplement to JCIH 2007 focuses on the practices of EI providers outside of the primary medical care and specialty medical care realms, rather than including the full spectrum of necessary medical, audiologic, and educational interventions. For more information about the recommendations for medical follow-up, primary care surveillance for related medical conditions, and specialty medical care and monitoring, the reader is encouraged to reference the year 2007 position statement of the JCIH as well as any subsequent revision. When an infant is confirmed to be D/HH, the importance of ongoing medical and audiologic management and surveillance both in the medical home and with the hearing health professionals, the otolaryngologist and the audiologist, cannot be overstated. A comprehensive discussion of those services is beyond the scope of this document. (3/13)

TIMING OF UMBILICAL CORD CLAMPING AFTER BIRTH

American College of Obstetricians and Gynecologists Committee on Obstetric Practice (12/12)

WEIGHING ALL PATIENTS IN KILOGRAMS

Emergency Nurses Association (9/16)

YEAR 2007 POSITION STATEMENT: PRINCIPLES AND GUIDELINES FOR EARLY HEARING DETECTION AND INTERVENTION PROGRAMS

Joint Committee on Infant Hearing

ABSTRACT. The Joint Committee on Infant Hearing (JCIH) endorses early detection of and intervention for infants with hearing loss. The goal of early hearing detection and intervention (EHDI) is to maximize linguistic competence and literacy development for children who are deaf or hard of hearing. Without appropriate opportunities to learn language, these children will fall behind their hearing peers in communication, cognition, reading, and social-emotional development. Such delays may result in lower educational and employment levels in adulthood. To maximize the outcome for infants who are deaf or hard of hearing, the hearing of all infants should be screened at no later than 1 month of age. Those who do not pass screening should have a comprehensive audiological evaluation at no later than 3 months of age. Infants with confirmed hearing loss should receive appropriate intervention at no later than 6 months of age from health care and education professionals with expertise in hearing loss and deafness in infants and young children. Regardless of previous hearing-screening outcomes, all infants with or without risk factors should receive ongoing surveillance of communicative development beginning at 2 months of age during well-child visits in the medical home. EHDI systems should guarantee seamless transitions for infants and their families through this process. (10/07)

APPENDIX 1

PPI: AAP Partnership for Policy Implementation

BACKGROUND

The American Academy of Pediatrics (AAP) develops policies that promote attainment of optimal physical, mental, and social health and well-being for all infants, children, adolescents, and young adults. These documents are valued highly not only by clinicians who provide direct health care to children but by members of other organizations who share similar goals and by parents, payers, and legislators. To increase clarity and action of AAP clinical guidance and recommendations for physicians at the point of care, the AAP formed the Partnership for Policy Implementation (PPI). The PPI is a group of pediatric medical informaticians who partner with authors of AAP clinical practice guidelines and clinical reports to help assure that clinical recommendations are stated with the precision needed to implement them in an electronic health record (EHR) system. Partnership for Policy Implementation volunteers focus on helping content experts develop clinical guidance that specifies exactly who is to do what, for whom, and under what circumstances.

VISION

The vision of the PPI is that all AAP clinical recommendations include clear guidance on how pediatricians can implement those recommendations into their patient care and that AAP clinical guidance can be easily incorporated within EHR decision-support systems.

MISSION

The mission of the PPI is to facilitate implementation of AAP recommendations at the point of care by ensuring that AAP documents are written in a practical, action-oriented fashion with unambiguous recommendations.

WHAT THE PPI IS

The PPI is a network of pediatric informaticians who work with AAP authors and clinical practice guideline subcommittees throughout the writing process.

Contributions of the PPI to the AAP writing process include disambiguation and specification; development of clear definitions; clearly defined logic; implementation techniques; action-oriented recommendations, including clinical algorithms; transparency of the evidence base for recommendations; and health information technology (HIT) standard development.

WHAT THE PPI HAS ACCOMPLISHED

Since inception of the PPI, more than 30 statements have been published using the PPI process, covering a wide variety of child health topics, including attention-deficit/hyperactivity disorder in children and adolescents (*Pediatrics.* 2019;144[4]:e20192528), influenza prevention and control (*Pediatrics.* 2019;144[4]:e20192478), infantile hemangiomas (*Pediatrics.* 2019;143[1]:e20183475), maintenance intravenous fluids (*Pediatrics.* 2018;142[6]:e20183083), child passenger safety (*Pediatrics.* 2018;142[5]:e20182460), and high blood pressure in children and adolescents (*Pediatrics.* 2018;142[3]:e20182096).

One example of how a statement developed using the PPI process has gained broader acceptance is the AAP annual influenza statement. Since 2007, the Centers for Disease Control and Prevention has adopted components of the PPI statement (specifically, the clinical algorithm) within its own statement on the same topic.

WHAT THE PPI IS DOING NOW

In addition to creating practical, action-oriented guidance that pediatricians can use at the point of care, the PPI works to make it easier for these recommendations to be incorporated into electronic systems. To date, the PPI has focused its involvement on the statement development process. Involvement of the PPI during the writing process helps produce a clear, more concise document. As these standards of care become well documented, the PPI can begin to focus on building or mapping pediatric vocabulary; once solidified, this vocabulary can be built into EHR systems. The standards of care can also be matched to various logical and functional HIT standards that already exist today. Through this work, the PPI improves AAP policy documents by providing specific guidance to pediatricians at the point of care, helping ensure that EHRs are designed to assist pediatricians in providing optimal care for children. The PPI developed a short video that provides an overview of its mission and process. This video is available on the PPI website (https://www.aap.org/en-us/professional-resources/quality-improvement/Pages/Partnership-for-Policy-Implementation.aspx) as well as the AAP YouTube channel at www.youtube.com/watch?v=woTfeoNcxn4.

The PPI continues to expand and mentor new members. For more information on the application process and about the PPI, please visit its website (https://www.aap.org/en-us/professional-resources/quality-improvement/Pages/Partnership-for-Policy-Implementation.aspx) or contact Kymika Okechukwu (kokechukwu@aap.org or 630/626-6317).

Appendix 2

American Academy of Pediatrics Acronyms

AACAP	American Academy of Child and Adolescent Psychiatry
AAFP	American Academy of Family Physicians
AAMC	Association of American Medical Colleges
AAOS	American Academy of Orthopaedic Surgeons
AAP	American Academy of Pediatrics
AAPD	American Academy of Pediatric Dentistry
ABM	Academy of Breastfeeding Medicine
ABMS	American Board of Medical Specialties
ABP	American Board of Pediatrics
ACCME	Accreditation Council for Continuing Medical Education
ACEP	American College of Emergency Physicians
ACGME	Accreditation Council for Graduate Medical Education
ACIP	Advisory Committee on Immunization Practices
ACMG	American College of Medical Genetics
ACO	Accountable Care Organization
ACOG	American College of Obstetricians and Gynecologists
ACOP	American College of Osteopathic Pediatricians
ACP	American College of Physicians
ADAMHA	Alcohol, Drug Abuse, and Mental Health Administration
AG-M	Action Group—Multidisciplinary (Section Forum)
AG-M1	Action Group—Medical 1 (Section Forum)
AG-M2	Action Group—Medical 2 (Section Forum)
AG-S	Action Group—Surgical (Section Forum)
AHA	American Heart Association
AHA	American Hospital Association
AHRQ	Agency for Healthcare Research and Quality
ALF	Annual Leadership Forum
AMA	American Medical Association
AMCHP	Association of Maternal and Child Health Programs
AMSA	American Medical Student Association
AMSPDC	Association of Medical School Pediatric Department Chairs
AMWA	American Medical Women's Association
APA	Academic Pediatric Association
APHA	American Public Health Association
APLS	Advanced Pediatric Life Support
APPD	Association of Pediatric Program Directors
APQ	Alliance for Pediatric Quality
APS	American Pediatric Society
AQA	Ambulatory Care Quality Alliance
ASHG	American Society of Human Genetics
ASTM	American Society of Testing and Materials
BHP	Bureau of Health Professions
BIA	Bureau of Indian Affairs
BLAST	Babysitter Lessons and Safety Training
BOD	Board of Directors
BPC	Breastfeeding Promotion Consortium
CAG	Corporate Advisory Group
CAMLWG	Children, Adolescents, and Media Leadership Workgroup
CAP	College of American Pathologists
CAQI	Chapter Alliance for Quality Improvement
CATCH	Community Access to Child Health
CDC	Centers for Disease Control and Prevention
CESP	Confederation of European Specialty Pediatrics
CFMC	Chapter Forum Management Committee
CFT	Cross Functional Team
CHA	Children's Hospital Association
CHIC	Child Health Informatics Center
CHIP	Children's Health Insurance Program
CISP	Childhood Immunization Support Program
CMC	Council Management Committee
CME	Continuing Medical Education
CMS	Centers for Medicare & Medicaid Services
CMSS	Council of Medical Specialty Societies
CnF	Council Forum
COA	Committee on Adolescence
COB	Committee on Bioethics
COCAN	Council on Child Abuse and Neglect
COCHF	Committee on Child Health Financing
COCIT	Council on Clinical Information Technology
COCM	Council on Communications and Media
COCME	Committee on Continuing Medical Education
COCN	Committee on Coding and Nomenclature
COCP	Council on Community Pediatrics
COCWD	Council on Children With Disabilities
COD	Committee on Drugs
CODe	Committee on Development
CODPR	Council on Disaster Preparedness and Recovery
COEC	Council on Early Childhood
COEH	Council on Environmental Health
CoF	Committee Forum
COFCAKC	Council on Foster Care, Adoption, and Kinship Care
COFGA	Committee on Federal Government Affairs
CoFMC	Committee Forum Management Committee
COFN	Committee on Fetus and Newborn
COG	Committee on Genetics
COGME	Council on Graduate Medical Education (DHHS/HRSA)
COHC	Committee on Hospital Care
COICFH	Council on Immigrant Child and Family Health
COID	Committee on Infectious Diseases
COIVPP	Council on Injury, Violence, and Poison Prevention

COMLRM	Committee on Medical Liability and Risk Management
COMSEP	Council on Medical Student Education in Pediatrics (AMSPDC)
CON	Committee on Nutrition
CONACH	Committee on Native American Child Health
COPA	Committee on Pediatric AIDS
COPACFH	Committee on Psychosocial Aspects of Child and Family Health
COPAM	Committee on Practice and Ambulatory Medicine
COPE	Committee on Pediatric Education
COPEM	Committee on Pediatric Emergency Medicine
COPR	Committee on Pediatric Research
COPW	Committee on Pediatric Workforce
COQIPS	Council on Quality Improvement and Patient Safety
CORS	Committee on Residency Scholarships
COSGA	Committee on State Government Affairs
COSH	Council on School Health
COSMF	Council on Sports Medicine and Fitness
COSUP	Committee on Substance Use and Prevention
CPS	Canadian Paediatric Society
CPTI	Community Pediatrics Training Initiative
CQN	Chapter Quality Network
CSHCN	Children With Special Health Care Needs
DHHS	Department of Health and Human Services
DOD	Department of Defense
DVC	District Vice Chairperson
EBCDLWG	Early Brain and Child Development Leadership Workgroup
EC	Executive Committee
ECHO	Expanding Capacity for Health Outcomes
ELWG	Epigenetics Leadership Workgroup
EMSC	Emergency Medical Services for Children
EPA	Environmental Protection Agency
EQIPP	Education in Quality Improvement for Pediatric Practice
eTACC	Electronic Translation of Academy Clinical Content
FAAN	Federal Advocacy Action Network
FASD	Fetal Alcohol Spectrum Disorder
FCF	Friends of Children Fund
FDA	Food and Drug Administration
FERPA	Family Educational Rights and Privacy Act
FOPE II	Future of Pediatric Education II
FOPO	Federation of Pediatric Organizations
FPN	Family Partnerships Network
FTC	Federal Trade Commission
GME	Graduate Medical Education
GSIPI	Gun Safety and Injury Prevention Initiative
HAAC	Historical Archives Advisory Committee
HBB	Helping Babies Breathe
HBSPG	Helping Babies Survive Planning Group
HCCA	Healthy Child Care America
HEDIS	Healthcare Effectiveness Data and Information Set
HHS	Health and Human Services
HIPAA	Health Insurance Portability and Accountability Act of 1996
HMO	Health Maintenance Organization
HOF	Headquarters of the Future
HQA	Hospital Quality Alliance
HRSA	Health Resources and Services Administration
HTC	Help the Children
HTPCP	Healthy Tomorrows Partnership for Children Program
IHS	Indian Health Service
IMG	International Medical Graduate
IPA	International Pediatric Association
IPC	International Pediatric Congress
IRB	Institutional Review Board
LLLI	La Leche League International
LWG	Leadership Workgroup
MCAN	Merck Childhood Asthma Network
MCH	Maternal and Child Health
MCHB	Maternal and Child Health Bureau
MCN	Migrant Clinicians Network
MHICSN-PAC	Medical Home Initiatives for Children With Special Needs Project Advisory Committee
MHLWG	Mental Health Leadership Work Group
MOC	Maintenance of Certification
MRT	Media Resource Team
MSAP	Medical Subspecialty Advisory Panel
NACHC	National Association of Community Health Centers
NAEMSP	National Association of EMS Physicians
NAEPP	National Asthma Education and Prevention Program
NAM	National Academy of Medicine
NAPNAP	National Association of Pediatric Nurse Practitioners
NASPGHAN	North American Society for Pediatric Gastroenterology, Hepatology, and Nutrition
NAWD	National Association of WIC Directors
NBME	National Board of Medical Examiners
NCBDDD	National Center on Birth Defects and Developmental Disabilities
NCE	National Conference & Exhibition
NCEPG	National Conference & Exhibition Planning Group
NCQA	National Committee for Quality Assurance
NHLBI	National Heart, Lung, and Blood Institute
NHMA	National Hispanic Medical Association
NHTSA	National Highway Traffic Safety Administration
NIAAA	National Institute on Alcohol Abuse and Alcoholism
NICHD	National Institute of Child Health and Human Development
NICHQ	National Initiative for Children's Health Quality
NIDA	National Institute on Drug Abuse
NIH	National Institutes of Health
NIMH	National Institute of Mental Health
NMA	National Medical Association
NNC	National Nominating Committee
NQF	National Quality Forum
NRHA	National Rural Health Association
NRMP	National Resident Matching Program
NRP	Neonatal Resuscitation Program
NSC	National Safety Council
NVAC	National Vaccine Advisory Committee
ODPHP	Office of Disease Prevention and Health Promotion
OED	Office of the Executive Director
OHISC	Oral Health Initiative Steering Committee
OLWG	Obesity Leadership Workgroup
P4P	Pay for Performance
PAAC	Payer Advocacy Advisory Committee
PAC	Project Advisory Committee
PAHO	Pan American Health Organization
PALS	Pediatric Advanced Life Support
PAS	Pediatric Academic Societies
PCO	*Pediatric Care Online*™

PCOC	Primary Care Organizations Consortium
PCPCC	Patient-Centered Primary Care Collaborative
PCPI	Physician Consortium on Performance Improvement
PEAC	Practice Expense Advisory Committee
PECOS	Pediatric Education in Community and Office Settings
PECS	Pediatric Education in Community Settings
PEPP	Pediatric Education for Prehospital Professionals
PIR	*Pediatrics in Review*
PLA	Pediatric Leadership Alliance
PPAAC	Private Payer Advocacy Advisory Committee (COCHF Subcommittee)
PPAC	Past President's Advisory Committee
PPC-PCMH	Physician Practice Connections—Patient-Centered Medical Home (NCQA)
PPI	Partnership for Policy Implementation
PPMA	Pediatric Practice Management Alliance
PREP	Pediatric Review and Education Program
PROS	Pediatric Research in Office Settings
PUPVS	Project Universal Preschool Vision Screening
QA	Quality Assurance
QI	Quality Improvement
QuIIN	Quality Improvement Innovation Network
RBPE	Resource-Based Practice Expense
RBRVS	Resource-Based Relative Value Scale
RCAC	Richmond Center Advisory Committee
RCE	Richmond Center of Excellence
RRC	Residency Review Committee (ACGME)
RUC	AMA/Specialty Society Relative Value Scale Update Committee
RVU	Relative Value Unit
SAM	Society for Adolescent Medicine
SAMHSA	Substance Abuse and Mental Health Services Administration
SAP	Surgical Advisory Panel
SCHIP	State Children's Health Insurance Program
SDBP	Society for Developmental and Behavioral Pediatrics
SF	Section Forum
SFMC	Section Forum Management Committee
SLGBTHW	Section on Lesbian, Gay, Bisexual, and Transgender Health and Wellness
SOA	Section on Anesthesiology and Pain Medicine
SOAC	Subcommittee on Access to Care
SOAH	Section on Adolescent Health
SOAI	Section on Allergy and Immunology
SOAPM	Section on Administration and Practice Management
SOATT	Section on Advances in Therapeutics and Technology
SOB	Section on Bioethics
SOBr	Section on Breastfeeding
SOCAN	Section on Child Abuse and Neglect
SOCC	Section on Critical Care
SOCCS	Section on Cardiology and Cardiac Surgery
SOCDRP	Section on Child Death Review and Prevention
SOCPT	Section on Clinical Pharmacology and Therapeutics
SOD	Section on Dermatology
SODBP	Section on Developmental and Behavioral Pediatrics
SOECP	Section on Early Career Physicians
SOEM	Section on Emergency Medicine
SOEn	Section on Endocrinology
SOEPHE	Section on Epidemiology, Public Health, and Evidence
SOGBD	Section on Genetics and Birth Defects
SOGHN	Section on Gastroenterology, Hepatology, and Nutrition
SOHCa	Section on Home Care
SOHM	Section on Hospital Medicine
SOHO	Section on Hematology/Oncology
SOHPM	Section on Hospice and Palliative Medicine
SOICH	Section on International Child Health
SOID	Section on Infectious Diseases
SOIM	Section on Integrative Medicine
SOIMG	Section on International Medical Graduates
SOIMP	Section on Internal Medicine/Pediatrics
SOMHEI	Section on Minority Health, Equity, and Inclusion
SOMP	Section on Medicine-Pediatrics
SONp	Section on Nephrology
SONPM	Section on Neonatal-Perinatal Medicine
SONS	Section on Neurological Surgery
SONu	Section on Neurology
SOOb	Section on Obesity
SOOH	Section on Oral Health
SOOHNS	Section on Otolaryngology—Head and Neck Surgery
SOOp	Section on Ophthalmology
SOOPe	Section on Osteopathic Pediatricians
SOOr	Section on Orthopaedics
SOPPSM	Section on Pediatric Pulmonology and Sleep Medicine
SOPS	Section on Plastic Surgery
SOPT	Section on Pediatric Trainees
SORa	Section on Radiology
SORh	Section on Rheumatology
SOSILM	Section on Simulation and Innovative Learning Methods
SOSM	Section on Senior Members
SOSu	Section on Surgery
SOTC	Section on Telehealth Care
SOTCo	Section on Tobacco Control
SOTM	Section on Transport Medicine
SOU	Section on Urology
SOUCM	Section on Urgent Care Medicine
SOUS	Section on Uniformed Services
SPR	Society for Pediatric Research
SPWG	Strategic Planning Work Group
TA	Technical Assistance
TA	Technology Assessment
TFOA	Task Force on Access (also known as Task Force on Health Insurance Coverage and Access to Care)
TFOABD	Task Force on Addressing Bias and Discrimination
TFOC	Task Force on Circumcision
TFODI	Task Force on Diversity and Inclusion
TFOSIDS	Task Force on Sudden Infant Death Syndrome
TIPP	The Injury Prevention Program
TJC	The Joint Commission
UNICEF	United Nations Children's Fund
UNOS	United Network for Organ Sharing
USDA	US Department of Agriculture
VIP	Value in Inpatient Pediatrics
WHO	World Health Organization
WIC	Special Supplemental Nutrition Program for Women, Infants, and Children

Subject Index

Page numbers followed by *f* indicate a figure.
Page numbers followed by *t* indicate a table.
Page numbers followed by *b* indicate a box.

A

B

C

D

E

F

G

H

I

J

K

L

M

N

O

P

Q

R

S

T

U

Pediatric Care Online provides 24/7 access to the most essential resources in pediatrics today.

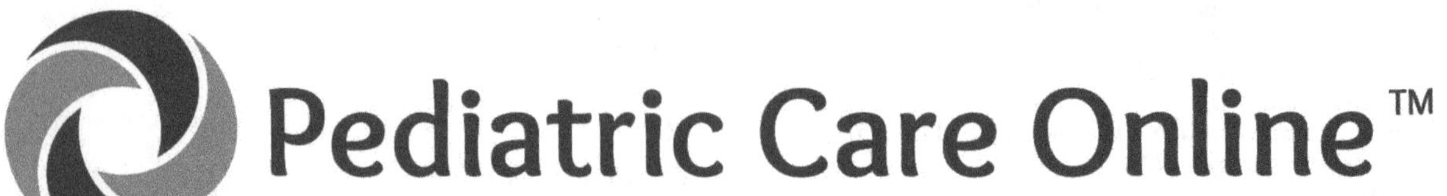

pediatriccare.solutions.aap.org

Pediatric Care Online is built to work the way you work at the point of care by providing expert help using the most essential AAP resources and tools, including

- **AAP Toolkits**—including Bright Futures, ADHD, and Autism.
- Just added to Pediatric Patient Education—**Schmitt Pediatric Care Advice** patient education collection of 280 handouts from Barton Schmitt, MD, FAAP, bringing the site total to **more than 800** age-based, symptom-based, and diagnosis-based resources.
- ***Red Book® Online***—keep current with infectious disease developments, simplify diagnosis and disease management; includes Red Book English and Spanish.
- **Point-of-Care Quick Reference**—Indispensable AAP information on 250+ topics streamlined for fast answers.
- ***AAP Textbook of Pediatric Care*, 2nd Edition**—375 chapters of expert guidance to diagnose, treat, and manage pediatric illnesses.
- **Clinical practice guidelines, policies, and reports**—The latest AAP recommendations on vaccine schedules, developmental screening, and more.
- **Visual Library**—Quickly search 2,700+ images for faster diagnosis.

DON'T WAIT—SUBSCRIBE TODAY!
FOR INDIVIDUAL (SINGLE-USER) ITEM#: PCO
Annual Subscription Price: $340 ***Member Price $272***

Provide anytime, anywhere access for all staff members and SAVE!
To learn more about practice or institutional site licenses, email **institutions@aap.org.**
EMR, EHR, and website integration and institutional licensing available. Call 888/227-1770 for details.

Members can request a **FREE 1-MONTH TRIAL!**
Visit **aap.org/pcotrial** today.

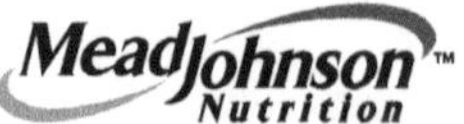

The American Academy of Pediatrics is the exclusive owner of the Pediatric Care Online™ Website and content. Mead Johnson Nutrition has no control over or responsibility for the Pediatric Care Online™ website and content.

American Academy of Pediatrics
DEDICATED TO THE HEALTH OF ALL CHILDREN®

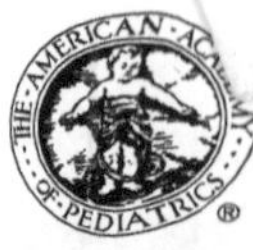

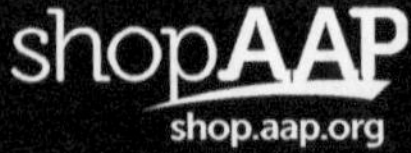

Visit **shop.aap.org/solutions** or call toll-free **888/227-1770.**